DRUG INTERACTIONS

Drug Interactions

A SOURCE BOOK OF ADVERSE INTERACTIONS,

THEIR MECHANISMS,

CLINICAL IMPORTANCE AND MANAGEMENT

IVAN H. STOCKLEY

BPharm, PhD, (Nott) FRPharmS (Lond), CBiol, MIBiol
University of Nottingham Medical School,
Nottingham, England

THIRD EDITION

OXFORD

BLACKWELL SCIENTIFIC PUBLICATIONS

LONDON EDINBURGH BOSTON
MELBOURNE PARIS BERLIN VIENNA

© 1981, 1991, 1994 Ivan Stockley

Published by
Blackwell Scientific Publications
Editorial Offices:
Osney Mead, Oxford OX2 0EL
25 John Street, London WC1N 2BL
23 Ainslie Place, Edinburgh EH3 6AJ
238 Main Street, Cambridge
    Massachusetts 02142, USA
54 University Street, Carlton
    Victoria 3053, Australia

Other Editorial Offices:
Librairie Arnette SA
1, rue de Lille
75007 Paris
France

Blackwell Wissenschafts-Verlag GmbH
Düsseldorfer Str. 38
D-10707 Berlin
Germany

Blackwell MZV
Feldgasse 13
A-1238 Wien
Austria

First published 1981
Second Edition 1991
Reissued in paperback 1993
Reprinted 1993
Third edition 1994

Set by Semantic Graphics, Singapore
Printed and bound in Great Britain
at The University Press, Cambridge

DISTRIBUTORS

Marston Book Services Ltd
PO Box 87
Oxford OX2 0DT
(*Orders*: Tel: 0865 791155
         Fax: 0865 791927
         Telex: 837515)

USA
Blackwell Scientific Publications, Inc.
238 Main Street
Cambridge, MA 02142
(*Orders*: Tel: 800 759-6102
         617 876-7000)

Canada
Times Mirror Professional Publishing, Ltd
130 Flaska Drive
Markham, Ontario L6G 1B8
(*Orders*: Tel: 800 268-4178
         416 470-6739)

Australia
Blackwell Scientific Publications Pty Ltd
54 University Street
Carlton, Victoria 3053
(*Orders*: Tel: 03 347-5552)

A catalogue record for this title
is available from the British Library

ISBN 0-632-03721-0

Library of Congress
Cataloging in Publication Data

Stockley, Ivan H.
    Drug interactions: a source book of
    adverse interactions, their mechanisms,
    clinical importance and management/
    Ivan H. Stockley.—3rd ed.
          p.   cm.
    Includes bibliographical references
    and index.
    ISBN 0-632-03721-0.
    1. Drug interactions. I. Title.
    [DNLM: 1. Drug Interactions—handbooks.
    QV 38 S865d1994]
    RM302.S76   1994
    615'.704—dc20

If you confess with your mouth, 'Jesus is Lord,' and believe in your heart that God raised him from the dead, you will be saved.

For it is with your heart that you believe and are justified, and it is with your mouth that you confess and are saved.

As the Scripture says, 'Anyone who trusts in him will never be put to shame.'

For there is no difference between Jew and Gentile—the same Lord is Lord of all and richly blesses all who call on him,

For, 'Everyone who calls on the name of the Lord will be saved.'

Romans 10: 9–13 (NIV)

Contents

Preface to the Third Edition

If you are familiar with the previous editions, you will see that the format of this one is little changed. The font has been altered from Palatino to Photina which is a little more compact and space-saving, but the general layout remains the same and the philosophy underlying the presentation of the data is as before.

The updating of the synopses and the writing of new ones has continued unabated since the publication of the second edition (1991) with the result that this edition contains almost a third more synopses. The spate of new information about interactions continues unchecked, and the intention is to continue to publish new and updated editions at approximately two to three-yearly intervals.

In the preparation of this edition I am indebted to a host of people. Diane Stevenson in particular has been a tower of strength in carrying out database searches for me and in keeping my filing system in apple-pie order. Drug information pharmacists in Hospital and Industry in the UK have continued to provide me with 'in house' data which is available nowhere else, or they have directed my attention to reports I might otherwise have missed. Users of previous editions have written and offered constructive and helpful criticisms. To all of these I am very grateful. It is always helpful for an author to know what readers like or dislike about a book, so please feel free to write and tell me what you think.

I continue to be grateful to Boehringer Ingelheim International with whom I collaborate in the production of the *Drug Interaction Alert* ready-reference chart which complements this book. I would like to acknowledge here both their continued generous support and their permission to reproduce the Alert on the cover of this book. The book is also intended to complement the *Drug Interaction Automatic Alerting System* which is used by John Richardson Pharmacy Computer systems in the UK. Users of both of these facilities will find that this book will give them the details of the interactions which both of these facilities provide in a summarized form.

Ivan H Stockley,
University of Nottingham
Medical School

Preface to the First Edition

Plans for this book were drawn up as long ago as 1971, but they were shelved in favour of writing a series of articles on interactions for *The Pharmaceutical Journal* at the invitation of the editor. Later in 1974 these articles were reprinted in facsimile form, with an index, and published under the title *Drug Interactions and their Mechanisms*, so there seemed little point at that time in writing another book on the same subject. A supplement on oral contraceptives was added to the 1978 reprint, but eventually it became clear that a complete rewrite was necessary, incorporating the old material as well as the mass of new data published since the articles were first written. This book is therefore the up-dated successor to the familiar yellow-backed reprinted series of articles.

My aim, as before, has been to present to the practising doctor, pharmacist, surgeon or nurse, or anyone else who has neither the time nor the facilities to carry out detailed literature searches of their own, what is known about the hundreds of drug interactions now on record. I have attempted not only to answer the question of what is likely to happen if two drugs are given concurrently, but also the important associated questions such as these: Is it a genuine, reported, interaction or is it still only theoretical? Has it been described many times or only once? Is the interaction, when it occurs, serious or not? Are all patients affected or only a few? Is it best to avoid the concurrent use of the drugs altogether, or can the interaction be accommodated in some way? And what alternative drugs can be used which do not interact?

So that these questions can be answered succinctly, the material has been organized into a series of individual drug-drug or drug-food synopses-600 or so in all—and categorized into 20 chapters. A very brief outline of the most common mechanisms of interaction has been included at the beginning of the book and a few chapters also include a very short pharmacological introduction for the benefit of those whose pharmacology is not as fresh as it might be. The synopses have a common format with a summary for rapid reading, but very extensive bibliographies are included for those who wish to study the original literature in depth. The synopses are assembled into chapters according to the drugs whose activity is changed, although where the same drug is the affecting or interacting agent, it is usually categorized elsewhere. For this reason the index *must* be used to ensure that the whole range of interactions can be identified.

Through the generosity of the Leverhulme Trust in particular, and a number of Pharmaceutical Companies—Boots, Geistlich, Glaxo, Janssen, Lepetit, Leo, Ortho, Pfizer, Roche, Upjohn and Warner-Lambert—I was able to accumulate sufficient funds for my University to pay a temporary replacement member of staff to undertake my teaching duties for a year, thus enabling me to take sabbatical leave to write this book. I am indebted to all of those, within and without the university, who in one way or another gave me the support I needed.

I also owe a debt of gratitude to many other people: the library staff of the Science and Medical Libraries in the University of Nottingham; the staff of the drug information and medical departments of many of the pharmaceutical companies in the UK; numerous individuals who have drawn my attention to obscure papers and articles which I might otherwise have missed; Dr JSB Stuart for some of the documentation of Chapter 12; Boehringer Ingelheim for allowing me to reproduce the *Drug Interaction Alert* chart on the jacket of this book; Mr Per Saugman and his staff at Blackwell Scientific Publications, in particular John Robson and Dominic Vaughan;

and my wife Bridget, and children Alex, Rosalind, Ben and Beth who with such good grace put up with my acquisition of an intended playroom for a study, and a house strewn, seemingly for ever, with papers.

Ivan H. Stockley
University of Nottingham

Before Using this Book...

...it is important to appreciate the extent and the limitations of our knowledge of drug interactions so that the information summarized here can be properly used.

What we know about interactions comes from a range of sources of widely varying quality and reliability. The best information comes from clinical studies carried out with large numbers of patients where the conditions are scrupulously controlled and results well analysed. With data of this kind a very good idea of the importance and the incidence of the interaction can be deduced.

However, what is known about very many interactions comes from much less reliable sources: from observations on only one or two patients, possibly in uncontrolled situations where it would be undesirable or unethical to re-challenge the patients with both drugs to confirm the interaction. It may be confined to the results of animal experiments or even based solely on theoretical considerations. Not that this kind of data is to be despised. Quite the contrary. Many of the now very well-confirmed interactions were initially detected in only one patient or even in laboratory animals, but such observations need careful confirmation before their clinical importance can be accurately assessed, and a clear distinction must be drawn between these possible interactions and those which are well-established.

It also needs to be remembered that patients are not like selected batches of laboratory animals, of the same age, weight, sex, and strain which can be expected to respond to drugs with some degree of uniformity. Every ward, surgery, office or clinic contains a mixture of individuals who will probably not respond uniformly to one or more drugs because their genetic make-up, sex, renal and hepatic func-

tions, diseases and nutritional states, ages and other parameters are all different. By the same token the drug dosages, their form, duration and order of administration can have a vital bearing on the way a patient responds, and on whether an interaction develops or not.

The sum of all these variables is that while it is possible to say what has already been seen to occur when drugs are given together, the outcome of giving the same drugs to other patients for the first time is never totally predictable because a new and unique 'experiment' is being undertaken. Despite this element of uncertainty, some idea of the probable outcome of using pairs of drugs in patients can be based on the clinical experience already available— the more extensive the data, the firmer the predictions.

The synopses in this book describe interactions of varying clinical importance. Some are life-threatening, while others range from the clearly important to those which are only moderately so. Yet others describe trivial interactions, or isolated cases, or even clear cases of 'no interaction'. All of these different synopses are included so that the reader has enough information to be able to make his or her own judgement about the safety of giving particular drugs together.

The 'importance and management' sections of the synopses are therefore intended to be broad assessments of the incidence and clinical importance of the interactions, with suggestions about how they can be managed. Readers should modify and refine what is written in these sections with the data they have about their own patients so that the measures taken can be individually tailored to fit their patient's needs.

Chapter 1
General Considerations and an Outline Survey of Some Basic Interaction Mechanisms

1 What is a drug interaction?

An interaction is said to occur when the effects of one drug are changed by the presence of another drug, food, drink or by some environmental chemical agent.

The outcome may be harmful if the interaction causes an increase in the efficacy or toxicity of the drug. For example, patients already taking warfarin may begin to bleed if given azapropazone or phenylbutazone unless the warfarin dosage is reduced appropriately. Patients taking monoamine oxidase inhibitor antidepressants may experience an acute and life-threatening hypertensive crisis if they eat tyramine-rich foods.

A reduction in efficacy as a result of an interaction may also be harmful. Thus patients on warfarin given rifampicin will need an increase in the dosage of warfarin to maintain adequate anticoagulation, and patients taking tetracycline antibiotics should avoid antacids and milky foods because the antibacterial effects can be drastically reduced.

These unwanted and unsought-for interactions are one kind of adverse drug reaction but there are other interactions which can be beneficial rather than adverse. Antihypertensive drugs and diuretics are commonly given together for the treatment of hypertension. Sulphamethoxazole is given with trimethoprim as Co-trimoxazole because the combined effects are greater than either drug alone. The mechanisms of both types of interaction, adverse or beneficial, are very similar, but only the adverse interactions form the subject of this book.

Sometimes the term 'drug interaction' is used for the physico-chemical reactions which can occur if drugs are mixed in intravenous fluids, causing precipitation or inactivation. It is also often used for the interference which drugs may have on biochemical and other assays carried out on body fluids which can invalidate the results. A long-established and less ambiguous term for the former is 'pharmaceutical incompatibilities'. There is no brief and widely accepted term for the drug–biochemical test interactions, but the simple term 'drug interactions' is possibly best reserved for the reactions which go on within, rather than outside, the body.

2 What is the incidence of drug interactions?

The more drugs a patient takes the greater the likelihood that an adverse reaction will occur. One hospital study found that the rate was 7% in those taking 6–10 drugs but 40% in those taking 16–20 drugs which represents a disproportionate increase.[1] A possible explanation is that the drugs were interacting together.

Some of the early studies on the frequency of interactions uncritically compared the drugs prescribed with lists of possible drug interactions, without appreciating that many interactions may be clinically trivial or totally theoretical. As a result an unrealistically high incidence was suggested. Most of the later studies have avoided this error by considering only potentially clinically important interactions and incidences of 4.7%,[2] 6.3%[3] and 8.8%[6] have been found. Even so, not all of these studies took into account the distinction which must be made between the incidence of potential interactions and the incidence of those where clinical problems actually arise. The simple fact is that some patients experience serious reactions while others appear not to react at all.

For example, a screening of 2422 patients over a total of 25 005 days revealed that 113 (4.7%) were taking combinations of drugs which could interact, but evidence of interactions was observed in only seven patients, representing 0.3%.[2] In another hospital study of 44 patients over a 5-day period taking 10–17 drugs, 77 potential drug interactions were identified, but only one probable and four possible adverse reactions (6.4%) were detected.[5] A further study among patients taking anticonvulsant drugs found that 6% of the cases of intoxication were due to drug interactions.[9] These figures are low compared with those of a hospital survey which monitored 927 patients who had had 1004 potentially interacting drug combinations. Changes in drug dosage were made in 44% of these cases.[4] A review of these and other studies found that the reported incidence rates ranged from 70.3 to 2.2%, and the percentage of patients actually experiencing problems ranged from 11.1 to 0%. Another review found a 37% incidence among 639 elderly patients.[12] Yet another review of 236 geriatric patients found an 88% incidence of clinically significant interactions, and a 22% incidence of potentially serious and life-threatening interactions.[14] A 4.1% incidence of drug interactions on prescriptions presented to community pharmacists in the USA was found in a further survey.[15] The incidence is likely to be higher in the elderly because ageing affects the functioning of the kidneys and liver so that many drugs are lost from the body much more slowly.[11,16]

These discordant figures need to be put into the context of under-reporting by doctors of adverse reactions of any kind, for reasons which include pressure of work, indifference, indolence or the fear of litigation. Both doctors and patients may not recognize adverse reactions and interactions, and many outpatients simply stop taking their drugs without saying why. None of these studies gives a clear answer to the question of how frequently drug interactions occur, but even if the incidence is as low as some of the studies suggest, it still represents a very considerable number of patients who appear to be at risk when one thinks of the large numbers of drugs administered and prescriptions handled every day by doctors and pharmacists.

3 How seriously should interactions be regarded and handled?

It would be very easy to conclude after leafing through this book that it is extremely risky to treat patients with more than one drug at a time, but this would be an over-reaction. The figures quoted in the previous section illustrate that many drugs which are known to interact in some patients simply fail to do so in others. This partially explains why some quite important drug interactions remained virtually un-noticed for many years, a good example of this being the effect which quinidine has on serum digoxin levels (see Fig. 1.1).

Examples of this kind suggest that patients apparently tolerate adverse interactions remarkably well and that many experienced physicians accommodate the effects (such as rises or falls in serum drug levels) without consciously recognizing that what they are seeing is the result of an interaction.

One of the reasons it is often difficult to detect an interaction is that, as already mentioned, patient variability is very considerable. We now know many of the predisposing and protective factors which determine whether an interaction occurs or not, but in practice it is still very difficult to predict what will happen when an individual patient is given two potentially interacting drugs. An easy solution to this practical problem is to choose a non-interacting alternative, but if none is available, it is frequently possible to give known interacting drugs provided appropriate precautions are taken. If the effects are well monitored and the dosages well adjusted, the effects of the interaction can often be allowed for. The reasons this can be done are that many interac-

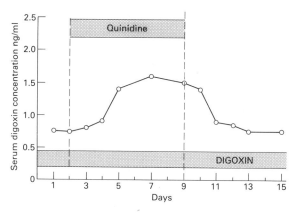

Fig. 1.1 A multiple-mechanism interaction. The effect of quinidine (1 mg daily) on the serum digoxin levels of five subjects taking constant doses of digoxin (after Doering W. N Engl J Med (1979) 301, 400, with permission). The mechanisms involved include changes in renal and non-renal (biliary) clearance, and possibly absorption and tissue binding.

tions are dose related so that if the dosage is reduced the effects will be reduced accordingly. For example, isoniazid causes the levels of phenytoin to rise, particularly in those individuals who are slow acetylators of isoniazid, and levels may climb into the toxic range. If the serum phenytoin levels are monitored and its dosage reduced appropriately, the concentrations can be kept within the therapeutic range. The dosage of the interacting drug may also be critical. Thus a small dosage of cimetidine may fail to inhibit the metabolism of warfarin, whereas a larger dose may have profound clinical effects.

Some interactions can be accommodated by using another member of the same group of drugs. For example, the serum levels of doxycycline can fall to subtherapeutic concentrations if phenytoin, barbiturates or carbamazepine are given, but other tetracyclines do not seem to be affected. Cimetidine causes serum warfarin levels to rise because it inhibits its metabolism, but not those of phenprocoumon because these two anticoagulants are metabolized in different ways. It is therefore clearly important not to extrapolate uncritically the interactions seen with one drug to all members of the same group.

The variability in patient response has lead to some extreme responses among prescribers. Some clinicians have become over-anxious about interactions so that their patients are denied useful drugs which they might reasonably be given if appropriate precautions are taken. This attitude is exacerbated by some of the more alarmist lists and charts of interactions which fail to make a distinction between interactions which are very well documented and well established, and those which have only been encountered in a single patient and which in the final analysis are probably totally idiosyncratic. 'One swallow does not make a summer', nor does a serious reaction in a single patient mean that the drugs in question should never again be administered to anyone else. At the other extreme there are a some clinicians who have personally encountered few interactions and therefore virtually disregard their existence so that some of their patients are potentially put at risk. The responsible position lies between these two extremes because a very substantial number of interacting drugs can be given together safely if the appropriate precautions are taken, whereas there are relatively few pairs of drugs which should always be avoided.

4 Mechanisms of drug interaction

Some drugs interact together in totally unique ways but, as the many examples in this book amply illustrate, there are certain mechanisms of interaction which are encountered time and time again. Some of these common mechanisms are discussed here in greater detail than space will allow in the individual synopses so that only the briefest reference need be made within the synopses.

Mechanisms which are unusual or peculiar to particular pairs of drugs are detailed within the synopses. Very many drugs which interact do so, not by a single mechanism, but often by two or more mechanisms acting in concert, although for clarity most of the mechanisms are dealt with here as though they occur in isolation. For convenience the mechanisms of interactions can be subdivided into those which involve the pharmacokinetics of a drug and those which are pharmacodynamic.

4.1 Pharmacokinetic interactions

Pharmacokinetic interactions are those which can affect the processes by which drugs are absorbed, distributed, metabolized and excreted (the so-called ADME interactions).

4.1.1 Drug absorption interactions

Most drugs are given orally for absorption through the mucous membranes of the gastrointestinal tract, and most of the interactions which go on within the gut result in reduced rather than increased absorption. A clear distinction must be made between those which decrease the *rate* of absorption and those which alter the *total* amount absorbed. For drugs which are given chronically on a multiple dose regimen (e.g. the oral anticoagulants) the rate of absorption is usually unimportant, provided the total amount of drug absorbed is not markedly altered. On the other hand for drugs which are given as single doses intended to be absorbed rapidly (e.g. hypnotics or analgesics) where a rapidly achieved high concentration is needed, a reduction in the rate of absorption may result in failure to achieve adequate serum levels. Table 1.1 lists some of the drug interactions which result from changes in absorption.

Table 1.1 Some drug absorption interactions

Drug affected	Interacting drugs	Effect of interaction
Digoxin	Metoclopramide Propantheline	Reduced digoxin absorption, increased digoxin absorption (due to changes in gut motility
Digoxin Thyroxine Warfarin	Cholestyramine	Reduced absorption of digoxin, thyroxine, warfarin due to binding/complexation with cholestyramine
Ketoconazole	Antacids, H_2-blockers	Reduced ketoconazole absorption due to reduced dissolution
Penicillamine	Al^{3+} and Mg^{2+} containing antacids, food, iron preparations	Formation of less soluble penicillamine chelates resulting in reduced absorption of penicillamine
Penicillin	Neomycin	Neomycin-induced malabsorption state
Quinolone antibiotics	Antacids containing Al^{3+}, Mg^{2+}, milk, Zn^{2+} (?), Fe^{2+}	Formation of poorly absorbed complexes
Tetracyclines	Antacids containing Al^{3+}, Ca^{2+}, Mg^{2+}, Bi^{2+}, milk, Zn^{2+}, Fe^{2+}	Formation of poorly soluble chelates resulting in reduced antibiotic absorption (see Fig. 1.2)

4.1.1.1 Effects of changes in gastrointestinal pH. The passage of drugs through mucous membranes by simple passive diffusion depends upon the extent to which they exist in the non-ionized, lipid-soluble form. Absorption is therefore governed by the pK_a of the drug, its lipid-solubility, the pH of the contents of gut and various other parameters relating to the pharmaceutical formulation of the drug. Thus the absorption of salicylic acid by the stomach is much higher at low pH than at high. On theoretical grounds it might be expected therefore that alterations in gastric pH caused by drugs such as antacids would have a marked effect on absorption, but in practice the outcome is often uncertain because a number of other mechanisms may also come into play such as chelation, adsorption and changes in gut motility which can considerably affect what actually happens. Rises in pH due to H_2-blockers and antacids which affect dissolution can, however,

markedly reduce the absorption of ketoconazole, and the absorption of enoxacin is also possibly reduced by rises in pH due to ranitidine.

4.1.1.2 Adsorption, chelation and other complexing mechanisms. Activated charcoal is intended to act as an adsorbing agent within the gut for the treatment of drug overdosage or to remove other toxic materials, but inevitably it can affect the absorption of drugs given in therapeutic doses. Antacids can also adsorb a very considerable number of drugs but often other mechanisms of interaction are also involved. For example the tetracycline antibiotics can chelate with a number of di- and trivalent metallic ions such as calcium, aluminium, bismuth and iron to form complexes which not only are poorly absorbed but have reduced antibacterial effects (see Fig. 1.2).

These metallic ions are found in dairy products and antacids. Separating the dosages by 2–3 h goes some way towards reducing the effects of this type of interaction. The marked reduction in the bioavailability of penicillamine by some antacids seems also to be due to chelation, although adsorption may have some part to play. Cholestyramine, an anionic exchange resin intended to bind bile acids and cholesterol metabolites in the gut, binds to a considerable number of drugs if co-administered (e.g.

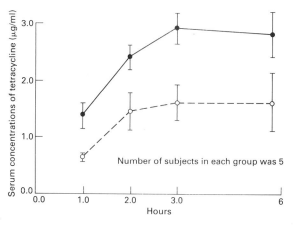

Fig. 1.2 A drug chelation interaction. Tetracycline forms a less-soluble chelate with iron if the two drugs are allowed to mix within the gut. This reduces the absorption and depresses the serum levels and the antibacterial effects (after Neuvonen PJ, Br Med J (1970) 4, 532, with permission). The same interaction can occur with other ions such as Al^{3+}, Ca^{2+}, Mg^{2+}, Bi^{2+} and Zn^{2+}.

digoxin, warfarin, thyroxine) thereby reducing their absorption. Table 1.1 lists these drugs which chelate or complex or adsorb other drugs thereby reducing their absorption.

4.1.1.3 Changes in gastrointestinal motility Since most drugs are largely absorbed in the upper part of the small intestine, drugs which alter the rate at which the stomach empties its contents can affect absorption. Propantheline, for example, delays gastric emptying and reduces paracetamol (acetaminophen) absorption whereas metoclopramide has the opposite effect; however the total amount of drug absorbed remains unaltered. These two drugs have quite the opposite effect on the absorption of hydrochlorothiazide and slowly dissolving brands of digoxin. Anticholinergic drugs decrease the motility of the gut, thus the tricyclic antidepressants can increase the absorption of dicoumarol probably because they increase the time available for dissolution and absorption, but in the case of levodopa they reduce the absorption possibly because the exposure time to intestinal mucosal metabolism is increased. The same reduced levodopa absorption has also been seen with homatropine. On the other hand benzhexol (another anticholinergic) reduces the absorption of chlorpromazine. Other examples of changes in motility which affect absorption include the reduced absorption caused by pethidine and diamorphine. These examples illustrate that what actually happens is sometimes unpredictable because the final outcome may be the result of several different mechanisms.

4.1.1.4 Malabsorption caused by drugs. Neomycin causes a malabsorption syndrome which is similar to that seen with non-tropical sprue. The effect is to impair the absorption of a number of drugs including digoxin and penicillin V.

4.1.2 Drug displacement (protein-binding) interactions

Following absorption, drugs are rapidly distributed around the body by the circulation. Some drugs are totally dissolved in the plasma water, but many others are transported with some proportion of their molecules in solution and the rest bound to plasma proteins, particularly the albumins. The extent of this binding varies enormously but some drugs are

extremely highly bound. For example, dicoumarol has only four out of every 1000 molecules remaining unbound at serum concentrations of 0.5 mg%. Drugs can also become bound to albumin in the interstitial fluid, and some such as digoxin can bind to the heart muscle tissue.

The binding of drugs to the plasma proteins is reversible, an equilibrium being established between those molecules which are bound and those which are not. Only the unbound molecules remain free and pharmacologically active, while those which are bound form a circulating but pharmacologically inactive reservoir which, in the case of 'restrictive' drugs, is temporarily protected from metabolism and excretion. As the free molecules become metabolized, so some of the bound molecules become unbound and pass into solution to exert their normal pharmacological actions, before they, in their turn are metabolized and excreted.

Depending on the concentrations and their relative affinities for the binding sites, one drug may successfully compete with another and displace it from the sites it is already occupying. The displaced (and now active) drug molecules pour into plasma water where their concentration rapidly rises. So, for example, a drug which reduces the binding from (say) 99 to 95% would thereby increase the unbound concentration of free and active drug from 1 to 4% (a fourfold increase). This displacement is only likely to raise the number of free and active molecules significantly if the majority of the drug is within the plasma rather than the tissues, so that only drugs with a low apparent volume of distribution (V_d) will be affected. Such drugs include the sulphonylureas such as tolbutamide (96% bound, V_d 10 l), oral anticoagulants such as warfarin (99% bound, V_d 9 l) and phenytoin (90% bound, V_d 35 l). Other highly bound drugs include diazoxide, ethacrynic acid, methotrexate, nalidixic acid, phenylbutazone and the sulphonamides.

Displacement of this kind happens when patients stabilized on warfarin are given chloral hydrate because its major metabolite, trichloroacetic acid, is a highly bound compound which successfully displaces warfarin, thereby increasing its anticoagulant effects. This effect is only very short-lived because the now free and active warfarin molecules become exposed to metabolism as the blood flows through the liver and the total amount of drug rapidly falls. A small but transient increase in the anticoagulant effects can be seen and the warfarin requirements fall briefly by about a third, but within about five days a new equilibrium becomes established with the same concentration of unbound warfarin, even though the free fraction has increased. Normally no change in the warfarin dosage is needed.[7]

In vitro many commonly used drugs are capable of being displaced by others, but in the body the effects seem almost always to be buffered so effectively that the outcome is normally clinically unimportant, and it would seem that the importance of this interaction mechanism has been grossly over-emphasized, despite statements made to the contrary in numerous papers, reviews and drug data sheets.[13] It is difficult to find an example of a clinically important interaction due to this mechanism alone. One possible example is the marked diuresis which was seen in patients with nephrotic syndrome when they were given clofibrate.[8] Usually this mechanism has a minor part to play compared with other mechanisms which are going on at the same time. However it may need to be taken into account in some circumstances.

Suppose, for example, an epileptic patient has a

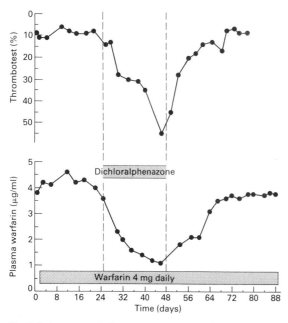

Fig. 1.3 An enzyme induction interaction. In this patient the hypnotic dichloralpenazone (Welldorm) increased the metabolism of the warfarin, thereby reducing its serum levels and its effects (thrombotest percentages) (after Breckenridge A et al., Clin Sci (1971) 40, 351, with permission).

total serum phenytoin concentration of 50 μmol/l of which 45 μmol/l is bound and 5 μmol/l free (i.e. 10% free). If now another drug is given which displaces a further 10%, more of the phenytoin thereby becomes exposed to metabolism and excretion so that the total serum phenytoin concentration is halved (to 25 μmol/l) with a free concentration of 20% but which still remains at 5 μmol/l. From the patient's point of view the effective amount of phenytoin stays the same, even though the total amount of phenytoin in circulation has halved. Under these circumstances there would be no need to change the phenytoin dosage, and to do so in order to accommodate the change in total levels might lead to overdosage.

Basic drugs as well as acidic drugs can be highly protein bound, but clinically important displacement interactions do not seem to have been described. The reasons seem to be that the binding sites within the plasma are different from those occupied by acidic drugs (alpha-1-acid glycoprotein rather than albumin) and, in addition, basic drugs have a large V_d with only a small proportion of the total amount of drug being within the plasma.

4.1.3 Drug metabolism (biotransformation) interactions

Although some drugs are lost from the body simply by being excreted unchanged in the urine, a very large number are chemically altered within the body to less lipid-soluble compounds which are more easily excreted by the kidneys. If this were not so, many drugs would remain in the body for extended periods of time and continue to exert their effects. This chemical change is called metabolism, biotransformation, biochemical degradation or sometimes detoxification. Some drug metabolism goes on in the serum, the kidneys, the skin and the intestines, but by far the greatest proportion is carried out by enzymes which are found in the membranes of the endoplasmic reticulum of the liver cells. If liver is homogenized and then centrifuged, the reticulum breaks up into small sacs called microsomes which carry the enzymes, and it is for this reason that the metabolizing enzymes of the liver are frequently referred to as the 'liver microsomal enzymes'.

4.1.3.1 Enzyme induction. A phenomenon familiar to prescribers is the 'tolerance' which develops to some drugs. For example, when barbiturates were widely

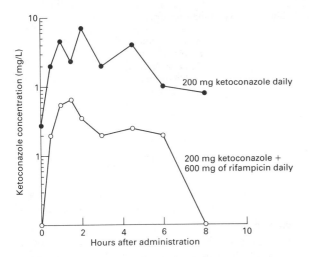

Fig. 1.4 An enzyme induction interaction. Rifampicin (600 mg daily plus isoniazid) increased the metabolism of the ketoconazole in this patient, thereby reducing the serum levels (after Brass C, Antimicrob Ag Chemother (1982) 21, 151, with permission).

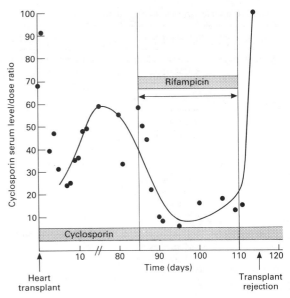

Fig. 1.5 An enzyme induction interaction. Rifampicin (600 mg daily) increased the metabolism of cyclosporin in this patient, thereby reducing the trough serum levels. He subsequently died because his heart transplant was rejected (after Van Buren D et al., Transplant Proc (1984) 16, 1642, with permission).

used as hypnotics it was found necessary to keep on increasing the dosage as time went by to achieve the same hypnotic effect, the reason being that the barbiturates increase the activity of the microsomal enzymes so that pace of metabolism and excretion increases. This phenomenon of enzyme stimulation or 'induction' not only accounts for the tolerance, but if another drug is present as well which is metabolized by the same range of enzymes (an oral anticoagulant for example), its enzymic metabolism is similarly increased and larger doses are needed to maintain the same therapeutic effect. Figure 1.3 shows the effects of an enzyme inducing agent, dichloralphenazone, on the metabolism and anticoagulant effects of warfarin. Figures 1.4 and 1.5 show the effects of another enzyme inducing agent, rifampicin (rifampin) on the serum levels of ketoconazole and cyclosporin. Table 1.2 lists some of the interactions due to enzyme induction and Table 1.3 contains some of the potent enzyme-inducing drugs.

A metabolic pathway which is commonly affected is Phase I oxidation, this term covering a number of metabolic biotransformations, all of which require the presence of NADPH and the haem-containing protein cytochrome P450. When enzyme induction occurs the amount of endoplasmic reticulum within the liver cells increases and the cytochrome P450 levels also rise. The extent of the enzyme induction depends on the drug and its dosage, but its development may take days or two–three weeks, and persist for a similar length of time after withdrawal of the inducing agent so that enzyme induction interactions are delayed in both starting and stopping. Enzyme induction is an extremely common mechanism of interaction and is not confined to drugs but is also caused by the chlorinated hydrocarbon insecticides such as dicophane and lindane, and after smoking tobacco. We now know that Cytochrome P450 is not one enzyme but a group of enzymes, and as these become individually characterized it is becoming increasingly possible to predict which drugs are likely to interact with which.[17]

These interactions can be accommodated by increasing the dose of the drug which is being affected, but the effects require thorough monitoring and there are obvious dangers if the inducing drug is withdrawn without reducing the dosage of the other drug. The raised drug dosage will be an overdose when the drug metabolism has returned to normal.

4.1.3.2 Enzyme inhibition. Just as some drugs can stimulate the activity of the microsomal enzymes, so

Table 1.2 Interactions due to enzyme induction

Drug affected	Inducing agent(s)	Effect of interaction
Anticoagulants (oral)	Aminoglutethimide Barbiturates Carbamazepine Dichloralphenazone Glutethimide Phenazone Rifampicin (rifampin)	Anticoagulant effects reduced (see Fig. 1.3)
Contraceptives (oral)	Barbiturates Carbamazepine Phenytoin Primidone Rifampicin	Contraceptive effects reduced. Break-through bleeding, contraceptive failures
Corticosteroids	Aminoglutethimide Barbiturates Carbamazepine Phenytoin Primidone Rifampicin	Corticosteroid effects reduced
Haloperidol	Tobacco smoke	Haloperidol effects reduced
Pentazocine	Tobacco smoke	Pentazocine effects reduced
Phenytoin	Rifampicin (rifampin)	Phenytoin effects reduced. Seizure-risk increased
Theophylline	Barbiturates Rifampicin Tobacco smoke	Theophylline effects reduced

Table 1.3 Enzyme inducing drugs

Aminoglutethimide
Barbiturates
Carbamazepine
Dichloralphenazone
Glutethimide
Phenazone (antipyrine)
Phenytoin
Primidone
Rifampicin (rifampin)
Tobacco smoke

there are others which have the opposite effect and act as inhibitors. The normal pace of drug metabolism is slackened so that the metabolism of other drugs given concurrently is also reduced and they begin to accumulate within the body, the effect being essentially the same as when the dosage is increased. Unlike enzyme induction which may take several days or even weeks to develop fully, enzyme inhibition can occur within two to three days resulting in the rapid development of toxicity. Figure 1.6 shows what happened when an epileptic patient on phenytoin was given chloramphenicol. The accumulating phenytoin was not detected until it reached levels at which the patient began to manifest toxicity.

Figure 1.7 illustrates the sharp and potentially hazardous rise in blood pressure which can occur if the normally protective monoamine oxidase within the gut wall and liver is inhibited by the presence of an MAO-inhibitory drug (tranylcypromine). Other mechanisms of interaction are also involved. Table 1.4 lists some other interactions due to the inhibition of microsomal and other enzymes, and Table 1.5 is a list of enzyme-inhibiting drugs. Numerous other examples are to be found throughout this book.

The clinical significance of many enzyme inhibition interactions depends on the extent to which the serum levels of the drug rise. If the serum levels remain within the therapeutic range the interaction may be advantageous. If not, the interaction be-

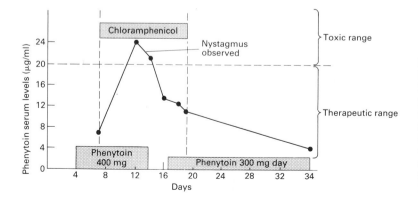

Fig. 1.6 An enzyme inhibition interaction. The chloramphenicol inhibited the metabolism of the phenytoin in this patient so that the serum levels climbed into the toxic range and intoxication developed (indicated by nystagmus). The problem was solved by stopping the phenytoin and later re-starting at a lower dosage (after Ballek RE et al., Lancet (1973) i, 150, with permission).

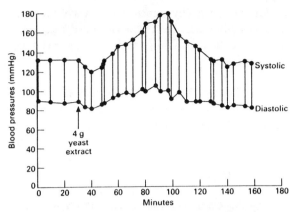

Fig. 1.7 An enzyme inhibition interaction. The effect of 4 g *Marmite* (a tyramine-rich yeast extract) on the diastolic and systolic blood pressures of a patient taking a Monoamine Oxidase Inhibitor (tranylcypromine) (after Blackwell B, Br J Psychiat (1967) 113, 349, with permission).

Table 1.4 Interactions due to enzyme inhibition

Drug affected	Inhibiting agent(s)	Clinical outcome
Alcohol	Chlorpropamide Disulfiram Latamoxef Metronidazole	Disulfiram-reaction due to a rise in blood acetaldehyde levels
Anticoagulants (oral)	Metronidazole Phenylbutazone Sulphinpyrazone	Anticoagulant effects increased. Bleeding possible
Azathioprine Mercaptopurine	Allopurinol	Azathioprine/ mercaptopurine effects increased; toxicity
Caffeine	Enoxacin Idrocilamide	Caffeine effects increased. Intoxication possible
Corticosteroids	Erythromycin Triacetyl- oleandomycin	Corticosteroid effects increased. Toxicity possible
Phenytoin	Chloramphenicol Isoniazid	Phenytoin effects increased. Intoxication possible (see Fig. 1.6)
Suxamethonium	Ecothiophate	Neuromuscular blockade increased. Prolonged apnoea possible
Tolbutamide Chloramphenicol	Azapropazone Phenylbutazone	Tolbutamide effects increased. Hypoglycaemia possible
Tyramine- containing foodstuffs	Monoamine oxidase inhibitors (MAOI)	Tyramine-induced hypertensive crisis (other mechanisms also involved; see Fig. 1.7)

Table 1.5 Some enzyme inhibitors

Allopurinol
Azapropazone
Chloramphenicol
Ciprofloxacin
Cimetidine
Disulfiram
Enoxacin
Erythromycin
Idrocilamide
Isoniazid
Ketoconazole
Phenylbutazone
Sulphinopyrazone
Triacetyloleandomycin

comes adverse as the serum levels climb into the toxic range.

4.1.3.3 Changes in blood flow through the liver

After absorption in the intestine, the portal circulation takes drugs directly to the liver before they are distributed by the blood flow around the rest of the body. A number of highly lipid-soluble drugs undergo substantial biotransformation during this 'first pass' through the gut wall and liver and there is evidence that some concurrently administered drugs can have a marked effect on the extent of first pass metabolism. Cimetidine (but not ranitidine) decreases hepatic blood flow and thereby increases the bioavailability of propranolol. Propranolol also reduces both its own clearance and that of other drugs such as lignocaine (lidocaine). A number of other drugs have the opposite effect and increase the flow of blood through the liver so that their metabolism is increased.

4.1.4 Interactions due to changes in excretion

With the exception of the inhalation anaesthetics, most drugs are excreted either in the bile or in the urine. Blood entering the kidneys along the renal arteries is, first of all, delivered to the glomeruli of the tubules where molecules small enough to pass through the pores of the glomerular membrane (e.g. water, salts, some drugs) are filtered through into the lumen of the tubules. Larger molecules, such as plasma proteins, and blood cells are retained. The blood flow then passes to the remaining parts of the kidney tubules where active energy-using transport systems are able to remove drugs and their metabolites from the blood and secrete them into the tubular filtrate. The tubule cells additionally possess active and passive transport systems for the reabsorption of drugs. Interference by drugs with kidney tubule fluid pH, with active transport systems and with blood flow to the kidney can alter the excretion of other drugs.

4.1.4.1 Changes in urinary pH. As with drug absorption in the gut, passive reabsorption of drugs depends upon the extent to which the drug exists in the non-ionized lipid-soluble form which in its turn depends on its pK_a and the pH of the urine. Only the un-ionized form is lipid-soluble and able to diffuse back through the lipid membranes of the tubule cells. Thus at high pH values (alkaline), weakly acid drugs (pK_a 3.0–7.5) largely exist as ionized lipid-insoluble molecules which are unable to diffuse into the tubule cells and will therefore be lost in the urine. The converse will be true for weak organic bases with pK_a values of 7.5–10.5. Thus pH changes which increase the amount in the un-ionized form (alkaline urine for acidic drugs, acid for bases) increase the loss of the drug, whereas moving the pH in the opposite directions will increase their retention. Figure 1.8 illustrates the situation with a weakly acidic drug. The clinical significance of this interaction mechanism is small because although a very large number of drugs are either weak acids or bases, almost all are largely metabolized by the liver to inactive compounds and few are excreted in the urine unchanged. In practice therefore only a handful of drugs seem to be affected by changes in urinary pH (the exceptions include changes in the excretion of quinidine and salicylate due to alterations in urinary pH caused by antacids). In cases of overdosage, deliberate urinary pH changes have been used to increase the loss of drugs such as phenobarbitone and salicylates.

4.1.4.2 Changes in active kidney tubule excretion. Drugs which use the same active transport systems in the kidney tubules can compete with one another for excretion. For example, probenecid reduces the excretion of penicillin and other drugs by successfully competing for an excretory mechanism, thus the 'loser' (penicillin) is retained. But even the 'winner' (probenecid) is also later retained because it is passively reabsorbed further along the kidney tubule (see Fig. 1.9). Table 1.6 contains some examples of drugs which interact in this way.

4.1.4.3 Changes in kidney blood flow. The flow of blood through the kidney is partially controlled by the production of renal vasodilatory prostaglandins. If the synthesis of these prostaglandins is inhibited (e.g. by indomethacin), the renal excretion of lithium is reduced and its serum levels rise as a result.

4.1.4.4 Biliary excretion and the entero-hepatic shunt. A number of drugs are excreted in the bile, either unchanged or conjugated (e.g. as the glucuronide) to make them more water soluble. Some of the conjugates are metabolized to the parent compound by the gut flora which are then reabsorbed. This recycling process prolongs the stay of the drug within the body, but if activity of the gut flora is decimated by the presence of an antibiotic, the drug is not recycled and is lost more quickly. This may possibly explain the rare failure of the oral contraceptives which can be brought about by the concurrent use of penicillins or tetracyclines.

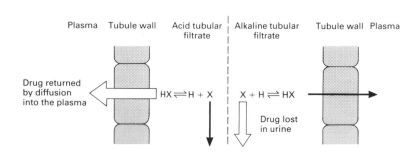

Fig. 1.8 An excretion interaction. If the tubular filtrate is acidified, most of the molecules of weakly acid drugs (HX) exist in an un-ionized lipid-soluble form and are able to return through the lipid membranes of the tubule cells by simple diffusion. Thus they are retained. In alkaline urine most of the drug molecules exist in an ionized non-lipid souble form (X). In this form the molecules are unable to diffuse freely through these membranes and are therefore lost in the urine.

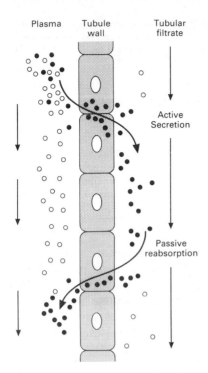

Plasma | Tubule wall | Tubular filtrate

Active Secretion

Passive reabsorption

Fig. 1.9 Competitive interaction between drugs for active tubular secretion. Probenecid (●) is able successfully to compete with some of the other drugs (○) for active secretory mechanisms in the kidney tubules which reduces their loss in the urine and raises serum levels. The probenecid is later passively reabsorbed.

4.2 Pharmacodynamic interactions

Pharmacodynamic interactions are those where the effects of one drug are changed by the presence of another drug at its site of action. Sometimes the drugs directly compete for particular receptors (e.g. beta-2 agonists such as salbutamol and beta-antagonists) but often the reaction is more indirect and involves the interference with physiological mechanisms. These interactions are much less easy to classify neatly than those which are pharmacokinetic.

4.2.1 Additive or synergistic interactions and combined toxicity

If two drugs which have the same pharmacological effect are given together, the effects can be additive. For example, alcohol depresses the central nervous system and, if taken in moderate amounts with normal therapeutic doses of any of a large number of

Table 1.6 Interactions due to changes in renal transport

Drug affected	Interacting drug	Result of interaction
Cephalosporins Dapsone Indomethacin Nalidixic acid Penicillin PAS (amino-salicylic acid)	Probenecid	Serum levels of drug affected raised; possibility of toxicity with some drugs. See Fig. 1.9
Methotrexate	Salicylates and some other NSAIDs	Methotrexate serum levels raised. Serious methotrexate toxicity possible
Acetohexamide Glibenclamide Tolbutamide	Phenylbutazone	Hypoglycaemic effects increased and prolonged due to reduced renal excretion

drugs (e.g. hypnosedatives, tranquillizers, etc.), the result may be excessive drowsiness. Strictly speaking these are not interactions within the definition given at the beginning of this chapter, nevertheless it is convenient to consider them within the broad context of the clinical outcome of giving two drugs together. Additive effects can occur with both the main effects of the drugs as well as their side-effects, thus an additive 'interaction' can occur with anticholinergic antiparkinson drugs (main effect) or butyrophenones (side effect) which can result in serious anticholinergic toxicity. Sometimes the additive effects are solely toxic (e.g. additive ototoxicity, nephrotoxicity or bone marrow depression). Examples of these reactions are listed in Table 1.7. It is common to use the terms 'additive', 'summation', 'synergy' or 'potentiation' to describe what happens if two or more drugs behave like this. These words have precise pharmacological definitions but they are often used rather loosely as synonyms because in practice in man it is often very difficult to know the extent of the increased activity, that is to say whether the effects are greater or smaller than the sum of the individual effects.

4.2.2 Antagonistic or opposing interactions

In contrast to additive interactions, there are some pairs of drugs with activities which are opposed to one another. For example the oral anticoagulants can prolong the blood clotting time by competitively

Table 1.7 Additive, synergistic or summation interactions

Drugs	Result of interaction
Anticholinergics + anticholinergics (anti-parkinsonian agents, butyrophenones, phenothiazines, tricyclic antidepressants, etc.)	Increased anticholinergic effects; heat stroke in hot and humid conditions; adynamic ileus; toxic psychoses
Antihypertensives + drugs causing hypotension (anti-anginals, vasodilators, phenothiazines)	Increased antihypertensive effects; orthostasis
CNS depressants + CNS depressants (alcohol, anti-emetics, antihistamines hypnosedatives, tranquillizers, etc.)	Impaired psychomotor skills, reduced alertness, drowsiness, stupor, respiratory depression, coma, death
Methotrexate + co-trimoxazole	Bone marrow megaloblastosis due to folic acid antagonism
Nephrotoxic drugs + nephrotoxic drugs (gentamicin or tobramycin with cephalothin)	Increased nephrotoxicity
Neuromuscular blockers + drugs with neuromuscular blocking effects (e.g. aminoglycoside antibiotics	Increased neuromuscular blockage; delayed recovery, prolonged apnoea
Potassium supplements + potassium-sparing diuretics (triamterene)	Marked hyperkalaemia

Table 1.8 Opposing or antagonistic interactions

Drug affected	Interacting drug	Results of interaction
Anticoagulants	Vitamin K	Anticoagulant effects opposed
Carbenoxolone	Spironolactone	Ulcer-healing effects opposed
Hypoglycaemic agents	Glucocorticoids	Hypoglycaemic effects opposed
Hypnotic drugs	Caffeine	Hypnosis opposed
Levodopa	Antipsychotics (those with Parkinson side effects)	Antiparkinsonian effects opposed

tensive effect is prevented. This is illustrated in Fig. 1.10. The tricyclic antidepressants also prevent the re-uptake of noradrenaline into peripheral adrenergic neurones so that its pressor effects are increased. The antihypertensive effects of clonidine are also prevented by the tricyclic antidepressants,

inhibiting the effects of dietary vitamin K. If the intake of vitamin K is increased the effects of the oral anticoagulant are antagonized and the prothrombin time can return to normal thereby cancelling out the therapeutic benefits of anticoagulant treatment. Other examples of this type of interaction are listed in Table 1.8.

4.2.3 Interactions due to changes in drug transport mechanisms

A number of drugs whose actions occur at adrenergic neurones can be prevented from reaching those sites of action by the presence of other drugs. Thus the uptake of guanethidine and related drugs (guanoclor, bethanidine, debrisoquine, etc.) is blocked by chlorpromazine, haloperidol, thiothixene, a number of indirectly-acting sympathomimetic amines and the tricyclic antidepressants so that the antihyper-

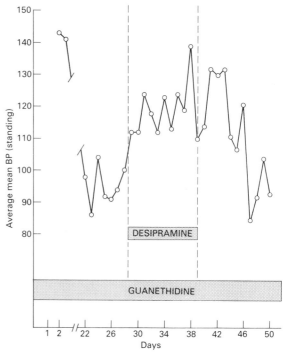

Fig. 1.10 A pharmacodynamic interaction. The desipramine (75–100 mg daily) inhibited the uptake of guanethidine (150 mg daily) into adrenergic neurones of the sympathetic nervous system thereby stopping its antihypertensive effects. As a result the blood pressure in this patient rose once again (after Oates JA et al., Ann NY Acad Sci (1971) 179, 302, with permission).

Table 1.9 Interactions due to changes in drug transport mechanisms

Drug affected	Interacting drug	Results of interaction
Clonidine	Tricyclic antidepressants	Antihypertensive effects opposed, possibly due to interference in CNS with clonidine uptake
Guanethidine-like antihypertensives (debrisoquine, guanoclor, etc.)	Tricyclic antidepressants Chlorpromazine Haloperidol Thiothixene Indirectly-acting sympathomimetics	Antihypertensive effects opposed, due to inhibition of uptake into adrenergic neurones. See Fig. 1.10
Noradrenaline (norepinephrine)	Tricyclic antidepressants	Pressor effects increased due to inhibition of noradrenaline uptake into adrenergic neurones

Table 1.10 Interactions due to disturbances in fluid and electrolyte balance

Drug affected	Interacting drug	Results of interaction
Digitalis	Potassium-depleting diuretics	Digitalis toxicity related to changes in ionic balance at the myocardium
Lithium chloride	Dietary salt restriction	Increased serum lithium levels; intoxication possible
	Increased salt intake	Reduced serum lithium levels
		Both changes related to changes in sodium excretion
Lithium chloride	Thiazide and related diuretics	Increased serum lithium levels. Intoxication possible
Guanethidine Chlorothiazide	Kebuzone Phenylbutazone	Antihypertensive effects opposed due to salt and water retention

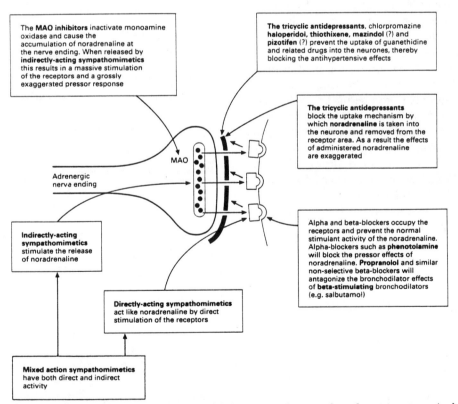

Fig. 1.11 Interactions at adrenergic neurones. A highly simplified composite diagram of an adrenergic neurone (molecules of noradrenaline (norepinephrine) indicated as (●) contained in a single vesicle at the nerve-ending) to illustrate in outline some of the different sites where drugs can interact. More details of these interactions are to be found in individual synopses.

one possible reason being that the uptake of cloni-dine within the CNS is blocked. Some of these interactions at adrenergic neurones are illustrated in Fig. 1.11. See also Table 1.9.

4.2.4 Interactions due to disturbances in fluid and electrolyte balance

An increase in the sensitivity of the myocardium to the digitalis glycosides, and resultant toxicity, can result from a fall in plasma potassium concentrations brought about by potassium-depleting diuretics such as frusemide. Plasma lithium levels can rise if thiazide diuretics are used because the clearance of the lithium by the kidney is changed, probably as a result of the changes in sodium excretion which can accompany the use of these diuretics. Table 1.10 lists some examples.

5 Conclusions

It is quite impossible to remember all the known clinically important interactions and how they occur, which is why this reference book has been written, but there are some broad general principles which need little memorizing. Be on the alert with any drugs which have a narrow therapeutic window or where it is necessary to keep serum levels at or above a suitable level (anticoagulants, anticonvulsants, cytotoxics, antihypertensives, anti-infectives, digitalis glycosides, hypoglycaemic agents, immunosuppressants, etc). Remember those drugs which are enzyme-inducing agents (phenytoin, barbiturates) and enzyme inhibitors (cimetidine), and keep in mind that the elderly are most at risk because of reduced liver and kidney function on which drug clearance depends. And think about the basic pharmacology of the drugs under consideration so that obvious problems (additive CNS depression for example) are not overlooked.

References

1 Smith JW, Seidl LG, Cluff LE. Studies on the epidemiology of adverse drug reactions. V. Clinical factors influencing susceptibility. Ann Intern Med (1969) 65, 629.

2 Puckett WH, Visconti JA. An epidemiological study of the clinical significance of drug-drug interaction in a private community hospital. Amer J Hosp Pharm (1971) 28, 247.

3 Shinn AF, Shrewsbury RP, Anderson KW. Development of a computerized drug interaction database (Medicom) for use in a patient specific environment. Drug Inform (1983) 17, 205.

4 Haumschild MJ, Ward ES, Bishop JM, Haumschild MS. Pharmacy-based computer system for monitoring and reporting drug interactions. Am J Hosp Pharm (1987) 44, 345.

5 Schuster BG, Fleckenstein L, Wilson JP, Peck CC. Low incidence of adverse reactions due to drug-drug interaction in a potentially high risk population of medical inpatients. Clin Res (1982) 30, 258A.

6 Ishikura C, Ishizuka H. Evaluation of a computerized drug interaction checking system. Int J Bio-Medical Computing (1983) 14, 311.

7 Boston Collaborative Drug Surveillance Program. Interaction between chloral hydrate and warfarin. N Eng J Med (1972) 286, 53.

8 Bridgeman JF, Rosem SM, Thorp JM. Complications during clofibrate treatment of nephrotic syndrome hyperlipoproteinaemia. Lancet (1972) ii, 506.

9 Manon-Espaillat R, Burnstine TH, Remler B, Reed RC, Osorio I. Antiepileptic drug intoxication: factors and their significance. Epilepsia (1991) 32, 96–100.

10 Jankel CA, Speedie SM. Detecting drug interactions: a review of the literature. DICP Ann Pharmacotherapy (1990) 24, 982–9.

11 Cadieux RJ. Drug interactions in the elderly. Postgrad Med (1989) 86, 179–86.

12 Manchon ND, Bercoff E, Lamarchand P, Chassagne P, Senant J, Bourreille J. Fréquence et gravité des interaction médicamenteuses dans une population âgée: étude prospective concernant 639 malades. Rev Med Interne (1989) 10, 521–5.

13 MacKichan JJ. Protein binding drug displacement interactions. Fact or fiction? Clin Pharmacokinetics (1989) 16, 65–73.

14 Lipton JL, Bero LA, Bird JA, McPhee SJ. The impact of clinical pharmacist' consultations on physicians' geriatric drug prescribing. Medical Care (1992) 30, 646–58.

15 Rupp MT, De Young M, Schondelmeyer SW. Prescribing problems and pharmacist interventions in community practice. Medical Care (1992) 30, 926–40.

16 Tinawi M, Alguire P. The prevalence of drug interactions in hospitalized patients. Clin Res (1992) 40, 773A.

17 Tucker GT. The rational selection of drug interaction studies: implications of recent advances in drug metabolism. Int J Clin Pharmacol Ther Toxicol (1992) 30, 550–3.

Chapter 2
Alcohol Interactions

For social and historical reasons alcohol is usually bought from a store or in a bar or restaurant, rather than from a Pharmacy because it is considered to be a drink and not a drug, but pharmacologically speaking it has much in common with medicinal drugs which depress the central nervous system. Objective tests show that as blood-alcohol levels rise, the ability to perform a number of skills gradually deteriorates as the brain becomes progessively disorganized. The myth that alcohol is a stimulant has

Table 2.1 Reactions to different concentrations of alcohol in the blood

Amount of alcohol drunk (units)			
Man 11 stones (70 kg)	Woman 9 stones (55 kg)	Blood–alcohol levels mg% (mg per 100 ml)	Reactions to different % of alcohol in the blood
2	1	25–30	Sense of well-being enhanced. Reaction times reduced
4	2	50–60	Mild loss of inhibition, judgement impaired, increased risk of accidents at home, at work and on the road; no overt signs of drunkenness
5	3	75–80	Physical co-ordination reduced, marked loss of inhibition; noticeably under the influence; at the legal limit for driving in the UK
7	4	100 +	Clumsiness, loss of physical control, tendency to extreme responses; definite intoxication
10	6	150	Slurred speech, possible loss of memory the following day, probably drunk and disorderly
24	14	360	Dead drunk, sleepiness, possible loss of consciousness
33	20	500	Coma and possibly death

1 unit	= half pint (300 ml medium strength beer)	= glass wine (100 ml)	= single single sherry or martini (a third of a gill (50 ml))	= single spirit one-sixth gill (25 ml)

3–4% alcohol	11% alcohol	17–20% alcohol	37–40% alcohol

After *Which?* October 1984, page 447 and others.

arisen because at parties and social occasions it helps people to lose some of their inhibitions and allows them to relax and unwind. Professor JH Gaddum put it amusingly and succinctly when, describing the early effects of moderate amounts of alcohol, he wrote that 'logical thought is difficult but after dinner speeches easy.' The expansiveness and locquaciousness which are socially acceptable, lead on, with increasing amounts of alcohol, to unrestrained behaviour in normally well-controlled individuals, through drunkenness, unconsciousness and finally death from respiratory failure. These effects are all a reflection of the progressive and deepening depression of the CNS.

Table 2.1 gives an indication in very broad terms of the reactions of men and women to different amounts and concentrations of alcohol. On the whole women are smaller than men, they have a higher proportion of fat in which alcohol is not very soluble, their body fluids represent a smaller proportion of their total body mass and their first-pass metabolism of alcohol is less than men because they have less alcohol dehydrogenase in their stomach wall. Consequently if a man and woman of the same weight matched each other, drink for drink, the woman would finish up with a blood alcohol level about 50% higher than the man. The values shown assume that the drinkers regularly drink, have had a meal and weigh between 9 and 11 stones (55–70 kg). Higher blood alcohol levels would occur if drunk on an empty stomach and lower values in much heavier individuals. The liver metabolizes about one unit per hour so that the values will fall with time.

Since alcohol impairs the skills needed to drive safely, almost all national and state authorities have imposed maximum legal blood-alcohol limits. In the UK and a number of other countries this is currently 80 mg/100 ml (35 μg per 100 ml in the breath) but impairment is clearly detectable at lower concentrations, for which reason some countries have imposed much lower legal limits. Since many countries express their statutory blood-alcohol limits for driving in mg/ml or g, and breath-alcohol limits in mg/L, all of the values in Table 2.2 have been expressed in the same way units for easy comparison.

Probably the most common drug interaction of all occurs if alcohol is drunk while taking other drugs which have CNS depressant activity, the result being even further CNS depression. Blood alcohol levels well within the legal driving limit may, in the pres-

Table 2.2 Maximum legally allowable blood alcohol limits when driving in various countries

100 mg%	Eire, Puerto Rico, Some of the States in the USA
90 mg%	Cyprus, Peru (0.99 ml%)
80 mg%	Austria, Belgium, Brazil, Canada, Ivory Coast, Denmark, France, Germany, Iceland, Ireland, Italy, Luxembourg, Mauritius, New Zealand, Northern Ireland, Singapore, South Africa, Spain, Switzerland, Thailand, United Kingdom, some of the States in the USA
54 mg%	Netherlands
50 mg%	Australia, Chile, Finland, Greece, Iceland, Japan, Norway, Portugal, Turkey, Yugoslavia
20 mg%	Poland, Sweden
0 mg%	Albania, Bahrain, Brunei, Bulgaria, Czech Republic, East Germany, Egypt, Hungary, Iran, Jordan, Pakistan, Romania, Saudi Arabia, Slovak Republic

Notes:

For easy comparison the legally allowable blood alcohol limits have all been expressed as mg%. Thus blood alcohol levels of 80 mg% = 80 mg of alcohol in 100 ml blood = 0.8 g/l. The breath level limit equivalent to 80 mg% can vary slightly: thus UK and Eire (35 μg/l), South Africa (38 μg/l).

Some of the Australian states have different rules for certain drivers (learners, bus drivers, etc.), and other countries have a two tier system with different penalties. Some of the former members of the Soviet Union do not have blood-alcohol levels specifically stated but it is an offence to drive while intoxicated. Muslim countries forbid alcohol entirely. Some of the legal limits are under review and likely to be reduced shortly to the next level (Austria, Eire, some states in the USA).

ence of other CNS depressants, be equivalent to blood alcohol levels at or above the legal limit (in terms of worsened driving and other skills). This can occur with some antihistamines, analgesics, antidepressants, cough, cold and influenza remedies, hypno-sedatives, psychotropics, tranquillizers, travel-sickness remedies and others (see Alcohol + CNS depressants). This chapter contains a number of synopses which describe the results of formal studies using alcohol with a number of recognized CNS depressants, but there are still many other drugs which await study of this kind and which undoubtedly represent a real hazard.

A less common interaction which can occur between alcohol and some drugs, chemical agents and fungi is the flushing (Antabuse) reaction. This is exploited in the case of disulfiram (Antabuse) as a drink deterrent, but it can occur unexpectedly with some other drugs and be both unpleasant and possibly frightening but it is not usually dangerous. See the Index.

Alcohol + Amphetamines

Abstract/Summary

Dexamphetamine (dextroamphetamine) can reduce to some extent the deleterious effects of alcohol on driving skills, but some impairment still occurs and it may be unsafe to drive.

Clinical evidence

Alcohol (0.85 g/kg–2 ml/kg 100 proof vodka in orange juice) worsened the performance of a SEDI task (Simulator Evaluation of Drug Impairment) in 12 normal subjects.[1] This task is believed to parallel the skills needed to drive safely and involves tests of attention, memory, recognition, decision making and reaction time. When additionally given 0.09 or 0.18 mg/kg dexamphetamine, the performance of the SEDI task was improved (dosage related) but the subjective assessment of intoxication was unchanged. Blood-alcohol levels reached a maximum of about 100 g/dl at an hour. The bioavailability of the alcohol was slightly increased.[1]

Earlier reports using different testing methods found that in some tests dexamphetamine modified the effects of alcohol, but the total picture was complex.[2,4–6] Another study found that dexamphetamine failed to improve attentive motor performance made worse by alcohol if the task was long and boring.[3]

Mechanism

Not understood. Although alcohol is a CNS depressant and the amphetamines are CNS stimulants, there is no simple antagonism between the two.

Importance and management

This interaction has been well studied, but the conclusions to be drawn from the results are not clear cut. Although there is some evidence that the effects of alcohol are modified or reduced, none of these reports should be used to support the uncritical use of amphetamines to sober up drinkers because their driving skills still remain impaired to some extent, particularly after a while when boredom or fatigue is likely to set in.

Reference

1 Perez-Reyes M, White WR, McDonald SA, Hicks RE. Interaction between ethanol and dextroamphetamines: effects of psychomotor performance. Alcoholism: clinical and Experimental Research (1992) 16, 75–81.
2 Kaplan HL, Forney RB, Richards AB, Hughes FW. Dextro-amphetamine, alcohol, and dextro-amphetamine-alcohol combination and mental performance. In Harger RN (Ed). Alcohol and traffic safety. Proc 4th Int Conf Alc Traffic Safety, Bloomington, Indiana. Indiana Univ Press (1966) 211–14.
3 Brown DJ, Hughes FW, Forney RB, Richards AB. Effect of d-amphetamine and alcohol on attentive motor performance in human subjects. In Harger RN (Ed). Alcohol and traffic safety. Proc 4th Int Conf Alc Traffic Safety, Bloomington, Indiana. Indiana Univ Press (1966) 215–19.
4 Huges FW, Forney RB. Dextro-amphetamine, ethanol and dextro-amphetamine-ethanol combinations on performance of human subjects

stressed with delayed auditor feedback (DAF). Psychopharmacologia (1964) 6, 234–8.
5 Newman HW, Newman EJ. Failure of dexedrine and caffeine as practical antagonists of the depressant effect of ethyl alcohol in man. Quart J Stud Alc (1956) 17, 406–10.
6 Wilson L, Taylor JD, Nash CW, Cameron DF. The combined effects of ethanol and amphetamine sulfate on performance of human subjects. Canad Med Ass J (1976) 94, 478–84.

Alcohol + Anticholinergics

Abstract/Summary

Propantheline and atropine appear not to affect blood alcohol levels but marked impairment of attention can occur if alcohol is taken in the presence of atropine or glycopyrrhonium, probably making driving more hazardous. No adverse interaction appears to occur with transdermal hyoscine (scopolamine) and alcohol.

Clinical evidence, mechanism, importance and management

Neither chronic oral propantheline (45–120 mg daily) nor single 3 mg doses of atropine 2 h before alcohol appears to affect blood alcohol levels.[3] However a study in healthy subjects of the effects of 0.5 mg atropine or 1.0 mg glycopyrrhonium, in combination with alcohol (0.5 mg/kg), showed that while reaction times and co-ordination were unaffected or even improved, there was a marked impairment of attention which was large enough to make driving more hazardous.[1] Patients should be warned.

A double-blind cross-over study in 12 normal subjects showed that a transdermal hyoscine (scopolamine) preparation (*Scopoderm-TTS*) did not alter the effects of alcohol on the performance of the psychometric tests used (Critical Flicker Fusion Frequency, Choice Reaction Tasks), nor was the loss of alcohol or hyoscine from the body changed. Blood alcohol levels up to 80 and 130 mg% were studied.[2] No special precautions seem necessary.

References

1 Linnoila M. Drug effects of psychomotor skills related to driving: interaction of atropine, glycopyrrhonium and alcohol. Eur J clin Pharmacol (1973) 6, 107.
2 Gleiter C H, Antonin K-H, Schoenleber W, Bieck P R. Interaction of alcohol and transdermally administered scopolamine. J Clin Pharmacol (1988) 28, 1123–7.
3 Gibbons DO, Lanet AF. Effects of intravenous and oral propantheline and metoclopramide on ethanol absorption. Clin Pharmacol Ther (1975) 17, 578–84.

Alcohol + Antihistamines

Abstract/Summary

Some antihistamines cause drowsiness which can be increased by alcohol. The detrimental effects of alcohol on driving skills are considerably increased by the use of the older more sedative antihistamines (promethazine, chlorpheniramine, diphenhydramine, etc.), but are much less marked with the less sedative antihistamines (clemastine, clemizole, cyclizine, cyprohepatadine, pheniramine, tripelennamine, triprolidine, etc.) and appear to be minimal or absent with the newer ones (acrivastine, astemizole, cetirizine, ebastine, loratadine, terfenadine). Some of the more sedative antihistamines occur in cough, cold and influenze remedies.

Clinical evidence

The antihistamines can be broadly subdivided into (a) the most sedative, (b) less sedative, and (c) those causing little or no sedation.

(a) Alcohol + the most sedative antihistamines (Chlorpheniramine, Diphenhydramine, Promethazine)

Alcohol (0.75 g/kg) and dexchlorpheniramine (4 mg/70 kg) given to 13 subjects significantly impaired their performance of a number of tests (standing steadiness, reaction time, manual dexterity, perception, etc.).[7] Significant impairment of psychomotor performance was also seen in other subjects given 12 mg chlorpheniramine with alcohol (0.5 mg/kg body weight).[19] Other studies also describe this interaction.[3] Diphenhydramine in doses of 25 or 50 mg was shown to increase the detrimental effects of alcohol on the performance of choice reaction and co-ordination tests by subjects who had taken 0.5 - 0.68 mg/kg alcohol; its interaction in doses of 50, 75 or 100 mg has been confirmed in other reports.[1,4,9,10,11,24] A marked interaction can also occur with promethazine,[8] and I am aware of a double motor fatality attributed to the overwhelming sedative effects of promethazine taken with alcohol and chlordiazepoxide. A very marked deterioration in driving skills was clearly demonstrated in a test of car drivers given 20 ml Beechams *Night Nurse* (promethazine + dextromethorphan), 10 ml *Benylin* (diphenhydramine + dextromethorphan), or 30 ml *Lemsip* Night time flu medicine (chlorpheniramine + dextromethorphan). Very poor scores were seen when they were additionally given a double scotch whiskey about one-and-a-half hours later.[23]

(b) Alcohol + less sedative antihistamines (Clemastine, Clemizole, Cyclizine, Cyprohepatadine, Mebhydrolin, Pheniramine, Tripelennamine, Triprolidine)

The effects of alcohol (blood levels about 50 mg%) and antihistamines, alone or together, on the performance of tests designed to assess mental and motor performance were examined in 16 subjects. Clemizole (40 mg), tripelennamine (50 mg), did not significantly affect the performance under the stress of delayed auditory feedback. Clemastine in 3 mg doses also affected co-ordination, whereas 1.5 mg and 1 mg did not.[2,4,5] A study[12] on five subjects showed that the detrimental effects of 100 ml whisky on the performance of driving tests on a racing car simulator (blood alcohol estimated as less than 80 mg%) were not increased by 50 mg cyclizine. However three of the

subjects experienced drowsiness after cyclizine, and other studies[13] have shown that cyclizine alone causes drowsiness in the majority. A study in 20 subjects of the effects of alcohol and mebhydrolin (0.71 mg/kg) found that the performance of a number of tests on perceptual, cognitive and motor functions was impaired to some extent.[14] No interaction was detected in one study of the combined effects of 4 mg pheniramine or 4 mg cyproheptadine and alcohol (0.7 g/kg),[6] however triprolidine (10 mg) impairs the deterioration in driving caused by alcohol.[17] A marked deterioration in driving skills has been demonstrated with 10 ml *Actifed Syrup* (triprolidine + pseudoephedrine) alone and with a double whisky.[23]

(c) Alcohol + least sedative antihistamines (Acrivastine, Astemizole, Cetirizine, Ebastine, Loratadine, Terfenadine)

A double blind study found that terfenadine alone (60–240 mg) did not affect psychomotor skills, nor did it affect the adverse effects of alcohol,[9] however a later study found that 240 mg slowed braking reaction times in the laboratory both alone and with alcohol.[21] Other studies have shown that astemizole (10–30 mg daily),[15,16,19] ebastine (20 mg),[22,26] terfenadine (60 mg) and loratadine (10–20 mg)[17] do not interact with alcohol. Acrivastine (4 and 8 mg) with and without alcohol was found in another study to behave like terfenadine.[18] 10 mg cetirizine also appeared not interact with alcohol in one study[20] but some slight additive effects were detected in another.[25]

Mechanism

When an interaction occurs it appears to be due to the combined or additive central nervous depressant effects of both the alcohol and the antihistamine.

Importance and management

An adverse interaction between alcohol and the most sedative antihistamines (diphenhydramine, chlorpheniramine, promethazine) is well established and clinically important. Marked drowsiness can occur if taken alone, making driving or handling other potentially dangerous machinery much more hazardous. This can be further worsened by alcohol. Remember that some of these antihistamines appear 'in disguise' as antiemetics, sedatives and as components of cough/cold and influenza remedies (eg *Benylin*, *Lemsip*, *Night Nurse*) which can be bought over the counter. Patients should be strongly warned.

The situation with some of the less sedative antihistamines (clemastine, clemizole, cyclizine, cyproheptadine, mebhydrolin, pheniramine, tripelennamine and triprolidine) is less clear cut, and tests with some of them failed to detect an interaction with normal doses and moderate amounts of alcohol, however it has been clearly seen with *Actifed Syrup* (containing triprolidine). It would therefore be prudent to issue some cautionary warning, particularly if the patient is likely to drive.

The newest antihistamines (acrivastine, astemizole, cetirizine, ebastine, loratadine, terfenadine) seem to cause little or no drowsiness in most patients and the risks if taken alone or with alcohol appear to be minimal or absent.

The effects of quite a number of antihistamines with alcohol do not seem to have been formally studied, but it seems almost certain that combined use will result in increased drowsiness and increased driving risks. These include azatadine, brompheniramine, dimethindene, diphenylpyraline, mequitazine, oxatomide, phenindamine, trimeprazine (and undoubtedly a number of others) all of which have some sedative effects. Patients should be warned.

References

1 Hughes FW, Forney RB. Comparative effect of three antihistamines and ethanol on mental and motor performance. Clin Pharmacol Ther (1961) 5, 414.
2 Linnoila M. Effects of drugs on psychomotor skills related to driving: antihistamines, chlormezanone and alcohol. Europ J Clin Pharmacol (1973) 5, 87.
3 Smith RB, Rossie GV, Orzechowski RF. Interactions of chlorpheniramine-ethanol combinations: acute toxicity and antihistamine activity. Toxicol Appl Pharmacol (1974) 28, 240.
4 Tang PC, Rosenstein R. Influence of alcohol and dramamine alone and in combination on psychomotor performance. Aerospace Med (1967) 38, 818.
5 Franks HM, Hensley VR, Hensley WJ, Starmer GA, Teo RKC. The interaction between ethanol and antihistamines. 2. Clemastine. Med J Aust (1979) 1, 185.
6 Landauer AA, Milner G. Antihistamines alone and together with alcohol in relation to driving safety. J Forens Med (1971) 18, 127.
7 Franks HM, Hensley VR, Hensley WJ, Starmer GA, Teo RKC. The interaction between ethanol and antihistamines. 1: Dexchlorpheniramine. Med J (1978) 1, 449.
8 Hedges A, Hills M, Maclay WP. Some drug and peripheral effects of meclastine, a new antihistamine drug in man. J Clin Pharmacol (1971) 11, 112.
9 Moser L, Huther KJ, Koch-Weser J, Lundt PV. Effects of terfenadine and diphenhydramine alone or in combination with diazepam or alcohol on psychomotor performance and subjective feelings. Europ J Clin Pharmacol (1978) 14, 417.
10 Baugh R, Calvert RT. The effects of diphenhydramine alone and in combination with ethanol on histamine skin response and mental performance. Europ J Clin Pharmacol (1977) 12, 201.
11 Burns M, Moskowitz H. Effects of diphenhydramine and alcohol on skills performance. Europ J Clin Pharmacol (1980) 17, 259.
12 Hughes DTD, Cramer F, Knight GJ. Use of a racing car simulator for medical research. The effects of marzine and alcohol on driving performances. Med Sci Law (1967) October, 200.
13 Brand JJ, Colquhoun WP, Gould AH, Perry WLM. (-)Hyoscine and cyclizine as motion sickness remedies. Br J Pharmac Chemother (1967) 30, 463.
14 Franks HM, Lawrie M, Schabinsky VV, Starmer GA, Teo RKC. Interaction of alcohol and antihistamines: 3. Mebhydrolin. Med J Aust (1981) 2, 447–9.
15 Bateman DN, Chapman PH, Rawlins MD. Lack of effect of astemizole on ethanol dynamics or kinetics. Eur J Clin Pharmacol (1983) 25, 567–8.
16 Moser L, Plum H, Bruckmann M. Interaktionen eines neuen Antihistaminikums mit Diazepam und Alkohol. Med Welt (1984) 35, 296–9.
17 Riedel WJ, Schoenmakers EAJM, O'Hanlon JF. The effects of loratadine alone and in combination with alcohol on actual driving performance. Institute for Drugs, Safety and Behaviour, University of Limburg, Maastricht, The Netherlands, August 1987.
18 Cohen AF, Hamilton MJ, Peck AW. The effects of acrivastine (BW825C), diphenhydramine and terfenadine in combination with alcohol on human CNS preformance. Eur J Clin Pharmacol (1987) 32, 279–88.
19 Hindmarch I, Bhatti JZ. Psychomotor effects of astemizole and chlorpheniramine, alone and in combination with alcohol. Int Clin Psychopharmacol (1987) 2, 117–19.
20 Doms M, Vanhulle G, Baelde Y, Coulie P, Dupont P, Rihoux J-P. Lack of potentiation by cetirizine of alcohol-induced psychomotor disturbances, Eur J Clin Pharmacol (1988) 34, 619–23.
21 Bhatti JZ, Hindmarch I. The effects of terfenadine with and without alcohol on an aspect of car driving performance. Clin Exp Allergy (1989) 19, 609–11.
22 Mattila MJ, Kuitunen T. Ebastine, a non-sedative H1-antihistamine without alcohol interaction. Eur J Pharmacol (1990) 183, 1653–4.
23 Carter N. Cold cures drug alert. Auto Express (1992) 218, 15–16
24 Burns M. Alcohol and antihistamines in combination: effects on performance. Alcoholism Clin Exp Res (1989) 13, 243.
25 Ramaekers JG, Uiterwijk MMC, O'Hanlon JF. Effects of loratadine and cetirizine on actual driving and psychometric test performance and EEG during driving. Eur J Clin Pharmacol (1992) 42, 363–9.
26 Mattila MJ, Kuitunen T, Plétan Y. Lack of pharmacodynamic and pharmacokinetic interactions of the antihistamine ebastine with ethanol in healthy subjects. Eur J Clin Pharmacol (1992) 43, 179–84.

Alcohol + Aspirin and Salicylates

Abstract/Summary

A small increase in the gastrointestinal blood loss caused by aspirin occurs in patients if they drink, but any increased damage to the lining of the stomach is small and appears usually to be of minimal importance in most normal individuals. Buffered aspirin, paracetamol and diflunisal do not interact in this way. Aspirin can elevate blood alcohol levels.

Clinical evidence

(a) Alcohol + Ubuffered aspirin: effect on blood loss

The mean daily blood loss from the gut of 13 men was 0.4 ml while taking no medication, 3.2 ml while taking 2100 mg of soluble unbuffered aspirin (*Disprin*) and 5.3 ml while also taking 180 ml Australian whisky (31.8% w/v ethanol). Alcohol alone did not cause gastrointestinal bleeding.[1]

A not dissimilar study showed that the daily blood loss increased from 2.15 to 5.32 ml when, in addition to 2400 mg aspirin daily, the subjects drank 140 ml vodka (40% alcohol) and 200 ml table wine.[5] An epidemiological study of patients admitted to hospital with gastrointestinal haemorrhage showed a statistical association between bleeding and the ingestion of aspirin with or without alcohol.[2] Endoscopic examination reveals that aspirin and alcohol have additive damaging effects on the gastric mucosa (not on the duodenum) but the extent is small.[7]

(b) Alcohol + Buffered aspirin: effect on blood loss

No increased gastrointestinal bleeding occurred in 22 normal subjects given three double whiskys (equivalent to 142 ml 40% ethanol) and 728 g sodium acetylsalicylate.[3]

(c) Alcohol + Aspirin: effect on blood alcohol levels

5 normal subjects were given a standard breakfast with and without 1 g aspirin, and an hour later they were given 0.3 g/kg alcohol. The aspirin increased the peak blood alcohol levels by

39% (from 5.44 to 7.56 mmol/L) and the AUC (area under the curve) by 26% (from 8.83 to 11.11 mmol/L.h).[8]

Mechanisms

(a & b). Aspirin and alcohol can damage the mucosal lining of the stomach, one measure of the injury being a fall in the gastric potential difference. An additive fall has been seen with unbuffered aspirin and alcohol, whereas an increase occurs with buffered aspirin.[4] Once the protective mucosal barrier is breached, exfoliation of the cells occurs and damage to the capillaries follows. Aspirin causes a marked prolongation in bleeding times, and this can be increased by alcohol.[6] The total picture is complex. (c) The increased blood alcohol levels in the presence of food and aspirin seem to occur because the aspirin reduces the enzymic oxidation of the alcohol by the gastric mucosa (by alcohol dehydrogenase), so that more remains available for absorption.[8]

Importance and management

The combined effect of aspirin and alcohol on the stomach wall is established. 3 g aspirin daily for a period of 3–5 days induces an average blood loss of about 5 ml or so. Some increased loss undoubtedly occurs with alcohol, but it seems to be quite small and unlikely to be of much importance in most normal individuals using moderate doses. In one study alcohol was found to be a mild damaging agent or a mild potentiating agent for other damaging drugs.[7] Buffered aspirin, paracetamol (acetaminophen) or diflunisal[5] are preferable because they do not interact with alcohol.[7] On the other hand it should be remembered that chronic and/or gross overuse of salicylates and alcohol may result in gastric ulceration.

Information about the increase in blood alcohol levels caused by aspirin after food is limited, but the interaction appears to be established. Its importance is uncertain, but the increases after 1 g aspirin and food are very broadly similar to those seen when alcohol alone is taken on an empty stomach.[9] A warning to patients may be appropriate.

References

1 Goulston K, Cooke AR. Alcohol, Aspirin and gastrointestinal bleeding. Brit Med J (1968) 4, 644.

2 Needham CD, Kyle J, Jones PF, Johnstone SJ, Kerridge DF. Aspirin and alcohol in gastrointestinal haemorrhage. Gut (1971) 12, 819.

3 Bouchier JAD, Williams HS. Determination of faecal blood-loss after combined alcohol and sodium acetylsalicylate intake. Lancet (1969) i, 178.

4 Murray HS, Strottman MP, Cooke AR. Effect of several drugs on gastric potential differences in man. Brit Med J (1974) 1, 19.

5 De Schepper PJ, Tjandramaga TB, De Roo M, Verhaest L, Daurio C, Steelman SL, Tempero KF. Gastrointestinal blood loss after diflunisal and after aspirin. Clin Pharmacol Ther (1978) 23, 669.

6 Rosove MH, Harwig SSL. Confirmation that ethanol potentiates aspirin-induced prolongation of the bleeding time. Thromb Res (1983) 31, 525–7.

7 Lanza FL, Royer GL, Nelson RS, Rack MF, Seckman CC. Ethanol, aspirin, ibuprofen, and the gastroduodenal mucosa: an endoscopic assessment. Gastroenterology (1985) 80, 767–9.

8 Roine R, Gentry T, Hernández-Munöz R, Baraona E, Lieber CS. Aspirin increases blood alcohol concentrations in humans after ingestion of alcohol. J Amer Med Ass (1990) 264, 2406–8.

9 DiPadova C, Worner TM, Julkuen RJK, Lieber CS. Effects of fasting and chronic alcohol consumption on the first-pass metabolism of ethanol. Gastroenterology (1987) 92, 1169–73.

Alcohol + Barbiturates

Abstract/Summary

Alcohol and the barbiturates are CNS depressants which together can have additive (possibly more than additive) effects. Activities requiring alertness and good co-ordination, eg driving a car or handling other potentially dangerous machinery, will be made more difficult and more hazardous. Alcohol may also continue to interact next day if the barbiturate has hangover effects.

Clinical evidence

A study in man of the effects of alcohol (0.5 mg/kg), taken the morning after using 100 mg amylobarbitone as a hypnotic the night before, showed that the performance of co-ordination skills was much more impaired than with either drug alone.[1]

This increased CNS depression due to combined use has been described in a number of other clinical studies,[2–4] and has featured very many times in coroners' reports of fatal accidents and suicides.[11] A study of the fatalities due to this interaction indicated that with some barbiturates the CNS depressant effects are more than additive.[9] There is also some evidence that blood alcohol levels may be reduced in the presence of a barbiturate.[3,5,7]

Mechanisms

Both alcohol and the barbiturates are CNS depressants, and simple additive CNS depression provides part of the explanation. The Ferguson principle may account for the more than additive effects.[10] Acute alcohol ingestion may inhibit the liver enzymes concerned with the metabolism of the barbiturates.[4,8]

Importance and management

Few formal studies in normal clinical situations have been made but the effects (particularly those which are fatal) are very well established, serious and of clinical importance. The most obvious hazards are increased drowsiness, lack of alertness and impaired co-ordination which make the handling of potentially dangerous machinery (e.g. car driving) more difficult and dangerous, but it has also been rightly pointed out that other risks are increased: '...many old people may have a whiskey nightcap with their barbiturate sleeping pill. They then have to get out of bed in the middle of the night to empty their bladder; they are unsteady, they fall, they are found in the morning with a fractured femur or in a hypothermic state. No figures are available to give a reliable idea of the scale of this problem...'[6] Only amylobarbitone is specifically referenced here but this interaction would be expected with all of the barbiturates (eg phenobarbitone, methylphenobarbitone, butobarbitone, quinalbarbitone. etc). Some barbiturate hangover effects may be present next morning and may therefore continue to interact significantly with alcohol. Patients should be warned.

References

1 Saario I, Linnoila M. Effect of subacute treatment with hypnotics alone or in combination with alcohol, on psychomotor skills relating to driving. Acta pharmacol et toxicol (1976) 38, 382.

2 Kielholz P, Goldberg L, Obersteg JI, Poldinger W, Ramseyer A, Schmid P. Fahrversuche zur Frage der Beeintrachtigung der Verkehrstuchtigkeit durch Alkohol, Tranquilizer und Hypnotika. Dtsch Med Wschr (1969) 94, 301.

3 Morrelli PL, Veneroni E, Zaccala M, Bizzi A. Further observations on the interaction betwen ethanol and psychotropic drugs. Arzneim-Forsch (Drug Res) (1971) 21, 20.

4 Wegener H, Kotter L. Analgetica und Verkehrstuchtigkeit Wirkung einer Kombination von 5-Allyl-5-isobutyl-saure. Dimethylaminophenazon und Coffeine nach einmaliger unter wiederholter Applikation. Arzneim-Forsch (Drug Res) (1971) 21, 47.

5 Mould GP, Curry SH, Binns TB. Interaction of glutethimide and phenobarbitone with ethanol in man. J Pharm Pharmac (1972) 24, 894.

6 Wilkes E. Are you still prescribing those outdated drugs? MIMS Magazine (1976) 27, 84.

7 Mezey E, Robles EA. Effects of phenobarbital administration on rates of ethanol clearance and on ethanol-oxidising enzymes in man. Gastroenterology (1974) 66, 248.

8 Rubin E, Lieber CS. Inhibition of drug metabolism by acute ethanol intoxication. A hepatic microsomal mechanism. Am J Med (1970) 49, 801.

9 Stead AH, Moffat AC. Quantification of the interaction between barbiturates and alcohol and interpretation of fatal blood concentrations. Human Toxicol (1983) 2, 5–14.

10 King LA. Thermodynamic interpretation of synergism in barbiturate/ethanol poisoning. Human Toxicol (1985) 4, 633–5.

11 Gupta RC, Kofoed J. Toxicological statistics for barbiturates, other sedatives, and tranquillizers in Ontario. Can Med Ass J (1966) 94, 863–5.

Alcohol + Benzodiazepines and related drugs

Abstract/Summary

Benzodiazepine and related tranquillizers increase the CNS depressant effects of alcohol to some extent, but usually less than other more obviously sedative drugs. The risks of car driving and handling other potentially dangerous machinery are increased. The risk is heightened because the patient may be unaware of being affected. Some hypnotic benzodiazepines used at night are still present in appreciable amounts next day and therefore may continue to interact if the patient drinks.

Clinical evidence

It is very difficult to assess and compare the results of the very many studies of this interaction because of the differences between the tests, their duration, the dosages of the benzodiazepines and alcohol, whether given chronically or acutely, and a number of other variables. However the overall picture seems to be that diazepam[6,8–13,16,21,26,27,37] has a more marked effect than chlordiazepoxide,[1–7] medazepam,[17] or oxazepam,[16] but

possibly the same as triazolam.[29,31] The effects of lormetazepam may be greater than diazepam.[38] The potencies of alpidem,[42] alprazolam[41,46] bromazepam,[14] clobazam,[15] lorazepam,[25,30,37,42] oxazolam,[39] metaclazepam,[40] potassium clorazepate[23] and zoplicone[45] are unclear, but brotizolam seems to have a small effect.[36] Those on lorazepam and triazolam may be unaware of the extent of the impairment which occurs[25,29] and the anxiolytic effects of lorazepam may be opposed by alcohol.[30] Alprazolam and alcohol together may possibly increase behavioural aggression.[44]

The hypnotic benzodiazepines flurazepam,[18,33,34] nitrazepam,[10,19] temazepam[33] and flunitrazepam[24,25,35] when taken the night before can interact with alcohol the next morning, but midazolam[28,43] triazolam[45] and zoplicone[45] appear not to do so. Loprazolam may mitigate the effects of alcohol and may possibly have less of a hangover effect.[32]

Mechanism

The CNS depressant actions of the benzodiazepines and alcohol are additive. Alcohol also increases the absorption and raises the serum levels of some benzodiazepines.[15,20,22]

Importance and management

Extensively studied and well established. The overall picture is that these drugs worsen the detrimental effects of alcohol. Up to a 20–30% increase has been suggested.[29] The extent will depend on the particular drug in question (see 'Clinical evidence' above), its dosage and the amounts of alcohol. Diazepam is high on the list and, with alcohol, is not infrequently found in the blood of car drivers involved in traffic accidents.[41] With modest amounts of alcohol the effects of the interaction may be quite small but patients taking any of these drugs should nevertheless be warned that their usual response to alcohol may be greater than expected, and their ability to drive a car or carry out other tasks requiring alertness may be impaired. They may also be unaware of the deterioration. The same warning applies to some of the hypnotic benzodiazepines taken the night before because the body may still contain significant amounts the next morning (see individual drugs discussed above).

References

1 Reggiani G, Hurlimann A, Theiss E. Some aspects of the experimental and clinical toxicology of chlordiazepoxide. Acta pharmacol et toxicol (1979) 45, 256.

2 Hughers FW, Forney RB, Richards AB, Comparative effect in human subjecds of chlordiazepoxide, diazepam and placebo on mental and physical performance. Clin Pharmacol Ther (1965) 6, 139.

3 Linnoila M. Effects of diazepam, chlordiazepoxide, thioridazine, haloperidol, flupenthixol and alcohol on psychomotor skills related to driving. Ann Med Exp Biol Fenn (1973) 51, 125.

4 Linnoila M, Saario I, Olkoniemi J, Liljequist R, Himberg JJ, Maki M. Effect of two weeks' treatment with chlordiazepoxide or flupenthixol alone or in combination with alcohol on psychomotor skills related to driving. Arzneim Forsch/Drug Res (1975) 25, 1088.

5 Hoffer A. Lack of potentiation by chlordiazepoxide (Librium) of depression of excitation due to alcohol. Canad Med Ass J (1962) 87, 920.

6 Dundee JW, Isaac M. Interaction of alcohol with sedatives and tranquil-

lizers (a study of blood levels at loss of consciousness following rapid infusion). Med Sci Law (1970) 10, 220.

7 Kielholz P, Goldberg L, Obersteg JI, Poldinger W, Ramseyer A, Schmid P. Fahrversuche zur Frage der Beeintrachtigung der Verkehrsuchtigkeit durch Alkohol Tranquilizer und Hypnotika. Dtsch Med Wsch (1969) 94, 301.

8 Morselli PL, Veneroni E, Zaccala M, Bizzi A. Further observations on the interaction between ethanol and psychotropic drugs. Arzneim-Forsch/Drug Res (1971) 21, 20.

9 Linnoila M, Hakkinen S. Effects of diazepam and codeine, alone and in combination with alcohol, on simulated driving. Clin Pharmacol Ther (1974) 15, 368.

10 Linnoila M. Drug interaction on psychomotor skills related to driving: hypnotics and alcohol. Ann Med Exp Biol Fenn (1973) 51, 118.

11 Missen AW, Cleary W, Eng L, McMillan S. Diazepam, alcohol and drivers. NZ Med J (1978) 87, 275.

12 Laisu U, Linnoil M, Seppala T, Himberg JJ, Mattila MJ. Pharmacokinetic and pharmacodynamic interactions of diazepam with different alcoholic beverages. Eur J clin Pharmacol (1979) 16, 263.

13 Palva ES, Linnoila M, Saario I, Mattila MJ. Acute and subacute effects of diazepam on psychomotor skills: interaction with alcohol. Acta pharmacol et toxicol (1979) 45, 257.

14 Seppala T, Saario I, Mattila MJ. Two weeks' treatment with chlorpromazine, thioridazine, sulpiride or bromazepam: actions and interactions with alcohol on psychomotor skills relating to driving. Mod Probl Pharmacopsych (1976) 11, 85.

15 Tauber K, Badian M, Brettell HF, Royen Th, Rupp K, Sitting W, Uihlein M. Kinetic and dynamic interaction of clobazam and alcohol. Br J clin Pharmacol (1979) 7, 91S.

16 Molander L, Durhok C. Acute effects of oxazepam, diazepam and methylperone, alone and in combination with alcohol on sedation, coordination and mood. Acta pharmacol et toxicol (1976) 38, 145.

17 Landauer AA, Pocock DA, Prott FW. The effect of medazepam and alcohol on cognitive and motor skills used in car driving. Psychopharmacologia (1974) 37, 159.

18 Saario I, Mattila M. Effect of subacute treatment with hypnotics alone or in combination with alcohol on psychomotor skills related to driving. Acta pharmacol et toxicol (1976) 38, 382.

19 Saario I, Linnoila M, Maki M. Interaction of drugs with alcohol on human psychomotor skills related to driving: effect of sleep deprivation or two weeks' treatment with hypnotics. J Clin Pharmacol (1975) 15, 52.

20 MacLeod SM, Giles HG, Patzalek G, Thiessen JJ, Sellers EM. Diazepam actions and plasma concentrations following ethanol ingestion. Eur J clin Pharmacol (1977) 11, 345.

21 Curry SH, Smith CM. Diazepam-ethanol interaction in humans: addition or potentiation? Comm Psychopharmacol (1979) 3, 101.

22 Laisi U, Linnoila M, Seppala T, Himberg J-J, Mattila MJ. Pharmacokinetic and pharmacodynamic interactions of diazepam with different alcoholic beverages. Eur J Clin Pharmacol (1979) 16, 263.

23 Staak M, Raff G, Nusser W. Pharmacopsychological investigations concerning the combined effects of dipotassium clorazepate and ethanol. Int J Clin Pharmacol Biopharm (1979) 17, 205.

24 Linnoila M, Erwin CW, Brendle A, Logue P. Effects of alcohol and flunitrazepam on mood and performance in healthy young men. J Clin Pharmacol (1981) 21, 430–5.

25 Sappala T, Aranko K, Mattila MJ, Shrotriya RC. Effects of alcohol on buspirone and lorazepam actions. Clin Pharmacol Ther (1982) 32, 201–7.

26 Smiley A, Moskowitz H. Effects of long-term administration of buspirone and diazepam on driver steering control. Am J Med (1986) 80 (Suppl 3B) 22–9.

27 Erwin CW, Linnoila M, Hartwell J, Erwin A, Guthrie S. Effects of buspirone and diazepam, alone and in combination with alcohol, on skilled performance and evoked potentials. J Clin Psychopharmacol (1986) 6, 199.

28 Hindmarch I, Subhanz Z. The effects of midazolam in conjunction with alcohol on sleep, psychomotor performance and car driving ability. Int J Clin Pharm Res (1983) III, 323–9.

29 Dorian P, Sellers EM, Kaplan HL, Hamilton C, Greenblatt DJ, Abernethy D. Triazolam and ethanol interaction: kinetic and dynamic consequences. Clin Pharmacol Ther (1985) 37, 558–62.

30 Lister RG, File SE. Performance impairment and increased anxiety resulting from the combination of alcohol and lorazepam. J Clin Psychopharmacol (1983) 3, 66–71.

31 Ochs HR, Greenblatt DJ, Arendt RM, Hubbel W, Shader RI. Pharmacokinetic noninteraction of triazolam and ethanol. J Clin Psychopharmacol (1984) 4, 106–7.

32 McManus IC, Ankier SI, Norfolk J, Phillips M, Priest RG. Effects of psychological performance of the benzodiazepine loprazolam alone and with alcohol. Br J clin Pharmac (1983) 16, 291–300.

33 Betts TA, Birtle J. Effect of two hypnotic drugs on actual driving performance next morning. Br Med J (1982) 285, 852.

34 Hindmarch I, Gudgeon AC. Lopirazolam (HR158) and flurazepam with ethanol compared on tests of psychomotor ability. Eur J Clin Pharmacol (1982) 23, 509–12.

35 Seppala T, Nuotto E, Dreyfus JF. Drug-alcohol interactions on psychomotor skills: zopiclone and flunitrazepam. Pharmacology (1983) 27, Suppl 2, 127–35.

36 Scavone JM, Greenblatt DJ, Harmatz JS, Shader RI. Kinetic and dynamic interaction of brotizolam and ethanol. Br J clin Pharmac (1986) 21, 197–204.

37 Aranko K, Seppala T, Pellinen J, Mattila MJ. Interaction of diazepam or lorazepam with alcohol. Psychomotor effects and bioassayed serum levels after single and repeated doses. Eur J Clin Pharmacol (1985) 28, 559–65.

38 Willumeit H-P, Ott H, Neubert W, Hemmerling J-G, Schratzer K, Fichte K. Alcohol interaction of lormetazepam, mepindol sulphate and diazepam measured by performance on the Driving simulator. Pharmacopsychiat (1984) 17, 36–43.

39 Hopes H, Debus G. Untersuchungen zu Kombinationseffekten von Oxazolam und Alkohol auf Leistung und Befinden bei gesunden Probanden. Arzneim-Forsch/Drug Res (1984) 34, 921–6.

40 Schmidt V. Experimentelle Untersuchunger zur Wechselwirkung zwischen Alkohol und Metaclazepam. Beitr Gerichtl Med (1983) 41, 413–7.

41 Chan AWK. Effects of combined alcohol and benzodiazepine: a review. Drug and Alcohol Dependence (1984) 13, 315–41.

42 Allen D, Baylav A, Lader M. A comparative study of the interaction of alcohol with alpidem, lorazepam and placebo in normal studies. Int Clin Psychopharmacol (1988) 3, 327–41.

43 Lichtor JL, Zacny J, Korttila K, Apfelbaum JL, Lane BS, Rupani G, Thisted RA, Dohrn C. Alcohol after midazolam sedation. Does it really matter ? Anesth Analg (1991) 72, 661–8.

44 Bond AJ, Silveira JC. Behavioural aggression following the combination of alprazolam and alcohol. J Psychopharmacology (1990) 4, 315.

45 Kuitunen T, Mattila MJ, Seppala T. Actions and interactions of hypnotics on human performance: single doses of zopiclone, triazolam and alcohol. Int Clin Psychopharmacol (1990) 5 (Suppl 2) 115–30.

46 Linnoila M, Stapleton JM, Lister R, Moss H, Lane E, Granger A, Eckardt MJ. Effects of single doses of alprazolam and diazepam, alone and in combination with ethanol, on psychomotor and cognitive performance and on autonomic nervous system reactivity in healthy volunteers. Eur J Clin Pharmacol (1990) 39, 21–8.

Alcohol + Binedaline

Abstract/Summary

Binedaline appears not to interact with alcohol.

Clinical evidence, mechanism, importance and management

A study in 12 normal subjects found that 100 mg of binedaline did not affect the performance of a number of tasks (alertness, attention, concentration etc) with or without alcohol (0.8 g/kg).[1]

References

1 Patat A, Klein MJ, Jones RW. Acute effects on psychomotor performance of binedaline alone and with alcohol. Meth and Find Exptl Clin Pharmacol (1988) 10, 393–99.

Alcohol + Bromvaletone or Ethinamate

Abstract/Summary

The detrimental effects of alcohol on the skills related to driving are made worse by bromvaletone, but the interaction with ethinamate is mild. Both showed hangover effects and can interact with alcohol next morning.

Clinical evidence, mechanism, importance and management

A study on a very large number of subjects given 1 g ethinamate or 0.6 g bromvaletone, either alone or with 0.5 g/kg alcohol, showed that the performance of a number of psychomotor skills related to driving was slightly impaired by ethinamate, but strongly impaired by bromvaletone. There was sufficient hangover for both drugs to interact with alcohol next morning after being used as hypnotics the night before.[1] The CNS depressant effects of these hypnotics and alcohol would seem to be additive. Patients should be warned.

Reference

1 Linnoila M. Drug interaction on psychomotor skills related to driving: hypnotics and alcohol. Ann Med Exp Biol Fenn (1973) 51, 118.

Alcohol + Butyraldoxime

Abstract/Summary

A disulfiram-like reaction can occur in those exposed to N-butyraldoxime if they drink alcohol.

Clinical evidence, mechanism, importance and management

Workers in a printing company complained of flushing of the face, shortness of breath, tachycardia and drowsiness very shortly after drinking quite small quantities of alcohol (one and a half ounces of whiskey), and were found to have increased levels of acetaldehyde in their blood. The reason appeared to be that the printing ink they were using contained N-butyraldoxime, an antioxidant which, like disulfiram, can inhibit the metabolism of alcohol so that acetaldehyde accumulates (see 'Alcohol + Disulfiram').[1] This reaction would seem to be more unpleasant and socially disagreeable than serious. No treatment normally seems necessary.

Reference

1 Lewis W, Schwartz L. An occupational agent (N-butyraldoxime) causing reaction to alcohol. Med Ann DC (1956) 25, 485–90.

Alcohol + Caffeine

Abstract/Summary

Despite popular belief, objective tests show that caffeine does not counteract the effects of alcohol. It does not sober up those who have drunk too much and may even make them more accident-prone.

Clinical evidence, mechanism, importance and management

A study on a large number of subjects given 300 mg caffeine, either alone or with alcohol (0.75 mg/kg), showed that the caffeine did not antagonize the deleterious effect of alcohol on the performance of psychomotor skill tests. Only reaction times were reversed.[1] Another investigation on eight subjects found that, contrary to expectations, caffeine increased the frequency of errors in the performance of a serial reaction task.[2] Yet another double-blind study clearly showed that caffeine did not antagonize the effects of alcohol.[3] A further study found no evidence that caffeine opposes the actions of alcohol, instead it appeared that it increases the detrimental effects.[4] The reasons for this are not understood.

Thus, despite the time-hallowed belief in the value of strong black coffee in sobering up those who have drunk too much, it is not effective. It not only does not make it safe for them to drive or handle dangerous machinery, it may even make them more accident-prone.

References

1 Franks HM, Hagedorn H, Hensley VR. The effect of caffeine on human performance, alone and in combination with alcohol. Pyschopharmacology (1975) 45, 177.
2 Lee DJ, Lowe G. Interaction of alcohol and caffeine in a perceptual-motor task. IRCS Med Sci: Libr Compend (1980) 8, 420.
3 Nuotto E, Mattila MJ, Sappala T, Konno K. Caffeine and coffee and alcohol effects on psychomotor function. Clin Pharmacol Ther (1982) 31, 68–76.
4 Osborne DJ, Rogers Y. Interactions of alcohol and caffeine on human reaction time. Aviat Space Environ Med (1983) 54, 528–34.

Alcohol + Calcium channel blockers

Abstract/Summary

Blood alcohol levels can be raised by verapamil and may remain elevated for a much longer period of time. Alcohol may also increase the bioavailability of nifedipine.

Clinical evidence

(a) Alcohol effects increased

10 normal subjects given 80 mg verapamil three times daily for six days were additionally given 0.8 mg/kg alcohol on day 6.

Peak serum alcohol levels were found to be raised by 16.7% (from 106.45 to 124.24 mg/dl) and the AUC_{0-12} (area under the 12 h curve) was raised by almost 30% (from 366 to 475 mg.hr/dl). The time that serum alcohol levels exceeded 100 mg/dl was prolonged from 0.2 to 1.3 h. and the subjects said they felt more intoxicated.[1] Another study carried out to find out if verapamil (80 or 160 mg) antagonizes the effects of alcohol found no evidence that it does so.[3]

(b) Nifedipine effects increased

0.8 mg/kg alcohol (75 ml 94% alcohol + 75 ml orange juice) given to ten normal subjects increased the AUC of single 20 mg doses of nifedipine by 54%, but no significant changes in heart rate or blood pressure were seen.[2] Another study carried out to find out if nifedipine (10 or 20 mg) antagonizes the effects of alcohol found no evidence that it does so.[3]

Mechanism

Not understood. It seems possible that the verapamil inhibits the metabolism of the alcohol by the liver, thereby reducing its loss from the body. Alcohol also appears to inhibit the metabolism of nifedipine.

Importance and management

Information seems to be limited to these reports and they need confirmation, but patients on verapamil should be warned that the effects of alcohol may possibly be increased. A rise of almost 17% is small but it could be enough to lift legal blood levels to illegal levels if driving. Moreover the intoxicant effects of alcohol may persist for a much longer period of time (by a factor of five in this instance).[1] The clinical significance of the nifedipine-alcohol interaction is uncertain,

References

1 Bauer LA, Schumock G, Horn J, Opheim K. Verapamil inhibits ethanol elimination and prolongs the perception of intoxication. Clin Pharmacol Ther (1992) 52, 6–10
2 Qureshi S, Laganiere S, Caille G, Gossard D, Lacasse Y, McGilveray I. Effect of an acute dose of alcohol on the pharmacokinetics of oral nifedipine in humans. Pharm-Res (1992) 9, 683–6.
3 Perez-Reyes M, White WR, Hicks RE. Interactions between ethanol and calcium channel blocketrs in humans. Alcohol Clin Exp Res (1992) 16, 769–75.

Alcohol + Cannabis

Abstract/Summary

Smoking cannabis (marijuana) alters the bioavailability of alcohol. The peak blood levels are reduced and delayed.

Clinical evidence, mechanism, importance and management

15 normal subjects given 0.7 g/kg alcohol developed peak blood alcohol levels of 78.25 mg/dl at 50 min, but if they smoked a cannabis cigarette 30 min after the drink, their peak blood alcohol levels were only 54.8 mg/dl and they occurred at 105 min. The duration of both the alcohol and the cannabis subjective effects were similarly reduced.[1]

Reference

1 Lukas SE, Benedikt R, Mendelson JH, Kouri E, Sholar M, Amass L. Marihuana attenuates the rise in plasma ethanol levels in human subjects. Neuropsychopharmacology (1992) 7, 77–81.

Alcohol + Cephalosporin antibiotics

Abstract/Summary

Disulfiram-like reactions can occur in those taking latamoxef (moxalactam), cephamandole, cefoperazone, cefmenoxime, cefotetan and possibly cefonicid after drinking alcohol or following an injection of alcohol. This is not a general reaction of the commonly used cephalosporins but is confined to those with particular chemical structures.

Clinical evidence

A young man with cystic fibrosis was given 2 g latamoxef (moxalactam) intravenously every 8 h for pneumonia. After three days' treatment he drank, as was his custom, a can of beer with lunch. He rapidly became flushed with a florid macular eruption over his face and chest. This faded over the next 30 min but he complained of severe nausea and headache. A woman patient also on latamoxef became flushed, diaphoretic and nauseated after drinking a cocktail of vodka and tomato juice.[1]

This reaction has been described in at least five other subjects who drank alcohol while receiving latamoxef.[6–8] The symptoms experienced have included flushing of the face, arms and neck, shortness of breath, headache, tachycardia, dizziness, hyper- and hypotension, and vomiting. Similar reactions have been described in patients on cephamandole,[2,5] cefoperazone,[3,12,14,17–20] cefmenoxime,[15] cefonicid[25] and cefotetan[23] after drinking wine, beer, or other alcoholic drinks,[4,11,13] and after the ingestion of an 8% alcoholic elixir.[15] It has also been seen following the injection of alcohol into the para-aortic space for celiac plexus block.[18]

Mechanism

These reactions appear to have the same pharmacological basis as the disulfiram-alcohol reaction (see appropriate synopsis). Studies in rats have shown that three of these antibiotics (latamoxef, cephamandole and cefoperazone) can raise blood acetaldehyde levels when alcohol is given, but to a lesser extent than disulfiram.[6,11] It appears that it normally only occurs with cephalosporins which possess a methyltetrazolethiol group in the 3-position on the cephalosporin molecule,[21] but it has also been seen with cefonicid which possesses a methylsulphonthiotetrazole group instead.[25]

Importance and management

An established interaction. The incidence appears to vary. One report[1] says that one out of 30 on latamoxef showed this reaction, and in another study only two out of 10 did so.[8] The incidence is possibly slightly higher with cefoperazone and it occurred in five out of eight subjects in a study of cefotetan.[23] It is usually more embarrassing or unpleasant and possibly frightening than serious, with the symptoms subsiding spontaneously after a few hours. There is evidence that the severity varies (cefoperazone >latamoxef >cefmetazole.[22]) Treatment is not usually needed but there are two reports[2,7] of two elderly patients who needed treatment for hypotension which was life-threatening in one case;[7] plasma expanders and dopamine have been used as treatment.[2,7]

Since the reaction is unpredictable, all patients on the antibiotics known to interact should be warned that it can occur during and up to three days after the course of treatment is over. Advise them to avoid alcohol. Those with kidney or liver disease in whom the drug clearance is prolonged should wait a week. It should not be forgotten that some foods and pharmaceuticals contain substantial amounts of alcohol, and a reaction with some topically applied products cannot be excluded (see 'Alcohol + Disulfiram').

This disulfiram-like reaction is not a general reaction of all the cephalosporins. There are no reports of reactions in those taking cefpirome,[26] cephalothin, cephradine, cefoxitin, cephazolin, or cefsulodin.[16] Ceftizoxime is reported not interact with alcohol in man.[9] No interaction was seen with cefonicid in one placebo-controlled study,[24] nevertheless a case report describes a disulfiram-reaction in one patient.[25] A number of less widely used cephalosporins and others which are still the subject of investigation are possible candidates for this reaction because they possess the methyltetrazolethiol group in the 3-position. These include cefazaflur,[11] cefotiam, ceforanide, cefpiramide (SM-1652, Yamanouchi), 7-methoxy cefazaflur (SKF 73678), SKF 80000, T-1982 (Toyoma), P-75123 (Pierrel), SQ 14359 and SQ 67590 (Squibb).[15,21]

References

1 Neu HC, Prince AS. Interaction between moxalactam and alcohol. Lancet (1980), i, 1422.
2 Portier H, Chalopin JM, Freysz M, Tanter Y. Interaction between cephalosporins and alcohol. Lancet (1980), ii, 263.
3 Foster TS, Raehl CL, Wilson HD. Disulfiram-like reaction associated with parenteral cephalosporin. Amer J Hosp Pharm (1980) 37, 858.
4 Reeves DS, Davies AJ. Alcohol-cephalosporin interaction. Lancet (1980) ii, 540.
5 Drummer S, Hauser WE, Remington JS. Antabuse-like effect of beta-lactam antibiotics. N Eng J Med (1980) 303, 1417.
6 Beuning MK, Wold JS, Isreal KS, Kammer RB. Disulfiram-like reaction to beta-lactams. J Amer Med Ass (1981) 245, 2027.
7 Brown KR, Guglielmo BJ, Pons VG, Jacobs RA. Theophylline elixir,

moxalactam and a disulfiram-like reaction. Ann Int Med (1982), 97, 621–2.
8 Elenbaas RM, Ryan JL, Robinson WA, Singsank MJ, Harvey MJ, Klaasen CD. Investigation of the disulfiram-like activity of moxalactam. Clin Pharmacol Ther (1982) 32, 347–55.
9 McMahon FG, Noveck RJ. Lack of disulfiram-like reactions with ceftizoxime. J Antimicrob Chemother (1982) Suppl C, 129–33.
10 Beuning MK, Wolds JS. Ethanol-moxalactam interactions in vivo. Rev Inf Dis (1982) 4, Suppl Nov/Dec S555–63.
11 Yanagihara M, Okada K, Nozaki M, Tsurumi K, Fujimura H. Cepheim antibiotics and alcohol metabolism. Disulfiram-like reaction resulting from intravenous administration of cepheim antibiotics. Fol Pharmacol Japon (1982) 79, 55–60.
12 Allaz AF, Dayer P, Fabre J, Rudhardt M, Balant L. Pharmacocinetique d'une novelle cephalosporine, la cefoperazone. Schweiz Med Wsch (1979), 109, 1999–2005.
13 McMahon FG. Disulfiram-like reaction to cephalosporin. J Amer Med Ass (1980), 243, 2397.
14 Kemmerich B, Lode H. Cefoperazone-another cephalosporin associated with a disulfiram type alcohol incompatibility. Infection (1981) 9, 110.
15 Uri JV, Parks DB. Disulfiram-like reaction to certain cephalosporins. Ther Drug Monit (1983) 5, 219–24.
16 McMahon FG. Quoted in 15 as personal communication.
17 Kannangara DW, Gallaagher K, Lefrock JL. Disulfiram-like reactions with newer cephalosporins: cefmenoxime. Amer J Med Sci (1984) 287, 45–7.
18 Umeda S, Arai T. Disulfiram-like reaction to moxalactam after celiac plexus block. Anesth Analg (1985) 65, 377.
19 Bailey RR, Peddie B, Blake E, Bishop V, Reddy J. Cefoperazone in the treatment of severe or complicated infections. Drugs (1981) 22 (Suppl 1), 76–86.
20 Ellis-Pegler RB, Lang SDR. Cefoperazone in Klebsiella Meningitis: A case report. Drugs (1981) 22 (Suppl 1), 69–71.
21 Norrby SR. Adverse reactions and interactions with newer cephalosporin and cephamycin antibiotics. Med Toxicol (1986) 1, 3246.
22 Nakamura K, Nakagawa A, Tanaka M. Effects of cephem antibiotics on ethanol metabolism. Fol Pharmacol Jap (1984) 83, 183–91.
23 Kline SS, Mauro VF, Forney RB, Freimer EH, Somani P. Cefotetan-induced disulfiram-type reactions and hypoprothrombinaemia. Antimicrob Ag Chemother (1987) 31, 1328–31.
24 McMahon FG, Ryan JR, Jain AK, LaCorte W, Ginzler F. Absence of disulfiram-type reactions to single and multiple doses of cefonicid: a placebo-controlled study. J Antimicrol Chemother (1987) 20, 913–8.
25 Marcon G, Spolaor A, Scevola M, Zolli M, Carlassara GB. Effetto disulfiram-simile da cefonicid: prima segnalazione. Recenti Progressi in Medicina (1990) 81, 47–8.
26 Lassman HB, Hubbard JW, Chen B-L, Puri SK. Lack of interaction between cefpirome and alcohol. J Antimicrob Chemother (1992) 29, Suppl A, 47–50.

Alcohol + Chloral hydrate

Abstract/Summary

Both alcohol and chloral are CNS depressants and their effects may be additive, possibly even more than additive. Some patients may experience a disulfiram-like flushing reaction if they drink after taking chloral for several days.

Clinical evidence

Studies in five subjects given chloral (15 mg/kg) and alcohol (0.5 mg/kg) found that both drugs given alone impaired their ability to carry out complex motor tasks. When taken together, the effects were additive, and possibly even more than additive. After taking chloral for seven days, one of the subjects experienced a disulfiram-like reaction (bright red-purple flushing of the face, tachycardia, hypotension, anxiety and persistent headache) after drinking alcohol.[1,2]

The disulfiram-like reaction has been described in other reports.[3,4] One of these was published more than a century ago in 1872 and describes two patients on chloral who experienced this reaction after drinking only half a bottle of beer.[3]

Mechanism

Alcohol, chloral and trichloroethanol (to which chloral is metabolized) are all CNS depressants. During concurrent use, the metabolic pathways used for their elimination are mutually inhibited: blood-alcohol levels rise because the trichloroethanol competitively depresses the oxidation of alcohol to acetaldehyde, while trichloroethanol levels also rise because its production from chloral is increased and its further conversion and clearance as the glucuronide is inhibited. As a result the rises in the blood levels of alcohol and trichloroethanol are exaggerated, and their effects are accordingly greater.[1,2,5,6] Blood levels of acetaldehyde are raised by only 50% during the use of chloral, so that the flushing reaction, despite its resemblance to the disulfiram reaction, may possibly have a partially different basis.[2]

Importance and management

A well-documented and established interaction. Only a few references are given here. A comprehensive bibliography is to found in references 1 and 2. Patients given chloral should be warned about the extensive CNS depression which can occur if they drink, and of the disulfiram-like reaction which may occur after taking chloral for a period of time. Its incidence is uncertain. The legendary Mickey Finn concocted of chloral and alcohol is reputed to be so potent that deep sleep can be induced in an unsuspecting victim within minutes of ingestion, but the evidence seems largely to be anecdotal. Very large doses of both would be likely to cause serious and potentially life-threatening CNS depression.

It seems likely that chloral betaine, triclofos and other compounds closely related to chloral hydrate will interact with alcohol in a similar manner, but this requires confirmation.

References

1 Sellers EM, Carr G, Bernstein JG, Sellers S, Koch-Weser J. Interaction of chloral hydrate and ethanol in man. II. Hemodynamic and performance. Clin Pharmacol Ther (1972) 13, 50.
2 Sellers EM, Lang M, Koch-Weser J, LeBlanc E, Kalant H. Interaction of chloral hydrate and ethanol in man. I. Metabolism. Clin Pharmacol Ther (1972) 13, 37.
3 Bjorstrom F. On the effect of alcoholic beverages and simultaneous use of chloral. Uppsala Lakareforenings Forhandlingar (1872) 8, 114.
4 Bardodej Z. Intolerance alkohlu po chloralhydratu. Ceskolov farm (1965) 14, 478.
5 Owens AH, Marshall EK, Brown GO. A comparative evaluation of the hypnotic potency of chloral hydrate and trichloroethanol. Bull Johns Hopkins Hosp (1955) 96, 71.
6 Wong LK, Biemann K. A study of drug interaction by gas chromatography-mass spectrometry. Synergism of chloral hydrate and ethanol. Biochem Pharmacol (1978) 27, 1019.

Alcohol + Cimetidine, Famotidine, Nizatidine or Ranitidine

Abstract/Summary

Although some studies have found that blood alcohol levels can be raised to some extent in those taking some H_2-blockers (cimetidine, ranitidine, nizatidine) and possibly remain elevated for longer than usual, others report that no significant interaction occurs. This interaction is not established. Drinking may worsen the gastrointestinal disease for which these H_2-blockers are being given.

Clinical Evidence

(a) Evidence of an interaction

A double-blind study on six volunteers showed that after taking 1200 mg cimetidine daily for seven days, their peak blood alcohol levels following the ingestion of 0.8 g/kg alcohol were raised about 12% (from 146 to 163 mg%). The AUC (area under the time/concentration curve) was increased about 7% (from 717 to 771 mg/100 ml/h). The subjects assessed themselves as being more intoxicated while taking cimetidine and alcohol than with alcohol alone.[1]

An essentially similar study[2,12] found that the blood alcohol levels were raised 17% (from 73 to 86 mg%) by cimetidine but not by ranitidine. A later study in six normal subjects found that 800 mg cimetidine daily for a week approximately doubled the AUC (from 0.89 to 1.64 mM.h) following a single 0.15 mg/kg oral dose of alcohol and raised peak levels about 33%. No changes were seen when the alcohol was given intravenously.[13] 2–3 fold rises in blood alcohol concentrations are described in another study using cimetidine or ranitidine.[19] Another study in subjects given cimetidine or ranitidine for only two days showed that peak blood alcohol levels were raised by 17 and 27% respectively, and the time for which blood levels remained above the 80 mg% mark (the legal driving limit in the UK and some other countries) was prolonged by about one-third.[3] Nizatidine was said to inhibit the metabolism of alcohol in man, but little detail was given in the report.[15] A further study in subjects given 0.75 g/kg alcohol found that single 800 mg doses of cimetidine, 300 mg nizatidine or 300 mg ranitidine raised blood alcohol levels at 45 min by 26% (from 75.5 to 95.2 mg%), 17.5% (from 75.5 to 88.7 mg%) and 3.2% (75.5 to 78.0%) respectively, and the AUCs at 120 min were increased by 25%, 20% and 9.8% respectively. Each of the subjects said they felt more inebriated after taking cimetidine or nizatidine.[17,20] Another study found that cimetidine almost doubled peak alcohol serum levels, whereas ranitidine raised the levels about 50%.[22]

(b) Evidence of no interaction

The makers of cimetidine (SKF) have on file three unpublished studies which failed to find any evidence that cimetidine or ranitidine significantly increased the blood levels of alcohol. One study was on six normal subjects given single 400 mg doses of cimetidine, another on six normal subjects given 1 g cimetidine daily for 14 days, and the last on 10 normal subjects given either 1 g cimetidine daily or 300 mg ranitidine daily.[7] A number of other studies also failed to demonstrate significant interactions involving either cimetidine, ranitidine or famotidine and a number of different alcoholic drinks.[5,6,8–11,14,16,18]

Three other studies found that famotidine had no significant effect on blood alcohol levels.[17,20,22]

Mechanism

It would appear that the interacting H_2-blockers inhibit the activity of alcohol dehydrogenase (ADH) in the gastric mucosa so that more alcohol passes unmetabolized into the circulation, thereby raising the levels.[19,21,23,24]

Importance and management

The contrasting and apparently contradictory results cited here clearly show that this interaction is by no means established. An extensive review of the data concluded that the interaction is clinically insignificant.[25] Until the situation is fully resolved, it might be prudent to tell patients who are starting H_2-blockers to be alert for any increase in their response to alcohol. In any case they should restrict their drinking because alcohol may worsen peptic ulcer and other diseases.

References

1 Feeley J, Wood AJJ. Effects of cimetidine on the elimination and actions of alcohol. J Amer Med Ass (1982) 247, 2819–21.
2 Seitz HK, Bosche J, Czygan P, Veith S, Simon B, Kommerell B. Increased blood ethanol levels following cimetidine but not ranitidine. Lancet (1983) i, 760.
3 Webster LK, Jones DB, Smallwood RA. Influence of cimetidine and ranitidine on ethanol pharmacokinetics. Aust NZ J Med (1985) 15, 359–60.
4 Couzigou P, Fleury B, Bourjac M, Betbeder A-M, Vincon G, Richard-Molard B, Albin H, Amouretti M, Beraud C. Pharmacocinetique de l'alcool apres perfusion intraveineuse de trois heures avec et sans cimetidine chez dix sujets sains non alcooliques. Gastroenterol Clin Biol (1984) 8, 103–8.
5 Dobrilla G, de Pretis G, Piazzi L, Chilovi F, Comberlato M, Valentini M, Pastorino A, Vallaperta P. Is ethanol metabolism affected by oral administration of cimetidine and ranitidine in therapeutic doses. Hepatogastroenterol (1984) 31, 35–7.
6 Johnston KI, Fenzl E, Hein B. Einfluss von Cimetidine auf den Abbau und die Wirkung des Alkohols. Arzneim-Forsch:Drug Res (1984) 34, 734–6.
7 Robson AS (Smith Kline and French). Personal communication (1989).
8 Tanaka E, Nakamura K. Effects of H_2-receptor antagonists on ethanol metabolism in Japanese volunteers. Br J Clin Pharmac (1988) 26, 96–9.
9 Tan OT, Stafford TJ, Sarkany I, Gaylarde PM, Tilsey C, Payne JP. Suppression of alcohol-induced flushing by a combination of H1 and H2 histamine antagonists. Br J Dermatol (1982) 107, 647–52.
10 Holtmann G, Singer MV. Histamine H_2-receptor antagonists and blood alcohol levels. Dig Dis Sci (1988) 33, 767–8.
11 Holtmann G, Singer MV, Knop D, Becker S, Goebell H. Effect of histamine H_2-receptor antagonists on blood alcohol levels. Gastroenterology (1988) 94, A190.
12 Seitz HK, Veith S, Czygan P, Bosche J, Simon B, Gugler R, Kommerell B. In vivo interactions between H_2-receptor antagonists and ethanol metabolism in man and in rats. Hepatology (1984) 4, 1231–4.
13 Caballeria J, Baraona E, Rodamilans M, Lieber CS. Effects of cimetidine on
gastric alcohol dehydrogenase activity and blood alcohol levels. Gastroenterology (1989) 96, 388–92.
14 Fraser AG. Ranitidine, cimetidine and famotidine have no effect on alcohol absorption in healthy volunteers. Gastroenterology (1991) 100, A66.
15 Palmer RH. Cimetidine and alcohol absorption. Gastroenterology (1989) 97, 1066.
16 Fraser AG, Prewett EJ, Hudson M, Sawyer AM, Rosalki SB, Pounder RE. The effect of ranitidine, cimetidine or famotidine on low-dose postprandial alcohol absorption. Aliment Pharmacol Ther (1991) 5, 263–72.
17 Guram M, Holt S. Are ethanol H_2-receptor antagonist interactions 'relevant'. Gastroenterlogy (1991) 100, 5 part 2, A749.
18 Jönsson K-Å, Jones AW, Boström T. No influence of omeprazole on the pharmacokinetics of ethanol in healthy men. World Congr Gastroenterology, Sydney, August 1990. Abstracts II, PD201.
19 Roine R, DiPadova C, Frezza M, Hernández-Muñoz R, Baraona E, Lieber CS. Effects of omeprazole, cimetidine and ranitidine on blood ethanol concentrations. Gastroenterology (1990) 98, A114.
20 Holt S, Gurum M, Howden CW. Evidence for an interaction between alcohol and certain H_2-receptor antagonists. Gut (1991) 32, A1220.
21 Caballeria J. Interactions between alcohol and gastric metabolizing enzymes: practical implications. Clin Therap (1991) 13, 511–20.
22 DiPadova C, Roine R, Frezza M, Gentry T, Baraona E, Lieber CS. Effects of ranitidine on blood alcohol levels after alcohol ingestion. Comparison with other H_2-receptor antagonists. J Amer Med Ass (1992) 267, 83–6.
23 Fiatarone JR, Bennett MK, Kelly P, James OFW. Ranitidine but not gastritis or female sex reduces the first pass metabolism of ethanol. Gut (1991) 32, A594.
24 Caballeria J, Baraona E, Deulofeu R, Hernández-Muñoz R, Rodés J, Lieber CS. Effects of H_2-receptor antagonists on gastric alcohol dehydrogenase activity. Dig Dis Sci (1991) 36, 1673–79.
25 Levitt MD. Review article: lack of clinical significance of the interaction between H_2-receptor antagonists and ethanol. Aliment Pharmacol Ther (1993) 7, 131–8.

Alcohol + Cisapride

Abstract/Summary

Cisapride possibly increases blood alcohol levels to some extent but the clinical importance of this is uncertain. It is probably small.

Clinical evidence, mechanism, importance and management

A preliminary study in 16 normal subjects given 0.7 mg/kg alcohol in orange juice found that 10 mg cisapride did not affect blood alcohol levels, but it was absorbed more quickly. The performance of a number of psychomotor tests was unaffected.[1] However a later study in five normal subjects given 10 mg cisapride, followed 1 h later by a standard meal, and then by 0.3 g/kg alcohol diluted in orange juice, found a 34% rise in maximum blood alcohol levels (from 5.2 to 7.0 mM) and a 24% increase in the AUC (area under the curve) over 4 h.[2] The reason appears to be that the cisapride speeds up the emptying of the stomach. The extent to which these modestly increased blood alcohol levels would affect the ability to drive or handle other dangerous machinery is uncertain, but until more information is available patients should be given some warning.

References

1 Idzikowski C, Welburn P. An evaluation of possible interactions between

ethanol and cisapride. Unpublished report N 49087 on file, Janssen Pharmaceuticals (1986).

2 Roine R, Heikkonen E, Salaspuro M. Cisapride enhances alcohol absorption and leads to high blood alcohol levels. Gastroenterol (1992) 102 (4 pt 2) A507.

Alcohol + Clovoxamine, Femoxetine, Fluoxetine and Fluvoxamine

Abstract/Summary

Clovoxamine, fluoxetine and femoxetine in therapeutic doses do not appear to interact with alcohol but some modest interaction possibly occurs with fluvoxamine.

Clinical evidence, mechanism, importance and management

(a) Clovoxamine, femoxetine, fluoxetine

Neither fluoxetine (30–60 mg) nor alcohol (4 oz whiskey) affected the pharmacokinetics of the other in normal subjects, and no changes in psychomotor activity were seen (stability of stance, motor performance, manual co-ordination).[1] Blood alcohol levels of 80 mg% (80 mg/dl) impaired the performance of a number of psychomotor tests in 12 subjects but the addition of 40 mg fluoxetine daily taken for six days had little further effect.[3] Another study also found no change in the performance of a number of psychophysiological tests when fluoxetine was combined with alcohol.[4] No significant interaction was seen in another study with femoxetine (200–600 mg) and alcohol (1 g/kg).[2] No sedation was seen in a study with 150 mg clovoxamine daily.[5] Another study in 12 subjects found no evidence that single doses of 50, 100 or 150 mg clovoxamine increased the effects of alcohol (0.8 g/kg) as measured by a number of psychomotor tests.[6] No special precautions would seem necessary with alcohol and any of these drugs.

(b) Fluvoxamine

One study found that 150 mg fluvoxamine daily with alcohol (0.5%) impaired alertness and attention more than alcohol alone,[7] whereas another study in subjects given 40 g alcohol (blood alcohol levels up to 70 mg/dl) failed to find evidence that the addition of 50 mg fluvoxamine twice daily worsened the performance of the psychomotor tests used, and even appeared to reverse some of the effects.[9,10] The pharmacokinetics of alcohol are hardly affected by fluvoxamine.[8] The situation with fluvoxamine is therefore less clear than with the related drugs listed in (a) above, but it would seem prudent to give patients some warning that the effects of alcohol may possibly be modestly increased.

References

1 Lemberger L, Rowe H, Bergstrom RF, Farid KZ and Enas GG. Effect of fluoxetine on psychomotor performance, physiologic response, and kinetics of ethanol. Clin Pharmacol Ther (1985) 37, 658–64.

2 Stromberg C and Mattila MJ. Acute and subacute effects on psychomotor performance of femoxetine alone and with alcohol. Eur J Clin Pharmacol (1985) 28, 641–7.

3 Allen D, Lader M, Curran HV. A comparative study of the interactions of alcohol with amitriptyline, fluoxetine and placebo in normal subjects. Prog Neuro-Psychopharmacol and Biol Psychiat (1988) 12, 63–80.

4 Schaffler K. Study on performance and alcohol interaction with the antidepressant fluoxetine. Int Clin Psychopharmacol (1989) 4, Suppl 1, 15–20.

5 Ochs HR, Greenblatt DJ, Verburg-Ochs B, Labedski L. Chronic treatment with fluvoxamine, clovoxamine and placebo: interaction with digoxin and effects on sleep and alertness. J Clin Pharmacol (1989) 29, 91–5.

6 Stromberg C, Mattila MJ. Acute comparison of clovoxamine and mianserin, alone and in combination with ethanol, on human psychomotor performance. Pharmacol Toxicol (1987) 60, 374–9.

7 Herberg K-W, Menke H. Study of the effects of the antidepressant fluvoxamine on driving skills and its interaction with alcohol. Duphar Laboratories. Data on file 1981.

8 van Harten J, Stevens LA, Raghoebar M. The influence of single-dose and multiple-dose administration of fluvoxamine on the pharmacokinetics of ethanol in man. Eur J Pharmacol (1990) 183, 2386–7.

9 van Harten J, Wesnes K, Raghoebar M. Negligible kinetic and dynamic interaction between fluvoxamine and alcohol. Clin Pharmacol Ther (1991) 49, 178.

10 van harten J, Stevens LA, Raghoebar M, Holland RL, Wesnes K, Cournot A. Fluvoxamine does not interact with alcohol or potentiate alcohol-related impairment of cognitive function. Clin Pharmacol Ther (1992) 52, 427–35.

Alcohol + CNS depressants

Abstract/Summary

The concurrent use of small or moderate amounts of alcohol and therapeutic doses of drugs which are CNS depressants can increase drowsiness and reduce alertness. These drugs include analgesics, anticonvulsants, antidepressants, antihistamines, antinauseants, narcotics, neuroleptics, tranquillizers, hypnosedatives and others. This increases the risk of accident when driving or handling other potentially dangerous machinery and may make the performance of everyday tasks more difficult and hazardous.

Clinical evidence, mechanism, importance and management

Alcohol is a CNS depressant (see the introduction to this chapter). With only small or moderate amounts of alcohol and blood alcohol levels well within legal driving limits, it may be quite unsafe to drive if another CNS depressant is being taken concurrently. The details of most of the drugs which have been tested are set out in the synopses in this chapter (see the Index), but there are others which nobody seems to have tested formally. The Abstract/Summary above lists some of those which commonly cause drowsiness. Quite apart from driving, almost everyone meets potentially dangerous situations every day at home, in the garden, in the street and at work. Crossing a busy street or even walking downstairs can become much more risky under the influence of drugs and drink. A cause for concern is that the patient may be partially or totally unaware of the extent of the deterioration in his skills. Patients should be warned.

Alcohol + Codeine

Abstract/Summary

Codeine in 50 mg doses, both alone and with alcohol, impairs the ability to drive safely but no interaction of importance would be expected with the relatively small amounts of codeine in most compound analgesic preparations.

Clinical evidence, mechanism, importance and management

Double blind studies on a very large number of professional army drivers found that 50 mg of codeine and alcohol (0.5 mg/kg), both alone and together, impaired their ability to drive safely on a static driving simulator. The number of 'collisions', neglected instructions and the times they 'drove off the road' were increased.[1,2] Codeine dosages of this order are given in the form of Codeine Phosphate Syrup (BPC 1973) and in Tablets of Codeine Phosphate BP so that these preparations, particularly with alcohol, could make drivers more accident-prone, but the increased hazard is difficult to quantify. Codeine phosphate in doses of 15, 25 or 30 mg occurs in some elixirs and linctuses, but only relatively small amounts (5–8 mg) are found in most proprietary compound analgesic tablets. Alcohol appears not to affect the pharmacokinetics of codeine.[3]

References

1 Linnoila M, Hakkinen S. Effects of diazepam and codeine, alone and in combination with alcohol, on simulated driving. Clin Pharmacol Ther (1974) 15, 368.
2 Linnoila M, Mattila MJ. Interaction of alcohol and drugs on psychomotor skills as demonstrated by a driving simulator. Br J Pharmac (1973) 47, 671P.
3 Bodd E, Beylich KM. Christopherson AS, Morland J. Oral administration of codeine in the presence of ethanol: a pharmacokinetic study in man. Pharmacol Toxicol (1987) 61, 297–300.

Alcohol + Dextropropoxyphene

Abstract/Summary

The central nervous depressant effects of alcohol are only modestly increased by dextropropoxyphene in normal therapeutic doses. In deliberate suicidal overdosage the CNS depressant effects appear to be additive and can be fatal.

Clinical evidence

Alcohol alone (blood levels of 50 mg%) impaired the performance of tests (motor co-ordination, mental performance and stability of stance) in eight volunteers more than 65 mg dextropropoxyphene alone. When given together there was some evidence that the effects were greater than with either alone, but in some instances the impairment was no greater than with just alcohol. The effect of alcohol clearly predominated.[1]

Another study found that the effects of 95 mg alcohol on the performance of two psychomotor tests were not altered in subjects who had also been given two tablets of *Distalgesic* (dextropropoxyphene 32.5 mg + paracetamol 325 mg in each tablet).[2] A further study found no change in the psychomotor effects of ethanol (0.5 mg/kg) following the addition of 130 mg dextropropoxyphene but the bioavailability of the dextropropoxyphene was raised by 25%.[6] Yet another found a 31% increase in bioavailability with blood alcohol levels of about 80 g/L.[3]

Mechanism

Not understood. Both drugs are CNS depressants and in overdosage the fatal dose of dextropropoxyphene is reduced by the presence of alcohol. Their effects seem to be additive.[4,5]

Importance and management

Numerous reports describe the severe and sometimes fatal respiratory depression which can follow alcohol/dextropropoxyphene overdosage, but information about moderate social drinking and therapeutic doses of dextropropoxyphene is limited. The objective evidence is that the interaction with moderate doses of both is quite small. Even so it would seem prudent (at the risk of being overcautious) to warn patients that dextropropoxyphene can cause drowsiness and this may be exaggerated to some extent by alcohol. They should be warned that driving or handling potentially hazardous machinery may be more risky, but total abstinence from alcohol does not seem to be necessary.

References

1 Kiplinger GF, Sokol G, Rodda BE. Effects of combined alcohol and propoxyphene on human performance. Arch int Pharmacodyn (1974) 212, 175.
2 Edwards C, Gard PR, Handley SL, Hunter M, Whittington RM. *Distalgesic* and ethanol-impaired funcdion. Lancet (1982) ii, 384.
3 Sellers EM, Hamilton CA, Kaplan HL, Degani NC, Foltz RL. Pharmacokinetic interaction of propoxyphene and alcohol. Br J clin Pharmac (1985) 19, 398–401.
4 Carson DJL, Carson ED. Fatal dextropropoxyphene poisoning in Northern Ireland. Review of 30 cases. Lancet (1977) i, 894–7.
5 Whittington RM, Barclay AD. The epidemiology of dextropropoxyphene (*Distalgesic*) overdose fatalities in Birmingham and the West Midlands. J Clin Hosp Pharm (1981) 6, 251–7.
6 Girre C, Hirschhorn M, Bertaux L, Palombo S, Dellatolas E, Ngo R, Moreno M, Fournier PE. Enhancement of proproxyphene bioavailability by ethanol. Relation to psychomotor performance and cognitive function in healthy volunteers. Eur J Clin Pharmacol (1991) 41, 147–52.

Alcohol + Dimethylformamide

Abstract/Summary

A disulfiram-like reaction can occur in about 20% of those who drink alcohol after being exposed to dimethylformamide (DMF) vapour.

Clinical evidence

A three-year study in a chemical plant where dimethylforma-mide (DMF) was used found that about 20% (19 out of 102 men) exposed to the vapour developed this reaction after drinking alcohol. Flushing of the face, and often of the neck, arms, hands and chest occurred after drinking alcohol, and sometimes dizziness, nausea and tightness of the chest. A single glass of beer was enough to induce a flush lasting 2 h. The majority of the men experienced the reaction within 24 h of exposure to DMF, but it could occur even after four days.[3]

Three further cases of this interaction are described in other reports.[1,2]

Mechanism

Men exposed to DMF vapour develop substantial amounts of DMF and its metabolite (N-methylformamide) in their blood and urine.[3] This latter compound in particular has been shown in rats given alcohol to raise their blood acetaldehyde levels by a factor of 5, so it would seem probable that the N-methyl-formamide is reponsible for this disulfiram-like reaction (see 'Alcohol + Disulfiram').[4]

Importance and management

An established interaction, the incidence being about 20%.[3] Those who come into contact with DMF, even in very low concentrations, should be warned of this possible interaction with alcohol. It would appear to be more unpleasant than serious in most instances, and normally requires no treatment.

References

1 Chivers CP. Disulfiram effect from inhalation of dimethylformamide. Lancet (1978) i, 331.
2 Reinl W, Urba HJ. Erkrankungen durch dimethylformamid. Int Arch Gewerbepath Gewerbehyg (1965) 21, 333.
3 Lyle WH, Spence TWM, McKinneley WM, Duckers K. Dimethylforma-mide and alcohol intolerance. Brit J Ind Med (1979) 36, 63.
4 Hanasono GK, Fuller RW, Broddle WD, Gibson WR. Studies on the effects of N,N-dimethylformamide on ethanol disposition and monoamine oxi-dase activity in rats. Toxicol Appl Pharmacol (1977) 39, 461.

Alcohol + Disulfiram

Abstract/Summary

The ingestion of alcohol while taking disulfiram will result in flushing and fullness of the face and neck, tachycardia, breathlessness, giddiness and hypotension, nausea and vom-iting. This is called the Disulfiram or Antabuse reaction. It is used to deter alcoholic patients from drinking. A mild skin flush reaction may possibly occur in particularly sensitive individuals if alcohol is applied to the skin or if the vapour is inhaled.

Clinical evidence

This toxic interaction was first observed in 1937 by Dr EE Williams amongst workers in the rubber industry who were handling tetraethylthiuram disulphide:

'Beer will cause a flushing of the face and hands, with rapid pulse, and some of the men describe palpitations and a terrible fullness of the face, eyes and head. After a glass of beer (six ounces) the blood pressure falls about 10 points, the pulse is slightly accelerated and the skin becomes flushed in the face and wrists. In 15 min the blood pressure falls another 10 points, the heart is more rapid, and the patient complains of fullness in the head.'[1]

The later observation[2] by Hald and his colleagues of the same reaction with the ethyl congener (disulfiram) led to its introduc-tion as a drink deterrent. Some patients also experience giddi-ness, sweating, nausea, vomiting, difficulty in breathing and headache. The severity of the reaction can depend upon the amount of alcohol ingested but some individuals are extremely sensitive. Respiratory depression, cardiovascular collapse, car-diac arrhythmias, unconsciousness and convulsions may occur. There have been fatalities.[4,5]

A mild disulfiram reaction is said to occur in some patients who apply alcohol to the skin. It has been reported after using after-shave lotion,[7] tar gel (33% alcohol)[6] and a beer-containing shampoo (3% alcohol).[8] A contact lens wetting solution (con-taining polyvinyl alcohol) used to irrigate the eye has also been implicated in a reaction.[14,15] It has also been described in a patient who inhaled vapour from paint in a poorly ventilated area and from the inhalation of 'mineral spirits'.[11] A woman on disulfiram reported vaginal stinging and soreness during sexual intercourse, and similar discomfort to her husband's penis which seemed to be related to the disulfiram dosage and how intoxicated her husband was.[13]

Mechanism

Partially understood. Alcohol is normally rapidly metabolized within the liver, firstly to acetaldehyde and then by a series of biochemical steps to water and carbon dioxide. Disulfiram inhibits the enzyme (acetaldehyde dehydrogenase) which is concerned with the metabolism of acetaldehyde and, as a result, the acetaldehyde accumulates. Prostaglandin release may also be involved.[16] Not all of the symptoms of the reaction can be reproduced by injecting acetaldehyde so that some other biochemical mechanism(s) must also be involved. For example, it is thought that the inhibition of dopamine-beta-hydroxylase may have some part to play. It has been suggested that the mild skin flush which can occur if alcohol is applied to the skin is not a true disulfiram reaction.[12]

Importance and management

An extremely well-documented and important interaction ex-ploited therapeutically to deter alcoholics from drinking. Initial treatment should be closely supervised because an extremely intense and potentially serious reaction occurs in a few individ-uals with even quite small doses of alcohol. Apart from the usual warnings about drinking, patients should also be warned about the unwitting ingestion of alcohol in some pharmaceutical preparations. The alcohol-content of nearly 500 American products has been published which is too extensive to be reproduced here.[10] The risk of a reaction is real. It has been seen following a single dose of an alcohol-containing cough mixture,[3] whereas the ingestion of small amounts of communion wine and the absorption of alcohol from a bronchial nebulizer spray are said not to result in any reaction.[9]

References

1 Williams EE. Effects of alcohol on workers with carbon disulfide. J Amer med Ass (1937) 109, 1472.

2 Hald J, Jacobssen E, Larsen V. The sensitizing effects of tetraethylthiuram disulphide (Antabuse) to ethyl alcohol. Acta Pharmacol (1948) 4, 285.

3 Koff RS, Popadimas I, Honig E. Alcohol in cough medicines: hazards to the disulfiram user. J Amer med Ass (1971) 215, 1988.

4 Garber RS, Bennett RE. Unusual reaction to antabuse: report of three cases. J Med Soc NJ (1950) 47, 168.

5 Kwentus J, Major LF. Disulfiram in the treatment of alcoholism. A review. J Stud Alc (1979) 40, 428.

6 Ellis CN, Mitchell AJ, Beardsley GR. Tar gel interaction with disulfiram. Arch Dermatol (1979) 115, 1367.

7 Mercurio F. Antabuse-alcohol reaction following the use of after-shave lotion. J Amer med Ass (1952) 149, 82.

8 Stoll D, King LE. Disulfiram-alcohol skin reaction to beer-containing shampoo. J Amer med Ass (1980) 244, 2045.

9 Rothstein E. Use of disulfiram (Antabuse) in alcoholism. N Eng J Med (1970) 283, 936.

10 Parker WA. Alcohol-containing pharmaceuticals. Am J Drug Alcohol Abuse (1982–3) 9, 195–209.

11 Scott GE, Little FW. Disulfiram reaction to organic solvents other than ethanol. N Eng J Med (1985) 312, 790.

12 Haddock NF, Wilkin JK. Cutaneous reactions to lower aliphatic alcohols before and during disulfiram therapy. Arch Dermatol (1982) 118, 157–9.

13 Chick JD. Disulfiram reaction during sexual intercourse. Br J Psychiatry (1988) 152, 438.

14 Newsom SR, Harper BS. Disulfiram-alcohol reaction caused by contact lens wetting solution. Contact and Intraocular Lens Med J (1980) 6, 407-8

15 Refojo MF. Letter to Editor. Contact and Intraocular Lens Med J (1981) 7, 172.

16 Truitt EB, Gaynor CR, Mehl DL. Aspirin attenuation of alcohol-induced flushing and intoxication in oriental and occidental subjects. Alcohol and Alcoholism (1987) 22 Suppl 1, 595–9.

Alcohol + Edible fungi

Abstract/Summary

A disulfiram-like reaction can occur if alcohol is taken after eating the smooth ink(y) caps fungus (*Coprinus atramentarius*), *Boletus luridus* and certain other edible fungi.

Clinical evidence

A man who drank three pints of beer 2 h after eating a meal of freshly picked and fried inky caps, developed facial flushing and a blotchy red rash over the upper half of his body. His face and hands swelled and he became breathless, sweated profusely, and vomited during the 3 h when the reaction was most severe. On admission to hospital he demonstrated tachycardia and some cardiac arrhythmia. The man's wife who ate the same

fungi but without alcohol did not show the reaction.[1]

This reaction has been described on many occasions in medical and pharmacological reports[9,11,13] and in books devoted to descriptions of edible and poisonous fungi.[10] Only a few are listed here. Mild hypotension and '...alarming orthostatic features...'[2,3] are said to be common symptoms but the arrhythmia seen in the case cited here[1] appears to be rare. Recovery is usually spontaneous and uncomplicated. A similar reaction has been described after eating *Boletus luridus*,[14] and other fungi including *Coprinus micaceus*, *Clitocybe claviceps* and certain morels.[14]

Mechanism

An early and attractive idea was that this reaction was due to disulfiram (one group of workers actually claimed to have isolated it from the fungus[4]), but this was not confirmed by later work[5,12] and it now appears that the active ingredient is coprine (N-5-(1-hydroxycyclopropyl)-glutamine).[6,7] This is metabolized in the body to 1-aminocyclopropanol which appears, like disulfiram, to inhibit aldehyde dehydrogenase (see 'Alcohol + Disulfiram'). The active ingredients of the other fungi are unknown.

Importance and management

An established and well documented interaction. It is said to occur up to 24 h after eating the fungi. The intensity depends upon the quantities of fungus and alcohol consumed, and the time interval between them.[1,2] Despite the widespread consumption of edible fungi and alcohol, reports of this reaction are few and far between, suggesting that even though it can be very unpleasant and frightening, the outcome is usually uncomplicated. Treatment appears normally not to be necessary.

The related fungus Coprinus comatus (the 'shaggy ink cap' or 'Lawyers wig') is said not to interact with alcohol,[3,8] nor is there anything to suggest that it ever occurs with the common field mushroom (*Agaricus campestris*) or the cultivated variety (*Agaricus bisporis*).[8]

References

1 Caley MJ, Clarke RA. Cardiac arrhythmias after mushroom ingestion. Brit Med J (1977) 2, 1633.

2 Buck RW. Mushroom toxins' brief review of literature. N Engl J Med (1961) 265, 681.

3 Broadhurst-Zingrich L. Ink caps and alcohol. Brit Med J (1978) 1, 511.

4 Simandl J, Franc J. Isolation of tetraethylthiuram disulfide from Coprinus atramentarius. Chem Listy (1956) 50, 1862.

5 Vanhaelen M, Vanhaelen-Fastre R, Hoyois J, Mardens Y. Reinvestigation of disulfiram-like activity of Coprinus atramentarius (Bull.ex Fr) Fr. extracts. J Pharm Sci (1976) 65, 1774.

6 Hatfield GM, Schaumberg IP. Isolation and structural studies of coprine, the disulfiram-like constituent of Coprinus atramentarius. Lloydia (1975) 38, 489.

7 Lindberg P, Bergman R, Wickberg B. Isolation and structure of coprine, a novel physiologically active cyclopropane derivative from Coprinus atramentarius and its synthesis via 1-amino-cyclo-propanol. J Chem Soc Chem Commun (1975) 946.

8 Radford AP. Ink caps and mushrooms. Brit Med J (1978) 1, 112.

9 Reynold WA, Lowe FH. Mushrooms and a toxic reaction to alcohol.

Report of four cases. N Engl J Med (1965) 189, 630.
10 Ramsbottom J. Mushrooms and Toadstools. Collins, London (1953) p 55.
11 Wildervanck LS. Alcohol en de kale inktzwam. Ned T Geneesk (1978) 122, 913.
12 Wier JK, Tyler VE. An investigation of *Coprinus atramentarius* for the presence of disulfiram. J Am Pharm Ass (1960) 49, 427.
13 Tottmar O, Marchner H, Lindberg P., in 'Alcohol and Aldehyde Metabolising Systems', ed Thuram RG, Williamson JR, Drott HR and Chance B. vol 2. Academic Press, NY. (1977) pp. 20–12.
14 Budmiger H, Kocher F. Hexenrohrling (*Boletus luridus*) mit alkohol. Ein Kasuistischer Beitrag. Schweiz med Wsch (1982) 112, 1179–81.

Alcohol + Fentanyl/Midazolam

Abstract/Summary

The residual effects of fentanyl/midazolam appear not to interact adversely with alcoholic drinks taken several hours later.

Clinical evidence, mechanism, importance and management

A study with 12 normal subjects concluded that the residual effects of fentanyl (2 µg/kg) and midazolam (0.1 mg/kg) given intravenously for surgery were unlikely to interact significantly in outpatients if they drank when they arrived home about 4 h later. The subjects were given enough alcohol to achieve blood levels of about 60 mg% (equivalent to 1.4 L of beer or 950 ml wine or 180 ml spirits).[1]

References

1 Lichtor JL, Zacny J, Apfelbaum JL, Lane BS, Rupani G, Thisted RA, Dohrn C, Korttila K. Alcohol after sedation with IV midazolam-fentanyl: effects on psychomotor functioning. Br J Anaesth (1991) 67, 579–84.

Alcohol + Furazolidone

Abstract/Summary

A disulfiram-like reaction may occur in patients taking furazolidone if they drink alcohol.

Clinical evidence

A patient taking 200 mg furazolidone four times daily complained of facial flushing, lacrimation, conjunctivitis, weakness and light-headedness within 10 min of drinking beer. It occurred on several occasions and lasted 30–45 min.[1]

A man prescribed 100 mg furazolidone four times daily and who had taken only three doses, developed intense facial flushing, wheezing and dyspnoea of an hour's duration within an hour of drinking 2 oz. of brandy. The same thing happened again the next day after drinking a martini cocktail. No treatment was given.[4] A report originating from the makers of furazolidone stated that by 1976, 43 cases of a disulfiram-like

reaction had been reported, of which 14 were produced experimentally using above normal doses of furazolidone.[3] A later study in 1986 described nine out of 47 patients (19%) who complained of a disulfiram-like reaction after drinking alcohol while taking 100 mg furazolidone four times daily for five days.[2] The report does not say whether all of them drank.[2]

Mechanism

Uncertain. It seems possible that furazolidone acts like disulfiram by inhibiting the activity of acetaldehyde dehydrogenase (see 'Alcohol + Disulfiram').

Importance and management

An established and clinically important interaction of uncertain incidence. One report suggests that possibly about 1 in 5 may be affected.[2] Reactions of this kind appear to be more unpleasant and possibly frightening than serious, and normally need no treatment, however patients should be warned about what may happen if they drink.

References

1 Calesnick B. Antihypertensive action of the antimicrobial agent furazolidone. Am J Med Sci (1958) 236, 736–46.
2 DuPoint HL, Ericsson CD, Reves RR, Galindo E. Antimicrobial therapy for travelers' diarrhea. Rev Infect Dis (1986) 8, Suppl 2, S217–22.
3 Chamberlain RE. (Eaton Laboratories, Norwich Pharmacal Co.) Chemotherapeutic properties of prominent nitrofurans. J Antimicrob Chemother (1976) 2, 325–336.
4 Kolodny AL. Side-effects produced by alcohol in a patient receiving furazolidone. Ma State Med J (1962) 11, 248.

Alcohol + Glutethimide

Abstract/Summary

The sedative effects of glutethimide are increased by alcohol and the performance of psychomotor skills is impaired. Driving or handling other potentially dangerous machinery is made more hazardous.

Clinical evidence, mechanism, importance and management

A double-blind study on normal subjects given 250 mg glutethimide, either alone or with alcohol (0.5 mg/kg), found that concurrent use both subjectively and objectively impaired the performance of a number of psychomotor skill tests related to driving (choice reaction, coordination, divided attention).[1] Both are CNS depressants and their effects would appear to be additive. It has also been reported that blood alcohol levels can be raised 11–30% by glutethimide and blood glutethimide levels are reduced,[2] but a later study was unable to confirm this.[1] It has also been claimed that effects of alcohol and glutethimide are antagonistic rather than additive.[2]

The information is limited and somewhat contradictory, nevertheless patients should be warned about the probable results of taking glutethimide and alcohol together. Driving, handling dangerous machinery or undertaking any task needing alertness and full coordination is likely to be made more difficult and hazardous. There is no evidence of a hangover effect which could result in an interaction with alcohol the next day.[1]

References

1 Saario I, Linnoila M. Effect of subacute treatment with hypnotics, alone or in combination with alcohol, on psychomotor skills related to driving. Acta pharmacol et toxicol (1976) 38, 382.
2 Mould GP, Curry SH, Binns TB. Interactions of glutethimide and phenobarbitone with ethanol in man. J Pharm Pharmac (1972) 24, 894.

Alcohol + Glyceryl trinitrate

Abstract/Summary

Patients who take glyceryl trinitrate (nitroglycerin) while drinking may feel faint and dizzy.

Clinical evidence, mechanism, importance and management

The results of studies[1,5] on the combined haemodynamic effects of alcohol and glyceryl trinitrate give support to claims made in 1965 and 1980 that concurrent use increases the risk of exaggerated hypotension and fainting.[2,3] Their vasodilatory effects[4] would appear to be additive. The greatest effect was seen when the glyceryl trinitrate was taken 1 h after starting to drink.[1] It is suggested that this increased susceptibility to postural hypotension should not be allowed to stop patients from using glyceryl trinitrate if they want to drink, but they should be warned and told what to do if they feel faint and dizzy.[1]

References

1 Kupari M, Heikkila J, Ylikahri R. Does alcohol intensify the hemodynamic effects of nitroglycerin. Clin Cardiol (1984) 7, 382–6.
2 Shafer N. Hypotension due to nitroglycerin combined with alcohol. N Engl J Med (1965) 272, 1169.
3 Opi LH. Drugs and the heart. Nitrates. Lancet (1980) i, 750–2.
4 Allison RD, Kraner JC, Roth GM. Effects of alcohol and nitroglycerin on vascular responses in man. Angiology (1971) 22, 211–222.
5 Abrams J, Schroeder K, Raizada V, Gibbs D. Potentially adverse effects of sublingual nitroglycerin during consumption of alcohol. J Amer Coll Cardiol (1990) 15, 226A.

Alcohol + Griseofulvin

Abstract/Summary

An increase in the intoxicant effects of alcohol has been reported to occur in a very small number of patients. A flushing reaction has also been described in one patient.

Clinical evidence, mechanism, importance and management

The descriptions of this interaction are very brief. One of them describes a man who had '...decreased tolerance to alcohol and emotional instability manifested by crying and nervousness so severe that the drug was stopped.'[1] Another states that '...a possible potentiation of the effects of alcohol has been noted in a very small number of patients.'[2] I am also personally aware of a man who experienced a marked increase in the intoxicant effects of alcohol while taking griseofulvin. A single case of flushing and tachycardia attributed to concurrent use has also been described.[2]

The documentation is extremely sparse which would seem to suggest that any interaction between alcohol and griseofulvin is uncommon. Normally concurrent use need not be avoided but patients should be warned.

References

1 Drowns BV, Fuhrman DL, Dennie CC. Use, abuse and limitations of griseofulvin. Missouri Med (1960) 57, 1473.
2 Simon HJ, Randz LA. Reactions to antimicrobial agents. Ann Rev Med (1961) 12, 119.

Alcohol + Hydromorphone

Abstract/Summary

A single case report describes a fatality due to the combined CNS depressant effects of hydromorphone and alcohol.

Clinical evidence, mechanism, importance and management

A young man died from the combined cardiovascular and respiratory depressant effects of hydromorphone (*Dilaudid*) and alcohol.[1] He fell into a sleep, the serious nature of which was not recognized by those around him. Post mortem analysis revealed alcohol and hydromorphone concentrations of 900 mg/l and 0.1 mg/l, neither of which is particularly excessive. This case emphasizes the importance of warning patients about the potentially hazardous consequences of drinking while taking potent CNS depressants of this kind.

Reference

1 Levine B, Saady J, Fierro M, Valentour J. A hydromophone and ethanol fatality. J Forensic Sci (1984) 29, 655–9.

Alcohol + Indomethacin or Phenylbutazone

Abstract/Summary

The skills related to driving are impaired by indomethacin and phenylbutazone. Further impairment occurs if patients drink while taking phenylbutazone, but this does not appear to occur with indomethacin.

Clinical evidence, mechanism, importance and management

A study on a large number of normal subjects showed that the performance of various psychomotor skills related to driving (choice reaction, coordination, divided attention tests) was impaired by 50 mg indomethacin or 200 mg phenylbutazone. The concurrent ingestion of alcohol (0.5 mg/kg) made things worse in those taking phenylbutazone, but the performance of those taking indomethacin was improved to some extent.[1] The reasons are not understood. The study showed that the subjects were subjectively unaware of the adverse effects of phenylbutazone. Information is very limited, but patients should be warned if they intend to drive.

Reference

1 Linnoila M, Seppala T, Mattila MJ. Acute effect of antipyretic analgesics, alone or in combination with alcohol, on human psychomotor skills related to driving. Br J clin Pharmac (1974) 1, 477.

Alcohol + Isoniazid

Abstract/Summary

Isoniazid increases the hazards of driving after drinking alcohol. Isoniazid-induced hepatitis may also possibly be increased by alcohol, but its effects are possibly reduced.

Clinical evidence, mechanism, importance and management

The effects of 750 mg isoniazid with 0.5 g/kg alcohol were examined in 100 volunteers given various psychomotor tests and using a driving simulator. No major interaction was seen in the psychomotor tests, but the number of drivers who 'drove off the road' on the simulator was increased.[1,2] There would therefore appear to be some extra risks for patients on isoniazid who drink and drive, but the effect does not appear to be large. Patients should nevertheless be warned. The incidence of severe progressive liver damage due to isoniazid is said to be higher in those who drink regularly,[3,4] and the clinical effects of isoniazid are also said to be reduced by heavy drinking in some patients.[3]

References

1 Linnoila M, Matilla MJ. Effects of isoniazid on psychomotor skills related to driving. J clin Pharmacol (1973) 13, 343.
2 Linnoila M, Matilla MJ. Interaction of alcohol and drugs on psychomotor skills as demonstrated by a driving simulator. Br J Pharmacol (1973) 47, 671 P.
3 Reynolds JEF (Ed). Martindale. The Extra Pharmacopoeia, edition 29. (1989) Pharmaceutical Press, London, pages 563–5.
4 Kopanoff DE, Snider DE, Caras GJ. Isoniazid-related hepatitis. Am Rev Resp Dis (1978) 117, 991–1001.

Alcohol + Jian Bu Wan

Abstract/Summary

Jian Bu Wan appears not to relieve or cure a hangover.

Clinical evidence, mechanism, importance and management

Jian Bu Wan is a Chinese traditional herbal medicine containing a bark which has anticholinergic, antibacterial, diuretic and choleretic properties. It is used to alleviate 'weakness', that is to say the cardiovascular and gastrointestinal symptoms after severe infections and acute alcohol intake. A controlled double-blind crossover study of 8 normal subjects who, the evening before, had drunk champagne and vodka (averaging 0.6 g/kg body weight), found no evidence that Jian Bu Wan was more effective than a placebo when given to treat a hangover the next morning. The subjects were given psychomotor function tests, a subjective evaluation of their symptoms, blood alcohol concentration tests, and their blood pressures and heart rates were measured.[1]

References

1 Frisk-Holmberg M, Kerth P, van der Kleyn E, Synavae P. Effects of Jian Bu Wan — a traditional Chinese medication on behavioural and cardiovascular parameters after acute alcohol intake in normal subjects. Fundam Clin Pharmacol (1990) 4, 11–15.

Alcohol + Ketoconazole

Abstract/Summary

Disulfiram-like reactions have been seen in a few patients taking ketoconazole after drinking alcohol.

Clinical evidence

One patient out of group of 12 taking 200 mg ketoconazole daily experienced a disulfiram-like reaction (nausea, vomiting, facial flushing) after drinking.[1] No further details are given and the report does not say whether any of the others drank alcohol. A woman on 200 mg ketoconazole daily developed a disulfiram-like reaction when she drank.[3] Another report describes a transient 'sunburn-like' rash or flush on the face, upper chest and back of a patient taking 200 mg ketoconazole daily when she drank modest quantities of wine or beer.[2] The reasons are not known but it seems possible that ketoconazole may act like disulfiram and inhibit the activity of acetaldehyde dehydrogenase (see 'Alcohol + Disulfiram'). The incidence of this reaction appears to be low (these appear to be the only reports) and its importance is probably small, but patients should be warned. Reactions of this kind are usually more unpleasant than serious, the disulfiram-alcohol reaction being the possible exception.

References

1 Fazio RA, Wickremesinghe PC, Arsura EL. Ketoconazole therapy of candida esophagitis — a prospective study of 12 cases. Am J Gastroenterol (1983) 79, 261–4.
2 Magnasco AJ, Magnasco LD. Interaction of ketoconazole and ethanol. Clin Pharm (1986) 5, 522–3.
3 Meyboom RHB, Pater BW. Overgevoeligheid voor alcoholische dranken tijdens behandeling met ketoconazol. Ned Tijdsch Geneeskd (1989) 133, 1463–4.

Alcohol + Lithium carbonate

Abstract/Summary

Some limited evidence suggests that lithium carbonate alone or combined with alcohol may make car driving more hazardous.

Clinical evidence, mechanism, importance and management

A study on 20 normal subjects given lithium carbonate to achieve blood levels of 0.75 meq/l and 0.5 g/kg alcohol, and who were subjected to various tests (choice reaction, coordination, attention) to assess any impairment of psychomotor skills related to driving, indicated that lithium both alone and with alcohol may increase the risk of accident.[1] Information is very limited but patients should be warned.

Reference

1 Linnoila M, Saario I, Maki M. Effects of treatment with diazepam or lithium and alcohol on psychomotor skills related to driving. Eur J clin Pharmacol (1974) 7, 337.

Alcohol + Liv.52

Abstract/Summary

Liv.52, an Ayurvedic herbal remedy, appears to reduce the hangover symptoms after drinking, reducing both urine and blood alcohol and acetaldehyde levels at 12 h. However it also raises the blood alcohol levels of moderate drinkers for the first few hours after drinking.

Clinical evidence

Nine volunteers who normally drank socially (40–100 g weekly) took six tablets of Liv.52 2 h before drinking alcohol (four 60 ml doses of whiskey, equivalent to 90 g alcohol). Their blood alcohol levels at 1 h were increased 15% (from 75.0 to 86.2 mg%). After taking three tablets of Liv.52 daily for two weeks, their 1 h blood alcohol levels were raised 27% (from 75% to 95.3 mg%).[1] The blood alcohol levels of eight other moderate drinkers were found to be raised over the first two hours by about 27–30% after taking three tablets of Liv.52 daily for two weeks, and by 16% and14% respectively over the following two hours.[2] Only a minor increase in the blood alcohol levels of occasional drinkers occurred.[2] Acetaldehyde levels in the blood and urine were markedly lowered at 12 hr, and hangover seemed to be reduced.[1]

Mechanisms

Not understood. Liv.52 contains the active principles from *Capparis sponosa*, *Cichorium intybus*, *Solanum nigrum*, *Cassia occidentalis*, *Terminalia arjuna*, *Achillea millefolium*, *Tamarix gallica* and *Phyllanthus amarus*.[1] These appear to increase the absorption of alcohol, or reduce its metabolism by the liver, thereby raising the blood-alcohol levels. It is suggested that the reduced hangover effects may possibly because it prevents the binding of acetaldehyde to cell proteins causing a more rapid elimination.[1]

Importance and management

Direct evidence experimental seems to be limited to these two studies.[1,2] Liv.52 appears to reduce the hangover effects after drinking, but at the same time it can significantly increase the blood alcohol levels of moderate drinkers for the first few hours after drinking. Increases of up to 30% may be enough to raise the blood alcohol from legal to illegal levels when driving. Moderate drinkers should be warned. Occasional drinkers appear to develop higher blood alcohol levels than moderate drinkers but Liv.52 seems not to increase them significantly.[1]

Reference

1 Chauhan BL, Kulkarni RD. Alcohol hangover and Liv.52. Eur J Clin Pharmacol (1991) 40, 187–8.
2 Chauhan BL, Kulkarni RD. Effect of Liv.52, a herbal preparation, on absorption and metabolism of ethanol in humans. Eur J Clin Pharmacol (1991) 40, 189–91.

Alcohol + Maprotiline

Abstract/Summary

The sedative effects of maprotiline and alcohol combined can possibly make car driving or handling dangerous machinery more hazardous.

Clinical evidence, mechanism, importance and management

A double blind cross-over trial in 12 normal subjects found that single 75 mg oral doses of maprotiline subjectively caused drowsiness which was increased by alcohol (1 g/kg) and worsened the performance of a number of tests.[1] However the same group later failed to find that 50 mg maprotiline twice daily increased the detrimental effects of alcohol. Nevertheless it would seem prudent (at the risk of being overcautious) to warn patients of the possible increased risk if they drive or handle potentially dangerous machinery.[2]

References

1 Stromberg C, Seppala T, Mattila MJ. Acute effects of maprotiline, doxepin and zimeldine with alcohol in healthy volunteers. Arch Int Pharmacodyn (1988) 291, 217–228.
2 Stromberg C, Suokas A, Seppälä T. Interaction of alcohol with maprotiline or nomifensine: echocardiographic and psychometric effects. Eur J Clin Pharmacol (1988) 35, 593–99.

Alcohol + Meprobamate

Abstract/Summary

The intoxicant effects of alcohol can be considerably increased by the presence of normal daily doses of meprobamate. Driving or handling other potentially dangerous machinery is made much more hazardous.

Clinical evidence

A study on 24 subjects, given 2.4 mg meprobamate daily for a week, showed that with blood alcohol levels of 50 mg% their performance of a number of co-ordination and judgement tests was much more impaired than with either drug alone. Some of the subjects were quite obviously drunk while taking both and showed '...marked muscular inco-ordination and little or no concern for the social proprieties....Two could not walk without assistance....Nothing approaching this was seen with alcohol alone.'[1]

Other studies confirm this interaction, although the effects appeared to be less pronounced.[2–7]

Mechanism

Both meprobamate and alcohol are CNS depressants which appear to have additive effects. There is also evidence that alcohol may inhibit or increase meprobamate metabolism, depending on whether it is taken acutely or chronically, but the contribution of this to the enhanced CNS depression is uncertain.[8,9]

Importance and management

A well-documented and potentially serious interaction. Normal daily dosages of meprobamate in association with relatively moderate blood-alcohol concentrations, well within the UK legal limit for driving, can result in obviously hazardous intoxication. Patients should be warned.

References

1 Zirkle GA, McAtee OB, King PD, Van Dyke R. Meprobamate and small amounts of alcohol. Effects on human ability, coordination and judgement. J Amer Med Ass (1960) 173, 1823.
2 Reisby N, Theilgaard A. The interaction of alcohol and meprobamate in man. Acta Psychiatr Scand (1969) Suppl 208, 192.
3 Forney RB, Hughes FW. Meprobamate, ethanol or meprobamate-ethanol combinations on performance of human subjects under delayed audio-feedback (DAF). J Psychol (1964) 57, 431.
4 Goldberg L. Behavioural and physiological effects of alcohol on man. Psychosom Med (1966) 28, 570.
5 Ashford JR, Cobby JM. Drug interactions. The effects of alcohol and meprobamate applied singly and jointly in human subjects. IV. J Stud Alc (1975) Suppl 7, 140.
6 Cobby JM, Ashford JR. Drug interactions. The effects of alcohol and meprobamate applied singly and jointly in human subjects. V. J Stud Alc (1975) Suppl 7, 162.
7 Ashford JR, Carpenter JA. Drug interactions. The effects of alcohol and meprobamate applied singly and jointly in human subjects. VI. J Stud Alc (1975) Suppl 7, 177.
8 Misra PS, Lefevre A, Ishi H, Rubin E, Lieber CS. Increase of ethanol, meprobamate and pentobarbital metabolism after chronic ethanol administration in man and in rats. Am J Med (1971) 51, 346.
9 Rubin E, Gang H, Misra PS, Lieber CS. Inhibition of drug metabolism by acute ethanol intoxication. A hepatic microsomal mechanism. Am J Med (1970) 49, 801.

Alcohol + Methaqualone or *Mandrax* (Methaqualone + Diphenhydramine)

Abstract/Summary

The CNS depressant effects of alcohol and its detrimental effects on the skills relating to driving or handling other potentially dangerous machinery are increased by the concurrent use of methaqualone or *Mandrax*.

Clinical evidence

(a) Alcohol + methaqualone

A retrospective study of drivers arrested for driving under the influence of drugs and/or drink showed that, generally speaking, those with blood-methaqualone levels of 1.0 mg/l or less showed no symptoms of sedation, whereas those above

2.0 mg/l demonstrated serious deterioration (staggering gait, drowsiness, incoherence and slurred speech). These effects were increased if the drivers had also been drinking. The authors write that '...the levels (of methaqualone) necessary for driving impairment are considerably lowered (by alcohol)...', but no precise measure of this is presented in the paper. A similar effect was seen in drivers taking methaqualone and diazepam.[3]

(b) Alcohol + Mandrax (Methaqualone 250 mg + Diphenhydramine 25 mg)

A double-blind study on 12 subjects given two *Mandrax* tablets showed that both mental and physical sedation and a reduction in cognitive skills were enhanced by alcohol (0.5 mg/kg). Residual amounts of *Mandrax* continued to interact as long as 72 h after a single dose. Methaqualone blood levels are also raised by regular moderate amounts of alcohol.[1]

Enhanced effects were also seen in another study.[2]

Mechanism

Alcohol, methaqualone and diphenhydramine are all CNS depressants, the effects of which are additive. The diphenhydramine-alcohol interaction is discussed under 'Alcohol + Antihistamines'. A hangover can occur because the elimination half-life of methaqualone is long (10–40 h).

Importance and management

An established interaction of importance. Those taking either methaqualone or *Mandrax* should be warned that handling machinery, driving a car, or any other task requiring alertness and full co-ordination, will be made more difficult and hazardous if they drink. Doses of alcohol below the legal driving limit with normal amounts of methaqualone may cause considerable intoxication. Patients should also be told that a significant interaction may possibly occur the following day because methaqualone taken on the previous day can have a hangover effect.

References

1 Roden S, Harvey P, Mitchard M. The effect of ethanol on residual plasma concentrations and behaviour in volunteers who have taken *Mandrax*. Br J clin Pharmac (1977) 4, 245.
2 Saario I, Linnoila M. Effect of subacute treatment with hypnotics, alone or in combination with alcohol, on psychomotor skills related to driving. Acta pharmacol et toxicol (1976) 38, 3382.
3 McCurdy HH, Solomons ET, Holbrook JM. Incidence of methaqualone in driving-under-the-influence (DUI) cases in the State of Georgia. J Anal Toxicol (1981) 5, 270–4.

Alcohol + Metoclopramide

Abstract/Summary

There is some evidence that metoclopramide can increase the rate of absorption of alcohol, raise maximum blood alcohol levels and possibly increase sedation.

Clinical evidence, mechanism, importance and management

A study in seven subjects found that 20 mg iv metoclopramide increased the rate of alcohol absorption, while the peak blood levels were raised from 55 to 86 mg/100 ml. Similar results were seen in two subjects given metoclopramide orally.[2] Another study in seven normal subjects found that 10 mg iv metoclopramide accelerated the rate of absorption of alcohol (70 mg/kg) given orally and increased its peak levels but not to a statistically significant extent. Blood alcohol levels remained below 12 mg%. More importantly the sedative effects of the alcohol were found to be increased.[1] The reasons are not fully understood but it appears to be related to an increase in gastric emptying. These studies were looking at intestinal absorption mechanisms rather than at daily practicalities so the importance of these findings is uncertain, but it seems possible that the effects of alcohol will be increased. More study is needed.

References

1 Bateman D, Kahn C, Mashiter K, Davies DS. Pharmacokinetic and concentration-effect studies with IV metoclopramide. Br J clin Pharmac (1978) 6, 401–5.
2 Gibbons DO, Lanet AF. Effects of intravenous and oral propanethline and metoclopramide on ethanol absorption. Clin Pharmacol Ther (1975) 17, 578–84.

Alcohol + Metronidazole

Abstract/Summary

A disulfiram-like reaction can develop in patients taking oral metronidazole who drink alcohol, and there is one report of its occurrence when applied as a vaginal insert. It can also occur if alcohol is present when metronidazole is given intravenously. The existence of this interaction is disputed in some reports.

Clinical evidence

A man who had been in a drunken stupor for three days was given two metronidazole tablets (total of 500 mg) 1 h apart by his wife in the belief that they might sober him up. 20 min after the first tablet he was awake and complaining that he had been given disulfiram (which he had had some months before). Immediately after the second tablet he took another drink and developed a classic disulfiram-like reaction with flushing of the face and neck, nausea and epigastric discomfort.[1]

All 10 alcoholic patients in a test of the value of metronidazole (250 mg twice daily) as a possible drink-deterrent experienced some disulfiram-like reactions of varying intensity (facial flushing, headaches, sensation of heat, fall in blood pressure, vomiting).[4] All of 60 other patients, given 250–750 mg daily, developed mild to moderate disulfiram-like reactions.[5] The incidence in other reports is said to be lower: 24%,[6] 10%[7] and 2%.[2] The reaction has been seen in a patient treated intravenously with metronidazole and a trimethoprim-sulphamethoxazole preparation containing 10% alcohol as a diluent,[11] and it has been reported in association with metabolic acidosis in an intoxicated man 4 h after being given metronidazole intravenously as prophylaxis following injury.[13] Another report describes a reaction when metronidazole was used as a vaginal insert.[12] Alcohol is also said to taste badly[1,4] or is less pleasurable[2] while taking metronidazole. Some drug abusers apparently exploit the reaction for 'kicks'.[10] In contrast, there are other reports which claim that metronidazole has no disulfiram-like effects whatsoever.[8,9]

Mechanism

Not fully understood. Metronidazole, like disulfiram, can inhibit the activity of acetaldehyde dehydrogenase, xanthine oxidase and aldehyde dehydrogenase.[3] The accumulation of acetaldehyde appears to be responsible for most of the symptoms (see 'Alcohol + Disulfiram').

Importance and management

An extensively studied and reported interaction, but it remains a somewhat controversial issue, the incidence being variously reported as between 0 and 100%. Nevertheless all patients given metronidazole by mouth should be warned what may happen if they drink. The reaction, when it occurs, normally seems to be more unpleasant and possibly frightening than serious, and usually requires no treatment, although one report describes a serious reaction when intravenous metronidazole was given to an intoxicated man.[13] The risk of a reaction with metronidazole used intravaginally seems to be small because the absorption is low (about 20% compared with about 100% orally) but evidently it can happen, even if rarely.[12] Patients should be warned.

References

1 Taylor JAT. Metronidazole-a new agent for combined somatic and psychic therapy for alcoholism. Bull Los Angeles Neurol Soc (1964) 29, 158.
2 Penick SB, Carrier RN, Sheldon JR. Metronidazole in the treatment of alcoholism. Amer J Psychiat (1969) 125, 1063.
3 Fried R, Fried LW. The effect of Flagyl on xanthine oxidase and alcohol dehydrogenase. Biochem Pharmacol (1966) 15, 1890.
4 Ban TA, Lehmann HE, Roy P. Preliminary report on the therapeutic effect of FLAGYL in alcoholism. L'Union Medicale du Canada (1966) 95, 147.
5 Sansoy OM, Vegas L. Evaluation of metronidazole in the treatment of alcoholism. J Ind Med Ass (1970) 55, 29.
6 de Mattos H. Relationship between alcoholism and the digestive system. Hospital (1968) 74, 281.
7 Channabasavanna SM, Kaliaperumal VG, Mathew G. Metronidazole in the treatment of alcoholism: a controlled trial. Ind J Psychiat (1979) 21, 90.
8 Goodwin DW. Metronidazole in the treatment of alcoholism. Amer J Psychiat (1968) 123, 1276–8.
9 Gelder MG, Edwards G. Metronidazole in the treatment of alcohol addiction. A controlled trial. Br J Psychiat (1968) 114, 473–5.
10 Giannini AJ, DeFrance DT. Metronidazole and alcohol — poential for combinative abuse. J Toxicol. Clin Toxicol (1983) 20, 509–15.
11 Edwards DL, Fink PC, Van Dyke PO. Disulfiram-like reaction associated with intravenous trimethoprim-sulphamethoxazole and metronidazole. Clin Pharm (1986) 5, 999–1000.
12 Plosker GL. Possible interaction between ethanol and vaginally administered metronidazole. Clin Pharm (1987) 6, 189–93.
13 Harries DP, Teale KFH, Sunderland G. Metronidazole and alcohol: potential problems. Scot Med J (1990) 35, 179–180.

Alcohol + Milk

Abstract/Summary

Blood levels of alcohol and its intoxicant effects are reduced if milk has been drunk.

Clinical evidence, mechanism, importance and management

10 subjects were given 25 ml alcohol (equivalent to a double whiskey) after drinking a pint and a half of water or milk during the previous 90 min. Blood alcohol levels 90 min later were reduced about 40% by the presence of the milk, and about 25% half an hour later. The intoxicant effects of the alcohol were also clearly reduced.[1] The reasons are not understood, but a possible explanation is that the absorption of the alcohol by the gut is reduced by the milk. These findings appear to confirm a long and widely-held belief among drinkers, but whether this interaction can be regarded as advantageous or undesirable is a moot point.

Reference

1 Miller DS, Stirling JL, Yudkin J. Effect of ingestion of milk on concentrations of blood alcohol. Nature (1966) 212, 1051.

Alcohol + Miscellaneous anxiolytics

Abstract/Summary

Buspirone does not appear to interact with alcohol directly, but it can cause drowsiness and weakness which may make driving more hazardous. Suriclone increases the CNS depressant effects of alcohol to some extent, but usually less than other more obviously sedative drugs.

Clinical evidence, mechanism, importance and management

Studies in 12 normal subjects showed that 10 or 20 mg buspirone did not appear to interact with alcohol (i.e. worsen the performance of certain psychomotor tests) but it did make them feel drowsy and weak. The tentative conclusion was drawn that patients might therefore be more aware of feeling 'under par' than with some other drugs (e.g. the benzodiazepines) and less likely to take risks.[1,2] Nevertheless it would seem prudent to warn patients of the potential hazards of driving or handling other potentially dangerous machinery.

Normal subjects on 0.2 or 0.4 mg suriclone three times a day showed modest changes in the performance of a number of tests when also taking alcohol (blood levels of 64–67 mg/dl), similar in many respects to those seen with diazepam, but the differences included increased irritability and antagonism, and some stomach troubles (indigestion, nausea, loss of appetite).[3] As with diazepam, warn patients of the possible increased risks of driving or handling other potentially dangerous machinery.

References

1 Mattila MJ, Aranko K, Sappala T. Acute effects of buspirone and alcohol on psychomotor skills. J Clin Psychiatry (1982) 43, 56–60.
2 Seppala T, Aranko K, Mattila MJ, Shrotriya RC. Effects of alcohol on buspirone and lorazepam actions. Clin Pharmacol Ther (1982) 32, 201–7.
3 Allen D, Lader M. The interactions of ethanol with single and repeated doses of suriclone and diazepam on physiological and psychomotor functions in normal subjects. Eur J Clin Pharmacol (1992) 42, 499–505.

Alcohol + Monosulfiram

Abstract/Summary

Disulfiram-like reactions have been seen in at least three patients who drank alcohol after using a solution of monosulfiram on the skin for the treatment of scabies.

Clinical evidence

A man who used undiluted *Tetmosol* (a solution of monosulfiram) for three days on the skin all over his body developed a disulfiram-like reaction (flushing, sweating, skin swelling, severe tachycardia and nausea) on the third day after drinking three double whiskeys. The same thing happened on two subsequent evenings after drinking.[1] Similar reactions have been described in two other patients after drinking while using *Tetmosol* or *Ascabiol* (also containing monosulfiram).[2,4]

Mechanism

Monosulfiram (tetraethylthiuram monosulphide) is closely related to disulfiram (tetraethylthiuram disulphide) and it appears that the pharmacological basis of the reaction[6] is similar to the disulfiram reaction (see 'Alcohol + Disulfiram').

Importance and management

An established interaction. The makers of monosulfiram preparations and others advise abstention from alcohol before, and for at least 48 h after, application, but this may not always be necessary. The writer of a letter, commenting on the first case cited, wrote that he had never encountered this reaction when using a diluted solution of *Tetmosol* on patients at the Dreadnought Seamen's Hospital in London who '...are not necessarily abstemious.'[3] This would suggest that the reaction is normally uncommon and unlikely to occur if the solution is correctly diluted (usually with 2–3 parts of water) thereby reducing the amount absorbed through the skin. However one unusually sensitive patient is said to have had a reaction (flushing, sweating, tachycardia) after using diluted *Tetmosol*, but without drinking alcohol. It was suggested that she reacted to the alcohol base of the formulation passing through her skin.[5] Patients should be warned.

References

1 Gold S. A skinful of alcohol. Lancet (1966) ii, 1417.
2 Dantas W. Monosulfiram como causa de sindrome do acetaldeido. Arq Cat Med (1980) 9, 29–30.
3 Erskine D. A skinful of alcohol. Lancet (1967) i, 54.
4 Blanc D, Deprez Ph. Unusual adverse reaction to an acaricide. Lancet (1990) 335, 1291.
5 Burgess I. Adverse reactions to monosulfiram. Lancet (1990) 336, 873.
6 Lipsky JJ, Nelson AN, Dockter EC. Inhibition of aldehyde dehydrogenase by sulfiram. Clin Pharmacol Ther (1992) 51, 184.

Alcohol + Nefazodone

Abstract/Summary, clinical evidence, mechanism, importance and management

400 mg nefazodone does not increase the sedative-hypnotic effects of alcohol.[1] No special precautions seem necessary.

Reference

1 Frewer LJ, Lader M. The effects of nefazodone, imipramine and placebo, alone and combined with alcohol, in normal subjects. Int Clin Psychopharmacol (1993) 8, 13–20.

Alcohol + Nitrofurantoin

Abstract/Summary, clinical evidence, mechanism, importance and management

Despite claims in some books and reviews, an extensive literature survey[1] failed to find any experimental or clinical evidence for an alleged disulfiram-like reaction between alcohol and nitrofurantoin. It was concluded that this 'interaction' is erroneous.

Reference

1 Rowles B, Worthen DB. Clinical drug information: a case of misinformation. New Eng J Med (1982) 306, 113–4.

Alcohol + Nitroimidazoles

Abstract/Summary

It is alleged that benznidazole, nimorazole, ornidazole and tinidazole can cause a disulfiram-like reaction with alcohol.

Clinical evidence, mechanism, importance and management

It has been claimed that all of the nitroimidazoles (benznidazole, metronidazole, nimorazole, ornidazole, tinidazole) can cause a disulfiram-like reaction with alcohol (flushing of the face and neck, palpitations, dizziness, nausea, etc.)[1,2] but so far I have been unable to find direct evidence confirming that this occurs, except with metronidazole (see 'Alcohol + Metronidazole'). Roche, the makers of benznidazole, say they have no record of this interaction on their drug database.[3] If a disulfiram-like reaction occurs it is usually more unpleasant and frightening than serious, and normally requires no treatment.

References

1 Bodino JAJ, Lopez EL. Schistosomiasis drugs. In 'Antimicrobial therapy in infants and children' edited by Koren G, Prober CG, Gold R, published by Marcel Dekker, NY (1988) pp 687–727.
2 Ralph ED. Nitroimidazoles. In 'Antimicrobial therapy in infants and children' edited by Koren G, Prober CG, Gold R, published by Marcel Dekker, NY (1988) pp 729–745.
3 Roche UK. Personal communication (1989).

Alcohol + Paraldehyde

Abstract/Summary

Both alcohol and paraldehyde have CNS depressant effects which can be additive. Their concurrent use in the treatment of acute intoxication has had a fatal outcome.

Clinical evidence, mechanism, importance and management

A report describes eight patients who died suddenly and unexpectedly after treatment for acute intoxication with 30–60 ml paraldehyde (normal dose range 3–30 ml; fatal dose 120 ml or more).[1] Both are CNS depressants and may therefore be expected to have additive effects at any dosage, although an animal study suggested that it may be less than additive.[2]

References

1 Kaye S, Haag HB. Study of death due to combined action of alcohol and paraldehyde in man. Toxicol Appl Pharmacol (1964) 6, 316.
2 Gessner PK, Shakarjian MP. Interactions of paraldehyde with ethanol and chloral hydrate. J Pharmacol Exp Ther (1985) 235, 32–6.

Alcohol + Phenothiazines, Butyrophenones and other psychotropic drugs

Abstract/Summary

The detrimental effects of alcohol on the skills related to driving are made worse by chlorpromazine, flupenthixol (possibly prochlorperazine?) and to a lesser extent by thioridazine. Any interaction with haloperidol, sulpiride or tiapride seems to be milder. There is evidence that drinking can precipitate the emergence of extrapyramidal side-effects in patients taking neuroleptics.

Clinical evidence

(a) Effect on driving skills

21 subjects showed a marked deterioration in the performance of a number of skills related to driving when given 200 mg chlorpromazine daily and alcohol (blood levels 42 mg%). Many complained of feeling sleepy, lethargic, dull, groggy and poorly coordinated and most considered themselves more unsafe to drive than with alcohol alone.[10] A later study confirmed these findings with 1 mg/kg chlorpromazine and blood alcohol levels of 80 mg%.[11] A double-blind study in subjects given 0.5 mg flupenthixol, three times a day for two weeks found that combined with 0.5 mg/kg alcohol their performance of a number of tests (choice reaction, coordination, attention) was impaired to such an extent that driving or handling other potentially dangerous machinery could be hazardous.[1,2] No interaction of any importance was seen with single 0.5 mg doses of haloperidol.[1,2] A study in 12 normal subjects found that 5 mg prochlorperazine three times daily for three days caused carelessness and slowing of a weaving test while driving a car, with little subjective appreciation of the deterioration. No changes could be detected in the performance of kinetic visual acuity or simple reaction time tests.[8] Alcohol would be expected to increase this impairment but nobody seems to have checked on this yet, nevertheless patients should be warned. In the same study 72 mg betahistidine daily for three days was found to have no detectable effect on driving performance.[8] Subjects given 150 mg sulpiride daily for two weeks demonstrated only a mild interaction with alcohol, whereas when given 30–60 mg thioridazine daily for two weeks some additive effects with alcohol were seen, with a moderately deleterious effect on attention.[2,3] Another study found that thioridazine and alcohol affected skills related to driving, but not as much as the effects seen with chlorpromazine.[11] Another study found no difference between the effects of thioridazine and a placebo.[12] A study in nine alcoholics given 400–600 mg tiapride daily showed that wakefulness was not impaired when combined with alcohol (0.5 mg/kg) and in fact appeared to be improved, but the effect on driving skills was not studied.[7]

(b) Precipitation of extra-pyramidal side-effects

A report[4] describes in detail seven patients who developed acute extrapyramidal side-effects (akathisia, dystonia) while taking trifluoperazine, fluphenazine and chlorpromazine when they drank alcohol. The author stated that these were examples of numerous such alcohol-induced neuroleptic toxicity reactions observed by him over an 18-year period involving phenothiazines and butyrophenones. Elsewhere he describes the emergence of drug-induced parkinsonism in a woman taking perphenazine and amitriptyline when she began to drink.[5] 18 cases of haloperidol-induced extrapyramidal reactions among young drug abusers, in most instances associated with the ingestion of alcohol, have also been described.[6]

(c) Reduced fluphenazine levels

A study in seven schizophrenics found that when given 40 g alcohol to drink at about the same time as their regular injection of fluphenazine decanoate (25–125 mg every two weeks), their serum fluphenazine levels were depressed by 30% at 2 h and by 16% at 12 h.[9]

Mechanisms

Uncertain. (a) Additive CNS depressant effects are one explanation of this interaction. (b) One suggestion to account for the emergence of the drug side-effects is that alcohol lowers the threshold of resistance to the neurotoxicity of these drugs. In addition is seems possible that alcohol impairs the activity of tyrosine hydroxylase so that the dopamine/acetylcholine balance within the corpus striatum is upset.[5]

Importance and management

The documentation is limited. (a) Warn patients that if they drink while on chlorpromazine, thioridazine or flupenthixol (probably other related drugs as well) they may become very drowsy, and should not drive or handle other potentially dangerous machinery. Some risk is possible with prochlorperazine as well, but the effects of alcohol with haloperidol, sulpiride and tiapride appear to be minimal. (b) The author of the reports describing the emergence of serious neuroleptic side-effects in those who drink, considers that patients should routinely be advised to abstain from alcohol during neuroleptic treatment. (c) The clinical importance of reduced fluphenazine levels is uncertain. This needs more study.

References

1 Linnoila M. Effects of diazepam, chlordiazepoxide, thioridazine, haloperidol, flupenthixol and alcohol on psychomotor skills related to driving. Ann Med Exp Biol Fenn (1973) 51, 125.
2 Linnoila M, Saario I, Olkonieme J, Liljequist R, Himberg JJ, Maki M. Effect of two weeks treatment with chlordiazepoxide or flupenthixol, alone or in combination with alcohol, on psychomotor skills related to driving. Arzneim-Forsch (Drug Res) (1975) 25, 1088.
3 Seppala T, Saario I, Matilla MJ. Two weeks' treatment with chlorpro-

mazine, thioridazine, sulpiride or bromazepam: actions and interactions with alcohol on psychomotor skills related to driving. Mod Probl Pharmacopsych (1976) 11, 85.
4 Lutz EG. Neuroleptic-induced akathisia and dystonia triggered by alcohol. J Amer Med Ass (1977) 236, 2422.
5 Lutz EG. Neuroleptic-induced parkinsonism facilitated by alcohol. J Med Soc NJ (1978) 75, 473–5.
6 Kenyon-David D. Haloperidol intoxication. NZ Med J (1981) 92, 165.
7 Vandel B, Bonim B, Vandel S, Blum D, Rey E, Volmat R. Etude de l'interaction entre le tiapride et l'alcool chez l'homme. Sem Hop Paris (1984) 60, 175–7.
8 Betts T, Harris D, Gadd E. The effects of two anti-vertigo drugs (betahistidine and prochlorperazine) on driving skills. Br J clin Pharmac (1991) 32, 455–8.
9 Soni SD, Bamrah JS, Krska J. Effects of alcohol on serum fluphenazine levels in stable chronic schizophrenics. Human Psychopharmacology (1991) 6, 301–6.
10 Zirkle GA, King PD, McAtee OB, Van Dyke R. Effects of chlorpromazine and alcohol on coordination and judgment. J Amer Med Ass (1959) 171, 1496–9.
11 Milner G, Landauer AA. Alcohol, thioridazine and chlorpromazine effects on skills related to driving behaviour. Brit J Psychiar (1971) 118, 351–2.
12 Saario I. Psychomotor skills during subacute treatment with thioridazine and bromazepam, and their combined effects with alcohol. Ann Clin Res (1976) 8, 117–23.

Alcohol + Procarbazine

Abstract/Summary

A flushing reaction has been seen in patients on procarbazine after drinking alcohol.

Clinical evidence, mechanism, importance and management

One report describes five patients taking procarbazine whose faces became very red and hot for a short time after drinking wine.[1] Another says that flushing occurred in three patients on procarbazine after drinking beer.[2] Two out of 40 patients in a third study complained of facial flushing after taking a small alcoholic drink, and one patient thought that the effects of alcohol were markedly increased.[3] Yet another describes a 'flush syndrome' in three out of 50 patients after drinking alcohol.[4] Whether this flushing reaction is related to the alcohol-disulfiram reaction (see 'Alcohol + Disulfiram') is not known. The evidence is very limited, but clearly this reaction is a possibility in patients on procarbazine who drink. It seems to be more embarrassing, possibly frightening, than serious, and if it occurs it is unlikely to require treatment, however patients should be warned.

References

1 Mathé G, Berumen L, Schweisguth O, Brule G, Schneider M, Cattan A, Amiel JL, Schwarzenberg L. Methyl-hydrazine in the treatment of Hodgkin's disease and various forms of haematosarcoma and leukaemia. Lancet (1963) ii, 1077.
2 Dawson WB. Ibenzmethyzin in the management of late Hodgkin's disease. In 'Natulan, Ibenzmethyzin'. Report of the proceedings of a symposium, Downing College, Cambridge, June 1965. Edited by Jelliffe AM and Marks J. John Wright, Bristol (1965) p 31.
3 Todd IDH. Natulan in the management of late Hodgkin's disease, other

lymphoreticular neoplasms, and malignant melanoma. Br Med J (1965) 1, 326–7.

4 Brulé G, Schlumberger JR, Griscelli C. N-isopropyl-alpha-(2-methyl-hydrazino)-p-toluamide, hydrochloride (NSC-77213) in treatment of solid tumors. Cancer Chemother Rep (1965) 44, 31–8.

Alcohol + Sodium cromoglycate

Abstract/Summary

No adverse interaction occurs between sodium cromoglycate and alcohol.

Clinical evidence, mechanism. importance and management

A double-blind crossover trial on 17 subjects found that 40 mg sodium cromoglycate had little or no effect on the performance of a number of tests on human perceptual, cognitive and motor skills, whether taken alone or with alcohol (0.75 g/kg). Nor did it affect blood alcohol levels.[1] This is in line with the common experience of patients, and no special precautions seem to be necessary.

Reference

1 Crawford WA, Frank HM, Hensley VR, Hensley WJ, Starmer GA, Teo RCK. The effect of sodium cromoglycate on human performance alone and in combination with ethanol. Med J Aust (1976) 2, 997.

Alcohol + Tetracyclic antidepressants

Abstract/Summary

Mianserin can cause drowsiness and impair the ability to drive or handle other dangerous machinery, particularly during the first few days of treatment. This impairment is increased by alcohol. Pirlindole appears not to interact with alcohol.

Clinical evidence

(a) Mianserin

A double-blind cross-over study in 13 normal subjects given 20–60 mg mianserin daily for eight days, with and without alcohol (1 g/kg), showed that their performance of a number of psychomotor tests (choice reaction, coordination, critical flicker frequency) were impaired by concurrent use. The subjects were aware of feeling drowsy and muzzy, and less able to carry out the tests.[1]

These results confirm the findings of other studies.[2,3,5]

(b) Pirlindole

A study in subjects given pirlindole indicated that it did not affect the performance of a number of psychomotor tests, with or without alcohol.[4]

Mechanism

The CNS depressant effects of mianserin appear to be additive with those of alcohol.

Importance and management

Drowsiness is a frequently reported side-effect of mianserin, particularly during the first few days of treatment. Patients should be warned that driving or handling dangerous machinery will be made more hazardous if they drink. Pirlindole appears not to interact.

References

1 Seppala T, Stromberg C, Bergman I. Effect of zimelidine, mianserin and amitriptyline on psychomotor skills and their interaction with alcohol. A placebo controlled study. Eur J Clin Pharmacol (1984) 27, 181–9.

2 Matilla MJ, Liljequist R, Seppala T. Effects of amitriptyline and mianserin on psychomotor skills and memory in man. Br J clin Pharmac (1978) 5, 53S.

3 Seppala T. Psychomotor skills during acute and two-week treatment with mianserin (Org GB 94) and amitriptyline and their combined effects with alcohol. Ann Clin Res (1977) 9, 66.

4 Ehlers T, Ritter M. Effects of the tetracyclic antidepressant pirlindole on sensorimotor performance and subjective condition in comparison to imipramine and during interaction with alcohol. Neuropsychobiology (1984) 12, 48–54.

5 Stromberg C, Mattila MJ. Acute comparison of clovoxamine and mianserin, alone and in combination with ethanol, on human psychomotor performance. Pharmacol Toxicol (1987) 60, 374–9.

Alcohol + Tolazoline

Abstract/Summary

A disulfiram-like reaction may occur in patients on tolazoline if they drink.

Clinical evidence, mechanism, importance and management

Seven normal subjects were given 500 mg tolazoline daily for four days. Within 15 and 90 min of drinking 90 ml port wine (18.2% alcohol) six of the seven experienced tingling over the head, and four developed warmth and fullness of the head.[1] The reasons are not understood, but this reaction is not unlike a mild disulfiram reaction and may possibly have a similar mechanism (see 'Alcohol + Disulfiram'). Patients given tolazoline should be warned about this reaction if they drink and advised to limit their consumption. Reactions of this kind with drugs other than disulfiram are usually more unpleasant or frightening than serious, and treatment is rarely needed.

Reference

1 Boyd EM. A search for drugs with disulfiram-like activity. QJ Stud Alcohol (1960) 21, 23–5.

Alcohol + Trazodone

Abstract/Summary

Trazodone makes driving or handling other dangerous machinery more hazardous, and further impairment may occur with alcohol.

Clinical evidence

A study in six normal subjects comparing the effects of amitriptyline (50 mg) and trazodone (100 mg) found that both drugs impaired the performance of a number of psychomotor tests, causing drowsiness and reducing 'clearheadedness' to approximately the same extent. Only manual dexterity was further impaired when the subjects on trazodone were given sufficient alcohol to give blood levels of about 40 mg%.[1]

Another study similarly found that the impairment of psychomotor performance by trazodone was increased by alcohol.[2]

Mechanism

Uncertain. Simple additive depression of the CNS seems a likely explanation.

Importance and management

An established interaction, and of practical importance. Patients should be warned that their ability to drive, handle dangerous machinery or to do other tasks needing complex psychomotor skills may be impaired by trazodone, and further worsened by alcohol.

References

1 Warrington SJ, Ankier SI, Turner P. Evaluation of possible interactions between ethanol and trazodone or amitriptyline. Neuropsychobiology (1986) 15 (Suppl 1) 31–7.
2 Tiller JWG. Antidepressants, alcohol and psychomotor performance. Acta Psychiatr Scand (1990) Suppl 360, 13–17.

Alcohol + Trichloroethylene

Abstract/Summary

A flushing skin reaction similar to a mild disulfiram reaction can occur in those exposed to trichloroethylene when they drink alcohol.

Clinical evidence

An engineer from a factory where trichloroethylene was being used as a degreasing agent, developed facial flushing, a sensation of increased pressure in the head, lacrymation, tachypnoea and blurred vision within 12 min of drinking 3 oz bourbon whiskey. The reaction did not develop when he was no longer exposed to the trichloroethylene. Other workers in the same plant reported the same experience.[1]

Vivid red blotches in a symmetrical pattern on the face, neck, shoulders and back were seen in other workers exposed for a few hours each day to 20–220 ppm trichloroethylene when they drank only half a pint (300 ml) of beer,[3] and it has also been reported elsewhere.[2] It has been described as the 'degreasers flush'. There is also some evidence that long-term exposure may possibly reduce mental capacity.[4]

Mechanism

Uncertain. One suggested mechanism is a disulfiram-like inhibition of acetaldehyde metabolism by trichloroethylene (see 'Alcohol + Disulfiram').

Importance and management

An established interaction. It would seem to be more unpleasant and socially disagreeable than serious, and normally requires no treatment. The whole question of whether long-term exposure to trichloroethylene is desirable does not seem to have been answered.

References

1 Pardys S, Brotman M. Trichloroethylene and alcohol: a straight flush. J Amer Med Ass (1974) 229, 521.
2 Smith GF. Trichloroethylene. A review. Brit J Industr Med (1966) 23, 249.
3 Stewart RD, Hake CL, Peterson JE. 'Degreasers Flush', dermal response to trichloroethylene and ethanol. Arch Environm Hlth (1974) 29, 1.
4 Windemuller FJB, Ettema JH. Effects of combined exposure to trichloroethylene and alcohol on mental capacity. Int Arch Occup Environ Hlth (1978) 41, 77.

Alcohol + Tricyclic antidepressants

Abstract/Summary

The ability to drive, to handle dangerous machinery or to do other tasks requiring complex psychomotor skills may be impaired by amitriptyline and to a lesser extent by doxepin, particularly during the first few days of treatment. This impairment is increased by alcohol. Amoxapine, clomipramine, desipramine, imipramine and nortriptyline appear to interact with alcohol only minimally. Information about other tricyclics appears to be lacking.

Clinical evidence

(a) Alcohol + Amitriptyline

Blood alcohol levels of about 80 mg% impaired the performance by 21 normal subjects of three motor skills tests related to driving. After additionally taking 0.8 mg/kg amitriptyline the performance was even further impaired.[1]

Similar results have been very clearly demonstrated in considerable numbers of subjects using a variety of psychomotor skill tests,[1-7] the interaction being most marked during the first few days of treatment, but tending to wane as treatment continued.[5] There is also some limited evidence from animal studies that amitriptyline may possibly enhance the fatty changes induced in the liver by alcohol,[8] but this still needs confirmation from human studies. Unexplained blackouts lasting a few hours have also been described in three women after drinking only modest amounts;[9] they had been taking amitriptyline or imipramine for only a month.

(b) Alcohol + Doxepin

A double-blind cross-over trial on 21 subjects given various combinations of alcohol and either doxepin or a placebo showed that with blood-alcohol levels of 40-50 mg% choice reaction test times were prolonged and the number of mistakes increased. Coordination was obviously impaired after seven days treatment with doxepin, but not after 14 days.[3]

In an earlier study doxepin appeared to cancel out the deleterious effects of alcohol on the performance of a simulated driving test.[10]

(c) Alcohol + Amoxapine, Clomipramine, Desipramine, Imipramine, Nortriptyline

Studies in subjects with blood-alcohol levels of 40-60 mg% showed that clomipramine and nortriptyline had only slight or no effects on various choice reaction, coordination, memory and learning tests.[3,11,12,17] The amoxapine-alcohol interaction was found to be slight[14] but two other patients have been described who experienced reversible extrapyramidal symptoms (parkinsonism, akathisia) while taking amoxapine, apparently caused by drinking.[16] Tests in subjects given 100 mg desipramine indicated that no significant interaction occurred with alcohol,[15] but 150 mg imipramine daily tends to increase the sedative-hypnotic effects of alcohol.[18]

Mechanisms

Part of the explanation is that both alcohol and some of the tricyclics, particularly amitriptyline, cause drowsiness and other CNS depressant effects which can be additive with the effects of alcohol.[6] The sedative effects in descending order are said in one review to be as follows: amitriptyline, doxepin, imipramine, nortriptyline, desipramine, protriptyline.[13] In addition, alcohol causes marked increases (+100-200%) in the plasma concentrations of amitriptyline, probably by inhibiting its metabolism during its first pass through the liver.[4]

Importance and management

The amitriptyline-alcohol interaction is well documented. Warn patients that driving or handling dangerous machinery may be made more hazardous if they drink, particularly during the first few days, but the effects of the interaction diminish during continued treatment. The alcohol-doxepin interaction is less well documented and the information is conflicting, but to be on the safe side a similar warning should be given. Amoxapine, clomipramine, desipramine, imipramine and nortriptyline appear to interact only minimally with alcohol. Direct information about other tricyclics seems to be lacking, but there appear to be no particular reasons for avoiding concurrent use. However prescribers may feel it appropriate to offer some precautionary advice because during the first 1-2 weeks of treatment many tricyclics (without alcohol) may temporarily impair the skills related to driving.[14]

References

1 Landauer AA, Milner G, Patman J. Alcohol and amitriptyline effects on skills related to driving behaviour. Science (1969) 163, 1467.

2 Seppala T. Psychomotor skills during acute and two-week treatment with mianserin (ORG GB 94) and amitriptyline and their combined effects with alcohol. Ann Clin Res (1977) 9, 66.

3 Seppala T, Linnoila M, Elonen E, Matilla MJ, Maki M. Effect of tricyclic antidepressants and alcohol on psychomotor skills related to driving. Clin Pharmacol Ther (1975) 17, 515.

4 Dorian P, Sellers EM, Reed KL, Warsh JJ, Hamilton C, Kaplan HL, Fan T. Amitriptyline and ethanol: pharmacokinetic and pharmacodynamic interaction. Eur J Clin Pharmacol (1983) 25, 325–331.

5 Seppala T, Stromberg C, Bergman I. Effects of zimelidine, mianserin and amitriptyline on psychomotor skills and their interaction with ethanol. A placebo controlled cross-over study. Eur J Clin Pharmacol (1984) 27, 181–9.

6 Scott DB, Fagan D, Tiplady B. Effects of amitriptyline and zimelidine in combination with alcohol. Psychopharmacology (1982) 76, 209–11.

7 Matilla M, Liljequist R, Seppala T. Effects of amitriptyline and mianserin on psychomotor skills and memory in man. Br J Clin Pharmacol (1978) 5, 53S.

8 Milner G, Kakulas K. The potentiation by amitriptyline of liver changes induced by ethanol in mice. Pathology (1969) 1, 113.

9 Hudson CJ. Tricyclic antidepressants and alcoholic blackouts. J Nerv Ment Dis (1981) 169, 381.

10 Milner G, Landauer AA. The effects of doxepin, alone and together with alcohol in relation to driving safety. Med J Aust (1978) 1, 837.

11 Hughes FW, Forney RB. Delayed audiofeedback (DAF) for induction of anxiety. Effect of nortriptyline, ethanol or nortriptyline-ethanol combinations on performance with DAF. J Amer Med Ass (1963) 185, 556.

12 Liljequist R, Linnoila M, Matilla M. Effect of two weeks' treatment with chlorimipramine and nortriptyline, alone or in combination with alcohol on learning and memory. Psychopharmacology (1974) 39, 181.

13 Marco LA, Randels RM. Drug interactions in alcoholic patients. Hillside J Clin Psychiatrq (1981) 3, 27–44.

14 Linnoila M, Seppala T. Antidepressants and driving. Accid Anal and Prev (1985) 17, 297–301.

15 Linnoila M, Johnsmn J, DuByoski K, Buchsbaum MS, Schneinin M, Kilts C. Effects of antidepressants on skilled performance. Br J clin Pharmac (1984) 18, 109–120S.

16 Shen WW. Alcohol, amoxapine and akathisia. Biol Psychiatry (1984) 19, 929–30.

17 Berlin I, Cournot A, Zimmer R, Pedarriosse AM, Manfredi R, Molinier P, Puech AJ. Evaluation and comparison of the interaction between alcohol and moclobemide or clomipramine in healthy subjects. Psychopharmacology (1990) 100, 40–5.

18 Frewer LJ, Lader M. The effects of nefazodone, imipramine and placebo, alone and combined with alcohol, in normal subjects. Int Clin Psychopharmacol (1993) 8, 13–20.

Alcohol + Viqualine (Ivoqualine)

Abstract/Summary

No adverse interaction occurs if alcohol and viqualine are taken together.

Clinical evidence, mechanism, importance and management

Alcohol (serum levels 17–22 mmol/l) had no effect on the steady-state serum levels of viqualine (75 mg twice daily for three days) in 16 normal subjects, nor was there any evidence of a disulfiram-like reaction. The deleterious effects of alcohol on a number of skills (word recall, manual tracking, body sway) and self-ratings of intoxication, sedation and performance were also not altered by the viqualine.[1] On the basis of this study there would seem to be no good reason for those taking viqualine to avoid alcoholic drinks.

Reference

1 Sullivan JT, Naranjo CA, Shaw CA, Kaplan HL, Kadlec KE, Sellers EM. Kinetic and dynamic interactions of oral viqualine and ethanol in man. Eur J Clin Pharmacol (1989) 36, 93–6.

Alcohol + Xylene

Abstract/Summary

Some individuals exposed to xylene vapour who subsequently drink alcohol may experience dizziness and nausea. A flushing skin reaction has also been seen.

Clinical evidence, mechanism, importance and management

Studies[1] in volunteers exposed to m-xylene vapour at concentrations of 140 or 250 ppm for 4 h who were then given alcohol to drink (0.8 g/kg) showed that about 10% experienced dizziness and nausea. One subject exposed to 300 ppm developed a conspicuous dermal flush on his face, neck, chest and back. He also showed some erythema on alcohol alone. The reasons for these reactions are not understood.

Reference

1 Riilimaki V, Laine A, Savolainene K, Sippel H. Acute solvent-ethanol interactions with special reference to xylene. Scand j work environ hlth (1982) 8, 77–9.

Chapter 3
Analgesic and Non-Steroidal
Anti-inflammatory Drug Interactions

The drugs dealt with in this chapter are listed in Table 3.1 with their proprietary names. In addition the list also contains other analgesic and non-steroidalanti-inflammatory drugs (NSAIDs) which act as interacting agents and which are dealt with in other chapters. The Index should be consulted for the full listing.

Table 3.1 Analgesics and non-steroidal anti-inflammatory drugs (NSAIDs)

Non-proprietary names	Proprietary names
Analgesics (non-narcotic)	
Alclofenac	*Allopydin, Argun, Darkeyfenac, Desiflam, Epinal, Mervan, Prinalgin, Vanadian, Zumaril*
Azapropazone	*Cinnamin, Pentosol, Prolixan, Rheumox, Tolyprin*
Clometacin	*Duperan*
Diclofenac	*Aflamin, Blesin, Delphimix, Dichronic, Diclo Attritin, -Phlogont, -Spondyril, Dicloreum, Dolobasan, Dolotren, Duravolten, Effekton, Flogofenac, Forgenac, Inflamac, Monoflam, Myogit, Neriodin, Novapirina, Panamor, Rheumavincin, Rhumalgan, Seecoren, Sofarin, Toryxil, Tsudohmin, Voltarol, Voltarene*
Diflunisal	*Adomal, Algobid, Antadar, Artrodol, Diflonid, Difludol, Diflunil, Diflusan, Dolisal, Dolobid, Dolobis, Donobid, Dopanone, Dorbid, Flulisin, Fluniget, Fluodonil, Flustar, Ilacen, Reuflos, Unisal*
Fenoprofen	*Fenopron, Fepron, Nalfon, Nalgesic, Progesic*
Feprazone	*Analud, Brotazona, Cocresol, Danfenona, Grisona, Impremial, Methrazone, Naloven, Nessazona, Nilatin, Prenakes, Prenazon, Rangozona, Represil, Tabien*
Floctafenine	*Idalon, Idarac*
Flufenamic acid	*Alfenamin, Ansatin, Arlef, Meralen, Sastridex, Surik*
Flurbiprofen	*Ansaid, Cebutid, Flugalin, Flurofen, Froben, Ocufen*
Glafenine	*Exidol, Glifan, Osodent, Privadol*
Ibuprofen	*Advul, Algofen, Anco, Artene, Brufen, Cuprofen, Emodin, Fenbid, Ibucasen, Inflam, Lidifen, Liptan, Migrafen, Motrin, Neobrufen, Novaprin, Novoprofen, Nurofen, Pacifene, Reclofen, Suspren, Uniprofen, Vesicum (incomplete list)*
Indobufen	*Ibustrin*
Indomethacin	*Agilex, Amuno, Arthrexin, Atracin, Boutycin, Confortid, Flexin, Indocid, Imbrilon, Inacid, Indomet,Indotard, Infrocin, Metindol, Sadeorum, Tannex, Vonum*
Isoxicam	*Maxicam, Pacyl, Vectren*
Kebuzone	*Chebutan, Chepirol, Chetopir, Gammachetone, Neo-panagyl, Neufenil*
Ketoprofen	*Alrheumat, Anaus, Arcental, Capisten, Fastum, Flexen, Ketalgin, Ketoartril, Ketoprosil, Meprofen, Orudis, Oruvail, Profenid, Reuprofen, Salient, Tafirol, Vasserprofen*
Meclofenamic acid	*Meclomen, Movens*
Mefenamic acid	*Bafameritin-m, Bonabol, Citronamic, Coslan, Lysalgo, Mefalgic, Mefedolo, Parkemed, Ponalar, Ponstan, Ponstil, Pontal*
Mofebutazone	*Chemiartrol, Monazone, Monbutina, Monoprine, Rheumatox*
Nabumetone	*Relifex, Relifen*

continued on p. 47

Table 3.1 *Continued*

Non-proprietary names	Proprietary names
Naproxen	*Alganil, Anaprox, Denaxpren, Floginax, Laraflex, Madaprox, Naprium, Naprorex, Naprosyn, Naproval, Piproxen, Proxen, Proxine, Rofanten, Xenar*
Nefopam	*Acupan, Doplitrone, Lenipan, Nefadol, Nefam, Oxadol, Sinalgico*
Oxametacin	*Dinulcid, Flogar, Restid*
Oxyphenbutazone	*Artroflog, Artzone, Butofen, Flogitolo, Oxibutol, Piraflogin, Rheumapax, Tandacote, Tandearil, Tanderil, Validil*
Paracetamol (acetaminophen)	
Penicillamine	*Artamin, Atamir, Cuprenil, Cuprimine, Depamine, Depen, Distamine, Mercatyl, Pendramine, Rhumantin, Sufortan, Trolovol, Vistamin*
Phenazone (antipyrine)	
Phenylbutazone	*Algoverine, Artrizin, Butacote, Butazolidin, Butalan, Butazina, Butoz, Ditrone, Denilbutina, Intrabutazone, Megazone, Panazone, Rheumaphen, Sinobutina*
Piroxicam	*Antiflog, Baxo, Dexicam, Doblexan, Feldene, Flogobene, Improntal, Larapram, Polipirox, Femoxicam, Reumagil, Roxene, Roxiden, Vitaxicam, Zamcam*
Salicylates	
Aspirin	
Aloxiprin	*Lyman tabs, Palaprin, Paloxin, Rumatral, Supperpyrin, Tiatral*
Benorylate	*Benoral, Benorile, Benortan, Benotamol, Bentum, Doline, Duvium, Salipran, Vetedol, Winolate*
Choline salicylate	
Sodium salicylate	
Sulindac	*Aflodac, Algocetil, Arthrocine, Citireuma, Clinoril, Clisundac, Lyndac, Reumofil, Sudac, Sulartrene, Sulen, Sulic, Sulindal, Sulindol*
Tiaprofenic acid	*Surgam (amyl), Surgamic, Tioprofen*
Tolfenamic acid	*Clotam*
Tolmetin	*Benetazon*

Analgesics (narcotic and related)

Alfentanil	*Alfenta, Rapifen*
Codeine	
(Dextro)propoxyphene	*Abalgin, Algafen, Antalvic, Daraphen, Depronal, Dolene, Dolocap, Dolorphen, Dolotard, Doloxene, Liberen, Novoproxyn, Proxagesic. Also contained in Cosalgesic, Distalgesic, Darvon Co*
Dextromoramide	*Jetriu, Palfium*
Diamorphine (heroin)	
Dihydrocodeine	*DF118*
Fentanyl	*Fentanest, Leptanal, Sublimaze, Thalamonal*
Hydromorphone	*Dilaudid*
Methadone	*Physeptone, Dolophine, Westalone, L-Polamidon*
Morphine	
Oxymorphone	*Numorphan*
Papaveretum	*Escopon, Omnopon*
Pentazocine	*Fortagesic, Fortral, Sosegon, Talwin, Fortal*
Pethidine (meperidine)	*Demerol*
Phenoperidine	
Sufentanil	

Alfentanil or Sufentanil + Erythromycin

Abstract/Summary

A few patients may experience prolonged and increased alfentanil effects if they are treated with erythromycin. Sufentanil appears not to interact.

Clinical evidence

(a) Alfentanil

A 32-year-old man undergoing exploratory laparotomy was given 1 g erythromycin and 1 g neomycin three times daily on the day before surgery. He was given pancuronium, alfentanil and thiopental for induction, followed by succinylcholine and N_2O/O_2. Anaesthesia was maintained with alfentanil. Altogether he received 20.9 mg of alfentanil. An hour after recovery he was found to be unarousable and with only 5 breaths per minute. He was successfully treated with naloxone.[1]

One gram of erythromycin daily for seven days increased the mean half-life of alfentanil in six subjects by 56% (from 84 to 131 min) and decreased the clearance from 3.9 to 2.9 ml/kg/min. Some of the subjects were much more sensitive than others: two showed marked changes; two showed little changes, and the other two showed intermediate effects. The two most sensitive subjects demonstrated considerable changes within a day of taking only 500 mg erythromycin.[2] Another patient given alfentanil and erythromycin is said to have developed respiratory arrest during recovery.[3]

(b) Sufentanil

Seven day's treatment with 500 mg erythromycin twice daily in six subjects was found not to affect the pharmacokinetics of intravenous sufentanil (3 µg/kg) in the nine hours following administration. Two of the subjects were the same as those who had shown an interaction with alfentanil cited above.[4]

Mechanism

Uncertain. Inhibition of the metabolism of the alfentanil by the erythromycin, resulting in increased alfentanil effects, is a likely explanation.[1,2]

Importance and management

Evidence is limited but the alfentanil/erythromycin interaction is established and clinically important. Be alert for evidence of prolonged alfentanil effects and respiratory depression, although the outcome of concurrent use is unpredictable. It has been advised that alfentanil should be only given in reduced amounts or avoided in patients who have recently had erythromycin.[2] Alternatively, sufentanil can be used instead in doses of 3 µg/kg or less, but much larger doses of sufentanil should only be given with caution.[4]

References

1 Bartkowski RR, McDonnell TE. Prolonged alfentanil effect following erythromycin administration. Anesthesiology (1990) 73, 566–8.
2 Bartkowski RR, Goldberg ME, Larijani GE, Boerner T. Inhibition of alfentanil metabolism by erythromycin. Clin Pharmacol Ther (1989) 46, 99–102.
3 Yate PM, Short TSM, Sebel PS, Morton J. Comparison of infusions of alfentanil or pethidine for sedation of ventilated patients on ITU. Br J Anaesth (1986) 58, 1091–9.
4 Bartkowski RR, Goldberg ME, Huffnagle S, Epstein RH. Sufentanil disposition. Is it affected by erythromycin administration? Anesthesiology (1993) 78, 260–5.

Alfentanil + Ondansetron

Abstract/Summary

Ondansetron appears not to interact adversely with alfentanil.

Clinical evidence, mechanism, importance and management

8 or 16 mg ondansetron in normal subjects was found to have no effect on the sedation or ventilatory depression due to alfentanil (a continuous infusion of 0.25–0.75 µg/kg following a 5 µg/kg bolus dose) and no effect on the rate of recovery.[1] No special precautions would seem to be necessary.

Reference

1 Dershwitz M, Di Biase PM, Rosow CE, Wilson RS, Sanderson PE, Joslyn AF. Ondansetron does not affect alfentanil-induced ventilatory depression or sedation. Anesthesiology (1992) 77, 447–52.

Alfentanil + Reserpine

Abstract/Summary

An isolated report describes ventricular dysrhythmias in a patient on reserpine when given alfentanil during anaesthesia.

Clinical evidence, mechanism, importance and management

A hypertensive woman on 0.25 mg reserpine daily was given 800 µg alfentanil intravenously before anaesthesia with thiopentone and suxamethonium, followed during the surgery with 900 µg alfentanil in 100 µg doses and 70% NO_2/O_2. Bradycardia developed and frequent unifocal premature ventricular contractions throughout the surgery, but they disappeared 3–4 h afterwards. The reasons are not understood.[1]

Reference

1 Jahr JS, Weber S. Ventricular dysrhythmias following an alfentanil anesthetic in a patient on reserpine for hypertension. Acta Anaesthesiol Scand (1991) 35, 788–9.

Antirheumatic agents + Mazindol

Abstract/Summary

Mazindol is reported not to interact adversely with indomethacin, salicylates and other analgesics and anti-inflammatory drugs.

Clinical evidence, mechanism, importance and management

A double-blind study of mazindol and a placebo was carried out on 26 obese arthritics, 15 of whom were on salicylates, 11 on indomethacin and one on dextropropoxyphene with paracetamol. Additional drugs used were ibuprofen (four patients), phenylbutazone (one patient), dextropropoxyphene (seven patients), paracetamol (three patients) and prednisone (nine patients). No adverse interactions were seen.[1]

Reference

1 Thorpe PC, Isaac PF, Rodgers JA. A controlled trial of mazindol (Sanjorex, Teronac) in the management of obese rheumatic patients. Curr Ther Res (1975) 17, 149.

Aspirin and Salicylates + Antacids, Urinary alkalinizers

Abstract/Summary

The serum salicylate concentrations of patients taking large doses of aspirin as an anti-inflammatory agent can be reduced to sub-therapeutic levels by concurrent use of some antacids.

Clinical evidence

A child with rheumatic fever taking 0.6 g aspirin five times daily had a serum salicylate concentration of between 8.2 and 11.8 mg/100 ml while taking 30 ml *Maalox* (aluminium and magnesium hydroxide suspension). When the *Maalox* was withdrawn, the urinary pH fell from a range of 7–8 to 5.0–6.4, whereupon the serum salicylate level rose to about 38 mg/100 ml, calling for a reduction in dosage.[1] An associated study in 13 normal subjects taking 4 g aspirin daily for a week showed that the concurrent use of 4 g sodium bicarbonate daily reduced serum salicylate levels from 27 to 15 mg/100 ml. This reflected a rise in the urinary pH from a range of 5.6–6.1 to 6.2–6.9.[1,7]

Similar changes have been reported in other studies.[3,5,6,8,9]

Mechanism

Aspirin and other salicylates are acidic compounds which are excreted by the kidney tubules and are ionized in solution. In alkaline solution, much of the drug exists in the ionized form which is not readily reabsorbed and therefore is lost in the urine. If the urine is made more acidic, much more of the drug exists in the un-ionized form which is readily reabsorbed so that less is lost in the urine and the drug is retained in the body.[8,9] Magnesium oxide also strongly adsorbs aspirin and sodium salicylate.[4]

Importance and management

A well-established and clinically important interaction for those on chronic treatment with large doses of salicylates because the serum salicylate may be reduced to sub-therapeutic levels. This interaction can occur with both 'systemic' antacids (e.g. sodium bicarbonate) as well as some 'non-systemic' antacids (e.g. magnesium-aluminium hydroxides), although some evidence suggests that some aluminium-containing antacids (*Amphojel* — aluminium hydroxide, and *Robalate* — aluminium aminoacetate) may have minimal effects on urinary pH.[1,2] Care should be taken to monitor serum salicylate levels if any antacid is started or stopped in patients where the control of salicylate levels is critical. No important interaction would be expected in those taking occasional doses of aspirin for analgesia.

References

1 Levy G. Interactions of salicylates with antacids. Clinical implications with respect to gastrointestinal bleeding and anti-inflammatory activity. Frontiers of Internal Medicine 1974, 12th Int Congr Intern Med, Tel Aviv, 1974, p 404, Karger, Basel (1975).
2 Muirden KR, Barraclough DRE. Drug interaction in the management of rheumatoid arthritis. Aust NZ J Med (1976) 6 (Suppl 1) 14.
3 Levy G, Lampman T, Kamath BL, Garrettson LK. Decreased serum salicylate concentration in children with rheumatic fever treated with antacid. N Engl J Med (1975) 293, 323.
4 Naggar VF, Khalil SA, Daabis NA. The in-vitro adsorption of some anti-rheumatics on antacids. Pharmazie (1976) 31, 461.
5 Hansten PD, Hayton WL. Effect of antacid and ascorbic acid on serum salicylate concentration. J Clin Pharmacol (1980) 24, 326.
6 Shastri RA. Effect of antacids on salicylate kinetics. Int J Clin Pharmacol ther Tox (1985) 23, 480–4.
7 Levy G, Leonard JR. Urine pH and salicylate therapy. J Amer Med Ass (1971) 217, 81.
8 Macpherson CR, Milne MD, Evans BM. The excretion of salicylate. Brit J Pharmacol (1955) 10, 484–9.
9 Hoffman WS, Nobe C. The influence of urinary pH on the renal excretion of salicyl derivatives during aspirin therapy. J Lab Clin Med (1950) 35, 237–48.

Aspirin and Salicylates + Caffeine

Abstract/Summary

Caffeine increases the bioavailability, the rate of absorption and the serum levels of aspirin.

Clinical evidence, mechanism, importance and management

120 mg caffeine increased the AUC (area under the curve) of a single 650 mg dose of aspirin in normal subjects by 36%, increased the rate of absorption, and increased the maximum serum levels by 15%.[1] This confirms the results of a previous study.[2] Both of these studies suggest that there may be merit in combining these two drugs if more rapid and effective analgesia is required. There would appear to be no reason for avoiding concurrent use.

References

1 Thithpandha A. Effect of caffeine on the bioavailability and pharmacokinetics of aspirin. J Med Assoc Thai (1989) 72, 562–6.
2 Yoovathawarn KC, Sriwatanakul K, Thithapandha A. Influence of caffeine on aspirin pharmacokinetics. Eur J Drug Metab Pharmacokinet (1986) 11, 71–6.

Aspirin and Salicylates + Carbonic anhydrase inhibitors

Abstract/Summary

A severe and even life-threatening toxic reaction can occur in those on high dose salicylate treatment if concurrently treated with carbonic anhydrase inhibitors (acetazolamide, dichlorphenamide).

Clinical evidence

A boy of eight with chronic juvenile arthritis, well controlled on prednisolone, indomethacin and aloxiprin, was admitted to hospital with drowsiness, vomiting and hyperventilation (diagnosed as metabolic acidosis) within a month of increasing the aloxiprin dosage from 3 to 3.5 g daily and adding 75 mg dichlorphenamide daily for glaucoma.[1]

Other cases of toxicity (metabolic acidosis) occurred in a 22-year-old woman on salsalate when additionally given 1000 mg acetazolamide daily,[1] and in two elderly women on large doses of aspirin when they were given acetazolamide or dichlorphenamide.[2] Poisoning developed in a man on dichlorphenamide within 10 days of starting to take 3.9 g aspirin daily.[4] Coma developed in an 85-year-old taking 3.9 g aspirin daily when the dosage of acetazolamide was increased from 0.5 to 1 g,[3] and toxicity in another very old man given both drugs.[5] Levels of unbound acetazolamide were found to be unusually high.[5]

Mechanism

Not fully established. One idea is that these carbonic anhydrase inhibitors (acetazolamide, dichlorphenamide) affect the plasma pH so that more of the salicylate exists in the non-ionized (lipid-soluble) form which can enter the CNS and other tissues more easily, leading to salicylate intoxication.[2] Animal studies confirm that carbonic anhydrase inhibitors increase the lethality of aspirin. An alternative suggestion is that because salicylate inhibits the plasma protein binding of acetazolamide and its excretion by the kidney, acetazolamide toxicity may occur which mimics salicylate toxicity.[5] It is not clear whether the increased salicylate clearance caused by the acetazolamide has any part to play.[6]

Importance and management

There are few clinical cases on record, but the interaction is established (well confirmed by animal studies) and potentially serious. Carbonic anhydrase inhibitors should probably be avoided in those on high dose salicylate treatment (a recommendation in one study[5]). If they are used, the patient should be well monitored for any evidence of toxicity (confusion, lethargy, hyperventilation, tinnitus) because the interaction may develop slowly and insidiously.[2] In this context other non-steroidal anti-inflammatory drugs may be safer. Naproxen proved to be a satisfactory substitute in one case.[1] The authors of one study suggest that methazolamide may possibly be a safer alternative to acetazolamide because it is minimally bound to plasma proteins.[5]

References

1 Cowan RA, Hartnell GG, Lowdell CP, McLean BI, Leak AM. Metabolic acidosis induced by carbonic anhydrase inhibitors and salicylates in patients with normal renal function. Brit Med J (1984) 289, 347–8.
2 Anderson CJ, Kaufman PL, Sturm RJ. Toxicity of combined therapy with carbonic anhydrase inhibitors and aspirin. Am J Ophthalmol (1978) 86, 516–19.
3 Chapron DJ, Brandt JL, Sweeny KR, Olesen-Zammett L. Interaction between acetazolamide and aspirin–a possible unrecognized cause of drug-induced coma. J Am Geriat Soc (1984) 32, S18.
4 Hurwitz GA, Wingfield W, Cowart TD, Jollow DJ. Toxic interaction between salicylates and a carbonic anhydrase inhibitor: the role of cerebral edema. Vet Hum Toxicol (1980) 22 (Suppl) 42–4.
5 Sweeney KR, Chapron DJ, Brandt JL, Gomolin IH, Feig PU, Kramer PA. Toxic interaction between acetazolamide and salicylate: case reports and a pharmacokinetic explanation. Clin Pharmacol Ther (1986) 40, 518–24.
6 Macpherson CR, Milne MD, Evans BM. The excretion of salicylate. Brit J Pharmacol (1955) 10, 484.

Aspirin and Salicylates + Cholestyramine

Abstract/Summary

Cholestyramine does not have a clinically important effect on the absorption of aspirin.

Clinical evidence, mechanism, importance and management

A study in three subjects and three patients, and a later study in seven subjects, found that 4 g cholestyramine delayed the absorption of a single 500 mg dose of aspirin (peak levels extended from 30 to 60 min) but the total amount absorbed was only reduced 5–6%. Some of the subjects had slightly higher serum aspirin levels while taking cholestyramine.[1] There would seem to be little reason for avoiding concurrent use unless rapid analgesia is needed.

Reference

1 Hahn K-J, Eiden W, Schettle M, Hahn M, Walter E, Weber E. Effect of cholestyramine on the gastrointestinal absorption of phenprocoumon and acetylosalicylic acid in man. Eur J clin Pharmacol (1972) 4, 142–5.

Aspirin and Salicylates + Corticosteroids, ACTH

Abstract/Summary

Concurrent use is very common but the incidence of gastrointestinal bleeding and ulceration may be increased. Serum salicylate levels are reduced by corticosteroids and therefore they may rise, possibly to toxic concentrations, if the corticosteroid is withdrawn without first reducing the salicylate dosage.

Clinical evidence

A 4-year-old boy chronically treated with at least 20 mg prednisone daily was additionally given 3.6 g choline salicylate daily, the prednisone gradually being tapered off to 2 mg daily over a three-month period. Severe salicylate intoxication developed, and in a retrospective investigation of the cause, using frozen serum samples drawn for other purposes, it was found that the serum salicylate levels had climbed from about 10 to 90 mg% during the withdrawal of the prednisone.[1] Later studies in three other patients on choline salicylate or aspirin and either prednisone or another unnamed corticosteroid, demonstrated similar but less spectacular rises (about threefold) during corticosteroid withdrawal.[1] Hydrocortisone was also found to increase the clearance of sodium salicylate in four other patients.[1]

A serum salicylate rise of similar proportions has been described in a patient on aloxiprin when prednisolone was withdrawn.[2] Other studies in considerable numbers of both adults and children show that prednisone, methylprednisolone, betamethasone and ACTH reduce serum salicylate levels.[4,5,8] Another study also found that intra-articular doses of steroids (dexamethasone, methylprednisolone, triamcinolone) reduced serum salicylate levels in patients given enteric-coated aspirin.[6] However one study in patients failed to show that 12–60 mg prednisone daily had any effect on the clearance of single doses of sodium salicylate.[9]

Mechanism

Uncertain. One idea is that the presence of the corticosteroid increases the glomerular filtration rate so that clearance of the salicylate is also increased. When the corticosteroid is withdrawn, the clearance returns to normal and the salicylate accumulates. Another suggestion is that the corticosteroids increase the metabolism of the salicylate.[4] Studies in mice have shown that cortisone protects them from the development of salicylism.[3]

Importance and management

A well-established interaction. Concurrent use is very common but patients should be monitored to ensure that salicylate levels remain adequate when corticosteroids are added[5] and do not become excessive if they are withdrawn. It should also be remembered that concurrent use may increase the incidence of gastrointestinal bleeding[7] and ulceration.

References

1 Klinenberg JR, Miller F. Effect of corticosteroids on blood salicylate concentration. J Amer Med Ass (1965) 194, 601.
2 Muirden KD, Barraclough DRE. Drug interactions in the management of rheumatoid arthritis. Aust NZ J Med (1976) 6 (Suppl 1) 14.
3 Montuori E. Accion de la cortisone sobre le toxicidad del salicilato di sodio. Rev Soc Argent Biol (1954) 30, 44.
4 Graham GG, Champion GD, Day RO, Paull PD. Patterns of plasma concentrations and urinary excretion of salicylate in rheumatoid arthritis. Clin Pharmacol Ther (1977) 22, 410–20.
5 Bardare M, Cislaghi GU, Mandelli M, Sereni F. Value of monitoring plasma salicylate levels in treating juvenile rheumatoid arthritis. Arch Dis Child (1978) 53, 381–5.
6 Edelman J, Potter JM, Hackett LP. The effect of intra-articular steroids on plasma salicylate concentrations. Br J clin Pharmac (1986) 21, 301–7.
7 Carson JL, Strom BL, Schinnar R, Sim E, Maislin G, Morse ML. Do corticosteroids really cause upper GI bleeding. Clin Res (1987) 35, 340A.
8 Koren G, Roifman C, Gelfand E, Lavi S, Suria D, Stein L. Corticosteroids-salicylate interaction in a case of juvenile rheumatoid arthritis. Ther Drug Monit (1987) 9, 177–9.
9 Day RO, Harris G, Brown M, Graham GG, Champion GD. Interaction of salicylate and corticosteroids in man. Br J clin Pharmac (1988) 26, 334–7.

Aspirin and Salicylates + Food

Abstract/Summary

Avoid food if rapid analgesia is needed because it delays the absorption of aspirin.

Clinical evidence, mechanism, importance and management

A study in 25 subjects given 650 mg aspirin in five different aspirin preparations showed that food roughly halved their serum salicylate levels when measured 10 and 20 min later, compared with those seen when the same dose was taken while fasting.[1] Similar results were found in another study in subjects given 1500 mg calcium aspirin.[2] In yet another study on eight subjects who were given 900 mg effervescent aspirin, their serum salicylate levels were roughly halved by food at 15 min, but were almost the same after an hour.[3] A possible reason for the reduced absorption is that the aspirin becomes adsorbed onto the food. Food also delays gastric emptying. Thus if rapid analgesia is needed, aspirin should be taken without food, but if aspirin is needed long-term, its administration with food can help to protect the gastric mucosa.

References

1 Wood JH. Effect of food on aspirin absorption. Lancet (1967) ii, 212.
2 Spiers ASD, Malone HF. Effect of food on aspirin absorption. Lancet (1967) i, 440.
3 Volans GN. Effects of food and exercise on the absorption of effervescent aspirin. Br J clin Pharmac (1974) 1, 137–41.

Aspirin and Salicylates + Kaolin-pectin

Abstract/Summary

Kaolin-pectin causes a small but clinically unimportant reduction in the absorption of aspirin.

Clinical evidence, mechanism, importance and management

The absorption of 975 mg aspirin in 10 normal subjects was reduced 5–10% by the concurrent use of 30 or 60 ml kaolin-pectin.[1] A likely explanation is that the aspirin becomes adsorbed by the kaolin so that the amount available for absorption through the gut wall is reduced. This small reduction in absorption is unlikely to be of clinical importance.

References

1 Juhl RP. Comparison of kaolin-pectin and activated charcoal for inhibition of aspirin absorption. Amer J Hosp Pharm (1979) 36, 1097–9.

Aspirin and Salicylates + Levamisole

Abstract/Summary

A rise in serum salicylate levels in a patient on aspirin when given levamisole was not confirmed in subsequent controlled studies.

Clinical evidence, mechanism, importance and management

A preliminary report of a patient who showed an increase in serum salicylate levels when levamisole was given with aspirin[1] prompted a study of this possible interaction. Nine normal subjects were given 3.9 g of sustained-release aspirin daily in two divided doses over a period of 3 weeks. During this period they were also given 50 mg levamisole three times a day for a week, each subject acting as his own control. No significant changes in serum salicylate levels were found.[2]

References

1 Laidlaw DA. Rheumatoid arthritis improved by treatment with levamisole and L-histidine. Med J Aust (1976) 2, 382.
2 Rumble RH, Brooks PM, Roberts MS. Interaction between levamisole and aspirin. Br J Clin Pharmac (1979) 7, 631.

Aspirin and Salicylates + Pentazocine

Abstract/Summary

Renal papillary necrosis occurred in man chronically taking large doses of aspirin when pentazocine was added.

Clinical evidence, mechanism, importance and management

An isolated report describes renal papillary necrosis in a man, regularly taking 1.8 to 2.4 g aspirin daily, within six months of additionally starting to take 800–850 mg pentazocine daily. He developed abdominal pain, nausea and vomiting, and passed tissue via his urethra. Before starting the pentazocine and when it was stopped, no necrosis was apparent. The postulated reason for this reaction is that the pentazocine-induced reduction in blood flow through the kidney potentiated the adverse effects of the chronic aspirin use.[1] The general importance of this case is uncertain, but it emphasises the risks of long-term use (possibly abuse) of aspirin with pentazocine. More study is needed.

Reference

1 Muhalwas KK, Shah GM, Winer RL. Renal papillary necrosis caused by long-term ingestion of pentazocine and aspirin. J Amer Med Ass (1981) 246, 867–8.

Aspirin and Salicylates + Phenylbutazone

Abstract/Summary

Phenylbutazone reduces the uricosuric effects of aspirin.

Clinical evidence

The observation that several patients given both drugs developed elevated serum urate levels, prompted a study on four patients without gout. This showed that 2 g aspirin daily had little effect on the excretion of uric acid in the urine, but marked uricosuria occurred with 5 g daily. When phenylbutazone was additionally given (200, 400 and then 600 mg daily over three days) the uricosuria was abolished. Serum uric acid levels rose from an average of 4 to 6 mg%. The interaction was confirmed in a patient with tophaceous gout. The retention of uric acid also occurs if the phenylbutazone is given first.[1]

Mechanism

Not understood. It seems almost certain that some interference occurs within the kidney tubules.

Importance and management

An established but sparsely documented interaction. If serum urate measurements are taken for diagnostic purposes, full account should be taken of this interaction. The potential problems arising from this interaction should also be recognized in any patient given both drugs.

Reference

1 Oyer JH, Wagner SL and Schmid FR. Suppression of salicylate-induced uricosuria by phenylbutazone. Am J Med Sci (1966) 225, 40–5.

Aspirin and Salicylates + Probenecid

Abstract/Summary

The uricosuric effects of aspirin or other salicylates and probenecid are not additive as might be expected but are mutually antagonistic.

Clinical evidence

A study showed that the urinary uric acid excretion in mg/average 24 h was found to be 673 mg with a single 3 g daily dose of probenecid, 909 mg with a 6 g daily dose of sodium salicylate, but only 114 mg when both drugs were used concurrently.[1]

Similar antagonism has been seen in other studies in patients given 2.6–5.2 g aspirin daily.[2–4] No antagonism is seen until serum salicylate levels of 5–10 mg/100 ml are reached.[4]

Mechanism

Not understood. The interference probably occurs at the site of renal tubular secretion, but it also seems that both drugs can occupy the same site on plasma albumins.

Importance and management

A well established and clinically important interaction. Regular dosing with substantial amounts of salicylates should be avoided if this antagonism is to be avoided, but small occasional analgesic doses probably do not matter. Serum salicylate levels of 5–10 mg/100 ml are necessary before this interaction occurs.

References

1 Seegmiller JE, Grayzel AI. Use of the newer uricosuric agents in the management of gout. J Amer Med Ass (1960) 173, 1076.

2 Pascale LR, Dubin A, Hoffman WS. Therapeutic value of probenecid (Benemid) in gout. J Amer Med Ass (1952) 149, 1188.
3 Gutman AB, Yu TF. Benemid (p-di-n-propylsulfamyl-benzoic acid) as uricosuric agent in chronic gout arthritis. Trans Ass Amer Phys (1951) 64, 279.
4 Pascale LR, Dubin A, Bronsky D, Hoffman WS. Inhibition of the uricosuric action of Benemid by salicylate. J Lab Clin Med (1955) 45, 771–7.

Aspirin and Salicylates + Sulphinpyrazone

Abstract/Summary

The uricosuric effects of the salicylates and sulphinpyrazone are not additive, as might be expected, but are mutually antagonistic.

Clinical evidence

6 g sodium salicylate with 600 mg sulphinpyrazone daily caused a urinary uric acid excretion in a patient of only 30 mg/average 24 h, whereas when each drug was used by itself in the same doses the excretion was 281 and 527 mg/av 24 h respectively.[1] A later study on five gouty men infused with sulphinpyrazone for about an hour (300 mg to prime followed by 10 mg/min) showed that the additional infusion with sodium salicylate (3 g to prime followed by 10–20 mg/min) virtually abolished the uricosuria. When the drugs were given in the reverse order to three other patients the same result was seen.[2] The uricosuria caused by 400 mg sulphinpyrazone was shown in another study to be completely abolished by 3.5 g aspirin.[3]

Mechanism

Not fully understood. Sulphinpyrazone competes successfully with salicylate for excretion by the kidney tubules so that salicylate excretion is reduced, but the salicylate blocks the inhibitory effect of sulphinpyrazone on the tubular reabsorption of uric acid so that the uric acid accumulates within the body.[2]

Importance and management

An established and clinically important interaction. Concurrent use for uricosuria should be avoided. Doses of aspirin as low as 700 mg can cause an appreciable fall in uric acid excretion[3] but the effects of an occasional small dose are probably of little practical importance.

References

1 Seegmiller JE, Grayzel AI. Use of the newer uricosuric agents in the management of gout. J Amer Med Ass (1960) 173, 1076.
2 Yu TF, Dayton PG, Gutman AB. Mutual suppression of the uricosuric effects of sulphinpyrazone and salicylate: a study in interaction between drugs. J Clin Invest (1963) 42, 1330.
3 Kersley GD, Cook ER, Tovey DCJ. Value of uricosuric agents and in particular of G 28315 in gout. Ann Rheum Dis (1958) 17, 326–33.

Azapropazone + Miscellaneous drugs

Abstract/Summary

The serum levels of azapropazone are not significantly changed by the concurrent use of chloroquine, dihydroxy-aluminium sodium carbonate, magnesium aluminium silicate, bisacodyl or anthraquinone laxatives.

Clinical evidence, mechanism, importance and management

A study in 12 subjects given 300 mg azapropazone three times a day found that the serum levels of azapropazone, measured at 4 h, were not affected by the concurrent use of chloroquine, 250 mg daily for 7 days.[1] Another study in 15 patients taking the same dosage of azapropazone found that the concurrent use of dihydroxy-aluminium sodium carbonate, magnesium aluminium silicate, bisacodyl or anthraquinone laxatives only caused a minor (5–6%) reduction in azapropazone serum levels.[2] No special precautions would seem to be needed if these drugs are given together.

References

1 Faust-Tinnefeldt G, Geissler HE. Azapropazon und rheumatologische Basistherapie mit Chloroquin unter dem Aspekt der Arzneimittelinteraktion. Arzneim-Forsch/Drug Res (1977) 27, 2170.
2 Faust-Tinnefeldt G, Geissler HE, Mutschler E. Azapropazon-Plasmaspiegel unter Begleitmedikation mit einem Antacidum oder Laxans. Arzneim-Forsch/Drug Res (1977) 27, 2411.

Buprenorphine, Oxycodone + Amitriptyline

Abstract/Summary

No marked increase in the CNS and respiratory depressant effects of buprenorphine occurs if amitriptyline is given concurrently. Oxycodone similarly appears not to interact adversely with amitriptyline.

Clinical evidence, mechanism, importance and management

A study in 12 normal subjects found that both 0.4 mg buprenorphine given sublingually and 50 mg amitriptyline given orally impaired the performance of a number of psychomotor tests (digit symbol substitution, flicker fusion, Maddox wing, hand-to-eye coordination, reactive skills) and the subjects felt drowsy, feeble, mentally slow and muzzy. When given together the effects were only moderately increased and the increase in the respiratory depressant effects of the buprenorphine was only mild.[1] A not dissimilar study using 0.28 mg/kg oxycodone and 50 mg amitriptyline found no major pharmacodynamic

interactions.[2] There seem to be no strong reasons for avoiding concurrent use.

References

1 Saarialho-Kere U, Mattila MJ, Paloheimo M, Seppala T. Psychomotor, respiratory and neuroendocrinological effects of buprenorphine and amitriptyline in healthy volunteers. Eur J Clin Pharmacol (1987) 33, 139–46.
2 Pöyhiä R, Kalso E, Seppälä T. Pharmacodynamic interactions of oxycodone and amitriptyline in healthy volunteers. Curr Ther Res (1992) 51, 739–49.

Butorphanol + Cimetidine

Abstract/Summary

Butorphanol and cimetidine appear not to interact.

Clinical evidence, mechanism, importance and management

The pharmacokinetics of transnasal butorphanol (1 mg) and cimetidine (300 mg 6-hourly) for 4 days were not significantly altered by concurrent use in 16 normal subjects.[1] There would seem to be no reason for avoiding combined use.

Reference

1 Shyu WC, Pittman KA, Barbhaiya RH. Pharmacokinetic (PK) interaction between transnasal burophanol (TNB) and cimetidine (C) in healthy subjects. Clin Pharmacol Ther (1993) 53, 163.

Codeine + Quinidine

Abstract/Summary

The analgesic effects of codeine are reduced or abolished by quinidine.

Clinical evidence

16 extensive metabolizers were given 100 mg codeine with and without single 200 mg doses of quinidine. The quinidine reduced the peak morphine levels by about 80% (from a mean of 18 to less than 4 nmol/l). Codeine alone increased the pain threshold (pin-prick pain test using an argon laser) but no significant analgesic effects were detectable when the quinidine was present.[2]

These studies confirm those of a previous study with 100 mg codeine and 50 mg doses of quinidine.[1] The quinidine reduced the peak morphine serum levels by more than 90% (by 92% in seven extensive metabolizers, and by 97% in one poor metabolizer) and similarly abolished the analgesic effects.[1]

Mechanism

Not fully understood. A possible reason is that the quinidine markedly reduces the metabolism of codeine to its active metabolite (morphine) by inhibiting the activity of liver cytochrome P450.

Importance and management

An established interaction. In practical terms it means that codeine will be virtually ineffective as an analgesic in those taking quinidine. An alternative analgesic should be used.

References

1 Desmeules J, Dayer P, Gascon M-P, Magistris M. Impact of genetic and environmental factors on codeine analgesia. Clin Pharmacol Ther (1989) 45, 122.
2 Sindrup SH, Arendt-Nielsen L, Brøfsen K, Bjerring P, Angelo HR, Erikson B, Gram LF. The effect of quinidine on the analgesic effect of codeine. Eur J Clin Pharmacol (1992) 42, 587–92.

Dextromoramide + Triacetyloleandomycin

Abstract/Summary

An isolated report describes a marked increase in the effects of dextromoramide and coma in a man when he was treated with triacetyloleandomycin.

Clinical evidence, mechanism, importance and management

A man on dextromoramide developed signs of overdosage (a morphine-like coma, mydriasis and depressed respiration) three days after starting treatment with triacetyloleandomycin for a dental infection. He recovered when treated with naloxone. A possible explanation is that the triacetyloleandomycin reduced the metabolism of the dextromoramide, thereby reducing its loss from the body and increasing its serum levels and effects.[1] The general importance of this interaction is uncertain but concurrent use should be well monitored. It is not clear whether other macrolide antibiotics can interact similarly.

Reference

1 Carry PV, Ducluzeau R, Jourdan C, Bourrat Ch, Vigneau C, Descotes J. De nouvelles interactions avec les macrolides. Lyon Med (1982) 248, 189–90.

Dextropropoxyphene + Food

Abstract/Summary

Food can delay the absorption of dextropropoxyphene, but the total amount absorbed may be slightly increased.

Clinical evidence, mechanism, importance and management

A study in normal subjects showed that, while fasting, peak serum dextropropoxyphene levels were reached after about 2 h. High fat and high carbohydrate meals delayed peak serum levels to about 3 h, and high protein to about 4 h. Both the protein and carbohydrate meals caused a small increase in the total amount of dextropropoxyphene absorbed.[1] Likely reasons for the delay in absorption are that food delays gastric emptying and possibly also physically prevents the dextropropoxyphene from coming into contact with the absorbing surface of the gut. Avoid food if rapid analgesic effects are needed.

Reference

1 Musa MN, Lyons LL. Effect of food and liquid on the pharmacokinetics of propoxyphene. Curr Ther Res (1976) 19, 669.

Dextropropoxyphene + Orphenadrine

Abstract/Summary

An alleged adverse interaction between dextropropoxyphene and orphenadrine which is said to cause mental confusion, anxiety, and tremors seems to be very rare, if indeed it ever occurs.

Clinical evidence, mechanism, importance and management

Riker, the makers of orphenadrine, used to state in their package insert that 'mental confusion, anxiety and tremors have been reported in patients receiving orphenadrine and dextropropoxyphene (propoxyphene) concurrently.' Eli Lilley, the makers of propoxyphene, issued a similar warning. However in correspondence with both manufacturers, two investigators of this interaction (Pearson and Salter[1]) were told that the basis of these statements consisted of either anecdotal reports from clinicians or cases where patients had received twice the recommended dose of orphenadrine, in all a total of 13 cases. In every case the adverse reactions seen were similar to those reported with either drug alone. A brief study on five patients given both drugs to investigate this alleged interaction failed to reveal an adverse interaction.[2]

The documentation is therefore sparse (to say the least) and no case of interaction has been firmly established. The investigators cited[1] calculated that the two drugs were probably being used together on three million prescriptions a year, and at that time (1970) a maximum of 13 doubtful cases had been reported. There seems therefore little reason for avoiding concurrent use, although prescribers should know that the advisability of using the two drugs together has been the subject of some debate.

References

1 Pearson RE, Salter FJ. Drug interaction? — Orphenadrine with propoxyphene. N Engl J Med (1970) 282, 1215.
2 Puckett WH, Visconti JA. Orphenadrine and propoxyphene (cont.) N Engl J Med (1970) 283, 544.

Dextropropoxyphene + Tobacco smoking

Abstract/Summary

Dextropropoxyphene is less effective as an analgesic in smokers than in non-smokers

Clinical evidence

A study on 835 patients who were given dextropropoxyphene hydrochloride for mild or moderate pain or headache showed that its efficacy as an analgesic was decreased by smoking. The drug was rated as ineffective in 10.1% of 335 non-smokers, 15% of 347 patients who smoked up to 20 cigarettes daily, and 20.3% of 153 patients who smoked more than 20 cigarettes daily.[1]

Mechanism

It is thought that tobacco smoke contains compounds which increase the activity of the liver enzymes concerned with the metabolism of dextropropoxyphene, thereby increasing its loss from the body and diminishing its effectiveness as an analgesic.[1]

Importance and management

The interaction appears to be well established. Prescribers should be aware that dextropropoxyphene is twice as likely to be ineffective (1 in 5) in those who smoke 20 cigarettes a day as in those who do not smoke (1 in 10).

Reference

1 Boston Collaborative Drug Surveillance Program. Decreased clinical efficacy of propoxyphene in cigarette smokers. Clin Pharmacol Ther (1973) 14, 259.

Diamorphine + Pyrithyldione

Abstract/Summary

A single case report describes a fatality due to the combined CNS depressant effects of diamorphine (heroin) and pyrithyldione.

Clinical evidence, mechanism, importance and management

A heroin (diamorphine) addict was found dead after taking pyrithyldione (a sedative and hypnotic) and heroin. His serum pyrithyldione and brain morphine levels were found to be 590 ng/ml and 0.06 ng/g respectively, suggesting that he had taken only a therapeutic dose of the pyrithyldione and a moderate dose of heroin. The presumed cause of death was the combined CNS depressant effects of both drugs. The authors of the report suggest that the pyrithyldione potentiated the effects of the heroin.[1]

Reference

1 Jorens PG, Coucke V, Selala MI, Schepens PJC. Fatal intoxication due to the combined use of heroin and pyrithyldione. Hum Exp Toxicol (1992) 11, 296–7.

Diclofenac + Miscellaneous drugs

Abstract/Summary

Aluminium hydroxide, digitoxin, doxycycline and cefadroxil do not interact with diclofenac. The biliary excretion of ceftriaxone is increased by diclofenac.

Clinical evidence, mechanism, importance and management

Two teaspoons of a 5.8% suspension of aluminium hydroxide had no effect on the bioavailability of a single 50 mg dose of diclofenac in nine normal subjects. The concurrent use of 0.1 mg digitoxin also had no effect on the serum levels of diclofenac (50 mg twice daily) of eight normal subjects.[1] In another study neither 2 g cefadroxil (eight patients) nor 200 mg doxycycline (seven patients) when taken daily for a week had any effect on the pharmacokinetics of 100 mg diclofenac.[2] No special precautions are needed while taking any of these drugs and diclofenac.

A pharmacokinetic study in eight patients who had undergone cholecystectomy and who had a T drain in the common bile duct, found that while taking diclofenac (50 mg 12-hourly) the excretion of ceftriaxone (2 g intravenously) in the bile was increased four-fold while the urinary excretion was approximately halved.[3] The clinical importance of this is uncertain, but probably small.

References

1 Schumacher A, Faust-Tinnefeldt G, Geissler HE, Gilfrich HJ, Mutschler E. Untersuchungen potentieller Interaktionen von Diclofenac-Natrium (Voltaren) mit einem Antazidum und mit Digitoxin. Therapiewoche (1983) 33, 2619–25.
2 Schumacher A, Geissler HE, Mutschler E, Osterburg M. Untersuchungen potentieller Interaktionen von Diclofenac-Natrium (Voltaren) mit Antibiotika. Z Rheumatol (1983) 42, 25–7.
3 Merle-Melet M, Brseler L, Lokiec F, Dopff C, Boissel P, Dureux JB. Effects

of diclofenac on ceftriaxone pharmacokinetics in humans. Antimicrob Ag Chemother (1992) 36, 2331–3.

Diclofenac + Pentazocine

Abstract/Summary

An isolated report describes grand mal seizures in a patient treated with diclofenac and pentazocine.

Clinical evidence, mechanism, importance and management

A man with Buerger's disease had a grand mal seizure while watching TV 2 h after being given a single 50 mg suppository of diclofenac. He was also taking 50 mg pentazocine three times daily. He may possibly have had a previous seizure some months before after taking a single 100 mg slow-release diclofenac tablet.[1] The reasons for this reaction are not known, but on rare occasions diclofenac alone has been associated with seizures (said to be 1 in 100,000[1]) and seizures have also been seen with pentazocine alone. It is not clear what part the disease itself, or watching TV, had a part to play in the development of this adverse reaction.[1]

No interaction between diclofenac and pentazocine is established, but be aware of this case if concurrent use is being considered, particularly in patients who are known to be seizure-prone.

Reference

1 Heim M, Nadvorna H, Azaria M. With comments by Straughan J, Hoehler HW. Grand mal seizures following treatment with diclofenac and pentazocine. S Afr Med J (1990) 78, 700–1.

Diflunisal + Antacids

Abstract/Summary

Aluminium- and magnesium-containing antacids can reduce the absorption of diflunisal by up to 40%, but no important interaction occurs if food is taken at the same time.

Clinical evidence, mechanism, importance and management

A study on four normal subjects found that when given three 15 ml doses of *Aludrox* (aluminium hydroxide), 2 h before, together with and 2 h after a single 500 mg oral dose of diflunisal, its absorption was reduced about 40%.[1] Another study[2] showed that the absorption of a single 500 mg dose of diflunisal was reduced 13% when given with 30 ml *Maalox* (aluminium-magnesium hydroxides), 21% when given 1 h later, and 32% when the antacid was given on a four-times-a-day schedule. Yet another study demonstrated a 26% reduction

in absorption by 15 ml aluminium hydroxide gel.[3] However the bioavailability of diflunisal was not significantly altered in those taking aluminium-magnesium hydroxides if also taken with food.[4] Just how these antacids cause a reduced absorption is not clear but adsorption has been suggested.[4] The clinical importance of this interaction is uncertain.

References

1 Verbeeck R, Tjandramaga TB, Mullie TB, Verbesselt R, De Shepper PJ. Effect of aluminium hydroxide on diflunisal absorption. Br J clin Pharmac (1979) 7, 519.
2 Holmes GI, Irvin JD, Schrogie JJ, Lavies RO, Breault GO, Rogers JL, Huber PB, Zinny MA. Effects of *Maalox* on the bioavailability of diflunisal. Clin Pharmacol Ther (1979) 25, 228.
3 Tobert JA, De Schepper P, Tjandramaga TB, Mullie A, Meisinger MAP, Buntinx AP, Huber PB, Yeh KC. The effect of antacids on the bioavailability of diflunisal. Clin Pharmacol Ther (1979) 25, 251.
4 Tobert JA, De Schepper P, Tjandramaga TB, Mullie A, Buntinx AP, Meisinger MAP, Huber PB, Hall TIP, Yeh KC. Effect of antacids on the bioavailabity of diflunisal in the fasting and prostprandial states. Clin Pharmacol Ther (1981) 30, 385.

Diflunisal and Oxaprozin + Miscellaneous drugs

Abstract/Summary, clinical evidence, mechanism, importance and management

The loss of difunisal from the body is faster in men than women, and is increased by smoking and oral contraceptives.[1] The pharmacokinetics of oxaprozin are only changed to a minor degree by conjugated oestrogens (*Pemarin*).[2,3] None of the changes appear to be large enough to be of clinical importance.

References

1 Macdonald JI, Herman RJ, Verbeeck RK. Sex-difference and the effects of smoking and oral contraceptive steroids on the kinetics of diflunisal. Eur J Clin Pharmacol (1990) 38, 175–9.
2 Scavone JM, Ochs HR, Greenblatt DJ, Matlis R. Pharmacokinetics of oxaprozin in women receiving conjugated estrogen. Eur J Clin Pharmacol (1988) 35, 105–8.
3 Scavone JM, Greenblatt DJ. Oxaprozin kinetics in women receiving conjugated estrogens. J Clin Pharmacol (1987) 27, 725.

Diflunisal + NSAIDs and Analgesics

Abstract/Summary

Aspirin can reduce serum diflunisal levels. Diflunisal raises serum indomethacin levels two-to-three-fold and concurrent use should be avoided. Paracetamol levels are increased by diflunisal but not those of naproxen.

Clinical evidence, mechanism, importance and management

(a) Diflunisal + Aspirin

The concurrent use of aspirin (600 mg four times daily) has been shown to cause a 15% fall in plasma diflunisal levels after two 250 mg doses daily over 3 days.[1],[2] This is probably clinically unimportant.

(b) Diflunisal + Indomethacin

A study in 16 normal subjects showed that diflunisal (500 mg twice daily) raised the steady-state serum levels and the AUC (area under the curve) of indomethacin (50 mg twice daily) two- to threefold.[8] Another study confirmed that serum indomethacin levels are approximately doubled and the CNS side-effects are increased (dizziness, nausea, tiredness, unsteadiness, light-headedness).[9] In yet another study it was found that two 250 mg doses of diflunisal daily with 75 mg indomethacin increased plasma indomethacin levels by 30–35%.[3] The reason appears to be that the diflunisal inhibits the glucuronidation of the indomethacin so that it is retained in the body longer.[8,9] The diflunisal appears to have no clear effect on the blood loss in the faeces.[8] Despite evidence that diflunisal protects the human gastric mucosa against the damaging effects of indomethacin,[6] fatal gastrointestinal haemorrhage has occurred in three patients concurrently treated with diflunisal and indomethacin, and the manufacturers advise avoidance.[5]

(c) Diflunisal + Paracetamol and Naproxen

Diflunisal raises serum paracetamol (acetaminophen) levels by 50% but the total bioavailability is unchanged.[7] Diflunisal has been found to have no effect on serum naproxen levels in daily doses of 500 mg.[4] Neither of these interactions has been shown to be clinically important.

References

1 Tempero KF, Cirillo VJ, Stellman SL. Diflunisal: a review of pharmacokinetic and pharmacodynamic properties, drug interactions and special tolerability studies in humans. Br J clin Pharmac (1977) 4, 31S.
2 Perrier CV. Unpublished observations quoted in ref.1.
3 De Schepper P. Unpublished observations quoted in ref.1.
4 Dresse A, Gerard MA, Quiraux N, Fischer P, Gerardy J. Effect of diflunisal on human plasma levels and on the urinary excretion of naproxen. Arch Int Pharmacodyn (1978) 236, 276.
5 Edwards IR. Medicines Adverse Reactions Committee: eighteenth annual report. NZ Med J (1984) 97, 729–32.
6 Cohen MM. Diflunisal protects human gastric mucosa against damage by indomethacin. Dig Dis Sci (1983) 28, 1070–77.
7 Diggins JB, (Merck Sharp Dohme). Personal communication (1988)
8 Van Hecken A, Verbesselt R, Tjandra-Maga TB, De Schepper PJ. Pharmacokinetic interaction between indomethacin and diflunisal. Eur J Clin Pharmacol (1989) 36, 507–12.
9 Eriksson L-O, Wahlin-Boll E, Liedholm H, Seidman P, Melander A. Influence of chronic diflunisal treatment on the plasma levels, metabolism and excretion of indomethacin. Eur J Clin Pharmacol (1989) 37, 7–15.

Etodolac + Antacid or Food

Abstract/Summary

Food delays the absorption of etodolac, but does not significantly reduce the amount absorbed. An un-named antacid did not interact.

Clinical evidence, mechanism, importance and management

A study in 18 normal subjects found that when given 400 mg etodolac after a high fat meal, peak concentrations were approximately halved (from 31 to 14 µg/ml) and delayed (from 1.4 to 3.8 h), but the total amount absorbed was not markedly changed (from 152 to 133 µg/h/ml). Thus food slows the rate but not the extent of absorption. When taken with an antacid (not named) neither the rate nor the extent of absorption was altered.[1]

Reference

1 Troy S, Sanda M, Dressler D, Chiang S, Latts J. The effect of food and antacid on etodolac bioavailability. Clin Pharmacol ther (1990) 47, 192.

Fenoprofen + Phenobarbitone

Abstract/Summary

Phenobarbitone increases the loss of fenoprofen from the body.

Clinical evidence, mechanism, importance and management

Pretreatment with 15 or 60 mg phenobarbitone 6-hourly for 10 days reduced the AUC of a single 200 mg dose of fenoprofen sodium in six normal subjects by 23% and 37% respectively.[1] The clinical importance of this awaits further study.

Reference

1 Hellberg L, Rubin A, Wolen RL, Rodda BE, Ridolfo AS, Gruber CM. A pharmacokinetic interaction in man between phenobarbitone and fenoprofen, a new anti-inflammatory agent. Br J clin Pharmac (1974) 1, 371–4.

Fentanyl + Anticonvulsants

Abstract/Summary

Patients on anticonvulsants appear to need more fentanyl than those not on anticonvulsants.

Clinical evidence, mechanism, importance and management

28 patients, undergoing craniotomy for seizure focus excision and on long term treatment with anticonvulsants in various combinations, needed 48–144% more fentanyl during anaesthesia than a control group of 22 patients who were not on anticonvulsants. The fentanyl maintenance requirements in µg/kg/h were 2.7 (control group), 4.0 (patients on carbamazepine), 4.7 (patients on carbamazepine, phenytoin or sodium valproate), and 6.3 (patients on carbamazepine, sodium valproate and either phenytoin or primidone).[1]

The suggested reason is that these anticonvulsants are potent enzyme inducing agents (with the exception of sodium valproate) which increase the metabolism of fentanyl by the liver so that it is cleared from the body more quickly.[1] A marked increase in the fentanyl requirements should be anticipated in any patient on long-term treatment with anticonvulsants, except possibly sodium valproate.

Reference

1 Tempelhoff R, Modica P, Spitznagel E. Increased fentanyl requirement in patients receiving long-term anticonvulsant therapy. Anaesthesiology (1988) 69, A594.

Fentanyl + Midazolam

Abstract/Summary

Serious hypotension has been seen in newly born babies treated with midazolam and fentanyl. Respiratory arrest occurred in a toddler.

Clinical evidence, mechanism, importance and management

A brief report describes hypotension in six newly born babies with respiratory distress who were given midazolam (a bolus of 200 µg/kg and/or 60 µg/kg/h infusion) for sedation during the first 12–36 h of life. Five of them were also given fentanyl either as an infusion (2 µg/kg/h) or a bolus (2.5 µg/kg), or both. Blood pressures fell to values in the range 38/28 to 31/19 mm Hg in five of them, and to less than 20 mm Hg in one.[1] Hypotension with this drug combination has also been seen in adult patients.[2] The reasons are not known. The authors of the first report[1] say that bolus doses of midazolam associated with fentanyl should be used with great caution in the newborn, especially if very premature or with unstable blood pressure. Another report describes respiratory arrest in a child of 14 months when given both drugs, but concludes that concurrent use is valuable and still acceptable provided they are given judiciously and with careful monitoring.[3]

References

1 Burtin P, Daoud P, Jacqz-Aigrain E, Mussat E, Moriette G. Hypotension with midazolam and fentanyl in the newborn. Lancet (1991) 337, 1545–6.

2 Heikkilä J, Arola M, Kanto J, Laaksonen V. Midazolam as adjunct to high dose fentanyl anaesthesia for coronary artery bypass grafting operation. Acta Anaesthesiol Scand (1984) 28, 683–89.

3 Yaster M, Nichols DG, Deshpande JK, Wetzel RC. Midazolam-fentanyl intravenous sedation in children: case report of respiratory arrest. Pediatrics (1991) 86, 463–6

Fentanyl + Cimetidine

Abstract/Summary

Some preliminary observations suggest that the effects of fentanyl may be increased by cimetidine.

Clinical evidence, mechanism, importance and management

The terminal half-life of fentanyl (100 µg/kg) is reported to be more than doubled (from 155 to 340 min) by pretreatment with cimetidine (10 mg/kg the night before and 5 mg/kg 90 min before). The possible reason is that the cimetidine inhibits the metabolism of the fentanyl by the liver, thereby delaying its clearance from the body.[1] The clinical importance of this interaction has not been assessed, but if both drugs are used concurrently, be alert for increased and prolonged fentanyl effects.

Reference

1 Unpublished data quoted by Maurer PM, Barkowski RR. Drug interactions of clinical significance with opioid analgesics. Drug Saf (1993) 8, 30–48.

Flufenamic, Mefenamic and Tolfenamic acids, Oxyphenbutazone or Phenylbutazone + Antacids

Abstract/Summary

The absorption of the fenamates is markedly accelerated by magnesium hydroxide but retarded by aluminium hydroxide. Sodium bicarbonate appears not to interact, and *in vitro* studies suggest that oxyphenbutazone and phenylbutazone are little affected.

Clinical evidence

Studies in six normal subjects given single 500 mg doses of mefenamic acid or 400 mg tolfenamic acid showed that magnesium hydroxide accelerated the absorption of both drugs (the mefanamic acid AUC after 1 h was increased three-fold and of tolfenamic acid seven-fold) but the total bioavailability was only slightly increased. Sodium bicarbonate had no significant effect, but aluminium hydroxide markedly retarded the rate of ab-

Table 3.2 These figures represent the percentage of antirheumatic drug adsorbed per gram of adsorbent. The figures in parentheses are the percentage eluted using either 0.01 N NCl (first figure) or 0.014 N NaHCO$_3$ (second figure)

	Magnesium trisilicate	Magnesium oxide	Aluminium hydroxide	Bismuth oxycarbonate	Calcium carbonate	Kaolin
Flufenamic acid	0	90 (26.-)	10	79	37	44
Mefenamic acid	0	95 (40.-)	69	26	2	90
Oxyphenbutazone	0	24 (100.-)	27	0	0	0
Phenylbutazone	0	12 (100.000)	0	0	0	0

sorption but no marked change in the total amount absorbed was seen.[2]

Table 3.2 summarizes some *in vitro* adsorption and elution studies undertaken with a number of antacids, designed to mimic the conditions which occur as drugs are moved through the intestinal tract.[1]

Mechanisms

A partially or totally reversible adsorption can occur with some of these antacids. It is not understood why the absorption of both mefenamic and tolfenamic acids is increased by magnesium hydroxide.

Importance and management

Information is very limited but it would appear that if rapid analgesia is needed with either mefenamic or tolfenamic acid, magnesium hydroxide can be given concurrently but aluminium hydroxide should be avoided. Aluminium hydroxide markedly retards the speed of absorption but only reduces the total absorption by about 20%. Sodium bicarbonate does not interact. The data in the table suggest that flufenamic acid is possibly similarly affected but whether the other antacids listed interact significantly is not known. There appears to be little problem with oxyphenbutazone or phenylbutazone, however the full significance of the data in the table needs to be evaluated clinically.

References

1 Naggar VF, Khalil SA, Daabis NA. The in vitro adsorption of some antirheumatics on antacids. Pharmazie (1976) 31, 461.
2 Neuvonen PJ, Kivisto KT. Effect of magnesium hydroxide on the absorption of tolfenamic and mefenamic acids. Eur J Clin Pharmacol (1988) 35, 495–502.

Flufenamic or Mefenamic acid + Cholestyramine

Abstract/Summary

The absorption of both flufenamic and mefenamic acid is markedly reduced in animals by the concurrent use of cholestyramine, but whether this is an important interaction in man is uncertain.

Clinical evidence, mechanism, importance and management

In vitro studies with physiological concentrations of bile salt anions have shown that chlolestyramine binds to both flufenamic and mefenamic acid, while reductions of 60–70% in the gastrointestinal absorption of both acids have been seen in the presence of cholestyramine in rats.[1] The same interaction seems a possibility in man, but so far nobody appears to have carried out a clinical study.

Reference

1 Rosenberg HA, Bates TR. Inhibitory effect of cholestyramine on the absorption of flufenamic and mefenamic acids in rats. Proc Soc Exp Biol Med (1974) 145, 93.

Ibuprofen + Alcohol

Abstract/Summary

Ibuprofen does not affect blood alcohol levels and appears only to have a very small damaging effect on the stomach wall when combined with alcohol. An isolated report describes acute renal failure in a young woman taking normal doses of ibuprofen when she drank a relatively large amount of rum.

Clinical evidence, mechanism, importance and management

Ibuprofen had no significant effect on blood alcohol levels of 19 normal subjects,[2] and in a comparative study with other analgesics (buffered aspirin, paracetamol, diflunisal), it was found to have only a small damaging effect on the stomach wall when combined with alcohol.[3] There would normally seem to be little reason for avoiding concurrent use.

After taking 400 mg ibuprofen the evening before, 400 mg the following morning, and then 375 ml of rum later in the day, followed by two further 400 mg tablets of ibuprofen, a normal healthy young woman with no history of renal disease developed acute renal failure.[1] The reason is not understood. One suggestion is that the alcohol may have made her normal kidneys susceptible to the adverse effects of ibuprofen which, like other NSAIDs, can block the synthesis of the vasodilatory prostaglandins by the kidneys. As a result her kidneys became starved of their normal blood flow.[1] This is an isolated case and not of general importance.

References

1 Elasser GN, Lopez L, Evans E, Barone EJ. Reversible acute renal failure associated with ibuprofen ingestion and binge drinking. J Fam Prac (1988) 27, 221–2.
2 Barron SE, Perry JR, Ferslew KE. The effect of ibuprofen on ethanol concentration and elimination rate. J Forensic Sci (1992) 37, 432–5.
3 Lanza FL, Royer GL, Nelson RS, Rack MF, Seckman CC. Ethanol, aspirin, ibuprofen, and the gastroduodenal mucosa: an endoscopic assessment. Gastroenterology (1985) 80, 767–9.

Ibuprofen or Flurbiprofen + Antacids

Abstract/Summary

Magnesium hydroxide increases the initial absorption of ibuprofen and flurbiprofen, but not if aluminium hydroxide is also present.

Clinical evidence, mechanism, importance and management

An antacid containing aluminium and magnesium hydroxides, given before, with and after a single 400 mg dose of ibuprofen, did not alter the ibuprofen pharmacokinetics in eight normal subjects.[1] Aluminium hydroxide may even delay its absorption.[2] Another study in six normal subjects found that 850 mg magnesium hydroxide increased the AUC_{0-1h} of a single 400 mg dose of ibuprofen by 65%, the peak concentration by 31%. The time to the peak was shorted by about 30 min. The total bioavailability was unchanged.[3]

30 ml *Maalox* (aluminium and magnesium hydroxides) taken 30 min before 100 mg flurbiprofen was found not to affect either the rate or extent of flurbiprofen absorption in a group of normal subjects.[4] Another study found that magnesium hydroxide increased the AUC over the first 2 h by 61%, but over 8 h the AUC was not changed.[5]

It would appear therefore that the initial absorption of both ibuprofen and flurbiprofen is increased by magnesium hydroxide, but not if aluminium hydroxide is present as well. Thus if rapid analgesia is needed, an antacid containing magnesium hydroxide but without aluminium hydroxide could be used.

References

1 Gontarz N, Small RE, Comstock TJ, Stalker DJ, Johnson SM, Willis HE. Effect of antacid suspension on the pharmacokinetics of ibuprofen. Clin Pharm (1987) 6, 413–16.
2 Laska EM, Sunshire A, Marrero I, Olson N, Siegel C, McCormick N. The correlation between blood levels of ibuprofen and clinical analgesic response. Clin Pharmac Ther (1986) 40, 1–7.
3 Neuvonen PJ. The effect of magnesium hydroxide on the oral absorption of ibuprofen, ketoprofen and diclofenac. Br J clin Pharmac (1991) 31, 263–6.
4 Caillé G, du Souich P, Vézina M, Pollock SR, Stalker DJ. Pharmacokinetic interaction between flurbiprofen and antacids in healthy volunteers. Biopharm Drug Disp (1989) 10, 607–15.

5 Rao TRK, Raviskhar K, Shobha JC, Sedkhar EC, Naido MUR, Krishna DR. Influence of magnesium hydroxide on the oral absorption of flurbiprofen. Drug Invest (1992) 4, 437–6.

Indomethacin + Allopurinol

Abstract/Summary

Allopurinol does not affect serum indomethacin levels.

Clinical evidence, mechanism, importance and management

Eight patients were treated for five days with 300 mg allopurinol and 50 mg indomethacin 8-hourly. The allopurinol had no significant effect on the AUC of indomethacin and the amounts of indomethacin excreted in the urine were not significantly altered.[1,2] There seems to be no reason for avoiding concurrent use.

References

1 Pullar T, Myall O, Dixon JS, Haigh JRM, Lowe JR, Bird HA. Allopurinol has no effect on steady-state concentrations of indomethacin. Br J clin Pharmac (1988) 23, 672P.
2 Pullar T, Myall O, Haigh JRM, Lowe JR, Dixon JS, Bird HA. The effect of allopurinol on the steady-state pharmacokinetics of indomethacin. Br J clin Pharmac (1988) 25, 755–7.

Indomethacin + Antacids

Abstract/Summary

The irritation of the gut caused by indomethacin can be relieved by the concurrent use of antacids, but serum indomethacin levels may be reduced to some extent as a result. This appears not to be clinically important.

Clinical evidence

The absorption of a single 50 mg dose of indomethacin in 12 normal subjects was reduced by 35% when taken with 80% *Mergel* (an antacid formulation of aluminium hydroxide, magnesium carbonate and hydroxide).[1]

In another study in normal subjects 700 mg aluminium hydroxide suspension caused a marked fall in peak indomethacin serum levels,[2] whereas in yet another study 30 ml magnesium-aluminium hydroxide caused only slight changes in the absorption of a 50 mg dose of indomethacin.[3]

Mechanism

In vitro studies have shown that indomethacin can be adsorbed by various antacids (magnesium trisilicate, magnesium oxide, magnesium hydroxide, bismuth oxycarbonate, calcium carbonate).[4] This may explain some of the reduction in gastrointestinal absorption, but other mechanisms may also be involved.

Importance and management

Adequately but not extensively documented. Some reduction in serum levels is possible. Despite this the makers of indomethacin recommend that it is taken with food, milk or an antacid to minimize gastrointestinal disturbances. Check that the indomethacin remains effective.

References

1 Galeazzi RL. The effect of an antacid on the bioavailability of indomethacin. Europ J clin Pharmacol (1977) 12, 65–8.
2 Garnham JC, Kaspi T, Kaye CM, Oh VMS. Different effects of sodium bicarbonate and aluminium hydroxide on the absorption of indomethacin in man. Postgrad Med J(1977) 53, 126–9.
3 Emori HW, Paulus H, Bluestone R, Champion GD, Pearson C. Indomethacin serum concentrations in man. Effects of dosage, food and antacid. Ann Rheum Dis(1976) 35, 333–8.
4 Naggar VF, Khalil SA, Daabis NA. The in-vitro adsorption of some antirheumatics on antacids. Pharmazie (1976) 31, 461.

Indomethacin + Cimetidine or Ranitidine

Abstract/Summary

Cimetidine can cause a small reduction in the serum levels of indomethacin but its anti-inflammatory effects do not seem to be significantly altered. Some evidence suggests that cimetidine but not ranitidine protects the duodenum from indomethacin damage.

Clinical evidence, mechanism, importance and management

Ten patients with rheumatoid arthritis on 100–200 mg indomethacin daily for over a year were additionally given 1 g cimetidine daily for a fortnight. Their serum indomethacin levels fell by an average of 18% (from 1.64 to 1.34 ng/ml) but there was no significant change in the clinical effectiveness of the anti-inflammatory treatment (as measured by articular index, pain, grip strength and ESR). The fall in indomethacin levels is thought to be due to some alteration in the absorption from the gut.[1] Another study found no changes in the pharmacokinetics of indomethacin in normal subjects given ranitidine.[5] No marked changes in the bioavailability of either cimetidine or ranitidine with indomethacin was seen in a single dose study of both drugs in normal subjects.[4]

No special precautions would therefore seem to be necessary during concurrent use of indomethacin and either of these H_2-blockers. Cimetidine appears to protect the duodenal, but not gastric, mucosa from the damaging effects of indomethacin,[2] but ranitidine seems not to give protection.[3] This needs confirmation.

References

1 Howes CA, Pullar T, Sourindhrin I, Mistra PC, Capel H, Lawson DH,

Tilstone WJ. Reduced steady-state plasma concentrations of chlorpromazine and indomethacin in patients receiving cimetidine. Eur J Clin Pharmacol (1983) 24, 99–102.
2 Stalnicowicz R, Pollack D, Ellakim A. Cimetidine significantly decreases indomethacin induced duodenal mucosal damage. Gut (1988) 29, 1578–82.
3 Stalnicowicz R, Goldin E, Fich A, Wengrower D, Eliakim R, LIgumsky M, Rachmilewitz D. Indomethacin-induced gastroduodenal damage is not affected by cotreatment with ranitidine. J Clin Gastroenterol (1989) 11, 178–82.
4 Delhotal-Landes B, Flouvat B, Liote F, Abel L, Meyer P, Vinceneux P, Carbon C. Pharmacokinetic interactions between NSAIDs (indomethacin or sulindac) and H₂-receptor antagonists (cimetidine or ranitidine) in human volunteers. Clin Pharmacol Ther (1988) 44, 442–52.
5 Kendall MJ, Gibson R, Walt RP. Co-administration of misoprostol or ranitidine with indomethacin: effects on pharmacokinetics, abdominal symptoms and bowel habit. Aliment Pharmacol Ther (1992) 6, 437–46.

Indomethacin + Cocaine

Abstract/Summary

An isolated report describes marked oedema, anuria and haematemesis in a premature child attributed to an interaction between the cocaine and indomethacin taken earlier by the mother before the birth.

Clinical evidence, mechanism, importance and management

A woman in premature labour was unsuccessfully treated with terbutaline and magnesium sulphate. Indomethacin proved to be more effective but after being given 400 mg over 2 days she gave birth to a boy estimated at 34–35 weeks. Before birth the child was noted to be anuric and at birth showed marked oedema, and later haematemesis. The suggested reasons are that the anuria and oedema were due to renal constriction of the foetus caused by the cocaine (the mother had been abusing cocaine), combined with some interference by the indomethacin with ADH-mediated water absorption. Both drugs can cause gastrointestinal bleeding which would account for the haematemesis. The authors of this report point out that one of the side-effects of cocaine is premature labour, and that the likelihood is high that indomethacin may be used to control it. They advise screening patients in premature labour for evidence of cocaine before indomethacin is given.[1]

Reference

1 Carlan SJ, Stromquist C, Angel JL, Harris M, O'Brien WF. Cocaine and indomethacin: fetal anuria, neonatal edema and gastrointestinal bleeding. Obst Gyn (1991) 78, 501–3

Indomethacin + Probenecid

Abstract/Summary

Serum indomethacin levels can be doubled by the concurrent use of probenecid. This can result in clinical improvement in patients with arthritic diseases, but indomethacin toxicity may also occur, particularly in those whose kidney function is impaired. The uricosuric effects of probenecid are not affected.

Clinical evidence

A study on 28 patients with osteoarthritis, taking 50–150 mg indomethacin daily, showed that 0.5–1.0 g probenecid daily roughly doubled their indomethacin serum levels and this paralleled the increased effectiveness (relief of morning stiffness, joint tenderness and raised grip strength indices). But four patients demonstrated indomethacin toxicity.[1]

Other studies have also demonstrated the marked rise in serum indomethacin levels caused by probenecid.[2–4] Clear signs of indomethacin toxicity (nausea, headache, tinnitus, confusion and a rise in blood urea) occurred in a woman with stable mild renal impairment when given probenecid.[5] The uricosuric effects of probenecid are not altered.[2]

Mechanism

Uncertain. It seems possible that the indomethacin and probenecid compete for the same kidney tubule secretory mechanisms, which leads to a decrease in the loss of the indomethacin.[2] There may also be some reduction in biliary excretion of indomethacin as well.[6]

Importance and management

An established and adequately documented interaction. Concurrent use should be well monitored because, while clinical improvement can undoubtedly occur, some patients may develop indomethacin toxicity (headache, dizziness, lightheadedness, nausea, etc.). This is particularly likely in those with some impaired kidney function. Reduce the indomethacin dosage as necessary.

References

1 Brooks PM, Bell MA, Sturrock RD, Famaey JP, Dick WC. The clinical significance of indomethacin-probenecid interaction. Br J clin Pharmac (1974) 1, 287.
2 Skeith MD, Simkin PA, Healey LA. The renal excretion of indomethacin and its inhibition by probenecid. Clin Pharmacol Ther (1968) 9, 89.
3 Emori W, Paulus HE, Bluestone R, Pearson CM. The pharmacokinetics of indomethacin in serum. Clin Pharmacol Ther (1973) 14, 134.
4 Baber N, Halliday L, Littler T, Orme ML'E, Sibeon R. Clinical studies of the interaction between indomethacin and probenecid. Br J Clin Pharmac (1978) 5, 364P.
5 Sinclair H, Gibson T. Interaction between probenecid and indomethacin. Brit J Rheumatol (1986) 25, 316–17.
6 Duggan DE, Hooke KF, White JD, Noll RM, Stevenson CR. The effects of probenecid upon the individual components of indomethacin elimination. J Pharmac Exp Ther (1977) 201, 463.

Indomethacin + Vaccines

Abstract/Summary

Some very limited evidence suggests that the response of the body to immunization with live vaccines may be more severe than usual in the presence of indomethacin.

Clinical evidence

A man with ankylosing spondylitis on 25 mg indomethacin three times a day had a strong primary type reaction 12 days after smallpox vaccination. He experienced 3 days of severe malaise, headache and nausea, as well as enlarged lymph nodes. The scab which formed was unusually large (3 cm diameter) but he suffered no long term ill-effects.[1]

Mechanism

Uncertain. The suggestion is that the indomethacin alters the response of the body to viral infections, whether originating from vaccines or not.[1] For example, a child taking indomethacin who developed haemorrhagic chickenpox during a ward outbreak of the disease suffered severe scarring.[2] The manufacturers (MSD) of indomethacin state that indomethacin may mask the signs and symptoms of infection.

Importance and management

Information is very sparse and the interaction is not adequately established, but be aware that a more severe reaction may possibly occur if live vaccines (e.g. rubella, measles, etc.) are used in patients using indomethacin.

References

1 Maddock AC. Indomethacin and vaccination. Lancet (1973) ii, 210–11.
2 Rodriguez RS, Barbabosa E. Haemorrhagic chicken pox after indomethacin. N Engl J Med (1971) 235, 690.

Isoxicam + Miscellaneous drugs

Abstract/Summary

Aspirin may possibly causes changes in the serum levels of isoxicam but the importance of this is uncertain. Blood loss is increased. Isoxicam is reported not to be affected by phenytoin.

Clinical evidence, mechanism, importance and management

200–300 mg isoxicam and 1800 mg aspirin daily for 14 days in normal subjects was found to cause small rises in the serum levels of both drugs. Gastrointestinal blood loss was significantly increased.[1] In contrast another study found that 3.9 g aspirin daily approximately halved the serum levels of isoxicam.[2] Reduced serum isoxicam levels were seen in another study.[3] Whether any of these changes has any important effect on the clinical efficacy of isoxicam is uncertain but the possible increase in gastrointestinal blood loss should not be overlooked.

Another study found that phenytoin does not change the pharmacokinetics of isoxicam.[4]

References

1 DJ Farnham. Studies of isoxicam in combination with aspirin, warfarin

sodium and cimetidine. Sem Arth Rheum (1982) 12 (Suppl 2), 179–183.

2 Grace EM, Mewa AAM, Sweeney GD, Rosenfeld JM, Darke AC, Buchanan WW. Lowering of plasma isoxicam concentrations with acetylsalicylic acid. J Rheumatol (1986) 13, 1119–21.

3 Esquivel M, Cussenot F, Ogilvie RI, East DS, Shaw DH. Interaction of isoxicam with acetylsalicylic acid. Br J clin Pharmac (1984) 18, 576–81.

4 Caille A. The effect of the administration of phenytoin on the pharmacokinetics of isoxicam. In preparation. Quoted by Downie WW, Gluckman MI, Ziehmer BA, Boyle JA. Clin Rheum Dis (1984) 10, 385–99.

Ketoprofen + Metoclopramide

Abstract/Summary

Metoclopramide reduces the bioavailability of ketoprofen.

Clinical evidence, mechanism, importance and management

Four normal subjects given 50 mg ketoprofen in capsule form (*Profenid*) showed reductions in their AUCs (areas under the curve) when concurrently given 10 mg metoclopramide. Both the AUC_{0-8h} and the AUC_{0-0} were reduced by about 28%. The maximum serum levels were almost halved and the time to reach this maximum was prolonged by 30%.[1] The probable reason is that the metoclopramide speeds up the gastric emptying so that the relatively poorly soluble ketoprofen spends less time in the stomach where it dissolves. As a result less is available for absorption in the small intestine.

The clinical importance of this interaction awaits assessment but the authors of this study recommend that ketoprofen (and possibly other NSAIDs which are poorly soluble) should be taken 1–2 h before the metoclopramide.

Reference

1 Etman MA, Ismail FA, Nada AH. Effect of metoclopramide on ketoprofen pharmacokinetics in man. Int J Pharmaceutics (1992) 88, 433–5.

Lornoxicam + Antacids

Abstract/Summary

Lornoxicam (chlortenoxicam) does not interact adversely with bismuth chelate, *Maalox* or *Solugastril*.

Clinical evidence, mechanism, importance and management

Neither 10 ml *Maalox* (aluminium and magnesium hydroxides) nor 10 g *Solugastril* (aluminium hydroxide and calcium carbonate) had any effect on the pharmacokinetic profile of lornoxicam in 18 normal subjects when given as a 4 mg film coated tablet.[1] A later study similarly found no changes in the absorption or pharmacokinetics of the same lornoxicam formulation when given with 120 mg bismuth chelate twice daily.[2] There

would seem to be no reason for avoiding concurrent use.

Reference

1 Dittrich P, Radhofer-Welte S, Magometschnigg D, Kukovetz WR, Mayerhofer S, Ferber HP. The effect of concomitantly administered antacids on the bioavailability of lornoxicam, a novel highly potent NSAID. Drugs Exptl Clin Res (1990) VXI, 57–62.

2 Ravic M, Johnston A, Turner P, Foley K, Rosenow D. Does bismuth chelate influence lornoxicam absorption ? Hum Exp Toxicol (1992) 11, 59–60.

Lornoxicam + Miscellaneous drugs

Abstract/Summary

Lornoxicam (chlortenoxicam) causes a small increase in the effects of glibenclamide and in the serum levels of digoxin but neither is probably clinically important.

Clinical evidence, mechanism, importance and management

(a) Digoxin

The concurrent use of 4 mg lornoxicam twice daily (taken for 14 days) and 0.25 mg digoxin daily (taken for 23 days) in 12 normal subjects had only a small effect on the pharmacokinetics of each drug. The apparent clearance of the digoxin was decreased by 14% while the maximum serum level of the lornoxicam was decreased by 21% and its elimination half-life increased by 40%.[2] None of these changes is probably clinically important, but until more is known it would seem prudent to monitor the effects if these two drugs are given to patients.

(b) Glibenclamide

4 mg lornoxicam twice daily for 6 days had no effect on the pharmacokinetics of a single 5 mg dose of glibenclamide in 15 normal subjects. The pharmacokinetics of lornoxicam also remained unchanged. However concurrent use significantly increased plasma insulin levels (AUC + 47%) and lowered serum glucose levels (– 8%), the suggested reason being that the lornoxicam displaces the glibenclamide from its plasma protein binding sites so that its unbound (and active) levels rise, thereby increasing the secretion of insulin. However the changes seen are believed to be too small to be clinically relevant.[1] This needs confirmation in diabetic patients.

References

1 Warrington SJ, Debbas NMG, Turner P, Ravic M. Chlortenoxicam and glibenclamide in normal subjects: interaction study. Charterhouse Clinical Research Unit. Internal study (1989). Unpublished data. Quoted by Ravic M, Johnston A, Turner P. Clinical pharmacological studies of some possible interactions of lornoxicam with other drugs. Postgrad Med J (1980) 66 (Suppl 4) S30–4.

2 Ravic M, Johnston A, Turner P, Ferber HP. A study of the potential

interaction of lornoxicam with digoxin in healthy volunteers. Quoted as 'in press' in reference 1 above.

Meclofenamic acid + Miscellaneous drugs

Abstract/Summary

Aspirin can cause a small and probably clinically unimportant reduction in serum meclofenamate levels, but intestinal bleeding is increased. Dextropropoxyphene and meclofenamate do not interact. Probenecid reduces the loss of meclofenamate from the body.

Clinical evidence, mechanism, importance and management

Ten normal subjects given 1.8 g aspirin daily and 300 mg sodium meclofenamate daily for 14 days showed no significant reductions in serum salicylate levels, but serum meclofenamate levels were depressed to some extent. The clinical significance of this is uncertain, but it is probably limited. The gastrointestinal blood loss was approximately doubled compared with either drug alone.[1] The concurrent use of 260 mg dextropropoxyphene daily and 400 mg sodium meclofenamate daily has no effect on the serum levels of either drug.[1] Single dose studies on the pharmacokinetics of 100 mg meclofenamate sodium in six normal subjects found that pretreatment with probenecid (dosage unstated) increased its AUC by an unstated amount and reduced its apparent plasma clearance to 40%, due primarily to a decrease in non-renal clearance.[2] The clinical importance of this is uncertain, but an increase in the effects, and possibly the toxicity, of meclofenamate sodium would be expected.

References

1 Baragar FD, Smith TC. Drug interaction studies with sodium meclofenamate (Meclomen®). Curr Ther Res (1978) 23, April Suppl. S51.
2 Waller ES. The effect of probenecid on the disposition of meclofenamate sodium. Drug Intell Clin Pharm (1983) 17, 453–4.

Methadone + Anticonvulsants

Abstract/Summary

Serum methadone levels can be reduced by the concurrent use of carbamazepine, phenobarbitone or phenytoin. An increase in the methadone dosage may be needed. Sodium valproate appears not to interact.

Clinical evidence

(a) Carbamazepine

A study in 37 patients on methadone maintenance found that only those on enzyme-inducing drugs (10 patients) had low trough methadone levels (less than 100 ng/ml). One was taking carbamazepine and he complained of daily withdrawal symptoms and had signs of opioid abstinence.[1] The other nine were taking phenobarbitone (five patients) or phenytoin (four patients).[1] Withdrawal symptoms were also seen in another patient given carbamazepine.[4]

(b) Phenobarbitone

In the study cited above, five patients on methadone maintenance who were on phenobarbitone had low trough serum methadone levels.[1] Another former heroin addict controlled with methadone complained of withdrawal symptoms when he started to take phenobarbitone. His methadone serum levels were found to be depressed.[5]

(c) Phenytoin

Methadone withdrawal symptoms developed in five patients within three to four days of starting to take 300–500 mg phenytoin daily. Methadone serum levels were depressed about 60%. The symptoms disappeared within 2–3 days of stopping the phenytoin and the serum methadone levels rapidly climbed to their former values.[2] Reduced serum methadone levels and withdrawal symptoms have been described in other patients taking phenytoin.[1,3,4] See also (a) and (d).

(d) Sodium valproate

Two patients who had had methadone withdrawal symptoms while on 300–400 mg phenytoin daily, and one of them later when on 600 mg carbamazepine daily, became free from withdrawal symptoms when given sodium valproate instead. It was also found possible virtually to halve their daily methadone dosage.[4]

Mechanism

Not fully established, but all of these anticonvulsants (except sodium valproate which does not interact) are recognized enzyme-inducing agents which can increase the metabolism of other drugs by the liver, thereby hastening their loss from the body. In one study it was found that while taking phenytoin the excretion into the urine of the main metabolite of methadone was increased.[2]

Importance and management

Information is limited but the interaction appears to be established and of clinical importance. Anticipate the need to increase the methadone dosage in patients taking carbamazepine, phenytoin or phenobarbitone. It may be necessary to give methadone twice daily to prevent withdrawal symptoms appearing towards the end of the day. Sodium valproate appears to be a non-interacting alternative.

References

1 Bell J, Seves V, Bowren P, Lewis J, Batey R. The use of serum methadone levels in patients receiving methadone maintenance. Clin Pharmacol Ther (1988) 43, 623–9.
2 Tong TG, Pond SM, Kreek MJ, Jaffery NF, Benowitz NL. Phenytoin-induced methadone withdrawal. Ann Intern Med (1981) 94, 349.
3 Finelli PF. Phenytoin and methadone tolerance. N Engl J Med (1976) 294, 227.
4 Saxon AJ, Whittaker S, Hawkes CS. Valproic acid, unlike other anticonvulsants, has no effect on methadone metabolism: Two cases. J Clin Psychiatry (1989) 50, 228–9.
5 Liu S-J, Wang RIH. Case report of barbiturate-induced enhancement of methadone metabolism and withdrawal syndrome. Am J Psychiatry (1984) 141, 1287–8.

Methadone + Fusidic acid, Zidovudine

Abstract/Summary

One report says that fusidic acid and zidovudine can reduce the effects of methadone. Others say that methadone is not affected by zidovudine but that the zidovudine serum levels can rise.

Clinical evidence

(a) Methadone effects reduced or unaffected

Two drug abusers with AIDS needed an increase in their methadone dosages, one from 40 to 60 mg daily, and the other from 60 to 80 mg daily, the first within a month of beginning treatment with 1 g zidovudine daily and the other within 6 months of starting to take 1500 mg fusidic acid daily.[1]

In contrast, two related studies found no evidence of any change in the pharmacokinetics of methadone in HIV-infected patients treated with zidovudine. No methadone withdrawal symptoms occurred.[2,3]

(b) Zidovudine effects increased

In the study already cited[2] and the earlier related study by the same workers,[3] the AUC (area under the curve) of the zidovudine was increased on average by 43% by the methadone, and in four of the nine patients it was doubled.[2]

Mechanism

(a) Both patients showed evidence of liver enzyme induction (using antipyrine as a marker of induction), from which it was concluded that these two drugs increase the metabolism and loss of methadone from the body.[1] (b) Methadone apparently reduces the glucuronidation of the zidovudine by the liver, resulting in an increase in its serum levels.[3]

Importance and management

Information appears to be limited to these somewhat inconsistent reports. Concurrent use need not be avoided but the outcome is uncertain. Be alert for any evidence of methadone underdosage and zidovudine toxicity.

References

1 Brockmeyer NH, Mertins L, Goos M. Pharmacokinetic interaction of antimicrobial agents with levomethadon in drug-addicted AIDS patients. Klin Wschr (1991) 69, 16–18.
2 Schwartz EL, Brechbuhl AB, Kahl P, Miller MA, Selwyn PA, Friedland GH. Pharmacokinetic interactions of zidovudine and methadone in intravenous drug-using patients with HIV infection. J Acquir Immune Defic Syndr (1992) 5, 619–26.
3 Schwartz EL, Brechbühl A-B, Kahl P, Miller MH, Selwyn PA, Friedland GH. Altered pharmacokinetics of zidovudine in former IV drug-using patients receiving methadone. 6th Int Conf AIDS, San Francisco (1990) Abstract SB432, p 194.

Methadone + Cimetidine

Abstract/Summary

Two elderly patients on methadone developed apnoea when additionally treated with cimetidine.

Clinical evidence, mechanism, importance and management

An elderly patient on 25 mg methadone daily developed apnoea 2 days after starting 1200 mg cimetidine daily.[1] Another elderly patient on methadone and morphine also developed apnoea (two breaths per minute) after taking 1200 mg cimetidine daily for 6 days.[2] This was controlled with naloxone.

Mechanism

Cimetidine inhibits the activity of the liver enzymes concerned with the N-demethylation of methadone (demonstrated in studies with liver microsomes taken from rats[1]) so that it accumulates in the body, thereby exaggerating its respiratory depressant effects. Both patients were elderly so that liver impairment might possibly have contributed to the development of this interaction.

Importance and mangement

Direct information seems to be limited to these two reports so that the general importance of this interaction is uncertain. Be alert for evidence of increased methadone effects in any patient. If the suggested mechanism of interaction is correct, ranitidine may prove to be a non-interacting alernative. This needs confirmation.

References

1 Dawson GW, Vestal RE. Cimetidine inhibits the in vitro N-demethylation of methadone. Res Comm Chem Pathol Pharmacol (1984) 46, 301–4.
2 Sorkin EM, Ogawa GS. Cimetidine potentiation of narcotic action. Drug Intell Clin Pharm (1983) 17, 60–1.

Methadone + Disulfiram

Abstract/Summary

No adverse interaction was seen in patients treated concurrently with methadone and disulfiram.

Clinical evidence, mechanism, importance and management

Seven opiate addicts, without chronic alcoholism or liver disease, and who were on methadone maintenance treatment (45–65 mg daily) showed an increase in the urinary excretion of the major pyrrolidine metabolite of methadone (an indicator of increased N-demethylation) when given 500 mg disulfiram daily for 7 days, but there was no effect on the degree of opiate intoxication, nor were withdrawal symptoms experienced.[1] No special precautions would seem to be necessary.

References

1 Tong TG, Benowitz NL, Kreek MJ. Methadone-disulfiram interaction during methadone maintenance. J Clin Pharmacol (1980) 20, 507.

Methadone + Rifampicin (Rifampin)

Abstract/Summary

Serum methadone levels can be markedly reduced by rifampicin. A dosage increase may be needed both for narcotic-dependent patients to prevent the development of withdrawal symptoms, and for patients given methadone as an analgesic.

Clinical evidence

Following the observation that former heroin addicts complained of withdrawal symptoms when given rifampicin, a study was made on 30 patients on methadone. 21 of them developed withdrawal symptoms within 1–33 days of starting 600–900 mg rifampicin and 300 mg isoniazid daily. Seven of the most severely affected developed symptoms within a week and their serum methadone concentrations fell by 33–68%. None of 56 other patients on methadone and other anti-tubercular treatment (which included isoniazid but not rifampicin) showed withdrawal symptoms.[1–3]

Other cases of this interaction have been reported.[4–6] Some patients needed a 50–100% increase in the dosage of methadone.[5,6] One needed an increase from 45 to 140 mg daily.[5]

Mechanism

Rifampicin is a potent enzyme-inducing agent which increases the activity of the liver enzymes concerned with the metabolism of methadone, as a result of which its clearance from the body is markedly increased. In the study cited the urinary excretion of the major metabolite of methadone rose by 250%.[1]

Importance and management

An established interaction of clinical importance. The incidence is high. Two-thirds (21) of the narcotic-dependent patients in the study cited[1] developed this interaction, 14 of whom were able with the support of counselling to tolerate the relatively mild symptoms. Withdrawal symptoms may develop within 24 h. The analgesic effects of methadone would also be expected to be reduced. Concurrent use need not be avoided, but the effects should be monitored and appropriate dosage increases (50–100% or more) made where necessary.

References

1 Kreek MJ, Garfield JN, Gutjah CL, Giusti LM. Rifampicin-induced methadone withdrawal. N Eng J Med (1976) 294, 1104–6.
2 Garfield JW, Kreek MJ, Giusti L. Rifampin-methadone relationship. 1. The clinical effects of rifampin-methadone interaction. Am Rev Resp Dis (1975) 111, 262.
3 Kreek MJ, Garfield JW, Gutjah CL, Bowen D, Field F, Rothschild M. Rifampin-methadone relationship. 2. Rifampin effects on plasma concentration, metabolism and excretion of methadone. Am Rev Resp Dis (1975) 111, 926–7.
4 Bending MR, Skacel PO. Rifampicin and methadone withdrawal. Lancet (1977) i, 1211.
5 Van Leeuwen DJ. Rifampicine leidt tot onthoudingsverschijnselen bij methadonegebruikers. Ned Tijdsch Geneeskd (1986) 130, 548–50.
6 Brockmeyer NH, Mertins L, Goos M. Pharmacokinetic interaction of antimicrobial agents with levomethadon in drug addicted AIDS patients. Klin Wschr (1991) 69, 16–18.

Methadone + Urinary acidifiers or alkalinizers

Abstract/Summary

The loss of methadone from the body in the urine is increased if the urine is made acid and reduced if it is made alkaline.

Clinical evidence

A study in patients on methadone found that the urinary clearance in those with urinary pHs of less than 6 was greater than those with higher urinary pHs.[1] When one subject's urinary pH was lowered from 6.2 to 5.5, the loss of unchanged methadone in the urine was doubled.[3]

A pharmacokinetic study in five normal subjects given 10 mg doses of methadone intramuscularly found that the plasma half-life was 19.5 h when the urine was made acidic (pH 5.2) with ammonium chloride compared with 42.1 h when the urine was made alkaline (pH 7.8) with sodium bicarbonate. The body clearance of the methadone fell from 134 to 91.9 ml/min when the urine was changed from acidic to alkaline.[4]

Mechanism

Methadone is eliminated from the body both by liver metabolism and excretion of unchanged methadone in the urine. Above pH 6 the urinary excretion is less important, but with urinary pH below 6 the half-life becomes dependent on both excretion (30%) and metabolism (70%).[2-4] Methadone is a weak base (pK_a 8.4) so that in acid urine little of the drug is in the un-ionized form and little is reabsorbed by simple passive diffusion. On the other hand in alkaline solution most of the drug is in the un-ionized form which is readily reabsorbed by the kidney tubules and little is lost in the urine.

Importance and management

An established interaction but of uncertain importance. Be alert for any evidence of reduced methadone effects in patients whose urine becomes acidic because they are taking large doses of ammonium chloride or acetazolamide. Lowering the pH to 5 with ammonium chloride to increase the clearance can also be used to treat intoxication.

References

1 Bellward GD, Warren DM, Howald W, Axelson JE, Abbott FS. Methadone maintenance; effect of urinary pH on renal clearance in chronic high and low doses. Clin Pharmacol Ther (1977) 22, 92–9.
2 Baselt RC, Casarett LJ. Urinary excretion of methadone in man. Clin Pharmacol Ther (1972) 13, 64.
3 Inturrisi CE, Verebeley K. Disposition of methadone in man after a single oral dose. Clin Pharmacol Ther (1972) 13, 923.
4 Nilsson M-I, Widerlöv E, Meresaar U, ĐAnggård E. Effect of urinary pH on the disposition of methadone in man. Eur J Clin Pharmacol (1982) 22, 337–42.

Morphine + Cimetidine or Ranitidine

Abstract/Summary

Clinically important interactions between morphine and these H_2-blockers appear to be rare. A slight and unimportant increase in respiratory depression may occur with cimetidine, and no interaction normally occurs with ranitidine. An isolated report describes an adverse reaction in one patient on morphine or papaveretum and cimetidine, and there is another isolated report involving morphine and ranitidine.

Clinical evidence

(a) Cimetidine

Cimetidine (1200 mg for four days) given to seven normal subjects had no effect on the pharmacokinetics of morphine. The extent and duration of the morphine-induced pupillary miosis was unchanged.[2] In other normal subjects it was found that 600 mg cimetidine 1 h before 10 mg morphine (IM) prolonged the respiratory depression due to morphine, but the extent was small and clinically insignificant.[3]

An acutely ill patient with grand mal epilepsy, gastrointestinal bleeding and an intertrochanteric fracture who was undergoing haemodialysis three times a week, was being treated with 900 mg cimetidine daily. After being given the sixth dose of morphine (15 mg 4-hourly) he became apnoeic (three respirations per minute) which was controlled with naloxone. He remained confused and agitated for the next 80 h with muscular twitching and further periods of apnoea controlled with naloxone. He had had nine 10 mg doses of morphine on a previous occasion in the absence of cimetidine without problems. About a month later he experienced the same adverse reactions when given papaveretum while still taking cimetidine.[1]

(b) Ranitidine

A man with terminal cancer on 150 mg ranitidine IV eight-hourly became confused, disorientated and agitated when given the ranitidine after an IV infusion of morphine (50 mg daily) was started. When the ranitidine was stopped his mental state improved but worsened when he was given ranitidine again 8 h and 16 h later. He improved when the ranitidine was stopped.[5]

Another report describes hallucinations in a patient given sustained-release morphine and ranitidine, but the author discounted the possibility of an interaction.[6]

Mechanism

Studies with human liver microsomal enzymes have shown that the metabolism of morphine is not affected by cimetidine or ranitidine.[4] The isolated cases of interaction remain unexplained.[1,5] It would seem that unidentified factors conspired to cause these reactions.

Importance and management

The virtual absence of a generally important morphine/cimetidine interaction is adequately documented. Concurrent use normally causes only a slight and normally unimportant prolongation of the respiratory depression due to morphine but it might possibly have some importance in patients with pre-existing breathing disorders. In vitro evidence suggests that ranitidine is unlikely to interact with morphine,[4] however the isolated cases cited here underline the importance of monitoring the concurrent use of morphine or papaveretum and any H_2-blocker.

References

1 Fine A, Churchill DN. Potential lethal interaction of cimetidine and morphine. Can Med Ass J (1981) 124, 1434.
2 Mojaverian P, Fedder IL, Vlasses PH, Rotmensch HH, Rocci ML, Swanson BN, Ferguson RK. Cimetidine does not alter morphine disposition. Br J clin Pharmac (1982) 14, 809–13.
3 Lam AM, Clement JL. Effect of cimetidine premedication on morphine-induced ventilatory depression. Can Anaesth Soc J (1984) 31, 36–43.
4 Knodell RG, Holtzman JL, Crankshaw DL, Steele NM, Stanley LN. Drug metabolism by rat and human hepatic microsomes in response to interaction with H_2-receptor antagonists. Gastroenterology (1982) 82, 84–7.
5 Martinez-Abad M, Gomis ᵀD, Ferrer JM. Ranitidine-induced confusion with concomitant morphine. ᴅ ᴜg Intell Clin Pharm (1988) 22, 914.
6 Jellema JG. Hallucinations during sustained-release morphine and methadone administration. Lancet (1987) ii, 392.

Morphine + Contraceptives (oral)

Abstract/Summary

The clearance of morphine is approximately doubled by the concurrent use of the oral contraceptives.

Clinical evidence, mechanism, importance and management

The clearance of morphine given intravenously (1 mg) was increased by 75%, and given orally (10 mg) by 120%, in six young women taking an oral contraceptive.[1] The suggested reason is that the oestrogen component of the contraceptive increases the activity of one of the liver enzymes (glucuronyl transferase) concerned with the metabolism of the morphine. This implies that the dosage of morphine would need to be virtually doubled to achieve the same degree of analgesia. Whether this is so in practice requires confirmation.

Reference

1 Watson KJR, Ghabrial H, Mashford ML, Harman PJ, Breen KJ, Desmond PV. The oral contraceptive pill increases morphine clearance but does not increase hepatic blood flow. Gastroenterol (1986) 90, 1779.

Morphine + Food

Abstract/Summary

Food increases the bioavailability of oral morphine and raises the serum levels.

Clinical evidence, mechanism, importance and management

12 patients with chronic pain were given 50 mg morphine hydrochloride by mouth in 200 ml water either while fasting or after a high fat breakfast (fried eggs and bacon, toast with butter, and milk). The maximum blood morphine concentrations and the time to achieve these concentrations were unaltered by the presence of the food, but the AUC (area under the curve) was increased by 34% and blood morphine levels were maintained at higher levels over the period from 4 to 10 h after being given the morphine.[1] The reasons are not understood. The inference to be drawn is that pain relief is likely to be increased if the morphine is given with food. This appears to be an advantageous interaction. More confirmatory study is needed.

Reference

1 Gourlay GK, Plummer JL, Cherry DA, Foate JA, Cousins MJ. Influence of a high-fat meal on the absorption of morphine from oral solutions. Clin Pharmacol Ther (1989) 46, 463–8.

Morphine + Metoclopramide

Abstract/Summary

Metoclopramide increases the rate of absorption of oral morphine and increases its sedative effects.

Clinical evidence

10 mg of oral metoclopramide markedly increased the extent and speed of sedation due to a 20 mg oral dose of morphine (*MST-Continus* Tablets — Napp Laboratories) over a period of 3–4 h in 20 patients undergoing surgery. Peak serum morphine levels and the total absorption remained unaltered.[1]

Mechanism

Metoclopramide increases the rate of gastric emptying so that the rate of morphine absorption from the small intestine is increased. An alternative idea is that both drugs act additively on opiate receptors to increase sedation.[1]

Importance and management

An established interaction which can be usefully exploited in anaesthetic practice, but the increased sedation may also represent a problem if the morphine is being given long-term.

Reference

1 Manara AR, Shelley MP, Quinn K, Park GR. The effect of metoclopramide on the absorption of oral controlled release morphine. Br J clin Pharmac (1988) 25, 518–21.

Morphine + Miscellaneous drugs

Abstract/Summary

Some supplemental drugs appear to increase the myoclonus caused by high doses of morphine. Diclofenac appears not to interact adversely with morphine.

Clinical evidence, mechanism, importance and management

The incidence of myoclonus (uncontrollable jerks of the arms, legs) in 19 patients with malignant disease on high doses of morphine (daily doses of 500 mg or more orally or 250 mg or more parenterally) appeared to be increased by the presence of other drugs including antidepressants (amitriptyline, doxepin), antipsychotics (chlorpromazine, haloperidol), non-steroidal anti-inflammatory drugs (indomethacin, naproxen, piroxicam, aspirin) and an antinauseant (thiethylperazine).[1] The reasons are not understood. The authors conclude that the best way to treat this problem is to change the supplemental drugs. More study is needed. Diclofenac does not significantly affect the pharmacokinetics of morphine, suggesting that they can be used together without any risk of morphine overdosage.[2]

Reference

1 Potter JM, Reid DB, Shaw RJ, Hackett P, Hickman PE. Myoclonus associated with treatment with high doses of morphine: the role of supplemental drugs. Br Med J (1989) 299, 165–3.
2 De Conno F, Ripamonti C, Bianchi M, Ventafridda V, Panerai AE. Diclofenac does not modify morphine bioavailability in cancer patients. Pain (1992) 48, 410–2.

Morphine + Tricyclic antidepressants

Abstract/Summary

The bioavailability and the degree of analgesia of oral morphine is increased by the concurrent use of clomipramine or amitriptyline. This is a useful interaction, but it also seems possible that the toxicity of morphine may be increased.

Clinical evidence, mechanism, importance and management

Clomipramine or amitriptyline in daily doses of 20 or 50 mg increased the AUC (area under the curve) of oral morphine by amounts ranging from 28 to 111% in 24 patients being treated for cancer pain. The half-life of morphine was also prolonged.[1] The reasons are not understood. The increased analgesia may not only be due to the increased serum levels of morphine, but may possibly involve an analgesic effect of the antidepressant. This is a useful interaction, but the possibility of increased morphine toxicity should also be borne in mind. Whether other tricyclic antidepressants behave similarly is uncertain.

Reference

1 Ventafridda V, Ripamonti C, De Conno F, Bianchi M, Pazzuconi F, Panerai AE. Antidepressants increase bioavailability of morphine in cancer patients. Lancet (1987) i, 1204.

Nabumetone + Miscellaneous drugs

Abstract/Summary

Nabumetone does not interact with warfarin and appears not to interact with antihypertensive drugs. It is not affected by aluminium hydroxide, paracetamol or aspirin but its absorption is increased by food and milk.

Clinical evidence, mechanism, importance and management

Nabumetone has been found not to affect significantly the anticoagulant effects of warfarin in normal subjects,[1] moreover it also appears not to affect bleeding time, platelet aggregation or prothrombin times in the absence of an anticoagulant.[4] Other single dose studies have shown that the absorption of nabumetone is also not significantly altered by aluminium hydroxide, aspirin or paracetamol but it is increased by food and milk.[2] No significant changes in blood pressure were seen in large numbers of hypertensive patients when given nabumetone.[3] Because the active metabolite of nabumetone is highly protein bound and can displace other highly protein bound drugs the makers of nabumetone say that the effects of hydantoin anticonvulsants (phenytoin) and the sulphonylureas may possibly be increased,[3] but the risk seems to be more theoretical than real and the makers say they have no reports of adverse interactions with either of these groups of drugs.[5]

References

1 Fitzgerald DE. Double blind study to establish whether there is any interaction between nabumetone and warfarin in healthy adult male volunteers. Roy Soc Med Int Congr Symp (1985) Series 69, 47–53.
2 Von Schrader HW, Buscher G, Dierdorf D, Mugge H, Wolf D. Nabumetone — a novel anti-inflammatory drug: the influence of food, milk, antacids, and analgesics on bioavailability of single oral doses. Int J Clin Pharmacol Ther Tox (1983) 21, 311–21.
3 Reliflex Product Booklet. Bencard (1987).
4 Al Balla S, Al Momen AK, Al Arfaj H, Al Sugair S, Gader AMA. Interaction between nabumetone — a new non-steroidal anti-inflammatory drug — and the haemostatic system ex vivo. Haemostasis (1990) 20, 270–5.
5 Bencard, Personnal Communication, September 1993.

Naproxen + Amoxycillin

Abstract/Summary

An isolated report describes acute interstitial nephritis with nephrotic syndrome associated with the use of naproxen and amoxycillin.

Clinical evidence, mechanism, importance and management

A man without any previous kidney problems developed acute interstitial nephritis with nephrotic syndrome after taking naproxen for 4 days (4 g) and amoxycillin for 10 days (24 g). He appeared to recover when the drugs were stopped, but 3 months later he developed kidney failure and needed haemodialysis. Some months later he had a kidney graft.[1] This is not only a rare syndrome (reported to be only 55 cases in the world literature in 1988)[1] but this is the first and only case involving both of these drugs. No special precautions would normally seem to be necessary.

Reference

1 Nortier J, Despierreux M, Bourgeois V, Dupont P. Acute interstitial nephritis with nephrotic syndrome after intake of naproxen and amoxycillin. Nephrol Dial Transplant (1990) 5, 1055–7.

Naproxen + Antacids

Abstract/Summary

There is evidence that the absorption of naproxen can be altered (increased or decreased) by some antacids, but the clinical importance of this is uncertain.

Clinical evidence, mechanism, importance and management

700 or 1400 mg sodium bicarbonate increased the rate and extent of absorption of single 300 mg doses of naproxen in 14 normal subjects, whereas 700 mg magnesium oxide or magnesium hydroxide had the opposite effect and reduced both. On the other hand when 15 or 60 ml *Maalox* were given, the rate and extent of absorption were slightly increased.[1] The reasons are not fully understood, but naproxen becomes more soluble as the pH rises which may account for the increased absorption with sodium bicarbonate, whereas magnesium and aluminium may form less soluble complexes.[2] The clinical importance of these observations is uncertain because single dose, short term studies (these studies only extended over 3 h) do not reliably predict what may happen when multiple doses are taken. Concurrent use need not be avoided but the effectiveness of the naproxen should be monitored if antacids are also given.

References

1 Segre EJ, Sevelius H, Varady J. Effects of antacids on naproxen absorption. N Engl J Med (1974) 291, 582.
2 Segre EJ. Drug interactions with naproxen. Eur J Rheumatol Inflamm (1979) 2, 12.

Naproxen + Cholestyramine

Abstract/Summary

Cholestyramine delays but does not reduce the absorption of naproxen.

Clinical evidence, mechanism, importance and management

The absorption of naproxen (a single 250 mg dose) was delayed but not reduced in eight normal subjects when given with cholestyramine (4 g in 100 ml orange juice). The amount absorbed after 2 h was reduced from 96 to 51%, but was complete after 5 h.[1] Since naproxen is given chronically, this delay is probably not important. This needs confirmation.

Reference

1 Calvo MV, Dominguez-Gil A. Interaction of naproxen with cholestyramine. Biopharm Drug Dis (1984) 5, 33–42.

Naproxen + diazepam

Abstract/Summary, clinical evidence, mechanism, importance and management

A double blind crossover study failed to find any clinically important changes in mood or attention in subjects given naproxen and diazepam.[1] No special precautions appear to be necessary.

Reference

1 Stitt FW, Latour R, Frane JW. A clinical study of naproxen-diazepam drug interaction on tests of mood and attention. Curr Ther Res (1977) 21, 149–56.

Naproxen + Sulglycotide

Abstract/Summary

Sulglycotide does not affect the absorption of naproxen.

Clinical evidence, mechanism, importance and management

200 mg sulglycotide had no significant effects on the pharmacokinetics of single 500 mg doses of naproxen in 12 normal subjects.[1] Sulglycotide may therefore be used to protect the gastric mucosa from possible injury by naproxen without altering its absorption.

Reference

1 Berte F, Feletti F, De Barnardi di Valserra M, Nazzari M, Cenedese A, Cornelli U. Lack of influence of suglycotide on naproxen bioavailability in healthy volunteers. Int J Clin Pharmacol Ther Tox (1988) 26, 125–8.

Narcotic analgesics + Benzodiazepines

Abstract/Summary

The respiratory depressant effects of opiates such as diamorphine and phenoperidine appear to be opposed by the presence of benzodiazepines. Patients on methadone who are given diazepam may experience increased drowsiness.

Clinical evidence, mechanism, importance and management

A 14-year-old boy with staphylococcal pneumonia secondary to influenza developed adult respiratory distress syndrome. It was decided to suppress his voluntary breathing with opiates and use assisted ventilation and he was therefore given phenoperidine and diazepam for 11 days, and later diamorphine with lorazepam. Despite very high doses (19.2 g diamorphine in 24 h) his respiratory drive was not suppressed. On day 17, despite serum morphine and lorazepam levels of 320 and 5.3 g/ml respectively, he remained conscious and his pupils were not constricted.[1] Later animal studies confirmed that lorazepam opposed the respiratory depressant effects of morphine.[1] In this situation this was an unwanted interaction, but under some circumstances it might be used to advantage. The effects on analgesia were not measured.

Four addicts, maintained on methadone for at least six months, were given 0.3 mg/kg diazepam for nine days. The pharmacokinetics were unaltered (confirmed in other studies[3,4]) and the opiate effects of the methadone remained unchanged, but all four were sedated.[2] The CNS depressant effects of both drugs would seem to be additive. Concurrent use need not be avoided but patients given both drugs are likely to experience increased drowsiness.

References

1 McDonald CF, Thomson SA, Scott NC, Scott W, Grant IWB, Crompton GK. Benzodiazepine — opiate antagonism — a problem in intensive care therapy. Intensive Care Med (1986) 12, 39–42.
2 Pond SM, Benowitz NL, Jacob P, Rigod J. Lack of effect of diazepam on methadone metabolism in methadone-maintained addicts. Clin Pharmacol Ther (1982) 31, 139–43.
3 Preston KL, Griffiths RR, Stitzer ML, Bigelow GE and Liebson IA. Diazepam and methadone interactions in methadone maintenance. Clin Pharmacol Ther (1984) 36, 534–41.
4 Preston KL, Griffiths RR, Cone EJ, Darwin WD, Gorodetzky CW. Diazepam and methadone blood levels following concurrent administration of diazepam and methadone. Drug Alc Dep (1986) 18, 195–202.

Narcotic analgesics + Promethazine

Abstract/Summary

Although promethazine can be used to reduce the dosage of many narcotic analgesics, it has potent sedative effects which would be expected to be additive with CNS depressant effects of the narcotics

Clinical evidence

The analgesic requirements of more than 300 patients treated with a variety of narcotic analgesics (morphine, pethidine, oxymorphone, hydromorphone, fentanyl, pentazocine) were reduced 28–44% when they were given promethazine, 50 mg/70 kg body weight.[1] This possible advantageous interaction would be expected to be accompanied by increased sedation since promethazine is a potent CNS depressant which would be additive with the CNS depressant effects of the narcotics. See also 'Pethidine (Meperidine) + Chlorpromazine and other Phenothiazines'.

Reference

1 Keeri-Szanto M. The mode of action of promethazine in potentiation of narcotic drugs. Br J Anaesth (1974) 46, 918–24.

Nefopam + Miscellaneous drugs

Abstract/Summary

Nefopam should not be given to patients taking anticonvulsants or the MAOI. Be cautious with tricyclic antidepressants, anticholinergics and sympathomimetics. The intensity and incidence of side-effects are somewhat increased when nefopam is given with codeine, pentazocine or dextropropoxyphene.

Clinical evidence, mechanism, importance and management

Detailed information about adverse interactions between nefopam and other drugs seems not to be available, but convulsions have been seen in a few patients and the makers say that nefopam is contraindicated in patients with a history of convulsive disorders. Caution should be exercised with the tricyclic antidepressants and other drugs with anticholinergic side-effects because the convulsive threshold may be lowered and the side-effects may be additive. The CSM has a number of reports of urinary retention caused by nefopam which would be expected to be worsened by drugs with anticholinergic activity.[3] Nefopam appears to have sympathomimetic activity and the makers say it should not be given with the MAOI. A controlled trial in 45 normal subjects divided into nine groups of five, each given 60 mg nefopam daily for three days with either 650 mg aspirin, 5 mg diazepam, 60 mg phenobarbitone, 65 mg dextropropoxyphene, 60 mg codeine, 50 mg pentazocine, 25 mg indomethacin or 50 mg hydroxyzine pamoate found that the only changes were possibly an additive increase in the intensity and incidence of side-effects with nefopam and codeine, pentazocine or dextropropoxyphene.[1] The incidence of sedation with nefopam is 20–30% which, depending on the circumstances, may present a problem if given with other sedative drugs.[2]

References

1 Lasseter KC, Cohen A, Back EL. Neofam HCl interaction study with eight other drugs. J Int Med Res (1976) 4, 195.
2 Heel RC, Brogden RN, Pakes GE, Speight TM, Avery GS. Nefopam: a review of its pharmacological properties and therapeutic efficacy. Drugs (1980) 19, 249–57.
3 Committee on the Safety of Medicines (CSM). Nefopam hydrochloride (Acupan). Current Problems no 24, January 1989.

Non-steroidal anti-inflammatory drugs + Antacids

Abstract/Summary

The absorption of suprofen, tolmetin and zomepirac is not significantly affected by the concurrent use of magnesium-aluminium hydroxide but a small reduction can occur with ketoprofen. Neither ketoprofen nor diclofenac are affected by magnesium hydroxide.

Clinical evidence, mechanism, importance and management

24 normal subjects were given 200 mg suprofen with either 8 oz water or 30 ml *Maalox* in water after an overnight fast. The bioavailability of the suprofen was not significantly affected by the antacid.[1] Neither single dose nor longer-term administration of 20 ml doses of *Maalox* affects the absorption or the plasma elimination half-life of 100 mg doses of zomepirac.[3] A detailed pharmacokinetic study on 24 subjects similarly showed that *Maalox*, given as single 20 ml doses four times a day over a three-day period, had no significant effect on the absorption from the gut of tolmetin given as single 400 mg doses.[4] Five normal subjects showed a 22% reduction in the absorption of 50 mg ketoprofen (as measured by the amount excreted in the urine) when given 1 g aluminium hydroxide, largely as a result of the adsorption of the ketoprofen by the antacid.[2] However in another study 850 mg magnesium hydroxide was found to have no significant effect on the absorption of 50 mg ketoprofen or 50 mg diclofenac.[5]

No particular precautions would seem to be needed if either of these antacids is given with diclofenac, suprofen, tolmetin or zomepirac, and it seems doubtful if the effects of ketoprofen will be reduced to any great extent by aluminium hydroxide.

References

1 Abrams LS, Marriott TB, Van Horn A. The effect of *Maalox* on the bioavailability of suprofen. Clin Res (1983) 31, 626A.
2 Ismail FA, Khalafallah N, Khalil SA. Adsorption of ketoprofen and bumadizone calcium on aluminium-containing antacids and its effect on ketoprofen bioavailability in man. Int J Pharmaceut (1987) 34, 189–96.
3 Nayak RK, Ng KT, Gottlieb S. Effect of chronic and acute antacid administration on zomepirac pharmacokinetics. Clin Pharmacol Ther (1980) 27, 275.
4 Ayres JW, Weidler DJ, Mackichan J, Sakmar E, Hallmark MB, Lemanowicz EF, Wagner JG. Pharmacokinetics of tolmetin with and without concomitant administration of antacid in man. Eur J Clin Pharmacol (1977) 12, 421.
5 Neuvonen PJ. The effect of magnesium hydroxide on the oral absorption of ibuprofen, ketoprofen and diclofenac. Br J clin Pharmac (1991) 31, 263–6.

Non-steroidal anti-inflammatory drugs + Food

Abstract/Summary

Gastric upset caused by indomethacin or suprofen can be minimized by taking them with food or milk. Any interaction seems to be of minimal importance.

Clinical evidence, mechanism, importance and management

Studies in patients and normal subjects, given single or multiple oral doses of indomethacin, have shown that food causes marked and complex changes in the immediate serum indo-

methacin levels (peak levels are delayed and altered), but fluctuations in levels are somewhat ironed out.[1] However another study comparing indomethacin concentrations in serum and synovial fluids found that they were about the same 5–9 h after taking the indomethacin,[2] so it would seem that the fluctuations and alterations which go on during the first 5 h are probably much less important than overall serum levels. Food also reduces the peak serum levels of suprofen (to 44%) and its bioavailability (to 81%).[3] The likelihood of an undesirable interaction with either of these NSAIDs seems to be small, whereas the advantages of taking them at meal times to avoid gastric upset (a makers recommendation) are considerable.

References

1 Emori HW, Paulus H, Bluestone R, Champion GD, Pearson C. Indomethacin serum concentrations in man. Effects of dosage, food and antacid. Ann Rheum Dis (1976) 35, 333–8.
2 Emori HW, Champion GD, Bluestone R, Paulus HE. The simultaneous pharmacokinetics of indomethacin in serum and synovial fluid. Ann Rheum Dis (1973) 32, 433.
3 Chaikin P, Marriott TB, Simon D, Weintraub HS. Comparative bioavailability of suprofen after coadministration with food or milk. J Clin Pharmacol (1988) 28, 1132–5.

Non-steroidal anti-inflammatory drugs + Gold

Abstract/Summary

Gold appears to increase the risk of aspirin-induced liver damage. Fenoprofen seems to be safer.

Clinical evidence, mechanism, importance and management

A study in rheumatoid patients given 3.9 g aspirin daily or 2.4 mg fenoprofen calcium suggested that concurrent gold induction therapy (sodium gold thiomalate, total dose 985 mg) can increase aspirin-induced hepatotoxicity. Levels of SGOT, LDH and alkaline phosphatase were raised. These indicators of liver dysfunction were not seen in the patients treated with fenoprofen suggesting that it is safer than aspirin in this context. Concurrent gold/NSAID treatment was more effective than the NSAIDs alone.[1] Fenoprofen would therefore seem to be preferable to aspirin.

Reference

1 Davis JD, Turner RA, Collins RL, Ruchte IR, Kaufmann JS. Fenoprofen, aspirin and gold induction in rheumatoid arthritis. Clin Pharmacol Ther (1977) 21, 52–61.

Non-steroidal anti-inflammatory drugs + H₂-blockers

Abstract/Summary

Cimetidine has no effect or causes only a modest and clinically unimportant rise in the serum levels of aspirin, ibuprofen, flurbiprofen, isoxicam, ketoprofen and naproxen. The importance of the increase in piroxicam levels and of ibuprofen in black subjects is uncertain. Ranitidine and nizatidine appear not to interact adversely with any of these NSAIDs. Famotidine raises the maximum serum levels of diclofenac and speeds up its absorption, and also has some effects on the absorption of aspirin. Diclofenac does not affect ranitidine.

Clinical evidence

(a) Aspirin and salicylates

Only a modest increase occurred in the serum salicylate levels of three out of six subjects given 1200 mg aspirin 1 h after 300 mg cimetidine.[1]

The total amount of aspirin absorbed was unaltered, but serum levels were slightly raised (from 161 to 180 μg/ml) in 13 patients with rheumatoid arthritis on enteric-coated aspirin after taking 1200 mg cimetidine daily for seven days.[2] Six normal subjects showed little change in the pharmacokinetics of a single 1 g dose of aspirin after being given 150 mg ranitidine twice daily for a week.[3] Famotidine has been found to cause some small changes in the pharmacokinetics of aspirin, but of doubtful clinical importance.[25]

(b) Diclofenac

40 mg famotidine raised the peak serum levels of diclofenac (100 mg in enteric-coated form) in 14 normal subjects from 5.48 to 7.04 mg/l and they occurred more rapidly (2.0 v 2.75 h). The extent of the absorption was unchanged.[21] Diclofenac does not affect the pharmacokinetics of ranitidine nor its ability to suppress gastric pH.[22] The pharmacokinetics of diclofenac are unaffected by ranitidine.[23]

(c) Flurbiprofen

300 mg cimetidine three times daily for two weeks increased the maximal serum level of flurbiprofen (150–300 mg daily) in 30 patients with rheumatoid arthritis, but 150 mg ranitidine twice daily had no effect. The efficacy of the flurbiprofen (assessed by Ritchie score, 50' walking time, grip strength) was not altered.[4] Another study in normal subjects taking single 200 mg doses of flurbiprofen found that serum flurbiprofen serum levels were very slightly raised by cimetidine and the AUC was raised 11%, but no significant interaction occurred with ranitidine.[6,8]

(d) Ibuprofen

1200 mg cimetidine daily raised the peak serum ibuprofen levels (single 600 mg dose) of 13 normal subjects by 14% (from 56 to 64 μg/ml) and AUCs by 6%. No changes were seen with 300 mg ranitidine daily.[4] Another study found larger changes (AUC for R-ibuprofen of +37%, for S-ibuprofen of +19% but these were not statistically significant).[20] However no changes were seen in three other studies with ibuprofen and cimetidine or ranitidine,[5,7,10–12] one of which also found no interaction between ibuprofen and nizatidine.[4] However analysis of the results of one study[6] showed that peak serum ibuprofen levels in black subjects (USA) were higher (+54%) and occurred sooner, whereas in white subjects (USA) they were lower (–27%) and delayed.[9,10]

(e) Isoxicam

200 mg cimetidine daily had no effect on the rate and extent of absorption of isoxicam.[13]

(f) Ketoprofen

1200 mg cimetidine twice daily was found not to affect the pharmacokinetics of 100 mg ketoprofen twice daily.[19]

(g) Naproxen

Naproxen and cimetidine do not interact together adversely nor does naproxen alter the beneficial effects of cimetidine on gastric acid secretion.[14] Nizatidine does not affect the pharmacokinetics of naproxen.[24]

(h) Piroxicam

1200 mg cimetidine daily for seven days slightly increased the half-life and the AUC of a single dose of piroxicam (by 7 and 16% respectively) in 10 normal subjects.[15] Another study also found a 16% rise in the AUC of piroxicam,[18] whereas yet another in 12 normal subjects found that the half-life and AUC of a single dose of piroxicam were increased by 41% and 31% respectively by 600 mg cimetidine daily, and the serum levels were raised accordingly.[16] For example, at 4 h they were raised almost 25%.[16] Ranitidine does not affect the pharmacokinetics of piroxicam.[17]

Mechanisms

Uncertain. Piroxicam serum levels are possibly increased because its metabolism is reduced by the cimetidine.[16]

Importance and management

None of the interactions between the NSAIDs and cimetidine, famotidine, nizatidine or ranitidine appear to be of particular clinical importance, except possibly those of piroxicam and ibuprofen in black subjects. These need further study. The H$_2$-blockers may protect the gastric mucosa from the irritant effects of the NSAIDs and concurrent use may therefore be advantageous.

References

1 Khoury W, Geraci K, Askari A, Johnson M. The effect of cimetidine on aspirin absorption. Gastroenterology (1979) 76, 1169.

2 Willoughby JS, Paton TW, Walker SE, Little AH. The effect of cimetidine on enteric-coated ASA disposition. Clin Pharmacol Ther (1983) 33, 268.

3 Corrocher R, Bambara LM, Caramaschi P, Testi R, Girelli M, Pellegatti M, Lomeo A. Effect of ranitidine on the absorption of aspirin. Digestion (1987) 37, 178–83.

4 Ochs HR, Greenblatt DJ, Matlis R, Weinbrenner J. Interaction of ibuprofen with the H$_2$-receptor antagonists ranitidine and cimetidine. Clin Pharmacol Ther (1985) 38, 648–51.

5 Conrad KA, Mayersohn M, Bliss M. Cimetidine does not alter ibuprofen kinetics after a single dose. Br J clin Pharmac (1984) 18, 624–6.

6 Sullivan KM, Small RE, Rock WL, Cox SR, Willis HE. Effects of cimetidine or ranitidine on the pharmacokinetics of flurbiprofen. Clin Pharm (1986) 5, 586–9.

7 Forsyth DR, Jayasinghe KSA, Roberts CJC. Do nizatidine and cimetidine interact with ibuprofen? Eur J Clin Pharmacol (1988) 35, 85–8.

8 Kreeft JH, Bellamy N, Freeman D. Do H2-antagonists alter the kinetics and effects of chronically administered flurbiprofen in rheumatoid arthritis? Clin Invest Med (1987) 10 (four Suppl B) B58.

9 Small RE, Wood JH. Influence of racial differences on effects of ranitidine and cimetidine on ibuprofen pharmacokinetics. Clin Pharm (1989) 8, 471–2.

10 Stephenson DW, Small RE, Wood JH. Effect of ranitidine and cimetidine on ibuprofen pharmacokinetics. Clin Pharm (1988) 7, 317–21.

11 Evans AM, Nation RL, Sansom LN. Lack of effect of cimetidine on the pharmacokinetics of R(–)- and S(+)-ibuprofen. Br J clin Pharmac (1989) 2, 143–9.

12 Small RE, Wilmot-Pater MG, McGee BA, Willis HE. Effects of misoprostol or ranitidine on ibuprofen pharmacokinetics. Clin Pharm (1991) 10, 870–2.

13 Farnham DJ. Studies of isoxicam in combination with aspirin, warfarin sodium and cimetidine. Sem Arth Rheum (1982) 12 (Suppl 2) 179–83.

14 Holford NHG, Riegelman S, Buskin JN, Upton RA. Pharmacokinetic and pharmacodynamic study of cimetidine administered with naproxen. Clin Pharmacol Ther (1981) 29, 251.

15 Mailhot C, Dahl SL, Ward JR. The effect of cimetidine on serum concentrations of piroxicam. Pharmacotherapy (1986) 6, 112–17.

16 Said SA, Foda AM. Influence of cimetidine on the pharmacokinetics of piroxicam in rat and man. Arzneim-Forsch/Drug Res (1989) 39, 790–2.

17 Dixon JS, Lacey LF, Pickup ME, Langley SJ, Page MC. A lack of pharmacokinetic interaction between ranitidine and piroxicam. Eur J Clin Pharmacol (1990) 39, 583–6.

18 Freeman DJ, Danter WR, Carruthers SG. Pharmacokinetic interaction between cimetidine and piroxicam in normal subjects. Clin Invest Med (1988) 11, (Suppl 4) c19.

19 Verbeeck RK, Corman CL, Wallace SM, Herman RJ, Ross SG, Le Morvan P. single and multiple dose pharmacokinetics of enteric coated ketoprofen: effect of cimetidine. Eur J Clin Pharmacol (1988) 35, 521–7.

20 Li G, Treiber G, Klotz U. The ibuprofen-cimetidine interaction. Stereochemical considerations. Drug Invest (1989) 1, 11–17.

21 Suraykumar J, Chakrapani T, Krishna DR. Famotidine affects the pharmacokinetics of diclofenac sodium. Drug Invest (1992) 4, 66–8.

22 Blum RA, Alioth C, Chan KKH, Furst DE, Ziehmer BA, Schentag JJ. Diclofenac does not affect the pharmacodynamics of ranitidine. Clin Pharmacol Ther (1992) 51, 192.

23 Dammann HG, Simon-Schultz J, Sallowsky E, Schmoldt A. The effects of misoprostol and of ranitidine on the pharmacokinetics of diclofenac. Gastroenterol (1992) 102, A55.

24 Satterwhite JH, Bowsher RR, Callaghen JT, Cerimele BJ, Levine LR. Nizatidine: lack of drug interaction with naproxen. Clin Res (1992) 40, 706A.

25 Domecq C, Fuentes A, Hurtado C, Arancibia A. Effect of famotidine on the bioavailability of acetylsalicylic acid. Med Sci Res (1993) 21, 219–20.

Non-steroidal anti-inflammatory drugs + Non-steroidal anti-inflammatory drugs

Abstract/Summary

Aspirin is reported to increase, decrease or have no effect on serum indomethacin levels. It reduces serum diclofenac, fenoprofen, flurbiprofen, ibuprofen, ketoprofen, naproxen, pirprofen, tenoxicam and tolmetin levels but not those of piroxicam or sudoxicam. Indomethacin and flubiprofen appear not to affect each other's pharmacokinetics but choline magnesium trisalicylate reduces serum naproxen levels. None of these changes has been clearly shown to be of significant clinical importance although concurrent use may possibly increase gastric irritation.

Clinical evidence

The overall picture with indomethacin is confusing and contradictory. Some studies report that aspirin reduces serum indomethacin levels and/or its effects.[1–3,10,12,29] Others claim that no interaction occurs[4–6,11] and no changes in clinical effectiveness take place.[6,7] Yet other studies using buffered aspirin claim that it increases the absorption of indomethacin and is associated with an increase in side-effects.[8,9] Aspirin has been found to more than halve the serum levels of ibuprofen[13,18] and tenoxicam,[30] and reduce the AUC of flurbiprofen to about a third[14] but without any clear changes in clinical effectiveness.[15] Aspirin also virtually halves the AUC of fenoprofen[1] and reduces the AUCs of ketoprofen,[20] diclofenac[19,21] and pirprofen[16] by about a third. Piroxicam[22] and sudoxicam[23] are not significantly affected by aspirin, and naproxen serum levels are only minimally depressed (AUC – 16%).[24,25] Salicylate levels are unaffected by piroxicam.[22] No clinically significant changes in the pharmacokinetics of either indomethacin or flurbiprofen occur if given concurrently.[17] Choline magnesium trisalicylate increases the clearance of naproxen by 56% and decreases its serum levels by 26%;[27] the value of concurrent use is debatable.[26,27] Serum tolmetin levels are slightly reduced by aspirin.[28]

Mechanism

Not resolved. Changes in the rates of absorption and renal clearance have been proposed.

Importance and management

Although extensively studied, there seems to be no clear evidence, one way or the other, that there are either marked advantages or disadvantages in using any of these drugs concurrently. It would be prudent to check on the effectiveness of concurrent use and possible adverse effects on the gastrointestinal tract since they can all cause irritation and bleeding.

References

1 Rubin A, Rodda BE, Warrack P, Gruber CM, Ridolfo AS. Interactions of aspirin with nonsteroidal antiinflammatory drugs in man. Arth Rheum (1973) 16, 635.

2 Kaldestad E, Hansen T, Brath HK. Interaction of indomethacin and acetylsalicylic acid as shown by the serum concentrations of indomethacin and salicylate. Eur J clin Pharmacol (1975) 9, 199.

3 Jeremy R, Towson J. Interaction between aspirin and indomethacin in the treatment of rheumatoid arthritis. Med J Aust (1970) 1, 127.

4 Champion D, Mongan E, Paulus H, Sarkissian E, Okun R, Pearson C. Effect of concurrent aspirin (ASA) administration on serum concentrations of indomethacin (I) Arth Rheum (1971) 14, 375.

5 Lindquist B, Jensen KM, Johansson H, Hansen T. Effect of concurrent administration of aspirin and indomethacin on serum concentrations. Clin Pharmacol Ther (1974) 15, 247.

6 Brooks PM, Walker JJ, Bell MA, Buchanan WW, Rhymer AR. Indomethacin-aspirin interaction: a clinical appraisal. Br Med J (1975) 2, 69.

7 The Cooperating Clinical Committee of the American Rheumatism Association. A three-month trial of indomethacin in rheumatoid arthritis with special reference to analysis and inference. Clin Pharmacol Ther (1967) 8, 11.

8 Turner P, Garnham JC. Indomethacin-aspirin interaction. Br Med J (1975) 2, 368.

9 Garnham JC, Raymond K, Shotton E, Turner P. The effect of buffered aspirin on plasma indomethacin. Eur J clin Pharmacol (1975) 8, 107.

10 Lei BW, Kwan KC, Duggan DE, Breault GO, Davis RL. The influence of aspirin on the absorption and disposition of indomethacin. Clin Pharmacol Ther (1976) 19, 110.

11 Barraclough DRE, Muirden KD, Laby B. Salicylate therapy and drug interaction in rheumatoid arthritis. Aust NZ J Med (1975) 5, 518–23.

12 Kwan KC, Breault GO, Davis RL, Lei BW, Czerwinski AW, Besselaar GH, Duggan DE. Effects of concomitant aspirin administration on the pharmacokinetics of indomethacin in man. J Pharmacokinet Biopharm (1978) 6, 451–76.

13 Albert KS, Gernaat CM. Pharmacokinetics of ibuprofen. Am J Med (1984) 77 (Suppl 1A), 40–46.

14 Kaiser DG, Brooks CD, Lomen PL. Pharmacokinetics of flurbiprofen. Am J Med (1986) 80, suppl 3A, 13–14.

15 Brooks PM, Khong TK. Flurbiprofen-aspirin interaction: a double-blind crossover study. Curr Med Res Opin (1977) 5, 53–7.

16 Luders RC, Bartlett MF, Maggio-Cavaliere MB, Chao DK, Gum OB, Proctor JD. Effect of aspirin on the disposition of pirprofen in man. Curr Ther Res (1982) 31, 413–21.

17 Rudge SR, Lloyd-Jones JK, Hind ID. Interaction between flurbiprofen and indomethacin in rheumatoid arthritis. Br J clin Pharmac (1982) 13, 448–51.

18 Grennan DM, Ferry DG, Ashworth ME, Kenny RE, Mackinnon M. The aspirin-ibuprofen interaction in rheumatoid arthritis. Br J clin Pharmac (1979) 8, 497–503.

19 Willis JV, Kendall MJ, Jack DB. A study of the effect of aspirin on the pharmacokinetics of oral and intravenous diclofenac sodium. Eur J Clin Pharmacol (1980) 18, 415–8.

20 Williams RL, Upton RA, Buskin JN, Jones RM. Ketoprofen-aspirin interactions. Clin Pharmacol Ther (1981) 30, 226–231.

21 Bird HA, Jill J, Leatham P, Wright V. A study to determine the clinical relevance of the pharmacokinetic interaction between aspirin and diclofenac. Agents-Action (1986) 18, 447–9.

22 Hobbs DV, Twomey TM. Piroxicam pharmacokinetics in man: aspirin and antacid studies. J Clin Pharmacol (1979) 270–281.

23 Wiseman EH, Chang Y-H, Hobbs DC. Interaction of sudoxicam and aspirin in animals and man. Clin Pharmacol Ther (1975) 18, 441.

24 Segre EJ, Chaplin M, Forchielli E, Runkel R, Sevelius H. Naproxen-aspirin interactions in man. Clin Pharmacol Ther (1974) 15, 374.

25 Segre E, Sevelius H, Chaplin M, Forchielli E, Runkel R, Rooks W. Interaction of naproxen and aspirin in the rat and in man. Scand J Rheumatol (1973) Suppl 2, 37.

26 Williken RF, Segre EJ. Combination therapy with naproxen and aspirin in rheumatoid arthritis. Arth Rheum (1976) 19, 677.

27 Furst DE, Sarkissian E, Blocka K, Cassell S, Dromgoole S, Harris ER, Hirschberg JM, Josephson N, Paulus HE. Arth Rheum (1987) 30, 1157–61.

28 Cressman WA, Wortham GF, Plostnieks J. Absorption and excretion of tolmetin in man. Clin Pharmacol Ther (1976) 19, 224–33.

29 Pawlotsky Y, Chales G, Grosbois B, Miane B, Bourel M. Comparative interaction of aspirin with indomethacin and sulindac in chronic rheumatic diseases. Eur J Rheumatol Inflamm (1978) 1, 18–20.

30 Day RO, Paull PD, Lam S, Swanson BR, Williams KM, Wade DN. The effect of concurrent aspirin upon plasma concentrations of tenoxicam. Br J clin Pharmac (1988) 26, 455–62.

Non-steroidal anti-inflammatory drugs + Probenecid

Abstract/Summary

Probenecid reduces the loss of carprofen, ketoprofen, ketorolac and naproxen from the body, and raises their serum levels. Increased effects would be expected and possibly increased toxicity. See index for other probenecid–NSAID interactions.

Clinical evidence

One gram probenecid approximately doubled the serum levels of carprofen in subjects after a single 100 mg dose and modestly increased its half-life, while the uricosuric effects of the probenecid remained virtually unchanged.[5] 500 mg probenecid six-hourly reduced the ketoprofen clearance in six subjects by 67% when given 50 mg 6-hourly.[1] 500 mg probenecid four times daily for 4 days increased the total AUC of a single 10 mg dose of ketorolac in eight subjects more than three-fold, increased its half-life from 6.6 to 15.1 h, raised its maximum serum levels by 19% and reduced its clearance by 67%.[6] 500 mg probenecid twice daily increased the serum naproxen levels of six subjects by 50% while taking 250 mg twice daily%.[2]

Mechanism

Probenecid possibly inhibits the metabolism (conjugation) of ketoprofen and apparently inhibits the loss of unchanged naproxen in the urine (half-life prolonged from 14 to 37 h). It also alters its metabolism by the liver.[3,4] The interactions with the other NSAIDs are not understood.

Importance and management

Information is limited but these interactions appear to be established. Their clinical importance is uncertain. There seem to be no reports of adverse effects due to these considerably increased NSAID serum levels but some caution would clearly be appropriate. Be alert for any evidence of increased side-effects. A dosage reduction may be necessary.

References

1 Upton RA, Williams RL, Buskin JN, Jones RM. Effects of probenecid on ketoprofen kinetics. Clin Pharmacol Ther (1982) 31, 705–12.

2 Runkel R, Mroszcak E, Chaplin M, Sevelius H, Segre E. Naproxen-probenecid interaction. Clin Pharmacol Ther (1978) 24, 706.

3 Runkel R, Forschielli E, Boost G, Chaplin M, Hill R, Sevelius H, Thompson G, Segre E. Naproxen metabolism, excretion and comparative pharmacokinetics, Scand J Rheumatol (1973) 2, 29.

4 Runkel R, Chaplin MD, Sevelius H, Ortega E, Segre E. Pharmacokinetics of naproxen overdoses. Clin Pharmacol Ther (1976) 20, 269.

5 Yü T-F, Perel J. Pharmacokinetic and clinical studies of carprofen in gout. J Clin Pharmacol (1980) 347–51.

6 Mroszczak EJ, Combs DL, Goldblum R, Yee J, McHugh D, Tsina I, Fratis T. The effect of probenecid on ketorolac pharmacokinetics after oral dosing of ketorolac tromethamine. Clin Pharmacol Ther 1992) 51, 154.

Non-steroidal anti-inflammatory drugs + Prostaglandins

Abstract/Summary

Isolated cases of adverse neurological side-effects have been seen with naproxen or phenylbutazone given with misoprostol. Misoprostol also increases the abdominal pain and other side-effects of diclofenac and indomethacin. Paracetamol (acetaminophen) intensifies pain if given with mifepristone and sulprostone used to induce abortion. No adverse or important pharmacokinetic interactions seem to occur between aspirin, ibuprofen and misoprostol, or between aspirin and arbaprostol or nocloprost.

Clinical evidence, mechanism, importance and management

(a) Aspirin, diclofenac, ibuprofen

No clinically important pharmacokinetic interactions have been found to occur between 975 mg aspirin and 200 μg misoprostol,[3] between ibuprofen and misoprostol,[6] or between aspirin and arbaprostil[4] or nocloprost.[11] No special precautions seem necessary.

(b) Indomethacin

One study found that 200 μg misoprostol raised steady-state indomethacin levels (50 mg three times daily) by about 30%,[7] whereas another found that 400 μg misoprostol reduced the AUC of indomethacin (50 mg twice daily) by 24% and reduced the maximum steady-state serum level by 13%. Concurrent use resulted in an increase in abdominal symptom severity, frequency of bowel movements and a decrease in faecal consistency.[10] Similar adverse effects were also seen in another study with 400 μg misoprostol twice daily and diclofenac.[9] These are probably of only minor importance. A combined diclofenac/misoprostol product is now available.

(c) Naproxen, phenylbutazone, etodolac

A man with rheumatoid arthritis on long-term naproxen developed ataxic symptoms a few hours after starting misoprostol. He said he 'felt like a drunk person, staggering all over and vomiting'. He rapidly improved when he stopped the misoprostol but the adverse symptoms recurred on two further occasions when he restarted misoprostol.[1] Three patients taking 200–400 mg phenylbutazone daily developed adverse effects when also given 400–800 μg misoprostol daily.[2] One had headaches, dizziness and ambulatory instability which disappeared and then reappeared when the misoprostol was stopped and then restarted. No problems occurred when the phenylbutazone was replaced by 400 mg etodolac daily. The other two developed symptoms including headache, tingles, dizziness, hot flushes and transient diplopia.[2,5] No problems developed when one of them was given naproxen and misoprostol.[5] The reasons are not understood (possibly a potentiation of the neurological side-effects of phenylbutazone ?). Although misoprostol appears to prevent gastric ulcers caused by the use of NSAIDs and concurrent use is usually uneventful, these adverse reports emphasise that good monitoring may be advisable.

(d) Paracetamol

A study in 45 women undergoing abortion with mifepristone and sulprostone found that paracetamol (acetaminophen) given as a 600 mg suppository intensified rather than reduced their pain, and approximately doubled its duration. The reason is not understood. The women had had the mifepristone two days earlier and the paracetamol was given 15 min before the intramuscular injection of 0.5 mg sulprostone.[8] Paracetamol is therefore not a satisfactory analgesic in the presence of these prostaglandins.

References

1 Huq M. Neurological adverse effects of naproxen and misoprostol combination. Br J Gen Prac (1990) 10, 432.

2 Jacquemier JM, Lassoued S, Laroche M, Mazières B. Neurosensory adverse effects after phenylbutazone and misoprostol combined treatment. Lancet (1989) 2, 1283.

3 Karim A, Rozek LF, Leese PT. Absorption of misoprostol (Cytotec), an antiulcer prostaglandin, or aspirin is not affected when given concomitantly to healthy human subjects. Gastroenterology (1987) 92, 1742.

4 Hsyu P-H, Cox JW, Pullen RH, Gee WL, Euler AR. Pharmacokinetic interactions between arbaprostil and aspirin in humans. Biopharm Drug Disp (1989) 10, 411–22.

5 Chassagne Ph, Humez C, Gourmelen O, Moore N, Le Loet X, Deshayes P. Neurosensory adverse effects after combined phenylbutazone and misoprostol. Br J Rheumatol (1991) XXX, 392.

6 Small RE, Wilmot-Pater MG, McGee B, Willis HE. Effects of misoprostol or ranitidine on ibuprofen pharmacokinetics. Clin Pharm (1991) 10, 870–2.

7 Rainsford KD, James C, Hunt RH, Stesko PI, Rischke JA, Karim A, Nicholson PA, Smith M, Hantsbargerr G. Effects of misoprostol on the pharmacokinetics of indomethacin in human volunteers. Clin Pharmacol Ther (1992) 51, 415–21.

8 Weber B, Fontan J-E. Acetaminophen as a pain enhancer during voluntary interruption of pregnancy with mifeprostone and sulprostone. Eur J Clin Pharmacol (1990) 39, 609.

9 Dammann HG, Simon-Schultz J, Sallowsky E, Schmoldt A. The effects of misoprostol and of ranitidine on the pharmacokinetics of diclofenac. Gastroenterol (1992) 102, A55.

10 Kendal MJ, Gibson R, Walt RP. Co-administration of misoprostol or ranitidine with indomethacin: effects on pharmacokinetics, abdominal symptoms and bowel habit. Aliment Pharmacol Ther (1992) 6, 437–46.

11 Siegmund W, Zschiesche M, Bohne M, Franke G, Amon I. Pharmacokinetic interactions between nocloprost, acetylsalicylic acid and ethanol. Int J Clin Pharmacol Ther Toxicol (1992) 30, 539–40.

Non-steroidal anti-inflammatory drugs + Sucralfate

Abstract/Summary

Sucralfate appears not to interact adversely with aspirin, choline-magnesium trisalicylate, diclofenac, ibuprofen, indomethacin, ketoprofen, piroxicam or naproxen, and may also possibly protect the gastric mucosa from damage.

Clinical evidence

Six normal subjects were given 2 g sucralfate half an hour before taking single doses of either 50 mg ketoprofen, 50 mg indomethacin or 500 mg naproxen. Some changes were seen (reduced maximal serum concentrations of ketoprofen, reduced rate of absorption of naproxen and indomethacin, increased time to achieve maximal serum concentrations with indomethacin) but no alterations in bioavailability occurred.[1] A delay, but no reduction in the total absorption of naproxen is described in two studies.[5,7] It is unlikely that its clinical efficacy will be reduced.[5] 2 g sucralfate daily for two days were found not to decrease the rate of absorption of single 400 mg doses of ibuprofen[2] nor of 650 mg doses of aspirin.[3] 5 g sucralfate in divided doses did not significantly alter the absorption of single 600 mg doses of ibuprofen.[4] 2 g of sucralfate was found not to affect significantly the pharmacokinetics of either 20 mg piroxicam or 50 mg diclofenac.[8] 4 g sucralfate daily was found not to affect the pharmacokinetics of 1.5 g choline-magnesium trisalicylate daily.[9] Sucralfate can protect human gastric mucosa from damage by aspirin.[6]

Mechanism

The protective effects of sucralfate may possibly be related to stimulation of prostaglandin production.

Importance and management

Single dose studies do not necessarily reliably predict what will happen when patients take drugs regularly, but the evidence available suggests that sucralfate is unlikely to have an adverse effect on treatment with any of these NSAIDs and may possibly have some protective effect on the gastric mucosa.

References

1 Caille G, Du Souich P, Gervais P, Besner J-G. Single dose pharmacokinetics of ketoprofen, indomethacin and naproxen taken alone or with sucralfate. Biopharm Drug Disp (1987) 8, 173–83.
2 Anaya AL, Mayersohn M, Conrad KA, Dimmitt DC. The influence of sucralfate on ibuprofen absorption in healthy adult males. Biopharm Drug Disp (1986) 7, 443–51.
3 Lau A, Chang C-W, Schlesinger P. Evaluation of a potential drug interaction between sucralfate and aspirin. Gastroenterology (1985) 88, 1465.
4 Pugh MC, Small RE, Garnett WR, Townsend RJ, Willis HE. Effect of sucralfate on ibuprofen absorption in normal volunteers. Clin Pharm (1984) 3, 630–3.
5 Caille G, du Souich P, Gervais P, Besner JG, Vezina M. Effects of concurrent sucralfate administration on pharmacokinetics of naproxen. Am J Med (1987) 83 (Suppl 3B) 67–73.
6 Stern AI, Ward F, Hartley G. Protective effect of sucralfate against aspirin-induced damage to human gastric mucosa. Am J Med (1987) 83 (Suppl 3B) 83–5.
7 Lafontaine D, Mailhot C, Vermeulen M, Bissonnette B, Lambert C. Influence of chewable sucralfate or a standard meal on the bioavailability of naproxen. Clin Pharm (1990) 9, 773–7.
8 Ungethüm W. Study on the interaction between sucralfate and diclofenac/piroxicam in healthy volunteers. Arzneim.-Forsch/Drug Res (1991) 41, 797–800.
9 Schneider DK, Gannon RH, Sweeney KR, DeFusco PA. Influence of sucralfate on trisilate bioavailability. J Clin Pharmacol (1991) 31, 377–9.

Oxyphenbutazone and Phenylbutazone + Anabolic steroids

Abstract/Summary

Serum oxyphenbutazone levels are raised about 40% by the use of methandienone (methandrostenolone). Phenylbutazone appears to be unaffected.

Clinical evidence

Oxyphenbutazone levels were raised 43% (range 5–100%) in six subjects on 300–400 mg oxyphenbutazone daily for 2–5 weeks when given 5 or 10 mg/kg methandienone. Neither 5 mg prednisone nor 1.5 mg dexamethasone daily was found to affect oxyphenbutazone levels.[1]

Two other studies confirm this interaction with oxyphenbutazone.[2,3] One of them found no interaction with phenylbutazone.[2]

Mechanism

Uncertain. One idea is that the anabolic steroids alter the distribution of oxyphenbutazone between the tissues and plasma so that more remains in circulation. There may also possibly be some changes in metabolism. Phenylbutazone possibly does not interact because it displaces oxyphenbutazone (its normal metabolite) from the plasma binding sites, thereby raising the levels of unbound oxyphenbutazone and obliterating the effect of the steroid.

Importance and management

The interaction is established but its importance is uncertain. There seem to be no reports of toxicity arising from concurrent use but the possibility should be borne in mind.

References

1 Weiner M, Siddiqui AA, Shahani RT, Dayton PG. Effect of steroids on disposition of oxyphenbutazone in man. Proc Soc Exp Biol Med (1976) 124, 1170.
2 Hvidberg E, Dayton PG, Read JM, Wilson CH. Studies of the interaction of phenylbutazone, oxyphenbutazone and methandrostenolone in man. Proc Soc Exp Biol Med (1968) 129, 438.

3 Weiner M, Siddiqui AA, Bostanci N, Dayton PG. Drug interactions. The effect of combined administration on the half-life of coumarin and pyrazolone drugs in man. Fed Proc (1965) 24, 153.

Paracetamol (Acetaminophen) + Alcohol

Abstract/Summary

Severe liver damage, fatal in some instances, can occur in alcoholics and persistent heavy drinkers who take only moderate doses of paracetamol. Moderate drinkers do not seem to be at risk.

Clinical evidence

Three chronic alcoholic patients developed severe liver damage after taking only slightly above recommended doses of paracetamol (acetaminophen). They demonstrated SGOT levels of 5000–10,000 iu. Two of them had taken only 10 g paracetamol over the two days prior to admission (normal dosage is up to 4 g daily). One of them died in hepatic coma and a post mortem revealed typical paracetamol toxicity. Two of them also developed renal failure.[1]

There are other reports of liver toxicity in a total of about 30 alcoholics attributed to the concurrent use of alcohol and paracetamol. About a third had been taking daily doses within the recommended daily maximum (4 g daily), and a third had had doses within the range 4–8 g daily.[2–18]

Mechanism

Paracetamol is normally predominantly metabolized by the liver to non-toxic sulphate and glucuronide conjugates. Persistent heavy drinking stimulates a normally minor biochemical pathway involving cytochrome P-450IIE1 which allows the production of unusually large amounts of highly hepatotoxic metabolites. Unless sufficient glutathione is present to detoxify these metabolites (alcoholics often have an inadequate intake of protein), they become covalently bound to liver macromolecules and damage results. In fact alcoholics may possibly be most susceptible to toxicity during alcohol withdrawal because, while drinking, alcohol may possibly compete with the paracetamol for metabolism and even inhibit it. Acute ingestion of alcohol by non-alcoholics appears to protect against damage because the damaging biochemical pathway is inhibited rather than stimulated.

Importance and management

An established and clinically important interaction. The incidence is uncertain, but possibly small, bearing in mind the very wide-spread use of paracetamol and alcohol. However damage, when it occurs, can be serious and therefore alcoholics and those who persistently drink heavily should be advised to avoid paracetamol or limit their intake considerably. The normal daily recommended 'safe' maximum of 4 g is almost certainly too high in some alcoholics. The risk for non-alcoholics, moderate drinkers and those who very occasionally drink a lot appears to be low.

References

1 McClain CJ, Kromhout JP, Peterson FJ, Holtzman JL. Potentiation of acetaminophen hepatotoxicity by alcohol. J Amer Med Ass (1980) 244, 251.
2 Emby DJ, Fraser BN. Hepatotoxicity of paracetamol enhanced by ingestion of alcohol. S Afr Med J (1977) 51, 208.
3 Goldfinger R, Ahmed KS, Pichumoni CS, Weseley SA. Concomitant alcohol and drug abuse enhancing acetaminophen toxicity. Am J Gastroenterol (1978) 70, 385.
4 Barker JD, de Carle DJ, Anuras S. Chronic excessive acetaminophen use and liver damage. Ann Intern Med (1977) 87, 299.
5 O'dell JR, Zetterman RK, Burnett DA. Centrilobular hepatic fibrosis following acetaminophen-induced necrosis in an alcoholic. J Amer Med Ass (1986) 255, 2636–7.
6 McJunkin B, Barwick KW, Little WC, Winfield JB. Fatal massive hepatic necrosis following acetaminophen overdosage. J Amer Med Ass (1976) 236, 1874–5.
7 LaBrecque DT, Mitros FA. Increased hepatotoxicity of acetaminophen in the alcoholic. Gastroenterology (1980) 78, 1310.
8 Johnson MW, Friedman PA, Mitch WE. Alcoholism, non-prescription drugs and hepatotoxicity. The risk of unknown acetaminophen ingestion. Am J Gastroenterol (1981) 76, 530–3.
9 Licht H, Seeff LB, Zimmerman HJ. Apparent potentiation of acetaminophen toxicity by alcohol. Ann Intern Med (1980) 92, 511.
10 Black M, Cornell JF, Rabin L, Schachter N. Late presentation of acetaminophen toxicity. Dig Dis Sci (1982) 27, 370–4.
11 Fleckenstein JL. Nyquil and acute hepatic necrosis. N Engl J Med (1985) 313, 48.
12 Gerber MA, Kaufmann H, Klion F, Alpert LI. Acetaminophen associated hepatic injury: report of two cases showing an unusual portal tract reaction. Human Pathol (1980) 11, 37–42.
13 Leist MH, Giuskin LE, Payne JA. Enhanced toxicity of acetaminophen in alcoholics. Report of three cases. J Clin Gastroenterol (1985) 7, 55–9.
14 Himmelstein DU, Woolandler SJ, Adler RD. Elevated SGOT/SGPT ratio in alcoholic patients with acetaminophen hepatotoxicity. Am J Gastroenterol (1984) 79, 718–20.
15 Levinson M. Ulcer, back pain and jaundice in an alcoholic. Hosp Prac (1983) 18, 48N, 48S.
16 Seeff LB, Cuccherini BA, Zimmerman HJ, Adler E, Benjamin SB. Acetaminophen hepatotoxicity in alcoholics. Ann Intern Med (1986) 104, 399–404.
17 Floren C-H, Thesleff P, Nilsson A. Severe liver damage caused by therapeutic doses of acetaminophen. Acta Med Scand (1987) 222, 285–8.
18 Edwards R, Oliphant J. Paracetamol toxicity in chronic alcohol abusers — a plea for greater consumer awareness. NZ Med J (1992) 105, 174–5.

Paracetamol (Acetaminophen) + Anticholinergic agents

Abstract/Summary

Anticholinergic drugs can delay gastric emptying so that the onset of analgesia with paracetamol may be delayed.

Clinical evidence, mechanism, importance and management

30 mg propantheline IV delayed the peak serum levels of

paracetamol (1.5 g) in six convalscent patients from about 1 h to 3 h. Peak concentrations were lowered by about a third, but the total amount of paracetamol absorbed was unchanged.[1] The reason is that propantheline is an anticholinergic drug which slows the rate at which the stomach empties so that the rate of absorption in the gut is reduced. The practical consequence of this is likely to be that rapid pain relief with single doses of paracetamol may be delayed and reduced by anticholinergics (e.g. some antiparkinson drugs, tricyclic antidepressants, some phenothiazines and antihistamines, etc.) but this needs clinical confirmation. Nobody seems to have studied any of these drugs except propantheline. If the paracetamol is being taken in repeated doses over extended periods it seems unlikely to be an important interaction because the total amount absorbed is unchanged.

Reference

1 Nimmo J, Heading RC, Tothill P, Prescott LF. Pharmacological modification of gastric emptying: effects of propantheline and metoclopramide on paracetamol absorption. Br Med J (1973) 1, 587.

Paracetamol (Acetaminophen) + Anticonvulsants

Abstract/Summary

The effects of paracetamol are possibly reduced in patients taking anticonvulsants (carbamazepine, phenytoin, phenobarbitone, primidone). Anticonvulsant serum levels are unaffected. Two isolated reports describe hepatotoxicity in two patients on phenobarbitone after taking normal doses of paracetamol. Paracetamol modestly increases the loss of lamotrigine from the body but appears not to affect phenytoin or carbamazepine.

Clinical evidence

(a) Paracetamol clearance increased

The AUC (area under the curve) of 1 g paracetamol taken orally was found to be 40% lower in six epileptic subjects than in six normal subjects (49.4 compared with 29.3 mg $l^{-1}h^{-1}$). Five of the epileptics were taking at least two of the following drugs: carbamazepine, phenobarbitone, primidone, phenytoin. One was taking only phenytoin.[1] Another study found that these anticonvulsants shortened the half-life of paracetamol.[7] Yet another found that the clearance of paracetamol was increased 46% by phenytoin and carbamazepine.[6]

(b) Anticonvulsant levels unaffected

The serum levels of phenytoin and carbamazepine in 10 epileptics were found not to be significantly affected by 1500 mg paracetamol daily for 3 days.[5]

(c) Heptatotoxicity

An epileptic on 100 mg phenobarbitone daily developed hepatitis after taking 1 g paracetamol daily for 3 months for headaches. Within 2 weeks of stopping the paracetamol her serum transaminase levels had fallen within the normal range which implied that her hepatitis was due to drug-induced liver damage.[2] Another patient on phenobarbitone developed liver and kidney toxicity after taking only 9 g paracetamol over 48 h.[8] Phenobarbitone also appeared to have increased the toxic effects of paracetamol in an adolescent who took an overdose.[3]

(d) Lamotrigine effects reduced

A study in eight normal subjects found that 2.7 g paracetamol (acetaminophen) daily reduced the AUC of a 300 mg dose of lamotrigine by 20% and reduced its half-life by 15%.[4]

Mechanisms

(a) The increased paracetamol clearance is due to the well-recognized enzyme inducing effects of the anticonvulsants which increase its metabolism (glucuronidation and oxidation) and loss from the body. (b) The liver enzyme induction caused by the phenobarbitone apparently resulted in an increase in the production of the hepatotoxic metabolites of paracetamol which exceeded the normal glutathione binding capacity, leading to liver damage. (c) It seems possible that paracetamol increases the metabolism of the lamotrigine.

Importance and management

Information is limited. The clinical importance of none of these interactions is established and further study is needed. Paracetamol is possibly a less effective analgesic in patients taking the interacting anticonvulsants. The risk of liver damage after overdosage is possibly increased, and perhaps after prolonged consumption[6] although only one case seems to have been reported (cited above).[3] The prolonged use of paracetamol should therefore probably be avoided by patients on these anticonvulsants. It is unlikely that the lamotrigine/paracetamol interaction is of practical importance, but this needs confirmation.

References

1. Perucca E, Richens A. Paracetamol disposition in normal subjects and in patients treated with antiepileptic drugs. Br J clin Pharmac (1979) 7, 201–6.

2 Pirotte JH. Apparent potentiation by phenobarbital of hepatotoxicity from small doses of acetaminophen. Ann Intern Med (1984) 101, 403.

3 Wilson JT, Kasantikul V, Harbison R, Martin D. Death in an adolescent following an overdose of acetaminophen and phenobarbital. Am J Dis Child (1978) 132, 466–73.

4 Depot M, Powell JR, Messenheimer JA, Cloutier G, Dalton MJ. Kinetic effects of multiple oral doses of acetaminophen on a single oral dose of lamotrigine. Clin Pharmacol Ther (1990) 48, 346–55.

5 Neuvonen PJ, Lehtovaara R, Bardy A, Elomaa E. Antipyretic analgesics in

patients on antiepileptic drug therapy. Eur J clin Pharmacol (1979) 15, 263–8.

6 Miners JO, Attwood J, Birkett DJ. Determinants of acetaminophen metabolism: effect of inducers and inhibitors of drug metabolism on acetaminophen's metabolic pathways. Clin Pharmacol Ther (1984) 35, 480–6.

7 Prescott LF, Critchley JAJH, Balali-Mood M, Pentland B. Effects of microsomal enzyme induction on paracetamol metabolism in man. Br J clin Pharmac (1981) 12, 149–53.

8 Marsepiol T, Mahassani B, Roudiak N, Sebbah JL, Caillard G. Potentialisation de la toxicité hépatique et rénale du paracétamol par le phénobarbital. JEUR (1989) 2, 118–20.

Paracetamol (Acetaminophen) + Cholestyramine

Abstract/Summary

The absorption of paracetamol may possibly be reduced if cholestyramine is given at the same time, but the reduction in absorption is small if given an hour later.

Clinical evidence

When four normal subjects took 12 g cholestyramine and 2 g paracetamol together the absorption of the paracetamol was reduced by 60% (range 30–98%) at 2 h but the results were said not to be statistically significant. When the cholestyramine was given 1 h after the paracetamol, the absorption was reduced by only 16%.[1]

Mechanism

Cholestyramine reduces the absorption, presumably because it binds with the paracetamol in the gut. Separating the dosages prevents mixing in the gut.

Importance and management

An established interaction. The cholestyramine should not be given within 1 h of the paracetamol if maximal analgesia is to be achieved.

Reference

1 Dorbnni B, Willcon RA, Thompson RPH, Williams R. Reduced absorption of paracetamol by activated charcoal and cholestyramine. Br Med J (1973) 3, 86.

Paracetamol (Acetaminophen) + Disulfiram

Abstract/Summary

Disulfiram does not appear to interact adversely with paracetamol.

Clinical evidence, mechanism, importance and management

After taking 200 mg disulfiram daily for 5 days, the clearance of paracetamol (a single 500 mg IV dose) was reduced by about 10% in five normal subjects without liver disease and five others with alcoholic liver cirrhosis.[1] The reason is uncertain. Among the conclusions drawn are that disulfiram does not interact adversely with paracetamol, and it might even reduce the risks of paracetamol overdose.[1,2]

References

1 Poulson HE, Ranek L, Jørgensen L. The influence of disulfiram on acetaminophen metabolism in man. Xenobiotica (1991) 21, 243–9.

2 Poulson HE, Loft S, Andersen JR, Andersen M. Disulfiram therapy — adverse drug reactions and interactions. Acta Psychiatr Scand (1992) 86 (Suppl 369) 59–66.

Paracetamol (Acetaminophen) + Food

Abstract/Summary, clinical evidence, mechanism, importance and management

Low and high protein meals appear to shorten the time to reach maximum serum paracetamol levels (from 28 to 16 min), but lower the peak concentrations by about 24%. The total amount of paracetamol absorbed is not affected.[1] Another study in South African subjects (Tswanas) found that a high fat meal delayed paracetamol absorption the most, while a high carbohydrate meal delayed it to a lesser extent.[2] The clinical importance of these findings is uncertain.

Reference

1 Robertson DRC, Higginson I, Macklin BS, Renwick AG, Waller DG, George CF. The influence of protein containing meals on the pharmacokinetics of levodopa in healthy volunteers. Br J clin Pharmac (1991) 31, 413–7.

2 Wessela JC, Koeleman HA, Boneschans B, Steyn HS. The influence of different types of breakfast on the absorption of paracetamol among members of an ethnic group. Int J Clin Pharmacol Ther Toxicol (1992) 30, 208–13.

Paracetamol (Acetaminophen) + H₂-blockers

Abstract/Summary, clinical evidence, mechanism, importance and management

No clinically important interaction has been seen when paracetamol and cimetidine are used concurrently.[1] Ranitidine does not affect the pharmacokinetics of paracetamol.[2] No special precautions would seem necessary.

References

1 Chen MM, Lee CS. Cimetidine-acetaminophen interaction in humans. J Clin Pharmacol (1985) 25, 227–9.

2 Thomas M, Michael MF, Andrew P, Scully N. A study to investigate the effects of ranitidine on the metabolic disposition of paracetamol in man. Br J clin Pharmac (1988) 25, 671P.

Paracetamol (Acetaminophen) + Isoniazid

Abstract/Summary

Two reports suggest that the toxicity of paracetamol, particularly in overdosage, may be increased by isoniazid.

Clinical evidence, mechanism, importance and management

A woman of 21 who had been taking 300 mg isoniazid for six months took ten 325 mg tablets of paracetamol for abdominal cramping. Within about 6 h she developed marked evidence of liver damage (prolonged prothrombin time, elevated ammonia, transaminases, hyperbilirubinaemia).[5]

A healthy young woman who had ingested not more than 11.5 g paracetamol in a suicide gesture, developed life-threatening hepatic and renal toxicity despite the fact that her serum paracetamol levels 13 h later were only 15 µmol/l (toxicity normally associated with levels 26 µmol/l.)[1]

Three other possible cases of this toxic interaction have been briefly described.[2,3]

Mechanism

Not established. A possible reason is that the isoniazid induces the mixed-function oxidase enzymes (P450IIE1) in both liver and kidneys, resulting in a greater proportion of the paracetamol being converted into toxic metabolites than would normally occur[1] (possibly similar to the increased toxicity of paracetamol seen in chronic alcoholics). The results of an experimental study contrasts with this suggestion because it has evidence that isoniazid actually reduces the formation of the toxic metabolite of paracetamol.[4]

Importance and management

Information is very limited, but it would now seem prudent to warn patients taking isoniazid not to take more than the recommended daily doses of paracetamol (4 g daily). More study is needed to clarify the situation.

References

1 Murphy R, Swartz R, Watkins P B. Severe acetaminophen toxicity in a patient receiving isoniazid. Ann Intern Med (1990) 113, 799–800.

2 Moulding TS, Redeker AG, Kanel GC. Twenty isoniazid-associated deaths

in one state. A, Rev Resp Dis (1989) 140, 700–5.

3 Moulding TS, Redeker AG. Acetaminophen, isoniazid, and hepatic toxicity. Ann Intern Med (1991) 114, 431.

4 Epstein MM, Nelson SD, Slattery JT, Kalhorn TF, Wall RA, Wright JM. Inhibition of the metabolism of paracetamol by isoniazid. Br J clin Pharmac (1991) 31, 139–42.

5 Crippin JS. Acetaminophen hepatotoxicity: potentiation by isoniazid. Am J Gastroenterol (1993) 88, 590–2.

Paracetamol (Acetaminophen) + Metoclopramide

Abstract/Summary

Metoclopramide increases the rate of absorption of paracetamol and raises its maximum serum levels.

Clinical evidence, mechanism, importance and management

10 mg metoclopramide IV increased the peak serum levels of paracetamol by 65% in five normal subjects after taking a single 1.5 g dose, and increased the rate of absorption (peak levels reached in 48 instead of 120 min), probably because the metoclopramide increases the rate of gastric emptying. The total amount absorbed remained virtually unchanged.[1,2] This suggests that the effectiveness and onset of analgesia by paracetamol would be quicker in the presence of metoclopramide. Concurrent use need not be avoided.

Reference

1 Nimmo J, Heading RC, Tothill P, Prescott LF. Pharmacological modification of gastric emptying: effects of propantheline and metoclopramide on paracetamol absorption. Br Med J (1973) 1, 587.

2 Nimmo J. The influence of metoclopramide on drug absorption. Postgrad Med J (1973) 49, July Suppl, 25–28.

Paracetamol (Acetaminophen) and Other drugs + Opiate analgesics

Abstract/Summary

Morphine and diamorphine delay gastric emptying so that the rate of absorption of other drugs given orally may be reduced.

Clinical evidence, mechanism, importance and management

The absorption of a single 20 mg/kg dose of paracetamol in eight normal subjects was markedly delayed and reduced 30 m after an IM injection of either pethidine (150 mg) or diamorphine (10 mg). Peak plasma paracetamol levels were reduced from 20 to 13.8 and 5.2 g/ml respectively, and delayed from 22 to 114 and 142 min respectively.[1] This interaction was also observed by the same authors in women in labour who had been given opiate analgesics.[2]

The underlying mechanism is that these opiate analgesics delay gastric emptying so that the rate of absorption of the paracetamol is reduced, but the total amount absorbed is not affected. In the study cited the paracetamol was principally being used as a model drug to identify the way in which these analgesics affect drug absorption, but it seems probable that other oral drugs intended to have a rapid effect may be affected similarly. One example is mexiletine (see 'Mexiletine + Morphine').

References

1 Nimmo WS, Heading RC, Wilson J, Tothill P, Prescott LF. Inhibition of gastric emptying and drug absorption by narcotic analgesics. Br J clin Pharmac (1975) 2, 509–13.
2 Nimmo WS, Wilson J, Prescott LF. Narcotic analgesics and delayed gastric emptying during labour. Lancet (1975) i, 890–3.

Paracetamol (Acetaminophen) + Oral contraceptives

Abstract/Summary

Paracetamol (acetaminophen) is cleared from the body more quickly in women taking oral contraceptives and the analgesic effects are expected to be reduced. Paracetamol also increases the absorption of ethinyloestradiol from the gut by about 20%.

Clinical evidence

(a) Effect of oral contraceptives on paracetamol

While taking oral contraceptives the plasma clearance of paracetamol in seven women, following a single 1.5 g dose, was increased by 63% (from 287 to 470 ml/min) and the elimination half-life decreased by 43% (from 2.40 to 1.67 h), when compared with women not taking oral contraceptives.[1]

Other studies have found increases in paracetamol clearance of 86%, 49% and 30%, and corresponding half-life decreases in women on oral contraceptives.[2–4]

(b) Effect of paracetamol on oral contraceptives

1 g paracetamol increased the AUC (area under the curve) of ethinyloestradiol by 21.6% in six normal women.[5,6]

Mechanism

The evidence suggests that the oral contraceptives increase the metabolism (both oxidation and glucuronidation) by the liver of the paracetamol so that it is cleared from the body more quickly.[3] The increased absorption of the ethinyloestradiol is probably because the paracetamol reduces its metabolism by the gut wall during absorption.[5,6]

Importance and management

The effect of the oral contraceptives on paracetamol is well-established. Its clinical importance has not been directly studied, but it seems likely that an increase in the dosage of paracetamol (acetaminophen) may be needed to achieve optimal analgesic effects in women on the pill. The clinical importance of the increased ethinyloestradiol absorption is uncertain.

References

1 Mitchell MC, Hanew T, Meredith CG, Schenker S. Effects of oral contraceptive steroids on acetaminophen metabolism and elimination. Clin Pharmacol Ther (1983) 34, 48–53.
2 Abernethy DR, Divoll M, Ochs HR, Ameer B, Greenblatt DJ. Increased metabolic clearance of acetaminophen with oral contraceptive use. Obst Gynecol (1982) 60, 338–41.
3 Miners JO, Attwood J, Birkett DJ. Influence of sex and oral contraceptive steroids on paracetamol metabolism. Br J Clin Pharmacol (1983) 16, 503–9.
4 Mucklow JC, Fraser HS, Bulpitt CJ, Kahn C, Mould G, Dollery CT. Environmental factors affecting paracetamol metabolism in London factory and office workers. Br J Clin Pharmacol (1980) 10, 67–74.
5 Rogers SM, Back DJ, Stevenson P, Grimmer SFM, Orme ML'E. Paracetamol interaction with oral contraceptive steroids. Br J Clin Pharmacol (1987) 23, 615 P.
6 Rogers SM, Back DJ, Stevenson P, Grimmer SFM, Orme ML'E. Paracetamol interaction with oral contraceptive steroids: increased plasma concentration of ethinyloestradiol. Br J clin Pharmac (1987) 23, 721–5.

Paracetamol (Acetaminophen) + Rifampicin (Rifampin), Sulphinpyrazone

Abstract/Summary

Sulphinpyrazone and rifampicin increase the loss of paracetamol from the body.

Clinical evidence, mechanism, importance and management

Sulphinpyrazone has been found to increase the clearance of paracetamol (+23%) as a result of increased metabolism (glucuronidation, oxidation) by the liver. It has been suggested that, as a result, the risk of liver damage may be increased after overdosage and perhaps during prolonged consumption, but this has yet to be confirmed.[1] Rifampicin (600 mg daily) was also found to increase the clearance of paracetamol in two patients but no precise data was given in the report.[2] The clinical importance of these findings awaits further study. There would seem to be little clear reason for avoiding concurrent use.

References

1 Miners JO, Attwood J, Birkett DJ. Determinants of acetaminophen metabolism: effect of inducers and inhibitors of drug metabolism on

acetaminophen's metabolic pathways. Clin Pharmacol Ther (1984) 35, 480–6.

2 Prescott LF, Critchley JAJH, Balali-Mood M, Pentland B. Effects of microsomal enzyme induction on paracetamol metabolism in man. Br J clin Pharmac (1981) 12, 149–53.

Paracetamol (Acetaminophen) + Sucralfate

Abstract/Summary, clinical evidence, mechanism, importance and management

No change in the bioavailability of 1 g paracetamol was found in six normal subjects when given 1 g sucralfate, using salivary paracetamol levels over 4 h as a measure.[1] Concurrent use need not be avoided.

Reference

1 Kamali F, Fry JR, Smart HL, Bell GD. A double-blind placebo-controlled study to examine effects of sucralfate on paracetamol absorption. Br J clin Pharmac (1985) 19, 113–4.

Penicillamine + Antacids

Abstract/Summary

The absorption of pencillamine from the gut can be reduced by 30–40% if antacids containing aluminium and magnesium hydroxides are taken concurrently.

Clinical evidence

30 ml *Maalox-plus* (aluminium hydroxide, magnesium hydroxide, simethicone) reduced the absorption of a single 500 mg dose of penicillamine in six normal subjects by a third.[1] Another study found that 30 ml *Aludrox* (aluminium and magnesium hydroxides) reduced the absorption by almost 40%.[2]

Mechanism

The most likely explanation is that the penicillamine forms less soluble chelates with magnesium and aluminium ions in the gut which reduces its absorption.[2] Another idea is that the penicillamine is possibly less stable at the higher pH values caused by the antacid.[1]

Importance and management

An established interaction of clinical importance. If maximal absorption is needed the administration of the two drugs should be separated to avoid mixing in the gut. Two hours or so has been found enough for most other drugs which interact similarly. There seems to be nothing documented about other antacids.

References

1 Osman MA, Patel RB, Schuna A, Sundstrom WR, Welling PG. Reduction in oral penicillamine absorption by food, antacid and ferrous sulphate. Clin Pharmacol Ther (1983) 33, 465–70.

2 Ifan A, Welling PG. Pharmacokinetics of oral 500-mg penicillamine: effect of antacids on absorption. Biopharm Drug Disp (1986) 7, 401–5.

Penicillamine + Food

Abstract/Summary

Food can reduce the absorption of penicillamine by as much as a half.

Clinical evidence

The presence of food reduced the serum penicillamine levels by about 50% (from 3.05 to 1.52 g/ml) in normal subjects given 500 mg. The total amount absorbed was reduced similarly (AUC_{0-12h} reduced from 14.7 to 7.16 h/ml).[1,3] These figures are in good agreement with previous findings.[2]

Mechanism

Uncertain. One suggestion is that food delays stomach emptying so that the penicillamine is exposed to more prolonged degradation in the stomach.[2] Another idea is that the protein in food increases the oxidation of the penicillamine to disulphides which are less easily absorbed.[2]

Importance and management

An established interaction. If maximal effects are required the penicillamine should not be taken with food.

References

1 Schuna A, Osman MA, Patel RB, Vellilf PG, Sundstrom WR. Reduction in oral penicillamine absorption by food, antacid and ferrous sulphate. J Rheumatol (1983) 10, 95–7.

2 Bergstrom RF, Kay DR, Harcom TM, Wagner JG. Penicillamine kinetics in normal subjects. Clin Pharmacol Ther (1981) 30, 404–13.

3 Osman MA, Patel RB, Schuna A, Sundstrom WR, Welling PG. Reduction in oral penicillamine absorption by food, antacid and ferrous sulphate. Clin Pharmacol Ther (1983) 33, 465–70.

Penicillamine + Iron preparations

Abstract/Summary

The absorption of penicillamine can be reduced as much as two-thirds by the concurrent use of iron preparations.

Clinical evidence

90 mg ferrous iron (*Fersamal*) reduced the absorption of 250 mg penicillamine in five normal subjects by about two-thirds (using the cupriuretic effects of penicillamine as a measure).[1]

A two-thirds reduction in absorption has been described in another study in subjects given 500 mg penicillamine and 300 mg ferrous sulphate.[5] Other studies confirm this interaction.[2,3] There is also evidence that withdrawal of iron from patients stabilized on penicillamine without a reduction in the dosage can lead to the development of toxicity (nephropathy).[4]

Mechanism

It is believed that the iron and penicillamine form a chemical complex or chelate within the gut which is less easily absorbed.

Importance and management

An established and clinically important interaction. For maximal absorption give the iron at least 2 h after the penicillamine. This should reduce their admixture in the gut.[1] Do not withdraw iron suddenly from patients stabilized on penicillamine because the marked increase in absorption which follows may precipitate penicillamine toxicity. The toxic effects of penicillamine seem to be dependent on the size of the dose and possibly also related to the rate at which the dosage is increased.[4] Only ferrous sulphate has been studied but other iron preparations would be expected to interact similarly.

References

1 Lyle WH. Penicillamine and iron. Lancet (1976) ii, 240.
2 Lyle WH, Pearcy DF, Hui M. Inhibition of penicillamine-induced cupiuresis by oral iron. Proc Roy Soc Med (1977) (Suppl 3) 48–9.
3 Hall ND, Blake DR, Alexander GJM, Vaisey C, Bacon PA. Serum SH reactivity: a simple assessment of D-penicillamine absorption. Rheumatol Int (1981) 1, 39–41.
4 Harkness JAL, Blake DR. Penicillamine nephropathy and iron. Lancet (1982) ii, 1368–9.
5 Osman MA, Patel RB, Schuna A, Sundstrom WR, Welling PG. Reduction in oral penicillamine absorption by food, antacid and ferrous sulphate. Clin Pharmacol Ther (1983) 33, 465–70.

Penicillamine + Miscellaneous drugs

Abstract/Summary

Penicillamine serum levels are increased by chloroquine and to a lesser extent by indomethacin. An increase in penicillamine toxicity is a possibility. An isolated report describes penicillamine-induced breast enlargement in a woman when given a combined oral contraceptive.

Clinical evidence, mechanism, importance and management

(a) Penicillamine + Chloroquine, Indomethacin

Studies in which chloroquine was given to patients on penicillamine found that it was more effective, less effective, or indistinguishable from penicillamine alone, however in some instances penicillamine toxicity was reported to be increased.[2] A pharmacokinetic study in patients with rheumatoid arthritis on 250 mg penicillamine daily found that single doses of chloroquine phosphate (250 mg) increased the AUC (area under the curve) by 34%, and raised the peak serum levels by about 55%.[1] It seems possible therefore that any increased toxicity is simply a reflection of increased serum penicillamine levels. Be alert for evidence of toxicity if both drugs are used. Indomethacin was also found in the last study cited to increase the AUC of penicillamine by 26% and the peak serum levels by about 22%.[1]

(b) Penicillamine + Oral contraceptives, Corticosteroids, Cimetidine.

A woman with Wilson's disease began to develop dark facial hair about 10 months after starting treatment with 1250–1500 mg penicillamine daily. When her testosterone levels were found to be slightly raised, after 20 months she was started on a combined oral contraceptive, but within a month her breasts began to enlarge and become more tender, and after a further six months the penicillamine was replaced by trientine hydrochloride.[2] The reasons are not understood, but the authors of the report suggest that the penicillamine was the prime cause of the macromastia, but it possibly needed the presence of a 'second trigger' (the oral contraceptive) to set things in motion.[2] There are eight other cases of macromastia on record associated with the use of penicillinamine, in some of which the second trigger may possibly have been a corticosteroid or cimetidine.[2] Macromastia appears to be an unusual side-effect of penicillamine and there would seem to be no general reason for patients taking penicillamine to avoid oral contraceptives.

References

1 Seideman P, Lindström B. Pharmacokinetic interactions of penicillamine in rheumatoid arthritis. J Rheumatol (1989) 16, 473–4.
2 Rose BI, Le Maire WJ, Jeffers LJ. macromastia in a woman treated with penicillamine and oral contraceptives. J Reprod Med (1990) 35, 43–5.

Pentazocine + Amitriptyline

Abstract/Summary

Concurrent use appears not to increase the impairment of psychomotor skills (such as those needed for driving) more than each drug given alone, but respiratory depression is increased.

Clinical evidence, mechanism, importance and management

Eleven normal subjects found that both pentazocine and amitriptyline caused them to feel drowsy, muzzy and clumsy, and both reduced the performance of a number of psychomotor tests. However when they were given 30 mg pentazocine IM after taking amitriptyline 50 mg daily for a week, the combination of drugs appeared not to impair driving or occupational skills more than either drug given alone.[1] Even so, patients should be warned of the side-effects of each drug. Respiratory depression was increased which may be undesirable in patients with a restricted respiratory capacity.[1]

Reference

1 Saarialho-Kere U, Mattila MJ, Sappälä T. Parenteral pentazocine: effects on psychomotor skills and respiration, and interactions with amitriptyline. Eur J Clin Pharmacol (1988) 35, 483–9.

Pentazocine + Tobacco smoking and Environmental pollution

Abstract/Summary

Those who smoke or who live in urban areas where the air is heavily polluted may need about 50% more pentazocine to achieve satisfactory analgesia than those who do not smoke or who live where the air is clean.

Clinical evidence, mechanism, importance and management

A study in which pentazocine was used to supplement nitrous oxide relaxant anaesthesia found that patients who came from an urban environment needed about 50% more pentazocine than those who lived in the country (3.6 compared with 2.4 g/kg/min). Roughly the same difference was seen between those who smoked and those who did not (3.8 compared with 2.5 g/kg/min).[1] In another study it was found that those who smoked metabolized 40% more pentazocine than non-smokers.[2]

The likely reason for these differences is that tobacco smoke and polluted city air contain chemical compounds which act as enzyme inducing agents which increase the rate at which the liver metabolizes pentazocine (and probably other drugs as well). Smokers and urban dwellers from polluted areas may need about 40–50% more pentazocine than country dwellers and non-smokers to achieve the equivalent amount of analgesia.

References

1 Keeri-Szanto M, Pomeroy JR. Atmospheric pollution and pentazocine metabolism. Lancet (1971) i, 947–9.
2 Vaughan DP, Beckett AH, Robbie DS. The influence of smoking on the intersubject variation in pentazocine elimination. Br J clin Pharmac (1976) 3, 279–83.

Pethidine (Meperidine) + Acyclovir

Abstract/Summary

An isolated report describes pethidine toxicity associated with the concurrent use of high dose acyclovir.

Clinical evidence, mechanism, importance and management

A man with Hodgkin's disease was treated with high dose acyclovir for localized herpes zoster, and with pethidine, methadone and carbidopa-levodopa for pain. On the second day he experienced nausea, vomiting and confusion, and later dysarthria, lethargy and ataxia. Despite vigorous treatment he later died. It was concluded that some of the adverse effects were due to pethidine toxicity arising from norpethidine accumulation, associated with renal impairment due to the acyclovir.[1]

Reference

1 Johnson R, Douglas J, Corey L, Krasney H. Adverse effects with acyclovir and meperidine. Ann Intern Med (1985) 103, 962–3.

Pethidine (Meperidine) + Barbiturates

Abstract/Summary

A single case report describes greatly increased sedation with severe CNS toxicity in a woman given pethidine after receiving phenobarbitone for a fortnight.

Clinical evidence

A woman whose pain had been satisfactorily controlled with pethidine without particular CNS depression, showed prolonged sedation with severe CNS toxicity when later given pethidine after being treated with 120 mg phenobarbitone daily for a fortnight as anticonvulsant therapy.[1]

Mechanism

Studies in the patient cited, in four other patients and in two normal subjects revealed that phenobarbitone stimulates the liver enzymes concerned with the metabolism (N-demethylation) of pethidine so that the production of its more toxic metabolite (norpethidine, normeperidine) is increased. The toxicity seen appears to be the combined effects of this compound and the directly sedative effects of the barbiturate.[1,2]

Importance and management

There is only one report of toxicity, but the metabolic changes described under 'Mechanism' were seen in other patients and subjects. The general clinical importance is uncertain but concurrent use should be undertaken with care. Since the metabolic product of pethidine is a less effective analgesic than the parent compound, the depth of analgesia may be reduced. It has also been suggested that if the pethidine is continued but the barbiturate suddenly withdrawn, the toxic concentrations of norpethidine might lead to convulsions in the absence of the anticonvulsant. Whether other barbiturates behave similarly is not clear, but it is possible. More study is needed to confirm these possibilities.

References

1 Stambaugh JE, Wainer IW, Hemphill DM, Schwartz I. A potentially toxic drug interaction between pethidine (meperidine) and phenobarbitone. Lancet (1977) i, 398.
2 Stambaugh JE, Wainer IW, Schwartz I. The effect of phenobarbital on the metabolism of meperidine in normal volunteers. J Clin Pharmacol (1978) 18, 482.

Pethidine (Meperidine) + Chlorpromazine or other Phenothiazines

Abstract/Summary

Pethidine (meperidine) and chlorpromazine can be used together for increased analgesia and for premedication before anaesthesia, but increased respiratory depression, sedation, CNS toxicity and hypotension can also occur. Other phenothiazines such as methotrimeprazine, promethazine, prochlorperazine, propiomazine and thioridazine may also interact to cause some of these effects.

Clinical evidence

A study in six normal subjects found that pethidine alone (100 mg/70 mg body weight) caused respiratory depression whereas chlorpromazine alone (25 mg/70 mg body weight) had no consistent effects. But together the respiratory depressant effects were greater than with pethidine alone. One subject showed marked respiratory depression, beginning about half an hour after receiving both drugs and lasting 2 h.[1]

No change in the pharmacokinetics of pethidine when chlorpromazine was given was found in a single dose study in normal subjects, but the excretion of the metabolites of pethidine was increased. The symptoms of lightheadedness, dry mouth and lethargy were significantly increased and four subjects experienced such marked debilitation that they required assistance to continue the study. Systolic and diastolic blood pressures were also depressed.[2]

A patient on chronic thioridazine treatment (100 mg daily) given premedication with pethidine, diphenhydramine and glycopyrrolate was very lethargic after surgery and stopped breathing. He responded to naloxone.[7] Studies with other phenothiazines have shown that promethazine increases the analgesic effects of pethidine,[3] and both propiomazine[5] and methotrimeprazine[8] can increase its respiratory depressant effects, but the effects of prochlorperazine[4] on respiration were not statistically significant.

Mechanism

There is evidence that chlorpromazine can increase the activity of the liver microsomal enzymes so that the metabolism of pethidine to normeperidine and normeperidinic acid are increased. These are toxic and probably account for the lethargy and hypotension seen in one study.[2] The effects of the phenothiazines on pethidine-induced respiratory depression may be related.

Importance and management

Lower doses of pethidine can be used if chlorpromazine is given,[6] but concurrent use is clearly not without its problems. A marked increase in respiratory depression can occur in some susceptible individuals.[1] The authors of one study offer the opinion that '...the debilitation observed after meperidine-chlorpromazine combinations again raises the question as to whether the clinical use of this combination is justified. The risks of increased CNS toxicity and hypotension outweigh the uncertain advantages, and the use of the combination as an analgesic should probably be discontinued.'[2]

Information about other adverse pethidine-phenothiazine interactions seems to be very limited. The pethidine-thioridazine interaction cited here seems to be the only one recorded.[7] Increased analgesia may occur but it may be accompanied by increased respiratory depression[3,5] which is undesirable in patients with existing respiratory insufficiency. One manufacturer of pethidine (Roche) advises that severe hypotension may take place with phenothiazines, but particular drugs are not named.

References

1 Lambertsen CJ, Wendel H, Longenhagen JB. The separate and combined respiratory effects of chlorpromazine and meperidine in normal men controlled at 46 mm Hg alveolar pCO$_2$. J Pharm Exptl Ther (1961) 131, 381–93.
2 Stambaugh JE, Wainer IW. Drug interaction: meperidine and chlorpromazine, a toxic combination. J Clin Pharmacol (1981) 21, 140.
3 Keeri-Szanto M. The mode of action of promethazine in potentiating narcotic drugs. Br J Anaesth (1974) 46, 918–24.
4 Steen SN, Yates M. The effects of benzquinamide and prochlorperazine separately and combined on the human respiratory centre. Anesthesiology (1972) 36, 519–20.
5 Hoffman JC, Smith TC. The respiratory effects of meperidine and propiomazine in man. Anesthesiology (1970) 32, 325–31.
6 Sadove MS, Levin MJ, Rose RF, Schwartz L, Witt FW. Chlorpromazine and narcotics in the management of pain of malignant lesions. J Amer Med Ass (1954) 155, 626–8.
7 Grothe DR, Ereshefsky L, Jann MW, Fidone GS. Clinical implication of the neuroleptic-opioid interaction. Drug Intell Clin Pharm (1986) 20, 75–7.
8 Zsigmond EK, Flynn K. The effect of methotrimeprazine on arterial blood gases in human volunteers. J Clin Pharmacol (1988) 28, 1033–7.

Pethidine (Meperidine) + Cimetidine or Ranitidine

Abstract/Summary

Cimetidine reduces the loss of pethidine from the body, but the extent to which this increases its analgesic and toxic effects is uncertain. It is probably not large. Ranitidine does not interact.

Clinical evidence

1200 mg cimetidine for week reduced the total body clearance of single 70 mg intravenous doses of pethidine in eight subjects by 22%.[1]

Mechanism

The probable reason is that the cimetidine inhibits the liver microsomal enzymes concerned with metabolism of the pethidine, because it was found that the production of the normal metabolite of pethidine, norpethidine, was reduced by 23%.[1] This is supported by other studies with both animal and human liver microsomes.[2]

Importance and management

Information about the pethidine/cimetidine interaction is very limited, and its clinical importance is uncertain. Since the effects of the pethidine, both analgesic and toxic, would be expected to be increased to some extent, concurrent use should be monitored. An alternative would be to use ranitidine which has been shown not to interact.[3]

References

1 Guay DRP, Meatherall RC, Chalmers JL, Grahame GR. Cimetidine alters pethidine disposition in man. Br J clin Pharmac (1984) 18, 907–14.
2 Knodell RG, Holtzman JL, Crankshaw DL, Steele NM, Stanley LN. Drug metabolism by rat and human hepatic microsomes in response to interaction with H$_2$-receptor antagonists. Gastroenterology (1982) 82, 84–8.
3 Guay DRP, Meatherall RC, Chalmers JL, Grahame GR, Hudson RJ. Ranitidine does not alter pethidine disposition in man. Br J clin Pharmac (1985) 20, 55–9.

Pethidine (Meperidine) + Furazolidine

Abstract/Summary

On the basis of animal experiments it has been suggested that if pethidine and furazolidone are used concurrently in man, a serious hyperpyrexic reaction may occur similar to that seen with the antidepressant MAOI. This has yet to be confirmed.

Clinical evidence, mechanism, importance and management

Fatal hyperpyrexia follows the injection of pethidine in rabbits given oral furazolidone for 4 days.[1] On the basis of this observation, linked with the known MAO-inhibitory properties of furazolidone in man[2] and the well-documented MAOI-pethidine interaction in man, there would seem to be the possibility of some risk if these two drugs are used together. More study is needed to find out if this is a clinically important interaction.

References

1 Eltayeb IB, Osman OH. Furazolidine-pethidine interactions in rabbits. Br J Pharmac (1975) 55, 497.
2 Pettinger WA, Soyangio FG, Oates JA. Monoamine oxidase inhibition by furazolidine in man. Clin Res (1966) 14, 258.

Pethidine (Meperidine) + Phenytoin

Abstract/Summary

An isolated report describes pethidine toxicity in a man taking phenytoin. Other studies confirm that phenytoin increases the production of the toxic metabolite of pethidine.

Clinical evidence

A man of 61 who was addicted to pethidine (5–10 g weekly) is reported to have developed repeated seizures and myoclonus despite, even possibly because, he was also taking phenytoin (see Mechanism below). The problem resolved when both drugs were stopped.[3]

Mechanism

It is known that phenytoin increases the production of nor-meperidine, the metabolic product of pethidine which is believed to be responsible for the neurotoxicity of pethidine (seizures, myoclonus, tremors etc). Studies[1,2] in normal subjects found that 300 mg phenytoin daily for nine days decreased the elimination half-life of pethidine (100 mg orally and 50 mg IV) from 6.4 to 4.3 h, and the systemic clearance increased from 14.3 to 18.2 ml/min/kg. Phenytoin is a well recognized and potent enzyme inducing agent.

Importance and management

This seems to be only report[3] of an adverse pethidine/phenytoin interaction so that its general importance is uncertain, however it would be prudent to monitor concurrent use in any patient. Since the studies cited[1,2] found that pethidine given orally produced more of the toxic metabolite (normeperidine) than when given intravenously, it may be preferable to give pethidine intravenously in patients taking phenytoin.

References

1 Pond SM, Kretzschmar KM. Decreased bioavailability and increased clearance of meperidine during phenytoin administration. Clin Pharmacol Ther (1981) 29, 273.
2 Pond SM, Kretzschmar KM. Effect of phenytoin on meperidine clearance and normeperidine formation. Clin Pharmacol Ther (1981) 30, 680.
3 Hochman MS. Meperidine-associated myoclonus and seizures in long-term hemodialysis patients. Ann Neurol (1983) 14, 593.

Phenazone (Antipyrine) + Miscellaneous drugs

Abstract/Summary

Changes in the half-life of phenazone (reduced by liver enzyme-inducers, prolonged by liver enzyme-inhibitors) are used to detect the possible effects of drugs on liver enzyme activity.

Clinical evidence, mechanism, importance and management

Phenazone (antipyrine) is metabolized by mixed function oxidase enzymes in the liver, for which reason it is extensively used as a model drug for studying whether other drugs stimulate (induce) or inhibit liver enzymes. For example, barbiturates reduce the half-life of phenazone. In one study amylobarbitone caused a 42% reduction thereby demonstrating that the liver enzymes were being stimulated to metabolize the phenazone more rapidly.[1] In contrast, other drugs which are enzyme inhibitors cause the half-life of phenazone to be prolonged which shows that the activity of the metabolizing enzymes is reduced. Equally it may be that the drug neither stimulates nor inhibits the enzymes which metabolize phenazone (for example, spiramycin[2]).

Thus phenazone often features in drug interaction studies because it provides predictive information about whether a particular drug is likely or not to stimulate or inhibit the metabolism of other drugs, but phenazone itself has only a minor role to play as an analgesic and antipyretic.

References

1 Vesell ES, Page JG. Genetic control of the phenobarbital-induced shortening of plasma antipyrine half-lives in man. J Clin Invest (1969) 48, 220.
2 Descotes J, Evreux J Cl. Drug interactions with spiramycin: lack of influence on antipyrine pharmacokinetics. Chimioterapia (1987) 6, 337–8.

Phenoperidine + Antacids

Abstract/Summary

An antacid has been shown to increase the serum levels of phenoperidine given intravenously.

Clinical evidence

Andursil (aluminium and magnesium hydroxides, magnesium carbonate, dimethicone) considerably increased the serum levels of phenoperidine in six normal subjects over the 20 min period following a 15 /kg IV dose. The peak level rose 60% (from 9.1 to 14.7 ng/ml) but fell after 20 min to about the same levels. The AUC (area under the curve) over this period was increased by 47%. The secondary peaks in the plasma concentrations were also ironed out.[1]

Mechanism

Uncertain. A possible reason is that changes in gastric pH caused by the antacid may alter the secretion of phenoperidine in the stomach (this also occurs with pethidine).

Importance and management

The clinical significance of this study is uncertain, but it seems possible that in the presence of antacids there may be an increase in both the analgesic and respiratory depressant effects of phenoperidine. More study is needed.

Reference

1 Calvey TN, Milne LA, Williams NE, Chan K, Murray GR. Effect of antacids on the plasma concentration of phenoperidine. Br J Anesth (1983) 55, 535–9.

Phenoperidine + Beta-blockers

Abstract/Summary

An isolated report describes a patient with tetanus who showed a very marked fall in blood pressure when given phenoperidine following a dose of propranolol.

Clinical evidence, mechanism, importance and management

A patient with tetanus was treated uneventfully with 2 mg phenoperidine on five occasions over 24 h. Later 2 mg propranolol IV was used to reduce the heart rate from 150 to 120 beats per minute, without any fall in blood pressure. When 2 mg phenoperidine was subsequently given, the systolic blood pressure fell to 30 mm Hg (heart rate 100–120 bpm) and this persisted for 5–10 min until reversed by naloxone.[1] The reasons for this marked hypotensive response are not understood. The general importance of this is uncertain because this incident occurred in the context of tetanus.

Reference

1 Woods KL. Hypotensive effect of propranolol and phenoperidine in tetanus. Br Med J (1978) 2, 1164.

Phenylbutazone + Allopurinol

Abstract/Summary

Allopurinol appears not to interact significantly with phenylbutazone.

Clinical evidence, mechanism, importance and management

The daily administration of 300 mg allopurinol to six normal subjects for a month had no effect on the elimination of a 200 mg daily dose of phenylbutazone, and no effect on the steady-state serum levels of phenylbutazone in three patients taking 200 or 300 mg daily.[1] In another study on six patients with acute gouty arthritis it was found that 300 mg allopurinol produced small but clinically unimportant effects on the half-life of phenylbutazone (6 mg/kg).[2] No special precautions would seem necessary if both drugs are given.

References

1 Rawlins MD, Smith SE. Influence of allopurinol on drug metabolism in man. Br J Pharmac (1973) 48, 693.
2 Horwitz D, Thorgeirsson SS, Mitchell JR. The influence of allopurinol and size of dose on the metabolism of phenylbutazone in patients with gout. Eur J Clin Pharmacol (1977) 12, 133.

Phenylbutazone + Barbiturates

Abstract/Summary

Some reduction in the serum levels of phenylbutazone may be expected if phenobarbitone is given concurrently, but the practical importance of this is uncertain.

Clinical evidence, mechanism, importance and management

The half-life of phenylbutazone is reduced (from 78 to 57 h) by the concurrent use of 90 mg phenobarbitone daily.[1] Other studies confirm that it increases the loss of phenylbutazone from the body.[2,3] The probable reason is that the phenobarbitone increases the metabolism of phenylbutazone by the liver, thereby hastening its clearance.

The clinical importance of this interaction is uncertain (probably small) but be alert for any evidence of reduced phenylbutazone effects if phenobarbitone is added. Other barbiturates are likely to behave similarly because they are all potent enzyme inducing agents.

References

1 Levi AJ, Sherlock S, Walker D. Phenylbutazone and isoniazid metabolism in patients with liver disease in relation to previous drug therapy. Lancet (1968) i, 1275.

2 Whittaker JA, Price Evans DA. Genetic control of phenylbutazone metabolism in man. Br Med J (1970) 3, 323.
3 Anderson KE, Peterson CM, Alvares AP, Kappas A. Oxidative drug metabolism and inducibility by phenobarbital in sickle cell anaemia. Clin Pharmacol Ther (1977) 22, 580.

Phenylbutazone + Cholestyramine

Abstract/Summary

Animal studies suggest that cholestyramine may delay the absorption of phenylbutazone, but the clinical importance of this is uncertain.

Clinical evidence, mechanism, importance and management

An *in vitro* study found that phenylbutazone becomes markedly bound (98%) to cholestyramine.[1] In rats it was found that 71.5 mg/kg and 357.5 mg/kg cholestyramine reduced phenylbutazone absorption by 32% and 49% respectively after 1 h, and by 22% and 47% after 2 h, but after 4 h the lower dose group showed a 29% increase in absorption and the higher dose group was the same as the control.[1] These results indicate that cholestyramine reduces the rate of absorption of phenylbutazone initially, however the total amount absorbed was not measured. Nobody seems to have checked on this interaction in man, but until more is known it would seem reasonable, and easy, to separate the dosages as much as possible to prevent admixture in the gut.

Reference

1 Gallo DG, Bailey KR, Sheffner A L. The interaction between cholestyramine and drugs. Proc Soc Exp Biol Med (1965) 120, 60–5.

Phenylbutazone + Indomethacin

Abstract/Summary, clinical evidence, mechanism, importance and management

An isolated report describes transient deterioration in renal function in a patient during recovery from phenylbutazone-induced renal failure when given 25 mg indomethacin three times a day.[1] A possible reason is that the indomethacin displaced the residual phenylbutazone from its plasma protein binding sites.[2] This possible interaction does not seem to be of general importance.

References

1 Kimberly R, Brandstetter RD. Exacerbation of phenylbutazone-related renal failure by indomethacin. Arch Intern Med (1978) 138, 1711.
2 Solomon HM, Schrogie JJ, Williams D. The displacement of phenylbutazone-^{14}C and warfarin-^{14}C from human albumin by various drugs and fatty acids. Biochem Pharmacol (1968) 17, 143.

Phenylbutazone + Methylphenidate

Abstract/Summary

Serum phenylbutazone levels are raised by methylphenidate.

Clinical evidence, mechanism, importance and management

Single dose and chronic studies in man using normal daily doses of phenylbutazone (200–400 mg) and methylphenidate showed that serum phenylbutazone levels were significantly increased in five out of six subjects, due, it is suggested to inhibition of liver metabolizing enzymes.[1] The clinical importance of this is uncertain.

Reference

1 Dayton PG, Perel JM, Israili ZH, Faraj BA, Rodewig K, Black N, Goldberg LI. Studies with methylphenidate: drug interactions and metabolism. Int Symp Alc Drug Addiction. Toronto, Ontario, October 1973. (Ed Sellers, EM) Clinical Pharmacology of Psychoactive Drugs, Addiction Res Foundation. ISBN-0-88868-007-4, pages 183–202.

Phenylbutazone + Pesticides

Abstract/Summary

Chronic exposure to lindane and other chlorinated pesticides can increase the rate of metabolism of phenylbutazone.

Clinical evidence, mechanism, importance and management

The plasma half-life of phenylbutazone in a group of men who regularly used chlorinated insecticide sprays (mainly lindane) as part of their work, was found to be shorter (51 h) than in a control group (64 h), due, it is believed, to the enzyme-inducing effects of the insecticides.[1] This is of doubtful direct clinical importance, but it illustrates the changed metabolism which can occur in those exposed to environmental chemical agents.

Reference

1 Kolomodin-Hedman B. Decreased plasma half-life of phenylbutazone in workers exposed to chlorinated pesticides. Eur J clin Pharmacol (1973) 5, 195.

Phenylbutazone + Tobacco smoking

Abstract/Summary

The loss of phenylbutazone from the body is greater in smokers than in non-smokers.

Clinical evidence, mechanism, importance and management

The half-life of a single dose of phenylbutazone was 37 h in a group of smokers (10 or more cigarettes daily for 2 years) compared with 64 h in a group of non-smokers. The metabolic clearance was approximately doubled.[1] The conclusion to be drawn is that those who smoke may possibly need larger or more frequent doses of phenylbutazone to achieve the same therapeutic response, but this needs confirmation.

Reference

1 Garg SK, Kiran TNR. Effect of smoking on phenylbutazone disposition. Int J Clin Pharmacol Ther Toxicol (1983) 20, 289–90.

Phenylbutazone or Oxyphenbutazone + Tricyclic antidepressants

Abstract/Summary

The tricyclic antidepressants can delay the absorption of phenylbutazone and oxyphenbutazone from the gut, but their antirheumatic effects are probably not affected.

Clinical evidence, mechanism, importance and management

When treated with 75 mg desipramine daily the absorption of phenylbutazone in four depressed women was considerably delayed, but the total amount absorbed (measured by the urinary excretion of oxyphenbutazone) remained unchanged.[1] In another five depressed women the half-life of oxyphenbutazone was found to be unaltered by 75 mg desipramine or nortriptyline daily.[2] Animal studies have confirmed that the absorption of phenylbutazone and oxyphenbutazone are delayed by the tricyclic antidepressants, probably because their anticholinergic effects reduce the motility of the gut,[3,4] but there seems to be no direct clinical evidence that the antirheumatic effects of either drug are reduced by this interaction. No particular precautions appear to be needed.

References

1 Consolo S, Morselli M, Zaccala M, Garattini S. Delayed absorption of phenylbutazone caused by desmethylimipramine in humans. Eur J Pharmacol (1970) 10, 239.
2 Hammer W, Martens S, Sjoqvist F. A comparative study of the metabolism of desmethylimipramine, nortriptyline and oxyphenbutazone in man. Clin Pharmacol Ther (1969) 10, 44.
3 Consolo S. An interaction between desipramine and phenylbutazone. J Pharm Pharmac (1968) 20, 574.
4 Consolo S and Garattini S. Effect of desipramine on intestinal absorption of phenylbutazone and other drugs. Eur J Pharmacol (1969) 6, 322.

Piroxicam + Antacids

Abstract/Summary, clinical evidence, mechanism, importance and management

A multiple dose study found that *Mylanta* and *Amphojel* did not significantly affect the bioavailability of piroxicam.[1] Concurrent use need not be avoided.

Reference

1 Hobbs DC, Twomey TM. Piroxicam pharmacokinetics in man: aspirin and antacid interaction studies. J Clin Pharmacol (1979) 270–81.

Piroxicam and Tenoxicam + Cholestyramine

Abstract/Summary

Cholestyramine increases the loss of both piroxicam and tenoxicam from the body and their therapeutic effects would be expected to be reduced accordingly.

Clinical evidence

A study on the enterohepatic recycling of these two analgesics in eight normal subjects found that when given 4 g cholestyramine three times a day, the clearances of 20 mg oral doses of piroxicam and 20 mg IV doses of tenoxicam were increased by 52% and 105% respectively, and their half-lives reduced by 40 and 52% respectively. The cholestyramine was not given until after the piroxicam had been absorbed.[1]

Another similar study confirmed these findings.[2] The elimination of both analgesics was approximately doubled by 24 g cholestyramine daily.[2]

Mechanism

Cholestyramine binds with other drugs in the gut. Since the cholestyramine was not given until the piroxicam had been absorbed and the tenoxicam was given intravenously,[1] it would seem probable that the cholestyramine binds with these drugs following their excretion in the bile, thereby preventing their reabsorption and increasing their loss.

Importance and management

Direct information appears to be limited to this study. Unlike the situation with a number of other drugs, this interaction can be reduced but not avoided by separating the dosages. Monitor the effects of concurrent use and increase the dosage of the piroxicam or tenoxicam as necessary. Alternatively use other NSAID's or hypolipidaemic drugs. Cholestyramine can be used

to speed the removal of piroxicam and tenoxicam following overdosage.[1,2]

Reference

1 Guentert TS, Defoin R, Mosberg H. Accelerated elimination of tenoxicam and piroxicam by cholestyramine. Clin Pharmacol Ther (1988) 43, 179.
2 Benveniste C, Striberni R, Dayer P. Indirect assessment of the enterohepatic recirculation of piroxicam and tenoxicam. Eur J Clin Pharmacol (1990) 38, 547–9.

Sulindac + Dimethyl sulfoxide (DMSO)

Abstract/Summary

A single case report describes a patient on sulindac who developed a serious peripheral neuropathy when he applied DMSO to his skin.

Clinical evidence, mechanism, importance and management

A man with a long history of degenerative arthritis was treated uneventfully with 400 mg sulindac daily for six months until, without his doctor's knowledge, he began regularly to apply a topical preparation containing 90% DMSO to his upper and lower extremities. Soon afterwards he began to experience pain, weakness in all his extremities, and difficulty in standing or walking. He was found to have both segmental demyelination and axonal neuropathy. He made a partial recovery but was unable to walk without an artificial aid.[1] The reason for this reaction is not known, but studies in rats have shown that DMSO can inhibit a reductase enzyme by which sulindac is metabolized,[2] and it may be that the high concentrations of unmetabolized sulindac increased the neurotoxic activity of the DMSO. Although there is only this case on record, its seriousness suggests that patients should not use sulindac and DMSO-containing preparations concurrently.

References

1 Reinstein L, Mahon R, Russo GL. Peripheral neuropathy after concomitant dimethylsulfoxide use and sulindac therapy. Arch Phys Med Rehabil (1982) 63, 581–4.
2 Swanson BN, Mojaverian P, Boppana VK, Dudash M. Dimethyl sulfoxide (DMSO) interaction with sulindac (SO). Pharmacologist (1981) 23, 196.

Sulphasalazine + Cimetidine

Abstract/Summary

Cimetidine does not interact with sulphasalazine.

Clinical evidence, mechanism, importance and management

A study in 14 patients with rheumatoid arthritis treated with sulphasalazine, nine also given 400 mg cimetidine three times daily, found that cimetidine for 18 weeks did not affect the plasma or urinary levels of the sulphasalazine and there were no changes in blood cell counts or haemoglobin levels. The conclusion was reached that no clinically important interaction occurs between these two drugs.[1]

Reference

1 Pirmohamed M, Coleman MD, Galvani D, Bucknall RC, Breckenridge AM, Park BK. Lack of interaction between sulphasalazine and cimetidine in patients with rheumatoid arthritis. Br J Rheumatol (1993) 32, 222–6.

Tenoxicam + Antacids

Abstract/Summary

Food and antacids appear not have a clinically important effect on the absorption of tenoxicam.

Clinical evidence, mechanism, importance and management

The bioavailability of 20 mg tenoxicam was found to be unaffected in 12 subjects by aluminium hydroxide (*Amphojel*) or aluminium/magnesium hydroxide (*Mylanta*) whether taken before, at the same time, or afterwards. Food delayed the achievement of peak serum levels.[1] No special precautions seem necessary.

Reference

1 Day RO, Lam S, Paull P, Wade D. Effect of food and various antacids on the absorption of tenoxicam. Br J clin Pharmac (1987) 24, 323–8.

Chapter 4
Antiarrhythmic Drug Interactions

This chapter is concerned with the Class I antiarrhythmic agents which possess some local anaesthetic properties, and with Class III drugs. Antiarrhythmic agents which fall into other classes are dealt with in the chapters devoted to specific groups of drugs (Beta-blockers, see Chapter 10; Calcium channel blockers, see Chapter 11; Digitalis Glycosides, see Chapter 14; (see also Table 4.2). Interactions in which the antiarrhythmic drug is the affecting agent, rather than the drug whose activity is altered, are dealt with in other chapters. Consult the Index for a full listing.

Table 4.1 Antiarrhythmic agents

Non-proprietary names	Proprietary names	Non-proprietary names	Proprietary names
Adenosine	*Ajmaline Aritmina, Cardiorhythmine, Gilurytmal, Nororytmina*	Pirmenol	
Amiodarone	*Atlansil, Coronovo, Cordarone (X), Trangorex*	Procainimide	*Bicoryl, Novacamid, Procamide, Procainamid Duriles, Procainamide Durettes, Procan SR, Procapan, Pronestyl*
Aprindine	*Amidonal, Fibocil, Fiboran*	Propafenone	—
Bretylium	*Bretylate, Bretylol*	Quinidine	*Biquin, Cardioquin(e), Chinidin-Duriles, Cin-Quin, Duraquin, Galactoquin, Galatturil-Chinidina, Gluquile, Kiditard, Kinichron, Kinidine Durettes, Kinidin Durules, Kinilentin, Longachin, Longacor, Naticardina, Natisedina, Natisedine, Neochinidin, Prosedyl, Optochinidin retard, Quinaglute, Quinate, Quincardina, Quinicardine, Quinidex, Quinidoxin, Quini Durules, Quinidurile, Quinobarb, Quinora, Ritmocor, Sedoquin, Systodin*
Cibenzoline (cifenline)	*Disopyramide Dicorynan, Dirythmin SA, Durbis, Norpace, Norpaso, Rhythmodan, Ritmodan, Ritmoforine, Rythmodul*		
Encainide	—		
Flecainide	—		
Lignocaine (lidocaine)	—		
Lorcainide	*Remivox*		
Mexiletine	*Mexitil*	Tocainide	*Tonocard*
Moricizine (ethmo(z/sine)			

Table 4.2 Modified Vaughan-Williams classification of the oral antiarrhythmic drugs

Class I: Membrane stabilizing drugs
    (a) Quinidine, procainamide, disopyramide
    (b) Lignocaine, Mexiletine, tocainide, phenytoin
    (c) Encainide, flecainide, propafenone
Difficult to classify — moricizine

Class II: Beta blockers
    Propranolol, atenolol

Class III: Inhibitors of depolarization
    Amiodarone, bretylium, sotalol

Class IV: Calcium channel blockers
    Verapamil, diltiazem

Adenosine + Caffeine, Nicotine, Theophylline

Abstract/Summary

On theoretical grounds both caffeine and theophylline might oppose the antiarrhythmic effects of adenosine. Nicotine appears to increase its circulatory effects.

Clinical evidence, mechanism, importance and management

(a) Caffeine, enprofylline, theophylline.

Experimental studies in man on the way xanthine drugs possibly interact with adenosine showed that caffeine and theophylline, but not enprofylline, reduce the increase in heart rate and the rise in systolic blood pressure caused by infusions of adenosine.[1–3] They appear to have opposite effects (vasoconstriction or vasodilation) on the circulatory system.[4] On theoretical grounds caffeine and theophylline might also possibly oppose the effects of adenosine used, for example, as an antiarrhythmic agent but this awaits clinical confirmation. Be alert for the need to use more adenosine in patients taking either of these drugs. One study concluded that adenosine infusion is unlikely to be of value in the management of theophylline toxicity.[6] More study is needed.

(b) Nicotine

2 mg nicotine chewing gum increased the circulatory effects of 0.07 mg/kg/min adenosine IV in 10 normal subjects. The increase in the heart rate rose from 5.5 to 14.9 beats/min while the diastolic pressure rise was reduced from 4.0 to 1.0 mm Hg.[5] What this means in practical terms is uncertain, but be aware that the effects of adenosine on the circulation may be modified to some extent by nicotine-containing products (tobacco smoking, nicotine gum, etc).

References

1 Smits P, Schouten J, Thien T. Cardiovascular effects of two xanthines and the relation to adenosine antagonism. Clin Pharmacol Ther (1989) 45, 593–9.
2 Smits P, Boekma P, De Abreu R, Thien T, van 't Laar A. Evidence for an antagonism between caffeine and adenosine in the human cardiovascular system. J Cardiovasc Pharmaco (1987) 10, 136–43.
3 Taddei S, Salvetti A, Pedrinelli R. Theophylline antagonizes the vasorelaxant action of adenosine in human forearm arterioles of hypertensive patients. Clin Pharmacol Ther (1990) 47, 144.
4 Fredholm BB. On the mechanism of action of theophylline and caffeine. Acta Med Scand (1985) 217, 149–53.
5 Smits P, Eijsbouts A, Thien T. Nicotine enhances the circulatory effects of adenosine in human beings. Clin Pharmacol Ther)1989) 46, 272–8.
6 Minton NA, Henry JA. Pharmacodynamic interactions between infused adosine and oral theophylline. Hum Exptl Toxicol (1991) 10, 411–8.

Adenosine + Dipyridamole

Abstract/Summary

Dipyridamole markedly reduces the dosage of adenosine necessary to control supraventricular tachycardia.

Clinical evidence

Adenosine by rapid IV bolus (10–200 µg/kg in stepwise doses) was found to restore sinus rhythm in 10 of 14 episodes of tachycardia in seven patients with supraventricular tachycardia. The mean dose was 8.8 mg compared with only 1.0 mg in two patients also taking oral dipyridamole.[1] Another study in six patients found that dipyridamole (0.56 mg/kg IV bolus, followed by a continuous infusion of 5 µg/kg/min) reduced fourfold the minimum effective dose of adenosine (from 68 to 17 µg/kg) to stop supraventricular tachycardia.[4]

Other studies in normal subjects have clearly shown that dipyridamole increases the cardiovascular effects of adenosine,[2,3] and increases its plasma levels.[5] A brief report describes a woman on dipyridamole (dosage not stated) with paroxysmal supraventricular tachcardia who lost ventricular activity for 18 s when given 6 mg adenosine IV.[6]

Mechanism

Not fully understood. Part of the explanation is that dipyridamole increases plasma levels of endogenous adenosine by inhibiting its uptake into cells.

Importance and management

An established interaction. Patients will need less adenosine to treat arrhythmias while taking dipyridamole. A four-fold reduction is suggested by one study.[4] Another report advises a dosage reduction from the usual 6 mg bolus dose initially to 3 mg adenosine in patients on dipyridamole.[6]

References

1 Watt AH, Bernard MS, Webster J, Passani SL, Stephens MR, Routledge PA. Intravenous adenosine in the treatment of supraventricular tachycardia: a dose-ranging study and interaction with dipyridamole. Br J clin Pharmac (1986) 21, 227–30.
2 Conradson T-BG, Dixon CMS, Clarke B, Barnes PJ. Cardiovascular effects of infused adenosine in man: potentiation by dipyridamole. Acta Physiol Scand (1987) 129, 387–91.
3 Biaggioni I, Onrot J, Hollister AS, Robertson D. Cardiovascular effects of adenosine infusion in man and their modulation by dipyridamole. Life Sci (1986) 39, 2229–36.
4 Lerman BB, Wesley RC, Belardinelli L. Electrophysiologic effects of dipyridamole on atrioventricular nodal conduction and supraventricular tachycardia. Role of endogenous adenosine. Circulation (1989) 80, 1536–43.
5 German DC, Kredich NM, Bjornsson TD. Oral dipyridamole increases plasma adenosine levels in human beings. Clin Pharmacol Ther (1989) 45, 80–4.
6 Mader TJ. Adenosine adverse interactions. Ann Emerg Med (1992) 21, 453.

Ajmaline + Miscellaneous drugs

Abstract/Summary

An isolated report describes cardiac failure in a patient given ajmaline and lignocaine concurrently. Quinidine causes a very considerable increase in the serum levels of ajmaline, and phenobarbitone appears to cause a marked reduction.

Clinical evidence, mechanism, importance and management

A woman of 67 showed marked aggravation of cardiac failure when treated with ajmaline orally and lignocaine intravenously for repeated ventricular tachycardias.[1] A study in four normal subjects found that if a single 200 mg oral dose of quinidine was given with a single 50 mg oral dose of ajmaline, the AUC (area under the curve) of ajmaline was increased 10- to 30-fold and the maximal serum concentrations increased from 0.018 to 0.141 g/ml.[2] Another study found that the metabolism of ajmaline was inhibited by quinidine, possibly because the quinidine becomes competitively bound to the metabolizing enzymes.[3] Yet another study found that phenobarbitone had the opposite effect and increased the clearance of ajmaline up to five times, so that its clinical effects would be expected to be markedly diminished.[4] The clinical importance of all of these interactions is uncertain but concurrent use should be well monitored.

References

1 Bleifeld W. Side effects of antiarrhythmics. Naunyn Schmiedbergs Arch Pharmakol (1971) 269, 282–97.
2 Hori R, Okumura K, Inui K-I, Yasuhara M, Yamada K, Sakurai T, Kawai C. Quinidine-induced rise in ajmaline plasma concentration. J Pharm Pharmacol (1984) 36, 205–7.
3 Köppel C, Tenczer J, Arndt I. Metabolic disposition of ajmaline. Eur J Drug Metab Pharmacokinet (1989) 14, 309–16.
4 Köppel C, Wagemann A, Martens F. Pharmacokinetics and antiarrhythmic efficacy of intravenous ajmaline in ventricular arrhythmia of acute onset. Eur J Drug Metab Pharmacokinet (1989) 14, 161–7.

Amiodarone + Anaesthetics

Abstract/Summary

There is evidence that the presence of amiodarone possibly increases the risk of complications and death during general anaesthesia.

Clinical evidence, mechanism, importance and management

One study reported that there is no increased risk if patients on amiodarone undergo general anaesthesia[1] whereas three others suggest that severe intra-operative complications may

occur.[2–4] A comparative retrospective review of patients undergoing cardio-pulmonary bypass surgery (16 patients with and 30 without amiodarone) showed that the incidence of slow nodal rhythm, complete heart block or pacemaker dependency rose from 17 to 66%. Intra-aortic balloon pump augmentation was 7% compared with 50%, and low SVR and high cardiac output rose from 0 to 13%. Mortality was 19% in the amiodarone group and 0% in the control group. Fentanyl and diazepam were used for most of the patients, but other anaesthetics included isoflurane, enflurane and halothane. Another study of 37 patients found no problems with eight non-cardiac surgery patients, but 29 cardiac surgery patients had dysrhythmic complications (52%), sometimes necessitating a pacemaker (24%). One patient had fatal vasoplegia after cardio-pulmonary bypass.[5] The authors of this report note that amiodarone persists in the body for many weeks which complicates any decision to withdraw the drug since there may be risks in delaying surgery. More study is needed.

References

1 Elliott PL, Schauble JF, Rogers MC, Reid PR. Risk of decompensation during anesthesia in the presence of amiodarone. Circulation (1983) 68, Suppl III-280.
2 Gallagher JD, Lieberman RW, Meranze J, Spielman SR, Ellison N. Amiodarone-induced complications during coronary artery surgery. Anesthesiology (1981) 55, 186–8.
3 MacKinnon G, Landymore R, Marble A. Should oral amiodarone be used for sustained ventricular tachycardia in patients requiring open-heart surgery? Can J Surg (1983) 26, 355–7.
4 Liberman BA, Teasdale SJ. Anesthesia and amiodarone. Can Anaesth Soc J (1985) 32, 629–38.
5 Van Dyck M, Baele Ph, Rennotte M Th, Matta A, Dion R, Kestens-Servaye Y. Should amiodarone by discontinued before cardiac surgery? Acta Anaesth Belg (1988) 39, 5–10.

Amiodarone + Beta-blockers

Abstract/Summary

Hypotension, bradycardia, ventricular fibrillation and asystole have been seen in a few patients given amiodarone with propranolol, metoprolol or sotalol.

Clinical evidence

A woman of 64 was treated for hypertrophic cardiomyopathy with amiodarone (1200 mg daily) and atenolol (50 mg daily). Five days later the atenolol was replaced by metoprolol (100 mg daily). Within 3 h she complained of dizziness, weakness and blurred vision. On examination she was found to be pale and sweating with a pulse rate of 20. Her systolic pressure was 60 mm Hg. She responded to atropine and isoprenaline (isoproterenol).[1] Severe hypotension has been reported in another patient on sotalol when given amiodarone.[4] Another report describes two cases of cardiac arrest in patients on amiodarone shortly after starting to take propranolol.[2] One developed ventricular fibrillation and the other asystole.

Mechanism

Not understood. The clinical picture is that of excessive beta-blockade. A possible explanation is that the amiodarone reduces the metabolism of some beta-blockers (propranolol, metoprolol) thereby markedly increasing their bradycardial effects which are additive with those of amiodarone. The effects of atenolol perhaps remained unaltered because it is largely cleared in the urine unchanged. Other pharmacodynamic effects may also come into play. Increased bradycardia and EEG changes have been seen with amiodarone and practolol.[3]

Importance and management

Concurrent use is not uncommon and may be therapeutically useful but the reports of adverse reactions cited here (they seem to be the only ones so far documented) emphasize the need for caution. Beta-blockers which are extensively metabolized by the liver (e.g. propranolol, metoprolol) may possibly be more risky than those which are not.

References

1 Leor J, Levartowsky D, Sharon C, Farvel Z. Amiodarone and beta-adrenergic blockers: an interaction with metoprolol but not with atenolol. Amer Heart J (1988) 116, 206–7.
2 Derrida JP, Ollagnier J, Benaim R, Haiat R, Chiche P. Amiodarone et propranolol; une association dangereuse? Nouv Presse Med (1979) 8, 1429.
3 Antonelli G, Cristallo E, Cesario S, Calabrese P. Modificazioni elettrocardiografiche indotte dalla somministrazione di amiodarone associato a practololo. Boll Soc Ital Cardiol (1973) 18, 236.
4 Warren R, Vohra J, Hunt D, Hamer A. Serious interactions of sotalol with amiodarone and flecainide. Med J Aust (1990) 152, 277.

Amiodarone + Calcium channel blockers

Abstract/Summary

Sinus arrest and serious hypotension occurred in a woman on diltiazem when given amiodarone.

Clinical evidence, mechanism, importance and management

A woman with compensated congestive heart failure, paroxysmal atrial fibrillation and ventricular arrhythmias was treated with frusemide and 90 mg diltiazem 6-hourly. Four days after starting additional treatment with amiodarone, 600 mg 12-hourly, she developed sinus arrest and a life-threatening low cardiac output state (systolic pressure 80 mm Hg) with oliguria. Both drugs were stopped and she was treated with pressor drugs and ventricular pacing. She had previously had no problems on diltiazem or verapamil alone, and later she did well on 400 mg amiodarone daily without diltiazem. The reason for this reaction is thought to be the additive effects of both drugs on myocardial contractility, and on sinus and atrioventricular nodal function.[1] Before this isolated case report was published, another author predicted this interaction on theoretical grounds and warned of the risks if dysfunction of the sinus node such as bradycardia or sick sinus syndrome is suspected, or if partial AV block exists.[2] Other calcium channel blockers such as verapamil could possibly interact similarly. Monitor concurrent use well.

References

1 Lee TH, Friedman PL, Goldman L, Stone PH, Antman EM. Sinus arrest and hypotension with combined amiodarone-diltiazem. Am Heart J (1985) 109, 163–4.
2 Marcus FI. Drug interactions with amiodarone. Am Heart J (1983) 106, 924–30.

Amiodarone + Carbimazole

Abstract/Summary

Carbimazole is effective in controlling amiodarone-induced thyrotoxicosis.

Clinical evidence, mechanism, importance and management

Five patients with amiodarone-induced thyrotoxicosis (100–200 mg daily) were successfully treated with carbimazole (20–60 mg daily) while continuing to take amiodarone.[1] Previous studies failed to find carbimazole effective.[2,3] Concurrent use need not be avoided.

References

1 Davies PH, Franklyn JA, Sheppard MC. Treatment of amiodarone induced thyrotoxicosis with carbimazole alone and continuation of amiodarone. Br Med J (1992) 305, 224–5.
2 Gammage MD, Franklyn JA. Amiodarone and the thyroid. Quart J med (1987) 283, 83–6.
3 Martino E, Aghini-Lombardi F, Mariotti S, Bartakeba K, Braverman L, Pinchera A. Amiodarone: a common source of amiodarone-induced thyrotoxicosis. Hormone Res (1987) 26, 158–71.

Amiodarone + Cholestyramine

Abstract/Summary

Cholestyramine binds with amiodarone within the gut and reduces its absorption.

Clinical evidence, mechanism, importance and management

When four 4 g doses of cholestyramine were given to 11 patients at 1.5 h intervals after a single 400 mg dose of amiodarone, the serum amiodarone levels 7 h later were depressed by about 50%. The amiodarone half-life was approximately halved.[1]

Mechanism

The probable reason is that the cholestyramine binds with the amiodarone in the gut, thereby reducing its absorption.[1]

Importance and management

Information is very limited but a reduced response to the amiodarone would be expected. It is uncertain whether separating the dosages to avoid mixing the gut would reduce or prevent this interaction because amiodarone is extensively secreted in the bile. Monitor the effects closely and raise the amiodarone dosage if necessary.

Reference

1 Nitsch J, Luderitz B. Beschleunigte Elimination von Amiodaron durch Colestyramin. Dtsch med Wschr (1986) 111, 1241–4.

Amiodarone + Cimetidine

Abstract/Summary

Cimetidine causes a rise in the serum levels of amiodarone.

Clinical evidence

The mean amiodarone serum levels of 12 patients on long-term treatment (200 mg daily) rose by an average of 38% (from 1.4 to 1.93 g/ml) when given 1200 mg cimetidine daily for a week. The desethyl-amiodarone levels rose by 54%. Only 8 of the 12 showed this effect.[1]

Mechanism

Not understood. Cimetidine is a well-recognized enzyme inhibitor which reduces the metabolism of many drugs (and possibly amiodarone) so that they are cleared more slowly.

Importance and management

Information seems to be limited to this study but it would appear to be of clinically important. Monitor the serum amiodarone levels if cimetidine is started, anticipating a rise. Not all patients appear to be affected. Remember that amiodarone is lost from the body very slowly (half-life 25–100 days) so that the results of the 1-week study cited here may possibly not adequately reflect the magnitude of this interaction. More study is needed.

Reference

1 Hogan C, Landau S, Tepper D, Somberg J. Cimetidine-amiodarone interaction. J Clin Pharmacol (1988) 28, 909.

Amiodarone + Disopyramide, Propafenone or Mexiletine

Abstract/Summary

The risk of atypical ventricular tachycardia or torsades de pointes seems to be increased if amiodarone is used with these antiarrhythmics.

Clinical evidence, mechanism, importance and management

A very brief report describes the concurrent use of amiodarone and disopyramide, propafenone or mexiletine in four patients, three of whom developed atypical ventricular contractions (AVT or torsades de pointes). Their QT intervals become markedly prolonged.[1] In another study five patients given amiodarone and disopyramide all had QT intervals of 0.60 sec immediately before developing torsades de pointes.[4] It has been suggested that, in general, class I antiarrhythmics should be avoided or used with caution if amiodarone is also used because of their additive effects in delaying conduction.[1,2] Concurrent use should be very well monitored. Prolongation of the QT interval rather than QT_c or QRS widening is thought to be a warning sign that the treatment needs modification.[4] The successful use of amiodarone (100–600 mg daily) with mexiletine (600 mg daily)[3,5] or disopyramide (300–500 mg daily)[6] has also been described.

References

1 Tartini R, Kappenberger L, Steinbrunn W, Meyer UA. Dangerous interaction between amiodarone and quinidine. Lancet (1982) i, 1327–9.
2 Tartini R, Kappenberger L, Steinbrunn W. Gefährliche interaktionen zwischen amiodaron und antiarrhythmika der klass I. Schweiz Med Wsch (1982)
3 Waleffe A, Mary-Rabine L, Legrand V, Demoulin JC, Kulbertus HE. Combined mexiletine and amiodarone treatment of refractory recurrent ventricular tachycardia. Am Heart J (1980) 100, 788–93.
4 Keren A, Tzivoni D, Gavish D, Levi J, Gottlieb S, Benhorin J, Stern S. Etiology, warning signs and therapy of Torsade de Pointes. Circulation (1981) 64, 1167–74.
5 Hoffman A, Follath F, Burckhardt D. Safe treatment of resistant ventricular arrhythmias with combination of amiodarone and quinidine or mexiletine. Lancet (1983) i, 704
6 James MA, Papouchado M and Vann Jonec J. Combined therapy with disopyramide and amiodarnne: a report of 11 cases. Int J Cabdiol (1986) 13, 248–52.

Aprindine + Amiodarone

Abstract/Summary

Serum aprindine levels can be increased by the concurrent use of amiodarone. Toxicity may occur unless the dosage is reduced.

Clinical evidence, mechanism, importance and management

The serum aprindine levels of two patients rose, accompanied by signs of toxicity (nausea, ataxia, etc.), when additionally treated with amiodarone. One of them on 100 mg aprindine daily showed a progressive rise in trough serum levels from 2.3 to 3.5 mg/l over a 5-week period when given 1200 mg and later 600 mg amiodarone daily. Even when the aprindine dosage was reduced, serum levels remained higher than before beginning the amiodarone.[1] The authors say that those given both drugs need less aprindine than those on aprindine alone. This interaction has been briefly reported elsewhere.[2] Its mechanism is not understood. Monitor the effects of concurrent use and reduce the dosage of aprinidine as necessary.

References

1 Southworthy W, Friday KJ and Ruffy R. Possible amiodarone-aprindine interaction. Amer Heart J (1982) 104, 323.
2 Zhang Z, Wang G, Wang H, Zhang J. Effect of amiodarone on the plasma concentration of aprindine. Zhongguo Yaoxue Zazhi (1991) 26, 156–9. Abstract 115: 197745u in Chemical Abstracts (1991) 115, 22.

Cifenline (cibenzoline) + Cimetidine or Ranitidine

Abstract/Summary

Cimetidine increases the serum levels of cifenline, but ranitidine does not interact.

Clinical evidence, mechanism, importance and management

1200 mg cimetidine daily raised the maximum serum levels of cifenline (single 160 mg doses) in 12 normal subjects by 27%, increased the AUC by 44%, and prolonged its half-life by 30%. 300 mg ranitidine daily had no effect.[1]The probable reason is that the cimetidine reduces the metabolism of the cifenline by the liver, whereas rantidine does not. The clinical importance of this interaction is not known. More study is needed.

Reference

1 Massarella JW, Defeo TM, Liguori J, Passe S, Aogaichi K. The effects of cimetidine and ranitidine on the pharmacokinetics of cifenline. Br J clin Pharmac (1991) 31, 481–3.

Disopyramide or Procainamide + Antacids and Antidiarrhoeals

Abstract/Summary

There is some inconclusive evidence that aluminium-containing antacids may possibly cause a small reduction in the absorption of these antiarrhythmic agents. Kaopectate reduces the bioavailability of procainamide.

Clinical evidence, mechanism, importance and management

An aluminium phosphate antacid had no statistically significant effect on the pharmacokinetics of a single 200 mg oral dose of disopyramide in 10 patients, but did affect the pharmacokinetics of a single 750 mg oral dose of procainamide. However the antacid appeared to reduce the absorption of both antiarrhythmic agents to a some extent in individual subjects.[1] An aluminium hydroxide antacid, but not magnesium oxide, has also been shown to reduce maximal procainamide serum levels in animals.[2] The clinical importance of these interactions is uncertain but probably small.

Kaopectate was found in one study to reduce the bioavailability of procainamide by 32%.[3] The clinical importance of this awaits further study.

References

1 Albin H, Vincon G, Bertolaso D, Dangoumau J. Influence du phosphate d'aluminium sur la biodisponibilie de la procainamide et du disopyramide. Therapie (1981) 36, 541–6.
2 Remon JP, Belpaire F, Van Severen R, Braeckman P. Interaction of antacids with antiarrhythmics.V. Effect of aluminium hydroxide and magnesium oxide on the bioavailability of quinidine, procainamide and propranolol in dogs. Arzneimittel Forsch (1983) 33, 117–120.
3 Al-Shora HI, Moustafa MA, Niazy EM, Gaber M, Gouda MW. Interactions of procainamide, verapamil, guanethidine and hydralazine with adsorbent antacids and antidiarrheal mixtures. Int J Pharmaceutics (1988) 47, 209–13.

Disopyramide + Beta-blockers

Abstract/Summary

Four patients treated for supraventricular tachycardia with intravenous disopyramide and practolol or pindolol developed severe bradycardia. One of them died. Other studies on patients and normal subjects suggest that adverse interactions between these drugs may be uncommon.

Clinical evidence

Two patients with supraventricular tachycardia (180 beat/min) were treated firstly with intravenous practolol (20 and 10 mg respectively) and shortly afterwards with disopyramide (150 and 80 mg respectively). The first patient rapidly developed sinus bradycardia of 25 beats/min, lost consciousness and became profoundly hypotensive. He failed to respond to 0.6 mg atropine but later his heart rate increased to 60 while a temporary pacemaker was being inserted.[1] Another patient similarly treated also developed severe bradycardia and asystole, despite the use of atropine. He was resuscitated with adrenaline but later died.[1]

Two other patients have been reported who developed severe bradycardia when treated for supraventricular tachycardia with either practolol[2] or pindolol[3] and disopyramide.

In contrast, studies in healthy subjects have shown that no adverse effects on left ventricular function occur if propranolol and disopyramide are used concurrently,[6,7] nor are the pharmacokinetics of either drug affected.[5] Atenolol (100 mg daily) has been shown to increase the serum disopyramide steady-state levels from 3.46 to 4.25 g/ml and reduce the clearance of disopyramide in healthy subjects and patients with ischaemic heart disease by 16% (from 1.9 to 1.59 ml/kg/min).[4] None of the subjects developed any adverse reactions or symptoms of heart failure, apart from one of the volunteers who showed transient first degree heart block.[4]

Mechanism

Not understood. Both drugs can depress the contractility and conductivity of the heart muscle.

Importance and management

The general clinical importance of this interaction is uncertain. The only clear risk seems to be in patients who are treated for supraventricular tachycardia with disopyramide and either practolol or pindolol given intravenously. Considerable caution should be exercised in these patients. More study is needed to find out the factors which contribute to the development of this potentially serious interaction.

References

1 Cumming AD, Robertson C. Interaction between disopyramide and practolol. Br Med J (1979) 2, 1264.
2 Gelipter D, Hazell M. Interaction between disopyramide and practolol. Br Med J (1980) 1, 52.
3 Pedersen C, Josephsen P, Lindvig K. Interaktion mellem disopyramide og pindolol efter oral indgift. Ugskr Laeg (1983) 145, 3266–7.
4 Bonde J, Bodtker S, Angelo H R, Svendsen T L, Kampmann J P. Atenolol inhibits the elimination of disopyramide. Eur. J. Clin. Pharmacol. (1986) 28, 41–3.
5 Karim A, Nissen C, Azarnoff DL. Clinical pharmacokinetics of disopyramide. J Pharmacokinet Biopharm (1982) 10, 465–94.
6 Cathcart-Rake WF, Coker JE, Atkins FL, Huffman DF, Hassanein KM, Shen DD, Azarnoff DL. The effect of concurrent oral administration of propranolol and disopyramide on cardiac function in healthy men. Circulation (1980) 61, 938–45.
7 Cathcart-Rake WF, Coker JE, Shen D, Huffman D, Azarnoff DL. The pharmacodynamics of concurrent disopyramide and propranolol. Clin Pharmacol Ther (1979) 25, 217.

Disopyramide + Erythromycin

Abstract/Summary

Two patients taking disopyramide developed cardiac arrhythmias when given erythromycin. Disopyramide serum levels were raised. Another patient given both drugs developed heart block.

Clinical evidence

A woman with ventricular ectopy taking disopyramide (300 mg alternating with 150 mg six-hourly) developed new arrhythmias (ventricular asystoles and later polymorphic ventricular tachycardia) within 36 h of starting 1 g erythromycin lactobionate IV 6-hourly and cephamandole. Her serum disopyramide level was found to be 16 mol/l. The problem resolved when the disopyramide was stopped and bretylium given, but it returned when the disopyramide was restarted. It resolved again when the erythromycin was stopped.[1]

Another patient with ventricular tachycardia, well controlled over five years with 200 mg disopyramide four times daily, developed ventricular tachycardia within a few days of starting 500 mg erythromycin base four times daily. His serum disopyramide levels were found to be elevated (30 mol/l). The problem resolved when both drugs were withdrawn.[1] Heart block is said to have developed in another patient treated with both drugs.[2]

Mechanism

Not fully established. An *in vitro* study using human liver microsomes indicated that erythromycin inhibits the metabolism (mono-N-dealkylation) of the disopyramide which, *in vivo*, would be expected to reduce its loss from the body and increase its serum levels.[3] Two of the patients developed high serum disopyramide levels.[1]

Importance and management

Information seems to be limited to these three cases[1,2] and the *in vitro* study cited.[3] The effects of concurrent use should be well monitored if erythromycin is added to disopyramide, being alert for the development of raised serum disopyramide levels. Information about other macrolides is lacking as yet but they too should be given with caution to patients taking disopyramide. More study is needed.

Reference

1 Ragosta M, Weihl AC, Rosenfeld LE. Potentially fatal interaction between erythromycin and disopyramide. Amer J Med (1989) 86, 465–6.
2 Beeley L, Cunningham H, Carmichael A, Brennan A. Bulletin of the W. Midlands Centre for Adverse Drug Reporting (1992) 35, 13.

3 Echizen H, Kawasaki H, Chiba K, Tani M. Ishizaki T. A potent inhibitory effect of erythromycin and other macrolide antibiotics on the mono-N-dealkylation metabolism of disopyramide with human liver microsomes. J Pharmacol Exp Ther (1993) 264, 1425–31.

Disopyramide + Phenobarbitone

Abstract/Summary

Serum disopyramide levels are reduced by the concurrent use of phenobarbitone (phenobarbital).

Clinical evidence

After taking 100 mg phenobarbitone daily for 21 days, the half-life and AUC (area under the time-concentration curve) of a single 200 mg dose of disopyramide in 16 normal subjects were reduced about 35%. No significant differences were seen between those who smoked and those who did not.[1]

Mechanism

It seems probable that the phenobarbitone (a known enzyme inducing agent) increases the metabolism of disopyramide by the liver, and thereby increases its loss from the body.

Importance and management

This interaction is not well established and its clinical importance is uncertain. The extent to it would reduce the control of arrhythmias by disopyramide in patients is unknown but monitor the effects and the serum levels of disopyramide if phenobarbitone is added or withdrawn. Other barbiturates would be expected to interact similarly.

Reference

1 Kapil RP, Axelson JE, Mansfield IL, Edwards DJ, McErlane B, Mason MA, Lalka D, Kerr CR. Disopyramide pharmacokinetics and metabolism: effect of inducers. Br J clin Pharmac (1987) 24, 781–91.

Disopyramide + Phenytoin

Abstract/Summary

Serum disopyramide levels are reduced by the concurrent use of phenytoin and may fall below therapeutic concentrations. Loss of arrhythmic control may occur.

Clinical evidence

Eight patients with ventricular tachycardia treated with disopyramide (600–2000 mg daily) showed a 54% fall in their serum disopyramide levels (from a mean of 3.99 to 1.82 g/ml) when concurrently treated with phenytoin (200–600 mg daily) for a week. Two of the patients who were monitored showed a 53- and 2000-fold increase in ventricular premature beat frequency as a result of this interaction.[1]

Falls in serum disopyramide levels (about 30%) which, in some instances, were then below the therapeutic range, have been described in other reports.[2,3,5] A marked fall in serum disopyramide levels (75% in one case) was seen in two patients after taking phenytoin (300–700 mg daily) for up to two weeks.[4] A pharmacokinetic study in normal subjects confirms this interaction.[5]

Mechanism

Phenytoin, which is a known enzyme-inducing agent, increases the metabolism of the disopyramide by the liver. The major metabolite (N-dealkyldisopyramide) also possesses antiarrhythmic activity neverthless the net effect is a reduction in arrhythmic control.[1]

Importance and management

An established interaction of clinical importance. Some loss of arrhythmic control can occur during concurrent use. Serum disopyramide levels and the antiarrhythmic response should be well monitored. An increase in the dosage of disopyramide may be necessary. Serum disopyramide levels return to normal within two weeks of withdrawing the phenytoin.

References

1 Matos JA, Fisher JD, Kim SG. Disopyramide-phenytoin interaction. Clin Res (1982) 29, 655A.
2 Aitio M-L, Vuorenmaa T. Enhanced metabolism and diminished efficacy of disopyramide by enzyme induction. Br J clin Pharmacol (1980) 9, 149–152.
3 Aitio M-L, Mansury L, Tala E, Haataja M, Aitio A. The effect of enzyme induction on the metabolism of disopyramide in man. Br J clin Pharmacol (1981) 279–85.
4 Kessler JM, Keys PW, Stafford RW. Disopyramide and phenytoin interaction. Clin Pharm (1982) 1, 263–4.
5 Nightingale J, Nappi JM. Effect of phenytoin on serum disopyramide concentrations. Clin Pharm (1987) 6, 46–50.

Disopyramide + Quinidine

Abstract/Summary

Disospyramide serum levels may be slightly raised by quinidine.

Clinical evidence, mechanism, importance and management

In the presence of quinidine the peak serum levels of disopyramide, given as single 150 mg doses to 16 normal subjects, were raised by 20% (from 2.68 to 3.23 g/ml), and by 14% when given chronically as 150 mg four times a day. Serum quinidine levels were decreased 26%. The frequency of adverse effects such as dry mouth, blurred vision, urine retention and nausea were also somewhat increased.[1] The mechanism of this interaction is not understood. Concurrent use would generally appear to be safe except in those whose disopyramide levels are already in the near-toxic range. The anticholinergic side-effects of disopyramide may be increased.

Reference

1 Baker BJ, Gammill J, Massengill J, Schubert E, Karin A, Doherty JE. Concurrent use of quinidine and disopyramide: evaluation of serum concentrations and electrocardiographic effects. Am Heart J (1983) 105, 12–15.

Disopyramide + Rifampicin (Rifampin)

Abstract/Summary

The serum levels of disopyramide can be markedly reduced by the concurrent use of rifampicin.

Clinical evidence

After taking rifampicin for 14 days the plasma levels of disopyramide in 12 patients with tuberculosis who had taken single 200 or 300 mg doses were approximately halved. The AUC's before and after were 20.3 and 8.22 g ml^{-1} h respectively, and the half-life was reduced from 5.9 to 3.25 h.[1] A woman already on rifampicin initially showed only subtherapeutic serum levels of disopyramide (0.9 μmol/L) when first started on 100 mg 8-hourly, and was found to need 250 mg 8-hourly to maintain adequate levels.[2]

Mechanism

The most probable explanation is that rifampicin (a well known enzyme inducer) markedly increases the metabolism of the disopyramide by the liver so that it is cleared from the body much more quickly.

Importance and management

Information seems to be limited to these studies, but they indicate that the dosage of disopyramide will need to be increased in most patients taking rifampicin.

References

1 Aito M-L, Mansury L, Tala E, Haataja M, Aitio A. The effect of enzyme induction on the metabolism of disopyramide in man. Br J clin Pharmac (1981) 11, 279–85.
2 Staum JM. Enzyme induction: rifampin-disopyramide interaction. DICP Ann Pharmacother (1990) 24, 701–3.

Encainide + Diltiazem

Abstract/Summary

Diltiazem causes a marked increase in the serum levels of encainide but the levels of its active metabolites are only slightly increased and no significant ECG changes occur.

Clinical evidence

A study in six normal subjects (extensive metabolizers) given 25 mg encainide 8-hourly for seven days showed that the concurrent use of 90 mg diltiazem eight-hourly for seven days increased the encainide AUC (area under the concentration-time curve) 2–3-fold (from 130 to 333 ng/h/ml), but the active metabolites of encainide were only slightly increased (+ 8–10%).[1]

Another study in normal subjects similarly found that there was little change in the AUC of the active metabolites of encainide when given diltiazem, and no ECG changes (QRS, QT_c or JT) were seen.[3]

Mechanism

Diltiazem appears to inhibit the metabolism of encainide by the liver, thereby increasing its serum levels.

Importance and management

Information is very limited. The active metabolites of encainide are largely responsible for its antiarrhythmic effects and these were little affected by this interaction. It seems very doubtful if any change in encainide dosage is needed when diltiazem is given, but further confirmation of this is needed. Nifedipine is reported not to interact.[2] There seems to be no information about other calcium channel blocking drugs.

References

1 Bottorff MB, Hoon TJ, Lalone RL, Kazierad DJ, Mirvis DM. Effects of diltiazem on the disposition of encainide and its active metabolites. Clin Pharmacol Ther (1988) 43, 195.
2 Quart BD, Gallo DG, Sami MH, Wood AJJ. Drug interaction studies and encainide use in renal and hepatic impairment. Am J Cardiol (1986) 58, 104–113C.
3 Kazierad DJ, Lalonde RL, Hoon TJ, Mirvis DM, Bottorff MB. The effect of diltiazem on the disposition of encainide and its active metabolites. Clin Pharmacol Ther (1989) 46, 668–73.

Encainide + Miscellaneous drugs

Abstract/Summary

No clinically significant interactions have been seen to occur between encainide and warfarin, acenocoumarol, sulphony-lureas, insulin, beta-blockers, nifedipine, diuretics, antipsychotics or amiodarone but the effects of cimetidine should be monitored.

Clinical evidence, mechanism, importance and management

A study in 13 normal subjects showed that the concurrent use of 1200 mg cimetidine daily for seven days while taking 75 mg encainide daily increased the AUC (area under the curve) of encainide by 32%, and of two metabolites of encainide (O-demethyl encainide and 3-methoxy-O-demethyl encainide) by 43 and 36% respectively. Despite the fact that a retrospective evaluation of 33 patients who had had both drugs revealed no evidence of any clinically significant interaction, the authors suggest that if cimetidine is added the effects should be monitored.[1] Retrospective analyses of large numbers of patients taking encainide and warfarin or nicoumalone (78 patients), oral sulphonylureas or insulin (40 patients), beta-blockers (88 patients), nifedipine (24 patients), un-named diuretics (229), and amiodarone and other anti-arrhythmics (118) and un-named antipsychotics (23 patients) revealed no clinically significant interactions.[1] See also 'Encainide + Quinidine'.

Reference

1 Quart BD, Gallo DG, Sami MH, Wood AJJ. Drug interaction studies and encainide use in renal and hepatic impairment. Am J Cardiol (1986) 58, 104–113C.

Encainide + Quinidine

Abstract/Summary

Quinidine causes a marked reduction in the clearance of encainide in those who are extensive metabolizers of encainide. The effects of encainide would be expected to be increased.

Clinical evidence

Seven normal subjects who were extensive metabolizers of encainide were given 60 mg encainide orally and 4.5 mg encainide C^{14} intravenously before and after taking 50 mg quinidine six-hourly for five days. The quinidine decreased the systemic clearance from 935 to 190 ml/min and the non-renal clearance from 782 to 95 ml/min. Serum encainide levels were markedly increased and the levels of the active metabolites of encainide were reduced. These changes were reflected to some extent in the ECG measurements made. A parallel study showed that no interaction occurred in four poor metabolizers of encainide.[1] A later study on 10 patients by the same workers found that the pharmacological effects of encainide were maintained or enhanced by quinidine.[2]

Mechanism

Quinidine causes a marked reduction in the metabolism of encainide by the liver in extensive metabolizers.

Importance and management

An established interaction which is expected to occur in most patients (most people are extensive metabolizers) but its clinical importance is uncertain. Monitor the encainide effects if quinidine is given concurrently, or withdrawn, adjusting the dosage as necessary.

Reference

1 Funck-Brentano C, Turgeon J, Woosely RL, Roden DM. Effect of low dose quinidine on encainide pharmacokinetics and pharmacodynamics. Influence of genetic polymorphism. J Pharmacol Exp Ther (1989) 249, 134–42.

2 Turgeon J, Pavlou HN, Wong W, Funck-Brentano C, Roden DM. Genetically determined steady-state interaction between enacainide and quinidine in patients with arrhythmias. J Pharm Exp Ther (1990) 255, 642–9.

Flecainide + Amiodarone

Abstract/Summary

Serum flecainide levels are increased by the concurrent use of amiodarone. The flecainide dosage should be reduced by a third. An isolated report describes torsades de pointe in a patient on amiodarone when given flecainide.

Clinical evidence

Seven patients on oral flecainide (200–500 mg daily) were given reduced doses when amiodarone was added (1200 mg loading doses, later reduced to 600 mg daily) because it was observed that the trough plasma levels of flecainide were increased. The flecainide dosage was reduced by a third (averaging a reduction from 325 to 225 mg daily) to keep the flecainide levels under control. Observations on two patients suggest that the interaction begins soon after the amiodarone is added, and it takes about two weeks to develop fully. Other reports confirm this interaction.[2,3] The authors of these two reports reduced the flecainide dosage by a half, but did not measure plasma levels. An isolated report describes torsades de pointe in a patient on amiodarone when given flecainide.[4]

Mechanism

Not understood

Importance and management

An established interaction, but the documentation is limited. A reduction in the flecainide dosage is necessary if the adverse effects of flecainide overdosage are to be avoided. A one-third reduction has proved to be satisfactory.[1] Remember that amiodarone is cleared from the body exceptionally slowly so that this interaction may persist for some time after it has been withdrawn. Also be aware that torsades de pointes has been seen.

References

1 Shea P, Roop L, Kim SS, Schechtman K, Ruffy R. Flecainide and amiodarone interaction. J Am Coll Cardiol (1986) 7, 1127–30.
2 Leclerq JF, Coumel P. La flecainide: un nouvel anti-arythmique. Arch Mal Coeur (1983) 76, 1218–30.
3 Fontaine G, Frank R, Tonet JL. Association amiodarone-flecainide dans le traitement des troubles du rythme ventriculaires graves. Arch Mal Coeur (1984) 77, 1421–2.
4 Andrivet P, Beasley V, Canh VD. Torsades de pointe with flecainide-amiodarone therapy. Int Care Med (1990) 16, 342–7.

Flecainide + Anticonvulsants

Abstract/Summary

No clinically important interaction appears to occur if phenytoin or phenobarbitone are given to patients on flecainide.

Clinical evidence, mechanism, importance and management

A controlled study with epileptic patients on phenytoin or phenobarbitone found that the pharmacokinetics of a single 2 mg/kg dose of flecainide were not statistically different from those in a group of normal subjects. The authors say that '...a modest reduction in flecainide half-life is possible, but may not require any adjustment in the flecainide dosage.'[1]

Reference

1 Pentikainen PJ, Halinen MO, Hiepakorpo S, Chang SF, Conard GJ, McQuinn RL. Pharmacokinetics of flecainide in patients receiving enzyme inducers. Acta Pharmacol Toxicol (1986) 59, Suppl 4, 91.

Flecainide + Cholestyramine

Abstract/Summary

An isolated report describes reduced serum flecainide levels in a patient given cholestyramine. Studies in other subjects failed to demonstrate any interaction.

Clinical evidence, mechanism, importance and management

A patient on 100 mg flecainide twice daily had unusually low trough serum levels (100 ng/ml). When he stopped taking cholestyramine (4 g three times daily) his plasma flecainide levels rose. However a later study on three normal subjects given 100 mg flecainide and 4 g cholestyramine three times daily, found little or no evidence of an interaction (steady-state flecainide levels of 63.1 and 59.1 ng/ml without and with cholestyramine). *In vitro* studies also failed to demonstrate any binding between flecainide and cholestyramine which might result in reduced absorption from the gut.[1]

Information seems to be limited to this report. Its general importance seems to be small, nevertheless the outcome of concurrent use should be monitored so that unusual cases can be identified.

Reference

1 Stein H, Hoppe U. Is there an interaction between flecainide and cholestyramine? Naunyn-Schmiedbergs Arch Pharmakol (1989) 339 (Suppl) R114.

Flecainide + Cimetidine

Abstract/Summary

Cimetidine can increase flecainide serum levels.

Clinical evidence

The flecainide serum levels of eight normal subjects taking 200 mg daily were raised 28% and the clearance reduced 27% after taking 1 g cimetidine daily for a week. 1 g cimetidine for five days almost doubled the serum flecainide levels (from 160–245 to 380–455 ng/ml) of 11 patients taking 200 mg flecainide daily.[4]

Mechanism

Uncertain, but it is thought that the cimetidine reduces both the renal clearance and the metabolism of the flecainide by the liver.[1-4]

Importance and management

An established but as yet not extensively documented interaction. Be alert for the need to reduce the flecainide dosage if cimetidine is added. More study is needed.

Reference

1 Tjandra Maga TB, Verbesselt R, Van Hecken A, Van Melle P, De Schepper PJ. Oral flecainide elimination kinetics: effects of cimetidine. Circulation (1983) 68, Supp III-416.
2 Tjandra Maga TB, Van Hecken A, Van Melle P, Verbesselt R, De Schepper PJ. Altered pharmacokinetics of oral flecainide by cimetidine. Br J clin Pharmac (1986) 22, 108–110.
3 Verbesselt R, Tjandra Maga TB, Van Hecken A, Van Melle P, De Schepper PJ. Effects of cimetidine on the elimination of oral flecainide. Eur Heart J (1984) 5, 136.
4 Nitsch J, Köhler U, Neyses L, L'9fderitz B. Flecainide-Plasmakonzentrazionen bei Hemmung des hepatischen Metabolismus durch Cimetidin. Klin Wschr (1987) 65 (Suppl IX) 250.

Flecainide + Food or Antacids

Abstract/Summary

The absorption of flecainide is not significantly altered if taken with food or an aluminium hydroxide antacid in adults, but it may possibly be reduced by milk in infants.

Clinical evidence, mechanism, importance and management

Neither food nor 15 ml of *Aludrox* (280 mg aluminium hydroxide per 5 ml) had any significant effect on the absorption of a single 200 mg dose of flecainide in normal adult subjects.[1] No special precautions seem necessary if taken together.

A premature baby being treated for refractory atrioventricular tachycardia with high doses of flecainide (40 mg/kg daily or 25 mg 6-hourly) developed flecainide toxicity (seen as ventricular tachycardia) when his milk feed was replaced by 5% dextrose. His serum flecainide levels approximately doubled, the conclusion being drawn that the milk had reduced the absorption.[2] Milk-fed infants on high doses may therefore possibly need a reduced flecainide dosage if milk is reduced or stopped. Monitor the effects.

Reference

1 Tjandra-Maga TB, Verbesselt R, Van Hecken A, Mullie A, De Schepper PJ. Flecainide: single and multiple oral dose kinetics, absolute bioavailability and effect of food and antacid in man. Br J clin Pharmac (1986) 22, 309–16.

Flecainide + Quinidine and Quinine

Abstract/Summary

Quinidine and quinine cause a modest reduction in the loss of flecainide from the body.

Clinical evidence, mechanism, importance and management

(a) Quinidine

50 mg oral quinidine given the night before decreased the clearance of a single 150 mg iv dose of flecainide acetate by 23% (from 0.64 to 0.49 l/h/kg) in six normal subjects.[1] Another related study found that the flecainide half-life was increased by 22% by a single 50 mg oral dose of quinidine.[5] Yet another study in six patients on chronic flecainide treatment found that when given 50 mg quinidine 6-hourly, the serum levels of S-(+)-flecainide were unchanged, but serum levels of R-(−)-flecainide increased approximately 15%. This is because the quinidine inhibits cytochrome P450IID6 in the liver which is concerned with the metabolism of the flecainide. The effects of

the flecainide were slightly but not significantly increased.[4] The importance of this interaction is uncertain, but it is probably small.

(b) Quinine

A single 500 mg dose of quinine increased the AUC of a single 150 mg IV dose of flecainide by 23% (from 189 to 232 mg/min/l) and reduced the systemic clearance by 19% (from 793 to 646 ml/min) in four normal subjects. Renal clearance remained unchanged.[2] Another study by the same workers found that 1500 mg quinine over 24 h decreased the total clearance of flecainide by about 20%,[3] and in normal subjects the increases in the PR and QRS intervals caused by both drugs appear to be additive.[3] The evidence suggests that quinine reduces the metabolism of flecainide.[2,3] The clinical importance of this interaction is uncertain but an increase in the serum levels of flecainide would be expected, accompanied by some, probably modest, changes in its effects.

References

1 Munafo A, Buclin T, Steinhäuslin Fl, Biollaz J. Disposition of flecainide in subjects taking quinidine. Clin Pharmacol Ther (1990) 47, 156.
2 Munafo A, Reymond-MIchel G, Borgeat J. Influence of quinine administration on flecainide kinetics. Clin Res (1988) 36, 368A.
3 Munafo A, Reymond-MIchel G, Biollaz J. Altered flecainide disposition in healthy volunteers taking quinine. Eur J Clin Pharmacol (1990) 38, 269–73.
4 Birgersdotter UM, Wong W, Turgeon J, Roden DM. Stereoselective genetically-determined interaction between chronic flecainide and quinidine in patients with arrhythmias. Br J clin Pharmac (1992) 33, 275–80.
5 Munafo A, Buclin T, Tuto D, Biollaz J. The effect of a low dose of quinidine on the disposition of flecainide in healthy volunteers. Eur J Cin Pharmacol (1992) 43, 441–3.

Flecainide + Tobacco smoking

Abstract/Summary

Tobacco smokers need larger doses of flecainide than non-smokers to achieve the same therapeutic effects.

Clinical evidence

Prompted by the chance observation that smokers appeared to have a reduced pharmacodynamic response to flecainide than non-smokers, a meta-analysis was undertaken of the findings of seven pharmacokinetic studies[2–4] and five multicentre efficacy trials[5] in which flecainide had been studied and in which the smoking habits of the subjects had been also been recorded: a total of 338 smokers and 288 non-smokers. This confirmed that smokers needed higher doses of flecainide to achieve the same steady-state serum levels. Trough serum plasma concentrations (ng/ml/mg dose) were 1.74 for the smokers and 2.18 for the non-smokers.[1]

Mechanism

The probable reason is that some components of the tobacco smoke stimulate the cytochrome P-450s in the liver concerned with the O-dealkylation of flecainide so that it is cleared from the body more quickly.

Importance and management

An established interaction. Anticipate the need to give smokers higher doses of flecainide than non-smokers to achieve the required therapeutic response.

References

1 Holtzman JL, Weeks CE, Kvam DC, Berry DA, Mottonen L, Ekholm BP, Chang SF, Conard GJ. Identification of drug interactions by meta-analysis of premarketing trials: The effect of smoking on the pharmacokinetic and dosage requirements of flecainide acetate. Clin Pharmacol Ther (1989) 46, 1–8.
2 Holtzman JL, Kvam DC, Berry DA, Borrell G, Harrison LI, Conard GJ. The pharmacodynamic and pharmacokinetic interaction of flecainide acetate with propranolol: effects on cardiac function and drug clearance. Eur J Clin Pharmacol (1987) 33, 97–9.
3 Conard GJ, Ober RE. Metabolism of flecainide. Am J Cardiol (1984) 53, 41–51B.
4 Holtzman JL, Finley D, Mottonen L, Berry DA, Ekholm BP, Kvam DC, McQuinn RL, Miller AM. The pharmacodynamic and pharmacokinetic interaction between single doses of flecainide acetate and verapamil: effects on cardiac function and drug clearance. Clin Pharmacol Ther (1989) 46, 26–32.
5 Morganroth J, Anderson JL, Gentzkow GD. Classification by type of ventricular arrhythmia predicts frequency of adverse cardiac events from flecainide. J Am Coll Cardiol (1986) 8, 607–15.

Flecainide + Verapamil

Abstract/Summary

Although flecainide and verapamil have been used together successfully, serious and potentially life-threatening cardiogenic shock and asytole have been seen in a few patients because their cardiac depressant effects can be additive.

Clinical evidence

A man with triple coronary vessel disease and on 200 mg flecainide daily for recurrent ventricular tachycardia, developed severe cardiogenic shock within two days of increasing the flecainide dosage to 300 mg daily and 1 day of starting 80 mg verapamil daily. His blood pressure fell to 60/40 mm Hg and he had an idioventricular rhythm of 88 beats per minute.[1] Another patient with atrial flutter and fibrillation was treated with digitalis and 120 mg verapamil three times daily. He was additionally given 120 mg flecainide daily for 10 days, but three days after the dosage was raised to 200 mg daily he fainted, and later developed severe bradycardia (15 beats per minute) and asystoles of up to 14 sec. He later died.[1]

Another report describes atrioventricular block in a patient with a pacemaker when treated with digoxin, flecainide and verapamil.[2]

Two studies in patients[4] and normal subjects[3] found that the kinetics of flecainide and verapamil were only minimally affected by concurrent use, but the PR interval was increased by both drugs and additive depressant effects were seen on heart contractility and AV conduction. No serious adverse responses occurred.

Mechanism

Flecainide and verapamil have little or no effects on the kinetics of each other,[3,4] but they can apparently have additive depressant effects on the heart (negative inotropic and chronotropic) in both patients and normal subjects.[3,4] Verapamil alone[10] and with beta-blockers[5,6] or digoxin,[8, 7] and flecainide alone[9,11] have been responsible for asystole and cardiogenic shock in a few patients. In the cases cited above[1–3] the depressant effects were serious because the patients already had compromised cardiac function.

Importance and management

An established interaction, but the incidence of serious adverse effects is probably not great. The additive depressant effects on heart function are probably of little importance in many patients, but may represent 'the last straw' in a few who have seriously compromised cardiac function. The authors of the reports cited[1] advise careful monitoring if both drugs are used and emphasize the potential hazards of combining IC antiarrhythmics and calcium channel blockers.

References

1 Buss J, Lasserre JJ, Heene DL. Asystole and cardiogenic shock due to combined treatment with verapamil and flecainide. Lancet (1992) 340, 546.
2 Tworek DA, Nazari J, Ezri M, Bauman JL. Interference by antiarrhythmic agents with function of electrical cardiac devices. Clin Pharm (1992) 11, 48–56.
3 Holtzman JL, Finley D, Mottonen L, Berry DA, Ekholm BP, Kvam DC, McQuinn RL, Miller AM. The pharmacodyamic and pharmacokinetic interaction between single doses of flecainide acetate and verapamil: Effects on cardiac function and drug clearance. Clin Pharmacol Ther (1989) 46, 26–32.
4 Landau S et al. The combined administration of verpamil and flecainide. J Clin Pharmacol (1988) 28, 909.
5 Benaim ME. Asystole after verapamil. Br Med J (1972) 2, 169–70.
6 Frierson J, Baily D, Shultz T, Sund S, Dimas A. Refractory cardiogenic shock and complete heart block after unsuspected verapamil-SR and atenolol overdose. Clin Cardiol (1992) 14, 933–5.
7 Kounis NG. Asystole after verapamil and digoxin. Br J Clin Pract (1980) 34, 57–8.
8 Perrot B, Danchin N, De La Chasie AT. Verapamil: a cause of sudden death in a patient with hypertrophic cardiomyopathy. Br Heart J (1984) 51, 532–4.
9 Forbes WP, Hee TT, Mohiuddin SM, Hillman DE. Flecainide-induced cardiogenic shock. Chest (1988) 94, 1121.
10 Cohen IL, Fein A, Nabi A. Reversal of cardiogenic shock and asystole in a septic patient with hypertrophic cardiomyopathy on verapamil. Crit Care Med (1990) 18, 775–6.
11 Echt DS, Liebson PR, Mitchell LB, Peters RW, Obias-Manno D, Barker AH, Arsensberg D, Baker A, Richardson DW, CAST investigators. Mortal-

ity and mobidity in patients receiving encainide, flecainide or placebo. N Engl J Med (1991) 324, 781–8.

in sick sinus syndrome during amiodarone administration. Am Heart J (1982) 104, 1384–5.

Lignocaine (Lidocaine) + Amiodarone

Abstract/Summary

An isolated report describes an elderly man who had a seizure, attributed to increased serum lignocaine levels, about two days after additionally starting to take amiodarone. Another patient with sick sinus syndrome had sinoatrial arrest when treated with both drugs.

Clinical evidence

(a) Increased lignocaine levels, seizure

An elderly man taking digoxin, enalapril, amitriptyline and temazepam was treated for monomorphic ventricular tachcardia, firstly with procainamide, later replaced by an infusion of lignocaine (2 mg/min), to which was added 600 mg amiodarone twice daily. After 12 h his lignocaine level was 5.4 mg/l (therapeutic levels 1.5–5 mg/l), but 53 h later he developed a seizure and his lignocaine level was found to have risen to 12.6 mg/l. A tomography brain scan showed no abnormalities which could have caused the seizure and it was therefore attributed to the toxic lignocaine levels.[1] The reason for the marked increase in serum lignocaine levels is not known.

(b) Sinoatrial arrest

An elderly man with long standing brady-tachycardia was successfully treated for atrial flutter firstly with a temporary pacemaker, later withdrawn, and 600 mg amiodarone daily. 10 days later and 25 min after a permanent pacemaker was inserted under local anaesthesia with 15 ml 2% lignocaine, when the braciocephalic vein was exposed, severe sinus bradycardia and long sinoatrial arrest developed. He was effectively treated with atropine plus isoprenaline, and cardiac massage.[2]

Mechanism

(a) Not known. (b) The authors of the report suggest a synergistic depression by both drugs of the sinus node.

Importance and management

Both reports are isolated and their general importance is very uncertain, however they clearly illustrate the need to monitor concurrent use closely, and to be aware of the possible risks.

References

1 Siegmund JB, Wilson JH, Imhoff TE. Amiodarone interaction with lidocaine. J Cardiovasc Pharmacol (1993) 21, 513–5.
2 Keidar S, Grenadier E, Palant A. Sinoatrial arrest due to lidocaine injection

Lignocaine (Lidocaine) + Barbiturates

Abstract/Summary

Serum lignocaine levels following intravenous infusion may be lower in those who are taking barbiturates.

Clinical evidence

Two tests were carried out on seven epileptic patients: firstly while taking their usual anti-epileptic drugs and sedatives (phenytoin, barbiturates, phenothiazines, benzodiazepines) and the other after taking only 300 mg phenobarbitone daily for four weeks. It was found that the phenobarbitone treatment caused a small increase (10–25%) in serum lignocaine levels given by infusion (2 mg/kg) but all of the levels were as much as 40% lower at 30 and 60 min than in the six control subjects who had not received any drugs.[1]

In a study in dogs, four out of six given lignocaine in therapeutic doses died from respiratory arrest when concurrently given a 30 mg/kg pentobarbitone infusion over 1 min. The other two showed apnoea.[2]

Mechanism

Not fully understood. One suggestion is that the barbiturates increase the activity of the liver microsomal enzymes, thereby increasing the rate of metabolism of the lignocaine.[1] The death of the dogs appeared to result from the additive depressant effects of the two drugs on the respiratory centre.

Importance and management

Direct information is very limited but the interaction in man appears to be established. It may be necessary to increase the dosage of lignocaine to achieve the desired therapeutic response in patients on phenobarbitone or other barbiturates. The clinical importance of the serious interaction seen in dogs is uncertain.

References

1 Heinonen J, Takki S, Jarho L. Plasma lidocaine levels in patients treated with potential inducers of microsomal enzymes. Acta anaesth Scandinav (1970) 14, 89–95.
2 LeLorier J. Lidocaine and pentobarbital: a potentially lethal drug-drug interaction. Toxicol Appl Pharmacol (1978) 44, 657.

Lignocaine (Lidocaine) + Beta-blockers

Abstract/Summary

The serum levels of lignocaine can be increased by the concurrent use of propranolol. Two cases of toxicity attributed to this interaction have been reported. Nadolol possibly interacts similarly, but there is uncertainty about metoprolol. Atenolol and pindolol appear not to interact but an increased loading dosage of lignocaine in the presence of penbutolol has been suggested.

Clinical evidence

(a) Lignocaine + Atenolol, Penbutolol, Pindolol

Studies with atenolol (50 mg daily),[5] pindolol and penbutolol[6] found that these beta-blockers appear not to affect the clearance of lignocaine, but the volume of distribution of penbutolol was altered so that it is possible that a higher loading dose of lignocaine may be needed.[6]

(b) Lignocaine + Metoprolol

A single dose study in normal subjects given 100 mg metoprolol twice daily for two days showed that it did not affect the pharmacokinetics of lignocaine,[7] and another study in seven normal subjects failed to find any changes in the pharmacokinetics of lignocaine after one week's treatment with metoprolol (100 mg 12-hourly).[5] In contrast another study found that lignocaine clearance was reduced 31% by metoprolol.[9]

(c) Lignocaine + Nadolol

A study in six normal subjects receiving 30-h infusions of lignocaine (2 mg/min) showed that three days' pretreatment with 160 mg nadolol daily raised the steady-state serum lignocaine levels by 28% (from 2.1 to 2.7 g/ml) and reduced the plasma clearance by 17% (from 1030 to 850 ml/min).[1]

(d) Lignocaine + Propranolol

A study on six normal subjects receiving 30 h infusions of lignocaine (2 mg/min) showed that 3 days' pretreatment with propranolol (80 mg 8-hourly) raised the steady-state serum lignocaine levels by 19% (from 2.1 to 2.5 g/ml) and reduced the plasma clearance by 15% (1030 to 866 ml/min).[1] Other studies found a 30%[8] and a 22.5%[2] increase in steady-state serum lignocaine levels and a 46%[9] fall in plasma clearance due to the concurrent use of propranolol. Another study found no significant differences in either total or free concentrations of lignocaine in patients on propranolol, but the adverse effects of lignocaine (bradycardias) were increased.[11] Two cases of lignocaine toxicity attributed to lignocaine-propranolol interaction occur in the FDA adverse drug reaction file.[10]

(e) Lignocaine + Un-named beta-blockers

A matched study in 50 patients showed that concurrent use of lignocaine and beta-blockers decreased arrhythmias and increased lignocaine toxicity, the mean serum lignocaine levels being raised by 39% (from 3.6 to 5.0 g/ml).[3]

Mechanism

Not fully agreed. There is some debate about whether the increased serum lignocaine levels largely occur because of the decreased cardiac output caused by the beta-blockers which decreases the flow of blood through the liver, thereby reducing the metabolism of the lignocaine,[1] or because of direct liver enzyme inhibition.[4]

Importance and management

The lignocaine-propranolol interaction is established and of clinical importance. Monitor the effects of concurrent use and reduce the lignocaine dosage if necessary to avoid toxicity. The situation with other beta-blockers is less clear. Nadolol appears to interact like propranolol, but it is uncertain whether metoprolol interacts or not. Atenolol, penbutolol and pindolol are reported not to interact, although it has been suggested that a higher loading dose (but not a higher maintenance dose) of lignocaine may be needed if penbutolol is used.[6] The suggestion has been made that a significant interaction is only likely to occur with non-selective beta-blockers without intrinsic sympathomimetic activity.[4] Until the situation is better defined it would seem prudent to monitor the effects of concurrent use with any beta-blocker.

Local anaesthetic preparations of lignocaine often contain adrenaline (epinephrine). See the index for 'Anaesthetics, local + Beta-blockers'.

References

1 Schneck DW, Luderer JR, Davis D, Vary J. Effects of nadolol and propranolol on plasma lidocaine clearance. Clin Pharmacol Ther (1984) 36, 584–7.
2 Svendsen TL, Tango M, Waldorff S, Steiness E, Trap-Jensen J. Effects of propranolol and pindolol on plasma lignocaine clearance. Br J clin Pharmac (1982) 13, 223–6S.
3 Wyse DG, Kellen J, Tam Y, Rademaker AW. Increased efficacy and toxicity of lidocaine in patients on beta-blockers. Circulation (1986) 74, II-43.
4 Bax NDS, Tucker GT, Lennard MS, Woods HF. The impairment of lignocaine clearance by propranolol-major contribution from enzyme inhibition. Br J clin Pharmac (1985) 19, 597–603.
5 Miners JO, Wing LMH, Lillywhite KJ, Smith KJ. Failure of 'therapeutic' doses of beta-adrenoceptor antagonists to alter the disposition of tolbutamide and lignocaine. Br J clin Pharmac (1984) 18, 853–60.
6 Ochs HR, Skanderra D, Abernethy DR, Greenblatt DJ. Effect of penbutolol on lidocaine kinetics. Arzneim-Forsch/Drug Res (1983) 33, 1680–1.
7 Jordo L, Johnsson G, Lundborg P, Regardh C-G. Pharmacokinetics of lidocaine in healthy individuals pretreated with multiple dose of metoprolol. Int J Clin Pharmacol Ther Tox (1984) 22, 312–15.
8 Ochs HR, Carstens G, Greenblatt DJ. Reduction of lidocaine clearance during continuous infusion and by co-administration of propranolol. N Engl J Med (1980) 303, 373.
9 Conrad KA, Byers JM, Finley PR, Burnham L. Lidocaine elimination:

effects of metoprolol and of propranolol. Clin Pharmacol Ther (1983) 33, 133–8.
10 Graham CM, Turner WM, Jones JK. Lidocaine-propranolol interactions. N Engl J Med (1981) 304, 1301.
11 Wyse DG, Kellen J, Tam Y, Rademaker AW. Increased efficacy and toxicity of ligocaine in patients on beta-blockers. Int J Cardiol (1988) 21, 59–70.

Lignocaine (Lidocaine) + Cimetidine or Ranitidine

Abstract/Summary

Cimetidine reduces the clearance of lignocaine and raises serum levels in some patients. Lignocaine toxicity may occur if the dosage is not reduced. Ranitidine appears to interact minimally. See also Anaesthetics, local + Cimetidine or Ranitidine in chapter 20.

Clinical evidence

(a) Studies with cimetidine in patients

15 patients were given 1 mg/kg lignocaine IV followed by a constant infusion of 2 or 3 mg/min until steady-state serum levels were established. 6 h later they were started on cimetidine (initial dose 300 mg IV, then 300 mg 6-hourly by mouth). After 12 h the lignocaine serum levels of 14 of the 15 had risen by an average of 75% (to 5.6 μg/ml) but only a 30% increase when compared with the control group (4.3 μg/ml). Six patients developed toxic serum levels (+ 5 μg/ml) and two experienced lethargy and confusion attributable to toxicity which disappeared when the lignocaine was stopped.[1]

A study in patients with suspected myocardial infarction given two 300 mg oral doses of cimetidine 4 h apart, starting 11–20 h after a 2 mg/min infusion of lignocaine began, showed that total lignocaine serum levels had risen by 28% after 24 h and unbound levels by 18%. In three of these patients whose diagnosis was subsequently confirmed, rises in total and unbound lignocaine serum levels of 24% and 9% occurred by 24 h.[3] In contrast, a study in six patients with suspected myocardial infarction given lignocaine infusions, followed later by a cimetidine infusion, failed to find a significant increase in the plasma accumulation of lignocaine.[6]

(b) Studies with cimetidine in normal subjects

A rise in peak serum lignocaine levels of 50% was seen in a study in six normal subjects given 300 mg cimetidine six-hourly for a day. Systemic clearance fell by 35% (from 766 to 576 ml/min) and five of the six experienced toxicity.[2] 18 normal subjects taking 1 g cimetidine daily for 3 days showed a 21% fall in lignocaine clearance.[4] An 18% and a 30% fall in lignocaine clearance was described in two studies in six and seven normal subjects.[10,5] In another study on six normal subjects the lignocaine clearance under steady-state conditions was reduced 34%.[7]

(c) Studies with ranitidine in normal subjects

A study in 10 normal subjects given 150 mg ranitidine twice daily for 5 days showed that it increased the systemic clearance of lignocaine (given orally or intravenously) by 9%.[8] Another study in six normal subjects given the same dose of ranitidine for one day found no change in the clearance of lignocaine given intravenously.[9]

Mechanism

Not established. It seems possible that the metabolism of the lignocaine is reduced both by a fall in blood flow to the liver and by direct inhibition of the activity of the liver microsomal J and enzymes. As a result its clearance is reduced and its serum levels rise.

Importance and management

The lignocaine-cimetidine interaction is well studied but controversial. It is confused by the differences between the studies (healthy subjects, patients with different diseases, different modes of drug administration, etc). A fall in the clearance of lignocaine (35% or more) and a resultant rise in the serum levels should be looked for if cimetidine is used, but a clinically significant alteration may not occur in every patient. It may possibly be of less importance in patients following a myocardial infarction because of the increased amounts of alpha-1-acid glycoprotein which alters the levels of bound and free lignocaine.[3] Monitor all patients closely for evidence of toxicity and check serum lignocaine levels regularly. A reduced infusion rate may be needed. Ranitidine would appear to be a suitable non-interacting alternative for cimetidine. See also Anaesthetics, local + Cimetidine or Ranitidine in chapter 20.

References

1 Knapp AB, Maguire W, Keren G, Karmen A, Levitt B, Miura DS, Somberg JC. The cimetidine-lidocaine interaction. Ann Intern Med (1983) 98, 174–7.
2 Feeley J, Wilkinson GR, McAllister CB, Wood AJJ. Increased toxicity and reduced clearance of lidocaine by cimetidine. Ann Intern Med (1982) 96, 592–4.
3 Berk SI, Gal P, Bauman JL, Douglas JB, McCue JD, Powell JR. The effect of oral cimetidine on total and unbound serum lignocaine concentrations in patients with suspected myocardial infarction. Int J Cardiol (1987) 14, 91–4.
4 Wing LMH. Miners JO, Birkett DJ, Foenander T, Lillywhite K, Wanwimolruk S. Lidocaine disposition-sex differences and effects of cimetidine. Clin Pharmacol Ther (1984) 35, 695–701.
5 Bauer LA, Edwards WAD, Randolph FP, Blouin RA. Cimetidine-induced decrease in lidocaine metabolism. Am Heart J (1984) 108, 413–15.
6 Patterson JH, Foster J, Powell JR, Cross R, Wargin W, Clark JL. Influence of a continuous cimetidine infusion on lidocaine plasma concentrations in patients. J Clin Pharmacol (1985) 25, 607–9.
7 Powell JR, Foster J, Patterson JH, Cross R, Wargin W. Effect of duration of lidocaine infusion and route of cimetidine administration on lidocaine pharmacokinetics. Clin Pharm (1986) 5, 993–8.J and
8 Robson RA, Wing LMH, Miners JO, Lilleywhite K, Birkett DJ. The effect of ranitidine on the disposition of lignocaine. Br J clin Pharmac (1985) 20, 170–3.
9 Feeley J, Guy E. Lack of effect of ranitidine on the disposition of lignocaine. Br J clin Pharmac (1983) 15, 378–9.

10 Jackson JE, Bentley JB, Glass SJ, Fukui T, Gandolfi AJ, Plachetka JR. Effects of histamine-2 receptor blockade on lidocaine kinetics. Clin Pharmacol Ther (1985) 37, 544–8.

Lignocaine (Lidocaine) + Disopyramide

Abstract/Summary

Laboratory studies show that disopyramide can increase the levels of unbound lignocaine, but whether in practice their combined effects have a clinically important depressant effect on the heart is not known.

Clinical evidence, mechanism, importance and management

An *in vitro* study using serum taken from nine patients receiving lignocaine for severe ventricular arrhythmias showed that there was an average 20% increase in its free (unbound) fraction when disopyramide in a concentration of 14.7 mol/l was added.[1] The reason would seem to be that disopyramide can displace lignocaine from its binding sites on plasma proteins (alpha-1-acid glycoprotein).

The importance of this possible displacement interaction in clinical practice uncertain. The suggestion made by the authors[1] is that a transient 20% increase in levels of free and active lignocaine plus the negative inotropic effects of the disopyramide might possibly be hazardous in patients with reduced heart function. More study is needed.

Reference

1 Bonde J, Jensen NM, Burgaard P, Angelo HR, Graudal N, Kampmann JP, Pedersen LE. Displacement of lidocaine from human plasma proteins by disopyramide. Pharmacol Toxicol (1987) 60, 151–5.

Lignocaine (Lidocaine) + Morphine

Abstract/Summary

Morphine given as an intravenous bolus does not alter lignocaine serum levels given as a continuous intravenous infusion.

Clinical evidence, mechanism, importance and management

A controlled study in 10 subjects who were receiving continuous lignocaine infusions during suspected myocardial infarction found that a 10 mg IV morphine sulphate bolus did not significantly alter the steady-state serum levels of lignocaine (about 2.45 g/ml).[1]

Reference

1 Vacek JL, Wilson DB, Hurwitz A, Gollub SB, Dunn MI. The effect of morphine sulphate on serum lidocaine levels. Clin Res (1988) 36) 325A.

Lignocaine (Lidocaine) + Phenytoin

Abstract/Summary

The incidence of central toxic side-effects may be increased following the concurrent intravenous infusion of lignocaine and phenytoin. Sinoatrial arrest has been reported in one patient. In patients taking phenytoin as an anticonvulsant, serum lignocaine levels are slightly reduced when given intravenously, but markedly reduced if given orally.

Clinical evidence

(a) Cardiac depression and increased side-effects

A study in five patients given 0.5–3.0 mg/min lignocaine intravenously for at least 24 h, followed by additional intravenous infusions of phenytoin, showed that serum levels of both drugs remained normal and unchanged but the incidence of side-effects (vertigo, nausea, nystagmus, diplopia, impaired hearing) were unusually high.[4]

Sinoatrial arrest occurred in a man following a suspected myocardial infarction with heart block, after receiving 1 mg/kg lignocaine infused intravenously in 1 min, followed 3 min later by 250 mg phenytoin over 5 min. The patient lost consciousness and his blood pressure could not be measured, but he responded to 200 mg isoprenaline.[1]

(b) Reduced serum lignocaine levels

A study found that the clearance of intravenous lignocaine is slightly greater in patients taking anticonvulsants than in normal subjects (0.85 compared with 0.77 l/min) but this difference was not statistically significant.[2] Other studies in epileptic patients and normal subjects showed that when taking phenytoin the bioavailability of lignocaine (lidocaine) given orally was halved.[2,3]

Mechanisms

(a) Phenytoin and lignocaine appear to have additive depressant actions on the heart. (b) The reduced lignocaine serum levels is possibly due to liver enzyme induction; when given orally the marked reduction results from the stimulation of hepatic first-pass metabolism phenytoin.[2,3]

Importance and management

Information is limited and the importance of the interactions is not well established. (a) The case of sinoatrial arrest emphasizes the need to exercise caution when giving two drugs which have depressant actions on the heart. (b) The reduction in serum lignocaine levels given intravenously to patients taking anticonvulsants, including phenytoin, is small and appears not to be of any clinical significance. Since lignocaine is not usually given orally, the practical importance of the marked reduction in bioavailability would also seem to be small.

References

1 Wood RA. Sinoatrial arrest: an interaction between phenytoin and lignocaine. Br Med J (1971) i, 645.
2 Perucca E, Richens A. Reduction of oral bioavailability of lignocaine by induction of first pass metabolism in epileptic patients. Br J clin Pharmac (1979) 8, 21–31.
3 Perucca E, Hedges A, Makki KA, Richens A. A comparative study of antipyrine and lignocaine disposition in normal subjects and in patients treated with enzyme-inducing drugs. Br J clin Pharmac (1980) 10, 491–7.
4 Karlsson E, Collste P, Rawlins ML. Plasma levels of lidocaine during combined treatment with phenytoin and procainamide. Europ J clin Pharmacol (1974) 7, 455

Lignocaine (Lidocaine) + Procainamide

Abstract/Summary

An isolated case of delerium has been described in a patient given lignocaine and procainamide.

Clinical evidence, mechanism, importance and management

A man with paroxysmal tachycardia, under treatment with oral procainamide and increasing doses of lignocaine by intravenous infusion, became restless, noisy and delerious when given a further intravenous dose of procainamide.[1] The reason is not understood but the symptoms suggest that the neurotoxic effects of the two drugs might be additive. Other studies in patients have shown that lignocaine plasma levels are unaffected by procainamide.[2]

References

1 Ilyas M, Owens D, Kvasnicka G. Delerium induced by a combination of anti-arrhythmic drugs. Lancet (1969) ii, 1368.
2 Karlsson E, Collste P, Rawlins MD. Plasma levels of lidocaine during combined treatment with phenytoin and procainamide. Eur J clin Pharmacol (1974) 7, 455.

Lignocaine (Lidocaine) + Propafenone

Abstract/Summary

Propafenone has miminal effects on the pharmacokinetics and pharmacodynamics of lignocaine, but the severity and duration of the CNS side-effects are increased.

Clinical evidence, mechanism, importance and management

12 normal subjects who had been taking 225 mg propafenone 8-hourly for 4 days were given a continuous infusion of lignocaine, 2 mg/kg/h for 22 h. The AUC (area under the curve) of the lignocaine was increased by 7% (from 76.3 to 81.7 µg/hr/ml) and the clearance was reduced by 7% (from 10.27 to 9.53 ml/min/kg). One poor metabolizer showed an increase in clearance. The pharmacodynamic changes seen were increases in the PR and QRS intervals of 10–20%. Combined use increased the severity and duration of adverse effects (lightheadedness, dizziness, parathesia, lethargy, somnolence). One subject withdrew from the study as a result.[1]

There would therefore appear to be no marked or important interactions (pharmacokinetic or pharmacodynamic) between these two drugs, but the increased side-effects may be poorly tolerated by some individuals which could limit their combined use.

Reference

1 Ujhelyi MR, O'Rangers EA, Fan C, Kluger J, Pharand C, Chow MSS. The pharmacokinetic and pharmacodynamic interaction between propafenone and lidocaine. Clin Pharmacol Ther (1993) 53, 38–48.

Lignocaine (Lidocaine) + Tocainide

Abstract/Summary

An isolated report describes a tonic-clonic seizure in a man which occurred during the period when his treatment for arrhythmia with lignocaine was being changed for tocainide.

Clinical evidence, mechanism, importance and management

An elderly man treated with frusemide and co-trimoxazole experienced a tonic-clonic seizure while his treatment with lignocaine was being changed to tocainide, although the serum levels of both antiarrhythmics remained within their therapeutic ranges. The patient became progressively agitated and disorientated about 2 h after taking the second of two 600 mg (six-hourly) oral doses of tocainide while still receiving 2 mg/min lignocaine IV, and about 1 h later he had the seizure. The patient subsequently tolerated each drug separately at concentrations similar to those which preceded the seizure without problems.[1] The reason for this reaction is not understood.

Reference

1 Forrence E, Covinsky JO, Mullen C. A seizure induced by concurrent lidocaine-tocainide therapy—Is it just a case of additive toxicity? Drug Intell Clin Pharm (1986) 20, 56–9.

Lorcainide + Rifampicin (Rifampin)

Abstract/Summary

A report describes a marked reduction in serum lorcainide concentrations and failure to control ventricular tachycardia in a man treated with rifampicin.

Clinical evidence, mechanism, importance and management

A 62-year-old on 600 mg rifampicin daily for tuberculosis had his treatment for ventricular tachycardia changed from lignocaine to lorcainide. It was found necessary to given him three times the normal dosage (800–900 mg daily instead of 200–300 mg) to control his condition and to achieve satisfactory serum levels (0.29 g/ml). The likely reason is that the rifampicin (a known, potent enzyme inducing agent) increased the metabolism of the lorcainide by the liver, thereby hastening its loss from the body and reducing the serum levels.[1] This seems to be the first and only report of this interaction, but be alert for it in any patient receiving these drugs and anticipate the need to increase the lorcainide dosage. The other inference to be drawn from this case is that lignocaine is not affected by rifampicin, but this needs confirmation.

Reference

1 Mauro VF, Somani P, Temesy-Armos PN. Drug interaction between lorcainide and rifampicin. Eur J Clin Pharmacol (1987) 31, 737–8.

Mexiletine + Antacids, Urinary acidifiers and Alkalinizers

Abstract/Summary

Changes in urinary pH caused by the concurrent use of acidifying or alkalinizing drugs do not normally have a marked effect on the plasma levels of mexiletine, but a few patients may be affected. The absorption is unaltered by the concurrent use of Gelusil.

Clinical evidence, mechanism, importance and management

Mexiletine is normally largely cleared from the body by liver metabolism[1] and only about 10% is excreted unchanged in the urine. Although changes in urinary pH can affect the amounts lost in the urine,[2,3,5] alterations brought about by diet or the concurrent use of alkalinizers or acidifiers (antacids, acetazolamide, etc.) would not be expected to have a marked effect on the plasma concentrations of mexiletine in most patients. There appear to be no reports of adverse interactions but concurrent use should be monitored. A single dose study showed that the bioavailability of mexiletine was unchanged by Gelusil.[4]

References

1 Beckett AH, Chidomere EC. The distribution, metabolism and excretion of mexiletine in man. Postgrad Med J (1977) 53 (Suppl 1) 60–6.
2 Kiddie MA, Kaye CM, Turner P. The influence of urinary pH on the elimination of mexiletine. Br J clin Pharmac (1974) 1, 229–32.
3 Johnston A, Burgess CD, Warrington SJ, Wadsworth J, Hamer NAJ. The effect of spontaneous changes in urinary pH on mexiletine plasma concentrations and excretion during chronic administration to healthy volunteers. Br J clin Pharmac (1979) 8, 349–52.
4 Herzog P, Holtermuller KH, Kasper W, Meinertz T, Trenk D, Jahnchen E. Absorption of mexiletine after treatment with gastric antacids. Br J clin Pharmac (1982) 14, 746–7.
5 Mitchell BG, Clements JA, Pottage A, Prescott LF. Mexiletine disposition: individual variation in response to urine acidification and alkalinization. Br J clin Pharmac (1983) 16, 281–4.

Mexiletine + Antiarrhythmic drugs

Abstract/Summary

The concurrent use of mexiletine and either propranolol or quinidine is reported to be beneficial, and side-effects may be reduced. The same is possibly also true for amiodarone. Quinidine raises mexiletine serum levels.

Clinical evidence, mechanism, importance and management

A study in patients showed that a combination of mexiletine and propranolol (240 mg daily) was more effective in blocking ventricular premature depolarizations (VPD) and ventricular tachycardia, without significant side-effects, than mexiletine alone.[1] A statistical decrease in VPDs in a considerable number of patients given combined treatment is described elsewhere.[2] Mexiletine and quinidine given concurrently are reported to be more effective than quinidine alone, and the incidence of side-effects is reduced.[3] Combined use is reported to prolong refractoriness and conduction time in the periinfarct zone.[5] The clinical consequences of the finding that quinidine reduces the metabolism and excretion of mexiletine in extensive metabolisers (total clearance reduced by 24%[7]) but not poor metabolisers, is uncertain. It is probably beneficial.[4,6,7] More study is needed.

References

1 Leahey EB, Heissenbuttel RH, Giardina EGV, Bigger JT. Combined mexiletine and propranolol treatment of refractory ventricular tachycardia. Br Med J (1980) 281, 357.
2 Quoted as unpublished data by Bigger JT. The interaction of mexiletine with other cardiovascular drugs. Am Heart J (1984) 107, 1079–85.
3 Duff HJ, Roden D, Primm RK, Oates JA, Woosley RL. Mexiletine in the treatment of resistant ventricular arrhythmias: enhancement of efficacy and reduction of dose-related side-effects by combination with quinidine. Circulation (1983) 67, 1124.
4 Broly F, Vandamme N, Caron J, Libersa C, Lhithermitte M. Single dose quinidine treatment inhibits mexiletine oxidation in extensive metabolisers of debrisoquine. Life Sci (1991) 48, PL-123–8.
5 Duff HJ, Rahmberg M, Sheldon RS. Role of quinidine in the mexiletine-quinidine interaction: electrophysiological correlates of enhanced antiarrhythmic efficacy. J Cardiovasc Pharmacol (1990) 16, 685–92.

6 Fiset C, Giguère R, Kroemer HK, Gilbert M, Rouleau JR, Mikus G, Nguyen NN, Eichelbaum M, Bélanger PM, Turgeon J. Genetically-determined pharmacokinetic interaction between mexiletine and quinidine in man. Clin Invest Med (1991) 4 Suppl A, A18.

7 Turgeon J, Fiset C, Giguère R, Gilbert M, Moerike K, Rouleau JR, Kroemer HK, Eichelbaum M, Grech-Bélanger O, Bélanger PM. Influence of debrisoquine phenotype and of quinidine on mexiletine disposition in man. J Pharmacol Exp Ther (1991) 259, 789–98.

Mexiletine + Cimetidine or Ranitidine

Abstract/Summary

No adverse interaction occurs if mexiletine and cimetidine or ranitidine are given concurrently. Cimetidine can reduce the gastric side-effects of mexiletine.

Clinical evidence, mechanism, importance and management

A study in 11 patients showed that their peak and trough serum mexiletine levels were unaltered when given cimetidine, 1 g daily for a week, and the frequency and severity of the ventricular arrhythmias for which they were receiving treatment remained unchanged. Moreover the gastric side-effects of mexiletine were reduced in half of the patients.[1] This study in patients confirms other single-dose studies[2-4] using cimetidine and ranitidine in normal subjects. There would seem to be no problems with giving these drugs concurrently, and some advantages.

References

1 Klein AL, Sami MH. Usefulness and safety of cimetidine in patients receiving mexiletine for ventricular arrhythmia. Am Heart J (1985) 109, 1281.

2 Klein A, Sami M, Selinger K. Mexiletine kinetics in healthy subjects taking cimetidine. Clin Pharmacol Ther (1985) 37, 669–73.

3 Brockmeyer NH, Breithaupt H, von Hattingberg MV, Ohnhaus EE. Metabolism of mexiletine alone and in combination with cimetidine and ranitidine in vivo and in vitro. Br J clin Pharmac (1987) 39, 246P.

4 Brockmeyer NH, Breithaupt H, Ferdinand W, von Hattingberg MV, Ohnhaus EE. Kinetics of oral and intravenous mexiletine: lack of effect of cimetidine and ranitidine. Eur J Clin Pharmacol (1989) 36, 375–8.

Mexiletine + Diamorphine or Morphine

Abstract/Summary

The absorption of mexiletine is depressed in patients following a myocardial infarction, and very markedly depressed and delayed if diamorphine or morphine is used concurrently. This can limit its value as an antiarrhythmic agent during the first few hours following an infarction.

Clinical evidence

A pharmacokinetic study in patients and normal subjects showed that the serum levels of mexiletine (400 mg orally followed by 200 mg 2 h later) in patients who had had a myocardial infarction and who had been given diamorphine (5–10 mg) or morphine (10–15 mg) were reduced as follows: at 2 h to 33%; 3 h 40%; 4 h 53%; 6 h 70% and 8 h 80%. The peak concentrations in the subjects and the patients occurred at 3 and 6 h respectively.[1,2]

Mechanism

The reduced absorption of mexiletine would seem to result from inhibition by the narcotics of gastric emptying. Other mechanisms probably contribute to its delayed clearance.

Importance and management

An established interaction although information is limited. The delay and reduction in the absorption would seem to limit the value of oral mexiletine during the first few hours after a myocardial infarction, particularly if these narcotic analgesics are used.

References

1 Prescott LF, Pottage A, Clements JA. Absorption, distribution and elimination of mexiletine. Postgrad Med J (1977) 53 (Suppl 1) 50–5.

2 Pottage A, Campbell RWF, Achuff SC, Murray A, Julian DC, Prescott LF. The absorption of oral mexiletine in coronary care patients. Eur J clin Pharmac (1978) 13, 393–9.

Mexiletine + Phenytoin

Abstract/Summary

Serum mexiletine levels are reduced by the concurrent use of phenytoin. An increase in the dosage may be necessary.

Clinical evidence

The observation of three patients who had unusually low serum mexiletine levels while taking phenytoin, prompted a pharmacokinetic study in six normal subjects. After taking 300 mg phenytoin daily for a week, the mean mexiletine AUC (area under the curve) and its half-life following single 400 mg doses were reduced by an average of about 50% (AUC reduced from 17.7 to 8.0 g/ml/h; half-life reduced from 17.2 to 8.4 h).[1]

Mechanism

The most likely explanation is that phenytoin, a potent liver enzyme-inducing agent, increases the metabolism and clearance of mexiletine from the body.

Importance and management

Information seems to be limited to this report,[1] but the interaction appears to be established. It seems possible that the fall in mexiletine levels will be clinically important in some individuals. Monitor the serum mexiletine levels and raise the dosage if necessary.

Reference

1 Begg EJ, Chinwah PM, Day RO, Wade DN. Enhanced metabolism of mexiletine after phenytoin administration. Br J clin Pharmac (1982) 14, 219–23.

Mexiletine + Rifampicin (Rifampin)

Abstract/Summary

The clearance of mexiletine from the body is increased by the concurrent use of rifampicin. An increase in the dosage of mexiletine may be necessary.

Clinical evidence, mechanism, importance and management

After taking 600 mg rifampicin daily for 10 days, the half-life of a single 400 mg dose of mexiletine was reduced in eight normal subjects by 40% (from 8.5 to 5 h).[1,2] The probable reason is that the rifampicin (a known, potent enzyme-inducing agent) increases the metabolism and clearance of the mexiletine from the body. It seems likely that the mexiletine dosage will need to be increased during concurrent use, but by how much is uncertain. More study is needed to confirm the clinical importance of this interaction.

References

1 Pentikainen PJ, Koivula IH, Hiltunen HA. Effect of enzyme induction on pharmacokinetics of mexiletine. Clin Pharmacol Ther (1982) 31, 260.
2 Pentikainen PJ, Koivula IH, Hiltunen HA. Effect of rifampicin treatment on the kinetics of mexiletine. Eur J Clin Pharmacol (1982) 23, 261–6.

Moricizine (Ethmozine) + Beta-blockers

Abstract/Summary

Moricizine appears not to interact adversely with propranolol.

Clinical evidence, mechanism, importance and management

No formal studies of the possible pharmacokinetic and pharmacodynamic interactions of propranolol and moricizine seem to have been carried out, but among patients given both drugs there seems to be no evidence of any adverse interactions, changes in blood pressure or heart rate.[1,2]

References

1 Pratt CM, Butman SM, Young JB, Knoll M, English LD. Antiarrhythmic efficacy of ethmozine (moricizine HCl) compared with disopyramide and propranolol. Am J Cardiol (1987) 60, 52–8F.
2 Butman SM, Knoll ML, Gardin JM. Comparison of ethmozine to propranolol and the combination for ventricular arrhythmias. Am J Cardiol (1987) 60, 603–7.

Moricizine (Ethmozine) + Cimetidine

Abstract/Summary

Cimetidine increases the serum levels of moricizine but the clinical importance of this is uncertain.

Clinical evidence, mechanism, importance and management

After taking 300 mg cimetidine four times daily for seven days, the clearance of a single 500 mg dose of moricizine in eight normal subjects was halved (from 38.2 to 19.7 ml/kg/min) and both its half-life and the AUC were increased (from 3.3 to 4.6 h and from 5.6 to 7.8 µg/ml/h respectively). It is believed that this is because the cimetidine reduces its metabolism by the liver.[1] Despite the increase in serum moricizine levels, the PR and QRS intervals were not further prolonged, possibly (so it is postulated) because some of the metabolites of moricizine are also pharmacologically active. Concurrent use should be well monitored but measuring serum moricizine levels may be of limited value. More study is needed. It seems unlikely that ranitidine will interact with moricizine.

Reference

1 Biollaz J, Shaheen O, Wood AJJ. Cimetidine inhibition of moricizine metabolism. Clin Pharmacol Ther (1985) 37, 665–8.

Pirmenol + Cimetidine

Abstract/Summary, clinical evidence, mechanism, importance and management

300 mg cimetidine four times daily for eight days in eight normal subjects had no significant effect on the pharmacokinetics of single 150 mg oral doses of pirmenol.[1] No clinically important interaction would therefore be expected in patients given both drugs.

Reference

1 Stringer KA, Lebsack ME, Cetnarowski-Cropp AB, Goldfarb AL, Radulovic LL, Broackbrader HN, Chang T, Sedman AJ. Effect of cimetidine

administration on the pharmacokinetics of pirmenol. J Clin Pharmacol (1992) 32, 91–2.

Pirmenol + Rifampicin (Rifampin)

Abstract/Summary

Rifampicin markedly increases the loss of pirmenol from the body. A reduction in its antiarrhythmic effects is likely to occur.

Clinical evidence

Fourteen days' treatment with 600 mg rifampicin daily markedly affected the pharmacokinetics of a single 150 mg dose of pirmenol in 12 normal subjects. The apparent plasma clearance increased seven-fold (from 12.8 to 88.2 l/h) and the AUC (area under the curve) decreased 83% (from 13.34 to 2.28 mg/h/l).[1,2]

Mechanism

The probable reason is that the rifampicin (a well-recognized enzyme inducer) increases the metabolism of the pirmenol by the liver, thereby increasing its loss from the body.

Importance and management

Direct information seems to be limited to this study but what occurred is consistent with the way rifampicin interacts with other drugs. Anticipate the need to increase the dosage of pirmenol if rifampicin is used concurrently.

References

1 Stringer KA, Thomas RW, Cetnarowski AB, Goldfarb AL. Effect of rifampin on the disposition of pirmenol. J Clin Pharmacol (1987) 27, 709.
2 Stringer KA, Cetnarowski AB, Goldfarb AB, Lebsack ME, Chang TS, Allen J. Enhanced pirmenol elimination by rifampin. J Clin Pharmacol (1988) 28, 1094–7.

Procainamide + Amiodarone

Abstract/Summary

Serum procainamide levels are increased by about 60% and of N-acetylprocainamide by about 30% if amiodarone is given concurrently. The dosage of procainamide will need to be reduced to avoid toxicity.

Clinical evidence

12 patients were stabilized on procainamide (2–6 g daily, or about 900 mg 6-hourly). When concurrently treated with amiodarone (600 mg loading dose 12-hourly for 5–7 days, then 600 mg daily) their mean serum procainamide levels rose by 57% (from 6.8 to 10.6 μg/ml) and their serum N-acetylprocainamide (NAPA) levels rose by 32% (from 6.9 to 9.1 μg/ml). Procainamide levels increased by more than 3.0 μg/ml in six patients. The increases usually occurred within 24 h, but in other patients as late as four or five days. Toxicity was seen in two patients. Despite lowering the procainamide dosages by 20%, serum procainamide levels were still higher (at 7.7 μg/ml) than before the amiodarone was started.[1]

An increase of 35% in trough serum procainimide level was seen in four other patients after four days treatment with amiodarone, 6–15 mg/kg.[2] A further study on eight patients by the same workers found that amiodarone decreased the clearance of procainamide by 23% and the electrophysiological actions of both drugs appeared to be additive.[3]

Mechanism

Not understood. An animal study found that the QT interval lengthening caused by N-acetylprocainamide was greatly increased by amiodarone.[4]

Importance and management

Information appears to be limited to these studies, but the interaction would seem to be established and clinically important. Its incidence is high (11 out of 12 in the report cited[1]), and it develops rapidly. The dosage of procainamide may need to be reduced 20–50% if amiodarone is given. Serum levels should be monitored and patients observed for side-effects.[1]

References

1 Saal AK, Werner JA, Greene HL, Sears GK, Graham EL. Effect of amiodarone on serum quinidine and procainamide levels. Am J Cardiol (1984) 53, 1265–7.
2 Windle JR, Prystowsky EN, Miles WM, Zipes DP, Heger JJ. Pharmacokinetic and pharmacodynamic interaction of amiodarone and procainamide. J Am Coll Cardiol (1985) 5, 481.
3 Windle J, Prystowsky EN, Miles WM, Heger JJ. Pharmacokinetic and electrophysiologic interactions of amiodarone and procainamide. Clin Pharmacol Ther (1987) 41, 603–10.
4 Xiaoquan L, Xiaolei Y, Shengkai H. Effect of steady state amiodarone on the pharmacokinetics and QT interval prolongation of N-acetylprocainamide. Zhongguo Yaoke Daxue Xuebao (1992) 23, 22–4.

Procainamide + Beta-blockers

Abstract/Summary

The pharmacokinetics of procainamide are little changed by either propranolol or metoprolol.

Clinical evidence, mechanism, importance and management

One study in six normal subjects found that long-term treatment with propranolol (period and dosage not stated) increased the procainamide half-life from 1.71 to 2.66 h and reduced the plasma clearance by 16%.[1] However a later study in eight normal subjects showed that the pharmacokinetics of a single 500 mg dose of procainamide hydrochloride were only slightly altered by the concurrent use of either 80 mg propranolol three times daily or 100 mg metoprolol twice daily. The procainamide half-life increased from 1.9 to 2.2 h with propranolol and to 2.3 h with metoprolol, but no significant changes in total clearance occurred. No changes in the AUC of N-acetyl procainamide were seen.[2] It seems unlikely that a clinically important adverse interaction normally occurs between these drugs. There seems to be no information about other beta-blockers.

References

1 Weidler DJ, Gang DC, Jalad NS, McFarland MA. The effect of long-term propranolol on the pharmacokinetics of procainamide in humans. Clin Pharmacol Ther (1981) 29, 289.

2 Ochs HR, Carstens G, Roberts G-M, Greenblatt DJ. Metoprolol or propranolol does not alter the kinetics of procainamide. J Cardiovasc Pharmacol (1983) 5, 392–5.

Procainamide + Cimetidine, Famotidine or Ranitidine

Abstract/Summary

Serum procainimide levels can be increased if cimetidine is given concurrently and toxicity may develop, particularly in those who have a reduced renal clearance such as the elderly. Raniditine and famotidine appear to interact only minimally or not at all.

Clinical evidence

(a) Cimetidine

36 elderly patients (65–90 years old) on sustained-release oral procainamide 6-hourly showed mean steady-state serum procainamide and N-acetylprocainamide levels rises of 55 and 36% respectively after taking 300 mg cimetidine 6-hourly for 3 days. 24 of them tolerated this without side-effects (serum procainamide and N-acetylprocainamide <12 and <15 mg/l respectively) but the other 12 had some adverse effects (nausea, weakness, malaise P-R intervals <20%) which was dealt with by stopping one or both drugs.[8] Another report describes an elderly man who developed procainamide toxicity when given 1200 mg cimetidine daily. His procainamide dosage was roughly halved (from 937 to 500 mg daily) to bring his serum procainamide and N-acetylprocainamide levels into the accepted therapeutic range.[1]

Other studies in normal subjects have found that cimetidine increases the procainamide AUC (area under the curve) by 35%-43%,[1-3,7,12] and decreases the loss through the kidneys by

35–36%.[4,12] A steady-state procainamide serum level increase of 45% has been seen following 1200 mg cimetidine daily.[6]

(b) Ranitidine and famotidine

One study found that ranitidine reduced the absorption of procainamide from the gut and the kidney excretion,[5] increasing the maximum procainamide levels by 16%, the AUC by 14% and the AUC of N-acetylprocainamide by 13%[5,9] whereas no change in the pharmacokinetics of procainamide by ranitidine was found in two other studies.[6,12] Yet another study found that 40 mg famotidine for five days did not affect the pharmacokinetics or pharmacodynamics of procainamide in normal subjects.[10,11]

Mechanism

Procainamide levels in the body are increased because the cimetidine reduces its kidney excretion by about a third or more,[1,4,12] but the precise mechanism is uncertain. One suggestion is that it interferes with the active secretion of procainamide by the kidney tubules.[3,4]

Importance and management

The procainamide-cimetidine interaction is established. Concurrent use should be undertaken with care because the safety margin of procainamide is low. Reduce the procainamide dosage as necessary. This is particularly important in the elderly because they have a reduced ability to clear both drugs. Ranitidine and famotidine appear not to interact to a clinically important extent, but it should be appreciated that what is known is based on studies in normal subjects rather than patients. Be alert for any of evidence of an adverse interaction.

References

1 Somogyi A, Heinzow B. Cimetidine reduces procainamide elimination. N Engl J Med (1982) 307, 1080.

2 Higbee MD, Wood JS, Mead RA. Case report. Procainamide-cimetidine interaction. A potential toxic interaction in the elderly. J Am Geriatr Soc (1984) 32, 162–4.

3 Somogyi A, McLean A, Heinzow B. Cimetidine-procainamide pharmacokinetic interaction in man: evidence of competition for tubular secretion of basic drugs. Eur J Clin Pharmacol (1983) 25, 339–45.

4 Christian CD, Meredith CG, Speeg KV. Cimetidine inhibits renal procainamide clearance. Clin Pharmacol Ther (1984) 36, 221–7.

5 Somogyi A, Bochner F. Dose and concentration dependent effect of ranitidine on procainamide disposition and renal clearance in man. Br J Clin Pharmac (1984) 18, 175–81.

6 Paloucek F, Rodvold K, Jang D, Gallestegui J. The effects of cimetidine and ranitidine on steady-state pharmacokinetics of procainamide. J Clin Pharmacol (1986) 26, 557.

7 Lai MY, Jiang FM, Chung CH, Chen HC, Chao PDL. Dose dependent effect of cimetidine on procainamide disposition in man. Int J Clin Phamacol Ther Toxicol (1988) 26, 118–21.

8 Bauer LA, Black D, Gensler A. Procainamide-cimetidine interaction in elderly male patients. J Amer Geriatr Soc (1990) 38, 467–9.

9 Somogyi A, Bochner F. Dose and concentration dependent effect of ranitidine on procainamide disposition and renal clearance in man. Br J Clin Pharmacol (1984) 18, 175–81.

10 Klotz U, Arvela P, Rosenkranz B. Interaction study of diazepam and

procainamide with the new H2-receptor antagonist famotidine. Clin Pharmacol Ther (1985) 37, 206.

11 Klotz U, Arvela P, Rosenkranz B. Famotidine, a new H2-receptor antagonist, does not affect hepatic elimination of diazepam or tubular secretion of procainamide. Eur J Clin Pharmacol (1985) 28, 671–5.

12 Rodvold KA, Paloucek FP, Jung D, Gallastegui J. Interaction of steady-state procainamide with H2-receptor anagonists cimetidine and ranitidine. Ther Drug Monit (1987) 9, 378–83.

Procainamide + Para-aminobenzoic acid (PABA)

Abstract/Summary

A single case report shows that para-aminobenzoic acid can reduce the metabolism of procainamide, increase its serum levels and reduce the production of N-acetylprocainamide.

Clinical evidence, mechanism, importance and management

A 61-year-old man, treated with procainamide for sustained ventricular tachycardia, was found to be a rapid acetylator of procainamide so that the serum levels of the procainamide metabolite (N-acetylprocainamide) were particularly high and he experienced some N-acetylprocainamide toxicity (this metabolite has some anti-arrhythmic properties but can also be toxic). When he was additionally given 1.5 g PABA 6-hourly for 30 h to suppress the production of this metabolite, the control of his arrhythmia improved.[1]

In this instance the interaction was exploited for the patient's benefit as part of an experimental study, but it draws attention to the possibility of increased procainamide levels in other patients concurrently treated with PABA. The importance of this is uncertain but the outcome should be monitored if PABA is added or withdrawn.

Reference

1 Nylen ES, Cohen AI, Wish MH, Lima JL, Finkelstein JD. Reduced acetylation of procainamide by para-aminobenzoic acid. J Amer Coll Cardiol (1986) 7, 185–7.

Procainamide + Probenecid

Abstract/Summary, clinical evidence, mechanism, importance and management

Probenecid appears not to interact with procainamide. The pharmacokinetics of procainamide and its effects on QT intervals are not altered by concurrent use.[1] No special precautions appear to be necessary.

Reference

1 Lam YWF, Boyd RA, Chin SK, Ghang D, Giacomini KM. Effect of

probenecid on the pharmacokinetics and pharmacodynamics of procainamide. J Clin Pharmacol (1991) 31, 429–32

Procainamide + Quinidine

Abstract/Summary

A single case report describes a marked increase in the serum procainamide levels of a patient when concurrently treated with quinidine.

Clinical evidence, mechanism, importance and management

A man with sustained ventricular tachycardia on high dose intravenous procainamide (2 g 8-hourly) showed a 70% increase (a rise from 9.1 to 15.4 ng/ml) in his steady-state serum procainamide levels when concurrently treated with 324 mg quinidine gluconate 8-hourly. The procainamide half-life increased from 3.7 to 7.2 h and its clearance fell from 27 to 16 l/h. The mechanism of interaction suggested by the authors of the report is that the quinidine interferes with one or more of renal pathways by which procainamide is cleared from the body.[1] Information so far seems to be limited to this report but it would seem prudent to monitor the effects if high-dose procainamide is given with quinidine. More study is needed to find out the general importance of this interaction.

Reference

1 Hughes B, Dyer JE, Schwartz AB. Increased procainamide plasma concentrations caused by quinidine: a new drug interaction. Am Heart J (1987) 114, 908–9.

Procainamide + Sucralfate

Abstract/Summary

Sucralfate appears not to affect the absorption of procainamide.

Clinical evidence, mechanism, importance and management

1 mg sucralfate taken 30 min before single 250 mg doses of procainamide reduced the mean maximum serum level in four normal subjects by 5.3%, but did not affect either the AUC (area under the curve) or the rate of absorption. The measurements were made on procainamide in the saliva.[1] These results need confirmation in patients taking long-term procainamide, but they suggest that a clinically significant interaction is unlikely.

Reference

1 Turkistani AAA, Gaber M, Al-Meshal MA, Al-Shora HI, Gouda MW. Effect of sucralfate on procainamide absorption. Int J Pharmaceutics (1990) 59, R1–3.

Procainamide + Trimethoprim

Abstract/Summary

Trimethoprim causes a marked increase in the serum levels of procainamide and its active metabolite, N-acetyl procainamide, with the risk of toxicity.

Clinical evidence

Eight normal subjects were given 500 mg procainamide 6-hourly for 3 days. The concurrent use of 200 mg trimethoprim daily increased the AUC (area under the curve) from 0 to 12 h of procainamide by 63% and of its active metabolite, N-acetyl procainamide, by 51%.[1,3] Another study found that 200 mg daily reduced the renal clearance of procainamide by 45% and of N-acetyl procainamide by 26%.[2]

Mechanism

Trimethoprim decreases the losses in the urine of both procainamide and its active metabolite by successfully competing for active secretion. It may also cause a small decrease in the metabolism of the procainamide.[1]

Importance and management

An established interaction but its documentation is limited. The need to reduce the procainamide dosage should be anticipated if trimethoprim is given to patients already controlled on procainamide. In practice the effects may be greater than the studies cited suggest because the elderly lose procainamide through the kidneys more slowly than normal young healthy subjects. Remember too that the daily dosage of trimethoprim in co-trimoxazole (trimethoprim 160 mg + sulphamethoxazole 800 mg) may equal or exceed the dosages used in the study cited.

References

1 Kosoglou T, Rocci ML, Vlasses PH. Evaluation of trimethoprim/procainamide interaction at steady-state in normal volunteers. Clin Pharmacol Ther (1988) 43, 131.
2 Vlasses PH, Kosoglou T, Chase SL, Greenspon AJ, Lottes S, Andress E, Ferguson RK, Rocci ML. Trimethoprim inhibition of the renal clearance of procainamide and N-acetylprocainamide. Arch Intern Med (1989) 149, 1350–3.
3 Kosoglou T, Rocci ML, Vlasses PH. Trimethoprim alters the disposition of procainamide and N-acetylprocainamide. Clin Pharmacol Ther (1988) 44, 467–77.

Propafenone + Barbiturates

Abstract/Summary

Phenobarbitone increases the loss of propafenone from the body, and reduces its serum levels.

Clinical evidence, mechanism, importance and management

After taking 100 mg phenobarbitone daily for 3 weeks the peak serum propafenone levels (following a single 300 mg dose) of seven subjects were reduced 26–87% and the AUC's were reduced 10–89%. The intrinsic clearance increased 11–849%. The results in four heavy smokers were similar.[1] The probable reason is that phenobarbitone (a potent stimulator of liver enzymes) markedly increases the metabolism of the propafenone and its loss from the body. The clinical importance of this awaits assessment but check that propafenone remains effective if phenobarbitone is added, and that toxicity does not occur if it is stopped. If the suggested mechanism is correct, other barbiturates would be expected to interact similarly. Study in patients is needed.

Reference

1 Chan GL-Y, Axelson JE, Kerr CR. The effect of phenobarbital on the pharmacokinetics of propafenone in man. Pharmaceut Res (1988) 5, S-153.

Propafenone + Cimetidine

Abstract/Summary

Cimetidine appears not to interact adversely with propafenone.

Clinical evidence, mechanism, importance and management

A study in 12 normal subjects given 225 mg propafenone 8-hourly showed that the concurrent use of 400 mg cimetidine eight-hourly caused some changes in the pharmacokinetics and pharmacodynamics of the propafenone. Raised peak and steady-state serum levels were seen but these were not statistically significant. A slight increase in the QRS duration also occurred.[1] None of the changes seems likely to be clinically important.

Reference

1 Pritchett ELC, Smith WM, Kirsten EB. Pharmacokinetic and pharmacodynamic interactions of propafenone and cimetidine. J Clin Pharmacol (1988) 28, 619–24.

Propafenone + Miscellaneous drugs

Abstract/Summary

Propafenone can oppose the effects of anticholinesterases used for myasthenia gravis and have anticholinergic effects which may possibly be additive with other anticholinergic drugs.

Shortness of breath and a worsening of the control of asthma have also been reported.

Clinical evidence, mechanism, importance and management

Propafenone is reported to aggravate myasthenia gravis, possibly due to its anticholinergic effects on nicotinic receptors on skeletal muscle. This was seen in a patient well controlled on pyridostigmine. Improvement occurred when the propafenone was withdrawn. Other cases have also been described. Avoidance of concurrent use has been advised.[1] Propafenone also has other anticholinergic effects (constipation, dry mouth, blurred vision)[1] which may possibly be additive with other drugs possessing anticholinergic effects (e.g. tricyclic antidepressants). Shortness of breath and a worsening of asthma have also been reported in a handful of cases, attributed to the beta-blocking effects of propafenone. Caution is advised in those with chronic airways disease.[1] See also 'Beta-blockers + Propafenone'.

Reference

1 Committee on the Safety of Medicines (CSM) Current Problems Series, No 29, August (1990).

Propafenone + Quinidine

Abstract/Summary

Quinidine doubles the serum levels of propafenone and halves the levels of its active metabolite in 'extensive' metabolizers, but the antiarrhythmic effects remain unaffected.

Clinical evidence

Nine patients on propafenone for frequent isolated ventricular ectopic beats, firstly had their dosage reduced to 150 mg 8-hourly and then four days later 50 mg quinidine daily was added. Four days later the steady-state serum propafenone levels in seven patients ('extensive' metabolizers) had more than doubled (from 408 to 1096 ng/ml) but the ECG intervals and arrhythmia frequency were unaltered. The steady-state serum propafenone levels remained unchanged in the other two patients ('poor' metabolizers).[1]

Mechanism

Quinidine inhibits the metabolism (cytochrome P450-dependent 5-hydroxylation) of propafenone by the liver in those who are 'extensive' metabolizers so that it is cleared more slowly. Its serum levels are doubled as a result, but the overall antiarrhythmic effects remain effectively unchanged because the production of its active antiarrhythmic metabolite (5-hydroxypropafenone) is simultaneously halved.[1] Whether one

is an 'extensive' or a 'poor' metabolizer is genetically predetermined.

Importance and management

An established interaction but apparently of little clinical importance, however until these results have been confirmed concurrent use should be well monitored. The patients described had their propafenone dosage approximately halved before the study began. The metabolic status of patients seems in this instance not to have been important.

Reference

1 Funck-Brentano C, Kroemer HK, Pavlou H, Woosley RL, Roden DM. Genetically determined interaction between propafenone and low dose quinidine: role of active metabolites in modulating net drug effect. Br J clin Pharmac (1989) 27, 435–44.

Propafenone + Rifampicin (Rifampin)

Abstract/Summary

Propafenone serum levels and its effects were markedly reduced in a patient when given rifampicin.

Clinical evidence, mechanism, importance and management

A man successfully treated with propafenone showed marked falls in his serum propafenone levels (from 993 to 176 ng/ml) and of its two active metabolites, 5-hydroxypropafenone (from 195 to 64 ng/ml) and N-depropylpropafenone (from 110 to to 64 ng/ml) within 12 days of starting to take 450 mg rifampicin twice daily. His arrhythmias returned. Two weeks after stopping the rifampicin his arrhythmias had disappeared and the propafenone and its metabolites had returned to acceptable levels (1411, 78 and 158 ng/ml respectively).[1] The probable reason is that the rifampicin (a potent enzyme inducing agent) increased the metabolism of the propafenone by the liver, thereby increasing its loss from the body and reducing its effects. This appears to be the first report of an interaction between these two drugs, but it is consistent with the way rifampicin affects other drugs. The authors of the report advise the use of another antibiotic if possible because of the probable difficulty in adjusting the propafenone dosage.

Reference

1 Castel JM, Cappiello E, Leopaldi D, Latini R. Rifampicin lowers plasma concentrations of propafenone and its antiarrhythmic effect. Br J Clin Pharmac (1990) 30, 155–6.

Quinidine + Amiodarone

Abstract/Summary

Serum quinidine levels can be approximately doubled by the concurrent use of amiodarone. Reduce the quinidine dosage appropriately to avoid quinidine toxicity and the risk of atypical ventricular tachycardia (AVT or torasades de pointes).

Clinical evidence

11 patients were stabilized on quinidine (daily doses of 4200–1200 mg). When concurrently treated with amiodarone (600 mg loading dose 12-hourly for 5–7 days, then 600 mg daily) their mean serum quinidine levels rose by an average of 32% (from 4.4 to 5.8 μg/ml). Three of them had a substantial increase (+ 2.0 μg/ml). Signs of toxicity (diarrhoea, nausea, vomiting, hypotension, etc.) were seen in some patients and the quinidine dosage was reduced in 9 of the 11 by an average of 37%. Even so, the quinidine serum levels were still higher (at 5.2 μg/ml) than before the amiodarone was started.[1]

A test on a normal subject showed that when 600 mg amiodarone was added to a daily quinidine dosage of 1200 mg, the serum quinidine levels doubled within three days and the QT interval was prolonged from 1.0 (no drugs) to 1.2 (quinidine alone) to 1.4 (quinidine + amiodarone).[2] This report also describes two patients with minor heart arrhythmias which developed into atypical ventricular tachycardia (AVT or 'torsades de pointes') when given both drugs.[2]

Mechanism

Not understood.

Importance and management

An established and clinically important interaction. It appears to occur in most patients, and to develop rapidly. It has been recommended that the dosage of quinidine should be reduced 30–50% if amiodarone is given, the serum levels should be monitored and patients observed closely for side-effects.[1] It has also been suggested that the ECG should be monitored for evidence of a prolongation of the QT interval.[2] An uncorrected QT interval greater than 0.60 sec may be an indication that the patient runs the risk of developing atypical ventricular tachycardia.[3] Successful and uneventful concurrent use is described in a report of patients on quinidine (dose not stated) and 200 mg amiodarone five times weekly.[4] Another describes successful and uneventful use for chronic atrial fibrillation without problems using small doses of quinidine (1100 mg daily) over two days.[5]

References

1 Saal AK, Werner JA, Greene HL, Sears GK, Graham EL. Effect of amiodarone on serum quinidine and procainamide levels. Am J Cardiol (1984) 53, 1265–7.

2 Tartini R, Kappenberger L, Steinbrunn W, Meyer UA. Dangerous interaction between amiodarone and quinidine. Lancet (1982) i, 1327–9.

3 Keren A, Tzivoni D, Gavish D, Levi J, Gottlieb S, Benhorin J, Stern S. Etiology, warning signs and therapy of Torsade de Pointes. Circulation (1981) 64, 1167–74.

4 Hoffman A, Follath F, Burckhardt D. Safe treatment of resistant ventricular arrhythmias with a combination of amiodarone and quinidine or mexiletine. Lancet (1983) i, 704.

5 Kerin NZ, Ansari-Leesar M, Faitel K, Narala C, Frumin H, Cohen A. The effectiveness and safety of the simultaneous administration of quinidine and amiodarone in the conversion of chronic atrial fibrillation. Am Heart J (1993) 125, 1017–21.

Quinidine + Anticonvulsants

Abstract/Summary

Serum quinidine levels can be reduced by the concurrent use of phenytoin, phenobarbitone or primidone. Loss of arrhythmia control is possible if the quinidine dosage is not increased.

Clinical evidence

When two patients appeared to have an increased quinidine clearance when given phenytoin and primidone, further study was made in four normal subjects. After 2 week's treatment with either phenytoin or phenobarbitone (in dosages adjusted to give 10–20 μg/ml) the elimination half-life of a single 300 mg dose of quinidine was reduced by about 50% and the total area under the time-concentration curve by about 60%.[1]

Similar results were found in another study in three normal subjects.[2] This interaction was observed in a patient with recurrent ventricular tachycardia.[3] Changes in quinidine levels due to pentobarbitone have been described in another report.[4] An estimated 70% reduction in the half-life of quinidine as a result of adding phenytoin to concurrent treatment with phenobarbitone is described in a 3-year-old child.[5] Difficulty in achieving adequate serum quinidine levels has been reported in a woman on phenytoin and primidone. Her quinidine half-life was approximately halved.[6]

Mechanism

The evidence suggests that phenytoin, primidone or phenobarbitone (all known enzyme-inducing agents) increase the metabolism by the liver of the quinidine and increase its loss from the body.

Importance and management

An established interaction of clinical importance although the documentation is not great. The concurrent use of phenytoin, primidone, phenobarbitone or any other barbiturate need not be avoided but be alert for the need to increase the quinidine dosage. If the anticonvulsants are withdrawn the quinidine dosage may need to be reduced to avoid quinidine intoxication. Quinidine serum levels should be monitored.

References

1 Data JL, Wilkinson GR, Nies AS. Interaction of quinidine with anticonvulsant drugs. N Engl J Med (1976) 294, 699.
2 Russo ME, Russo J, Smith RA, Pershing LK. The effect of phenytoin on quinidine pharmacokinetics. Drug Intell Clin Pharm (1982) 16, 480.
3 Urbano AM. Phenytoin-quinidine interaction in a patient with recurrent ventricular tachyarrhythmias. N Engl J Med (1983) 308, 225.
4 Chapron DJ, Mumford D, Pitegoff GJ. Apparent quinidine-induced digoxin toxicity after withdrawal of pentobarbital. A case of sequential drug interactions. Arch Intern Med (1979) 139, 363.
5 Rodgers GC, Blackman MS. Quinidine interaction with anticonvulsants. Drug Intell Clin Pharm (1983) 17, 819–20.
6 Kroboth FJ, Kroboth PD, Logan T. Phenytoin-theophylline-quinidine interaction. N Engl J Med (1983) 308, 725.

Quinidine + Aspirin

Abstract/Summary

A patient and two normal subjects given quinidine and aspirin showed a two- to three-fold increase in bleeding times. The patient bled.

Clinical evidence, mechanism, importance and management

A patient with a prolonged history of paroxysmal atrial tachycardia was given quinidine (800 mg daily) and aspirin (325 mg twice daily). After a week he showed generalized petechiae and blood in his faeces. His prothrombin and partial prothrombin times were normal but the template bleeding time was more than 35 min (normal 2–10 min). Further study in two normal subjects showed that quinidine alone (975 mg daily for five days) and aspirin alone (650 mg three times a day for five days) prolonged bleeding times by 125% and 163% respectively; given together the bleeding times were prolonged by 288%.[1] The underlying mechanism is not totally understood but it is believed to be the outcome of the additive effects of two drugs, both of which can reduce blood platelet aggregation.

This seems to be the only study of this adverse interaction, but what is known from other studies about the effects of both drugs on platelet function when given alone supports this report. Concurrent use in other patients should be well monitored to check that bleeding does not occur.

Reference

1 Lawson D, Mehta J, Mehda P, Lipman BC, Imperi GA. Culmulative effects of quinidine and aspirin on bleeding time and platelet alpha-2-adrenoceptors: potential mechanism of bleeding diathesis in patients receiving this combination. J Lab Clin Med (1986) 108, 581–6.

Quinidine + Beta-blockers

Abstract/Summary

Normally an advantageous interaction. Relatively modest doses of quinidine and propranolol can control atrial fibrilla-

tion in patients resistant to high doses of quinidine. Propranolol serum levels are raised. An isolated report describes a patient on quinidine who developed marked bradycardia (36 beats/min) when using timolol eye drops. Another describes orthostatic hypotension with quinidine and propranolol.

Clinical evidence

(a) Advantageous interactions

A man with atrial fibrillation of 10 year's duration which was totally resistant to large doses of quinidine, returned to sinus rhythm after treatment with 80 mg propranolol daily for 10 days, to which was then added 0.2 g quinidine three times a day. He was later maintained on the same dose of quinidine with only 20 mg propranolol.[1]

Similar successes with combined treatment are described elsewhere: 9 out of 10 responded favourably in one study,[2] 34 out of 48 in another,[3] and 13 out of 17 in yet another.[4]

A pharmacokinetic study showed that concurrent use can double the AUC and the peak serum levels of propranolol. Maximum heart rates during exercise were significantly more suppressed.[5] Another study found that propranolol AUCs were approximately tripled.[12] Peak serum quinidine levels were found in one study to be raised by over 50% and its clearance reduced by almost 40% by the presence of propranolol,[6] but this was not confirmed in two other studies.[7,8]

(b) Adverse interactions

An elderly man who for 6 months had been uneventfully taking 500 mg quinidine three times a day for atrial premature beats, was hospitalized with dizziness after starting to use 0.5% timolol eye drops for open-angle glaucoma. He was found to have a sinus bradycardia of 36 beats/min. The symptoms abated when the drugs were withdrawn and normal sinus rhythm returned after 24 h. The same symptoms developed within 30 h of re-starting concurrent use, but disappeared when the quinidine was withdrawn.[7] In another report a man on quinidine and propranolol is described who felt dizzy and faint when standing, which worsened with exercise but disappeared when sitting or lying down.[10]

Mechanism

Both propranolol and quinidine increase the refractory period and reduce the conduction velocity of heart muscle. Together they appear to be better than quinidine alone in the control of arrhythmias. Quinidine appears to increase propranolol serum levels largely by inhibiting the debrisoquin isoenzyme.[11] The adverse quinidine-timolol interaction possibly arose because the negative chronotropic effects of the quinidine and the timolol-induced reduction in sinus rates were additive.[9] Other unidentified factors may also have had a part to play.

Importance and management

The propranolol-quinidine is normally an advantageous interaction. Combined use can be exploited in the treatment of atrial fibrillation. Prescribers who intend to use quinidine and timolol eye drops concurrently should be aware of the adverse interaction report cited above, and of the possibility of orthostatic hypotension.

References

1 Stern S. Synergistic action of propranolol with quinidine. Am Heart J (1962) 72, 569.
2 Stern S, Borman JB. Early conversion of atrial fibrillation after open-heart surgery by combined propranolol and quinidine treatment. Isr J med Sci (1969) 5, 102.
3 Fors WJ, Vanderark CR, Reynolds JW. Evaluation of propranolol and quinidine in the treatment of quinidine-resistant arrhythmias. Amer J Cardiol (1971) 27, 190.
4 Stern S. Conversion of chronic atrial fibrillation to sinus rhythm with a combined propranolol and quinidine treatment. Amer Heart J (1967) 74, 170.
5 Sakurai T, Kawai C, Yasuhara M, Okumura K, Hori R. Increased plasma concentration of propranolol by a pharmacokinetic interaction with quinidine. Jap Circ J (1983) 47, 872.
6 Kessler KM, Humphries WC, Black M, Spann JF. Quinidine pharmacokinetics in patients with cirrhosis or receiving propranolol. Amer Heart J (1978) 96, 627–35.
7 Kates RE, Blandford MF. Disposition kinetics of oral quinidine when administered concurrently with propranolol. J Clin Pharmacol (1979) 19, 378.
8 Fenster P, Perrier D, Mayersohn M, Marcus FI. Kinetic evaluation of the propranolol-quinidine combination. Clin Pharmacol Ther (1980) 27, 450–3.
9 Dinai Y, Sharir M, Naveh N, Floman N, Halkin H. Bradycardia induced by interaction between quinidine and ophthalmic timolol. Ann Intern Med (1985) 103, 890–1.
10 Loon NR, Wilcox CS, Folger W. Orthostatic hypotension due to quinidine and propranolol. Am J Med (1986) 81, 1101–4.
11 Zhou H-H, Anthony LB, Roden DM, Wood AJJ. Quinidine reduces clearance of (+)-propranolol more than (–)-propranolol through marked reduction in 4-hydroxylation. Clin Pharmacol Ther (1990) 47, 686–93.
12 Yasuhara M, Yatsuzuka A, Yamada K, Okumura K, Hori R, Sakura T, Kawai C. Alteration of propranolol pharmacokinetics and pharmacodynamics by quinidine in man. J Pharmacobio-Dyn (1990) 13, 681–7.

Quinidine + Calcium channel blockers

Abstract/Summary

A few patients have shown depressed serum quinidine levels while taking nifedipine, but others have shown no interaction. In contrast, verapamil reduces the clearance of quinidine and in one patient the serum quinidine levels doubled and quinidine toxicity developed. Acute hypotension has also been seen in three patients on quinidine when given verapamil intravenously. Diltiazem and felodipine appear not to interact.

Clinical evidence

(a) Diltiazem

A study in 10 normal subjects given 0.6 mg quinidine twice daily and 120 mg diltiazem daily for seven days showed that the pharmacokinetics of neither drug was affected by the presence of the other.[4]

(b) Felodipine

A study in 12 normal subjects found that felodipine had no clinically significant effect on the pharmacokinetics or antiarrhythmic effects of quinidine.[9,11]

(c) Nifedipine

Two patients taking 300–400 mg quinidine six-hourly and 10 mg nifedipine 6 or 8-hourly showed a doubling of their serum quinidine levels (from 2–2.5 to 4.6 µg/ml and from 1.8–1.6 to 3.5 µg/ml respectively) when the nifedipine was withdrawn. The increased serum quinidine levels were reflected in a prolongation of the QT_c interval. Four other patients failed to demonstrate this interaction.[1]

Two other reports describe the same response:[2,3] the quinidine serum level doubled in one patient when the nifedipine was stopped,[2] and in the other it was found difficult to achieve adequate serum quinidine levels during concurrent use, even when the quinidine dosage was increased threefold. When the nifedipine was withdrawn, the quinidine levels rose once again.[3] A study in 12 patients found that no significant change occurred in serum quinidine levels in the group as a whole when given nifedipine, but one patient showed a 41% decrease.[8,9,11] An experimental study found that quinidine has a small inhibitory effect on the metabolism of nifedipine (half-life prolonged 40%).[10]

(d) Verapamil

A cross-over study in six normal subjects showed that after taking 80 mg verapamil daily for three days the clearance of a single 400 mg dose of quinidine was decreased by 32% (from 17 to 11.69 l/h) and the half-life was increased by 35% (from 6.87 to 9.29 h).[5]

A patient given 648 mg quinidine bisulphate six-hourly showed an increase in serum levels from 2.3 to 5.6 g/ml when given 80 mg verapamil 8-hourly for a week. He became dizzy and had blurred vision. In a subsequent study in this patient it was found that the verapamil halved the quinidine clearance and almost doubled the serum half-life.[6] Three other patients given quinidine orally showed marked hypotension (falls in systolic pressures to 80 and 60 mm Hg were seen in two patients, and in the other patient a systolic/diastolic pressure fall from 130/70 to 80/50 mm Hg) when given verapamil intravenously.[7]

Mechanism

Not understood. One suggestion is that the quinidine-nifedipine interaction is due to changes in cardiovascular haemodynamics.[1] The quinidine-verapamil interaction is possibly due to an inhibitory effect of verapamil on the metabolism of quinidine. The marked hypotension[7] observed may be related to the antagonistic effects of the two drugs on catecholamine-induced alpha-receptor induced vasoconstriction.

Importance and management

The quinidine-nifedipine interaction is established and clinically important but it only appears to affect a few individuals. Concurrent use should be well monitored. An increase in the dosage of quinidine may be needed. What is known about the quinidine-verapamil interaction suggests that a reduction in the dosage of the quinidine may be needed to avoid toxicity. If the verapamil is given intravenously, be alert for evidence of acute hypotension. Monitor the effects of concurrent use closely. No interaction apparently occurs between quinidine and diltiazem or felodipine.

References

1 Farringer JA, Green JA, O'Rourke RA, Linn WA, Clementi WA. Nifedipine-induced alterations in serum quinidine concentrations. Am Heart J (1984) 108, 1570–2.

2 Van Lith RM, Appleby DH. Quinidine-nifedipine interaction. Drug Intell Clin Pharm (1985) 19, 829–30.

3 Green JA, Clementi WA, Porter C, Stigelman W. Nifedipine-quinidine interaction. Clin Pharm (1983) 2, 461–5.

4 Matera MG, De Santis D, Vacca C, Fici F, Romano AR, Marrazzo R, Marmo E. Quinidine-diltiazem: pharmacokinetic interaction in humans. Curr Ther Res (1986) 40, 653–6.

5 Lavoie R, Blevins RD, Rubenfire M, Edwards DJ. The effect of verapamil on quinidine pharmacokinetics in man. Drug Intell Clin Pharm (1986) 20, 457.

6 Trohman RG, Estes DM, Castellanos A, Palomo AR, Myerburg RJ, Kessler KM. Increased plasma concentrations during administration of verapamil; a new quinidine-verapamil interaction. Am J Cardiol (1986) 57, 706–7.

7 Maisel AS, Motulsky HJ, Insel PA. Hypotension after quinidine plus verapamil. Possible additive competition at alpha-adrenergic receptors. N Engl J Med (1985) 312, 167–70.

8 Munger MA, Jarvis RC, Nair R, Kasmer RJ, Nara AR, Urbanic A, Green JA. Elucidation of the nifedipine-quinidine interaction. Clin Pharmacol Ther (1989) 45, 411–16.

9 Bailey DG, Melendez L, Freeman DJ, Kreeft J Carruthers SG. Evaluation of the interaction between quinidine and the calcium channel antagonists nifedipine and felodipine. Clin Invest Med (1991) 14, 4 Suppl A, A19.

10 Schellens JHM, Ghabrial H, van der Wart HHF, Bakker EN, Wilkinson GR, Breimer DD. Differential effects of quinidine on the disposition of nifedipine, sparteine and mephenytoin in humans. Clin Pharmacol Ther (1991) 50, 520–8.

11 Bailey DG, Freeman DJ, Melendez LJ, Kreeft JH, Edgar B, Carruthers SG. Quinidine interaction with nifedipine and felodipine: pharmacokinetic and pharmacodynamic evaluation. Clin Pharmacol Ther (1993) 53, 354–9.

Quinidine + Cimetidine and Ranitidine

Abstract/Summary

Quinidine serum levels can rise and intoxication may develop in some patients when concurrently treated with cimetidine. An isolated case of ventricular bigeminy occurred in a patient on quinidine and ranitidine.

Clinical evidence

1200 mg cimetidine for seven days prolonged the elimination half-life of a single dose of quinidine by 55% (from 5.8 to 9.0 h) in six normal subjects. Peak serum levels were raised by 21%. These changes were reflected in ECG changes (+ 50% and + 28% respectively in the mean areas under the QT and QT_c time curves), but these were said not to be statistically significant.[1]

A later study, prompted by the observation of two patients who developed toxic quinidine levels when given cimetidine, found essentially the same. The AUC and half-life of quinidine were increased by 14.5 and 22.6% respectively, and the clearance was decreased by 25%.[2] A study in four normal subjects found that 1200 mg cimetidine daily for five days prolonged the elimination half-life of quinidine by 54% and decreased the body clearance by 36%. Cimetidine prolonged the QT by 30% above quinidine's effect alone.[5,6,8] Another single case report describes marked increases in both quinidine and digoxin concentrations in a woman when given cimetidine.[3] Ventricular bigeminy occurred in a man on quinidine when given ranitidine. His serum quinidine levels remained unchanged.[4]

Mechanism

It was originally believed that the cimetidine depressed the metabolism of the quinidine by the liver so that it is cleared more slowly, as a result its effects are increased.[2] However more recent data suggest that cimetidine successfully competes with quinidine for its excretion by the kidneys.[7]

Importance and management

This interaction is established and of clinical importance. The incidence is unknown. Be alert for changes in the response to quinidine if cimetidine is started or stopped. Ideally the quinidine serum levels should be monitored and the dosage reduced as necessary. Reductions of 25% (oral) and 35% (intravenous) have been recommended.[6] Those at greatest risk are likely to be patients with impaired kidney function, the elderly and those with serum quinidine levels already at the top end of the range.[2] The situation with ranitidine is uncertain.

References

1 Hardy BG, Zador IT, Golden L, Lalka D, Schentag JJ. Effect of cimetidine on the pharmacokinetics and pharmacodynamics of quinidine. Amer J Cardiol (1983) 52, 172–5.

2 Kolb KW, Garnett WR, Small RE, Vetrovec GW, Kline BJ, Fox T. Effect of cimetidine on quinidine clearance. Ther Drug Monitor (1984) 6, 306–12.

3 Polish LB, Branch RA, Fitzgerald GA. Digitoxin-quinidine interaction: potentiation during administration of cimetidine. South Med J (1981) 74, 633–4.

4 Iliopoulou A, Kontogiannis D, Tsoutsos D, Mouloupoulos S. Quinidine-ranitidine adverse reaction. Eur Heart J (1986) 7, 360.

5 Boudoulas H, MacKichan JJ, Schall SF. Effect of cimetidine on quinidine pharmacokinetics and pharmacodynamics. Clin Res (1987) 35, 874A.

6 MacKichan JJ, Boudoulas H, Schaal SF. Effect of cimetidine on quinidine bioavailability. Biopharm Drug Dis (1989) 10, 121–5.

7 Hardy BG, Schentag JJ. Lack of effect of cimetidine on the metabolism of quinidine: effect on renal clearance. Int J Clin Pharmacol Ther Tox (1988) 26, 388–91.
8 Boudoulas H, MacKichan JJ, Schaal SF. Effect of cimetidine on the pharmacodynamics of quinidine. Med Sci Res (1988) 16, 713–4.

Quinidine + Kaolin–pectin

Abstract/Summary

There is some evidence that kaolin–pectin can reduce the absorption of quinidine and lower its serum levels.

Clinical evidence, mechanism, importance and management

When given 30 ml of *Kaopectate* (kaolin + pectin), the maximal salivary quinidine concentration after a single 100 mg oral dose was reduced in four normal subjects by 54% and the AUC by 58%.[1] There is a correlation between salivary and serum concentrations after a single dose of the drug.[2] This is consistent with an *in vitro* study in which 40 ml of a 40 mg/100 ml solution were mixed with 1 g kaolin. The amount of quinidine adsorbed onto 1 g kaolin rose from 3.54 to 5.81 mg over the pH range 2 to 5.5–7.5 (i.e. those occurring within the gut).[1] Quinidine is also bound by pectin.[3] More study is needed to confirm these two studies but be alert for the need to increase the quinidine dosage if kaolin–pectin is used concurrently.

References

1 Moustafa MA, Al-Shora HI, Gaber M, Gouda MW. Decreased bioavailability of quinidine sulphate due to interactions with adsorbent antacids and antidiarrhoeal mixtures. Int J Pharmaceutics (1987) 34, 207–11.
2 Narang PK, Carliner NH, Fisher ML, Crouthamel WG. Quinidine saliva concentrations; absence of correlation with serum concentrations at steady-state. Clin Pharmacol Ther (1983) 34, 695–702.
3 Bucci AJ, Myre SA, Tan HSI, Shenouda LS. In vitro interaction of quinidine with kaolin and pectin. J Pharm Sci (1981) 70, 999–1002.

Quinidine + Ketoconazole

Abstract/Summary

An isolated report describes a marked increase in serum quinidine levels in man when additionally treated with ketoconazole.

Clinical evidence, mechanism, importance and management

An elderly man with chronic atrial fibrillation, treated with 300 mg quinidine four times daily, was additionally given 200 mg ketoconazole daily for candidal oesophagitis. Within seven days his serum quinidine levels had risen from a range of 1.4–2.7 mg/l to 6.9 mg/l but he showed no evidence of toxicity. The elimination half-life of quinidine was found to be 25 h

(normal values in healthy subjects 6.7 h). The quinidine dosage was reduced to 200 mg twice daily but it needed to be increased to its former value by the end of a month. The reasons for this reaction are not understood.[1]

This is an isolated case so that its general importance is uncertain, but it draws attention to the need to monitor serum quinidine levels in any patient if ketoconazole is added.

Reference

1 McNulty RM, Lazor JA, Sketch M. Transient increase in plasma quinidine concentrations during ketoconazole-quinidine therapy. Clin Pharm (1989) 8, 222–5.

Quinidine + Laxatives

Abstract/Summary

Quinidine serum levels can be reduced by the concurrent use of an anthraquinone-containing laxative.

Clinical evidence, mechanism, importance and management

Studies on patients with heart arrhythmias taking 500 mg quinidine bisulphate 12-hourly showed that concurrent use of an anthraquinone-containing laxative (*Liquedepur*, Fa.Natterman, Cologne) reduced serum quinidine levels measured 12 h after the last dose of quinidine by about 25%.[1] This might be of clinical importance in patients whose serum levels are barely adequate to control their arrhythmia.

Reference

1 Guckenbiehl W, Gilfrich HJ, Just H. Einfluss von Laxantien und Metoclopramid auf die Chindin-Plasmakonzentration wahrend Langzeittherapie bei Patienten mit Herzrhythmusstorungen. Med Welt (1976) 27, 1273.

Quinidine + Lignocaine (Lidocaine)

Abstract/Summary

A single case report describes a man on quinidine who had sinoatrial arrest when he was given lignocaine.

Clinical evidence, mechanism, importance and management

A man with Parkinson's disease was given 300 mg quinidine six-hourly for the control of ventricular ectopic beats. After receiving 600 mg he was given lignocaine as well, initially a bolus of 80 mg, followed by an infusion of 4 mg/min because persistent premature ventricular beats developed. Within 2.5 h the patient complained of dizziness and weakness, and was found to have sinus bradycardia, SA arrest and atrioventricular escape rhythm. Normal sinus rhythm resumed when the lignocaine was stopped. The reasons for this reaction are not understood.[1]

Reference

1 Jerestay RM, Kahn AH, Landry AB. Sinoatrial arrest due to lidocaine in a patient receiving quinidine. Chest (1972) 61, 683.

Quinidine + Metoclopramide

Abstract/Summary

Metoclopramide can reduce the absorption of quinidine from a sustained-release formulation but may increase the absorption with other preparations.

Clinical evidence

A study of this interaction was prompted by the case of a patient on sustained-release quinidine (*Quinidex*) whose arrhythmia failed to be controlled when metoclopramide was added. Five normal subjects were given 10 mg metoclopramide 6-hourly 24 h before and 48 h after a single oral dose of 600 mg or 900 mg quinidine. Five others received the quinidine but not the metoclopramide. It was found that the metoclopramide caused a mean decrease in the quinidine absorption of 10%, but two subjects had decreases of 22.5 and 28.1%.[1] Another study in patients taking 500 mg quinidine 12-hourly found that 30 mg daily doses of metoclopramide increased the mean serum levels measured 3.5 h after the last dose of quinidine by almost 20% (from 1.6 to 1.9 µg/ml) and at 12 h by about 16% (from 2.4 to 2.8 µg/ml).[2]

Mechanism

Not understood. Metoclopramide alters both the gastric emptying time and gastrointestinal motility which can affect absorption.

Importance and management

Direct information seems to be limited to these studies using different quinidine preparations. Since the outcome of concurrent use is uncertain, the effects should be well monitored. More study is needed.

References

1 Yuen GJ, Hansten PD, Collins J. Effect of metoclopramide on the adsorption of an oral sustained-release product. Clin Pharm (1987) 6, 722–5.
2 Guckenbiehl W, Gilfrich HJ, Just H. Einfluss von Laxantien und Metoclopramid auf die Chindin-Plasmakonzentration wahrend Langzeittherapie bei Patienten mit Herzrhythmusstorungen. Med Welt (1976) 27, 1273.

Quinidine + Quinolone antibiotics

Abstract/Summary

Ciprofloxacin appears not to interact with quinidine.

Clinical evidence, mechanism, importance and management

The pharmacokinetics of a single 400 mg oral dose of quinidine and the ECG parameters measured (QRS and QT_c prolongation) were unchanged in seven normal subjects after taking 750 mg ciprofloxacin daily for 6 days. One subject showed a 10% fall in quinidine clearance but this is unlikely to increase steady-state serum quinidine levels by more than 11%.[1] There would seem to be little reason for avoiding concurrent use. There seems to be no information as yet about the effects of other quinolone antibiotics.

Reference

1 Bleske B E, Carver P L, Annesley T M, Bleske J R M, Morady F. The effect of ciprofloxacin on the pharmacokinetic and ECG parameters of quinidine. J Clin Pharmacol (1990) 30, 911–5.

Quinidine + Rifampicin (Rifampin)

Abstract/Summary

The serum levels of quinidine and its therapeutic effects can be markedly reduced by the concurrent use of rifampicin.

Clinical evidence

It was noted that control of ventricular dysrhythmia with quinidine was lost in a patient when he was given rifampicin. Further study in normal subjects showed that concurrent treatment with 600 mg rifampicin daily reduced the mean half-life of the quinidine by almost 60% (from 6.1 to 2.3 h), and the AUC fell from 20.1 to 3.4 g/ml/h.[1,2]

Another report described a patient taking 800–1200 mg quinidine daily who showed a reduction in serum levels from 4.0 to 0.5 µg/ml within two weeks of starting 600 mg rifampicin daily.[3] Yet another patient failed to achieve adequate serum quinidine levels despite large daily doses of quinidine (3200 mg) while taking rifampicin. When the rifampicin was stopped, the quinidine dosage was reduced 44% (to 1800 mg daily) but the serum levels rose 43% (from 1.4 to 2 µg/ml).[4] A 'double interaction' was seen in a patient on quinidine and digoxin when given rifampicin: the quinidine levels fell, resulting in a fall in digoxin levels.[5]

Mechanism

Rifampicin is a potent enzyme-inducing agent which increases the metabolism of the quinidine by the liver three–four-fold, thereby increasing its loss from the body and reducing its effects. It has been suggested that two of the quinidine metabolites (3-hydroxyquinidine and 2-oxoquinidinone) may be as potent as quinidine itself which might offset to some extent the effects of this interaction.[6]

Importance and management

An established and clinically important interaction. The dosage of quinidine will need to be increased if rifampicin is given concurrently. Monitor the serum levels. Doubling the dose may not be enough.[2,5] An equivalent dosage reduction will be needed if the rifampicin is stopped.

References

1 Twum-Barima Y, Carruthers SG. Evaluation of rifampicin-quinidine interaction. Clin Pharmacol Ther (1980) 27, 290.
2 Twum-Barima Y, Carruthers SG. Quinidine-rifampicin interaction. N Engl J Med (1981) 304, 1466.
3 Ahmad D, Mathur P, Ahunjma S, Henerson R, Carruthers G. Rifampicin-quinidine interaction. Br J dis Chest (1979) 73, 409.
4 Schwartz A, Brown JR. Quinidine-rifampin interaction. Am Heart J (1984) 107, 789–90.
5 Bussey HI, Merritt GJ, Hill EG. The influence of rifampin on quinidine and digoxin. Arch Intern Med (1984) 144, 1021–3.
6 Bussey HI, Farringer J, Merritt GJ. Influence of rifampin on quinidine and digoxin. Drug Intell Clin Pharm (1983) 17, 436.

Quinidine + Sucralfate

An isolated report describes a marked reduction in serum quinidine levels in a patient attributed to the concurrent use of sucralfate.

Abstract/Summary

Clinical evidence, mechanism, importance and management

An elderly woman on multiple therapy which included warfarin, quinidine and digoxin developed subtherapeutic levels of all three while taking sucralfate, even when the dosages were separated from the sucralfate by 2 h. When the sucralfate was stopped her serum quinidine levels rapidly climbed from 0.31 to 5.55 μmol/l.[1] The suggestion is that the sucralfate can bind with quinidine within the gut. The general importance of this interaction is uncertain, but be alert for any evidence of reduced effects if both drugs are given.

Reference

1 Rey AM, Gums JG. Altered absorption of digoxin, sustained-release quinidine, and warfarin with sucralfate absorption. DICP Ann Pharmacotherapy (1991) 25, 745–6

Quinidine + Urinary alkalinizers and Antacids

Abstract/Summary

Large rises in urinary pH due to the concurrent use of some antacids, diuretics or alkaline salts can cause the retention of quinidine which may lead to quinidine intoxication. The outcome of using many antacids with quinidine is uncertain but apart from one patient who was also taking large amounts of citrus fruit juice there seem to be no reports of clinically important interactions.

Clinical evidence

The urinary excretion of quinidine in four normal subjects taking 200 mg 6-hourly by mouth was reduced by an average of 50% (from 53 to 26 ml/min) when their urine was made alkaline (i.e. changed from pH 6–7 to pH 7–8) with sodium bicarbonate and acetazolamide (0.5 g every 12 h). Below pH 6 their serum quinidine excretion averaged 115 mg/l, whereas when urinary pH values rose above 7.5 their average excretion fell to 13 mg/l. The quinidine excretion rate decreased from 103 to 31 g/min. In six other subjects the rise in serum quinidine levels was reflected in a prolongation of the QT interval. Raising the urinary pH from about 6 to 7.5 in one individual increased serum quinidine levels from about 1.6 to 2.6 μg/ml.[1]

A patient on quinidine who took about eight *Mylanta* tablets daily (aluminium hydroxide gel 200 mg, magnesium hydroxide 200 mg) for a week and large amounts of citrus fruit juice developed quinidine intoxication.[2]

Mechanism

In acid urine much of the quinidine excreted by the kidney tubules is in the ionized (lipid-insoluble) form which is unable to diffuse freely back into the cells and so is lost in the urine. In alkaline urine more of the quinidine is in the un-ionized (lipid-soluble) form which freely diffuses back into the cells and is retained. In this way the pH of the urine determines how much quinidine is lost or retained and thereby governs the serum levels. Changes in pH and adsorption effects within the gut due to antacids may also possibly affect the absorption of quinidine.[4,5]

Importance and management

An established interaction. Monitor the effects of drugs which can markedly change urinary pH are started or stopped. Reduce the quinidine dosage accordingly. Acetazolamide and sodium bicarbonate can both raise the urinary pH significantly, depending on the dosages used.[1] Other urinary alkalinizers are expected to behave similarly.

The effects of those antacids which are known to raise the urinary pH is less certain because there is some indirect evidence that the interaction is possibly offset by reductions in absorption from the gut.[4,5] There is a single case report of quinidine intoxication due to *Mylanta* (aluminium-magnesium hydroxide) but the patient was also taking large amounts of fruit juice.[2] *Maalox* can raise the pH by 1.0 and could possibly interact similarly.[3] *Milk of magnesia* (magnesium hydroxide) and *Titralac* (calcium carbonate-glycine) in normal doses raise the pH by 0.5 so that a smaller effect is likely.[3] *Amphogel* (aluminium hydroxide) and *Robalate* (dihydroxyaluminium glycinate) are reported to have no effect on urinary pH.[3] Aluminium hydroxide gel is reported on average not to alter the absorption of quinidine sulphate[6] or quinidine gluconate[7] from the gut, but the bioavailability in some individuals is reported to have changed by + 35 and – 18%.[7] In those instances where the antacids do not affect urinary pH at all but reduce the quinidine absorption from the gut (magnesium trisilicate?),[5] an increase in the quinidine dosage may possibly be needed. However much more study is needed to find out which, if any, of these antacids normally interacts significantly, and by how much.

References

1 Gerhardt RE, Knouss RF, Thyrium PT, Luchi RJ, Morris JJ. Quinidine excretion in aciduria and alkaluria. Ann Intern Med (1969) 71, 927.
2 Zinn MB. Quinidine intoxication from alkali ingestion. Texas med (1970) 66, 64.
3 Gibaldi M. Effect of antacids on pH of urine. Clin Pharmacol Ther (1974) 16, 520.
4 Remon JP, Van Severen R, Braeckman P. Interaction entre antiarrythmiques, antiacides et antidiarrheques. III. Influence d'antacides et d'antidiarrheques sur la reabsorption in vitro de sels de quinidine. Pharm Acta Helv (1979) 54, 19.
5 Moustafa MA, Al-Sora HI, Gaber M, Gouda MW. Decreased bioavailability of quinidine sulphate due to interactions with adsorbent antacids and antidiarrhoeal mixtures. Int J Pharmaceutics (1987) 34, 207–11.
6 Romankiewicz JA, Reidenberg M, Drayer D. The non-interference of aluminium hydroxide gel with quinidine sulfate absorption: an approach to control quinidine-induced diarrhea. Am Heart J (1978) 96, 518–20.
7 Mauro VF, Mauro LS, Fraker TD, Temesy-Armos PN, Somani P. Effect of aluminium hydroxide gel on quinidine gluconate absorption. DICP Ann Pharmacotherapy (1990) 24, 252–4.

Tocainide + Antacids or Urinary alkalinizers

Abstract/Summary

Raising the pH of the urine can reduce the loss of tocainide in the urine.

Clinical evidence

When five normal subjects took 30 ml of an un-named antacid four times a day for 48 h before and 58 h after a single 600 mg dose of tocainide, the urinary pH rose from 5.9 to 6.9. The total clearance fell by 28% (from 2.55 to 1.85 ml/kg/min). Peak serum levels rose by 24% (from 4.2 to 3.4 g/ml), the half-life and AUC (area under the curve) rose from 13.2 to 15.4 h and from 51.7 to 68.5 g.h/ml respectively.[1]

Mechanism

Tocainide is a weak base so that its loss in the urine will be affected by the pH of the urine. Alkalinization of the urine increases the number of un-ionized molecules available for passive reabsorption, thereby reducing the urinary loss and raising the serum levels.

Importance and management

Information is limited and the clinical importance uncertain, but be alert for any evidence of increased tocainide effects and possible toxicity if other drugs are given which can alter urinary pH. Reduce the tocainide dosage if necessary. Aluminium-magnesium hydroxide (*Mylanta*) and *Maalox* can raise urinary pH by 1.0 whereas *Milk of magnesia* (magnesium hydroxide) and *Titralac* (calcium carbonate-glycine) in normal doses raise the pH by only 0.5.[2] *Amphogel* (aluminium hydroxide) and *Robalate* (dihydroxy aluminium glycinate) are reported to have no effect on urinary pH.[2] More study is needed.

References

1 Meneilly GP, Scavone JM, Meneilly GS, Wei JY. Tocainide: pharmacokinetic alterations during antacid-induced urinary alkalinization. Clin Pharmacol Ther (1987) 41, 178.
2 Gibaldi M. Effect of antacids on pH of urine. Clin Pharmacol Ther (1974) 16, 520.

Tocainide + Cimetidine

Abstract/Summary

There is some evidence that cimetidine can reduce the bioavailability and serum levels of tocainide but ranitidine appears not to interact.

Clinical evidence, mechanism, importance and management

Four days treatment with cimetidine (dose not stated) in 11 normal subjects had an effect on the pharmacokinetics of 500 mg tocainide given intravenously over 15 min (half-life increased, clearance decreased), but too small to be clinically important.[1] However 1200 mg cimetidine daily for two days reduced the AUC (area under the curve) of a single 400 mg oral dose of tocainide in seven other normal subjects by about a third (from 31.6 to 23.1 µg/ml) and reduced peak serum levels from 2.4 to 1.7 µg/ml, but no changes in the half-life or renal clearance occurred.[2,3] The reasons for this and its clinical importance are uncertain, but be alert for evidence of a reduced response to tocainide in the presence of cimetidine. 150 mg ranitidine twice daily was found not to interact.[2]

References

1 Holmes GI, Antonello J, Yeh KC, Demstriades J, Irvin JD, McMahon FG. Intravenous tocainide maintains safe therapeutic levels when administered concomitantly with cimetidine. Clin Pharmacol Ther (1987), 41, 237.

2 Lalonde RL, North DS, Mattern AL, Kapil RP. Tocainide pharmacokinetic after H-2 antagonists. Clin Pharmacol Ther (1987) 41, 241.

3 North DS, Mattern AL, Kapil RP, Lalonde RL. The effect of histamine-2 receptor antagonists on tocainide pharmacokinetics. J Clin Pharmacol (1988) 28, 640–3.

Tocainide + Rifampicin (Rifampin)

Abstract/Summary

The loss of tocainide from the body is increased by the concurrent use of rifampicin.

Clinical evidence

The AUC of a single 600 mg oral dose of tocainide was reduced by almost 30% (from 76.8 to 55 mg/h/l) and the half-life was also reduced about 30% (from 13.2 to 9.4 h) in eight normal subjects given 300 mg rifampicin twice daily for 5 days.[1]

Mechanism

This response is consistent with the well-recognized enzyme inducing effects of rifampicin which increase the metabolism of drugs by the liver, thereby increasing their loss from the body and reducing their serum levels.

Importance and management

Information is limited to this single dose study in normal subjects but the interaction would seem to be established and likely to be of clinical importance. Monitor patients if given rifampicin for evidence of reduced tocainide serum levels and reduced effects. Increase the dosage as necessary. Reduce the tocainide dosage if the rifampicin is withdrawn. More study is needed.

Reference

1 Rice TL, Patterson JH, Celestin C, Foster JR, Powell JR. Influence of rifampin on tocainide pharmacokinetics in humans. Clin Pharm (1989) 8, 200.

Chapter 5
Antibiotic and Anti-Infective Agent
Drug Interactions

'Most physicians...have the vague feeling that if one anti-microbial drug is good, two should be better, and three should cure almost everybody of almost every ailment.'

This 'vague feeling' has proved to be valid in a number of instances, but there is also good evidence that sometimes the very opposite is true. This situation has fuelled a keen debate about the desirability or otherwise of combining antimicrobial agents which has gone on for many years, and various schemes have been published which try to provide a logical framework for predicting the likely outcome. One of the serious difficulties is the often poor correlation between in vitro and in vivo studies so that it is difficult to get a thoroughly reliable indication of how antimicrobial agents will behave together in clinical practice. Some of the synopses in this chapter illustrate these difficulties very clearly.

Some of the arguments in favour of combining antimicrobial agents are as follows. Where the infections are acute and undiagnosed the presence of more than one drug increases the chance that at least one effective antimicrobial is present. This may be especially important if the patient is infected by more than one organism. The possibility of the emergence of resistant organisms is decreased by the use of more than one drug, and in some cases two drugs acting at different sites may be more effective than one drug alone. It may also be that two drugs administered below their toxic thresholds may be as

effective and less toxic than one drug at a higher concentration.

In contrast there are other arguments against using antimicrobials together. One serious objection is that two drugs may actually be less effective than one on its own. In theory this could arise if a bactericidal drug, which requires actively dividing cells for it to be effective, were used with a bacteriostatic drug. However in practice this seems to be less important than might be supposed and there are relatively few well-authenticated clinical examples. Another objection is that some broad-spectrum drugs may be sub-optimal for particular organisms and may inadequately control the infection. Toxic side-effects may possibly also be increased by the use of more than one drug.

An indiscriminate and 'blunderbuss' approach to the treatment of infections is no longer in favour, the general consensus of informed opinion being that the advantages of combined antimicrobial treatment are balanced by a number of clear disadvantages, and that usually one drug alone, properly chosen, is likely to be equally effective.

Some of the synopses in this chapter are concerned with the adverse effects of combining antimicrobials together but most of them deal with the interactions caused by non-infective agents. Interactions where the antimicrobials are the affecting or interacting agent are dealt with in other chapters. A complete listing is to be found in the Index.

Table 5.1 Antibiotics

Aminoglycosides	*Cephalosporins*	*Cephaloridine*	*Penicillins*	*Polypeptide*
Amikacin	Cefacetrile	Cephradine	Amoxycillin	Bacitracin
Dibekacin	Cefaclor	Cephaloglycin	Ampicillin	Colistin
Dihydrosteptomycin	Cedfadroxil	Cephalothin	Azlocillin	Polymyxin B
Framycetin	Cefamandole	Cephamandole	Bacampicillin	Vancomycin
Gentamicin	Cefazaflur	Cephapirin	Benzylpenicillin	
Kanamycin	Cefmetazole	Cephazolin	Carbenicillin	*Quinolones*
Neomycin	Ceforanide		Ciclacillin	Ciprofloxacin
Netilmicin	Cefotaxime	Chloramphenicol	Cloxacillin	Enoxacin
Paromomycin	Cefotetan	Clindamycin	Dicloxacillin	Nalidixic acid
Ribostamycin	Cefotiam	Fusidic acid	Flucloxacillin	Norfloxacin
Sissomycin	Cefoxitin	Lincomycin	Methicillin	Ofloxacin
Streptomycin	Cefpiramide		Mezlocillin	Pefloxacin
Tobramycin	Cefsulodin	*Macrolides*	Nafcillin	
	Cefuroxime	Erythromycin	Oxacillin	Rifampicin (rifampin)
Antifungals	Ceftazidine	Josamycin	Phenethicillin	
Amphotericin B	Ceftizoxime	Midecamycin	Piperacillin	*Tetracyclines*
Fluconazole	Ceftriaxone	Miocamycin	Pivampicillin	Chlortetracyline
Griseofulvin	Cephalexin	Spiramycin	Ticarcillin	Demeclocycline
Ketoconazole	Cephaloflycin	Triacetyloleandomycin	Phenoxymethyl-	Doxycycline
Miconazole	Cephacetrile		penicillin	Methacycline
			(penicillin V)	Minocycline
				Oxytetracycline
				Rolitetracycline
				Tetracycline

Table 5.2 Non-antibiotic anti-infectives

Antimarlarials	*Antiprotozoals*	*Antituberculars and antileprotics*	*Antivirals*	*Sulphonamides*
Chloroquine	Metronidazole	Aminosalicyclic acid	Acyclovir	Co-trimoxazole
Hydroxychloroquine		(PAS)	Interferon	Sulphadiazine
Mepacrine Pamaquine	*Anthelmintics*	Clofazimine	Vidarabine	Sulphamethoxine
Primaquine	Levamisole	Cycloserine	Zidovudine	Sulphadimidine
Proguanil	Metriphonate	Dapsone		(-methazine
Pyrimethamine	Piperazine	Ethambutol	Furazolidone	-merazine)
	Praziquantel	Isoniazid	Hexamine	Sulphafurazole
		Prothionamide	(methenamine)	(sulfisoxazole)
		Pyrazinamide	Nitrofurantoin	Sulphamerazine
			Sulphasalazine	Sulphamethizole
				Sulphamethoxazole
				Sulphamethoxypryridazine
				Sulphametopyridazine
				Sulphaphenazole
				Sulphasomidine
				Sulphathiazole

Aminoglycoside antibiotics + Amphotericin

Abstract/Summary

Nephrotoxicity attributed to the concurrent use of gentamicin and amphotericin has been described in four patients.

Clinical evidence, mechanism, importance and management

Four patients given moderate doses of gentamicin showed renal deterioration when additionally given amphotericin. Both antibiotics in sufficiently high doses are known to be nephrotoxic and it is suggested, on the basis of what was seen, that low doses of each may have additive nephrotoxic effects.[1] The documentation seems to be limited to this report. Until more is known it would be prudent to monitor renal function carefully if these two antibiotics are used.

Reference

1 Churchill DN, Seeley J. Nephrotoxicity associated with combined gentamicin-amphotericin B. Nephron (1977) 19, 176.

Aminoglycoside antibiotics + Cephalosporins

Abstract/Summary

The nephrotoxic effects of gentamicin and tobramycin can be increased by the concurrent use of cephalothin. This may possibly be true for other aminoglycosides, but some cephalosporins (cited below) appear not to interact adversely.

Clinical evidence

A randomized double-blind trial in patients with sepsis showed the following incidence of definite nephrotoxicity: gentamicin + cephalothin 30% (seven of 23); tobramycin + cephalothin 21% (five of 24); gentamicin + methicillin 10% (two of 20); tobramycin + methicillin 4% (one of 23).[1]

A very considerable number of studies and case reports confirm this increase in the incidence of nephrotoxicity when gentamicin[2-12,22] or tobramycin[13,14] are used with cephalothin. However the opposite conclusion has been reached by a few others.[15-17] Cefuroxime[18] and cefotaxime[19] are reported not to increase the nephrotoxic effects of tobramycin. No clinically important adverse interaction occurs if ceftazidime and tobramycin[21] or cefepime and amikacin[23] are used together. Hypokalaemia has also been described in patients taking cytotoxic drugs for leukaemia when they were given gentamicin and cephalexin.[20]

Mechanism

Uncertain. The nephrotoxic effects of gentamicin and tobramycin are well documented and it appears that these effects can be additive with cephalothin in some patients. Doses which are well tolerated separately can be nephrotoxic when given together.[12]

Importance and management

The gentamicin-cephalothin interaction is very well documented and potentially serious, but there is less information about tobramycin with cephalothin. The risk of nephrotoxicity is probably greatest if high doses are used in those with some existing renal impairment. Concurrent use is not totally contraindicated (see the report cited above[1]) but renal function should be very closely monitored and dosages kept to a minimum. One study suggests that short-lasting treatment is sometimes justified.[22] The combination of gentamicin or tobramycin and cephalothin is probably best avoided in high risk patients wherever possible. Possible alternatives with a much reduced risk of nephrotoxicity are gentamicin or tobramycin with methicillin,[1] or tobramycin with cefuroxime,[18] cefotaxime[19] or ceftazidime,[21] or amikacin with cefepime.[23] Whether other aminoglycosides interact similarly is uncertain, but the possibility should be borne in mind.

References

1 Wade JC, Smith CR, Petty BG, Lipsky JJ, Conrad G, Ellner J, Lietman PS. Cephalothin plus an aminoglycoside is more nephrotoxic than methicillin plus an aminoglycoside. Lancet (1978) ii, 604.
2 Opitz A, Herrman I, von Harrath D, Schaefer K. Akute niereninsuffizienz nach Gentamycin-cephalosporin-Kombinationstherapie. Med Welt (1971) 22, 434.
3 Plager JE. Association of renal injury with combined cephalothin-gentamicin therapy among patients severely ill with malignant disease. Cancer (1976) 37, 1937.
4 Burck HC, Sorgel G. Nephrotoxicity of the combined application of cephalothin and gentamicin, in, Proceedings of 6th International Congress of Nephrology. Int Congr Nephrology, Florence, Italy. (1975) Abstract 700.
5 EORTC International Antimicrobial Therapy Project Group. The antibiotic regimens in the treatment of infection in febrile granulocytopenic patients with cancer. J Infect Dis (1978) 137, 14.
6 Kleinknecht D, Ganeval D, Droz D. Acute renal failure after high doses of gentamicin and cephalothin. Lancet (1973) i, 1129.
7 Noone P, Pattison JR, Shafi MS. Renal failure in combined gentamicin and cephalothin therapy. Br Med J (1973) 2, 777.
8 Bobrow SN, Jaffe E, Young RC. Anuria and acute tubular necrosis associated with gentamicin and cephalothin. J Amer Med Ass (1972) 222, 1546.
9 Fillastre JP, Laumonier R, Humbert G, Dubois D, Metayer J, Delpech A, Leroy J, Robert M. Acute renal failure associated with combined gentamicin and cephalothin therapy. Br Med J (1973) 2, 396.
10 Zazgornik J, Schmidt P, Lugscheider R, Kopsa H. Akutes Nierenversagen bei kombinierter Cephaloridin-Gentamycin-Therapie. Wien Klin Wsch (1973) 85, 839.
11 Cabanillas F, Burgos RC, Rodriguez RC, Baldizon C. Nephrotoxicity of combined cephalothin-gentamicin regimen. Arch Intern Med (1975) 135, 850.
12 Tvedgaard E. Interaction between gentamicin and cephalothin as cause of acute renal failure. Lancet (1976) ii, 581.
13 Tobias JS, Whitehouse JM, Wrigley PF. Severe renal dysfunction after tobramycin/cephalothin therapy. Lancet (1976) i, 425.

14 Klastersky J, Hensgens C, Debusscher L. Empiric therapy for cancer patients: comparative study of ticarcillin-tobramycin, ticarcillin-cephalothin, and cephalothin-tobramycin. Antimicrob Ag Chemother (1975) 7, 640.

15 Fanning WL, Gump D, Jick H. Gentamicin- and cephalothin-associated rises in blood urea nitrogen. Antimicrob Ag Chemother (1976) 10, 80.

16 Stille W, Arndt I. Argumente gegen eine Nephrotoxizitat von Cephalothin und Gentamcyin. Med Welt (1972) 23, 1603.

17 Wellwood JM, Simpson PM, Tighe JR, Thompson EE. Evidence of gentamicin nephrotoxicity in patients with renal allografts. Br Med J (1975) 3, 278.

18 Trollford B, Alestig K, Rodjer S, Sandberg T, Westin J. Renal function in patients treated with tobramycin-cefuroxime or tobramycin-penicillin G. J Antimicrob Chemother (1983) 12, 641–5.

19 Kuhlmann J, Seidl G, Richter E, Grotsch H. Tobramycin nephrotoxicity: failure of cefotaxime to potentiate injury in patient. Naunyn Schmied Arch Pharmakol (1981) 316, R80.

20 Young GP, Sullivan J, Hurley A. Hypokalaemia due to gentamicin/cephalexin in leukaemia. Lancet (1973) ii, 855.

21 Aronoff GR, Brier RA, Sloan RS, Brier ME. Interactions of ceftazidime and tobramycin in patients with normal and impaired renal function. Antimicrob Ag Chemother (1990) 34, 1139–42.

22 Hansen MM, Kaaber K. Nephrotoxicity in combined cephalothin and gentamicin therapy. Acta Med Scand (1977) 201, 463–7.

23 Barbhaiya RH, Knupp CA, Pfeffer M, Pittman KA. Lack of pharmacokinetic interaction between cefepime and amikacin in humans. Antimicrob Ag Chemother (1992) 36, 1382–6.

Aminoglycosides + Clindamycin, Lincomycin

Abstract/Summary

Three cases of acute renal failure have been tentatively attributed to the concurrent use of gentamicin and clindamycin. Lincomycin does not affect the pharmacokinetics of gentamicin.

Clinical evidence, mechanism, importance and management

Three patients with normal renal function developed acute renal failure when they were concurrently treated with gentamicin (4–5 mg/kg/day for 13–18 days) and clindamycin (0.9–1.8 mg/kg/day for 7–13 days). They recovered within 3–5 days of discontinuing the antibiotics.[1] The reasons for the renal failure are not known, but clindamycin has been shown to produce lysosomal changes in the kidney cells of rats which are similar to those produced by gentamicin.[2] Until more is known it would be prudent to monitor renal function carefully if these antibiotics are used together. Tobramycin with clindamycin is reported not to be nephrotoxic.[3] The pharmacokinetics of gentamicin (single IM doses) were found to be unchanged by the presence of lincomycin in normal subjects, but their safety when combined was not assessed.[4]

References

1 Butkus DE, de Torrente A, Terman DS. Renal failure following gentamicin in combination with clindamycin. Gentamicin nephrotoxicity. Nephron (1976) 17, 307.

2 Gray JE, Purmalis A, Purmalis B, Mathews J. Ultrastructural studies of the hepatic changes brought about by clindamycin in animals. Toxicol Appl Pharmacol (1971) 19, 217.

3 Gillett P, Wise R, Melkian V, Falk R. Tobramycin/cephalothin nephrotoxicity. Lancet (1976) i, 547.

4 Gong R, Chen S, Pan H, Xiao G. The effect of lincomycin on the pharmacokinetics of gentamicin. Zhongguo Yiyuan Yaoxue Zazhi (1992) 12, 265–7.

Aminoglycosides + Dimenhydrinate

Abstract/Summary

The manufacturers of dimenhydrinate (diphenhydramine) suggest that it may possibly undesirably mask the ototoxic effects of streptomycin and other aminoglycoside antibiotics.

Clinical evidence, mechanism, importance and management

Dimenhydrinate can block the dizziness, nausea and vomiting which can occur during treatment with streptomycin.[1,2] However Searle, the manufacturers of dimenhydrinate, have warned that '...caution should be used when Dramamine (dimenhydrinate) is given in conjunction with certain antibiotics which may cause ototoxicity, since Dramamine is capable of masking ototoxic symptoms and an irreversible state may be reached.'[1,3] There seems to be no direct clinical evidence to confirm this, but there would seem to be an obvious hazard in not taking enough notice of the warning signs of developing ototoxicity with streptomycin or any other aminoglycoside.

References

1 Titche LL, Nady A. Control of vestibular toxic effects of streptomycin by Dramamine. Dis Chest (1950) 18, 386.

2 Cohen AC, Glinsky GC. Hypersensitivity to streptomycin. J Allergy (1951) 22, 63.

3 Physicians Desk Reference (1972), p 1246. Medical Economics Inc., USA.

Aminoglycosides + Ethacrynic acid

Abstract/Summary

The concurrent use of aminoglycoside antibiotics and ethacrynic acid should be avoided because their damaging actions on the ear can be additive. Intravenous administration and renal impairment are additional causative factors. Even sequential administration may not be safe.

Clinical evidence

Four patients with some renal impairment became permanently deaf after treatment with 1.0–1.5 g kanamycin and 50–150 mg ethacrynic acid. One of them was given the drugs 2 h apart and was deaf within 30 min. Another showed deafness which took almost a fortnight to develop. He was given kanamycin on the first and fifth days of treatment and ethacrynic acid on the second.[1]

There are other reports describing temporary, partial or total permanent deafness in man as a result of giving ethacrynic acid with gentamicin,[5] kanamycin,[3,5,7,10] streptomycin,[1,2,6,10] or neomycin.[2,8,10] This interaction has been very extensively demonstrated in animals.

Mechanism

Both the aminoglycosides and ethacrynic acid given singly can damage the ear and cause deafness, the site of action of the aminoglycosides being the hair cell and that of ethacrynic acid the stria vascularis. Animal studies have shown that neomycin can cause a fivefold increase in the concentration of ethacrynate in cochlear tissues, and it is possible that the aminoglycoside has some effect on the tissues which allows the ethacrynic acid to penetrate more easily.[4] Similar results have been found with gentamicin.[9]

Importance and management

A well-established and well-documented interaction. Concurrent and sequential use should be avoided because permanent deafness may result. Patients with renal impairment seem to be particularly at risk, probably because the drugs are less rapidly cleared. Most of the reports describe deafness after intravenous administration but it has also been seen when given orally. If it is deemed absolutely necessary to use both drugs, minimal doses should be used and the effects on hearing should be monitored continuously. Not every aminoglycoside has been implicated, but their ototoxicity is clearly established and they may be expected to interact in a similar way.

References

1 Johnson AH, Hamilton CA. Kanamycin ototoxicity - possible potentiation by other drugs. S Med J (1970) 63, 511.

2 Mathog RH, Klein WJ. Ototoxicity of ethacrynic acid and aminoglycoside antibiotics in uremia. N Engl J Med (1969) 280, 1223.

3 Ng PS, Conley CE, Ing TS. Deafness after ethacrynic acid. Lancet (1969) i, 673.

4 Orsulakova A, Schacht J. A biochemical mechanism of the ototoxic interaction between neomycin and ethacrynic acid. Acta Otolaryngol (1981) 93, 43–8.

5 Meriwether WD, Mangi RJ, Serpick AA. Deafness following standard intravenous dose of ethacrynic acid. J Amer Med Ass (1971) 216, 795–8.

6 Schneider WJ, Becker EL. Acute transient hearing loss after ethacrynic acid therapy. Arch Intern Med (1966) 117, 715–17.

7 Slone D, Jick H, Lewis GP, Shapiro S, Miettinen OS. Intravenously given ethacrynic acid and gastrointestinal bleeding. J Amer Med Ass (1969) 209, 1668–71.

8 Matz GJ, Beal DDC, Krames L. Ototoxicity of ethacrynic acid. Demonstrated in a human temporal bone. Arch Otolaryngol (1969) 90, 152–5.

9 Tran Ba Huy P, Meulemans A, Manuel Ch, Sterkers O, Wassef M. Critical appraisal of the experimental studies on the ototoxic interaction between ethacrynic acid and aminoglycoside antibiotics. A pharmacokinetic analysis. In 'Ototoxic side-effects of diuretics' (ed by Klinke R, Lahn W, Querfurth H, Scholtholt J) Scand Audiol (1981) Suppl 14, 225–32.

10 Johnson AH, Hamilton CH. Kanamycin ototoxicity - possible potentiation by other drugs. South Med J (1970) 63, 511–13.

Aminoglycosides + Extended spectrum penicillins

Abstract/Summary

Gentamicin, netilmicin, tobramycin and sisomicin are chemically inactivated if mixed in intravenous fluids with carbenicillin, ticarcillin, azlocillin, piperacillin or mezlocillin. Some inactivation can occur if both drugs are given to patients with severe renal impairment or those undergoing haemodialysis, but no interaction of importance appears to occur in those with normal renal function.

Clinical evidence

(a) Aminoglycosides + penicillins in vitro

In vitro studies with solutions of gentamicin (5 μg/ml) and carbenicillin (200 μg/ml) found that the gentamicin became inactivated. These studies were undertaken to check on clinical observations of suspected inactivation.[1]

Inactivation has also been described in other reports involving carbenicillin with gentamicin,[2–6] netilmicin,[12] tobramycin[5] or sisomicin;[5] ticarcillin with gentamicin,[5,6] tobramycin[5] or sisomicin;[5] azlocillin with gentamicin, tobramycin and netilmicin;[12] mezlocillin with gentamicin, tobramycin and netilmicin;[12] and piperacillin with amikacin, gentamicin and tobramycin.[20]

(b) Aminoglycosides + penicillins in patients with renal impairment

A study in six patients with severe renal failure who were receiving carbenicillin (1.5–15 g daily) administered in divided doses 3–6 times daily by IV infusion, showed that the presence of the penicillin prevented the achievement of serum gentamicin levels above 4 μg/ml even though large doses were given.[7] A similar interaction was seen with carbenicillin and tobramycin.[7]

Other reports similarly describe the adverse interaction of gentamicin with carbenicillin,[2,6,11,23] ticarcillin,[6,23] and piperacillin;[19] and tobramycin with ticarcillin.[16] A reduction in the half-life of gentamicin to about a half or a third has been described as well.[6,9]

(c) Aminoglycosides + penicillins in patients undergoing haemodialysis

When given 4 g piperacillin 12-hourly, the pharmacokinetics of netilmicin (2 mg/kg) in six chronic haemodialysis patients were unchanged, whereas the clearance of tobramycin (2 mg/kg) was more than doubled (from 3.6 to 8.3 ml/min) and the half-life reduced from 73 to 22 h.[21] A patient showed a reduction in tobramycin half-life from an expected 70 h to 10.5 h when also treated with piperacillin.[22]

(d) Aminoglycosides + penicillins in patients with normal renal function

A patient with normal renal function was given 80 mg gentamicin intravenously, with and without 4 g carbenicillin. The serum gentamicin concentration profiles in both cases were very similar, with only a fraction of depression due to the carbenicillin.[2]

No interaction was seen in 10 patients with normal renal function given tobramycin and piperacillin,[18] and only minimal changes in 9 normal subjects given tobramycin with piperacillin/tazobactam.[24]

(e) Aminoglycosides + Imipenem/cilastin

The suspicion that low tobramycin serum levels seen in a patient might have been due to an interaction with imipenem/cilastin were not confirmed in a later *in vitro* study.[25] It has also been suggested that the nephrotoxic effects of imipenem and the aminoglycosides might possibly be additive but this awaits confirmation.[26]

Mechanism

These penicillins interact chemically with the aminoglycoside antibiotics to form biologically inactive amides by a reaction between the amino groups on the aminoglycosides and the beta-lactam ring on the penicillins.[8] Thus both antibiotics are inactivated.

Importance and management

These interactions are well documented and of clinical importance. Gentamicin, netilmicin, tobramycin and sisomicin should not be mixed with carbenicillin, ticarcillin, azlocillin, piperacillin or mezocillin in infusion fluids before administration because inactivation occurs. Inactivation can also occur in patients with renal failure. In those cases where concurrent use is thought necessary, it has been recommended that the penicillin dosage should be adjusted to renal function and the serum levels of both antibiotics closely monitored.[7] There is some *in vitro* evidence that minimal inactivation occurs in serum between amikacin and ticarcillin or carbenicillin,[5] and the authors of another study suggest using amikacin with piperacillin, keeping the latter at concentrations of 250 µg165/ml or lower.[15] However this requires confirmation and it would be prudent to monitor concurrent use very closely. Piperacillin appears to affect tobramycin in patients on haemodialysis, but not netilmicin.

There would seem to be no reason for avoiding concurrent use in patients with normal renal function because no significant *in vivo* inactivation appears to occur. Moreover there is good clinical evidence that concurrent use is valuable in the treatment of Pseudomonas infections.[2,10] Tobramycin appears not to be affected by imipenem/cilastin.[25]

It has been shown that significant inactivation of tobramycin in particular, and gentamicin and amikacin to a lesser extent

by carbenicillin, ticarcillin, penicillin and ampicillin, can occur in samples of serum taken for laboratory assay if left at room temperature (losses up to 25% after 12 h) or even frozen (losses up to 20% after 24 h).[13,14,17] It has been suggested that samples which cannot be assayed at once should have 50 mega units per litre of penicillinase added.[13]

References

1 McLaughlin JE, Reeves DS. Clinical and laboratory evidence for the inactivation of gentamicin by carbenicillin. Lancet (1971) i, 261.
2 Eykyn S, Phillips I, Ridley M. Gentamicin plus carbenicillin. Lancet (1971) i, 545.
3 Levison ME, Kaye D. Carbenicillin plus gentamicin. Lancet (1971) ii, 45.
4 Lynn B. Carbenicillin plus gentamicin. Lancet (1971) i, 653.
5 Holt HA, Broughall JM, McCarthy M, Reeves DS. Interactions between aminoglycoside antibiotics and carbenicillin or ticarcillin. Infection (1976) 4, 109.
6 Davies M, Morgan JR, Anand C. Interactions of carbenicillin and ticarcillin with gentamicin. Antimicrob Ag Chemother (1975) 7, 431.
7 Weibert R, Keane W, Shapiro F. Carbenicillin inactivation of aminoglycosides in patients with severe renal failure. Trans Amer Soc Artif Int Organs (1976) 22, 439.
8 Perenyi T, Graber H, Arr M. Uber die Wechselwirkung der Penizilline und Aminoglykosid-Antibiotika. Int J Clin Pharmacol Ther Toxicol (1974) 10, 50.
9 Riff LJ, Jackson GG. Laboratory and clinical conditions for gentamicin activation by carbenicillin. Arch Intern Med (1972) 130, 887.
10 Kluge RM, Standiford HC, Tatem B, Young VM, Schimpff SC, Greene WH, Calia FM, Hornick RB. The carbenicillin-gentamicin combination against pseudomonas aeruginosa. Correlation of effect with gentamicin sensitivity. Ann Intern Med (1974) 81, 584.
11 Weibert RT, Keanse WF. Carbenicillin-gentamicin interaction in acute renal failure. Am J Hosp Pharm (1977) 43, 1137.
12 Henderson JL, Polk RE, Kline BJ. In vitro inactivation of gentamicin, tobramycin and netilmicin by carbenicillin, azlocillin or mezlocillin. Amer J Hosp Pharm (1981) 38, 1167.
13 Edwards DJ, Schentag JJ. In vitro interactions between beta-lactam antibiotics and tobramycin. Clin Chem (1981) 27, 341.
14 Polk RE, Kline BJ. Mail order tobramycin serum levels: low values caused by ticarcillin. Amer J Hosp Pharm (1980) 37, 920.
15 Hale DC, Jenkins R, Matsen JM. In vitro inactivation of aminoglycoside antibiotics by piperacillin and carbenicillin. Amer J Clin Pathol (1980) 74, 316.
16 Chow MSS, Quintiliani R, Nightingale CH. In vivo inactivation of tobramycin by ticarcillin. A case report. J Amer Med Ass (1982) 247, 658–65.
17 Tindula RJ, Ambrose PJ, Harralson AF. Aminoglycoside inactivation by penicillins and cephalosporins and its impact on drug level monitoring. Drug Intell Clin Pharm (1983) 17, 906–8.
18 Lau A, Lee M, Flascha S, Prasad R, Sharifi R. Effect of piperacillin on tobramycin pharmacokinetics in patients with normal renal function. Antimicrob Ag Chemother (1983) 24, 533–7.
19 Thompson MIB, Russo ME, Saxon BJ, Atkin-Thor E, Matsen JM. Gentamicin inactivation by piperacillin or carbenicillin in patients with end-stage renal disease. Antimicrob Ag Chemother (1982) 21, 268–73.
20 Hale DC, Jenkins R, Matsen JM. In vitro inactivation of aminoglycoside anibiotics by piperacillin and carbenicillin. Am J Clin Pathol (1980) 74, 316–19.
21 Halstenson CE, Heim KL, Abraham PA, Keane WF. Netilmicin disposition is not altered by concomitant piperacillin administration. Clin Pharmacol Ther (1985) 41, 210.
22 Uber WE, Brundage RC, White RL, Brundage DM, Bromley HR. In vivo inactivation of tobramycin by piperacillin. DICP Ann Pharmacother (1991) 25, 357–9.
23 Kradjan WA, Burger R. In vivo inactivation of gentamicin by carbenicillin and ticarcillin. Arch Intern Med (1980) 140, 1668–70.
24 Lathia C, Sia L, Lane R, Greene D, Kuye O, Batra A, Yacobi A, Faulkner R. Pharmacokinetics of piperacillin/tazobactam IV with and without tobramycin IV in healthy adult male volunteers. Pharm Res (1991) 8, (10 Suppl) S-303.

25 Ariano RE, Kassum DA, Meatherall RC, Patrick WD. Lack of *in vitro* inactivation of tobramycin by imipenem/cilastin. Ann Pharmacother (1992) 26, 1075–7.
26 Albrecht LM, Rybak MJ. Combination imipenem-aminoglycoside therapy. Drug Intell Clin Pharm (1986) 20, 506.

Aminoglycosides + Frusemide (Furosemide) or Bumetanide

Abstract/Summary

Although some patients have developed nephrotoxicity and/or ototoxicity while taking both drugs, it has not been established that the damage resulted from an interaction, nevertheless concurrent use should be well monitored.

Clinical evidence

An analysis of three prospective, controlled, randomized and double blind trials showed that the concurrent use of amino-glycosides (gentamicin, tobramycin, amikacin) and frusemide did not increase either aminoglycoside-induced nephrotoxicity or ototoxicity. Nephrotoxicity developed in 20% (10 of 50 patients) given frusemide and 17.1% (38 of 222) not given frusemide. Auditory toxicity developed in 21.7% (five of 23) given frusemide and 23.5% (28 of 119) not given frusemide.[1]

A clinical study evaluating a possible interaction found that frusemide increased the aminoglycoside-induced renal damage, whereas two other clinical studies found no interaction.[2–4] There are clinical reports claiming that concurrent use results in ototoxicity, but usually only small numbers of patients were involved and control groups were not included.[5–8] A retrospective study of neonates suggested the possibility of increased ototoxicity but no firm conclusions could be drawn.[15] A patient has been described on gentamicin who rapidly developed deafness only when frusemide was replaced by ethacrynic acid.[1] There seem to be no clinical reports of an amino-glycoside-bumetanide interaction, but it has been described in animals.[12,13]

Mechanism

Normally none, although both the aminoglycosides and frusemide given singly are associated with ototoxicity. Studies in patients and normal subjects have shown that frusemide reduces the renal clearance of gentamicin and can cause both a rise in serum gentamicin[9,10] and tobramycin levels.[11]

Importance and management

Although there is ample evidence of an adverse interaction in animals,[14] the weight of evidence suggests that frusemide does not normally increase either the nephrotoxicity or ototoxicity of the aminoglycosides in man. Nevertheless as there is still some uncertainty about the safety of concurrent use it would be prudent to monitor for any evidence of changes in aminoglyco-side serum levels or of kidney or ear damage. The authors of the major study cited[1] suggest that an interaction may possibly exist if high dose infusions of frusemide are used. See also 'Mechanism' above. The same precautions would also be appropriate with bumetanide.

References

1 Smith CR, Lietman PS. Effect of furosemide on aminoglycoside-induced nephrotoxicity and auditory toxicity in humans. Antimicrob Ag Chemother (1983) 23, 133–7.
2 Bygbjerg IC, Moller R. Gentamicin-induced nephropathy. Scand J Infect Dis (1976) 8, 203–8.
3 Prince RA, Ling MH, Hepler CD, Rainville EC, Kealey GP, Doivta ST, LeFrock JL, Kowalsky SF. Factors associated with creatinine clearance changes following gentamicin therapy. Am J Hosp Pharm (1980) 37, 1489–95.
4 Smith CR, Maxwell RR, Edward CQ, Rogers JF, Lietman PS. Nephrotoxicity induced by gentamicin and amikacin. Johns Hopkins MJ (1978) 142, 85–90.
5 Gallagher KL, Jones JK. Furosemide-induced ototoxicity. Ann Intern Med (1979) 91, 744–5.
6 Noel P, Levy V-G. Toxicite renale de l'association gentamicine-furosemide. Une observation. Nouv Presse Med (1978) 7, 351.
7 Brown CB, Ogg CS, Cameron JS, Bewick M. High dose frusemide in acute reversible intrinsic renal failure. Scot med J (1974) 19, 35.
8 Thomsen J, Bech P, Szpirt W. Otological symptoms in chronic renal failure. The possible role of aminoglycoside-furosemide interaction. Arch Oto-Rhino-Laryng (1976) 214, 71.
9 Lawson DH, Tilstone WJ, Semple PF. Furosemide interactions: studies in normal volunteers. Clin Res (1976) 24, 3.
10 Lawson DH, Tilstone WJ, Gray JMB, Srivastava PK. Effect of furosemide on the pharmacokinetics of gentamicin in patients. J Clin Pharmacol (1982) 22, 254–8.
11 Kak JS, Lyman C, Kilarski DJ. Tobramycin-furosemide interaction. Drug Intell Clin Pharm (1984) 18, 235–8.
12 Ohtani I, Ohtsuki K, Omata T, Ouchi J, Saito T. Interaction of bumetanide and kanamycin. Oto-Rhino-Laryngol (1978) 40, 216.
13 Brummett RE, Bendrick T, Himes D. Comparative ototoxicity of bumet-anide and furosemide when used in combination with kanamycin. J Clin Pharmacol (1981) 21, 628–36.
14 Ohtani I, Ohtsuki K, Omata T, Ouchi J, Saito T. Potentiation and its mechanism of cochlear damage resulting from furosemide and aminogly-coside antibiotics. Oto-Rhino-Laryngol (1978) 40, 53–63.
15 Salamy A, Eledridge L, Tooley WH. Neonatal status and hearing loss in high-risk infants. J Pediatr (1989) 114, 847–52.

Aminoglycosides + Indomethacin

Abstract/Summary

Conflicting reports claim that serum gentamicin and amikacin levels are, or are not, raised in premature babies when given indomethacin to treat patent ductus arteriosis.

Clinical evidence

(a) Aminoglycoside serum levels increased

A study in 22 preterm (premature) infants with gestational ages ranging from 25 to 34 weeks, showed that the use of indo-methacin (0.2 mg/kg) caused a rise in the serum levels of either gentamicin or amikacin which they were being given concurrently. Trough and peak levels of gentamicin were raised 48 and 32% respectively, and of amikacin 28 and 17%.[1]

(b) Aminoglycoside serum levels unchanged

Eight out of 13 infants showed no increase in serum gentamicin levels when given 0.2–0.25 mg/kg indomethacin, four showed slight to moderate rises and one had a substantial rise.[2] In another study in 31 preterm babies given 0.2 mg/kg parenteral indomethacin, no significant changes in serum gentamicin levels were seen.[3]

Mechanism

Indomethacin reduces the filtration rate of the kidney tubules. Since the aminoglycosides are lost from the body by kidney filtration, the effect of the indomethacin is possibly to cause the retention of the antibiotic in the body.

Importance and management

Information seems to be limited to these studies[1–3] although supporting evidence comes from the fact that indomethacin also causes the retention of digoxin in premature babies. The authors of the second study[2] suggest that the different results may be because their aminoglycoside serum levels were lower before the indomethacin was given, and also because they measured the new steady-state levels after 40–60 h instead of 24 h. Whatever the explanation, concurrent use should be very closely monitored because toxicity is associated with raised aminoglycoside serum levels. The authors of the first study[1] suggest that the aminoglycoside dosage should be reduced before giving indomethacin and the serum levels and kidney function well monitored during concurrent use. Other aminoglycosides possibly behave similarly. This interaction does not seem to have been studied in adults.

References

1 Zarfin Y, Koren G, Maresky D, Perlman M, MacLeod S. Possible indomethacin-aminoglycoside interaction in pre-term infants. J Pediatr (1985) 106, 511–13.
2 Jerome M, Davis JC. The effects of indomethacin on gentamicin serum levels. Proc West Pharmacol Soc (1987) 30, 85–7.
3 Grylack LJ, Scanlon JW. Interaction of indomethacin and gentamicin in preterm newborns. Pediatric Res (1988) 23, 409A.

Aminoglycosides + Magnesium salts

Abstract/Summary

Respiratory arrest occurred in a baby with elevated serum magnesium levels when given gentamicin.

Clinical evidence

A baby girl born to a woman whose pre-eclampsia had been treated with magnesium sulphate was found to have muscle weakness and a serum magnesium concentration of 4.3 mg/dl. When 12 h old the baby was given ampicillin, 100 mg/kg IV and gentamicin 2.5 mg/kg IM every 12 h. Soon after the second dose of gentamicin she stopped breathing and needed intubation. The gentamicin was stopped and the baby improved.[1] Animal studies confirm this interaction.[1]

Mechanism

Magnesium ions and the aminoglycoside antibiotics have neuro-muscular blocking activity which can be additive (see also 'Neuromuscular blockers + Magnesium salts and and/or 'Anaesthetics + Aminoglycoside antibiotics'). In the case cited it was enough to block the actions of the respiratory muscles.

Importance and management

Direct information about this interaction is very limited, but it is well supported by the well-recognized pharmacological actions of magnesium and the aminoglycosides, and their interactions with conventional neuromuscular blockers. The aminoglycosides as a group should be avoided in hypermagnesemic infants needing antimicrobial treatment. If this is not possible, the effects on their respiration should be closely monitored.

Reference

1 L'Hommedieu CS, Nicholas D, Armes DA, Jones P, Nelson T, Pickering LK. Potentiation of magnesium sulfate-induced neuromuscular weakness by gentamicin, tobramycin and amikacin. J Pediatr (1983) 102, 629–31.

Aminoglycosides + Miconazole

Abstract/Summary

A report describes a reduction in serum tobramycin levels due to miconazole.

Clinical evidence, mechanism, importance and management

Intravenous miconazole significantly lowered the peak serum tobramycin levels (from 9.1 to 6.7 µg/ml) of nine patients undergoing bone marrow transplantation. Six of them needed dosage adjustments.[1] The reasons are not understood. Concurrent use should be monitored. More study is needed.[1]

Reference

1 Hatfield SM, Crane LR, Duman K, Karanes C, Kiel RJ. Miconazole-induced alteration in tobramycin pharmacokinetics. Clin Pharm (1986) 5, 415–19.

Aminoglycosides + Penicillin V

Abstract/Summary

The serum levels of penicillin V (phenoxymethylpenicillin) when given orally can be halved by the concurrent use of neomycin.

Clinical evidence, mechanism, importance and management

The serum concentrations of penicillin V in five normal subjects, given 250 mg oral doses, were reduced by 50% while also taking 12 g neomycin daily, a return to normal not being achieved until six days after the neomycin was withdrawn.[1] The probable reason is that neomycin causes a reversible malabsorption syndrome which affects the absorption of several drugs. It seems possible that kanamycin and paromomycin might do the same, but this needs confirmation. Parenteral administration of the penicillin or an increase in the oral dosage would seem to be logical answers to this problem, but whether these are effective seems not to have been documented. This study appears to be the only direct evidence of this interaction.

Reference

1 Cheng SH, White A. Effect of orally administered neomycin on the absorption of penicillin V. N Engl J Med (1962) 267, 1296.

Aminoglycosides + Vancomycin

Abstract/Summary

Most but not all of the evidence suggests that the nephrotoxicity of the aminoglycosides and vancomycin may be additive.

Clinical evidence, mechanism, importance and management

Although the combination of an aminoglycoside and vancomycin can possibly be valuable in the treatment of resistant staphylococcal infections, a retrospective study of 94 patients found a high incidence of nephrotoxicity in patients given both drugs (35%) compared with either drug given alone (2–10%).[1,2] Another study in 229 patients found that nephrotoxicity was 15–18% with vancomycin or the aminoglycoside (not named) alone, or when given together; however in patients with trough serum vancomycin levels of 10 µg/ml or more the incidence rose to 27% in those on vancomycin alone and to 42% in those taking both drugs.[4] A study using changes in alanine aminopeptidase in the urine as a possible indicator of kidney toxicity found a five-fold increase in patients given gentamicin and vancomycin.[6] 28 out of 105 (27%) patients given vancomycin and aminoglycosides (not named) developed nephrotoxicity. 22 of the 28 had other factors known to contribute to renal failure.[7] A very brief report describes renal impairment in two patients in whom vancomycin and gentamicin had been used concurrently.[8] Additive nephrotoxicity has been clearly demonstrated in rats.[3]

In contrast to these reports, another study failed to find that concurrent use significantly increased the incidence of nephrotoxicity above the 17% seen with vancomycin alone (aminoglycoside not named).[5]

The picture is not totally clear but what is currently known suggests that it would certainly be prudent to monitor concurrent use carefully for nephrotoxicity, particularly in those with raised trough serum antibiotic levels or other associated risk factors (age, liver disease, peritonitis, use of amphotericin B, male sex).[8]

References

1 Farber B, Moellering R. Retrospective study of the toxicity of preparations of vancomycin from 1974–1981. Antimicrob Ag Chemother (1981) 23, 138–41.
2 Hewitt W. Gentamicin toxicity in perspective. Postgrad Med J (1974) 50 (Suppl 7) 55–9.
3 Wold J, Turnipseed A. Toxicity of vancomycin in laboratory animals. Rev Infect Dis (1981) 3 (Suppl) 224–9.
4 Cimino MA, Rotstein C, Slaughter RL, Emrich LJ. Relationship of serum antibiotic concentrations to nephrotoxicity in cancer patients receiving concurrent aminoglycoside and vancomycin therapy. Am J Med (1987) 83, 1091–7.
5 Downs NJ, Neihart RE, Dolezal JM, Hodges GR. Mild nephrotoxicity associated with vancomycin use. Arch intern Med (1989) 149, 1777–81.
6 Rybak MJ, Frankowski JJ, Edwards DJ, Albrecht LM. Alanine aminopeptidase and 'a72-microglobulin excretion in patients receiving vancomycin and gentamicin. Antimicrob Ag Chemother (1987) 31, 1461–4
7 Pauly DJ, Musa DM, Lestico MR, Lindstrom MJ, Hetsko CM. Risk of nephrotoxicity with combination vancomycin-aminoglycoside antibiotic therapy. Pharmacotherapy (1990) 10, 378–82.
8 Beeley L, Cunningham H, Brennan A. Bulletin W Midlands Centre for Adverse Drug Reaction Reporting. (1993) 36, 17.

Aminosalicylic acid (PAS) + Alcohol

Abstract/Summary

Alcohol can completely nullify the blood-lipid-lowering effects of PAS

Clinical evidence, mechanism, importance and management

A study was made in a group of 65 patients of the effectiveness of PAS-C (purified PAS recrystallized in vitamin C) and diet on the treatment of hyperlipidaemia types IIa and IIb. When three of them drank unstated amounts of beer, the effects of the PAS-C on lowering serum cholesterol, triglyceride and LDL-cholesterol levels were completely abolished.[1] The reasons are not understood. Patients given PAS to reduce blood-lipid levels should avoid alcohol. There seems to be no evidence that alcohol affects the treatment of tuberculosis with PAS.

Reference

1 Kuo PT, Fan WC, Kostis JB, Hayase K. Combined para-aminosalicylic acid and dietary therapy in long term control of hypercholesterolemia and hypertriglyceridemia (types II'02a and II'02b hyperlipoproteinaemia). Circulation (1976) 53, 338–41.

Aminosalicylic acid (PAS) + Aspirin and Salicylates

Abstract/Summary

Additive gastrointestinal irritation is possible with these drugs, but whether other adverse interactions occur is uncertain.

Clinical evidence, mechanism, importance and management

There seems to be little or no direct evidence of adverse interactions between these drugs although Martindale's Extra Pharmacopoeia states that the adverse effects of aminosalicylic acid and the salicylates may be additive. No clinical details or references are given.[1] However since a common problem with both aminosalicylic acid and aspirin is gastrointestinal irritation and even gastric bleeding, it might be prudent to avoid regular concurrent use. Occasional use probably does not matter.

Reference

1 Reynolds JEF (ed). Martindale. The Extra Pharmacopoeia. 29th Edtn. Pharm Press, London (1989) p 554.

Aminosalicylic acid (PAS) + Diphenhydramine

Abstract/Summary

Diphenhydramine can cause a small reduction in the absorption of aminosalicylic acid from the gut.

Clinical evidence, mechanism, importance and management

A study in nine subjects (and in rats) showed that when 50 mg diphenhydramine was injected intramuscularly 10 min before giving 2 g aminosalicylic acid by mouth, the mean peak serum aminosalicylic acid levels were reduced about 15%, and the total amount absorbed over 2 h was reduced about 10%.[1] The possible reason is that the diphenhydramine reduces peristalsis in the gut which in some way reduces aminosalicylic acid absorption. The extent to which diphenhydramine or any other anticholinergic drug diminishes the therapeutic response to long-term treatment with aminosalicylic acid is uncertain, but it is probably small.

Reference

1 Lavigne J-G, Marchand C. Inhibition of the gastrointestinal absorption of p-aminosalicylate (PAS) in rats and humans by diphenhydramine. Clin Pharmacol Ther (1973) 14, 404–12.

Aminosalicylic acid (PAS) + Probenecid

Abstract/Summary

The serum levels of aminosalicylic acid can be raised two- to fourfold by the concurrent use of probenecid.

Clinical evidence, mechanism, importance and management

When 0.5 g probenecid was administered 6-hourly, the serum levels of aminosalicylic acid in man following single 4 g doses were increased two- to four-fold.[1] Similar results are described in another report.[2] The reasons are uncertain but it seems probable that the probenecid successfully competes with the aminosalicylic acid for active excretion by the kidney tubules, resulting in its retention and accumulation in the body.

The documentation of this interaction is limited but it appears to be established. Such large increases in serum aminosalicylic acid levels would be expected to lead to toxicity and it also seems possible that the dosage of aminosalicylic acid could be reduced without losing the required therapeutic response. This needs confirmation. Concurrent use should be undertaken with caution.

References

1 Boger WP, Pitts FW. Influence of p-(di-N-propylsulfamyl)-benzoic acid, 'Benemid' on para-aminosalicylic (PAS) plasma concentrations. Amer Rev Tuberc (1950) 61, 682.
2 Carr DT, Karlson AG, Bridge EV. Concentration of PAS and tuberculo-static potency of serum after administration of PAS with and without Benemid. Proc Staff Meet Mayo Clin (1952) 27, 209.

Amoxycillin + Nifedipine

Abstract/Summary

Nifedipine increases the absorption of amoxycillin from the gut but this is unlikely to be clinically important.

Clinical evidence, mechanism, importance and management

When 1 g amoxycillin was given half-an-hour after 20 mg nifedipine, peak serum amoxycillin levels in eight normal subjects were raised by 33%, the bioavailability was raised 21% and the absorption rate was raised by 70%.[1] Suggested reasons are that the nifedipine slows the movement through the gut so that more time is available for absorption, or that the uptake through the gut wall is increased in some way.[1] There would seem to be no good reason for avoiding concurrent use.

Reference

1 Westphal J-F, Trouvin J-H, Deslande A, Carbon C. Nifedipine enhances amoxicillin absorption kinetics and bioavailability in humans. J Pharmacol Exp Ther (1990) 255, 312–7.

Amphotericin + Corticosteroids

Abstract/Summary

Amphotericin and the corticosteroids can cause both potassium loss and salt and water retention which can have adverse effects on cardiac function.

Clinical evidence

Four patients treated with amphotericin and 25–40 mg hydrocortisone daily developed cardiac enlargement and congestive heart failure. The cardiac size decreased and the failure disappeared within two weeks of stopping the hydrocortisone. The amphotericin was continued successfully with the addition of potassium supplements.[1]

Mechanism

Amphotericin causes potassium to be lost in the urine. Hydrocortisone can cause potassium to be lost and salt and water to be retained. Working in concert these could account for the hypokalaemic cardiopathy and the circulatory overload which was seen.

Importance and management

Information is limited but the interaction would seem to be established. Monitor the electrolyte and fluid balance and the cardiac function during concurrent use. The elderly would seem to be particularly at risk. Corticosteroids can be used to control the immediate side-effects of amphotericin (fever, chills, headache, nausea, vomiting) but bear in mind that the corticosteroids can also reduce the resistance to infection.

Reference

1 Chung D-K, Koenig MG. Reversible cardiac enlargement during treatment with amphotericin B and hydrocortisone. Report of three cases. Am Rev Resp Dis (1971) 103, 831–41.

Amphotericin + Low salt diet

Abstract/Summary, clinical evidence, mechanism, importance and management

The renal toxicity of amphotericin B can be associated with sodium depletion. When the sodium is replaced the renal function improves.[1,2]

References

1 Feeley J, Heidemann H, Gerkens J, Roberts LJ, Branch RA. Sodium depletion enhances nephrotoxicity of amphotericin B. Lancet (1981) i, 1422–3.
2 Heidemann HT, Gerkens JF, Spickard WA, Jackson EK, Branch RA. Amphotericin B nephrotoxicity in humans decreased by salt repletion. Am J Med (1983) 75, 476–81

Amphotericin + Miconazole or Ketoconazole

Abstract/Summary

There is evidence that amphotericin with either miconazole or ketoconazole may possibly be less effective than amphotericin alone.

Clinical evidence, mechanism, importance and management

Studies in a few patients and *in vitro* experiments suggest that the antifungal effects of amphotericin and miconazole used together may be antagonistic, and not additive as might be expected.[1,4] In another study, four out of six patients failed to respond to amphotericin treatment while concurrently receiving ketoconazole, whereas it was successful in 5/6 others who stopped taking either miconazole or ketoconazole.[3] Other *in vitro* studies similarly suggest that amphotericin and ketoconazole may be less effective than amphotericin alone.[2] whereas yet another *in vitro* study indicates that the antifungal effects may be increased.[5]

The reasons are not understood. Until more is known it might be better to avoid concurrent use (or at least the outcome should be very well monitored).

References

1 Schachter LP, Owellen RJ, Rathbun HK, Buchanan B. Antagonism between miconazole and amphotericin B. Lancet (1976) ii, 318.
2 Sud IJ, Feingold DS. Effect of ketoconazole on the fungicidal action of amphotericin B in *Candida albicans*. Antimicrob Ag Chemother (1983) 23, 185–7.
3 Meunier-Carpentier F, Cruciani M, Klastersky J. Oral prophylaxis with miconazole or ketoconazole of invasive fungal disease in neutropenic cancer patients. Eur J Cancer Clin Oncol (1983) 19, 43–8.
4 Cosgrove RF, Beezer AE, Miles RJ. In vitro studies of amphotericin B in combination with the imidazole antifungal compounds clotrimazole and miconazole. J Infect Dis (1979) 138, 681–5.

5 Odds FC. Interactions among amphotericin B, 5-fluorocytosine, ketoconazole, and miconazole against pathogenic fungi *in vitro*. Antimicrob Ag Chemother (1982) 22, 763–70.

Amphotericin + Pentamidine

Abstract/Summary

There is evidence that acute renal failure may develop in patients on amphotericin if pentamidine is given concurrently.

Clinical evidence, mechanism, importance and management

A retrospective study over the 1985–88 period of patients with AIDS showed that 101 of them had been treated with amphotericin B for various systemic mycoses. They were given 0.6–0.8 mg/kg/day for 7–10 days, followed by thrice-weekly dosing for about 9 weeks. Out of nine also concurrently treated for *Pneumocystis carinii* pneumonia, only the four who had been given pentamidine parenterally developed acute and rapid reversible renal failure. No renal failure was seen in two others given the pentamidine by inhalation or three given iv cotrimoxazole.[1] All recovered when the drugs were withdrawn. The reason for the kidney damage would appear to be the additive nephrotoxic effects of both drugs. The reason no toxicity occurred when the pentamidine was given by inhalation is possibly because the serum levels achieved were low. The authors of the study advise caution if both drugs are used. More study is needed.

Reference

1 Antoniskis D, Larsen RA. Acute, rapidly progressive renal failure with simultaneous use of amphotericin B and pentamidine. Antimicrob Ag Chemother (1990) 34, 470–2.

Ampicillin or Amoxycillin + Allopurinol

Abstract/Summary

The incidence of skin rashes among those taking either ampicillin or amoxycillin is increased by the concurrent use of allopurinol.

Clinical evidence

A retrospective search through the records of 1324 patients, 67 of whom were taking allopurinol and ampicillin, showed that 15 of them (22%) developed a skin rash compared with 94 (7.5%) of the rest not taking allopurinol.[1] The types of rash were not defined.

Another study[2] showed similar results: 35 out of 252 patients (13.9%) compared with 251 out of 4434 (5.9%). A parallel study revealed that eight out of 36 patients (22%) on amoxycillin and allopurinol developed a rash, whereas only 52 out of 887 (5.9%) did so on amoxycillin alone.[2]

Mechanism

Not understood. One suggestion is that the allopurinol itself was responsible.[1] Another is that hyperuricaemic individuals may possibly have an altered immunological reactivity.[3]

Importance and management

An established interaction of limited importance. There would seem to be no strong reason for avoiding concurrent use, but prescribers should recognize that the development of a rash is by no means unusual. Whether this also occurs with penicillins other than ampicillin or amoxycillin is uncertain. It appears not to have been reported.

References

1 Boston Collaborative Drug Surveillance Programme. Excess of ampicillin rashes associated with allopurinol or hyperuricaemia. N Engl J Med (1972) 286, 505.
2 Jick H, Porter JB. Potentiation of ampicillin skin reactions by allopurinol or hyperuricaemia. J Clin Pharmacol (1981) 21, 456.
3 Fessel WJ. Immunological reactivity in hyperuricaemic patients. N Engl J Med (1972) 286, 1218.

Antibiotics + Alcohol

Abstract/Summary

No adverse or undesirable interaction normally occurs between alcohol and most antibiotics, with the exception of some cephalosporins, griseofulvin and possibly doxycycline and erythromycin succinate.

Clinical evidence, mechanism, importance and management

A long-standing and very common belief among members of the general public (presumably derived from advice given by doctors and pharmacists) is that alcohol should be strictly avoided while taking any antibiotic. This belief was expressed in 1965 by Dr W Kitto of Chicago who, in answer to a question posed in the Journal of the American Medical Association, claimed that alcohol increases the degradation of penicillin in the gut and reduces the amount available for absorption.[2] However a much later study in 1987 showed that the pharmacokinetics of phenoxymethylpenicillin were unaffected by alcoholic drinks.[1] Another study found that alcohol delayed the absorption of amoxycillin but did not affect the total amount absorbed.[3]

It is difficult to know how this clinical folklore arose because there is little to support it for most antibiotics. The few exceptions include latamoxef, cephamandole, cefoperazone, cefmenoxime, a few other uncommon cephalosporins, and griseofulvin, all of which sometimes cause an unpleasant disulfiram-like reaction with alcohol. This does not happen with most of the commonly prescribed cephalosporins. It is also recognized that serum doxycycline levels may be significantly reduced by alcohol in alcoholics, but not in normal subjects. The absorption of erythromycin succinate is also reduced by alcohol. Details of these interactions are to be found in the appropriate synopses. See the Index.

References

1 Lindberg RLP, Huupponen RK, Viljanen S, Pihlajamaki KK. Ethanol and the absorption of oral penicillin in man. Int J Clin Pharmacol Ther Toxicol (1987) 25, 536–8.
2 Kitto W. Antibiotics and alcohol ingestion. J Amer Med Ass (1965) 193, 411.
3 Morasso MI, Hip A, Marquez M, *Gonzalez* C, Arancibia A. Amoxicillin kinetics and ethanol ingestion. Int J Clin Pharmacol Ther Toxicol (1988) 26, 428–31.

Antibiotics + Antacids, Anticholinergics, H$_2$-blockers

Abstract/Summary

Aluminium-magnesium hydroxide (*Maalox*), pirenzepine and ranitidine do not significantly affect the bioavailability of amoxycillin or amoxycillin-clavulanic acid. Ranitidine does not have a clinically important effect on the bioavailability of doxycycline but *Maalox* does.

Clinical evidence, mechanism, importance and management

Maalox (aluminium magnesium hydroxide, 10 doses of 10 ml), pirenzepine (50 mg for 4 doses) and ranitidine (150 mg for 3 doses) have only small and therapeutically unimportant effects on the pharmacokinetics of 1 g amoxycillin or 500 mg amoxycillin/125 mg clavulanic acid.[1] The bioavailabity of 200 mg doxycycline was not altered by either pirenzepine or ranitidine. There would seem to be no reason for avoiding the concurrent use of any of these drugs, however the bioavailability of doxycycline was markedly reduced (85%) by *Maalox*. See also 'Tetracyclines + Antacids'.

Reference

1 Depperman K-M, Lode H, Höffken G, Tschink G, Kalz C, Koeppe P. Influence of ranitidine, pirenzepine, and aluminium magnesium hydroxide on the bioavailability of various antibiotics, including amoxycillin, cephalexin, doxycycline and amoxycillin-clavulanic acid. Antmicrob Ag Chemother (1989) 33, 1901–7.

Antibiotics + Immunoglobulins

Abstract/Summary

Animal studies suggest that concurrent use may be much less effective than the antibiotic alone.

Clinical evidence, mechanism, importance and management

A study in newborn rats infected with group B streptococcal infection found the following mortalities: 100% with immuno-globulin (2 g/kg) alone, 51% with penicillin G alone, 88% with immunoglobulin + penicillin G. Not dissimilar results were found when the penicillin was replaced by ceftriaxone.[1] More study is needed to find out if this unexpected adverse effect also occurs in man.

Reference

1 Kim KS. High-dose intravenous immune globulin impairs antibacterial activity of antibiotics. J Allergy Clin Immunol (1989) 84, 579–88.

Anti-infective agents + Cimetidine

Abstract/Summary, clinical evidence, mechanism, importance and management

Human studies show that cimetidine does not adversely affect the bioavailability of ampicillin or co-trimoxazole.[1] The bio-availability of benzylpenicillin may even be increased.[2]

References

1 Rogers HJ, James CA, Morrison PJ, Bradbrook ID. Effect of cimetidine on oral absorption of ampicillin and co-trimoxazole. J Antimicrob Chemother (1980) 6, 297.
2 Fairfax AJ, Adam J, Pagan FS. Effect of cimetidine on absorption of oral benzylpenicillin. Br Med J (1977) 2, 820.

Antimalarials + Antacids, Antidiarrhoeals

Abstract/Summary

The absorption of chloroquine can be reduced about 20% by the concurrent use of magnesium trisilicate, and about 30% by kaolin. *In vitro* studies suggest that pyrimethamine may possibly be similarly affected.

Clinical evidence

Six normal subjects were given 1 g chloroquine with either 1 g magnesium trisilicate or 1 g kaolin after an overnight fast. The magnesium trisilicate reduced the AUC (area under the curve) of the chloroquine by 18.2% and the kaolin reduced it by 28.6%.[1]

Related *in vitro* studies by the same authors using segments of everted rat intestine showed that the absorption of chloroquine and pyrimethamine respectively were decreased as follows: magnesium trisilicate (-31.3 and – 37.5%), kaolin (-46.5 and – 49.9%), calcium carbonate (-52.8 and – 31.5%), and gerdiga (-36.1 and – 38.0%). Gerdiga is a clay containing hydrated silicates with sodium and potassium carbonates and bicarbonates. It is used in rural areas of the Sudan as an antacid and is similar to attapulgite.[2]

Mechanism

These anticid and antidiarrhoeal compounds adsorb chloroquine thereby reducing the amount available for absorption by the gut. Pyrimethamine appears to be similarly affected.

Importance and management

The chloroquine/magnesium trisilicate and chloroquine/kaolin interactions are established. Whether the therapeutic effects of the chloroquine are significantly reduced is uncertain, nevertheless it would seem prudent to separate the doses as much as possible to reduce admixture in the gut. Nobody seems to have checked if other antacids interact similarly. There does not seem to be any direct evidence from clinical studies that the effects of pyrimethamine are significantly reduced by antacids and antidiarrhoeals, however its *in vitro* absorption pattern in animal studies is similar to chloroquine.[2]

References

1 McElnay JC, Mukhtar HA, D'Arcy PF, Temple DJ, Collier PS. The effect of magnesium trisicate and kaolin on the *in vivo* absorption of chloroquine. J Trop Med Hyg (1982) 85, 159–63.
2 McElnay JC, Mukhtar HA, D'Arcy PF and Temple DJ. *In vitro* experiments on chloroquine and pyrimethamine absorption in the presence of antacid constituents of kaolin. J Trop Med Hyg (1982) 85, 153–8.

Azithromycin + Miscellaneous drugs

Abstract/Summary

Azithromycin appears not to interact with carbamazepine, cimetidine, methylprednisolone, theophylline, warfarin, zidovudine or a number of other drugs used for analgesia, anxiety, arthritis, asthma, hypnosis or sedation. Food appears to halve its absorption and antacids may reduce its peak serum levels.

Clinical evidence, mechanism, importance and management

A large-scale study in a total of almost 4000 patients treated with azithromycin found no evidence that 1.5 g for five days had any effect on the prothrombin time response to a single dose of warfarin, nor on the plasma levels of single IV or oral does of theophylline.[1] No adverse effects were reported in another clinical study of patients on azithromycin and theophylline.[3] No pharmacokinetic interactions occurred with carbamazepine[1,5] or methylprednisolone.[1] No interaction problems occurred with those patients (45%) who received concurrent treatment with bronchodilators, analgesics, hypnotics/sedatives/anxiolytics or anti-arthritic drugs (none of them specifically named).[1] 1 g oral azithromycin weekly 2 h before zidovudine for five weeks was found not to alter the pharmacokinetic profile of zidovudine.[4] However until more data has accumulated it would be prudent to monitor the concurrent use of any of these drugs.

The peak serum levels, but not the total absorption, of azithromycin is reduced by aluminium and magnesium antacids. It is not affected by 800 mg cimetidine given 2 h previously,[2] but the absorption is reduced approximately 50% by the presence of food.[2] It is suggested therefore that azithromycin should not be given with antacids or 1 h before or 2 h after a meal.[1] The author of the report also advises the avoidance of ergot alkaloids, and suggests caution with cyclosporin and digoxin because clinically important interactions have been seen between these drugs and related macrolide antibiotics,[1] but so far there is no direct evidence of any adverse interactions between these drugs and azithromycin.

Reference

1 Hopkins S. Clinical toleration and safety of azithromycin. Am J Med (1991) 91, (Suppl 3A) 3A-40–5S.
2 Foulds G, Hilligoss DM, Henry EB et al. The effects of an antacid or cimetidine on the serum concentrations of azithromycin. J Clin Pharmacol (1991) 31, 164–7.
3 Davies BI, Maesen FPV, Gubbelman R. Azithromycin (CP-62,993) in acute exacerbations of chronic bronchitis: an open, clinical, microbiological and pharmacokinetic study. J Antimicrob Chemother (1989) 23, 743–51.
4 Chave JP, Manuafo A, Chatton J-Y, Dayer P, Glauser MP, Biollaz J. Once-a-week azithromycin in AIDS patients: tolerability, kinetics, and effects of zidovudine disposition. Antimicrob Ag Chemother (1992) 36, 1013–8.
5 Rapeport WG, Dewland PM, Muirhead DC, Forster PL. Lack of an interaction between azithromycin and carbamazepine. Br J clin Pharmac (1992) 26, 551P.

Bacampcillin + Miscellaneous drugs

Abstract/Summary

Bacampicillin appears not to be affected by food, but a reduction its bioavailability may possibly occur if the gastric pH is increased.

Clinical evidence, mechanism, importance and management

Bacampicillin is a prodrug, without appreciable antibacterial of its own which is hydrolysed in the body to active ampicillin.

Although direct clinical evidence is largely lacking, it would be expected to interact like ampicillin (see the index). One very limited study[1] suggested that food decreases the bioavailability of bacampicillin about 26% but these results have been criticised[2] and on the basis of other work which suggests that no important interaction occurs[3] the makers say that '..it (bacampicillin) can be given without regard to time of food intake.' When given with 300 mg ranitidine and 4 g sodium bicarbonate, without and with breakfast, the bioavailabilities were reduced by 55% and 84% respectively but these observations remain unconfirmed and their clinical significance is uncertain.

Reference

1 Sommers De K, van Wyk M, Moncrieff J, Schoeman HS. Influence of food and reduced gastric acidity on the bioavailability of bacampicillin and cefuroxime axetil. Br J clin Pharmac (1984) 18, 535–9.

2 Heyda BM (Upjohn). Personal communication 1993.

3 Magni L, Sjöberg B, Sjövall J, Wessman J. Clinical pharmacological studies with bacampicillin, in Chemotherapy (1976) 5, 109–114, edited by Williams JD, Geddes AM. Plenum Publishing Corp, NY.

Cefprozil + Food, propantheline, metoclopramide

Abstract/Summary, clinical evidence, mechanism, importance and management

Food, propantheline and metoclopramide have minimal effects on the pharmacokinetics of cefprozil,[1] none of which is likely to be clinically important. No special precautions would seem to be necessary.

Reference

1 Shukla UA, Pittman KA, Barbhaiya RH. Pharmacokinetic interactions of cefprozil with food, propantheline, metoclopramide, and probenecid in healthy volunteers. J Clin Pharmacol (1992) 32, 725–31.

Cephalosporins + Antacids, H$_2$-blockers, Pirenzepine

Abstract/Summary

No clinically significant interactions appear to occur between *Maalox* and cephalexin, cefixime or cefprozil; between *Alka-Seltzer* and cefixime; between cefditoren pivoxil and either aluminium hydroxide or cimetidine, or between ranitidine or pirenzepine and cephalexin. *Maalox* and famotidine reduce the bioavailability of cefpodoxime proxetil, while ranitidine with sodium bicarbonate reduces the bioavailability of cefuroxime axetil. *Maalox* and cimetidine also cause a small reduction in the bioavailability of cefaclor AF.

Clinical evidence, mechanism, importance and management

(a) Cefaclor + Maalox

A study of cefaclor AF (a formulation with a slower rate of release) found that 800 mg cimetidine the night before reduced its maximum serum concentration by 12%, whereas *Maalox* given one hour after the cefaclor in the fed state reduced the AUC by 17%.[9] These reductions are small and unlikely to be clinically important, but this needs confirmation.

(b) Cefditoren pivoxil + Aluminium hydroxide, Cimetidine

The pharmacokinetics of cefditoren pivoxil were found to be unchanged by aluminium hydroxide or cimetidine.[8] No special precautions seem to be needed if given concurrently.

(c) Cefixime, Cephalexin, Cefprozil + Maalox, Pirenzepine, Alka-Seltzer

Maalox (10 doses of 10 ml), ranitidine (150 mg for 3 doses) or pirenzepine (50 mg for 4 doses) had only small and therapeutically unimportant effects on the pharmacokinetics of 1 g cephalexin.[7] *Maalox* and *Alka-Seltzer* do not significantly affect the absorption of cefixime,[4,5] and *Maalox* does not·affect the bioavailability of cefprozil.[6] No special precautions would seem necessary if any of these drugs is used concurrently.

(d) Cefpodoxime proxetil, Cefuroxime axetil + Maalox, Famotidine, Ranitidine, Sodium bicarbonate

10 ml *Maalox* or 40 mg famotidine reduced the bioavailability of cefpodoxime proxetil in 10 normal subjects by about 40%, (possibly due to reduced dissolution at increased gastric pH values) but not when the dosages were separated by 2 hr.[2] This confirms the findings of a previous study.[3] It has been recommended that cefpodoxime is given at least 2 h after antacids or H$_2$-blockers which can raise the gastric pH.[2]

300 mg ranitidine with 4 g sodium bicarbonate reduced the AUC of 1 g cefuroxime axetil in one study by over 60% and the urinary recovery fell by 35%.[1] It would seem reasonable to follow the same precautions with cefuroxime as those recommended for cefpodoxime (see above), although the clinical importance of neither of these two interactions seems to have been studied. Other anti-ulcer drugs (cimetidine, ranitidine, nizatidine, omeprazole, antacids etc) which can raise the pH would be expected to interact similarly

References

1 Sommers De K, Van Wyk M, Moncrieff J, Schoeman HS. Influence of food and reduced gastric acidity on the bioavailability of bacampicillin and cefuroxime axetil. Br J clin Pharmac (1984) 18, 535–9.

2 Saathoff N, Lode H, Neider K, Depperman KM, Borner K, Koeppe P. Pharmacokinetics of cefpodoxime proxetil and interactions with an antacid and an H2 receptor antagonist. Antimicrob Ag Chemother (1992) 36, 796–800.

3 Hughes GS, Heald DS, Barker KB, Patel RK, Spillers CR, Watts KC. The effects of gastric pH and food on the pharmacokinetics of a new oral cephalosporin, cefpodoxime proxetil. Clin Pharmacol Ther (1989) 6, 674–85.

4 Petitjean O, Brion N, Tod M, Montagne A, Nicolas P. Étude de l'interaction pharmacocinétique entre le céfixime et deux antiacids. Résultats préliminaires. La Presse Méd (1989(18, 1596–8.

5 Healey DP, Sahai JV, Sterling LP, Racht EM. Influence of an antacid containing aluminium and magnesium on the pharmacokinetics of cefixime. Antimicrob Ag Chemother (1989) 33, 1994–7.

6 Shyu WC, Wilber RB, Pittman KA, Barbhaiya RH. Effect of antacid on the bioavailability of cefprozil. Antimicrob Ag Chemother (1992) 36, 962–5.

7 Depperman K-M, Lode H, Höffken G, Tschink G, Kalz C, Koeppe P. Influence of ranitidine, pirenzepine, and aluminium magnesium hydroxide on the bioavailability of various antibiotics, including amoxycillin, cephalexin, doxycycline and amoxycillin-clavanulanic acid. Antmicrob Ag Chemother (1989) 33, 1901–7.

8 Shiba K, Maezawa H, Yoshida M, Sakai O. Effects of antacids on pharmacokinetics of cefditoren pivoxil and its metabolism in humans. Chemotherapy (Tokyo) (1992) 40, 1310–19.

9 Satterwhite JH, Cerimele BJ, Coleman DL, Hatcher BL, DeSante KA. Pharmacokinetics of cefaclor AF: effects of age, antacids and H2-receptor antagonists. Postgrad Med J (1992) 68 (Suppl 3) S3–9.

Cephalosporins + Calcium channel blockers

Abstract/Summary

Nifedipine increases the serum levels of cefixime but this is unlikely to be clinically important.

Clinical evidence, mechanism, importance and management

The AUC of a single 200 mg dose of cefixime was increased by about 70% in eight normal subjects and the peak serum levels increased almost 50% when taken 30 min after a 20 mg dose of nifedipine. The rate of absorption was also increased. No adverse responses were seen. One suggested reason is that the nifedipine increases the absorption of the cefixime by affecting the carrier system across the epithelial wall of the gut.[1] It seems doubtful if this increased cefixime bioavailability is clinically important and no particular precautions would seem to be necessary. There seems to be no information about other cephalosporin and calcium channel blockers.

Reference

1 Duverne C , Bouten A, Deslandes, Westphal J-F, Trouvin J-H, Farinotti R, Carbon C.. Modification of cefixime bioavailability by nifedipine in humans: involvement of the dipeptide carrier system. Antimicrob Ag Chemother (1992) 36, 2462.

Cephalosporins + Cholestyramine

Abstract/Summary

Cholestyramine binds with cefadroxil and cephalexin in the gut which delays their absorption. The importance of this is uncertain but probably small.

Clinical evidence

The peak serum levels of cefadroxil (after a 500 mg oral dose) were reduced and delayed in four normal subjects when the antibiotic was taken with 10 g cholestyramine, but the total amount absorbed was not affected.[1] Similar results were found in a study involving cephalexin and cholestyramine.[2]

Mechanism

Cholestyramine is an ion-exchange resin which binds with these two cephalosporins in the gut. This prevents the early and rapid absorption of the antibiotic, but as the cholestyramine-cephalosporin complex passes along the gastro-intestinal tract, the antibiotic is progressively released and eventually virtually all of it becomes available for absorption.[1]

Importance and management

Direct information seems to be limited to the studies cited. The clinical significance is uncertain, but as the total amount of antibiotic absorbed is not reduced it is probably of little importance. This needs confirmation. Information about other cephalosporins seems to be lacking.

References

1 Marino EL, Vicente MT, Dominguez-Gil A. Influence of cholestyramine on the pharmacokinetic parameters of cefadroxil after simultaneous administration. Int J Pharmaceutics (1983) 16, 23–30.

2 Parson RL, Paddock GM, Hossack GM. Cholestyramine-induced antibiotic malabsorption. Chemotherapy 4. In Williams JD and Geddes AM. (eds) Pharmacology of Antibiotics. Plenum Press, New York, London (1975) pp 191–8.

Cephalosporins + Frusemide (Furosemide)

Abstract/Summary

The nephrotoxic effects of cephaloridine appear to be increased by the concurrent use of frusemide. It is uncertain whether cephalothin and cephacetrile are similarly affected. Cephradine levels in the brain are reduced by frusemide.

Clinical evidence

Nine out of 36 patients who developed acute renal failure while taking cephaloridine had also been treated with a diuretic, frusemide being used in seven cases. Other factors such as age and dosage may also have been involved. The authors of this report related their observations to previous animal studies which showed that potent diuretics such as frusemide and ethacrynic acid enhanced the incidence and extent of tubular necrosis.[1,2]

Several other reports describe nephrotoxicity in patients given both drugs.[3,4,6] Brain concentrations of cephradine are markedly reduced by frusemide.[13] A single report describes nephrotoxicity in a patient on cephalothin given frusemide.[3]

Mechanism

Cephaloridine is nephrotoxic, but why this should be increased by frusemide is not understood. Its clearance is reduced by frusemide.[7,12] One clinical study showed that frusemide (80 mg) increased the serum half-life of cephaloridine by 25%,[8] but whether this has any bearing on the matter is uncertain.

Importance and management

The cephaloridine/frusemide interaction is not well-established, but there is enough evidence to suggest that concurrent use should be undertaken with caution. Age and/or renal impairment may possibly be predisposing factors. Renal function should be checked frequently. A pharmacokinetic study suggests that the development of this adverse interaction may possibly depend on the time relationship of drug administration, and it has been recommended that frusemide should be avoided 3 or 4 h before the cephaloridine.[11]

Most other cephalosporins appear not to interact with frusemide with a few possible exceptions: There is a question mark hanging over cephalothin and cephacetrile because animal studies have demonstrated increased nephrotoxicity.[9,10] Nephrotoxicity has been seen in a patient on cephalothin and frusemide.[3] Frusemide is also reported markedly to reduce brain concentrations of cephradine.[12] On the other hand studies in man have shown that cefoxitin seems to be relatively free of nephrotoxicity alone or combined with frusemide.[5] Ceftriaxone does not interfere with the diuretic effects of frusemide.[14]

References

1 Foord RD. Cephaloridine and the kidney. Proc VIth Int Congr Chemother, Tokyo (1969)1, 597.
2 Dodds MG and Foord RD. Enhancement by potent diuretics of renal tubular necrosis induced by cephaloridine. Br J Pharmacol (1970) 4, 227
3 Simpson IJ. Nephrotoxicity and acute renal failure associated with cephalothin and cephaloridine, NZ Med J (1971) 74, 312.
4 Kleinknecht D, Jungers P and Fillastre J-P. Nephrotoxocity of cephaloridine. Ann Intern Med (1974) 80, 421
5 Trolifors B. Effects on renal function of treatment with cefoxitin alone or in combination with furosemide. Scand J Inf Dis (1978) (Suppl) 13, 73.
6 Lawson DH, Macadam RF, Singh H, Gavras H and Linton AL. The nephrotoxicity of cephaloridine. Postgrad Med J (1970) 46 (Suppl) 36.

7 Lawson DH, Tilstone WJ and Semple PF. Furosemide interaction studies in normal volunteers. Clin Res (1976) 24, 3.
8 Norrby R, Stenqvist K and Elgefors B. Interaction between cephaloridine and furosemide in man. Scand J Inf Dis (1976) 8, 209.
9 Lawson DH, Macadam RF, Singh H, Gavras H, Hartz S, Tumbu and Linton A. Effect of furosemide on antibiotic induced renal damage in rats. J Inf Dis (1972)126, 593.
10 Luscombe DK and Nichols PJ. Possible interaction between cephacetrile and frusemide in rabbits and rats. J Antimicrob Chemother (1972) 1, 67.
11 Kosmidis J, Polyzos A and Daikos GK. Pharmacokinetic interactions between cephalosporins and furosemide are influenced by administration time relationships. Curr Chemother Infect Dis. PISF Int Congr Chemother 11th (1979 and 1980) p 673.
12 Tilstone WJ, Semple PF, Lawson DH and Boyle JA. Effects of furosemide on glomerular filtration rate and clearance practolol, digoxin, cephaloridine and gentamicin. Clin Pharmacol Ther (1976) 22, 389.
13 Adam D, Jacoby W and Ralf WK. Beeinflusung der Antibiotika-Konzentration im Gewebe durch ein Saluretikum. Klin Wsch (1978) 56, 247.
14 Korn H, Eichler H G and Gasic S. A drug interaction study of ceftriaxone and frusemide in healthy volunteers. Int J Clin Pharmacol Ther Tox (1986) 24, 262–4.

Cephalosporins + Penicillins

Abstract/Summary

Mezlocillin reduces the loss of cefotaxime from the body

Clinical evidence, mechanism, importance and management

When cefotaxime (30 mg/kg) and mezlocillin (50 mg/kg) were infused together over 30 min in eight normal subjects, the kinetics of the mezlocillin were unchanged but the clearance of the cefotaxime was reduced by 40–42%. The clinical significance of this is uncertain.[1,2]

Reference

1 Flaherty J, Barriere S, Gambertoglio J. Interaction between cefotaxime and mezlocillin. Clin Pharmacol Ther (1985) 41, 196.
2 Rodondi LC, Flaherty JF, Schoenfeld P, Barriere SL, Gambertoglio JG. Influence of coadministration on the pharmacokinetics of mezlocillin and cefotaxime in healthy volunteers and in patients with renal failure. Clin Pharmacol Ther (1989) 45, 527–34.

Cephalosporins + Phenobarbitone

Abstract/Summary

A marked increase in serious skin reactions has been seen in children given cefotaxime and phenobarbitone.

Clinical evidence, mechanism, importance and management

A 30-month study observed a very marked increase in drug-induced reactions in children in intensive care who were treated with high-dose phenobarbitone and beta-lactam antibiotics, mainly cefotaxime. 24 out of 49 children developed mainly exanthematous skin reactions.[1] The reasons are not known. More study is needed to confirm these findings.

Reference

1 Harder S, Schneider W, Bae ZU, Bock U, Zielens. Unerwünschte Arzneimittelreaktionen bei gleichzeitiger Gabe von hochdosiertem Phenobarbital und Betalaktam-Antibiotika. Klin Pädiatr (1990) 202, 404–7.

Cephalosporins + Probenecid

Abstract/Summary

The serum levels of many but not all cephalosporins are raised by probenecid. This can be exploited in the treatment of some conditions but it may also possibly increase the risk of nephrotoxicity with cephaloridine and cephalothin.

Clinical evidence

10 normal subjects given single 500 mg oral doses of cephradine or cefaclor developed markedly raised serum antibiotic concentrations when given probenecid (500 mg doses taken 25, 13 and 2 h before the antibiotic). Peak serum levels were very roughly doubled.[1] Probenecid also raises the serum levels and prolongs the half-life of cefmetazole,[15] cefprozil,[17] cephaloridine,[2] cephazolin,[3] cephacetrile,[4] cephradine,[5] cephaloglycin,[6] cephalothin,[7] cephamandole,[8] cefoxitin,[9,11,16] ceftizoxime[12] and cephalexin.[10] Probenecid is reported to lack any effect on the pharmacokinetics of ceftriaxone[13] and ceforanide.[14]

Mechanism

Probenecid inhibits the excretion of the cephalosporins by the kidney tubules by successfully competing for the excretory mechanisms. A fuller explanation of this mechanism is set out in the introductory chapter. Thus the cephalosporin is retained in the body and its serum levels rise. The extent of the rise cannot be fully accounted for by this mechanism alone and it is suggested that some change in tissue distribution may also sometimes have a part to play.[1]

Importance and management

An extremely well-documented interaction, only a few representative references being listed here. The serum levels of many cephalosporins will be higher if probenecid is used concurrently, but no special precautions are normally needed. This interaction has been exploited in the treatment of gonorrhoea. Elevated serum levels of some cephalosporins, in particular cephaloridine and cephalothin, may increase the risk of nephrotoxicity.

References

1 Welling PG, Dean S, Selen A, Kendall MJ, Wise R. Probenecid: an unexplained effect on cephalosporin pharmacology. Br J clin Pharmac (1979) 8, 491.
2 Kaplan KS, Reisberg BE, Weinstein L. Cephaloridine: antimicrobial activity and pharmacologic behaviour. Amer J Med Sci (1967) 253, 667.
3 Duncan WC. Treatment of gonorrhoea with cefazolin plus probenecid. J Infect Dis (1974) 120, 398.
4 Wise R, Reeves DS. Pharmacological studies on cephacetrile in human volunteers. Curr Med Res Opin (1974) 2, 249.
5 Mischler TW, Sugerman AA, Willard SA, Bannick LJ, Neiss ES. Influence of probenecid and food on the bioavailability of cephradine in normal male subjects. J Clin Pharmacol (1974) 14, 604.
6 Applestein JM, Crosby EB, Johnson WD, Kaye D. In-vitro antimicrobial activity and human pharmacology of cephaloglycin. Appl Microbiol (1968) 16, 1006.
7 Tuano SB, Brodie JL, Kirby WMM. Cephaloridine versus cephalothin: relation of the kidney to blood level differences after parenteral administration. Antimicrob Ag Chemother (1966) 101.
8 Griffith RS, Black HR, Brier GL, Wolney JD. Effect of probenecid on the blood levels and urinary excretion of cefamandole. Antimicrob Ag Chemother (1977) 11, 809.
9 Bint AJ, Reeves DS, Holt HA. Effect of probenecid on serum cefoxitin concentrations. J Antimicrob Chemother (1977) 3, 627.
10 Taylor WA and Holloway WJ. Cephalexin in the treatment of gonorrhoea. Int J Clin Pharmacol (1972) 6, 7.
11 Reeves DS, Bullock DW, Bywater MJ, Holt HA, White LO, Thornhill DP. The effect of probenecid on the pharmacokinetics and distribution of cefoxitin in healthy volunteers. Br J clin Pharmac (1981) 11, 353.
12 LeBel M, Paone RP and Lewis GP. Effect of probenecid on the pharmacokinetics of ceftizoxime. J Antimicrob Chemother (1983) 12, 147–55.
13 Stockel K, McNamara PJ, Brandt R, Ziegler WH. The influence of protein binding on the pharmacokinetics of 'Rocephin' Roche. 12th Int Congr Chemother, Florence. (1981) 987.
14 Jovanovich JF, Saravolatz LD, Burch K, Pohlod DJ. Failure of probenecid to alter the pharmacokinetics of ceforanide. Antimicrob Ag Chemother (1981) 20, 530–2.
15 Ko H, Cathcart KS, Griffith DL, Peters GR, Adams WJ. Pharmacokinetics of intravenously administered cefmetazole and cefoxitin and effects of probenecid on cefmetazole elimination. Antimicrob Ag Chemother (1989) 33, 356–61.
16 Vlasses PH, Holbrook AM, Schrogie JJ, Rogers JD, Ferguson RK, Abrams WB. Effect of orally administered probencid on the pharmacokinetics of cefoxitin. Antimicrob Ag Chemother (1980) 17, 847–55.
17 Shukla UA, Pittman KA, Barbhaiya RH. Pharmacokinetic interactions of cefprozil with food, propantheline, metoclopramide, and probenecid in healthy volunteers. J Clin Pharmacol (1992) 32, 725–31.

Cephalothin + Colistin sulphomethate sodium

Abstract/Summary

Renal failure has been attributed to the concurrent use of cephalothin and colistin sulphomethate sodium (colistimethate sodium).

Clinical evidence, mechanism, importance and management

Four patients developed acute renal failure during treatment with colistin sulphomethate sodium. Three were given cephalothin concurrently and the fourth had previously been treated with this antibiotic.[1] An increase in renal toxicity associated with concurrent use has been described in another report.[2] The reason for this reaction is not known. What is know suggests that renal function should be closely monitored if these antibiotics are given concurrently or sequentially.

References

1 Adler S, Segal DP. Nonoliguric renal failure secondary to sodium colis-timethate. A report of four cases. Amer J Med Sci (1971) 262, 109.
2 Koch-Weser J, Sidel VW, Federman EB, Karnarek F, Finer DC, Eaton AE. Adverse effects of sodium colistimethate. Manifestations and specific reaction rates during 317 courses of therapy. Ann Intern Med (1970) 72, 857.

Chloramphenicol + Cimetidine

Abstract/Summary, clinical evidence, mechanism, importance and management

An isolated report describes the development of pancytopenia and aplastic anaemia in a man on cimetidine within 6 days of being given intravenous chloramphenicol. It proved to be fatal.[1] A possible reason is that their bone marrow depressant effects were additive. The general importance of this is uncertain.

Reference

1 Farber BF, Brody JP. Rapid development of aplastic anemia after intrave-nous chloramphenicol and cimetidine therapy. S Med J (1981) 74, 1257–8.

Chloramphenicol + Paracetamol (Acetaminophen)

Abstract/Summary

Paracetamol is reported to increase, decrease or to have no effect on chloramphenicol serum levels. The outcome of con-current use is therefore uncertain.

Clinical evidence, mechanism, importance and management

Following an initial observation that the half-life of chloram-phenicol in children with kwashiorkor was prolonged by parac-etamol, a study on six adults found that the half-life of chloram-phenicol (1 g intravenously) was increased from 3.25 to 15 h by 100 mg paracetamol (given intravenously 2 h later). The reason is not understood.[1] Later studies in 18 child patients,[2] and eight[3] and five[5] normal adults failed to confirm the existence of this interaction. Another study[4] in five child patients paradoxically found that the clearance of chloramphenicol was increased and its half-life was reduced from 3 to 1.2 h.

These contradictory reports make the whole situation con-fusing. The outcome of concurrent use is uncertain, but it would clearly be prudent to monitor serum chloramphenicol

levels closely. A reversible form of bone marrow depression which is dose-related can take place when chloramphenicol concentrations reach the 25–35 µg/ml range. More study is needed.

References

1 Buchanan N, Moodley GP. Interaction between chloramphenicol and paracetamol. Br Med J (1979) 2, 307.
2 Kearns GL, Bocchini JA, Brown RD, Cotter DL, Wilson JT. Absence of a pharmacokinetic interaction between chloramphenicol and acetami-nophen in children. J Pediatr (1985) 107, 134–9.
3 Rajpurohit R, Krishnaswamy K. Lack of effect of paracetamol on the pharmacokinetics of chloramphenicol in adult human subjects. Ind J Pharmac (1984) 16, 124–8.
4 Spika JS, Davis DJ, Martin SR, Beharry K, Rex J, Aranda JV. Interaction between chloramphenicol and acetaminophen. Arch Dis Child (1986) 61, 1121–4.
5 Stein CM, Thornhill DP, Neill P, Nyazema NZ. Lack of effect of paraceta-mol on the pharmacokinetics of chloramphenicol. Br J clin Pharmac (1989) 27, 262–4.

Chloramphenicol + Penicillins, Streptomycin or Cephalosporins

Abstract/Summary

Antagonism between chloramphenicol and other antibiotics has been described in a case of staphylococcal endocarditis, in bacterial meningitis in a large group of patients and in an infant, and in experimental pneumococcal meningitis in dogs. In contrast, no antagonism and even additive antibiotic effects have been described in other infections.

Clinical evidence

(a) Antibiotic antagonism

A study on 264 patients (adults and children of more than two months) with acute bacterial meningitis showed that on ampi-cillin alone the case-fatality ratio was 4.3% compared with 10.5% on a combination of ampicillin, chloramphenicol and streptomycin. The neurological sequelae (hemiparesis, deaf-ness, cranial nerve palsies) were also markedly increased by the use of the combined drugs.[6]

A man with acute *Staphylococcus aureus* endocarditis showed clinical deterioration and positive blood culture when chloram-phenicol was added to methicillin. The patient's serum inhib-ited the infecting organism at a dilution of 1 in 64, but was not bactericidal even at 1 in 2. After withdrawal of the chloram-phenicol, methicillin alone was successful. The patient's serum was then still inhibitory at 1 in 64 but had become bactericidal at 1 in 32.[4]

Antibiotic antagonism was clearly seen in an infant of two-and-a-half months with meningitis due to *Salmonella enter-itidis* when treated with chloramphenicol and ceftazidime,[7] and in experimental pneumococcal meningitis in dogs treated with chloramphenicol and penicillin.[1]

(b) Lack of antagonism and increased antibiotic effects

A report claims that no antagonism was seen in 65 of 66 patients given chloramphenicol and benzylpenicillin for bronchitis or bronchopneumonia.[2] Ampicillin with chloramphenicol is more effective than chloramphenicol alone in the treatment of typhoid,[3] and benzyl procaine penicillin with chloramphenicol is more effective than chloramphenicol alone in the treatment of gonorrhoea (failure rates of 1.8 compared with 8.5%).[8] In a study on premature, newborn children and infants it was found that the presence of pencillin markedly raised the serum concentrations of concurrently administered chloramphenicol.[5]

Mechanism

By no means fully understood. Chloramphenicol inhibits bacterial protein synthesis and can change an actively growing bacterial colony into a static one. Thus the effects of a bactericide, such as penicillin, which interferes with cell wall synthesis, are blunted, and the death of the organism occurs more slowly. This would seem to explain the antagonism seen with some organisms.

Importance and management

Proven cases of antibiotic antagonism in patients seem to be few in number (although *in vitro* evidence is available). Some practitioners totally avoid concurrent use, but there is certainly insufficient evidence to impose a general prohibition because (depending on the organism) they have sometimes been used together with clear advantage.[3,8] The authors of one report[1] point out that where the diagnosis of the meningitis is still not clear, and when chloramphenicol is thought to be necessary because the condition could be due to *H. influenzae* or one of the enterobacteriaceae, it would seem reasonable to use the penicillin or other bactericide first of all, withholding treatment with the bacteriostat for at least an hour.

References

1 Wallace JF, Smith RH, Garcia M, Petersdorf RG. Studies on the pathogenesis of meningitis. VI. Antagonism between penicillin and chloramphenicol in experimental pneumococcal meningitis. J Lab Clin Med (1967) 70, 408.
2 Ardalan P. Zur frage des Antagonismus von Penicillin und Chloramphenicolus Klinischer sicht. Prax Pneumol (1969) 23, 722.
3 De Ritis R, Giammanco G, Manzillo G. Chloramphenicol combined with ampicillin in the treatment of typhoid. Br Med J (1972) 4, 17.
4 Percival A. In Antibiotic Interactions. Williams JD (ed) (1979) Academic Press.
5 Windorfer A, Pringsheim W. Studies on the concentrations of chloramphenicol in the serum and cerebrospinal fluid of neonates, infants and small children. Europ J Pediatr (1977) 124, 129–38.
6 Mathies AW, Leedom JM, Ivler D, Wehrle PF, Portnoy B. Antibiotic antagonism in bacterial meningitis. Antimicrob Ag Chemother (1967) 218–24.
7 French GL, Ling TKW, Davies DP, Leung DTY. Antagonism of ceftazidime by chloramphenicol *in vitro* and *in vivo* during treatment of Gram negative meningitis. Br Med J (1985) 291, 636–7.
8 Gjessing HC, Odegaard K. Oral chloramphenicol alone and with intramus-

cular procaine penicillin in the treatment of gonorrhoea. Br J Ven Dis (1967) 43, 133–6.

Chloramphenicol + Phenobarbitone

Abstract/Summary

Studies in children show that phenobarbitone can markedly depress serum chloramphenicol levels. There is a single report of markedly increased serum phenobarbitone levels in a man caused by the use of chloramphenicol.

Clinical evidence

(a) Decreased serum chloramphenicol concentrations

Two children of three and 7 months treated for *H. influenzae* meningitis with 100 mg/kg/day chloramphenicol, initially intravenously but later orally, failed to achieve the expected peak serum levels of 15–25 mg/l while concurrently receiving phenobarbitone (10 mg/kg/day) to prevent convulsions. One child had serum chloramphenicol levels of only 5 mg/l or less until the chloramphenicol dosage was doubled, when they rose to 7–11 mg/l.[1] This interaction has been described in another single case report of a child who was also being treated with phenytoin.[6] Other studies in neonates (20 patients) confirm that this interaction can occur, but no statistically significant effect was confirmed in infants (40 patients).[7]

(b) Decreased serum phenobarbitone concentrations

A man admitted to hospital on numerous occasions for pulmonary complications associated with cystic fibrosis, had average serum phenobarbitone concentrations of 35 mg/l while taking 200 mg phenobarbitone daily and chloramphenicol. When the antibiotic was withdrawn, his serum phenobarbitone levels fell by a third (to 24 mg/l) even though the phenobarbitone dosage was increased from 200 to 300 mg daily.[4]

Mechanism

Phenobarbitone is a potent liver enzyme inducing agent which can increase the metabolism and clearance of chloramphenicol (clearly demonstrated in rats[2]) so that its serum levels fall and its effects are reduced. Chloramphenicol has the opposite effect and inhibits the metabolism of the phenobarbitone (also demonstrated in animals[5]) so that the effects of the barbiturate are increased.

Importance and management

The documentation of these interactions is limited. Their incidence is not known. Concurrent use should be well monitored to ensure that chloramphenicol serum levels are adequate, and that phenobarbitone levels do not become too high. Make appropriate dosage adjustments as necessary. Other barbiturates also act like phenobarbitone and may be expected to interact similarly. Sodium valproate has little or no enzyme-inducing activity and may be a suitable anticonvulsant alternative for phenobarbitone.[3]

References

1 Bloxham RA, Durbin GM, Johnson T, Winterborn MH. Chloramphenicol and phenobarbitone-a drug interaction. Arch Dis Child (1979) 54, 76.
2 Bella DD, Ferrari V, Marca G, Bonanomi L. Chloramphenicol metabolism in the phenobarbital-induced liver. Comparison with thiamphenicol. Biochem Pharmacol (1960) 17, 2381.
3 Oxley J, Hedges A, Makki KA, Monks A, Richens A. Lack of hepatic enzyme-inducing effect of sodium valproate. Br J clin Pharmac (1979) 8, 189.
4 Koup JR, Gibaldi M, McNamara P, Hilligoss DM, Colburn W, Bruck E. Interaction of chloramphenicol with phenytoin and phenobarbital. Case report. Clin Pharmacol Ther (1978) 24, 571.
5 Adams HR. Prolonged barbiturate anaesthesia by chloramphenicol in animals. J Amer Vet Med Assoc (1970) 157, 1908.
6 Powell DA, Nahala MC, Durrell DC, Glazer JP, Hilty MJ. Interactions among chloramphenicol, phenytoin and phenobarbitone in a pediatric patient. J Pediatr (1981) 98, 1001.
7 Windorfer A, Pringsheim W. Studies on the concentrations of chloramphenicol in the serum and cerebrospinal fluid of neonates, infants and small children. Eur J Pediat (1977) 124, 129–38.

Chloramphenicol + Rifampicin (Rifampin)

Abstract/Summary

The chloramphenicol serum levels of four children were markedly lowered when additionally treated with rifampicin.

Clinical evidence

Two children aged two and five with *Haemophilus influenzae* meningitis were given 100 mg/kg/day chloramphenicol in four divided doses by slow infusion. Within three days of starting rifampicin (20 mg/kg/day) their peak serum chloramphenicol levels were depressed by 85 and 64% respectively, and only returned to the therapeutic range when the chloramphenicol dosage was increased to 125 mg/kg/day.[1]

Two other children of 5 and 18 months with *Haemophilus influnzae* infections are also reported to have shown marked reductions (75% and 94% respectively) in serum chloramphenicol levels when given rifampicin (20 mg/kg daily) for 4 days, despite increases in the chloramphenical dosages of 20–25%.[2]

Mechanism

It is thought that rifampicin, a potent enzyme inducing agent, markedly increased the metabolism of the chloramphenicol by the liver, thereby lowering its serum levels.[1,2] An increased clearance of chloramphenicol in the presence of rifampicin has also been demonstrated in chimpanzees.[2]

Importance and management

Even though so far only four cases have been reported, the evidence is sufficiently strong for this interaction to be taken seriously. There is a risk that the serum chloramphenicol will fall to sub-therapeutic levels. The authors of the second report point out that raising the chloramphenicol dosage may possibly expose the patient to a greater risk of bone marrow aplasia. They suggest delaying rifampicin prophylaxis in patients with invasive HIB infections until the end of chloramphenicol treatment. More study is needed.

References

1 Prober CG. Effect of rifampin on chloramphenicol levels. N Engl J Med (1985) 312, 788–9.
2 Kelly HW, Couch RC, Davis RL, Cushing AH, Knott R. Interaction of chloramphenicol and rifampin. J Pediatrics (1988) 112, 817–20.

Chloroquine + Cholestyramine

Abstract/Summary

Cholestyramine can reduce the absorption of chloroquine, but the clinical importance of this is uncertain.

Clinical evidence, mechanism, importance and management

4 g cholestyramine reduced the absorption of 10 mg/kg chloroquine by about 30% in five children aged 6–13. Considerable individual differences were seen.[1] This reduced absorption is consistent with the way cholestyramine interacts with other drugs by binding to them in the gut. The clinical importance is uncertain but separating the dosages by a few hours is effective in reducing the effects of this interaction with other drugs. More study is needed.

Reference

1 Gendrel D, Verdier F, Richard-Lenoble D, Nardou M. Interaction entre cholestyramine et chloroquine. Arch Fr Pediatr (1990) 47, 387–8.

Chloroquine + Cimetidine or Ranitidine

Abstract/Summary

Cimetidine reduces the metabolism and the loss of chloroquine from the body. The clinical importance of this is still uncertain. Ranitidine appears not to interact.

Clinical evidence, mechanism, importance and management

400 mg cimetidine daily for four days approximately halved (from 0.49 to 0.23 l/d/kg) the clearance of a single dose of chloroquine (600 mg base) in 10 normal subjects. The elimination half-life was prolonged from 3.11 to 4.62 days.[1] The suggested reason is that the cimetidine inhibits the metabolism of the chloroquine by the liver, thereby reducing its loss from the body. The clinical importance of this interaction is uncertain, but since the main metabolite of chloroquine has pharmacological activity it would seem prudent to be alert for any signs of chloroquine toxicity during concurrent use. A similar study by the same authors found that ranitidine does not interact with chloroquine.[2]

References

1 Ette EI, Brown-Awala EA, Essien EE. Chloroquine elimination in humans: effect of low-dose cimetidine. J Clin Pharmacol (1987) 27, 813–16.
2 Ette EI, Brown-Awala EA, Essien EE. Effect of ranitidine on chloroquine disposition. Drug Intell Clin Pharm (1987) 21, 732–4.

Chloroquine + Imipramine

Abstract/Summary, clinical evidence, mechanism, importance and management

No pharmacokinetic interaction was seen in six normal subjects given single doses of 300 mg chloroquine and 50 mg imipramine.[1] No special precautions would seem necessary during concurrent use.

Reference

1 Onyeji CO, Toriola TA, Ogunbona FA. Lack of pharmacokinetic interaction between chloroquine and imipramine. Ther Drug Monit (1993) 15, 43–6.

Co-trimoxazole + Folic acid

Abstract/Summary

The effects of folic acid used to treat megaloblastic anaemia can be reduced or abolished by co-trimoxazole.

Clinical evidence

Four patients failed to respond to their treatment for megaloblastic anaemia with folic acid while concurrently taking co-trimoxazole. The expected reticulocyte response failed to occur in three of the patients and the fourth showed no clinical improvement until the co-trimoxazole was withdrawn.[1] This interaction has been described in other reports.[2,3]

Mechanism

Not understood. In theory neither sulphamethoxazole nor trimethoprim should disturb folate metabolism in man. Along with other mammmals we rely on folate in the diet rather than on an ability to synthesize it from PABA. Moreover mammalian dihydrofolate reductase is about 50,000 times less sensitive to trimethoprim than the bacterial enzyme. But in practice haematological changes can occur in man.

Importance and management

An established interaction. The 'antifolate' effects of co-trimoxazole are well documented. In normal individuals the effects are usually mild and relatively unimportant, but in patients with megaloblastic anaemia the effects are much more serious and co-trimoxazole should therefore be avoided.

References

1 Chanarin I, England JM. Toxicity of trimethoprim-sulphamethoxazole in patients with megaloblastic anaemia. Br Med J (1972) 1, 651.
2 Rooney PJ, Housley E. Trimethoprim-sulphamethoxazole in folic acid deficiency. Br Med J (1972) 2, 656.
3 Hill AVL, Kerr DNS. Toxicity of co-trimoxazole in nutritional haematinic deficiency. Postgrad Med J (1973) 49, 596.

Co-trimoxazole + Kaolin-pectin

Abstract/Summary

Kaolin-pectin can cause a small but probably clinically unimportant reduction in serum co-trimoxazole levels.

Clinical evidence, importance and management

Eight normal subjects were given 20 ml co-trimoxazole suspension (160 mg trimethoprim + 800 mg sulphamethoxazole, *Septran paediatric*) with and without 20 ml kaolin–pectin suspension. The kaolin–pectin reduced the AUC of the trimethoprim by 12% and of the sulphamethoxazole by 9.5%. The maximal serum levels were reduced by 20% and 7.6% respectively.[1] The probable reason is that the drugs are adsorbed onto the the kaolin–pectin which reduces their bioavailability. These reductions are small and unlikely to be clinically relevant, but this needs confirmation.

Reference

1 Gupta KC, Desai NK, Satoskar RS, Gupta C, Goswami SN. Effect of pectin and kaolin on bioavailability of co-trimoxazole suspension. Int J Clin Pharmacol Ther Tox (1987) 25, 320–1.

Co-trimoxazole + Prilocaine-lignocaine (Lidocaine) cream

Abstract/Summary

Methaemoglobinaemia developed in a baby treated with co-trimoxazole when a prilocaine-lignocaine cream was applied to his skin.

Clinical evidence, mechanism, importance and management

A 12-week-old child on co-trimoxazole (sulphamethoxazole + trimethoprim) for two months for pyelitis was treated with 5 g of EMLA cream (25 mg prilocaine + 25 mg lidocaine per gram) applied to the back of his hands and in the cubital regions. This cream allows pain-free venipuncture. 5 h later, just before an operation began, his skin was noted to be pale and his lips had a brownish cyanotic colour. This was found to be due to the presence of 28% methaemoglobin.[1] The authors of the report suggest that the prilocaine together with the sulphamethoxazole (both known to be able to cause methaemoglobin formation) suppressed the activity of two enzymes (NADH-dehydrogenase and NADP-diaphorase) which normally keep blood levels of methaemoglobin to a minimum.[1] Other studies in children confirm that EMLA cream can increase methaemoglobin levels up to 2%.[2,3]

The report cited[1] appears to be unusual, but it has been suggested that there may be a special risk of methaemoglobinaemia with EMLA in children with pre-existing anaemia, reduced renal excretion of the metabolites of prilocaine, or the concurrent use of sulphonamides.[2]

References

1 Jakobson B, Nilsson A. Methaemoglobinaemia associated with a prilocaine-lidocaine cream and trimethoprim-sulphamethoxazole. A case report. Acta Anaesthesiol Scand (1985) 29, 453–55.
2 Frayling IM, Addison GM, Chattergee K, Meakin G. Methaemoglobinaemia in children treated with prilocaine-lignocaine cream. Br Med J (1990) 301, 153–4.
3 Engberg G, Danielson S, Henneberg S, Nilsson A. Plasma concentrations of prilocaine and lidocaine and methaemoglobin formation in infants after epicutaneous application of a 5% lidocaine-prilocaine cream (EMLA). Acta Anaesthesiol Scand (1987) 31, 624–8.

Cycloserine + Alcohol, Isoniazid, Phenytoin

Abstract/Summary

Cycloserine is reported to increase the effects of alcohol and phenytoin. Its CNS side-effects are increased by isoniazid.

Clinical evidence, mechanism, importance and management

A brief report describes an enhancement of the actions of alcohol in two patients on cycloserine.[1] Patients should be warned. In a report about the concurrent use of cycloserine and isoniazid, both increased and decreased serum cycloserine levels were seen but the mean values were not significantly changed. Only one out of 11 on cycloserine alone developed CNS effects (drowsiness, dizziness, unstable gait), but when given in conjunction with isoniazid, nine of the 11 developed these effects.[2] Lilley who market cycloserine also say that it reduces the metabolism of phenytoin so that the risk of phenytoin intoxication is increased, but the documentation for this is uncertain.

References

1 Glass F, Mallach HJ, Simsch A. Beobachtungen und Untersuchungen uber die gemeinsame wirkung von Alkohol und D-Cycloserin. Arzneim-Forsch (Drug Res) (1965) 15, 684.
2 Mattila MJ, Nieminen E, Tiitinen H. Serum levels, urinary excretion, and side-effects of cycloserine in the presence of isoniazid and p-aminosalicylic acid. Scand J Resp Dis (1969) 50, 291–300.

Dapsone + Cimetidine, Omeprazole, Ranitidine

Abstract/Summary

Cimetidine raises serum dapsone levels but the theoretically expected increase in toxicity appears to be offset by a reduction in the production of the toxic metabolite of dapsone.

Clinical evidence, mechanism, importance and management

The AUC of a single 100 mg dose of dapsone was increased by 40% (from 31 to 43.3 ml/h) in seven normal subjects after taking 1200 mg cimetidine daily for 3 days.[1] The probable reason is that the cimetidine (a known enzyme inhibitor) inhibits the metabolism of the dapsone by the liver. This might be expected to increase the risk of haematological side-effects of dapsone by raising its serum levels, but the cimetidine also apparently markedly reduces the production of dapsone hydroxylamine (peak serum levels reduced from 2.5 to 0.98%) which appears to be responsible for the methaemoglobinaemia and haemolysis, so that the outcome may possibly be more favourable than adverse.[1] Another report on a small number of patients failed to find that cimetidine, ranitidine or omeprazole affected the outcome of dapsone prophylaxis for *Pneumocystis carinii* pneumonia in HIV patients.[2] More study is needed to confirm these findings

References

1 Coleman MD, Scott AK, Breckenridge AM, Park BK. The use of cimetidine as a selective inhibitor of dapsone N-hydroxylation in man. Br J clin Pharmac (1990) 30, 761–7.
2 Huengsberg M, Castelino S, Sherrard J, O'Farrell N, Bingham J. Does drug interaction cause failure of PCP prophylaxis with dapsone ? Lancet (1993) 341, 48.

Dapsone + Clofazimine

Abstract/Summary

Dapsone can reduce the anti-inflammatory effects of clofazimine but it does not affect its pharmacokinetics.

Clinical evidence, mechanism, importance and management

Clofazimine does not affect the pharmacokinetics of dapsone.[2-4] 14 out of 16 patients with severe recurrent erythema nodosum leprosum (ENL) failed to respond adequately when given dapsone and clofazimine and needed additional therapy with corticosteroids. When the dapsone was stopped the patients responded to clofazimine alone and in some instances they were controlled on smaller doses.[1] Further evidence of this interaction comes from a laboratory study which suggests that the actions of clofazimine may be related to its ability to inhibit neutrophil migration (resulting in decreased numbers of neutrophils in areas of inflammation), whereas dapsone can have the opposite effect.[1] Although the information is very limited, it would seem prudent to avoid concurrent use in the treatment of ENL. The authors of the report cited[1] are at great pains to emphasize that what they describe only relates to the effects of dapsone on the anti-inflammatory effects of clofazimine, and not to the beneficial effects of combined use when treating drug-resistant *Mycobacterium leprae*.

References

1 Imkamp FMJH, Anderson R, Gatner EMS. Possible incompatibility of dapsone with clofazimine in the treatment of patients with erythema nodosum leprosum. Lepr Rev (1982) 53, 148–53.
2 Venkatesan K, Mathur A, Girdhar BK, Bharadwaj VP. The effect of clofazimine on the pharmacokinetics of rifampicin and dapsone in leprosy. J Antimicrob Chemother (1986) 18, 715–18.
3 Pieters FAJ, Woonink F, Zuidema J. Influence of once-monthly rifampicin and daily clofazimine on the pharmacokinetics of dapsone in leprosy patients in Nigeria. Eur J Clin Pharmacol (1988) 34, 73–6.
4 Venkatesan K, Bharadwaj VP, Ramu R, Desikan KV. Study on drug interactions. Leprosy in India (1980) 52, 229–35.

Dapsone + Didanosine

Abstract/Summary

The prophylactic effects of dapsone in preventing pneumocystis infection may be reduced or abolished in the presence of
oral didanosine because of the formulation of the latter. Separating their administration may possibly be effective.

Clinical evidence

Dapsone (25 mg four times daily) is normally very effective in preventing pneumocystis infection in HIV patients, however one report describes failure in 11 out of 28 HIV patients while also taking didanosine. Four of them died from respiratory failure.[1] A later report on a small number of patients failed to confirm this interaction.[2]

Mechanism

One suggestion is this. Didanosine (*Videx*) is formulated with a citrate-phosphate buffer intended to facilitate its absorption at pH7–8. At these high pH values the dapsone becomes very insoluble and therefore fails to be absorbed sufficiently to be effective. Other mechanisms of interaction possibly have some part to play as well.

Importance and management

Information is very limited. The authors of the report cited[1] suggest that the administration of the two drugs should be separated by at least 2 hours.[1] This is effective with didanosine and ketoconazole (also dependent on a low pH for its absorption) but confirmatory study is needed. An alternative would be to use co-trimoxazole (800 mg sulphamethoxazole-trimethoprim 160 mg) twice daily which in this same study[1] was 100% effective in 17 patients, however see also 'Dapsone + Trimethoprim'.

References

1 Metroka CE, McMechan MF, Andrada R, Laubenstein LJ, Jacobus DP. Failure of prophylaxis with dapsone in patients taking dideoxyinosine. N Engl J Med (1992) 325, 737.
2 Huengsbert M, Castelino S, Sherrard J, O'Farrell N, Bingham J. Does drug interaction cause failure of PCP prophylaxis with dapsone ? Lancet (1993) 341, 48.

Dapsone + Probenecid

Abstract/Summary

The serum levels of dapsone can be markedly raised by the concurrent use of probenecid.

Clinical evidence

A study in 12 men given 500 mg dapsone with 300 mg probenecid, and 3 h later another 500 mg dapsone, showed that the dapsone serum levels were raised about 50% when measured at 4 h. The urinary excretion of dapsone and its metabolites were found to be reduced.[1]

Mechanism

Not fully examined. It seems probable that the probenecid inhibits the renal excretion of dapsone by the kidney.

Importance and management

The documentation is very limited, but it seems to be an established interaction. It is likely that the probenecid will raise the serum levels of dapsone given chronically. The importance of this is uncertain, but the extent of the rise and the evidence that the haematological toxicity of dapsone may be dose-related[2] suggests that it may well have some clinical importance. This needs confirmation.

References

1 Goodwin CS, Sparell G. Inhibition of dapsone excretion by probenecid. Lancet (1969) ii, 884.
2 Ellard GA. Dapsone acetylation in dermatitis herpetiformis. Br J Derm (1974) 90, 441.

Dapsone + Rifampicin (Rifampin)

Abstract/Summary

Rifampicin increases the excretion of dapsone and lowers its serum levels.

Clinical evidence, mechanism, importance and management

A study in seven patients with leprosy given single doses of dapsone (100 mg) and rifampicin (600 mg), alone or together, showed that while the pharmacokinetics of rifampicin were not significantly changed by dapsone, the half-life of the dapsone was halved and the AUC was reduced by about 20%.[1] This confirms previous studies in patients given both drugs for several days who had reduced dapsone serum levels and an increased urinary excretion.[2-4]

Mechanism

It seems probable that the rifampicin, well recognized as a potent liver-enzyme inducing agent, increases the metabolism and loss of dapsone from the body.

Importance and management

This interaction is established, but its clinical importance is uncertain. Concurrent use should be well monitored to confirm that treatment is effective. It may be necessary to raise the dosage of dapsone. It has been pointed out that there is the risk of treatment failures for *Pneumocystis carinii* pneumonia as well as for leprosy.[5]

References

1 Krishna DR, Appa Rao AVN, Ramanakar TV, Prabhakar MC. Pharmacokinetic interaction between dapsone and rifampicin (rifampin) in leprosy patients. Drug Dev Ind Pharmacy (1986) 12, 443–9.
2 Balakrishnan S, Seshadri PS. Drug interactions, the influence of rifampicin (rifampin) and clofazimine on the urinary excretion of DDS. Lepr India (1970) 53, 17–22.
3 Peters JH, Murray JF, Gordon GR, Gelber RH, Levy L, Laing ABG, Waters MFR. Tissue levels of dapsone in mice, rats and man. Int J Lepr (1976) 44, 545.
4 Peters JH, Murray JF, Gordon GR. Effect of rifampicin on the disposition of dapsone in Malayan leprosy patients. Fed Proc (1977) 36, 996.
5 Jorde UP, Horowitz HW, Wormser GP. Significance of drug interactions with rifampin in Pneumocystis carinii pneumonia prophylaxis. Arch Intern Med (1992) 152, 2348.

Dapsone + Trimethoprim

Abstract/Summary

The serum levels of each drug are raised by the presence of the other. Both increased efficacy and dapsone toxicity have been seen.

Clinical evidence

18 patients with AIDS, under treatment for *Pneumocystiis carinii* pneumonia and taking dapsone (100 mg daily), were compared with 30 other patients taking dapsone and trimethoprim (20 mg/kg daily). The latter developed serum dapsone levels which were 40% higher (a rise from 1.5 to 2.1 μg/ml) at 7 days. Dapsone toxicity (methaemoglobinaemia) and efficacy were also increased. The trimethoprim serum levels were also 48.4% higher in those given dapsone + trimethoprim than in another group of 30 patients given dapsone + co-trimoxazole (trimethoprim + sulphamethoxazole), even so the incidence of toxicity was paradoxically higher in the latter group.[1]

Mechanism

Not understood. Dapsone and trimethoprim appear to have mutually inhibitory effects on clearance. Steady-state serum levels were reached after 7 days.

Importance and management

Information is limited but the interaction appears to be established. Concurrent use appears to be an effective form of treatment, but be alert for evidence of increased dapsone toxicity (methaemoglobinaemia).

References

1 Lee B L, Medina I, Benowitz N L, Jacob P, Wofsy C B, Mills J. Dapsone, trimethoprim and sulfamethoxazole plasma levels during treatment of pneumocystis pneumonia in patients with acquired immunodeficiency syndrome (AIDS). Ann Intern Med (1989) 110, 606–11.

Didanosine + Food

Abstract/Summary

Food can reduce the bioavailability of didanosine, possibly causing a loss in efficacy.

Clinical evidence, mechanism, importance and management

Eight subjects were given 375 mg didanosine chewable tablets (*Videx*) alone or five minutes after breakfast. The food reduced the didanosine AUC by 45% and the maximum serum level by 54%.[1] Another study using sachets containing didanosine, sucrose and a buffer found that food reduced the bioavailability from 29 to 17%.[2] The reason would appear to be that food delays gastric emptying so that the didanosine is exposed to prolonged contact with gastric acid which causes decomposition with a resultant fall in bioavailability. This is an established interaction but its effect on the efficacy of didanosine does not seem to have been studied. To achieve maximum bioavailability the didanosine should be taken while fasting.

References

1 Shyu WC, Knupp CA, Pitman KA, Dunkle L, Barbhaiya RH. Food-induced reduction in bioavailability of didanosine. Clin Pharmacol Ther (1991) 50, 503–7.
2 Hartman NR, Yarchoan R, Luda JM, Thomas RV, Wyvill KM, Flora KP, Broder S, Johns DG. Pharmacokinetics of 2′,3′-dideoxyinosine in patients with severe human immunodeficiency infection. II. The effects of different formulations and the presence of other medications. Clin Pharmacol Ther (1991) 50, 278–85.

Didanosine + Ganciclovir

The pharmacokinetics of didanosine are not altered by ganciclovir.[1]

Reference

1 Hartman NR, Yarchoan R, Luda JM, Thomas RV, Wyvill KM, Flora KP, Broder S, Johns DG. Pharmacokinetics of 2′,3′-dideoxyinosine in patients with severe human immunodeficiency infection. II. The effects of different formulations and the presence of other medications. Clin Pharmacol Ther (1991) 50, 278–85.

Didanosine + Ranitidine

Concurrent use results in a minor increase in the serum levels of didanosine, and a minor decrease in the serum levels of ranitidine.

Clinical evidence, mechanism, importance and management

Twelve HIV-positive patients were given 375 mg didanosine either alone or 2 h after 150 mg ranitidine. The didanosine AUC (area under the curve) was increased 14% by the ranitidine.[1] The reason is not known but the ranitidine possibly enhances the effects of the citrate-phosphate buffer with which the didanosine is formulated. The ranitidine AUC was reduced by 16% for reasons which are not understood.[1] These bioavailability changes (didanosine + 14%, ranitidine – 16%) appear to be too small to matter and no particular precautions would seem necessary if the drugs are taken in this way. It is not known whether other H_2-blockers or omeprazole behave similarly.

Reference

1 Knupp CA, Dixon RM, Graziano F, Dunkle LM, Barbhaiya RH. Pharmacokinetic interaction study of didanosine and ranitidine in patients seropositive for human immunodeficiency virus. Antimicrob Ag Chemother (1992) 36, 2075–9.

Didanosine + Rifabutin (Ansamycin)

Abstract/Summary, clinical evidence, mechanism, importance and management

300–600 mg rifabutin (ansamycin) daily for 11 days was found not to affect the pharmacokinetics of didanosine (167 or 250 mg twice daily) in 11 patients with AIDS.[1] No special precautions would seem necessary if both drugs are given.

Reference

1 Sahai J, Foss N, Li R, Narang PK, Cameron DW. Rifabutin (R) and didanosine (ddi) interaction in AIDS patients. Clin Pharmacol Ther (1993) 53, 197.

Erythromycin + Alcohol

Abstract/Summary

Alcohol can cause a moderate reduction in the absorption of erythromycin ethylsuccinate.

Clinical evidence, mechanism, importance and management

When single 500 mg doses of erythromycin ethylsuccinate were taken by nine subjects with 150 ml of an alcoholic drink, followed 160 min later by another 150 ml, the erythromycin AUC was decreased by 27% and the absorption delayed. One subject showed a paradoxical 185% increase in absorption. The alcoholic drink was pisco sour which contains lemon juice, sugar and pisco (alcohol obtained by distilling grape juice). Blood alcohol levels achieved were about 50 mg% (0.5 g/l).[1] The reason for the reduced absorption is not understood but it is suggested that the slight delay is because alcohol delays gastric emptying so that the erythromycin reaches its absorption site in the duodenum a little later. The extent to which the reduced absorption might affect the control of an infection is uncertain. More study is needed to assess the clinical importance of this interaction.

Reference

1 Morasso MI, Chávez J, Gai MN, Arancibia A. Influence of alcohol consumption on erythromycin ethylsuccinate kinetics. Int J Clin Pharmacol Ther Toxicol (1990) 28, 426–9.

Erythromycin + Antacids

Abstract/Summary

Mylanta can prolong the absorption of erythromycin but the clinical importance of this is uncertain.

Clinical evidence, mechanism, importance and management

30 ml *Mylanta* (aluminium hydroxide, magnesium hydroxide, dimethicone) given with 500 mg erythromycin stearate to eight normal subjects had no significant effect on the AUC, peak serum concentration, or time to peak serum concentration of the erythromycin, but the mean elimination rate constant was 0.44 compared with 0.2 h.$^{-1}$ Thus the total amount of erythromycin absorbed remained unaltered but its absorption appeared to be prolonged.[1] The reason for this is not clear nor is its clinical importance known but it is probably small.

Reference

1 Yamreudeewong W, Scavone JM, Paone RP, Lewis GP. Effect of antacid co-administration on the bioavailability of erythromycin stearate. Clin Pharmacy (1989) 8, 352–4.

Erythromycin + Other antibiotics

Abstract/Summary

There is evidence that the effectiveness of concurrent treatment with erythromycin and other antibiotics (e.g. penicillin, ampicillin, lincomycin) may sometimes be more, and sometimes less, effective than with only one antibiotic.

Clinical evidence, mechanism, importance and management

The penicillins and erythromycin have a similar range of antibacterial activity so that so that it is fairly unusual to use them together and not much is known about the effectiveness of concurrent use. A large scale clinical study of uncomplicated scarlatina showed that penicillin was more effective than erythromycin, while the two antibiotics together were slightly less effective, as judged by the duration of the fever and the disappearance of the haemolytic streptococci.[1] This antagonism was seen in an *in vitro* study.[2] It has been suggested that combined treatment may possibly be more effective in the case of double infections with penicillinase-producing staphylococci.[1] There is also evidence that erythromycin with ampicillin is effective in pulmonary nocardiosis.[3] *In vitro* antagonism has been seen when a strain of staphylococci (resistant to erythromycin but sensitive to lincomycin) was exposed to both antibiotics together.[4] Whether this is likely to occur *in vivo* is uncertain. The general points for and against concurrent treatment with antibiotics and anti-infective agents are outlined in the introduction to this chapter.

References

1 Strom J. Penicillin and erythromycin singly and in combination in scarlatina therapy and the interference between them. Antibiot Chemotherap (1961) 11, 694.
2 Manten A. Synergism and antagonism between antibiotic mixtures containing erythromycin. Antibiot Chemotherap (1954) 4, 1228.
3 Bach MC, Monaco AP, Finland M. Pulmonary nocardiosis: therapy with minocycline and with erythromycin plus ampicillin. J Amer Med Ass (1973) 224, 1378.
4 Griffint LJ, Ostrande WE, Mullins CG, Beswick DE. Drug antagonism between lincomycin and erythromycin. Science (1964) 147, 746.

Erythromycin + Sucralfate

Abstract/Summary

Sucralfate appears not to interact adversely with erythromycin.

Clinical evidence, mechanism, importance and management

The pharmacokinetics (elimination rate constant, half-life, AUC) of erythromycin (single 400 mg dose) were not significantly altered by 1 g sucralfate in 6 normal subjects when given single 400 mg doses of erythromycin ethylsuccinate. It was concluded that the therapeutic effects of erythromycin are unlikely to be affected by concurrent use.[1]

Reference

1 Miller LG, Prichard JG, White CA, Vytla B, Feldman S, Bowman C. Effect of concurrent sucralfate administration on the absorption of erythromycin. J Clin Pharmacol (1990) 30, 39–40.

Erythromycin + Urinary acidifiers or Alkalinizers

Abstract/Summary

In the treatment of urinary tract infections, the antibacterial activity of erythromycin is maximal in alkaline urine and minimal in acid urine.

Clinical evidence

Urine taken from seven volunteers taking 1 g erythromycin, four times a day, was tested against five genera of Gram-negative bacilli (*Escherichia coli*, *Klebsiella pneumoniae*, *P. mirabilis*, *Ps. aeruginosa* and *Serrata sp.*) both before and after treatment with acetazolamide or sodium bicarbonate. A direct correlation was found between the activity of the antibiotic and the pH of the urine. Normally acid urine had little or no antibacterial activity, whereas alkalinized urine had activity.[1] Clinical studies have confirmed the increased antibacterial effectiveness of erythromycin in the treatment of bacteriuria when the urine is made alkaline.[2,3]

Mechanism

The pH of the urine does not apparently affect the way the kidney handles the antibiotic (most of it is excreted actively rather than passively) but it does have a direct influence on the way the antibiotic affects the micro-organisms. Mechanisms suggested include effects on bacterial cell receptors, induction of active transport mechanisms on bacterial cell walls, and changes in ionization of the antibiotic which enables it to enter the bacterial cell more effectively.

Importance and management

An established interaction which can be exploited. The effectiveness of the antibiotic in treating urinary tract infections can be maximized by making the urine alkaline (for example with acetazolamide or sodium bicarbonate). Treatment with urinary acidifiers will minimize the activity of the erythromycin and should be avoided.

References

1 Sabath LD, Gerstein DA, Loder PB, Finland M. Excretion of erythromycin and its enhanced activity in urine against gram-negative bacilli with alkalinization. J Lab Clin Med (1968) 72, 916.
2 Zinner SH, Sabath LD, Casey JI, Finland M. Erythromycin and alkalization of the urine in the treatment of urinary tract infections due to gram-negative bacilli. Lancet (1971) i, 1267.
3 Zinner SH, Sabath LD, Casey JI, Finland M. Erythromycin plus alkalization in the treatment of urinary infection Antimicrob Ag Chemother (1969) 9, 413

Ethambutol + Antacids

Abstract/Summary

Aluminium hydroxide can cause a small, and probably clinically unimportant, reduction in the absorption of ethambutol in some patients.

Clinical evidence, mechanism, importance and management

A study in 13 patients with tuberculosis, given single 50 mg/kg doses of ethambutol, showed that when they were also given 1.5 g aluminium hydroxide at the same time and repeated 15 and 30 min later, their serum ethambutol levels were delayed and reduced. The average urinary excretion of ethambutol over a 10 h period was reduced about 15%. There were marked variations. Some showed no interaction and others an increased absorption. No interaction was seen in six normal subjects similarly treated.[1] Just why this interaction occurs is not understood, but aluminium hydroxide can affect gastric emptying. The reduction in absorption is generally small and variable, and it seems doubtful if it will have a significant effect on the treatment of tuberculosis.

Reference

1 Mattila MJ, Linnoila M, Seppala T, Koskinen R. Effect of aluminium hydroxide and glycpyrrhonium on the absorption of ethambutol and alcohol in man. Br J clin Pharmacol (1978) 5, 161.

Ethionamide + Miscellaneous drugs

Abstract/Summary

Ethionamide has been associated in a few cases with mental depression, psychiatric disturbances, hypoglycaemia, hypothyroidism and alcohol-related psychotoxicity.

Clinical evidence, mechanism, importance and management

Ethionamide can cause depression, mental disturbances and hypoglycaemia.[1,4,5] Caution has been advised in patients under treatment for these psychiatric conditions, epilepsy and diabetes mellitus.[1] Hypothyroidism and thyroid enlargement have also been reported in a few patients treated with ethionamide and particular care may therefore be necessary in patients under treatment for thyroid malfunction.[2] A psychotoxic reaction has also been seen in a patient on ethionamide attributed to the heavy consumption of alcohol.[3] The incidence and importance of all of these reactions is uncertain, but prescribers should take them into account if ethionamide is prescribed with other drugs.

References

1 Martindale. The Extra Pharmacopoeia, edition 28 (1982).
2 Moulding T, Fraser R. Hypothyroidism related to ethionamide. Amer Rev Resp Dis (1970) 101, 90.
3 Lansdown FS, Beran M, Litwak T. Psychotoxic reaction during ethionamide therapy. Am Rev Resp Dis (1967) 95, 1053.
4 Narang RK. Acute psychotic reaction probably caused by ethionamide. Tubercle (1972) 53, 137.
5 Sharma GS, Gupta PK, Jain NK, Shanker A, Nanawati V. Toxic psychosis to isoniazid and ethionamide in a patient with pulmonary tuberculosis. Tubercle (1979) 60, 171.

Famciclovir + Cimetidine

No clinically important interaction appears to occur if famciclovir and allopurinol or cimetidine are given concurrently.

Abstract/Summary, clinical evidence, mechanism, importance and management

No clinically relevant changes in the pharmacokinetics of either allopurinol or famciclovir were seen in 12 normal subjects given 500 mg famciclovir after taking 300 mg allopurinol daily for 5 days.[2] 800 mg cimetidine daily for 6 days increased the AUC of 500 mg famiciclovir in 12 subjects by 18%, but this small change is unlikely to be of clinical importance.[1] No special precautions would seem necessary if either of these drugs is used with famciclovir.

Reference

1 Pratt SK, Fowles SE, Pierce DM, Prince WT. An investigation of the potential interaction between cimetidine and famciclovir in non-patient volunteers. Br J clin Pharmac (1991) 32, 656P.
2 Fowles SE, Pierce D, Laroche J, Pratt SK, Prince WT, Thomas D, Woodward A. An investigation into the potential interaction between allopurinol and oral famciclovir in non-patient volunteers. Br J clin Pharmac (1992) 34, 449–50P.

Fansidar + Zidovudine

Abstract/Summary, clinical evidence, mechanism, importance and management

A study in patients with AIDS found that 250 mg zidovudine four times daily did not adversely affect the prevention of toxoplasma encephalitis with *Fansidar* (pyrimethamine + sulphadoxine), 1 tablet twice weekly for up to 8 months.[1]

Reference

1 Eljaschewitsch J, Schürmann D, Pohle HD, Ruf B. Zidovudine does not antagonized *Fansidar* in preventing toxoplasma encephalitis in HIV infected patients. Istituto Superiore di Sanita. VII Inf Conf on AIDS, Florence, Italy, June 16–21 (1991), 4, 265B.

Fluconazole + Hydrochlorothiazide

Abstract/Summary, Clinical evidence, mechanism, importance and management

A very brief report describes a 40% increase in fluconazole serum levels in a small group of normal subjects when given hydrochlorothiazide.[1] It is suggested that no change in the fluconazole dosage is needed.[1]

Reference

1 Quoted as unpublished data on file, Pfizer, by Grant SM, Clissold SP. Fluconazole. A review of its pharmacodynamic and pharmacokinetic properties, and therapeutic potential in superficial and system mycoses. Drugs (1990) 39, 877–916.

Fluconazole, Itraconazole or Ketoconazole + Antacids, H₂-blockers, sucralfate

Abstract/Summary

Antacids, cimetidine and ranitidine which reduce the acidity of the stomach can very markedly reduce the gastrointestinal absorption of ketoconazole. Sucralfate has a much smaller effect. Antacids, cimetidine and ranitidine appear not to interact significantly with fluconazole or itraconazole.

Clinical evidence

(a) Fluconazole

20 ml *Maalox forte* (aluminium and magnesium hydroxides) did not affect the absorption of single 100 mg doses of fluconazole in 14 normal subjects.[7] The AUC $_{0-48}$ (area under the concentration-time curve over 48 h) of 100 mg fluconazole given to 6 normal subjects was reduced by only 13% when a single 400 mg dose cimetidine was given.[8] Another study found that cimetidine did not significantly affect fluconazole absorption.[9]

(b) Itraconazole

12 normal subjects were given 400 mg cimetidine twice daily or 150 mg ranitidine twice daily for 3 days before and after single 200 mg doses of itraconazole. The AUC and maximum serum levels of the itraconazole were reduced, but not significantly. The largest changes were 20% reductions in the AUC and maximum serum levels due to ranitidine.[6]

(b) Ketoconazole

A patient failed to respond to treatment with ketoconazole

while on cimetidine, sodium bicarbonate and aluminium oxide. Even when the ketoconazole dosage was raised to 400 mg daily her serum levels remained less than 1 µg/ml (normally 2 µg/ml 2–4 h after a 200 mg dose). A later study in three normal subjects found that when 200 mg ketoconazole was taken 2 h after 400 mg cimetidine, the absorption was considerably reduced (AUC reduced by 60%). When this was repeated but with 0.5 g sodium bicarbonate as well, the absorption was reduced to about 5%. In contrast, when this was repeated once more but with the ketoconazole in an acidic solution, the absorption was increased by 50%.[1]

Another study in 24 subjects found iv cimetidine titrated to give a gastric pH of 6 or more reduced the absorption by 95%.[9] A study in six subjects found that 150 mg ranitidine given 2 h before 400 mg ketoconazole reduced its AUC (area under the curve) by almost 96% (from 37.05 to 1.64 µg.h/L).[4,5] 1 g sucralfate caused a much smaller reduction (21%).[4,5] A study on four patients showed that the concurrent use of *Maalox* reduced the absorption of ketoconazole (AUC reduced by 40%) but the authors of the paper state that it had no statistical significance.[2] An anecdotal report suggested that giving ketoconazole 2 h before a stomatitis cocktail containing *Maalox* seemed to improve its effectiveness.[10]

Mechanism

Ketoconazole is a poorly soluble base which must be transformed by the acid in the stomach into the soluble hydrochloride salt. Agents which reduce gastric secretion, such as H_2 blockers or antacids, raise the pH in the stomach so that the dissolution of the ketoconazole and its absorption are reduced. Conversely, anything which increases the gastric acidity increases the dissolution and the absorption.[2,3] The sucralfate interaction is not fully understood. The absorption of fluconazole and itraconazole is minimally affected by changes in gastric pH.

Importance and management

The interactions with ketoconazole are clinically important but not extensively documented. Advise patients to take antacids and/or cimetidine or ranitidine not less than 2–3 h after the ketoconazole so that absorption can take place before the pH of the gastric contents is changed.[1] Monitor the effects to confirm that the ketoconazole is effective. It seems probable that other H_2-blockers will interact similarly but this needs confirmation. Also monitor the effects of sucralfate, but a much more modest interaction is expected. Fluconazole and itraconazole are alternative antifungals which only interact to a small and clinically irrelevant extent with H_2-blockers and would not be expected to be affected by antacids.

References

1 Van der Meer JW, Keuning JJ, Scheigrond HW, Heykants J, Van Cutsem J, Brugmans J. The influence of gastric acidity on the bioavailability of ketoconazole. J Antimicrob Chemother (1980) 6, 552–4.
2 Brass C, Galgiani JN, Blaschke TF, Defelice R, O'Reilly RA, Stevens DA. Disposition of ketoconazole, an oral antifungal in humans. Antimicrob Agents Chemother (1982) 21, 151–8.
3 Sutherland CH, Murphy JE, Schlefifer NH. The effects of two gastric acidifying agents on the pharmacokinetics of ketoconazole. 18th Annual Midyear Clinical Meeting of the American Society of Hospital Pharmacists, Atlanta, Georgia, Dec 4–8, 1983, p. 141.
4 Goss TF, Piscitelli SC, Schentag JJ. Evaluation of ketoconazole bioavailability interactions with sucralfate and ranitidine using gastric pH monitoring. Clin Pharmacol Ther (1991) 49, 128.
5 Piscitelli SC, Goss TF, Wilton JH, D'Andrea DT, Goldstein H, Schentag JJ. Effects of ranitidine and sucralfate on ketoconazole bioavailability. Antimicrob Ag Chemother (1991) 35, 1765–71.
6 Stein AG, Daneshmend TK, Warnock DW, Bhaskar N, Burke J, Hawkey CJ. The effects of H2-receptor antagonists on the pharmacokinetics of itraconazole, a new oral antifungal. Br J clin Pharmac (1989) 27, 104–5P.
7 Thorpe JE, Baker N, Bromet-Petit M. Effect of oral antacid administration on the pharmacokinetics of oral fluconazole. Antimicrob Ag Chemother (1990) 34, 2032–3.
8 Lazar JD, Wilner KD. Drug interactions with fluconazole. Rev Infect Dis (1990) 12 (Suppl 3) S327–33.
9 Blum RA, D'Andrea DT, Florentino BM, Wilton JH, Hilligoss DM, Gardner MJ, Henry EB, Goldstein H, Schentag JJ. Increased gastric pH and the bioavailability of fluconazole and ketoconazole. Ann Intern Med (1991) 114, 755–7.
10 Franklin MG. Nizoral and stomatitis cocktails may not mix. Oncol Nurs Forum (1991) 18, 1417.

Fluconazole + Rifampicin (Rifampin), Rifabutin (Ansamycin)

Abstract/Summary

Although rifampicin causes only a modest increase in the loss of fluconazole from the body, the reduction in its effects may possibly be clinically important. The situation with rifabutin is uncertain (no effect and reduced effects seen),

Clinical evidence

(a) Rifampicin

Normal subjects taking 600 mg rifampicin daily for 20 days were given 200 mg fluconazole on day 14. The AUC of the fluconazole was decreased by 23% and the half-life decreased by 22%.[1] 600 mg rifampicin daily for 19 days in another 16 subjects reduced the fluconazole AUC by 23%.[3]

Three patients with AIDS being treated for cryptococcal meningitis with fluconazole (400 mg daily) relapsed when rifampicin was added.[2] Another undetailed report says that one of five patients on fluconazole needed an increased dosage or a replacement antifungal when given rifampicin. It also occurred in two of four receiving rifabutin.[4]

(b) Rifabutin (ansamycin)

12 HIV patients were given 500 mg zidovudine daily from day 1–44, 200 mg fluconazole daily from days 3–30 and 300 mg rifabutin from days 17–44. No significant changes in the pharmacokinetics of fluconazole occurred between days 16 and 30.[5] This differs from the report cited in (a) above.[4]

Mechanism

A possible reason is that rifampicin increases the metabolism of the fluconazole by the liver, thereby increasing its loss from the body.[3] However fluconazole (unlike ketoconazole) is mainly excreted unchanged in the urine so that changes in its metabolism would not be expected to have a marked effect. The situation with rifabutin is uncertain.

Importance and management

Information is very limited. Although rifampicin has only a relatively small effect on fluconazole (compared with its considerable effects on ketoconazole),[1,3] the cases of relapse cited above[2] and the need for an increased dosage[4] indicate that this interaction may possibly be clinically important. Monitor concurrent use and increase the fluconazole dosage if necessary. The situation with rifabutin is uncertain but the effects should be monitored similarly.

References

1 Lazar J D, Wilner K D. Drug interactions with fluconazole. Rev Infect Dis (1990) 12 (Suppl 3) S327–33.
2 Coker R J, Tomlinson D R, Parkin J, Harris J, Pinching A J. Interaction between fluconazole and rifampicin. Br Med J (1990) 301, 818.
3 Apseloff G, Hilligoss M, Gardner MJ, Henry EB, Inskeep PB, Gerber N, Lazar JD. Induction of fluconazole metabolism by rifampin: in vivo study in humans. J Clin Pharmacol (1991) 31, 358–61.
4 Tett S, Carey D, Lee H-S. Drug interactions with fluconazole. Med J Aust (1992) 156, 365.
5 Trapnell CB, Lavelle JP, O'Leary CR, James DS, Li R, Colburn D, Woosely RL, Narang PK. Rifabutin does not alter fluconazole pharmacokinetics. Clin Pharmacol Ther (1993) 53, 196.

Fluconazole + Zidovudine

Abstract/Summary, clinical evidence, mechanism, importance and management

Twelve HIV patients were given 500 mg zidovudine daily from day 1–44, 200 mg fluconazole daily from days 3–30 and 300 mg rifabutin from days 17–44. No significant changes in the pharmacokinetics of fluconazole occurred between days 16 and 30.[1] No special precautions would seem necessary if fluconazole is given to patients taking zidovudine.

Reference

1 Trapnell CB, Lavelle JP, O'Leary CR, James DS, Li R, Colburn D, Woosely RL, Narang PK. Rifabutin does not alter fluconazole pharmacokinetics. Clin Pharmacol Ther (1993) 53, 196.

Flucytosine + Cytarabine

Abstract/Summary

Some very limited evidence suggests that cytarabine may oppose the activity of 5-flucytosine.

Clinical evidence, mechanism, importance and management

A man with Hodgkin's disease treated for cryptococcal meningitis with 100 mg/kg 5-flucytosine daily showed a fall in his serum and CSF levels from 30–40 mg/l to undetectable levels when given cytarabine intravenously. *In vitro* tests showed that 1 mg/l cytarabine completely abolished the activity of up to 50 mg/l 5-flucytosine against the patient's strain of cryptococcus, whereas procarbazine did not. When the cytarabine was replaced by procarbazine in the patient, his body fluid levels of 5-flucytosine returned to their former values.[1] In another study in a patient with myeloid leukaemia it was found that the predose and postdose 5-flucytosine levels fell from 65 and 80 mg/l to 42 and 53 mg/l respectively while concurrently receiving cytarabine and daunorubicin.[2] This was attributed to an improvement in renal function rather than antagonism between the two drugs.[2] No changes in the activity of 5-flucytosine against 14 out of 16 wild isolates of cryptococcus in the presence of cytarabine was seen in an *in vitro* study, although an increase was seen in one and a decrease in the other.[2]

The evidence for this interaction is therefore very limited indeed and its general clinical importance remains uncertain, but the manufacturers warn against concurrent use. It has been suggested that if both drugs are used, the flucytosine should be given 3 h or more after the cytarabine when the serum levels will have fallen.[3]

References

1 Holt RJ. Clinical problems with 5-flucytosine. Mykosen (1978) 21, 363–9.
2 Wingfield HJ. Absence of fungistatic antagonism between flucytosine and cytarabine in vitro and in vivo. J Antimicrob Chemother (1987) 20, 523–7.
3 Scoffield RE (Pfizer). Personal communication (1988).

Flucytosine + Miscellaneous drugs

Abstract/Summary

The interactions of flucytosine with amphotericin B and aluminium hydroxide-magnesium hydroxide do not appear to be of clinical importance.

Clinical evidence, mechanism, importance and management

The combined use of flucytosine and amphotericin B is more effective than flucytosine alone in the treatment of cryptococcal meningitis, but the amphotericin causes some deterioration in kidney function which can result in raised flucytosine blood levels and some increase in toxicity. Nevertheless combined use is thought to be useful.[1] Aluminium hydroxide-magnesium hydroxide delays the absorption of flucytosine from the gut, but the total amount absorbed remains unaffected.[2]

References

1 Bennett JE, Dismukes WE, Duma RJ, Medoff G, Sande MA, Gallis A, Leonard J, Fields BT, Bradshaw M, Haywood H, McGee ZA, Cate TR, Cobbs CG, Warner JF, Alling DW. A comparison of amphotericin B alone and combined with flucytosine in the treatment of cryptococcal meningitis. N Engl J Med (1979) 301, 126–31.

2 Cutler RE, Blair AD and Kelly MR. Flucytosine kinetics in subjects with normal and impaired renal function. Clin Pharmacol Ther (1978) 24, 333–42.

Foscarnet + Miscellaneous drugs

Abstract/Summary

Four patients showed marked hypocalcaemia when concurrently treated with foscarnet and pentamidine. One of them died. Foscarnet and zidovudine do not have a pharmacokinetic interaction.

Clinical evidence, mechanism, importance and management

(a) Pentamidine

Four patients with suspected AIDS-related cytomegaloviral infections of the chest developed signs of hypocalcaemia within 10 days of starting treatment with foscarnet and pentamidine (dosages not stated.) All four had paraesthesiae of the hands and feet, and three of them had Chvosteks's and Trousseau's signs. The serum calcium levels of three of them fell but normalized when the drugs were stopped. The fourth patient died with severe hypocalcaemia (1.42 mmol/l). Both drugs have been associated with hypocalcaemia in HIV patients and in these four patients their effects appear to have been additive. The authors of the report advise very close monitoring if both drugs are used.[1] Martindale's Extra Pharmacopoeia also suggests that extreme caution is needed if administered together because both are potentially nephrotoxic.[3]

(b) Zidovudine

The antiviral effects of foscarnet and zidovudine appear to be additive or synergistic, but no significant alteration in the pharmacokinetics of either drug was seen in a 14-day study of five AIDS patients given both drugs which might possibly have provided some explanation.[2] Concurrent use would seem to be valuable.

References

1 Youle MS, Clarbour J, Gazzard B, Chanas A. Severe hypocalcaemia in AIDS patients treated with foscarnet and pentamidine. Lancet (1988) 1, 1455–6.

2 Aweeka FT, Gambertoglio JG, Van der Horst C, Raasch R, Jacobson MA. Pharmacokinetics of concomitantly administered foscarnet and zidovudine for treatment of human immunodeficiency virus infection (AIDS clinical trials group protocol 053). Antimicrob Ag Chemother (1992) 36, 1773–8.

3 Reynolds JEF (ed). Martindale. The Extra Pharmacopoeia, edn 30 (1993) p 545.

Fosfomycin trometamol + Cimetidine or Metoclopramide

Abstract/Summary

Cimetidine does not affect the pharmacokinetics of fosfomycin trometanol. Metoclopramide reduces its bioavailability but the evidence suggests that this probably does not affect the control of urinary tract infections.

Clinical evidence, mechanism, importance and management

Cimetidine (400 mg on the night before and 400 mg 30 min before) had almost no effect on the pharmacokinetics of 50 mg/kg fosfomycin trometamol in nine normal subjects, whereas 20 mg metoclopramide 30 min before reduced the peak serum levels by 42% and the AUC by 27%. The reason seems to be that the metoclopramide speeds the transit through the gut so that less time is available for good absorption. However despite these reductions, the urinary concentrations remained above the minimum levels required for common urinary pathogens for at least 36 h after giving the antibiotic.[1] This suggests that the interaction may not be of clinical importance.

Reference

1 Bergan T, Mastopaolo G, Di Mario F, Naccarato R. Pharmacokinetics of fosfomycin and influence of cimetidine and metoclopramide on the bioavailability of fosfomycin trometamol, in New Trends in Urinary Tract Infections (eds Neu and Williams) Int Symp Rome 1987, pp 157–66.

Furazolidone + Sympathomimetic amines (directly and indirectly-acting)

Abstract/Summary

After 5–10 days' use furazolidone has MAO-inhibitory activity approximately equivalent to the antidepressant and antihypertensive MAOIs. The concurrent use of sympathomimetic amines with indirect activity (amphetamines, phenylpropanolamine, ephedrine, etc.) or tyramine-rich foods and drinks may be expected to result in a potentially serious rise in blood pressure, although direct evidence of accidental adverse reactions of this kind seem not to have been reported. The pressor effects of noradrenaline (norepinephrine) are unchanged.

Clinical evidence

After 6 days' treatment with 400 mg furazolidone daily, the

pressor responses to tyramine or dexamphetamine in four hypertensive patients had increased two- to threefold, and after 13 days about ten-fold. These responses were approximately the same as those found in two other patients on pargyline.[1] The MAO-inhibitory activity of furazolidone was confirmed by measurements taken on jejunal specimens. The pressor effects of noradrenaline were unchanged.[1]

Mechanism

The MAO-inhibitory activity of furazolidone is not immediate and may in fact be due to a metabolite of furazolidone.[4] It develops gradually so that, after 5–10 days' use, indirectly-acting sympathomimetics will interact with furazolidone in the same way as they do in the presence of other MAOI's.[2,3] More details of the mechanisms of this interaction are to be found elsewhere (see (MAOI + Tyramine-rich foods), (MAOI + Indirectly-acting sympathomimetics)).

Importance and management

The MAO-inhibitory activity of furazolidone after 5–10 days' use is established, but reports of hypertensive crises either with sympathomimetics or tyramine-containing foods or drinks appear to be lacking. Notwithstanding, it would seem prudent to warn patients given furazolidone not to take any of the drugs, foods or drinks which are prohibited to those on antidepressant or antihypertensive MAOI (e.g. cough, cold and influenza remedies containing phenylpropanolamine, phenylephrine, pseudoephedrine, etc., appetite-suppressants containing sympathomimetics, or tyramine-rich foods or drinks). See the appropriate synopses for more detailed lists of these drugs, foods and drinks ('MAOI + Tyramine-rich foods', 'MAOI + Tyramine-rich alcoholic drinks.'). No adverse interaction would be expected with noradrenaline (norepinephrine).

References

1 Pettinger WA, Oates JA. Supersensitivity to tyramine during monoamine oxidase inhibition in man. Mechanism at the level of the adrenergic neurone. Clin Pharmacol Ther (1968) 9, 341.
2 Pettinger WA, Soyangco FG, Oates JA. Monoamine oxidase inhibition by furazolidone in man. Clin Res (1966) 14, 258.
3 Pettinger WA, Soyangco F, Oates JA. Inhibition of monoamine oxidase in man by furazolidone. Clin Pharmacol Ther (1968) 9, 442.
4 Stern IJ, Hollifield RD, Wilk S, Buzard JA. The anti-monoamine oxidase effects of furazolidone. J Pharmacol Exp Ther (1967) 156, 492–9.

Griseofulvin + Phenobarbitone

Abstract/Summary

The antifungal effects of griseofulvin can be reduced or even abolished by the the concurrent use of phenobarbitone (phenobarbital).

Clinical evidence

Two epileptic children of seven and eight, taking 40 mg phenobarbitone daily, failed to respond to long-term treatment for *tinea capitis* with griseofulvin, 400 mg daily, until the barbiturate was withdrawn.[7]

Two other patients have been reported who similarly failed to respond to griseofulvin while taking phenobarbitone.[3,6] Two studies, one in six and the other in eight normal subjects, found that while taking 90 mg phenobarbitone daily the absorption of griseofulvin given orally was reduced by 45% and 33% respectively. The peak serum levels after 8 h were reduced 33% (from 1.35 to 0.9 μg/ml) in the latter study.[1,2]

Mechanism

Not fully understood. Initially it was thought[4] that the phenobarbitone increased the metabolism and clearance of the griseofulvin but it now seems that it reduces the absorption of griseofulvin from the gut.[2] One idea is that the phenobarbitone increases peristalsis so that the opportunity for absorption is diminished.[2] Another suggestion is that the phenobarbitone forms a complex with the griseofulvin which makes an already poorly soluble drug even less soluble, and therefore less readily absorbed.[5]

Importance and management

An established interaction of clinical importance, although the evidence seems to be limited to the reports cited. If the barbiturate must be given, it has been suggested that the griseofulvin should be given in divided doses three times a day to give it a better chance of being absorbed.[2] The effect of increasing the dosage of griseofulvin appears not to have been studied. An alternative is to exchange the phenobarbitone for a non-interacting anticonvulsant such as sodium valproate. This proved to be successful in one of the cases cited.[7]

References

1 Busfield D, Child KJ, Atkinson RM, Tomich EG. An effect of phenobarbitone on blood levels of griseofulvin in man. Lancet (1963) ii, 1042.
2 Riegleman S, Rowland M, Epstein WL. Griseofulvin-phenobarbital interaction in man. J Amer Med Ass (1970) 213, 426.
3 Lorenc E. A new factor in griseofulvin treatment failures. Missouri Med (1967) 64, 32.
4 Busfield D, Child KJ, Tomich EG. An effect of phenobarbitone on griseofulvin metabolism in the rat. Brit J Pharmacol (1964) 22, 137.
5 Abougela IKA, Bigford DJ, McCorquodale K, Grant DJW. Complex formation and other physico-chemical interactions between griseofulvin and phenobarbitone. J Pharm Pharmac (1976) 28, 44P.
6 Stepanova Zh V, Sheklahova AA. Liuminal kak prichina neudachi griseoful'vinoterapii bol'nogo mikrospoviei. (Luminal as a cause of failure of griseofulvin therapy of a patient with microsporosis). Vestn Dermatol Venereol (1975) 12, 63–5.
7 Beurey J, Weber M, Vignaud J-M. Traitment des teignes microsporiques. Interference metabolique entre phenobarbital et griseofulvine. Ann Dermatol Venereol (Paris) (1982) 109, 567–70.

Hetacillin + Miscellaneous drugs

Abstract/Summary, clinical evidence, mechanism, importance and management

No changes in serum antibiotic levels were seen in 12 patients concurrently treated with hetacillin and anticonvulsants (carbamazepine, clonazepam, diazepam, phenytoin, phenobarbitone, primidone, sodium valproate) or in 12 other patients treated with chlorpromazine.[1] No special precautions would seem to be necessary.

Reference

1 Galanopoulou P, Karageorgiou Ch, Dimakopoulou K. Effect of enzyme induction on bioavailability of hetacillin in patients treated with anticonvulsants and chlorpromazine. Eur J Drug Metab Pharmacokinet (1990) 15, 15–18.

Hexamine compounds + Urinary acidifiers or Alkalinizers and Sulphonamides

Abstract/Summary

Urinary alkalinizers (e.g. potassium citrate) and those antacids which can raise the urinary pH above 5 should not be used during treatment with hexamine compounds (methenamine). If some of the older less-soluble sulphonamides are also used there is the risk of kidney damage due to crystalluria at low urinary pH values.

Clinical evidence, mechanism, importance and management

(a) Hexamine + urinary acidifiers or alkalinizers

Hexamine (methenamine) and hexamine mandelate are only effective as urinary antiseptics if the pH is about 5 or lower when formaldehyde is released. This is normally achieved by giving urinary acidifiers such as ammonium chloride or sodium acid phosphate. In the case of hexamine hippurate, the acidification of the urine is achieved by the presence of hippuric acid. The concurrent use of compounds which raise the urinary pH such as acetazolamide, sodium bicarbonate, potassium citrate, etc. is clearly contraindicated.[1] Potassium citrate mixture BPC at normal therapeutic doses has been shown to raise the pH by more than 1 thereby making the urine sufficiently alkaline to interfere with the activation of methenamine to formaldehyde.[2] Concurrent use should therefore be avoided. Some antacids can also cause a very significant rise in the pH of the urine.[1]

(b) Hexamine + urinary acidifiers + sulphonamides

At pH values of 5 and below at which hexamine is effective, many of the older sulphonamides (sulphapyridine, sulphadiazine, sulphamethizole, etc.) are insoluble and can crystallize out in the kidney tubules causing physical damage.[1] Although this is much less likely to occur with the newer, more soluble sulphonamides, it would seem preferable to avoid the problem by using some other form of treatment.

References

1 Levy C. Interactions of salicylates with antacids. Clinical implications with respect to gastrointestinal bleeding and anti-inflammatory activity. Frontiers of Internal Medicine 1974, 12th Int Congr Intern Med, Tel Aviv 1974. Karger, Basel (1975) p 404.
2 Lipton JH. Incompatibility between sulfamethizole and methenamine mandelate. N Engl J Med (1963) 268, 92.

8-Hydroxyquinoline + Zinc oxide

Abstract/Summary

The presence of zinc oxide inhibits the therapeutic effects of 8-hydroxyquinoline in ointments.

Incompatibility

The observation that a patient had an allergic reaction to 8-hydroxyquinoline in ointments with a paraffin base, but not a zinc oxide base, prompted further study of a possible incompatibility. A study in 13 patients confirmed that zinc oxide reduces the eczematogenic (allergic) properties of the 8-hydroxyquinoline, but it also inhibits its antibacterial and antimycotic effects as well, and appears to stimulate the growth of *Candida albicans*.[1]

Mechanism

It seems almost certain that the zinc ions form chelates with 8-hydroxyquinoline which have little or no antibacterial properties.[1,2]

Importance and management

The documentation is limited but the reaction appears to be established. There is no point in using zinc oxide to reduce the allergic properties of the 8-hydroxyquinoline if, at the same time, the therapeutic effects disappear.

References

1 Fischer T. On 8-hydroxyquinoline-zinc oxide incompatibility. Dermatologica (1974) 149, 129.
2 Alberta A, Rubbo SD, Goldacre RJ, Balfour BJ. The influence of chemical constitution on antibacterial activity III. A study of 8-hydroxyquinoline (oxine) and related compounds. Brit J exp Path (1974) 28, 69.

Influenza vaccine + Paracetamol (Acetaminophen), Alprazolam and Lorazepam

Abstract/Summary

Paracetamol does not affect the vaccine and appears to reduce its side-effects. The pharmacokinetics of alprazolam, lorazepam and paracetamol are not affected by influenza vaccine.

Clinical evidence, mechanism, importance and management

The pharmacokinetics of single doses of 650 mg paracetamol (acetaminophen) given IV, alprazolam 1 mg orally or lorazepam 2 mg IV remained unaffected in normal subjects when measured 7 and 14 days after 0.5 ml influenza vaccine given intramuscularly.[1] 1 g paracetamol four times daily for two days had no effect on the production of *H. influenzae* antibodies in a group of 29 elderly patients concurrently given inactivated influenza virus vaccine, and appeared to reduce the adverse effects of the vaccine (fever etc).[2] There would seem to be no reason for avoiding the concurrent use of these drugs and, in the case of paracetamol, some advantage.

References

1 Scavone JM, Blyden GT, LeDuc BW, Greenblatt DJ. Effect of influenza vaccine on acetaminophen, alprazolam, antipyrine and lorazepam pharmacokinetics. J Clin Pharmacol (1986) 26, 556.

2 Gross P, Bonelli J, Weksler M, Russo C, Munk G, Dran S, Levandrowski R. Acetaminophen prevents adverse effects but does not reduce antibody responses to inactivated influenza virus vaccine in the elderly. Int Sci Conf Antimicrob Ag Chemother (1992) Abstracts, p 179.

Interferon + Aspirin, Paracetamol or Prednisone

Abstract/Summary

Aspirin and paracetamol (acetaminophen) appear neither to reduce the effects of interferon nor its side-effects. Prednisone also does not reduce its side-effects but it may possibly reduce its biological activity.

Clinical evidence

Studies were made in eight normal subjects given a single IM dose of 18×10^6 U interferon (rHuIFN alpha 2a*) alone or after 24 h of an 8-day course of either aspirin (650 mg four-hourly), paracetamol (acetaminophen) (650 mg 4-hourly) or prednisone (40 mg daily). None of these additional drugs reduced the interferon side-effects (fever or chills, headache or myalgia) nor was the activity of the interferon affected as measured by a virus yield inhibition assay with vesicular stomatitis virus. However the prednisone reduced the AUC of 2'-5'-oligoadenylate synthetase activity (a measure of the activity of the interferon) by almost 40%.[1]

Mechanism

Not understood.

Importance and management

Information seems to be limited to this study, on the basis of which there would seem to be no point in using either aspirin or paracetamol to reduce the side-effects of interferon, but apparently no adverse interaction occurs either. In the case of prednisone (and possibly other corticosteroids) the reduction in the biological activity of the interferon would seem to be a disadvantage but more confirmatory study of this is needed.

Reference

1 Witter FR, Woods AS, Griffin MD, Smith CR, Nadler P, Lietman PS. Effects of prednisone, aspirin and acetaminophen on an *in vivo* biologic response to interferon in humans. Clin Pharmacol Ther (1988) 44, 239–43.

Isoniazid + Aminosalicylic acid (PAS)

Abstract/Summary

Isoniazid serum levels are raised by the concurrent use of aminosalicylic acid. A generally advantageous interaction.

Clinical evidence, mechanism, importance and management

A study in man showed that the concurrent administration of aminosalicylic acid significantly increased the serum levels and half-lives of isoniazid due, it is suggested, to the inhibition of the isoniazid metabolism by the aminosalicylic acid. The effect was most marked among the 'fast' acetylators of isoniazid.[1] No precise figures were stated. There seem to be no reports of isoniazid toxicity arising from this interaction and the outcome would appear to be advantageous.

Reference

1 Boman G, Borga O, Hanngren A, Malmborg A-S, Sjoqvist F. Pharmacokinetic interactions between the tuberculostatics rifampicin (rifampin), para-aminosalicylic acid and isoniazid. Acta Pharmac Toxicol (1970) 28 (suppl 1) 15.

Isoniazid + Antacids

Abstract/Summary

The absorption of isoniazid from the gut is reduced by the concurrent use of aluminium hydroxide. The isoniazid should be given at least an hour before the antacid to minimize the effects of this interaction.

Clinical evidence

Ten patients with tuberculosis were given 45 ml aluminium hydroxide (*Amphojel*) at 6, 7 and 8 am, followed immediately by isoniazid and any other medication they were receiving. 1 h serum isoniazid levels and the AUC (area under the curves) were depressed, and peak serum concentrations occurring between 1 and 2 h after ingestion were reduced about 16%, or expressed in μg/ml/mg or isoniazid/kg body weight to allow for different dosages, by 25%.[1] The effect of magaldrate (hydrated magnesium aluminate) was less.[1]

Mechanism

Aluminium hydroxide delays gastric emptying (demonstrated in man and rats[2,3]), causing retention of the isoniazid in the stomach. Since isoniazid is largely absorbed from the intestine, the decrease in serum isoniazid concentrations is explained. It also appears to inhibit absorption as well.

Importance and management

This interaction appears to be established, although information is limited. Its clinical importance is uncertain, but as single high doses of isoniazid are more effective in arresting tuberculosis than the same amount of drug in divided doses[4,5] it would seem wise to avoid this interaction by following the recommendations made in the study cited, namely to give the isoniazid at least an hour before the aluminium hydroxide.[1] There seems to be no information about the effects of other antacids.

References

1 Hurwitz A, Schlozman DL. Effects of antacids on gastrointestinal absorption of isoniazid in rat and man. Amer Rev Resp Dis (1974) 109, 41.
2 Hava M, Hurwitz A. The relaxing effect of aluminium hydroxide on rat and human gastric smooth muscle *in vitro*. Europ J Pharmac (1973) 7, 156.
3 Vats TS, Hurwitz A, Robinson RG, Herrin W. Effects of antacids on gastric emptying in children. Pediatr Res (1973) 22, 340.
4 Fox W. General considerations in intermittent drug therapy of pulmonary tuberculosis. Postgrad med J (1971) 47, 729.
5 Hudson LD, Sharbara JA. Twice weekly tuberculosis chemotherapy. J Amer Med Ass (1973) 223, 139.

Isoniazid + Cheese or Fish

Abstract/Summary

Patients taking isoniazid who eat histamine-rich foods (e.g. cheese, certain tropical fish such as tuna) may experience a flushing reaction with headache, difficulty in breathing, nausea and tachycardia.

Clinical evidence

Three months after starting to take 300 mg isoniazid daily, a woman experienced a series of unpleasant reactions 10–30 min after eating cheese. These reactions included chills, headache (sometimes severe), itching of the face and scalp, slight diarrhoea, flushing of the face and on one occasion the whole body, variable and mild tachycardia and a bursting sensation in the head. Blood pressure measurements showed only a modest rise (from 95/65 to 110/80 mm Hg). No physical or biochemical abnormalities were found.[1]

Headache, dizziness, blurred vision, tachycardia, flushing of the skin and redness of the eyes, burning sensation of the body, difficulty in breathing, abdominal colic, diarrhoea, vomiting, sweating and wheezing have all been described in other patients on isoniazid after eating cheese[3,5,9,12] and certain tropical fish including tuna (skipjack or bonito-*Katsuwanus pelamis*),[4,6,7,11] *Sardinella (Amblygaster) sirm*,[8] *Rastrigella kanagurta*[2] and others.[10] There are well over 300 cases of this reaction on record.

Mechanism

The most likely explanation is that these samples of food contained unusually large amounts of histamine produced by the decarboxylating activity of certain bacteria on the amino acid histidine. Normally this is inactivated by histaminase in the body, but in the presence of isoniazid which is a potent inhibitor of this enzyme, it can be absorbed largely unchanged and histamine intoxication develops. Histamine survives all but very prolonged cooking. Tuna fish contains 180–500 mg histamine per 100 g.[11]

Importance and management

An established and well-documented interaction. The incidence appears to be small. With the exception of one patient who appeared to have had a cerebrovascular accident,[7] the reactions experienced by the others were unpleasant and alarming but not serious or life-threatening, and required little or no treatment. Two reports say that treatment with antihistamines was effective.[10,11] Isoniazid has been in use since 1956 and there would seem little need now to introduce any general dietary restrictions, but if any of these reactions is experienced, it would be worthwhile examining the patient's diet and advising the avoidance of probable offending foodstuffs. Very mature cheese and fish which is not fresh are to be treated with suspicion, but there is no way one can guess the likely histamine content of food without undertaking a detailed analysis.

References

1 Smith CK, Durack DT. Isoniazid and cheese reaction. Ann Intern Med (1978) 88, 520.
2 Uragoda CG. Histamine intoxication with isoniazid and a species of fish. Ceylon Med J (1978) 23, 109–10.
3 Uragoda CG, Lodha SC. Histamine intoxication in a tuberculous patient after ingestion of cheese. Tubercle (1979) 60, 59.
4 Uragoda CG, Kottegoda SR. Adverse reactions to isoniazid on ingestion of fish with a high histamine content. Tubercle (1977) 58, 83.
5 Lejonc JL, Gusmini D, Brochard P. Isoniazid and reaction to cheese. Ann Intern Med (1979) 91, 793.
6 Uragoda CG. Histamine poisoning in tuberculous patients after ingestion of tuna fish. Amer Rev Resp Dis (1980) 121, 157.
7 Senanayake N, Vyravanthan S, Kanagasuriyama S. Cerebrovascular accident after a 'skipjack' reaction in a patient taking isoniazid. Brit Med J (1978) 2, 1127.
8 Uragoda CG. Histamine poisoning in tuberculous patients on ingestion of tropical fish. J Trop Med Hyg (1978) 81, 243–5.
9 Hauser MJ, Baier H. Interactions of isoniazid with foods. Drug Intell Clin Pharm (1982) 16, 617–8.
10 Diao Y et al. Histamine like reaction in tuberculosis patients taking fishes containing much of histamine under treatment with isoniazid in 277 cases. Chin J Tubercul Resp Dis (Chung Hua Chieh Ho Ho Hu Hsi Hsi Chi Ping Tsa Chih) (1986) 9, 267–9, 317–18.
11 Senanayake N, Vryavanthan S. Histamine reactions due to ingestion of tuna fish (Thunnus argentivittatus) in patients on antituberculous therapy. Toxicon (1982) 19, 184–5.
12 Toutoungi M, Carroll R, Dick P. Isoniazide (INH) and tyramine-rich food. Chest (1986) 89 (Suppl 6) 540S.

Isoniazid + Cimetidine or Ranitidine

Abstract/Summary

Pharmacokinetic evidence suggests that neither cimetidine nor ranitidine interact with isoniazid.

Clinical evidence, mechanism, importance and management

400 mg cimetidine or 300 mg ranitidine, three times a day, for three days had no effect on the pharmacokinetics of single 10 mg/kg doses of isoniazid in 12 normal subjects. Neither the absorption nor the metabolism of isoniazid were changed.[1] The absence of an interaction indicated by this study needs clinical confirmation.

Reference

1 Paulsen O, Hoglund P, Nilsson L-G, Gredeby H. No interaction between H_2 blockers and isoniazid. Eur J Respir Dis (1986) 68, 286–90.

Isoniazid + Corticosteroids

Abstract/Summary

Prednisolone can lower serum isoniazid levels, but this may not be clinically important.

Clinical evidence, mechanism, importance and management

26 patients with tuberculosis were treated with 10 mg/kg isoniazid daily. The 13 slow inactivators of isoniazid showed a 23% fall in serum isoniazid levels when given 20 mg prednisolone, while the 13 rapid inactivators showed a 38% fall over 8.5 h. The reasons are not understood, but changes in the metabolism and/or the excretion of the isoniazid by the kidney are possibilities. Despite these changes, the response to treatment was excellent.[1] In another group of 49 patients, both slow and rapid inactivators, the additional use of 12 mg/kg rifampicin largely counteracted the isoniazid-lowering effects of the prednisolone.[1]

None of these interactions was of clinical importance, but the authors point out that if the dosage of isoniazid had been lower, its effects might have been reduced. Be alert for any evidence of a reduced response during concurrent use, and raise the isoniazid dosage if necessary. There seems to be no information about other corticosteroids.

Reference

1 Sarma GR, Kailasam S, Nair NGK, Narayana ASL, Tripathy SP. Effect of prednisolone and rifampin on isoniazid metabolism in slow and rapid inactivators of isoniazid. Antimicrob Ag Chemother (1980) 18, 661–6.

Isoniazid + Disulfiram

Abstract/Summary

Seven patients on isoniazid have been described who experienced difficulties in co-ordination and changes in affect and behaviour after taking disulfiram concurrently. Four others became drowsy.

Clinical evidence

Seven patients with tuberculosis who had been taking 0.6–1.0 g isoniazid daily for not less than 30 days, without problems, experienced adverse reactions within 2–8 days of starting to take 0.5 g disulfiram daily. Among the symptoms were dizziness, disorientation, a staggering gait, insomnia, irritable and querulous behaviour, listlessness and lethargy. One patient showed hypomania. Most of them were also taking chlordiazepoxide and other drugs including PAS, streptomycin and phenobarbitone. The adverse reactions decreased or disappeared when the disulfiram was either reduced to 0.25–

0.125 g daily, or withdrawn. These seven patients represented less than a third of those who received both drugs. Four other patients given only isoniazid and disulfiram also showed drowsiness and depression.[1]

Mechanism

Not understood. One idea is that some kind of synergy occurred between the two drugs because both can produce not dissimilar side-effects if given in high doses. The authors of the report[1] speculate that isoniazid and disulfiram together inhibit two of three biochemical pathways concerned with the metabolism of dopamine. One of these metabolizes dopamine by dopamine beta-hydroxylase to noradrenaline, and then by MAO to 3,4-dihydroxyphenyl acetic acid. This leaves a third pathway open, catalyzed by COMT, which produces a number of methylated products of dopamine. These may possibly have been responsible for the mental and physical reactions seen.

Importance and management

Information about this interaction appears to be limited to the report cited[1] and one other.[2] Its incidence is uncertain, but two-thirds of the group failed to show this interaction and no interaction occurred in another patient taking both drugs and rifampicin (rifampin).[2] If concurrent use is undertaken, the response should be closely monitored and where necessary the dosage of disulfiram should be reduced, or withdrawn.

References

1 Whittington HG, Grey L. Possible interaction between disulfiram and isoniazid. Amer J Psychiat (1969) 125, 1725.
2 Rothstein E. Rifampin with disulfiram. J Amer Med Ass (1972) 219, 1216.

Isoniazid + Ethambutol

Abstract/Summary

There is experimental evidence that ethambutol does not affect serum isoniazid levels but there is also some evidence which suggests that the optic neuropathy of ethambutol may be increased by the concurrent use of isoniazid.

Clinical evidence, mechanism, importance and management

The mean serum levels of isoniazid after taking a single 300 mg dose were not significantly changed in 10 patients with tuberculosis when they were also given a single 20 mg/kg dose of ethambutol.[1] The possible effects of concurrent use over a period of time were not studied. However there is some evidence that the optic neuropathy of ethambutol may be increased by the concurrent use of isoniazid.[2-5]

References

1 Singhai KC, Varshney DP, Rathi R, Kishore K, Varshney SC. Serum concentration of isoniazid administered with and without ethambutol in pulmonary tuberculosis patients. Indian J Med Res (1986) 83, 360–2.
2 Renard G, Morax PV. Nevrite optique au cours des traitements antituberculeux. Ann Oculist (Paris) (1977) 210, 53–61.
3 Karmon G, Savir H, Zevin D, Levi J. Bilateral optic atrophy due to combined ethambutol and isoniazid treatment. Ann Ophthalmol (1979) 11, 1013–17.
4 Garret CR. Optic neuritis in a patient on ethambutol and isoniazid evaluated by visual evoked potentials. Case report. Mil Med (1985) 150, 43–6.
5 Jumenez-Lucho VE, Del Busto R, Odel J. Isoniazid and ethambutol as a cause of optic neuropathy. Eur J Respir Dis (1987) 71, 42–5.

Isoniazid + Fluconazole

Abstract/Summary

Fluconazole appears not to interact with isoniazid.

Clinical evidence, mechanism, importance and management

A double blind crossover study in 16 normal subjects (8 'fast' and 8 'slow' acetylators of isoniazid) found that 400 mg fluconazole daily for a week had no clinically significant effect on the pharmacokinetics of isoniazid.[1] No special precautions would appear necessary during concurrent use.

Reference

1 Buss DC, Routledge PA, Hutchings A, Brammer KW, Thorpe JE. The effect of fluconazole on the acetylation of isoniazid. Hum & Exp Toxicol (1991) 10, 85–6.

Isoniazid + Food

Abstract/Summary

The absorption of isoniazid is markedly reduced if taken with food. (See also 'Isoniazid + Cheese or Fish'.)

Clinical evidence

A study in nine normal subjects given 10 mg/kg body weight isoniazid showed that when taken with breakfast, rather than when fasting, the mean peak isoniazid serum concentrations were delayed and reduced to 30%, and the AUC (area under the curve) was reduced to 57%.[1] Similar results were found in another study.[4]

Mechanism

Uncertain. The presence of food delays the gastric emptying so that the absorption further along the gut is also delayed, but the reduced absorption is not understood.

Importance and management

Information is limited but the interaction seems to be established. As single high doses of isoniazid are more effective in arresting tuberculosis than the same amount of drug in divided doses[2-4] it seems probable that this interaction is clinically important. For maximal absorption isoniazid should be taken without food. See also 'Isoniazid + Cheese or Fish'.

References

1 Melander A, Danielson F, Hanson A, Jansson L, Rerup C, Schersten B, Thulin T, Wahlin E. Reduction of isoniazid bioavailability in normal men by concomitant intake of food. Acta Med Scand (1976) 200, 93–7.
2 Fox W. General considerations in intermittent drug therapy of pulmonary tuberculosis. Postgrad med J (1971) 47, 727.
3 Hudson LD, Sharbara JA. Twice weekly tuberculosis chemotherapy. J Amer Med Ass (1973) 223, 139.
4 Mannisto P, Mantyla R, Klinge R. Influence of various diets on the bioavailability of isoniazid. J Antimicrob Chemother (1982) 10, 427–34.

Isoniazid + Levodopa

Abstract/Summary

An isolated case report describes hypertension, tachycardia, flushing and tremor in a patient attributed to the concurrent use of isoniazid and levodopa.

Clinical evidence, mechanism, importance and management

A patient being treated with levodopa developed hypertension, agitation, tachycardia, flushing and severe non-parkinsonian tremor after starting to take isoniazid. He recovered when the isoniazid was stopped.[1] The reasons are not understood. The author suggested that it might be related in some way to the MAOI–levodopa interaction, but the MAO-inhibitory properties of isoniazid are small. Some of the symptoms seen were not dissimilar to those experienced by patients on isoniazid who ate cheese or fish (see 'Isoniazid + Cheese or Fish'). Concurrent use should be monitored.

Reference

1 Morgan JP. Isoniazid and levodopa. Ann Intern Med (1980) 92, 434.

Isoniazid + Pethidine (Meperidine)

Abstract/Summary

An isolated case report describes hypotension and lethargy in a patient following the concurrent use of isoniazid and pethidine (meperidine).

Clinical evidence, mechanism, importance and management

A patient became lethargic and his blood pressure fell from 124/68 to 84/50 mm Hg within 20 min of being given 75 mg pethidine (meperidine) intramuscularly. An hour before he had been given 30 mg isoniazid. There was no evidence of fever or heart arrhythmias, and his serum electrolytes, glucose levels and blood gases were normal. His blood pressure returned to normal over the next 3 h. He had previously had both pethidine and isoniazid separately without incident. He was subsequently treated with morphine sulphate, 4 mg every 2–4 h intravenously, uneventfully.[1] The authors of the report attribute this reaction to the MAO-inhibitory properties of the isoniazid and equate it with the severe and potentially fatal MAOI-pethidine interaction, but in fact this reaction was mild and lacked many of the characteristics of the more serious reaction. Moreover isoniazid possesses little MAO-inhibitory properties and does not normally interact like the potent antidepressant and anti-hypertensive MAOI. There is too little evidence to forbid concurrent use, but clearly it should be undertaken with caution.

Reference

1 Gannon R, Pearsall W, Rowley R. Isoniazid, meperidine and hypotension. Ann Intern Med (1983) 99, 415.

Isoniazid + Propranolol

Abstract/Summary

Propranolol causes a small reduction in the clearance of isoniazid from the body. It seems unlikely to be of much practical importance.

Clinical evidence, mechanism, importance and management

The clearance of single 600 mg intravenous doses of isoniazid was found in six normal subjects to have been reduced by 21% (from 16.4 to 13.0 l/h) after they had been taking 120 mg propranolol daily for three days,[1] a suggested reason being that the propranolol inhibits the metabolism of the isoniazid.[1] However the increase in isoniazid levels is likely to be only modest, and this interaction is probably of little clinical importance.

Reference

1 Santoso B. Impairment of isoniazid clearance by propranolol. Int J Clin Pharmacol Ther Toxicol (1985) 23, 134–6.

Isoniazid + Rifabutin (Ansamycin)

Abstract/Summary

Rifabutin does not alter the pharmacokinetics of isoniazid

Clinical evidence, mechanism, importance and management

300 mg rifabutin daily for seven days had no significant effect on the plasma pharmacokinetics of isoniazid (after a single 300 mg dose) or acetylisoniazid in six normal subjects. Two of the six were rapid acetylators of isoniazid.[1] Although both drugs have been effectively used together in the treatment of tuberculosis,[2] it is not clear is whether concurrent use increases the incidence of hepatotoxicity, as occurs with isoniazid and rifampicin. Combined use should therefore be well monitored.

References

1 Breda M, Painezzola E, Benedetti MS, Efthymiopoulos C, Carpentieri M, Sassella D, Rimoldi R. A study of the effects of rifabutin on isoniazid pharmacokinetics and metabolism in healthy volunteers. Drug Metab Drug Interact (1993) 10, 323–40.
2 McGregor MM, Van den Merve MP. The use of rifabutin for pulmonary TB in Southern Africa. Am Rev Resp Dis (1990) 141, A432.

Isoniazid + Rifampicin (Rifampin)

Abstract/Summary

Although concurrent use is common and therapeutically valuable, there is evidence that the incidence of isoniazid hepatotoxicity, particularly in slow acetylators, may be increased.

Clinical evidence, mechanism, importance and management

Both drugs used together have a valuable part to play in short-course chemotherapy of tuberculosis. Studies in man have shown that the serum levels and half-lives of both drugs are unaffected,[1,7] however there is now some evidence that the incidence of heptatotoxicity rises if both drugs are used concurrently.[5] Reports from India suggest that the incidence can be as high as 8–10% while much lower figures, 2–3%, are reported in the West.[2] The reasons for the hepatotoxicity are not fully understood but rifampicin alone can cause liver damage by its own toxic action. One suggestion is that the rifampicin increases the metabolism of isoniazid, resulting in the formation of hydrazine which is a proven hepatotoxic agent.[2,4] Higher plasma levels of hydrazine are said to occur in slow acetylators of isoniazid,[2] but one study failed to confirm that this is so.[6]

Concurrent use need not be avoided, but it would be prudent to be on the watch for signs of liver damage if both drugs are given, and especially in patients also exposed to other potent enzyme inducers such as phenytoin and the barbiturates.[3]

References

1 Boman G. Serum concentration and half-life of rifampicin (rifampin) after simultaneous oral administration of aminosalicylic acid or isoniazid. Europ J clin Pharmacol (1974) 7, 217.
2 Gangadharam PJ. Isoniazid, rifampin and hepatotoxicity. Am Rev Respir Dis (1986) 133, 963–5. (Review).
3 Lenders JWM, Bartelink AKM, van Herwaarden CLA, van Haelst UJGM, van Tongeren JHM. Dodelijke levercelnecrose na kort durende toediening van isoniazide en rifampcin (rifampin)e aan een patient die reeds werd behandeld met anti-epileptika. Ned Tijd Geneeskund (1983) 127, 420–3.
4 Pessayre D, Bentata M, Degott C, Nonel O, Miguet J-P, Rueff B, Nehamour J-P. Isoniazid-rifampicin (rifampin) fulminant hepatitis. A possible consequence of the enhancement of isoniazid hepatotoxicity by enzyme induction. Gastroenterology (1977) 72, 284.
5 Steele MA, Burk RF, DesPrez RM. Toxic hepatitis with isoniazid and rifampin. A meta-analysis. Chest (1991) 99, 465–71.
6 Jenner PJ, Ellard GA. Isoniazid-related hepatotoxicity: a study of the effect of rifampicin administration on the metabolism of acetylisoniazid in man. Tubercle (1989) 70, 93–101.
7 Sarma GR, Kailasam S, Nair NGK, Narayana SL, Tripathy SP. Effect of prednisolone and rifampin on isoniazid metabolism in slow and rapid inactivators of isoniazid. Antimicrob Ag Chemother (1980) 18, 661–6.

Isoniazid + Sodium valproate

An isolated report describes liver toxicity attributed to the concurrent use of isoniazid and sodium valproate.

Abstract/Summary, clinical evidence, mechanism, importance and management

A girl of 13 with epilepsy and tuberculosis was treated with 300 mg isoniazid and 750 mg primidone daily. Within two days of adding 600 mg sodium valproate daily she developed stomach ache, loss of appetite, vomiting and drowsiness. Her liver enzymes (SGOT, SGPT, GGT) were found to have risen and her fibrinogen levels fell. The sodium valproate was stopped and recovery from these adverse effects occurred while taking only phenobarbitone. She had previously had both isoniazid alone and sodium valproate alone without problems.[1] Just why concurrent use should cause liver toxicity of this kind is not understood. The general importance of this reaction is uncertain but be alert for any evidence of an adverse response in any patient given both drugs.

Reference

1 Dockweiler U. Isoniazid-induced valproic acid toxicity, or vice versa. Lancet (1987) 2, 152.

Itraconazole + Anticonvulsants

Abstract/Summary

Phenytoin and carbamazepine can reduce serum itraconazole levels, thereby reducing or abolishing its antifungal effects.

Clinical evidence, mechanism, importance and management

Two patients on phenytoin and two on phenytoin and carbamazepine failed to respond to treatment with 400 mg itraconazole daily for aspergillosis, coccidioidomycosis or cryptococcosis, or suffered a relapse. All of them had undetectable or substantially reduced serum itraconazole levels compared with other patients on itraconazole alone.[1] The probable reason is that these anticonvulsants increase the metabolism and clearance of the antifungal, thereby reducing its effects. Although direct evidence of this interaction is very limited indeed, it appears to be clinically important. Be alert for the need to increase the itraconazole dosage in the presence of either of these anticonvulsants.

Reference

1 Tucker RM, Denning DW, Hanson LH, Rinaldi MG, Graybill JR, Sharkey PK, Pappagianis D, Stevens DA. Interaction of azoles with rifampin, phenytoin and carbamazepine: *in vitro* and clinical observations. Clin Infect Dis (1992) 14, 165–74.

Itraconazole + Anti-tubercular drugs

Abstract/Summary

Rifampicin markedly reduces serum itraconazole serum levels. This can reduce or abolish the antifungal effects of the itraconazole, depending on the infection being treated.

Clinical evidence

A patient on 600 mg rifampicin and 300 mg isoniazid daily was additionally started on 200 mg itraconazole daily. After two weeks his serum itraconazole levels were negligible (0.011 mg/l). Even when the dosage was doubled the levels only reached a maximum of 0.056 mg/l. Later when the antitubercular drugs had been stopped and while taking 300 mg itraconazole daily, his serum itraconazole level was 3.23 mg/l. On 200 mg daily it was 2.35–2.60 mg/l.[1]

A later study in eight other patients given both drugs confirmed that the itraconazole levels were reduced but the clinical outcome depended on the mycosis being treated. Four out of five responded to treatment for *Cryptococcus neoformans* infection, despite undetectable itraconazole levels, apparently because there is synergy between the two drugs. In contrast, two patients with coccidioidomycosis failed to respond, and two others with cryptococcosis suffered a relapse or persistence of seborrheic dermatitis (possibly due to *M. furfur*) while taking both drugs.[2] Reduced serum itraconazole levels have also been seen in normal subjects.[3]

Mechanism

The suggested reason is that the rifampicin increased the metabolism of the itraconazole, and hastened its loss from the body. This is consistent with the way rifampicin interacts with many other drugs.

Importance and management

An established and clinically important interaction. Monitor the effects of concurrent use, being alert for the need to increase the itraconazole dosage. The clinical importance of this interaction apparently depends on the mycosis being treated.

References

1 Blomely M, Teare EL, De Belder A, Thway Y, Weston M. Itraconazole and anti-tuberculosis drugs. Lancet (1990) 2, 1255.
2 Tucker RM, Denning DW, Hanson LH, Rinaldi MG, Graybill JR, Sharkey PK, Pappagianis D, Stevens DA. Interaction of azoles with rifampin, phenytoin and carbamazepine: *in vitro* and clinical observations. Clin Infect Dis (1992) 14, 165–74.
3 Meunier F. Serum fungistatic and fungicidal activity in volunteers receiving antifungal agents. Eur J Clin Microbiol (1986) 5, 103–9.

Itraconazole + Didanosine

Abstract/Summary

A single case report describes reduced itraconazole effects and reduced serum levels (apparently due to reduced absorption) in a patient when given didanosine.

Clinical evidence

A patient previously successfully treated for cryptococcal meningitis and on maintenance treatment with itraconazole, relapsed when his HIV treatment was changed from zidovudine to didanosine. An interaction between the didanosine and itraconazole was suspected so that over the next two days he was given the itraconazole, firstly with the didanosine, and then without it. With the didanosine his itraconazole serum levels were undetectable at 2 h and reached a peak of 1.4 µg/ml after 8 hr. Without the didanosine the 2 h level was 1.6 µg/ml.[1]

Mechanism

Didanosine is extremely acid labile at pH values below 3 so that it has to be formulated with buffering agents (dihydroxyaluminium sodium carbonate, sodium citrate and magnesium hydroxide) to keep the pH as high as possible to minimize the acid-induced hydrolysis. Itraconazole on the other hand depends for its absorption on stomach acidity. The raised pH due to the buffers would therefore appear to have reduced the itraconazole absorption in this patient. It seems probable that the didanosine itself had no part to play in this interaction.

Importance and management

Information seems to be limited to this single report. Its general importance is uncertain, but it would now be prudent to monitor the effects of concurrent use for any evidence of an inadequate response to the itraconazole. If the suggested mechanism of interaction is true, then giving the itraconazole at least 2 h before the didanosine should go a long way towards solving the problem.

Reference

1 Moreno F, Hardin TC, Rinaldi MG, Graybill JR. Itraconazole-didanosine excipient interaction. J Amer Med Ass (1993) 269, 1508.

Ketoconazole + Didanosine

Abstract/Summary

Ketoconazole causes a small reduction in the bioavailability of didanosine, but provided ketoconazole is given at least two hours before didanosine, no clinically relevant interaction appears to occur between these two drugs.

Clinical evidence, mechanism, importance and management

12 HIV-positive patients were given 375 mg didanosine twice daily either alone or 2 h after 200 mg ketoconazole, four times daily, for four days. The steady-state serum didanosine levels were reduced by 12% and the AUC by 8%, but no changes in the pharmacokinetics of the ketoconazole were seen.[1] The minor fall in didanosine levels is probably too small to matter. It appears that a two-hour separation is enought to prevent the citrate-phosphate buffer (with which the didanosine is formulated) from affecting the gastric pH which could possibly alter the bioavailability of the ketoconazole. Provided the ketoconazole is given at least 2 h before the didanosine, there would seem to be no reason for avoiding concurrent use.

Reference

1 Knupp CA, Brater DC, Relue J, Dunkle LM, Barbhaiya RH. A pharmacokinetic interaction study between didanosine and ketoconazole in HIV patients. Clin Pharmacol Ther (1992) 51, 155.

Ketoconazole or Itraconazole + Food

Abstract/Summary

Itraconazole should be taken with or after food to achieve the best results from treatment. The manufacturers also advise taking ketoconazole with food, but the background evidence supporting this is confusing and contradictory.

Clinical evidence

(a) Itraconazole

A study in 24 patients with superficial dermatophyte, *Candida albicans* and pityriasis versicolor infections given 50 or 100 mg doses of itraconazole daily showed that taking the drug with or after breakfast produced higher serum levels and gave much better treatment results than taking it before.[4]

(b) Ketoconazole

One study found that the AUC and peak serum concentrations of a single 200 mg dose of ketoconazole was reduced by about 40% (from 14.4 to 8.6 µg/h/ml and from 4.1 to 2.3 µg/ml respectively) when taken by 10 normal subjects after a standardized meal.[2] Another study found that high carbohydrate and fat diets tended to reduce the rate and extent of ketoconazole absorption of ketoconazole.[3] This contrasts with another investigation which found that the absorption of single 200 or 800 mg doses of ketoconazole in eight normal subjects was not altered when taken after a standardized breakfast although the peak serum levels were delayed. The absorption of single 400 and 600 mg doses were somewhat increased.[1]

Importance and management

Information about itraconazole is limited but on the basis of the study cited it should be taken with food to get the best results. A confusing and conflicting picture is presented by the studies with ketoconazole, however the manufacturers say that 'absorption of ketoconazole is maximal when taken during a meal, as it depends on stomach acidity' and 'should always be taken with meals'. Two (680 mg) or more glutamic acid hydrochloride capsules can be used to enhance the absorption of ketoconazole in patients with reduced gastric acidity.[3]

References

1 Daneshmend TK, Warnock DW, Ene MD, Johnson EM, Potten MR, Richardson MD, Williamson PJ. Influence of food on the pharmacokinetics of ketoconazole. Antimicrob Ag Chemother (1984) 25, 1–3.
2 Mannisto PT, Mantyla R, Nykanen S, Lamminsivu U, Ottoila P. Impairing effect of food on ketoconazole absorption. Antimicrob Ag Chemother (1982) 21, 730–33.
3 Lelawongs P, Barone JA, Colaizzi JL, Hsuan AT, Mechlinski W, Legendre R, Guarnieri J. Effect of food and gastric acidity on absorption of orally administered ketoconazole. Clin Pharmacy (1988) 7, 228–35.
4 Wishart JM. The influence of food on the pharmacokinetics of itraconazole in patients with superficial fungal infection. J Am Acad Dermatol (1987) 17, 220–3.

Ketoconazole + Phenytoin

Abstract/Summary

Three patients have been described who showed reduced serum ketoconazole levels and reduced antifungal effects while taking phenytoin. Ketoconazole appears not to affect serum phenytoin levels.

Clinical evidence

A man being treated for coccidioidal meningitis with ketoconazole relapsed when he was given 300 mg phenytoin daily. A pharmacokinetic study showed that his peak serum ketoconazole levels and AUC were reduced compared with the values seen before the phenytoin was started (even though the dosage was increased from 400 to 600 mg, and later 1200 mg), and compared with other patients taking half the dose of ketoconazole (400 or 600 mg).[1] Coccidioidomycosis in another patient progressed despite the use of ketoconazole while taking phenytoin.[4] Low serum ketoconazole levels were seen in another patient treated with phenytoin and phenobarbitone.[2] It appears that ketoconazole does not affect the serum levels of phenytoin.[3]

Mechanism

Not established, but a likely explanation is that the phenytoin, a known potent enzyme-inducing agent, increases the metabolism and clearance of the ketoconazole from the body.

Importance and management

Information appears to be limited to these reports but be alert for any signs of a reduced antifungal response in any patient. It may be necessary to increase the dosage of the ketoconazole. It is not yet clear whether the phenobarbitone taken by one patient also interacted with the ketoconazole.[2]

References

1 Brass C, Galgiani JN, Blaschke TF, Deflice R, O'Reilly RA, Stevens DA. Disposition of ketoconazole, an oral antifungal, in humans. Antimicrob Ag Chemother (1982) 21, 151–8.
2 Stockley RJ, Daneshmend TK, Bredow MT, Warnock DW, Richardson MD, Slade RR. Ketoconazole pharmacokinetics during chronic dosing in adults with haematological malignancy. Eur J Clin Microbiol (1986) 5, 513–7.
3 Touchette MA, Chandrasekar PH, Millad MA, Edwards DJ. Differential effects of ketoconazole and fluconazole on phenytoin and testosterone concentrations in man. Pharmacotherapy (1991) 11, 275.
4 Tucker RM, Denning DW, Hanson LH, Rinaldi MG, Graybill JR, Sharkey PK, Pappagianis D, Stevens DA. Interaction of azoles with rifampin, phenytoin and carbamazepine: *in vitro* and clinical observations. Clin Infect Dis (1992) 14, 165–74.

Ketoconazole + Rifampicin (Rifampin) and Isoniazid

Abstract/Summary

The serum levels of ketoconazole can be markedly reduced (50–90%) by the concurrent use of rifampicin and/or isoniazid. Serum rifampicin levels can be halved by the concurrent use of ketoconazole, but are possibly unaffected if the drugs are given 12 h apart.

Clinical evidence

(a) Effect on serum ketoconazole levels

The serum ketoconazole levels of a patient taking 200 mg daily were approximately halved (area under the curve reduced from 17.33 to 9.19 µg/h/ml) when concurrently treated with 600 mg rifampicin. After five months of concurrent use with rifampicin and 300 mg isoniazid daily, there was a tenfold decrease in peak serum levels (AUC reduced from 17.33 to 2.02 µg/h/ml)[1]. A study in a 3-year-old child who had responded poorly to treatment showed that peak serum ketoconazole levels were reduced 65–80% by the concurrent use of rifampicin and/or isoniazid, and the AUCs were similarly reduced. The interaction also occurred when the dosages were separated by 12 h. When all three drugs were given together the ketoconazole serum levels were undetectable.[3] Other reports confirm this interaction can occur.[2,4–10] One of them found an 80% reduction in the AUC of ketoconazole but no reduction in rifampicin levels.[6]

(b) Effect on serum rifampicin levels

A study in the child cited above showed that rifampicin serum levels were approximately halved by the concurrent use of ketoconazole, but when given 12 h after the ketoconazole, the serum levels remained unaffected.[3]

Mechanisms

It seems probable that rifampicin reduces the serum levels of ketoconazole by increasing its rate of metabolism within the liver, thereby hastening its clearance from the body. Just how isoniazid interacts is uncertain. It is suggested that ketoconazole impairs the absorption of rifampicin from the gut.

Importance and management

The ketoconazole-rifampicin interactions appear to be established and of clinical importance, but there is less information about the ketoconazole-isoniazid interaction. The effects on rifampicin can apparently be avoided by giving the ketoconazole at a different time (12 h apart is known to be effective) but this does not solve the problem of the effects on ketoconazole. The dosage of at least one of the drugs will need to be increased to achieve both good antitubercular and antifungal responses. Concurrent use should be well monitored and dosage increases made if necessary.

References

1 Brass C, Galgiani JN, Blaschke TF, Defelice R, O'Reilly RA, Stevens DA. Disposition of ketoconazole, an oral antifungal, in humans. Antimicrob Ag Chemother (1982) 21, 151–8.

2 Drouhet E, Dupont B. Laboratory and clinical assessment of ketoconazole in deep seated mycoses. Am J Med (1983) 74, (1B) 30- 47.

3 Engelhard D, Stutman MR, Marks MI. Interaction of ketoconazole with rifampin and isoniazid. N Engl J Med (1984) 311, 1681–3.

4 Meunier-Carpentier F, Heymans C, Snoeck R. Interaction of rifampin and ketoconazole and Bayer n7133 (Bay) in normal volunteers. Presented at the 23rd Interscience Conference on Antimicrobial Agents and Chemotherapy, Las Vegas, October 24–6, 1983.

5 Doble H, Hykin P, Shaw R, Keal EE. Pulmonary mycobacterium tuberculosis in acquired immune deficiency syndrome. Br Med J (1985) 291, 849–50.

6 Doble H, Shaw R, Rowland-Hill C, Lush M, Warnock DW, Keal EE. Pharmacokinetic study of the interaction between rifampin and ketoconazole. J Antimicrob Chemother (1988) 21, 633–5.

7 Abadie-Kemmerly S, Pankey GA, Dalvisio JR. Failure of ketoconazole treatment of Blastomyces dermatidis due to interaction of isoniazid and rifampin. Ann Intern Med (1988) 109, 844–5.

8 Pilheu JA et al. Interaction of ketoconazole with isoniazid and rifampicin. Eur Resp J (1988) 1 (Suppl 2) 274s.

9 Tucker RM, Denning DW, Hanson LH, Rinaldi MG, Graybill JR, Sharkey PK, Pappagianis D, Stevens DA. Interaction of azoles with rifampin, phenytoin and carbamazepine: in vitro and clinical observations. Clin Infect Dis (1992) 14, 165–74.

10 Pilheu JA, Glati MR, Yunis AS, De Salvo M, Negroni R, Fernandez JGC, Mingolla L, Rubio MC, Masana M, Acevedo C. Interaccion farmacocinetica entre ketoconazol, isoniacida y rifampicina. Medicina (Buenos Aires) (1989) 49, 43–7.

Lincomycin or Clindamycin + Food or Drinks

Abstract/Summary

The serum levels of lincomycin are markedly depressed (by up to two-thirds) if taken in the presence of food, but clindamycin is not significantly affected. Cyclamate sweeteners can also reduce the absorption of lincomycin.

Clinical evidence

The mean peak serum levels of lincomycin achieved after single 500 mg oral doses in 10 normal subjects were approximately 3 μg/ml when taken 4 h before breakfast, 2 μg/ml when taken 1 h before breakfast, and less than 1 μg/ml when taken after breakfast. The mean total amounts of lincomycin recovered from the urine were respectively 40.4, 23.8 and 8.9 mg. There were considerable individual variations.[1]

Depressed serum lincomycin levels due to the presence of food have been described in other reports,[2,3] but the absorption of clindamycin is not affected.[3,4] Sodium cyclamate used as an artificial sweetener in diet foods, drinks and some pharmaceuticals can also markedly reduce the absorption of lincomycin (reduction in AUC of 75% using 1 Molar equivalent with 500 mg lincomycin).[5]

Mechanism

Not understood.

Importance and management

The interaction with lincomycin is well established and of clinical importance. Lincomycin should not be taken with food or within several hours of eating a meal if adequate serum levels are to be achieved. An alternative is clindamycin, a synthetic derivative of lincomycin, which has the same antibacterial spectrum but the absorption of which is not affected by the presence of food. The interaction with sodium cyclamate is an unlikely occurrence because cyclamates have been banned in the UK (and many other countries as well) as a sweetener in foods and drinks, but it is still sometimes found in pharmaceuticals.

References

1 McCall CE, Steigbigel NH, Finland M. Lincomycin: activity in vitro and absorption and excretion in normal young men. Amer J Med Sci (1967) 254, 144.

2 Kaplan K, Chew WH, Weinstein L. Microbiological, pharmacological and clinical studies of lincomycin. Amer J Med Sci (1965) 251, 137.

3 McGehee RF, Smith CB, Wilcox C, Finland M. Comparative studies of antibacterial activity in vitro and absorption and excretion of lincomycin and clinimycin. Amer J Med Sci (1968) 256, 279.

4 Wagner JG, Novak E, Patel NC, Chidester CG, Lummis WL. Absorption, excretion and half-life of clinimycin in normal adult males. Amer J Med Sci (1968) 256, 25.

5 Wagner JC. Aspects of pharmacokinetics and biopharmaceutics in relation to drug activity. Amer J Pharm (1969) 141, 5.

Lincomycin or Clindamycin + Kaolin

Abstract/Summary

Kaolin-containing anti-diarrhoeal preparations can markedly reduce the absorption of lincomycin by the gut. This can be avoided by giving the linocomycin 2 h after the kaolin. Lincomycin-induced diarrhoea is a potential hazard. The rate but not the extent of clindamycin absorption is altered by kaolin-pectin.

Clinical evidence

3 fl oz of Kaopectate (kaolin–pectin) reduced the absorption of 0.5 g lincomycin by about 90% in eight normal subjects. Giving the Kaopectate 2 h before the antibiotic had little or no effect on its absorption, whereas when given 2 h after, the absorption was reduced about 50%.[1]

This interaction is described in another report.[3] The absorption rate of clindamycin is markedly prolonged by kaolin, but the extent of its absorption remains unaffected.[4]

Mechanism

It seems probable that the lincomycin becomes adsorbed onto the kaolin, thereby reducing its bioavailability. The kaolin also coats the lining of the gut and acts as a physical barrier to absorption.[1,2]

Importance and management

Information seems to be limited to this study, but the lincomycin–kaolin interaction appears to be an established and of clinical importance. For good absorption and a good antibiotic response separate their administration as much as possible, ideally giving the kaolin 2 h before the antibiotic. Remember that lincomycin itself can cause diarrhoea in a fairly large proportion of patients which, in some cases, has lead to the development of fatal pseudomembraneous colitis. Marked diarrhoea, according to the makers, is an indication that the lincomycin should be stopped immediately. Clindamycin appears to be a suitable alternative to lincomycin.

References

1 Wagner JG. Design and data analysis of biopharmaceutical studies in man. Can J Pharm Sci (1966) 1, 55.
2 Rowe EL. Quoted in 1 above.
3 Wagner JG. Pharmcokinetics. I. Definitions, modelling and reasons for measuring blood levels and urinary excretion. Drug Intell (1968) 2, 38.
4 Albert KS, De Sante KA, Welch RD, Di Santo AR. Pharmacokinetic evaluation of a drug interaction between kaolin-pectin and clindamycin. J Pharm Sci (1978) 67, 1579.

Macrolide antibiotics + Antacids, Ranitidine

Abstract/Summary, clinical evidence, mechanism, importance and management

Maalox (aluminium and magnesium hydroxides) and ranitidine are reported not to affect the pharmacokinetics of clarithromycin or roxithromycin.[1,2,3] There would seem to be no reason for avoiding concurrent use.

Reference

1 Nilsen OG. Roxithromycin. A new molecule, a new pharmacokinetic profile. Drug Invest (1991) 3, Suppl 3, 28–32.
2 Zündorf H, Wischmann L, Fassenbender M, Lode H, Borner K, Koeppe P. Pharmacokinetics of clarithromycin and possible interaction with H_2-blockers and antacids. 31st Intersci Conf Antimicrob Ag Chemother (1991) Abstracts, 185.
3 Boeckh M, Lode H, Hoffken G, Daeschlein S, Koeppe P. Pharmacokinetics of roxithromycin and influence of H_2-blockers and antacids on gastrointestinal absorption. Eur J clin Microbiol Infect Dis (1992) 11, 465–8.

Mebendazole + Miscellaneous drugs

Abstract/Summary

Cimetidine raises serum mebendazole levels and increases its effectiveness. Phenytoin and carbamazepine, but not sodium valproate, lower serum mebendazole levels.

Clinical evidence, mechanism, importance and management

(a) Mebendazole + Anticonvulsants

The same study cited above found that both phenytoin and carbamazepine (but not sodium valproate) lowered serum mebendazole levels, presumably due to their well-recognized enzyme inducing effects which increase the metabolism and loss of mebendazole from the body.[1] It may be necessary to increase the mebendazole dosage in the presence of these two anticonvulsants. Monitor the outcome of concurrent use. This interaction is only likely to be important when treating organisms within the tissues which are affected by drug serum levels, rather than when treating infections in the gut.

(b) Mebendazole + Cimetidine

A study in eight patients (five with peptic ulcers and three with hydatid cysts) taking 1.5 mg mebendazole daily found that cimetidine (400 mg three times daily for 30 days) raised the maximum serum mebendazole levels by 48%, due, it is believed, to the enzyme inhibitory effects of the cimetidine.[1] The previously unresponsive hepatic hydatid cysts resolved totally. This is a therapeutically valuable interaction, but be alert for any evidence of mebendazole toxicity (allergic reactions, leucopenia, alopecia). A previous study had suggested that the rises in serum mebendazole levels were too small be useful.[2]

References

1 Bekhti A, Pirotte J. Cimetidine increases serum mebendazole concentrations. Implications for treatment of hepatic hydatic cysts. Br J clin Pharmac (1987) 24, 390–2.
2 Luder PJ, Siffert B, Witassek F, Meister F, Bircher J. Treatment of hydatid disease with high oral doses of mebendazole. Long-term follow up of plasma mebendazole levels and drug interactions. Eur J clin Pharmac (1986) 31, 443–8.

Mefloquine + Antimalarials

Abstract/Summary

Pamaquine can increase both the serum levels of mefloquine and its side-effects. Mefloquine serum levels may possibly be increased by quinine but not by primaquine.

Clinical evidence, mechanism, importance and management

(a) Pamaquine

A randomized crossover study in 14 subjects given 1 g mefloquine found that the addition of 15 mg or 30 mg pamaquine raised the peak serum levels of mefloquine respectively by 48% (from 1.64 to 2.42 µg/ml) and 28% (from 2.52 to 3.24 µg/ml).

Those taking the larger dose of pamaquine showed a transient increase in peak pamaquine serum levels, and its conversion to its inactive carboxyl metabolite also increased. Significant CNS symptoms were also experienced by those taking the larger dose of pamaquine.[1] The clinical significance of this interaction is uncertain, but combined used can apparently increase the mefloquine side-effects.

(b) Primaquine

No pharmacokinetic interaction was seen in eight subjects given single oral doses of 750 mg mefloquine and 45 mg primaquine, and no increased side-effects attributable to concurrent use.[3] No special precautions seem to be needed.

(b) Quinine

In vitro data and unpublished clinical observations[2] suggest that quinine may inhibit the metabolism of mefloquine, thereby raising its serum levels. The clinical importance of this awaits further study.

References

1 Macleod CM, Trenholme GM, Nora MV, Bartley EA, Frischer H. Interaction of primaquine with mefloquine in healthy males. 30th Ann Intersc Conf Antimicrob Ag Chemother, Atlanta, GA, October 23rd, 1990, 213.
2 Bangchang KN, Karbwang J, Back DJ. Mefloquine metabolism by human liver microsomes. Effect of other antimalarial drugs. Biochem Pharmacol (1992) 43, 1957–61.
3 Karbwang J, Bangchang KN, Thanavibul A, Back DJ, Bunnag D. Pharmacokinetics of mefloquine in the presence of primaquine. Eur J Clin Pharmacol (1992) 42, 559–60.

Mefloquine + Metoclopramide

Abstract/Summary

Although metoclopramide increases the rate of absorption of mefloquine and increases its peak blood levels, its side-effects are reduced.

Clinical evidence, mechanism, importance and management

When 10 mg metoclopramide was taken 15 min before a single 750 mg dose of mefloquine, the absorption half-life in seven normal subjects was reduced from 3.2 to 2.4 h and the peak blood levels were raised from 1196 to 1570 ng/ml, but the total amount absorbed was unchanged. Despite these changes, the toxicity of mefloquine (dizziness, nausea, vomiting, abdominal pain) were reduced.[1] There would therefore seem to be some advantage in taking these drugs concurrently.

Reference

1 Na Bangchang K, Karbwang J, Bunnag D, Harinasuta T. The effect of metoclopramide on mefloquine pharmacokinetics. Br J clin Pharmac (1991) 32, 640–1.

Mefloquine + Tetracycline

Abstract/Summary

Mefloquine serum levels are increased by tetracycline.

Clinical evidence, mechanism, importance and management

The maximum serum levels of mefloquine following a single 750 mg dose were increased by 27.5% (from 1160 to 1600 ng/ml) in 20 normal Thai men after taking 250 mg tetracycline four times daily for a week. The AUC (0–7 days) was increased 30% and the terminal half-life reduced from from 19.3 to 14.4 days, without evidence of an increase in side-effects. The suggested reason for the increased mefloquine levels is that its enterohepatic recycling is reduced.[1] The authors of the report conclude that concurrent use may be valuable for treating multi-drug resistant falciparum malaria because higher mefloquine levels are associated with a more effective response.[2] There would seem to be advantages in combined use.

References

1 Karbwang J, Bangchang KN, Back DJ, Bunnag D, Rooney W. Effect of tetracycline on mefloquine pharmacokinetics in Thai males. Eur J Clin Pharmacol (1992) 43, 567–9.
2 Karbwang J. Unpublished observations quoted in ref 1.

Mesalazine + Ispaghula, Lactitol or Lactulose

Abstract/Summary

On theoretical grounds, delayed-release formulations designed to release mesalazine in the colon when the pH rises should not be given with lactulose, lactitol or other preparations which lower the pH in the colon. However ispaghula which lowers colonic pH appears not to affect the bioavailability of mesalazine.

Clinical evidence, mechanism, importance and management

Asacol is a preparation of mesalazine (mesalamine, 5-aminosalicylic acid, 5-ASA) coated with an acrylic based resin (*Eudragit S*) which disintegrates above pH 7 and releases the mesalazine into the terminal ileum and colon.[1] Since the disintegration depends upon this pH rise, the makers of *Asacol* say that the concurrent use of preparations which lower the pH in the lower part of the gut should be avoided.

Those preparations which affect colonic pH include lactulose and lactitol which are metabolized by the gut bacteria to a number of acids (acetic, butyric, propionic, lactic). In normal subjects lactulose (30–80 g/24 h) can cause falls in the pH of the right colon from 6.0 to 4.85,[1] 6.51 to 5.63[2] and from 6.36 to 5.1;[3] and in the left colon from 7.0 to 6.7.[1,2,3] Lactitol (40–180 g/24 h) can cause falls in the pH of the right colon from 6.36–5.78[2] and from 6.51 to 5.18.[3] Ispaghula supplements can similarly lower colonic pH (from 6.5 to 5.8 in the right colon, and from 7.3 to 6.6 in the left colon).[4] However a study in patients given mesalazine found that despite this colonic acidification by ispaghula husk (*Fybogel*), the release of mesalazine appeared not to be affected.[5]

Thus although on theoretical grounds isphagula husk would be expected to reduce the effects of mesalazine, no interaction of clinical importance seems to occur, and none has yet been shown to occur with either lactulose or lactitol. More study is needed to find out what actually happens in practice.

References

1 Bown R L, Gibson J A, Sladen G E, Hicks B, Dawson A M. Effects of lactulose and other laxatives on ileal and colonic pH as measured by a radiotelemetry device. Gut (1974) 15, 999–1004.
2 Patil D H, Westaby D, Mahida Y R, Palmter K R, Rees R, Clark M L, Dawson A M, Silk D B A. Comparative modes of action of lactitol and lactulose in the treatment of hepatic encephalopathy. Gut (1987) 28, 255–9.
3 Patil D H, Westaby D, Mahida Y R, Palmter K R, Rees R, Clark M L, Dawson A M, Silk D B A. Comparison of lactulose and lactitol on ileal and colonic pH. Gut (1985) 26/120 A1125.
4 Evans DF, Crompton J, Pye J, Hardcastel JD. The role of dietary fibre on acidification of the colon in man. Gastroenterology (1988) 94, A118.
5 Riley SA, Tavares IA, Bishai PM, Bennett A, Mani V. Mesalazine release from coated tablets: effect of dietary fibre. Br J clin Pharmac (1991) 32, 248–50.

Metronidazole + Antacid, Kaolin-pectin and Cholestyramine

Abstract/Summary

The absorption of metronidazole from the gut is unaffected by kaolin-pectin, but a small reduction occurs if an aluminium hydroxide antacid or cholestyramine given concurrently.

Clinical evidence, mechanism, importance and management

The bioavailability of single 1 g doses of metronidazole in five normal subjects was not significantly changed by 30 ml of a kaolin-pectin antidiarrhoeal mixture, but a 14.5% reduction occurred with 30 ml of an aluminium hydroxide and simethicone suspension, and a 21.3% reduction with 4 g cholestyramine.[1] The clinical importance of these reductions is uncertain, but probably small, however clinical studies are needed to confirm this. Separating the dosages as much as possible is an effective way of preventing the admixture of drugs within the gut. More study is needed to find out whether repeated doses have a clinically relevant effect.

Reference

1 Molokhia AM, Al-Rahman S. Effect of concomitant oral administration of some adsorbing drugs on the bioavailability of metronidazole. Drug Dev Ind Pharm (1987) 13, 1229–37.

Metronidazole + Barbiturates

Abstract/Summary

Phenobarbitone markedly increases the loss of metronidazole from the body so that larger doses are needed. Conventional doses of metronidazole failed to clear up trichomoniasis in a woman, and giadiasis or amoebiasis in children while taking phenobarbitone.

Clinical evidence

A woman with vaginal trichomoniasis was given metronidazole on several occasions over the course of a year, but the infection flared up again as soon as it was stopped. When it was realized that she was also taking 100 mg phenobarbitone daily, the metronidazole dosage was doubled (to 500 mg three times daily for 7 days) and she was cured.[1] A pharmacokinetic study found that the metronidazole was being cleared from her body much more rapidly than usual (half-life 3.5 h compared with the normal 8–9 h).[1]

A retrospective study in children who had failed to respond to metronidazole for giardiasis or amoebiasis found that 80% of them had been on long-term phenobarbitone treatment, and in a prospective study in 36 children the normal recommended dosage had to be increased threefold (to 60 mg/kg) to achieve a cure. The half-life of metronidazole in 15 other children was found to be 3.5 h compared with the normal 8–9 h.[4] 120 mg phenobarbitone daily reduced the metronidazole AUC in six patients with Crohn's disease by about one-third.[2] and in another seven normal subjects 100 mg phenobarbitone for seven days increased the clearance of metronidazole 1.5-fold.[3]

Mechanism

Phenobarbitone is a known and potent liver enzyme-inducing agent which increases the metabolism and loss of metronidazole from the body.

Importance and management

An established and clinically important interaction. Monitor the effects of concurrent use and anticipate the need to increase the metronidazole dosage two- to three-fold if phenobarbitone or any other barbiturate (all are potent enzyme-inducing agents) is given concurrently.

References

1 Mead PB, Gibson M, Schentag JJ, Ziemniak JA. Possible alteration of

metronidazole metabolism by phenobarbital. N Engl J Med (1982) 306, 1490.

2 Eradiri O, Jamali F, Thomson ABR. Interaction of metronidazole with cimetidine and phenobarbital in Crohn's disease. Clin Pharmacol Ther (1987) 41, 235.

3 Loft S, Sonne J, Poulsen HE, Petersen KT, Jorgensen BG, Dossing M. Inhibition and induction of metronidazole and antipyrine metabolism. Eur J Clin Pharmacol (1987) 32, 35–41.

4 Gupte S. Phenobarbital and metabolism of metronidazole. N Engl J Med (1983) 308, 529.

Metronidazole + Chloroquine

Abstract/Summary

An isolated report describes acute dystonia in a patient on metronidazole when given a single dose of chloroquine.

Clinical evidence, mechanism, importance and management

A patient given a 7-day course of metronidazole (400 mg three times daily) and ampicillin, following a laparoscopic investigation, developed acute dystonic reactions (facial grimacing, coarse tremors, etc.) on day 6 within 10 min of being given a single dose of chloroquine (5 ml of the phosphate, equivalent to 200 mg base, plus 25 mg promethazine IM). She had had chloroquine before without problems. The symptoms subsided within 15 min of being given 5 mg diazepam intravenously. Although extrapyramidal reactions to chloroquine appear to be rare the authors of the report suggest that sulphadoxine/pyrimethamine should be used for malarial prophylaxis in patients on metronidazole.[1]

Reference

1 Achumba JI, Ette EI, Thomas WOA, Essien EE. Chloroquine-induced acute dystonic reactions in the presence of metronidazole. Drug Intell Clin Pharm (1988) 22, 308–10.

Metronidazole + Cimetidine

Abstract/Summary

A study found that cimetidine reduces the loss of metronidazole from the body to some extent, but the clinical importance of this is probably small.

Clinical evidence, mechanism, importance and management

The half-life of metronidazole (400 mg IV dose) in six normal subjects was increased from 6.2 to 7.9 h after taking cimetidine daily for 6 days. The total plasma clearance was reduced almost 30%.[1] It is believed that this is due to inhibition by cimetidine of the metabolism of the metronidazole by the liver. However in another study in six patients with Crohn's disease, cimetidine was found not to affect either the AUC or the half-life of metronidazole,[2] and no evidence of an interaction was found in a further study in six normal subjects.[3]

The effect of this interaction, if and when it occurs, is not large and it seems unlikely that clinical effects will be marked. There appear to be no reports of metronidazole toxicity during concurrent use.

References

1 Gugler R, Jensen JC. Interaction between cimetidine and metronidazole. N Engl J Med (1983) 309, 1518–19.

2 Eradiri O, Jamali F, Thomson ABR. Interaction of metronidazole with cimetidine and phenobarbital in Crohn's disease. Clin Pharmacol Ther (1987) 41, 235.

3 Loft S, Dossing M, Sonne J, Dalhof K, Bjerrum K, Poulsen HE. Lack of effect of cimetidine on the pharmacokinetics and metabolism of a single oral dose of metronidazole. Eur J Clin Pharmacol (1988) 35, 65–8.

Metronidazole + Corticosteroids

Abstract/Summary

Prednisone increases the loss of metronidazole from the body. An increase in the dosage of metronidazole may be needed.

Clinical evidence

When given 20 mg prednisone daily for 6 days, the AUC of metronidazole (250 mg twice daily) in six patients with Crohn's disease was reduced by 31% (from 78.6 to 53.8 mg/h).[1]

Mechanism

Prednisone appears to increase the metabolism of metronidazole by enzyme induction, thereby increasing its clearance from the body.[1]

Importance and management

Information appears to be limited to this report, but the interaction would seem to be of moderate clinical importance. Be alert for the need to increase the metronidazole dosage. Information about other corticosteroids is lacking.

Reference

1 Eradiri O, Jamali F, Thomson ABR. Interaction of metronidazole with phenobarbital, cimetidine, prednisone, and sulfasalazine in Crohn's disease. Biopharm Drug Disp (1988) 9, 219–27.

Metronidazole + Disulfiram

Abstract/Summary

Acute psychoses and confusion can result from the concurrent use of metronidazole and disulfiram.

Clinical evidence, mechanism, importance and management

In a double-blind study on 58 hospitalized chronic alcoholics being treated with disulfiram, half of them were given 750 mg metronidazole daily for a month, and then 250 mg daily. Six of the 29 developed acute psychoses or confusion, five had paranoid delusions and three experienced visual and auditory hallucinations. The symptoms increased when the drugs were withdrawn, but disappeared at the end of a fortnight and did not reappear when disulfiram alone was restarted.[1] Similar reactions have been described in two other reports.[2,3]

The reasons for these reactions are not understood but this appears to be an established interaction. The incidence is high. Concurrent use should be avoided or very well monitored.

References

1 Rothstein E, Clancy DD. Toxicity of disulfiram combined with metronidazole. N Engl J Med (1969) 280, 1006.
2 Goodhue WW. Disulfiram-metronidazole (well-identified) toxicity. N Engl J Med (1969) 280, 1482.
3 Scher JM. Psychotic reaction to disulfiram. J Amer Med Ass (1967) 201, 1051.

Metronidazole + Rifampicin (Rifampin)

Abstract/Summary

Rifampicin increases the clearance of metronidazole from the body, but the clinical importance of this is uncertain.

Clinical evidence

10 normal subjects were given 500 or 1000 mg metronidazole IV before and after taking 450 mg rifampicin daily for seven days. The rifampicin reduced the metronidazole AUC (area under the curve) by 33% and increased its clearance by 44%. There was a slight (10%) difference between the clearances of the 500 and the 1000 mg metronidazole doses.[1] The reason for this interaction is almost certainly because the rifampicin (a well-recognized and potent enzyme inducer) increases the metabolism of the metronidazole by the liver, thereby increasing its loss from the body.

The effectiveness of the metronidazole would be expected to be reduced by this interaction, but nobody seems to have checked on whether this is of real clinical importance. In the absence of definite reports, it would now clearly be prudent to monitor the outcome of adding rifampicin to metronidazole. More study is needed.

Reference

1 Djojasaputro M, Mustafo SS, Donatus IA, Santoso B. The effects of doses and pretreatment with rifampicin on the elimination kinetics of metronidazole. Eur J Pharmacol (1990) 183, 1870–1.

Nalidixic acid + Nitrofurantoin

Abstract/Summary

In vitro studies have demonstrated antagonistic antibacterial effects when the two drugs are used together, but whether this also happens in clinical practice is uncertain.

Clinical evidence, mechanism, importance and management

The antibacterial activity of nalidixic acid can be inhibited by sub-inhibitory concentrations of nitrofurantoin. 44 out of 53 strains of *Escherichia coli*, *Salmonella* and *Proteus* showed antagonism.[1] Another study confirmed these findings.[2] Whether this similarly occurs if both antibacterials are given to patients is uncertain, but the advice[1] that concurrent use should be avoided when treating urinary tract infections seems sound.

References

1 Stille W, Ostner KH. Antagonismus Nitrofurantoin-Nalidixinsaure. Klin Wsch (1966) 44, 155.
2 Piguet D. In vitro inhibitive action of nitrofurantoin on the bacteriostatic activity of nalidixic acid. Ann Inst Pasteur (Paris) (1969) 116, 43.

Niclosamide + Alcohol

Abstract/Summary

Alcohol may possibly increase the side-effects of niclosamide.

Clinical evidence, mechanism, importance and management

The makers of niclosamide (Bayer) advise the avoidance of alcohol while taking niclosamide. The reasoning behind this is that while niclosamide is virtually insoluble in water, it is slightly soluble in alcohol which might possibly increase its absorption by the gut resulting an increase in its side-effects. There are no formal reports of this but Bayer has some anecdotal information which is consistent with this suggestion.[1]

Reference

1 Berryman KD (Bayer). Personnal communication (1992).

Nitrofurantoin + Antacids

Abstract/Summary

The antibacterial effectiveness of nitrofurantoin in the treatment of urinary tract infections is possibly reduced by magnesium trisilicate, but aluminium hydroxide is reported not to interact. Whether other antacids interact adversely is uncertain.

Clinical evidence

5 g magnesium trisilicate in 150 ml water reduced the absorption of single 100 g oral doses of nitrofurantoin in six normal subjects by more than 50%. The time during which the concentration of nitrofurantoin in the urine was at, or above, the minimal antibacterial inhibitory concentration of 32 µg/ml was also reduced.[1] The amounts of nitrofurantoin adsorbed by other antacids in *in vitro* tests were as follows: magnesium trisilicate and charcoal 99%, bismuth oxycarbonate and talc 50–53%, kaolin 31%, magnesium oxide 27%, aluminium hydroxide 2.5% and calcium carbonate 0%.[1]

A cross-over study in six subjects confirmed that aluminium hydroxide gel does not affect the absorption of nitrofurantoin from the gut (as measured by its excretion into the urine).[2]

Mechanism

Antacids can, to a greater or lesser extent, adsorb nitrofurantoin onto their surfaces, as a result less is available for absorption by the gut and for excretion into the urine.

Importance and management

Whether in clinical practice the concurrent use of magnesium trisilicate significantly reduces the antibacterial effectiveness of nitrofurantoin awaits confirmation. The response should be well monitored. It may be necessary to increase the dosage of the nitrofurantoin. The results of the *in vitro* studies suggest that the possible effects of the other antacids are smaller, and aluminium hydroxide is reported not to interact.

References

1 Naggar VF, Khalil SA. Effect of magnesium trisilicate on nitrofurantoin absorption. Clin Pharmacol Ther (1979) 25, 857.
2 Jaffe JM, Hamilton BH, Jeffers S. Nitrofurantoin-antacid interaction. Drug Intell Clin Pharm (1976) 10, 419.

Nitrofurantoin + Anticholinergics and Diphenoxylate

Abstract/Summary

Diphenoxylate and anticholinergic drugs such as propantheline can double the absorption of nitrofurantoin in some patients, but the clinical importance of this is uncertain.

Clinical evidence, mechanism, importance and management

30 mg propanethline approximately doubled the absorption of 100 mg nitrofurantoin (as measured by the urinary excretion) in six normal subjects.[1] Two out of six men in another study similarly showed a nearly doubled nitrofurantoin absorption when given 200 mg diphenoxylate daily, but the other four showed little effect.[2] The suggested mechanism is that the reduced motility of the gut caused by these drugs allows the nitrofurantoin to dissolve more completely so that it is absorbed by the gut more easily. Whether this is of any clinical importance is uncertain but it would be expected to be accompanied by an increase in the therapeutic effects of nitrofurantoin and possibly in the incidence of dose-related adverse reactions. So far there appear to be no reports of any problems arising from concurrent use.

References

1 Jaffe JM. Effect of propantheline on nitrofurantoin absorption. J Pharm Sci (1975) 64, 1729.
2 Callahan M, Bullock FJ, Braun J, Yesair DW. Pharmacodynamics of drug interactions with diphenoxylate. Fed Proc (1974) 33, 513.

Penicillins + Chloroquine

Abstract/Summary

The absorption of ampicillin is reduced by the concurrent use of chloroquine, but bacampicillin is not affected.

Clinical evidence, mechanism, importance and management

1 g chloroquine reduced the absorption of single 1 g doses of oral ampicillin in seven normal subjects by about a third (from 29 to 19%), as measured by its excretion in the urine.[1] A likely reason is that the chloroquine irritates the gut so that the ampicillin is moved through more quickly and less time is available for absorption. A reasonable solution to the problem would seem to be to increase the dosage of the ampicillin or possibly to separate the administration of the drugs. Not less than 2 h has been suggested.[1] This needs confirmation. An

alternative is to use bacampicillin (an ampicillin pro-drug) the bioavailability of which is not affected by chloroquine.[2]

References

1 Ali HM. Reduced ampicillin bioavailability following oral coadministration with chloroquine. J Antimicrob Chemother (1985) 15, 781–4.
2 Ali HM. The effect of Sudanese food and chloroquine on the bioavailability of ampicillin from bacampicillin tablets. Int J Pharmacy (1981) 9, 185–90.

Penicillins + Dietary fibre

Abstract/Summary

Dietary fibre can reduce the absorption of amoxycillin.

Clinical evidence, mechanism, importance and management

The AUC of single 500 mg oral doses of amoxycillin in 10 subjects was found to be 12.17 µg/ml/h while taking a low fibre diet (7.8 g daily) but only 9.65 µg/ml/h while on a high fibre diet (36.2 g daily). Peak serum levels were the same and occurred at 3 h. The subjects used were slum-dwellers in Santiago and the two diets represented the amounts of fibre normally eaten during the winter and summer seasons. A possible reason for the reduced absorption is that the amoxycillin becomes trapped within the fibre. The clinical importance of this interaction is uncertain but it may be necessary to increase the dosage of this antibiotic in those who have a high fibre diet to accommodate the reduced absorption.[1]

Reference

1 Lutz M, Espinoza J, Arancibia A, Araya M, Pacheco I, Brunser O. Effect of structured dietary fibre on bioavailability of amoxycillin. Clin Pharmacol Ther (1987) 42, 220–4.

Penicillin + Guar gum

Abstract/Summary

Guar gum reduces the absorption of phenoxymethyl penicillin.

Clinical evidence, importance and management

5 g guar gum (*Guarem* 95% guar gum) significantly reduced the absorption of a single 1980 mg dose of potassium phenoxymethyl penicillin when taken together by 10 normal subjects. Peak serum penicillin levels were reduced by 25% and the AUC 0–6 h by 28%.[1] The reasons are not understood. The clinical significance of this finding is uncertain, but it would clearly be important if the reduced amount of penicillin absorbed was inadequate to control infection. The effect of guar gum on other penicillins seems not to have been studied.

Reference

1 Huupponen R, Seppälä P, Iisalo E. Effect of guar gum, a fibre preparation, on digoxin and penicillin absorption in man. Eur J Clin Pharmacol (1984) 26, 279–81.

Penicillins + Miscellaneous drugs

Abstract/Summary

Aspirin, indomethacin, probenecid, phenylbutazone, sulphaphenazole and sulphinpyrazone prolong the half-life of benzyl penicillin (penicillin G) significantly, whereas chlorothiazide, sulphamethizole and sulphamethoxypyridazine do not. These interactions do not seem to present any problems in practice. The interaction of probenecid with some of the penicillins is exploited therapeutically. Some sulphonamides reduce oxacillin blood levels.

Table 5.3 Changes in half-life of Penicillin G

Drug	Number of patients	Change in half life in minutes		Significance P
		From	To	
Aspirin (3 g)	11	44.5	72.4	<0.05
Chlorothiazide (2 g)	6	53.5	62.3	NS
Indomethacin (75 mg)	11	42.7	52.2	<0.05
Phenylbutazone(600 mg)	12	42.8	102.2	<0.01
Probenecid (2 g)	22	40.4	104.3	<0.001
Sulphamethizole (4 g)	5	58.6	70.6	NS
Sulphamethoxypyridazine (500 mg)	6	60.0	50.8	NS
Sulphaphenazole (1 g)	7	34.9	50.4	<0.05
Sulphinpyrazone (600 mg)	8	42.6	70.3	<0.001

Clinical evidence

Studies in patients given the following drugs for 5–7 days showed the following changes in the half-life of benzyl penicillin (penicillin G):

Probenecid also increases the serum concentrations of other penicillins including nafcillin[2] and ticarcillin[6] but not piperacillin.[4] 3 g sulphamethoxypyridazine given eight hours before 1 g oral oxacillin to normal subjects reduced the 6 h urinary recovery by 54%. 3.9 g sulphaethylthiadiazole given three hours before the oxacillin reduced the 6 h urinary recovery by 42%.[5]

Mechanisms

In many cases it seems likely that the interacting drugs successfully compete with penicillin for excretion by the kidney tubules so that the pencillin is retained in the body. This is certainly true for probenecid.

Importance and management

None of the interactions listed in Table 5.3 appears to be adverse and some may be exploited. The penicillin-probenecid interaction can be used to achieve higher and more prolonged plasma concentrations of the penicillins (ampicillin, amoxycillin, ticarcillin) in the treatment of gonorrhoea, the prevention of diphtheria and endocarditis and other conditions, or even simply to save money.[3] No particular precautions would seem necessary during concurrent use of these drugs and the penicillins, except to ensure that the levels of the antibiotic do not become excessive. The importance of the oxacillin-sulphonamide interaction is uncertain, but it can easily be avoided by choosing alternative drugs.

References

1 Kampmann H, Hansen JM, Siersboek-Nielsen K, Laursen H. Effect of some drugs on penicillin half-life in blood. Clin Pharmacol Ther (1972) 13, 516–19.
2 Waller ES, Sharanevych MA, Yakatan GJ. The effect of probenecid on nafcillin disposition. J Clin Pharmacol (1982) 22, 482–9.
3 Allen MB, Fitzpatrick RW, Barratt A, Cole RB. The use of probenecid to increase the serum amoxycillin levels in patients with bronchiectasis. Resp Med (1990) 84, 143–6.
4 Ganes D, Bastra V, Faulkner R, Greene D, Haynes J, Kuye O, Ruffner A, shin K, Tonelli A, Yacobi A. Effect of probenecid on the pharmacokinetics of piperacillin and tazobactam in healthy volunteers. Pharm Res (1991) 8 (Suppl 10) S-299.
5 Kunin CM. Clinical pharmacology of the new penicillins. II Effect of drugs which interfere with binding to serum proteins. Clin Pharmacol Ther (1966) 7, 180–88.
6 Corvaia L, Li SC, Ioannides-Demos LL, Bowes G, Spicer WJ, Spelman DW, Tong NM, Mclean AJ. A prospective study of the effects of oral probenecid on the pharmacokinetics of intravenous ticarcillin in patients with cystic fibrosis. J Antimicrob Chemother (1992) 30, 875–8.

Penicillins + Tetracyclines

Abstract/Summary

Tetracyclines can reduce the effectiveness of penicillin in the treatment of pneumococcal meningitis and probably scarlet fever. It is uncertain whether a similar interaction occurs with other infections. It may possibly only be important with those infections where a rapid kill is essential.

Clinical evidence

In patients with pneumococcal meningitis it was shown that penicillin alone (one million units every 2 h) was more effective than penicillin with chlortetracycline (0.5 g every 6 h). Out of 14 patients given penicillin alone, 70% recovered compared with only 20% in another group of essentially similar patients who had had both antibiotics.[1]

Another report about the treatment of pneumococcal meningitis with penicillin and tetracyclines (chlortetracycline, oxytetracycline, tetracycline) confirmed that the mortality was much less in those given only pencillin.[2] In the treatment of scarlet fever (Group A beta-haemolytic streptococci), no difference was seen in the initial response, but spontaneous reinfection occurred more frequently in those who had had penicillin and chlortetracycline.[3]

Mechanism

The generally accepted explanation is that bactericides, such as penicillin which inhibits bacterial cell wall synthesis, require cells to be actively growing and dividing to be maximally effective, a situation which will not occur in the presence of bacteriostatic antibiotics such as the tetracyclines.

Importance and management

An established and important interaction when treating pneumococcal meningitis, and probably scarlet fever as well. The documentation seems to be limited to the reports cited. Concurrent use should be avoided in these infections, but the importance of this interaction with other infections is uncertain. It demonstrably does not occur when treating pneumococcal pneumonia.[4] It has been suggested that antagonism, if it occurs, may only be significant when it is essential to kill bacteria rapidly.[4] The antibiotics implicated in the interaction are penicillin, tetracycline, chlortetracycline and oxytetracycline, but any penicillin and tetracycline would be expected to behave similarly. Among the general rules which should be applied if concurrent use is thought appropriate are: to give the bactericidal penicillin a few hours before the bacteriostatic tetracycline (see 'Mechanism' above), and to ensure that the doses are well above minimally effective levels.

References

1 Lepper MH, Dowling HF. Treatment of pneumococcic meningitis with penicillin compared with penicillin plus aureomycin: studies including observations on an apparent antagonism between penicillin and aureomycin. Arch Intern Med (1951) 88, 489.

2 Olsson RA, Kirby JC, Romansky MJ. Pneumococcal meningitis in the adult. Clinical, therapeutic and prognostic aspects in forty-three patients. Ann Intern Med (1961) 55, 545.

3 Strom J. The question of antagonism between penicillin and chlortetracycline illustrated by therpeutical experiments in Scarlatina. Antibiot Med (1955) 1,6.

4 Ahern JJ, Kirby WMM. Lack of interference of aureomycin in treatment of pneumoccoal pneumonia. Arch Intern Med (1953) 91, 197.

Piperazine + Phenothiazines

Abstract/Summary

An isolated case of convulsions in a child was attributed to the use of chlorpromazine following piperazine.

Clinical evidence, mechanism, importance and management

A child given piperazine for pin worms developed convulsions when treated with chlorpromazine several days later.[1] In a subsequent animal study using 4.5 or 10 mg/kg chlorpromazine, many of the animals died from respiratory arrest after severe clonic convulsions.[1] However a later study failed to confirm these findings so that it is by no means certain whether the adverse reaction was due to an interaction or not.[2] Nevertheless there is enough evidence to warrant some caution if these drugs are used concurrently.

References

1 Boulos BM, Davis LE. Hazard of simultaneous administration of phenothiazine and piperazine. N Engl J Med (1969) 280, 1245.

2 Armbrecht BH. Reaction between piperazine and chlorpromazine. N Engl J Med (1970) 282, 149.

Praziquantel + Anticonvulsants

Abstract/Summary

Phenytoin and carbamazepine markedly reduce the serum levels of praziquantel. Neurocysticercosis treatment failures may occur as a result.

Clinical evidence, mechanism, importance and management

A comparative study of patients on chronic anticonvulsant treatment and healthy subjects given oral doses of 25 mg/kg praziquantel found that serum phenytoin and carbamazepine levels of 11 µg/ml and 7 µg/ml respectively, reduced the peak serum praziquantel levels and AUC (area under the curve) at 12 h by 75 and 90% respectively.[1] The probable reason is that these anticonvulsants increase the metabolism and loss of praziquantel by the liver, thereby hastening its loss from the body. The authors postulate that these marked reductions could explain some of the treatment failures in patients with active neurocysticercosis.[1]

Information is very limited but it may be necessary to raise the praziquantel dosage to compensate for this increased loss in patients on these anticonvulsants. More study is needed.

Reference

1 Bittencourt PRM, Gracia CM, Martins R, Fernandes AG. Praziquantel is almost inactivated by carbamazepine and phenytoin. Epilepsia (1991) 322, Suppl 1, 104.

Praziquantel or Albendazole + Corticosteroids

Abstract/Summary

The continuous use of dexamethasone can reduce serum praziquantel levels by 50%, but raise those of albendazole by 50%.

Clinical evidence

8 patients with parenchymal brain cysticercosis treated with praziquantel (50 mg/kg divided into three doses 8-hourly) showed a 50% reduction in steady-state serum levels (from 3.13 to 1.55 µg/ml) when given 8 mg dexamethasone 8-hourly.

Mechanism

Not understood.

Importance and management

Information about praziquantel seems to be limited to this study[1] but the interaction would appear to be established. How much it affects the outcome of treatment for cysticercosis is unknown because the optimum praziquantel dosage is still uncertain but a reduction in efficacy seems probable. The authors of the report suggest that dexamethasone should not be given continuously with praziquantel but only used transiently for the treatment of the adverse effects arising from the inflammatory response to the dead and dying parasites in the CNS. This interaction is only likely to be important for infections where treatment depends upon the maintenance of adequate serum levels. There seems to be no information about other corticosteroids.

An alternative cysticidal is albendazole (15 mg/kg), the plasma levels of which were found in a study in eight patients to be increased about 50% by the use of 8 mg dexamethasone 8-hourly.[2]

References

1 Vazquez ML, Jung H, Sotelo J. Plasma levels of praziquantel decrease when dexamethasone is given simultaneously. Neurology (1987) 37, 1561–2.

2 Jung H, Hurtado M, Medina M T, Sanchez M, Sotelo J. Dexamethasone increases plasma levels of albendazole. J Neurol (1990) 237, 279–80.

Primaquine + Mepacrine (Quinacrine)

Abstract/Summary

Primaquine appears not to interact adversely with mepacrine although theoretically it might be expected to do so.

Clinical evidence, mechanism, importance and management

Patients given pamaquine, a predecessor of primaquine, showed grossly elevated serum levels when concurrently treated with mepacrine.[1,2] The probable reason is that the mepacrine occupies binding sites in the body normally also used by the pamaquine and, as a result, the latter fails to become sequestered at these sites and the serum levels become very high. On theoretical grounds primaquine might be expected to interact with mapacrine similarly, but there seem to be no reports confirming that a clinically important interaction actually takes place.

References

1 Zubrod CG, Kennedy TJ, Shannon JA. Studies on the chemotherapy of the human malarias. VIII. The physiological disposition of pamaquine. J Clin Invest (1948) 27 (Suppl) 114–120.

2 Earle DP, Bigelow FS, Zubrod CG, Kane CA. Studies on the chemotherapy of the human malarias. IX. Effect of pamaquine on the blood cells of man. J Clin Invest (1948) 27, (Suppl) 121–9.

Proguanil + Chloroquine

Abstract/Summary

Chloroquine appears almost to double the incidence of mouth ulcers among those taking proguanil prophylactically.

Clinical evidence, mechanism, importance and management

Following the observation that mouth ulcers appeared to be common amongst those taking prophylactic antimalarials, an extensive study was undertaken in 628 servicemen in Belize. 24% of those on 200 mg proguanil daily developed mouth ulcers, and 37% developed ulcers while also taking 150– 300 mg chloroquine base weekly. The incidence of diarrhoea was also increased (from 63 to 82%) among those who developed the ulcers. The reasons are not understood. The authors of the study suggest that these two drugs should not be given together unnecessarily for prophylaxis against *Pl. falciparum*.[1]

Reference

1 Drysdale SF, Phillips-Howard PA, Behrens RH. Proguanil, chloroquine and mouth ulcers. Lancet (1990) 1, 164.

Prothionamide + Rifampicin (Rifampin) and/or Dapsone

Abstract/Summary

Prothionamide appears to be very hepatotoxic, which is possibly increased by the concurrent use of rifampicin or isopiperazinylrifamycin SV. Prothionamide does not affect the pharmacokinetics of either dapsone or rifampicin.

Clinical evidence

39% of 39 patients with leprosy became jaundiced after 24–120 days treatment with dapsone (100 mg daily), prothionamide (300 mg daily) and isopiperazinylrifamycin SV (300–600 mg monthly). Laboratory evidence of liver damage occurred in a total of 56% and despite the withdrawal of the drugs from all the patients, two of them died.[1] All the patients except two had had dapsone before, alone, for 3–227 months without reported problems.[1] 22% of 50 other leprosy patients also showed liver damage after treatment with dapsone (100 mg) and prothionamide (300 mg) daily, with rifampicin (900 mg), prothionamide (500 mg) and clofazimine (300 mg) monthly for 30–50 days. One patient died.[1] Most of the patients recovered within 30–60 days after withdrawing the treatment. Jaundice, liver damage and deaths have occurred in other leprosy patients given rifampicin and prothionamide or ethionamide.[2–4] Prothionamide does not affect the pharmacokinetics of either dapsone or rifampicin.[5]

Mechanism

Although not certain, it seems probable that the liver damage was primarily caused by the prothionamide, possibly exacerbated by the rifampicin or the isopiperazinylrifamycin SV.

Importance and management

This serious and potentially life-threatening hepatotoxic reaction to prothionamide is established, but the part played by the other drugs, particularly the rifampicin, is uncertain. Strictly speaking this may not be an interaction. If prothionamide is given the liver function should be very closely monitored in order to detect toxicity as soon as possible.

References

1 Baohong J, Jiakun C, Chenmin W, Guang X. Hepatotoxicity of combined therapy with rifampicin and daily prothionamide for leprosy. Lepr Rev (1984) 55, 283–9.
2 Lesobre R, Ruffine J, Teyssier L, Achard F, Brefort G. Les icterus en cours du traitment par la rifampicine. Rev Tuberc Pneumol (1969) 33, 393–403.
3 Report of the Third Meeting of the Scientific Working Group on Chemotherapy of Leprosy (THELEP) of the UNDP/World Bank/WHO Special Programme for Research and Training in Tropical Diseases. Int J Lepr (1981) 49, 431–6.
4 Cartel JL, Millan J, Guelpa-Lauras CC, Grosset JH. Hepatitis in leprosy patients treated by a daily combination of dapsone, rifampicin and a thioamide. Int J Lepr (1983) 51, 461–5.
5 Mathur A, Venkatesan K, Girdhar BK, Bharadwaj VP, Girdhar A, Bagga AK. A study of drug interactions in leprosy - 1. Effect of simultaneous administration of prothionamide on metabolic disposition of rifampicin and dapsone. Lepr Rev (1986) 57, 33–7.

Pyrantel + Piperazine

Abstract/Summary

Piperazine opposes the anthelmintic actions of pyrantel.

Clinical evidence, mechanism, importance and management

Pyrantel acts as an anthelmintic because it depolarizes the neuromuscular junctions of some intestinal nematodes causing the worms to contract. This paralyzes the worms so that they are dislodged by peristalsis and expelled in the faeces. Piperazine also paralyzes nematodes but it does so by causing hyperpolarization of the neuromuscular junctions. These two pharmacological actions oppose one another, as was shown in two *in vitro* pharmacological studies. Strips of whole *Ascaris lumbricoides* which contracted when exposed to pyrantel (1.5 ng/ml) failed to do so when also exposed to piperazine (1 mg/ml).[1] Parallel electrophysiological studies using Ascaris cells confirmed that the depolarization due to pyrantel (which causes the paralysis) was opposed by piperazine.[1]

In practical terms this means that piperazine does not add to the anthelmintic effect of pyrantel on *Ascaris* as might be expected, but opposes it. For which reason it is usually recommended that concurrent use should be avoided, but direct clinical evidence confirming that combined use is ineffective seems to be lacking. It seems reasonable to extrapolate the results of these studies on *Ascaris lumbricoides* (roundworm) to the other gastrointestinal parasites for which pyrantel is used, i.e. *Enterobius vermicularis* (threadworm or pinworm), *Ancylostoma duodenale*, *Necator americanus* (hookworm), *Trichuris trichiura* (whipworm), *Trichostrongylus colubriformis* and *orientalis*, but no one seems to have checked on this directly.

Reference

1 Aubry ML, Cowell P, Davey MJ, Shevde S. Aspects of the pharmacology of a new anthelmintic: pyrantel. Br J Pharmac (1970) 38, 332–44.

Pyrazinamide + Miscellaneous drugs

Abstract/Summary

Pyrazinamide should be used with caution with other potentially hepatotoxic drugs. It may cause hyperuricaemia which is modestly reduced by aminosalicylic acid or probenecid, but more extensively by aspirin. Pyrazinamide may possibly adversely affect the control of diabetes.

Clinical evidence, mechanism, importance and management

Hepatotoxicity is the most common side-effect of pyrazinamide[1,2] and it should therefore be used with caution with other potentially hepatotoxic drugs. It has been used with good effect in the treatment of tuberculosis in combination with other agents such as rifampicin, isoniazid and streptomycin.[1] Pyrazinamide can decrease the urinary output of uric acid by a third to a half, resulting in a rise in the serum levels of urate in the blood (hyperuricaemia).[3,4] This hyperuricaemia is inhibited to some extent by aminosalicyclic acid, but probenecid is no more effective and the response is short-lived.[3,4] On the other hand it is reduced by aspirin (2.4 g daily).[4] Pyrazinamide is contraindicated in patients with existing hyperuricaemia or gouty arthritis.[1] The control of diabetes mellitus is reported to be more difficult in some patients taking pyrazinamide.[1,2]

References

1 Data Sheet Compendium 1985–86, Datapharm Publications 1985. p 942
2 Martindale. The Extra Pharmacopoeia, 28th Edition. Pharmaceutical Press 1982.
3 Cullen JH, LeVine M, Fiore JM. Studies of hyperuricaemia produced by pyrazinamide. Amer J Med (1957) 23, 587–95.
4 Shapiro M, Hyde L. Hyperuricaemia due to pyrazinamide. Amer J Med (1957) 23, 596–9.

Pyrimethamine + Co-trimoxazole or Sulphonamides

Abstract/Summary

Serious pancytopenia and megaloblastic anaemia have been described in patients under treatment with pyrimethamine and either co-trimoxazole or other sulphonamides.

Clinical evidence

A woman taking 50 mg pyrimethamine weekly as malarial prophylaxis, developed petechial haemorrhages and widespread bruising within 10 days of starting to take co-trimoxazole (320 mg trimethoprim + 800 mg sulphamethoxazole daily). She was found to have gross megaloblastic changes and pancytopenia in addition to being obviously pale and ill. After withdrawal of the two drugs she responded rapidly to hydroxycobalamin and folic acid, with chloroquine as malarial prophylaxis.[1]

Similar cases have been described in other patients taking pyrimethamine with co-trimoxazole[2,4–6] or sulphafurazole.[3] Another case has been referred to elsewhere involving a sulphonamide.[7]

Mechanism

Uncertain, but a reasonable surmise can be made. Pyrimethamine and trimethoprim are both 2 : 4 diaminopyrimidines and both selectively inhibit the actions of the enzyme dihydrofolate reductase which is concerned with the eventual synthesis, amongst other compounds, of the nucleic acids needed for the production of new cells. The sulphonamides inhibit another part of the same synthetic chain. The adverse reactions seen would seem to reflect a gross depression of the normal folate metabolism caused by the combined actions of both drugs. Megaloblastic anaemia and pancytopenia are among the adverse reactions of pyrimethamine and, more rarely, of co-trimoxazole taken alone. In theory this should not occur (see 'Co-trimoxazole + Folic acid') but in practice it clearly does so occasionally.

Importance and management

Information seems to be limited to the reports cited, but the interaction appears to be established. Its incidence is unknown. Concurrent use need not be avoided but the authors of the report cited[1] advise that co-trimoxazole should be prescribed '...with caution and haematological cover...' to patients given pyrimethamine or proguanil for malarial prophylaxis, and '...further caution...' in the tropics because of the folate deficiency associated with pregnancy and malnutrition in children. The manufacturers of co-trimoxazole support this in advising that if the dosage of pyrimethamine is high the blood picture should be monitored regularly.

References

1 Fleming AF, Warrell DA, Dickmeiss H. Co-trimoxazole and the blood. Lancet (1974) ii, 284.

2 Andsell VE, Wright SG, Hutchinson DBA. Megaloblastic anaemia associated with combined pyrimethamine and co-trimoxazole administration. Lancet (1976) ii, 1257.

3 Waxman S, Herbert V. Mechanism of pyrimethamine induced megaloblastosis in human bone marrow. N Engl J Med (1969) 280, 1316.

4 Malfatti S, Piccini A. Anemia megaloblastica pancitopenica in corso di trattemento con pirimetamina, trimethoprim e sulfametossazolo. Haematologica (1976) 61, 349.

5 Borgstein A, Tozer RA. Infectious mononucleosis and megaloblastic anaemia associated with Daraprim and Bactrim. Centr Afr J Med (1974) 20, 185.

6 Whitman EN. Effects in man of prolonged administration of trimethoprim and sulfisoxazole. Postgrad Med J (1969) 45 (Suppl) 46.

7 Weissbach G. Auswirkongen Kombinierter Behaudlung der Kindlichen. Tosoplasmose mit Pyrimethamin (Daraprim) und Sulfornamiden auf Blut und Knochenmark/ Zschrärztl Fortbilld (1965) 59, 10–22.

Quinine + Miscellaneous drugs

Abstract/Summary

The loss of quinine from the body is reduced by the concurrent use of cimetidine, but not ranitidine. A single case report describes a reduction in the serum levels and therapeutic effects of quinine in a patient when rifampicin was given. Urinary alkalinizers can increase the retention of quinine in man, and antacids can reduce the absorption in animals. Doxycycline does not alter the pharmacokinetics of quinine. None of these interactions appears to be of general clinical importance.

Clinical evidence, mechanism, importance and management

(a) Cimetidine and ranitidine

1 g cimetidine daily for a week reduced the clearance of quinine in six subjects by 27% (from 0.182 to 0.133 l/h/kg) while its half-life was increased by 49% (from 7.6 to 11.3 h) and the AUC was increased by 42% (53.9 to 76.8 mg/l/h). Peak levels were unchanged. No interaction was seen when cimetidine was replaced by ranitidine.[1] The probable reason is that cimetidine (a recognized enzyme inhibitor) reduces the metabolism of the quinine by the liver so that it is lost from the body more slowly, whereas ranitidine does not. The clinical importance of this is uncertain, but prescribers should be alert for any evidence of quinine toxicity during concurrent use (the increase in AUC was 75% in one subject[1]).

(b) Doxycycline

The pharmacokinetics of quinine were found to be unchanged by doxycycline in patients with acute falciparum malaria.[2] No special precautions would seem to be necessary.

(c) Rifampicin

A patient with myotonia controlled with quinine reported a worsening of the symptoms within three weeks of starting to take rifampicin for the treatment of tuberculosis. Peak quinine levels were found to be low, but rose again when the rifampicin was stopped. Control of the myotonia was restored after six weeks.[3] The probable reason is that rifampicin (a potent liver enzyme-inducing agent) increases the metabolism of the quinine by the liver, thereby hastening its clearance from the body and thereby reducing its effects. Information appears to be limited to this report but it is consistent with the way rifampicin affects a number of other drugs. Monitor the effects of concurrent use and anticipate the need to raise the quinine dosage as necessary. Reduce the dosage when the rifampicin is stopped.

(d) Urinary alkalinizers and acidifiers

The excretion of unchanged quinine in man is virtually halved (from 17.4 to 8.9%) if the urine is changed from acid to alkaline with agents such as acetazolamide or sodium bicarbonate.[1,6] The reason is that at alkaline pH values more of the quinine exists in the un-ionized (lipid soluble) form which is more easily reabsorbed by the kidney tubules.[4] However there seem to be no reports of adverse effects arising from changes in excretion due to this interaction. Magnesium and aluminium hydroxide gel depresses the absorption of quinine from the gut of rats and reduces blood quinine levels by 50–70%.[2,5] The reason appears to be that aluminium hydroxide slows gastric emptying which reduces absorption, and magnesium hydroxide also forms an insoluble precipitate with quinine. However there seem to be no clinical reports of a reduction in the therapeutic effectiveness of quinine due to the concurrent use of antacids.

References

1 Wanwimolruk S, Sunbhanich M, Pongmarutai M and Patamasucon P. Effects of cimetidine and ranitidine on the pharmacokinetics of quinine. Br J clin Pharmac (1986) 22, 346–50.

2 Couet W, Laroche R, Floch JJ, Istin B, Fourtillan JB, Sauniere JF. Pharmacokinetics of quinine and doxycycline in patients with acute faciparum malaria: a study in Africa. Ther Drug Monit (1991) 13, 496–501.

3 Osborn JE, Pettit MJ, Graham P. Interaction between rifampicin and quinine: case report. Pharm J (1989) 243, 704.

4 Haag HB, Larson PS, Schwartz JJ. The effect of urinary pH on the elimination of quinine in man. J Pharmacol Exp Ther (1943) 79, 136.

5 Hurwitz A. The effects of antacids on gastrointestinal drug absorption. II. Effect of sulfadiazine and quinine. J Pharmacol Exp Ther (1971) 179, 485.

6 Haag HB, Larson PS, Schwartz JJ. The effect of urinary pH on the elimination of quinine in man. J Pharmacol Exp Ther (1943) 79, 136–9.

Quinolone antibiotics + Antacids

Abstract/Summary

Serum amifloxacin, ciprofloxacin, enoxacin, levofloxacin, lomefloxacin, norfloxacin, ofloxacin and pefloxacin levels can be reduced below therapeutic concentrations by the concurrent use of aluminium and magnesium antacids. Separating the dosages as much as possible goes some way towards reducing this interaction but it may be difficult to avoid it entirely with some of the quinolones. Norfloxacin appears not to interact with bismuth subsalicylate.

Clinical evidence

(a) Amifloxacin + Antacids

30 ml of *Maalox* (aluminium-magnesium hydroxides) reduced the bioavailability and peak serum levels of a single 200 mg dose of amifloxacin in 16 normal subjects by about 85%.[17]

(b) Ciprofloxacin + Antacids

10 patients on dialysis (CAPD) because of renal failure were given 250 mg ciprofloxacin four times daily. The steady-state serum ciprofloxacin levels of three of them concurrently taking aluminium-containing antacids (*Maalox*, *Malinal*) as phosphate binders were reduced by approximately two-thirds (peak serum levels fell from 3.69 to 1.25 μg/ml), whereas the serum levels of three others taking a calcium carbonate containing antacid (*Titralac*) were unaffected.[1] Similar results were found in another study in patients undergoing peritoneal dialysis.[24]

Other studies clearly show that peak serum ciprofloxacin levels and its bioavailability are reduced about 80–90% when aluminium hydroxide or *Maalox* (aluminium and magnesium hydroxides) antacids are given with, or within 2 h of, the ciprofloxacin.[2,11,18,20] Two studies found that the bioavailability was reduced 40–50% with calcium carbonate antacids,[10,18,33] while another found that calcium carbonate given 2 h before did not affect the bioavailability.[19] A single dose study found that 100 ml magnesium citrate solution (8 g) reduced the AUC of a single 500 mg dose of ciprofloxacin by 80%.[15]

(c) Enoxacin, Levofloxacin (DR-3355), Lomefloxacin, Norfloxacin, Ofloxacin, Pefloxacin + Antacids

Reductions in absorption of 50–98% in serum enoxacin, lomefloxacin, norfloxacin, ofloxacin and pefloxacin have been described in studies and case reports involving antacids containing aluminium and magnesium hydroxides or magnesium trisilicate. A reduction of about a third was seen when *Maalox* was given 2 h after the norfloxacin.[16] A smaller reduction (about 50–60%) was seen with norfloxacin and calcium carbonate (*Titralac*).[13,14,16] No clinically important interaction was seen in a study of ofloxacin with a chewing tablet of *Maalox*[8] but two studies found that the AUC was reduced by about two-thirds by aluminium and magnesium hydroxides.[73,20,31] Norfloxacin is not affected by bismuth subsalicylate[23,28] while only a small reduction (– 31% AUC, – 19% maximum serum levels) occurs with ciprofloxacin.[30] Aluminium hydroxide and magnesium oxide reduced the bioavailability of levofloxacin by 55 and 78% respectively, but calcium carbonate had no effect.[29]

Mechanism

It is believed that certain functional groups (3-carbonyl and 4-oxo) on the antibiotics form insoluble chelates with aluminium and magnesium ions in the gut which reduces absorption.[2,6,32] In addition these chelates appear to be relatively inactive as antibacterials.[4] Enoxacin also appears to be less soluble as the pH rises.[12]

Importance and management

The aluminium/magnesium antacid-ciprofloxacin interaction is established and clinically important. Serum antibiotic levels may become subtherapeutic against organisms such as *staphy-*

lococci and *Pseudomonas aeruginosa.*[5,11] Do not give these antacids and ciprofloxacin at the same time. Separating the dosages as much as possible reduces the effects of this interaction but it is difficult to assess the best time scheduling. Giving the antacid 2–4 h before the antibiotic to reduce mixing in the gut can still result in reductions in absorption of 30–75%.[6,11] One study suggests that the absorption is reduced 20–40% if the antacid is given 2–4 h after the antibiotic,[6] whereas another suggests that no interaction occurs if given 2 h after the antibiotic.[11] The makers of ciprofloxacin advise avoidance within 4 h of these antacids, but with calcium carbonate it seems that giving it 2 h after the ciprofloxacin may avoid the interaction.[19] Remember also that some antacids can raise the urinary pH. The solubility of ciprofloxacin decreases as the pH rises and excessive urinary alkalinity should be avoided to prevent crystalluria and possible kidney damage.

Less is known about amifloxacin, enoxacin, levofloxacin, lomefloxacin, norfloxacin, ofloxacin and pefloxacin but the evidence is that they interact like ciprofloxacin and the same general precautions should be followed. If *Maalox* is given 4–8 h before enoxacin no interaction occurs, whereas some reduction in absorption occurs (up to 30%) if given up to 2–3 h afterwards.[22,12] Three other studies found that if *Maalox* was given 2 h after lomefloxacin or norfloxacin the absorption was only reduced about 20–33%.[13,16,25] Yet another found that 15 ml aluminium-magnesium hydroxide and 5 ml calcium carbonate 2 h before of after ofloxacin did not interfere with its absorption.[21] There is also some evidence that sodium bicarbonate does not interact significantly with norfloxacin.[14]

References

1 Fleming LW, Moreland TA, Stewart WK, Scott AC. Ciprofloxacin and antacids. Lancet (1986) ii, 248.

2 Hoffken G, Borner K, Glatzel PD, Koeppa P, Lode H. Reduced enteral absorption of ciprofloxacin in the presence of antacids. Eur J Clin Microbiol (1985) 4, 345.

3 Preheim LC, Cuevas TA, Roccaforte JS, Mellencamp MA, Bittner MJ. Ciprofloxacin and antacids. Lancet (1986) ii, 48.

4 Machka K, Braveny J. Inhibitorische wirkung verschiedener faktoren auf die aktivitat von gyrasehemmern. FAC (1985) 3, 557–62.

5 Rubinstein E, Segev S. Drug interactions with ciprofloxacin and with other non-antibiotics. Am J Med (1987) 82 (Suppl 4A) 119–23.

6 Schentag JJ, Watson WA, Nix DE, Sedman AJ, Frost RW, Letteri J. The dependent interactions between antacids and quinolone antibiotics. Clin Pharmacol Ther (1988) 43, 135.

7 Vinceneux Ph, Weber Ph, Gaudin H, Boussougant Y. Diminution de l'absorption de la pefloxacin par les pansements gastriques. La Presse Med (1986) 15, 1826.

8 Maesen FPV, Davies BI, Geraedts WH, Shmajow CA. Ofloxacin and antacids. J Antimicrob Chemother (1987) 19, 848–9.

9 Noyes M, Polk RE. Norfloxacin and absorption of magnesium-aluminium. Ann Intern Med (1988) 109, 168–9.

10 Polk RE. Influence of chronic administration of calcium on the bioavailability of oral ciprofloxacin. 29th Int Conf Antimicrob Ag Chemother, Houston, Texas (1989), 211.

11 Nix DE, Watson WA, Lener ME, Frost RW, Krol G, Goldstein H, Letterei J, Schentag JJ. Effects of aluminium and magnesium antacids and ranitidine on the absorption of ciprofloxacin. Clin Pharmacol Ther (1989) 46, 700–5.

12 Grasela TH, Schentag JJ, Sedman AJ, Wilton JH, Thomas DJ, Schultz RW, Lebsack ME, Kinkel AW. Inhibition of enoxacin absorption by antacids and ranitidine. Antimicrob Ag Chemother (1989) 33, 615–7.

13 Nix DE, Wilton JH, Ronald B, Distlerath L, Williams VC, Norman A. Inhibition of norfloxacin absorption by antacids. Antimicrob Ag Chemother (1990) 34, 432–5.

14 Okhamafe AO, Akerele JO, Chukuka CS. Pharmacokinetic interactions of norfloxacin with some metallic medicinal agents. Int J Pharmaceutics (1991) 68, 11–18.

15 Brouwers JRBJ, van der Kam HJ, Sijtsma J, Proost JH. Important reduction of ciprofloxacin absorption by sucralfate and magnesium citrate solution. Drug Invest (1990) 2, 197–9.

16 Nix DE, Wilton JH, Schentag JJ, Parpia SH, Norman A, Goldstein HR. Inhibition of norfloxacin absorption by antacids and sucralfate. Rev Inf Dis (1989) II, Suppl 5, S1096.

17 Stroshane RM, Brown RR, Cook JA, Wissel PS. Effect of food, milk and antacid on the absorption of orally administered amifloxacin. Rev Inf Dis (1989) II, Suppl 5, S1018.

18 Frost RW, Lettieri JT, Noe A, Shamblen EC, Lasseter K. Effect of aluminium hydroxide and calcium carbonate antacids on ciprofloxacin bioavailability. Clin Pharmacol Ther (1989) 45, 165.

19 Lomaestro BM, Bailie GR. Effect of staggered dose of calcium on the bioavailability of ciprofloxacin. Antimicrob Ag Chemother (1991) 35, 1004–7.

20 Höffken G, Lode H, Wiley R, Glatzel TD, Sievers D, Olschewski T, Borner K, Koeppe T. Pharmacokinetics and bioavailability of ciprofloxacin and ofloxacin: effect of food and antacid intake. Rev Infect Dis (1988) 10 Suppl 1, S138–9.

21 Flor S, Guay DR, Opsahl JA, Tack K, Matzke GR. Effects of magnesium-aluminium hydroxide and calcium carbonate antacids on bioavailability of ofloxacin. Antimicrob Ag Chemother (1990) 34, 2436–8.

22 Misiak P, Toothaker R, Lebsack M, Sedman A, Colburn W. The effect of dosing-time intervals on the potential pharmacokinetic interaction between oral enoxacin and oral antacid. Program and Abstracts of 28th Interscience Conf on Antimicrob Ag Chemother, Los Angeles, October 1988, p 367.

23 Campbell NRC, Kara M, Hasinoff BB, McKay DW. Clinical and chemical interactions between norfloxacin and clinically used metal ions. Clin Invest Med (1991) 14, A18.

24 Golper TA, Hartstein AI, Morthland VH, Christensen JM. Effects of antacids and dialysate dwell times on multiple dose pharmacokinetics of oral ciprofloxacin in patients on continuous ambulatory peritoneal dialysis. Antimicrob Ag Chemother (1987) 31, 1787–90.

25 Forster T, Blouin R. The effect of antacid timing on lomefloxacin bioavailability. Proc 29th Intersci Conf Antimicrob Ag Chemother (1989) Houston, Texas, Abstracts, page 318.

26 Shiba K, Saito A, Miyahara T, Tachizawa H, Fujimoto T. Effect of aluminium hydroxide, an antacid, on the pharmacokinetics of new quinolones in humans. Proc 15th Int Congr Chemother, Istanbul 1987, 168.

27 Metz R, Jaehde U, Wiesemann H, Gottschalk B, Stephan U, Schunack W. Pharmacokinetic interactions and non-interactions of pefloxacin. Proc 15th Int Congr Chemother, Istanbul, 1987, 997.

28 Campbell NRC, Kara M, Hasinoff BB, Haddara WM, McKay DW. Norfloxacin interaction with antacids and minerals. Br J clin Pharmac (1992) 33, 115–6.

29 Shiba K, Sakai O, Shimada J, Okazaki O, Aoki H, Hakusui H. Effects of antacids, ferrous sulphate and ranitidine on absorption of DR-3355 in humans. Antimicrob Ag Chemother (1992) 36, 2270–4.

30 Sahai J, Oliveras L, Garber G. Effect of bismuth subsalicylate (Peptobismol, PB) on ciprofloxacin absorption: a prelminary investigation. 17th Int Congr Chemother, June 1991, Berlin. Abst 414

31 Shiba K, Yoshida M, Kachi M, Shimade J, Saito A, Sakai N. Effects of peptic ulcer-healing drugs on the pharmacokinetics of new quinolone. 17th Int Congr Chemother, June 1991, Berlin, Abstract 415.

32 Shimada J, Shiba K, Oguma T, Miwa H, Yoshimura Y, Nishikawa T, Okabayashi Y, Kitagawa T, Yamamoto S. Effect of antacid absorption of the quinolone lomefloxacin. Antimicrob Ag Chemother (1992) 36, 1219–24.

33 Sahai J, Healey DP, Stotka J, Polk RE. The influence of chronic administration of calcium carbonate on the bioavailability of oral ciprofloxacin. Br J clin Pharmac (1993) 35, 302–4.

Quinolone antibiotics + Cetraxate

Abstract/Summary, clinical evidence, mechanism, importance and management

A single dose study found that cetraxate (dose not stated) does not affect the pharmacokinetics of a single 200 mg dose of ofloxacin.[1] No special precautions would seem to be necessary.

Reference

1 Shiba K, Yoshida M, Kachi M, Shimada J, Saito A, Sakai N. Effects of peptic ulcer-healing drugs on the pharmacokinetics of new quinolone. 17th Int Congr Chemother, June 1991, Berlin, Abstract 415.

Quinolone antibiotics + Cytotoxic agents

Abstract/Summary

The absorption of ciprofloxacin can be halved by the concurrent use of some cytotoxic agents.

Clinical evidence

Six patients with newly diagnosed haematological malignancies (five with acute myeloid leukaemia and one with non-Hodgkinson's lymphoma) were treated with 500 mg ciprofloxacin twice daily to control possible infections when neutropenic. It was found that after 13 days chemotherapy their mean maximum serum ciprofloxacin levels had fallen by 46% (from 3.7 to 2.0 mg/l) and the AUC_{0-4} (area under the concentration-time curve over 4 h) by 53% (10.7 to 5.7 mg/l/h). There were large individual differences between the patients. The cytotoxic agents used were cyclophosphamide, cytosine arabinoside, daunorubicin, doxorubicin, mitozantrone and vincristine.[1]

Mechanism

Uncertain. It seems to result from a reduction in absorption of the ciprofloxacin by the small intestine, possibly related to the damaging effect these cytoxic agents have on the rapidly dividing cells of the intestinal mucosa.

Importance and management

Direct information seems to be limited to this report, but it is consistent with the way cytotoxic agents can reduce the absorption of some other drugs. The authors point out that the antibiotic levels achieved are probably adequate for most infections,[1] but clearly the outcome of concurrent use should be well monitored to confirm that this is so. If the suggested mechanism of interaction is correct, no interaction should occur if the ciprofloxacin is given by injection. Nothing appears to be documented about any of the other quinolone antibiotics.

Reference

1 Johnson EJ, MacGowan AP, Potter MN, Stockley RJ, White LO, Slade R R, Reeves DS. Reduced absorption of oral ciprofloxacin after chemotherapy for haematological malignancy. J Antimicrob Chemother (1990) 25, 837–42.

Quinolone antibiotics + Didanosine

Abstract/Summary

An extremely marked reduction in the serum levels of ciprofloxacin occurs if it is given at the same time as didanosine. Separating the dosages may go some way towards reducing this interaction.

Clinical evidence

When 750 mg ciprofloxacin was given at the same time as two didanosine tablets to 12 normal subjects, the AUC of the ciprofloxacin and its maximum serum levels were reduced by 98% (from 15.50 to 0.26 µg/h/ml) and 93% (from 3.38 to 0.25 µg/ml) respectively.[1]

Mechanism

Not fully established, but the reason is almost certainly because of an interaction between the buffering agents in the didanosine formulation and the ciprofloxacin. Didanosine is extremely acid labile at pH values below 3 so that it has to be formulated with buffering agents (such as aluminum and magnesium hydroxides) to keep the pH as high as possible to minimize the acid-induced hydrolysis. Ciprofloxacin forms insoluble non-absorbable chelates with these ions so that its bioavailability is markedly reduced. See 'Quinolone antibiotics + Antacids'.

Importance and management

An established and clinically important interaction. Such drastic reductions in serum ciprofloxacin levels mean that minimal inhibitory concentrations against a considerable number of organisms are unlikely to be achieved. The authors of the report suggest that the ciprofloxacin should be given at least 2 h before or 6 h after the didanosine. The effectiveness of this needs confirmation. Other quinolone antibiotics which interact with antacids seem likely to interact similarly, but so far reports are lacking.

Reference

1 Sahai J, Gallicano K, Oliveras L, Khaliq S, Hawley-Foss N, Garber G. Cations in the didanosine tablet reduce ciprofloxacin bioavailability. Clin Pharmacol Ther (1993) 53, 292–7.

Quinolone antibiotics + Fenbufen

Abstract/Summary

Convulsions have occurred in a very small number of patients given enoxacin and fenbufen.

Clinical evidence, mechanism, importance and management

A very small number of Japanese patients with no previous history of seizures developed convulsions when treated with enoxacin and fenbufen in normal doses,[1-3] as a result of which the Japanese Welfare Ministry advised physicians to avoid prescribing these two drugs together.

The reasons for this adverse reaction are by no means fully understood but there are a few clues. Convulsions have been seen in a few patients taking other quinolones, some of whom were epileptics and some who were not (see 'Anticonvulsants + Quinolone antibiotics'). Experiments in mice have shown that quinolones (including enoxacin) competitively inhibit the binding of gamma-amino butyric acid to its receptors, an inhibitory transmittor in the CNS which is believed to be involved in the control of convulsive activity. Both enoxacin and fenbufen affect the gamma-aminobutyric acid$_A$ receptor site in the hippocampus and frontal cortex of mice, which is associated with convulsive activity,[4] and it could be that the fenbufen simply lowers the amount of enoxacin needed to precipitate convulsions.

In practical terms this means that there is a finite (though probably very small) risk if enoxacin and fenbufen are given together. However it would seem prudent to avoid the concurrent use of these drugs, particularly in patients with a history of convulsions, because it is not possible to predict which patients are likely to be affected. There are many alternative antibiotics and NSAIDs available.

References

1 Takeo G, Shibuya N, Motomura M, Kanazawa H, Shishido H. A new DNA gyrase inhibitor induces convulsions: a case report and animal experiments. Chemotherapy (Tokyo) (1989) 37, 1159.
2 Morita H, Maemura K, Sakai Y, Kaneda Y. Exoxacin and feubufen Nippon Naika Gakkai Zasshi (1988) 77, 744–5.
3 Morikawa K, Nagata O, Kubo S. Unusual CNS toxic action of new quinolones. Paper presented to 27th Interscience Conference on Antimicrobial agents and Chemotherapy, New York, NY; October 5th 1987.
4 Motomura M, Kataoka Y, Takeo G, Shibayama K, Ohishi K, Nakamura T, Niwa M, Tsujihata M, Nagataki S. Hippocampus and frontal cortex are the potential mediatory sites for convulsions induced by new quinolones and non-steroidal anti-inflammatory drugs. Int J Clin Pharmacol Ther Toxicol (1991) 29, 223–7.

Quinolone antibiotics + H$_2$-blockers

Abstract/Summary

Most quinolones are not affected by H$_2$-blockers, but cimetidine increases the bioavailability of pefloxacin and intravenous enoxacin, and ranitidine reduces the bioavailability of enoxacin, but none of these changes has been shown to be clinically important.

Clinical evidence, mechanism, importance and management

Neither cimetidine nor ranitidine appear to have a clinically important effect on the pharmacokinetics of ciprofloxacin,[1,2,5,8-10] nor ranitidine on the pharmacokinetics of levofloxacin[17] or lomefloxacin.[12] Cimetidine also appears not to interact with ofloxacin.[15] A study of the concurrent use of cimetidine and pefloxacin showed that the AUC was increased about 40% (from 49 to 69 µg/h/ml), the half-life increased from 10.3 to 15.3 h and the clearance was reduced from 151 to 110 ml/min.[3,13]

50 mg ranitidine given intravenously 2 h before a single 400 mg oral dose of enoxacin was found to have reduced the absorption by 26–40%[4,6,7,16] which seemed to be related to change in gastric pH caused by the ranitidine.[6] but 150 mg ranitidine twice daily did not to affect the pharmacokinetics of a single 400 mg intravenous dose of enoxacin.[11] Enoxacin plasma levels were higher following a 400 mg intravenous doses after taking 300 mg cimetidine four times daily. Renal clearance and systemic clearance were reduced 26% and 20% respectively, and the elimination half-life was increased 30%.[11]

Famotidine given 8 h before norfloxacin significantly reduced its maximum serum concentrations in six normal subjects, but the bioavailability (AUC) and urinary recovery rate were unchanged.[14] No changes in the absorption of norfloxacin were seen in the same subjects when given troxipide.[14]

Although the pharmacokinetic changes seen in a few of these studies are not small, none have been shown to affect the outcome of treatment and they are probably only of modest clinical importance, nevertheless it would be prudent to monitor the outcome of concurrent use. On the whole combined use would seem likely to be advantageous.

References

1 Hoffken G, Lode H, Wiley P-D. Pharmacokinetics and interaction in the bioavailability of new quinolones. In: Proc Int Symp on New Quinolones, Geneva 1986, 141.
2 Wingender W, Foerster D, Beerman D. Effect of gastric emptying on rate and extent of the systemic availability of ciprofloxacin. In: Proc 14th Int Congr Chemother, Kyoto, Japan 1986.
3 Søfrgel F, Koch U, Metz R, Stephan V. Cimetidine inhibits the hepatic metabolism of pefloxacin. In: Proc 26th Interscience Conference on Antimicrobial Agents and Chemotherapy, New Orleans, Louisiana 1986.
4 COMPRECIN (enoxacin) Clinical Information Manual (Parke Davis) April 1989, references 222 and 223: Schentag JJ, Sedman AJ and Wilton DJ. Interaction between enoxacin, ranitidine and antacids. 3rd European Congress of Clinical Microbiology, The Hague (1987). Thomas D, Latts J, Sedman A, Kinkel A. A study to examine potential pharmacokinetic interaction of enoxacin (CI-919) with antacids or ranitidine, (Protocol 919–66), RR-764–00840, 1987.
5 Nix DE, Watson WA, Lener ME, Frost RW, Krol G, Goldstein H, Letterei J, Schentag JJ. Effects of aluminium and magnesium antacids and ranitidine on the absorption of ciprofloxacin. Clin Pharmacol Ther (1989) 46, 700–5.
6 Lebsack M, Nix D, Schentag J, Welage L, Ryerson B, Totthaker R, Sedman A. Impact of gastric pH on ranitidine-enoxacin drug-drug interaction. J Clin Pharmacol (1988) 28, 939.

7 Grasela TH, Schentag JJ, Sedman AJ, Wilton JH, Thomas DJ, Schultz RW, Lebsack ME, Kinkel AW. Inhibition of enoxacin absorption by antacids and ranitidine. Antimicrob Ag Chemother (1989) 33, 615–7.

8 Höffken G, Lode H, Wiley R, Glatzel TD, Sievers D, Olschewski T, Borner K, Koeppe T. Pharmacokinetics and bioavailability of ciprofloxacin and ofloxacin: effect of food and antacid intake. Rev Infect Dis (1988) 10 Suppl 1, S138–9.

9 Ludwig E, Graber H, Székely É, Csiba A. Metabolic interactions of ciprofloxacin. Diag Microbiol Infect Dis (1990) 13, 135–41.

10 Prince RA, Liou W-S, Kasik JE. Effect of cimetidine on ciprofloxacin pharmacokinetics. Pharmacotherapy (1990) 10, 233.

11 Misiak PM, Eldon MA, Toothaker RD, Sedman AJ. Effects of oral cimetidine or ranitidine on the pharmacokinetics of intravenous enoxacin. J Clin Pharmacol (1993) 33, 53–6.

12 Nix D, Schentag J. Lomefloxacin absorption kinetics when administered with ranitidine and sucralfate. 29th Interscience Conf Antimicrob Ag Chemother (1989) 136.

13 Sörgel F, Mahr G, Koch HU, Stephan U, Wiesemann HG, Malter U. Effects of cimetidine on the pharmacokinetics of pefloxacin in healthy volunteers. Rev Infect Dis (1988) 10, Suppl 1, S137.

14 Shimada J, Hori S. Effect of antiulcer drugs on gastrointestinal absorption of norfloxacin. Chemotherapy (Tokyo) (1992) 40, 1141–7.

15. Shiba K, Yoshida M, Kachi M, Shimade J, Saito A, Sakai N. Effects of peptic ulcer-healing drugs on the pharmacokinetics of new quinolone. 17th Int Congr Chemother, June 1991, Berlin, Abstract 415.

16 Lebsack ME, Nix D, Ryerson B, Toothaker RD, Welage L, Norman AM, Schentag JJ, Sedman AJ. Effect of gastric acidity on enoxacin absorption. Clin Pharmacol Ther (1992) 52, 252–6.

17 Shiba K, Sakai J, Shimada J, Okazaki O, Aoki H, Hakusui H. Effects of antacids, ferrous sulphate and ranitidine on absorption of DR-3355 in humans. Antimicrob Ag Chemother (1992) 36, 2270–4.

Quinolone antibiotics + Iron and zinc preparations

Abstract/Summary

Iron preparations such as ferrous fumarate, gluconate and sulphate can markedly reduce the absorption of ciprofloxacin, levofloxacin, norfloxacin and ofloxacin from the gut. Zinc interacts to a lesser extent.

Clinical evidence

200 mg iron (in the form of an iron-glycine-sulphate complex) reduced the bioavailability of the ciprofloxacin (500 mg) in 12 normal subjects by 48% and that of (400 mg) ofloxacin by 36%.[1]

325 mg ferrous sulphate three times a day reduced the absorption of ciprofloxacin in normal subjects by 64% (range 39–81%),[3,8] while a multivitamin with zinc preparation (*Stresstabs 600 with zinc*) reduced it by 24% (ranged 2–50%).[8] Another study reported that zinc reduced norfloxacin absorption by an unspecified amount.[9] A patient on ciprofloxacin (peak serum levels of 1.5 mg/l) developed reduced levels (0.3–0.5 mg/l) when given ferrous sulphate, and increased levels again (5.2 mg/l) when the ferrous sulphate was stopped.[4] 200 mg ferrous fumarate reduced the bioavailability of a single 200 mg dose of ciprofloxacin in eight normal subjects to 30%.[6] A further study found that ferrous sulphate, ferrous gluconate and *Centrum Forte* reduced the AUC of ciprofloxacin by 46%,

67% and 56% respectively, and the peak serum concentrations by 37%, 57% and 53% respectively.[7] *Centrum Forte* is a multi-mineral preparation containing iron, magnesium, zinc, calcium, copper and manganese.[7]

A very marked reduction (96%) in bioavailability was seen in a single dose study with ferrous sulphate and norfloxacin.[5] Another study by the same authors found that ferrous sulphate and zinc sulphate reduced the absorption of norfloxacin by 55–56%.[10] Ferrous sulphate was found to reduce the bioavailability of levofloxacin (DR-3355) by 79%.[11]

Mechanism

Uncertain, but the suggestion is that a quinolone-iron or -zinc complex is formed (chelation between the metal and the 4-oxo- and adjacent carboxyl groups) which is less easily absorbed. An *in vitro* study also showed that antibacterial effects of ciprofloxacin, ofloxacin and norfloxacin are markedly reduced by ferric chloride or ferrous sulphate when tested against *Salmonella typhimurium* and *Shigella sonnei*.[2]

Importance and management

The quinolone/iron interaction is established and would appear to be clinically important. Avoid the concurrent use of ciprofloxacin, levofloxacin, ofloxacin or norfloxacin and iron preparations. Alternatively, separate the dosages as much as possible to avoid mixing in the gut and monitor the effectiveness of the antibiotic treatment. There seems to be no direct information about other quinolones but, since many of them are known to interact with the metal ions found in a number of antacids, an interaction with iron would also be expected. The importance of the interaction with zinc is uncertain but monitor concurrent use and be alert for any evidence of a reduced antibiotic response.

References

1 Lode H, Stuhlert P, Deppermann KH, Mainz D. Pharmacokinetic interactions between ciprofloxacin/ofloxacin and ferro-salts. 29th Int Conf Antimicrob Ag Chemother, Houston Tex (1989), 136.

2 Smith JT. Oral iron, 4-quinolones and enteric infection. 29th Int Conf Antimicrob Ag Chemother, Houston Tex (1989) 149.

3 Polk RE. Effect of ferrous sulfate and multivitamins with zinc on the absorption of ciprofloxacin in normal volunteers. 29th Int Conf Antimicrob Ag Chemother, Houston Tex (1989) 136.

4 LePennec M P, Kitzis M D, Terdjman M, Foubard S, Garbarz E, Hanania G. Possible interaction of ciprofloxacin with ferrous sulphate. J Antimicrob Chemother (1990) 25, 184–5.

5 Okhamafe AO, Akerele JO, Chukuka CS. Pharmacokinetic interactions of norfloxacin with some metallic medicinal agents. Int J Pharmaceutics (1991) 68, 11–18.

6 Brouwers JRBJ, Van der Kam HJ, Sijtsma J, Proost JH. Decreased ciprofloxacin absorption with concomitant administration of ferrous fumarate. Pharm Weekbl [Sci] 1990, 12, 182–3.

7 Kara M, Hasinoff BB, McKay DW, Campbell NRC. Clinical and chemical interactions between iron preparations and ciprofloxacin. Br J clin Pharmac (1991) 31, 257–61.

8 Polk RE, Healey DP, Sahai J, Drwal L, Racht E. Effect of ferrous sulfate and multivitamins with zinc on the absorption of ciprofloxacin in normal volunteers. Antimicrob Ag Chemother (1989) 33, 1841–4.

9 Campbell NRC, Kara M, Hasinoff BB, McKay DW. Clinical and chemical

interactions between norfloxacin and clinically used metal ions. Clin Invest Med (1991) 14, A18.

10 Campbell NRC, Kara M, Hasinoff BB, Haddara WM, McKay DW. Norflox-acin interaction with antacids and minerals. Br J clin Pharmac (1992) 33, 115–6.

11 Shiba K, Okazaki O, Aoki H, Sakaj O, Shimada J. Inhibition of DR-3355 absorption by metal ions. 31st Intersci Conf Antimicrob Ag Chemother (1991) Abstracts, 198.

Quinolone antibiotics + Metronidazole

Abstract/Summary, clinical evidence, mechanism, importance and management

Metronidazole appears not to affect the pharmacokinetics of ciprofloxacin[1,2] or pefloxacin[3] but the clearance of metronida-zole may be reduced.[1] There seem to be no adverse interac-tions.

References

1 Ludwig E, Graber H, Székely É, Csiba A. Metabolic interactions of ciprofloxacin. Diag Microbiol Infect Dis (1990) 13, 135–41.

2 Boeckh M, Grineisen S, Shokry F. Pharmacokinetics and serum bacteri-cidal activity of ciprofloxacin and ofloxacin alone and in combination with metronidazole or clindamycin. In Abstract book of the 28th Interscience Conf Antimicrob Ag Chemotherapy, Los Angeles, Calif. (1988) Abstr 770.

3 Metz R, Jaehde U, Wiesemann H, Gottschalk B, Stephan U, Schunack W. Pharmacokinetic interactions and non-interactions of pefloxacin. Proc 15th Int Congr Chemother, Istanbul, 1987, 997.

Quinolone antibiotics + Non-steroidal anti-inflammatory drugs (NSAIDs)

Abstract/Summary, clinical evidence, mechanism, importance and management

A study on more than 1500 patients on ofloxacin found that the incidence of psychotic side-effects (euphoria, hysteria, psychosis) was not increased by the concurrent use of NSAIDs (aspirin, diclofenac, dipyrone indomethacin, paracetamol).[1] No special precautions are necessary.

Reference

1 Jüngst G, Weidmann E, Breitstadt A, Huppertz E. Does ofloxacin interact with NSAID's to cause psychotic side-effects ? 17th Int Congr Chemother, Berlin, June 23–8, 1991, 408.

Quinolone antibiotics + Other antibiotics

Abstract/Summary

Rifampicin (rifampin) appears not to have a clinically impor-tant effect on either ciprofloxacin, fleroxacin or pefloxacin. Azlocillin reduces the clearance of ciprofloxacin. Piperacillin, ceftazidime and tobramycin appear not to affect the pharmaco-kinetics of pefloxacin, nor amoxycillin the absorption of ofloxacin. Clindamycin appears not to affect the pharmacoki-netics of ciprofloxacin but it may antagonize its effects on *S. aureus.*

Clinical evidence, mechanism, importance and management

(a) Quinolones + Rifampicin (Rifampin)

Ciprofloxacin (750 mg 12-hourly) and rifampicin (300 mg 12-hourly) for 2 weeks did not significantly affect the pharmacok-inetics of either drug in 12 elderly patients (aged 67–95).[2] This confirms two other pharmacokinetic studies, one of which also reported that combined use provided excellent serum bacteri-cial activity against *S. aureus* strains, although somewhat lower than rifampicin alone.[1,6]

A study in eight normal subjects found that 900 mg rifampi-cin daily for 10 days decreased the half-life and AUC_{0-12} of pefloxacin (400 mg twice daily) by about 30% due to a 35% increase in total plasma clearance.[4] Despite these changes the serum pefloxacin levels still remained well above the minimal inhibitory concentrations (0.50 mg/l) for 90% of strains of methicillin-sensitive strains of *S. aureus* and *S. epidermis*.[4] An-other study in 13 normal subjects found that after taking 600 mg rifampicin daily for a week, the clearance of fleroxacin (400 mg daily) was increased by 18% but the fleroxacin levels remained above the MIC_{90} of susceptible *S. aureus* for at least 24 h.[7] No special precautions would seem necessary if rifampi-cin is given with any of these quinolones.

(b) Quinolones + Other antibiotics

A single dose study found that azlocillin (60 mg/kg IV) increased the AUC of ciprofloxacin (4 mg/kg IV) by 35%.[3] Another study found that single IV doses of 4 g piperacillin, 2 g ceftazidime or 100 mg tobramycin had no effect on the pharmacokinetics of pefloxacin.[5] The absorption of ofloxacin is not altered by amoxycillin.[8]

One study found that the pharmacokinetics of ciprofloxacin are not affected by clindamycin and there is evidence that combined use may possibly enhance the antibacterial activity against streptococci and staphylococci,[8] while another found that the serum bacterial activity of ciprofloxacin against *S. aureus* was completely antagonised by clindamycin if the strains were susceptible to the latter.[9]

References

1 Rubin J et al, unpublished observations quoted by Polk RE, Drug-drug interactions with ciprofloxacin and other fluoroquinolones. Am J Med (1989) 87 (Suppl 5A) 76–81S.

2 Chandler MHH, Toler SM, Rapp RP, Muder RR, Korvick JA. Multiple-dose pharmacokinetics of concurrent oral ciprofloxacin and rifampin therapy in elderly patients. Antimicrol Ag Chemother (1990) 34, 442–7.

3 Barriere SL, Catlin DH, Orlando PLK, Noe A, Frost RW. Alteration in the

pharmacokinetic disposition of ciprofloxacin by simultaneous administration of azlocillin. Antimicrob Ag Chemother (1990) 34, 823–6.

4 Humbert G, Brumpt I, Montay G, Le Liboux A, Frydman A, Borsa-Lebas F, Moore N. Influence of rifampin on the pharmacokinetics of pefloxacin. Clin Pharmacol Ther (1991) 50, 682–7.

5 Metz R, Jaehde U, Wiesemann H, Gottschalk B, Stephan U, Schunack W. Pharmacokinetic interactions and non-interactions of pefloxacin. Proc 15th Int Congr Chemother, Istanbul, 1987, 997.

6 Paintaud G, Alván G, Hellgren U, Nilsson-Ehle I. Lack of effect of amoxicillin on the absorption of ofloxacin. Eur J Clin Pharmacol (1993) 44, 207–9.

7 Schrenzel J, Dayer P, Weidekamm E, Portmann R, Lew DP. Influence of rifampin on the pharmacokinetics of fleroxacin. Int Sci Conf Antimicrob Ag Chemother (1992) Abstracts, p 355.

8 Deppermann K-M, Boeckh M, Grineisen S, Shokry F, Borner K, Koeppe P, Krasemann C, Wagner J, Lode H. Brief report: combination effects of ciprofloxacin, clindamycin and metronidazole intravenously in volunteers. Amer J Med (1989) 87 (Suppl 5A) 5A-46–8S.

9 Weinstein MP, Deeter RG, Swanson KA, Gross JS. Crossover assessment of serum bacterial activity and pharmacokinetics of ciprofloxacin alone and in combination in healthy volunteers. Antimicrob Ag Chemother (1991) 35, 2352–8.

Quinolone antibiotics + Pancreatic enzyme supplements

Abstract/Summary

Ciprofloxacin is not affected by pancreatic enzyme supplements.

Clinical evidence, mechanism, importance and management

Six patients with cystic fibrosis, chronically infected with *P. aeruginosa* and treated with a range of drugs including ceftazidime, tobramycin, ticarcillin and salbutamol, demonstrated no significant changes in the pharmacokinetics of single 750 mg doses of ciprofloxacin when given standard doses of pancreatic enzymes (seven *Pancrease* capsules).[1] No special precautions would seem to be necessary during concurrent use.

Reference

1 Mack G, Cooper PJ, Buchanan N. Effects of enzyme supplementation on oral absorption of ciprofloxacin in patients with cystic fibrosis. Antimicrob Ag Chemother (1991) 35, 1484–5.

Quinolone antibiotics + Pirenzepine or dairy products

Abstract/Summary

Pirenzepine and most foods delay but do not reduce the absorption of amifloxacin, ciprofloxacin, enoxacin, lomefloxacin or ofloxacin. Dairy products reduce the bioavailability of ciprofloxacin and norfloxacin, but not ofloxacin or amifloxacin.

Clinical evidence, mechanism, importance and management

(a) Dairy products

A study in seven normal subjects given single 500 mg doses of ciprofloxacin found that 300 ml milk or yoghourt reduced the serum levels at 30 min by 70% and 92%, peak levels by 36% and 47%, and the AUC by 30% and 36% respectively.[3] Another study found that 300 ml milk of yoghourt reduced the absorption and the peak serum levels of a single 500 mg dose of norfloxacin by about 50%.[7] The reason is that the calcium in from the milk and yoghourt combines with the ciprofloxacin and norfloxacin to produce insoluble chelates. The effect of these changes on the control of infection are uncertain but until the situation is clear patients should be advised not to take these dairy products within 1–2 h of the antibiotic to prevent admixture in the gut.

In contrast, a study in 21 normal subjects found that 8 ozs (about 250 ml) milk had no clinically significant effects on the absorption of ofloxacin.[4] Another study confirmed this lack of interaction with both milk and yoghurt.[8] The bioavailability of amifloxacin is also minimally altered by milk.[5]

(b) Other food or pirenzepine

Four 50 mg oral doses of pirenzepine or food delayed the absorption of ciprofloxacin and ofloxacin in 10 subjects, but their bioavailabilities remain unchanged.[1] A study using a high fat and high calcium meal found no important change in the absorption of ciprofloxacin.[5] Another study confirmed that a delay occurs with ofloxacin but the bioavailability is unchanged.[4] Food delays the time when peak serum levels of lomefloxacin are achieved, but peak levels and the amount absorbed are unaltered.[2] Food similarly has little effect on amifloxacin.[5] Food also has no effect on the absorption of enoxacin, but high carbohydrate meals cause a delay (almost an hour) in the achievement of peak serum levels.[6] All of these changes are probably of minimal clinical importance.

References

1 Höffken G, Lode H, Wiley R, Glatzel TD, Sievers D, Olschewski T, Borner K, Koeppe T. Pharmacokinetics and bioavailability of ciprofloxacin and ofloxacin: effect of food and antacid intake. Rev Infect Dis (1988) 10 Suppl 1, S138–9.

2 Hooper WD, Dickinson RG, Eadie MJ. Effect of food on absorption of lomefloxacin. Antimicrob Ag Chemother (1990) 34, 1797–9.

3 Neuvonen PJ, Kivistö KT, Lehto P. Interference of dairy products with the absorption of ciprofloxacin. Clin Pharmacol Ther (1991) 50, 498–502.

4 Dudley MN, Marchbanks CR, Flor SC, Beals B. The effect of food or milk on the absorption kinetics of ofloxacin. Eur J Clin Pharmacol (1991) 41, 569–71.

5 Stroshane RM, Brown RR, Cook JA, Wissel PS, Silverman MH. Effect of food, milk and antacid on the absorption of orally administered amifloxacin. Rev Infect Dis (1989) 11, Suppl 5, S1018–9.

6 Somogyi AA, Bochner F, Keal JA, Rolan PE, Smith M. Effect of food on enoxacin absorption. Antimicrob Ag Chemother (1987) 31, 638–9.

7 Kivistö KT, Ojala-Karlsson P, Neuvonen PJ. Inhibition of norfloxacin absorption by dairy products. Antimicrob Ag Chemother (1992) 36, 489–91.

8 Neuvonen PJ, Kivistö KT. Milk and yoghurt do not impair the absorption of ofloxacin. Br J clin Pharmac (1992) 33, 346–8.

Quinolone antibiotics + Probenecid

Abstract/Summary

Serum cinoxacin, enoxacin and nalidixic acid levels are markedly increased by the concurrent use of probenecid but fleroxacin levels are only moderately increased and those of ciprofloxacin are unaffected.

Clinical evidence

(a) Cinoxacin

A study in six subjects found that while taking 0.5 g probenecid three times daily the serum levels of cinoxacin following an infusion were approximately doubled.[4]

(b) Ciprofloxacin

1 g probenecid given 30 min before 500 mg ciprofloxacin was found to reduce the renal clearance by up to 50%, but since other pharmacokinetic parameters (maximum serum levels, AUC) were unchanged, no accumulation of ciprofloxacin appears to occur.[7]

(c) Enoxacin

The renal clearance of 600 mg enoxacin was halved (from 374 to 171 ml/min) in one subject and the half-life increased from 3 to 7 h after taking 2.5 g probenecid.[6]

(d) Fleroxacin

A study in normal subjects given a single 200 mg dose of fleroxacin, followed by 500 mg probenecid at 0.5, 12, 24 and 36 h later, found that the fleroxacin AUC was increased by 37% (from 32.6 to 44.7 mg/h/l), the maximal serum levels were slightly but not significantly increased, and its unchanged urinary excretion was decreased by 22%.[3] Another study found that probenecid had no significant effects of its urinary excretion.[5]

(e) Nalidixic acid

Following the observation of a man who had ingested unknown amounts of several drugs including nalidixic acid and probenecid and who showed grossly elevated nalidixic acid serum levels, the possible interaction between these two drugs was studied. Two volunteers, acting as their own controls, ingested 0.5 g nalidixic acid with and without 0.5 g probenecid. Their peak serum nalidixic acid levels were unaffected at 2 h, but at 8 h the levels were increased three-fold by the presence of probenecid.[1]

Another study in five women with urinary tract infections treated with nalidixic acid showed that the concurrent use of probenecid increased the maximal serum nalidixic acid concentrations and the AUC by 43% (from 33 to 48 µg/ml) and 74% (from 82 to 143 µg.h.ml^{-1}) respectively.[2]

Mechanism

The reasons are not well understood but a suggested explanation is that probenecid successfully competes with these quinolones for excretion by the kidney tubules so that they are retained in the body. Some changes in metabolism are also possible.

Importance and management

The importance of the interactions between cinoxacin, enoxacin or nalidixic acid and probenecid is uncertain, but the increase in the serum antibiotic levels is probably advantageous. There seems to be no good reason for avoiding the concurrent use of probenecid and any of these quinolones.

References

1 Dash H, Mills J. Severe metabolic acidosis associated with nalidixic acid overdose. Ann Intern Med (1976) 84, 570.
2 Ferry N, Cuisinaud G, Pozet N, Zech PY, Sassard J. Influence du probenecid sur la pharmacocinetique de l'acide nalidixique. Therapie (1982) 37, 645–9.
3 Shiba K, Saito A, Shimada J, Hori S, Kaji M, Miyahara T, Kusajima H, Kaneko S. Interactions of fleroxacin with dried aluminium hydroxide gel and probenecid. Rev Infect Dis (1989) II (Suppl 5), S1097–8.
4 Rodriguez N, Madsen PO, Welling PG. Influence of probenecid on serum levels and urinary excretion of cinoxacin. Antimicrob Ag Chemother (1979) 15, 465–69.
5 Weidekamm E, Portmann R, Suter K, Partos C, Dell D, Lücker PW. Single- and multiple dose pharmacokinetics of fleroxacin, a trifluorinated quinolone, in humans. Antimicrob Ag Chemother (1987) 31, 1909–14.
6 Wijnands WJA, Vree TB, Baars AM, van Herwaarden CLA. Pharmacokinetics of enoxacin and its penetration into brochial secretions and lung tissue. J Antimicrob Ag Chemother (1988) 21, Suppl B, 67–77.
7 Wingender W, Beerman D, Förster D, Graefe K-H, Kuhlmann J. Interactions of ciprofloxacin with food intake and drugs. Curr Clin Pract Ser (1986) 34, 136–140.

Quinolone antibiotics + Sucralfate

Abstract/Summary

Sucralfate causes only a modest reduction in fleroxacin levels whereas a very marked reduction occurs in the absorption of ciprofloxacin, enoxacin, lomefloxacin, ofloxacin and norfloxacin if taken together. The interaction is very much reduced if the sucralfate is given 2–6 h after the antibiotic.

Clinical evidence

(a) Ciprofloxacin + Sucralfate

The absorption of 500 mg ciprofloxacin in 8 normal subjects was reduced by 91% (from 8.8 to 1.1 µg/h/ml) and the maximum serum concentration by 90% (from 2.0 to 0.2 µg/ml) while taking 1 g sucralfate four times daily.[5]

A patient given 1 g sucralfate four times daily had serum ciprofloxacin levels which were 85–90% lower than five other patients who were not taking sucralfate.[3] A single dose study found a 60% reduction in the AUC of ciprofloxacin following a 2 g dose of sucralfate.[6] A study in 12 normal subjects found that a 1 g dose of sucralfate 6 and 12 h before a single 750 mg dose of ciprofloxacin, reduced the ciprofloxacin AUC (area under the concentration-time curve) by 30%. Three of the subjects showed little or no changes but a decrease of more than 50% was seen in four others.[2] A related study in 12 subjects found that the bioavailabilites of 750 mg ciprofloxacin were 4%, 82% and 96% respectively when given at the same time, 2 h and 6 h before the sucralfate.[7]

(b) Enoxacin + Sucralfate

1 g sucralfate given to eight normal subjects 2 h before or with 400 mg enoxacin reduced the bioavailability by 54% and 88% respectively. When given 2 h after the enoxacin no changes occurred.[9]

(c) Fleroxacin + Sucralfate

The bioavailability of 400 mg fleroxacin was reduced to 76% in 20 normal subjects taking 1 g sucralfate six-hourly.[12,13]

(d) Lomefloxacin + Sucralfate

A study in 12 normal subjects found that when 400 mg lomefloxacin was given 2 h after 1 g sucralfate the lomefloxacin AUC was reduced by 25% and the maximal serum concentration by 30%.[10]

(e) Norfloxacin + Sucralfate

A study in eight normal subjects showed that while taking sucralfate (1 g four times daily) the bioavailability of single 400 mg doses of norfloxacin as measured by changes in the AUC was markedly reduced: to 1.8% when taken with the sucralfate and to 56.6% when taken 2 h afterwards.[1,4,8]

(f) Ofloxacin + Sucralfate

A single dose study found that sucralfate (dose not stated) reduced the maximum serum levels and the AUC of a single dose of ofloxacin to about one-third.[11]

Mechanism

Not fully established, but a likely explanation is that the aluminium hydroxide component of sucralfate (200 mg in each g) forms an insoluble chelate with the quinolone which reduces its absorption. See 'Quinolones and Antacids'.

Importance and management

Established and clinically important interactions. As it seems likely that serum ciprofloxacin, enoxacin, lomefloxacin, ofloxacin and norfloxacin levels will be reduced to subtherapeutic concentrations if given with the sucralfate, separate the dosages as much as possible (by 2 h or more) giving the quinolone first. More study is needed to confirm both these findings and the effectiveness of separating the dosages. The interaction with fleroxacin is only modest (bioavailability reduced 24%) and probably not clinically important, but some separation of the dosages might improve matters. This needs confirmation. Pefloxacin also interacts with antacids containing aluminium hydroxide (see Quinolones + Antacids) and may therefore possibly interact with sucralfate.

References

1 Parpia SH, Nix DE, Hejmanowski LG, Wilton JH, Goldstein HR, Schentag JJ. The effect of sucralfate on the oral bioavailability of norfloxacin. Pharmacotherapy (1988) 8, 140.

2 Nix DE, Watson WA, Handy L, Frost RW, Rescott DL, Goldstein HR. The effect of sucralfate pretreatment on the pharmacokinetics of ciprofloxacin. Pharmacotherapy (1989) 9, 377–80.

3 Yuk JH, Nightingale CN, Quintiliani R. Ciprofloxacin levels when receiving sucralfate. J Amer Med Ass (1989) 262, 901.

4 Parpia S H, Nix D E, Hejmanowski L G, Goldstein HR, Witton JH, Schentag JJ. Sucralfate reduces the gastrointestinal absorption of norfloxacin. Antimicrob Ag Chem (1989) 33, 99–102.

5 Garrelts JC, Godley PJ, Peterie JD, Gerlach EH, Yakshe CC. Sucralfate significantly reduces ciprofloxacin concentrations in serum. Antimicrob Ag Chemother (1990) 34, 931–3.

6 Brouwers JRBJ, van der Kam HJ, Sijtsma J, Proost JH. Important reduction of ciprofloxacin absorption by sucralfate and magnesium citrate solution. Drug Invest (1990) 2, 197–9.

7 Van Slooten AD, Nix DE, Wilton JH, Love JH, Spivey JM, Goldstein HR. Combined use of ciprofloxacin and sucralfate. DICP Ann Pharmacother (1991) 25, 578–82.

8 Nix DE, Wilton JH, Schentag JJ, Parpia SH, Norman A, Goldstein HR. Inhibition of norfloxacin absorption by antacids and sucralfate. Rev Inf Dis (1989) II, Suppl 5, S1096.

9 Ryerson B, Toothaker R, Schleyer I, Sedman A, Colburn W. Effect of sucralfate on enoxacin pharmacokinetics. 29th Intersci Conf Antimicrob Ag Chemotherapy (1989) 136.

10. Nix D, Schentag J. Lomefloxacin absorption kinetics when administered with ranitidine and sucralfate. 29th Interscience Conf Antimicrob Ag Chemother (1989) 136.

11 Shiba K, Yoshida M, Kachi M, Shimade J, Saito A, Sakai N. Effects of peptic ulcer-healing drugs on the pharmacokinetics of new quinolone. 17th Int Congr Chemother, June 1991, Berlin, Abstract 415.

12 Lubowski TJ, Nightingale CH, Sweeney K, Quintiliani R. An unusually marginal interaction between fleroxacin and sucralfate. Int Sci Conf Antimicrob Ag Chemother (1992) Abstracts, p 355.

13 Lubowski TJ, Nightingale CH, Sweeney K, Quintiliani R. Effect of sucralfate on pharmacokinetics of fleroxacin in healthy volunteers. Antimicrob Ag Chemother (1992) 36, 2785–60.

Rifampicin (Rifampin) + Aminosalicylic acid (PAS)

Abstract/Summary

The serum levels of rifampicin are halved if aminosalicylic acid in granular form containing bentonite is used concurrently. This interaction may be avoided by separating the dosages by 8–12 h or by using an aminosalicylic acid formulation which does not contain bentonite.

Clinical evidence

A study in 30 patients with tuberculosis found that their serum rifampicin levels (doses 10 mg/kg) were reduced more than 50% (from 6.06 to 2.91 µg/ml) at 2 h by the concurrent use of PAS-Granulate (*Ferrosan*).[1] Subsequent studies by the same workers on six normal subjects showed that this interaction was not due to the aminosalicylic acid itself but to the bentonite which was the main excipient of the granules.[2] Other studies confirm this marked reduction in serum rifampicin levels in the presence of aminosalicylic acid granules.[3,4]

Mechanism

The bentonite excipient in aminosalicylic acid granules adsorbs the rifampicin so that much less is available for absorption by the gut, resulting in reduced serum levels.

Importance and management

Well documented and clinically important. Separating the administration of the two drugs by 8–12 h to prevent their mixing in the gut has been suggested as an effective way to prevent this interaction.[1] An alternative is to give aminosalicylic acid preparations which do not contain bentonite or any other substances which can adsorb rifampicin.

References

1 Boman G, Hanngren A, Malmborg A-S, Borga O, Sjoqvist F. Drug Interaction: decreased serum concentrations of rifampicin when given with PAS. Lancet (1971) i, 800.
2 Boman G, Lundgren P, Stjernstrom G. Mechanism of the inhibitory effect of PAS granules on the absorption of rifampicin: absorption of rifampicin by an excipient, bentonite. Eur J clin Pharmacol (1975) 8, 293.
3 Boman G. Serum concentrations and half-life of rifampicin after simultaneous oral administration of aminosalicylic acid or isoniazid. Eur J clin Pharmacol (1974) 7, 217.
4 Boman G, Borga O, Hanngren A, Malmborg A-S, Sjoqvist F. Pharmacokinetic interactions between the tuberculostatics rifampicin, para-aminosalicylic acid and isoniazid. Acta Pharmac Toxicol (1970) 28, (Suppl 1) 15.

Rifampicin (Rifampin) + Antacids

Abstract/Summary

The absorption of rifampicin can be reduced up to 36% by the concurrent use of antacids but the clinical importance of this is uncertain.

Clinical evidence

When single 600 mg doses of rifampicin were taken with different antacids and 200 ml of water by five normal subjects, the absorption of the rifampicin was reduced as follows (as measured by the fall in the urinary excretion): with 15 or 30 ml aluminium hydroxide gel (20–31% reduction); with 2 or 4 g magnesium trisilicate (32–36% reduction); and with 2 g sodium carbonate (21% reduction).[1]

Mechanism

The rise in the pH within the stomach caused by these antacids reduces the dissolution of the rifampicin thereby inhibiting its absorption. In addition aluminium ions may form less soluble chelates with rifampicin, and magnesium trisilicate can adsorb rifampicin, both of which would also be expected to reduce bioavailability.[1]

Importance and management

Direct information seems to be limited to this report. No one seems to have assessed the effects of a 20–35% reduction in absorption on rifampicin treatment, but if antacids are given it would be prudent to be alert for any evidence that it is less effective than expected.

Reference

1 Khalil SAH, El-Khordagui LK, El-Gholmy ZA. Effect of antacids on oral absorption of rifampicin. Int J Pharmaceut (1984) 20, 99–106.

Rifampicin (Rifampin) + Clofazimine

Abstract/Summary

Rifampicin appears not to interact adversely with clofazimine.

Clinical evidence, mechanism, importance and management

The pharmacokinetics of rifampicin were not altered by clofazimine in a multidose study,[1] confirming a single dose study which found that the bioavailability of clofazimine remained unaltered, although a reduction in the rate of absorption was seen.[2] No special precautions would seem to be necessary.

References

1 Venkatesan K, Mathur A, Girdhar BK, Bharadwaj VP. The effect of clofazimine on the pharmacokinetics of rifampicin and dapsone in leprosy. J Antimicrob Chemother (1986) 18, 715–18.
2 Mehta J, Gandhi IS, Sane SB, Wamburkar MN. Effect of clofazimine and dapsone on rifampicin (Lostril) pharmacokinetics in multibacillary and paucibacillary leprosy cases. Indian J Lepr (1985) 57, 297–310.

Rifampicin (Rifampin) + Co-trimoxazole

Abstract/Summary

Co-trimoxazole can increase rifampicin serum levels.

Clinical evidence, mechanism, importance and management

Co-trimoxazole (two tablets 12-hourly) for 5–10 days in 15 patients with tuberculosis increased the AUC of rifampicin (450 mg daily) by 62% and the peak levels by 31%. The reasons are not understood. No adverse effects were seen but the authors of the report point out that while concurrent use may be beneficial there is also the risk that hepatotoxicity may be increased.[1] Good monitoring is advised.

Reference

1 Bhatia RS, Uppal R, Malhi R, Behera D, Jindal SK. Drug interaction between rifampicin and co-trimoxazole in patients with tuberculosis. Hum Exptl Toxicol (1991) 10, 419–21.

Rifampicin (Rifampin) + Dipyrone

Abstract/Summary

The pharmacokinetics of rifampicin are not significantly changed by dipyrone.

Clinical evidence, mechanism, importance and management

A study in untreated patients with leprosy showed that the pharmacokinetics of a single 600 mg dose of rifampicin were not statistically significantly changed by 1 g dipyrone, but peak serum rifampicin levels occurred sooner (at 3 instead of 4 h) and were about 50% higher.[1] However it should be emphasized that dipyrone is often considered an unsafe drug because, like the related amidopyrine, it can cause potentially fatal agranulocytosis. It has been stated that it should only be used in serious and life-threatening situations where alternative antipyretics are not available.[2]

References

1 Krishna DR, Ramankar TV, Prabhakar MC. Pharmacokinetics of rifampin in the presence of dipyrone in leprosy patients. Drug Dev Ind Pharm (1984) 10, 101–10.
2 Reynolds JEF (ed). Martindale. The Extra Pharmacopoeia Edition 28, Pharmaceutical Press, London (1982) p 251.

Rifampicin (Rifampin) + Food

Abstract/Summary

Food delays and reduces the absorption of rifampicin from the gut.

Clinical evidence

When a single 10 mg/kg dose of rifampicin was taken by six normal subjects with a standard Indian breakfast (125 g wheat, 10 g visible fat, 350 g vegetables) the absorption of the rifampicin was reduced. The AUC after 8 h was reduced by 26%. and the peak serum levels were reduced by 30% (from 11.84 µg/ml at 2 h to 8.35 µg/ml at 4 h).[1]

Mechanism

Not understood.

Importance and management

An established interaction. The recommendation is that rifampicin should be taken on an empty stomach or 30 min before a meal, or 2 h after a meal to ensure rapid and complete absorption.

Reference

1 Polasa K, Krishnaswamy K. Effect of food on bioavailability of rifampicin. J Clin Pharmacol (1983) 23, 433–7.

Rifampicin (Rifampin) + Probenecid

Abstract/Summary

Whether or not the serum levels of rifampicin are increased by the concurrent use of probenecid is unpredictable.

Clinical evidence, mechanism, importance and management

A study in five normal subjects given probenecid before and after taking single 300 mg doses of rifampicin showed that mean peak serum rifampicin levels were raised 86%. At 4, 6 and 9 h the percentage increases were 118, 90 and 102% respectively.[1] However subsequent studies in patients, taking either 600 or 300 mg rifampicin plus 2 g probenecid taken 30 min before, showed that the latter group achieved serum rifampicin levels which were only about half those achieved by those on 600 g rifampicin.[2] Similar results were found in another study on patients given 450 mg rifampicin. The reasons for these discordant results are not understood.

Rifampicin is effective but expensive, so that the idea of giving smaller doses with probenecid to raise serum levels is attractive because the cost of treatment might hopefully be reduced. But the response of patients is so inconsistent and unpredictable that these drugs cannot be used together routinely for this purpose. It should however be borne in mind that the occasional patient may show elevated rifampicin levels.

References

1 Kenwright S, Levi AJ. Impairment of hepatic uptake of rifamycin antibiotics by probenecid, and its therapeutic implications. Lancet (1973) ii, 1401.
2 Fallon RJ, Lees AE, Allan GW, Smith J, Tyrrell WF. Probenecid and rifampicin serum levels. Lancet (1975) ii, 792.

Rifampicin (Rifampin) + Ranitidine

Abstract/Summary

Rantidine appears not to interact with rifampicin.

Clinical evidence, mechanism, importance and management

A controlled study in 112 patients with pulmonary tuberculosis treated with a daily regimen of rifampicin (10 mg/kg), isoniazid (300 mg) and ethambutol (20 mg/kg) found that 150 mg ranitidine twice daily did not affect the pharmacokinetics of the rifampicin (as measured by the total and unchanged urinary excretion). No changes occurred in the incidence of adverse hepatic reactions, while gastrointestinal reactions were reduced.[1] There would seem to be no reason for avoiding the concurrent use of these drugs. Ranitidine also appears not to interact with isoniazid (see Isoniazid + Cimetidine or Ranitidine).

Reference

1 Purohit SD, Johri SC, Gupta PR, Mehta YR, Bhatnagar M. Ranitidine-rifampicin interaction. J Assoc Phys India (1992) 40, 308–10.

Rifampicin (Rifampin) + Triacetyloleandomycin (Troleandomycin)

Abstract/Summary

Cholestatic jaundice has been attributed to the concurrent use of these two antibiotics.

Clinical evidence, mechanism, importance and management

Two cases of cholestatic jaundice have been reported in patients treated with both rifampicin and triacetyloleandomycin.[1,2] Both antibiotics are potentially hepatotoxic and it seems possible that their liver damaging effects can be additive. As a general rule the concurrent use of hepatotoxic drugs should be avoided.

References

1 Piette F, Peyrard P. Ictere benin medicamenteux lors d'un traitement associant rifampicin-triacetyloleandomycine. Nouv Presse med (1979) 8, 368.
2 Givaudan JF, Gamby Th, Privat Y. Ictere cholestatique apres association rifampicine-troleandomycin: une nouvelle observation. Nouv Presse med (1979) 8, 2357.

Rifapentine + Other drugs

Abstract/Summary, clinical evidence, mechanism, importance and management

Rifapentine (MDL 473) is a derivative of rifampicin with a similar antibacterial spectrum, approximately a ten times greater potency, and a longer half-life. Like rifampicin it is a potent liver enzyme inducing agent.[1] Although so far no clinically important interactions have been documented, it would be expected to interact with many of the drugs with which rifampicin interacts (see Index).

Reference

1 Durand DV, Hampden C, Boobis AR, Park BK, Davies DS. Induction of mixed function oxidase activity in man by rifapentine (MDL 473), a long-acting rifamycin derivative. Br J clin Pharmac (1986) 21, 1–7.

Rimantadine + Cimetidine

Abstract/Summary

Cimetidine causes a small but probably clinically unimportant rise in the serum levels of rimantadine.

Clinical evidence, mechanism, importance and management

After taking 300 mg cimetidine four times daily for 6 days, the AUC of a single 100 mg dose of rimantadine in 23 normal subjects was increased by 20% and the apparent total clearance reduced by 17%. The authors of the study suggest that these changes are likely to have little, if any, clinical consequences,[1] however this needs confirmation in patients who are actually being treated with rimantadine.

Reference

1 Holazo AA, Choma N, Kucera V, Sniezak B. The effect of cimetidine on the disposition of rimantadine in healthy subjects. J Clin Pharmacol (1988) 28, 908–59.

Sulphamethoxazole + Salbutamol (Albuterol)

Abstract/Summary

Salbutamol reduces the rate but increases the extent of absorption of sulphamethoxazole.

Clinical evidence, mechanism, importance and management

A study in six normal subjects found that 4 mg oral salbutamol (albuterol) four times daily for 2 weeks had no effect on the most of the pharmacokinetic parameters of a single 400 mg oral dose of sulphamethoxazole (in co-trimoxazole), except that the absorption rate constant was reduced about 40% (from 1.168 to 0.688/h) while the extent of absorption over 72 h was increased by 22.6%.[1] A possible reason is that the stimulation of the beta-receptors by the salbutamol in the gut causes relaxation which allows an increased contact time for the sulphamethoxazole.[1] The clinical significance of this interaction awaits assessment, but it seems unlikely to be of importance. No interaction would be expected with salbutamol given by inhalation.

Reference

1 Adebayo GI, Ogundipe TO. Effects of salbutamol on the absorption and disposition of sulphamethoxazole in adult volunteers. Eur J Drug Metab Pharmacokinet (1989) 14, 57–60.

Sulphasalazine + Antibiotics

Abstract/Summary

The release in the colon of the active drug (5-aminosalicylic acid) from sulphasalazine is markedly reduced by the concurrent use of ampicillin and rifampicin which reduce the activity of the gut bacteria. This interaction seems likely with any other oral antibiotic which similarly reduces the gut microflora.

Clinical evidence

(a) Sulphasalazine + Ampicillin

The conversion and release by the bacterial microflora within the gut of the active metabolite of sulphasalazine (5-aminosalicylic acid) was reduced by a third in five normal subjects (taking 2 g over 72 h) when they were also given 250 mg ampicillin four times daily.[1]

(b) Sulphasalazine + Rifampicin (Rifampin)

A crossover trial on 11 patients with Crohn's disease, on long term treatment with sulphasalazine, showed that while concurrently taking rifampicin (10 mg/kg/day) and ethambutol (15 mg/kg/day) their plasma levels of both 5-aminosalicylic acid and sulphapyridine fell by 60%.[2]

Mechanism

The azo link of sulphasalazine is split by the anaerobic bacteria in the colon to release sulphapyridine and 5-aminosalicylic acid, the latter being the active metabolite which acts locally in the treatment of Crohn's disease. Antibiotics which decimate the gut flora can apparently reduce this conversion and this is reflected in lower plasma levels. Rifampicin also possibly increased the metabolism of the sulphapyridine.

Importance and management

Information is limited but the interaction appears to be established. The extent to which these antibiotics reduce the effectiveness of sulphasalazine in the treatment of Crohn's disease or ulcerative colitis seems not to have been assessed, but it would clearly be prudent to be on the alert for evidence of a reduced effect if ampicillin, rifampicin or any other oral antibiotic (demonstrated with neomycin in animals[3]) is given which affects the activity of the gut microflora.

References

1 Houston JB, Day J, Walker J. Azo reduction of sulphasalazine in healthy volunteers. Br J clin Pharmac (1982) 14, 395–8.
2 Shaffer JL, Houston JB. The effect of rifampicin on sulphapyridine plasma concentrations following sulphasalazine administration. Br J clin Pharmac (1985) 19, 526–8.
3 Peppercorn MA, Goldman P. The role of intestinal bacteria in the metabolism of salicylazosulfapyridine. J Pharmacol Exp Ther (1972) 181, 555–62.

Sulphasalazine or Sodium Fusidate + Cholestyramine

Abstract/Summary

Animal studies show that cholestyramine can bind with these two drugs in the gut, thereby reducing their activity, but whether this also occurs in man awaits confirmation.

Clinical evidence, mechanism, importance and management

In vitro and *in vivo* studies with rats have shown that cholestyramine binds with sodium fusidate in the gut, thereby reducing the amount available for absorption.[1] Another study in rats found that cholestyramine binds with sulphasalazine so that the azo-bond is protected against attack by the bacteria within the gut. As a result the active 5-aminosalicylic acid is not released and the faecal excretion of intact sulphasalazine increases 30-fold.[2] It seems possible that both of these interactions could also occur in man, but confirmation of this is as yet lacking. Separating the dosages to prevent admixture in the gut has proved effective with other drugs which bind with cholestyramine.

References

1 Johns WE, Bates TR. Drug-cholestyramine interactions. I. Physicochemical factors affecting *in vitro* binding of sodium fusidate to cholestyramine. J Pharm Sci (1972) 61, 730.
2 Pieniaszek HJ, Bates TR. Cholestyramine-induced inhibition of salicylazosulfapyridine (sulfasalazine) metabolism by rat intestinal microflora. J Pharmacol Exp Ther (1976) 198, 240.

Sulphasalazine + Iron salts

Abstract/Summary

Sulphasalazine and iron appear to bind together in the gut, but whether this reduces the therapeutic response to either compound is uncertain.

Clinical evidence, mechanism, importance and management

400 mg ferrous iron reduced the serum levels of sulphasalazine in five normal subjects taking single 50 mg/kg doses. At 5 h the serum levels were reduced about 40%. The reasons are not known, but it seems likely that the sulphasalazine chelates with the iron in the gut which interferes with its absorption.[1] The extent to which this suggested chelation affects the ability of the intestinal bacteria to split the sulphasalazine and release its locally active metabolite (5-aminosalicylic acid) and thereby affects the therapeutic response, seems not to have been studied. More study is needed.

Reference

1 Das KM, Eastwood MA. Effect of iron and calcium on salicylazosulphapyridine metabolism. Scott Med J (1973) 18, 45–56.

Sulphasalazine + Metronidazole

Abstract/Summary

Metronidazole appears not to interact adversely with sulphasalazine.

Clinical evidence, mechanism, importance and management

A study in 10 patients (seven with Crohn's disease and five with ulcerative colitis) on long-term sulphasalazine treatment found no statistically significant changes in serum sulphapyridine levels while taking 400 mg metronidazole twice daily for 8–14 days.[1] There seems to be no good reason for avoiding concurrent use.

Reference

1 Shaffer JL, Kershaw A, Houston JB. Disposition of metronidazole and its effects on sulphasalazine metabolism in patients with inflammatory bowel disease. Br J clin Pharmac (1986) 21, 431–5.

Sulphonamides + Barbiturates

Abstract/Summary

The anaesthetic effects of thiopentone (thiopental) are increased but shortened by pretreatment with sulphafurazole (sulfisoxazole). Phenobarbitone appears not to interact signficantly with sulphafurazole or sulphasomidine. There seem to be no reports of any adverse sulphonamide-barbiturate interactions.

Clinical evidence

(a) Thiopentone (Thiopental) + Sulphafurazole (Sulfisoxazole)

A study in 48 patients showed that the prior intravenous administration of sulphafurazole (sulfisoxazole), 40 mg/kg, reduced the required anaesthetic dosage of thiopentone (thiopental) by 40%, but the awakening time was shortened.[1]

This interaction has also been observed in animal experiments.[2]

(b) Sulphafurazole or Sulphasomidine + Phenobarbitone (Phenobarbital)

A study in children showed that phenobaritone did not affect the pharmacokinetics of sulphfurazole (sulfisoxazole) or sulphasomidine.[3]

Mechanism

It is suggested that sulphafurazole successfully competes with the thiopentone for the plasma protein binding sites,[4] the result being that more free and active barbiturate molecules remain in circulation to exert their anaesthetic effects and a smaller dose is therefore required.

Importance and management

The evidence for the sulphfurazole-thiopentone interaction is limited, but it appears to be strong. Less thiopentone than usual may be required to achieve adequate anaesthesia, but since the awakening time is shortened repeated doses may be needed. Information about other sulphonamide-barbiturate interactions are also very limited, but none so far reported seems to be of clinical importance.

References

1 Csogor SI, Kerek SF. Enhancement of thiopentone anaesthesia by sulphafurazole. Br J Anaesth (1970) 42, 988.
2 Csogor SI, Palfy B, Feztz G. Influence du sulfathiazol sur l'effet narcotique du thiopental et de l'hexobarbital. Rev Roum Physiol (1971) 8, 81.
3 Krauer B. Comparative investigations of elimination kinetics of two sulphonamides in children with and without phenobarbital administration. Schweiz Med Wsch (1971) 101, 668.
4 Csogor SI, Papp J. Competition between sulphonamides and thiopental for binding sites on plasma proteins. Arzneim-Forsch (1970) 20, 1925.

Sulphonamides + Local anaesthetics

Abstract/Summary

The para-aminobenzoic acid (PABA) derived from certain local anaesthetics can reduce the effects of the sulphonamides and allow the development of local and even generalized infections.

Clinical evidence

Four patients on sulphonamides developed local infections in areas where procaine had been injected prior to diagnostic taps in meningitis, or draining procedures in empyema. Extensive cellulitis of the lumbar region occurred in one case, and the patient died of meningitis despite continued therapy with sulphadiazine.[1]

A study in man[2] demonstrated that the amount of procaine in pleural fluid after anaesthesia for thoracentesis was sufficient to inhibit the antibacterial activity of 5% sulphapyridine against type III pneumococci. Other studies in animals confirm that antagonism can occur both *in vitro*[6] and *in vivo*[3-5] with local anaesthetics which are hydrolyzed to PABA.

Mechanism

The ester type of local anaesthetic is hydrolyzed within the body to produce PABA which antagonizes the effects of the sulphonamides by competitive inhibition. A fuller explanation of the sulphonamide-PABA interaction is given in the 'Sulphonamide + PABA' synopsis.

Importance and management

Clinical examples of this interaction seem to be few but the supporting evidence (human, animal and *in vitro* studies dating back to the mid-1940s) is strong. This would seem to be an interaction of clinical importance. Local anaesthetics of the ester type which are hydrolyzed to PABA (e.g. amethocaine,

procaine, benzocaine) should be avoided in patients using sulphonamides, whereas those of the amide type (bupivacaine, cinchocaine [dibucaine], lignocaine [lidocaine], mepivacaine and prilocaine) do not interact adversely.

References

1 Peterson OL, Finland M. Sulfonamide inhibiting action of procaine. Amer J Med Sci (1944) 207, 166.
2 Boroff DA, Cooper A, Bullowa JGM. Inhibition of sulfapyridine by procaine in chest fluids after procaine anaesthesia. Proc Soc Exp Biol Med (1941) 47,182.
3 Pfeiffer CC, Grant CW. The procaine-sulfonamide antagonism: an evaluation of local anesthetics for use with sulfonamide therapy. Anesthesiology (1944) 5, 605.
4 Casten D, Fried JJ, Hallman FA. Inhibitory effect of procaine on bacteriostatic activity of sulfathiazole. Surg Gyn Obst (1943) 76, 726.
5 Powell HM, Krahl ME, Clowes GHA. Inhibition of chemotherapeutic action of sulfapyridine by local anesthetics. J Indiana Med Ass (1942) 35, 62.
6 Walker BS, Derow MA. The antagonism of local anesthetics against the sulfonamides. Amer J Med Sci (1945) 210, 585.

Sulphonamides + Para-aminobenzoic acid (PABA)

Abstract/Summary

The antibacterial effects of the sulphonamides are reduced or abolished by para-aminobenzoic acid (PABA).

Clinical evidence and mechanism

Many micro-organisms can synthesize their own folate if provided with para-aminobenzoic acid (PABA), whereas man needs preformed folate in his diet. The molecular structure of the sulphonamides is sufficiently like PABA for micro-organisms to incorporate them into the synthetic biochemical pathways concerned with making folate, but sufficiently dissimilar for the synthesis to fail. Starved of folate in this way, the organism ceases to grow and multiply, and it is in this way that the sulphonamides act as bacteriostatic agents. The term 'competitive antagonist' is used to describe this situation because PABA and the sulphonamide compete with one another to take part in the synthetic reactions, the relative concentrations of each molecule being among the factors which determine the 'winner', hence the clinical importance of achieving adequate concentrations of the sulphonamide and of avoiding the introduction of additional PABA molecules.

Importance and management

The interaction between PABA and the sulphonamides has been very extensively studied and is very well documented. PABA should not be given to patients taking sulphonamides. Although PABA features in both the BP and USP, it is now used largely in topical preparations as a sunscreen agent and it is most unlikely to be absorbed through the skin. Oral administration is probably not common. However potassium amino-benzoate is given orally and is therefore expected to interact with the sulphonamides just like PABA.

Temafloxacin + Miscellaneous drugs

Abstract/Summary, clinical evidence, mechanism, importance and management

Temfloxacin was withdrawn worldwide in the Summer of 1992 because of its adverse reactions which included hypogly-caemia and haemolytic anaemia, but for the sake of complete-ness its interactions are very briefly summarized here. A very marked reduction in bioavailability (– 60%) occurs if given with antacids such as *Maalox* (aluminium and magnesium hydroxide),[1,13] while a modest increase (22%) occurs with cimetidine.[1,12] The pharmacokinetics of caffeine are unaf-fected by temafloxacin,[2,14] and it has only minor effects on theophylline.[2–6,11] It causes no significant changes in the effects of oral contraceptives,[7,8] warfarin[9] or heparin.[10,15]

References

1 Seelmann R, Mahr G, Sörgel F, Gottschalf B, Granneman R, Sylvester J, Muth P, Stephan U. The effect of antacids and cimetidine on the pharmacokinetics of temafloxacin. 29th Interscience Conf Antimicrob Ag Chemother (1989) 136.

2 Sörgel F, Mahr G, Kinzig M, Buchal G, Noje M, Wiesemann HG, Stephan U, Granneman R. The influence of temafloxacin and ciprofloxacin on the elimination of caffeine in human volunteers. 31st Intersci Conf Antimi-crob Ag Chemother (1991) Abstracts, 197.

3 Mahr G, Seelmann R, Granneman R, Sylvester J, Gottschalf B, Jürgens C, Muth P, Stephan U, Sörgel F. The effect of temafloxacin and enoxacin on the pharmacokinetics of theophylline. Proc 29th Intersci Conf Antimicrob Ag Chemother (1989) Houston, Texas, p 137.

4 Santais M-C, Grossriether H, Callens E, Chauvin JP, Ruff F. Effect of temafloxacin on the pharmacokinetics of theophylline. 31st Intersci Conf Antimicrob Ag Chemother (1991) Abstracts, 196.

5 Chodosh S, Siepman N. Influence of quinolones on theophylline levels in patients with lower respiratory tract infections. 31st Intersci Conf Antimi-crob Ag Chemother (1991) Abstracts, 245.

6 Ruff F, Santais MC, Callens E, Chauvin J-P, Hazebroucq J. Effect of temafloxacin on the pharmacokinetics of theophylline. Am J Med (1991) 91, Suppl 6A, 76S-80S.

7 Orme M, Back DJ, Tjia J, Martin C, Millar E, Mant T, Morrison P. The lack of interaction between temafloxacin and oral contraceptive steroids. Br J Clin Pharmac (1991) 31, 228P.

8 Back DJ, Tjia J, Martin C, Millar E, Mant T, Morrison P, Orme M. The lack of interaction between temafloxacin and combined oral contraceptives. Contraception (1991) 43, 317–23.

9 Millar E, Coles S, Wyld P, Nimmo W. Temafloxacin does not potentiate the anticoagulant effect of warfarin in healthy subjects. Clin Pharmacokinet (1992) 22 (Suppl 1) 102–6.

10 Mant T, Morrison P, Millar E. The lack of interaction between temafloxa-cin and the acute administration of heparin. 17th Int Congr Chemother, June 1991, Berlin. Abstract 413.

11 Sörgel F, Mahr G, Granneman GR, Stephan U, Nickel P, Muth P. Effects of 2 quinolone antibacterials, temafloxacin and enoxacin, on theophylline pharmacokinetics. Clin Pharmacokinet (1992) 22 (Suppl 1) 65–74.

12 Sörgel F, Granneman GR, Stephan U, Locke C. Effect of cimetidine on the pharmacokinetics of temafloxacin. Clin Pharmacokinet (1992) 22 (Suppl 1) 75–82.

13 Granneman GR, Stephan U, Birner B, Sørgel F, Mukherjee D. Effect of antacid medication on the pharmacokinetics of temafloxacin. Clin Phar-macokinet (1992) 22 (Suppl 1) 83–89.

14 Mahr G, Sörgel F, Granneman GRR, Kinzig M, Muth P, Patterson K, Fuhr U, NIckel P, Stephan U. Effects of temafloxacin and ciprofloxacin on the pharmacokinetics of caffeine. Clin Pharmacokinet (1992) 22 (Suppl 1) 90–7.

15 Mant T, Morrison P, Millar E. Absence of drug interaction between temafloxacin and low dose heparin. Clin Pharmacokinet (1992) 22 (Suppl 1) 98–101.

Terbinafine + Miscellaneous drugs

Abstract/Summary

Cimetidine can raise serum terbinafine levels, whereas ri-fampicin lowers its serum levels. Terbinafine appears not to induce or inhibit liver enzymes and therefore is unlikely to interact with drugs susceptible to enzyme induction or inhibi-tion. Terbinafine causes a small and almost certainly clinically unimportant fall in cyclosporin serum levels.

Clinical evidence, mechanism, importance and management

(a) Terbinafine + Cimetidine

800 mg cimetidine twice daily for five days increased the AUC of a single 250 mg dose of terbinafine in 12 subjects by 34% and reduced its clearance by 30%.[1] The likely reason is that cimetidine (a known enzyme inhibitor) reduces the metabolism of the terbinafine by the liver, so that it is cleared from the body more slowly. It seems doubtful if this modest increase in the serum levels of terbinafine is of much clinical importance, but until more information is available it would be prudent to monitor concurrent use.

(b) Terbinafine + Cyclosporin

A study in 20 normal subjects found that after taking 250 mg terbinafine daily for 6–7 days the mean AUC of single 300 mg doses of cyclosporin was decreased by 12%. The maximum serum concentration of the cyclosporin was reduced 14%. The reason is not understood.[6] This study confirms a previous *in vitro* work with human liver microsomal enzymes showing that terbinafine does not inhibit cyclosporin metabolism.[5] This small change in the pharmacokinetics of cyclosporin is unlikely to be clinically important.

(c) Terbinafine + Rifampicin

In the study cited above, 600 mg rifampicin daily for 6 days reduced the AUC of terbinafine by 51% and increased its clearance by 106%.[1] Rifampicin is a potent enzyme inducing agent which increases the metabolism and loss from the body of many drugs. Be alert, therefore, for the need to increase the dosage of terbinafine if rifampicin is given.

(d) Terbinafine + Other drugs

Terbinafine has been found not to affect the metabolism of antipyrine (phenazone) which is used a 'marker' drug to find out if enzyme induction or inhibition occurs,[2] nor does it appear to interact with cytochrome P-450 isoenzymes *in vitro*,[3] suggesting that terbinafine is unlikely to interact with many drugs which are known to be affected by enzyme inducers and inhibitors. Direct studies are needed to confirm the absence of clinically important interactions, but in their datasheet the manufacturers of terbinafine reasonably suggest that, on the basis of studies with human liver microsomes, cyclosporin, coumarin anticoagulants, tolbutamide and the oral contraceptives are unlikely to be affected by terbinafine.[4]

References

1 Jensen JC. Pharmacokinetics of Lamisil in humans. J Dermatol Treat (1990) 1 (Suppl 2) 15–8.
2 Seyffer R, Eichelbaum M, Jensen JC, Klotz U. Antipyrine metabolism is not affected by terbinafine, a new antifungal agent. Eur J Clin Pharmacol (1989) 37, 321–3.
3 Back DJ, Stevenson P, Tija JF. Comparative effects of two antimycotic agents, ketoconazole and terbinafine, on the metabolism of tolbutamide, ethinyloestradiol, cyclosporine and ethoxcoumarin by human-liver microsome *in vitro*. Br J clin Pharmac (1989) 28, 166–70.
4 Lamisil datasheet. Sandoz January 1991.
5 Back DJ, Tjia JF. Comparative effects of the antimycotic drugs ketoconazole, fluconazole, itraconazole and terbinafine on the metabolism of cyclosporin by human liver microsomes. Br J clin Pharmac (1991) 32, 624–6.
6 Long CC, Hill SA, Thomas RC, Holt DW, Finlay AY. The effect of terbinafine on the pharmacokinetics of cyclosporin *in vivo*. Skin Pharmacol (1992) 5, 200–1.

Tetrachlorethylene + Alcohol

Abstract/Summary

Alcohol can increase the toxicity of tetrachlorethylene.

Clinical evidence, mechanism, importance and management

Tetrachlorethylene used as an anthelmintic is normally only slightly absorbed by the gut. This is increased by alcohol, leading to increased toxicity (CNS depression, liver and other toxicity).[1] Alcohol should therefore be avoided.

Reference

1 Reynolds JEF (Ed). Martindale. The Extra Pharmacopoeia, Edition 30. Pharm Press, London (1993) p 54.

Tetracyclines + Alcohol

Abstract/Summary

The serum levels of doxycycline may fall below minimal therapeutic concentrations in alcoholic patients, but tetracycline itself is not affected and it seems likely that the other tetracyclines are also not affected. There is nothing to suggest that moderate amounts of alcohol will significantly affect the serum levels of doxycycline or any other tetracycline in normal non-alcoholic subjects.

Clinical evidence

A study found that the half-life of doxycycline was 10.5 h in six alcoholics compared with 14.7 h in six normal healthy volunteers. The serum levels of two of the alcoholic patients fell well below what is generally accepted as the minimum therapeutic concentrations. The half-life of tetracycline was the same in both groups. All of them were given 100 mg doxycycline daily after a 200 mg loading dose, and 500 mg tetracycline twice daily after an initial 750 mg loading dose.[1]

In another study in normal subjects it was found that cheap red wine (but not whiskey) postponed the absorption of doxycycline, probably because of the acetic acid content which slows gastric emptying, but did not affect its total absorption. The authors concluded that '..the acute intake of alcoholic beverages generally does not interfere with the kinetics of doxycycline to an extent which would jeopardise therapeutic levels in tissues.'[4]

Mechanism

Heavy drinkers can metabolize some drugs much more quickly than non-drinkers due to the enzyme-inducing effects of alcohol,[2,3] and this interaction with doxycycline would seem to be due to this effect, possibly associated with some reduction in absorption from the gut.

Importance and management

Information is limited, but the doxycycline-alcohol interaction appears to be established. It seems to be clinically significant in alcoholic subjects but not in normal individuals. One suggested solution to the problem is to dose alcoholic subjects twice daily instead of only once. Alternatively tetracycline could be used because it appears not to be affected. There is nothing to suggest that moderate or even occasional heavy drinking affects any of the tetraclines in normal subjects.

References

1 Neuvonen PJ, Pentilla O, Roos M, Tirkkonen J. Effect of long-term alcohol consumption on the half-life of tetracycline and doxycycline in man. Int J Clin Pharmacol (1976) 14, 306.
2 Misra PS, Leferre A, Ishii H, Rubin E, Lieber CS. Increase of ethanol, meprobamate and pentobarbital metabolism after chronic ethanol admin-

istration in man and rats. Amer J Med (1971) 51, 346.

3 Neuvonen PJ, Pentilla O, Lehtovaara K, Aho K. Effect of antiepileptic drugs on the elimination of various tetracycline derivatives. Europ J Clin Pharmacol (1975) 9, 147.

4 Mattila MJ, Laisi U, Linnoila M, Salonen R. Effect of alcoholic beverages on the pharmacokinetics of doxycycline in man. Acta pharmacol et toxicol (1982) 50, 370–3.

Tetracyclines + Antacids

Abstract/Summary

The serum levels and, as a consequence, the therapeutic effectiveness of the tetracycline antibiotics can be markedly reduced or even abolished by the concurrent use of antacids containing aluminium, bismuth, calcium or magnesium. Other antacids such as sodium bicarbonate which raise the gastric pH may also reduce the bioavailability of some tetracycline preparations. Even the serum levels of intravenous doxycycline can be reduced.

Clinical evidence

(a) Aluminium-containing antacids

Two teaspoonfuls of aluminium hydroxide gel (*Amphogel*) given with 500 mg chlortetracycline to five patients and six normal subjects every 6 h reduced the serum antibiotics levels by 80–90% within 48 h. One patient had a recurrence of her urinary tract infection which only subsided when the antacid was withdrawn.[1] This was confirmed in another study.[2]

Other studies in man showed that 30 ml aluminium hydroxide reduced oxytetracyline serum levels by more than 50%;[3] 20 ml caused a 75% reduction in demeclocycline serum levels;[4] 15 ml caused a 100% reduction in serum doxycycline levels; and 30 ml magnesium-aluminium hydroxide (*Maalox*) caused a 90% reduction in tetracyline serum levels.[6] The mean serum levels of an intravenous dose of doxycycline was also found to be reduced by 36% when aluminium hydroxide was taken orally.[15]

(b) Calcium, magnesium or bismuth-containing antacids

Bismuth subsalicylate markedly reduces the absorption of tetracycline[13] and a 50% reduction in serum doxycycline levels can occur.[14] Bismuth carbonate interacts with the tetracyclines *in vitro*.[9] Magnesium sulphate certainly interacts with tetracycline, but in the clinical study on record[6] the amount of magnesium was much higher than would normally be found in the usual dose of antacid. Magnesium oxide interacted in an *in vitro* study.[9] There seem to be no direct clinical studies with calcium-containing antacids but a clinically important interaction seems an almost certainty, based on an *in vitro* study with calcium carbonate,[9] studies of calcium in milk (see synopsis on 'Tetracyclines + Milk and Dairy products') and as dicalcium phosphate,[7] and as an excipient in tetracycline capsules.[8]

(c) Sodium-containing antacids

2 g sodium bicarbonate reduced the absorption of a 250 mg capsule of tetracycline hydrochloride in eight subjects by 50%. If however the tetracycline was dissolved before administration, the absorption was unaffected by the sodium bicarbonate.[10]

Another study stated that 2 g sodium bicarbonate had an insignificant effect on tetracycline absorption.[12]

Mechanism

Work in the mid-1950s demonstrated that the tetracyclines bind with aluminium, bismuth, calcium, magnesium and other metallic ions to form compounds (chelates) which are much less soluble and therefore much less readily absorbed by the gut.[11] In addition the solubility of the tetracylines is a hundred times greater at pH 1–3 than at pH 5–6, so that an antacid which raises the gastric pH above about 4 for 20–30 min could prevent up to 50% of the tetracycline from being fully dissolved in the stomach.[10] Once the undissolved drug is emptied out of the stomach, the pH in the duodenum (5–6) and in the rest of the gut are unfavourable for full dissolution, so that a good proportion of the tetracycline may never dissolve and so it remains unavailable for absorption. This may also explain why sodium bicarbonate interacts with tetracycline. A third reason for the reduced absorption may be because the tetracyclines are adsorbed onto the antacid.[13]

Importance and management

Extremely well-documented, long and well-established interactions. Their clinical importance depends on how much the serum tetracycline levels are lowered, but with normal antacid dosages the reductions cited above (50–100%) are so large that many organisms will not be exposed to minimum inhibitory concentrations (MIC). As a general rule none of the aluminium, bismuth, calcium or magnesium containing antacids, or others such as sodium bicarbonate which can markedly alter gastric pH, should be given at the same time as the tetracycline antibiotics. If they must be used, separate the dosages maximally to prevent their admixture in the gut. Sodium bicarbonate and other antacids which only affect the extent of absorption by altering gastric pH will only interact with tetracycline preparations which are not already dissolved before ingestion (e.g. those in capsule form). Patients should be warned about taking any over-the-counter antacids and indigestion preparations.

Instead of using antacids to minimize the gastric irritant effects of the tetracyclines it is usually recommended that tetracyclines are taken before food, however it is not entirely clear how much this affects their absorption. One study demonstrated that food reduced the absorption of demeclocycline,[4] whereas another claimed that it did not.[5]

References

1 Waisbren BA, Hueckel JS. Reduced absorption of Aureomycin caused by

aluminium hydroxide gel (*Amphojel*). Proc Soc Exp Biol Med NY (1950) 73, 73.

2 Seed JC, Wilson CE. The effect of aluminium hydroxide on serum Aureomycin concentrations after simultaneous oral administration. Bull Johns Hopkins Hosp (1950) 86, 415.

3 Michel JC, Sayer RJ, Kirby WMM. Effect of food and antacids on blood levels of Aureomycin and Terramycin. J Lab Clin Med (1950) 36, 632.

4 Scheiner J, Altemeier WA. Experimental study of factors inhibiting absorption and effective therapeutic levels of declomycin. Surg Gynec Obstet (1962) 114, 9.

5 Rosenblatt JE, Barrett JE, Brodie JL, Kirby WMM. Comparison of *in vitro* activity and clinical pharmacology of doxycycline with other tetracyclines. Antimicrob Ag Chemother (1966) 134.

6 Harcourt RS, Hamburger M. The effect of magnesium sulphate in lowering tetracycline blood levels. J Lab Clin Med (1957) 50, 464.

7 Boger WP, Gavin JJ. An evaluation of tetracycline preparations. N Engl J Med (1959) 261, 827.

8 Sweeney WM, Hardy SM, Dornbush AC, Ruegsegger JM. Absorption of tetracycline in human beings as affected by certain excipients. Antibiot Med Clin Ther (1957) 4, 642.

9 Christensen EKJ, Kerckhoffs HPM, Huizinga T. De invloed van antacida op de afgifte *in vitro* van tetracycline-hydrochloride. Pharm Weekblad (1967) 102, 463.

10 Barr WH, Adir J, Garrettson L. Decrease of tetracycline absorption in man by sodium bicarbonate. Clin Pharmacol Ther (1971) 12, 779.

11 Albert A, Rees CW. Avidity of the tetracyclines for the cations of metals. Nature (1956) 177, 433.

12 Garty M, Hurwitz A. Effect of cimetidine and antacids on gastrointestinal absorption of tetracycline. Clin Pharmacol Ther (1980) 28, 203.

13 Albert KS, Welch RD, De Sante KA, Disanto AR. Decreased tetracycline bioavailability caused by bismuth subsalicylate antidiarrhoeal mixture. J Pharm Sci (1979) 68, 586.

14 Ericsson CD, Feldman S, Pickering LK, Cleary TG. Influence of subsalicylate bismuth on absorption of doxycycline. J Amer Med Ass (1982) 247, 2266.

15 Nguyen VX, Nix DE, Gillikin S, Schentag JJ. Effect of oral antacid administration on the pharmacokinetics of intravenous doxycycline. Antimicrob Ag Chemother (1989) 33, 434–6.

Tetracyclines + Anticonvulsants

Abstract/Summary

The serum levels of doxycycline are reduced and may fall below the accepted therapeutic minimum in patients on long-term treatment with barbiturates, phenytoin or carbamazepine. Other tetracyclines appear to be unaffected.

Clinical evidence

A study in 14 patients taking phenytoin (200–500 mg daily) and/or carbamazepine (300–1000 mg daily) showed that the half-life of doxycycline was approximately half that of nine other patients not taking anticonvulsants (7.1 compared with 15.1 h).[1]

Similar results were found in 16 other patients on anticonvulsant therapy with phenytoin, carbamazepine and phenobarbitone. The serum doxycycline levels of almost all of them fell below 0.5 µg/ml during the 12–24 h period following their last dose of doxycycline (100 mg). Tetracycline, methacycline, oxytetracycline, demeclocycline and chlortetracycline were not significantly affected by these anticonvulsants.[2] Other studies confirm this interaction between the anticonvulsant barbiturates (and in one case the hypnotic amylobarbitone) and doxycycline.[3,4]

Mechanism

Uncertain. These anticonvulsants are known enzyme-inducing agents and it seems probable that they increase the metabolism of the doxycycline by the liver, thereby hastening its clearance from the body.

Importance and management

The doxycycline-anticonvulsant interactions are established. The extent to which concurrent use affects treatment with doxycycline seems not to have been studied, but serum doxycycline levels below 0.5 µg/ml are less than the accepted minimum inhibitory concentration (MIC). It seems likely that the antibiotic will fail to be effective. The suggestion has been made that the interaction can be accommodated by increasing the doxycycline dosage or by giving it twice daily.[2] Alternatively, tetracyclines which are reported not to be affected by the anticonvulsants could be used: tetracycline, methacycline, oxytetracycline, demeclocycline and chlortetracycline.[2]

References

1 Pentilla O, Neuvonen PJ, Aho K, Lehtovaara R. Interaction between doxycycline and some antiepileptic drugs. Br Med J (1974) 2, 470.

2 Neuvonen PJ, Pentilla O, Lehtovaara R, Aho K. Effect of antiepileptic drugs on the elimination of various tetracycline derivatives. Eur J clin Pharmacol (1975) 9, 147.

3 Neuvonen PJ, Pentilla O. Interaction between doxycycline and barbiturates. Br Med J (1974) 1, 535.

4 Alestig K. Studies on the intestinal excretion of doxycycline. Scand J Infect Dis (1974) 6, 265.

Tetracyclines + Cimetidine

Abstract/Summary

Cimetidine seems not to affect the serum levels of tetracycline.

Clinical evidence, mechanism, importance and management

A study in five normal subjects showed that cimetidine reduced the absorption of a single dose of tetracycline (500 mg) in capsule form by about 30%, but not when the tetracyline was given in solution.[1] A similar reduction was seen in another single dose study,[3] but no interaction was found in a third single dose study.[2] However when tetracycline in either tablet or suspension form was given to six subjects with 1200 mg cimetidine daily for six days, no changes in the serum levels of tetracycline were seen.[3] So it seems that in practice cimetidine has little or no effect on serum tetracycline levels. No special precautions would seem necessary. Information about other tetracyclines seems to be lacking.

References

1 Cole JJ, Charles BG, Ravenscroft PJ. Interaction of cimetidine with tetracycline absorption. Lancet (1980) ii, 536.
2 Garty M, Hurwitz A. Effect of cimetidine and antacids on gastro-intestinal absorption of tetracycline. Clin Pharmacol Ther (1980) 28, 203.
3 Fisher P, House F, Inns P, Morrison PJ, Rogers HJ, Bradbrook ID. Effect of cimetidine on the absorption of orally administered tetracycline. Br J Clin Pharmac (1980) 9, 153–8.

Tetracyclines + Coffee or Orange Juice

Abstract/Summary

Orange juice and coffee do not interact with tetracycline.

Clinical evidence, mechanism, importance and management

A study in 9 normal subjects found that 200 ml of orange juice or coffee did not significantly affect the bioavailability of a single 250 mg dose of tetracycline, despite the fact that orange juice contained 35–70 mg calcium per 100 ml which might be expected to combine with tetracycline to produce poorly absorbable chelates (see 'Tetracyclines + Antacids'). The reason seems to be that at the relevant pH values in the gut, the calcium is bound to components within the orange juice (citric, tartaric and ascorbic acids) and is not free to combine with the tetracycline.[1] Nobody seems to have checked with other tetracylines, but it seems likely that they will behave similarly.

Reference

1 Jung H, Rivera O, Reguero M T, Rodríguez J M, Moreno-Esparza R. Influence of liquids (coffee and orange juice) on the bioavailability of tetracycline. Biopharm Drug Disp (1990) 11, 729–34.

Tetracyclines + Colestipol

Abstract/Summary

Colestipol can markedly reduce the absorption of tetracycline.

Clinical evidence

A study in nine subjects found that 30 g colestipol taken either in 180 ml water or orange juice reduced the absorption of a single 500 mg dose of oral tetracycline hydrochloride by 54–56% (as measured by recovery in the urine).[1] This confirms a previous study which found a 50–60% reduction in the bioavailability of tetracycline.[2]

Mechanism

Colestipol binds to bile acids in the gut and can also bind with some drugs, thereby reducing their availability for absorption.

An *in vitro* study found a 30% binding.[3] The presence of citrate ions in the orange juice which can also bind to colestipol appears not to have a marked effect on the binding of the tetracycline.

Importance and management

Direct information seems to be limited to the reports cited but it is consistent with the way colestipol interacts with other drugs. In practice colestipol is normally given in 15–30 g daily doses, divided into two or four doses, and tetracycline in 250–500 mg doses six-hourly which means that it is difficult to avoid some mixing in the gut. It seems very probable that a clinically important interaction will occur, but by how much the steady-state serum tetracycline levels are affected seems not to have been determined. Tell patients to separate the dosages as much as possible. Monitor the outcome well. It may be necessary to increase the dosage of tetracycline. It also seems likely that other tetracylines will interact similarly.

References

1 Friedman H, Greenblatt DJ, LeDuc BW. Impaired absorption of tetracycline by colestipol is not reversed by orange juice. J Clin Pharmacol (1989) 29, 748–51.
2 Brown RK. The effect of concomitant administration of colestipol hydrochloride on the bioavailability of orally administered tetracycline hydrochloride. Report on file Upjohn Co (1975).
3 Ko H, Royer ME. In vitro binding of drugs to colestipol hydrochloride. J Pharmac Sci (1974) 63, 1914.

Tetracyclines + Diuretics

Abstract/Summary

It has been recommended that the concurrent use of tetracyclines and diuretics should be avoided because of their association with rises in blood urea nitrogen levels.

Clinical evidence, mechanism, importance and management

A retrospective study of patient records as part of the Boston Collaborative Drug Surveillance Program showed that a strong association existed between tetracycline administration with diuretics (not named) and rises in blood urea nitrogen (BUN) levels.[1] The suggested reasons are that the tetracyclines have anti-anabolic effects, whereas diuretics can decrease the glomerular filtration rate and increase the reabsorption of filtered urea, both of which can result in rises in BUN levels.[2] The recommendation was made that tetracyclines should be avoided in patients on diuretics when alternative antibiotics could be substituted.[1] This would seem to be particularly appropriate for patients with existing renal impairment, however it has been claimed that doxycycline may be used in those with renal failure.[2]

References

1 Boston Collaborative Drug Surveillance Program. Tetracycline and drug-attributed rises in blood urea nitrogen. J Amer Med Ass (1972) 220, 377.
2 Tannenberg AM. Tetracyclines and rises in urea nitrogen. J Amer Med Ass (1972) 221, 713–14.

Tetracyclines + Ethinyloestradiol

Abstract/Summary

There is some evidence that preparations containing ethinyloestradiol may accentuate the facial pigmentation which can be caused by minocycline.

Clinical evidence

Two teenage sisters taking minocycline for severe acne vulgaris (50 mg four times daily, later reduced to twice daily), developed dark-brown pigmentation in the acne scars when also given *Dianette* (cyproterone acetate and ethinyloestradiol) for about 15 months.[1] The type of pigmentation was not identified because they both declined to have a biopsy, but in other cases it has been found to consist of haemosiderin, iron, melanin and a metabolic degradation product of minocycline.[1] Two other reports describe facial pigmentation in other patients on minocycline, two of whom were taking oral contraceptives containing ethinyloestradiol.[2,3] Other young women who have developed minocycline pigmentation may also have been taking oral contraceptives because they fall into the right age-group, but this is not specifically stated in any of the reports.

Mechanism

Not understood. It seems possible that the facial pigmentation (melasma, chloasma) which can occur with oral contraceptives may have been additive with the effects of the minocycline.[1]

Importance and management

Evidence is very limited but it has been suggested that everyone on long-term minocycline treatment should be well screened for the development of pigmentation, particularly if they are taking other drugs such as the oral contraceptives which are know to induce hyperpigmentation.[1] See also 'Contraceptives, oral + Antibiotics and Anti-infective agents.'

References

1 Eedy DJ, Burrows D. Minocycline-induced pigmentation occurring in two sisters. Clin Exptl Dermatol (1991) 16, 55–7.
2 Ridgeway HA, Sonnex TS, Kennedy CTC. et al. Hyperpigmentation associated with oral minocycline. Br J Dermatol (1982) 107, 95–102.
3 Prigent F, Cavalier-Balloy B, Tollenacre C, Civatte J. Pigmentation cutane induite par la minocycline: deux cas. Ann Dermatol Vénérol (1986) 113, 227–33.

Tetracyclines + Iron preparations

Abstract/Summary

The absorption from the gut of both the tetracylines and of iron salts is markedly reduced by concurrent use, leading to depressed drug serum levels. Their therapeutic effectiveness may be reduced or even abolished. If both must be given, their administration should be separated as much as possible to prevent mixing in the gut.

Clinical evidence

(a) Effect of iron on absorption of the tetracyclines

An investigation in 10 normal adults given single oral doses of tetracyclines (200–500 mg) showed that the concurrent use of 200 mg ferrous sulphate decreased the serum antibiotic levels as follows: tetracycline reduced 40–50%; oxytetracycline 50–60%; methacycline and doxycycline 80–90%.[1] Another study found that 300 mg ferrous sulphate reduced the absorption of tetracycline by 81% and of minocycline by 77%.[10]

Other studies found that in some instances the iron caused the tetracycline serum levels to fall below minimal bacterial inhibitory concentrations (MIC).[2–5,10] If the iron was given 3 h before or 2 h after the tetracycline the serum levels were not significantly depressed,[2–4] with the exception of doxycycline.[4] Even when the iron was given up to 11 h after the doxycycline, serum concentrations were still lowered 20–45%.[4]

(b) Effect of tetracyclines on the absorption of iron

When 250 mg ferrous sulphate (equivalent to 50 mg Fe^{2+}) was given with 500 mg tetracycline, the absorption of iron in normal subjects was reduced 37–78%, and in those with depleted iron stores 40–65%.[8,9]

Mechanism

The tetracyclines have a strong affinity for iron and form poorly soluble tetracycline-iron chelates which are much less readily absorbed by the gut, and as a result the serum tetracycline levels achieved are much lower.[6,7] There is also less free iron available for absorption. Separating the administration of the two prevents their admixture,[2,3] but in the case of doxycycline some of the antibiotic is returned into the gut in the bile which tends to thwart any attempt to keep the iron and antibiotic apart.[4] The different extent to which iron salts interact with the tetracyclines appears to be a reflection of their ability to liberate ferrous and ferric ions which are free to combine with the tetracycline.[5]

Importance and management

Well-documented and well-established interactions of clinical importance. Reductions in serum tetracycline levels of the order of 30–90% due to the presence of iron are so large that levels may fall below those which inhibit bacterial growth (MIC).[3] However the extent of the reductions depends on a number of factors. (a) The particular tetracycline used: tetracycline itself in the study cited above was affected the least;[1] (b) the time-interval between the administration of the two drugs: giving iron 3 h before or 2 h after the antibiotic is satisfactory with tetracycline itself[2] but 11 h is inadequate for doxycycline; (c) the particular iron preparation used: with tetracycline the reduction in serum levels with ferrous sulphate was 80–90%, with ferrous fumarate, succinate and gluconate 70–80%; with ferrous tartrate 50%; and with ferrous sodium edetate 30%.[5] The interaction can therefore be accommodated by separating the dosages as much as possible, avoiding the use of doxycycline, and choosing one of the iron preparations causing minimal interference.

One suggestion is a schedule in which 500 mg tetracycline is given 30–60 min before breakfast and dinner (total daily dose 1 g), and 50 mg Fe^{2+} before lunch and 2 h after dinner.[9] This provides the patient with tetracycline serum concentrations of about 3–5 µg/ml and a daily iron absorption of 25 mg, sufficient to allow optimal haemoglobin regeneration values of 0.2–0.3 g%/day.

Only tetracycline, oxytetracycline, methacycline, minocycline and doxycycline have been shown to interact with iron, but it seems reasonable to expect that the others will behave in a similar way.

References

1 Neuvonen PJ, Gothoni G, Hackman R, Bjorkjsten K. Interference of iron with the absorption of tetracyclines in man. Br Med J (1970) 4, 532.
2 Mattila MJ, Neuvonen PJ, Gothoni G, Hackman CR. Interference of iron preparations and milk with the absorption of tetracyclines. Excerpta Medica Int Congr Series No. 254 (1972). Toxicological problems of drug combinations, 128.
3 Gothoni G, Neuvonen PJ, Mattila M, Hackman R. Iron-tetracycline interaction: effect of time interval between the drugs. Acta Med Scand (1972) 191, 409.
4 Neuvonen PJ, Pentilla O. Effect of oral ferrous sulphate on the half-life of doxycycline in man. Eur J Clin Pharmacol (1974) 7, 361.
5 Neuvonen PJ, Pentilla O. Inhibitory effect of various iron salts on the absorption of tetracycline in man. Eur J clin Pharmacol (1974) 7, 357.
6 Albert A, Rees CW. Avidity of the tetracyclines for the cations of metals. Nature (1956) 177, 433.
7 Albert A, Rees CW. Incompatibility of aluminium hydroxide and certain antibiotics. Br Med J (1955) 2, 1027.
8 Heinrich HC, Oppitz KH, Gabbe EE. Hemmung der Eisenabsorption beim Menschen durch Tetracyclin. Klin Wsch (1974) 52, 493.
9 Heinrich HC, Oppitz KH. Tetracycline inhibits iron absorption in man. Naturwissenschaften (1973) 60, 524.
10 Leyden JJ. Absorption of minocycline hydrochloride and tetracycline hydrochloride. Effects of food, milk and iron. J Am Acad Dermatol (1985) 12, 308–12.

Tetracyclines + Kaopectate

Abstract/Summary

Kaopectate reduces the absorption of tetracycline.

Clinical evidence, mechanism, importance and management

Healthy human subjects were given 250 ml tetracycline hydrochloride as a solution or as a capsule, with and without 30 ml Kaopectate. The absorption was reduced about 50% by the Kaopectate. Even when the Kaopectate was given 2 h before or after the tetracycline, the drug absorption was still reduced about 20%.[1] A likely reason is that tetracycline becomes adsorbed onto the Kaopectate so that less is available for absorption.

If these two drugs are given together, consider separating the dosages more than 2 h to minimize admixture in the gut. It may even be necessary to increase the tetracycline dosage. Information about other tetracyclines is lacking but be alert for them to interact similarly.

Reference

1 Gouda MW. Effect of an antidiarrhoeal mixture on the bioavailability of tetracycline. Int J Pharmaceut (1993) 89, 75–7.

Tetracyclines + Metoclopramide

Abstract/Summary, clinical evidence, mechanism, importance and management

20 mg metoclopramide was found to double the rate of absorption of tetracycline in four convalescent patients and slightly reduce the maximum serum levels following a single 500 mg dose.[1] This appears to be of no clinical importance.

Reference

1 Nimmo J. The influence of metoclopramide on drug absorption. Postgrad Med J (1973) 49, July Suppl, 25–8.

Tetracyclines + Milk and Dairy products

Abstract/Summary

The absorption of the tetracyclines can be markedly reduced (up to 70–80%) if they are allowed to come into contact in the gut with milk or other dairy products. As a result their therapeutic effects may be diminished or even abolished. Doxycycline and minocycline are less affected (25–30%).

Clinical evidence

The serum levels of 12 normal subjects given single 300 mg oral doses of demeclocyline were reduced 70–80% when ingested with either 8 oz (a little over a third of a pint) of fresh pasteurized milk, 8 oz buttermilk or 4 oz cottage cheese, when compared with four other subjects given the same amount of antibiotic but with a meal containing no dairy products.[1] A 50% reduction was seen in other subjects given 300–500 mg tetracycline, methacycline or oxytetracycline with 300 ml (about half a pint) of milk. Doxycycline was not affected.[2]

Similar results were found in other studies.[3,4] A 20% reduction in serum doxycycline levels (from 1.79 to 1.45 µg/ml) was found 2 h after a single 100 mg oral dose with 240 ml milk.[3] Another study found a 30% reduction in the absorption of 200 mg doxycycline when taken with 300 ml fresh milk, and a 24% reduction in peak serum levels.[11] 6 oz (about 180 ml) homogenized milk reduced the absorption of 100 mg minocycline by 27%.[12]

Mechanism

The tetracyclines have a strong affinity for the calcium ions which are found in abundance in milk and dairy products.[5,6] The tetracycline-calcium chelates formed are much less readily absorbed from the gastrointestinal tract, and as a result the serum levels achieved are much lower. It has also been shown *in vitro* that these chelates have a very much reduced antibacterial activity.[8] Doxycycline[7] and minocycline have a lesser tendency to form chelates which explains why their serum levels are reduced to a smaller extent than other tetracyclines.

Importance and management

Well-documented and very well-established interactions of clinical importance. Reductions in serum tetracycline levels of 50–80% are so large that their antibacterial effects may become minimal or even nil. For this reason tetracyclines should not be taken with milk or dairy products such as yoghourt or cheese. Separate the ingestion of these foods and the administration of the tetracycline as much as possible. In the case of iron which interacts by the same mechanism, 2–3 h is enough. The small amounts of milk in coffee appear not to matter[13], and this is probably true for tea as well. Doxycycline[11,14] and minocycline[10,12] are not affected as much by dairy products (reductions of about 25–30%) and in this respect have some advantages over other tetracyclines. The manufacturers of tetracycline phosphate (*Tetrex*) claim that the phosphate combines with the calcium leaving more free tetracycline available for absorption. This form also appears to have advantages.[9]

It is common practice to advise patients to take the tetracyclines before food to overcome the gastric irritant effects, but it is not entirely clear whether, or how much, this affects the amount available for absorption. One study with demeclocycline demonstrated that food reduced the absorption,[1] whereas another claimed that it did not.[3]

References

1 Scheiner J, Altemeier WA. Experimental study of factors inhibiting absorption and effective therapeutic levels of declomycin. Surg Gynec Obstet (1962) 114, 9.

2 Neuvonen P, Matilla M, Gothoni H, Hackman R. Interference of iron and milk with absorption of tetracycline. Scand J Clin Lab Invest (1971) 116 (Suppl 27) 76.
3 Rosenblatt JE, Barrett JE, Brodie JL, Kirby WMM. Comparison of *in vitro* activity and clinical pharmacology of doxycycline with other tetracyclines. Antimicrob Ag Chemother (1966) 134.
4 Matilla MJ, Neuvonen PJ, Gothoni G, Hackman CR. Interference of iron preparations and milk with the absorption of tetracyclines. Excerpta Medica Int Congr Series (1972) 254, 128.
5 Albert A, Rees CW. Avidity of the tetracyclines for the cations of metals. Nature (1956) 177, 433.
6 Albert A, Rees CW. Incompatibility of aluminium hydroxide and certain antibiotics. Br Med J (1955) 2, 1027.
7 Schach von Wittenau M. Some pharmacokinetic aspects of doxycycline metabolism in man. Chemotherapy (1968) 13 (Suppl) 41.
8 Weinberg ED. The mutual effects of antimicrobial compounds and metallic ions. Bacteriol Rev (1957) 21, 46.
9 ABPI Data Sheet Compendium 1985–6, Datapharm Publications London (1985) p 266.
10 Ibid p 728.
11 Meyer FP, Specht H, Quednow B, Walther H. Influence of milk on bioavailability of doxycycline - New aspects. Infection (1989) 17, 245–6.
12 Leyden J J. Absorption of minocycline hydrochloride and tetracycline hydrochloride. Effects of food, milk and iron. J Am Acad Dermatol (1985) 12, 308–12.
13 Jung H, Rivera O, Reguero M T, Rodríguez J M, Moreno-Esparza R. Influence of liquids (coffe and orange juice) on the bioavailability of tetracycline. Biopharm Drug Disp (1990) 11, 729–34.
14 Siewert M, Blume H, Stenzhorn G, Kieferndorf U. Zur Qualitätsbeurteilung von doxycyclinhaltigen Fertigarzneimitteln. 3 Mittelung: Vergleichende Bioverfügbarkeitsstudie unter Berücksichtigung einer Einnahme mit Milch. Pharm Ztg Wiss (1990) 3, 96–102.

Tetracyclines + Phenothiazines

Abstract/Summary

An isolated report describes black galactorrhoea in a woman treated with minocycline, perphenazine, amitriptyline and diphenhydramine.

Clinical evidence, mechanism, importance and management

A woman taking 200 mg minocycline daily for four years to control pustulocystic acne, developed irregular darkly pigmented macules in the areas of acne scarring and later began to produce droplets of darkly coloured milk which was found to contain macrophages filled with particles of iron and haemosiderin. The situation resolved when the drugs were withdrawn.[1] Galactorrhoea is a known side-effect of the phenothiazines and is due to an elevation of serum prolactin levels caused by the blockade of dopamine receptors in the hypothalamus. The dark colour appeared to be a side-effect of the minocycline which can cause hemosiderin to be deposited in cells, and in this instance to be scavenged by the macrophages which were then secreted in the milk.

Reference

1 Basler RS, Lynch PJ. Black galactorrhoea as a consequence of minocycline and phenothiazine therapy. Arch Dermatol (1985) 121, 417–18.

Tetracyclines + Rifampicin (Rifampin)

Abstract/summary

Some patients show a marked fall (50%) in serum doxycycline levels if given rifampicin.

Clinical evidence

A pharmacokinetic study in seven patients given 200 mg doxycycline daily showed that the concurrent use of 10 mg/kg rifampicin daily caused a considerable reduction in the serum doxycycline levels. The reduction was very marked in four patients but not significant in the other three. A mean fall of 36% (from 14.18 to 9.11 h) occurred in the doxycycline half-life in the whole group of seven, a 106% increase in clearance (from 4.7 to 9.67 l/h) and a reduction in the AUC of 54% (from 54.38 to 24.77 mg.h.l^{-1}).[1]

Mechanism

Uncertain. It seems probable that the rifampicin (a known potent enzyme inducing agent) increases the metabolism of the doxycycline thereby increasing its loss from the body.

Importance and management

Information seems to be limited to this study. This interaction would appear to be clinically important in some patients but not others. More confirmatory study is needed. Monitor the effects of concurrent use and increase the doxycycline dosage as necessary. The study revealed that before the rifampicin was given, the doxycycline half-life in those patients who were affected by this interaction was longer (17.8 h) than in the others (9.2 h). This would seem to be a way of identifying those patients likely to be at risk.

Reference

1 Garraffo R, Dellamonica P, Fournier JP, Lapalaus Ph, Bernard E, Beziau H, Chichmanian RM. Effet de la rifampicine sur la pharmacocinetique de la doxycycline. Path Biol (1987) 35, 746–9.

Tetracyclines + Thiomersal

Abstract/Summary

Patients being treated with tetracyclines who use contact lens solutions containing thiomersal (thimerosal, thiomersalate, mercuriothiolate) may experience an inflammatory ocular reaction.

Clinical evidence, mechanism, importance and management

The observation of two patients who had ocular reactions (red eye, irritation, blepharitis) when they used a 0.004% thiomersal-containing contact-lens solution while taking a tetracycline, prompted further study of this interaction. A questionnaire sent to other patients revealed nine other cases which suddenly began shortly after starting to use a tetracycline, and which cleared when the thiomersal or the tetracycline was stopped. The same reaction was also clearly demonstrated in rabbits.[1] The reasons are not understood.

Reference

1 Crook TG, Freeman JJ. Reactions induced by the concurrent use of thimerosal and tetracycline. Amer J Opt Physiol Optics (1983) 60, 759–61.

Tetracyclines + Zinc sulphate

Abstract/Summary

The absorption of tetracycline can be reduced by as much as 50% if zinc sulphate is taken concurrently. Separating their administration as much as possible minimizes the effects of this interaction. Doxycycline interacts minimally with zinc.

Clinical evidence

Seven subjects given 500 mg tetracycline, either alone or with zinc sulphate (200 mg containing 45 mg Zn^{2+}), had tetracycline serum concentrations which were reduced 30–40% by the presence of the zinc. The AUCs were similarly reduced.[1]

A more than 50% reduction was seen in another study,[2] and this interaction was confirmed in yet another.[7] The reduction in serum zinc concentrations was found to be minimal.[2]

Mechanism

Zinc (like iron, calcium, magnesium and aluminium) forms a relatively stable and poorly absorbed chelate with tetracycline within the gut which results in a reduction in the amount of antibiotic available for absorption.[3,4]

Importance and management

An established and moderately well documented interaction of clinical importance. Separate the administration of tetracycline and zinc sulphate as much as possible to minimize admixture in the gut (in the case of iron which interacts by the same mechanism, 2–3 h is enough.[5]) An alternative is to use doxycycline which has been shown to interact minimally with zinc.[1] Other tetracyclines would be expected to interact like tetracycline itself, but this needs confirmation. The small reduction in serum zinc concentrations is likely to be of little practical importance.[2,6]

References

1 Penttila O, Hurme H, Neuvonen PJ. Effect of zinc sulphate on the absorption of tetracycline and doxycycline in man. Eur J Clin Pharmacol (1975) 9, 131.
2 Andersson K-E, Bratt L, Dencker H, Kamure C, Lanner E. Inhibition of tetracycline absorption by zinc. Eur J Clin Pharmacol (1976) 10, 59.
3 Albert A, Rees CW. Avidity of the tetracyclines for cations of metals. Nature (1956) 177, 433.
4 Doluisio JT, Martin AN. Metal complexation of the tetracycline hydrochlorides. J Med Chem (1963) 16, 16.
5 Gothoni G, Neuvonen PJ, Mattila M, Hackman R. Iron-tetracycline interaction: effect of time interval between drugs. Acta med Scand (1972) 191, 409.
6 Andersson K-E, Bratt L, Dencker H, Lanner E. Some aspects of the intestinal absorption of zinc in man. Eur J Clin Pharmacol (1975) 9, 423.
7 Mapp RK, McCarthy TJ. The effect of zinc sulphate and of bicitropeptide on tetracycline absorption. S Afr Med J (1976) 50, 1829.

Tinidazole + Cimetidine

Abstract/Summary

Cimetidine reduces the loss of tinidazole from the body. The clinical importance of this is uncertain.

Clinical evidence, mechanism, importance and management

After taking 800 mg cimetidine daily for seven days the peak serum levels of tinidazole in six normal subjects following a single 600 mg dose were raised by 21% (from 14.1 to 17.1 µg/ml), the 24 h AUC was increased by 40% (from 150 to 210 µg/ml/h) and the half-life increased by 47% (from 7.66 to 11.23 h).[1] The probable reason is that the cimetidine inhibits the metabolism of the tinidazole by the liver, thereby reducing its loss from the body. Some increase in both the therapeutic and the toxic effects of tinidazole would be expected, but the clinical importance of this is uncertain. It appears not to have been studied.

Reference

1 Patel RB, Shah GF, Raval JD, Gandhi TP, Gilbert RN. The effect of cimetidine and rifampicin on tinidazole kinetics in healthy human volunteers. Indian Drugs (1986) 23, 338–41.

Tinidazole + Rifampicin (Rifampin)

Abstract/Summary

Rifampicin increases the loss of tinidazole from the body. The clinical importance of this is uncertain.

Clinical evidence, mechanism, importance and management

After taking 600 mg rifampicin daily for seven days the peak serum levels of tinidazole in six normal subjects following a single 600 mg dose were reduced by 21% (from 14.1 to 11.1 µg/ml), the 24 h AUC was reduced by 30% (from 150 to 105 ug/ml/h) and the half-life reduced by 27% (from 7.66 to 5.6 h).[1] The probable reason is that the rifampicin increases the metabolism of the tinidazole by the liver, thereby increasing its loss from the body. Some reduction in the therapeutic effects of tinidazole would be expected, but the clinical importance of this is uncertain. It appears not to have been studied.

Reference

1 Patel RB, Shah GF, Raval JD, Gandhi TP, Gilbert RN. The effect of cimetidine and rifampicin on tinidazole kinetics in healthy human volunteers. Indian Drugs (1986) 23, 338–41.

Trimethoprim + Antacids

Abstract/Summary

Magnesium trisilicate and kaolin-pectin reduce the bioavailability of trimethoprim in rats, but the clinical importance of this is uncertain.

Clinical evidence, mechanism, importance and management

A study in rats showed that magnesium trisilicate and kaolin-pectin reduced the peak serum levels (at 1 h) of oral trimethoprim by 50 and 30% respectively, and the AUC's (areas under the curve) by 30 and 21%.[1] Whether this interaction affects the clinical effectiveness of trimethoprim in man has not been assessed, but the possibility should be borne in mind.

Reference

1 Babhair SA, Tariq M. Effect of magnesium trisilicate and kaolin-pectin on the bioavailability of trimethoprim. Res Comm Chem Pathol Pharmacol (1983) 40, 165–8.

Trimethoprim + Guar or Food

Abstract/Summary

Guar gum and food can reduce the absorption of trimethoprim from a suspension.

Clinical evidence, mechanism, importance and management

A study over a 24 h period in 12 normal subjects given a single

3 mg/kg oral dose of a trimethoprim suspension showed that mean peak serum levels were depressed 22% and 16% respectively by food and food with guar. Both reduced the AUC by 22%.[1] The greatest individual reductions were 44% (peak serum levels) and 47% (AUC) with food, and 47% (peak serum levels) and 38% (AUC) with food + guar.[1] The reasons are not understood but it may be due to adsorption of the trimethoprim onto the food and guar.

The clinical importance of this interaction is still uncertain but since a marked reduction in absorption can occur in some individuals it would seem sensible to take trimethoprim suspension between meals. Whether the same interaction occurs with other trimethoprim formulations is not known.

Reference

1 Hoppu K, Tuomisto J, Koskimies O, Simell O. Food and guar decrease absorption of trimethoprim. Eur J Clin Pharmacol (1987) 32, 427–9.

Trimethoprim + Rifampicin

Abstract/Summary, clinical evidence, mechanism, importance and management

An advantageous drug combination. More than additive antibacterial activity occurs. After 4–5 days the loss of trimethoprim increases because of the enzyme inducing activity of the rifampicin,[1,2] but this does not appear to be of clinical importance.

References

1 Buniva G, Palminteri R, Berti M. Kinetics of a rifampicin-trimethoprim combination. Int J Clin Pharmacol Biopharm (1979) 17, 256–9.
2 Emmerson AM, Grüneberg RN, Johnson ES. The pharmacokinetics in man of a combination of rifampicin and trimethoprim. J Antimicrob Chemother (1978) 4, 523–31.

Vancomycin + Indomethacin

Abstract/Summary

Indomethacin reduces the loss of vancomycin from the body in premature babies.

Clinical evidence, mechanism, importance and management

The half-life of vancomycin (15–20 mg/kg IV given over 1 h) was found to be 24.6 h in six neonates with patent ductus arteriosus given indomethacin compared with only 7.0 h in five other control neonates, without patent ductus arteriosus and not given indomethacin.[1] The reason is uncertain but it seems possible that the indomethacin reduces the clearance of the vancomycin (and other drugs) by the kidneys. The authors of this report suggest that the usual vancomycin maintenance dosage should be halved if indomethacin is also being used. It is not known whether indomethacin has the same effect on vancomycin in adult patients.

Reference

1 Spivey JM, Gal P. Vancomycin pharmacokinetics in neonates. Am J Dis Child (1986) 140, 859.

Vidarabine + Allopurinol

Abstract/Summary

There is evidence that if allopurinol and vidarabine (adenine arabinoside) are used concurrently the toxicity of vidarabine may be increased.

Clinical evidence

Two patients with chronic lymphocytic leukaemia treated with 300 mg allopurinol daily developed severe neurotoxicity (coarse rhythmic tremors of the extremities and facial muscles, and impaired mentation) four days after vidarabine was added for the treatment of viral infections.[1] A retrospective search to find other patients who had had both drugs for four days revealed a total of 17 patients, five of whom had experienced adverse reactions including tremors, nausea, pain, itching and anaemia.[1]

Mechanism

Uncertain. One suggestion is that the allopurinol allows hypoxanthine arabinoside, the major metabolite of vidarabine, to accumulate. A study with rat liver cytosol showed that allopurinol increased the half-life of this metabolite from 40 min to 4 h.[2]

Importance and management

Information seems to be limited to this study so that the general clinical importance of this possible interaction is uncertain, but it would be prudent to exercise particular care if these drugs are used together. More study is needed.

References

1 Friedman HM, Grasela T. Adenine arabinoside and allopurinol-possible adverse drug interaction. N Engl J Med (1981) 304, 423.
2 Drach JC, Rentea RG, Cowen ME. The metabolic degradation of 9B-D-arabinofuranosyladenine (ara-A) *in vitro*. Fed Proc (1973) 32, 777.

Zalcitabine + Didanosine

Abstract/Summary

An isolated report describes increased neuropathy in a patient given both drugs. Both can cause peripheral neuropathy.

Clinical evidence, mechanism, importance and management

The commonest serious toxicity of both didanosine and zalcitabine is peripheral neuropathy, with up to a third of patients taking either drug being affected.[2,3] The usual advice to avoid the concurrent use of drugs which share this serious side-effect seems a sensible precaution, but there is only one report attributing an exacerbation of zalcitabine neuropathy to the additional use of didanosine.[1] There is no proof that the frequency or severity of the neuropathy is normally increased if the two are combined.

References

1 LeLacheur SF, Simon GL. Exacerbation of dideoxycytidine-induced neuropathy with dideoxydidanosine. J AIDS (1991) 4, 538–9.
2 Yarchoan R, Mitsuya H, Pluda J M et al. The National Cancer Institute phase I study of 2',3'-dideoxyinosine administration in adults with AIDS or AIDS-related complex: analysis of activity and toxicity profiles. Rev Infect Dis (199) 12 (Suppl 5) S522–33.
3 Yarchoan R, Perno CF, Thomas RV et al. Phase I studies of 2',3'-dideoxycytidine in severe human immunodeficiency virus infection as a single agent and alternating with zidovudine (AZT). Lancet (1988) 1, 76–81.

Zidovudine (Azidothymidine) + Benzodiazepines

Abstract/Summary

Oxazepam causes a modest increase in the bioavailability of zidovudine, and can increase the incidence of headaches.

Clinical evidence, mechanism, importance and management

A pharmacokinetic study in six HIV-infected patients found that oxazepam increased the bioavailability of zidovudine by 23%. All of them were sleepy and fatigued while taking oxazepam, and five of the six complained of headaches while taking both drugs. The authors of the report suggest that if headaches occur during concurrent use, the benzodiazepine should be stopped before concluding that the headaches are due solely to the zidovudine or an HIV-related pathology.[1]

Reference

1 Mole L, Israelski D, Bubp J, O'Hanley P, Merigan T, Blaschke T. Pharmacokinetics of zidovudine alone and in combination with oxazepam in HIV infected patients. J Acq Imm Def Syndr (1993) 6, 56–60.

Zidovudine (Azidothymidine) + Food

Abstract/Summary

The absorption of zidovudine is markedly reduced if taken with food.

Clinical evidence, mechanism, importance and management

13 patients with AIDS showed increases in zidovudine AUCs and maximal serum level increases of 280 and 140% respectively when taken fasting than when taken with breakfast.[1] The reasons are not understood. The practical consequences of these changes are also uncertain.

Reference

1 Lotterer E, Ruhnke M, Trautmann M, Beyer R, Bauer FE. Decreased and variable systemic availability of zidouvidine in patients with AIDS if administered with a meal. Eur J Clin Pharmacol (1991) 40, 305–8.

Zidovudine (Azidothymidine) + Ganciclovir

Abstract/Summary

A marked increase in haematological toxicity occurs if zidovudine and ganciclovir are used concurrently, without any increase in efficacy.

Clinical evidence

The efficacy of zidovudine (600–1200 mg daily) alone or combined with ganciclovir (5 mg/kg IV twice daily for 14 days, then once daily five days per week) was assessed in 40 patients for the treatment of AIDS-related cytomegalovirus (CMV) disease. Severe haematological toxicity occurred in all of the patients given 1200 mg zidovudine daily. Even with reduced zidovudine dosages (600 mg) 82% of the patients experienced profound and rapid toxicity (anaemia, neutropenia, leukopenia, gastrointestinal disturbances). Zidovudine dosage reductions to 300 mg daily were needed by many patients. No increased efficacy was seen, instead the CMV disease progressed (worsening opthalmologic findings) and new infections developed.[1]

Another study in 16 AIDS patients with cytomegalovirus retinitis given both drugs found increased bone marrow toxicity but no improved efficacy over ganciclovir alone.[3]

Mechanism

Not understood. No changes in the pharmacokinetics of either drug were seen.[1] The toxicity of the two drugs may be simply additive. *In vitro* studies with three human cell lines showed synergistic cytotoxicity when both drugs were used.[2]

Importance and management

An established and clinically important interaction. Concurrent use should be avoided because of the severe toxicities. The authors of one of the studies say that '.. we consider that the toxic effects of concurrent therapy with ganciclovir and zidovudine are unacceptable..'.[3]

References

1 Hochster H, Dieterich D, Bozzette S, Reichman RC, Connor JD, Liebes L, Sonke RL, Spector SA, Valentine F, Pettinelli C, Richman DD. Toxicity of combined ganciclovir and zidovudine for cytomegalovirus disease associated with AIDS. An AIDS clinical trials group study. Ann Intern Med (1990) 113, 111–6.
2 Prichard MN, Prichard LE, Baguley WA, Nassiri MR, Shipman C. Three-dimensional analysis of the synergistic cytotoxicity of ganciclovir and zidovudine. Antimicrob Ag Chemother (1991) 35, 1060–5.
3 Millar AB, Miller RF, Patou G, Mindel A, Marsh R, Semple SJG. Treatment of cytomegalovirus retinitis with zidovudine and ganciclovir in patients with AIDS: outcome and toxicity. Genitourin Med (1990) 66, 156–8.

Zidovudine (Azidothymidine) + Interferon

Abstract/Summary

Interferon causes a marked increase in the serum levels of zidovudine.

Clinical evidence

AIDS patients who had been taking 200 mg zidovudine four-hourly for 8 weeks were additionally given 90×10^6 Units of recombinant beta interferon subcutaneously. After 3 days the zidovudine metabolism was reduced by 66% (from 1.18 to 0.4/h) and after 15 days by 93% (to 0.08/h). By day 15 the zidovudine half-life was increased two- to three-fold.[1]

Mechanism

Beta interferon appears to inhibit the metabolism (glucuronidation) of the zidovudine by the liver.

Importance and management

Information seems to be limited to this report. The zidovudine dosage should be reduced if beta interferon is added in order to avoid increased zidovudine toxicity. A dosage reduction of two-thirds or even more would seem possible. More study is needed to confirm these observations.

Reference

1 Nokta M, Loh JP, Douidar SM, Snodgrass WR, Ahmed EA, Pollard RB. Molecular interaction of recombinant beta interferon and zidovudine: alterations of AZT pharmacokinetics in HIV-infected patients. 5th Int Conf AIDS Montreal (1989) p 278.

Zidovudine (Azidothymidine) + Lithium carbonate

Abstract/Summary

Lithium can apparently oppose the neutropenic effects of zidovudine.

Clinical evidence, mechanism, importance and management

A study in five patients with AIDS found that serum lithium carbonate levels of 0.6–1.2 mmol/l increased their neutrophil counts sufficiently to allow the re-introduction of zidovudine previously withdrawn due to neutropenia. Withdrawal of the lithium resulted in a rapid fall in neutrophil levels in two patients.[1] The reasons for this effect on neutrophil production are not understood.

This report suggests that no adverse reaction occurs in patients taking zidovudine who are given lithium, and that there are some advantages. More study is needed.

Reference

1 Roberts DE, Berman SM, Nakasato S, Wyle FA, Wishnow RM, Segal GP. Effect of lithium carbonate on zidovudine-associated neutropenia in the acquired immunodeficiency syndrome. Amer J Med (1988) 85, 428.

Zidovudine (Azidothymidine) + Miscellaneous drugs

Abstract/Summary

Acyclovir, aspirin and ketoconazole appear not to increase the haematological toxicity of zidovudine but overwhelming fatigue is reported in one patient given acyclovir. Marked neutropenia occurred in four patients given zidovudine and vancomycin. Some *in vitro* evidence suggests that chloramphenicol and ethinyloestradiol might increase the effects and toxicity of zidovudine. Trimethoprim and dapsone increase the serum levels of zidovudine whereas clarithromycin reduces its levels. Clindamycin, interleukin-2, itraconazole, indomethacin and naproxen appear not to interact. Zidovudine appears not to interact adversely with antitubercular drugs.

Clinical evidence, mechanism, importance and management

(a) Acyclovir, aspirin, co-trimoxazole, itraconazole, ketoconazole

A study of zidovudine use in 282 AIDS patients found that haematological abnormalities (anaemia, leukopenia, neutropenia) were very common indeed and 21% needed multiple red cell transfusions. Some of the patients also received acyclovir, aspirin, ketoconazole, co-trimoxazole and paracetamol (acetaminophen) but only the paracetamol increased the haematological toxicity (neutropenia) by an unstated amount.[1] A report says that overwhelming fatigue occurred in a patient when given zidovudine and acyclovir on two occasions.[2] 200 mg itraconazole daily for two weeks was reported in a study to have no effect on the pharmacokinetics of zidovudine in seven patients, but the serum levels in two patients were reported as being higher.[4]

(b) clarithromycin

Fifteen HIV infected patients were given oral zidovudine (100 mg four-hourly for five days) and oral clarithromycin (500, 1000 or 2000 mg 12-hourly) both individually and concurrently. The pharmacokinetics of the clarithromycin were not substantially changed but the serum zidovudine levels and AUCs were reduced 32–46% and 12–26% respectively. It was not seen in all patients.[12] The clinical importance of these reductions is uncertain.

(b) Ethambutol, isoniazid, pyrazinamide, rifampicin

A comparative study in HIV infected patients given zidovudine and antitubercular treatment (isoniazid, rifampicin, pyrazinamide, ethambutol) found no evidence of an adverse interaction although marked anaemia occurred in those given both groups of drugs. The authors advise careful monitoring for haematological toxicity.[8]

(c) Indomethacin, naproxen, clindamycin, chloramphenicol and ethinyloestradiol

An *in vitro* study using human liver microsomes found that indomethacin, naproxen, chloramphenicol and ethinyloestradiol inhibited the glucuronidation of zidovudine by 50% or more.[7] This suggested that some of these drugs might possibly increase the effects and the toxicity of zidovudine, however three studies found no changes in the kinetics of zidovudine by indomethacin (50 mg daily for 3 days) or naproxen (0.5–1 g daily for three or 4 days) or clindamycin in HIV patients.[5,6,9] No special precautions would seem necessary with these three drugs but the effects of the concurrent use of the other drugs in patients awaits assessment.

(d) Interleukin-2

A study in patients found that a four week course of interleukin-2 (0.25 x 10^6 units/m^2/ day) by continuous infusion had no clinically significant effect on the pharmacokinetics of zidovudine (100 mg IV bolus doses).[11] No special precautions would seem necessary.

(e) Trimethoprim, dapsone

Five HIV patients showed a zidovudine AUC rise of 30% when given trimethoprim (no dosage stated) and a 40% rise when given dapsone as well (no dosage stated), but dapsone alone had no effect.[10] It seems unlikely that these changes are clinically important, but concurrent use should nevertheless be monitored.

(f) Vancomycin

Another report describes marked neutropenia in four HIV patients on zidovudine when given vancomycin (which also can have neutropenic effects).[3] On theoretical grounds any drug causing bone marrow suppression might be additive with the effects of zidovudine.

References

1 Richman DD, Fischl MA, Grieco MH, Gottlieb MS, Volberding PA, Laskin OL, Leedom JM, Groopman JE, Mildvan D, Hirsch MS, Jackson GG, Durack DT, Nusinoff-Lehrman S, the AZT Collaborative Working Group. The toxicity of azidothymidine (AZT) in the treatment of patients with AIDS and AIDS-related complex. A double-blind, placebo-controlled trial. N Engl J Med (1987) 317, 192–7.
2 Bach MC. Possible drug interaction during therapy with azidothymidine and acyclovir for AIDS. N Engl J Med (1987) 316, 547.
3 Kitchen LW, Clark RA, Hanna BJ, Pollock B, Valainis GT. Vancomycin and neutropenia in AZT-treated AIDS patients with staphylococcal infections. J Acquir Imm Def Syndrom (1990) 3, 925.
4 Henrivaux Ph, Fairon Y, Fillet G. Pharmacokinetics of AZT among HIV infected patients treated by itraconazole. 5th int Conf AIDS Montreal (1989), p 278.
5 Jones DR, Black JR. Evaluation of pharmacokinetic interactions between the combination of primaquine plus clindamycin and ziodovudine. In Programme and Abstracts of the 17th Int Conf AIDS (1990) p222.
6 Barry M, Howe J, Back D, Breckenridge A, Brettle R, Mitchell R, Beeching N, Nye F. Effect of non-steroidal anti-inflammatory drugs on zidovudine pharmacokinetics. Br J clin Pharmac (1992) 34, 446P.
7 Sim SM, Back DJ, Breckenridge AM. The effect of various drugs on the glucuronidation of zidovudine (azidothymidine; AZT) by human liver microsomes. Br J clin Pharmac (1991) 32, 17–21.
8 Antoniskis D, Easley AC, Espin BM, Davidson PT, Barnes PF. Combined toxicity of zidovudine and antituberculous chemotherapy. Am Rev Respir Dis (1992) 145, 430–4.
9 Sahai J, Gallicano K, Garber G, Pakuts A, Hawlwy-Foss N, Huang L, McGilveray I, Cameron DW. Evaluation of the *in vivo* effect of naproxen on zidovudine pharmacokinetics in patients infected with human immuno-deficiency virus. Clin Pharmacol Ther (1992) 52, 464–70.
10 Lee BL, Safrin S, Makrides V, Benowitz NL, Gembertoglio JG, Mills J. Trimethoprim decreases the renal clearance of zidovudine. Clin Pharmacol Ther (1992) 51,183.
11 Skinner MH, Pauloin D, Schwartz D, Merigan TC, Blaschke TF. Il-2 does not alter zioduvidine kinetics. Clin Pharmacol Ther (1989) 45, 128.
12 Gustayson LE, Chu S-y, Mackenthun A, Gupta SD, Craft JC. Drug interaction between clarithromycin and oral zidovudine in HIV-1 infected patients. Clin Pharmacol Ther (1993) 53, 163.

~ Zidovudine (Azidothymidine) + Paracetamol (acetaminophen)

Abstract/Summary

Limited and unconfirmed evidence suggests that paracetamol possibly increases the bone marrow suppressant effects of zidovudine. A single case report describes severe liver toxicity.

Clinical evidence

A study of zidovudine use in 282 AIDS patients found that haematological abnormalities (anaemia, leukopenia, neutropenia) were very common indeed and 21% needed multiple red cell transfusions. Some of the patients also received acyclovir, aspirin, ketoconazole, co-trimoxazole and paracetamol (acetaminophen) but only the paracetamol increased the haematological toxicity (neutropenia) by an unstated amount.[1] A patient on zidovudine and co-trimoxazole developed severe hepatotoxicity within a day of taking 2 g paracetamol.[6]

Clinical studies using up to 650 mg paracetamol four hourly found that it either had no effect at all on the pharmacokinetics of zidovudine and did not increase its clearance.[2-5]

Mechanism

Not understood. Paracetamol does not increase the serum levels of zidovudine[2-5] which might have provided an explanation for the apparent increased toxicity. Paracetamol does not affect the glucuronidation of zidovudine.[7]

Importance and management

There is very little hard evidence to go on at the moment, but it would clearly be prudent to monitor any patient taking both drugs for any evidence of bone marrow or liver toxicity. More study is needed.

References

1 Richman DD, Fischl MA, Grieco MH, Gottlieb MS, Volberding PA, Laskin OL, Leedom JM, Groopman JE, Mildvan D, Hirsch MS, Jackson GG, Durack DT, Nusinoff-Lehrman S, the AZT Collaborative Working Group. The toxicity of azidothymidine (AZT) in the treatment of patients with AIDS and AIDS-related complex. A double-blind, placebo-controlled trial. N Engl J Med (1987) 317, 192–7.
2 Sattler FR, Ko R, Antoniskis D, Shields M, Cohen J, Nicoloff J, Leedom J Koda R. Acetaminophen does not impair clearance of zidovudine. Ann Intern Med (1991) 114, 937–40.
3 Steffe EM, King JH, Inciardi JF, Flynn NF, Goldstein E, Tonjes TS, Benet LZ. The effect of acetaminophen on zidovudine metabolism in HIV-infected patients. J Acq Imm Def Syndr (1990) 3, 691–4.
4 Ptachcinski J, Pazin G. The effect of acetaminophen on the pharmacokinetics of zidovudine. Pharmacotherapy (1989) 9, 190.
5 Pazin GJ, Ptachcinski RJ, Sheehan M. Ho M. Interactive pharmacokinetics of ziodovudine and acetaminophen. 5th int Conf AIDS Montreal (1989), p 278.
6 Shriner K, Goetz MB. Severe hepatotoxicity in a patient receiving both acetaminophen and zidovudine. Amer J Med (1992) 93, 94–6.
7 Kamali F, Rawlins MD. Influence of probenecid and paracetamol (acetaminophen) on zidovudine glucuronidation in human liver in vitro. Biopharm Drug Disp (1992) 13, 403–9.

Zidovudine (Azidothymidine) + Probenecid

Abstract/Summary

Probenecid halves the loss of zidovudine from the body and raises its serum levels. The incidence of rashes is reported to be very much increased by concurrent use.

Clinical evidence

The concurrent use of zidovudine 4-hourly and 500 mg probenecid 8-hourly for three days increased the zidovudine AUC in 12 patients with AIDS or AIDS-related complex by an average of 80% (range 14–192%).[4]

Three other studies with seven patients and two patients found that 500 mg probenecid 6-hourly doubled the AUC of zidovudine (2 mg/kg three times daily).[1,5] Similar results were found in a study in normal subjects.[7] However another report describes a very high incidence of rashes in six out of eight men with HIV infections when given both drugs. The rash and constitutional symptoms were sufficiently severe for the probenecid to be withdrawn from two of them.[3]

Mechanism

Experimental clinical evidence indicates that probenecid reduces the metabolism (glucuronidation) of the zidovudine by the liver enzymes, thereby reducing its loss from the body.[2,4,6-8]

Importance and management

An established and clinically important interaction. Concurrent use should be well monitored to ensure that zidovudine levels do not rise excessively. Reduce the zidovudine dosage as necessary. It has been suggested that the same dose of zidovudine could be given 8-hourly instead of 4-hourly for convenience and to save costs,[4] however the apparent increase in serious rashes during concurrent use (cited above[3]) should be borne in mind. The safety of combined use needs further assessment.

References

1 Hedaya MA, Elmquist WF, Sawchuk RJ. Probenecid inhibits the metabolic and renal clearances of zidovudine (AZT) in human volunteers. Pharmaceutical Res (1990) 7, 411–7.
2 Kawali F, Rawlins MD. Inhibition of zidovudine glucuronidation by probenecid in human liver microsomes. Clin Sci (1990) 79, 27P.
3 Petty BG, Kornhauser DM, Lietman PS. Zidovudine with probenecid: a warning. Lancet (1990) 1, 1044–5.
4 Kornhauser DM, Petty BG, Hendrix CW, Woods AS, Nerhood LJ, Bartlett

JG, Lietman PS. Probenecid and zidovudine metabolism. Lancet (1989) 2, 473–5.

5 de Miranda P, Good SS, Yarchoan R, Thomas RV, Blum MR, Myers CE, Broder S. Alteration of zidovudine pharmacokinetics by probenecid in patients with Aids or Aids-related complex. Clin Pharmacol Ther (1989) 46, 494–500.

6 Sim SM, Back DJ, Breckenridge AM. The effect of various drugs on the glucuronidation of zidovudine (azidothymidine; AZT) by human liver microsomes. Br J clin Pharmac (1991) 32, 17–21.

7 Campion JJ, Bawdon RE, Baskin LB, Bartoon CI. Effect of probenecid on the pharmacokinetics of zidovudine and zidovudine glucuronide. Pharmacotherapy (1990) 10, 235.

8 Kamali F, Rawlins MD. Influence of probenecid and paracetamol (acetaminophen) on zidovudine glucuronidation in human liver *in vitro*. Biopharm Drug Disp (1992) 13, 403–9.

Zidovudine (Azidothymidine) + Sodium valproate

Abstract/Summary

Sodium valproate raises serum zidovudine levels.

Clinical evidence, mechanism, importance and management

Six asymptomatic HIV-infected patients given 100 mg zidovudine 8-hourly showed a 72% increase in the zidovudine plasma AUC while taking 250–500 mg sodium valproate 8-hourly. The evidence indicated that the metabolism (glucuronidation) of the zidovudine was inhibited by the sodium valproate so that its bioavailability was increased.[1] Concurrent use should be well monitored for evidence of increased zidovudine effects and toxicity.

Reference

1 Lertora JJ, Greenspan DL, Rege AB, Akula S, George WJ, Hyslop NE, Agrawal KC. Valproic acid inhibits glucuronidation of zidovudine (AZT) in HIV infected patients. Clin Pharmacol Ther (1993) 53, 197.

Zidovudine (Azidothymidine) + Trimethoprim, Co-trimoxazole

Abstract/Summary

Trimethoprim alone or in co-trimoxazole reduces the loss of zidovudine in the urine, but the extent appears to be too small to be clinically important. No increased toxicity would be expected.

Clinical evidence

A study in nine HIV patients given 3 mg/kg zidovudine by constant rate infusion over 1 h found that neither trimethoprim alone nor co-trimoxazole (sulphamethoxazole + trimethoprim) affected the metabolic clearance of the zidovudine, but the renal clearance was reduced by 58 and 48% respectively, and that of its glucuronide by 27 and 39% respectively.[1]

Five other HIV patients showed a zidovudine AUC rise of 30% when also given trimethoprim (no dosage stated).[2]

Mechanism

A likely reason is that the trimethoprim inhibits the secretion of both zidovudine and its glucuronide by the kidney tubules.

Importance and management

Information is very limited. Since renal clearance represents only 20–30% of the total clearance of zidovudine, the authors of one of these reports[1] suggest that this interaction is unlikely to be clinically important unless the glucuronidation by the liver is impaired by liver disease or other drugs. This needs confirmation. It is consistent with the results of another study in which co-trimoxazole (amongst a number of other drugs) did not appear to increased the haematological toxicity of zidovudine,[3] however concurrent use should be well monitored. It should however also be pointed out that co-trimoxazole alone has been associated with a high incidence of adverse effects in patients with AIDS.[4]

References

1 Chatton JY, Munafo A, Chave JP, Steinhäuslin F, Roch-Ramel F, Glauser MP, Biollas J. Trimethoprim, alone of in combination with sulphamethoxazole, decreases the renal excretion of zidovudine and its glucuronide. Br J clin Pharmac (1992) 34, 551–4.

2 Lee BL, Safrin S, Makrides V, Benowitz NL, Gembertoglio JG, Mills J. Trimethoprim decreases the renal clearance of zidovudine. Clin Pharmacol Ther (1992) 51,183.

3 Richman DD, Fischl MA, Grieco MH, Gottlieb MS, Volberding PA, Laskin OL, Leedom JM, Groopman JE, Mildvan D, Hirsch MS, Jackson GG, Durack DT, Nusinoff-Lehrman S, the AZT Collaborative Working Group. The toxicity of azidothymidine (AZT) in the treatment of patients with AIDS and AIDS-related complex. A double-blind, placebo-controlled trial. N Engl J Med (1987) 317, 192–7.

4 Medina I, Mills J, Leoung G, Hopefull PC, Lee B, Modin G, Benowitz N, Wopsy CB. Oral therapy for Pneumocystis carinii peneumonia in the acquired immunodeficiency syndrome: a controlled trial of trimethoprim-sulphamethoxazole versus dapsone-trimethoprim. N Engl J Med (199) 323, 776–82.

Chapter 6
Anticoagulant Drug Interactions

The blood clotting process

When blood is shed or clotting is initiated in some other way, a complex cascade of biochemical reactions is set in motion which ends in the formation of a network or clot of insoluble protein threads enmeshing the blood cells. These threads are produced by the polymerization of the molecules of fibrinogen (a soluble protein present in the plasma) into threads of insoluble fibrin. The penultimate step in the chain of reactions requires the presence of an enzyme, thrombin, which is produced from its precursor prothrombin, already present in the plasma. Figure 6.1 is a highly simplified diagram to illustrate the final stages of this cascade of reactions.

Mode of action of the anticoagulants

The oral anticoagulants extend the time taken for blood to clot and, it is believed, also inhibit the pathological formation of blood clots within blood vessels by reducing the concentrations within the plasma of a number of components necessary for the cascade to proceed, namely factors VII, IX, X and II (prothrombin). The parts played by three of these

four are not shown in the simplified diagram illustrated but they are essential for the production of the so-called 'thromboplastins'.

The synthesis of normal amounts of these four factors takes place within the liver with vitamin K as one of the essential ingredients, but, in the presence of an oral anticoagulant, the rate of synthesis of all four is retarded. One of the early theories to explain why this happens was based on the observed resemblance between the molecular shapes of vitamin K and the oral anticoagulants. It was suggested that the molecules were sufficiently similar for the anticoagulant actually to take part in the biochemical reactions by which all four are synthesized, but sufficiently dissimilar to prevent the completion of these reactions. The term 'competitive antagonist' is used to describe this situation because vitamin K and the oral anticoagulants compete with one another to take part in the reactions, their relative concentrations being among the factors which determine the 'winner'. This theory is now known to be too simple, but the basic principle of a concentration competition between the two types of molecules remains perfectly valid. A reduction in the concentrations and activity of all four factors is embraced by the portmanteau term 'hypoprothrombinaemia'.

The therapeutic use of the oral anticoagulants

During anticoagulant therapy it is usual to depress the levels of the prothrombin and factors VII, IX and X to those which are believed to give protection against intravascular clotting, without running the risk of excessive depression which leads to bleeding. To achieve this each patient is individually titrated with doses of anticoagulant until the desired response is attained, a procedure which normally takes

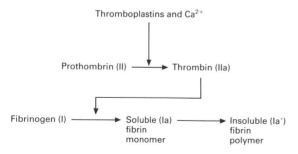

Fig 6.1 A highly simplified flow diagram of the final stages of the blood clotting process.

several days because the oral anticoagulants do not act directly on the blood clotting factors already in circulation, but on the rate of synthesis of new factors by the liver. The 'end point' of the titration is determined by one of a number of different but closely related laboratory in vitro tests which measure the extension in the time taken for the blood to clot (e.g. the so-called 'one-stage prothrombin time') although the result of the test may be expressed, not in seconds, but as a ratio or a percentage of normal values. The normal plasma clotting time, using the Quick one-stage prothrombin time test, is about 12 s, an extension to about 24–30 s or so is usually regarded as adequate in anticoagulant therapy. Other tests include the thrombotest and the prothrombin-proconvertin (P-P) test.

Anticoagulant interactions

Therapeutically desirable prothrombin levels can be upset by a number of factors including diet, disease and the use of other drugs. In the case of drugs, either the addition or the withdrawal may upset the balance in a patient already well stabilized on the anticoagulant. Some drugs increase the activity of the anticoagulants and can cause bleeding if the dosage of the anticoagulant is not reduced appropriately. Others reduce the activity and return the prothrombin time to normal. If one believes in the therapeutic value of the oral anticoagulants, both situations are serious and may be fatal, although excessive hypoprothrombinaemia manifests itself more obviously and immediately as bleeding and is usually regarded as the more serious.

Bleeding and its treatment

When prothrombin times become excessive, bleeding can occur. In order of decreasing frequency the bleeding shows itself as ecchymoses, blood in the urine, uterine bleeding, black faeces, bruising, nosebleeding, haematoma, gum bleeding, coughing and vomiting blood.

If minor bleeding occurs, the anticoagulant should be stopped at once and 10–20 mg vitamin K1 (phy-

Table 6.1 Anticoagulants. Not all of the anticoagulants listed are in the text

Non-proprietary names	Proprietary names
Oral anticoagulants	
Coumarins	
Cumetharol	*Dicoumoxyl*
Cyclocoumarol	
Dic(o)umarol (bishydroxycoumarin)	*Apekumarol, Baracoumin, Dicumerol, Dicumol, Dufalone*
Ethylbiscoumacetate	*Stabilene, Tromexan(e), Tromexano*
Ethylidene dicoumarin	*Pertromban*
Nicoumalone (acenocoumarol)	*Sint(h)rom(e)*
Phenprocoumon	*Liquamar, Marcoumar, Marcumar*
Tioclomarol	*Apegmone*
Warfarin potassium and sodium	*Aldocumar, Athrombin-K, Coumadan Sodico, Coumadin(e), Marevan, Panwarfin, Sofarin, Warfarin, Warfilone, Warnerin*
Indanediones	
Anisindione	*Miradon, Unidone*
Bromindione	*Fluidane*
Clorindione (chlorphenindione)	*Indalitan*
Diphenadione	*Dipaxin(e)*
Flurindione	*Previscan*
Phenindione	*Danilone, Dindevan, Emandione, Hedulin, Pindione, Trombantin*
Parenteral anticoagulants	
Heparin	

tonadione) given orally. This should return the prothrombin time to normal within about 24 h and the bleeding should cease. If the bleeding is more severe, at least 50 mg vitamin K1 should be given intravenously. If bleeding is not reduced significantly within a few hours, more vitamin K1 should be given and transfusion with fresh whole blood, fresh frozen plasma or plasma concentrates of factors II, IX and V should be undertaken.

This chapter is concerned with those drugs which affect the activity of the anticoagulants. When the anticoagulant is the affecting agent the interaction is dealt with elsewhere in this book. The Index should be consulted.

Anticoagulants + ACE inhibitors

Abstract/Summary

No ACE-inhibitor has so far been shown to interact significantly with an oral anticoagulant.

Clinical evidence, mechanism, importance and management

5 mg ramipril daily for seven days in eight subjects had no effect on the pharmacokinetics or anticoagulant effects of phenprocoumon.[1] 20 mg benazepril daily has been found not affect the serum levels of either warfarin or nicoumalone. The anticoagulant activity of nicoumalone was not altered, but the effects of warfarin were slightly reduced, but not enough to be clinically important.[2] 20 mg enalapril for five days is reported not to affect the anticoagulant effects of warfarin (2.5–7.5 mg daily),[3] and 2.5 mg cilazapril daily for three weeks had no effect on the thrombotest times or coagulation factors II, VII and X in 28 patients on long-term nicoumalone or phenprocoumon treatment.[4]

No special precautions would seem necessary if any of these anticoagulants and ACE-inhibitors are used concurrently. There seems to be nothing documented about any other anticoagulants and ACE-inhibitors and it seems unlikely that an interaction will occur with any of them.

References

1 Verho M, Malerczyk V, Grotsch H, Zenbil I. Absence of interaction between ramipril, a new ACE-inhibitor, and phenprocoumon, an anticoagulant agent. Pharmacotherapeutica (1989) 5, 392–9.
2 Van Hecken A, De Lepeleire I, Verbesselt R, Arnout J, Angehrn J, Youngberg C, De Schepper PJ. Effect of benazepril, a converting enzyme inhibitor, on plasma levels and activity of acenocoumarol and warfarin. Int J Clin Pharm Res (1988) VIII, 315–19.
3 Merck, Sharpe & Dohme. Unpublished data on file quoted by Gomez HJ, Cirillo VJ, Irvin JD. Enalapril: a review of human pharmacology. Drugs (1985) 30 Suppl 1, 13–24.
4 Boeijinga JK, Breimer DD, Kraay CJ, Kleinbloesem CH. Absence of interaction between the ACE inhibitor cilazapril and coumarin derivatives in elderly patients on long term oral anticoagulants. Br J Clin Pharmacol (1992) 33, 553P.

Anticoagulants + Acemetacin or Oxametacin

Abstract/Summary

The anticoagulant effects of warfarin and nicoumalone (acenocoumarol) can be increased by the concurrent use of oxametacin. An anticoagulant dosage reduction may be needed. Acemetacin does not interact with phenprocoumon.

Clinical evidence, mechanism, importance and management

Oxametacin (100 mg three times a day) for 14 days reduced the thrombotest percentages of 12 anticoagulated patients (11 on warfarin and one on nicoumalone) from 11.2 to 7.8%. A third needed a reduction in their anticoagulant dosage or its withdrawal.[1] Concurrent use should be monitored, reducing the anticoagulant dosage if necessary. Apply the same precautions with any other anticoagulant but direct information is lacking. A study in 20 patients on phenprocoumon found no interaction with 60 mg acemetacin three times daily.[2]

References

1 Baele G, Rasquin K, Barbier F. Effects of oxametacin on coumarin anticoagulation and on platelet function in humans. Arzneim.-Forsch/Drug Res (1983) 33, 149–52.
2 Hess H, Koeppen R. Kontrollierte Doppelblindstudie zur Frage einer möglichen Interferenz von Acemetacin mit einer laufenden Antikoagulanzien-Therapie. Arzneim-Forsch/Drug Res (1980) 30, 1421–3.

Anticoagulants + Acitretin or Etretinate

Abstract/Summary

A single case report describes reduced warfarin effects in a patient when given etretinate. Acitretin does not significantly alter the anticoagulant effects of phenprocoumon.

Clinical evidence

(a) Phenprocoumon + Acitretin

50 mg acitretin daily for 10 days slightly increased the prothrombin complex activity of 10 subjects on phenprocoumon (1.5–3.0 mg daily) from 22 to 24% (corresponding INR's of 2.91 and 2.71), but there were no important changes in Quick values.[1]

(b) Warfarin + Etretinate

A man with T-cell lymphoma who had recently had chemotherapy (cyclophosphamide, adriamycin, vincristine and prednisolone) was anticoagulated with warfarin after developing a pulmonary embolism. When he was started on 40 mg etretinate daily it was found necessary to increase his warfarin dosage from 7 to 10 mg daily. His liver function tests were normal.[2] This report is a little confused by the other drugs being taken concurrently (co-proxamol, tolbutamide, 8-methoxypsoralen, prednisone, brompheniramine, cimetidine), some of which can interact with warfarin.

Mechanism

Not understood.

Importance and management

Information appears to be limited to these reports. Monitor the concurrent use of warfarin and etretinate in any patient, increasing the anticoagulant dosage as necessary. Follow the same precautions with acitretin which is a metabolite of etretinate, because it seems possible that it may interact similarly. No special precautions seem necessary if acitretin is given to patients on phenprocoumon but the outcome should be monitored. There seems to be no information about other anticoagulants.

References

1 Hartmann D, Mosberg H, Weber W. Lack of effect of acitretin on the hypoprothrombinemic action of phenprocoumon in healthy volunteers. Dermatologica (1989) 178, 33–6.
2 Ostlere LS, Langtry JAA, Jones S, Staughton RCD. Reduced therapeutic effect of warfarin caused by etretinate. Br J Dermatol (1991) 124, 505–10.

Anticoagulants + Alcohol

Abstract/Summary

The effects of the oral anticoagulants are unlikely to be changed in those with normal liver function who drink small or moderate amounts of alcohol, but heavy drinkers or patients with some liver disease may show considerable fluctuations in their prothrombin times.

Clinical evidence

(a) Patients and subjects free from liver disease

Twenty ounces (one pint or 56.4 g ethanol) of a Californian white table wine a day, given over a 3-week period at meal times to eight normal subjects anticoagulated with warfarin, were found to have no significant effects on either the serum warfarin levels nor the anticoagulant response.[8]

Other studies in both patients and normal subjects on either warfarin or phenprocoumon have very clearly confirmed the absence of an interaction with alcohol.[1,2,9,10] In one study the subjects were given almost 600 ml of a table wine (12% alcohol) or 300 ml of a fortified wine (20% alcohol).[9–11]

(b) Chronic alcoholics or those with liver disease

A study[3] in 15 alcoholics given a single dose of warfarin who had been drinking heavily (250 g ethanol or more daily) for at least three months, confirmed the results of a previous investigation that the half-life of warfarin was reduced from 40.1 to 26.5 h but, surprisingly, a comparison of their prothrombin times with those of normal subjects showed no differences.[4]

Other reports have shown that prothrombin times and war-

farin levels of those with liver cirrhosis and other dysfunction can rise markedly after they have been on the binge, but restabilize soon afterwards when the drinking stops.[2,5]

Mechanism

It seems probable that in man, as in rats,[6] continuous heavy drinking stimulates the hepatic enzymes concerned with the metabolism of warfarin, leading to its more rapid elimination.[3] As a result the half-life shortens. The fluctuations in prothrombin times in those with liver dysfunction[2,5] may possibly occur because sudden large amounts of alcohol exacerbate the general malfunction of the liver and this affects the way it metabolizes warfarin. It may also change the ability of the liver to synthesize the blood clotting factors.[7]

Importance and management

The absence of an interaction in those free from liver disease is well documented and well established. It appears to be quite safe for patients on oral anticoagulants to drink small or moderate amounts of alcohol. Even much less conservative amounts (up to 8 oz/250 ml of spirits[1] or a pint of wine[8]) do not create problems with the anticoagulant control, so that there appears to be a good margin of safety even for the less than abstemious. Only warfarin and phenprocoumon have been investigated but other anticoagulants may be expected to behave similarly. On the other hand those who drink heavily may possibly need above-average doses of the anticoagulant, while those with liver damage who continue to drink may experience marked fluctuations in their prothrombin times. This typically occurs in alcoholics after going on the binge over the weekend. An attempt to limit their intake of alcohol is desirable from this as well as from other points of view.

References

1 Waris E. Effect of ethyl alcohol on some coagulation factors in man during anticoagulant therapy. Ann Med Exp Biol Fenn (1965) 115, 53.
2 Udall JA. Drug interference with warfarin therapy. Clin Med (1970) 77, 20.
3 Kater RMH, Roggin G, Tobon F, Zieve P, Iber FL. Increased rate of clearance of drugs from the circulation of alcoholics. Amer J Med Sci (1969) 258, 35.
4 Kater RM, Carruli N, Iber FL. Differences in the rate of ethanol metabolism in recently drinking alcoholic and non-alcoholic subjects. Amer J Clin Nutrition (1969) 14, 21.
5 Breckenridge A, Orme M. Clinical implications of enzyme induction. Ann NY Acad Sci (1971) 179, 421.
6 Rubin E, Hutterev F, Lieber CS. Ethanol increases hepatic smooth endoplasmic reticulum and drug metabolising enzymes. Science (1968) 159, 1469.
7 Riedler G. Einfluss des Alkohols auf die Antikoagulantien Therapie. Thromb Diath Haemorr (1966) 16, 613.
8 O'Reilly RA. Warfarin and wine. Clin Res (1978) 26, 145A.
9 O'Reilly RA. Lack of effect of mealtime wine on the hypoprothrombinaemia of oral anticoagulants. Amer J Med Sci (1979) 277, 189.
10 O'Reilly RA. Lack of effect of fortified wine ingested during fasting and anticoagulant therapy. Arch Int Med (1981) 141, 458.
11 O'Reilly RA. Effect of wine during meals and fasting on the hypoprothrombinaemia of oral anticoagulants. Clin Pharmacol Ther (1980) 27, 277.

Anticoagulants + Allopurinol

Abstract/Summary

Most patients on oral anticoagulants given allopurinol do not develop an adverse interaction, but because excessive hypoprothombinaemia and bleeding can occur quite unpredictably in a few individuals it is important to monitor the initial anticoagulant response in all patients.

Clinical evidence

An extensive multi-hospital study of the adverse effects of allopurinol identified three patients who developed excessive anticoagulation while concurrently taking warfarin and allopurinol. One of them developed extensive intrapulmonary haemorrhage and had a prothrombin time of 71 s.[6]

A sharp increase in prothrombin times was seen in a very elderly woman on warfarin when given allopurinol.[3] Two patients on long-term treatment with phenprocoumon began to bleed when started on allopurinol.[5] A man on warfarin demonstrated a 42% increase in his prothrombin ratio after taking 100 mg allopurinol for 2 days.[7] 2.5 mg/kg allopurinol twice daily for 14 days increased the mean half-life of a single dose of dicoumarol in six normal subjects from 51 to 152 h,[1] whereas three other subjects showed an increase from only 13 to 17 h.[4] The disposition of warfarin remained unaltered.[4] No change was seen in the prothrombin ratios of two patients on warfarin who took allopurinol for 3 weeks,[2] whereas one out of six subjects taking allopurinol for a month demonstrated a 30% reduction in the elimination of warfarin.[2] Another report describes a case of an interaction with allopurinol.[8]

Mechanism

It has been suggested that, as in rats, allopurinol inhibits the metabolism of the anticoagulants by the liver, thereby prolonging their effects and half-lives.[1,4,7] There is a wide individual variability in the effects of allopurinol on drug metabolism in man,[2] so that only a few individuals are affected.

Importance and management

An established and clinically important interaction. Its incidence is unknown, but it appear to be quite small. Since it is impossible to predict who is likely to be affected, monitor the prothrombin times of all patients on anticoagulants when allopurinol is added. The interaction has only been reported with warfarin, phenprocoumon and dicoumarol, but apply the same precautions with any anticoagulant.

References

1 Vesell ES, Passananti GT, Greene FF. Impairment of drug metabolism in man by allopurinol and nortriptyline. N Eng J Med (1970) 283, 1484.
2 Rawlins MD, Smith SE. Influence of allopurinol on drug metabolism in man. Br J Pharmac (1973) 48, 693.
3 Self TH, Evans WE, Ferguson T. Drug enhancement of warfarin activity. Lancet (1975) ii, 557.
4 Pond SM, Graham GG, Wade DN, Sudlow G. The effect of allopurinol and clofibrate on the elimination of coumarin anticoagulants in man. Aust NZ J Med (1975) 5, 324.
5 Jahnchen E, Meinertz T, Gilfrich MJ. Interaction of allopurinol in man. Klin Wsch (1977) 55, 759.
6 McInnnes GT, Lawson DH, Jick H. Acute adverse reactions attributed to allopurinol in hospitalized patients. Ann Rheum Dis (1981) 40, 245–9.
7 Barry M, Feeley J. Allopurinol influences aminophenazone elimination. Clin Pharmacokinet (1990) 19, 167–9.
8 Weart CW. Coumarin and allopurinol. A drug interaction case report. 32nd Annual Meeting, American Society of Hospital Pharmacists (1975).

Anticoagulants + Aminoglutethimide

Abstract/Summary

The anticoagulant effects of warfarin and nicoumalone (acenocoumarol) can be markedly reduced by the concurrent use of aminoglutethimide.

Clinical evidence

Three patients on nicoumalone needed a doubled dosage to maintain adequate anticoagulation while taking 250 mg aminoglutethimide four times daily for 3–4 weeks.[1]

Two other patients needed a three- to four-fold increase in warfarin dosage while taking 250 mg aminoglutethimide four times a day.[2] The increased requirement persisted for two weeks after the aminoglutethimide was stopped, and then declined. Brief mention of the need to take 'much larger doses' of warfarin while on aminoglutethimide is reported elsewhere.[3]

Mechanism

Uncertain, but the most likely explanation is that aminoglutethimide, like glutethimide, stimulates the activity of the liver enzymes concerned with the metabolism of the anticoagulants, thereby increasing their loss from the body. Some effect on blood steroid levels which might affect coagulation has also been suggested.[2]

Importance and management

Information appears to be limited to the reports cited but the interaction would seem to be established. Monitor the effects if aminoglutethimide is given to patients already on either warfarin or nicoumalone and increase the anticoagulant dosage as necessary. Reduce the dosage if it is withdrawn. Information about other anticoagulants is lacking but it would be prudent to apply the same precautions.

References

1 Bruning PF, Bonfrer JG M. Aminoglutethimide and oral anticoagulant therapy. Lancet (1983) ii, 582.
2 Lonnong PE, Kvinnsland S, Jahren G. Aminoglutethimide and warfarin. A

new important drug interaction. Cancer Chemother Pharmacol (1984) 12, 10–12.

3 Murray RML, Pitt P, Jerums G. Medical adrenalectomy with aminoglutethimide in the management of advanced breast cancer. Med J Aust (1981) 1, 179–81.

Anticoagulants + Aminoglycoside antibiotics

Abstract/Summary

If the intake of vitamin K is normal, either no interaction occurs or only a small and clinically unimportant increase in the effects of the oral anticoagulants takes place during concurrent treatment with neomycin, kanamycin or paromomycin. No interaction of any importance is likely with other aminoglycoside antibiotics administered parenterally.

Clinical evidence

Six out of 10 patients on warfarin who were given 2 g neomycin daily over a 3-week period showed a gradual increase in their prothrombin times averaging 5.6 s.[1] The author of this report also describes another study on 10 patients taking warfarin given 4 g neomycin daily which produced essentially similar results.[2]

A small increase in the effects of an un-named anticoagulant was seen in five patients given neomycin with bacitracin, three patients on 1 g streptomycin daily, and two patients on 1 g streptomycin with 1 Mu of penicillin daily.[3] No interaction was found in other long-term studies of warfarin with neomycin,[4,5] or dicoumarol with paromomycin.[5]

Mechanism

Not understood. One idea is that these antibiotics increase the anticoagulant effects by decimating the bacterial population in the gut, thereby reducing their production of vitamin K. However this incorrectly supposes that the gut bacteria are normally an essential and important source of the vitamin.[5] Another suggestion is that these antibiotics decrease the vitamin K absorption as part of a general antibiotic-induced malabsorption syndrome.[6]

Importance and management

A sparsely documented interaction but common experience seems to confirm that normally no interaction of any significance occurs. Concurrent use need not be avoided. Occasionally vitamin K deficiency and/or spontaneous bleeding[7,8] is seen after the prolonged use of gut-sterilizing antibiotics, a totally inadequate diet, starvation or some other condition in which the intake of vitamin K is very limited. Under these circumstances the effects of the oral anticoagulants would be expected to be significantly increased and appropriate precautions should be taken. Only warfarin and dicoumarol feature in the reports cited but it seems probable that the other anticoagulants will behave similarly. There is nothing to suggest that an adverse interaction occurs between the oral anticoagulants and aminoglycosides administered parenterally.

References

1 Udall JA. Drug interference with warfarin therapy. Clin Med (1970) 77, 20
2 Udall JA. Human sources and absorption of vitamin K in relation to anticoagulation stability. J Amer Med Ass (1965) 194, 107.
3 Magid E. Tolerance to anticoagulants during antibiotic therapy. Scand J Lab Invest (1962) 14, 565.
4 Schade RWB. A comparative study of the effects of cholestyramine and neomycin in the treatment of type II hyperlipoprotinaemia. Acta Med Scand (1976) 199, 175.
5 Messinger WJ, Samet CM. The effect of bowel sterilizing antibiotic on blood coagulation mechanisms. The anticholesterol effect of paromomycin. Angiology (1965) 16, 29.
6 Faloon WW, Paes IC, Woolfolk D, Nankin H, Wallace K, Haro EN. Effect of neomycin and kanamycin upon intestinal absorption. Ann NY Acad Sci (1966) 132, 879.
7 Haden HT. Vitamin K deficiency associated with prolonged antibiotic administration. Arch Int Med (1957) 100, 986.
8 Frick PG, Riedler G, Brogli H. Dose response and minimal daily requirements for vitamin K in man. J Appl Physiol (1967) 23, 387.

Anticoagulants + Aminosalicylic acid (PAS) and/or Isoniazid

Abstract/Summary

A report attributes a bleeding episode in a patient on warfarin to the concurrent use of isoniazid. Another report describes a markedly increased anticoagulant response in a patient when given aminosalicylic acid and isoniazid.

Clinical evidence

A man on warfarin and taking 300 mg isoniazid daily began to bleed (haematuria, bleeding gums, etc.) within 10 days of accidentally doubling his dosage of isoniazid. His prothrombin time had increased from 26.3 s to 53.3 s.[1]

Another patient taking digoxin, potassium chloride, dioctyl calcium sulfosuccinate, diazepam and warfarin, was additionally given 12 g aminosalicylic acid, 300 mg isoniazid and 100 mg pyridoxine daily. His prothrombin time increased from 18 to 130 s over 20 days but no signs of haemorrhage were seen.[2] Two patients on isoniazid, aminosalicylic acid and streptomycin (but not taking anticoagulants) developed haemorrhage attributed to the anticoagulant effects of isoniazid.[3]

Mechanism

Not understood. The small depressant effect which aminosalicylic acid has on prothrombin formation in man is unlikely to have been responsible. Isoniazid can increase the anticoagulant effects of dicoumarol in dogs[4] but not of warfarin in rabbits.[5] In dogs the effect is thought to be due to inhibition by the isoniazid of the liver enzymes concerned with the metabolism of the anticoagulant, resulting in a slower clearance from the body.[4]

Importance and management

The interactions of warfarin with isoniazid and aminosalicylic acid are not established. Concurrent use need not be avoided, but prescribers should be aware of these cases and monitor the effects.

References

1 Rosenthal AR, Self TH, Baker ED, Londen RA. Interaction of isoniazid and warfarin. J Amer Med Ass (1977) 238, 2177.
2 Self TH. Interaction of warfarin and aminosalicylic acid. J Amer Med Ass (1973) 223, 1285.
3 Castell FA. Accion anticoagulante de la isoniazide. Enfermedaders de Torax (1969) 69, 153.
4 Eade NR, McLeod PJ, MacLeod SM. Potentiation of bishydroxycoumarin in dogs by isoniazid and p-aminosalicylic acid. Amer Rev Resp Dis (1971) 103, 792.
5 Kiblawi SS. Influence of isoniazid on the anticoagulant effect of warfarin Clin Ther (1979) 2, 235.

Anticoagulants + Amiodarone

Abstract/Summary

The anticoagulant effects of warfarin, phenprocoumon and nicoumalone (acenocoumarol) are increased by amiodarone and bleeding may occur if the dosage of the anticoagulant is not reduced. Reduce the dosage by one to two-thirds with warfarin and phenprocoumon and by a third to a half with nicoumalone. The onset of this interaction may be slow, but it may also persist long after the amiodarone has been withdrawn.

Clinical evidence

Five out of nine patients well stabilized on warfarin showed signs of bleeding (four had microscopic haematuria and one had diffuse ecchymoses) within 3–4 weeks of starting to take amiodarone (dosage not stated). All nine showed increases in their prothrombin times averaging 21 s. It was necessary to decrease the warfarin dosage by an average of a third (range 16–45%) to return their prothrombin times to the therapeutic range. The effects of amiodarone persisted for 6 to 16 weeks in four of the patients from whom it was withdrawn.[1]

A prolongation in prothrombin times and/or bleeding has been described in other patients on warfarin given 600–800 mg amiodarone daily.[2–4,6,8,10,13,18–20,22] Amiodarone similarly interacts with phenprocoumon[5] and nicoumalone.[9,11,14–16,21]

Mechanism

Experimental evidence suggests that amiodarone inhibits P4502C9 (an isoenzyme of P450 concerned with the metabo-

lism of (S)-warfarin) so that the loss of the anticoagulant from the body is decreased and its effects are thereby increased.[24]

Importance and management

A well documented, established and clinically important interaction. It appears to occur in most patients.[1,6,17,20] The dosage of either warfarin or phenprocoumon should be reduced by one-third to two-thirds[1,5,12,13,20] in order to avoid bleeding. One report[13] suggests an average 35% reduction with warfarin in a 70 kg patient on 200 mg amiodarone daily, 50% on 400 mg and 65% on 600 mg and above. The dosage of nicoumalone should be reduced by a third to a half.[9,21,22] These suggested reductions are very broad generalizations and individual patients may need more or less.[23] The interaction develops within two weeks and may persist for many weeks after the withdrawal of the amiodarone because up to a third may still be present a month after treatment has ceased.[7] Prothrombin times should be very closely monitored both during and after treatment. One study advises weekly monitoring for the first four weeks.[20] It would seem prudent to assume that other anticoagulants interact similarly, but so far there is no direct evidence that they do so.

References

1 Martinowitz U, Rabinovici J, Goldfarb D, Many A, Bank H. Interaction between warfarin sodium and amiodarone. N Eng J Med (1981) 304, 671.
2 Rees A, Dalal JJ, Reid PG, Henderson AH, Lewis MJ. Dangers of amiodarone and anticoagulant treatment. Br Med J (1981) 282, 1756.
3 Serlin MJ, Sibeon RG, Green GJ. Dangers of amiodarone and anticoagulant treatment. Br Med J (1981) 283, 58.
4 Simpson WT. In 'Amiodarone in Cardiac Arrhythmias'. Simpson WT, Caldwell ADS (eds). Roy Soc Med Int Congr Ser 16. Royal Society of Medicine/Academic Press/Grune and Stratton, London (1979) p 50–2.
5 Broekmans AW, Meyboom RHB. Bijwerkingen van geneesmiddelen. Potentiering van het cumarine-effekt door amiodaron (Cordarone). Ned Tijd Geneesk (1982) 126, 1415.
6 Hamer A, Peter T, Mandel WJ, Scheinman MM, Weiss D. The potentiation of warfarin anticoagulation by amiodarone. Circulation (1982) 65, 1025–29.
7 Broekhuysen J, Laruel R, Slon R. Recherches dan la serie des benzofuranes. XXXVIII. Etude comparee du transit et du metabolisme de l'amiodarone chez diverses especes d'animaux et chez l'homme. Arch Int Pharmacodyn Ther (1969) 177, 340.
8 Ugovern B, Garan H, Kelly E, Ruskin JN. Adverse reactions during treatment with amiodarone. Br Med J (1983) 287. 175–80.
9 Arboix M, Frati ME, Laporte J-R. The potentiation of acenocoumarol anticoagulant effects by amiodarone. Br J clin Pharmac (1984) 18, 355–60.
10 Raeder EA, Podrid PJ, Lown B. Side effects and complications of amiodarone therapy. Am Heart J (1985) 109, 975–83.
11 El Allaf D, Sprynger M, Carlier J. Potentiation of the action of oral anticoagulants by amiodarone. Acta Clin Belg (1984) 39, 306–8.
12 Watt AH, Buss DC, Stephens MR, Routledge PA. Amiodarone reduced plasma warfarin clearance in man. Br J clin Pharmac (1985) 19, 591P.
13 Almog S, Shafran N, Halkin H, Weiss P, Farfel Z, Martinowitz U, Bank H. Mechanism of warfarin potentiation by amiodarone: dose- and concentration-dependent inhibition of warfarin elimination. Eur J Clin Pharmacol (1985) 28, 257–261.
14 Richard C, Riou B, Fournier C, Rimailho A, Auzepy P. Depression of vitamin K-dependent coagulation by amiodarone. Circulation (1983) 68, Suppl III, 278.
15 Richard C, Riou B, Berdeaux A, Forunier C, Khayat D, Rimailho A, Giudicelli JF, Auzepy P. Prospective study of the potentiation of aceno-

coumarol by amiodarone. Eur J Clin Pharmacol (1985) 28, 625–9.

16 Pini M, Manotti C, Quintavalla R. Interaction between amiodarone and acenocoumarin. Thromb Haem (1985) 54, 549.
17 Kerin N, Blevins R, Goldman L, Faitel K, and Rubenfire M. The amiodarone-warfarin interaction: incidence, time course and clinical significance. JACC (1986) 7, 91A.
18 Watt AH, Stephens MR, Buss DC, Routledge PA. Amiodarone reduces plasma warfarin clearance in man. Br J clin Pharmac (1985) 20, 707–9.
19 O'Reilly RA, Trager WF, Kettie AE, Goulart DA. Interaction of amiodarone with racemic warfarin and its separate enantiomorphs in humans. Clin Pharmacol Ther (1987) 42, 290–4.
20 Kerin NZ, Blevins RD, Goldman L, Faitel K, Rubenfire M. The incidence, magnitude and time course of the amiodarone-warfarin interaction. Arch InternMed (1988) 148, 1779–81.
21 Fondevila C, Meschengieser S, Lazzari MA. Amiodarone potentiates acenocoumarin. Thromb Res (1988) 52, 203–8.
22 Caraco Y, Shajek-Shaul T. The incidence and clinical significance of amiodarone and acenocoumarol interaction. Thromb Haemostasis (1989) 62, 906–8.
23 Fondevila C, Meschengieser S, Lazzari M. Amiodarone-acenocoumarin interaction. Thromb Haemstasis (1991) 65, 328.
24 Heimark LD, Wienkers L, Kunze K, Gibaldi M, Eddy AC, Trager WF, O'Reilly RA, Goulart DA. The mechanism of the interaction between amiodarone and warfarin in humans. Clin Pharmacol Ther (1992) 51, 398–407.

Anticoagulants + Anabolic steroids and Related sex hormones

Abstract/Summary

The anticoagulant effects of bromindione, dicoumarol, nicoumalone (acenocoumarol), phenindione, phenprocoumon and warfarin are markedly increased by the concurrent use of danazol, ethyloestrenol, oxymetholone, methandienone (methandrostenolone), methyltestosterone, norethandrolone and stanozolol. Bleeding may occur if the anticoagulant dosage is not reduced appropriately.

Clinical evidence

Six patients stabilized on warfarin or phenindione were started on 15 mg oxymetholone daily. One patient developed extensive subcutaneous bleeding and another had haematuria. After 30 days on oxymetholone all six patients had thrombotests of less than 5% which returned to the therapeutic range within a few days of its withdrawal.[1]

Similarly increased anticoagulant effects and bleeding have been described in studies and case reports involving warfarin with danazol,[13,14,20,21] oxymetholone,[4–6] methandienone[2,4,7,8] or stanozolol;[15,17–19] dicoumarol with norethandrolone[2,4] or stanozolol;[12] bromindione with methandienone;[2,4] phenindione with ethyloestrenol;[9] phenprocoumon with methyltestosterone;[10] and nicoumalone with oxymetholone.[11]

One report[6] says that three patients on warfarin given Sustanon (containing four combined esters of testosterone) developed no changes in their anticoagulant requirements, whereas another report[16] describes a woman who showed a 78% and a 65% increase in prothrombin times on two occasions when using a 2% testosterone propionate vaginal oint-

ment twice daily. A 25% reduction in warfarin dosage was needed.

Mechanism

Not understood. Various theories have been put forward including increased metabolic destruction of the blood clotting factors, or decreased synthesis;[2,3] reduced levels of plasma triglycerides which might reduce vitamin-K availability (though this is disputed);[4,7] and increased concentrations of the anticoagulant at the receptor site or increased receptor affinity.

Importance and management

Well documented, well established and clinically important interactions which develop rapidly, possibly within 2–3 days. Most, if not all, patients are affected.[1,3] If concurrent use cannot be avoided, the dosage of the anticoagulant should be appropriately reduced. One recommendation is that the initial dosage of danazol[14] should be halved, but the size of the reduction with other steroids is uncertain. After withdrawal of the steroid the anticoagulant dosage will need to be increased. It seems probable that all the anticoagulants will interact with any 17-alkyl substituted steroid such as fluoxymesterone and oxandrolone, but as yet there is no direct evidence that they do so. The situation with testosterone and other non 17-alkylated steroids is not clear (see cases cited above).[6,16]

References

1 Longridge RGM, Gilliam PMS and Barton GMG. Decreased anticoagulant tolerance with oxymetholone. Lancet (1971) ii, 90.
2 Pyorala K, Kekki M. Decreased anticoagulant tolerance during methandrostenolone therapy. Scand J Clin Lab Invest (1963) 15, 367.
3 Schrogie JJ, Solomon HM. The anticoagulant response to bishydroxycoumarin. II. The effect of D-thyroxine, clofibrate and norethandrolone. Clin Pharmacol Ther (1967) 8, 70.
4 Murakami M, Odake K, Matsuda T, Onchi K, Umeda T, Nishuro T. Effects of anabolic steroids on anticoagulant requirements. Jap Circ J (1965) 29, 243.
5 Robinson BHB, Hawkins JB, Ellis JE, Moore-Robinson M. Decreased anticoagulant tolerance with oxymetholone. Lancet (1971) i, 1356.
6 Edwards MS, Curtis JR. Decreased anticoagulant tolerance with oxymetholone. Lancet (1971) ii, 221.
7 Dresdale FC, Hayes JC. Potential dangers in the combined use of methandrostenolone and sodium warfarin. J Med Soc New Jersey (1967) 64, 609.
8 McLaughlin GE, McCarty DJ, Segal BL. Hemarthrosis complicating anticoagulant therapy. A report of three cases. J Amer Med Ass (1966) 196, 1020.
9 Vere DW, Fearnley GR. Suspected interaction between phenindione and ethyloestrenol. Lancet (1968) ii, 281.
10 Husted S, Andreasen F, Foged L. Increased sensitivity to phenprocoumon during methyltestosterone therapy. Europ J clin Pharmacol (1976) 10, 209.
11 De Oyda JC, del Rio A, Noya M, Villeneuva A. Decreased anticoagulant tolerance with oxymetholone in paroxysmal noctural haemoglobinuria. Lancet (1971) ii, 259.
12 Howards CW, Hanson SG, Wahed MA. Anabolic steroids and anticoagulants. Brit Med J (1977) i, 1659.
13 Goulbourne IA, MacLeod DAD. An interaction between danazol and warfarin. Brit J Obst Gyn (1981) 88, 950–1.
14 Small M, Peterkin M, Lowe GDO, McCune G, Thomson JA. Danazol and oral anticoagulants. Scott Med J (1982) 27, 331–2.

15 Acomb C, Shaw PW. A significant interaction between warfarin and stanozolol. Pharm J (1985) 234, 73–4.

16 Lorentz S Mc and Weibert RT. Potentiation of warfarin anticoagulation by topical testosterone ointment. Clin Pharm (1985) 4, 332–4.

17 Cleverly CR. Personal communication (1987).

18 Shaw PW, Smith AM. Possible interaction of warfarin and stanozolol. Clin Pharm (1987) 6, 500–2.

19 Elwin C-E, Törngren M. Samtidigt intag av warfarin och stanozolol orsak till blödningar hos patienten. Läkartidningen (1988) 85, 3290.

20 Meeks ML, Mahaffey KW, Katz MD. Danazol increases the anticoagulant effect of warfarin. Ann Pharmacother (1992) 26, 641–2.

21 Booth CD. A drug interaction between danazol and warfarin. Pharm J (1993) 250, 439.

Anticoagulants + Antacids

Abstract/Summary

Aluminium hydroxide does not interact with either warfarin or dicoumarol, and magnesium hydroxide does interact with warfarin. There is some evidence that the absorption of dicoumarol may be increased by magnesium hydroxide and warfarin by magnesium trisilicate, but there is no direct evidence that this is clinically important.

Clinical evidence

(a) Dicoumarol + Aluminium or Magnesium hydroxide

15 ml of magnesium hydroxide (Milk of Magnesia) taken with dicoumarol, and a further dose 3 h later, was found to raise serum dicoumarol levels of six subjects by 75% and the area under the curve by 50%. No interaction occurred with aluminium hydroxide.[2]

(b) Warfarin + Aluminium or Magnesium hydroxide, or Magnesium trisilicate.

30 ml aluminium/magnesium hydroxide (*Maalox*) given with warfarin, and four subsequent doses at 2 h intervals, had no effect on the plasma warfarin levels or on the anticoagulant response of six subjects.[1] No interaction occurs with warfarin and aluminium hydroxide (*Amphogel*),[2] but an *in vitro* study suggests that the absorption of warfarin may be increased by magnesium trisilicate.[4]

Mechanism

It is suggested that dicoumarol forms a more readily absorbed chelate with magnesium so that its effects are increased.[1,3]

Importance and management

No special precautions need be taken if aluminium or magnesium hydroxide antacids are given to patients on warfarin, or if aluminium hydroxide is given to those on dicoumarol. Choosing these antacids avoids the possibility of an adverse interaction. Despite the evidence from the studies cited, there seems to be no direct clinical evidence of an adverse interaction between any anticoagulant and an antacid.

References

1 Robinson DS, Benjamin DM, McCormack JJ. Interaction of warfarin and nonsystemic gastrointestinal drugs. Clin Pharmacol Ther (1971) 12, 491.

2 Ambre JJ, Fischer LJ. Effect of coadministration of aluminium and magnesium hydroxides on absorption of anticoagulants in man. Clin Pharmacol Ther (1973) 12, 231.

3 Akers MA, Lach JL and Fischer LJ. Alterations in the absorption of bishydroxycoumarin by various excipient materials. J Pharm Sci (1973) 62, 391.

4 McElnay JC, Harron DWG, D'Arcy PF, Collier PS. Interaction of warfarin with antacid constituents. Br Med J (1978) 2, 1166.

Anticoagulants + Ascorbic acid (Vitamin C)

Abstract/Summary

Four controlled studies with large numbers of patients failed to demonstrate any interaction, although two isolated cases have been reported in which the effects of warfarin were reduced by ascorbic acid.

Clinical evidence

The prothrombin time of a woman, stabilized on 7.5 mg warfarin daily, who began to take regular amounts of ascorbic acid (dose not stated), fell steadily from 23 s to 19, 17 and then 14 s with no response to an increase in the dosage of warfarin to 10, 15 and finally 20 mg daily. The prothrombin time returned to 28 s within two days of stopping the ascorbic acid.[1] A woman who had been taking 16 g ascorbic acid daily proved to be unusually resistant to the actions of warfarin and required 25 mg daily before a significant increase in prothrombin times was achieved.[2]

In contrast, no changes in the effects of warfarin were seen in five patients given 1 g ascorbic acid daily for a fortnight,[3] 84 patients given an unstated amount for 10 weeks,[4] 11 patients given up to 4 g daily for 2 weeks,[10] or 19 patients given up to 5–10 g daily for one or 2 weeks.[5] In this last study a mean fall of 17.5% in total plasma warfarin concentrations was seen.

Mechanism

Not understood. Some animal studies have demonstrated this interaction[6,7] and others have not,[8,9] but none of them has provided any definite clues about why it ever occurs, and then only rarely. One suggestion is that high doses of ascorbic acid can cause diarrhoea which might prevent adequate absorption of the anticoagulant.

Importance and management

Well-controlled clinical studies in large numbers of patients on warfarin have failed to confirm this interaction, even using very large doses (up to 10 g daily) of ascorbic acid. There is no good reason for avoiding the concurrent use. Information about other anticoagulants is lacking, but it seems likely that they will behave similarly. Check on any patient particularly resistant to the warfarin to confirm that ascorbic acid is not being taken.

References

1 Rosenthal G. Interaction of ascorbic acid and warfarin. J Amer Med Ass (1971) 215, 1671.
2 Smith EC, Skalski RJ, Johnson GC, Rossi GV. Interaction of ascorbic acid with warfarin. J Amer Med Ass (1972) 221, 1166.
3 Hume R, Johnstone JMS and Weyers E. Interaction of ascorbic acid and warfarin. J Amer Med Ass (1972) 219, 1479.
4 Dedichen J. Effect of ascorbic acid given to patients on chronic anticoagulant therapy. Boll Soc Ital Cardiol (1973) 18, 690.
5 Feetam CL, Leach RH, Meynell MJ. Lack of clinical important interaction between warfarin and ascorbic acid. Toxicol Appl Pharmacol (1975) 31, 544.
6 Sigell LT and Flessa HC. Drug interactions with anticoagulants. J Amer Med Ass (1970) 214, 2035.
7 Sullivan WR, Gangstad EO, Link KP. Studies on the haemorrhagic sweet clover disease. J Biol Chem (1943) 151, 477.
8 Weintraub M, Griner PF. Warfarin and ascorbic acid: lack of evidence for a drug interaction. Toxicol Appl Pharmacol (1974) 28, 53.
9 Deckert FW. Ascorbic acid and warfarin. J Amer Med Ass (1973) 223, 440.
10 Blakely JA. Interaction of warfarin and ascorbic acid. 1st Florence Conf Haemostasis and Thrombosis (1977) May. Abstracts p 99.

Anticoagulants + Aspirin and other Salicylates

Abstract/Summary

Aspirin in doses of only 500 mg daily increases the likelihood of bleeding 3–5 times in those taking anticoagulants. Aspirin damages the stomach wall, prolongs bleeding times and in 2–4 g daily doses can increase prothrombin times, but there seems to be little reason for avoiding low-dose aspirin (75 mg daily). Increased warfarin effects have been seen when methylsalicylate and trolamine salicylate were used on the skin.

Clinical evidence

A study in 534 patients with artificial heart valves found that three times as many bled (requiring blood transfusion or hospitalization) among those on 500 mg aspirin daily (14%) as among those on warfarin alone (5%). Bleeding was mainly gastrointestinal or cerebral. All of those with intracerebral bleeding died.[1]

This finding broadly confirms two other studies on a total of 270 patients in whom bleeding was found to be about five times more common in anticoagulated patients taking aspirin (0.5–1.0 g daily) than among those taking only the anticoagulant.[2,3] A further study found that 1 g aspirin daily increased the bleeding episodes in those on anticoagulants (un-named) from 4.7 to 13.9 per 100 patients per year.[15]

Other studies in patients taking dicoumarol, nicoumalone or warfarin found that 2–4 g aspirin daily increased the anticoagulant effects. The anticoagulant dosage could be reduced about 30%.[4,5] However another investigator using 3 g aspirin daily failed to find any effect on prothrombin times.[10] Methyl salicylate ointment applied to the skin has been found to increase the effects of warfarin; bleeding and bruising associated with raised INR's have been seen.[12-14] A raised prothrombin time has also been reported with topical trolamine salicylate.[14]

Low-dose aspirin (75 mg daily) doubles the normal blood loss from the gastric mucosa but it still remains very small (compared with the 14-fold increase with 2.4 g daily) and warfarin does not increase it.[11] Only minor episodes of bleeding (nose bleeds, bruising) occur with low dose aspirin and low intensity warfarin (INR 1.5).[16]

Mechanism

Aspirin has a direct irritant effect on the stomach lining and can cause gastrointestinal bleeding. It also decreases platelet aggregation and prolongs bleeding times, all of which would seem to account for the bleeding described.[1-3] In addition, larger doses (2–4 g daily) of aspirin alone are known to have a direct hypoprothrombinaemic effect, like the anticoagulants, which is reversible by vitamin K.[6-9]

Importance and management

The anticoagulant/aspirin interaction is well documented and clinically important. Patients should avoid self-prescribed aspirin in normal analgesic and anti-inflammatory doses while taking any anticoagulant, although only dicoumarol, acenocoumarol and warfarin appear to have been investigated. Low-dose aspirin (75 mg daily) used for its platelet anti-aggregant effects appears not to matter. Warn patients that many proprietary over-the-counter analgesic, antipyretic, cold and influenza preparations may contain substantial amounts of aspirin. Paracetamol (acetaminophen) is a safer analgesic substitute. Some of the other salicylates are less irritant and have a smaller effect on platelet function than aspirin so that, on theoretical grounds, the avoidance of concurrent use may be less important. Remember too that topical methyl salicylate and trolamine salicylate may cause problems.

References

1 Chesebro JH, Fuster V, Elveback LR, Ugoon DC, Pluth JR, Puga FJ, Wallace RB, Danielson GK, Orszulak TA, Piehler JM, Schaff HV. Trial of combined warfarin plus dipyridamole or aspirin therapy in prosthetic heart valve replacement: danger of aspirin compared with dipyridamole. Amer J Cardiol (1983) 51, 1537–41.
2 Altman R, Boullon F, Rouvier J, Rada R, de la Fuente L and Favaloro R. Aspirin and prophylaxis of thrombo-embolic complications in patients with substitute heart valves. J Thoracic Cardiovasc Surg (1976) 72, 127–9.
3 Dale J, Myhre E, Storstein O, Stormorken H, Efkind L. Prevention of arterial thromboembolism with acetylsalicylic acid: a controlled clinical study in patients with aortic ball valves. Am Heart J (1977) 94, 101–111.
4 Watson RM, Pierson NJ. Effect of anticoagulant therapy upon aspirin-induced gastrointestinal bleeding. Circulation (1961) 24, 613.
5 O'Reilly RA, Sahud MA, Aggeler PM. Impact of aspirin and chlorthalidone

on the pharmacodynamics of oral anticoagulants drugs in man. Ann NY Acad Sci (1971) 179, 173.

6 Shapiro S. Studies on prothrombin. VI. The effect of synthetic vitamin K on the prothrombinopenia induced by salicylate in man. J Amer Med Ass (1944) 125, 546.

7 Quick AJ, Clesceri L. Influence of acetylsalicylic acid and salicylamide on the coagulation of the blood. J Pharmac Exp Ther (1960) 128, 95.

8 Meyer OO, Howard B. Production of hypoprothrombinaemia and hypocoagulability of the blood with salicylates. J Pharmac Exp Ther (1943) 53, 251.

9 Park BK, Leck JB. On the mechanisms of salicylate-induced hypoprothrombinaemia. J Pharm Pharmacol (1981) 33, 25.

10 Udall JA. Drug interference with warfarin therapy. Amer J Cardiol (1969) 23, 143.

11 Pritchard PJ, Kitchingham GK, Walt RP, Daneshmend TK, Hawkey CJ. Human gastric mucosal bleeding induced by low dose aspirin but not warfarin. Br Med J (1989) 298, 493–6.

12 Chow WH, Cheung KL, Ling HM, See T. Potentiation of warfarin anticoagulation by topical methylsalicylate ointment. J Roy Soc Med (1989) 82, 501–2.

13 Yip ASB, Chow WH, Tai YT, Cheung KL. Adverse effect of topical methylsalicylate ointment on warfarin anticoagulation: an unrecognized potential hazard. Postgrad Med J (1990) 66, 367–9.

14 Littleton F. Warfarin and topical salicylates. J Amer Med Ass (1990) 263, 2888.

15 Dale J, Myhre E, Loew D. Bleeding during acetylsalicylic acid and anticoagulant therapy in patients with reduced platelet reactivity after aortic valve replacement. Am Heart J (1980) 99, 746–52.

16 Meade TW, Roderick PJ, Brennan PJ, Wiles HC, Kelleher CC. Extra-cranial bleeding and other symptoms due to low dose aspirin and low intensity oral anticoagulation. Thromb Haem (1992) 68, 1–6.

Anticoagulants + Azapropazone

Abstract/Summary

The anticoagulant effects of warfarin are markedly increased by azapropazone. Bleeding will occur if the dosage of warfarin is not considerably reduced.

Clinical evidence

A woman on digoxin, frusemide, spironolactone, allopurinol, and stabilized on warfarin (prothrombin ratio 2.8) developed haematemesis within four days of starting to take 300 mg azapropazone four times a day. Her prothrombin ratio was found to have risen to 15.7 (prothrombin time of 220 s). Subsequent gastroscopic examination revealed a benign ulcer, the presumed site of the bleeding.[1]

At least 12 other patients are reported to have developed this interaction. Bruising or bleeding (melaena, epistaxes, haematuria etc) and prolonged prothrombin times occurred within a few days of starting azapropazone.[2,6,7,9–11] Three died.[7,9,10] Another patient on warfarin and azapropazone and also taking diclofenac and co-proxamol showed an increase in prothrombin times.[8] This interaction has been experimentally confirmed in two normal subjects.[3]

Mechanism

Not understood. Azapropazone displaces warfarin from its plasma protein binding sites[3–5] thereby increasing the amount

of free and pharmacologically active molecules, but it is almost certain that this on its own does not fully account for the clinical effects reported. Changes in the metabolism of the warfarin are possibly mainly responsible.

Importance and management

The warfarin/azapropazone interaction is established and clinically important. The incidence is uncertain. Concurrent use should be avoided.[10] If it is essential to give azapropazone, the manufacturers advise that it should only be given to patients if the warfarin dosage has been reduced to a very low level, after which daily prothrombin determinations and dosage adjustments should be carried out. Information about other anticoagulants is lacking but it would be prudent to assume that they interact similarly.

References

1 Powell-Jackson PR. Interaction between azapropazone and warfarin. Br Med J (1977) 1, 1193.

2 Green AE, Hort JF, Korn HET and Leach H. Potentiation of warfarin by azapropazone. Br Med J (1977) 1, 1532.

3 McElnay JC, D'Arcy PF. Interaction between azapropazone and warfarin. Br Med J (1977) 2, 773.

4 McElnay JC, D'Arcy PF. The effect of azapropazone on the binding of warfarin to human serum proteins. J Pharm Pharmac (1978) 30 (Suppl) 73P.

5 McElnay JC, D'Arcy PF. Interaction between azapropazone and warfarin. Experientia (1978) 34, 1320.

6 Beeley L. Bulletin of the West Midlands Adverse Drug Reaction Study Group. University of Birmingham, England. January 1980, no 10.

7 Anon. Interactions. Doctors warned on warfarin dangers. Pharm J (1983) 230, 676.

8 Beeley L, Stewart P, Hickey FL. Bulletin of West Midlands Centre for Adverse Drug Reaction Reporting (1988) 27, 27.

9 Win N, Mitchell DC, Jones PAE, French EA. Azapropazone and warfarin. Br Med J (1991) 302, 969–70.

10 Beeley L, Cunningham H, Carmichael AE, Brennan A. Bulletin of West Midlands Centre for Adverse Drug Reaction Reporting (1991) 33, 19.

11 Beeley L, Magee P, Hickey FM. Bulletin of West Midlands Centre for Adverse Drug Reaction Reporting (1989) 28, 34.

Anticoagulants + Barbiturates

Abstract/Summary

The effects of the anticoagulants are reduced by the concurrent use of barbiturates. Full therapeutic anticoagulation may only be achieved by raising the anticoagulant dosage about 30–60%. If the barbiturate is later withdrawn, the anticoagulant dosage should be reduced to avoid the risk of bleeding.

Clinical evidence

Two examples from many:

A study on 16 patients on long-term warfarin treatment showed that when they were also given 2 g/kg phenobarbitone (phenobarbital), their average daily warfarin requirements rose over a 4-week period by 25% (from 5.7 to 7.1 mg daily).[1]

An investigation on 12 patients taking either warfarin or phenprocoumon demonstrated that when concurrently given secbutobarbitone sodium (butabarbital), 60 mg daily for the first week and 120 mg daily for the next two weeks, their anticoagulant requirements rose by 35–60%, reaching a maximum after 4–5 weeks.[2]

This interaction has been described in man between warfarin and amylobarbitone (amobarbital),[3,4,23] butobarbitone (butobarbital),[5] heptabarbitone (heptabarbital),[6,7] phenobarbitone (phenobarbital),[8–12] quinalbarbitone (secobarbital)[3,4,12–14,24] and secbutobarbitone (butabarbital);[2] between dicoumarol and aprobarbitone (aprobarbital),[15] heptabarbitone (heptabarbital),[16,17] phenobarbitone (phenobarbital),[18–20] and vinbarbitone (vinbarbital);[15] between ethylbiscoumacetate and amylobarbitone (amobarbital),[16,21] pentobarbitone (pentobarbital),[22] and phenobarbitone (phenobarbital);[21] between phenprocoumon and secbutobarbitone (butabarbital);[2] and between nicoumalone (acenocoumarol) and pentobarbitone (pentobarbital)[27] and heptabarbitone (heptabarbital).[17]

Mechanism

Studies in man and animals[4,6,8,11,14] clearly show that the barbiturates are potent liver enzyme inducing agents which increase the metabolism and clearance of the anticoagulants from the body. They may also reduce the absorption of dicoumarol from the gut.[17]

Importance and management

This interaction is clinically important and overwhelmingly well documented. The reduction in the effects of the anticoagulant exposes the patient to the risk of thrombus formation if the dosage is not increased appropriately. A very large number of anticoagulant/barbiturate pairs have been found to interact, and the others may be expected to behave similarly. The only known exception is quinalbarbitone (secobarbital) which in daily doses of 100 mg appears to have little[12] or no[13,14] effect on dicoumarol or warfarin, but in daily doses of 200 mg interacts like the other barbiturates.[13] The barbiturates interact less with R warfarin than S warfarin, but in practice R warfarin appears to have little advantage over the usual RS racemic mixture.[25,26]

The reduction in the anticoagulant effects begins within a week, sometimes within 2–4 days, reaching a maximum after about three weeks, and it may still be evident up to six weeks after stopping the barbiturate.[2] Patients' responses can vary considerably. Stable anticoagulant control can be re-established[23] in the presence of the barbiturate by increasing the anticoagulant dosage by about 30–60%.[1,2,10,20] This may be necessary for epileptic patients.[23] Care must be taken not to withdraw the barbiturate without also reducing the anticoagulant dosage, otherwise bleeding will occur.[1,10,23] Alternative non-interacting sedative and hypnotic drugs which are safer (?) and easier to use include nitrazepam, chlordiazepoxide, diazepam, and flurazepam. See 'Anticoagulants + Benzodiazepines'. Information is lacking about anticoagulants other than those cited, but they are expected to interact similarly.

References

1 Robinson DS, McDonald MG. The effect of phenobarbital administration on the control of coagulation achieved during warfarin therapy in man. J Pharmacol Exp Ther (1966) 153, 250.

2 Antlitz AM, Tolentino M, Kosal MF. Effect of butabarbital on orally administered anticoagulants. Curr Ther Res (1968) 10, 70.

3 Breckenridge A, Orme M. Clinical implications of enzyme induction. Ann NY Acad Sci (1971) 179, 421.

4 Robinson DS, Sylwester D. Interaction of commonly prescribed drugs and warfarin. Ann Int Med (1970) 72, 853.

5 MacGregor AG, Petrie JC, Wood RA. Therapeutic conferences. Drug interaction. Br Med J (1971) 1, 389.

6 Levy G, O'Reilly RA, Aggeler PM, Keech GM. Pharmacokinetic analysis of the effect of barbiturate on the anticoagulant action of warfarin in man. Clin Pharmacol Ther (1970) 11, 372.

7 O'Reilly RA, Aggeler PM. Effect of barbiturates on oral anticoagulants in man. Clin Res (1969) 17, 153.

8 MacDonald MG, Robinson DS, Sylwester D, Jaffe JJ. The effects of phenobarbital, chloral betaine and glutethimide administration on warfarin plasma levels and hypoprothrombinemic responses in man. Clin Pharmacol Ther (1969) 10, 80.

9 Seller K, Duckert F. Properties of 3-(1-phenyl-propyl)-4-oxycoumarin (Marcoumar) in the plasma when tested in normal cases and under the influence of drugs. Thromb Diath Haemorrh (1969) 19, 89.

10 MacDonald MG, Robinson DS. Clinical observations of possible barbiturate interference with anticoagulation. J Amer Med Ass (1968) 204, 97.

11 Corn M. Effect of phenobarbital and glutethimide on biological half-life of warfarin. Thromb Diath Haemorrh (1966) 16, 606.

12 Udall JA. Clinical implications of warfarin interactions with five sedatives. Am J Cardiol (1975) 35, 67.

13 Feuer DJ, Wilson WR, Ambre JJ. Duration of effect of secobarbital on the anticoagulant effect and metabolism of warfarin. The Pharmacologist (1971) 3, 195.

14 Breckenridge AM, Orme ML'E, Davies L, Thorgeirsson SS, Davis DS. Dose-dependent enzyme induction. Clin Pharmacol Ther (1973) 14, 514.

15 Johansson S-A. Apparent resistance to oral anticoagulant therapy and influence of hypnotics on some coagulation factors. Acta Med Scand (1968) 184, 297.

16 Dayton PG, Tarcan Y, Chenkin T, Weiner M. The influence of barbiturates on coumarin plasma levels and prothrombin response. J Clin Invest (1961) 40, 1797.

17 Aggeler PM, O'Reilly RA. Effect of heptabarbital on the response to bishydroxycoumarin in man. J Lab Clin Med (1969) 74, 229.

18 Corn M, Rockett JF. Inhibition of bishydroxycoumarin activity by phenobarbital. Med Ann DC (1965) 34, 578.

19 Cucinell SA, Conney AH, Sansur M, Burns JJ. Drug interactions in man. One lowering effect phenobarbital on plasma levels of bishydroxycoumarin (Dicumarol) and diphenylhydantoin (Dilantin). Clin Pharmacol Ther (1965) 6, 420.

20 Goss JE, Dickhaus DW. Increased bishydroxycoumarin requirements in patients receiving phenobarbital. N Eng J Med (1965) 273, 1094.

21 Avellaneda M. Interferencia de los barbituricos en la accion del Tromexan. Medicina (1955) 15, 109.

22 Reverchon F, Sapir M. Constatation clinique d'un antagonism entre barbituriques et anticoagulants. La Presse Med (1961) 96, 1570.

23 Williams JRB, Griffin JP, Parkins A. Effect of concomitantly administered drugs on the control of long term anticoagulant therapy. Quart J Med (1976) 45, 63.

24 Cucinell SA, Odessky L, Weiss M, Dayton PG. The effect of chloral hydrate on bishydroxycoumarin metabolism. A fatal outcome. J Amer Med Ass (1966) 197, 360.

25 Orme M, Breckenridge A. Enantiomers of warfarin and phenobarbital. N Eng J Med (1976) 295, 1482.

26 O'Reilly RA, Trager WF, Motley CH, Howald W. Interaction of secobarbital with warfarin pseudoracemates. Clin Pharmacol Ther (1980) 28, 187.

27 Kroon C, De Boer A, Hoogkamer JFW, Schoemaker HC, vd Meer FJM, Edelbroek PM, Cohen AF. Detection of drug interactions with single dose acenocoumarol: new screening method ? Int J Clin Pharmacol Ther Toxicol (1990) 28, 355–60.

Anticoagulants + Benfluorex

Abstract/Summary

Benfluorex does not alter the anticoagulant effects of phenprocoumon.

Clinical evidence, mechanism, importance and management

25 patients on phenprocoumon showed no significant changes in their prothrombin times while taking 450 mg benfluorex daily for nine weeks when compared with equivalent periods before and after while not taking benfluorex.[1] There seems to be no information about other anticoagulants.

Reference

1 De Witte P, Brems HM. Co-administration of benfluorex with oral anticoagulant therapy. Curr Med Res Opin (1980) 6, 478.

Anticoagulants + Benziodarone

Abstract/Summary

The anticoagulant effects of ethylbiscoumacetate, diphenadione, nicoumalone (acenocoumarol) and warfarin are increased by benziodarone. The dosage of anticoagulant should be reduced appropriately. Chlorindione, dicoumarol and phenindione do not interact, but the situation with phenprocoumon is not clear.

Clinical evidence

90 patients on anticoagulants were given 200 mg benziodarone three times a day for two days and 100 mg three times a day thereafter. To maintain constant PP percentages the anticoagulant dosages were reduced as follows: ethylbiscoumacetate 17% (nine patients), diphenadione 42% (eight patients), nicoumalone 25% (seven patients) and warfarin 46% (15 patients). No changes were needed in those taking chlorindione (five patients), dicoumarol (nine patients), phenindione (10 patients) or phenprocoumon (eight patients). A parallel study on 12 normal subjects confirmed the interaction with warfarin.[1]

The absence of an interaction with dicoumarol confirms a previous study,[2] however another study found that 300–600 mg benziodarone daily increased the anticoagulant effects of phenprocoumon in nine out of 29 patients and the ecchymoses observed were more frequent and larger.[3] The metabolism of ethylbiscoumacetate appears to be increased by benziodarone.[3]

Mechanism

Not understood. Benziodarone alone has no definite effect on activity of prothrombin or factors VII, IX or X.

Importance and management

Information appears to be limited to the studies cited, but the interaction would seem to be established. The dosages of the interacting anticoagulants and possibly of phenprocoumon should be reduced appropriately to prevent bleeding. No particular precautions are necessary with the non-interacting anticoagulants.

References

1 Pyorala K, Ikkala E, Siltanen P. Benziodarone (Amplivix) and anticoagulant therapy. Acta Med Scand (1963) 173, 385.
2 Gillot P. Valeur therapeutique du L 2329 dans l'angine de poitrine. Acta Cardiol (1959) 14, 494.
3 Verstraete M, Vermylen J, Claeys H. Dissimilar effect of two anti-anginal drugs belonging to the benzofuran group on the action of coumarin derivatives. Arch int Pharmacodyn (1968) 176, 33–41.

Anticoagulants + Benzodiazepines

Abstract/Summary

The anticoagulant effects of warfarin are not affected by chlordiazepoxide, diazepam, flurazepam, nitrazepam or triazolam. The effects of phenprocoumon are not affected by nitrazepam or oxazepam, nor ethylbiscoumacetate by chlordiazepoxide. An interaction between any oral anticoagulant and a benzodiazepine is unlikely, but there are three unexplained and unconfirmed cases attributed to an interaction.

Clinical evidence

A number of studies on a very large number of patients administered anticoagulants and benzodiazepines for extended periods confirm the lack of an interaction between warfarin and chlordiazepoxide,[1–4,7] diazepam,[1,4,7] and flurazepam,[5] nitrazepam[1,4,6] or triazolam;[13] between ethylbiscoumacetate and chlordiazepoxide;[8] and between phenprocoumon, oxazepam[12] and nitrazepam.[9]

There are three discordant reports: A patient on warfarin showed an increased anticoagulant response when given diazepam.[10] A patient on dicoumarol developed multiple ecchymoses and a prothrombin time of 53 s within a fortnight of starting to take 20 mg diazepam daily.[11] And a patient showed a fall in serum warfarin levels and in the anticoagulant response when given chlordiazepoxide.[6] It is by no means certain that these responses were due to an interaction.

Mechanism

The three discordant reports are not understood. Enzyme

induction is a possible explanation in one case[6] because increases in the urinary excretion of 6-beta-hydroxycortisol have been described during chlordiazepoxide use.[1,6]

Importance and management

Well documented and well established. The weight of evidence, including common experience, shows that benzodiazepines can safely be given to patients taking anticoagulants. Not all of the anticoagulant/benzodiazepine pairs been examined, but none of them would be expected to interact.

References

1 Orme M, Breckenridge A, Brooks RV. Interactions of benzodiazepines with warfarin. Br Med J (1972) 3, 611.
2 Lackner H, Hunt VE. The effect of Librium on hemostasis. Amer J Med Sci (1986) 256, 368.
3 Robinson DS, Sylwester D. Interaction of commonly prescribed drugs and warfarin. Ann Int Med (1970) 72, 853.
4 Breckenridge A, Orme E. Interaction of benzodiazepines with oral anticoagulants. In 'The Benzodiazepines'. Garattini S, Mussini E, Randall LO (eds) Raven Press, NY. (1973) p 647.
5 Robinson DS, Amidon EI. Interaction of benzodiazepines with warfarin in man. Ibid p 641.
6 Breckenridge A, Orme M. Clinical implications of enzyme induction. Ann NY Acad Sci (1971) 179, 421.
7 Solomon HM, Barakat MJ, Ashley CJ. Mechanisms of drug interaction. J Amer Med Ass (1971) 216, 1997.
8 Van Dam FE, Gribnau-Overkamp MJH. The effect of some sedatives (phenobarbital, glutethimide, chlordiazepoxide, chloral hydrate) on the rate of disappearance of ethylbiscoumacetate from the plasma. Folia Med Neerl (1967) 10, 141.
9 Bieger R, De Jonge H, Loeliger EA. Influence of nitrazepam on oral anticoagulation with phenprocoumon. Clin PharmacolTher (1972) 13, 361.
10 McQueen EG. New Zealand Committee on Adverse Drug Reactions. 9th Annual Report 1974. NZ Med J (1974) 80, 305.
11 Taylor PJ. Haemorrhage while on anticoagulant therapy precipitated by drug interaction. Arizona Med (1967) 24, 697.
12 Schneider J und Kamm G. Beeinflusst Oxazepam (Adumbran) die Antikoagulanzientherapie mit Phenprocoumon? Med Klin (1978) 73, 153.
13 Cohon MS. (Upjohn) Quoted as In-house data in 'Triazolam human pharmacokinetic review, Halcion® tablets,' Drug Information Services Unit, January 1990, pp 24–5.

Anticoagulants + Benzydamine Hydrochloride

Abstract/Summary

Benzydamine does not alter the anticoagulant effects of phenprocoumon.

Clinical evidence, mechanism, importance and management

14 patients on phenprocoumon showed no significant changes in their anticoagulant response while taking 150 mg benzydamine daily for two weeks, although there was some evidence of a fall in blood levels of the anticoagulant.[1] No particular precautions would seem necessary during concurrent use. Information about other anticoagulants is lacking.

Reference

1 Duckert F, Widmer LK and Madar G. Gleichzeitige Behandlung mit oraler Antikoagulantien und Benzydamin. Schweiz med Wsch (1974) 104, 1069.

Anticoagulants + Beta-blockers

Abstract/Summary

The effects of the oral anticoagulants are not normally affected by the concurrent use of beta-blocking drugs.

Clinical evidence, mechanism, importance and management

No clinically important changes in prothrombin times were found in nine patients anticoagulated with nicoumalone (acenocoumarol) or warfarin who were given metoprolol or atenolol.[1] Similarly, no interaction was seen in six subjects on warfarin and propranolol,[2] in 15 patients on phenprocoumon and pindolol,[4] in five patients on warfarin and acebutalol,[8] in eight subjects on warfarin and betaxolol,[9] in 10 men on warfarin and esmolol,[10] or six subjects on warfarin and bisoprolol.[11] Single dose studies in six subjects on warfarin and propranolol, metoprolol or atenolol also demonstrated no significant interaction.[3] A transient increase in phenprocoumon levels was seen in single dose studies in subjects given metoprolol,[5] but not when given atenolol[5] or carvedilol.[12] In contrast, a patient on warfarin has been reported who showed a marked rise in his British Corrected Ratio when given propranolol.[6] Haemorrhagic tendencies without any changes in Quick time or any other impairment of coagulation have been described in two patients on phenindione and propranolol.[7]

These findings confirm the general clinical experience that the effects of the anticoagulants are not normally affected by the concurrent use of the beta-blockers, but very rarely (and quite unpredictably) some change may be seen.

References

1 Mantero F, Procidano M, Vicariotto MA, Girolami A. Effect of atenolol and metoprolol on the anticoagulant activity of acenocoumarin. Br J clin Pharmac (1984) 17, 94–6S.
2 Scott AK, Park BK, Breckenridge AM. Interaction between warfarin and propranolol. Br J clin Pharmac (1984) 17, 86S.
3 Bax NDS, Lennard MS, Tucker GT, Woods HF, Porter NR, Malia RG, Preston FE. The effect of beta-adrenoceptor antagonists on the pharmacokinetics and pharmacodynamics of warfarin. Br J clin Pharmac (1984) 17, 85S.
4 Vinazzer H. Effect of the beta-receptor blocking agent Visken on the action of coumarin. Int J Clin Pharmacol (1975) 12, 458.
5 Spahn H, Kirch W, Mutschler E, Ohnhaus EE, Kitteringham NR, Logering HJ, Paar D. Pharmacokinetic and pharmacodynamic interactions between phenprocoumon and atenolol or metoprolol. Br J clin Pharmac (1984) 17, 97–102S.
6 Bax NDS, Lennard MS, Al-Asady S, Deacon CS, Tucker GT, Woods HF.

Inhibition of drug metabolism by beta-adrenoceptor antagonists. Drugs (1983) 25 (Suppl 2) 121–6.

7 Neilson GH, Seldon WA. Propranolol in angina pectoris. Med J Aust (1969) 1, 856.

8 Ryan JR. Clinical pharmacology of acebutolol. Am Heart J (1985) 109, 1131.

9 Thiercelin JF, Warrington SJ, Thenot JP, Orofiamma B. Lack of interaction of betaxolol on warfarin induced hypocoagulability. In Proc 2nd Eur. Cong Biopharm Pharmacokinet. Vol III: Clinical Pharmacokinetics (published by Imprimerie de l'Universite de Clermont Ferrant, 1984) edited by Aiache JM, Hirtz J, pp 73–80.

10 Lowenthal DT, Porter RS, Saris SD, Bies CM, Slegowski MB, Staudacher A. Clinical pharmacology, pharmacodynamics and interactions of esmolol. Am J Cardiol (1985) 56, 14–17F.

11 Warrington SJ, Johnston A, Lewis Y, Murphy M. Bisoprolol: studies of potential interactions with theophylline and warfarin in healthy volunteers. J Cardiovasc Pharmacol (1990) 16, (Suppl 5) S164–8.

12 Caspary S, Merz P-G, Brei R, Harder S. Interaction profile of carvedilol: investigations with digitoxin and phenprocoumon. Int J Clin Pharmacol Ther Toxicol (1992) 30, 537–8.

Anticoagulants + 5-Bromo-2′-deoxyuridine (BUDR)

Abstract/Summary

The anticoagulant effects of warfarin were markedly increased in a patient after receiving a number of courses of BUDR.

Clinical evidence, mechanism, importance and management

A 65-year-old man with grade III anaplastic astrocytoma under treatment with warfarin was given a number of courses of 1400 mg BUDR daily IV as a radiosensitizer. His prothrombin times were unaffected by the first 4-day course of BUDR, but they became more prolonged with successive courses and after the fourth course his prothrombin time climbed to about 45 s which was treated with 10 mg vitamin K. A significant increase also took place when a fifth cycle of 990 mg BUDR was given and the warfarin had to be stopped.[1] The reason for this reaction is not understood. Those using BUDR should be aware that this adverse interaction may occur.

Reference

1 Oster SE, Lawrence HJ. Potentiation of anticoagulant effect of coumadin by 5-bromo-2'-deoxyuridine (BUDR). Cancer Chemother Pharmacol (1988) 22, 181.

Anticoagulants + Calcium channel blockers

Abstract/Summary

Diltiazem appears not to affect the anticoagulant effects of warfarin, nor prenylamine the effects of phenprocoumon.

Clinical evidence, mechanism, importance and management

A study in 30 patients with angina treated with phenprocoumon found that the addition of 60 mg prenylamine three times a day for three weeks had no effect on their prothrombin times.[1] In another study ten men were given racemic warfarin, eight R-warfarin and ten S-warfarin as single 1.5 mg/kg IV doses. After taking 120 mg diltiazem three times a day for four days the clearance of R-warfarin was decreased by about 20% but the more potent S-warfarin remained unaffected. The total anticoagulant response remained unchanged.[2] No special precautions would seem to be necessary during concurrent use. There seems to be no information about other anticoagulants with calcium channel blockers.

References

1 Bohm C, Denes G. Untersuchung zur Erfassung eventueller Klinischer Interaktionene zwichsen Phenprocoumon und Prenylamin (Ergebnisse einer Multizenterstudie). Acta Ther (1987) 13, 333–43.

2 Abernethy DR, Kaminsky LS, Dickinson TH. Selective inhibition of warfarin metabolism by diltiazem in humans. J Pharmacol Exp Ther (1991) 257, 411–5.

Anticoagulants + Carbamazepine, Oxcarbazepine

Abstract/Summary

The anticoagulant effects of warfarin can be markedly reduced by carbamazepine. The warfarin dosage may need to be approximately doubled to accommodate this interaction. Oxcarbazepine appears not to interact with warfarin.

Clinical evidence

Two patients on warfarin given carbamazepine (200 mg daily for the first week, 400 mg daily for the second and 600 mg for the third) showed an approximately 50% fall in serum warfarin levels which was reflected in sharp rises in their PP percentages.[1] The half-life of warfarin in three other patients fell by 53, 11 and 60% respectively when similarly treated.[1]

This interaction has been described in six other reports.[2–7] One of them describes a patient stabilized on both drugs who developed widespread dermal ecchymoses and a prothrombin time of 70 s a week after stopping the carbamazepine. She was restabilized on approximately half the dose of warfarin in the absence of the carbamazepine.[7]

A study in 10 subjects on warfarin found that 450 mg oxcarbazepine twice daily for a week increased the Quick values from 41 to only 46.[8] A very similar study by the same workers found a change in Quick values from 36.6 to 38.1% due to oxcarbazepine.[9]

Mechanism

Uncertain, but the available evidence suggests that carbamazepine increases the metabolism of warfarin by the liver, thereby increasing its loss from the body and reducing its effects.[1,2]

Importance and management

The warfarin-carbamazepine interaction is moderately well-documented, established and clinically important. The incidence is uncertain. Monitor the anticoagulant response if carbamazepine is added to established treatment with warfarin and anticipate the need to double the dosage. Information about other anticoagulants is lacking but it would be prudent to apply the same precautions. Oxcarbazepine appears to be a non-interacting alternative.

References

1 Hansen JM, Siersbaek-Nielsen K, Skovsted L. Carbamazepine-induced acceleration of diphenylhydantoin and warfarin metabolism in man. Clin Pharmacol Ther (1971) 12, 539.
2 Ross JR, Beeley L. Interaction between carbamazepine and warfarin. Br Med J (1980) 1, 1415.
3 Kendall AG, Boivin M. Warfarin-carbamazepine interaction. Ann Intern Med (1981) 94, 280.
4 Massey EW. Effect of carbamazepine on coumarin metabolism. Ann Neurol (1983) 13, 691–2.
5 Penry JK, Newmark ME. The use of antiepileptic drugs. Ann Intern Med (1981) 94, 280.
6 Beeley L, Stewart P, Hickey FM. Bulletin of the West Midlands for Adverse Drug Reaction Reporting (1988) 26, 18.
7 Denbow CE, Fraser HS. Clinically significant haemorrhage due to warfarin-carbamazepine interaction. South Med J (1990) 83, 981.
8 Krämer G, Tettenborn B, Klosterkov-Jensen P, Mainz FRG. Oxcarbazepine-warfarin drug interaction study in healthy volunteers. Epilepsia (1991) 32 Suppl 1, 70.
9 Krämer G, Tettenborn B, Klosterkov Jensen P, Menge GP, Stoll KD. Oxcarbazepine does not affect the anticoagulant activity of warfarin. Epilepsia (1992) 33, 1145–8.

Anticoagulants + Carbon tetrachloride

Abstract/Summary

A single case report describes an increase in the anticoagulant effects of dicoumarol in a patient who accidentally drank some carbon tetrachloride.

Clinical evidence, mechanism, importance and management

A patient, well stabilized on dicoumarol, accidentally drank 0.1 ml carbon tetrachloride. Next day his prothrombin time had risen to 41 s (prothrombin activity fall from 18 to 10%). These values were approximately the same next day although the dicoumarol had been withdrawn, and marked hypoprothrombinaemia persisted for another 5 days.[1]

The probable reason for this reaction is that carbon tetra-chloride is very toxic to the liver, the changed anticoagulant response being a manifestation of this. Carbon tetrachloride, once used as an anthelmintic in man, is no longer used in human medicine, but is still employed as an industrial solvent and degreasing agent. On theoretical grounds it would seem possible for anticoagulated patients exposed to substantial amounts of the vapour to experience this interaction but this has not been reported.

Reference

1 Luton EF. Carbon tetrachloride exposure during anticoagulant therapy. Dangerous enhancement of hypoprothrombinemic effect. J Amer Med Ass (1966) 194, 120.

Anticoagulants + Carnitine

Abstract/Summary

An isolated report describes gastrointestinal bleeding and a marked increase in the anticoagulant effects of nicoumalone in a patient given L-carnitine.

Clinical evidence, mechanism, importance and management

A woman who had taken nicoumalone (acenocoumarol) for 17 years, because of aortic and mitral prosthetic valves, was admitted to hospital with melaena within five days of starting to take 1 g L-carnitine daily. Her INR had risen from 2.1 to 7. Endoscopy and colonoscopy revealed diffuse bleeding from superficial erosions in the gut. She was discharged 10 days later on the same dose of nicoumalone with an INR of 2.1, but without the carnitine.[1] The reason for this marked increase in the anticoagulant effects of the nicoumalone is not known.

This seems to the first and only recorded case of an interaction between an oral anticoagulant and carnitine, but it would now be prudent to monitor the outcome if carnitine is added to a stable regime with any oral anticoagulant, being alert for an increased response.

Reference

1 Martinez E, Domingo P, Roca-Cusachs A. Potentiation of acencoumarol action by L-carnitine. J Int Med (1993) 233, 94.

Anticoagulants + Cephalosporins

Abstract/Summary

Cefamandole can increase the anticoagulant effects of warfarin. Hypoprothrombinaemia (without an anticoagulant) and/or bleeding has been seen with cefoperazone, cephazolin, cephalothin and latamoxef (moxalactam). It is suggested that it may also occur with cephaloridine. If these cephalosporins and oral anticoagulants are used together it seems possible that their anticoagulant effects might be additive.

Clinical evidence

(a) Warfarin + cefamandole

A study of a possible interaction was prompted by two patients who developed unusually high prothrombin times (one of them bled) when given both drugs. 60 other patients undergoing heart valve replacement surgery were given antibiotics prophylactically before the chest incision was made, and at six-hourly intervals thereafter for about 72 h. Those given 2 g cefamandole (44 patients) showed a much greater anticoagulant response than those given 500 mg vancomycin (16 patients).[1] A later study by the same workers confirmed these findings.[15] They recommend that those aged over 60 undergoing this kind of surgery, who have a baseline prothrombin time of 14 s or more, should be started on no more than 5 mg warfarin daily if they are to be given cefamandole. Serious bleeding (in the absence of an anticoagulant) following the use of cephamandole has been described in 3 out of 37 patients in another report,[10] and seven other cases are described elsewhere.[11]

(b) Cefoperazone, cephaloridine, cefazolin, cephalothin and latamoxef

It has been claimed that cephaloridine given alone can induce an extension of prothrombin times, but no evidence is given.[2,3] A patient has been described who, 12 days after starting to take 0.5 g cephazolin eight-hourly, was noted to have increased prothrombin and partial thromboplastin times.[4] These returned to normal within 48 h of withdrawing the antibiotic, and recurred 10 days after it was restarted. Increased prothrombin times were found in another study.[15] 17 cases of hypoprothrombinaemia and/or bleeding have been described with latamoxef (moxalactam),[5] and several other cases have been reported with cefoperazone.[6–9,16] Cephalothin has also been implicated.[13]

Mechanism

Not fully understood.[14] One suggestion is that the hypoprothrombinaemia associated with these antibiotics is due to vitamin K deficiency caused by a combination of low vitamin K intake and a suppression of the intestinal bacterial flora which normally act as a supplementary source of vitamin K (cefamandole is secreted in the bile). As a result bleeding occurs because the vitamin K-dependent blood clotting factors fall to very low levels. There is also evidence that these cephalosporins have a direct coumarin-like effect.[16] Latamoxef also inhibits platelet aggregation.[12] The presence of an anticoagulant is an additional factor.

Importance and management

It is well established that bleeding can occur in some patients if

these antibiotics are given in the absence of an anticoagulant, but there are few reports of bleeding in patients also taking anticoagulants. Patients most at risk would seem to be those whose intake of vitamin K is restricted (poor diet, malabsorption syndromes, etc.) and those with renal failure. The use of an anticoagulant represents just another factor which may precipitate bleeding. Concurrent use should be well monitored. Excessive hypoprothrombinaemia can be controlled with vitamin K.

References

1 Angaran DM, Dias VC, Arom KV, Northrup WF, Kersten TE, Lindsay WG, Nicoloff DM. The influence of prophylactic antibiotics on the warfarin anticoagulation response in the post-operative prosthetic cardiac valve patient. Ann Surg (1984) 199, 107–111.
2 Council on Drugs. Evaluation of a new antibacterial agent, cephaloridine (Loridine). J Amer Med Ass (1986) 206, 1289.
3 Wade A. Martindales Extra Pharmacopoeia 27th ed. Pharmaceutical Press, London (1977) p 1099.
4 Lerner PI, Lubin A. Coagulopathy with cefazolin in uremia. N Eng J Med (1974) 290, 1324.
5 Beeley L, Beadle R, Lawrence R. Bulletin of the West Midlands Centre for Adverse Drug Reaction Reporting (1984) 19, 15.
6 Meisel S. Hypoprothrombinaemia due to cefoperazone. Drug Intell Clin Pharm (1984) 18, 316.
7 Cristiano P. Hypoprothrombinaemia associated with cefoperazone treatment. Drug Intell Clin Pharm (1984) 18, 314–6.
8 Osborne JC. Hypoprothrombinaemia and bleeding due to cefoperazone. Ann InternMed (1985) 102, 721–2.
9 Freedy HR, Cetnarowski AB, Lumish RM, Schafer FJ. Cefoperazone-induced coagulopathy. Drug Intell Clin Pharm (1986) 20, 281–3.
10 Hooper CA, Haney BB, Stone HH. Gastrointestinal bleeding due to vitamin K deficiency in patients on parenteral cefamandole. Lancet (1980) i, 39–40.
11 Rymer W, Greenlaw CW. Hypoprothrombinaemia associated with cefamandole. Drug Intell Clin Pharm (1980) 14, 780–3.
12 Bang NU, Tessler SS, Heidenreich RO, Marks CA, Mattler LE. Effects of moxalactam on blood coagulation and platelet function. Rev Infect Dis (1982) 4 (Suppl) S546–54.
13 Natelson EA, Brown CH, Bradshaw MW. Influence of cephalosporin antibiotics on blood coagulation and platelet function. Antimicrob Ag Chemother (1976) 9, 91–3.
14 Babiak LM and Rybak MJ. Hematological effects associated with beta-lactam use. Drug Intell Clin Pharm (1986) 20, 833–6.
15 Angaran DM, Dias VD, Arom KV, Northrup WF, Kersten TG, Lindsay WG, Nicoloff DM. The comparative influence of prophylactic antibiotics on the prothrombin response to warfarin in the postoperative prothetic cardiac valve patients. Ann Surg (1987) 206, 155–61.
16 Andrassy K, Kodersich J, Fritz S, Bechtold H, Sonntag H. Alteration of hemostasis associated with cefoperazone treatment. Infection (1986) 14, 27–31.

Anticoagulants + Chloral hydrate

Abstract/Summary

The anticoagulant effects of warfarin are transiently increased by chloral hydrate, but this is normally of little or no clinical importance. Chloral betaine, petrichloral and triclofos may be expected to have a similar effect.

Clinical evidence

A retrospective study on 32 patients just starting on warfarin showed that while the loading doses of warfarin in the control and chloral-treated groups were the same, the warfarin requirements of the chloral group during the first four days fell by about a third, but rose again to normal by the 5th day.[1]

A study on 10 patients and four normal subjects taking warfarin showed that when given 1 g chloral hydrate each night, there was a minor, clinically unimportant and short-lived increase in the prothrombin times of five of them during the first few days of concurrent treatment, but no change in the overall long-term anticoagulant control.[2]

Similar results have been described in other studies on large numbers of patients taking warfarin and chloral[3-5,8,10,11] or triclofos.[7] Chloral betaine appears to behave similarly.[9] An isolated and by no means fully explained case of fatal hypoprothrombinaemia has been reported[6] in a patient on dicoumarol who was given chloral for 10 days, later replaced by secobarbital. Another patient on dicoumarol and chloral showed a reduction in prothrombin times.[6]

Mechanism

Chloral hydrate is mainly metabolized to trichloroacetic acid which then successfully competes with warfarin for its binding sites on plasma proteins.[8] As a result, free and active molecules of warfarin flood into plasma water by displacement so that the effects of the warfarin are increased. But this is only short-lived because the warfarin molecules become exposed to metabolism by the liver, so that their effects are reduced once more.

Importance and management

A well-documented and well understood interaction, normally of little or no clinical importance. There is very good evidence that concurrent use need not be avoided.[1-5,8,10,11] The ultra-cautious might wish to keep an eye on the anticoagulant response during the first 4–5 days. It is uncertain whether other anticoagulants behave in the same way because the evidence is sparse, indirect and inconclusive,[6,12,13] but what is known suggests that they probably do.

Triclofos[7] and chloral betaine[9] appear to behave like chloral, and petrichloral may also be expected to do so. Dichloral-phenazone on the other hand interacts quite differently (see 'Anticoagulants + Dichloralphenazone').

References

1 Boston Collaborative Drug Surveillance Program. Interaction between chloral hydrate and warfarin. N Eng J Med (1972) 286, 53.
2 Udall JA. Warfarin-chloral hydrate interaction. Pharmacological activity and significance. Ann Int Med (1974) 81, 341.
3 Griner PF, Raisz LG, Rickles FR. Wiesner PJ, Odoroff CL. Chloral hydrate and warfarin interaction: clinical significance? Ann Intern Med (1971) 74, 540.
4 Udall JA. Clinical implications of warfarin interactions with five sedatives. Amer J Cardiol (1975) 35, 67.
5 Udall JA. Warfarin interactions with chloral hydrate and glutethimide. Curr Ther Res (1975) 17, 67.
6 Cucinell SA, Odessky K, Weiss M, Dayton PG. The effect of chloral hydrate on bishydroxycoumarin metabolism. A fatal outcome. J Amer Med Ass (1966) 197, 366.
7 Sellers EM, Lang M, Koch-Weser J. Enhancement of warfarin-induced hypoprothrombinaemia by triclofos. Clin PharmacolTher (1972) 13, 911.
8 Sellers EM, Koch-Weser J. Kinetics and clinical importance of displacement of warfarin from albumin by acidic drugs. Ann NY Acad Sci (1971) 179, 213.
9 McDonald MG, Robinson DS, Sylwester D, Jaffe JJ. The effects of phenobarbital, chloral betaine and glutethimide administration on warfarin plasma levels and hypoprothrombinaemic responses in man. Clin PharmacolTher (1969) 10, 80.
10 Breckenridge A, Orme ML'E, Thorgeirsson S, Davies DS, Brooks RV. Drug interactions with warfarin: studies with dichloralphenazone, chloral hydrate and phenazone (antipyrine). Clin Sci (1971) 40, 351.
11 Breckenridge A, Orme M. Clinical implications of enzyme induction. Ann NY Acad Sci (1971) 179, 421.
12 Dayton PG, Tarcam Y, Chenkin Th and Wiener M. The influence of barbiturates on coumarin plasma levels on prothrombin response. J Clin Invest (1961) 40, 1797.
13 Van Dam FE, Gribnau-Overkamp MJH. The effects of some sedatives (phenobarbital, glutethimide, chlordiazepoxide, chloral hydrate) on the rate of disappearance of ethylbiscoumacetate from the plasma. Folia Med Neerl (1967) 10, 141.

Anticoagulants + Chloramphenicol

Abstract/Summary

The anticoagulant effects of dicoumarol and nicoumalone (acenocoumarol) and possibly ethylbiscoumacetate can be increased by the concurrent use of chloramphenicol.

Clinical evidence

A study in four patients showed that the half-life of dicoumarol was increased on average by a factor of three (from 8 to 25 h) when treated with 2 g chloramphenicol daily for 5–8 days.[1]

Three out of nine patients taking an unnamed anticoagulant showed a fall in their Prothrombin-Proconvertin values from a range of 10–30% down to less than 6% when given 1–2 g chloramphenicol daily for 4–6 days.[2] One patient showed a smaller reduction.

There is another report of an increased anticoagulant response involving nicoumalone, and a brief comment implicating, but not confirming, an interaction involving dicoumarol and ethylbiscoumacetate.[3] Hypoprothrombinaemia and bleeding have been described in patients on chloramphenicol in the absence of an anticoagulant.[4,5]

Mechanism

Uncertain. One suggestion is that the chloramphenicol inhibits the liver enzymes concerned with the metabolism of the anticoagulants so that their effects are prolonged and increased.[1] Another is that the antibiotic decimates the gut bacteria thereby decreasing a source of vitamin K, but it is doubtful if these bacteria are normally an important source of the vitamin except in exceptional cases where dietary levels are very inadequate.[6] A third suggestion is that chloramphenicol blocks production of prothrombin by the liver.[4]

Importance and management

The documentation is very sparse indeed, but what is known suggests that the concurrent use of dicoumarol or nicoumalone and chloramphenicol should be avoided. If concurrent use is undertaken, the anticoagulant dosage should be reduced and the prothrombin time monitored closely. Direct evidence of an interaction with any other anticoagulant is lacking (except possibly ethylbiscoumacetate). It is noteworthy that there is nothing on record about warfarin and chloramphenicol which might imply that no clinically important interaction occurs (?). All of the cases cited above involved the use of normal oral doses of chloramphenicol. There is nothing to suggest that the small doses used in eye drops would interact with any of the anticoagulants.

References

1 Christensen LK and Skovsted L. Inhibition of drug metabolism by chloramphenicol. Lancet (1969) ii, 1397.
2 Magid E. Tolerance to anticoagulants during antibiotic therapy. Scand J Lab Clin Invest (1962) 14, 565.
3 Johnson R, David A, Chartier Y. Clinical experience with G-23350 (Sintrom). Can Med Ass J (1957) 77, 760.
4 Klippel AP, Pitsinger B. Hypoprothrombinaemia secondary to antibiotic therapy and manifested by massive gastrointestinal haemorrhage. Arch Surg (1968) 96, 266.
5 Matsniotis N, Messaritakis J, Vlachou C. Hypoprothrombinaemia bleeding in infants associated with diarrhoea and antibiotics. Arch Dis Child (1970) 45, 586.
6 Udall JA. Human sources and absorption of vitamin K in relation to anticoagulant stability. J Amer Med Ass (1965), 194, 107.

Anticoagulants + Cholestyramine or Colestipol

Abstract/Summary

The anticoagulant effects of phenprocoumon and warfarin can be reduced by cholestyramine. Separating the dosages as much as possible may help to minimize the effects of this interaction. No important interaction occurs between phenprocoumon or warfarin and colestipol.

Clinical evidence

(a) Phenprocoumon or Warfarin + Cholestyramine

10 subjects were treated for one-week periods either with warfarin alone or warfarin with 8 g cholestyramine given three times a day. With warfarin alone peak serum levels reached 5.6 g/ml and prothrombin times were prolonged by 11 s. With cholestyramine given 30 min after the warfarin, peak levels were reduced to 2.7 μg/ml and the prothrombin times were prolonged by 8 s, whereas when the cholestyramine was given 6 h after the warfarin, peak levels reached 4.7 μg/ml and prothrombin times were again prolonged by 11 s.[1]

Comparable results have been found in other studies using single doses of warfarin or phenprocoumon.[2]

(b) Phenprocoumon or Warfarin + Colestipol

Phenprocoumon serum levels and the prothrombin response were unaffected in four normal subjects by the simultaneous administration of 8 g colestipol.[13] No changes in the absorption of single 10 or 40 mg doses of warfarin in the presence of 10 g colestipol were seen in another study.[12]

Mechanism

Cholestyramine binds to bile acids within the gut and also to anticoagulants, thereby preventing their absorption.[2,3,5–7] As both warfarin and phenprocoumon undergo entero-hepatic recycling, continuous further contact with the cholestyramine can occur.[4,8] Cholestyramine also reduces the absorption of fat-soluble vitamins such as vitamin K so that it can have some direct hypoprothrombinaemic effects of its own.[10,11] This may offset to some extent the full effects of its interaction with anticoagulants. Colestipol on the other hand appears not to bind to any great extent at the pH values in the gut.[13]

Importance and management

The anticoagulant/cholestyramine interaction is established, but its magnitude and clinical importance is still uncertain. If concurrent use is thought necessary, prothrombin times should be monitored and the dosage of the anticoagulant increased appropriately. Giving the cholestyramine 3–6 h after the anticoagulant has been shown to minimize the effects of this interaction.[1,9] Information about other anticoagulants is lacking but as cholestyramine interacts with dicoumarol and ethylbiscoumacetate in animals[7] it would be prudent to expect that they all interact similarly in man.

No special precautions appear necessary if warfarin or phenprocoumon and colestipol are given concurrently. There seems to be no information about other anticoagulants.

References

1 Kventzel WP, Brunk SF. Cholestyramine-warfarin interaction. Clin Res (1970) 18, 594.
2 Robinson DA, Benjamin DM, McCormack JJ. Interaction of warfarin and non-systemic gastrointestinal drugs. Clin Pharmacol Ther (1971) 12, 491.
3 Benjamin D, Robinson DS, McCormack JJ. Cholestyramine binding to warfarin in man and in vitro. Clin Res (1970) 18, 336.
4 Jahnchen E, Meinertz T, Gilfrich H-J, Kersting F, Groth U. Enhanced elimination of warfarin during treatment with cholestyramine. Br J clin Pharmac (1978) 5, 437.
5 Hahn KJ, Eiden W, Schettle M, Hahn M, Walter E, Weber E. Effect of cholestyramine on the gastrointestinal absorption of phenprocoumon and acetylsalicylic acid in man. Europ J Clin Pharmacol (1972) 4, 142.
6 Gallo DG, Bailey KK, Sheffner AL. The interaction between cholestyramine and drugs. Proc Soc Exp Biol Med (1965) 120, 60.
7 Tembo AV, Bates TR. Impairment by cholestyramine of dicumarol and tromexan absorption in rats: a potential drug interaction. J Pharmacol Exp Ther. (1974) 191, 53.
8 Meinertz T, Gilfrich H-J, Groth N, Jonen HG, Jahnchen E. Interruption of

the enterohepatic circulation of phenprocoumon by cholestyramine. Clin Pharmacol Ther (1977) 147, 166.

9 Cali TJ. Combined therapy with cholestyramine and warfarin. Am J Pharm (1975) 72, 759.

10 Casdorph HR. Safe uses of cholestyramine. Ann Int Med (1970) 72, 759.

11 Gross L and Brotman M. Hypoprothrombinaemia and haemorrhage associated with cholestyramine therapy. Ann Int Med (1970) 72, 95.

12 Hannigan JJ. Colestipol-warfarin drug interaction study. A comparison of plasma warfarin concentrations following oral administration of 10 mg warfarin with and without an ionic exchange resin (colestipol hydrochloride or cholestyramine). On file Upjohn (1975). Quoted by Heel RC, Brogden RN, Pakes GE, Speight TM, Avery GS. Colestipol: a review of its pharmacological properties and therapeutic effects in patients with hypercholesterolaemia. Drugs (1980) 19, 161–80.

13 Harvengt C, Desager JP. Effects of colestipol, a new bile acid sequestrant, on the absorption of phenprocoumon in man. Europ J clin Pharmacol (1973) 6, 19.

Anticoagulants + Cimetidine, Famotidine, Nizatidine, Ranitidine or Roxatidine

Abstract/Summary

The anticoagulant effects of warfarin can be increased if cimetidine is given concurrently. Severe bleeding has occurred in a few patients but some show no interaction at all. Nicoumalone (acenocoumarol) and phenindione seem to interact similarly but not phenprocoumon. Famotidine, nizatidine, ranitidine and roxatidine normally appear to be non-interacting alternative H_2-blockers but bleeding has been reported in a handful of cases.

Clinical evidence

(a) Cimetidine

A very brief report in 1978, published as a letter by the makers of cimetidine, stated that at that time they were aware of 17 cases worldwide indicating that 1 g cimetidine daily could cause a prothrombin time rise of about 20% in those stabilized on warfarin.[1]

A number of studies and case reports have confirmed this interaction with warfarin.[2–5,9–12] Serum warfarin levels are reported to rise (25–80%),[6,11] and prothrombin times can be increased (>30 s). Severe bleeding (haematuria, internal haemorrhages, etc.) and very prolonged prothrombin times have been seen in few patients.[2,4,9,10,12] However one study found that only half of the group of 14 patients studied demonstrated this interaction,[18] and another on 27 patients found that although the AUC of warfarin increased by 21–39% and the clearance fell by 22–28%, prothrombin times only increased by 2–2.6 s.[15] Nicoumalone and phenindione appear to interact like warfarin,[3] but not phenprocoumon.[8]

(b) Famotidine

A study in 8 subjects taking subtherapeutic doses of warfarin (mean 4 mg daily) showed that seven days treatment with 40 mg famotidine did not affect prothrombin times, thrombotest coagulation times or steady-state serum warfarin levels.[20] No changes in prothrombin times were seen in three patients on nicoumalone or flunidione when given famotidine.[26] In another report two patients on warfarin are said to have bled and had prolonged prothrombin times attributed to the concurrent use of famotidine.[22]

(c) Nizatidine

Nizatidine appears to behave like ranitidine and normally does not interact with warfarin,[19,25] but an isolated case of bleeding and markedly prolonged prothrombin times have been seen.[22]

(d) Ranitidine

The concurrent use of 400 mg ranitidine daily for two weeks had no effect on warfarin concentrations or on prothrombin times in five subjects. In another study with 11 subjects it was found that 300 mg ranitidine daily for three days had no effect on the pharmacodynamics or pharmacokinetics of a single dose of warfarin.[2] In contrast, a third study[16,17] on five subjects reported that 300 mg ranitidine daily for a week reduced the clearance of a single dose of warfarin by almost 30%, but the half-life was not significantly changed and prothrombin times were not measured. 750 mg ranitidine daily given to two subjects was also reported to have reduced the warfarin clearance by more than 50%. A number of aspects of this last study are open to doubt and the validity of the results is questionable. There is however an isolated report where 600 mg ranitidine daily, but not 300 mg, appeared to have been the cause of hypoprothrombinaemia and bleeding in a patient on warfarin.[21]

(e) Roxatidine

12 normal subjects anticoagulated with warfarin showed no changes in pharmacokinetics of the warfarin or the prothrombin ratio when given 150 mg roxatidine daily for four days.[24]

Mechanism

Cimetidine can inhibit the liver enzymes concerned with the metabolism (phase one hydroxylation) and clearance of warfarin so that its effects are prolonged and increased.[7] This also appears to be true for nicoumalone and phenindione, but not phenprocoumon which is metabolized by different enzymes using another biochemical pathway (phase two glucuronidation).[8] The warfarin-cimetidine interaction has been found to be stereoselective, that is to say the cimetidine interacts with the R(+) isomer but not with the S(−) isomer.[13,14,23] The other H_2- blockers normally do not act as enzyme inhibitors.

Importance and management

The warfarin-cimetidine interaction is well documented, well established and clinically important. Although many patients (probably up to 50%) may not develop this interaction, if bleeding is to be avoided with certainty the effects should be monitored closely when cimetidine is first added, being alert for the need to reduce the warfarin dosage. Nicoumalone and phenindione are reported to interact similarly but the documentation is much more limited. Expect other anticoagulants to behave in the same way, with the possible exception of phenprocoumon. Famotidine, nizatidine, ranitidine and roxatidine normally appear not to interact with oral anticoagulants, but concurrent use should be monitored because quite unpredictably and rarely, bleeding and extended prothrombin times have been seen.

References

1 Flind AC. Cimetidine and oral anticoagulants. Lancet (1978) ii, 1054.
2 Silver BA, Bell WR. Cimetidine potentiation of the hypoprothrombinaemic effect of warfarin. Ann Intern Med (1979) 90, 348.
3 Serlin MJ, Sibeon RG, Mossman S, Breckenridge AM, Williams JR B, Atwood JL and Willoughby JMT. Cimetidine interaction with oral anticoagulants in man. Lancet (1979) ii, 317.
4 Hetzel D, Birkett D, Miners J. Cimetidine interaction with warfarin. Lancet (1979) ii, 639.
5 Breckenridge AM, Challiner M, Mossman S, Park BK, Serlin MJ, Sibeon RG, Williams JRB and Willoughby JMT. Cimetidine increases the action of warfarin in man. Br J Clin Pharmac (1979) 8, 392 P.
6 Serlin MJ, Sibeon RG, Breckenridge AM. Lack of effect of ranitidine on warfarin action. Br J Clin Pharmac (1981) 12, 791.
7 Henry DA, MacDonald IA, Kitchingman G, Bell GD, Langman MJS. Cimetidine and ranitidine: comparison of effects on hepatic metabolism. Br Med J (1980) 281, 775.
8 Harenberg J, Staiger Ch, de Vries JX, Walter E, Weber E, Zimmerman R. Cimetidine does not increase the anticoagulant effect of phenprocoumon. Br J Clin Pharmac (1982) 14, 292–3.
9 Wallin BA, Jacknowitz A, Raich PC. Cimetidine and effect of warfarin. Ann Inter Med (1979) 90, 993.
10 Kerly B, Ali M. Cimetidine potentiation of warfarin action. Can Med Ass J (1982) 126, 116.
11 O'Reilly RA. Comparative interaction of cimetidine and ranitidine with racemic warfarin in man. Arch Intern Med (1984) 144, 989–91.
12 Davanesen S. Prolongation of prothrombin time with cimetidine. Med J Aust (1981) 1, 537.
13 Choonara IA, Cholerton S, Haynes BP, Breckenridge AM, Park BK. Stereoselective interaction between the R enantiomer of warfarin and cimetidine. Br J Clin Pharmac (1986) 21, 271–77.
14 Toon S, Hopkins KJ, Garstang FM, Diquet B, Gill TS, Rowland M. The warfarin-cimetidine interaction: stereochemical considerations. Br J clin Pharmac (1986) 21, 245–6.
15 Sax MJ, Randolph WC, Peace KE, Chretien S, Frank WO, Braverman AJ, Gray DR, McCree LC, Wyle F, Jackson BJ, Beg MA, Young MD. Effect of two cimetidine regimens on prothrombin time and warfarin pharmacokinetics during long-term warfarin therapy. Clin Pharm (1987) 6, 492–5.
16 Desmond PV, Breen KJ, Harman PJ, Mashford ML and Morphett BJ. Decreased clearance of warfarin after treatment with cimetidine or ranitidine. Aust NZJ Med (1983) 13, 327.
17 Desmond PV, Breen KJ, Harman PJ, Mashford ML and Morphett BJ. Decreased oral warfarin clearance after ranitidine and cimetidine. Clin Pharmacol Ther (1984) 35, 338–41.
18 Bell WR, Anderson KC, Noe DA, Silver BA. Reduction in the plasma clearance rate of warfarin induced by cimetidine. Arch Intern Med (1986) 146, 2325–8.
19 Callaghan JT, Nyhart EH. Drug interactions between H_2-blockers and theophylline or warfarin. Pharmacologist (1988) 30, A14.
20 De Lepeleire I, van Hecken A, Verbesselt R, Tjandra-Maga TB, Buntix A, Distlerath L, De Schepper PJ. Lack of interaction between famotidine and warfarin. Int J Clin Pharm Res (1990) X,167–71.
21 Baciewicz AM, Morgan PJ. Ranitidine-warfarin interaction. Ann Intern Med (1990) 112, 76–7.
22 Shinn AF. Unrecognized drug interactions with famotidine and nizatidine. Arch intern Med (1991) 151, 810–4.
23 Niopas J, Toon S, Rowland M. Further insight into the stereoselective interaction between warfarin and cimetidine in man. Br J clin Pharmac (1991) 32, 508–11.
24 Labs RA. Interaction of roxatidine acetate with antacids, food and other drugs. Drugs (1988) 35, Suppl 3, 82–9.
25 Cournot A, Berlin I, Sallord JC, Singlas E. Lack of interaction between nizatidine and warfarin during concurrent use. J Clin Pharmacol (1988) 28, 1120–2.
26 Chichmanian RM, Mignot G, Spreux A, Jean-Girard C, Hofliger P. Tolérance de la famotidine. Étude due réseau médecins sentinelles en pharmacovigilance. Therapie (1992) 47, 239–43.

Anticoagulants + Cinchophen

Abstract/Summary

The anticoagulant effects of dicoumarol, ethylbiscoumacetate and phenindione are markedly increased by cinchophen. Bleeding will occur if the anticoagulant dosage is not reduced appropriately.

Clinical evidence

A patient taking an un-named anticoagulant was given a total of 4 g cinchophen over a period of two days, at the end of which his prothrombin levels were found to be less than 5%. The next day he had haematemeses and died. This prompted a study in three patients taking phenindione, ethylbiscoumacetate and dicoumarol. Within two days of starting to take 4 g cinchophen daily, the prothrombin levels of two of them fell sharply from a range of 10–25% to less than 5%. A smaller fall occurred in the third patient.[1]

Mechanism

Cinchophen by itself appears to have a direct effect on the liver, like the oral anticoagulants, which reduces the synthesis of prothrombin.[2] There is a latent period similar to that of dicoumarol before the fall in blood prothrombin levels begins, and a short delay after its withdrawal before the prothrombin levels rise again.[1] Its effects can be reversed by the administration of vitamin K.[3] This interaction would therefore seem to result from the additive effects of two anticoagulant drugs.

Importance and management

Direct information about this interaction seems to be limited to the report cited,[1] but what is known suggests that it is of clinical importance. Its incidence is uncertain. Cinchophen should not be given to patients on any anticoagulant unless the prothrombin times can be well monitored and the dosage reduced appropriately.

References

1 Jarnum S. Cinchophen and acetylsalicylic acid in anticoagulant treatment. Scand J Lab Invest (1974) 6, 91.

2 Hueper WC. Toxicity and detoxication of cinchophen. Arch Pathol (1946) 41, 592.
3 Rawls A. Prevention of cinchophen toxicity by use of vitamin K. NY State J Med. (1942) 42, 2021.

Anticoagulants + Cisapride

Abstract/Summary

Cisapride causes a small increase in the anticoagulant effects of nicoumalone (acenocoumarol) but appears not to affect phenprocoumon or warfarin.

Clinical evidence, mechanism, importance and management

22 patients on nicoumalone showed an increase in thrombotest values while on cisapride (10 mg three times daily for 3 weeks) due, it is suggested, to the increase in gastrointestinal motility caused by cisapride which increases nicoumalone absorption. These values fell when the cisapride was stopped.[1] Another study in 12 normal subjects on warfarin showed that 10 mg cisapride daily for 25 days had no statistically significant effects on prothrombin times (expressed as international normalized ratios).[2] A further study in 24 normal subjects found that 10 mg cisapride four times daily did not affect the anticoagulant effects of phenprocoumon.[3] There seems to be no information about other anticoagulants but until more is known it would seem advisable to monitor the effects for at least a week after starting or stopping cisapride so that the anticoagulant dosage can be modified if necessary.[1]

References

1 Jonker JJ C. Effect of cisapride on anticoagulant treatment with aceno-coumarol. Clinical Research Report, R 51619-NL, August (1985). Janssen unpublished data.
2 Daneshmend TK, Mahida YR, Bhaskar NK, Hawkey CJ. Does cisapride alter the anticoagulant effect of Warfarin? A pharmacodynamic assessment. British Society of Gastroenterology Spring Meeting-12–14 April 1989.
3 Wesermeyer D, Mönig H, Gaska T, Masuch S, Seiler KU, Huss H, Bruhn HD. Der Einflu??? von Cisaprid und Metoclopramid auf die Bioverfüg-barkeit von Phenprocoumon. Hämostaseologie (1991) 11, 95–102.

Anticoagulants + Clofibrate, Bezafibrate, Fenofibrate or Gemfibrozil

Abstract/Summary

The fibrates increase the effects of oral anticoagulants. This has been reported to occur with bezafibrate, nicoumalone and phenprocoumon; with clofibrate, dicoumarol, phenindione and warfarin; with fenofibrate and nicoumalone; and with gemfibrozil and warfarin. Bleeding is possible if the anticoagulant dosage is not reduced appropriately (a third to a half).

Clinical evidence

(a) Anticoagulants + Clofibrate

A study in three hospitals of 42 patients taking either phenini-done or warfarin showed that when additionally given either clofibrate or *Atromid* (clofibrate with androsterone) it was necessary to reduce the anticoagulant dosages. 10 out of 15 in Belfast needed a 25% reduction and five of them bled. All nine in Edinburgh needed a 33% reduction, and 14 out of 18 in Johannesburg also needed a reduction.[1]

This interaction has been confirmed in other studies on a considerable number of patients anticoagulated with warfarin,[2–4,7,10,11] phenindione[5,6,8] or dicoumarol.[9] Bleeding has been described frequently, and death due to haemorrhage has occurred in at least two cases.[7,8]

(b) Anticoagulants + Bezafibrate

A study on 15 patients with hyperlipidaemia on phenprocoumon found that it was necessary to reduce the anticoagulant dosage by 20% when given 450 mg bezafibrate daily, and by 33% when given 600 mg.[15] In another study in 22 patients taking 400 mg bezafibrate daily the dosage of nicoumalone also needed to be reduced by 20% to maintain a constant INR .[18] Severe hypoprothrombinaemia and gastrointestinal bleeding occurred in a patient with hypoalbuminaemia due to nephrotic syndrome and chronic renal failure on nicoumalone (aceno-coumarol) when bezafibrate was added without a suitable adjustment of the anticoagulant dosage.[19]

(c) Anticoagulants + Fenofibrate (Procetofene)

Two patients on nicoumalone needed a 30% reduction in their dosage to maintain the same prothrombin time when given 200 mg fenofibrate in the morning and 100 mg in the evening.[20] Six patients taking coumarin anticoagulants (not specifically named) needed an average dosage reduction of 12% (range 0–21%) when treated with fenofibrate.[21] In another study it was found that fenofibrate increased the effects of un-named anticoagulants in four patients by the same amount as that seen with clofibrate (i.e. by about one-third[23]). A patient on an un-named anticoagulant developed haematuria when treated with fenofibrate.[22]

(d) Anticoagulants + Gemfibrozil

A brief report describes bleeding ('..menstrual cycle prolonged and lots of blood clots..') and much higher prothrombin times (values not given) in a woman on warfarin within two weeks of starting to take 1200 mg gemfibrozil daily. Halving the warfarin dosage resolved the problem.[17] Gemfibrozil causes haemostatic changes very similar to those seen with clofibrate.[16]

Mechanism

Uncertain. Clofibrate can displace warfarin from its plasma

protein binding sites,[12-14] but this does not adequately explain the interaction. Another suggestion is that the fibrates increase the affinity of the anticoagulant for the receptor sites.[9,15]

Importance and management

The anticoagulant/clofibrate interactions are well-documented, established and clinically important. The incidence is reported to be between 20 and 100%,[2,15] but it would be wise to assume that all patients will be affected. The anticoagulant dosage should be reduced initially by a third to a half to avoid the risk of bleeding. Information about other anticoagulants not cited is lacking, but expect them to interact similarly until the contrary is proved.

Much less is know about bezafibrate, fenofibrate and gemfibrozil but it would be prudent to follow the same precautions with any of these fibrates and any oral anticoagulant. More study is needed.

References

1 Oliver MF, Roberts SD, Hayes D, Pantridge JF, Suzman MM, Bersohn I. Effect of *Atromid* and ethyl chlorophenoxy-isobutyrate on anticoagulant requirements. Lancet (1963) i, 143.
2 Udall JA. Drug interference with warfarin therapy. Clin Med (1970) 77, 20.
3 Eastham RD. Warfarin dosage, clofibrate and age of patient. Lancet (1973) ii, 554.
4 Roberts SD, Pantridge JF. Effect of *Atromid* on requirements of warfarin. J Atheroscler Res (1963) 3, 655.
5 Williams GEO, Meynell MJ, Gaddie R. Atromid and anticoagulant therapy. J Atheroscler Res (1963) 3, 658.
6 Rogen AS, Ferguson JC. Clinical observations on patients treated with *Atromid* and anticoagulants. J Atheroscler Res (1963) 3, 671.
7 Solomon RB, Rosner F. Massive haemorrhage and death during treatment with clofibrate and warfarin. NY State J Med (1973) 73, 2002.
8 Rogen AS, Ferguson JC. Effect of *Atromid* on anticoagulant requirements. Lancet (1963) i, 272.
9 Schrogie JJ, Solomon HM. The anticoagulant response to bishydroxycoumarin. II. The effect of D-thyroxine, clofibrate and norethandrolone. Clin Pharmacol Ther (1967) 8, 70.
10 Bjornsson TD, Meffin PJ, Blaschke TF. Interaction of clofibrate with the optical enantiomorphs of warfarin. Pharmacologist (1976) 18, 207.
11 Counihan TB, Keelan P. *Atromid* in high cholesterol states. J Atherscler Res (1963) 3, 580.
12 Solomon HM, Schrogie JJ, Williams D. The displacement of phenylbutazone-C[14] and warfarin-C[14] from human albumin by various drugs and fatty acids. Biochem Pharmacol(1968) 17, 143.
13 Solomon HM, Schrogie JJ. The effect of various drugs on the binding of warfarin-C[14] to human albumin. Biochem Pharmacol(1967) 16, 1219.
14 Bjornsson TD, Meffin PJ, Swezy S, Blaschke TF. Clofibrate displaces warfarin from plasma proteins in man: an example of a pure displacement interaction. J PharmacolExp Ther (1979) 210, 316.
15 Zimmerman R, Ehlers W, Walter E, Hoffrichter A, Lang PD, Andrassy K, Schlierf G. The effect of bezafibrate on the fibrinolytic system and the drug interaction with phenprocoumon. Atherosclerosis (1978) 29, 477–85.
16 Rasi VPO and Torstila I. The effect of gemfibrozil upon platelet function and blood coagulation. Preliminary report. Proc Roy Soc Med (1976) 69, Suppl 2. 109–11.
17 Ahmad S. Gemfibrozil interaction with warfarin sodium (coumadin). Chest (1990) 98, 1041–2.
18 Manotti C, Quintavalla R, Pini M, Tomasini G, Vargiu G, Dettori AG. Interazione farmacologica tra bezafibrato in formulazione retard ed acenocoumarolo. Studio clinico. G della Arteriosclerosi (1991) 16, 49–52.
19 Blum A, Seligman H, Livneh A, Ezra D. Severe gastrointestinal bleeding induced by a probable hydroxycoumarin-bezafibrate interaction. Isr J Med Sci (1992) 28, 47–9.
20 Harvengt C, Heller F, Desager JP. Hypolipidemic and hypouricemic action of fenofibrate in various types of hyperlipoproteinemias. Artery (1980) 7, 73–82.
21 Stahelin HB, Seiler W, Pult N. Erfahrungen mit dem Lipidsenker Procetofen (Lipanthyl). Schweiz Rundschau Med (Praxis) (1979) 68, 24–8.
22 Lauwers PL. Effect of procetofene on blood lipids of subjects with essential hyperlipidaemia. Curr Ther Res (1979) 26, 30–8.
23 Raynaud Ph. Un nouvel hypolipidemiant: le procetofene. Revue de Medecine de Tours (1977) 11, 325–30.

Anticoagulants + Contraceptives (oral) and Related sex hormones

Abstract/Summary

The anticoagulant effects of dicoumarol and phenprocoumon can be decreased, and the effects of nicoumalone (acenocoumarol) increased, by the concurrent use of oral contraceptives. A modest dosage adjustment may be necessary.

Clinical evidence

(a) Dicoumarol + oral contraceptives

A study on four healthy subjects given single 150 or 200mg doses of dicoumarol after a 20-day course of *Enovid* (norethynodrel and mestranol) showed that the anticoagulant effects were decreased in three of the four, although the dicoumarol half-life remained unaltered.[1]

(b) Nicoumalone (acenocoumarol) + oral contraceptives

A survey on 12 patients taking nicoumalone showed that, while taking oral contraceptives, over an average of 2 years their anticoagulant dosage requirements were reduced by about 20%. Even then they were anticoagulated to a higher degree (prothrombin ratio of 1.67 compared with 1.50) than with the anticoagulant alone. The contraceptives used were *Neogynona*, *Microgynon*, *Eugynon* (ethinyloestradiol with D-norgestrel) or *Topasel* (IM ampoules of oestradiol enanthate with dihyroxyprogesterone acetophenide).[2]

(c) Phenprocoumon

A controlled study in 14 women showed that while taking combined oral contraceptives the clearance of a single 0.22 mg/kg dose of phenprocoumon was increased by 25% (from 1.61 to 1.96 ml/min/kg).[5]

(d) Unnamed anticoagulants

Megestrol is reported to increased bleeding times with anticoagulants (un-named) in a very brief report about one patient.[4]

Mechanism

Not understood. The oral contraceptives increase plasma levels of some blood clotting factors (particularly factor X and fibrinogen) and reduce levels of antithrombin III.[6] They can apparently increase the metabolism (glucuronidation) of phenprocoumon.[5,7]

Importance and management

Direct information seems to be limited to these reports. Concurrent use need not be avoided, but some modest adjustment in the anticoagulant dosage may be necessary. Information about other anticoagulants is lacking. One study suggests that the progestogen-only contraceptives may not affect the coagulability of the blood as much as the oestrogen/progestogen types, but whether this is reflected in an absence of an interaction with the oral anticoagulants is not documented.[3]

References

1 Schrogie JJ, Solomon HM, Zieve PD. Effect of oral contraceptives on vitamin K dependent clotting activity. Clin Pharmacol Ther (1967) 8, 670
2 de Teresa E, Vera A, Ortigosa J, Pulpon LA, Arus AP and de Artaza M. Interaction between anticoagulants and contraceptives: an unsuspected finding. Br Med J (1979) 2, 1260.
3 Poller L, Thomson JM, Tabiowo A, Priest CM. Progesterone oral contraception and blood coagulation. Br Med J (1969) 1, 554.
4 Beeley L, Stewart P, Hickey FM. Bull W Midlands Centre for Adverse Drug Reaction Reporting (1988) 27, 24.
5 Mönig H, Baese C, Heidemann HT, Ohnhaus EE, Schulte HM. Effect of contraceptive steroids on the pharmacokinetics of phenprocoumon. Br J clin Pharmac (1990) 30, 115–8.
6 Robinson GE, Burren T, Mackie IJ, Bounds W, Walshe K, Faint R, Guillebaud J, Machin SJ. Changes in haemostasis after stopping the combined contraceptive pill: implications for major surgery. Br Med J (1991) 302, 269–71.
7 Mönig H, Baese C, Heidemann HT, Schulte HM. The use of oral contraceptive steroids effects the pharmacokinetics of phenprocoumon. Acta Endocrinol (1989) 120, Suppl, 180

Anticoagulants + Corticosteroids or ACTH

Abstract/Summary

Unpredictable but probably small changes (increases or decreases) in the effects of the oral anticoagulants may occur during concurrent treatment with corticosteroids or ACTH.

Clinical evidence

(a) Increased anticoagulant effects

Ten out of 14 patients on long-term treatment with either dicoumarol or phenindione showed a small but definite increase in their anticoagulant responses when treated with ACTH for 4–9 days.[1] A patient controlled on ethylbiscoumacetate began to bleed from the gut and urinary tract within three days of starting treatment with 20 mg ACTH daily.[4]

(b) Decreased anticoagulant effects

A study on 24 patients anticoagulated for several days with dicoumarol showed that 2 h after receiving 10 mg prednisone their silicone coagulation time had decreased from 28 to 24 min, and 2 h later was down to 22 min.[2] A decrease in the anticoagulant effects of ethyl biscoumacetate is described in two patients given ACTH and cortisone.[3]

Mechanism

Not understood. Corticosteroids can increase the coagulability of the blood in the absence of anticoagulants.[5,6] Increased effects have been described in animals.[4]

Importance and management

Very poorly documented. The interaction is not established. Nothing of any consequence seems to have been reported in the last 30 years or so which suggests that any interaction is usually not very important. The most constructive thing that can be said is that if either ACTH or any corticosteroid is given to patients taking anticoagulants, the effects should be monitored. But it is impossible to predict whether any dosage adjustments will be upward or downward.

References

1 Hellem AJ, Solem JH. The influence of ACTH on prothrombin-proconvertin values in blood during treatment with dicumarol and phenylindandione. Acta Med Scand (1954) 150, 389.
2 Menczel J, Dreyfuss F. Effect of prednisone on blood coagulation time in patients on dicumarol therapy. J Lab Clin Med (1960) 56, 14.
3 Chatterjea JB, Salomon L. Antagonistic effects of ACTH and cortisone on the anticoagulant activity of ethylbiscoumacetate. Br Med J (1954) 2, 790.
4 van Cauwenberge H, Jacques LB. Haemorrhagic effects of ACTH with anticoagulants. Can Med Ass J (1958) 79, 536.
5 Cosgriff SW, Diefenbach AF, Vogt W. Hypercoagulability of the blood associated with ACTH and cortisone therapy. Amer J Med (1950) 9, 752.
6 Ozsoylu S, Strauss HS, Diamond LK. Effects of corticosteroids on coagulation of the blood. Nature (Lond) (1962) 195, 1214.

Anticoagulants + Cytotoxic (antineoplastic) agents

Abstract/Summary

A number of case reports describe an increase in the effects of warfarin, accompanied by bleeding in some cases, caused by the concurrent use of cytotoxic drug regimens containing cyclophosphamide, doxorubicin, etoposide, 5-fluorouracil (5-FU), ifosfamide/mesna, methotrexate, mustine (methchlorethamine), procarbazine, sulofenur, vincristine and vindesine. A decrease in the effects of warfarin has been seen with regimens of azathioprine, cyclophosphamide, mercaptopurine and mitotane.

Clinical evidence

(a) Anticoagulant effects increased

A woman stabilized on warfarin developed an iliopsoas hae-matoma three weeks after starting treatment with cyclophos-phamide, methotrexate, 5-FU, vincristine and prednisone.[1] The prothrombin times of two women on warfarin approximately doubled, accompanied by bleeding, on day 15 of each cycle of adjuvant treatment with CMF (cyclophosphamide, methotrex-ate and 5-FU).[2] A man on warfarin showed a progressive rise in prothrombin times when given a continuous infusion of 5-FU.[12] Three out of 25 patients developed blood loss from the gut when treated with warfarin and rapid iv 5-FU which was controlled by adjusting the warfarin dosage.[13] An elderly man on warfarin showed a marked increase in prothrombin times (prolongation of 8–15 s) on two occasions when given 500 mg etoposide and 5 mg vindesine.[3] The prothrombin times of an elderly man given warfarin increased 50–100% in the middle of three cycles of treatment with ProMace-Mopp (cyclophospha-mide, doxorubicin, etoposide, methchlorethamine, vincristine, procarbazine, methotrexate and prednisone), and he developed a subconjunctival haemorrhage during the first cycle.[3] Three patients on warfarin showed a marked and very rapid increase in INRs when treated with ifosfamide/mesna.[9] Three patients developed a marked increase in prothrombin times while receiving warfarin and sulofenur (LY186641).[10]

(b) Anticoagulant effects decreased

A woman who was resistant to warfarin (7–14 mg daily) while taking azathioprine began to bleed (epistaxes, haematemesis) when the azathioprine was stopped. She was restabilized on 5 mg warfarin daily.[11] A man well stabilized on warfarin showed a marked reduction in his anticoagulant response on two occasions when treated with mercaptopurine,[4] but no changes occured when given busulfan, cyclophosphamide, cytarabine or mephalan. A woman on warfarin showed a marked rise in prothrombin times when her treatment with cyclophosphamide was withdrawn.[5] The anticoagulant effects of warfarin were progressively reduced in a woman while receiving mitotane.[8] Later this effect began to reverse.

Mechanisms, importance and management

Just why these responses occurred is not understood (except possibly with mercaptopurine which appears to increase the synthesis or activation of prothrombin[14]). It is not even possible in some cases to identify precisely the drug (or drugs) responsi-ble. The absence of problems in studies using warfarin as an adjunct to chemotherapy[6,7] and the small number of reports describing difficulties suggest that many of these interactions may be uncommon events. The concurrent use of most of these drugs need not be avoided but there is clearly a need to monitor the effects of warfarin closely both during and after treatment with these and other cytotoxic agents to ensure that prothrom-bin times are well controlled. The anticoagulant dosages may need adjustment. It has been suggested that subcutaneous heparin should be given rather than warfarin to patients on sulofenur.[10]

References

1 Booth BW, Weiss RB. Venous thrombosis during adjuvant chemotherapy. N Engl J Med (1982) 305, 170.

2 Seifter EJ, Brooks BJ, Urbs WJ. Possible interactions between warfarin and antineoplastic drugs. Cancer Treat Rep (1985) 69, 244–5.

3 Ward K, Bitran JD. Warfarin, etoposide and vindesine interactions. Cancer Treat Rep (1984) 68, 817–18.

4 Spiers ASD and Misbashan RS. Increased warfarin requirement during mercaptopurine therapy: a new drug interaction. Lancet (1974) ii, 221.

5 Tashima CK. Cyclophosphamide effect on coumarin anticoagulation. South Med J (1979) 72, 633.

6 Zacharski LR, Henderson WG, Rickles FR, Forman WB, Cornell CJ, Forcier RJ, Edwards RL, Headley E, Kim S-E, O'Donnell JF, O'Dell R, Tornyos K, Kwaan HC. Effect of warfarin anticoagulation on survival in carcinoma of the lung, colon, head and neck, and prostate. Cancer (1984) 53, 2046–52.

7 Ibid. Effect of warfarin on survival in small cell carcinoma of the lung. J Amer Med Ass (1981) 245, 831–5.

8 Cuddy PG, Loftus LS. Influence of mitotane on the hypoprothrombinemic effect of warfarin. South Med J (1986) 79, 387–8.

9 Hall G, Lind MJ, Huang M, Moore A, Gane A, Robert JT, Cantwell BMJ. Intravenous infusions of ifosfamide/mesna and perturbation of warfarin anticoagulant control. Postgrad Med J (1990) 66, 860–1.

10 Fossella FV, Lippman SM, Seitz DE, Alberts DS, Taylor CW, Wiltshaw E, Hardy J, O'Brien M, Haynes TR, Wolen RL. Hypoprothrombinaemia from coadministration of sulofenur (LY 186641) and warfarin: report of three cases. Invest New Drugs (1991) 9, 357–9.

11 Singleton JD, Conyers L. Warfarin and azathioprine: an important drug interaction. Am J Med (1992) 92, 217.

12 Wajima T, Mukhopadhyay P. Possible interaction between warfarin and 5-fluorouracil. Amer J Hematol (1992) 40, 238–43.

13 Chelobowski RT, Gota CH, Chann KK, Weiner JM, Block JB, Batemen JR. Clinical and pharmacokinetic effects on combined warfarin and 5-fluorouracil in advanced colon cancer. Cancer Res (1982) 42, 4827.

14 Martini A, Jähnchen E. Studies in rats on the mechanisms by which 6-mercaptopurine inhibits the anticoagulant effect of warfarin. J Pharma-col Exp Ther (1977) 201, 547–53.

Anticoagulants + Dextropropoxyphene

Abstract/Summary

Five patients on warfarin have shown a marked increase in prothrombin times and/or bleeding when given *Distalgesic* (dextropropoxyphene/paracetamol (acetaminophen)), but the interaction seems to be an uncommon. Other patients on unnamed anticoagulants have been reported not to develop this interaction.

Clinical evidence

A man on 6 mg warfarin daily developed marked haematuria within six days of starting to take two tablets of *Distalgesic* (dextropropoxyphene 32.5 mg, paracetamol (acetaminophen) 325 mg per tablet) three times a day. His plasma warfarin levels had risen by a third (from 1.8 to 2.4 g/ml).[1] Another patient controlled for six weeks on warfarin showed gross haematuria within only 5 h of taking six tablets of *Distalgesic* over a 6 h period. Her prothrombin time increased from about 30/40 s to 130 s.[1]

This interaction has been seen in four other patients on warfarin.[2,4,7,8] The prothrombin time of one of them rose from 28/44 s to 80 s within three days of substituting paracetamol (acetaminophen) by two tablets of *Distalgesic* four times a day.[4] Another developed a prothrombin time of more than 50 s after taking 30 tablets of *Darvocet-N 100* (dextropropoxyphene 100 mg, paracetamol (acetaminophen) 650 mg) and possibly an unknown amount of ibuprofen over a 3-day period. Increased warfarin effects leading to severe retroperitoneal haemorrhage has also been briefly reported in a patient taking co-proxamol (dextropropoxyphene + paracetamol). Methocarbamol may have been a contributory factor.[8] Death due to unknown causes in a patient on warfarin and dextropropoxyphene has also been described.[3]

In contrast, a double-blind trial on 23 patients anticoagulated with un-named coumarol derivatives and given 450 mg dextropropoxyphene daily for 15 days failed to show any change in prothrombin times.[6]

Mechanism

Not understood. It seem possible that in man, as in animals,[5] dextropropoxyphene inhibits or competes with the liver enzymes concerned with the metabolic clearance of warfarin, thereby prolonging and increasing its effects. There is also the possibility that the paracetamol (acetaminophen) component of the *Distalgesic* and *Darvocet* had some part to play (see 'Anticoagulants + Paracetamol').

Importance and management

Information is very limited but what is known suggests that only a few patients are likely to develop this interaction. Concurrent use need not be avoided but it would be prudent to monitor the effects, whether using warfarin or any other anticoagulant, because the occasional patient may show a marked response.

References

1 Orme M, Breckenridge A. Warfarin and *Distalgesic* interaction. Br Med J (1976) i, 200.
2 Jones RV. Warfarin and *Distalgesic* interaction. Br Med J (1976) i, 460.
3 Udall JA. Drug interference with warfarin therapy. Clin Med (1970) 77, 20.
4 Smith R, Pruden D, Hawkes C. Propoxyphene and warfarin interaction. Drug Intell Clin Pharm (1984) 18, 822.
5 Breckenridge A, Orme ML'E, Thorgeirsson S, Davies DS, Brooks RV. Drug interactions with warfarin: studies with dichloralphenazone, chloral hydrate and phenazone (antipyrine). Clin Sci (1971) 40, 351.
6 Franchimont P, Heden G. Comparative studies of ibuprofen and dextropropoxyphene in scapulo-humeral periarthritis following myocardial infarction. XIII Int Cong Rheumatol 30th Sept-6th Oct 1973, Kyoto, Japan.
7 Justice JL and Kline SS. Analgesics and warfarin. A case that brings up questions and cautions. Postgrad Med (1988) 83, 217.
8 Beeley L, Magee P, Hickey FN. Bulletin of the West Midlands Centre for Adverse Drug Reaction Reporting (1990) 30, 32.

Anticoagulants + Dichloralphenazone

Abstract/Summary

The anticoagulant effects of warfarin are reduced by the concurrent use of dichloralphenazone. Other anticoagulants probably interact similarly.

Clinical evidence

Five patients on long-term warfarin treatment showed an approximately 50% (20.2–68.5%) reduction in plasma warfarin levels, and a fall in the anticoagulant response, when given 1.3 g doses of dichloralphenazone each night for 2 weeks. Another patient given the same doses nightly over a month showed a 70% fall in plasma warfarin levels and a thrombotest percentage rise from 9 to 55%. These values returned to normal when the hypnotic was withdrawn.[2] Similar results have been described in other reports.[1,3]

Mechanism

The phenazone (antipyrine) component of the hypnotic is a potent liver enzyme inducing agent which increases the metabolism and clearance of the warfarin, thereby reducing its effects.[2,3] The effects of the chloral appear to be minimal, (see 'Anticoagulants + Chloral hydrate').

Importance and management

Information is limited, but it appears to be an established and clinically important interaction, probably affecting most patients. The dosage of warfarin will need to be increased to accommodate this interaction. Non-interacting alternatives for dichloralphenazone may be found among the benzodiazepines (see 'Anticoagulants + Benzodiazepines'). If the dosage of warfarin has been disturbed by using dichloralphenazone, it may take up to a month for it to restabilize.

References

1 Breckenridge A, Orme ML'E, Davies DS, Thorgeirsson S, Dollery CT. Induction of drug metabolising enzymes in man and rat by dichloralphenazone. 4th Int Congr Pharmacol(1969) Basel.
2 Breckenridge A, Orme ML'E, Thorgeirrson S, Davies DS, Brooks RV. Drug interaction with warfarin: studies with dichloralphenazone, chloral hydrate and phenazone (antipyrine). Clin Sci (1971) 40, 351.
3 Breckenridge A, Orme M. Clinical implications of enzyme induction. NY Acad Sci (1971) 179, 421.

Anticoagulants + Diflunisal

Abstract/Summary

There is some limited evidence that diflunisal can increase the anticoagulant effects of nicoumalone (acenocoumarol) and possibly warfarin, but phenprocoumon appears not to be affected. Prothrombin times should be checked if diflunisal is given to patients taking any anticoagulant, and when the diflunisal is withdrawn.

Clinical evidence

The serum warfarin levels of five normal subjects on subtherapeutic doses fell by about a third (from 741 to 533 ng/ml) when given 500 mg diflunisal for two weeks, but the anticoagulant response was unaffected.

When the diflunisal was withdrawn, the serum warfarin levels rose once more while the anticoagulant response fell.[1] Another report very briefly describes an increased INR during concurrent use.[4]

A brief report states that three out of six subjects on nicoumalone experienced significant increases in prothrombin times when given 750 mg diflunisal daily, but no interaction was seen in two subjects on phenprocoumon.[3]

Mechanism

Uncertain. Diflunisal can displace warfarin from its plasma protein binding sites[1] but this on its own is almost certainly not the full explanation.

Importance and management

This interaction is neither well defined nor well documented. Its importance is uncertain, however the reports cited and the manufacturers literature suggest that an increased anticoagulant effect should be looked for if diflunisal is added to established treatment with any anticoagulant. A decreased effect would be expected if diflunisal is withdrawn. Phenprocoumon is possibly an exception and appears not to interact. The risk of bleeding (because of changes in platelet activity or gastrointestinal irritation) appears to be less than with aspirin.[2]

References

1 Serlin MJ, Mossman S, Sibeon RG, Tempero KF, Breckenridge AM. Interaction between diflunisal and warfarin. Clin Pharmacol Ther (1980) 28, 493.
2 Tempero KF, Cirillo VJ, Steelman SL. Diflunisal: a review of pharmacokinetic and pharmacodynamic properties, drug interactions, and special tolerability studies in humans. Br J clin Pharmac (1977) 4, 31S.
3 Caruso I et al. Unpublished observations quoted in ref. 2.
4 Beeley L, Cunningham H, Carmichael A, Brennan A. Bulletin of the W. Midlands Centre for Adverse Drug Reporting (1992) 35, 13.

Anticoagulants + Dipyridamole

Abstract/Summary

Mild bleeding can sometimes occur if anticoagulants and dipyridamole are used concurrently even though prothrombin times remain stable and well within the therapeutic range.

Clinical evidence

Thirty patients stabilized on either warfarin (28 patients) or phenindione (two patients) showed no significant changes in prothrombin times when given dipyridamole in doses up to 400 mg daily for a month, but three patients developed mild bleeding (epistaxis, bruising, haematuria) which resolved when either drug was withdrawn or the dosage reduced.[1]

Two other reports state that prothrombin ratios remain unaltered when dipyridamole is given with warfarin, and claim that there is no risk of bleeding.[2,3] No bleeding problems were described in a study of the value of combined use (300 mg dipyridamole daily) in patients with heart valve replacements.[4]

Mechanism

Uncertain. A reduction in platelet adhesiveness or aggregation induced by the dipyridamole may have been responsible.[1]

Importance and management

Information seems to be very limited. Since bleeding can sometimes occur even when prothrombin values are within the therapeutic range, some caution is appropriate. The authors of the study cited suggest that prothrombin activity should be maintained at the upper end of the therapeutic range as a precaution.[1] Only warfarin and phenindione have been implicated, but it would be sensible to apply the same precautions with any anticoagulant.

References

1 Kalowski S, Kincaid-Smith P. Interaction of dipyridamole with anticoagulants in the treatment of glomerulonephritis. Med J Aust (1973) 2, 164.
2 Rajah SM, Sreeharan N, Rao S, Watson D. Warfarin versus warfarin plus dipyridamole on the incidence of arterial thromboembolism in prosthetic heart valve patients. VII Int Cong Thromb Haem London (1979) Abstr 379.
3 Donaldson DR, Sreeharan N, Crow MJ, Rajahs SM. Assessment of the interaction of warfarin with aspirin and dipyridamole. Thromb Haemostas (Stuttgart) (1982) 47, 77.
4 Kawazoe K, Fujita T, Manabe H. Dipyridamole combined with anticoagulant in prevention of early postoperative thromboembolism after cardiac valve replacement. Thromb Res (1991) Suppl XII, 27–33.

Anticoagulants + Dipyrone (Metamizole)

Abstract/Summary

One report claims that no interaction occurs with phenprocoumon or ethylbiscoumacetate, whereas another describes a rapid but transient increase in the effects of ethylbiscoumacetate.

Clinical evidence, mechanism, importance and management

The concurrent use of 1 g dipyrone daily did not alter the anticoagulant effects of either phenprocoumon (five subjects) or ethylbiscoumacetate (six subjects).[1] Another report describes a short-lived but rapid increase (within 4 h) in the effects of ethylbiscoumacetate caused by dipyrone.[2] The reasons are not understood. Monitor the effects if concurrent use is thought appropriate. Dipyrone is believed to cause serious blood dyscrasias including agranulocytosis so that the advisability of its use is uncertain

References

1 Badian M, Le Normand Y, Rupp W, Zapf R. There is no interaction between dipyrone (metamizol) and the anticoagulants, phenprocoumon and ethylbiscoumacetate, in normal caucasian subjects. Int J Pharmaceut (1984) 18, 9–15.
2 Mehvar SR, Jamali F. Dipyrone-ethylbiscoumacetate interaction in man. Ind J Pharm (1981) 7, 293–9.

Anticoagulants + Disopyramide

Abstract/Summary

The anticoagulant effects of warfarin are reduced to some extent by disopyramide in many patients, but there are two reports of patients who needed less warfarin while taking disopyramide.

Clinical evidence

(a) Reduced warfarin effects

A study in 10 patients with recent atrial fibrillation scheduled for electroconversion, maintained on warfarin and with a British Corrected Ratio of 2–3, found that disopyramide increased the clearance of warfarin by 21% (from 166.3 to 201.1 ml/h).[5] Another study found that two out of three patients needed a warfarin dosage increase of about 10% when concurrently treated with disopyramide (600 mg daily) for atrial fibrillation.[2]

(b) Increased warfarin effects

A report describes a patient who following a myocardial infarction was given 3 mg warfarin daily and 100 mg disopyramide 6-hourly with digoxin, frusemide and potassium supplements. When the disopyramide was withdrawn his warfarin requirements doubled over a 9-day period.[1] An increased response to warfarin in the presence of disopyramide has been seen in another patient.[4]

Mechanism

Unknown. One idea is that when the disopyramide controls

fibrillation, changes occur in cardiac output and in the flow of blood through the liver which might have an effect on the synthesis of the blood clotting factors.[2,3] But the discordant response in the two patients remains unexplained.

Importance and management

Very poorly documented and not established. The outcome of concurrent use is uncertain. It would be prudent to monitor the response to any anticoagulant if disopyramide is given or withdrawn, and appropriate dosage adjustments made if necessary.

References

1 Haworth E, Burroughs AK. Disopyramide and warfarin interaction. Br Med J (1977) 2, 866.
2 Sylven C, Anderson P. Evidence that disopyramide does not interact with warfarin. Br Med J (1983) 286, 1181.
3 Ryll C, Davis LJ. Warfarin-disopyramide interactions. Drug Intell Clin Pharm (1979) 13, 260.
4 Marshall J. Personal communication 1987.
5 Woo KS, Chan K, Pun CO. The mechanisms of warfarin-disopyramide. Circulation (1987) 76, Suppl IV-520.

Anticoagulants + Disulfiram

Abstract/Summary

The anticoagulant effects of warfarin are increased by disulfiram and bleeding can occur if the anticoagulant dosage is not reduced appropriately. Bad breath smelling of bad eggs has also been described during concurrent treatment.

Clinical evidence

Haemorrhage in a patient given warfarin and disulfiram prompted study of this interaction.[1] Eight normal subjects anticoagulated with warfarin were given 500 mg disulfiram daily for 21 days. The plasma warfarin levels of seven of them rose by an average of 20% and their prothrombin activity fell by about 10%.

Other experiments with single doses of warfarin confirm these results,[2–4] and the interaction has been described in other reports.[5,6] Bad breath reminiscent of the smell of bad eggs has also been described in patients taking warfarin and disulfiram.[6]

Mechanism

Not fully understood. The suggestion[2–4] that disulfiram inhibits the liver enzymes concerned with the metabolism of warfarin has not been confirmed by later studies.[7] It is now postulated[7] that disulfiram may chelate with the metal ions necessary for the production of active thrombin from prothrombin, thereby augmenting the actions of warfarin.

Importance and management

An established interaction, although direct information about patients is very limited. What is known suggests that most individuals will demonstrate this interaction. If concurrent use is thought appropriate, the effects of warfarin or any other anticoagulant should be monitored and suitable dosage adjustments made when adding or withdrawing disulfiram. Patients already on disulfiram should be started on a small dose of anticoagulant.

References

1 Rothstein E. Warfarin effect enhanced by disulfiram. J Amer Med Ass (1968) 206, 1574.

2 O'Reilly RA. Interaction of sodium warfarin and disulfiram. Ann Int Med (1973) 78, 73.

3 O'Reilly RA. Potentiation of anticoagulant effect by disulfiram. Clin Res (1971) 19, 180.

4 O'Reilly RA. Interaction of warfarin and disulfiram in man. Fed Proc (1972) 31, 248.

5 Rothstein E. Warfarin effect enhanced by disulfiram (Antabuse). J Amer Med Ass (1972) 221, 1051.

6 O'Reilly RA, Mothley CH. Breath odor after disulfiram. J Amer Med Ass (1977) 238, 2600.

7 O'Reilly RA. Dynamic interaction between disulfiram and separated enantiomorphs of racemic warfarin. Clin Pharmacol Ther (1981) 29, 332.

Anticoagulants + Ditazole

Abstract/Summary

Ditazole does not alter the anticoagulant effects of nicoumalone.

Clinical evidence, mechanism, importance and management

Fifty patients with artificial heart valves taking nicoumalone (acenocoumarol) showed no changes in their prothrombin times while taking 800 mg ditazole daily.[1] No special precautions are needed. There seems to be no information about other anticoagulants.

Reference

1 Jacovella G, Milazzotto F. Ricerca di interazioni fra ditazolo e anticoagulanti in portatori di protesi valvolari intracardache. Clinica Terapeutica (1977) 80, 425.

Anticoagulants + Diuretics

Abstract/Summary

The anticoagulant effects of warfarin are not affected by the concurrent use of bumetanide, frusemide or chlorothiazide. Frusemide also appears not to affect phenprocoumon. A small reduction in the effects of warfarin, clorindione and phenprocoumon, but not of nicoumalone, occurs with chlorthalidone. Spironolactone reduces the effects of warfarin similarly. On rare occasions a marked increase has been seen with ethacrynic acid. In contrast the anticoagulant effects of ethylbiscoumacetate, nicoumalone and warfarin can be increased by tienilic acid (ticrynafen) and bleeding may occur.

Clinical evidence

(a) Ethylbiscoumacetate, Nicoumalone and Warfarin + Tienilic acid

Two patients taking ethylbiscoumacetate began to bleed spontaneously (haematuria, ecchymoses of the legs and gastrointestinal bleeding) when they started to take 250 mg tienilic acid daily. The thrombotest percentage of one of them was found to have fallen below 10%.[10] Increased anticoagulant effects and/or bleeding, beginning within a few days, have been described in patients or subjects given tienilic acid while taking ethylbiscoumacetate,[10,16] nicoumalone (acenocoumarol)[11,12] or warfarin.[14,16,17]

(b) Nicoumalone, Phenprocoumon or Warfarin + Chlorthalidone

Six normal subjects given single 1.5 mg/kg doses of warfarin showed reduced hypoprothrombinaemia (from 77 to 58 u) when also given 100 mg chlorthalidone daily, although the plasma warfarin levels remained unaltered.[3] Similarly reduced anticoagulant effects have been described with phenprocoumon, and clorindione but no significant effects were seen on the activity of nicoumalone.[4]

(c) Phenprocoumon + Frusemide

A pharmacokinetic study in 17 normal subjects showed that 40 mg frusemide twice daily had no effect on the pharmacokinetics of single oral doses of phenprocoumon (022 mg/kg).[18]

(d) Warfarin + Frusemide or Bumetanide

A study in 10 normal subjects showed that their response to single 0.8 mg/kg doses of warfarin were unaffected by taking 1 mg bumetanide daily for 14 days.[1] This confirms a previous study in 11 normal subjects given 2 mg daily.[2] A study on six normal subjects showed that warfarin plasma levels, half-lives and prothrombin times in response to a 50 mg oral dose were not significantly altered by the presence of frusemide (80 mg daily).[2]

(e) Warfarin + Ethacrynic acid

A case report describes a marked increase in the anticoagulant effects of warfarin in a woman on two occasions when administered doses of ethacrynic acid ranging from 50 to 300 mg. She had hypoalbuminaemia.[5] A therapeutically significant interaction between warfarin and ethacrynic acid is reported elsewhere, but no details are given.[6]

(f) Warfarin + Spironolactone

A study in nine subjects given single 1.5 mg/kg doses of warfarin showed that the concurrent use of 200 mg spironolactone reduced the prothrombin time (expressed as a percentage of the control activity with warfarin alone) from 100 to 76%. Plasma warfarin levels remained unchanged.[8]

(g) Warfarin + Thiazides

A study on eight normal subjects given single 40–60 mg oral doses of warfarin and 1 g chlorothiazide daily showed that the mean half-life of the anticoagulant was increased slightly (from 39 to 44 h) but the prothrombin time was barely affected (from 18.9 to 18.6 s).[7]

Mechanism

It has been suggested that the diuresis induced by chlorthalidone and spironolactone reduces plasma water which leads to a concentration of the blood clotting factors.[3,8] Ethacrynic acid can displace warfarin from its plasma protein binding sites,[9] but it is almost certain that this, on its own, does not explain the marked interaction described.[5,6] Tienilic acid reduces the metabolism of S-warfarin (but not R-warfarin) thereby prolonging its stay in the body and increasing its effects.[17] It was originally thought that this was a drug displacement interaction.[10,13,15]

Importance and management

The documentation relating to diuretics other than tienilic acid is very limited indeed and seems to be confined to the reports cited, most of which were single dose studies. This evidence suggests that most of these diuretics either do not interact with the anticoagulants at all, or they do so only to a small extent. This is in general agreement with common experience. Prothrombin times should be monitored if chlorthalidone or spironolactone is started or withdrawn, and the anticoagulant dosages adjusted if necessary. Somewhat greater caution should be exercised with ethacrynic acid, particularly in those with hypoalbuminaemia or kidney dysfunction. Information about other anticoagulants is lacking.

The anticoagulant-tienilic acid interaction is established and of clinical importance. The incidence is uncertain. Concurrent use should be avoided. If that is not possible, prothrombin times should be closely monitored and the anticoagulant dosage reduced as necessary. There seems to be no information about other anticoagulants but it would be prudent to assume that they will interact similarly. Tienilic acid has been withdrawn in many countries because of its hepatotoxicity.

References

1 Nipper H, Kirby S, Iber FL. The effect of bumetanide on the serum disappearance rate of warfarin sodium. J Clin Pharmacol (1981) 21, 654–6.
2 Nilsson CM, Horton ES, Robinson DS. The effect of furosemide and bumetanide on warfarin metabolism and anticoagulant response. J Clin Pharmacol (1978) 18, 91.
3 O'Reilly RA, Sahud MA, Aggeler PM. Impact of aspirin and chlorthalidone on the pharmacodynamics of oral anticoagulant drugs in man. Ann NY Acad Sci (1971) 179, 173.
4 Vinazzer H. Die Beeinflussungen der Antikoagulantientherapie durch ein Diuretikum. Wien Z Inn Med Ihre Grenzge (1963) 44, 323.
5 Petrick RJ, Kronacher N, Alcena V. Interaction between warfarin and ethacrynic acid. J Amer Med Ass (1975) 231, 843–4.
6 Koch-Weser J. Hemorrhagic reactions and drug interactions in 500 warfarin-treated patients. Clin Pharmacol Ther (1973) 14, 139.
7 Robinson DS, Sylwester D. Interaction of commonly prescribed drugs and warfarin. Ann Int Med (1970) 72, 853.
8 O'Reilly RA. Spironolactone and warfarin interaction. Clin Pharmacol Ther (1980) 27, 198.
9 Sellers EM, Koch-Wester J. Kinetics and clinical importance of displacement of warfarin from albumin by acidic drugs. Ann NY Acad Sci (1971) 179, 213–25.
10 Detilleux M, Caquet R, Laroche C. Potentialisation de l'effet des anticoagulantes comariniques par un nouveaux diuretique, l'acide tienilique. Nouv Presse med (1976) 36, 2395.
11 Portier H, Destaing F, Chavve L. Potentialisation de l'effet des anticoagulantes coumariniques par l'acide tienilique: un nouvelle observation. Nouv Presse med (1977) 6, 468.
12 Grand A, Drouin B, Arche GJ. Potentialisation de l'action anticoagulante des antivitamines K par l'acide tienilique. Nouv Presse med (1977) 6, 2691.
13 Slattery JT, Levy G. Ticrynafen effect on warfarin protein binding in human serum. J Pharm Sci (1979) 68, 393.
14 McLain DA, Garriga FJ, Kantor OS. Adverse reactions associated with ticrynafen use. J Amer Med Ass (1980) 243, 763.
15 Prandota J, Albengres E, Tillement JP. Effect of tienilic acid (Diflurex) on the binding of warfarin ^{14}C to human plasma proteins. Int J Clin Pharmacol Ther Toxicol (1980) 18, 158.
16 Prandota J, Pankow-Prandota L. Klinicznie znamienna interakcja nowego leku moczopednego kwasu tienylowego z lekami przeciwzakrzepowymi pochodnymi kumaryny. Przeglad Lek (1982) 39, 385–8.
17 O'Reilly RA. Ticrynafen-racemic warfarin interaction: hepatotoxic or stereoselective? Clin Pharmacol Ther (1982) 32, 356–61.
18 Mönig H, Böhm M, Ohnhaus EE, Kirch W. The effects of frusemide and probenecid on the pharmacokinetics of phenprocoumon. Eur J Clin Pharmacol (1990) 39, 261–5.

Anticoagulants + Erythromycin

Abstract/Summary

A marked increase in the effects of warfarin with bleeding has been seen in a small number of patients when concurrently treated with erythromycin, but most patients are unlikely to develop a clinically important interaction. This interaction has also been seen in a patient on nicoumalone (acenocoumarol).

Clinical evidence

(a) Warfarin

A case report describes an elderly woman on warfarin, digoxin, hydrochlorothiazide and quinidine who developed haematuria and bruising within a week of starting to take 2 g erythromycin stearate daily. Her prothrombin time had risen to 64 s.[1]

Eight other cases of bleeding and/or hypoprothrombinaemia have been described in patients on warfarin when given erythromycin (as ethylsuccinate, stearate, estolate, lactobionate or base).[2-8,13] A study in 12 normal subjects showed that the clearance of a single dose of warfarin was reduced by an average of 14% (range zero to almost one-third) after taking 1 g erythromycin daily for 8 days.[9] Erythromycin caused only a small increase in the effects of warfarin in another study on eight patients.[11,12]

(b) Nicoumalone (acenocoumarol)

Haemorrhage occurred in a patient on nicoumalone when treated with erythromycin.[10]

Mechanism

It is believed that erythromycin can stimulate the liver enzymes to produce metabolites which bind to cytochrome P450 to form inactive complexes, the result being that the metabolism of warfarin is reduced and its effects are thereby increased.[9] But why it only happens in a few individuals is not clear.

Importance and management

An established interaction, but unpredictable. The incidence is uncertain but the paucity of reports suggests that it is low. The effect in a few patients is evidently considerable, but in most it is likely to be small and unimportant. Concurrent use need not be avoided but it would be prudent to monitor the effects, especially in those who clear warfarin slowly and who therefore only need low doses. The elderly in particular would seem to fall into this higher risk category. Information about anticoagulants other than warfarin and nicoumalone seems not to be available but the same precautions would be advisable.

References

1 Bartle WR. Possible warfarin-erythromycin interaction. Arch Intern Med (1980) 140, 985.
2 Schwartz JI, Bachmann K. Erythromycin-warfarin interaction. Arch Intern Med (1984) 144, 2094.
3 Husserl FE. Erythromycin-warfarin interaction. Arch Intern Med (1983) 143, 1831–2.
4 Sato RI, Gray DR, Brown SE. Warfarin interaction with erythromycin. Arch Intern Med (1984) 144, 2413–4.
5 Friedman HS, Bonventre MV. Erythromycin-induced digoxin toxicity. Chest (1982) 82, 202.
6 Hansten PD, Horn JR. Erythromycin and warfarin. Drug Interactions Newsletter (1985) 5, 37–40.
7 Hassell D, Utt JK. Suspected interaction: warfarin and erythromycin. South Med J (1985) 78, 1015–16.
8 Bussey HI, Knodel LC and Boyle DA. Warfarin-erythromycin interaction. Arch Intern Med (1985) 145, 1736–7.
9 Bachmann K, Schwartz JI, Forney R, Frogameni A, Jauregui LE. The effect of erythromycin on the disposition kinetics of warfarin. Pharmacology (1984) 28, 171–6.
10 Grau E, Fontenberta J, Felez J. Erythromycin-oral anticoagulants interaction. Arch Intern Med (1986) 146, 1639.
11 Weibert RT. Effect of erythromycin in patients receiving long term warfarin therapy. Clin Pharmacol Ther (1987) 41, 224.
12 Weibert RT, Lorentz SM, Townsend RJ, Cook CE, Klauber MR, Jagger PI. Effect of erythromycin on patients receiving long-term warfarin. Clin Pharmacy (1989) 8, 210–14.
13 O'Donnell D. Antibiotic-induced potentiation of oral anticoagulant agents. Med J Aust (1989) 150, 163–4.

Anticoagulants + Ethchlorvynol

Abstract/Summary

The anticoagulant effects of dicoumarol and warfarin (probably other anticoagulants as well) are reduced by the concurrent use of ethchlorvynol.

Clinical evidence

Six patients on dicoumarol showed a rise in their Quick index from 38 to 55% while taking 1 g ethchlorvynol daily over an 18-day period. Another patient on dicoumarol became overanticoagulated and developed haematuria on two occasions when the ethchlorvynol was withdrawn, once for 6 days and the other for 4 days.[1] A marked reduction in the anticoagulant effects of warfarin occurred in another patient when given ethchlorvynol.[2]

Mechanism

Uncertain. The idea that ethchlorvynol increases the metabolism of the anticoagulants by the liver is not confirmed by studies in dogs and rats.[3]

Importance and management

Information is very sparse and limited to dicoumarol and warfarin, but the interaction seems to be established. Be alert for other anticoagulants to behave similarly. Anticipate the need to alter the anticoagulant dosage if ethchlorvynol is started or stopped. An alternative non-interacting substitute may be found among the benzodiazepines.

References

1 Cullen SI, Catalano PM. Griseofulvin-warfarin antagonism. J Amer Med Ass (1967) 199, 582.
2 Johansson SA. Apparent resistance to oral anticoagulant therapy and influence of hypnotics on some coagulation factors. Acta med Scand (1968) 184, 297.
3 Martin YC. The effect of ethchlorvynol on the drug-metabolising enzymes of rats and dogs. Biochem Pharmacol (1967) 16, 2041.

Anticoagulants + Feprazone

Abstract/Summary

The anticoagulant effects of warfarin are increased by feprazone which can lead to bleeding.

Clinical evidence

Five patients on long term warfarin treatment showed a mean prothrombin time rise from 29 to 38 s after 5 days treatment with 300 mg feprazone daily, despite a 40% reduction in their warfarin dosage (from 5 to 3 mg daily). Four days after withdrawal of the feprazone, their prothrombin times were almost back to pretreatment levels.[1]

Mechanism

Unknown. Feprazone is highly bound to plasma proteins so that some of the interaction may be due to displacement from plasma protein binding sites, but this is certainly not the whole story.

Importance and management

Although information is limited to the study quoted, the interaction would appear to be established. Concurrent use should be avoided to prevent bleeding. If that is not possible, the anticoagulant response should be closely monitored and suitable reductions made to the warfarin dosage. Other anticoagulants may be expected to behave similarly.

Reference

1 Chierichetti S, Bianchi G, Cerri B. Comparison of feprazone and phenylbutazone interaction with warfarin in man. Curr Ther Res (1975) 18, 568.

Anticoagulants + Floctafenine or Glafenine

Abstract/Summary

The anticoagulant effects of nicoumalone (acenocoumarol) and phenprocoumon are increased by floctafenine. The anticoagulant effects of phenprocoumon are increased by glafenine but no interaction occurs with nicoumalone (acenocoumarol), ethylbiscoumacetate or 'indanedione'.

Clinical evidence, mechanism, importance and management

(a) Glafenine

A double-blind study on 20 patients stabilized on phenprocoumon showed that a significant increase in thrombotest times occurred within a week of starting to take 600 mg glafenine daily.[2] Another report states that five out of seven patients needed an anticoagulant dosage reduction while taking glafenine.[3] The reason is not understood. Monitor the effects of concurrent use and reduce the anticoagulant dosage appropriately. 10 subjects on nicoumalone (acenocoumarol), ethylbiscoumacetate or 'indanedione' showed no changes in their anticoagulant response when given 800 mg glafenine daily over a 4-week period.[4]

(b) Floctafenine

A double-blind study[1] on 10 patients on nicoumalone (acenocoumarol) or phenprocoumon showed that concurrent treatment with 800 mg floctafenine daily prolonged their Thrombotest times by an average of approximately one-third. The anticoagulant dosage of some of the patients was reduced. The reasons are not understood. The effects of concurrent use should be monitored and the anticoagulant dosage reduced as necessary. Information about other anticoagulants is lacking, but the same precautions would seem to be appropriate.

References

1 Boejinga JK, van de Broeke RN, Jochemsen R, Breimer DD, Hoogslag MA, Jeleticka-Bastiaanse A. De invloed van floctafenine (Idalon) op antistollingsbehandeling met coumarinederivaten. Ned T Geneesk (1981) 125, 1931–5.
2 Boejinga JK and van der Vijgh WJF. Double blind study of the effect of glafenine (Glifanan) on oral anticoagulant therapy with phenprocoumon (Marcumar). Europ J clin Pharmacol (1977) 12, 291.
3 Boejinga JK, Gan TB and van der Meer J. De invloed van glafenine (Glifanan) op antistollingsbehandeling met coumarinederivaten. Ned T Geneesk (1974) 118, 1895.
4 Raby C. Recherches sur une eventuelle potentialisation de l'action des anticoagulants de synthese par la glafenine. Therapie (1977) 32, 293.

Anticoagulants + Flosequinan

Abstract/Summary

Flosequinan normally appears not to interact to a clinically significant extent with warfarin.

Clinical evidence, mechanism, importance and management

20 patients anticoagulated with warfarin showed statistically significant increases in INR, PTT and prothrombin times, and a decrease in factor VII when given 50 mg flosequinan twice daily for two weeks, but the values remained within acceptable clinical levels and none of the changes was considered to be clinically relevant.[1] Isolated reports of decreased warfarin requirements have been reported to the makers of flosequinan, but no causal link has been established.[2] No special precautions seem necessary during concurrent use except that it has been suggested that INRs should be well monitored in those with severe heart failure who are given flosequinan and warfarin. Flosequinan was withdrawn in July 1993.

References

1 Anon. An investigation into the effect of warfarin on warfarin-induced anticoagulation. Boots Unpublished protocol (1993).
2 Glodkowski PE (Boots). Personnal communication 1993.

Anticoagulants + Fluconazole

Abstract/Summary

The anticoagulant effects of warfarin and nicoumalone (acenocoumarol) are increased by fluconazole.

Clinical evidence

A study in seven patients on warfarin found that when 100 mg fluconazole daily was added, their prothrombin times progressively increased from 15.8 s on day 1 to 18.9 s on day 5, and to 21.9 s on day 8. The fluconazole was stopped early in three patients due to high prothrombin times, but none exceeded an increase of 9.7 s and no bleeding occurred.[9]

A cross-over study in 13 subjects given 200 mg fluconazole daily for 7 days and then a single 15 mg dose of warfarin found that the changes in the prothrombin time curve over 168 h were increased about 10% in 10 subjects, by about 13% in 2 subjects, and doubled in one other subject. The last subject was given vitamin K.[1] 400 mg fluconazole daily for a week increased the prothrombin time AUC following a single dose of pseudo-racemic warfarin in six subjects by 44%.[3] Increased prothrombin times and INRs have been reported in other patients and subjects on warfarin when treated with fluconazole.[2,4 – 6,8] Two patients bled.[2,8]

A patient on nicoumalone suffered an intracranial haemorrhage (prothrombin time 170 s) 5 days after starting to take 200 mg fluconazole daily.[7]

Mechanism

Not understood. It seems possible that just as fluconazole inhibits fungal cytochrome P-450, it similarly inhibits the metabolism of the anticoagulants by the liver, thereby increasing their effects.

Importance and management

An established and clinically important interaction. If fluconazole is added to treatment with warfarin or nicoumalone, the prothrombin times should be well monitored and the anticoagulant dosage reduced as necessary. There seems to be no information about other anticoagulants, but it would be prudent to follow the same precautions with any of them.

References

1 Lazar J D, Wilner K D. Drug interactions with fluconazole. Rev Infect Dis (1990) 12 (Suppl 3) S327–33.
2 Seaton TL, Cleum CL, Black DJ. Possible potentiation of warfarin by fluconazole. DICP Ann Pharmacother (1990) 24, 1177–8.
3 Black DJ, Gidal BE, Seaton TL, McDonnell ND, Kunze KL, Evans BS, Bauwens JE, Petersdorf SH, Trager WF. An evaluation of the effect of fluconazole on the stereoselective metabolism of warfarin. Clin Pharmacol Ther (1992) 51, 184.
4 Tett S, Carey D, Lee H-S. Drug interactions with fluconazole. Med J Aust (1992) 156, 365.

5 Beeley L, Cunningham H, Brennan A. Bull W Midlands Centre of Adverse Drug Reporting. (1993) 36, 17.
6 Rieth H, Sauerbrey N. Interaktionsstudien mit Fluconazol, einem neuen Triazolantimykotikum. Wien Med Wchsch (1989) 139, 370–4.
7 Isalska BJ, Stanbridge TN. Fluconazole in treatment of candidal prothetic valve endocarditis. Br Med J (1988) 297, 178–9.
8 Kerr HD. Case report: potentiation of warfarin by fluconazole. Am J Med Sci (1993) 305, 164–5.
9 Crussell-Porter LL, Rindone JP, Ford MA, Jaskar DW. Low-dose fluconazole therapy potentiates the hypoprothrombinemic response to warfarin sodium. Arch Intern Med (1993) 153, 102–4.

Anticoagulants + Flutamide

Abstract/Summary

Flutamide can increase the anticoagulant effects of warfarin.

Clinical evidence

Five patients with prostatic cancer and taking warfarin showed increases in their prothrombin times when given flutamide. For example one patient needed reductions in his warfarin dosage from 35 to 22.5 mg weekly over a 2-month period. Another showed a prothombin time rise from 15 to 37 s within four days of starting 750 mg flutamide daily.[1]

Mechanism

Not understood. Flutamide sometimes causes liver dysfunction.

Importance and management

Information is very limited but the interaction would seem to be established. Monitor prothrombin times if flutamide is given to patients on warfarin, reducing the dosage when necessary. Nothing seems to be known about the effects on other anticoagulants but it would seem prudent to follow the same precautions.

Reference

1 Chandler R (Schering-Plough). Reports on Company files. Personal communication (1990).

Anticoagulants + Food

Abstract/Summary

The rate of absorption of dicoumarol can be increased by food. Two reports describe antagonism of the effects of warfarin by ice-cream, and another attributes an increase in prothrombin time to the use of aspartame. Avocado and soy may also reduce the effects of warfarin. See also 'Anticoagulants + Netto', and 'Anticoagulants + Vitamin K'.

Clinical evidence

(a) Dicoumarol + Food

A study with 10 normal subjects showed that the peak serum concentrations of dicoumarol, following a single 250 mg dose, were increased on average by 85% when taken with food. Two subjects showed increases of 242 and 206%.[1]

(b) Warfarin + Asparatame, Avocados, Ice-cream, Soy

A very brief report states that a patient on warfarin showed a raised prothrombin time, possibly due to the use of aspartame.[3] Two women on warfarin showed falls in their international normalized ratios (from 2.5 to 1.6 and from 2.7 to 1.6 respectively) when they started to eat 100 g avocado or more daily. Their INRs climbed again when the avocado was stopped.[6] A woman taking 22.5 mg warfarin in single daily doses failed to show the expected prolongation of her prothrombin times. It was then discovered that she took the warfarin in the evening and she always ate ice-cream before going to bed. When the warfarin was taken in the mornings, the prothrombin times increased.[2] Another patient's warfarin requirements almost doubled when she started to eat very large quantites of ice cream (1 litre each evening) but not while taking normal amounts. She took the warfarin at 6 pm and the ice cream at about 10 pm.[5] A study in 10 patients with hypercholesterolaemia found that two weeks' treatment with a soy-protein cholesterol-lowering diet caused a marked reduction (Quick time increase of 114%) in the anticoagulant effects of warfarin.[4] 'Warfarin resistance' was seen in another patient when given a constant intravenous infusion of soybean oil emulsion (*Intralipid*).[7]

Mechanisms

Not understood. One suggestion for the dicoumarol/food reaction[1] is that prolonged retention of dicoumarol with food in the upper part of the gut, associated with increased tablet dissolution, may have been responsible for the increased absorption. Soy protein possibly increases the activity of vitamin K at its liver receptors, thereby reducing the effects of warfarin. Avocado contains too little vitamin K (8 µg/100 g) for it to affect warfarin by competitive inhibition.

Importance and management

None of these interactions is very well documented, however they clearly demonstrate that some foods and intravenous preparations can sometimes affect the response to the oral anticoagulants, and may account for otherwise unexplained fluctuations or changes in the anticoagulant response which some patients show. There is not enough evidence to indicate that these foods or preparations should be avoided unless problems develop.

References

1 Melander A, Wahlin E. Enhancement of dicoumarol bioavailability by concomitant food intake. Europ J Clin Pharmacol (1978) 14, 441.
2 Simon LS and Likes KE. Hypoprothrombinaemic response due to ice-cream. Drug Intell Clin Pharm (1978) 12, 121.
3 Beeley L, Beadle F, Lawrence R (eds). Bulletin of the West Midlands Centre for Adverse Drug Reaction Reporting, Birmingham, England. (1974) 19, 9.
4 Gaddi A, Sangiorigi Z, Ciarrocchi A, Braiato A, Descovich GC. Hypocholesterolemic soy protein diet and resistance to warfarin therapy. Curr Ther Res (1989) 45, 1006–10.
5 Blackshaw C A, Watson V A. Interaction between warfarin and ice cream. Pharm J (1990) 244, 318.
6 Blickstein D, Shaklai M, Inbal A. Warfarin antagonism by avocado. Lancet (1991) 337, 914–5.
7 Lutomski DM, Palascak JE, Bower RH. Warfarin resistance associated with intravenous lipid administration. J Parenter Enteral Nutr (1987) 11, 316–8.

Anticoagulants + Glucagon

Abstract/Summary

The anticoagulant effects of warfarin are rapidly and markedly increased by glucagon in large doses (50 mg or more over two days) and bleeding can occur if the warfarin dosage is not reduced appropriately.

Clinical evidence

Eight out of nine patients on warfarin showed a marked increase in the anticoagulant effects (prothrombin times of 30–50 s or more) when given 50 mg glucagon over 2 days. Three of them bled. Eleven other patients given a total of 30 mg glucagon over 1–2 days failed to show this interaction.[1]

Mechanism

Unknown. Changes in the production of blood clotting factors and an increase in the affinity of warfarin for its site of action have been proposed.[1] A study in guinea pigs using nicoumalone suggested that changes in warfarin metabolism or its absorption from the gut are not responsible.[2]

Importance and management

This appears to be an established interaction of clinical importance, although direct information is limited to the report cited.[1] Its authors recommend that if 25 mg glucagon per day or more is given for two or more days, the dosage of warfarin should be reduced in anticipation and prothrombin times closely monitored. Smaller doses (total 30 mg) are reported not to interact.[1] Information about other anticoagulants is lacking, but it would be prudent to assume that they will interact similarly.

References

1 Koch-Weser J. Potentiation by glucagon of the hypoprothrombinemic action of warfarin. Ann Intern Med (1970) 72, 331.
2 Weiner M, Moses D. The effect of glucagon and insulin on the prothrombin response to coumarin anticoagulants. Proc Soc Biol Med (1968) 127, 761.

Anticoagulants + Glutethimide

Abstract/Summary

The anticoagulant effects of warfarin and dicoumarol are decreased by the concurrent use of glutethimide in many but not all patients.

Clinical evidence

10 subjects on warfarin, with prothrombin times of 18–22 s, showed a mean reduction of 4 s in their prothrombin times after taking 500 mg glutethimide daily for four weeks.[5,6] Other studies have shown that 1 g glutethimide daily for three weeks reduces the half-life of warfarin by a third to a half.[1,4] 750 mg glutethimide daily for 10 days can reduce the half-life of dicoumarol by about a third.[2,3] In contrast, an early study on 25 patients found no evidence of an interaction with dicoumarol.[7] Another unexplained report describes a paradoxical increase in prothrombin times and haemorrhage in a patient on warfarin after taking 3.5 g glutethimide over a 5-day period.[8]

Mechanism

Glutethimide is a liver enzyme inducing agent which increases the metabolism and clearance of the anticoagulants from the body, thereby reducing their effects.[1–6] There is no obvious explanation for the reports of 'no interaction'[7] and of an 'increased effect'[8] cited above.

Importance and management

An established interaction but of uncertain incidence. In one study[1] 40% of the subjects failed to show the interaction, and in another[6] one out of 10 did not. Monitor concurrent use and increase the anticoagulant dosage as necessary. The interaction can develop within a few days and persist for up to three weeks or more after the glutethimide has been withdrawn.[4] Information about anticoagulants other than warfarin and dicoumarol is lacking, but it would be prudent to assume that they will interact similarly. A non-interacting substitute for glutethimide may possibly be found among the benzodiazepines.

References

1 Corn M. Effect of phenobarbital and glutethimide on the biological half-life of warfarin. Thromb Diath Haemorrh (1966) 16, 606.
2 van Dam, FE, Overkamp MJH. The effect of some sedatives (phenobarbital,

glutethimide, chlordiazepoxide, chloral hydrate) on the rate of disappearance of ethylbiscoumacetate from the plasma. Folia medica Neerlandica (1967) 10, 141.
3 van Dam FE, Overkamp M, Haanen C. The interaction of drugs. Lancet (1966) ii, 1027.
4 Macdonald MG, Robinson DS, Sylwester D, Jaffe JJ. The effects of phenobarbital, chloral betaine and glutethimide administration on warfarin plasma levels and hypoprothrombinaemic responses in man. Clin Pharmacol Ther (1969) 10, 80.
5 Udall JA. Clinical implications of warfarin interactions with five sedatives. Amer J Cardiol (1975) 35, 67.
6 Udall JA. Warfarin interactions with chloral hydrate and glutethimide. Curr Ther Res (1975) 17, 67.
7 Grilli H. Glutethimide y tiempo de prothrombina. Su aplicion en la terapeutica anticoagulante. Pren med argent (1959) 46, 2867.
8 Taylor PJ. Haemorrhage while on anticoagulant therapy precipitated by drug interaction. Arizona Med (1967) 24, 697.

Anticoagulants + Griseofulvin

Abstract/Summary

The anticoagulant effects of warfarin can be reduced by the concurrent use of griseofulvin in some but not all patients.

Clinical evidence

The anticoagulant effects of warfarin were markedly reduced in three out of four individuals (two of them patients) when they were given 1–2 g griseofulvin daily. The fourth subject (a volunteer) showed no interaction, even when the griseofulvin dosage was raised to 4 g daily for two weeks.[1]

In another study[2] only four out of 10 patients on warfarin showed this interaction after taking 1 g griseofulvin daily for two weeks.[2] The average reduction in prothrombin time was 4.2 s. A very brief report describes a coagulation defect in a patient on warfarin and griseofulvin.[3] Yet another describes this interaction in man which took 12 weeks to develop fully.[4] He eventually needed a 41% increase in his daily dose of warfarin.

Mechanism

Not understood. It has been suggested that the griseofulvin acts as a liver enzyme inducer which increases the metabolism of the warfarin, thereby reducing its effects.[1,4]

Importance and management

An established interaction but not well documented. It affects some but not all patients (three out of four, and four out of ten).[1,2] Because of its unpredictability, the prothrombin times of all patients on warfarin who are given griseofulvin should be monitored, and suitable warfarin dosage increases made as necessary. Information about other anticoagulants is lacking, but it would be prudent to assume that they will interact similarly.

References

1 Cullen SI, Catalano PM. Griseofulvin-warfarin antagonism. J Amer Med Ass (1967) 199, 582.

2 Udall JA. Drug interference with warfarin therapy. Clin Med (1970) 77, 20.

3 McQueen EG. New Zealand Committee on Adverse Drug Reactions: 14th Annual Report. NZ Med J (1980) 91, 226.

4 Okino K, Weibert RT. Warfarin-griseofulvin interaction. Drug Intell Clin Pharm (1986) 20, 291–3.

Anticoagulants + Halofenate

Abstract/Summary

An isolated case report describes a marked increase in the anticoagulant effects of warfarin caused by the concurrent use of halofenate.

Clinical evidence, mechanism, importance and management

A patient, controlled on 10 mg warfarin daily, showed a dramatic increase in his prothrombin time to 103 s when he was given 10 mg/kg halofenate daily. His prothrombin times returned to normal when the warfarin dosage was reduced to 2.5 mg daily.[1] A similar interaction has been seen in dogs and it is suggested that halofenate can affect both the synthesis and destruction of prothrombin, the net effect being a prolongation of the prothrombin time.[2] Although this interaction appears to be of little general importance, it should be borne in mind if these drugs are used together.

References

1 McMahon FG, Jaqin A, Ryan JR, Hague D. Some effects of MK 185 on lipid and uric acid metabolism in man. Univ Mich Med Centre J (1970) 36, 247.

2 Weintraub M, Griner PF. Alterations in the effects of warfarin in dogs by halofenate. An influence upon the kinetics of prothrombin. Thromb Diath Haemorrh (1975) 34, 445.

Anticoagulants + Haloperidol

Abstract/Summary

A single case report describes a marked reduction in the anticoagulant effects of phenindione caused by the concurrent use of haloperidol.

Clinical evidence, mechanism, importance and management

A man, stabilized on 50 mg phenindione daily, was given haloperidol by injection (5 mg 8-hourly for 24 h) followed by 3 mg twice daily by mouth. Adequate anticoagulation was not achieved even when the phenindione dosage was increased to 150 mg. When the haloperidol dosage was halved, the necessary dose of anticoagulant was 100 mg, and only when the haloperidol was withdrawn was it possible to return to the original anticoagulant dosage.[1] The reasons for this are not understood. Concurrent use need not be avoided, but prescribers should be aware of this case.

Reference

1 Oakley DP, Lautch H. Haloperidol and anticoagulant treatment. Lancet (1963) ii, 1229.

Anticoagulants + Heparinoids

Abstract/Summary

An isolated case report describes bleeding in a patient on nicoumalone after using a heparinoid-impregnated bandage. Some of the normal tests of anticoagulation are unreliable for a few hours after giving lomoparan to patients already taking nicoumalone (acenocoumarol).

Clinical evidence, mechanism, importance and management

A man who was well stabilized on nicoumalone (acenocoumarol) and also taking metoprolol, dipyridamole and isosorbide dinitrate began to bleed within about three days of starting to use a medicated bandage on an inflamed lesion on his hand, probably caused by a mosquito bite. His prothrombin percentage was found to have fallen to less than 10%. The bandage was impregnated with a compound based on xylane acid polysulphate which is a semi-synthetic heparinoid.[1] It would appear that enough of the heparinoid had been absorbed through his skin to increase his anticoagulation to the point where he began to bleed.

A study in six normal subjects, anticoagulated with nicoumalone (steady-state thrombotest values of 10–15%), found that a single IV bolus injection of 3250 anti-Xa units of lomoparan (Org 10172) prolonged the Prothrombin time, activated partial thromboplastin time and Stypven time more than would have been expected by the simple addition of the effects of both drugs. These effects were seen up to 1 h. The Thrombotest was affected up to 5 h.[2] The results of these clinical tests may therefore be unreliable during these periods. There is no suggestion that concurrent use should be avoided.

References

1 Potel G, Maulaz B, Paboeuf C, Touze MD, Baron D. Potentialisation de l'acenocoumarol apres application cutanee d'un heparinoide semi-synthetique. Therapie (1989) 44, 67–70.

2 Stiekema JCJ, de Boer A, Danhof M, Kroon C, Broekmans AW, van Dinther ThG, Voerman J, Breimer DD. Interaction of the combined medication with the new low-molecular-weight heparinoid lomoparan (Org 10172) and acenocoumarol. Haemostasis (1990) 20,136–46.

Anticoagulants + Herbal remedies

Abstract/Summary

An isolated report attributes an increase in the anticoagulant effects of warfarin in two patients to the ingestion of medicinal garlic. Some herbal remedies such as tonka beans, melilot and sweet woodruff contain naturally occurring anticoagulants which may be expected to increase the effects of the anticoagulant drugs.

Clinical evidence, mechanism, importance and management

(a) Garlic

The INR of a patient stabilized on warfarin more than doubled and haematuria occurred eight weeks after starting to take three *Höfels* garlic pearls daily. The situation resolved when the garlic was stopped. The INR rose on a later occasion while taking two *Kwai* garlic tablets daily. The INR of another patient also more than doubled while taking six *Kwai* garlic tablets daily.[1,3] It would therefore seem prudent to monitor the effects and adjust the anticoagulant dosage if medicinal garlic is added to established treatment.

(b) Tonka, Melilot, Sweet Woodruff

A woman with unexplained abnormal menstrual bleeding was found to have a prothrombin time of 53 s, and laboratory tests showed that her blood clotting factors were abnormally low. When given parenteral vitamin K her prothrombin time rapidly returned to normal. She strongly denied taking any anticoagulant drugs, but it was eventually discovered that she had been drinking large quantities of a herbal tea containing among other ingredients tonka beans, melilot and sweet woodruff, all of which contain natural coumarins that can be converted into anticoagulants by moulds.[2] The anticoagulant effects of these compounds may have been increased by the paracetamol (acetaminophen) and dextropropoxyphene which she was taking concurrently. The effects of conventional anticoagulants would be expected to be increased by herbal remedies of this kind if taken in sufficient quantities.

References

1 Sunter W. Warfarin and garlic. Pharm J (1991) 246, 722.
2 Hogan RP. Hemorrhagic diathesis caused by drinking an herbal tea. J Amer Med Ass (1983) 249, 2679–80.
3 Sunter W. Personnal communication 1991.

Anticoagulants + Hydrocodone

Abstract/Summary

The anticoagulant effects of warfarin have been shown to be increased by hydrocodone in a patient and in a normal subject.

Clinical evidence, mechanism, importance and management

A patient, well stabilized on warfarin (and also taking digoxin, propranolol, clofibrate and spironolactone) showed a rise in his prothrombin time from about twice to three times his control value when he began to take *Tussionex* (hydrocodone + phenyltoloxamine) for a chronic cough. When the cough syrup was discontinued, his prothrombin time fell. In a subsequent study in a volunteer the equivalent dosage of hydrocodone increased the elimination half-life of warfarin from 30 to 42 h.[1] The reason is not known. Concurrent use need not be avoided but monitor the effects and reduce the warfarin dosage if necessary.

Reference

1 Azarnoff DL. Drug interactions: the potential for adverse effects. Drug Inf J (1972) 6, 19.

Anticoagulants + Indomethacin

Abstract/Summary

The anticoagulant effects of warfarin, phenprocoumon, nicoumalone (acenocoumarol) and clorindione are not normally affected by the concurrent use of indomethacin, but some caution is still necessary because indomethacin can irritate the gut and cause bleeding.

Clinical evidence

100 mg indomethacin daily for five days had no effect on the anticoagulant effects of warfarin in 16 normal subjects. When taken for 11 days by 19 normal subjects, neither the anticoagulant effects nor the half-life of warfarin were affected.[1]

Other studies in normal subjects and patients anticoagulated with phenprocoumon,[2–4] clorindione[2] or nicoumalone[5] similarly showed that the anticoagulant effects were not changed by indomethacin.

In contrast a handful of somewhat equivocal reports describe possible interactions in patients taking warfarin. One patient was also taking allopurinol which is known to interact occasionally with anticoagulants.[6] Another patient appeared to be inadequately stabilized on the anticoagulant before the indomethacin was given.[7] No details are given in the third case,[8] and two other isolated cases appear to result from unexplained interactions.[9,10]

Mechanism

None. Indomethacin reduces platelet aggregation and thereby prolongs bleeding when it occurs.

Importance and management

It is well established that normally indomethacin does not alter the anticoagulant effects of warfarin, nicoumalone, phenprocoumon or clorindione. Other anticoagulants would be expected to behave similarly. Concurrent use need not be avoided but some caution is still appropriate because indomethacin, like other NSAIDs, can cause gastrointestinal irritation, ulceration and bleeding which may be prolonged. In one case this is reported to have had a fatal outcome.[9]

References

1 Vesell ES, Passananti GT, Johnson AO. Failure of indomethacin and warfarin to interact in normal human volunteers. J Clin Pharmacol (1975) 19, 486.
2 Muller G, Zollinger W. The influence of indomethacin on blood coagulation, particularly with regard to the interference with anticoagulant treatment. Die Entzundung-Grundlagen und Pharmakologische Beeinflussung. International Symposium on Inflammation. Freiburg in Breisgau, May 4–6, 1966. Heister R, Hofmann HF (eds), Urban and Schwarzenburg, Munich (1966).
3 Frost H, Hess H. Concomitant administration of indomethacin and anticoagulants. Ibid.
4 Muller KH, Herrman K. Is simultaneous therapy with anticoagulant and indomethacin feasible? Med Welt (1966) 17, 1553.
5 Gaspardy, Von G, Balint G, Gapsardy G. Wirkung der Kombination Indomethacin under Syncumar (acenocoumarol) auf die Prothrombinspiegel im Blutplasma. Z Rheumaforsch (1967) 26, 332.
6 Odegaard AE. Undersokelse av interaksjon mellom antikoagulantia og indometacin. Tidsskr Norske Laegeforen (1974) 94, 2313.
7 Koch-Weser J. Haemorrhagic reactions and drug interactions in 500 warfarin-treated patients. Clin Pharmacol Ther (1973) 14, 139.
8 McQueen EG. New Zealand Committee on Adverse Reactions. NZ Med J (1980) 91, 226.
9 Self TH, Soloway MS, Vaughan D. Possible interaction of indomethacin and warfarin. Drug Intell Clin Pharm (1978) 12, 580.
10 Beeley L and Stewart P. Bulletin of the West Midlands Centre for Adverse Drug Reaction Reporting (1987) 25, 28.

Anticoagulants + Influenza vaccines

Abstract/Summary

The concurrent use of warfarin and influenza vaccine is usually safe and uneventful, but there are reports of bleeding in a handful of patients (life-threatening in one case) attributed to an interaction. Nicoumalone (acencoumarol) also does not normally interact.

Clinical evidence

(a) Evidence of no interaction

After vaccination with 1982/3 Trivalent influenza vaccines, Types A and B, the prothrombin times of 21 men on long-term warfarin treatment were not significantly altered.[3] Other studies[4,6] on 13 and 19 elderly men and women, 24, 26 and 33 other patients,[10–12] found no evidence of an adverse warfarin-influenza vaccine interaction, although a small increase in the prothrombin ratio (from 1.68 to 1.81) was seen in one study[11] and a small prothrombin time decrease in another.[12] No interaction was seen in other studies on four volunteer subjects[7] or on seven and 33 residents in nursing homes.[5,8] One case of gross but transient haematuria occurred, but it was not possible to link this firmly with the vaccination.[5] Trivalent influenza vaccine has also been shown not to affect anticoagulation with nicoumalone (acenocoumarmol).[14]

(b) Evidence of an interaction

A very brief report describes a patient on long-term warfarin treatment who '...almost bled to death after receiving a 'flu shot...'.[1] No further details are given.[1] An elderly man on long-term warfarin treatment developed bleeding (haematemesis and melaena) shortly after being given an influenza vaccine. His prothrombin time was found to be 36 s. A subsequent study on eight patients showed that vaccination (with Trivalent types A and B) prolonged their prothrombin times by 40%, but no signs of bleeding were seen.[2] A man well-stabilized on warfarin developed diffuse gastric bleeding and a massive gastrointestinal haemorrhage (prothrombin time of 48 s) within 10 days of influenza vaccination.[9] Another patient on warfarin showed INR increases from 2.5 to 6.0 and 7.0 on two successive years when vaccinated against influenza.[13]

Mechanism

Not understood. One suggestion is that when an interaction occurs the synthesis of the blood clotting factors is altered.[2] There is no evidence that the vaccine changes the metabolism of the warfarin[2] although the metabolism of aminopyrine (used as an indicator of changes in metabolism) is reduced.[9]

Importance and management

A well-investigated interaction. The weight of evidence shows that influenza vaccination in those taking warfarin is normally safe and uneventful, nevertheless it would be prudent to be on the alert because very occasionally and unpredictably bleeding may occur. Nicoumalone appears to behave like warfarin. Information about other anticoagulants is lacking but it seems probable that they too will not interact.

References

1 Sumner HW, Holtzman JL and McLain CJ. Drug-induced liver diseases. Geriatrics (1981) 36, no.10, 83.
2 Kramer P, Tsuru M, Cook CE, McLain CJ, Holtzman JL. Effect of influenza vaccine on warfarin anticoagulation. Clin Pharmacol Ther (1984) 35, 416–8.
3 Lipsky BA, Pecoraro RE, Roben NJ, de Baquiere P, Delaney CJ. Influenza vaccination and warfarin anticoagulation. Ann Int Med (1984) 100, 835–7.
4 Gomolin IH, Chapron DJ, Luhan PA. Effects of influenza virus vaccine on theophylline and warfarin clearance in institutionalized elderly. J Amer Ger Soc (1984) 32, April Suppl. S21.
5 Patriara PA, Kendal AP, Stricof RL, Weber JA, Meissner MK, Dateno B. Influenza vaccination and warfarin or theophylline toxicity in nursing home residents. N Eng J Med (1983) 308, 1601–2.
6 Gomolin IH, Chapron DJ, Luhan PA. Lack of effect of influenza vaccine on theophylline levels and warfarin anticoagulation in the elderly. J Am Geriatr Soc (1985) 33, 269.
7 Scott AK, Cannon J, Breckenridge AM. Lack of effect of influenza

vaccination on warfarin in healthy volunteers. Br J Clin Pharmacol (1985) 19, 144P.

8 Gomolin IH. Lack of effect of influenza vaccine on warfarin anticoagulation in the elderly. Canada Med Ass J (1986) 135, 39–41.

9 Kramer P, McClain CJ. Depression of aminopyrine metabolism by vaccination. N Engl J Med (1981) 21, 1262–4.

10 Bussey HI, Saklad JJ. Influence of influenza vaccine on warfarin therapy. Drug Intell Clin Pharm (1986) 20, 460.

11 Weibert RT, Lorentz SM, Norcross WA, Klauber MR, Jagger PI. Effect of influenza vaccine in patients receiving long-term warfarin therapy. Clin Pharm (1986) 5, 499–503.

12 Bussey HI, Saklad JJ. Effect of influenza vaccine on chronic warfarin therapy. Drug Intell Clin Pharm (1988) 21, 198–201.

13 Beeley L, Cunningham H, Carmichael AE, Brennan A. Newsletter of the West Midlands Centre for Adverse Drug Reaction Reporting, (1991), 33, 19.

14 Souto JC, Oliver A, Montserrat I, Mateo J, Sureda A, Fontcurberta J. Lack of effect of influenza vaccine on anticoagulation by acenocoumarol. Ann Pharmacother (1993) 27, 365–8.

Anticoagulants + Insecticides

Abstract/Summary

A single case has been reported of a patient who totally failed to respond to warfarin after very heavy exposure to an insecticide.

Clinical evidence, mechanism, importance and management

A rancher in the USA on warfarin showed a very marked reduction in his anticoagulant response after dusting his sheep with an insecticide containing 5% camphechlor (toxaphene) and 1% lindane (gamma-benzene hexachloride). Normally 7.5 mg warfarin daily maintained his prothrombin time at 35 s (control 12 s), but after exposure to the insecticide even 15 mg daily failed to have any effect at all.[1] The dusting was done by putting the insecticide in a sack and hitting the sheep with it in an enclosed barn. These compounds are known liver enzyme inducing agents[2] which increase the metabolism and clearance of the warfarin, thereby reducing and even abolishing its effects. Intense exposure of this kind is unusual, but it serves to illustrate the interaction potentialities of the chlorinated hydrocarbon insecticides, particularly for farm workers and others who may be exposed to considerable concentrations over long periods of time.

References

1 Jeffery WH, Ahlin TA, Goreen C, Hardy WR. Loss of warfarin effect after occupational insecticide exposure. J Amer Med Ass (1976) 236, 2881.

2 Conney AH. Environmental factors influencing drug metabolism. In Fundamentals of Drug Metabolism and Disposition. LaDu BN, Mandel HG, Way EL (eds). Williams and Wilkins Co (1971) p 253.

Anticoagulants + Isoxicam and Piroxicam

Abstract/Summary

Isoxicam and piroxicam can increase the effects of warfarin and nicoumalone (acenocoumarol). Bleeding may occur if the anticoagulant dosage is not reduced.

Clinical evidence

(a) Isoxicam

Six patients stabilized on warfarin needed a reduction in their warfarin dosage, averaging 20% (range 10–30%) when given 200 mg isoxicam daily over a 6 week period. The effects of the interaction appeared in the second week and almost reached a maximum after 4 weeks.[2]

(b) Piroxicam

A man stabilized on warfarin showed a fall in his prothrombin time from 1.7–1.9 times his control value to a value of 1.3 when he stopped taking piroxicam, 20 mg daily. The prothrombin times rose again when he re-started the piroxicam, and fell and rose again when the piroxicam was again stopped and re-started.[1] Another patient on warfarin showed increases and then decreases in prothrombin times when 20 mg piroxicam daily was started and then stopped.[5]

20 mg piroxicam daily increased the effects of nicoumalone (acenocoumarol) in four out of 11 subjects, three being considered mild and one being significant.[3] An increased prothrombin ratio has been seen in another patient.[4] A further patient on nicoumalone developed gastrointestinal bleeding 3 days after starting to take 20 mg piroxicam daily. His INR rose from 2.2 to 6.5.[6]

Mechanism

Not understood.

Importance and management

Established but not well documented interactions. The incidence is uncertain. Concurrent use need not be avoided but monitor the outcome well and reduce the anticoagulant dosage as necessary. Remember too that isoxicam and piroxicam can cause gastrointestinal irritation and reduce platelet aggregation. It is probably easier to use an alternative non-interacting NSAID. Information about other anticoagulants is lacking but it would be prudent to assume that they will interact similarly.

References

1 Rhodes RS, Rhodes PJ, Klein C, Sintek CD. A warfarin-piroxicam drug interaction. Drug Intell Clin Pharm (1985) 19, 556–8.

2 Farnham DJ. Studies of isoxicam in combination with aspirin, warfarin

sodium and cimetidine. Sem Arth Rheum (1982) 12 (Suppl 2) 179–83.

3 Jacotot B. Interaction of piroxicam with oral anticoagulants. IXth Eur Congr Rheumatol, Wiesbaden, September 1979, pp 46–82.

4 Beeley L and Stewart P. Bulletin of the W. Midlands Centre for Adverse Drug Reaction Reporting (1987) 25, 28.

5 Mallet L, Cooper JW. Prolongation of prothrombin time with the use of piroxicam and warfarin. Can J Hosp Pharm (1991) 44, 93–4.

6 Desprez D, Blanc P, Larrey D, Michel H. Hémorragie digestive favorisée par une hypocoagulation excessive due à une interaction médicamenteuses piroxicam — antagonisme de la vitamine K. Gastroenterol Clin Biol (1992) 16, 906–7.

Anticoagulants + Itraconazole

Abstract/Summary

An isolated report describes a very marked increase in the anticoagulant effects of warfarin, accompanied by bruising and bleeding, in a patient when given itraconazole.

Clinical evidence, mechanism, importance and management

A woman stabilized on warfarin (5 mg daily) and also taking ipratropium bromide, salbutamol, budesonide, quinine sulphate and omeprazole, was additionally started on 200 mg itraconazole twice daily for oral candidiasis caused by the inhaled steroid. Within 4 days she developed generalized bleeding and recurrent nose bleeds. Her international normalized ratio (INR) had risen to more than 8. The warfarin and itraconazole were stopped, but next day she was admitted to hospital for intractable bleeding and increased bruising, for which she was treated with fresh frozen plasma. Two days later when the bleeding had stopped and her INR had returned to 2.4, she was restarted on warfarin and later restabilized on her original dosage.[1] The reasons for this reaction are not understood.

This seems to be the first and only report of this interaction so that its general importance is uncertain, but it would clearly to sensible to monitor the concurrent use of warfarin and itraconazole. Warn patients to seek informed advice if any unexplained bruising or bleeding occurs.

Reference

1 Yeh J, Soo S-C, Summerton C, Richardson C. Potentiation of action of warfarin by itraconazole. Br Med J (1990) 310, 669.

Anticoagulants + Ketoconazole

Abstract/Summary

Three elderly patients showed an increase in the anticoagulant effects of warfarin when given ketoconazole. There is other evidence which shows that not all individuals will demonstrate this interaction.

Clinical Evidence

An elderly woman, stabilized on warfarin for 3 years, complained of spontaneous bruising 3 weeks after starting a course of ketoconazole (200 mg twice daily). Her British comparative ratio was found to have risen from 1.9 to 5.4. Her liver function was normal. She was restabilized on her previous warfarin dosage three weeks after the ketoconazole was withdrawn.[1]

The British Committee on the Safety of Medicines has a report of a man of 84 taking warfarin whose British comparative ratio rose to 4.8 when given ketoconazole, and fell to 1.4 when it was withdrawn.[1] Janssen, the makers of ketoconazole, also have a report of an elderly man on warfarin whose prothrombin time climbed from 26–39 s to over 60 s when given 400 mg ketoconazole daily.[3] In contrast, two volunteers showed no changes in their anticoagulant response to warfarin when concurrently treated with ketoconazole (200 mg daily) over a 3 week period.[2]

Mechanism

Uncertain. It has been suggested[4] that, as in rats,[5] ketoconazole may inhibit human liver enzymes concerned with the metabolism of warfarin so that its effects are increased. It is perhaps noteworthy that all of the cases involved elderly patients whose liver function may already have been poor.

Importance and management

Information about this interaction seems to be limited to the reports cited. Its general importance and incidence is therefore uncertain, but it is probably quite small. However it would now seem prudent to monitor the anticoagulant response of any patient given both drugs, particularly the elderly, to ensure that excessive hypoprothrombinaemia does not occur. Information about other anticoagulants is lacking.

References

1 Smith AG, Potentiation of oral anticoagulants by ketoconazole. Br Med J (1984) 288, 188–9.

2 Stevens DA, Stiller RL, Williams PL and Sugar AM. Experience with ketoconazole in three major manifestations of progressive coccidiomycosis. Am J Med (1983) 74 (1B), 58–63.

3 Simonite J. Janssen Pharmaceuticals. Personnal communication (1986).

4 Simpson JG, Cunningham C, Whiting P. Potentiation of oral anticoagulants by ketoconazole. Br Med J (1984) 288, 646.

5 Niemegeers CJE, Levron JC, Awouters F, Janssen PAJ. Inhibition and induction of microsomal enzymes in the rat. A comparative study of four antimycotics: miconazole, econazole, clotrimazole and ketoconazole. Arch Int Pharmacodynam (1961) 251, 26–38.

Anticoagulants + Ketorolac

Abstract/Summary

Ketorolac appears not to interact with warfarin, but it may possibly cause serious gastrointestinal bleeding and is considered by the CSM as contraindicated in patients taking anti-coagulants.

Clinical evidence, mechanism, importance and management

After taking 10 mg ketorolac four times daily for 6 days, no major changes occurred in the pharmacokinetics of (R) or (S) warfarin, nor in the pharmacokinetic profile of a single 25 mg dose of racemic warfarin in 12 normal subjects.[1] This suggests that ketorolac is normally unlikely to affect the anticoagulant response of patients taking warfarin chronically, but this needs confirmation. However the CSM in the UK has had five reports of post-operative haemorrhage and four reports of gastrointestinal haemorrhage (one fatal) in patients taking ketorolac. A US study also identified an increased risk of gastrointestinal bleeding with ketorolac. On the basis of this evidence the CSM now say that ketorolac is contraindicated with anticoagulants, including low doses of heparin.[2]

References

1 Toon S, Holt B L, Mullins F G P, Bullingham R, Aarons L, Rowland M. Investigations into the potential effects of multiple dose ketorolac on the pharmacokinetics and pharmacodynamics of racemic warfarin. Br J clin Pharmac (1990) 30, 743–50.
2 Committee on the Safety of Medicines, Current Problems in Pharmacovigilance (1993) 19, 5–6.

Anticoagulants + Laxatives, Liquid paraffin or Psyllium

Abstract/Summmary

The theoretical possibility that laxatives or liquid paraffin might affect the response to oral anticoagulants appears to be unconfirmed. Psyllium (ispaghula) has been shown not to affect either the absorption or the anticoagulant effects of warfarin.

Clinical evidence, mechanism, importance and management

A study in six normal subjects showed that psyllium, given as a 14 g dose of colloid (*Metamucil*) in a small amount of water with a single 40 mg dose of warfarin, and three further doses of psyllium at 2 h intervals thereafter, did not affect either the absorption or the anticoagulant effects of the warfarin.[1] In theory, laxatives and liquid paraffin (mineral oil) which shorten the transit time along the gut might be expected to decrease the absorption of both vitamin K and the oral anticoagulants. Liquid paraffin might also be expected to impair the absorption of the lipid-soluble vitamin, but despite warnings in various books, reviews and lists of drug interactions, there appears to be no direct evidence, as yet, that this is an interaction of any practical importance.

Reference

1 Robinson DS, Benjamin DM, McCormack JJ. Interaction of warfarin and nonsystemic gastrointestinal drugs. Clin Pharmacol Ther (1971) 12, 491.

Anticoagulants + Lornoxicam (Chlortenoxicam)

Abstract/Summary

Lornoxicam can raise serum warfarin levels to a moderate extent and increase its anticoagulant effects.

Clinical evidence, mechanism, importance and management

12 normal subjects were firstly given 4 mg lornoxicam twice daily for 5 days, then warfarin was added until a stable prothrombin time, averaging 23.58 s, was achieved. The period to achieve this varied from 9–24 days, depending on the subject. The lornoxicam was then withdrawn but the warfarin continued, whereupon the mean prothrombin time fell to 19.5 s and the serum warfarin levels fell by 25% (from 1.02 to 0.77 μg/ml). The INR fall was from 1.48 to 1.23.[1,2] The mechanism of this interaction is not known but it is possible that the lornoxicam inhibits the liver metabolism and loss of warfarin from the body.

Information seems to be limited to these studies, but it would now be prudent to monitor the outcome if lornoxicam is added to warfarin, reducing the warfarin dosage as necessary. Adopt the same precautions with any other anticoagulant.

References

1 Ravic M, Turner P. Study of a potential effect of chlortenoxicam on the anticoagulant activity of warfarin. Eur J Pharmacol (1990) 183, 1030.
2 Ravic M, Johnston A, Turner P, Ferber HP. A study of the interaction between lornoxicam and warfarin in healthy volunteers. Hum Exp Toxicol (1990) 9, 413–4.

Anticoagulants + Lovastatin

Abstract/Summary

The anticoagulant effects of warfarin can be increased by lovastatin in some patients. Bleeding may occur unless the anticoagulant dosage is reduced.

Clinical evidence

Two patients on warfarin approximately doubled their prothrombin times (from 18–24 s to 42–48 s) within 10–21 days of starting to take 20 mg lovastatin daily. One developed minor rectal bleeding and the other had haematuria and epistaxes. The problem rapidly resolved when the warfarin dosage was reduced from 5 to 2 mg daily.[3] A prothrombin time increase from 15 to 24 s occurred in another patient on warfarin after taking 20 mg lovastatin daily for 2 weeks.[4]

The makers of lovastatin have 10 other reports on record of bleeding and/or increased prothrombin times in patients on warfarin when given lovastatin, but no details are given.[1,2]

Mechanism

Uncertain. Inhibition of the metabolism of the warfarin which results in its accumulation has been suggested.[3]

Importance and management

Information seems to be limited to these reports but the interaction is established. The incidence is uncertain but prothrombin times should be monitored in all patients if warfarin or any other anticoagulant is started, stopped or its dosage changed. A 60% dosage reduction was effective in one case.[3]

References

1 Tobert JA, Shear CL, Chremos AN, Mantell GE. Clinical experience with lovastatin. Am J Cardiol (1990) 65, 23–6F.
2 Tobert JA. Efficacy and long term adverse effect pattern of lovastatin. Am J Cardiol (1988) 62, 28–34J.
3 Ahmad S. Lovastatin. Warfarin interaction. Arch Intern Med (1990) 150, 2407.
4 Hoffman HS. The interaction of lovastatin and warfarin. Conn Med (1992) 56, 107.

Anticoagulants + Macrolide antibiotics

Abstract/Summary

An isolated case of fatal bleeding occurred in a patient on warfarin when given clarithromcyin. Ponsinomycin (miocamycin) appears not to interact with nicoumalone (acenocoumarol), nor roxithromycin with warfarin. See also Anticoagulants + Erythromycin.

Clinical evidence, mechanism, importance and management

(a) Nicoumalone + Ponsinomycin

The pharmacokinetics of a single oral dose of nicoumalone were not significantly changed in six subjects after taking 800 mg ponsinomycin twice daily for 4 days.[2] This suggests that no interaction is likely in patients but confirmation of this is needed. There seems to be no information as yet about other anticoagulants.

(b) Warfarin + Clarithromycin

The CSM has an isolated case on record of a woman taking warfarin for mitral valve disease who suffered a fatal cerebrovascular bleed three days after starting to take clarithromycin. Her INR was above 10.[3] It would now be prudent to monitor the response if clarithromycin is given to any patient taking an anticoagulant.

(c) Warfarin + Roxithromycin

150 mg roxithromycin twice daily for two weeks had no significant effect on the thrombotest percentages of 21 normal subjects given enough warfarin to maintain the values at 10–20%. Serum roxithromycin levels also remained unchanged.[1] No special precautions are needed during concurrent use. There is as yet no information about other anticoagulants.

References

1 Paulsen O, Nilsson L-G, Saint-Salvi B, Manuel C, Lunell E. No effect of roxithromycin on pharmacokinetic or pharmacodynamic properties of warfarin and its enantiomers. Pharmacol Toxicol (1988) 63, 215–20.
2 Couett W, Istin B, Decourt JP, Ingrand I, Girault J, Fourtillan JB. Lack of effect of ponsinomycin on the pharmacokinetics of nicoumalone enantiomers. Br J clin Pharmac (1990) 30, 616–20.
3 Committee on the Safety of Medicines. Current Problems No 35, November (1992) p 4.

Anticoagulants + Meclofenamic acid or Mefenamic acid

Abstract/Summary

The anticoagulant effects of warfarin are increased to some extent by meclofenamic acid and a modest reduction in the warfarin dosage may be needed. Mefenamic acid appears not to interact significantly.

Clinical evidence

(a) Meclofenamic acid

After taking sodium meclofenamate (200–300 mg daily) for seven days, the average dose of warfarin required by seven patients fell from 6.5 to 4.25 mg daily, and by the end of four weeks it was 5.5 mg (a 16% reduction with a 0–25% range).[5]

(b) Mefenamic acid

After taking 2 g mefenamic acid daily for a week the mean prothrombin concentrations (20.03%) of 12 normal subjects on warfarin fell by 3.49%.[1] Microscopic haematuria were seen in three of them, but no overt haemorrhage. Their prothrombin concentrations were 15–25% of normal, well within the accepted anticoagulant range.

Mechanisms

Mefenamic acid can displace warfarin from its plasma protein binding sites,[2–4] and *in vitro* studies have shown that therapeutic concentrations (equivalent to 4 g daily) can increase the unbound and active warfarin concentrations by 140–340%.[2,3] But this interaction mechanism alone is only likely to have a transient effect.

Importance and management

The warfarin-meclofenamic acid interaction is established but of only moderate clinical importance. A modest reduction in warfarin dosage may be needed. Mefenamic acid appears not to interact significantly, but bear in mind that both of these NSAIDs may irritate the gut. There seems to be no information about other anticoagulants.

References

1 Holmes EL. Pharmacology of the fenamates: IV. Toleration by normal human subjects. Ann Phys Med (1966) 9 (Suppl) 36.

2 Sellers EM, Koch-Weser J. Displacement by warfarin from human albumin by diazoxide and ethacrynic, mefenamic and nalidixic acids. Clin Pharmacol Ther (1969) 11, 524.

3 Sellers EM, Koch-Weser J. Kinetics and clinical importance of displacement of warfarin from albumin by acidic drugs. Ann NY Acad Sci (1971) 179, 213.

4 McElnay JC, D'Arcy PFD. Displacement of albumin-bound warfarin by anti-inflammatory agent *in vitro*. J Pharm Pharmacol (1980) 32, 709.

5 Baragar FD, Smith TC. Drug interaction studies with sodium meclofenamate (Meclomen). Curr Ther Res (1978) 23, April Suppl. S51.

Anticoagulants + Meprobamate

In vitro

Abstract/Summary

The anticoagulant effects of warfarin are not significantly altered by the concurrent use of meprobamate.

Clinical evidence, mechanism, importance and management

Nine men stabilized on warfarin were given 1600 mg meprobamate daily for 2 weeks. Three of them showed a small increase in prothrombin times, five a small decrease and one remained unaffected.[1] 10 patients on warfarin showed only a small clinically unimportant reduction in prothrombin times when given 2400 mg meprobamate daily for four weeks.[2] Similar results were found in another study.[3] No particular precautions seem necessary. Other anticoagulants would be expected to behave similarly, but this requires confirmation.

References

1 Udall JA. Warfarin therapy not influenced by meprobamate. A controlled study in nine men. Curr Ther Res (1970) 12, 724.

2 Gould I, Michael A, Fisch S, Gomprecht RF. Prothrombin levels main-

tained with meprobamate and warfarin. A controlled study. J Amer Med Ass (1972) 220, 1460.

3 DeCarolis PP, Gelfland ML. Effect of tranquillizers on prothrombin times response to coumarin. J Clin Pharmacol (1975) 15, 557.

Anticoagulants + Meptazinol

Abstract/Summary

The anticoagulant effects of warfarin are not altered by meptazinol.

Clinical evidence, mechanism, importance and management

800 mg meptazinol daily for seven days had no significant effect on the prothrombin times of six elderly patients on warfarin (approximately 5 mg daily).[1] No special precautions seem to be necessary. Information about other anticoagulants is lacking.

Reference

1 Ryd-Kjellen E, Alm A. Effect of meptazinol on chronic anticoagulant therapy. Human Toxicol (1986) 5, 101–2.

Anticoagulants + Methaqualone

Abstract/Summary

Methaqualone can cause a small but clinically unimportant reduction in the anticoagulant effects of warfarin.

Clinical evidence, mechanism, importance and management

10 patients on warfarin given 300 mg methaqualone at bedtime for three weeks showed a small but clinically unimportant fall in their prothrombin times. Their average prothrombin times before, during and after concurrent treatment were 20.9, 20.4 and 19.6 s respectively.[1] Another report describes a patient whose warfarin plasma levels were unaffected by the concurrent use of methaqualone,[2] although there was some evidence that enzyme induction had occurred. It seems probable that the small change in prothrombin times reflects a limited degree of enzyme induction which results in the metabolism and clearance of warfarin being slightly increased. Methaqualone has certainly been shown to have some enzyme-inducing effects in man.[2,3] However no special precautions seem to be necessary during the concurrent use of warfarin and methaqualone. Other anticoagulants are expected to behave similarly.

References

1 Udall JA. Clinical implications of warfarin interactions with five sedatives. Amer J Cardiol (1975) 35, 67.
2 Whitfield JB, Moss DW, Neale G, Orme M, Breckenridge A. Changes in plasma gamma-glutamyl transpeptidase activity associated with alterations in drug metabolism in man. Br Med J (1973) i, 316.
3 Nayak RK, Smyth RD, Chamberlain AP. Methaqualone pharmacokinetics after single and multiple dose administration in man. J Pharmacokinet Biopharmaceut (1974) 2, 107.

Anticoagulants + Methylphenidate

Abstract/Summary

Despite some evidence to the contrary, the anticoagulant effects of ethylbiscoumacetate are not normally affected by the concurrent use of methylphenidate. No interaction is expected with any of the other anticoagulants.

Clinical evidence, importance and management

After taking 20 mg methylphenidate daily for 3–5 days, the half-life of ethyl biscoumacetate in four normal subjects was on average approximately doubled, due, it was suggested, to the enzyme inhibitory effects of the methylphenidate.[1] However a subsequent double-blind study on 12 subjects failed to confirm that any interaction occurs.[2]

This interaction has not been confirmed and there seems to be no reason for avoiding concurrent use. Other anticoagulants are not expected to interact.

References

1 Garrettson LK, Perel JM, Dayton PG. Methylphenidate interaction with both anticonvulsants and ethyl biscoumacetate. J Amer Med Ass (1969) 207, 2053.
2 Hague DE, Smith ME, Ryan JR, McMahon FG. The interaction of methylphenidate and prolintane with ethyl biscoumacetate metabolism. Fed Proc (1971) 30, 336 (Abs).

Anticoagulants + Metoclopramide

Abstract/Summary

Metoclopramide causes a small change in the pharmacokinetics of phenprocoumon, but no important changes in the anticoagulant effects seem to occur.

Clinical evidence, mechanism, importance and management

10 days treatment with 30 mg metoclopramide daily reduced the AUC of a single dose of phenprocoumon in 12 normal subjects by 16%, but no significant changes in the anticoagulant effects were seen.[1] There seems to be no other information about phenprocoumon or any other anticoagulant

Reference

1 Wesermeyer D, Mönig H, Gaska T, Masuch S, Seiler KU, Huss H, Bruhn HD. Der Einfluß von Cisaprid und Metoclopramid auf die Bioverfügbarkeit von Phenprocoumon. Hämostaseologie (1991) 11, 95–102.

Anticoagulants + Metronidazole

Abstract/Summary

The anticoagulant effects of warfarin are markedly increased by metronidazole. Bleeding can occur if the dosage of warfarin is not reduced appropriately.

Clinical evidence

750 mg metronidazole daily for a week increased the half-life of racemic warfarin (i.e. the normal ordinary mixture of R(+) and S(−) by about one-third (from 35 to 46 h) in eight normal subjects.[1] The anticoagulant effects of S(−) warfarin were virtually doubled and the half-life increased by 60%, but no change in the response to R(+) was seen (except in one subject).

Bleeding has been seen in two patients taking warfarin and metronidazole.[2,3] One of them had severe pain in one leg, ecchymoses and haemorrhage of the legs, and an increase in her prothrombin time from 17/19 s to 147 s within 17 days of starting the metronidazole.[2]

Mechanism

It is suggested[1] that the metronidazole inhibits the activity of the enzymes responsible for the metabolism (ring oxidation) of the S(−) warfarin, but not the R(+) warfarin. As a result the racemate with the more potent activity is retained within the body, and its actions are increased and prolonged.

Importance and management

An established and clinically important interaction, although the documentation is small. If concurrent use cannot be avoided, reduce the warfarin dosage appropriately. What is known suggests that a reduction of about one-third to a half may be necessary. Information about other anticoagulants is lacking, but it would be prudent to expect them to behave similarly. Some indirect evidence suggests that metronidazole may possibly not interact with phenprocoumon.[4]

References

1 O'Reilly RA. The stereoselective interaction of warfarin and metronidazole in man. N Engl J Med (1976) 295, 354.
2 Kazmier FJ. A significant interaction between metronidazole and warfarin. Mayo Clin Proc (1976) 51, 782.
3 Dean RP, Talbert RL. Bleeding associated with concurrent warfarin and metronidazole therapy. Drug Intell Clin Pharm (1980) 14, 864.
4 Staiger Von Ch, Wang NS, de Vries J, Weber E. Untersuchungen zur

Wirkung von Metronidazol auf den Phenazon-Metabolismus. Arzneim.-Forsch./Drug Res (1984) 34, 89–91.

Anticoagulants + Miconazole

Abstract/Summary

The anticoagulant effects of nicoumalone (acenocoumarol), ethylbiscoumacetate, fluindione, phenindione, phenprocoumon, tioclomarol and warfarin can be markedly increased if miconazole is given orally. Bleeding can occur if the anticoagulant dosage is not reduced appropriately (halving the dose may be sufficient). It is doubtful if an interaction occurs if miconazole pessaries or creams are used, but it can occur with buccal gel formulations.

Clinical evidence

Two patients with prosthetic heart valves, well stabilized for several months on warfarin, developed haemorrhagic complications within 10 days of starting to take miconazole (250 g four times a day). One of them developed blood blisters and bruised easily. Her prothrombin ratio was found to have risen from 2–3 to 16. The other patient was found to have a prothrombin ratio of 23.4. He developed two haematomas soon after both drugs were withdrawn. Both patients were subsequently restabilized in the absence of miconazole on their former doses of warfarin. None of the other drugs being taken is likely to have been responsible for the increased anticoagulant effects.[1]

The Centres de Pharmacovigilance Hospitaliere in Bordeaux have on record five cases where miconazole (500 g daily) was responsible for a marked increase in prothrombin times and/or bleeding (haematomas, haematuria, gastrointestinal bleeding) in patients taking nicoumalone (two cases), ethylbiscoumacetate (one case), tioclomarol (one case) and phenindione (one case).[2] Other cases have been described elsewhere involving nicoumalone, fluindione, warfarin and phenprocoumon.[3–10]

Mechanism

There is evidence that miconazole inhibits the metabolism of warfarin by the liver (inhibition of P4502C9) thereby reducing its loss from the body and increasing its effects.[12] Just why other anticoagulants are affected is still uncertain.

Importance and management.

An established interaction of clinical importance. The incidence is not known. In three cases[1,2] the bleeding began within 10–13 days of starting the miconazole whereas another patient bled within only three days.[4] Oral miconazole should not be given to patients taking any of the anticoagulants cited unless the prothrombin times can be closely monitored and suitable dosage reductions made. Two reports indicate that halving the dose may be sufficient[2,5] but in some instances the reduction needed may be much greater. One patient required an increase in her nicoumalone dosage from 2 mg twice weekly to 3–4 mg daily when miconazole (dose not stated) was withdrawn.[3] An interaction with miconazole as a cream or pressary is unlikely because the concentrations used are low and the systemic absorption is small, however this needs confirmation. Absorption from a buccal gel can apparently be substantial because five patients taking either warfarin, nicoumalone or fluindione bled or showed prolonged prothrombin times as a result of an interaction.[6–9,11] Information about other anticoagulants is lacking, but it would be prudent to assume that they will interact similarly.

References

1 Watson PG, Lochan RG, Redding VJ. Drug interaction with coumarin derivative anticoagulants. Br Med J (1982) 285, 1044–5.
2 Loupi E, Descotes J, Lery N, Evreux J Cl. Interactions medicamenteuses et miconazole. Therapie (1982) 37, 437–41.
3 Anon. New Possibilities in the treatment of systemic mycoses. Reports on the experimental and clinical evaluation of miconazole. Round table discussion and Chairman's summing up. Proc Roy Soc Med (1977), 70, Suppl l, 52.
4 Ponge T, Barrier J, Spreux A, Guillou B, Larousse Cl and Grolleau JY. Potentialisation des effets de l'acenocoumarol par le miconazole. Therapie (1982) 37, 217–24.
5 Goenen M, Reynaert M, Jaumin P, Chalant Ch.H and Tremoreaux J. A case of candida albicans endocarditis three years after an aortic valve replacement. J Cardiovasc Surg (1977) 18, 391–6.
6 Ducroix JP, Smail A, Sevenet F, Adrejak M, Baillet J. Hématome oesophagien secondaire à une potentialisation des effets de l'acénocoumarol par le gel buccal de miconazole. Rev Med Interne (1989) 10, 557–9.
7 Marotel C, Cerisay D, Vasseur P, Rouvier B, Chabanne JP. Potentialisation des effets de l'acenocoumarol par le gel buccal de miconazole. La Presse Med (1986) 15, 1684–5.
8 Colquhoun MC, Daly M, Stewart P, Beeley L. Interaction between warfarin and miconazole oral gel. Lancet (1987) i, 695.
9 Ponge T, Rapp MJ, Fruneau P, Ponge A, Wassen-Hove L, Larousse Cl and Cottin S. Interaction medicamenteuse impliquant le miconazole en gel et la fluindione. Therapie (1987) 42, 412–3.
10 Beeley L, Magee P, Hickey FM. Bulletin of West Midlands Centre for Adverse Drug Reaction Reporting (1989) 29, 33.
11 Shenfield GM, Page M. Potentiation of warfarin action by miconazole oral gel. Aust NZ J Med (1991) 21, 928.
12 O'Reilly RA, Goulart DA, Kunze KL, Neal J, Gibaldi M, Eddy AC, Trager WF. Mechanisms of the stereoselective interaction between miconazole and racemic warfarin in human subjects. Clin Pharmacol Ther (1992) 51, 656–7.

Anticoagulants + Monoamine oxidase inhibitors

Abstract/Summmary

The theoretical possibility that the concurrent use of MAOI might increase the effects of the oral anticoagulants has not been confirmed in man. Moclobemide does not interact with phenprocoumon nor brofaromine with warfarin.

Clinical evidence, mechanism, importance and management

A number of studies[1–4] have shown that the monoamine

oxidase inhibitors can increase the effects of some oral anti-coagulants in animals, but reports of this interaction in man are lacking and no special precautions seem to be necessary. A study in normal subjects found that 200 mg moclobemide three times daily for seven days had no effect on the anticoagulant effects of phenprocoumon.[5,6] Another study in 12 normal subjects also found no evidence that brofaromine alters the anticoagulant effects of warfarin.[7]

References

1 Fumarola D, De Rinaldis P. Ricerche sperimentali sugli inibitori della mono-aminossidasi. Influenza della nialmide sulla attivita degli anticaogu-lanti indiretti. Haematolgica (1964) 49, 1263.

2 Reber K, Studer A. Beeinflussung der Wirkung einiger indirekter Antiko-agulantien durch Monoaminoxydase-Hemmer. Thromb Diath Haemorrh (1965) 14, 83.

3 De Nicola P, Fumarola D, De Rinaldis P. Beeinflussung der gerinnungs-hemmenden Wirkung der indirekten Antikoagulantien durch die MAO-Inhibitoren. Thromb Diath Haemorrh (1964) 12 (Suppl), 125.

4 Hrdina P, Rusnakova M, Kovalcik V. Changes of hypoprothrombinaemic activity of indirect anticoagulants after MAO inhibitors and reserpine. Biochem Pharmacol (1953) 12 (Suppl), 241.

5 Zimmer R, Gieschke R, Fischbach R, Gasic S. Interaction studies with moclobemide. Acta Psychiatr Scand (1990) Suppl 360, 84–6.

6 Amrein R, Güntert TW, Dingemanse J, Lorscheid T, Stabl M, Schmid-Burgk W. Interactions of moclobemide with concomitantly administered medication: evidence from pharmacological and clinical studies. Psychoph-armacology (1992) 106, S24–31.

7 Harding SR, Conly J, Lawrin-Workewych M, D'Souza J. A study of the interaction between brofaromine and warfarin in healthy volunteers. Clin Invest Med (1992) 15, Suppl A18.

Anticoagulants + Moricizine (Ethmozine)

Abstract/Summary

An isolated report describes bleeding in a patient on warfarin when given moricizine, but most patients do not seem to be affected.

Clinical evidence

The prothrombin time of a woman on warfarin, digoxin, captopril and prednisone rose from 15–20 s to 41 s within four days of starting 300 mg moricizine three times daily. She bled (haematemesis, haematuria). She responded rapidly to with-drawal of the warfarin and moricizine, and the administration of phytonadione.[2]

This report contrasts with two others: 250 mg moricizine 8-hourly for 14 days caused little or no change in the pharma-cokinetics of single 25 mg doses of warfarin in 12 normal subjects. There was only a slight decrease in the warfarin elimination half-life (from 37.6 to 34.2 h) and no change in prothrombin times.[1,3] In 51 patients receiving warfarin chron-ically, no significant changes in warfarin dosage requirements were needed after moricizine was started.[1]

Mechanism

Not understood.

Importance and management

Information appears to be limited to these reports. Although most patients seem unlikely to be affected, it would be prudent to monitor the outcome of giving moricizine to patients receiv-ing warfarin. As yet information about other anticoagulants does not appear to be available.

References

1 Quoted as data on file, Du Pont Pharmaceuticals, by Siddoway LA, Schwartz SL, Barbey JT, Woosley RL. Clinical Pharmacokinetics of moricizine. Am J Cardiol (1990) 65, 21–25D.

2 Serpa MD, Cosslias J, McGreevy MJ. Moricizine-warfarin: a possible interaction. Ann Pharmacother (1992) 26, 127.

3 Benedek IH, King S-YP, Powell RJ, Agra AM, Schary WL, Pieniaszek HJ. Effect of moricizine on the pharmacokinetics and pharmacodynamics of warfarin in healthy subjects. J Clin Pharmacol (1992) 32, 558–63.

Anticoagulants + Nalidixic acid

Abstract/Summary

Three patients, two on warfarin and the other on nicoumalone, developed hypoprothrombinaemia when given nalidixic acid. One of them bled.

Clinical evidence

A patient, well stabilized on warfarin (prothrombin ratio 2.0), developed a purpuric rash and bruising within 6 days of starting to take 2 g nalidixic acid daily. Her prothrombin time was found to have risen to 45 s.[1] Another, previously well controlled on warfarin, developed a prothrombin time of 60 s 10 days after starting to take 3 g nalidixic acid daily.[5] Yet another patient on nicoumalone (acenocoumarol) developed hypoprothrombinaemia after receiving 1 g nalidixic acid daily.[2]

Mechanism

Uncertain. In vitro experiments[3,4] have shown that nalidixic acid can displace warfarin from its binding sites on human plasma albumin, but this mechanism on its own is almost certainly not the full explanation.

Importance and management

Information seems to be limited to the reports cited. It seems to be an established interaction but apparently uncommon. Con-current use need not be avoided but it would be prudent to monitor the effects closely, particularly during the first week.

References

1 Hoffbrand BI. Interaction of nalidixic acid and warfarin. Br Med J (1974) 2, 666.
2 Potasman I, Bassan H. Nicoumalone and nalidixic acid interaction. Ann Intern Med (1980) 92, 572.
3 Sellers EM, Koch-Weser J. Kinetics and clinical importance of displacement of warfarin from albumin by acidic drugs. Ann NY Acad Sci (1971) 179, 213.
4 Sellers EM, Koch-Weser J. Displacement of warfarin from human albumin by diazoxide and ethacrynic, mefenamic and nalidixic acids. Clin Pharmacol Ther (1970) 11, 524.
5 Leor J, Levartowsky D, Sharon C. Interaction between nalidixic acid and warfarin. Ann Intern Med (1987) 107, 601.

Anticoagulants + Natto

Natto, a Japanese food made from fermented soyabean, can reduce the effects of warfarin.

Clinical evidence

A retrospective study of 10 patients on warfarin who had had heart valve replacements found that eating natto caused the thrombotest values to rise from a range of 12–25% to 33–100%. The extent of the rise appeared to be related to the amount eaten. The values fell again when the natto was stopped. A healthy subject on warfarin with a thrombotest value of 40%, showed no changes 5 h after eating 100 g natto, but demonstrated a rise to 86% after 24 h and to 90% after 48 hr.[1] Similar rises were seen in animals.[1]

Mechanism

Not fully established. Natto appears not to contain significant amounts of vitamin K, but there is evidence that, after ingestion, the activity of *Bacillus natto* on the natto in the gut causes a marked increase in the synthesis and subsequent absorption of vitamin K.[1] This would oppose the actions of the warfarin (see 'Anticoagulants + vitamin K').

Importance and management

Information appears to be limited to this study[1] and a previous one by the same author,[2] however the interaction appears to be established. Patients on warfarin should be advised to avoid natto. Other oral anticoagulants would be expected to be similarly affected (assuming that the proposed mechanism of interaction is correct).

Reference

1 Kudo T. Warfarin antagonism of natto and increase in serum vitamin K by intake of natto. Artery (1990) 17, 189–201.
2 Kudo T, Uchibori Y, Astumi K, Numao K, Miura M, Shigara M, Hashimoto A. Warfarin antagonism by intake of natto under anticoagulant therapy. Igaku no Ayumi (1978) 104, 36.

Anticoagulants + Nizatidine

Abstract/Summary

Nizatidine does not interact with warfarin.

Clinical evidence, mechanism, importance and management

Seven normal subjects given enough warfarin (about 5–6 mg daily) to increase prothrombin times from 11.5 to 17.6 s showed no significant changes in their prothrombin times, kaolin-cephalin clotting times, the activity of factors II, VII, XI and X, or on their steady-state serum warfarin levels when given 300 mg nizatidine daily for 2 weeks.[1] This failure of nizatidine to affect warfarin levels is consistent with the fact that it does not inhibit the activity of liver microsomal enzymes, unlike cimetidine. No particular precautions appear to be necessary during concurrent use. There seems to be no direct information about other anticoagulants, but they would be expected to behave similarly.

Reference

1 Cournot A, Berlin I, Sallord JC, Singlas E. Lack of interaction between nizatidine and warfarin during concurrent use. J Clin Pharmacol (1988) 28, 1120–2.

Anticoagulants + Nomifensine

Abstract/Summary

A very brief single case report describes a marked increase in the anticoagulant effects of warfarin attributed to the concurrent use of nomifensine.[1] Nomifensine was withdrawn worldwide in 1986.

Reference

1 Beeley L. Bulletin of the West Midlands Adverse Drug Reaction Study Group. University of Birmingham, England. January (1980) no 10.

Anticoagulants + Non-steroidal antiinflammatory drugs (NSAIDs)

Abstract/Summary

The effects of the anticoagulants can be increased by flurbiprofen in a few patients and they may bleed. No interaction normally occurs with ibuprofen in normal doses, and this also would appear to be true for diclofenac, fenbufen, indoprofen, ketoprofen, naproxen, nimesulide, oxaprozin, pirprofen and tolmetin, but isolated cases have been described with diclofenac, ketoprofen, tiaprofenic acid and tolmetin. The man-

ufacturers of fenoprofen say that an interaction is possible, but there seems to be no direct clinical evidence that it actually occurs. All NSAIDs cause some gastrointestinal irritation and possible bleeding. Other NSAIDs are discussed individually elsewhere. See Index.

Clinical evidence

(a) Diclofenac

Studies in 32 patients and a further 20 patients on nicoumalone (acenocoumarol) showed that the concurrent use of 100 mg diclofenac daily normally does not alter its anticoagulant effects.[22] Other studies similarly confirm that diclofenac normally does not interact with either nicoumalone, phenprocoumon or warfarin.[23–5,32] However an unexplained case of pulmonary haemorrhage associated with a very prolonged prothrombin time has been described,[20] and another report states that the INR of a patient on warfarin rose from 2.8 to 5.8 after only three doses of diclofenac.[34]

(b) Fenbufen

A study in five subjects on warfarin showed that when given 800 mg fenbufen daily for a week, their prothrombin times within two days were increased by 1.9 s, and the serum warfarin levels fell by 14%.[9] These changes are unlikely to be clinically significant but this needs confirmation.

(c) Fenoprofen

In vitro evidence shows that the phenylalkanoic acid derivatives can displace anticoagulants from plasma protein binding sites, but there is no direct clinical evidence that this results in a clinically important interaction with fenoprofen.

(d) Flurbiprofen

19 patients on phenprocoumon given 150 mg flurbiprofen daily showed a small but significant fall in prothrombin times. Two patients bled (haematuria, epistaxis, haemorrhoidal bleeding) and three patients showed a fall in prothrombin times below the therapeutic range.[1]

Two patients on nicoumalone showed a rise in thrombotest times and bled (haematuria, melaena, haematomas) within 2–3 days of starting to take 150–300 mg flurbiprofen daily.[2] A necrotising purpuric rash accompanied by an increase in the thrombotest values was seen in two patients on warfarin treated with flurbiprofen.

(e) Ibuprofen

Studies with 19 patients[3,4] and 24 patients[5] on phenprocoumon, and 36 subjects,[6] 50 patients and 30 subjects,[7] and 40 patients[13] on warfarin showed that the effects of these anticoagulants were not altered while concurrently taking 600–2400 mg ibuprofen daily for 7–14 days. However one study on 20 patients taking warfarin showed that 1800 mg ibuprofen daily significantly prolonged bleeding times (4 cases above the normal range) and microscopic haematuria and haematoma were seen.[33] A raised INR occurred in one patient on warfarin who used topical ibuprofen.[34]

(f) Indoprofen

A study on 18 patients on warfarin given 600 mg indoprofen daily for seven days showed that no changes occurred in any of the blood coagulation measurements made.[8]

(g) Ketoprofen

A study in 15 normal subjects stabilized on warfarin found that 100 mg ketoprofen twice daily for 7 days had no effect on their prothrombin times or coagulation cascade parameters, and there was no evidence of bleeding.[35] This contrasts with an isolated case of bleeding in a patient on warfarin (prothrombin time increased from 18 to 41 s) a week after starting to take 75 mg ketoprofen daily.[18]

(h) Naproxen

A study on 10 subjects showed that 17 days treatment with naproxen (750 mg daily) did not alter the pharmacokinetics of a single dose of warfarin, or its anticoagulant effects.[17] Similar results were found in another study.[14] Yet another study in patients on phenprocoumon showed that 500 mg naproxen daily transiently increased the anticoagulant effects and caused an unimportant change in primary bleeding time.[15]

(i) Nimesulide

10 patients on 5 mg warfarin daily showed no significant changes in their prothrombin times, partial thromboplastin time or bleeding times when concurrently treated with 100 mg nimesulide twice daily for a week.[21]

(j) Oxaprozin

A study in 10 normal subjects stabilized on warfarin for an average of 13 days showed that while taking 1200 mg oxaprozin daily for 7 days their prothrombin times were not significantly altered.[31]

(k) Pirprofen

A study in 18 patients on long-term treatment with phenprocoumon showed that there was no change in the anticoagulant effects while taking 600 mg pirprofen daily. Bleeding time was prolonged by about 50%.[12]

(l) Tolmetin

15 subjects on warfarin showed no changes in prothrombin times while taking 1200 mg tolmetin daily over a 3-week

period.[26] 15 subjects on phenprocoumon similarly showed no changes in prothrombin times when given 800 mg tolmetin daily for 10 days.[27] Bleeding times are also reported not to be significantly altered in subjects or patients on phenprocoumon[27] or nicoumalone[28] when given 800 mg tolmetin daily. However there is a single unexplained case report of a diabetic patient on insulin, digoxin, theophylline, ferrous sulphate, frusemide and sodium polystyrene sulphonate who bled after taking three 400 mg doses of tolmetin. His prothrombin time had risen from 15–22 s to 70 s.[29] The manufacturers of tolmetin and the FDA also have 10 other cases on record.[29,30] However the manufacturers of tolmetin point out that over a 10-year period approximately 10 million patients have received tolmetin so that the risk of an interaction appears to be very small indeed.[30]

(m) Tiaprofenic acid

A study in six subjects on phenprocoumon showed that while taking 800 mg tiaprofenic acid daily for two days the anticoagulant effects and the pharmacokinetic profiles of both drugs remained unchanged.[10,11] No significant interaction occurred in nine patients on nicoumalone given 600 mg tiaprofenic acid daily for two weeks, but a 'rebound' rise in prothrombin percentages occured following its withdrawal.[16] However an elderly man on nicoumalone had severe epistaxis and bruising 4–6 weeks after starting to take 600 mg tiaprofenic acid daily. His prothrombin time had risen to 129 s.[19]

Mechanism

Drug displacement and enzyme inhibition do not seem to explain the anticoagulant/flubiprofen interactions.[1] Most of the phenylalkanoic acid derivatives can displace the anticoagulants from plasma protein binding sites to some extent, but this mechanism on its own is rarely, if ever, responsible for a clinically important drug interaction.

Importance and management

It is well established that no adverse interaction normally occurs between ibuprofen and either warfarin or phenprocoumon. Other anticoagulants would be expected to behave similarly. The absence of an interaction also normally appears to be true with indoprofen, fenbufen, ketoprofen, naproxen, nimesulide, oxaprozin and pirprofen although the documentation is more limited, but a few patients have bled when given diclofenac, flurbiprofen or tolmetin. As this is unpredictable and occasionally serious it is important to monitor the effects of concurrent use in all patients. There also seems to be a slight possibility of an interaction with tiaprofenic acid, but with fenoprofen it appears at present to be only theoretical. However some caution is appropriate with every non-steroidal anti-inflammatory drug because, to a greater or lesser extent, they irritate the stomach lining and have effects on platelet activity which can affect bleeding times[33] and which may result in gastrointestinal bleeding. See the index for interactions with other NSAIDs.

References

1 Marbert GA, Duckert F, Walter M, Six P, Airenne H. Interaction study between phenprocoumon and flurbiprofen. Curr Med Res Opin (1977) 5, 26.

2 Stricker BHCh and Delhez JL. Interaction between flurbiprofen and coumarins. Br Med J (1982) 285, 812–13.

3 Thilo D, Nyman F, Duckert F. A study of the effect of the anti-rheumatic drugs ibuprofen (Brufen) on patients being treated with the oral anticoagulant phenprocoumon (Marcoumar). J Int Med Res (1974) 2, 276.

4 Duckert F. The absence of effect of the antirheumatic drug ibuprofen on oral anticoagulation with phenprocoumon. Curr Med Res Opin (1975) 3, 556.

5 Bockhout-Musser MJ, Loeliger EA. Influence of ibuprofen on oral anticoagulation with phenprocoumon. J Int Med Res (1974) 2, 279.

6 Penner JA, Abbreht PH. Lack of interaction between ibuprofen and warfarin. Curr Ther Res (1975) 18, 862.

7 Goncalves L. Influence of ibuprofen on haemostasis in patients on anticoagulant therapy. J Int Med Res (1973) 1, 180.

8 Jacono A, Passo P, Gualtieri S, Raucci D, Bianchi A, Vigorito C, Bergamini N, Iadevaia V. Clinical study of the possible interactions between indoprofen and oral anticoagulants. Eur J Rheumatol Inflamm (1981) 4, 32–5.

9 Savitsky JP, Terzakis T, Bina P, Chiccarelli F, Hayes J. Fenbufen-warfarin interaction in healthy volunteers. Clin Pharmacol Ther (1980) 27, 284.

10 von Durr J, Pfeiffer MH, Wetzelsberger K, Lucker PW. Untersuchung zur Frage einter Interaktion von Tiaprofensaure und Phenprocoumon. Arzneim.-Forsch/Drug Res (1981) 31, 2163–7.

11 Luckner PW, Penth B, Wetzelberger K. Pharmacokinetic interaction between tiaprofenic acid and several other compounds for chronic use. Rheumatology (1982) 7, 99–106.

12 Marbet GA, Duckert F, Schonenberger PM. Eine Untersuchung uber Wechselwirkung zwischen Pirprofen und Phenprocoumon. Fortsch Med (1985) 163, 207–9.

13 Marini U, Cecchi A, Venturino M. Mancanza di interazione tra ibuprofen lisinato e anticoagulanti orali. Clin Ter (1985) 112, 25–9.

14 Jain A, McMahon FG, Slattery JT, Levy G. Effect of naproxen on the steady-state serum concentration and anticoagulant activity of warfarin. Clin Pharmacol Ther (1979) 25, 61.

15 Angelkort B. Zum einfluss von Antikoagulantien-behandlung mit Phenprocoumon. Forschrift Med (1978) 96, 1249.

16 Meurice J. Interaction of tiaprofenic acid and acenocoumarol. Rheumatol (1982) 7, 111–7.

17 Slattery JT, Levy G, Jain A, McMahon FG. Effect of naproxen on the kinetics of elimination and anticoagulant activity of a single dose of warfarin. Clin Pharmacol Ther (1979) 25, 51.

18 Flessner MF, Knight H. Prolongation of prothrombin time and severe gastrointestinal bleeding associated with combined use of warfarin and ketoprofen. J Amer Med Ass (1988) 259, 353.

19 Whittaker SJ, Jackson CW, Whorwell PJ. A severe, potentially fatal, interaction between tiaprofenic acid and nicoumalone. Br J Clin Prac (1986) 40, 440.

20 Gomez LMC, Beato EP, Venegas JP, Moro EP. Hemorragia pulmonar debido a la interaccion de acenocoumarina y diclofenac sodico. Rev clin esp (1987) 181, 227–8.

21 Auteri A, Bruni F, Blardi P, Di Renzo M, Pasqui AL, Saletti M, Verzuri MS, Scaricabarozzi I, Vargiu G, Di Perri T. Clinical study on pharmacological interaction between nimesulide and warfarin. Int J Clin Pharmacol Res, (1991), 11, P 267–70.

22 Michot F, Ajdacic K, Glaus L. A double-blind clinical trial to determine if an interaction exists between diclofenac sodium and the oral anticoagulant acenocoumarol (nicoumalone). J Int Med Res (1975) 3, 153.

23 Wagenhauser F. Research findings with new, non-steroidal antirheumatic agents. Scand J Rheum (1975) 4 (Suppl 8) S05–01.

24 Krzywanek HJ, Breddin K. Beeinflusst Diclofenac die orale Antikoagulantientherapie und die Plattchenaggregation? Med Welt (1977) 28, 1843.

25 Breddin K (1975) Cited as personal communication in 22 above.

26 Whitsett TL, Barry JP, Czerwinski AW, Hall WH, Hampton JW. Tolmetin and warfarin. A clinical investigation to determine if interaction exists. In 'Tolmetin, A New Non-steroidal Anti-Inflammatory Agent.' Ward JR (ed). Proceedings of a Symposium, Washington DC, April 1975, Excerpta Medica, Amsterdam, New York, p. 160.

27 Rust O, Biland L, Thilo D, Nyman D, Duckert F. Prufung des Antirheumatikums Tometin auf Interaktionen mit oralen Antikoagulantien. Schweiz med Wsch (1975) 105, 752.

28 Malbach E. Uber die Beeinflussung der Blutungzeit durch Tolectin. Schweiz Rundschau Med (Praxis) (1978) 67, 161.

29 Koren JF, Cochran DL and Janes RL. Tolmetin-warfarin interaction. Am J Med (1987) 82, 1278–9.

30 Santopolo AC. Tolmetin-warfarin interaction. Am J Med (1987) 82, 1279–80.

31 Davis LJ, Kayser SR, Hubscher J, Williams RL. Effects of oxaprozin on the steady-state anticoagulant activity of warfarin. Clin Pharm (1984) 3, 295–7.

32 Fitzgerald DE, Russell JG. Voltarol and warfarin, an interaction? In Current Themes in Rheumatology, Chiswell RJ, Birdwood GFB (Eds). Cambridge Medical Publications p 26.

33 Schulman S, Henriksson K. Interaction of ibuprofen and warfarin on primary haemostasis. Br J Rheumatol (1989) 28, 46–9.

34 Beeley L, Cunningham H, Carmichael AE, Brennan A. Newsletter of the West Midlands Centre for Adverse Drug Reaction Reporting, (1991), 33, 18.

35 Mieszczak C, Winther K. Lack of interaction of ketoprofen with warfarin. Eur J Clin Pharmacol (1993) 44, 205–6.

Anticoagulants + Omeprazole

Abstract/Summary

Omeprazole causes a small but apparently clinically trivial change in the anticoagulant effects of warfarin, but it may possibly decrease the prothrombin time in the presence of heparin.

Clinical evidence, mechanism, importance and management

Twenty-one normal subjects anticoagulated with warfarin had a statistically significant though small decrease in their mean thrombotest percentage (from 21.1 to 18.7%) after taking 20 mg omeprazole daily for 2 weeks. (S)-warfarin serum levels remained unchanged but a slight (12%) rise in (R)-warfarin levels was seen.[1] 28 patients anticoagulated with warfarin given 20 mg omeprazole daily for three weeks had no significant changes in their coagulation times or thrombotest values. (S)-warfarin levels were unchanged while a 9.5% increase in (R)-warfarin levels occurred.[2] The reasons are not understood.

These results indicate that no special precautions are necessary if this dosage of omeprazole is given to patients on warfarin. There seems to be no information about other oral anticoagulants, however a very brief report describes a decrease in the prothrombin time in a patient treated with heparin and omeprazole. The general importance of this is uncertain.[3] More study is needed.

Reference

1 Sutfin T, Balmer K, Bostrom H, Eriksson S, Hoglund P, Paulsen O. Stereoselective interaction of omeprazole with warfarin in healthy men. Ther Drug Monit (1989) 11, 176–84.

2 Unge P, Svedberg L-E, Nordgren A, Blom H, Andersson T, Lagerström P-O, Idström J-P. A study of the interaction of omeprazole and warfarin in anticoagulated patients. Br J clin Pharmac (1992) 34, 509–12.

3 Beeley L, Cunningham H, Brennan A. Bulletin W Midlands Centre for Adverse Drug Reaction Reporting. (1993) 36, 9.

Anticoagulants + Oxaceprol

Abstract/Summary

An isolated report describes a marked fall in the response to fluindione in a patient when given oxaceprol.

Clinical evidence, mechanism, importance and management

A woman of 77 with hypertension and atrial fibrillation, under treatment with propafenone, frusemide, enalapril and fluindione (15 mg daily), was additionally started on 300 mg oxaceprol daily. Within 2 days her Quick Time had risen from 26 to 57% and by the end of the week to 65%. When the oxaceprol was withdrawn, her Quick Time returned to its previous values (23–30%).[1] The mechanism is not understood. The general importance of this interaction is uncertain, but the concurrent use of oxaceprol and any anticoagulant should be very well monitored; be alert for the need to modify the anticoagulant dosage.

Reference

1 Bannwarth B, Tréchot P, Mathieur J, Froment J, Netter P. Interaction oxacéprol-fluindione. Therapie (1990) 45, 162–3.

Anticoagulants + Oxpentifylline

Abstract/Summary

The anticoagulant effects of phenprocoumon are not significantly altered by the concurrent use of oxpentifylline (pentoxifylline).

Clinical evidence, mechanism, importance and management

The anticoagulant effects of phenprocoumon were slightly but not significantly altered by the concurrent use of 1600 mg oxpentifylline daily for 27 days in 10 patients.[1] No special precautions would seem to be necessary. Information about other anticoagulants seems to be lacking.

Reference

1 Ingerlsev J, Mouritzen C, Stenbjerg S. Pentoxifylline does not interfere with stable coumarin anticoagulant therapy: a clinical study. Pharmatherapeutica (1986) 4, 595–600.

Anticoagulants + Oxyphenbutazone

Abstract/Summary

The anticoagulant effects of warfarin are markedly increased by oxyphenbutazone which can lead to serious bleeding.

Clinical evidence, mechanism, importance and management

A man on warfarin developed gross haematuria within nine days of starting to take 400 mg oxyphenbutazone daily. His prothrombin time had increased to 68 s. A subsequent study on him confirmed that the hypoprothrombinaemia was due to the oxyphenbutazone.[1] Two similar cases have been described elsewhere.[2,3] A clinical study has also shown that oxyphenbutazone slows the clearance of dicoumarol.[4]

Oxyphenbutazone is the major metabolite of phenylbutazone within the body and it may be presumed that the explanation for the anticoagulant/phenylbutazone interaction equally applies to oxyphenbutazone (see 'Anticoagulants + Phenylbutazone'). Direct evidence of this interaction seems to be limited to the reports cited, but it would appear to be established and of clinical importance. It would be prudent to apply all the precautions suggested for phenylbutazone.

References

1 Hobbs CB, Miller AL and Thornley JH. Potentiation of anticoagulant therapy by oxyphenbutazone. A probable case. Postgrad Med J (1965) 41, 563.
2 Fox SL. Potentiation of anticoagulants caused by pyrazole compounds. J Amer Med Ass (1964) 188, 320.
3 Taylor PJ. Haemorrhage while on anticoagulant therapy precipitated by drug interaction. Arizona Med (1967) 24, 697.
4 Weiner M, Siddiqui AA, Bostanci N, Dayton PG. Drug interactions: the effect of combined administration on the half-life of coumarin and pyrazolone drugs in man. Fed Proc (1965) 24, 153.

Anticoagulants + Paracetamol (Acetaminophen)

Abstract/Summary

The anticoagulant effects of anisindione, dicoumarol, phenprocoumon and warfarin are normally not affected, or only increased to a small extent, by small doses of paracetamol (acetaminophen), but if larger doses are taken regularly a reduction in the anticoagulant dosage may be needed. There is an isolated case of bleeding with warfarin and paracetamol.

Clinical evidence

(a) Prothrombin times unchanged

10 patients on warfarin showed no changes in their prothrombin times when given 3.0 g paracetamol daily for two weeks.[3] A further study on 10 patients given warfarin or phenprocoumon found that two 650 mg doses of paracetamol similarly had no effect on prothrombin times measured over the following 48 h.[2]

(b) Prothrombin times increased

The prothrombin times of 50 patients taking anisindione, dicoumarol, phenprocoumon or warfarin were increased by an average of 3.7 s after taking 2.6 g paracetamol daily for two weeks.[1]

2 g paracetamol daily for three weeks increased the thrombotest times of 10 patients on un-named coumarin anticoagulants by approximately 20%. The anticoagulant dosage was reduced in five out of the 10 patients and in one of the 10 control patients.[4]

15 normal subjects, given enough warfarin to increase their prothrombin times by 1.35–1.50, were additionally given 4 g paracetamol daily for two weeks. The prothrombin times of seven rose by more than 20% (to 1.75) compared with one subject taking placebo, and by more than 33% (to 2.0) in five others. The increases were seen from about day seven and were maximal after 12.5 days.[6]

An isolated report describes bleeding (haematuria, gum bleeding) in a woman on warfarin after taking about 1.6 g paracetamol daily in a compound paracetamol-codeine preparation for 10 days. Her prothrombin time rose to 96 s.[5,7] See also 'Anticoagulants + Dextropropoxyphene' because paracetamol is a component of *Distalgesic* and *Darvocet*.

Mechanism

Not understood.

Importance and management

An established interaction although there are unexplained inconsistencies in the evidence. The weight of clinical evidence and common experience suggests that occasional small doses of paracetamol (possibly up to about 2 g daily) for a few days are normally unlikely to cause important increases in prothrombin times, but if larger amounts are taken (2–4 g daily) for longer than a few days it would be prudent to monitor prothrombin times so that any anticoagulant dosage reductions can be made. Anticoagulants other than those specifically cited would be expected to interact similarly. In this context paracetamol is safer than aspirin because it does not affect platelets or cause gastric bleeding.

References

1 Antlitz AM, Mead JA ,Tolentino MA. Potentiation of oral anticoagulant therapy by acetaminophen. Curr Ther Res (1968) 10, 501.
2 Antlitz AM, Awalt LF. A double blind study of acetaminophen used in conjunction with oral anticoagulant therapy. Curr Ther Res (1969) 11, 360.
3 Udall JA. Drug interference with warfarin therapy. Clin Med (1978) 77, 20.

4 Boejinga JJ, Boerstra EE, Ris P, Breimer DD, Jeletich-Bastiaanse A. Interaction between paracetamol and coumarin anticoagulants. Lancet (1982) i, 506.

5 Kwan D, Bartle WR. Drug interactions with warfarin. Med J Aust (1993) 158, 574.

6 Rubin RN, Mentzer RL, Budzynski AZ. Potentiation of anticoagulant effect of warfarin by acetaminophen (Tylenol®). Clin Res (1984) 32, 698A.

7 Bartle WR, Blakey JA. Potentiation of warfarin anticoagulation by acetaminophen. J Amer Med Ass (1991) 265, 1260.

Anticoagulants + Penicillins

Abstract/Summary

The effects of the oral anticoagulants are not normally altered by the penicillins but isolated cases of increased prothrombin times and bleeding have been seen in patients given penicillin G, talampicillin and ampicillin/flucloxacillin. Carbenicillin in the absence of an anticoagulant can prolong prothrombin times and might therefore also do so in the presence of an anticoagulant. In contrast, a handful of cases of reduced warfarin effects have been reported with amoxycillin, nafcillin and dicloxacillin.

Clinical evidence

(a) Decreased anticoagulant effects

The prothrombin time of a patient stabilized on warfarin fell from a range of 20–25 s down to 14–17 s (despite a doubling of the warfarin dosage) when given 12 g nafcillin daily given intravenously.[1] A few months after the nafcillin was discontinued, the half-life of the warfarin was found to have climbed from 11 to 44 hours. Six other cases of this 'warfarin resistance' with high dose nafcillin have been reported.[15-18] Seven days treatment with 500 mg dicloxacillin sodium four times daily and at bedtime reduced the mean prothrombin times of seven patients on warfarin by 1.9 s. One patient showed a 5.6 s reduction.[14] A very brief report states that amoxycillin caused an unspecified decrease in prothrombin times in five patients, but by implication it was small and of limited clinical importance.[19]

(b) Increased anticoagulant effects

Hypoprothrombinaemia has been described in one patient on warfarin given 24 million units of penicillin G daily intravenously.[2] Penicillin G is also known to be able to increase bleeding times and cause bleeding in the absence of an anticoagulant.[5] The prothrombin time of a patient on warfarin increased when treated with ampicillin and flucloxacillin, and both bleeding and an increase in the prothrombin ratio have been described in a patient on warfarin given talampicillin.[3] Increases in bleeding times, bleeding,[4-7,9,12] and extended prothrombin times[9,12] have been described with carbenicillin in the absence of an anticoagulant. Ampicillin, methicillin and ticarcillin are also reported to prolong bleeding times,[8,10,11,13] and in theory they might also increase the effects of both

heparin and the oral anticoagulants, but reports of such interactions seem to be lacking.

Mechanisms

The nafcillin-warfarin interaction is possibly due to increases in the metabolism of warfarin by the liver. Changes in bleeding times caused by the other penicillins appear to result from changes in Antithrombin III activity, blood platelet changes and alterations in the fibrinogen-fibrin conversion.

Importance and management

Documented reports of interactions between anticoagulants and penicillins are relatively rare, bearing in mind how frequently these drugs are used. Normally no changes occur, however individual physicians say that they have seen changes and this is reflected in a statement in the British National Formulary which says that '...common experience in anticoagulant clinics is that prothrombin times can be prolonged by a few seconds following a course of broad-spectrum antibiotic e.g. ampicillin.' Concurrent use should therefore be monitored so that the very occasional and unpredictable cases (increases or decreases in the anticoagulant effects) can be identified and handled accordingly.

References

1 Qureshi GD, Reinders TP, Somori GJ, Evans HJ. Warfarin resistance with nafcillin therapy. Ann Int Med (1984) 100, 527–9.

2 Brown MA, Korschinski ED, Miller DR. Interaction of penicillin-G and warfarin? Can J Hosp Pharm (1979) 32, 18–19.

3 Beeley L and Daly M. Bull W Mid Centre for Adverse Drug Reaction Reporting (1986) 23, 13.

4 Brown CH, Natelson EA, Bradshaw MW, Williams TW, Alfrey CP. The hemostatic defect produced by carbenicillin, N Engl J Med (1974) 291, 265–70.

5 Roberts PL. High dose penicillin and bleeding. Ann Intern Med (1974) 81, 267–8.

6 McClure PD, Casserly JG, Monsier C, Crozier D. Carbenicillin-induced bleeding disorder. Lancet (1970) ii, 1307–8.

7 Waisbren BA, Evani SV, Ziebert AP. Carbenicillin and bleeding. J Amer Med Ass (1971) 217, 1243.

8 Andrassy K, Ritz E, Weisschedel E. Bleeding after carbenicillin administration. N Engl J Med (1975) 292, 109–10.

9 Yudis M, Mahood WH, Maxwell R. Bleeding problems with carbenicillin. Lancet (1972) ii, 599.

10 Brown CH, Bradshaw MJ, Natelson EA, Alfrey CP, Williams TW. Defective platelet function following the administration of penicillin compounds. Blood (1976) 47, 949.

11 Brown CH, Natelson EA, Bradshaw MW, Alfrey CP, Williams TW. Study of the effects of ticarcillin on blood coagulation and platelet function. Antimicrob Ag Chemother (1975) 7, 652.

12 Lurie A, Ogilvie M, Townsend R, Gold C, Meyers AM, Goldberg B. Carbenicillin-induced coagulopathy. Lancet (1970) i, 1114–15.

13 Beeley L and Stewart P. Bull W Mid Centre for Adverse Drug Reaction Reporting (1987) 25, 16.

14 Krstenansky PM, Jones WN, Garewal HS. Effect of dicloxacillin sodium on the hypoprothrombinemic response to warfarin sodium. Clin Pharm (1987) 6, 804–6.

15 Fraser GL, Miller M, Kane K. Warfarin resistance associated with nafcillin therapy. Am J Med (1989) 87, 237–8.

16 Du Pont Pharmaceuticals (1988). Quoted in ref 15 as personal communication.

17 Davis RL, Berman W, Wernly JA, Kelly HW. Warfarin-nafcillin interaction. J Pediat (1991) 118, 300–3.
18 Shovick VA, Rihn TL. Decreased hypoprothrombinemic response to warfarin secondary to the warfarin-nafcillin interaction. DICP Ann Pharmacother (1991) 25, 598–9.
19 Radley AS, Hall J. Interactions. Pharm J (1992) 249, 81.

Anticoagulants + Phenazone (Antipyrine)

Abstract/Summary

The anticoagulant effects of warfarin are reduced by the concurrent use of phenazone.

Clinical evidence

The plasma warfarin concentrations of five patients were halved (from 2.93 to 1.41 μg/ml) and the anticoagulant effects accordingly reduced after taking 600 mg phenazone daily for 50 days.[1] The prothrombin percentage of one patient rose from five to 50%. In an associated study it was found that 600 mg phenazone daily for 30 days caused falls in the warfarin half-lives in two patients from 47 to 27 h and from 69 to 39 h respectively.[1–3]

Mechanism

Phenazone is an enzyme inducing agent which increases the metabolism and clearance of warfarin from the body, thereby reducing its effects.[1–3]

Importance and management

An established interaction. The effects of concurrent use should be monitored and the dosage of warfarin increased appropriately. Other anticoagulants may be expected to behave similarly.

References

1 Breckenridge A, Orme M. Clinical implication of enzyme induction. Ann NY Acad Sci (1971) 179, 421.
2 Breckenridge A, Orme ML'E, Thorgeirsson S, Davies DS, Brooks RV. Drug interactions with warfarin: studies with dichloralphenazone, chloral hydrate and phenazone (Antipyrine). Clin Sci (1971) 40, 351.
3 Breckenridge A, Orme ML'E, Thorgeirsson S, Dollery CT. Induction of drug metabolising enzymes in man and rat by dichloralphenazone. 4th Int Congr Pharmacol (Basel) July 14–18 (1969) p 182.

Anticoagulants + Phenothiazines

Abstract/Summary

Chlorpromazine does not interact significantly with nicoumalone.

Clinical evidence, mechanism, importance and management

Although chlorpromazine in doses of 40–100 mg is said to have '...played a slightly sensitizing role...' in two out of eight patients on nicoumalone[1] and is reported to increase its anticoagulant effects in animals,[2] there is nothing to suggest that special precautions should be taken during concurrent use in man. No important interactions appear to occur between the oral anticoagulants and other phenothiazines.

References

1 Johnson R, David A, Chartier Y. Clinical experience with G-23350 (Sintrom). Can Med Ass J (1957) 77, 760.
2 Weiner M. Effect of centrally active drugs on the action of coumarin anticoagulants. Nature (1966) 212, 1599.

Anticoagulants + Phenylbutazone

Abstract/Summary

The anticoagulant effects of warfarin are markedly increased by phenylbutazone. Concurrent use should be avoided because serious bleeding can occur. Bleeding has been seen in patients on phenindione or phenprocoumon when given phenylbutazone, but successful concurrent use has been achieved with both phenprocoumon and nicoumalone (acenocoumarol) apparently achieved by careful reduction of the anticoagulant dosage.

Clinical evidence

(a) Phenylbutazone added to stabilized warfarin treatment

A man, stabilized on warfarin following mitral valve replacement, was later given phenylbutazone for back pain by his general practitioner. On admission to hospital a week later he had epistaxis, and his face, legs and arms had begun to swell. He showed extensive bruising of the jaw, elbow and calves, some evidence of gastrointestinal bleeding, and a prothrombin time of 98 s.[2]

(b) Warfarin added to treatment with phenylbutazone

A man, hospitalized following a myocardial infarction, was given a single 600 mg dose of phenylbutazone. Next day, when coagulation studies were done, his prothrombin time was 12 s and he was given 40 mg warfarin to initiate anticoagulant therapy. Within 48 h he developed massive gastrointestinal bleeding and was found to have a prothrombin time exceeding 100 s.[3]

There are numerous other reports of this interaction in man involving warfarin,[4–11] phenprocoumon[1.15.20] and nicoumalone.[16] A single unconfirmed report describes this interaction in two patients taking phenindione.[14]

Mechanism

Phenylbutazone inhibits the metabolism of S(-) warfarin (the more potent of the two isomers) so that it is cleared from the body more slowly and its effects are increased and prolonged.[12] Phenylbutazone also very effectively displaces the anticoagulants from their plasma protein binding sites, thereby increasing the concentrations of free and active anticoagulant molecules in plasma water,[4,9,13,17,18] but the importance of this latter mechanism is probably small.

Importance and management

The warfarin/phenylbutazone interaction is very well established and clinically important. Serious bleeding can occur and concurrent use should be avoided. Much less is known about phenindione with phenylbutazone but it is probably equally unsafe.[14] Direct evidence of a serious phenprocoumon/phenylbutazone interaction seems to be limited to two reports,[1,20] and there is good evidence[19] that successful and apparently uneventful concurrent use is possible, presumably because the response and the anticoagulant dosages carefully controlled. A study in 357 patients given 600 mg phenylbutazone to which was added nicoumalone (acenocoumarol) from day five onwards found that 25% less nicoumalone was needed than in control group on nicoumalone alone. Evidently concurrent their use is possible. Information about other anticoagulants is lacking, but until there is clear evidence to the contrary, expect them to behave like warfarin. Remember too that phenylbutazone affects platelet aggregation and can cause gastrointestinal bleeding, whether an anticoagulant is present or not. Alternative non-interacting NSAID's include ibuprofen and naproxen. See Index.

References

1 Sigg A, Pestalozzi H, Clauss A, Koller F. Verstarkung der Antikoagulantienwirkung durch Butazolidin. Schweiz med Wsch (1956) 86, 1194.

2 Bull J, Mackinnon J. Phenylbutazone and anticoagulant control. Practitioner (1975) 215, 767.

3 Robinson DS. The application of basic principles of drug interaction to clinical practice. J Urology (1975) 113, 100.

4 Aggeler PM, O'Reilly RA, Leong I, Kowitz PE. Potentiation of anticoagulant effect of warfarin by phenylbutazone. N Engl J Med (1967) 476, 196.

5 Udall JA. Drug interference with warfarin therapy. Clin Med (1970) 77, 20.

6 McLaughlin GE, McCarty DJ, Segal BL. Hemarthrosis complicating anticoagulant therapy: report of three cases. J Amer Med Ass (1966) 196, 1020.

7 Hoffbrand BI, Kininmonth DA. Potentiation of anticoagulants. Br Med J (1967) 2, 838.

8 Eisen MJ. Combined effect of sodium warfarin and phenylbutazone. J Amer Med Ass (1964) 189, 64.

9 O'Reilly RA. The binding of sodium warfarin to plasma albumin and its displacement by phenylbutazone. Ann NY Acad Sci (1973) 226, 293.

10 Schary WL, Lewis RJ, Rowland M. Warfarin-phenylbutazone interaction in man. A long-term multiple-dose study. Res Comm Chem Pathol Pharmacol (1975) 10, 663.

11 Chierichetti S, Bianchi G, Cerri B. Comparison of feprazone and phenylbutazone intraction with warfarin in man. Curr Ther Res (1975) 18, 568.

12 Lewis RJ, Trager WF, Chan KK, Breckenridge A, Orme M, Rowland M, Schary W. Warfarin. Stereochemical aspects of its metabolism and the interaction with phenylbutazone. J Clin Invest (1974) 53, 1607.

13 Tillement J-P, Zini R, Mattei C, Singlas E. Effect of phenylbutazone on the binding of vitamin K antagonists to albumin. Europ J clin Pharmacol (1973) 6, 15.

14 Kindermann A. Vasculares Allergid nach Butalidon und Gefahren Kombinierter Anwendung mit Athrombon (Phenylindandion) Dermatol Wsch (1961) 143, 172.

15 Seiler K, Duckert F. Properties of 3-(1-phenyl-propyl)-4-oxycoumarin (Marcoumar) in the plasma when tested in normal cases under the influence of drugs. Thromb Diath Haemorrh (1968) 19, 389.

16 Guggisberg W, Montigel C. Erfahrungen mit kombinierter Butazolidin-Sintrom-Prophylaxe und Butazolidin-prophylaxe thromboembolischer Erkrangungen. Ther Umsch (1958) 15, 227.

17 Solomon HM, Schrogie JJ. The effect of various drugs on the binding of warfarin-^{14}C to human albumin. Biochem Pharmacol (1967) 16, 1219.

18 O'Reilly RA. Interaction of several coumarin compounds with human and canine plasma albumin. Mol Pharmacol (1970) 7, 209.

19 Kaufmann P. Vergleich zwischen einer Thromboembolie-prophylaxe mit Antikoagulantien und mit Butazolidin. Schweiz Med Wsch (1957) (Suppl 24) 87, 755.

20 O'Reilly RA. Phenylbutazone and sulfinpyrazone interaction with oral anticoagulant phenproumon. Arch Int Med (1982) 142, 1634.

Anticoagulants + Phenyramidol

Abstract/Summary

The anticoagulant effects of warfarin, dicoumarol and phenindione are increased by phenyramidol. Bleeding can occur if the anticoagulant dosage is not reduced appropriately.

Clinical evidence

Two patients on warfarin showed a marked increase in their prothrombin times when given 1.2–1.6 mg phenyramidol daily. One of them bled. Further study on eight other patients taking warfarin, dicoumarol, or phenindione showed that a marked increase in their prothrombin times occurred within 3–7 days of starting to take 0.8–1.6 g phenyramidol daily. No marked change occurred in a patient on phenprocoumon, but he only took the phenyramidol for 3 days.[1]

Mechanism

Studies in man, mice and rabbits suggest that phenyramidol inhibits the metabolism of the anticoagulants so that they are cleared from the body more slowly and their effects are thereby increased and prolonged.[2]

Importance and management

An established interaction although the documentation is very limited. Monitor prothrombin times and reduce the anticoagulant dosage as necessary to avoid bleeding. Anticoagulants other than those cited may be expected to behave similarly. The failure to demonstrate an interaction with phenprocoumon may have been because the phenyramidol was given for such a short time.

References

1 Carter SA. Potentiation of the effect of orally administered anticoagulants by phenyramidol hydrochloride. N Engl J Med (1965) 273, 423.
2 Solomon HM, Schrogie JJ. The effect of phenyramidol on the metabolism of bishydroxycoumarin. J Pharmacol Exp Ther (1966) 154, 660.

Anticoagulants + Picotamide

Abstract/Summary

Picotamide does not alter the anticoagulant effects of warfarin.

Clinical evidence, mechanism, importance and management

300 mg picotamide daily for 10 days had no effect on the serum levels of warfarin or its anticoagulant effects in 10 patients with aortic or mitral valve prostheses.[1] No special precautions would seem necessary. There seems to be no information about other anticoagulants.

Reference

1 Parise P, Gresele P, Viola E, Ruina A, Migliacci R, Nenci GG. La picotamide non interferisce con l'attività anticoagulante del warfarin in pazienti portatori di protesi valvolari cardiache. La Clinica Terapeutica (1990) 135, 479–82.

Anticoagulants + Piracetam

Abstract/Summary

A single case report describes a woman on warfarin who began to bleed within a month of starting to take piracetam.

Clinical evidence, mechanism, importance and management

A woman patient on regular treatment with warfarin, insulin, thyroxine and digoxin began to bleed (menorrhagia) within a month of starting to take 600 mg piracetam (*Nootropil*) daily. Her British Corrected Ratio (BCR) was found to have risen to 4.1 (normal range 2.3 to 2.8). Within 2 days of withdrawing both the warfarin and piracetam her BCR had fallen to 2.07.[1] The reason for this apparent interaction is not known. There is far too little evidence to forbid concurrent use, but be alert for this reaction if both drugs are used.

Reference

1 Pan HYM, Ng RP. The effect of Nootropil in a patient on warfarin. Eur J Clin Pharmacol (1983) 24, 711.

Anticoagulants + Pirmenol

Abstract/Summary

The anticoagulant effects of warfarin are not changed by pirmenol.

Clinical evidence, mechanism, importance and management

The prothrombin times of 10 patients on warfarin were not significantly changed when they were additionally given 150 mg pirmenol twice daily by mouth for 14 days.[1] No special precautions would therefore seem to be necessary. There seems as yet to be no information about other anticoagulants.

References

1 Stringer K A, Switzer D F, Abadier R, Lebsack M E, Sedman A J,Chrymko M. The effect of pirmenol administration on the anticoagulant activity of warfarin. J Clin Pharmacol (1991) 31, 607–10.

Anticoagulants + Ponalrestat

Abstract/Summary

Ponalrestat does not alter the anticoagulant effects of warfarin.

Clinical evidence, mechanism, importance and management

Twelve diabetics stabilized on warfarin showed no changes in warfarin serum levels or prothrombin ratios when concurrently treated with 600 mg ponalrestat daily for 2 weeks.[1] No special precautions seem necessary. There seems to be no information about other anticoagulants.

Reference

1 Moulds RFW, Fullinfaw RO, Bury RW, Plehwe WE, Jacka N, McGrath KM, Martin FIR. Ponalrestat does not cause a protein binding interaction with warfarin in diabetic patients. Br J clin Pharmac (1991) 31, 715–8.

Anticoagulants + Pravastatin

Abstract/Summary

Pravastatin does not interact with warfarin

Clinical evidence, mechanism, importance and management

Ten normal subjects were given 20 mg pravastatin alone twice daily for 3½ days, 5 mg warfarin alone twice daily for six days, and then both pravastatin and warfarin together for six days. The warfarin did not alter the pharmacokinetics of pravastatin, nor were the anticoagulant effects or the plasma protein binding of the warfarin significantly changed.[1] No changes in prothrombin times were seen in extensive clinical trials in patients, some of whom were on warfarin and pravastatin.[2] No special precautions would therefore seem necessary if pravastatin is given to patients taking warfarin. There appears to be nothing documented about any of the other anticoagulants.

References

1 Light RT, Pan HY, Glaess SR, Bakry D. A report on the pharmacokinetic and pharmacodynamic interaction of pravastatin and warfarin in healthy male volunteers. Unpublished report on file of ER Squibb. Protocol No 27, 201–59 (1988).
2 Catalano P. Pravastatin safety: an overview. In: Wood C, ed. Lipid management: pravastatin and the differential pharmacology of HMG-CoA reductase inhibiators. Roy Soc Med Round Table Ser No.16. Oxford, Alden Press (1990) 26–31.

Anticoagulants + Probenecid

Abstract/Summary

Some preliminary evidence suggests that probenecid increases the loss of phenprocoumon from the body. The anticoagulant effects would be expected to be decreased.

Clinical evidence, mechanism, importance and management

500 mg probenecid four times daily for seven days reduced the AUC (area under the curve) of a single 0.22 mg/kg dose of phenprocoumon in 17 normal subjects by 48%.[1] The reasons are not understood, but one possibility is that while probenecid inhibits the glucuronidation of phenprocoumon (its normal route of metabolism) it may also increase the formation of hydroxylated metabolites so that its overall loss is increased.[1] This study suggests that, in the presence of probenecid, the dosage of phenprocoumon may need to be increased, but this awaits formal clinical confirmation in patients. There seems to be nothing documented about other anticoagulants.

Reference

1 Mönig H, Böhm M, Ohnhaus EE, Kirch W. The effects of frusemide and probenecid on the pharmacokinetics of phenprocoumon. Eur J Clin Pharmacol (1990) 39, 261–5.

Anticoagulants + Proguanil

Abstract/Summary

An isolated report describes bleeding in a woman patient on warfarin after taking proguanil for about 5 weeks.

Clinical importance, mechanism, importance and management

A woman stabilized on warfarin developed haematuria, bruising and abdominal and flank discomfort about 5 weeks after starting to take 200 mg proguanil daily. Her prothrombin ratio was found to be 8.6. Within 12 h of being treated with fresh frozen plasma and vitamin K her prothrombin ratio had fallen to 2.3.[1] The mechanism of this interaction is unknown. Its general importance is uncertain, but it would now seem prudent to monitor the response to any anticoagulant if proguanil is added.

Reference

1 Armstrong G, Beg MF, Scahill S. Warfarin potentiation by proguanil. Br Med J (1991) 303, 789.

Anticoagulants + Prolintane

Abstract/Summary

The anticoagulant effects of ethyl biscoumacetate are not affected by the concurrent use of prolintane. Information about other anticoagulants is lacking.

Clinical evidence, mechanism, importance and management

The responses to single 20 mg/kg doses of ethylbiscoumacetate were examined in 12 subjects before and after four days' treatment with 20 mg prolintane daily. The mean half-life of the anticoagulant and prothrombin times remained unchanged.[1] Other anticoagulants probably behave similarly, but this requires confirmation.

Reference

1 Hague DE, Smith ME, Ryuan JR, McMahon FG. The interaction of methylphenidate and prolintane with ethylbiscoumacetate metabolism. Fed Proc (1971) 30, 336 (Abs).

Anticoagulants + Propafenone

Abstract/Summary

The anticoagulant effects of warfarin and possibly fluindione and phenprocoumon are increased by the concurrent use of propafenone. A reduction in the anticoagulant dosage may be necessary.

Clinical evidence

The mean steady-state serum levels of warfarin in eight normal subjects taking 5 mg daily rose by 38% (from 0.98 to 1.36 μg/ml) after taking 225 mg propafenone three times daily for a week. Five of the eight showed prothrombin time increases of 4–6 s.[1] Two further reports describe marked increases in the anticoagulant effects of fluinidione and phenprocoumon in two patients treated with propafenone.[2,3]

Mechanism

A possible reason is that the propafenone reduces the metabolism and loss from the body of these anticoagulants, thereby increasing their effects.

Importance and management

Information seems to be limited to these reports but they indicate that prothrombin times should be well monitored if propafenone is given to patients on fluindione, warfarin or phenprocoumon, and the anticoagulant dosage reduced where necessary. It would be prudent to apply the same precautions with any other anticoagulant.

References

1 Kates RE, Yee Y-G and Kirsten EB. Interaction between warfarin and propafenone in healthy volunteers. Clin Pharmacol Ther (1987) 42, 305–11.
2 Korst HA, Brandes JW, Littmann KP. Cave: Propafenon potenziert Wirkung von oralen Antikaogulantien. Med Klin (1981) 72, 349–50.
3 Welsch M, Heitz C, Stephan D, Imbs JL. Potentialisation de l'effet anticoagulant de la fluindione par la propafénone. Therapie (1991) 46, 253–6.

Anticoagulants + Proquazone

Abstract/Summary

The anticoagulant effects of phenprocoumon are not affected by the concurrent use of proquazone.

Clinical evidence, mechanism, importance and management

300 mg proquazone daily for 14 days had no effect on the plasma levels of factors II, VII, X, or prothrombin times or platelet aggregation in 20 patients on phenprocoumon.[1] Other anticoagulants probably behave similarly but this requires confirmation.

Reference

1 Vinazzer H. On the interaction between the anti-inflammatory substance proquazone (RU 43–715) and phenprocoumon. Int J Pharmacol (1977) 15, 214.

Anticoagulants + Quinidine

Abstract/Summary

The anticoagulant effects of warfarin can be increased (bleeding has been seen), decreased or remain unaltered when quinidine is given concurrently. A decrease in the effects of dicoumarol has also been reported.

Clinical evidence

(a) Anticoagulant effects increased

Three patients stabilized on warfarin with prothrombin levels within the range 18–25% began to bleed within 7–10 days of starting to take 800–1400 mg quinidine daily. Their prothrombin levels were found to have fallen to 6–8%. Bleeding ceased when the warfarin was withdrawn.[3] There are other reports of haemorrhage associated with the concurrent use of warfarin and quinidine.[2,4,9]

(b) Anticoagulant effects decreased

Four patients on warfarin or dicoumarol needed dosage increases of 7–23% to maintain adequate anticoagulation while receiving 1200 mg quinidine daily.[8]

(c) Anticoagulant effects unaltered

Ten patients on long-term treatment with warfarin (2.5–12.5 mg daily) showed no significant alteration in their prothrombin times when given 800 mg quinidine daily for 2 weeks.[5–7] Another study on eight patients also failed to find evidence of an interaction.

Mechanism

Quinidine can depress the synthesis of the vitamin-K dependent blood clotting factors and has a direct hypoprothrombinaemic effect of its own.[2] This would account for its additive effects with warfarin,[3] but does not explain why it can apparently also have antagonistic effects,[8] or no effect at all.[5–7]

Importance and management

Since increases[1–4] (with subsequent bleeding) and decreases[8] in the effects of warfarin, as well as the absence of an interaction[5–7,9] have been described, the outcome of concurrent use is clearly very uncertain. It would therefore be prudent to monitor the effects of quinidine closely to ensure that prothrombin times remain within the therapeutic range. The same precautions should apply with all the other anticoagulants, although nothing seems to be documented about any but dicoumarol, cited above.[8]

References

1 Sopher IM, Ming SC. Fatal corpus luteum haemorrhage during anticoagulant therapy. Obst Gynecol (1971) 37, 695.
2 Beaumont JL and Tarrit A. Les accidents haemorrhagiques survenus au cours de 1500 traitements anticoagulants. Sang (1955) 26, 680.
3 Gazzaniga AB, Stewart DR. Possible quinidine-induced haemorrhage in a patient on warfarin sodium. N Engl J Med (1969) 280, 711.
4 Koch-Weser J. Quinidine-induced hypoprothrombinemic haemorrhage in patients on chronic warfarin therapy. Ann Intern Med (1968) 68, 511.
5 Udall J. Quinidine and hypoprothrombinaemia. Ann Intern Med (1968) 69, 403.
6 Udall J. Drug interference with warfarin therapy. Amer J Cardiol (1969) 23, 143.
7 Udall J. Drug interference with warfarin therapy. Clin Med (1970) 77, 20.
8 Sylven C, Anderson P. Evidence that disopyramide does not interact with warfarin. Brit Med J (1983) 286, 1181.
9 Jones FL. More on quinidine induced hypoprothrombinaemia. Ann Intern Med (1986) 69, 1074.

Anticoagulants + Quinine

Abstract/Summary

The effects of the oral anticoagulants appear normally only to be slightly increased by quinine, however an isolated report describes bleeding in a man on phenprocoumon attributed to concurrent use.

Clinical evidence

Two studies[1,3] using the Page method[4] to measure prothrombin times showed that marked increases (up to 12 s) could occur when normal doses of quinine (330 mg) were given in man in the absence of an anticoagulant, but other studies[2,3] using the conventional Quick method showed that the prothrombin times were only prolonged by 0–2.1 s.

In contrast a patient on chronic phenprocoumon treatment repeatedly developed extensive haematuria within 24 h of drinking 1 litre of 'Indian tonic water' containing 30 mg quinine.[5]

Mechanism

Not understood. In the studies in man it was found that prothrombin time changes could be completely reversed by vitamin K (menadiol sodium diphosphate)[1,3] which suggests that quinine, like the oral anticoagulants, is a competitive inhibitor of vitamin K. The increase in prothrombin times and their decrease in response to vitamin K took several days, which is consistent with a pharmacological action involving changes in the synthesis by the liver of blood clotting factors. The isolated case of bleeding is not understood.

Importance and management

Common experience would seem to confirm that any increase in the effects of oral anticoagulants is normally very small and of little or no clinical importance. Concurrent use need not be avoided, however the case cited shows that very exceptionally

bleeding can occur even with quite a small dose (30 mg). Quinine can be given in doses of up to 2 g daily for the treatment of malaria.

References

1 Pirk LA and Engelberg R. Hypoprothrombinemic action of quinine sulfate. J Amer Med Ass (1945) 128, 1093.
2 Quick AJ. Effect of synthetic vitamin K and quinine sulphate on the prothrombin level. J Lab Clin Med (1946) 31, 79.
3 Pirk LA and Engelberg R. Hypoprothrombinemic action of quinine sulfate. Amer J Med Sci (1947) 213, 593.
4 Page RC, de Beer EJ, Orr ML. Prothrombin studies using Russell viper venom: relation of clotting time to prothrombin concentration in human plasma. J Lab Clin Med (1941) 27, 197.
5 Iven H, Lerche L, Kascube M. Influence of quinine and quinidine on the pharmacokinetics of phenprocoumon in rat and man. Eur J Pharmacol (1990) 183, 662.

Anticoagulants + Quinolone antibiotics

Abstract/Summary

The quinolone antibiotics appear normally not to increase the effects of anticoagulants in most patients, but some increased effects and even bleeding has been seen in a few individuals on warfarin when given ciprofloxacin, norfloxacin, or ofloxacin, or when given pefloxacin while on nicoumalone.

Clinical evidence

(a) Anticoagulants + Ciprofloxacin

Bayer, the UK manufacturers of ciprofloxacin, have in their records reports of no significant changes in prothrombin times in 40 patients chronically treated with ethyl-biscoumacetate or nicoumalone when ciprofloxacin was used concurrently.[2] No effects on warfarin anticoagulation were seen in three studies in nine and 16 patients given 500 mg ciprofloxacin twice daily for seven or 10 days,[10,20] or in 13 patients given 750 mg twice daily for 12 days.[17]

In contrast there are eight published reports (and possibly others) where ciprofloxacin has been responsible for increased prothrombin times and/or bleeding in patients on warfarin. Two reports describe marked increases in prothrombin times and/or bleeding in two patients on warfarin, associated with taking 750 mg ciprofloxacin twice daily.[9,12] The FDA has on record two cases of increased prothrombin times, one showing haematuria, in patients on warfarin given 1 g ciprofloxacin daily.[11] There are also other cases (not detailed) on the FDA files.[11] Elevated warfarin levels in another patient and prolonged prothrombin times in seven others on warfarin have also been observed.[2,13–16,19]

(b) Anticoagulants + Enoxacin

400 mg enoxacin twice daily did not affect the pharmacokinetics of S-warfarin in six normal subjects, whereas the clearance of R-warfarin was decreased from 0.22 to 0.15 l/h and its

elimination half-life was prolonged from 36.8 to 52.2 h. The overall anticoagulant (hypoprothrombinaemic) response to the warfarin was unaltered.[1] Another report about one patient is in agreement with these findings.[6]

(c) Anticoagulants + Fleroxacin

The pharmacokinetics and pharmacodynamics (prothrombin time and factor VII clotting time) of single 25 mg doses of racemic warfarin were unaffected in 12 normal subjects after taking 400 mg fleroxacin four times daily for nine days.[18]

(d) Anticoagulants + Norfloxacin

Six days' treatment with 400 mg norfloxacin twice daily was found not to alter either the pharmacokinetics or anticoagulant effects of warfarin in 10 normal subjects.[8]

In contrast, a 91-year-old woman on warfarin and digoxin developed a serious brain haemorrhage within 11 days of starting to take norfloxacin (precise dose not stated but said to be 'full'). Her prothrombin times had risen from 21.6 to 36.5 s. The manufacturers of norfloxacin (MSD) are said to have other reports of a warfarin/norfloxacin interaction but no details are given.[5] The FDA also has on record three cases of increased prothrombin times in patients on warfarin (two of them bled) when given 800 mg norfloxacin daily.[11]

(e) Anticoagulants + Ofloxacin

200 mg ofloxacin daily for week did not significantly affect the prothrombin times of seven subjects on phenprocoumon.[4] However a woman with a mitral valve replacement and under treatment with digoxin, frusemide, spironolactone, verapamil and 5 mg warfarin daily, showed a marked increase in her international normalized ratio (from 2.5 to 4.4) within two days of starting to take 200 mg ofloxacin three times daily. Two days later the ratio had risen to 5.8.[7] An increased INR has been briefly described in another patient.[17]

(f) Anticoagulants + Pefloxacin

A patient showed a marked increase in the effects of nicoumalone (Quick time reduced from 26 to less than 5%) within five days of starting to take pefloxacin (800 mg daily) and rifampicin (1200 mg daily).[3] Rifampicin is an enzyme inducer which normally causes a reduction in the effects of the anticoagulants, which would suggest that the pefloxacin was responsible for this reaction.

Mechanism

Uncertain. It is not clear what other factors might have been responsible in those cases where the effects of the anticoagulants were increased.

Importance and management

Moderately well documented. The overall picture is that no

adverse interaction normally occurs with these quinolones, but very occasionally and unpredictably increased anticoagulant effects and bleeding occurs. It would therefore be prudent to monitor the effects of adding any quinolone antibiotic to treatment with any oral anticoagulant. So far there appears to be no information about any of the other quinolones not cited here.

References

1 Toon S, Hopkins KJ, Garstang FM, Aarons L, Sedman A, Rowland M. Enoxacin-warfarin interaction: pharmacokinetic and stereochemical aspects. Clin Pharmacol Ther (1987) 42, 33–41.

2 Ansell PJ. Bayer UK Limited. Personal communication (1988).

3 Pertek JP, Helmer J, Vivin P, Kipper R. Potentialisation d'une antivitamine K par l'association pefloxacine-rifampicine. Ann Fr Anesth Reanim (1986) 5, 320–1.

4 Verho M, Malerczyk V, Rosenkrantz B, Grotsch H. Absence of interaction between ofloxacin and phenprocoumon. Curr Med Res Opin (1987) 10, 474–9.

5 Linville T, Matanin D. Norfloxacin and warfarin. Ann Intern Med (1989) 110, 751.

6 McLeod AD, Burgess C. Drug interaction between warfarin and enoxacin. NZ Med J (1988) 101, 216.

7 Leor J, Matetzki S. Ofloxacin and warfarin. Ann Intern Med (1988) 109, 761.

8 Rocci ML, Vlasses PH, Distlerath LM, Gregg MH, Wheeler SC, Zing W, Bjornsson TD. Norfloxacin does not alter warfarin's disposition or anticoagulant effect. J Clin Pharmacol (1990) 30, 728–32.

9 Mott FE, Murphy S, Hunt V. Ciprofloxacin and warfarin. Ann Intern Med (1989) 110, 542–3.

10 Rindone JP, Keuey CL, Jones WN, Garewal HS. Hypoprothrombinemic effect of warfarin not influenced by ciprofloxacin. Clin Pharmacy (1991) 10, 136–8.

11 Jolson HM, Tanner LA, Green L, Grasela TH. Adverse reaction reporting of interaction betweeen warfarin and fluoroquinolones. Arch Intern Med (1991) 151, 1003–4.

12 Linville D, Emory C, Graves L. Ciprofloxacin and warfarin interaction. Am J Med (1991) 90, 765.

13 Beeley L, Cunningham H, Carmichael AE, Brennan A. Newsletter of the West Midlands Centre for Adverse Drug Reaction Reporting, (1991), 33, 36

14 Kamada AK. Possible interaction betwen ciprofloxacin and warfarin. DICP Ann Pharmacotherapy (1990) 24, 27–8.

15 Johnson KC, Joe RH, Self TH. Drug interaction. J Fam Prac (1991) 33, 338.

16 Renzi R, Finkbeiner S. Ciprofloxacin interaction with warfarin: a potentially dangerous side-effect. Am J Emerg Med (1991) 9, 551–2.

17 Israel DS, Stotka JL, Rock WL, Polk RE. Effect of ciprofloxacin administration on warfarin response in adult subjects. 31st Intersci Conf Antimicrob Ag Chemother (1991). 199.

18 Holazo AA, Soni PP, Kachevsky V, Min BH, Townsend L, Patel IH. Fleroxacin-warfarin interaction in humans. 30th Intersci Conf Antimicrob Ag Chemother, October (1990) Atlanta, Georgia, p 253.

19 Dugoni-Kramer BM. Ciprofloxacin-warfarin interaction. Ann Pharmacother (1991) 25, 1397.

21 Bianco TM, Bussey HI, Farnett LE, Linn WD, Roush MK, Wong YWJ. Potential warfarin-ciprofloxacin interaction in patients receiving long-term anticoagulation. Pharmacotherapy (1992) 12, 435–9.

Anticoagulants + Rifampicin (Rifampin)

Abstract/Summary

The anticoagulant effects of warfarin, nicoumalone (acenocoumarol) and phenprocoumon are markedly reduced by the concurrent use of rifampicin. The anticoagulant dosage will need to be increased (possibly two-threefold) to accommodate this interaction.

Clinical evidence

The dosage of nicoumalone (acenocoumarol) needed to be markedly increased in 18 patients to maintain the Quick value within the therapeutic range after being given 900 mg rifampicin daily for seven days.[1] There are numerous other reports and studies of this interaction in man involving a considerable number of patients and subjects on nicoumalone,[6] phenprocoumon[7,14] or warfarin.[2-5,8-11,13]

Mechanism

Rifampicin is a potent liver enzyme inducing agent which increases the metabolism and clearance of the anticoagulants from the body, thereby reducing their effects.[12] Other mechanisms may also be involved.[13] One study found that the serum levels of warfarin and the prothrombin response were approximately halved.[3]

Importance and management

A well-documented and clinically important interaction which will occur in most patients. A marked reduction in the anticoagulant effects may be expected within 5–7 days,[1,2] persisting for about the same length of time or longer after the rifampicin has been withdrawn. With warfarin there is evidence that the dosage may need to be doubled[2] or tripled[8] to accommodate this interaction, and reduced by an equivalent amount following withdrawal of the rifampicin.[2,5,13] It seems probable that other anticoagulants will behave similarly.

References

1 Michot F, Burgi M, Buttner J. Rimactan (Rifampizin) und Antikoagulantientherapie. Schweiz med Wsch (1970) 100, 583.
2 Romankiewicz JA, Ehrman M. Rifampin and warfarin: a drug interaction. Ann Intern Med (1975) 82, 224.
3 O'Reilly RA. Interaction of sodium warfarin and rifampin. Ann Intern Med (1974) 81, 337.
4 O'Reilly RA. Interaction of rifampicin in man. Clin Res (1973) 21, 207.
5 Self TH, Mann RB. Interaction of rifampicin and warfarin. Chest (1975) 67, 490.
6 Sennwalt G. Etude de l'influence de la rifampicine sur l'effet anticoagulant de l'acenocoumarol. Rev medicale Suisse Romande (1974) 94, 945.
7 Boekhout-Mussert RJ, Bieger R, van Brummelen A, Lemkes HHD. Inhibition by rifampicin of the anticoagulant effect of phenprocoumon. J Amer Med Ass (1974) 229, 1903.
8 Fox P. Warfarin-rifampicin interaction. Med J Aust (1982) 1, 60.
9 O'Reilly RA. Interaction of chronic daily warfarin therapy and rifampin. Ann Intern Med (1975) 83, 506.
10 Felty P. Warfarin-rifampicin interaction. Med J Aust (1952) 62, 60.
11 Beeley L, Daly M, Stewart P. Bull W Med Centre for Adverse Drug Reaction Reporting (1987) 24, 23.
12 Heinmark LD, Gibaldi M, Trager WF, O'Reilly RA, Goulart DA. The mechanism of the warfarin-rifampicin drug interaction in humans. Clin Pharmacol Ther (1987) 42, 388–94.
13 Almog S, Martinowitz U, Halkin H, Bank HZ, Farfel Z. Complex interaction of rifampin and warfarin. South Med J (1988) 81, 1304–6.
14 Ohnhaus EE, Kampschultze J, Mönig H. Effect of propranolol and rifampicin on liver blood flow and phenoprocoumon elimination. Acta Pharmacol Toxicol (1986) 59, Suppl 4, 92.

Anticoagulants + Rioprostil

Abstract/Summary

Rioprostil can reduce the effects of the oral anticoagulants to some extent but the clinical importance of this is uncertain.

Clinical evidence, mechanism, importance and management

The effects of seven days pretreatment with rioprostil (0.3 mg twice daily) on the anticoagulant effects of single doses of nicoumalone (10 mg) or phenprocoumon (0.2 mg/kg) were examined on 13 subjects. The pharmacokinetics of these anticoagulants remained unchanged but their effects were reduced. The thrombotest and factor VII activity percentages rose for reasons which are not understood. For example those on phenprocoumon showed a rise in the thrombotest percentages on day three from a range of 18–50% (no rioprostil) to 26–100% (on rioprostil). However the authors of this report say that 'the observed interaction can be classed with the pharmacological curiosities because there is poor clinical relevancy.'[1] Until this is confirmed the effects of the concurrent use of rioprostil and any anticoagulant should be monitored for evidence of a reduced anticoagulant effect.

Reference

1 Thijssen HHW, Hamulyak K. The interaction of the prostaglandin E derivative rioprostil with oral anticoagulant agents. Clin Pharmacol Ther (1989) 46, 110–16.

Anticoagulants + Simvastatin

Abstract/Summary

Simvastatin normally causes a small, clinically unimportant, increase in the anticoagulant effects of warfarin, but more marked effects and bruising have been seen in one patient.

Clinical evidence, mechanism, importance and management

20 normal subjects on 5–13 mg warfarin daily and with prothrombin times averaging 19 s, had an increase in their prothrombin times of less than 2 s after taking 40 mg simvastatin daily for seven days.[1] A patient on warfarin with Type III hyperlipoproteinaemia showed no changes in her INR over 20 weeks when concurrently treated with 20 mg simvastatin daily.[3] However a single case report describes bruising, haematuria and a raised INR in one patient.[2]

Information is limited but it would seem that no important interaction normally occurs, however it would be prudent to monitor concurrent use so that any rare and unpredictable cases can be safely managed.

References

1 Zocor (simvastatin) product monograph, Merck Sharpe and Dhome (1988), 25.
2 Beeley L, Cunningham H, Carmichael AE, Brennan A. Newsletter of the West Midlands Centre for Adverse Drug Reaction Reporting, (1991) 33, 20.
3 Gaw A, Wosornu D. Simvastatin during warfarin therapy in hyperlipoproteinaemia. Lancet (1992) 340, 979–80.

Anticoagulants + Sucralfate

Abstract/Summary

Four case reports describe a marked reduction in the effects of warfarin in three patients given sucralfate. Other evidence suggests that this interaction is uncommon.

Clinical Evidence

A man on multiple therapy (digoxin, frusemide, chlorpropamide, potassium chloride and warfarin) had serum warfarin levels depressed about two-thirds when given sucralfate. When the sucralfate was withdrawn, his serum warfarin levels rose to their former levels accompanied by the expected prolongation of prothrombin times.[2] The prothrombin times of another patient remained subtherapeutic while taking sucralfate, despite warfarin doses of up to 17.5 mg warfarin daily. When the sucralfate was stopped his prothrombin time rose to 1.5 times his control, even though the warfarin dose was reduced to 10 mg daily.[4] Two other patients showed reduced responses to warfarin while taking sucralfate.[5,6]

In contrast, an open cross-over study on eight elderly patients taking warfarin found that their anticoagulant response and serum warfarin levels remained unchanged while taking sucralfate (1 g three times a day) over a period of two weeks.[1] No interaction was found in another study.[3]

Mechanism

Unknown. It is suggested that the sucralfate may possibly adsorb the warfarin so that its bioavailability is reduced.[4]

Importance and management

The documentation appears to be limited to the reports cited. Any interaction would therefore seem to be uncommon. Concurrent use need not be avoided but be alert for evidence of a reduced anticoagulant response to warfarin. Information about other anticoagulants is lacking, but it would seem prudent to take the same precautions. Ranitidine is an alternative non-interacting anti-ulcer agent.

References

1 Neuvonen PJ, Jaakkola A, Totterman J, Penttila O. Clinically significant sucralfate-warfarin interaction is not likely. Br J clin Pharmac (1985) 20, 178–9
2 Mungall D, Talbert RL, Phillips C, Jaffe D, Ludden TM. Sulcrate and warfarin. Ann Int Med (l983) 98, 557.
3 Talbert RL, Dalmady-Israel C, Bussey HI, Crawford MH, Ludden TM. Effect of sucralfate on plasma warfarin concentration in patients requiring chronic warfarin therapy. Drug Intell Clin Pharm (1985) 19, 456.
4 Braverman SE, Marino MT. Sucralfate-warfarin interaction. Drug Intell Clin Pharm (1988) 22, 913.
5 Rey AM, Gums JG. Altered absorption of digoxin, sustained-release quinidine, and warfarin with sucralfate absorption. DICP Ann Pharmacotherapy (1991) 25, 745–6.
6 Parrish RH, Waller B, Gondalia BG. Sucralfate-warfarin interaction. Ann Pharmacother (1992) 26, 1015–6.

Anticoagulants + Sulindac

Abstract/Summary

Five patients have shown a marked increase in the anticoagulant effects of warfarin when given sulindac (two of them bled), but it seems probable that only the occasional patient will develop this interaction.

Clinical evidence

A patient on warfarin, ferrous sulphate, phenobarbitone and sulphasalazine showed a marked increase in his prothrombin times (more than three times the control value) after taking 200 mg sulindac daily for five days.[1,2,4] There are four similar cases of this interaction on record.[3,4,7] Two of the patients bled, one of whom did so after taking only three 100 mg doses of sulindac.[3]

In contrast, studies in patients and normal subjects on warfarin or phenprocoumon and given sulindac failed to demonstrate this interaction.[4–6]

Mechanism

Not understood.

Importance and management

An established but uncommon and unpredictable interaction affecting only the occasional patient.[4,5] Monitor the effects if sulindac is added to warfarin or any other anticoagulant, bearing in mind that all NSAIDs can irritate the gastric mucosa, affect platelet activity and cause gastrointestinal bleeding. Alternative anti-inflammatory drugs which do not interact include ibuprofen and naproxen (see Index).

References

1 Beeley L (ed). Bulletin of the West Midlands Adverse Reaction Group, University of Birmingham, England. (1978) No. 6.
2 Beeley L and Baker S. Personal communication (1978).

3 Carter SA. Potential effect of sulindac on response of prothrombin time to oral anticoagulants. Lancet (1979) ii, 698.

4 Ross JRY and Beeley L. Sulindac, prothrombin time and anticoagulants. Lancet (1979) ii, 1075.

5 Loftin JP, Vessell ES. Interaction between sulindac and warfarin: different results in normal subjects and in an unusual patient with a potassium-losing renal tubular defect. J Clin Pharmacol (1979) 11–12, 733.

6 Schenk H, Klein G, Haralambus J, Goebel R. Coumarintherapie unter dem antirheumaticum sulindac. Z Rheumatol (1980) 39, 102.

7 McQueen EG. New Zealand Committee on Adverse Drug Reactions. 17th Annual Report 1982. NZ Med J (1983) 96, 95–9.

Anticoagulants + Suloctidil or Zomepirac

Abstract/Summary

Suloctidil does not significantly alter the anticoagulant effects of phenprocoumon, nor zomepirac the effects of warfarin.

Clinical evidence, mechanism, importance and management

Eight patients showed no significant changes in the anticoagulant effects of phenprocoumon when treated with 300 mg suloctidil three times a day.[1] The anticoagulant effects of warfarin were similarly unaltered in 16 subjects given 150 mg zomepirac four times a day.[2] No special precautions seem to be necessary. Information about other anticoagulants is lacking.

References

1 Verhaeghe R, Vanhoof A. The concomitant use of suloctidil and a long-acting oral anticoagulant. Acta Clin Belg (1977) 32, 1.

2 Minn FL and Zinny MA. Zomepirac and warfarin: a clinical study to determine if interaction exists. J Clin Pharmacol (1980) 12–13, 418.

Anticoagulants + Sulphinpyrazone

Abstract/Summary

The anticoagulant effects of warfarin and nicoumalone (acenocoumarol) are markedly increased by sulphinpyrazone. Serious bleeding can occur if the anticoagulant dosage is not reduced appropriately. Phenprocoumon does not interact significantly.

Clinical evidence

The prothrombin ratios of five patients on warfarin rose rapidly over 2–3 days after 800 mg sulphinpyrazone was added. The average warfarin requirements fell by 46% and two patients needed vitamin K to combat the excessive hypoprothrombinaemia. When the sulphinpyrazone was withdrawn, the warfarin requirements rose to their former levels within 1–2 weeks.

This interaction has been described in numerous studies and case reports in those taking warfarin[2,3,6–12,17] and nicou-malone.[13] Severe bleeding occurred in some instances. An increased effect followed by an unexplained reduced effect has been described in one report.[8] In a trial using nicoumalone it was found possible to reduce the anticoagulant dosage by an average of 20% while taking 800 mg sulphinpyrazone daily.[13] Phenprocoumon is reported not to interact.[16,19]

Mechanism

Some early *in vitro* evidence[4,5] suggested that plasma protein binding displacement might explain this interaction, but more recent clinical studies[1,14,15,18] indicate that sulphinpyrazone also inhibits the metabolism of the anticoagulants (the more potent S(–) isomer in the case of warfarin) so that the anticoagulant is cleared from the body more slowly and its effects are increased and prolonged.

Importance and management

A well established interaction of clinical importance. If sulphinpyrazone is added, Prothrombin Times should be well monitored and suitable anticoagulant dosage reductions made. Halving the dosage of warfarin[1,4,17] and reducing the nicoumalone dosage by 20%[13] has proved to be adequate in patients taking 600–800 mg sulphinpyrazone daily. Phenprocoumon is reported not to interact,[16,19] but it would be prudent to expect other anticoagulants to behave like warfarin and nicoumalone. It has been recommended that because of the difficulties of monitoring this interaction and of making the necessary dosage adjustments, concurrent use should not be undertaken unless the patient is hospitalized.[3]

References

1 Miners JO, Foenander T, Wanwimolruk S, Gallus AS, Birkett DJ. Interaction of sulphinpyrazone with warfarin. Europ J Clin Pharmacol (1982) 22, 327–31.

2 Weiss M. Potentiation of coumarin effect by sulphinpyrazone. Lancet (1979) i, 609.

3 Mattingly D, Bradley M, Selley PJ. Hazards of sulphinpyrazone. Br Med J (1978) 2, 1786.

4 Tulloch JA, Marr TCK. Sulphinpyrazone and warfarin after myocardial infarction. Br Med J (1979) ii, 133.

5 Seiler K, Duckert F. Properties of 3-(1-phenyl-propyl)-4-oxycoumarin (Marcoumar) in the plasma when tested in normal cases and under the influence of drugs. Thromb Diath Haemorrh (1968) 19, 389.

6 Davis JW, Johns LE. Possible interaction of sulphinpyrazone with coumarins. N Engl J Med (1978) 299, 955.

7 Bailey RR, Reddy J. Potentiation of warfarin action by sulphinpyrazone. Lancet (1980) i, 254.

8 Nenci GG, Agnelli G, Berretini M. Biphasic sulphinpyrazone-warfarin interaction. Br Med J (1981) 282, 1361.

9 Gallus A, Birkett D. Sulphinpyrazone and warfarin: a probable interaction. Lancet (1980) i, 535.

10 Jamil A, Reid JM, Messer M. Interaction between sulphinpyrazone and warfarin. Chest (1981) 79, 375.

11 Girolami A, Schivazappa L, Fabris F, Randi ML. Biphasic sulphinpyrazone interaction. Br Med J (1981) 283, 1338.

12 Thompson PL and Serjeant C. Potentially serious interaction of warfarin with sulphinpyrazone. Med J Aust (1981) 1, 41.

13 Michot F, Holt NF, Fontanilles F. Uber die beeinflussung der gerinnung-shemmenden Wirkungen von Acenocoumarol durch Sulphinpyrazon. Schweiz med Wsch (1981) 111, 255.

14 O'Reilly RA, Goulart DA. Comparative interaction of sulphinpyrazone and phenylbutazone with racemic warfarin: alteration in vivo of free fraction of plasma albumin. J Pharmacol Exp Ther (1981) 219, 691.

15 O'Reilly RA. Stereoselective interaction of sulfinpyrazone with racemic warfarin and its separated enantiomorphs in man. Circulation (1982) 65, 202–7.

16 O'Reilly RA. Phenylbutazone and sulphinpyrazone interaction with oral anticoagulant phenprocoumon. Arch Intern Med (1982) 142, 1634.

17 Girolami A, Fabris F, Casonata A, Randi ML. Potentiation of anticoagulant response to warfarin by sulphinpyrazone: a double-blind study in patients with prosthetic heart valves. Clin Lab Haemat (1982) 4, 23–6.

18 Toon S, Lawrence KL, Gibaldi M, Trager WF, O'Reilly RA, Motley CH, Goulart DA. The warfarin-sulfinpyrazone interaction: stereochemical considerations. Clin Pharmacol Ther (1986) 39, 15–24.

19 Heimark LD, Toon S, Gibaldi M, Trager WF, O'Reilly RA, Goulart DA. The effect of sulfinpyrazone on the disposition of pseudoracemic phenprocoumon in humans. Clin Pharmacol Ther (1987) 42, 312–19.

Anticoagulants + Sulphonamides

Abstract/Summary

The anticoagulant effects of warfarin are increased by co-trimoxazole (sulphamethoxazole/trimethoprim). Bleeding may occur if the dosage of the warfarin is not reduced appropriately. Phenindione does not interact with co-trimoxazole. There is also evidence that sulphaphenazole, sulphafurazole (sulfisoxazole) and sulphamethizole may interact like co-trimoxazole.

Clinical evidence

(a) Co-trimoxazole (sulphamethoxazole/trimethoprim)

Six out of 20 patients taking warfarin showed an increase in their prothrombin ratios within 2–6 days of starting to take two tablets of co-trimoxazole daily (each tablet contains 400 mg sulphamethoxazole and 80 mg trimethoprim).[9] One patient bled and needed to be given vitamin K. The warfarin was temporarily withdrawn from four patients and the dosage was reduced in the last patient to control excessive hypoprothrombinaemia.[9] An increase in the effects of warfarin caused by co-trimoxazole has been described in numerous other reports.[10–12,14–24] In some cases bleeding occurred. Phenindione is reported not to interact.[13]

(b) Sulphafurazole (sulfisoxazole)

A man taking digitalis, diuretics, antacids and warfarin was later started on 500 mg sulphafurazole (sulfisoxazole) six-hourly. After 9 days his prothrombin time had risen from 20 to 28 s, and after 14 days he bled (haematuria, haemoptysis, gum bleeding). His prothrombin time had risen to 60 s.[5] Two other patients bled and demonstrated prolonged prothrombin times when given warfarin and sulphafurazole (sulfisoxazole).[7,8]

(c) Sulphamethizole

The half-life of warfarin was increased over 40% (from 65 to 93 h) in two patients after taking 4 g sulphamethizole daily for a week.[6]

(d) Sulphaphenazole

16 patients given single oral doses of phenindione and 500 mg sulphaphenazole showed prothrombin time increases after 24 h of 16.8 s compared with 10.3 s in 12 other patients who had only had phenindione.[2] These patients almost certainly had some hypoalbuminaemia.

Mechanism

Not fully understood. Plasma protein binding displacement can occur, but on its own it does not provide an adequate explanation.[3,4] Sulphonamides can drastically reduce the intestinal bacterial synthesis of vitamin K, but this is not normally an essential source of the vitamin unless dietary sources are exceptionally low.[1] Evidence suggesting that the metabolism of the anticoagulants is decreased appears not to be fully established.[3,6] It has been shown that co-trimoxazole largely affects the more potent S-warfarin.[22]

Importance and management

The warfarin/co-trimoxazole interaction is well documented and well established. The incidence appears to be high. If bleeding is to be avoided the warfarin dosage should be reduced and prothrombin times monitored. Information about other anticoagulants is lacking, apart from phenindione which is said not to interact.

The phenidione/sulphaphenazole, warfarin/sulphafurazole (sulfisoxazole) and warfarin/sulphamethizole interactions are poorly documented, but it would seem prudent to follow the precautions suggested for co-trimoxazole if any of these sulphonamides is given. Some caution would be appropriate with any sulphonamide, but direct information is lacking.

References

1 Udall JA. Human sources and absorption of vitamin K in relation to anticoagulation stability. J Amer Med Ass (1965) 194, 107.

2 Varma DR, Gupta RK, Gupta S, Sharma KK. Prothrombin response to phenindione during hypoalbuminaemia. Br J clin Pharmac (1975) 2, 467.

3 Seiler K, Duckert F. Properties of 3-(1-phenyl-propyl)-4-oxycoumarin (Marcoumar) in the plasma when tested in normal cases and under the influence of drugs. Thromb Diath Haemorrh (1968) 19, 389.

4 Solomon HM, Schrogie JJ. The effect of various drugs on the binding of warfarin C[14] to human albumin. Biochem Pharmacol (1967) 16, 1219.

5 Self TH, Evans W, Ferguson T. Interaction of sulfisoxazole and warfarin. Circulation (1975) 52, 528.

6 Lumholtz B, Siersbaek-Nielsen K, Skovsted L, Kampmann J, Hansen JM. Sulphamethizole-induced inhibition of diphenylhydantoin, tolbutamide and warfarin metabolism. Clin Pharmacol Ther (1975) 17, 731.

7 Sioris LJ, Weibert RT, Pentel PR. Potentiation of warfarin anticoagulation by sulfisoxazole. Arch Int Med (1980) 140, 546–7.

8 Kayser S. Warfarin-sulfonamide interaction. Hospital Pharmacy Bulletin, University of California at San Francisco Hospitals 1978.

9 Hassall C, Feetam CL, Leach RH, Meynell MJ. Potentiation of warfarin by co-trimoxazole. Lancet (1975) ii, 1155.
10 Barnett DB, Hancock BW. Anticoagulant resistance: an unusual case. Br Med J (1975) i, 608.
11 O'Reilly RA, Motley CH. Racemic warfarin and trimethoprim-sulfamethoxazole interaction in humans. Ann Int Med (1979) 91, 34.
12 Hassal C, Feetam CL, Leach RH, Meynell MJ. Potentiation of warfarin by co-trimoxazole. Br Med J (1975) 2, 684.
13 De Swiet J. Potentiation of warfarin by co-trimoxazole. Br Med J (1975) 3, 491.
14 Tilstone WJ, Gray JMB, Nimmo-Smith RH, Lawson DH. Interaction between warfarin and sulphamethoxazole. Postgrad Med J (1977) 53, 388.
15 Kaufman JM, Fauver HE. Potentiation of warfarin by trimethoprim-sulfamethoxazole. Urology (1980) 16, 601.
16 Beeley L, Ballantine N, Beadle F. Bulletin West Midlands Centre for Adverse Drug Reaction Reporting (1983) 16, 7.
17 McQueen EG. New Zealand Committee on Adverse Drug Reactions. 17th Annual Report 1982. NZ Med J (1983) 96, 95–9.
18 Greenlaw CW. Drug interaction between cotrimoxazole and warfarin. Am J Hosp Pharm (1978) 35, 1399.
19 Errick JK, Keyes PW. Co-trimoxazole and warfarin: case report of an interaction. Am J Hosp Pharm (1979) 36, 1155.
20 O'Donnell D. Antibiotic-induced potentiation of oral anticoagulant agents. Med J Aust (1989) 150, 163–4.
21 Keys PW. Drug interaction between co-trimoxazole and warfarin. Am J Hosp Pharm (1979) 36, 1155–6.
22 O'Reilly RA. Stereoselective interaction of trimethoprim-sulfamethoxazole with the separated enantiomorphs of racemic warfarin in man. N Eng J Med (1980) 302, 33–5.
23 Beeley L, Magee P, Hickey FM. Bulletin of West Midlands Centre for Adverse Drug Reaction Reporting (1989) 28, 29.
24 Wolf R, Elman M, Brenner S. Sulfonamide-induced bullous hemorrhagic eruption in a patient with low prothrombin time. Isr J Med Sci (1992) 28, 882–4.

Anticoagulants + Tamoxifen

Abstract/Summary

The anticoagulant effects of warfarin are markedly increased by tamoxifen. A dosage reduction (about a half, or even more) may be needed to avoid bleeding.

Clinical evidence

A woman on warfarin needed a dosage reduction from 5 to 1 mg daily to keep her prothrombin time within the range 20–25 s when given 40 mg tamoxifen daily. A retrospective study of the records of five other patients on tamoxifen revealed that two had shown marked increases in prothrombin times and bleeding shortly after starting warfarin. The other three needed warfarin doses which were about one-third of those taken by other patients not on tamoxifen.[1]

This confirms the first report of this interaction in a woman on warfarin who developed haematemesis, abdominal pain and haematuria 6 weeks after starting 20 mg tamoxifen daily. Her prothrombin time had risen from 39 to 206 s. She was restabilized on a little over half the warfarin dosage while continuing to take the tamoxifen.[2] The Aberdeen Hospitals Drug File has on record 22 patients given both drugs. 17 of them had no problems but two developed grossly elevated warfarin levels and three haemorrhaged.[3] The manufacturers (ICI) of tamoxifen have another report of this interaction on their files.[2]

Mechanism

Uncertain. It seems possible that these drugs compete for the same metabolizing systems in the liver, the result being that the loss of the warfarin is reduced and its effects are increased and prolonged.

Importance and management

An established and clinically important interaction. Monitor the effects closely if tamoxifen is added to treatment with warfarin and reduce the dosage appropriately. The reports cited here indicate a reduction of a half to two-thirds but some patients may need much larger reductions. The warfarin dosage will need to be increased if the tamoxifen is later withdrawn. The authors of one of the reports[1] postulate that the anti-tumour effects of the tamoxifen may also possibly be reduced. This needs further study. The effect of tamoxifen on other anticoagulants is uncertain but be alert for the same reaction.

References

1 Tenni P, Lalich DL and Byrne MJ. Life threatening interaction between tamoxifen and warfarin. Br Med J (1989) 298, 93.
2 Lodwick R, McConkey B, Brown AM, Beeley L. Life threatening interaction between tamoxifen and warfarin. Br Med J (1987) 295, 1141.
3 Ritchie LD, Grant SM. Tamoxifen-warfarin interaction: the Aberdeen hospitals drug file. Br Med J (1989) 298, 1253.

Anticoagulants + Tenoxicam

Abstract/Summary

Tenoxicam does not alter the anticoagulant effects of warfarin. Preliminary data also indicates that it does not interact with phenprocoumon.

Clinical evidence, mechanism, importance and management

Single dose and steady-state studies in 14 subjects found that 20 mg tenoxicam daily for 14 days had no significant effect on the anticoagulant effects of warfarin or on bleeding times.[1] Case studies in a small number of patients and subjects similarly found no significant effect on the anticoagulant effects of phenprocoumon.[2] No special precautions would seem to be necessary.

Reference

1 Eichler H-G, Jung M, Kyrle PA, Rotter M, Korn A. Absence of interaction between tenoxicam and warfarin. Eur J Clin Pharmacol (1992) 42, 227–9.
2 Quoted as data on file, Hoffmann-Laroche & Co, Basel, Switzerland in reference 1.

Anticoagulants + Terodiline

Abstract/Summary

Terodiline does not alter the anticoagulant effects of warfarin.

Clinical evidence, mechanism, importance and management

22 normal subjects were given enough warfarin (2.5–9.4 mg daily) to achieve thrombotest percentages within the 10–20% range. When additionally given 25 mg terodiline twice daily for two weeks, the serum levels and anticoagulant effects of the warfarin were unchanged.[1] No special precautions would seem necessary during concurrent use. There seems to be nothing documented about other anticoagulants.

Reference

1 Hoglund P, Paulsen O, Bogentoft S. No effect of terodiline on anticoagulation effect of warfarin and steady-state plasma levels of warfarin enantiomers in healthy volunteers. Ther Drug Monit (1989) 11, 667–73.

Anticoagulants + Tetracyclic, Tricyclic and other antidepressants

Abstract/Summary

The effects of the oral anticoagulants are not normally altered by the concurrent use of tricyclic antidepressants, nor by maprotiline or mianserin, but the anticoagulant control in the occasional patient may become more difficult. A single case report describes a patient on warfarin whose prothrombin times were increased when given mianserin, and two others given lofepramine.

Clinical evidence

A study[1,2] in six volunteers given nortriptyline (0.6 mg/kg daily) for eight days indicated that the mean half-life of dicoumarol was increased from 35 to 106 h, but a later study failed to find a consistent effect of either nortriptyline (40 mg daily) or amitriptyline (75 mg daily) taken over nine days on the half-lives or elimination of either dicoumarol or warfarin in 12 normal subjects. The half-lives were shortened, prolonged or remained unaffected.[3]

Two reports have briefly noted that the control of anticoagulation may be more difficult in patients taking amitriptyline and other tricyclic antidepressants.[4,5] Two other very brief reports suggest the possibility of increased warfarin effects in patients given lofepramine.[11]

The anticoagulant effects of nicoumalone (20 patients) have been shown to be unaffected by the use of maprotiline (150 mg daily),[6] and the effects of phenprocoumon (60 patients) were not affected by mianserin (30–60 mg daily).[7] A single case

report describes a man on warfarin whose prothrombin time rose from 20 to 25 s after taking 10 mg mianserin daily for seven days.[8]

Mechanism

Not understood. One suggestion is that the tricyclic antidepressants inhibit the metabolism of the anticoagulant (seen in animals with nortriptyline and amitriptyline on warfarin,[9] but not with desipramine or nicoumalone[10]). Another idea is that the tricyclics slow intestinal motility thereby increasing the time available for the dissolution and absorption of dicoumarol.

Importance and management

No general clinically important interaction has been established. There would therefore appear to be no good reason for avoiding the concurrent use of the oral anticoagulants and either the tricyclic antidepressants, maprotiline or mianserin but the outcome should be monitored because the occasional patient may show an altered anticoagulant response.

References

1 Vesell ES, Passananti GT, Greene FE. Impairment of drug metabolism in man by allopurinol and nortriptyline. N Engl J Med (1970) 283, 1484.
2 Vesell ES, Passananti GT, Aurori KC. Anomalous results of studies on drug interaction in man. Pharmacology (1975) 13, 101.
3 Pond SM, Graham GG, Birkett DJ, Wade DN. Effects of tricyclic antidepressants on drug metabolism. Clin Pharmacol Ther (1975) 18, 191.
4 Koch-Weser J. Haemorrhagic reactions and drug interactions in 500 warfarin treated patients. Clin Pharmacol Ther (1973) 14, 139.
5 Williams JRB, Griffin JP, Parkins A. Effect of concomitantly administered drugs on the control of long term anticoagulant therapy. Quart J Med (1976) 45, 63.
6 Michot F, Glaus K, Jack DB, Theobald W. Antikoagulatorische Wirkung von Sintrom und Konzentration von Ludiomil in Blut bei gleichzeitiger Verabreichung beider Praparate. Med Klin (1975) 70, 626.
7 Kopera H, Schenk H, Stulmeijer S. Phenprocoumon requirement, whole blood coagulation time, bleeding time and plasma gamma-GT in patients receiving mianserin. Europ J clin Pharmacol (1978) 13, 351.
8 Warwick HMC and Mindham RHS. Concomitant administration of mianserin and warfarin. Br J Psychiat (1983) 143, 308.
9 Loomis CW, Racz WJ. Drug interactions of amitriptyline and nortriptyline with warfarin in the rat. Res Commun Chem Pathol Pharmacol (1980) 30, 41.
10 Weiner M. Effect of centrally active drugs on the action of coumarin anticoagulants. Nature (1966) 212, 1599.
11 Beeley L, Stewart P, Hickey FM. Bulletin W. Midlands Centre for Adverse Drug Reaction Reporting (1988) 26, 21.

Anticoagulants + Tetracyclines

Abstract/Summary

The effects of the anticoagulants are not usually altered by concurrent treatment with the tetracycline antibiotics, but a few patients have shown increases and even bleeding.

Clinical evidence

Six out of nine patients on an un-named anticoagulant showed a fall in their PP% from a range of 10–30% to less than 6% when treated with 250 mg chlortetracycline four times a day for 4 days.[1] One patient out of another 20 patients taking dicoumarol bled when given tetracycline.[2] An increased anticoagulant effect is briefly mentioned in two other reports,[3,4] and a single report describes a woman on warfarin who bled (menorrhagia) after taking 200 mg doxycycline daily for 8 days.[5] A patient on warfarin bled (right temporal lobe haematoma) and had an extended prothrombin time a week after starting to take a tetracycline/nystatin.[11] Another patient on warfarin also bled (epistaxis, haematemesis, melaena) 3 weeks after starting to take a tetracycline/nystatin.[11] A patient on warfarin showed a marked increase in INR (from about 2.0 to 7.66) 6 weeks after starting to take 250 mg tetracycline four times daily, with changes in INR over the next few months which broadly paralleled the decreases in the tetracyline dosage.[12] Two patients on nicoumalone (acenocoumarol) or warfarin developed markedly increased prothrombin ratios with bruising, haematomas and bleeding when treated with doxycycline.[14] These reports contrast with another in which tetracycline was found not to affect the prothrombin times of patients on chronic warfarin treatment.[13]

Mechanism

Not understood. Tetracyclines in the absence of anticoagulants can reduce prothrombin activity,[6,15] and both hypoprothrombinaemia and bleeding have been described.[7,8] It seems possible that very occasionally the anticoagulant and the tetracycline have additive hypoprothrombinaemic effects. The idea that antibiotics can decimate the intestinal flora of the gut thereby depleting the body of an essential source of vitamin K has been shown to be incorrect, apart from exceptional cases where normal dietary sources are extremely low.[9,10]

Importance and management

A sparsely documented and apparently uncommon interaction, bearing in mind the wide-spread use of the tetracyclines. Concurrent use need not be avoided, but as the occasional patient may show increased anticoagulant effects and even bleeding, the effects should be monitored.

References

1 Magid E. Tolerance to anticoagulants during antibiotic therapy. Scand J clin Lab Invest (1962) 14, 565.
2 Chiavazza F, Merialdi A. Sulle interferenze fra dicumarolo e antibiotici. Minerva Ginecol (1973) 25, 630.
3 Wright IS. Pathogenesis and treatment of thrombosis. Circulation (1952) 5, 178.
4 Scarrone LA, Beck DF, Wright IS. Tromexan and dicumarol in thromboembolism. Circulation (1952) 6, 489.
5 Westfall LK, Mintzer DL and Wiser TH. Potentiation of warfarin by tetracycline. Amer J Hosp Pharm (1980) 37, 1624.
6 Searcy RL, Craig RG, Foreman JA, Bergqvist LM. Blood clotting anomalies

associated with intensive tetraycycline therapy. Clin Res (1964) 12, 230.
7 Rios JF. Haemorrhagic diathesis induced by antimicrobials. J Amer Med Ass (1968) 205, 142.
8 Kippel AP, Pitsinger B. Hypoprothrombinaemia secondary to antibiotic therapy and manifested by massive gastrointestinal haemorrhage. Arch Surg (1968) 96, 266.
9 Udall JA. Human sources and absorption of vitamin K in relation to anticoagulation stability. J Amer Med Ass (1965) 194, 107.
10 Pineo GF, Gallus AS, Hirsh J. Unexpected vitamin K deficiency in hospitalized patients. Can Med Ass J (1973) 109, 880–3.
11 O'Donnell D. Antibiotic-induced potentiation of oral anticoagulant agents. Med J Aust (1989) 150, 163–4.
12 Danos EA. Apparent potentiation of warfarin activity by tetracycline. Clin Pharmacy (1992) 11, 806–8.
13 Messinger WJ, Samet CM. The effect of a bowel sterilizing antibiotic on blood coagulation mechanisms. Angiology (1965) 29–36.
14 Caraco Y, Rubinow A. Enhanced anticoagulant effect of coumarin derivatives induced by doxycline coadministration. Ann Pharmacother (1992) 26, 1084–6.
15 Searcy RL, Simms NM, Foreman JA, Bergquist LM. Evaluation of the blood-clotting mechanism in tetracycline-treated patients. Antimicrob Ag Chemother (1965) 179–83.

Anticoagulants + Thyroid or Antithyroid compounds

Abstract/Summary

The anticoagulant effects of warfarin, dicoumarol, nicoumalone (acenocoumarol) and phenindione are increased by the concurrent use of thyroid compounds. Bleeding can occur if the anticoagulant is not reduced appropriately. A reduction in the anticoagulant effects may be expected if anti-thyroid compounds are used.

Clinical evidence

Hypothyroidic patients are relatively resistant to the effects of the oral anticoagulants and need larger doses than hyperthyroidic patients who are relatively sensitive.[6,8,11,14] Drug-induced changes in thyroid status (even in those who are euthyroidic but who are taking thyroxine for hypercholesterolaemia) will alter the response to the oral anticoagulants.

(a) Anticoagulants + Thyroid compounds

A patient with myxoedema required a gradual reduction in his dosage of phenindione from 200 to 75 mg daily as his thyroid status was restored by the administration of liothyronine.[3] Seven out of 11 euthyroidic patients on warfarin showed lengthening prothrombin times and needed a small weekly dosage reduction in warfarin (by 2.5 mg to 30 mg) during the first four weeks of treatment with 4–8 mg d-thyroxine daily for hypercholesterolaemia. One patient bled.[1] Hypoprothrombinaemia and bleeding have been described in two patients on warfarin when their thyroid replacement therapy was started or increased.[13] Similar responses have been described in other reports and studies involving warfarin,[4,12,15] dicoumarol[2] and nicoumalone.[3]

(b) Anticoagulants + Antithyroid compounds

A hyperthydroidic patient on warfarin showed a marked increase in his prothrombin times on two occasions when his treatment with methimazole was stopped and he became hyperthyroidic again.[6]

Mechanism

In hypothyroidic patients the catabolism (destruction) of the blood clotting factors (II, VII, IX and X) is low and this tends to cancel to some extent the effects of the anticoagulants which reduce blood clotting factor synthesis. Conversely, in hyperthyroidic patients in whom the catabolism is increased, the net result is an increase in the effects of the anticoagulants.[5] It has also been suggested that the thyroid hormones may increase the affinity of the anticoagulants for its receptor sites.[7,4]

Importance and management

A clearly documented and clinically important interaction occurs if oral anticoagulants and thyroid compounds are taken concurrently. Hypothyroidic patients taking an anticoagulant who are subsequently treated with thyroid as replacement therapy will need a changing downward adjustment of the anticoagulant dosage as treatment proceeds if excessive hypoprothrombinaemia and bleeding are to be avoided. Some adjustment may be necessary with euthyroidic (normal) patients given dextrothyroxine for hypercholesterolaemia. All of the oral anticoagulants may be expected to behave similarly.

As the thyroid status of hyperthyroidic patients returns to normal by the use of antithyroid drugs (e.g. carbimazole, methimazole, propylthiouracil) an increase in the anticoagulant requirements would be expected. Propylthiouracil in the absence of an anticoagulant has very occasionally been reported to cause hypoprothrombinaemia and bleeding.[9,10]

References

1 Owens JC, Neeley WB, Owen WR. Effect of sodium dextrothyroxine in patients receiving anticoagulants. N Engl J Med (1962) 266, 76.
2 Jones RJ, Cohen L. Sodium dextrothyroxine in coronary disease and hypercholesterolemia. Circulation (1961) 24, 164.
3 Walters MB. The relationship betwen thyroid function and anticoagulant therapy. Amer J Cardiol (1963) 11, 112.
4 Solomon HM, Schrogie JJ. Change in receptor site affinity: a proposed explanation for the potentiating effect of D-thyroxine on the anticoagulant response to warfarin. Clin Pharmacol Ther (1967) 8, 797.
5 Loeliger EA, van der Esch B, Mattern MJ, Hemker HC. The biological disappearance rate of prothrombin, factors VII, IX and X from plasma in hypothyroidism, hyperthyroidism and during fever. Thromb Diath Haemorrh (1964) 10, 267.
6 Vagenakis AG. Enhancement of warfarin-induced hypoprothrombinemia by thyrotoxicosis. Johns Hopkins Med J (1972) 131, 69.
7 Schrogie JJ, Solomon HM. The anticoagulant reponse to bishydroxycoumarin. II. The effect of D-thyroxine, clofibrate and norethandrolone. Clin Pharmacol Ther (1967) 8, 70.
8 Self TH, Straughan AB, Weisburst MR. Effect of hyperthyroidism on hypoprothrombinemic reponse to warfarin. Amer J Hosp Pharm (1976) 33, 387.
9 D'Angelo G, LeGresley L. Severe hypoprothrombinemia after propylthiouracil therapy. Can Med Ass J (1959) 71, 479.
10 Gotta AW, Sullivan CA, Seaman J, Jaen-Giles B. Prolonged intra-operative bleeding caused by propylthiouracil-induced hypoprothrombinemia. Anesthesiology (1972) 37, 562.
11 McIntosh TJ, Brunk SF, Kolln I. Increased sensitivity to warfarin thyrotoxicosis. J Clin Invest (1970) 49, 63A.
12 Winters WL amd Soloff LA. Observations on sodium d-thyroxine as a hypercholesterolemic agent in persons with hypercholesterolemia with and without ischemic heart disease. Amer J Med Sci (1962) 103, 458.
13 Hansten PD. Oral anticoagulants and drugs which alter thyroid function. Drug Intell Clin Pharm (1980) 14, 331.
14 Rice AJ, McIntosh TJ, Fouts JR, Brunk SF, Wilson WR. Decreased sensitivity to warfarin in patients with myxedema. Amer J Med Sci (1971) 262, 211.
15 Costigan DC, Freedman MH, Ehrlich RM. Potentiation of oral anticoagulant effect of L-thyroxine. Clin Pediatr (1984) 23, 172.

Anticoagulants + Ticlopidine

Abstract/Summary

The concurrent use of warfarin and ticlopidine may possible cause liver damage.

Clinical evidence, mechanism, importance and management

A Japanese study has found evidence that warfarin and ticlopidine together can sometimes cause cholestatic liver injury and severe jaundice. Four out of 132 patients (3%) given both drugs after cardiovascular surgery demonstrated this toxicity. The authors conclude that '...close attention should be paid to the concomitant use of these drugs.'[1]

Reference

1 Takase K, Fujioka H, Ogasawara M, Aonuma H, Tameda Y, Nakano T, Kosaka Y. Drug-induced hepatitis during combination therapy of warfarin potassium and ticlopidine hydrochloride. Mie Med J (1990) 40, 27–32.

Anticoagulants + Trazodone

Abstract/Summary

An isolated case report describes a woman who needed an increase in her warfarin dosage while taking trazodone, but other studies suggest that concurrent use can be uneventful.

Clinical evidence, mechanism, importance and management

A woman needed a 17% increase (from 6.4 to 7.5 mg) in her daily dosage of warfarin when given 300 mg trazodone daily in order to maintain her prothrombin time at 20 s. Her warfarin requirements fell when the trazodone was later withdrawn.[1] The reasons for this reaction are not understood. In contrast, six anticoagulated patients on heparin or a coumarin anticoagulant showed no significant changes in prothrombin times when given 75 mg trazodone daily.[2] Check the prothrombin times if trazodone is given.

References

1 Hardy J-L and Sirois A. Reduction of prothrombin and partial thromboplastin times with trazodone. Canad Med Ass J (1986) 135, 1372.
2 Cozzolino G, Pazzaglia I, De Gaetano V, Macri M. Clinical investigation on the possible interaction between anticoagulants and a new psychotropic drug (Trazodone). Clin Europa (1972) 11, 593.

Anticoagulants + Vinpocetine

Abstract/Summary

Preliminary evidence suggests that the anticoagulant effects of warfarin may possibly be reduced to a small extent by vinpocetine.

Clinical evidence, mechanism, importance and management

A study in 18 normal subjects compared the effects of single 25 mg doses of warfarin before and while taking 10 mg vinpocetine daily.[1] A small reduction in the anticoagulant effects occurred, but more study is needed to find out whether this is clinically important. Monitor the effects of concurrent use.

Reference

1 Hitzenberger G, Sommer W, Grandt R. Influence of vinpocetine on warfarin-induced inhibition of coagulation. Int J Clin Pharmacol Ther Toxicol (1990) 28, 323–8 .

Anticoagulants + Vitamin E

Abstract/Summary

There is some very limited evidence that the effects of warfarin may be increased, and of dicoumarol reduced, by the concurrent use of large doses of vitamin E.

Clinical evidence, mechanism, importance and management

A patient on warfarin (and also taking digoxin, frusemide, clofibrate, potassium chloride and phenytoin, later substituted by quinidine) began to bleed as a result of secretly taking 1200 iu vitamin E daily over a period of 2 months. His prothrombin time was found to be 36 s. A later study showed that 800 iu vitamin E daily reduced his blood clotting factor levels and caused bleeding.[1] Another study on three normal subjects showed that 42 iu vitamin E daily for a month reduced the response to a single dose of dicoumarol after 36 h from 52 to 33%.[2] The reasons are not fully understood. One suggestion is

that vitamin E interferes with the activity of vitamin K in producing the blood clotting factors[1] Another idea is that it increases the dietary requirements of vitamin K.[3,4] This interaction is poorly documented and its importance uncertain. There seems to be no clear reason for avoiding vitamin E in normal doses, but large doses may cause problems.[1] The effects should be monitored.

References

1 Corrigan JJ, Marcus FI. Coagulopathy associated with vitamin E ingestion. J Amer Med Ass (1974) 230, 1300.
2 Schrogie JJ. Coagulopathy and fat-soluble vitamins. J Amer Med Ass (1975) 232, 341.
3 Anon. Vitamin K, vitamin E and the coumarin drugs. Nutr Rev (1982) 40, 180.
4 Anon. Megavitamin E supplementation and vitamin K-dependent carboxylation. Nutr Rev (1983) 41, 268–70.

Anticoagulants + Vitamin K

Abstract/Summary

The effects of the anticoagulants can be reduced or abolished by the concurrent use of vitamin K. This can be used as an effective antidote for overdosage, but unintentional and unwanted antagonism has occurred in patients after taking some proprietary chilblain preparations, health foods, food supplements, enteral feeds or exceptionally large amounts of some green vegetables (such as spinach, brussel sprouts or broccoli) which contain significant amounts of vitamin K. See also 'Anticoagulants + Food' and 'Anticoagulants + Netto'.

Clinical evidence

A woman on nicoumalone showed a fall in her British corrected anticoagulant ratio to 1.2 (normal range 1.8–3.0) within two days of starting to take an over-the-counter chilblain preparation (*Gon*) containing 10 mg acetomenaphthone per tablet. She took a total of 50 mg vitamin K over 48 h.[1]

Similar antagonism has been described in patients on warfarin taking liquid dietary supplements such as *Ensure*,[2,7,14,16] *Ensure-Plus*,[6,9] *Isocal*,[12] *Nutrilite 330*[21] and *Osmolite*.[8,13,15,22] A reduction in the effects of dicoumarol, nicoumalone and warfarin (described as 'warfarin resistance') has been seen in those whose diets contained exceptionally large amounts of green vegetables (up to 0.75–1.1 lb daily)[3,4,10] such as spinach,[5,17] brussel sprouts[18,20] or broccoli[17,23] or liver[19,23] which are rich in vitamin K.

Mechanism

The oral anticoagulants compete with the normal supply of vitamin K from the gut to reduce the synthesis by the liver of blood clotting factors. If this supply is boosted by an unusually large intake of vitamin K, the competition swings in favour of the vitamin and the synthesis of the blood clotting factors begins to return to normal. As a result the prothrombin time also begins to fall to its normal value. Brussel sprouts increase the metabolism of warfarin to a small extent which would also decrease its effects.[20] There is also some evidence that a physico-chemical interaction (possibly binding to protein) may possibly occur between warfarin and enteral foods in the gut.[22,24]

Importance and management

A very well established, well documented and clinically important interaction expected to occur with every oral anticoagulant because they have a common mode of action. The drug intake and diet of any patient who shows 'warfarin resistance' should be investigated for the possibility of this interaction. It can be accommodated either by increasing the anticoagulant dosage, or by reducing the intake of vitamin K. In one case separating the administration of the warfarin and an enteral food by 3 h or more was effective.[22] However patients on vitamin K rich diets should not change their eating habits without at the same time reducing the anticoagulant dosage because excessive anticoagulation and bleeding may occur.[23] It is estimated that a normal Western diet contains 300–500 µg vitamin K daily, and that the minimum daily requirement is 0.30–1.50 µg/kg body weight (about 100 µg in a 10 stone/140 lb/63 kg individual). Table 6.2 gives the vitamin K content of some foods. Other tables listing the vitamin K content of the enteral feeds have been published,[12–14,18,21] but the situation is continually changing as manufacturers reformulate their products, in some instances to accommodate the problem of this interaction.

References

1 Heald GE, Poller L. Anticoagulants and treatment for chilblains. Br Med J (1974) 2, 455.
2 O'Reilly RA, Ryland DA. 'Resistance' to warfarin due to unrecognized vitamin K supplementation. N Engl J Med (1980) 303, 160.
3 Quick AJ. Leafy vegetables in diet alter prothrombin time in patients taking anticoagulant drugs. J Amer Med Ass (1964) 187 (11) 27.
4 Qureshi GD, Reinders P, Swint JJ, Slate MB. Acquired warfarin resistance and weight-reducing diet. Arch Intern Med (1981) 141, 507.
5 Udall JA, Krock LB. A modified method of anticoagulant therapy. Curr Ther Res (1968) 10, 207.
6 Zallman JA, Lee DP, Jeffrey PL. Liquid nutrition as a cause of warfarin resistance. Amer J Hosp Pharm (1981) 38, 1174.
7 Westfall LK. An unrecognized cause of warfarin resistance. Drug Intell Clin Pharm (1981) 15, 131.
8 Lader EW, Yang L and Clarke A. Warfarin dosage and vitamin K in *Osmolite*. Ann Intern Med (1980) 93, 373.
9 Michaelson R, Kempson SJ, Naria B, Gold JWM. Inhibition of the hypoprothrombinemic effect of warfarin (Coumadin) by *Ensure-Plus*, a dietary supplement. Clin Bull (1980) 10, 171–2.
10 Kempin SJ. Warfarin resistance caused by broccoli. N Engl J Med (1983) 308, 1229–30.
11 Olson RE. Vitamin K. In: Modern nutrition in health and disease. Goodhart RS, Shils ME (eds.) Lea and Febiger, Philadelphia (1980) p 170–180.
12 Watson AJM, Pegg M, Green JRB. Enteral feeds may antagonize warfarin. Br Med J (1984) 288, 557.
13 Parr MD, Record KE, Griffith GL, Zeok JV, Todd EP. Effect of enteral nutrition on warfarin therapy. Clin Pharm (1982) 1, 274–6.
14 Howards PA, Hannaman KN. Warfarin resistance linked to enteral nutrition products. J Amer Diet Ass (1985) 85, 713–15.
15 Lee M, Schwart RN, Sharifi R. Warfarin resistance and vitamin K. Ann Intern Med (1981) 94, 140.
16 McIntire B, Wright RA. Enteral alimentation: an update on new products. Nutr Supp Serv (1981) 1, 7.
17 Karlson B, Leijd B, Hellstrom A. On the influence of vitamin K-rich vegetables and wine on the effectiveness of warfarin treatment. Acta Med Scand (1986) 220, 347–50.
18 Kutsop JJ. Update on vitamin K content of enteral products. Am J Hosp Pharm (1984) 41, 1762.
19 Kalra PA, Cooklin M, Wood G, O'Shea GM, Holmes AM. Dietary modification as a cause of anticoagulation instability. Lancet (1988) ii, 803.
20 Ovesen L, Lyduch S, Idorn ML. The effect of diet rich in brussel sprouts on warfarin pharmacokinetics. Eur J Clin Pharmacol (1988) 34, 521–4.
21 Oren B, Shvartzman P. Unsuspected source of vitamin K in patients treated with anticoagulants: a case report. Fam Prac (1989) 6, 151–2.
22 Petretich DA. Reversal of *Osmolite*-warfarin interaction by changing warfarin administration time. Clin Pharm (1990) 9, 93.
23 Chow WH, Chow TC, Tse TM, Tai YT, Lee WT. Anticoagulation instability with life-theatening complication after dietary modification. Postgrad Med J (1990) 66, 855–7.
24 Allen J, Penrod LE, Vickery WE. Warfarin resistance and enteral feedings: an *in vitro* study. Arch Phys Med Rehabil (1991) 72, 832.

Table 6.2 Vitamin K content of some meat and vegetables

Foods	Vitamin K content (µg/100 g)
Turnip greens	650
Beetroot	650
Broccoli	200
Cabbage	125
Green beans	14
Lettuce	129
Liver, pig	25
Liver, beef	92
Potatoes	3
Spinach	89

Data from Olson[11] and others.[23]

Heparin + Aprotinin

Abstract/Summary

Aprotinin-treated patients also given protamine may subsequently need increased doses of heparin.

Clinical evidence, mechanism, importance and management

One report suggested that patients who had been treated with aprotinin needed considerably more heparin than usual, the suggested reason being that aprotinin has an effect on antithrombin III.[1] A later report however pointed out that the more likely reason is that these aprotinin-treated patients had also been given protamine which would oppose the effects of the heparin.[2] Whatever the explanation, be alert for the need to use more heparin after aprotinin has been used.

References

1 Fisher AR, Bailey CR, Shannon CN, Wielogorski AK. Heparin resistance after aprotinin. lancet (1992) 340, 1230–1.
2 Hunt BJ, Murkin JM. Heparin resistance after aprotinin. Lancet (1993) 341, 126.

Heparin + Aspirin

Abstract/Summary

Although concurrent use is effective in the prevention of post-operative thromboembolism, the risk of bleeding in patients receiving heparin is increased almost two-and-a-half times by the use of aspirin.

Clinical evidence

Eight out of 12 patients developed serious bleeding when treated with heparin (5000 u subcutaneously every 12 h) and aspirin (600 mg twice daily) as prophylaxis for deep vein thrombosis following operations for fracture of the hip. Haematomas of the hip and thigh occurred in three patients, bleeding through the wound in four, and uterine bleeding in the other patient.[1] An epidemiological study of 2656 patients given heparin and aspirin (doses not stated) revealed that the incidence of bleeding was almost 2.5 times that which was seen in patients not given aspirin.[2] A striking prolongation of bleeding times is described elsewhere[3] in patients on heparin after treatment with aspirin.

Mechanism

Heparin suppresses the normal blood clotting mechanisms and prolongs bleeding times.[3] Aspirin decreases platelet aggregation so that any heparin-induced bleeding is exaggerated and prolonged.[3]

Importance and management

An established and important interaction. Although concurrent use is effective in the prevention of post-operative thromboembolism,[4] the risks of this interaction need to be very carefully considered, and the advantages and disadvantages carefully weighed. The assertion[5] made in 1969 that aspirin '...should be scrupulously avoided in patients on heparin...' is an overstatement, but it emphasises the need for care. Concurrent use should certainly be carefully monitored. If an analgesic is required, paracetamol (acetaminophen) is a safer substitute.

References

1 Yett HS, Skillman JJ, Salzman EW. The hazards of aspirin plus heparin. N Engl J Med (1978) 298, 1092.
2 Walker AM, Jick H. Predictors of bleeding during heparin therapy. J Amer Med Ass (1980) 244, 1209.
3 Heiden D, Rodrien R, Mieckle CH. Heparin bleeding, platelet dysfunction and aspirin. J Amer Med Ass (1981) 246, 330.

4 Vinazzer H, Loew D, Simma W, Brucke P. Prophylaxis of postoperative thromboembolism by low dose heparin and by acetylsalicylic acid given simultaneously: a double blind study. Thromb Res (1980) 17, 177.
5 Deykin D. The use of heparin. N Engl J Med (1976) 294, 1122.

Heparin + Dextran

Abstract/Summary

Although concurrent use can be successful and uneventful, there is evidence that the anticoagulant effects of heparin can be increased by some dextrans. It has been suggested that the heparin dosage may need to be reduced to a third or a half during concurrent use to prevent bleeding.

Clinical evidence

A study on nine patients with peripheral vascular disease showed that the mean clotting time 1 h after the infusion of 10,000 u heparin was increased from 36 to 69 s when given at the same time as 500 ml dextran. Dextran alone had no effect, but the mean clotting time after 5,000 u heparin with dextran was almost the same as after 10,000 u heparin alone.[1,2] The abstract quoted[1] contains some confusing typographical errors but the correct text has been confirmed.[2] This study would seem to explain two other reports of an increase in the incidence of bleeding in those given both heparin and dextran.[3,4]

Mechanism

Both heparin and dextran prolong coagulation time, but by a number of different and independent mechanisms. When given together their effects would seem to be additive.[3]

Importance and management

Direct documentation is limited, but the interaction seems to be established. Uneventful concurrent use[5,6] has been described with dextran 40 which suggests that the interaction may possibly be confined to the use of dextran 70, but this requires confirmation. If concurrent use is undertaken the effects should be very closely monitored and the dosage of heparin reduced as necessary (a third to a half has been recommended[1]).

References

1 Atik M. Potentiation of heparin by dextran and its clinical implication. Thromb Haemorrh (1977) 38, 275.
2 Atik M. Personal communication (1980).
3 Bloom WL and Brewer SS. The independent yet synergistic effects of heparin and dextran. Acta Chir Scand (1968) 387 (Suppl) 53.
4 Morrison N D, Stephenson CBS, Maclean D, Stanhope JM. Deep vein thrombosis after femoropopliteal bypass grafting with observations on the incidence of complications following the use of dextran 70. NZ Med J (1976) 84, 233.
5 Schondorf TH, Weber V. Prevention of deep venous thrombosis in orthopedic surgery with the combination of low dose heparin plus either

dihydroergotamine or dextran. Scand J Haematol (1980) 36 (Suppl) 126.

6 Serjeant JCB. Mesenteric embolus treated with low-molecular weight dextran. Lancet (1965) i, 139.

Heparin + Miscellaneous drugs

Abstract/Summary

Changes in the protein binding of several drugs (diazepam, propranolol, quinidine and verapamil) by heparin appears to be an artefact of the assay method used and not of clinical importance. Patients who smoke may possibly need fractionally more heparin than non-smokers.

Clinical evidence, mechanism, importance and management

(a) Diazepam, propranolol, quinidine and verapamil

A number of studies have found that heparin reduces the plasma protein binding in man and animals of several drugs including diazepam,[1] propranolol,[1] quinidine[4] and verapamil.[5] For example, three patients on oral propranolol and three given 10 mg diazepam im were given 3000 iu heparin just before cardiac catheterization. Five minutes after the heparin, the free fraction of diazepam was found to have risen four-fold (from 1.8 to 7.9%) while the free levels had risen from 2.0 to 8.4 ng/ml. The free fraction of the propranolol rose from 7.4 to 12.5% and the free levels rose from 1.7 to 2.7 ng/ml.[1]

The postulated reason for these changes was that the heparin displaces these drugs from their binding sites on the plasma albumins with additionally some changes in free fatty acid levels. It was also suggested that these changes in protein binding might possibly have some clinical consequences. For example, would there be sudden increases in sedation or respiratory depression because of the rapid increase in the active (free) fraction of diazepam ?

The answer seems to be these changes are not likely to be of clinical importance. One study suggested that the heparin-induced protein binding changes are an artefact of the study methods used,[3] and this would seem to be supported by an experimental study which failed to find that heparin had any effect on the beta-blockade of propanolol.[2] Moreover there seem to be no other reports confirming that these interactions are of real clinical importance. No special precautions would seem to be necessary.

(b) Tobacco smoking

A study of the factors affecting the sensitivity of individuals to heparin found that its half-life in smokers was 0.62 compared with 0.97 h in non-smokers. The dosage requirements of the smokers was slightly increased (18.8 compared with 16.0 U/hr/lean body weight).[6] These differences would seem to be too small to be of practical importance.

Reference.

1 Wood AJJ, Robertson D, Robertson RM, Wilkinson GR, Wood M. Elevated plasma free drug concentrations of propranolol and diazepam during cardiac catheterization. Circulation (1980) 62, 1119–22.

2 De Leve LD, Piafasky KM. Lack of heparin effect on propranolol-induced beta-adrenoceptor blockade. Clin Pharmacol Ther (1982) 31, 216.

3 Brown JE, Kitchell BB, Bjornsson TD, Shand DG. The artifactual nature of heparin-induced drug protein-binding alterations. Clin Pharmacol Ther (1981) 30, 636–43.

4 Kessler KM, Leech RC, Spann JF. Blood collection techniques, heparin and quinidine protein binding. Clin Pharmacol Ther (1979) 25, 204–10.

5 Keefe DL, Yee YG, Kates RE. Verapamil protein binding in patients and normal subjects. Clin Pharmacol Ther (1981) 29, 21–6.

6 Cipolle RJ, Seifert RD, Neilan BA, Zaske DE, Haus E. Heparin kinetics: variables related to disposition and dosage. Clin Pharmacol Ther (1981) 30, 387–93.

Heparin + Glyceryl trinitrate (Nitroglycerin) or Isosorbide dinitrate

Abstract/Summary

Some studies claim that the effects of heparin can be reduced by the concurrent infusion of nitrates, but others have failed to confirm this interaction.

Clinical evidence

(a) Heparin effects reduced

While receiving intravenous glyceryl trinitrate, seven patients with coronary artery disease needed an increased dose of intravenous heparin to achieve satisfactory anticoagulation (activated partial thromboplastin times (APTT) of 1.5–2.5 x control values). When the glyceryl trinitrate was stopped six out of the eight showed a marked increase in APTT values to 3.5. One patient had transient haematuria.[1]

This study confirms a previous report, the authors of which attributed this response to an interaction with the propylene glycol diluent of the glyceryl trinitrate infusion.[2] However it still occurred when glyceryl trinitrate was given without propylene glycol.[1] The partial thromboplastin time (PTT) of 27 patients given heparin was approximately halved (from 130 to about 60 s) when additionally given 2–5 mg/h glyceryl trinitrate intravenously. The heparin levels measured in nine patients were unchanged. The PTT rose again when the glyceryl trinitrate was stopped.[4,5] The PTT in eight out of 10 patients treated with heparin was reduced by 2–5 mg/h glyceryl trinitrate.[8] Yet another study found that concurrent use had no effect at 2 h, but heparin levels were markedly reduced (by 56%) at 4 h, and the APTT ratio was accordingly lower.[10] Reduced heparin effects have been described in other studies.[7,15,16]

(b) Heparin effects unchanged

A study in 10 patients following angioplasty found no significant APTT changes over a 30 min period following the addition of intravenous glyceryl trinitrate (41–240 g/ml) to infusions of heparin.[3] A 60-minute infusion of 5 mg glyceryl trinitrate in eight normal subjects had no effect on the APTT or prothrombin time following a 5000 u iv injection of heparin.[6] A further study in 24 patients failed to find any effects on APTT in 17 of the patients on heparin infused with 1–5 mg glyceryl trinitrate or isosorbide dinitrate, and only three had increases of more than 17 s when the nitrate was stopped.[9] No evidence of any change in the anticoagulant effect of a 40 u/kg bolus of heparin by 100 µg/min infusion of glyceryl trinitrate was found in seven normal subjects.[11] Another study in 22 patients failed to find a significant change in APTT due to heparin and glyceryl trinitrate.[13] The authors of another brief report also question the existence of this interaction.[12] Yet another study found that a glyceryl trinitrate infusion of 1 µg/kg/min had no effect on the activity of heparin (40–180 u/kg) in 13 patients on chronic nitrate treatment.[14]

Mechanism

Not understood. One study suggests that what occurs is related to a glyceryl trinitrate-induced antithrombin III abnormality.[8] Another says that heparin levels are lowered.[10]

Importance and management

The discord between these reports is not understood. Until the situation is fully resolved it would be prudent to monitor the effects of concurrent use, being alert for the need to use higher doses of heparin. If this occurs, remember to reduce the heparin dosage when the glyceryl trinitrate infusion is stopped. More study is needed.

References

1 Habbab MA, Haft JI. Heparin resistance induced by intravenous nitroglycerin. A word of caution when both drugs are used concomitantly. Arch Intern Med (1987) 147, 857–60.
2 Col J, Col-Debeys C, Lavenne-Pardonge E. Propylene glycol-induced heparin resistance. Am Heart J (1985) 110, 171–3.
3 Lepor NE, Amin DK, Berberian L and Shah PK. Does nitroglycerin induce heparin resistance? Clin Cardiol (1989) 12, 432–4.
4 Pizzulli L, Nitsch J, Luederitz B. Nitroglycerin inhibition of the heparin effect. Eur Heart J (1989) 10 (Abstr Suppl) 116.
5 Pizzulli L, Nitsch J, Luederitz B. Hemmung der Heparinwirkung durch Glyceroltrinitrat. Dtsch Med Wochensch (1988) 113, 1837–40.
6 Bode V, Welzel D, Franz G, Polensky U. Absence of drug interaction between heparin and nitroglycerin. Arch Intern Med (1990) 150, 2117–9.
7 Dascalov TN, Chaushev AG, Petrov AB, Stancheva LG, Stanachcova SD, Ivanov AA. Nitroglycerin inhibition of the heparin effect in acute myocardial infarction patients. Eur Heart J (1990) 11, (Suppl) 321.
8 Becker RC, Corrao JM, Bovill EG, Gore JM, Baker SP, Miller ML, Lucan FV, Alpert JA. Intravenous nitroglycerin-induced heparin resistance: a qualitative antithrombin III abnormality. Am Heart J (1990) 119, 1254–61.
9 Pye M, Olroyd KG, Conkie J, Hutton I, Cobbe SM. Is there an interaction between IV nitrate therapy and heparin anticoagulation ? Eur heart J (1991) 12 (Abst suppl) 80.
10 Brack MJ, Gershlick AH. Nitrate infusion even in lower dose decreases the anticoagulant effect of heparin through a direct effect on heparin levels. Eur heart J (1991) 12 (Abst suppl) 80.
11 Schoenenberger RA, Ménat L, Weiss P, Marbett GA, Ritz R. Absence of nitrogluycerin-induced heparin resistance in healthy volunteers. Eur heart J (1992) 13, 411–4.
12 Day MW, Absher RK. We don't observe the same heparin-nitroglycerin reactions. Critical Care Nurse (1992) 12, 18.
13 Gonzalez ER, Jones HD, Graham S, Elswick RK. Assessment of the drug interaction between intravenous nitroglycerin and heparin. Ann Pharmacother (1992) 26, 1512–4.
14 Reich DL, Hammerschlag BC, Rand JH, Perucho-Powell MH, Thys DM. Modest doses of nitroglycerin do not interfere with beef lung heparin anticoagulation in patients taking nitrates. J Cardiothoracic & Vasc Anesthesia (1992) 6, 677–9
15 Pizzulli L, Nitsch J, Lüderitz B. Nitroglycerin inhibition of the heparin effect. Eur Heart J (1989) 10, Abstr Suppl, 116.
16 Brack MJ, More RS, Hubner PJ, Gerschlick AH. The effect of low dose nitrogycerin on plasma heparin concentrations and activated partial thromboplastin times. Blood Coag & Fibrinolysis (1993) 4, 183–6. .

Heparin + Probenecid

Abstract/Summary

Some very limited evidence suggests that the effects of heparin may be possibly increased by probenecid and bleeding may occur.

Clinical evidence, mechanism, importance and management

In 1950 (but not reported[1] until 1975) a woman with subacute bacterial endocarditis was treated with probenecid orally and penicillin by intravenous drip, kept open with minimal doses of heparin. After a total of 215 mg (about 20,000 u) heparin had been given over a 3-week period, increasing epistaxes developed and the clotting time was found to be 24 min (normal 5–60). This was controlled with protamine. It had previously been observed that carinamide, the predecessor of probenecid, prolonged clotting times in the presence of heparin.[2] The general importance of this possible interaction is uncertain, but it would seem prudent to monitor the effects of concurrent use.

References

1 Sanchez G. Enhancement of heparin effects by probenecid. N Engl J Med (1975) 292, 48.
2 Sirka HD, McCleery RS, Artz CP. The effect of carinamide with heparin on the coagulation of human blood: a preliminary report. Surgery (1948) 24, 811.

Heparin + Streptokinase

Abstract/Summary

Patients previously treated with streptokinase appear to be partially resistant to the anticoagulant effects of heparin.

Clinical evidence, mechanism, importance and management

50 patients given streptokinase (750,000–1,500,000 u) for acute myocardial infarction needed approximately 24% more

heparin (37755 compared with 30294 u/day) in order to achieve the desired APTT than other patients who had not had streptokinase. Even then their APTTs were 15% lower. Anticoagulation was also delayed (5 days compared with 3). The reasons are not understood. On the basis of this study, anticipate the need to use higher heparin doses and to make more frequent dosage adjustments if streptokinase has been given.[1]

These patients also needed more warfarin (+12%) but this value was not statistically significant.[1] More study is needed.

Reference

1 Zagher D, Maaravi Y, Matzner Y, Gilon D, Gotsman MS, Weiss T. Partial resistance to anticoagulation after streptokinase treatment for acute myocardial infarction. Am J Cardiol (1990) 66, 28–30.

Chapter 7
Anticonvulsant Drug Interactions

The anticonvulsant drugs listed in Table 7.1 find their major application in the treatment of various kinds of epilepsy, although some of them are also used for other conditions. The list is not exclusive by any means, but it contains the anticonvulsant drugs which are discussed either in this chapter or elsewhere in this book. In addition, some of the barbiturates which are not used as anticonvulsants are also included in this chapter. The Index should be consulted for a full list of interactions involving all of these drugs.

Table 7.1 Anticonvulsant drugs

Generic or non-proprietary names	Proprietary names
Acetazolamide	*Acetamide, Atenezol, Diamox, Defiltran, Didoc, Diuramid, Diurawas, Edemox, Glaucomide, Glauconox, Glaupax, Inidrase, Oratrol*
Carbamazepine	*Convuline, Hermolepsin, Karbamazepin, Nordotold, Tegretal, Tegretol, Timonil*
Clonazepam	*Clonopin, Iktorivil, Rivotril*
Ethosuximide	*Emeside, Ethymal, Petinimid, Petnidan, Pyknolepsinum, Simatin, Suxinutin, Thetamid, Zarodan, Zarontin*
Felbamate	
Flunarizine	
Gabapentin	*Neurontin*
Lamotrigine	*Lamictal*
Methsuximide (mesuximide)	
Methylphenobarbitone (mephobarbital)	
Oxcarbazepine	*Trileptal*
Pheneturide	*Benuride*
Phenobarbitone (phenobarbital)	
Phenytoin (diphenylhydantoin)	*Antisacer, Apamin, Dantoin, Difhydan, Di-Hydan, Dilantin, Dintoina, Diphantoine, Diphenylan, Ditan, Epanutin, Epilantin, Epinat, Fenantoin, Fenytoin, Hydantol, Labopal, Lehydan, Neosidantoina, Phenhydan, Phentoin, Pyoredol, Solantyl, Tacosal, Toin Unicelles, Zentropil*
Primidone	*Dilon, Liskantin, Majdolsin, Midone, Mylepsin, Mylepsinum, Mysoline, Prosoline, Resimatil, Sertan*
Progabide	
Sodium valproate (valproic acid, dipropylacetate)	*Convulex, Convulexette, Depakene, Depakin, Depakine, Deprakine, Epilim, Logical (magnesium valproate), Orfiril, Propymal*
Stiripentol	
Sulthiame	*Ospolot*
Valpromide (dipropylacetamide)	*Depamide, Vistora*
Vigabatrin	

Anticonvulsants + Acetazolamide

Abstract/Summary

Severe osteomalacia and rickets have been seen in patients on phenytoin, phenobarbitone and primidone when concurrently treated with acetazolamide. A marked reduction in serum primidone levels with a loss in seizure control, and rises in serum carbamazepine levels with toxicity have also been described in a very small number of patients.

Clinical evidence

(a) Osteomalacia

Two young women on phenytoin, primidone or phenobarbitone developed severe osteomalacia while taking 750 mg acetazolamide daily, despite a normal intake of calcium. When the acetazolamide was withdrawn, the hyperchloraemic acidosis shown by both patients abated and the high urinary excretion of calcium fell by 50%.[1] This interaction has been described in two adults[3] and three children[2] who developed rickets.

(b) Reduced serum primidone levels

A patient on primidone showed an increased fit-frequency and a virtual absence of primidone (or phenobarbitone) in the serum when treated with 250 mg acetazolamide daily. Primidone absorption recommenced when the acetazolamide was withdrawn. A subsequent study in two other patients found that acetazolamide had a small effect on the primidone in one, and no effect in the other.[5]

(c) Increased serum carbamazepine levels

A girl of 9 and two teenage boys of 14 and 19, all of them on the highest dosages of carbamazepine tolerable without side-effects, developed signs of toxicity after taking acetazolamide (250–750 mg daily) and were found to have serum carbamazepine levels which were elevated 30–50%. In one instance toxicity appeared within 48 h.[6]

Mechanisms

Uncertain. (a) Mild osteomalacia induced by anticonvulsants is a recognized phenomenon.[4] This, it seems, is exaggerated by acetazolamide which increases urinary calcium excretion, possibly by causing systemic acidosis which results from the reduced absorption of bicarbonate by the kidney. (b and c) Not understood.

Importance and management

The documentation of all of these interactions is very limited, and their incidence uncertain. Concurrent use should be monitored for the possible development of these adverse interactions and steps taken to accommodate them. Withdraw the acetazolamide if necessary, or in the case of the anticonvulsants, adjust the dosage appropriately. In the case of the children cited[2] the acetazolamide was withdrawn and 10,000 U of vitamin D were given. It seems possible that other carbonic anhydrase inhibitors may behave like acetazolamide.

References

1 Mallette LE. Anticonvulsants, acetazolamide and osteomalacia. N Engl J Med (1975) 292, 668.
2 Matsuda I, Takekoshi Y, Shida N, Fujieda K, Nagai B, Arashima S, Anakura M, Oka Y. Renal tubular acidosis and skeletal demineralization in patients on long-term anticonvulsant therapy. J Pediatr (1975) 87, 202.
3 Mallette LE. Acetazolamide-accelerated anticonvulsant osteomalacia. Arch Intern Med (1977) 137, 1013.
4 Anast CS. Anticonvulsant drugs and calcium metabolism. N Engl J Med (1975) 292, 567.
5 Syversen GB, Morgan JP, Weintraub M, Myers GJ. Acetazolamide-induced interference with primidone absorption. Arch Neurol (1977) 34, 80.
6 McBride MC. Serum carbamazepine levels are increased by acetazolamide. Ann Neurol (1984) 16, 393.

Anticonvulsants + Aspartame

Abstract/Summary

Aspartame can cause convulsions in some susceptible individuals.

Clinical evidence, mechanism, importance and management

Grand mal seizures have been reported in 80 people associated with the consumption of aspartame (*Nutrasweet*) as a sweetening agent. Three of them were taking phenytoin. Petit mal and psychomotor attacks were also seen in another 18 subjects taking aspartame.[1] Another 149 cases of aspartame-associated convulsions have been reported to the FDA.[1] The reasons for this adverse reaction are not understood. It would seem prudent for patients taking anticonvulsants to avoid aspartame.

Reference

1 Roberts HJ. Aspartame (*Nutrasweet*)-associated epilepsy. Clin Res (1988) 36, 349A.

Anticonvulsants + Calcium channel blockers

Abstract/Summary

(A) Anticonvulsant and toxic effects increased: both diltiazem and verapamil (but not nifedipine) can increase serum carbamazepine levels causing intoxication. Diltiazem can also increase serum phenytoin levels. A single case report describes

intoxication with nifedipine but usually it appears not to interact.

(B) Calcium channel blocker effects reduced: the serum levels of felodipine and nimodipine are very markedly reduced by carbamazepine, phenobarbitone and phenytoin, but felodipine levels are only modestly reduced by oxcarbazepine. Verapamil levels may also be very much reduced by phenobarbitone and phenytoin. Nimodipine levels are raised by sodium valproate.

Clinical evidence

(A) Anticonvulsant and toxic effects increased

(a) Carbamazepine + Diltiazem or Nifedipine

An epileptic patient on 1 g carbamazepine daily developed signs of toxicity (dizziness, nausea, ataxia and diplopia) within two days of starting to take 60 mg diltiazem three times a day. His serum carbamazepine levels had risen about 50% (from 13 to 21 mg/l) but fell once again when the diltiazem was stopped. No interaction occurred when the diltiazem was replaced by nifedipine, 20 mg three times a day.[1] Five other reports describe carbamazepine toxicity in a total of about 12 patients given diltiazem.[3,10,12,15,16] One developed a 50% rise in carbamazepine serum levels,[3] and others two to three-fold rises.[10,12,15] Another patient showed a marked fall in serum carbamazepine levels (−54%) when diltiazem was stopped.[11] A retrospective study of patients suggested that nifedipine does not usually interact.[12]

(b) Carbamazepine + Verapamil

Six epileptic patients developed mild carbamazepine intoxication within 36–96 h of starting 120 mg verapamil three times a day. The symptoms disappeared when the verapamil was withdrawn. Total carbamazepine serum levels had risen by 46% (33% in free plasma carbamazepine concentrations). Rechallenge of two of the patients with less verapamil (120 mg twice a day) caused a similar rise in serum verapamil levels. This report also describes another patient with elevated serum carbamazepine levels while taking verapamil.[2] Two reports describe carbamazepine toxicity in three patients caused by verapamil. The verapamil was successfully replaced by nifedipine in one patient.[4,8]

(c) Phenytoin + Diltiazem

Two out of 14 patients on phenytoin developed elevated serum phenytoin levels and signs of toxicity when given diltiazem.[12]

(d) Phenytoin + Nifedipine

An isolated report describes intoxication in a man on phenytoin three weeks after starting to take 30 mg nifedipine daily. His serum phenytoin levels had risen to 30.4 μg/ml. Two weeks after stopping the nifedipine his serum phenytoin levels had fallen to 10.5 μg/ml and all the symptoms had gone two weeks later.[5] A retrospective study of patients suggested that nifedipine does not usually interact.[12]

(B) Calcium channel blocker effects reduced

(a) Felodipine + Carbamazepine, Oxcarbazepine, Phenobarbitone and Phenytoin

After taking 10 mg felodipine daily for four days, 10 epileptics on carbamazepine or phenytoin or phenobarbitone, or carbamazepine with phenytoin, had markedly reduced serum felodipine levels (peak levels of 1.6 nmol/l compared with 8.9 nmol/l in 12 control subjects). The AUC (area under the curve) was reduced by about 94%.[7] Another study in eight subjects found that the AUC of felodipine was reduced much less (by 28%) while taking 600–900 mg oxcarbazepine daily for a week.[17]

(b) Nifedipine + Phenobarbitone

A study in 15 normal subjects showed that after taking 100 mg phenobarbitone daily for two weeks the clearance of a single 20 mg dose of nifedipine in a 'cocktail' also containing sparteine, mephenytoin and antipyrine was increased almost threefold (from 1088 to 2981 ml/min) and the nifedipine AUC was reduced about 60% (from 343 to 135 ng.h/ml).[9]

(c) Nimodipine + Carbamazepine, Phenobarbitone, Phenytoin, Sodium valproate.

A study eight epileptic patients on chronic treatment with phenobarbitone, carbamazepine with phenobarbitone, or carbamazepine with phenytoin found that the AUC of a single 60 mg oral dose of nimodipine was more than seven-fold lower than in a group of normal subjects (9.4 compared with 104.9 ng/ml/h). In another group of epileptic patients on sodium valproate, the AUC of nimodipine was about 50% higher than in the control group.[14]

(c) Verapamil + Phenobarbitone

A study in seven normal subjects showed that after taking 100 mg phenobarbitone daily for 3 weeks the clearance of verapamil (80 mg orally 6-hourly) was increased fourfold (from 22 to 91 ml/min/kg) and the bioavailability was reduced fivefold (from 0.59 to 0.12).[6]

(d) Verapamil + Phenytoin

A woman on phenytoin showed persistently subnormal serum verapamil levels (<50 ng/ml) despite increases in the verapamil dosage. When the phenytoin was stopped, her serum verapamil levels rose to expected concentrations.[13]

Mechanism

It would appear that the calcium channel blockers inhibit the metabolism of carbamazepine and phenytoin by the liver, thereby reducing their loss from the body and increasing serum levels. In contrast, the anticonvulsants are well recognized as enzyme inducers which can increase the metabolism of the calcium channel blockers by the liver, resulting in a very rapid loss from the body.

Importance and management

(A) Information about the effects of calcium channel blockers on anticonvulsants is limited, but what is known indicates that if verapamil or diltiazem are given with carbamazepine, or diltiazem with phenytoin, the anticonvulsant dosage will need to be reduced to avoid intoxication. (about 50% with carbamazepine/diltiazem has been suggested)[15] Nifedipine normally appears to be a non-interacting alternative, but there is an isolated case with phenytoin. There appears to be no information about the effects of calcium channel blockers on other anticonvulsants.

(B) Carbamazepine, phenobarbitone and phenytoin markedly reduce felodipine and nimodipine levels, and both phenobarbitone and phenytoin can have the same effect on verapamil, and possibly on nifedipine also. A considerable increase in the dosage of these calcium channel blockers will be needed in epileptic patients taking these drugs, but oxcarbazepine has only a moderate effect. The nimodipine dosage may need to be reduced with sodium valproate. There is no direct information of interactions with other calcium channel blockers, but be alert for evidence of reduced effects with others metabolized in a similar way (nifedipine, nicardipine, nitrendipine).

References

1 Brodie MJ, Macphee GJA. Carbamazepine neurotoxicity precipitated by diltiazem. Brit Med J (1986) 292, 1170–1.
2 Macphee GJA, McInnes GT, Thompson GG, Brodie MJ. Verapamil potentiates carbamazepine neurotoxicity: a clinically important inhibitory interaction. Lancet (1986) i, 700–3.
3 Eimer M, Carter BL. Elevated serum carbamazepine concentrations following diltiazem initiation. Drug Intell Clin Pharm (1987) 21, 340–2.
4 Beattie B, Biller J, Mehlaus B, Murray M. Verapamil-induced carbamazepine neurotoxicity. Eur Neurol (1988) 28, 104–5.
5 Ahmad S. Nifedipine-phenytoin interaction. J Am Coll Cardiol (1984) 3, 1582.
6 Rutledge DR, Pieper JA, Sirmans SM, Mirvis DM. Verapamil disposition after phenobarbital treatment. Clin Pharmacol Ther (1987) 41, 245.
7 Capewell S, Freestone S, Critchely JAJH, Pottage A, Prescott LF. Reduced felodipine bioavailability in patients taking anticonvulsants. Lancet (1988) ii, 480–2.
8 Price WA, Di Marzio LR. Verapamil-carbamazepine neurotoxicity. J Clin Psychiatry (1988) 49, 80.
9 Schellens JHM, van der Wart JHF, Brugman M, Breimer DD. Influence of enzyme induction and inhibition on the oxidation of nifedipine, sparteine, mephenytoin and antipyrine in humans assessed by a 'cocktail' study design. J Pharmacol Exp Ther (1989) 249, 638–45.
10 Ahmad S. Diltiazem-carbamazepine interaction. Am Heart J (1990) 120, 1485.
11 Gadde K, Calabrese JR. Diltiazem effect on carbamazepine levels in manic depression. J Clin Psychopharmacol (1990) 10, 378–9.
12 Bahls FH, Ozuna J, Ritchie DE. Interactions between clacium channel blockers and the anticonvulsants carbamazepine and phenytoin. Neurology (1991) 41, 740–2.
13 Woodcock BG, Kirsten R, Nelson K, Rietbrock S, Hopf R, Kaltenbach M. A reduction in verapamil concentrations with phenytoin. N Eng J Med (1990) 325, 1179.
14 Tartara A, Galimberti CA, Manni R, Parietti L, Zucca C, Baasch H, Caresia L, Mück W, Barzaghi N, Gatti G, Perucca E. Differential effects of valproic acid and enzyme-inducing anticonvulsants on nimodipine pharmacokinetics in epileptic patients. Br J clin Pharmac (1991) 32, 335–40.
15 Shaughnessy AF, Mosley MR. Elevated carbamazepine levels associated with diltiazem use. Neurology (1992) 42, 937–8.
16 Maoz E, Grossman E, Thaler M, Rosenthal T. Carbamazepine neurotoxic reaction after administration of diltiazem. Arch Intern med (1992) 152, 2503–4.
17 Zaccara G, Gangemi PW, Bendoni L, Menge GP, Schwabe S, Monza GC. Influence of single and repeated doses of oxcarbazepine on the pharmcokinetic profile of felodipine. Ther Drug Monit (1993) 15, 39–42.

Anticonvulsants + Cinromide

Abstract/Summary

Cinromide can depress the serum levels of phenytoin, carbamazepine and sodium valproate.

Clinical evidence, mechanism, importance and management

A very brief report states that during concurrent use cinromide was seen to reduce serum concentrations of phenytoin by 18%, of carbamazepine by 31% and (in one patient) of sodium valproate by 41%.[1] The clinical importance of these interactions is uncertain.

Reference

1 Cramer JA, Mattson RH. Cinromide pharmacokinetics and interactions. Epilepsia (1981) 22, 235.

Anticonvulsants + Cytotoxic drugs

Abstract/Summary

Carbamazepine, phenytoin and sodium valproate serum levels can fall during concurrent treatment with several cytotoxic drug regimens and seizures can occur if the anticonvulsant dosages are not raised appropriately. In contrast, both UFT and tegafur have been responsible for causing acute phenytoin intoxication. The effects of some cytotoxics are reduced or changed by anticonvulsants (details in Chapter 12).

Clinical evidence

(a) Anticonvulsant levels reduced

A retrospective study of 26 patients who had had three or more cycles of either cisplatin or carmustine, or both, showed that an average 41% increase in phenytoin dosage was needed (range 20–100%).[11] Two reports[1,2] describe two patients who showed a marked fall in serum phenytoin levels (from an estimated 15 to 2 μg/ml in one case accompanied by seizures) when concurrently treated with bleomycin, cisplatin, and vinblastine. The phenytoin absorption from the gut was reduced to 22–32%.[1] Another report described a similar interaction in a patient on carmustine, vinblastine and methotrexate.[3,4] On two occasions an epileptic woman treated with phenytoin, carbamazepine and sodium valproate had seizures within 2–3 days of starting a Chap-V course (intravenous doxorubicin, 35 mg/m² on day 1 and cisplatin 20 mg/m² for days 1–5). The serum levels of all three anticonvulsants fell below therapeutic levels.[5] On a third occasion the trough serum levels of carbamazepine and sodium valproate from days 5/7 to 13 were seen to decrease from 3.6 to 1.2 and from 40.9 to 10 mg/l respectively when given these cytotoxic drugs.[5] A child with lymphoblastic leukaemia needed a 100% increased in his phenytoin dosage after treatment with high-dose methotrexate, folinic acid, vincristine, daunorubicin, colaspase and prednisone.[10] The carbamazepine serum levels of a child with malignant lymphoblastic lymphoma fell when given chemotherapy, often falling below therapeutic concentrations, and convulsions occurred. They rose again when the chemotherapy was stopped.[9] The chemotherapy included cytarabine/vincristine, hydroxyurea/daunorubicin, methotrexate/lomustine and thioguanine/cyclophosphamide.[9]

(b) Anticonvulsant levels raised

Three patients with malignant brain tumours developed acute phenytoin intoxication associated with raised serum phenytoin levels when concurrently treated with UFT (uracil and tegafur, a masked compound of 5-FU). One of the patients showed no interaction when the UFT was replaced by 5-FU.[6] Acute phenytoin intoxication has been described with UFT in another report,[7] and in a further report involving tegafur alone.[8]

(c) Cytotoxic effects reduced or altered

See 'Doxorubicin + Barbiturates', 'Ifosfamide + Barbiturates', 'Streptozocin + Phenytoin', 'Teniposide + Anticonvulsants' in Chapter 12. Use the index.

Mechanisms

Not fully established, but a suggested reason for the fall in serum anticonvulsant levels is that these cytotoxic drugs damage the intestinal wall which reduces the absorption of the anticonvulsants. Other mechanisms may also have some part to play. The raised serum phenytoin levels possibly occur because the liver metabolism of the phenytoin is reduced by these cytotoxics. Changes in plasma protein binding may also have be involved.

Importance and management

Information is scattered and incomplete, but the interactions appear to be established. Serum anticonvulsant levels should be closely monitored during treatment with any of these cytotoxics, making dosage adjustments as necessary.

References

1 Sylvester RK, Lewis FB, Caldwell KC, Lobell M, Perri R, Sawchuk RA. Impaired phenytoin bioavailability secondary to cisplatinum, vinblastine and bleomycin. Ther Drug Monit (1984) 6, 302–5.

2 Fincham RW, Schottelius DD. Case report. Decreased phenytoin levels in antineoplastic therapy. Ther Drug Monit (1979) 1, 277.

3 Riva R, Albani F, Baruzzi A. On the interaction between phenytoin and antineoplastic agents. Ther Drug Monit (1985) 7, 123–6.

4 Bollini P, Riva R, Albani F, Ida N, Cacciari L, Bollini C, Baruzzi A. Decreased phenytoin level during antineoplastic therapy: a case report. Epilepsia (1983) 24, 75–8.

5 Neef C, de Voogd-van der Straaten I. An interaction between cytostatic and anticonvulsant drugs. Clin Pharmacol Ther (1988) 43, 372–5.

6 Wakisaka S, Shimauchi M, Kaji Y, Nonaka A, Kinoshita K. Acute phenytoin intoxication associated with the antineoplastic agent UFT. Fukuoka Acta med (1990) 81, 192–6.

7 Japanese Ministry of Health and Welfare: Report of Adverse Effects of Drugs, no 85, June (1987).

8 Hara T, Ichimiya A. Acute phenytoin intoxication caused by drug interaction with an antitumour agent, tegafur. 20th Jap Conf Epilepsia, Tokyo, Nov 1986.

9 Nahum MP, Ben Arush MW, Robinson E. Reduced plasma carbamazepine level during chemotherapy in a child with malignant lymphoma. Acta Paed Scand (1990) 79, 873–5.

10 Jarosinski PF, Moscow JA, Alexander MS. Altered phenytoin clearance during intensive treatment for acute lymphoblastic leukemia. J Pediatr (1988) 112, 996–99.

11 Grossman SA, Sheidler VR, Gilbert MR. Decreased phenytoin levels in patients receiving chemotherapy. Am J Med (1989) 87, 505–10.

Anticonvulsants + Denzimol

Abstract/Summary

Very marked and rapid rises in the serum levels of carbamazepine and phenytoin occur, accompanied by acute toxicity, if denzimol is given concurrently. No interaction seems to occur with either sodium valproate or primidone.

Clinical evidence, mechanism, importance and management

All six patients on carbamazepine showed very marked rises in serum concentrations within 5–30 days and acute toxicity when concurrently treated with denzimol (150–450 mg daily). Despite a reduction in the carbamazepine dosage in four of the six, serum levels rose by 114% (range 50–142%). Two patients on phenytoin showed rises of 97 and 174% respectively over a five-week period. Seven other patients taking sodium valproate or primidone showed no significant changes in their serum levels.[1] It is suggested that the rises in serum anticonvulsant levels occur because denzimol inhibits the metabolism of carbamazepine and phenytoin by the liver. More study is needed to assess whether it can safely be given routinely with these two anticonvulsants.

Reference

1 Patsalos PN, Shorvon SD, Elyas AA, Smith G. The interaction of denzimol (a new anticonvulsant) with carbamazepine and phenytoin. J Neurol Neurosurg Psychiatry (1985) 48, 374–7.

Anticonvulsants + Dextromethorphan

Abstract/Summary

Dextromethorphan appears not to affect the serum levels of carbamazepine or phenytoin, but some increase in seizure frequency may occur.

Clinical evidence, mechanism, importance and management

A double-blind cross-over study in epileptic patients with severe complex partial seizures, five on carbamazepine and four on phenytoin, found that the concurrent use of dextromethorphan (120 mg daily) in liquid form (*Delsym*) over three months had no effect on the serum anticonvulsant levels. Complex partial seizure frequency rose by 25% but this was said not to be clinically significant.[1]

Reference

1 Fisher RS, Cysyk BJ, Lesser RP, Pontecorvo MJ, Ferkany JT, Schwerdt PR, Hart J, Gordon B. Dextromethorphan for treatment of complex partial seizures. Neurology (1990) 40, 547–8.

Anticonvulsants + Dextropropoxyphene

Abstract/Summary

Carbamazepine serum levels can be raised by the concurrent use of dextropropoxyphene. Toxicity may develop unless suitable dosage reductions are made. A trivial or only modest rise in serum phenytoin or phenobarbitone levels may occur so that the development of toxicity is unlikely in most patients. Oxcarbazepine appears not to interact.

Clinical evidence

(a) Carbamazepine + Dextropropoxyphene

The observation of toxicity (headache, dizziness, ataxia, nausea, tiredness) during the concurrent use of carbamazepine and dextropropoxyphene prompted further study. Five subjects given 65 mg dextropropoxyphene three times a day showed a mean rise in serum carbamazepine levels of 65%. Three of them showed evidence of carbamazepine toxicity.[1–2] In another study the same workers found a 66% rise in other subjects after six days treatment with dextropropoxyphene.[3]

Intoxication due to this interaction is reported elsewhere.[4,5,7,8] 69–600% rises in trough serum carbamazepine levels have been described.[8]

(b) Oxcarbamazepine + Dextropropoxyphene

6 days treatment with 65 mg dextropropoxyphene three times daily did not affect the steady-state levels of the active metabolite of oxcarbamazepine (750–2700 mg daily) in seven patients with epilepsy or trigeminal neuralgia.[9]

(c) Phenobarbitone + Dextropropoxyphene

Four epileptics averaged a 20% rise in serum phenobarbitone levels after taking dextropropoxyphene 65 mg three times a day for a week.[3]

(d) Phenytoin + Dextropropoxyphene

Only a very small rise in serum phenytoin levels occurred in six patients when concurrently treated with dextropropoxyphene (65 mg three times a day) for 6–13 days.[3] In contrast, one patient is reported to have experienced a marked elevation in serum phenytoin levels while taking dextropropoxyphene.[6]

Mechanisms

Uncertain. It is suggested that the dextropropoxyphene inhibits the metabolism of the carbamazepine by the liver enzymes, leading to its accumulation in the body,[1–2] and this may also be true to a much lesser extent for the phenobarbitone.

Importance and management

The carbamazepine-dextropropoxyphene interaction is well established and clinically important. Avoid concurrent use. If dextropropoxyphene is absolutely necessary, monitor the serum carbamazepine levels and make suitable dosage reductions to prevent the development of intoxication. In most cases it would seem simpler to use a non-interacting analgesic, although the occasional single dose may not matter. The concurrent use of dextropropoxyphene and either phenytoin or phenobarbitone need not be avoided, but since rises in the serum levels of both anticonvulsants can occur it would be prudent to monitor the outcome. No special precautions seem necessary with oxcarbazepine.

References

1 Dam M, Christiansen J. Interaction of propoxyphene with carbamazepine. Lancet (1977) ii, 509.
2 Dam M, Kristensen B, Hansen BS, Christiansen J. Interaction between carbamazepine and propoxyphene in man. Acta Neurol Scand (1977) 56, 603.
3 Hansen BS, Dam M, Brandt J, Hvidberg EF, Angelo H, Christensen JM, Lous P. Influence of dextropropoxyphene on steady state serum levels and protein binding of three anti-epileptic drugs in man. Acta Neurol Scand (1980) 61, 357.

4 Yu YL, Huang CY, Chin E, Woo E, Chang CM. Interaction between carbamazepine and dextropropoxyphene. Postgrad Med J (1986) 62, 231–3.

5 Kubacka RT, Ferrante JA. Carbamazepine-propoxyphene interaction. Clin Pharm (1983) 2, 104.

6 Kutt H. Biochemical and genetic factors regulating Dilantin metabolism in man. Ann NY Acad Sci (1971) 179, 704.

7 Risinger MW. Carbamazepine toxicity with concurrent use of propoxyphene: a report of five cases. Neurology (1987) 37 (Suppl 1) 87.

8 Oles KS, Mirza W, Penry JK. Catastrophic neurologic signs due to drug interaction: Tegretol and Darvon. Surg Neurol (1989) 32, 144–51.

9 Mogensen PH, Jorgensen L, Boas J, Dam M, Vesterager A, Flesch G, Jensen PK. Effects of dextropropoxyphene on the steady-state kinetics of oxcarbazepine and its metabolites. Acta Neurol Scand (1992) 85, 14–17.

Anticonvulsants + Disulfiram

Abstract/Summary

Phenytoin serum levels are markedly and rapidly increased by the concurrent use of disulfiram. Phenytoin intoxication can develop. There is evidence that phenobarbitone and carbamazepine are not affected by disulfiram, and that calcium carbimide does not interact with phenytoin.

Clinical evidence

The serum phenytoin levels of four patients on long-term treatment showed rises of 100–500% over a 9-day period when concurrently treated with 400 mg disulfiram daily, with no signs of levelling off until the disulfiram was withdrawn. Two of them developed signs of mild intoxication.[1] In a follow-up study on two patients, one of them showed ataxia and a serum phenytoin rise of 55% (from 18 to 28 μg/ml) within five days.[1,2] Disulfiram increased the half-life of phenytoin in 10 normal subjects from 11 to 19 h.[3] There are other case reports describing this interaction.[4–7]

Mechanism

The disulfiram inhibits the liver enzymes concerned with the metabolism of the phenytoin, thereby prolonging its stay in the body and resulting in a rise in its serum levels (to toxic concentrations in some instances). One study concluded that the inhibition was non-competitive.[7]

Importance and management

An established, moderately well documented, clinically important and potentially serious interaction. It seems to occur in most patients and develops rapidly. Recovery may take 2–3 weeks when the disulfiram is withdrawn. Olesen[1,2] offers the opinion that the dosage of phenytoin '...could of course be reduced [to accommodate the interaction] but it would be difficult to maintain the precise balance required...'.

Alternative anticonvulsants include phenobarbitone which in one study[2,3] (paralleling those cited above) showed only minor serum level fluctuations (10%) with disulfiram. Three of the patients were taking primidone and one phenobarbitone. Carbamazepine also appears not to interact. Signs of toxicity disappeared in a patient when phenytoin was replaced by carbamazepine,[6] and this observation was confirmed in a study on five non-alcoholic patients.[8]

A different solution is to replace the disulfiram with calcium carbimide. A study in four patients showed that 50 mg daily for a week followed by 100 mg for two weeks had no effect on serum phenytoin levels.[2]

References

1 Olesen OV. Disulfiramum (Antabuse) as inhibitor of phenytoin metabolism. Acta pharmacol et toxicol (1966) 24, 317.

2 Olesen OV. The influence of disulfiram and calcium carbimide on the serum diphenylhydantoin excretion of HPPH in the urine. Arch Neurol (1967) 16, 642.

3 Svendsen TL, Kristensen MB, Hansen JM, Skovsted L. The influence of disulfiram on the half-life and metabolic clearance rate of diphenylhydantoin and tolbutamide in man. Europ J clin Pharmacol (1976) 9, 439.

4 Kiorboe E. Phenytoin intoxication during treatment with Antabuse. Epilepsia (1966) 7, 246.

5 Kiorboe E. Antabus som arsag til forgiftning med fenytoin. Ugeskr laeg (1966) 128, 1531.

6 Dry J, Pradalier A. Intoxication par la phenytoin au cours d'une association therapeutique avec le disulfirame. Therapie (1973) 28, 799.

7 Taylor JW, Alexander B, Lyon LW. Mathematical analysis of a phenytoin-disulfiram interaction. Amer J Hosp Pharm (1981) 38, 93.

8 Krag B, Dam M, Helle A, Christensen JM. Influence of disulfiram on the serum concentrations of carbamazepine in patients with epilepsy. Acta neurol Scand (1981) 63, 395.

Anticonvulsants + Erythromycin

Abstract/Summary

Carbamazepine serum levels can very rapidly rise to toxic concentrations if erythromycin is given concurrently. Intoxication has been described in many reports. An isolated report describes sodium valproate intoxication in a woman given erythromycin. Erythromycin appears not to interact with oxcarbazepine or phenytoin.

Clinical evidence

(a) Carbamazepine

A girl of eight on 50 mg phenobarbitone and 800 mg carbamazepine daily was additionally given 500 mg and later 1000 mg erythromycin daily. Within two days she began to experience balancing difficulties and ataxia which were eventually attributed to carbamazepine intoxication. Her serum carbamazepine levels were found to have risen from a little below 10 μg/ml to over 25 μg/ml (therapeutic range 2–10 μg/ml).[1]

Marked rises in serum carbamazepine levels (two to fourfold) and/or intoxication within 24–72 h of starting erythromycin have been described in children and adults. At least 30 cases of carbamazepine intoxication have been reported.[3–11,13–17,19–22] Sinus arrest and AV block developed in a child.[21] 1 g erythromycin daily for five days in eight normal subjects reduced the clearance of carbamazepine by an average of 20% (range 5–41%).[2] Another study confirmed this interaction.[18]

(b) Oxcarbazepine

The pharmacokinetics of single 600 mg doses of oxcarbazepine in eight normal subjects were unaffected by seven day's treatment with 500 mg erythromycin twice daily.[24]

(c) Phenytoin

Single dose studies show that the clearance of phenytoin is unchanged by erythromycin treatment.[12]

(d) Sodium valproate

A woman taking lithium and 3500 mg sodium valproate daily developed fatigue and walking difficulties a day after starting 250 mg erythromycin four times daily, and within a week she had slurred speech, confusion, difficulty in concentrating and a worsening gait. Her serum valproate levels had risen from 88 mg/l (measured 2 months before) to 260 mg/l. She recovered rapidly when the valproate and erythromycin were withdrawn. Her serum lithium levels remained unchanged.[23]

Mechanism

It is suggested that erythromycin has a high affinity for the active site on the liver enzymes concerned with the metabolism of the carbamazepine so that the metabolism of the latter is rapidly and markedly inhibited, resulting in its rapid accumulation which leads to toxicity.[11]

Importance and management

The carbamazepine/erythromycin interaction is very well-documented and established. Its incidence is uncertain. Concurrent use should be avoided unless the effects can be very closely monitored (measurement of serum carbamazepine levels) and suitable dosage reductions made. Toxic symptoms (ataxia, vertigo, drowsiness, lethargy, confusion, diplopia) can develop very rapidly (within 24 h), and serum carbamazepine levels can return to normal within 8–12 h of withdrawing the antibiotic.[10] It has been suggested that '...the interaction may be more intense at higher erythromycin dosing rates (for instance 500 mg every 6 h).'[2] There is only a single case report of erythromycin interacting with sodium valproate, but it would be prudent to monitor concurrent use. Erythromycin appears not to interact with oxcarbazepine or phenytoin.

References

1 Amedee-Manesme O, Rey E, Brussieux J, Goutieres F, Aicardi J. Antibiotiques a ne jamais associer a la carbamazepine. Arch Fr Pediatr (1982) 39, 126.
2 Wong YY, Ludden TM, Bell RD. Effect of erythromycin on carbamazepine kinetics. Drug Intell Clin Pharm (1983) 16, 484.
3 Straughan J. Erythromycin-carbamazepine interaction. S Afr Med J (1982) 61, 420–1.
4 Mesdjian E, Dravet C, Cenraud B, Roger J. Carbamazepine intoxication due to triacetyloleandomycin administration in epileptic patients. Epilepsia (1980) 21, 489–96.
5 Vajda FJE and Bladin PF. Carbamazepine-erythromycin base interaction. Med J Aust (1984) 2, 81.
6 Hedrick R, Williams F, Morin R, Lamb WA, Cate JC. Carbamazepine-erythromycin interaction leading to carbamazepine toxicity in four epileptic children. Ther Drug Monit (1983) 5, 405–7.
7 Miller SL. The association of carbamazepine intoxication and erythromycin use. Ann Neurol (1985) 18, 413.
8 Berrettini WH. A case of erythromycin-induced carbamazepine toxicity. J Clin Psychiatry (1986) 47, 147.
9 Carranco E, Kareus J, Co S, Peak V, Al-Rajeh S. Carbamazepine toxicity induced by concurrent erythromycin therapy. Arch Neurol (1985) 42, 187–8.
10 Goulden KJ, Camfield P, Dooley JM, Fraser A, Meek DC, Renton KW, Tibbles JAR. Severe carbamazepine intoxication after coadministration of erythromycin. J Pediatr (1986) 109, 135–8.
11 Wroblewski BA, Singer WD, Whyte J. Carbamazepine-erythromycin interaction. Case studies and clinical significance. J Amer Med Ass (1986) 255, 1165–7.
12 Bachmann K, Schwartz JI, Forney RB, Jauregui L. Single dose phenytoin clearance during erythromycin treatment. Res Comm Chem Path Pharmacol (1984) 46, 207–17.
13 Kessler JM. Erythromycin-carbamazepine interaction. S Afr Med J (1985) 67, 1038.
14 Jaster PJ, Abbas D. Erythromycin-carbamazepine interaction. Neurology (1986) 36, 594–5.
15 Loiseau P, Guyot M, Pautrizel B, Vincon G, Albin H. Intoxication par la carbamazepine due a l'interaction carbamazepine-erythromycine. La Presse Med (1985) 14, 162.
16 Zitelli BJ, Howrie DL, Altman H, Marcon TJ. Erythromycin-induced drug interactions. Clin Ped (1987) 26, 117–19.
17 Beeley L, Magee P, Hickey FM. Bulletin of West Midlands Centre for Adverse Drug Reaction Reporting (1989) 29, 24.
18 Miles MV, Tennison MB. Erythromycin effects on multiple-dose carbamazepine kinetics. Ther Drug Monit (1989) 11, 47–52.
19 Goldhoorn PB, Hofstee N. Een interactie tussen erytromycine en carbamazepine. Ned Tijdschr Geneeskd (1989) 133, 1944.
20 Mitsch RA. Carbamazepine toxicity precipitated by intravenous erythromycin. DICP Ann Pharmacotherapy (1989) 23, 878–9.
21 Macnab AJ, Robinson JL, Adderley RJ, D'Orsogna L. Heart block secondary to erythromycin-induced carbamazepine toxicity. Paediatrics (1987) 80, 951–3.
22 Woody RC, Kearns GL, Bolyard KJ. Carbamazepine intoxication following the use of erythromycin in children. Ped Infect Dis J (1987) 6, 578–9.
23 Redington K, Wells C, Petito F. Erythromycin and valproate interaction. Ann Intern Med (1992) 116, 877–8.
24 Keränen Y, Jolkkonen T, Jensen J, Menge GP, Andersson P. Absence of interaction between oxcarbazepine and erythromycin. Acta Neurol Scand (1992) 86, 120–3.

Sodium valproate + Felbamate

Abstract/Summary

Felbamate can raise sodium valproate serum levels

Clinical evidence, mechanism, importance and management

The steady-state sodium valproate levels in eight epileptics were raised 28% (from 66.9 to 85.4 μg/ml) by 1200 mg felbamate daily, and by 54% (from 66.9 to 103.0 μg/ml) by

2400 mg daily.[1] The reasons are not understood. It may be necessary to reduce the sodium valproate dosage to avoid toxicity if felbamate is given. More study is needed to establish the clinical importance of this interaction.

Reference

1 Wagner ML, Graves NM, Leppik IE, Remmel RP, Ward DL, Shumaker RC. The effect of felbamate on valproate disposition. Epilepsia (1991) 32, Suppl 3, 15.

Anticonvulsants + Fluzinamide

Abstract/Summary

Phenytoin reduces serum fluzinamide levels, while fluzinamide raises serum phenytoin levels. Neurotoxicity has been seen when fluzinamide was given with phenytoin and carbamazepine.

Clinical evidence

(a) Fluzinamide serum levels reduced

A double-blind multiple dose study in 12 normal subjects taking 200 mg fluzinamide 8-hourly showed that the concurrent use of 100 mg phenytoin 8-hourly for 7 days reduced the fluzinamide AUC by a third (from 24 to 16 μg/h/ml).[1] The AUCs of the three metabolites were also reduced.

(b) Phenytoin serum levels increased

A parallel study in 12 other normal subjects taking 100 mg phenytoin 8-hourly found that the concurrent use of 200 mg fluzinamide 8-hourly for 7 days increased the phenytoin AUC by 50% (from 64 to 97 μg/h/ml).[1]

Mechanisms

Not understood. No marked changes in plasma protein binding were seen in this study.[1]

Importance and management

Information appears to be limited to this study. The clinical importance of these findings is uncertain, but it is clear that concurrent use should be well monitored. The authors of the report say that patients in previous studies with partial seizures demonstrated neurotoxicity when fluzinamide was given with phenytoin and carbamazepine.[1]

Reference

1 Carchman S H, Crowe J T, Wright G J. Steady-state interactions between antiepileptic drugs fluzinamide and phenytoin. Clin Pharmacol Ther (1986) 39, 185.

Anticonvulsants + Folic acid

Abstract/Summary

If folic acid supplements are given to treat the folate deficiency which can be caused by the use of anticonvulsants (phenytoin, phenobarbitone, primidone and possibly pheneturide), the serum anticonvulsant levels may fall, leading to decreased seizure control in some patients.

Clinical evidence

A study on 50 folate-deficient epileptics (taking phenytoin with phenobarbitone and primidone) found that after one month's treatment with 5 mg folic acid daily, the serum phenytoin levels of one group (10 patients) had fallen from 20 to 10 μg/ml, and of another group taking 15 mg daily from 14 to 10 μg/ml. Only one patient showed a marked increase in fit frequency and severity.[1]

Another long-term study on 26 patients with folic acid deficiency (less than 5 ng/ml) due to anticonvulsant treatment with two or more drugs (phenytoin, phenobarbitone, primidone) found that when they were given 15 mg folic acid daily the mental state of 22 of them improved to a variable degree, but the frequency and severity of fits in 13 (50%) increased to such an extent that the vitamin had to be withdrawn.[2] Similar results have been described in other studies and reports.[2,3,8,10]

Mechanism

Patients on anticonvulsants not infrequently have subnormal serum folic acid levels (frequencies of 27–58% have been reported[4]) due, so it is believed, to the enzyme-inducing characteristics of the anticonvulsants which make excessive demands on folate for the synthesis of the cytochromic enzymes concerned with drug metabolism. Ultimately drug metabolism becomes limited by the lack of folate, and patients may also develop a depression in their general mental health[2] and even frank megaloblastic anaemia.[7] If however folic acid is given to treat this deficiency, the metabolism of the anticonvulsant increases once again,[9] resulting in a reduction in serum anticonvulsant levels which, in some instances, may become so low that seizure control is partially or totally lost.

Importance and management

A very well documented and clinically important interaction (only a few references are listed here). Reductions in serum phenytoin levels of 16–50% after taking 5–15 mg folic acid daily for 2–4 weeks have been described.[2–5] The incidence is uncertain (reports range from 0–50%[1,2,6]). Folic acid supplements should only be given to folate-deficient epileptics taking phenytoin, phenobarbitone, primidone and possibly pheneturide if their serum anticonvulsant levels can be well monitored so that suitable dosage increases can be made.

References

1 Baylis EM, Crowley JM, Preece JM, Sylvester PE, Marks V. Influence of folic acid on blood-phenytoin levels. Lancet (1971) i, 62.

2 Reynolds EH. Effects of folic acid on the mental state and fit-frequency of drug-treated epileptics. Lancet (1967) i, 1086.

3 Strauss RG, Bernstein R. Folic acid and Dilantin antagonism in pregnancy. Obstet Gynecol (1974) 44, 345.

4 Davis RE, Woodliff HJ. Folic acid deficiency in patients receiving anticonvulsant drugs. Med J Aust (1971) 2, 1070.

5 Furlanut M, Benetello P, Avogaro A, Dainese R. Effects of folic acid on phenytoin kinetics in healthy subjects. Clin Pharmacol Ther (1978) 24, 294.

6 Grant RHE and Stores OPR. Folic acid in folate-deficient patients with epilepsy. Brit Med J (1970) 4, 644.

7 Ryan GMS and Forshaw JWB. Megaloblastic anaemia due to phenytoin sodium. Brit Med J (1955) 11, 242.

8 Latham AN, Millbank L, Richens A, Rowe DJF. Liver enzyme induction by anticonvulsant drugs, and its relationship to disturbed calcium and folic acid metabolism. J Clin Pharmacol (1973) 13, 337.

9 Berg MJ, Fischer LJ, Rivey MP, Vern BA, Lantz RK, Schottelius DD. Phenytoin and folic acid interaction: a preliminary report. Ther Drug Monit (1983) 5, 389–94.

10 Berg MJ, Fincham RW, Ebert BE, Schottelius DD. Phenytoin pharmacokinetics: before and after folic acid administration. Epilepsia (1992) 33, 712–20.

Anticonvulsants + Gabapentin

Abstract/Summary

Gabapentin does not affect the pharmacokinetics of carbamazepine, phenytoin, phenobarbitone or sodium valproate.

Clinical evidence, mechanism, importance and management

The pharmacokinetics of both phenytoin and gabapentin remained unchanged in eight epileptics when given 400 mg gabapentin three times daily for eight days. The patients had been taking phenytoin for at least two months.[1] Gabapentin also does not affect phenobarbitone levels, or be affected by phenobarbitone.[2] Other studies confirm that the steady-state pharmacokinetics of carbamazepine, phenobarbitone, phenytoin and sodium valproate are unaffected by gabapentin, and that the pharmacokinetics of gabapentin are similarly unaffected by these anticonvulsants.[3,4] No dosage adjustments are therefore needed if gabapentin is added to treatment with these anticonvulsants.

References

1 Anhut H, Leppik I, Schmidt B, Thomann P. Drug interaction study of a new anticonvulsant gabapentin with phenytoin in epileptic patients. Naunyn-Schmied Arch Pharmacol (1988) 337, Suppl R127.

2 Hooper WD, Kavanagh MC, Herkes GK, Eadie MJ. Lack of a pharmacokinetic interaction between phenobarbitone and gabapentin. Br J clin Pharmac (1991) 31, 171–4.

3 Brockbrader HN, Radulovic LL, Loewen G, Chang T, Welling PG, Reece PA, Underwood B, Sedman AJ. Lack of drug-drug interactions between neurontin (gabapentin) and other antiepileptic drugs. 20th Int Epilepsy Congress, Oslo, Norway, July 1993 (Abstract).

4 Richens A. Clinical pharmacokinetics of gabapentin, in 'New Trends in Epilesy Management: The Role of Gabapentin' (ed D. Chadwick). Proceedings of a satellite symposium, Epilepsy Europe 1992. Int Congress and Symposium Series No 198, Roy Soc Med Services, London, NY 1993. p 41–6

Anticonvulsants + Influenza vaccines

Abstract/Summary

Influenza vaccine can cause a rise in serum phenobarbitone levels, but carbamazepine is unaffected. See also 'Phenytoin + Influenza vaccines'.

Clinical evidence, mechanism, importance and management

Serum phenobarbitone levels rose by 30% in 11 out of 27 children (very prolonged in some individuals) when given 0.5 ml of an influenza vaccine, USP, types A and B, whole virus (Squibb), but no significant changes occurred in the serum carbamazepine levels of another 20 children.[1] The suggested reason is the vaccine inhibits the liver enzymes concerned with the metabolism of phenobarbitone, thereby reducing its loss from the body. Information is very limited but it now seem prudent to monitor the effect of giving influenza vaccines to patients treated with phenobarbitone. See also 'Phenytoin + Influenza vaccines'.

Reference

1 Jann MW, Fidone GS. Effect of influenza vaccine on serum anticonvulsant concentrations. Clin Pharm (1986) 5, 817–20.

Anticonvulsants + Lamotrigine

Abstract/Summary

Lamotrigine increases the serum levels of the active metabolite of carbamazepine. Toxicity may develop if the carbamazepine dosage is not reduced. Sodium valproate reduces the loss of lamotrigine from the body. Phenobarbitone, phenytoin and primidone are reported not to be affected by lamotrigine.

Clinical evidence, mechanism, importance and management

(a) Carbamazepine

A study in three epileptics on carbamazepine found that the addition of lamotrigine increased the serum levels of the active metabolite of carbamazepine (carbamazepine epoxide), but carbamazepine levels remain unchanged. One patient had carbamazepine epoxide serum levels of 2.0–2.2 µg/ml while on 1100 mg carbamazepine daily which rose to 4.7–8.7 µg/ml when lamotrigine was added. Toxicity occurred in two of the patients (dizziness, double vision, sleepiness, nausea).[1] In another study in 10 patients the addition of 200 mg lamotrigine increased the the mean serum carbamazepine-epoxide serum levels by 47%. Toxicity was seen (dizziness, nausea, diplopia).[2,7] The reasons for the reaction are not known. No changes in carbamazepine levels were seen in another study.[5] Information is still very limited, but in practical terms it means that serum carbamazepine epoxide levels should be well monitored if lamotrigine is added. Be alert for the need to reduce the carbamazepine dosage.

(b) Phenobarbitone, phenytoin, primidone

No changes in the serum levels of these anticonvulsants were seen in a study in patients concurrently treated with 75 to 400 mg lamotrigine daily.[5] No special precautions seem necessary.

(c) Sodium valproate

200 mg sodium valproate 8-hourly reduced the clearance of lamotrigine in six subjects by 20% (from 0.372 to 0.297 ml/min/kg) and increased the AUC by 30%. It is thought that the two drugs compete for glucuronidation by the liver.[3,6] A meta-analysis of large numbers of epileptics found that although patients on both drugs tended to be taking lower doses of lamotrigine than other patients, the mean serum levels achieved were roughly doubled. If at the same time they were also taking enzyme-inducing anticonvulsants, their serum levels of lamotrigine were only raised about 40%.[4] The general picture is that the combined use of lamotrigine and sodium valproate is therapeutically valuable but should be well monitored.[8]

References

1 Graves NM, Ritter FJ, Wager ML, Floren KL, Alexander BJ, Campbell JI, Leppik E. Effect of lamotrigine on carbamazepine epoxide concentrations. Epilepsia (1991) 32, Suppl 3, 13.
2 Warner T, Patsalos PN, Prevett M, Elyas AA, Duncan JS. Lamotrigine-induced carbamazepine toxicity: a pharmacokinetic interaction. Epilepsia (1991) 32, Suppl 1, 95.
3 Yuen AWC, Land G, Weatherley BC, Peck AW. Sodium valproate inhibits lamotrigine metabolism. Fundam Clin Pharmacol (1991) 5, 468.
4 Betts T, Goodwin G, Withers RM, Yuen AWC. Human safety of lamotrigine. Epilepsia (1991) 32, Suppl 2, S17–21.
5 Jawad S, Richens A, Goodwin G, Yuen WC. Controlled trial of lamotrigine (Lamictal) for refractory partial seizures. Epilepsia (1989) 30, 356–63.
6 Yuen AWC, Land G, Weatherley BC, Peck AW. Sodium valproate acutely inhibits lamotrigine metabolism. Br J clin Pharmac (1992) 33, 511–3.
7 Warner T, Patsalos PN, Prevett M, Elyas AA, Duncan JS. Lamotrigine-induced carbamazepine toxicity: an interaction with carbamazepine-10,11-epoxide. Epilepsy Res (1992) 11, 147–50.
8 Panayiotopoulos CP, Ferrie CD, Knott C, Robinson RO. Interaction of lamotrigine with sodium valproate. Lancet (1993) 341, 445.

Anticonvulsants + Mefloquine

Abstract/Summary

An epileptic controlled on sodium valproate developed convulsions when given mefloquine. Mefloquine is normally contraindicated in epileptics.

Clinical evidence, mechanism, importance and management

An isolated report describes a woman of 20, with a 7-year history of epilepsy (bilateral myoclonus and generalized tonic-clonic seizures) currently treated with 1300 mg sodium valproate daily, who developed tonic-clonic seizures eight hours after taking the second of three prophylactic doses of 250 mg mefloquine.[1] It is not clear whether this resulted from a drug-drug or a drug-disease interaction, but the makers of mefloquine advise its avoidance in those with a history of convulsions

Reference

1 Besser R, Krämer G. Verdacht auf anfallfördernde Wirkung von Mefloquin (Lariam®). Nervenarzt (1991) 62, 760–1.

Anticonvulsants + Nafimidone

Abstract/Summary

Nafimidone causes a marked rise in the serum levels of carbamazepine and phenytoin. Dosage reductions are necessary to prevent toxicity.

Clinical evidence

Two epileptics with intractable partial seizures, stabilized on carbamazepine and phenytoin, showed a rise in the serum levels of both drugs within a day of additionally starting to take nafimidone (3 mg/kg daily in three divided doses). By the second day carbamazepine toxicity had developed. In four other patients, similarly treated, the dosages of carbamazepine and phenytoin were reduced to prevent excessively high serum levels. Carbamazepine elimination was reduced 76–87% and phenytoin elimination by 38–77% while taking nafimidone. Serum levels fell to normal within a day of stopping the nafimidone.[1]

Mechanism

Not understood. It seems possible that nafimidone inhibits the metabolism of carbamazepine and phenytoin by the liver, thereby reducing their loss from the body.

Importance and management

Information is limited but the interaction would appear to be established. The dosages of carbamazepine and phenytoin will need to be markedly reduced if nafimidone is added, and increased when it is withdrawn.

Reference

1 Treiman DM, Ben-Menachem E. Inhibition of carbamazepine and phenytoin metabolism by nafimidone, a new antiepileptic drug. Epilepsia (1987) 28, 699–705.

Anticonvulsants + Non-steroidal anti-inflammatory drugs

Abstract/Summary

Phenytoin toxicity has been seen in one patient on phenytoin while concurrently taking aspirin and another taking ibuprofen, but other evidence suggests that these reactions are rare. Carbamazepine is unaffected by aspirin, and both phenytoin and carbamazepine are unaffected by tolfenamic acid. See index for other anticonvulsants and NSAIDs.

Clinical evidence, mechanism, importance and management

(a) Anticonvulsants + Aspirin

It has been claimed that if a '...patient has been taking large quantities of aspirin for headache...the dilantin (phenytoin) is potentiated',[1] but this remains unconfirmed apart from an isolated report of phenytoin toxicity in one patient associated with taking 975 mg of an enteric-coated aspirin.[5] While it is known that the salicylates are able to displace phenytoin from its plasma protein binding sites,[2–7] a study in 10 epileptics on phenytoin given 1500 mg aspirin daily for three days found no evidence of significant changes in serum phenytoin levels or its effects.[8] Bearing in mind the extremely common use of aspirin, the almost total silence in the literature about an adverse phenytoin-aspirin interaction implies that no special precautions are normally needed. No changes in carbamazepine serum levels were seen in the same patients while taking 1500 mg aspirin for three days.[8]

(b) Anticonvulsants + Ibuprofen

Studies[9,10] in normal subjects have shown that the pharmacokinetics of single doses of phenytoin (300–900 mg) are not altered by 1200–2400 mg ibuprofen daily, however a single report describes a woman stabilized on 300 mg phenytoin daily who developed phenytoin intoxication within a week of starting to take 1600 mg ibuprofen daily.[11] Her serum phenytoin levels had risen from a range of 40–70 to 101 mmol/l. The reasons

are not understood. Her phenytoin serum levels fell when the ibuprofen was withdrawn. Both phenytoin and ibuprofen have been available for a number of years and this case seems to be the first and only report of an adverse interaction.

(c) Anticonvulsants + Tolfenamic acid

300 mg tolfenamic acid for three days had no significant effect on the serum levels of phenytoin or carbamazepine in 11 patients.[8] No special precautions seem necessary if taken concurrently.

References

1 Toakley JG. Dilantin overdosage. Med J Aust (1968) 2, 639.
2 Ehrnebo M, Odar-Cederlof I. Distribution of phenobarbital and diphenylhydantoin between plasma and cells in blood: effect of salicylic acid, temperature and total drug concentration. Eur J clin Pharmacol (1977) 11, 37.
3 Fraser DG, Ludden TM, Evans RP, Sutherland EW. Displacement of phenytoin from plasma binding sites by salicylate. Clin Pharmacol Ther (1980) 27, 165.
4 Paxton JW. Effects of aspirin on salivary and serum phenytoin kinetics in healthy subjects. Clin Pharmacol Ther (1980) 27, 170.
5 Leonard RF, Knott PJ, Rankin GO, Melnick DE. Phenytoin-salicylate interaction. Clin Pharmacol Ther (1981) 29, 260.
6 Olanow CW, Finn A, Prussak C. The effect of salicylate on phenytoin pharmacokinetics. Trans Am Neurol Ass (1979) 104, 109.
7 Inoue F, Walsh RJ. Folate supplements and phenytoin-salicylate interaction. Neurology (1983) 33, 115–16.
8 Neuvonen PJ, Lehtovaara R, Bardy A, Elomaa E. Antipyretic analgesics in patients on anti-epileptic drug therapy. Eur J Clin Pharmacol (1979) 15, 263.
9 Bachmann KA, Schwartz JI, Forney RB, Jauregui L and Sullivan TJ. Inability of ibuprofen to alter single dose phenytoin disposition. Br J clin Pharmac (1986) 21, 165–9.
10 Townsend R, Fraser DG, Scavone JM, Cox SR. The effects of ibuprofen on phenytoin pharmacokinetics. 6th Annual Meeting of the American College of Clinical Pharmacy (Abstract) 1985.
11 Sandyk R. Phenytoin toxicity induced by interaction with ibuprofen. S Afr Med J (1982) 62, 592.

Anticonvulsants + Oxcarbazepine

Abstract/Summary

Sodium valproate and phenytoin serum levels are modestly increased in patients when carbamazepine is replaced by oxcarbazepine.

Clinical evidence, mechanism, importance and management

A double-blind crossover comparison of oxcarbazepine and carbamazepine in 48 epileptics found that when carbamazepine was replaced by oxcarbazepine, the serum levels of sodium valproate rose by 32%, of phenytoin by 23%, and of both when taken together by 21–25%. The trial extended over 12 weeks to establish steady-state levels.[1] The reasons are not known but the suggestion is that the oxcarbazepine causes less enzyme induction than carbamazepine. The clinical importance of these increases in valproate and phenytoin levels is uncertain but good monitoring would be appropriate.

Reference

1 Houtkooper MA, Lammertsma A, Meyer JWA, Goedhart DM, Meinardi H, van Oorschot CAEH, Blom GF, Höppener RJEA, Hulsman JARJ. Oxcarbazepine (GP 47.680): a possible alternative to carbamazepine? Epilepsia (1987) 28, 693–8.

Anticonvulsants + Oxiracetam

Abstract/Summary

Oxiracetam does not affect the serum levels of sodium valproate, carbamazepine, clobamazam or desmethylclobazam, but the loss of oxiracetam from the body may be increased so that some change in its dosage may possibly be needed.

Clinical evidence, mechanism, importance and management

800 mg oxiracetam twice daily for 14 days given to four epileptics did not affect the serum levels of sodium valproate, carbamazepine, clobazam and desmethylclobazam, but it was noted that the oxiracetam half-life was shorter (2.8–7.56 h) than in a previous study (5.6–11.7 h) with normal subjects given 2 g oxiracetam.[1,2] There would seem to be no reason for avoiding concurrent use in patients taking these anticonvulsants, but it may be necessary to raise the oxiracetam dosage or give it more frequently. More study is needed to confirm these findings.

References

1 van Wieringen A, Meijer J W A, van Emde Boas W, Vermeij T A C. Pilot study to determine the interaction of oxiracetam with antiepileptic drugs. Clin Pharmacokinet (1990) 18, 332–8.
2 Perucca E, Albrici A, Gatti G, Spalluto R, Visconti M. Pharmacokinetics of oxiracetam following intravenous and oral administration in healthy volunteers. Eur J Drug Metab Pharmacokinetic (1984) 9, 267–74.

Anticonvulsants + Progabide

Abstract/Summary

Serum phenytoin levels can rise if progabide is used concurrently. A reduction in the dosage of phenytoin may be required. A small rise in serum phenobarbitone levels has been seen. Changes in the serum levels of other anticonvulsants (carbamazepine, sodium valproate, clonazepam) caused by progabide and their effects on serum progabide levels appear to be only moderate or small.

Clinical evidence

(a) Carbamazepine, clonazepam, phenobarbitone, sodium valproate

Information about these anticonvulsants is limited, but progabide is reported to reduce (-10%[10])[12], increase[12] or not to change carbamazepine[3,4,7,8] sodium valproate,[4,7,8] or clonazepam levels significantly,[5] while a small increase in serum phenobarbitone levels has been seen.[4,7,9,12] An increase in carbamazepine-epoxide levels of up to 24% has been reported.[9,10] Some reduction in serum progabide levels is reported with sodium valproate.[8]

(b) Phenytoin

Marked increases in serum phenytoin levels have been seen in a few patients given progabide concurrently.[1,2] In one study in epileptic patients, 17 out of 26 needed a reduction in the dosage of phenytoin to keep the levels within $+25\%$ of the serum levels before progabide was given, and this occurred within 4–10 weeks of starting concurrent treatment. Most of the patients needing a dosage reduction showed a maximum increase of 40% or more.[3,6] Other studies also describe increased phenytoin levels and intoxication.[11,12] In contrast only small changes were seen in another study.[7] Yet another described a small increase in the clearance of progabide in the presence of phenytoin.[8]

Mechanism, importance and management

Uncertain. Established interactions. The overall picture is that concurrent use should be well monitored. Be alert for the need to reduce the dosage of phenytoin and phenobarbitone if progabide is used concurrently. The significance of the increased levels of carbamazepine-epoxide is uncertain.

References

1 Dam M, Gram L, Philbert A, Hansen BS, Blatt Lyon B, Christensen JM, Angelo HR. Progabide: a controlled trial in partial epilepsy. Epilepsia (1983) 24, 127–34.
2 Van der Linden GJ, Meinardi H, Meijer JWA, Bossi L and Gomeni C.A double-blind cross-over trial with progabide (SL 76002) against placebo in patients with secondary generalized epilepsy. In: Advances in Epileptology: XIIth Epilepsy Int Symp. Dam M, Gram L and Penry JK (eds). Raven Press, New York. (1981) pp 141–4.
3 Cloyd JC, Brundage RC, Leppik IE, Graves NM, Welty TE. Effect of progabide on serum phenytoin and carbamazepine concentrations: a preliminary report. In: LERS Monograph series, volume 3. Edited by Bartholini G. Epilepsy and GABA receptor agonists: basic and therapeutic research. Meeting, Paris, March 1984. Raven Press, New York. (1985) pp 271–8.
4 Thenot JP, Bianchetti G, Abriol C, Feuerstein J, Lambert D, Thebault JJ, Warrington SJ, Rowland M. Interactions between progabide and antiepileptic drugs. Ibid (1985) pp 259–69.
5 Warrington SJ, O'Brien C, Thiercelin JF, Orofiamma B, Morselli PL. Evaluation of pharmacodynamic interaction between progabide and clonazepam in healthy men. Ibid (1985) pp 279–86.
6 Cloyd JC, Brundage RC, Leppik IE, Graves NM, Welty TE. Effect of progabide on phenytoin pharmacokinetics. Epilepsia (1984) 5, 656–7.
7 Bianchetti G, Thiercelin JF, Thenot JP, Feuerstein D, Lambert D, Rulliere JJ, Thebault JJ, Morselli PL. Effect of progabide on the phamacokinetics of various antiepileptic drugs. Neurology (1984) 34 (Suppl 1) 213.
8 Thiercelin JF, Padovani P, Thenot JP, Rowland M, Warrington S, Morselli PL. Effect of various antiepileptic drugs on the pharmacokinetics of progabide and its acid metabolite. Neurology (1984) 34 (Suppl 1) 266.
9 Bianchetti G, Padovani P, Thenot JP, Thiercelin JF, Morselli PL. Pharmacokinetic interactions of progabide with other antiepileptic drugs. Epilepsia (1987) 28, 68–73.

10 Graves NM, Fuerst RH, Cloyd JC, Brundage RC, Welty TE, Leppik IE. Progabide-induced changes in carbamazepine metabolism. Epilepsia (1988) 29, 775–80.
11 Crawford P, Chadwick D. A comparative study of progabide, valproate and placebo as add-on therapy in patients with refractory epilepsy. J Neurol Neurosurg Psychiatry (1986) 49, 1251–7.
12 Schmidt D, Utech K. Progabide for refractory partial epilepsy: a controlled add-on trial. Neurology (1986) 36, 217–221.

Anticonvulsants + Pyridoxine

Abstract/Summary

Large doses of pyridoxine (200 mg daily) can cause marked reductions (40–50%) in the serum phenytoin and phenobarbitone levels of some patients.

Clinical evidence

200 mg pyridoxine daily for 4 weeks reduced the phenobarbitone serum levels of five epileptics by about 50%. Reductions in serum phenytoin levels of almost 40% (range 8–66%) were also seen when given pyridoxine (80–200 mg daily) for 2–4 weeks. A number of other patients were not affected.[1]

Mechanism

It is suggested that the pyridoxine increases the activity of the liver enzymes concerned with the metabolism of the these anticonvulsants.[1]

Importance and management

Information seems to be limited to just one report, but what is known suggests that concurrent use should be monitored if large doses of pyridoxine like this are used, being alert for the need to increase the anticonvulsant dosage. It seems unlikely that small doses (as in multivitamin preparations) will interact to any great extent.

Reference

1 Hansson O, Sillanpaa M. Pyridoxine and serum concentrations of phenytoin and phenobarbitone. Lancet (1976) i, 256.

Anticonvulsants + Quinolone antibiotics

Abstract/Summary

Ciprofloxacin, enoxacin and nalidixic acid very occasionally cause convulsions and the makers advise caution or avoidance in epileptic subjects. Norfloxacin and ofloxacin have also been associated with seizures in two patients. An isolated report

describes a fall in serum phenytoin levels when ciprofloxacin was started.

Clinical evidence, mechanism, importance and management

The makers of ciprofloxacin and enoxacin suggest that these antibiotics should be used with caution or avoided in epileptics because a very small number of patients have developed convulsions. Ciprofloxacin has been associated with convulsions in both epileptic and non-epileptic patients.[1-3,5,10] Two of the patients were also being treated with theophylline.[5,6] Blood levels of phenytoin and valproic acid normally appear to be unaffected by ciprofloxacin,[1] but an isolated case report describes a marked fall in phenytoin serum levels in an elderly man when ciprofloxacin was started.[11] Enoxacin,[4] ofloxacin [10] and norfloxacin[7,8,10] may also possibly lower the convulsive threshold in patients predisposed to seizures. During the period 1964–75 The Committee on the Safety of Medicines in the UK received eight reports of convulsions associated with nalidixic acid. Another was reported in 1977, and three have been described in Australia.[9]

These reports illustrate that care should be exercised if any of these antibiotics is given to epileptic patients. Most of the reactions seem to be disease-drug interactions rather than drug-drug interactions.

References

1 Slavich IL, Gleffe R, Haas EJ. Grand mal seizures during ciprofloxacin therapy. J Amer Med Ass (1989) 261, 558–9.
2 Beeley L, Magee P, Hickey F. Newsletter of the W.Midlands Centre for Adverse Drug Reaction Reporting, January (1989).
3 Schacht P, Arcieri G, Branolte J, Bruck H, Chysky V, Griffith E, Gruenwald G, Hullmann R, Konopka CA, O'Brien B, Rahm V, Ryoki T, Westwood A, Weuta H. Worldwide clinical data on efficacy and safety of ciprofloxacin. Eur J Clin Study Treat Infect (1988) Suppl 1, 29–43.
4 Comprecin (enoxacin) Clinical Information Manual. Parke Davis (1989).
5 Karki SD, Bentley DW, Raghavan M. Seizure frequency with ciprofloxacin and theophylline combined therapy. DICP Ann Pharmacotherapy (1990) 24, 595–6.
6 Arcieri G, Griffith E, Gruenwaldt G. Ciprofloxacin: an update on clinical experience. Am J Med (1987) 84 (Suppl 4A), 381–6.
7 Simpson KJ, Brodie M. Convulsions related to enoxacin. Lancet (1985) 2, 161.
8 Anastasio GD, Menscer D, Little JM. Norfloxacin and seizures. Ann Intern Med (1988) 109, 169–70.
9 Fraser AG, Harrower ADB. Convulsions and hyperglycaemia associated with nalidixic acid. Br Med J (1977) 2, 1518.
10 Committee on the Safety of Medicines. Current Problems (1991) 32, 2.
11 Dillard ML, Fink RM, Parkerson R. Ciprofloxacin-phenytoin interaction. Ann Pharmacother (1992) 26, 263.

Anticonvulsants + Stiripentol

Abstract/Summary

Stiripentol causes marked rises in the serum levels of carbamazepine, phenobarbitone and phenytoin. Reduce their dosages to avoid the development of toxicity.

Clinical evidence

Six epileptic patients taking two or three anticonvulsants (phenytoin, phenobarbitone, carbamazepine, primidone, nitrazepam) were additionally given stiripentol (600–2400 mg daily). All five on phenytoin showed a reduction in the phenytoin clearance from 29.5 to 18.5 litre daily while taking 1200 mg stiripentol daily, and to 6.48 litre daily while on 2400 mg stiripentol. These changes in clearance were reflected in marked rises in the steady-state serum levels of the anticonvulsants: for example the serum phenytoin levels of one patient rose from 14.4 mg/l to 27.4 mg/l over 30 days while taking stiripentol, despite a halving of his phenytoin dosage. Phenytoin toxicity was seen in two subjects.[1]

The clearance of carbamazepine in one subject fell from 209 to 128 litre daily while on 1200 mg stiripentol daily and to 61 litre daily while on 2400 mg stiripentol daily. Phenobarbitone clearance in two subjects fell from 3.8 and 5 litre daily to 2.3 and 3.4 litre daily respectively while taking 2400 mg stiripentol daily.[1] Two other studies in adults and children confirmed that stiripentol reduces the clearance of carbamazepine to a half or a third.[2–4]

Mechanism

It seems that stiripentol inhibits the activity of the liver enzymes concerned with the metabolism of these anticonvulsants so that their loss from the body is reduced and their serum levels rise accordingly.[3]

Importance and management

Established and clinically import interactions. Phenytoin, phenobarbitone and carbamazepine dosages should be reduced to avoid the development of elevated serum levels and possible toxicity during the concurrent use of stiripentol. In the case of phenytoin, halving the dose may not be enough. One study suggests that the carbamazepine dosage should be decreased incrementally over 7–10 days as soon as the stiripentol is started and, regardless of age, the maintenance dose of carbamazepine should be 4.4 to 8.7 mg/kg/day to give serum levels of 5–10 μg/ml.[3]

References

1 Levy RH, Loiseau P, Guyot M, Blehaut HM, Tor J, Morland TA. Stiripentol kinetics in epilepsy: non-linearity and interactions. Clin Pharmacol Ther (1984) 36, 661–9.

2 Levy RH, Kerr BM, Farwell J, Anderson GD, Martinez-Lage M, Tor J. Carbamazepine/stiripentol interaction in adult and paediatric patients. Epilepsia (1989) 30, 701.

3 Kerr BM, Martinez-Lage JM, Viteri C, Tor J, Eddy C, Levy RH. Carbamazepine dose requirements during stiripentol therapy: influence of cytochrome P-450 inhibition by stiripentol. Epilepsia (1991) 32, 267–4.

4 Levy RH, Martinez-Lage JM, Tor J, Blehaut H, Gonzalez I, Bainbridge B. Stiripentol level-dose relationship and interaction with carbamazepine in epileptic patients. Epilepsia (1985) 26, 545–6.

Anticonvulsants + Terfenadine

Abstract/Summary

An isolated report describes carbamazepine toxicity apparently caused by the addition of terfenadine. Terfenadine does not alter the pharmacokinetics of phenytoin.

Clinical evidence, mechanism, importance and management

(a) Carbamazepine

A woman of 18 taking carbamazepine after treatment for brain metastases, developed confusion, disorientation, visual hallucinations, nausea and ataxia (interpreted as carbamazepine intoxication) shortly after starting 60 mg terfenadine twice daily for rhinitis. The symptoms disappeared when the tefenadine was stopped. Her total carbamazepine serum levels (8.9 mg/l) were within the normal range, but the levels of free carbamazepine were found to be 6.0 mg/l (almost three times the upper limit of normal). The authors speculate that the terfenadine had displaced the carbamazepine from its plasma protein binding sites, thereby increasing the levels of free and active carbamazepine.[1] The report is very brief and does not say whether any other drugs were being taken.

The general importance of this interaction is uncertain, but it is probably small. However until more information is available it would seem prudent to monitor the outcome of adding terfenadine to treatment with carbamazepine.

(b) Phenytoin

Single and chronic daily doses of 60 mg terfenadine twice daily for two weeks had no effect on the pharmacokinetics of phenytoin in 12 epileptics.[2] No special precautions are needed if both drugs are used.

References

1 Hirschfeld S, Jarosinski. Drug interaction of terfenadine and carbamazepine. Ann Intern Med (1993) 118, 907–8.

2 Coniglio AA, Garnett WR, Pellock JH, Tsidonis O, Hepler CD, Serafin R, Small RE, Driscoll SM, Karnes HT. Effect of acute and chronic terfenadine on free and total serum phenytoin concentrations in epileptic patients. Epilepsia (1989) 30, 611–16.

Anticonvulsants + Tobacco smoking

Abstract/Summary

Smoking appears to have no important effect on the serum levels of phenytoin, phenobarbitone or carbamazepine.

Clinical evidence, mechanism, importance and management

A comparative study in 88 epileptic patients taking anticonvulsants (phenobarbitone, phenytoin and carbamazepine alone and in combination) found that although smoking had a tendency to lower the steady-state serum concentrations of these drugs, a statistically significant effect was only shown on the concentration-dose ratios of the phenobarbitone-treated patients.[1] In practical terms smoking appears to have only a negligible effect on the serum levels of these anticonvulsants and epileptics are unlikely to need higher doses than non-smokers.

Reference

1 Benetello P, Furlanut M, Pasqui L, Carmillo L, Perlotto N, Testa G. Absence of effect of cigarette smoking on serum concentrations of some anticonvulsants in epileptic patients. Clin Pharmacokinetics (1987) 12, 302–4.

Anticonvulsants + Vigabatrin

Abstract/Summary

Vigabatrin modestly lowers serum phenytoin, phenobarbitone and primidone levels but not those of carbamazepine or sodium valproate. The phenytoin dosage may need to be increased.

Clinical evidence, mechanism, importance and management

A study in epileptic patients showed that 2–3 g vigabatrin daily did not change the serum levels of phenobarbitone (26 patients), carbamazepine (12 patients) or sodium valproate (two patients), but the mean serum phenytoin levels (19 patients) were about 20% lower during concurrent use (for reasons which are not understood) and in two patients they fell below the therapeutic range. Seizure-frequency generally remained unaltered.[1] The combined use of Vigabatrin and sodium valproate to 16 children with refractory epilepsy was found not to affect the steady-state serum levels of either drug and it reduced the frequency of seizures.[6] Another study found reductions of – 20% with phenytoin, – 7% with phenobarbitone and – 11% with primidone. The frequency of complex partial seizures was halved but in this study seizure-frequency increased with phenytoin and its dosage had to be increased.[5] This confirms the findings of three other studies.[2–4]

Vigabatrin would therefore appear to be a valuable drug but some increase in the dosage of phenytoin may possibly be necessary. No dosage changes seem necessary with the other anticonvulsants cited.

References

1 Tassinari CA, Michelucci R, Ambrosetto G, Salvi F. Double-blind study of vigabatrin in the treatment of drug-resistant epilepsy. Arch Neurol (1987) 44, 907–10.

2 Rimmer EM, Richens A. Double-blind study of gamma-vinyl GABA in patients with refractory epilepsy. Lancet (1984) i, 189–90.

3 Browne TR, Mattson RH, Penry JK, Smith DB, Treimann DM, Wilder BJ, Ben-Menachem E, Napolieloo MJ, Sherry KM, Szabo GK. Vigabatrin for refractory complex partial seizures; multicenter single-blind study with long-term follow up. Neurology (1987) 37, 184–9.

4 Rimmer EM, Richens A. Interaction between vigabatrin and phenytoin. Br J clin Pharmac (1989) 27, 27–33S.

5 Browne TR, Mattson RH, Penry JK, Smith DB, Treiman DM, Wilder BJ, Ben-Menachem E, Miketta RM, Sherry KM, Szabo GK. A multicentre study of vigabatrin for drug-resistant apilepsy. Br J clin Pharmac (1989) 95–100S.

6 Armijo JA, Arteaga R, Valdizan EM, Herranz JL. Coadministration of vigabatrin and valproate in children with refractory epilepsy. Clin Neuropharmacol (1992) 15, 459–69.

Anticonvulsants + Viloxazine

Abstract/Summary

Viloxazine can cause a 50% rise in serum carbamazepine levels. Intoxication may occur if the carbamazepine dosage is not reduced appropriately. Viloxazine can also raise serum phenytoin to toxic levels. Oxcarbazepine levels are unaffected by viloxazine.

Clinical evidence

(a) Carbamazepine + Vloxazine

Seven patients on carbamazepine showed a 50% rise (from 8.1 to 12.1 µg/ml) in their serum carbamazepine levels after taking 300 mg viloxazine daily for 3 weeks.[1] Five developed signs of mild intoxication (dizziness, ataxia, fatigue, drowsiness). These symptoms disappeared and the serum carbamazepine levels fell when the viloxazine was withdrawn.[1] Another study confirmed this interaction. Intoxication was seen.[4] The pharmacokinetics of viloxazine are unaffected by carbamazepine.[3]

(b) Oxcarbazepine + Viloxazine

The steady-state serum oxcarbazine levels of six patients with simple or partial seizures on 1200–1400 mg daily were unaffected by 200 mg viloxazine daily for 10 days. No adverse side-effects were seen.[5]

(c) Phenytoin + Viloxazine

Ten epileptic patients taking phenytoin (200–400 mg daily) showed a 37% rise (from18.8 µg/ml to 25.7 µg/ml) in serum phenytoin levels over three weeks when 150–300 mg viloxazine daily was added. The rise ranged from 7 to 94%. Signs of toxicity (ataxia, nystagmus) developed in four of the patients 12–16 days after starting the viloxazine. Their serum phenytoin levels had risen to between 32.3 and 41 µg/ml.[2] The symptoms disappeared and phenytoin levels fell when the viloxazine was withdrawn.[2] The pharmacokinetics of viloxazine are unaffected by phenytoin.[3]

Mechanism

Uncertain. What is known suggests that the viloxazine inhibits the metabolism of some anticonvulsants, thereby reducing their clearance from the body and raising their serum levels.

Importance and management

Information seems to be limited to the reports cited. If concurrent use is undertaken, both serum carbamazepine and phenytoin levels should be monitored closely and suitable dosage reductions made as necessary to avoid the possible development of intoxication. No special precautions seem necessary with oxcarbazepine.

References

1 Pisani F, Narbone MC, Fazio A, Cristafulli P, Primerano G, D'Angostino AA, Oteri G, Perri R. Effect of viloxazine on serum carbamazepine levels in epileptic patients. Epilepsia (1984) 25, 482–5.
2 Pisani F, Fazio A, Artesi C, Russo M, Trio R, Oteri G, Perucca E, Di Perri R. Elevation of plasma phenytoin by viloxazine in epileptic patients: a clinically significant interaction. J Neurol Neurosurg Psychiat (1992) 55, 126–7.
3 Pisani F, Fazio A, Spina E, Artesi C, Pisani B, Russo M, Trio R, Perucca E. Pharmacokinetics of the antidepressant drug viloxazine in normal subjects and in epileptic patients receiving chronic anticonvulsant treatment. Psychopharmacology (1986) 90, 295–8.
4 Pisani F, Fazio A, Oteri G, Perucca E, Russo M, Trio R, Pisani B, Di Perri R. Carbamazepine-viloxazine interaction in patients with epilepsy. J Neurol Neurosurg Psychiatry (1986) 49, 1142–5.
5 Pisani F, Oteri G, Russo M, Trio A, D'Agostino AA, Di Perri R, Flesch G, Monza GC. Double-blind, within-patient study to evaluate the influence of viloxazine on the steady-state plasma levels of oxcarbazepine and its metabolites. Epilepsia (1991) 32, Suppl 1, 70

Barbiturates + Caffeine

Abstract/Summary

The hypnotic effects of pentobarbitone (pentobarbital) are reduced or abolished by the concurrent use of caffeine. Caffeine-containing drinks should be avoided at bedtime if satisfactory hypnosis is to be achieved.

Clinical evidence

A controlled study on 42 patients given either a placebo, or 250 mg caffeine, or 100 mg pentobarbitone, or both caffeine and pentobarbitone, showed that the caffeine totally abolished the hypnotic effects of the barbiturate. The effects of the pentobarbitone-caffeine combination were indistinguishable from the placebo.[1]

Mechanism

Caffeine stimulates the cerebral cortex and impairs sleep, whereas pentobarbitone depresses the cortex and promotes sleep. These mutually opposing actions would seem to explain this interaction.

Importance and management

There seems to be only one direct study of this interaction, but it is well supported by common experience and the numerous studies of the properties of each of these compounds. Patients given barbiturate hypnotics should avoid caffeine-containing drinks (tea, coffee, *Coca-Cola*, etc.) at or near bedtime if the hypnotic is to be effective. The same is probably true for other non-barbiturate hypnotics, but this needs confirmation.

Reference

1 Forrest WH, Bellville JW, Brown BW. The interaction of caffeine with pentobarbital as a night-time hypnotic. Anesthesiology (1972) 36, 37.

Barbiturates + Cimetidine

Abstract/Summary

Phenobarbitone reduces the absorption of cimetidine, and cimetidine reduces the metabolism of pentobarbitone, but both interactions seem to be of very limited clinical importance.

Clinical evidence, mechanism, importance and management

In vitro studies with human liver microsomes showed that cimetidine in above clinical concentrations reduced the metabolism of pentobarbitone, whereas ranitidine did not interact.[2] A study on eight normal subjects showed that 100 mg phenobarbitone daily for three weeks reduced the AUC of a single 400 mg oral dose of cimetidine by 15%, and the time during which the plasma concentrations of the cimetidine exceeded 0.5 µg/ml (regarded as therapeutically desirable) was reduced by 11%.[1] The mechanisms underlying these interactions are that cimetidine is an enzyme inhibitor which reduces the rate of metabolism of pentobarbitone, whereas phenobarbitone apparently stimulates the enzymes in the gut wall so that the metabolism of the cimetidine is increased. Thus the amount absorbed and released into the circulation is reduced.

Direct information is limited. Mutual interactions take place between these drugs but the effects are small and unlikely to be of clinical importance. No special precautions seem to be necessary. Direct information about other barbiturates is lacking but it seems probable that they will behave similarly.

References

1 Somogyi A, Thielscher S, Gugler R. Influence of phenobarbital treatment on cimetidine kinetics. Eur J clin Pharmacol (1981) 19, 343.
2 Knodell RG, Holtzmann JL, Crankshaw DL, Steele NM, Stanley LN. Drug metabolism by rat and human hepatic microsomes in response to interaction with H_2-receptor antagonists. Gastroenterol (1982) 82, 84–88.

Barbiturates + Miconazole

Abstract/Summary

Miconazole increases serum pentobarbitone levels.

Clinical evidence, mechanism, importance and management

Five patients in intensive care given pentobarbital to decrease intracranial pressure showed marked rises in serum pentobarbital levels, and falls in total plasma clearance of 50–90% when concurrently treated with miconazole. The reason is thought to be that the miconazole inhibits the liver enzymes concerned with the metabolism of the barbiturate, thereby reducing its clearance from the body.[1] It would be prudent to monitor the effects of concurrent use to ensure that serum barbiturate levels do not rise too high. There seems to be no information about other barbiturates.

Reference

1 Heinemeyer G, Roots I, Schultz H, Dennhardt R. Hemmung der Pentobarbital-Elimination durch Miconazol bei Intesivtherapie des erhohten intracraniellen Druckes. Intensivmed (1988) 22, 164–7.

Barbiturates + Rifampicin (Rifampin)

Abstract/Summary

Rifampicin markedly increases the clearance of hexobarbitone (hexobarbital) from the body, and phenobarbitone possibly increases the clearance of rifampicin. The effects of each drug may be expected to be reduced.

Clinical evidence

(a) Effect of rifampicin on hexobarbitone

A study in six healthy subjects found that 1200 mg rifampicin daily for 8 days decreased the average elimination half-life of hexobarbitone from 407 to 171 min, and increased the metabolic clearance three-fold.[1] Similar results have been found in other studies with normal subjects[2] and those with cirrhosis or cholestasis.[3] Other studies with hexobarbitone enantiomers found that 600 mg rifampicin daily for 6 days caused a six-fold increase in the clearance of S-(+) hexobarbitone in both young

and old (71 years) subjects, but the clearance of R-(–) hexobarbitone was increased 89-fold in the young and only 19-fold in the old.[6]

(b) Effect of phenobarbitone on rifampicin

Conflicting evidence. One study showed no effect[4] whereas another indicated that the serum levels of rifampicin were reduced.[5]

Mechanism

Rifampicin is a potent liver enzyme inducing agent which accelerates the metabolism of the hexobarbitone. Whether phenobarbitone (also a potent enzyme inducing agent) can affect the metabolism of rifampicin in a similar way is not clear.

Importance and management

The documentation for both of these interactions is very limited, but the effects seen are consistent with what is known about these drugs. Concurrent use need not be avoided, but be alert for a reduced response to both drugs. Be aware of the differences between old and young patients and increase the dosages as necessary. Whether rifampicin interacts with other barbiturates is uncertain.

References

1 Breimer DD, Zilly W, Richter E. Influence of rifampicin on drug metabolism: differences between hexobarbital and antipyrine. Clin Pharmacol Ther (1977) 21, 470.
2 Breimer DD, Zilly W, Richter E. Induction of drug metabolism in man after rifampicin treatment measured by increased hexobarbital and tolbutamide clearance. Eur J Clin Pharmacol (1975) 9, 219.
3 Breimer DD, Zilly W, Richter E. Stimulation of drug metabolism by rifampicin in patients with cirrhosis or cholestasis measured by increased hexobarbital and tolbutamide clearance. Eur J Clin Pharmacol (1977) 11, 287.
4 Acocella G, Bonollo L, Mainardi M, Margaroli P, Nicolis FB. Kinetic studies on rifampicin. III. Effect of phenobarbital on the half-life of the antibiotic. Tijdschrift Gastro-Enterologie (1974) 17, 151.
5 De la Roy Y de R, Beauchant G, Breuil K and y Patte F. Diminution de taux serique de rifampicine par le phenobarbital. Presse Med (1971) 79, 350.
6 Smith DA, Chandler MHH, Shedlofsky SI, Wedlund PJ, Blouin RA. Age-dependent stereoselective increase in the oral clearance of hexobarbitone isomers caused by rifampicin. Br J clin Pharmac (1991) 32, 735–9.

Barbiturates + Sodium valproate

Abstract/Summary

Serum phenobarbitone levels can be increased by the concurrent use of sodium valproate which may result in excessive sedation and lethargy. A reduction in the dosage of the phenobarbitone by a third to a half can be safely carried out without loss of seizure control.

Clinical evidence

A 9-month study in 11 epileptics on phenobarbitone (90–400 mg daily) showed that when they were additionally given sodium valproate (11–42 mg/kg/day) they complained of sedation and, on average, the dosage of phenobarbitone could be reduced to 54% with continued good seizure control. Two other patients on a constant dose of phenobarbitone showed significantly increased phenobarbitone levels (12 and 48% respectively).[1]

Another study showed that 1200 mg sodium valproate raised serum phenobarbitone levels by an average of 27%.[2] This interaction has been described in numerous other reports.[3–17,19] Sodium valproate levels are also reported to be reduced about 25%.[18]

Mechanism

The evidence indicates that sodium valproate inhibits the metabolism of the phenobarbitone by the liver, leading to its accumulation in the body.

Importance and management

An extremely well documented and well established interaction of clinical importance. The incidence seems to be high. The effects of concurrent use should be well monitored and suitable phenobarbitone dosage reductions made when necessary to avoid toxicity (sedation and lethargy). It would seem that the dosage can be safely reduced by a third to a half with full seizure control.[1]

References

1 Wilder BJ, Willmore LJ, Bruni J, Villarreal HJ. Valproic acid: interaction with other anticonvulsant drugs. Neurology (1978) 28, 892.
2 Richens A, Ahmad S. Controlled trial of sodium valproate in severe epilepsy. Brit Med J (1975) 3, 255.
3 Meinardi H, Bongers E. Analytical data in connection with the clinical use of di-n-propylacetate. In Clinical Pharmacology of Antiepileptic Drugs, edited by Schneider H et al. Springer-Verlag, NY and Berlin (1975) p. 235.
4 Schobben F, Van der Kleijn E, Gabreels FJM. Pharmacokinetics of di-n-propylacetate in epileptic patients. Eur J clin Pharmacol (1975) 8, 97.
5 Gram L, Wulff K, Rasmussen KE. Valproate sodium: a controlled clinical trial including monitoring of drug levels. Epilepsia (1977) 18, 141.
6 Jeavons PM, Clark JE. Sodium valproate in treatment of epilepsy. Brit Med J (1974) 2, 584.
7 Volzke E, Doose H. Dipropylacetate (Depakine, Ergenyl) in the treatment of epilepsy. Epilepsia (1973) 14, 185.
8 Millet Y, Sainty JM, Galland MC, Sidoine R, Jonglard J. Problemes poses par l'association therapeutique phenobarbital de sodium a propos d'un cas. Eur J Toxicol (1976) 9, 381.
9 Jeavons PM, Clark JE, Maheshwari MC. Treatment of generalized epilepsies of childhood and adolescence with sodium valproate ('Epilim'). Dev Med Child Neurol (1977) 19, 9.
10 Vakil SD, Critchley EMR, Phillips JC, Haydock C, Cocks A, Dyeb T. The effect of sodium valproate (Epilim) on phenytoin and phenobarbitone blood levels. In Clinical and Pharmacological Aspects of Sodium Valproate (Epilim) in the Treatment of Epilepsy. Proceedings of a Symposium held at the University of Nottingham, September 1975, p75.
11 Scott DF, Boxer CM, and Herzberg JL. A study of the hypnotic effects of Epilim and its possible interaction with phenobarbitone. Ibid p 155.
12 Richens A, Scoular IT, Ahamad S, Jordan BJ. Pharmacokinetics and

efficacy of Epilim in patients receiving long-term therapy with other antiepileptic drugs. Ibid p 78.
13 Loiseau P, Orgogozo JM, Brachet-Liermain A, Morselli PL. Pharmacokinetic studies on the interaction between phenobarbital and valproic acid. In Adv Epileptol Proc Cong Int League Epilepsy 13th. Edited by Meinardi H and Rowan A. (1977/8) p 261.
14 Fowler GW. Effect of dipropylacetate on serum levels of anticonvulsants in children. Proc West Pharmacol (1978) 21, 37.
15 Patel IH, Levy RH, Cutler RE. Phenobarbital-valproic acid interaction. Clin Pharmacol Ther (1980) 27, 515.
16 Coulter DL, Wu H, Allen RJ. Valproic acid therapy in childhood epilepsy. J Amer Med Ass (1980) 244, 785.
17 Kapetanovic IM, Kupferberg HJ, Porter RJ, Theodore W, Schulman E, Penry JK. Mechanism of valproate-phenobarbital interaction. Clin Pharmacol Ther (1981) 29, 480.
18 May T, Rambeck B. Serum concentrations of valproic acid: influence of dose and comedication. Ther Drug Monit (1985) 7, 387–90.
19 de Gatta MRF, Gonzalez ACA, Sanchez MJC, Hurle AD-G, Borbujo JS, Corral LM. Effect of sodium valproate on phenobarbital serum levels in children and adults. Ther Drug Monitor (1986) 8, 416–20.

Barbiturates + Triacetyloleandomycin

Abstract/Summary

A patient showed a fall in his serum phenobarbitone levels when concurrently treated with triacetyloleandomycin.

Clinical evidence, mechanism, importance and management

A patient on phenobarbitone and carbamazepine showed a fall in serum phenobarbitone levels (from about 40 to 31 μg/ml) over a 3 -day period when treated with triacetyloleandomycin.[1] The general importance of this single report is uncertain, but it would now seem prudent to be alert for changes in seizure control if this antibiotic is used.

Reference

1 Dravet C, Mesdjian E, Cenraud B, Roger J. Interaction between carbamazepine and triacetyloleandomycin. Lancet (1977) i, 810.

Carbamazepine + Acetazolamide

Abstract/Summary

Carbamazepine serum levels and seizure control can be increased by acetazolamide, but a few patients may need a reduction in the carbamazepine dosage to avoid side-effects.

Clinical evidence, mechanism, importance and management

A study in 54 children with grand mal and temporal lobe epilepsy found that seizure control was improved when acetazolamide (10 mg/kg/day) was added to carbamazepine. 60% of them showed carbamazepine serum level rises of 1–6 mg/l. Ten children developed side-effects within 1–10 days of starting the acetazolamide which responded to a reduction in the carbamazepine dosage, although three children whose serum carbamazepine levels rose by 10–23 mg/l paradoxically failed to develop side-effects.[1] This is generally speaking an advantageous interaction, however it is clearly important to monitor the outcome and to adjust the drug dosage as necessary.

Reference

1 Forsythe WI, Ownes JR, Toothill C. Effectiveness of acetazolamide in the treatment of carbamazepine-resistant epilepsy in children. Develop Med Child Neurol (1981) 23, 761–9.

Carbamazepine + Allopurinol

Abstract/Summary

Allopurinol can raise serum carbamazepine levels by about a third. Some reduction in the carbamazepine dosage may be needed.

Clinical evidence

A study in seven epileptic patients on anticonvulsants which included carbamazepine, showed that when 100 mg allopurinol three times daily was added for 2 months, followed by 200 mg three times daily for 3 months, the mean trough steady-state serum carbamazepine levels of six of the patients rose by 30% or more. Three of them needed a reduction in the carbamazepine dosage because of the symptoms which developed. The carbamazepine clearance fell by 14% during months 1 and 2, and by 32% during the last 3-month period.[1]

Mechanism

Uncertain. A possible explanation is that allopurinol can act as a liver enzyme inhibiting agent which reduces the metabolism and clearance of other drugs by the liver.

Importance and management

Information is limited to this study, but be alert for the need to reduce the dosage of carbamazepine if allopurinol is added. More study is needed.

Reference

1 Mikat M, Erba G, Skousteli H, Gadia C. Pharmacokinetic study of allopurinol in resistant epilepsy: evidence for significant drug interactions. Neurology (1990) 40 (Suppl 1) 138.

Carbamazepine + Cholestyramine or colestipol

Abstract/Summary

Colestipol causes only a minor reduction in the absorption of carbamazepine. Cholestyramine does not interact.

Clinical evidence, mechanism, importance and management

A study in six normal subjects found that 8 g cholestyramine did not affect the absorption of 400 mg carbamazepine, whereas 10 g colestipol reduced it by 10%.[1] This small reduction is unlikely to be clinically important, but monitor concurrent use nonetheless.

Reference

1 Neuvonen P J, Kivistö K, Hirvisalo E L. Effects of resins and activated charcoal on the absorption of digoxin, carbamazepine and frusemide. Br J clin Pharmac (1988) 25, 229–33.

Carbamazepine or Oxcarbazepine + Cimetidine or Ranitidine

Abstract/Summary

Epileptic patients and subjects chronically treated with carbamazepine show a transient increase in serum levels, possibly accompanied by an increase in side-effects, for the first few days after starting to take cimetidine, but these side-effects rapidly disappear. Ranitidine appears not to interact. Oxcarbazepine is not affected by cimetidine.

Clinical evidence

(a) Carbamazepine

The steady-state carbamazepine levels of eight normal subjects on 900 mg daily increased by 17% within two days of starting 1200 mg cimetidine daily. Six experienced side-effects, but after seven day's treatment the carbamazepine levels had fallen again and the side-effects disappeared.[8]

The steady-state carbamazepine levels of seven epileptic patients on chronic treatment remained unaltered when given 1 g cimetidine daily for a week.[6] No interaction was also seen in another study in 11 epileptic patients.[7] A very elderly woman, aged 89, developed signs of carbamazepine toxicity within two days of starting to take 400 mg cimetidine daily, and showed a rise in serum carbamazepine levels which fell once again when the cimetidine was withdrawn.[5]

The results of these studies in patients and subjects taking carbamazepine chronically and quoted above differ from the single dose studies and short-term studies in normal subjects. For example, a 33% rise in serum levels,[1] a 20% fall in clearance[2] and a 26% increase in the AUC[3] have been reported.

(b) Oxcarbazepine

Eight normal subjects showed no changes in the pharmacokinetics of a single 600 mg oral dose of oxcarbazepine after taking 1200 mg cimetidine daily for seven days.[9]

Mechanism

Not fully understood. It is thought that cimetidine can inhibit the activity of the liver enzymes concerned with the metabolism of carbamazepine, resulting in its reduced clearance from the body, but the effect is short-lived because it is opposed by the auto-inducing effects of the carbamazepine. This would explain why the single-dose and short-term studies in normal subjects suggest that a clinically important interaction could occur, but in practice in patients on long-term treatment it causes few problems.

Importance and management

The carbamazepine-cimetidine interaction is established but of minimal importance. Patients on chronic treatment with carbamazepine should be warned that for the first few days after starting to take cimetidine they may experience some increase in the carbamazepine side-effects (nausea, headache, dizziness, fatigue, drowsiness, ataxia, an inability to concentrate, a bitter taste) because the serum levels are transiently increased, but these side-effects normally subside and disappear by the end of a week. Ranitidine appears to be a non-interacting alternative to cimetidine.[4] Oxcarbazepine appears not to interact with cimetidine.

References

1 Macphee GJA, Thompson GG, Scobie G, Agnew E, Parke BK, Murray T, McColl KEL and Brodie MJ. Effects of cimetidine on carbamazepine auto- and hetero-induction in man. Br J clin Pharmac (1984) 18, 411–19.
2 Webster LK, Mihaly GW, Jones DB, Smallwood RA, Phillips JA, Vajda FJ. Effect of cimetidine and rantidine on carbamazepine and sodium valproate pharmacokinetics. Eur J Clin Pharmacol (1984) 27, 341–3.
3 Dalton MJ, Powell JR, Messenheimer JA. The influence of cimetidine on single dose carbamazepine pharmacokinetics. Epilepsia (1985) 26, 127–30.
4 Dalton MJ, Powell JR, Messenheimer JA. Ranitidine does not alter single-dose carbamazepine pharmacokinetics in healthy adults. Drug Intell Clin Pharm (1985) 19, 941–4.
5 Telerman-Topet N, Duret ME, Coers C. Cimetidine interaction with carbamazepine. Ann Intern Med (1981) 94, 544.
6 Sonne J, Luhdorf K, Larsen NE, Andreasen PB. Lack of interaction between cimetidine and carbmazepine. Acta Neurol Scand (1983) 68, 253–6.
7 Levine M, Jones MW, Sheppard I. Differential effect of cimetidine on serum concentrations of carbamazepine and phenytoin. Neurology (1985) 35, 562–5
8 Dalton MJ, Powell JR, Messenheimer JA, Clark J. Cimetidine and carbamazepine: a complex drug interaction. Epilepsia (1986) 27, 553–8.
9 Keränen T, Jolkkonen J, Klosterskov-Jensen P, Menge GP. Oxcarbazepine

does not interact with cimetidine in healthy volunteers. Acta Neurol Scand (1992) 85, 239–42.

Carbamazepine + Danazol

Abstract/Summary

Serum carbamazepine levels can be doubled by the concurrent use of danazol. Carbamazepine toxicity may occur unless the dosage is reduced appropriately.

Clinical evidence

The serum carbamazepine levels of six epileptics approximately doubled within 7–30 days of being treated with danazol (500 mg). Acute carbamazepine toxicity (dizziness, drowsiness, blurred vision, ataxia, nausea) was experienced by five out of the six.[2] Other reports similarly describe rises in serum carbamazepine levels of 50–100% when danazol was added.[1,3,4]

Mechanism

Danazol inhibits the metabolism of the carbamazepine by the liver, thereby reducing its loss from the body.[1,4,5] During danazol treatment the clearance of carbamazepine was found to be reduced by 60% and the half-life doubled.[4]

Importance and management

This interaction is established and of clinical importance. Concurrent use should be avoided unless the carbamazepine serum levels can be monitored and the dosage reduced as necessary.

References

1 Kramer G, Besser R, Theisohn M, Eichelbaum M. Carbamazepine-danazol drug interaction: mechanism and usefulness. Acta Neurol Scand (1984) 70, 249.
2 Zielinski JJ, Lichten EM, Haidukewych D. Clinically significant danazol-carbamazepine interaction. Ther Drug Monit (1987) 9, 24–7.
3 Ramsy RE, McJilton JS, Vasquez D, Marcos J. Increase in the protein binding of carbamazepine from danazol co-administration. Abstracts of the 16th Epilepsy International Congress, Hamburg, Sept 6–9, 1986.
4 Kramer G, Theisohn M, von Unruh GE, Eichelbaum M. Carbamazepine-danazol interaction: its mechanism examined by a stable isotope technique. Ther Drug Monitor (1986) 8, 387–92.
5 Kramer G, Theisohn M. Therapeutische nutzbare Arzneimittelinteraktionen mit Carbamazepin. Psycho (1983) 9, 366–8.

Carbamazepine + Diuretics

Abstract/Summary

Two patients on carbamazepine developed hyponatraemia when given hydrochlorothiazide or frusemide.

Clinical evidence, mechanism, importance and management

Two epileptic patients developed symptomatic hyponatraemia while on carbamazepine, one while taking hydrochlorothiazide and the other while taking frusemide.[1] The reasons are uncertain but all three drugs can cause sodium to be lost from the body. This seems to be an uncommon interaction but be aware that it can occur.

Reference

1 Ramzy Y, Nastase C, Camille Y, Henderson M, Belzile L and Beland F. Carbamazepine, diuretics and hyponatremia: a possible interaction. J Clin Psychiatry (1987) 48, 281–3.

Carbamazepine + Felbamate

Abstract/Summary

Felbamate reduces serum carbamazepine levels and increases serum carbamazepine-epoxide levels. Felbamate levels may fall. The importance of these changes is uncertain.

Clinical evidence

The serum carbamazepine levels (4–12 µg/ml) of 22 patients fell by 25% (range 10–42%) when additionally given felbamate (3000 mg/day). It occurred within a week, reaching a plateau after 2–4 weeks, and returning to the original levels within 2–3 weeks of stopping the felbamate.[3]

Other studies in epileptics have found reductions in carbamazepine levels of between 18 and 31%.[1,2,5,6] when felbamate was given. The carbamazepine-epoxide serum levels were also found in these studies to have risen by between 33% and 57%.[3,5,6] Carbamazepine also increases the clearance of felbamate to some extent.[4]

Mechanism

Not established. It is thought that the felbamate increases the metabolism of the carbamazepine.[3]

Importance and management

This interaction is established, but its clinical importance is uncertain because the modest fall in serum carbamazepine levels would seem to be offset by the rise in levels of its metabolite, carbamazepine-epoxide, which also has anticonvulsant activity. There is probably no need to alter the carbamazepine dosage, but be alert for any changes in the anticonvulsant control. More study is needed.

References

1 Fuerst RH, Graves NM, Leppik IE, Remmel RP, Rosenfeld WE, Sierzant

TL. A preliminary report on alteration of carbamazepine and phenytoin metabolism by felbamate. Drug Intell Clin Pharm (1986) 20, 465–6.
2 Fuerst RH, Graves NM, Leppik IE, Brundage RC, Holmes GB, Remmel RP. Felbamate increases phenytoin but decreases carbamazepine concentrations. Epilepsia (1988) 29, 488–91.
3 Albani F, Theodore WH, Washington P, Devinsky O, Bromfield E, Porter RJ, Nice FJ. Effect of Felbamate on plasma levels of carbamazepine and its metabolites. Epilepsia (1991) 32, 130–2.
4 Wagner ML, Graves NM, Marienau K, Holmes GB, Remmel RP, Leppik IE. Discontinuation of phenytoin and carbamazepine in patients receiving felbamate. Epilepsia (1991) 32, 398–406.
5 Howard JR, Dix RK, Shumaker RC, Perhach JL. The effect of felbamate on carbamazepine pharmacokinetics. Epilepsia (1992) 33, Suppl 3, 84–5.
6 Wagner ML, Remmel RP, Graves NM, Leppik IE. Effect of felbamate on carbamazepine and its major metabolites. Clin Pharmacol Ther (1993) 53, 536–43.

Carbamazepine + Fluoxetine

Abstract/Summary

Increased serum carbamazepine levels (possibly with toxicity) may occur if fluoxetine is additionally given. Parkinson-like symptoms have also been seen during concurrent use in two patients.

Clinical evidence

(a) Carbamazepine effects increased

An epileptic well controlled on 1 g carbamazepine daily for 3 years developed signs of toxicity (diplopia, blurred vision, tremor, vertigo) within a week of starting to take 20 mg fluoxetine daily. Her serum carbamazepine levels after a fortnight had risen by 33% (from 36 to 48 µmol/l). The toxicity resolved when the carbamazepine dosage was reduced to 800 mg daily. Another patient on 600 mg carbamazepine daily also developed toxic symptoms (nausea, vomiting, vertigo, tinnitus) within 10 days of starting to take 20 mg fluoxetine daily. Her serum carbamazepine levels had risen by over 60% (from 27 to 44 µmol/l). The toxic symptoms resolved when the fluoxetine was stopped.[1]

A study in six normal subjects found that seven day's treatment with 20 mg fluoxetine daily increased the AUC of carbamazepine (400 mg daily for three weeks) by 42% (from 199.7 to 284.1 µg/ml.h) and of its active epoxide metabolite by 16% (from 30.5 to 35.6 µg/ml/h). The clearance of the carbamazepine was decreased by 36% (from 38.1 to 24.4 ml/min).[2] Another study by the same group of workers found increases in the AUCs of carbamazepine and its epoxide of 27 and 31% respectively in the presence of fluoxetine.[3]

(b) Development of parkinsonism

Two patients on carbamazepine (200 mg twice daily) developed severe parkinsonism within 3–9 days of starting to take 20 mg fluoxetine daily. Carbamazepine levels were within the range 6.0–7.4 mg/l [4]

Mechanism

The evidence suggests that fluoxetine inhibits the metabolism of carbamazepine by the liver, so that its loss from the body is reduced and its serum levels rise.[2,3] The parkinsonism is not understood.

Information and management

Information appears to be limited to these reports, but the interactions appear to be established. Monitor the effects of concurrent use in any patient, anticipating the need to reduce the dosage of the carbamazepine to prevent the development of toxicity. Be alert for any evidence of parkinsonian symptoms. More study is needed.

References

1 Pearson HJ. Interaction of fluoxetine with carbamazepine. J Clin Psychiat (1990) 51, 126.
2 Grimsley SR, Jann MW, D'Mello AP, Carter GC, D'Souza MJ. Pharmaco-dynamics and pharmacokinetics of fluoxetine/carbamazepine interaction. Clin Pharmacol Ther (1991) 49, 135.
3 Grimsley SR, Jann MW, Carter GC, D'Mello AP, D'Souza MJ. Increased carbamazepine plasma concentrations after fluoxetine coadministration. Clin Pharmacol Ther (1991) 50, 10–5.
4 Gernaat HBPE, van de Woude J, Touw DJ. Fluoxetine and parkinsonism in patients taking carbamazepine. Am J Psychiatry (1991) 148, 1604–5.

Carbamazepine + Fluvoxamine

Abstract/Summary

Carbamazepine serum levels are increased by fluvoxamine. The dosage will need to be reduced to avoid toxicity.

Clinical evidence

Three patients on constant doses of carbamazepine developed increased serum levels and signs of carbamazepine toxicity (nausea, vomiting) when additionally treated with fluvoxamine. Carbamazepine levels doubled in one of them within 10 days of starting to take 50–100 mg fluvoxamine daily. The interaction was accommodated by reducing the carbamazepine dosage by 200 mg daily in all three (from 1000 to 800 mg in one of them, and from 800 to 600 mg daily in the other two).[1]

A patient taking 600 mg carbamazepine daily showed a rise in her serum carbamazepine levels from 7.3 to 12.4 µg/ml when additionally given 600 mg fluvoxamine daily.[2] No toxicity occurred but the patient felt more tired. Even when the carbamazepine dosage was reduced to 400 mg daily her serum levels remained between 10.9 and 11.8 µg/ml.[2]

Mechanism

The presumed reason for this reaction is that the fluvoxamine reduces the metabolism of the carbamazepine by the liver, resulting in a reduced loss from the body.[1,2]

Importance and management

Information appears to be limited to these reports but it appears to be a clinically important interaction. Monitor the effects of concurrent use, anticipating the need to reduce the carbamazepine dosage.

Reference

1 Fritze J, Unsorg B, Lanczik M. Interaction between carbamazepine and fluvoxamine. Acta Psychiatr Scand (1991) 84, 583–4.
2 Bonnet P, Vandel S, Nezelof S, Sechter D, Bizouard P. Carbamazepine, fluvoxamine. Is there a pharmacokinetic interaction? Therapie (1992) 47, 165–7.

Carbamazepine + Gemfibrozil

Abstract/Summary

Two patients with hyperlipoproteinaemia showed rises in carbamazepine serum levels when gemfibrozil was added.

Clinical evidence, mechanism, importance and management

Two patients with type IV hyperlipoproteinaemia showed rises in serum carbamazepine levels when given 300 mg gemfibrozil daily. One showed a rise from 8.8 to 11.4 µg/ml within four days. A rise from 8.3 µg/ml to 13.7 µg/ml was found in the other patient three months after starting to take 300 mg gemfibrozil twice daily. The suggested reason[1] is that those with elevated cholesterol and total lipids clear carbamazepine from the body more quickly[2] so that when this condition is treated with gemfibrozil the carbamazepine clearance becomes more normal and its serum levels rise accordingly. The clinical importance of this interaction is uncertain but be alert for any evidence of carbamazepine toxicity if gemfibrozil is added.

References

1 Denio L, Drake ME,, Pakalnis A. Gemfibrozil-carbamazepine interaction in epileptic patients. Epilepsia (1988) 29, 654.
2 Wichlínski LM, Sieradzki E, Gruchala M. Correlation between the total cholesterol serum concentration data and carbamazepine steady-state blood levels in humans. DICP (1983) 17, 812–4.

Carbamazepine + Isoniazid

Abstract/Summary

Carbamazepine serum levels are markedly and very rapidly increased by the concurrent use of isoniazid. Intoxication can occur if the carbamazepine dosage is not reduced appropriately.

Clinical evidence

Ten out of 13 patients, stabilized on carbamazepine developed disorientation, listlessness, aggression, lethargy and, in one case, extreme drowsiness when concurrently treated with 200 mg isoniazid daily. Serum carbamazepine levels were measured in three of the patients and they were found to have risen above the normal therapeutic range.[3]

Carbamazepine toxicity, associated with marked rises in serum carbamazepine levels, has been described in other reports.[1,2,4,5,8] Some of the patients were also taking sodium valproate or in one case[8] cimetidine. An unexplained report describes carbamazepine toxicity in a patient when given isoniazid but only when rifampicin was present as well.[7] There is also some evidence that carbamazepine increases the hepatotoxicity of isoniazid.[6]

Mechanism

It seems probable that the isoniazid inhibits the activity of the liver enzymes concerned with the metabolism and clearance of carbamazepine, so that it accumulates in the body.

Importance and management

The documentation is limited, but a clinically important and potentially serious interaction is established. Toxicity can develop quickly (the reports indicate within 1–5 days) and also disappear quickly if the isoniazid is withdrawn. Concurrent use should not be undertaken unless the effects can be closely monitored and suitable downward dosage adjustments made (a reduction to a half or a third can be effective[3]). It seems probable that those who are 'slow' metabolizers of isoniazid may show this interaction more quickly and to a greater extent than fast metabolizers.[1]

References

1 Wright JM, Stokes EF, Sweeney VP. Isoniazid-induced carbamazepine toxicity and vice versa: a double drug interaction. N Engl J Med (1982) 307, 1325–7.
2 Block SH. Carbamazepine-isoniazid interaction. Pediatr (1982) 69, 494–5.
3 Valsalan VC, Cooper GL. Carbamazepine intoxication caused by interaction with isoniazid. Br Med J (1982) 285, 261–2.
4 Arguelles PP, Riera JMS, Tahull JMG and Bori AV. Interaccion carbamacepina-tuberculostaticos. Med Clin (1984) 83, 867–8.
5 Beeley L and Ballantine N. Bulletin of the West Midlands Adverse Drug Reaction Group. (1981) 13, 8.
6 Barbare JC, Lallement PY, Vorhauer W, Veyssier P. Hepatotoxicite de l'isoniazide: influence de la carbamazepine? Gastroenterol Clin Biol (1986) 10, 523–4.
7 Fleenor ME, Harden JW, Curtis G. Interaction between carbamazepine and antituberculous agents. Chest (1991) 6, 1554.
8 Garcia B, Zaborras E, Aveas V, Obeso G, Jiménez I, De Juane P, Bermejo T. Interaction between isoniazid and carbamazepine potentiated by cimetidine. Ann Pharmacother (1992) 26, 841.

Carbamazepine + Isotretinoin

Abstract/Summary

A study in one patient found that isotretinoin reduces the serum levels of carbamazepine and its anticonvulsant metabolite.

Clinical evidence, mechanism, importance and management

A study in an epileptic patient with severe acne found that the carbamazepine AUC while taking 600 mg daily was reduced by 10% while taking 0.5 mg/kg/day isotretinoin, and by 24% by 1.0 mg/kg/day. The AUCs of carbamazepine-epoxide (the active metabolite of carbamazepine) were reduced by 21 and 44% respectively. The patient showed no adverse effects but the author of the report suggests that concurrent use should be monitored.[1] Be alert for any evidence of reduced epileptic control if isotretinoin is added.

Reference

1 Marsden JR. Effect of isotretinoin on carbamazepine pharmacokinetics. Br J Dermatol (1988) 119, 403–11.

Carbamazepine + Macrolide antibiotics

Abstract/Summary

Carbamazepine serum levels are markedly and very rapidly increased by the concurrent use of triacetyloleandomycin. Intoxication can often develop within 1–3 days. Clarithromycin, flurithromycin, josamycin and ponsinomycin appear to interact to a lesser extent but roxithromycin not at all. See also 'Carbamazepine + Erythromycin'.

Clinical evidence

(a) Clarithromycin

A cross-over trial in 12 subjects found that 500 mg clarithromycin 12-hourly for 5 days increased the AUC of a single 400 mg dose of carbamazepine by 26%, and reduced that of its active metabolite by 16%.[12] A patient showed an approximately 50% rise in serum carbamazepine levels while taking 500 mg clarithromycin daily for 10 days, despite a reduction in his carbamazepine dosage from 800 to 600 mg daily.[13]

(b) Flurithromycin, Josamycin, Ponsinomycin (Miocamycin)

Josamycin (2 g daily for a week) and flurithromycin (500 mg daily for a week) have been found to reduce the clearance of carbamazepine by about 20%.[6–9] A single dose study in 14 subjects found that after taking 1600 mg ponsinomycin daily for 8 days the AUC of a single 200 mg dose of carbamazepine was increased by 13%, and the AUC of its active metabolite (10,11-epoxycarbamazepine) was reduced 26%.[10] Another study in patients on carbamazepine found that the addition of 600 mg ponsinomycin twice daily caused a small increase in the trough serum levels of carbamazepine, and only an 11.6% increase in the area under the curve.[11]

(c) Triacetyloleandomycin

Eight epileptics on carbamazepine developed signs of intoxication (dizziness, nausea, vomiting, excessive drowsiness) within 24 h of starting to take triacetyloleandomycin. The only two patients available for examination showed a sharp rise in serum carbamazepine levels (from 5 to 28 μg/ml) over 3 days, and a rapid fall following withdrawal.[1,5] Another report[2] by the same authors describes a total of 17 similar cases of intoxication caused by triacetyloleandomycIn. Some of the patients demonstrated three or fourfold increases in serum carbamazepine levels. Other cases have been described elswhere.[3,4] In most instances the serum carbamazepine levels returned to normal within about 3–5 days of withdrawing the antibiotic.[2]

Mechanism

It seems probable that triacetyloleandomycin, and to a much lesser extent some of the other macrolides, slow the rate of metabolism of the carbamazepine by the liver enzymes so that the anticonvulsant accumulates within the body. Triacetyloleandomycin forms a complex with cytochrome P-450 in the liver.[14]

Importance and management

The carbamazepine-triacetyloleandomycin interaction is established, clinically important and potentially serious. The incidence is high. The rapidity of its development (24 h in some cases) and the extent of the rise in serum carbamazepine levels suggest that it would be difficult to control carbamazepine levels by reducing its dosage. Concurrent use should be avoided if possible.

Clarithromycin, josamycin, flurithromycin and ponsinomycin appear to be safer alternatives to either triacetyloleandomycin or erythromycin, nevertheless a small or modest reduction in the dosage of the carbamazepine may be needed (with clarithromycin an approximately 25% reduction has been suggested[13]) with subsequent good monitoring. Roxithromycin has been shown not to interact.[8]

References

1 Dravet C, Mesdjian E, Cenraud B, Roger J. Interaction between carbamazepine and triacetyloleandomycin. Lancet (1977) i, 810.

2 Mesdjian E, Dravet C, Cenraud B, Roger J. Carbamazepine intoxication due to triacetyloleandomycin administration in epileptic patients. Epilepsia (1980) 21, 489–496.

3 Amedee-Manesme O, Rey E, Brussieux J, Gontiers F, Aicardi J. Antibiotiques a ne jamais associer a la carbamazepine. Arch Fr Pediatr (1982) 39, 126.

4 Bavoux F, Dreyfus-Brisac C, Lanfranchi C, Ponsot G. Interaction carbamazepine-troleandomycine et interaction carbamazepine-erythromycine. BIR Creteil (1980) 4, 1.

5 Dravet C, Mesdjian E, Cenraud B, Roger J. Interaction carbamazepine triacetyloleandomycine: une nouvelle interaction medicamenteuse? Nouv Presse Med (1977) 6, 467.

6 Albin H, Vincon G, Pehourcq F, Dangoumau J. Influence de la josamycine sur la pharmacocinetique de la carbamazepine. Therapie (1982) 37, 151–6.

7 Vincon G, Albin H, Demotes-Mainard F, Guyot M, Brachet-Liermain A, Loiseau P. Pharmacokinetic interaction between carbamazepine and josamycin. Proc Eur Congr Biopharmaceutics Pharmacokinetics vol III: Clinical Pharmacokinetics. Edited by Aiache JM, Hirtz J. Published by Imprimerie de l'Universite de Clermont-Ferrand. (1984) pp 270–6.

8 Saint-Salvie B, Tremblay D, Surjus A, Lefebvre MA. A study of the interaction of roxithromycin with theophylline and carbamazepine. J Antimicrob Chemother (1987) 20, Suppl B, 121–9.

9 Barzaghi N, Gatti G, Crema F, Faja A, Monteleone E, Amione C, Leone L and Perucca E. Effect of flurithromycin, a new macrolide antibiotic, on carbamazepine disposition in normal subjects. Int J Clin Pharm Res (1988) VIII, 101–5.

10 Couet W, Istin B, Ingrand I, Girault J, Fourtillan J-B. Effect of ponsinomycin on single dose kinetics and metabolism of carbamazepine. Ther Drug Monit (1990) 12, 144–9.

11 Zagnoni PG, DeLuca M, Casini A. Carbamazepine-miocamycin interaction. Epilepsia (1991) 32, Suppl 1, 28.

12 Richens A, Chu S-Y, Sennello LT, Sonders RC. Effect of multiple doses of clarithromycin on the pharmacokinetics of carbamazepine. 30th Ann Intersc Conf Antimicrob Ag Chemother, Atlanta, GA, October 23rd, 1990, 213.

13 Albani F, Riva R, Baruzzi A. Clarithromycin-carbamazepine interaction: a case report. Epilepsia (1993) 34, 161–2.

14 Pessayre D, Larrey D, Vitaux J, Breil P, Belghiti J, Benhamou J-P. Formation of an inactive cytochrome P-450 Fe(II) metabolite complex after administration of troleandomycin in humans. Biochem Pharmacol (1982) 31, 1699–1704.

Carbamazepine + Miconazole

Abstract/Summary

An isolated report describes an adverse response in a patient on carbamazepine when given miconazole.

Clinical evidence, mechanism, importance and management

A patient on long-term treatment with carbamazepine (400 mg daily) developed malaise, myoclonia and tremor within three days of being given 1.125 g miconazole, and on each subsequent occasion when given miconazole. These toxic effects disappeared when the miconazole was withdrawn.[1] The general importance of this reaction is unknown.

Reference

1 Loupi E, Descotes J, Lery N, Evreux JCl. Interactions medicamenteuses et miconazole. A propos de 10 observations. Therapie (1982) 37, 437–41.

Carbamazepine + Monoamine oxidase inhibitors (MAOI)

Abstract/Summary

Phenelzine, moclobemide and tranylcypromine appear not to interact adversely with carbamazepine.

Clinical evidence, mechanism, importance and management

There appear to be no reports of adverse reactions during concurrent treatment but the makers of carbamazepine say that concurrent use should be avoided because of the close structural similarity between carbamazepine and the tricyclic antidepressants (and the theoretical risk of an adverse interaction). However a report describes a woman taking 600 mg carbamazepine daily (blood level 9.7 mg/l) who was additionally given up to 40 mg tranylcypromine daily. After 2 weeks her carbamazepine levels were 6.3 mg/l and her depressive symptoms improved substantially.[1] Two other patients similarly treated also experienced no adverse effects and no substantial changes in the serum levels of carbamazepine were seen.[1,2] Another report describes the successful and uneventful use of carbamazepine and phenelzine in an elderly patient with no changes in carbamazepine serum levels.[3] No adverse effects were seen in three patients concurrently treated with moclobemide and carbamazepine for four weeks.[4] Bearing in mind that the MAOI and the tricyclics can be administered together under certain well controlled conditions without problems (see 'Monoamine oxidase inhibitors + Tricyclic antidepressants'), the warning about the risks may prove to be overcautious. As yet there seems to be no direct information about other MAOIs.

References

1 Lydiard RB, White D, Harvey B, Taylor A. Lack of pharmacokinetic interaction between tranylcypromine and carbamazepine. J Clin Psychopharmacol (1987) 7, 360.
2 Joffe RT, Post RM, Uhde TW. Lack of pharmacokinetic interaction of carbamazepine and tranylcypromine. Arch Gen Psychiatry (1985) 42, 738.
3 Yatham LN, Barry S, Mobayed M, Dinan TG. Is the carbamazepine-phenelzine combination safe ? Am J Psychiatry (1990) 147, 367.
4 Amrein R, Güntert TW, Dingemanse J, Lorscheid T, Stabl M, Schmid-Burgk W. Interactions of moclobemide with concomitantly administered medication: evidence from pharmacological and clinical studies. Psychopharmacol (1992) 106, S24–31.

Carbamazepine + Neuroleptics

Abstract/Summary

Toxicity due to an increase in the serum levels of carbamazepine-epoxide have been reported in two patients on carbamazepine when given loxapine or chlorpromazine with amoxapine, but thioridazine appears not to interact. Carbamazepine can lower fluphenazine serum levels. Some preliminary evidence also suggests that the use of neuroleptics with carbamazepine may possibly increase the risk of the development of Stevens-Johnson syndrome.

Clinical evidence, mechanism, importance and management

(a) Raised carbamazepine-epoxide levels, or no changes

Two patients, one on 500 mg loxapine daily and the other on 350 mg chlorpromazine and 300 mg amoxapine daily, developed toxicity (ataxia, nausea, anxiety) when given 600–900 mg carbamazepine daily although their serum carbamazepine levels were low to normal. The toxicity appeared to be due to elevated carbamazepine-epoxide levels (the metabolite of carbamazepine). The problem resolved when the carbamazepine dosages were reduced. The authors of this report advise monitoring the serum levels of both carbamazepine and its metabolite if toxicity develops.[5] 100–200 mg thioridazine daily was found in another study to have no effect on the steady-state levels of carbamazepine or carbamazepine-epoxide in eight epileptic patients.[7]

(b) Stevens-Johnson syndrome

Three patients on various neuroleptics (fluphenazine, haloperidol, trifluoperazine, chlorpromazine, amitriptyline, diazepam) developed Stevens-Johnson syndrome within 8–14 days of starting to take carbamazepine. All three had erythema multiforme skin lesions and involvement of at least two mucous membranes.[1] After treatment, all three were restarted on all their previous drugs, except carbamazepine, without problems. Another case has been reported in a patient on carbamazepine, lithium carbonate, haloperidol and benzhexol.[2] The reasons are not understood. Stevens-Johnson syndrome with carbamazepine is rare and appears only to have been described in two other patients on carbamazepine alone.[3,4] It is not yet clear whether the concurrent use of neuroleptics increases the risk of its development, but until more is known it would be prudent to monitor the outcome, particularly during the first two weeks. More study is needed.

(c) Reduced fluphenazine levels

A patient on 37.5 mg fluphenazine decanoate weekly showed a serum level rise from 0.51 ng/ml to 1.17 ng/ml six weeks after stopping 800 mg carbamazepine daily. A moderate improvement in his schizophrenic condition occurred.[6]

References

1 Wong KE. Stevens-Johnson syndrome in neuroleptic-carbamazepine combination. Singapore Med J (1990) 31, 432–3.
2 Fawcett RG. Erythema multiforme major in a patient treated with carbamazepine. J Clin Psychiatry (1987) 48, 416–7.
3 Coombes BM. Stevens-Johnson syndrome associated with carbamazepine ('Tegretol'). Med J Aust (1965) 1, 895–6.
4 Patterson J. Stevens-Johnson syndrome associated with carbamazepine. Clin Psychopharmacol (1985) 5, 185.
5 Pitterle ME, Collins M. Carbamazepine-10,11-epoxide evaluation with coadministration of loxitane and amoxapine. Epilepsia (1988) 29, 654,12.
6 Jann MW, Fidone GS, Hernandez JM, Amrung S, Davis CM. Clinical implications of increased antipsychotic plasma concentrations upon anticonvulsant cessation. Psychiatry Res (1989) 28, 153–9.
7 Spina E, Amendola D'Agostino AM, Ioculano MP, Oteri G, Fazio A, Pisani F. No effect of thioridazine on plasma concentrations of carbamazepine and its active metabolite carbamazepine-10,11-epoxide. Ther Drug Monit (1990) 12, 511–3.

Carbamazepine + Phenobarbitone

Abstract/Summary

Carbamazepine serum levels are reduced to some extent by the concurrent use of phenobarbitone, but seizure control remains unaffected.

Clinical evidence

A comparative study in epileptic patients showed that on average those taking both carbamazepine and phenobarbitone (44 patients) had carbamazepine serum levels which were 18% lower than those taking only carbamazepine (43 patients).[1] Similar results were found in other studies in both adult and child patients treated with both drugs.[2,3] The seizure control remained unaffected. Carbamazepine-epoxide levels are increased.[4]

Mechanism

It seem probable that phenobarbitone stimulates the liver enzymes concerned with the metabolism of the carbamazepine, resulting in its more rapid clearance from the body.

Importance and managment

An established interaction, but of little practical importance since the seizure control is not diminished, despite the small fall in serum carbamazepine levels, because its metabolite (carbamazepine-epoxide) also has anticonvulsant activity.

References

1 Christiansen J, Dam M. Influence of phenobarbital and diphenylhydantoin on plasma carbamazepine levels in patients with epilepsy. Acta Neurol Scandinav (1973) 49, 543–6.
2 Cereghino JJ, Brock JT, Van Meter JC, Penry JK, Smith LD and White BG. The efficacy of carbamazepine combinations in epilepsy. Clin Pharmacol Ther (1975) 18, 733.
3 Rane A, Hojer B, Wilson JT. Kinetics of carbamazepine and its 10,11-epoxide metabolite in children. Clin Pharmacol Ther (1976) 19, 276.
4 Dam M, Jensen A, Christiansen J. Plasma level and effect of carbamazepine in grand mal and psychomotor epilepsy. Acta Neurol Scand (1975) 75, Suppl 51, 33–8.

Carbamazepine + Primidone

Abstract/Summary

A single case report describes markedly reduced serum carbamazepine levels, accompanied by poor seizure control, in a patient concurrently treated with primidone.

Clinical evidence

The complex partial seizures of a 15-year-old boy failed to be controlled despite treatment with primidone (12 mg/kg daily in three doses) and carbamazepine (10 mg/kg daily in three doses). Even when the carbamazepine dosage was increased from 10 to 20 and then to 30 mg daily his serum carbamazepine levels only rose from 3.5 to 4.0 and then to 4.8 μg/ml, and his seizures continued. When the primidone was gradually withdrawn his serum carbamazepine levels climbed to 12 μg/ml and his seizures completely disappeared.[1]

Mechanism

When the primidone was stopped, the clearance of the carbamazepine decreased by about 60%. This is consistent with the known enzyme-inducing effects of primidone (converted in the body to phenobarbitone) which can increase the metabolism of other drugs by the liver.

Importance and management

Direct information seems to be limited to this report so that its general importance is uncertain, but be alert for evidence of reduced carbamazepine levels in any patient given primidone. More study is needed.

Reference

1 Benetello P, Furlanut M. Primidone-carbamazepine interaction: clinical consequences. Int J Clin Pharm Res (1987) VII, 165–8.

Carbamazepine + Sodium valproate

Abstract/Summary

The serum levels of carbamazepine may fall by 20–25% (or remain unaffected) during concurrent use, and those of sodium valproate fall by 60% or more, but the rise in the levels of carbamazepine-epoxide which also has anticonvulsant activity may possibly offset the effects of this interaction (but also cause side-effects). There is also some very limited evidence that concurrent use may possibly increase the incidence of sodium valproate induced hepatotoxicity

Clinical evidence

(a) Serum carbamazepine levels reduced, unchanged.

A study on seven adult epileptics who had been taking carbamazepine (8.3–13.3 mg/kg) for more than two months showed that their steady-state serum carbamazepine levels fell by an average of 24% (range 3–59%) over a 6-day period when concurrently treated with sodium valproate (2 g daily). The levels fell in six of the patients and remained unchanged in one.[1,2]

Other reports state that falls,[4,5,7] no changes[5,6,9,19] and even a slight rise[7] have been seen in some patients. Three reports describe very marked rises in the serum levels of carbamazepine-10,11-epoxide which may cause the development of marked side-effects such as blurred vision, dizziness, vomiting, tiredness and even nystagmus.[9,18,20] Rises of 50% or more in epoxide levels were seen.[20] Acute psychosis occurred in one patient when carbamazepine was added to sodium valproate treatment.[10]

(b) Serum sodium valproate levels reduced

A study on the kinetics of sodium valproate in six normal subjects showed that the concurrent use of carbmazepine, 200 mg daily, over a three week period reduced the minimum steady-state sodium valproate levels by about 20% and increased the clearance by 30%.[3] Other reports have described reductions in serum sodium valproate levels of 62–66% when carbamazepine was added,[8,14] and rises of 50–65% when the carbamazepine was withdrawn.[15,16] The rise appears to reach a plateau after about 4 weeks.[16]

(c) Increased sodium valproate induced heptatoxicity

Some very limited evidence from epidemiological studies suggests that polytherapy increases the incidence of sodium valproate induced hepatotoxicity,[11] whereas monotherapy reduces it.[12]

Mechanism

The evidence suggests that each drug increases the metabolism of the other so that both are cleared from the body more quickly. The levels of the metabolite of carbamazepine, carbamazepine-epoxide, increase during concurrent use, probably by inhibiting its metabolism.[17] Carbamazepine may also possibly increase the formation of a minor but heptatotoxic metabolite of sodium valproate (2-propyl-4-pentenoic acid or 4-ene-VPA).[13]

Importance and management

Moderately well documented interactions, both of which seem to be established. Be alert for falls in the serum levels of both drugs. However the clinical importance of this is uncertain because the metabolite of carbamazepine (carbamazepine-epoxide) also has anticonvulsant activity so that it may not be necessary to increase the dosages of the drugs to maintain adequate seizure control. Be alert for evidence of high levels of carbamazepine-epoxide and its associated toxicity. Also bear in mind the evidence that concurrent use may possibly increase the incidence of sodium valproate induced liver toxicity.

References

1 Levy RH, Morselli PL, Bianchetti G, Guyot M, Brachet-Liermain A, Loiseau P. Interaction between valproic acid and carbamazepine in epileptic patients. In 'Metabolism of Antiepileptic Drugs' edited by RH Levy et al. Raven Press, New York (1984) pp 45–51.

2 Levy RH, Moreland TA, Morselli PL, Guyot M, Brachet-Liermain A and Loiseau P. Carbamazepine/valproic acid interaction in man and rhesus monkey. Epilepsia (1984) 25, 338–45.

3 Bowdle TA, Levy RH, Cutler RE. Effects of carbamazepine on valproic acid kinetics in normal subjects. Clin Pharmacol Ther (1979) 26, 629.

4 Jeavons PM, Clark JE. Sodium valproate in the treatment of epilepsy. Brit Med J (1974) 2, 584.

5 Wilder BJ, Willmore LJ, Bruni J, Villarreal HJ. Valproic acid: interaction with other anticonvulsant drugs. Neurology (1978) 28, 892.

6 Fowler GW. Effects of dipropylacetate on serum levels of anticonvulsants in children. Proc West Pharmacol Soc (1978) 21, 37.

7 Varma R, Michos GA, Varma RS, Hoshino AY. Clinical trials of Depakene (valproic acid) coadministered with anticonvulsants in epileptic patients. Res Comm Psychol Psychiat Behav (1980) 5, 265.

8 Reunanen MI, Luoma P, Myllyla VV, Hokkanen M. Low serum valproic acid concentrations in epileptic patients on combination therapy. Curr Ther Res (1980) 28, 455–62.

9 Pisani F, Fazio A, Oteri G, Ruello C, Gitto C, Russo R, Perucca E. Sodium valproate and valpromide: differential interactions with carbamazepine in epileptic patients. Epilepsia (1986) 27, 548–52.

10 McKee RJW, Larkin JG, Brodie MJ. Acute psychosis with carbamazepine and sodium valproate. Lancet (1989) i, 167.

11 Dreifuss FE, Santilli N, Langer DH, Sweeney KP, Moline KA, Menander KB. Valproic acid fatalities: a retrospective review. Neurology (1987) 37, 379–85.

12 Dreifuss FE, Langer DH, Moline KA, Maxwell DE. Valproic acid hepatic fatalities. II. US experience since 1984. Neurology (1989) 39, 201–7.

13 Levy RH, Rettenmeier AW, Anderson GD, Wilensky AJ, Friel PN, Bailiie TA, Acheampong A, Tor J, Guyot M, Poiseau P. Effects of polytherapy with phenytoin, carbamazepine, and stiripentol on formation of 4-ene-valproate, a hepatotoxic metabolite of valproic acid. Clin Pharmacol Ther (1990) 48, 225–35.

14 May T, Rambeck B. Serum concentrations of valproic acid; influence of dose and comedication. Ther Drug Monit (1985) 7, 387–90.

15 Henriksen O, Johannessen SI. Clinical and pharmacokinetic observations on sodium valproate — a 5 year follow-up study in 100 children with epilepsy. Acta Neurol Scand (1982) 65, 504–23.

16 Jann MW, Fidone GS, Israel MK, Bonadero P. Increased valproate serum concentrations upon carbamazepine cessation. Epilepsia (1988) 29, 578–81.

17 Pisani F, Caputo M, Fazio A, Oteri G, Russo M, Spina E, Perucca E, Bertilsson L. Interaction of carbamazepine-10,11-epoxide, an active metabolite of carbamazepine, with valproate: a pharmacokinetic study. Epilepsia (1990) 31, 339–42.

18 Rambeck B, Sälke-Treumann A, May Th, Boenigk HE. Valproic acid-induced carbamazepine-10,11-epoxide toxicity in children and adolescents. Eur Neurol (1990) 30, 79–83.

19 Sunaoshi W, Miura H, Takanashi S, Shira H, Hosoda N. Influence of concurrent administration of sodium valproate on the plasma concentrations of carbamazepine and its epoxide and diol metabolites. Jap J Psychiat Neurol (1991) 45, 474–7.

20 Kutt H, Solomon G, Peterson H, Dhar A, Caronna J. Accumulation of carbamazepine epoxide caused by valproate contributing to intoxication syndromes. Neurology (1985) 35 (Suppl 1) 286.

Carbamazepine + Valnoctamide

Abstract/Summary

Carbamazepine intoxication may develop if valnoctamide is taken concurrently.

Clinical evidence, mechanism, importance and management

A preliminary study in epileptics on carbamazepine found that valnoctamide caused a 1.5 to six-fold increase in the serum levels of carbamazepine-epoxide (an active metabolite), associated in some instances with clinical signs of carbamazepine intoxication. A further study in six normal subjects found that 600 mg valnoctamide daily for eight days increased the half-life of a single 100 mg dose of carbamazepine-epoxide threefold (from 6.7 to 19.7 h) and decreased its oral clearance fourfold (from 109.6 to 28.8 ml/h/kg.[1,2]

Mechanism

The reason appears to be that the valnoctamide inhibits the enzyme (epoxide hydrolase) which is concerned with the metabolism and elimination of carbamazepine and its metabolite.

Importance and management

Information is limited but the interaction appears to be established. Patients on carbamazepine who additionally take valnoctamide (available as an over-the-counter tranquillizer in some countries) could rapidly develop carbamazepine toxicity because the metabolism of its major metabolite (carbamazepine-epoxide) is inhibited. There may also be other risks relating to the detoxification of a number of other compounds. This is very similar to the interaction which can occur between carbamazepine and valpromide (an isomer of valnoctamide). Valnoctamide should be avoided unless the carbamazepine dosage can be reduced appropriately.

References

1 Pisiani F, Fazio A, Artesi C, Oteri G, Spina E, Tomson T, Perucca E. Impairment of carbamazepine-10,11-epoxide elimination by valnoctamide, a valpromide isomer, in healthy subjects. Br J clin Pharmac (1992) 34, 85–7.

2 Pisiani et al, unpublished data, quoted in reference 1.

Carbamazepine + Valpromide

Abstract/Summary

Carbamazepine intoxication can occur if valpromide is substituted for sodium valproate in patients taking carbamazepine. The serum levels of carbamazepine may not rise but the levels of its active metabolite, carbamazepine-epoxide, can be markedly increased. It has been suggested that this may possibly increase the teratogenic, mutagenic and carcinogenic risks.

Clinical evidence

Five out of seven epileptic patients on carbamazepine developed symptoms of carbamazepine intoxication when concurrent treatment with sodium valproate was replaced by valpromide (*Depamide*), despite the fact that their serum carbamazepine

levels did not increase.[1] The intoxication appeared to be connected with a four-fold increase in the serum levels of the metabolide of carbamazepine (carbamazepine-10,11-epoxide) which rose to 8.5 μg/ml.[1]

In another study on six epileptic patients the serum levels of this metabolite rose threefold (range two- to nine-fold) within a week of concurrent use and two of the patients developed confusion, dizziness and vomiting. The symptoms disappeared and serum carbamazepine-epoxide levels fell when the valpromide dosage was reduced to two-thirds.[2]

Mechanism

Valpromide reduces the metabolism by the liver of carbamazepine and its metabolite, carbamazepine-epoxide, because it inhibits epoxide hydrolase.[4] This metabolite has anticonvulsant activity but it may also be toxic if its serum levels become excessive.[2,3]

Importance and management

An established interaction. It is suggested that both carbamazepine and carbamazepine-epoxide serum levels should be monitored during concurrent use.[3] The dosages should be reduced appropriately if necessary. There is also some debate about whether this combination should be avoided, not only because of the risk of intoxication but also because inhibition of epoxide hydrolase may be undesirable.[1] This enzyme is thought to be important for the detoxification of a number of teratogenic, mutagenic and carcinogenic epoxides.[1,3]

References

1 Meijer JWA, Binnie CD, Debets RMChr, Van Parys JAP and de Beer-Pawlikowski NKB. Possible hazard of valpromide-carbamazepine combination therapy in epilepsy. Lancet (1984) i, 802.

2 Pisani F, Fazio A, Oteri G, Ruello C, Gitto C, Russo R, Perucca E. Sodium valproate and valpromide: differential interactions with carbamazepine in epileptic patients. Epilepsia (1986) 27, 548–52.

3 Levy RH, Kerr BM, Loiseau P, Guyot M, Wilensky AJ. Inhibition of carbamazepine epoxide elimination by valpromide and valproic acid. Epilepsia (1986) 27, 592.

4 Pisani F, Fazio A, Oteri G, Spina E, Perucca E, Bertilsson L. Effect of valpromide on the pharmacokinetics of carbamazepine-10,11-epoxide. Br J Clin Pharmac (1988) 25, 611–13.

Ethosuximide + Barbiturates, Phenytoin or Primidone

Abstract/Summary

Falls in serum ethosuximide levels can occur if primidone or phenytoin are used concurrently, whereas methylphenobarbitone (mephobarbital) can cause a rise. Ethosuximide is also reported to have caused phenytoin intoxication.

Clinical evidence, mechanism, importance and management

A study[1] on 198 epileptic patients showed that the concurrent use of phenytoin or primidone depressed serum ethosuximide levels, whereas a report describes a rise when methylphenobarbitone was used.[2] Three cases have occurred in which ethosuximide appeared to have been responsible for the development of phenytoin intoxication,[3–5] but primidone serum levels are reported not to be affected.[6] The concurrent use of anticonvulsant agents is common and often advantageous, but these reports emphasize the need to monitor the effects to ensure that seizure control remains good and that toxicity does not develop.

References

1 Battino D, Cusi C, Franceschetti S, Moise A, Spina S, Avanzini G. Ethosuximide plasma concentrations: influence of age and concomitant therapy. Clin Pharmacokinet (1982) 7, 176–80.
2 Smith GA, McKauge L, Dubetz D, Tyrer JH, Eadie MJ. Factors influencing plasma concentrations of ethosuximide. Clin Pharmacokinet (1979) 4, 38.
3 Lander CM, Eadie MJ, Tyrer JH. Interactions between anticonvulsants. Proc Aust Assoc Neurol (1975) 12, 111.
4 Dawson GW, Brown HW, Clark BG. Serum phenytoin after ethosuximide. Ann Neurol (1978) 4, 583.
5 Franzten E, Hansen JM, Hansen OE. Phenytoin (Dilantin) intoxication. Acta Neurol Scand (1967) 43, 440.
6 Schmidt D. The effect of phenytoin and ethosuximide on primidone metabolism in patients with epilepsy. J Neurol (1975) 209, 115.

Ethosuximide + Carbamazepine

Abstract/Summary

Serum ethosuximide levels are reduced by carbamazepine, but whether this adversely affects seizure control is uncertain.

Clinical evidence

A study in normal subjects taking 500 mg ethosuximide daily showed that the mean serum levels were reduced by 17% (from 32 to 27 μg/ml) after taking 200 mg carbamazepine daily for 18 days. One patient showed a 35% reduction.[1] A reduction in serum levels has also been described in patients.[3] In contrast, no interaction was seen in another study on epileptic patients taking several anticonvulsants.[2] The most probable explanation for this interaction is that the carbamazepine (a recognized enzyme inducing agent) increases the metabolism and clearance of the ethosuximide. The evidence for this interaction is very limited and its clinical importance is uncertain, but until it is more clearly defined it would be prudent to be alert for any signs of reduced seizure control.

References

1 Warren JW, Benmaman JD, Wannamaker BBB and Levy RH. Kinetics of a carbamazepine-ethosuximide interaction. Clin Pharmacol Ther (1980) 28, 646.

2 Smith GA, McKauge L, Dubetz D, Tyrer JH, Eadie MJ. Factors influencing plasma concentrations of ethosuximide. Clin Pharmacokinet (1979) 4, 38.
3 Battino D, Cusi C, Franceschetti S, Moise A, Spina S, Avanzini G. Ethosuximide plasma concentrations: influence of age and associated concomitant therapy. Clin Pharmacokinet (1982) 7, 176–80.

Ethosuximide + Isoniazid

Abstract/Summary

A single report describes a patient who developed psychotic behaviour and signs of ethosuximide intoxication when concurrently treated with isoniazid.

Clinical evidence, mechanism, importance and management

An epileptic patient, well controlled on ethosuximide and sodium valproate for 2 years, developed persistent hiccoughing, nausea, vomiting, anorexia and insomnia within a week of starting to take 300 mg isoniazid daily. Psychotic behaviour gradually developed over the next five weeks. The appearance and subsequent disappearance of these symptoms appeared to be related to the sharp rise (up to 198 ug/ml) and later the fall in serum ethosuximide levels.[1] It is suggested that the isoniazid may have inhibited the metabolism of the ethosuximide, leading to accumulation and intoxication. The general importance of this reaction is uncertain, but it would now seem prudent to monitor concurrent use in any patient.

Reference

1 Van Wieringen A, Vrijlandt CM. Ethosuximide intoxication caused by interaction with isoniazid. Neurology (1983) 33, 1227–8.

Ethosuximide + Sodium valproate

Abstract/Summary

Some studies have shown that ethosuximide serum levels can rise significantly if sodium valproate is given concurrently. Other studies have failed to demonstrate this interaction.

Clinical evidence

Four out of five patients taking ethosuximide (averaging 27 mg/kg) showed an approximately 50% increase in serum levels (from an average of 73 to 112 μg/ml) within three weeks of starting to take sodium valproate (averaging 42 mg/kg). Sedation occurred. Other anticonvulsants being taken included phenytoin, phenobarbitone, primidone and clonazepam.[1] Nine days treatment with sodium valproate is reported in a single dose study in six normal subjects to have raised serum ethosuximide levels, the clearance being reduced by 15%,[2] but other studies have described no changes[3,4] or even reduced serum levels.[5] The reason for these discordant results is not understood. The concurrent use of anticonvulsant agents is common and often advantageous, but these reports emphasize the need to monitor the effects to ensure that toxicity does not develop and that good seizure control is maintained.

References

1 Mattson RH, Cramer JA. Valproic acid and ethosuximide interaction. Ann Neurol (1980) 7, 583.
2 Pisani F, Narbone MC, Trunfio C, Fazio A, La Rosa G, Oteri G, Di Perri R. Valproic acid-ethosuximide interaction: a pharmacokinetic study. Epilepsia (1984) 23, 229–33.
3 Fowler GW. Effect of dipropylacetate on serum levels of anticonvulsants in children. Proc West Pharmacol Soc (1978) 21, 37.
4 Bauer LA, Harris C, Wilensky AJ, Raisys VA, Levy RH. Ethosuximide kinetics: possible interaction with valproic acid. Clin Pharmacol Ther (1982) 31, 741–5.
5 Battino D, Cusi C, Franceschetti S, Moise A, Spina S, Avanzini G. Ethosuximide plasma concentrations: influence of age and associated concomitant therapy. Clin Pharmacokinet (1982) 7, 176–80.

Flunarizine + Anticonvulsants

Abstract/Summary

Phenytoin, carbamazepine and sodium valproate can reduce serum flunarizine levels.

Clinical evidence, mechanism, importance and management

A study of the value of flunarizine in treating epilepsy found that other anticonvulsants (carbamazepine, phenytoin, sodium valproate) reduced the serum levels of flunarizine (possibly by enzyme induction). The more drugs were used, the greater the reduction. Flunarizine did not affect the serum levels of these other anticonvulsants.[1] There would seem to be no reason for avoiding concurrent use, but the outcome should be monitored.

Reference

1 Binnie CD, de Beukelaar F, Meijer JWA, Meinardi H, Overweg J, Wauquier A, van Wieringen A. Open dose-ranging trial of flunarizine as add-on therapy in epilepsy. Epilepsia (1985) 26, 424–8.

Gabapentin + Miscellaneous drugs

Abstract/Summary

Gabapentin appears not to interact to a clinically important extent with cimetidine, oral contraceptives, *Maalox* or probenecid.

Clinical evidence, mechanism, importance and management

Gabapentin has been found not to induce or inhibit hepatic mixed function enzymes (as determined by its lack of effect on antipyrine (phenazone) and is therefore unlikely to interact with drugs which are affected by enzyme inducers or inhibitors. The steady-state pharmacokinetics of ethinyl oestradiol and norethindrone (in *Norlestrin*, an oral contraceptive) were unaffected by repeated administration of gabapentin so that the reliability of combined oral contraceptives of this type would not be expected to altered. *Maalox TC* reduced the bioavailability of gabapentin by less than 20% and cimetidine decreased the renal clearance of gabapentin by 12%, whereas probenecid had no effect on renal clearance.[1,2] Neither of these modest changes is expected to be of clinical importance. There would seem to be no need to take special precautions if any of these drugs is used concurrently.

Reference

1 Busch JA, Bockbrader HN, Randinitis J Chang T, Elling PG, Reece PA, Underwood B, SEdman AJ, Vollmer KO, Türck D. Lack of clinically significant drug interactions with Neurontin (Gabapentin). 20th Int Epilepsy Congress, Oslo, Norway, July 1993.
2 Richens A. Clinical pharmacokinetics of gabapentin, in 'New Trends in Epilesy Management: The Role of Gabapentin' (ed D. Chadwick). Proceedings of a satellite symposium, Epilepsy Europe 1992. Int Congress and Symposium Series No 198, Roy Soc Med Services, London NY 1993. p 41–6

Methsuximide + Felbamate

Abstract/Summary

Preliminary information indicates that methsuximide toxicity can develop if its dosage is not reduced while taking felbamate.

Clinical evidence, mechanism, importance and management

Three adolescent epileptics on methsuximide developed mild side-effects within three days of starting to take felbamate, which became more serious by the end of a month (decreased appetite, nausea, weight loss, insomnia, dizziness, hiccups, slurred speech). During this time the normethsuximide levels in two of them rose 26 and 46%. Despite a reduction in the methsuximide dosage of 15%, the normethsuximide levels rose by 5%. The adverse effects disappeared and the normethsuximide levels fell when the methsuximide dosage was further reduced. Other anticonvulsants being taken were carbamazepine (1), ethotoin (1) and sodium valproate (1).

The reasons for the rise in normethsuximide levels are not known, but it seems possible that felbamate inhibits its metabolism. There would seem to be no reason to avoid concurrent use, but dosage adjustments are clearly needed.

Reference

1 Patrias J, Espe-Lillo J, Ritter FJ. Felbamate-methsuximide interaction. Epilepsia (1992) 33, Suppl 3, 84.

Methsuximide + Phenobarbitone, Phenytoin, Primidone.

Abstract/Summary

The serum levels of phenobarbitone, phenytoin and of the active metabolite of methsuximide, are increased by concurrent use. Dosage reductions may be necessary to prevent undesirable side-effects.

Clinical evidence, mechanism, importance and management

A study in 94 hospitalized patients with petit mal epilepsy found that when methsuximide was given to patients on phenobarbitone or primidone, the mean serum levels of phenobarbitone rose by 38 and 40% respectively. Phenytoin serum levels rose by 78%. It was also found that the concurrent use of either phenobarbitone or phenytoin increased the serum levels of the active anticonvulsant metabolite of methsuximide (N-desmethyl-methsuximide). The suggested reason is that all of these drugs compete for the same metabolic mechanisms (hydroxylation) in the liver. As a result each one is metabolized more slowly and is therefore is lost from the body more slowly. The authors of this study conclude that the undesirable side-effects of mesuximide on combined therapy partly arise from these increases in serum anticonvulsant levels. This, they suggest, can be avoided, or at least reduced, if serum levels are regularly monitored and the dosages reduced where necessary.[1]

References

1 Rambeck B. Pharmacological interactions of mesuximide with phenobarbital and phenytoin in hospitalized epileptic patients. Epilepsia (1979) 20, 147–56.

Phenytoin + Alcohol

Abstract/Summary

Chronic heavy drinking reduces serum phenytoin concentrations and above-average doses of phenytoin may be needed to maintain adequate levels. Excessive drinking also seems to increase the frequency of seizures in epileptics. Moderate and occasional drinking has little effect.

Clinical evidence

A comparative study showed that blood phenytoin levels measured 24 h after the last dose of phenytoin of a group of 15 drinkers (consuming a minimum of 200 g ethanol daily for at least three weeks) was approximately half that of 76 non-drinkers. The phenytoin half-life was reduced 30% (from 23.5 to 16.3 h).[1]

Another study confirmed that alcoholics have lower than usual plasma levels of phenytoin after taking standard doses while drinking,[2] and a report describes a chronic alcoholic who was resistant to large doses of phenytoin.[3] The metabolism of phenytoin is not affected by acute ingestion of alcohol.[4]

Mechanism

Supported by animal data,[5] the evidence suggests that alcohol induces liver microsomal enzymes so that the rate of metabolism and clearance of phenytoin from the body is increased.

Importance and management

An established interaction although the documentation is limited. Those who drink heavily may need above average doses of phenytoin to maintain adequate serum levels. Epileptics should be encouraged to limit their drinking because heavy drinking appears to increase the frequency of seizures.[6] Occasional moderate drinking appears to be safe.

References

1 Kater RMH, Roggin G, Tobon F, Zieve P, Iber FL. Increased rate of clearance of drugs from the circulation of alcoholics. Amer J Med Sci (1969) 258, 35.
2 Sandor P, Sellers EM, Dumbrell M, Khouw V. Effect of short- and long-term alcohol use on phenytoin kinetics in chronic alcoholics. Clin Pharmacol Ther (1981) 30, 390–7.
3 Birkett DJ, Graham GG, Chinwah PM, Wade DN, Hickie JB. Multiple drug interactions with phenytoin. Med J Aust (1977) 2, 467–8.
4 Schmidt D. Effect of ethanol intake on phenytoin metabolism on volunteers. Experentia (1975) 31, 1313.
5 Rubin E, Lieber CS. Hepatic microsomal enzymes in man and rat: induction and inhibition by ethanol. Science (1968) 162, 690.
6 Lambie DG, Stanaway L and Johnson RH. Factors which influence the effectiveness of treatment of epilepsy. Aust NZ Med J (1986) 16, 779–84.

Phenytoin + Allopurinol

Abstract/Summary

A single case report describes phenytoin intoxication in a boy when given allopurinol.

Clinical evidence, mechanism, importance and management

A 13-year-old boy with Lesch-Nyhan syndrome who was taking phenobarbitone, clonazepam, sodium valproate and phenytoin (200 mg daily) became somnolent within seven days of starting to take allopurinol (150 mg daily). His serum phenytoin levels were found to have almost tripled (from 7.5 to 20 μg/ml).[1]

The reason for this reaction is not known (possibly inhibition of liver enzymes ?) and its general importance is uncertain — probably very small — but it might be prudent to monitor the effects of concurrent use to confirm that no toxic effects develop.

Reference

1 Yokochi K, Yokochi A, Chiba K, Ishizaki T. Phenytoin-allopurinol interaction: Michaelis-Menten kinetic parameters of phenytoin with and without allopurinol in a child with Lesch-Nyhan syndrome. Ther Drug Monit (1982) 4, 353–7.

Phenytoin + Amiodarone

Abstract/Summary

Serum phenytoin levels can be raised, markedly so in some individuals, by the concurrent use of amiodarone. Phenytoin intoxication may occur if the dosage of phenytoin is not reduced appropriately. Amiodarone serum levels are reduced.

Clinical evidence

(a) Phenytoin serum levels increased

Three patients showed a marked rise in serum phenytoin levels when concurrently treated with amiodarone (400–1200 mg daily). One of them developed phenytoin intoxication (ataxia, lethargy, vertigo) within four weeks of starting to take amiodarone and had a serum phenytoin level of 40 µg/ml, representing a three- to four-fold rise. Levels restabilized when the phenytoin dosage was reduced from 400 to 200 mg daily. The serum phenytoin levels of the other two were approximately doubled by the amiodarone.[1]

A threefold rise in serum phenytoin levels with toxicity caused by amiodarone (400 mg daily) described in another report,[2] and a study in normal subjects showed that after taking 200 mg amiodarone daily for 3 weeks the AUC of phenytoin was increased by 31%.[3] A pharmacokinetic study found that 200 mg amiodarone daily for 6 weeks raised the peak serum phenytoin levels by 33% and the AUC by 40%.[6] An elderly man showed evidence of intoxication within 2 weeks of starting to take amiodarone.[4]

(b) Amiodarone serum levels reduced

A study in five subjects given 200 mg amiodarone daily showed that over a 5-week period the serum amiodarone levels gradually increased. When phenytoin (3–4 mg/kg daily) was added for a period of 2 weeks, the serum amiodarone levels fell to concentrations which were 32.5%–48.7% below those predicted.[5,7]

Mechanisms

Uncertain. (a) It seems possible that amiodarone inhibits the liver enzymes concerned with the metabolism of phenytoin,

resulting in a rise in its serum levels. Amiodarone also binds extensively to serum and tissue proteins and a displacement interaction may have had some part to play. (b) Phenytoin is an enzyme-inducing agent which possibly increases the metabolism of the amiodarone by the liver.

Importance and management

Information seems to be limited to the reports cited but both interactions appear to be clinically important. Concurrent use should not be undertaken unless the effects can be well monitored. (a) The phenytoin dosage should be reduced as necessary. A 25–30% reduction has been recommended for those taking 2–4 mg/kg/day.[6,8] The phenytoin levels in some individuals can be doubled after only 10 days concurrent use.[1] One of the patients described above was restabilized on half the dosage of phenytoin.[1] Amiodarone is cleared from the body very slowly so that this interaction will persist for weeks after its withdrawal. Continued monitoring is important. Be aware that ataxia due to phenytoin intoxication may be confused with amiodarone-induced ataxia.[1,4] (b) It is not clear whether the amiodarone dosage should be increased or not to accommodate this interaction because the metabolite of amiodarone (N-desmethylamiodarone) also has important antiarrhythmic effects.[7]

References

1 McGovern B, Geer VR, LaRaia PJ, Garan H, Ruskin JN. Possible interaction between amiodarone and phenytoin. Ann Intern Med (1984) 101, 650–1.
2 Gore JM, Haffajee CI, Alpert JS. Interaction of amiodarone and diphenylhydantoin. Amer J Cardiol (1984) 54, 1145.
3 Nolan PE, Marus FI, Hoyer G, Bliss M, Mayersohn MP, Gear K. Pharmacokinetic interaction between amiodarone and phenytoin. J Amer Coll Cardiol (1987) 9, (2 Suppl A) 47A.
4 Shackleford EJ, Watson FT. Amiodarone-phenytoin interaction. Drug Intell Clin Pharm (1987) 21, 921.
5 Nolan PE, Marcus FI, Karol MD, Hoyer GL and Gear K. Evidence for an effect of phenytoin on the pharmacokinetics of amiodarone. Pharmacotherapy (1988) 8, 121.
6 Nolan PE, Erstad BL, Hoyer GL, Bliss M, Gear K, Marcus FI. Steady-state interaction between amiodarone and phenytoin in normal subjects. Amer J Cardiol (1990) 65, 1252–7.
7 Nolan PE, Marcus FI, Karol MD, Hoyer GL, Gear K. Effect of phenytoin on the clinical pharmacokinetics of amiodarone. J Clin Pharmacol (1990) 30, 1112–9.
8 Nolan PE, Eerstad BL, Hoyer GL, Bliss M, Gear K, Marcus FI. Interaction between amiodarone and phenytoin. Am J Cardiol (1991) 67, 328–9.

Phenytoin + Antacids

Abstract/Summary

Some, but not all, studies have shown that antacids can reduce phenytoin serum levels and this may have been responsible for some loss of seizure control in a few patients, but usually no clinically important interaction occurs.

Clinical evidence

(a) Evidence of an interaction

Three patients taking phenytoin were found to have low serum phenytoin levels (2–4 µg/ml) when given phenytoin and un-named antacids at the same time, but when the antacid administration was delayed 2–3 h the serum phenytoin levels rose 2–3-fold.[1]

A controlled study in six epileptics showed that *Gelusil* (magnesium trisilicate and aluminium hydroxide) could cause a 12% reduction in serum phenytoin levels.[2] Two epileptics are reported elsewhere to have shown inadequate seizure control which coincided with their ingestion of antacids for dyspepsia.[3] Reduced levels of phenytoin (AUC's reduced about one-third) occurred in eight subjects given either aluminium hydroxide, magnesium hydroxide or calcium carbonate,[5] and a reduction (greater than 30%) occurred in three subjects given *Asilone* (dimethicone, aluminum hydroxide, magnesium oxide).[6]

(b) Evidence of no interaction

A study in six normal subjects given aluminium hydroxide or magnesium hydroxide failed to show any change in the rate or extent of absorption of a single dose of phenytoin.[3] Another study on two subjects[4] found no alteration in the absorption of phenytoin due to magnesium hydroxide, aluminium hydroxide-magnesium trisilicate mixture or calcium carbonate. No statistically significant decrease in absorption was seen in six subjects given *Asilone*.[6]

Mechanism

Not understood. One suggestion is that diarrhoea and a general increase in peristalsis caused by some antacids may cause a reduction in phenytoin absorption. Another is that antacids may cause changes in gastric acid secretion which could affect phenytoin solubility.

Importance and management

This possible interaction is fairly well documented, but the results are conflicting. In practice it appears not to be important in most patients, although some loss of seizure control has been seen to occur in a few. The interaction is unpredictable because it seems to depend on the individual patient and the antacid being taken. Concurrent use need not be avoided but if there is any hint that an epileptic patient is being affected, separation of the dosages by 2–3 h may minimize the effects.

References

1 Pippinger L. Quoted by Kutt H in 'Interactions of antiepileptic drugs.' Epilepsia (1975) 16, 393.
2 Kulshreshtha VK, Thomas M, Wadsworth J, Richens A. Interaction between phenytoin and antacids. Br J clin Pharmac (1978) 6, 177.
3 O'Brien LS, Orme ML'E and Breckenridge AM. Failure of antacids to alter the pharmacokinetics of phenytoin. Br J clin Pharmac (1978) 6, 176.
4 Chapron DJ, Kramer PA, Mariano SL and Hohnadel DC. Effect of calcium and antacids on phenytoin bioavailability. Arch Neurol (1979) 36, 436.
5 Carter BL, Garnett WR, Pellock JM, Stratton MA, Howell JR. Effect of antacids on phenytoin bioavailability. Ther Drug Monit (1981) 3, 333–40.
6 McElnay JC, Uprichard G, Collier PS. The effect of activated dimethicone and a proprietary antacid preparation containing this agent on the absorption of phenytoin. Br J clin Pharmac (1982) 13, 501.

Phenytoin + Anticoagulants

Abstract/Summary

The serum levels of phenytoin can be increased by dicoumarol (intoxication seen) and phenprocoumon, but they are usually unchanged by warfarin and phenindione. However a single case of phenytoin intoxication has been seen with warfarin. Phenytoin can reduce the anticoagulant effects of dicoumarol and increase the effects of warfarin, whereas the effects of phenprocoumon normally appear to be unaltered.

Clinical evidence

Effects of oral anticoagulants on phenytoin

(i) Phenytoin + Dicoumarol

A study on six subjects taking 300 mg phenytoin daily showed that when additionally given dicoumarol (doses adjusted to give prothrombin values of about 30%) their serum phenytoin levels rose on average over 7 days by almost 10 µg/ml (+126%).[4] Similar results are described in another study.[7] A patient on dicoumarol developed phenytoin intoxication within only 6 days of starting to take 300 mg phenytoin daily.[6]

(ii) Phenytoin + Phenprocoumon or Pheninidione

A study in four patients on 300 mg phenytoin daily showed that when additionally given phenprocoumon (doses adjusted to give PP values within the therapeutic range) their serum phenytoin levels rose from 10 to 14 µg/ml over 7 days.[7] The phenytoin half-life increased from 9.9 to 14 h. No changes were seen in an associated study when pheninidione was used instead of phenprocoumon.[7]

(iii) Phenytoin + Warfarin

A study in two patients on 300 mg phenytoin daily found that serum phenytoin levels were unaffected by the concurrent use of warfarin over seven days, and the half-life of phenytoin in four other patients was unaffected.[7] However a patient on 300 mg phenytoin daily has been described who developed signs of intoxication within a short time of starting to take warfarin.[5]

Effects of phenytoin on oral anticoagulants

(i) Dicoumarol + Phenytoin

Six subjects on constant daily doses of dicoumarol (40–160 mg) were given 300 mg phenytoin daily for a week. Serum dicoumarol levels started to fall within 5 days and continued to do so for five days after the phenytoin was stopped. They fell from 29 to 21 µg/ml. No significant changes in the PP% occurred until three days after stopping the phenytoin when it climbed from 20 to 50%. Four other subjects on 60 mg dicoumarol daily showed a fall in serum levels from 20 to 5 µg/ml over a 6 week period while taking 300 mg phenytoin daily for the first week and then 100 mg daily for 5 weeks. The PP% after 2 weeks had risen from 20 to 70% and only fell to previous levels 5½ weeks after stopping the phenytoin.[1]

(ii) Phenprocoumon + Phenytoin

An investigation in patients on long-term phenprocoumon treatment showed that in the majority of cases phenytoin had no significant effect on either serum phenprocoumon levels or the anticoagulant control, although a few patients showed a fall and others a rise in serum anticoagulant levels.[2]

(iii) Warfarin + Phenytoin

The prothrombin time of a patient on warfarin increased from 21 to 32 s over a month when given 300 mg phenytoin daily, despite a 22% reduction in the warfarin dosage. He was restabilized on the original warfarin dosage when the phenytoin was withdrawn. Another patient is said to have shown this interaction but no details are given.[8] Four other reports describe this interaction.[9–12] One of them[11] describes a patient who had an increased anticoagulant response for 6 days, after which it was reduced.

Table 7.2 Summary of interactions between phenytoin and anticoagulants

Concurrent treatment with phenytoin and anticoagulant	Effect on serum anticoagulant levels	Effect on serum phenytoin levels
Dicoumarol	Reduced[1]	Markedly increased[4,6,7]
Phenprocoumon	Usually unchanged[2]	Increased[7]
Warfarin	Increased[8–12] Single case of increase followed by decrease[11]	Usually unchanged[7] Single case of increase[5]
Phenindione	Not documented	Usually unchanged[4,7]
Other anticoagulants	Not documented	Not documented

Mechanisms

Multiple and complex. Dicoumarol and phenprocoumon (but not normally warfarin) appear to inhibit the metabolism of phenytoin by the liver so that its loss from the body is reduced. Phenytoin appears to increase the metabolism of dicoumarol, reduce the metabolism of warfarin, but has no effect on the metabolism of phenprocoumon. Phenytoin possibly also has a diverse depressant effect on the liver which lowers blood clotting factor production.[3]

Importance and management

None of these interactions has been extensively studied, but what is known suggests that the use of dicoumarol with phenytoin should be avoided. Serum phenytoin levels should be well monitored if phenprocoumon is used, and both the phenytoin levels and anticoagulant control should be well monitored if warfarin is given. Dosage adjustments may be needed to accommodate these interactions. Information about other anticoagulants (apart from phenindione) appears to be lacking, but it would clearly be prudent to monitor the effects of concurrent use. See Table 7.2 for a summary.

References

1 Hansen JM, Siersbaek-Nielsen K, Kristensen M, Skovsted L and Christensen LK. Effect of diphenylhydantoin on the metabolism of dicoumarol in man. Acta Med Scand (1971) 189, 15.
2 Chrishe HW, Tauchert M, Hilger HH. Effect of phenytoin on the metabolism of phenprocoumon. Eur J Clin Invest (1974) 4, 331.
3 Solomon GE, Hilgartner MW, Kutt H. Coagulation defects caused by diphenylhydantoin. Neurology (1972) 22, 1165.
4 Jansen JM, Kristensen M, Skovsted L and Christensen LK. Dicoumarol induced diphenylhydantoin intoxication. Lancet (1966) ii, 265.
5 Rothermich NO. Diphenylhydantoin intoxication. Lancet (1966) ii, 640.
6 Franzten E, Hansen JM, Hansen OE, Kristensen M. Phenytoin (Dilantin) intoxication. Acta Neurol Scand (1967) 43, 440.
7 Skovsted L, Kristensen M, Hansen JM, Siersbaek-Nielsen K. The effect of different oral anticoagulants on diphenylhydantoin (DPH) and tolbutamide metabolism. Acta Med Scand (1976) 199, 513.
8 Nappi JM. Warfarin and phenytoin interaction. Ann Intern Med (1979) 90, 852.
9 Koch-Weser J. Haemorrhagic reactions and drug interactions in 500 warfarin treated patients. Clin Pharmacol Ther (1973) 14, 139.
10 Taylor JW, Lyon LW. Oral anticoagulant-phenytoin interactions. Drug Intell Clin Pharm (1980) 14, 669–73.
11 Levine M, Sheppard I. Biphasic interaction of phenytoin and warfarin. Clin Pharm (1984) 3, 200–3.
12 Panegyres PK, Rischbieth RH. Fatal phenytoin warfarin interaction. Postgrad Med J (1991) 67, 98.

Phenytoin + Azapropazone

Abstract/Summary

Serum phenytoin levels can be markedly increased by the concurrent use of azapropazone. Phenytoin intoxication can develop rapidly. It is inadvisable for patients to take these drugs concurrently.

Clinical evidence

When a patient developed phenytoin intoxication within two weeks of starting 1200 mg azapropazone daily, further study was made in five normal subjects given 15–250 mg phenytoin daily. When additionally given 1200 mg azapropazone daily, their mean serum phenytoin levels fell briefly from 5 to 3.7 µg/ml before rising steadily over the next seven days to 10.6 µg/ml. At this point the phenytoin was withdrawn because two subjects complained of severe drowsiness.[1,4] An extension of this study is described elsewhere.[3] Another report describes phentyoin intoxication in a woman when fenclofenac was replaced by 1200 mg azapropazone daily.[2]

Mechanism

The most likely explanation is that azapropazone inhibits the liver enzymes concerned with the metabolism of phenytoin, resulting in its accumulation in the body. It also seems possible that azapropazone displaces phenytoin from its plasma protein binding sites so that levels of unbound (and active) phenytoin are increased. This means that intoxication might occur at serum levels which would be well tolerated in the absence of azapropazone.

Importance and management

Information seems to be limited to the reports cited, but it appears to be a clinically important interaction. The incidence is uncertain, but it was demonstrated by all the five subjects examined in the study cited.[1,3] As intoxication may possibly occur at serum levels which would be well tolerated in the absence of azapropazone, concurrent use is potentially hazardous and the manufacturers (Robins) state that azapropazone should not be given to patients taking phenytoin.

References

1 Geaney DP, Carver JG, Aronson JK, Warlow CP. Interaction of azapropazone with phenytoin. Brit Med J (1982) 284, 1373.
2 Roberts CJC, Daneshmend TK, Macfarlane D, Dieppe PA. Anticonvulsant intoxication precipitated by azapropazone. Posdgrad Med J (1981) 57, 191.
3 Geaney DP, Carver JG, Davies CL and Aronson JK. Pharmacokinetic investigation of the interaction of azapropazone with phenytoin. Br J clin Pharmac (1983) 15, 727–34.
4 Aronson JK, Hardman M, Reynolds DJM. ABC of monitoring drug therapy. Phenytoin. Brit Med J (1992) 305, 1215–8.

Phenytoin + Barbiturates

Abstract/Summary

Concurrent use is common, advantageous and normally uneventful. Changes in serum phenytoin levels (often decreases but sometimes increases) can occur if phenobarbitone is added but seizure control is not usually affected. Phenytoin intoxication following barbiturate withdrawal has been seen.

Increased phenobarbitone levels and possibly toxicity may result from the addition of phenytoin to phenobarbitone treatment.

Clinical evidence

(a) Phenytoin treatment to which phenobarbitone is added

A study in 12 epileptics treated with phenytoin (3.7 to 6.8 mg/kg daily) showed that while taking phenobarbitone (1.4–2.5 mg/kg daily) their serum phenytoin levels were depressed. Five patients showed a mean reduction of two thirds (from 15.7 to 5.7 µg/ml). In most cases phenytoin levels rose again when the phenobarbitone was withdrawn. In one patient this was so rapid and steep that he developed ataxia and a cerebellar syndrome with phenytoin levels up to 60 µg/ml, despite a reduction in phenytoin dosage.[1]

This interaction has been described in other reports.[2–6] However a rise[4–7] or no alteration[3–6,8] in serum phenytoin levels have also been described.

(b) Phenobarbitone treatment to which phenytoin is added

Elevated serum phenobarbitone levels occurred in 40 epileptic children when additionally given phenytoin. In five patients illustrated the phenobarbitone levels approximately doubled. In some cases mild ataxia was seen but the relatively high barbiturate levels were well tolerated.[2] A long-term study in six adult epileptics found that when phenytoin was added to phenobarbitone, the level/dose ratio of the phenobarbitone gradually rose from an average of 8.66 to a maximum of 13.8 day/kg/l at the end of a year, and then gradually fell again over the next 2 years.[9]

Mechanism

Phenobarbitone can have a dual effect on phenytoin metabolism: it may cause enzyme induction which results in a more rapid clearance of the phenytoin from the body, or with large doses it may inhibit metabolism by competing for enzyme systems. The total effect will depend on the balance between the two. The reason for the elevation of serum phenobarbitone levels is not fully understood.

Importance and management

Concurrent use is common and can be therapeutically valuable. Some manufacturers market fixed-dose combinations of both drugs (e.g. *Epanutin* with *Phenobarbitone, Garoin*). Changes in dosage or the addition or withdrawal of either drug need to be monitored to ensure that drug intoxication does not occur, or that seizure control is worsened. The contradictory reports cited here do not provide a clear picture of what is likely to happen. Other barbiturates are also enzyme-inducing agents and may be expected to interact similarly.

References

1 Morselli PL, Rizzo M, Garattini S. Interaction between phenobarbital and diphenylhydantoin in animals and in epileptic patients. Ann NY Acad Sci (1971) 179, 88.
2 Cucinell SA, Conney AH, Sansur M, Burns JJ. Drug interactions in man. I. Lowering effect of phenobarbital on plasma levels of bishydroxycoumarin (Dicumarol) and diphenylhydantoin (Dilantin). Clin Pharmacol Ther (1965) 6, 420.
3 Buchanan RA, Heffelfinger JC, Weiss CF. The effect of phenobarbital on diphenylhydantoin metabolism in children. Paediatrics (1969) 43, 114.
4 Kutt H, Hayes J, Verebeley K, McDowell F. The effect of phenobarbital on plasma diphenylhydantoin level and metabolism in man and rat liver microsomes. Neurology (1969) 19, 611.
5 Diamond WD, Buchanan RA. A clinical study of the effect of phenobarbital on diphenylhydantoin plasma levels. J Clin Pharmacol (1970) 10, 306.
6 Garrettson LK and Dayton PG. Disappearance of phenobarbital and diphenylhydantoin from serum of children. Clin Pharmacol Ther (1970) 11, 674.
7 Booker HE, Tormay A, Toussaint J. Concurrent administration of phenobarbital and diphenylhydantoin: lack of interference effect. Neurology (1971) 21, 383.
8 Browne TR, Szabo GK, Evans J, Greenblatt DJ, Mikati MA. Phenobarbital does not alter phenytoin steady-state serum concentration of pharmacokinetics. Neurology (1988) 38, 639–42.
9 Encinas MP, Buegla DS, González CA, Sánchez MJC, Hurlé AD-G. Influence of length of treatment on the interaction between phenobarbital and phenytoin. J Clin Pharmaco Ther (1992) 17, 49–50.

Phenytoin + Benzodiazepines

Abstract/Summary

Reports are inconsistent: benzodiazepines can cause serum phenytoin levels to rise (intoxication has been seen), fall, or remain unaltered. In addition phenytoin may cause clonazepam, oxazepam and diazepam serum levels to fall.

Clinical evidence

(a) Serum phenytoin levels increased

The observation of intoxication in patients on phenytoin when given chlordiazepoxide or diazepam prompted more detailed study. 25 patients on 300–400 mg phenytoin daily and one of these benzodiazepines demonstrated serum phenytoin levels which were 80–90% higher than those not taking a benzodiazepine. Some individuals demonstrated even greater increases.[1] Increased phenytoin serum levels and intoxication have also been attributed in other reports to the concurrent use of diazepam,[4,5,11,12] clonazepam,[2,7,15,16] chlordiazepoxide[3] and possibly, but not certainly, to nitrazepam.[6]

(b) Serum phenytoin levels decreased

24 patients given phenytoin and 4–6 mg clonazepam daily over a two month period showed a mean 18% fall in their serum phenytoin levels.[9] Other studies describe similar findings with clonazepam[13,20] and diazepam.[8,10]

(c) Serum phenytoin levels unaltered and/or serum benzodiazepine levels reduced

Clonazepam is reported not to alter serum phenytoin levels.[13,14] In addition, a study in patients given 250–400 mg phenytoin daily showed that serum clonazepam levels were reduced by more than 50% (from 183 to 81 ng/ml).[17] Diazepam and oxazepam may be similarly affected in epileptic patients given phenytoin or phenobarbitone.[18,19] Alprazolam does not appear to affect serum phenytoin levels.[21]

Mechanisms

The inconsistency of these reports is not understood. Benzodiazepine-induced changes in the metabolism of the phenytoin, both enzyme induction and inhibition,[9,10,13] as well as alterations in the apparent volume of distribution have been discussed. Enzyme induction may possibly account for the fall in serum benzodiazepine levels.

Importance and management

A confusing picture. Concurrent use certainly need not be avoided (it has proved to be valuable in many cases) but the serum phenytoin levels should be monitored so that undesirable changes can be detected. Only diazepam, chlordiazepoxide, nitrazepam and clonazepam have been implicated, but it seems possible that other benzodiazepines will interact similarly.

References

1 Vajda FJ E, Prineas RJ, Lovell RRH. Interaction between phenytoin and the benzodiazepines. Lancet (1971) i, 346.
2 Eeg-Oloffson O. Experiences with Rivotril in treatment with epilepsy-particular minor motor epilepsy-in mentally retarded children. Acta Neurol Scand (1973) 49 (Suppl 530 29.
3 Kutt H, McDowell FJ. Management of epilepsy with diphenylhydantoin sodium. J Amer Med Ass (1968) 203, 969.
4 Rogers HJ, Halsam RA, Longstreth J, Lietman PS. Diphenylhydantoin-diazepam interaction: a pharmacokinetic analysis. Pediatr Res (1975) 9, 286.
5 Ibid. Phenytoin intoxication during concurrent diazepam therapy. J Neurol Neurosurg Psychiat (1977) 40, 890.
6 Treasure T, Toseland PA. Hyperglycaemia due to phenytoin toxicity. Arch Dis Child (1971) 46, 563.
7 Windorfer C. Drug interactions during anticonvulsive therapy. Int J Clin Pharmacol (1976) 14, 231.
8 Siris JH, Pippenger CE, Werner WL and Masland RI. Anticonvulsive drug serum levels in psychiatric patients with seizure disorders. NY State J Med (1974) 74, 1554.
9 Edwards VE, Eadie MJ. Clonazepam-a clinical study of its effectiveness as an anticonvulsant. Proc Aus Assoc Neurol (1973) 10, 61.
10 Houghton GW, Richens A. The effects of benzodiazepines and pheneturide on phenytoin metabolism in man. Br J Clin Pharmacol (1974) 1, P344.
11 Kaviks J, Berry SW, Wood D. Serum folic acid and phenytoin levels in permanently hospitalized patients receiving anticonvulsant therapy. Med J Aust (1971) 2, 369.
12 Shuttleworth E, Wise G, Paulson G. Choreoathetosis and diphenylhydantoin intoxication. J Amer Med Ass (1974) 230, 1170.
13 Huang CY, McLeod JG, Sampson D, Hensley WJ. Clonazepam in the treatment of epilepsy. Med J Aust (1974) 2, 5.
14 Johannessen SI, Strandjord EE, Munthe-Kaas AW. Lack of effect of clonazepam on serum levels of diphenylhydantoin, phenobarbital and

carbamazepine. Acta Neurol Scand (1977) 55, 506.

15 Janz D, Schneider H. Bericht uber Wodadiboff II. In 'Antiepileptische Langzeitmedikation'. Biblthea Psychiatr (1975) 151, 55. Karger Verlag, Basel.

16 Windorfer A, Sauer W. Drug interactions during anticonvulsant therapy in childhood: diphenylhydantoin, primidone, phenobarbitone, clonazepam, nitrazepam, carbamazepine and dipropylacetate. Neuropaediatr (1977) 8, 29.

17 Sjo O, Hvidberg EF, Naestroft J, Lund M. Pharmacokinetics and side-effects of clonazepam and its 7-amino metabolite in man. Europ J Clin Pharmacol (1975) 8, 249.

18 Hepner GW, Vesell ES, Lipton A, Harvey HA, Wilkinson GR, Schenker S. Disposition of aminopyrine, antipyrine, diazepam and indocyanin green in patients with liver disease or on anticonvulsant therapy: diazepam breath test and correlations in drug elimination. J Lab Clin Med (1977) 90, 440–56.

19 Scott AK, Khir ASM, Steele WH, Hawksworth GM, Petrie JC. Oxazepam pharmacokinetics in patients with epilepsy treated long-term with phenytoin alone or in combination with phenobarbitone. Br J clin Pharmacol (1983) 16, 441–4.

20 Saavedra IN, Aguilera LI, Faure E, Galdames DG. Case report. Phenytoin/clonazepam interaction. Ther Drug Monit (1985) 7, 481.

21 Patrias JM, DiPiro JT, Cheung RPF, Townsend RJ. Effect of alprazolam on phenytoin pharmacokinetics. Drug Intell Clin Pharm (1987) 21, 2A.

Phenytoin + Carbamazepine

Abstract/Summary

The reports are inconsistent. Some describe rises in serum phenytoin levels (with toxicity) whereas others describe falls in both phenytoin and carbamazepine serum levels. Concurrent use should be monitored.

Clinical evidence

(a) Reduced serum phenytoin levels

600 mg carbamazepine daily for 4–14 days reduced the serum phenytoin levels of three out of seven patients from 15 to 7 µg/ml, 18 to 12 µg/ml and 16 to 10 µg/ml respectively. Phenytoin serum levels rose again 10 days after withdrawal of the carbamazepine.[1] Reduced serum phenytoin levels have been described in other reports.[2–6]

(b) Raised serum phenytoin levels

A study in six epileptics treated with phenytoin (350–600 mg daily) showed that the addition of carbamazepine (600–800 mg daily) increased the phenytoin serum levels by 35%, increased its half-life by 41% and reduced its clearance by 36.5% over a 12-week period. Five of the six showed developed additional signs of toxicity (sedation, ataxia, nystagmus, etc). Neurotoxicity increased by 204%. The phenytoin dosage remained unchanged throughout the period of the study.[15]

Increases in serum phenytoin levels have been described in other reports.[4,9–14] Rises of 81% and up to 100% have been reported.[12,9]

(c) Reduced serum carbamazepine levels

A series of multiple regression analyses on data from a large number of patients (precise number is not clear from the report), showed that phenytoin reduces serum carbamazepine on average by 0.9 µg/ml for each 2 mg/kg phenytoin taken each day.[4] Reduced serum carbamazepine levels have been described in other studies.[7,8,13,17] Two studies found that phenytoin markedly increases the levels of the active metabolite of carbamazepine, the 10–11 epoxide.[16,18]

Mechanisms

Not understood. A reduction in phenytoin metabolism and increases in carbamazepine metabolism have been suggested.[14,16]

Importance and management

These contradictory reports makes assessment of this interaction difficult. What is known indicates that it would be wise to monitor anticonvulsant levels during concurrent use (including the active metabolite of carbamazepine, carbamazepine-epoxide) so that steps can be taken to avoid the development of toxicity. Not all patients appear to demonstrate an adverse interaction, but it is not possible to identify those potentially at risk. The risk of carbamazepine-induced water intoxication is reported to be reduced in patients concurrently taking phenytoin.[8]

References

1 Hansen JM, Siersboek-Nielsen K, Skovsted L. Carbamazepine-induced acceleration of diphenylhydantoin and warfarin administration in man. Clin Pharmacol Ther (1971) 12, 539.

2 Cereghino JJ, van Meter JC, Brock JT, Penry JK, Smith LD and White BG. Preliminary observations of serum carbamazepine concentration in epileptic patients. Neurology (1973) 23, 357.

3 Hooper WD, Dubetz DK, Eadie MJ, Tyrer JH. Preliminary observations on the clinical pharmacology of carbamazepine ('Tegretol'). Proc Aust Ass Neurol (1974) 11, 189.

4 Lander CM, Eadie MJ, Tyrer JH. Interactions between anticonvulsants. Proc Aust Ass Neurol (1975) 12, 111.

5 Lai M-L, Huang JD. Effect of single- and multiple-dose carbamazepine on the pharmacokinetics of diphenylhydantoin. Eur J Clin Pharmacol (1992) 43, 201–3.

6 Windorfer A, Sauer W. Drug interactions during anticonvulsant therapy in childhood: diphenylhydantoin, primidone, phenobarbitone, clonazepam, nitrazepam, carbamazepine and dipropylacetate. Neuropadiatrie (1977) 8, 29.

7 Cereghino JJ, Block JT, van Meter JC, Penry JK, Smith LD and White BG. The efficacy of carbamazepine combinations in epilepsy. Clin Pharmacol Ther (1975) 18, 733.

8 Perucca E, Richens A. Reversal by phenytoin of carbamazepine-induced water intoxication: a pharmacokinetic interaction. J Neurol Neurosurg Psychiat (1980) 43, 540.

9 Gratz ES, Theodore WH, Newmark ME, Kuppferberg HJ, Porter RJ, Qu Z. Effect of carbamazepine on phenytoin clearance in patients with complex partial seizures. Neurology (1982) 32, A223.

10 Browne TR, Evans JE, Szabo GK, Evans BA, Greenblatt DJ. Effect of carbamazepine on phenytoin pharmacokinetics determined by stable isotope technique. J Clin Pharmacol (1984) 24, 396.

11 Leppik IE, Pepin SM, Jacobi J, Miller KW. Effect of carbamazepine on the Michaelis-Menten parameters of phenytoin. In Metabolism of Antiepileptic Drugs (ed Levy RH et al) Raven Press, New York. (1984) pp 217–22.

12 Zielinski JJ, Haidukewych D, Leheta BJ. Carbamazepine-phenytoin interaction: elevation of plasma phenytoin concentrations due to carbamazepine comedication. Ther Drug Monit (1985) 7, 51–3.

13 Hidano F, Obata N, Yahaba Y, Unno K, Fukui R. Drug interactions with phenytoin and carbamazepine. Fol Psych Neurol Japon (1983) 37, 342–4.

14 Zielinski JJ, Haidukewych D. Dual effects of carbamazepine-phenytoin interaction. Ther Drug Monitor (1987) 9, 21–3.

15 Browne TR, Szabo GK, Evans JE, Evans BA, Greenblatt DJ, Mikati MA. Carbamazepine increases phenytoin serum concentration and reduces phenytoin clearance. Neurology (1988) 38, 1146–50.

16 Hagiwara M, Takahashi R, Watabe M, Amanuma I, Kan R, Takahashi Y, Kumashiro H. Influence of phenytoin on metabolism of carbamazepine. Neurosciences (1989) 15, 303–9.

17 Ramsay RE, McManus DQ, Guterman A, Briggle TV, Vazquez D, Perhalski R, Yost RA, Wong P. Carbamazepine metabolism in humans: effect of concurrent anticonvulsant therapy. Ther Drug Monit (1990) 12, 235–41.

18 Dam M, Jensen A, Christiansen J. Plasma level and effect of carbamazepine in grand mal and psychomotor epilepsy. Acta Neurol Scand (1975) 75, Suppl 51, 33–8.

Phenytoin + Chloramphenicol

Abstract/Summary

Serum phenytoin levels can be raised by the concurrent use of chloramphenicol. Phenytoin toxicity may occur unless the phenytoin dosage is reduced appropriately. Other evidence indicates that phenytoin may reduce or raise serum chloramphenicol levels in children.

Clinical evidence

(a) Serum phenytoin levels increased

A man on phenytoin (400 mg daily) developed signs of toxicity within a week of additionally taking chloramphenicol (four six-hourly doses of 1 g intravenously followed by 2 g six-hourly). His serum phenytoin levels had risen approximately threefold (from about 7 to 24 μg/ml).[2] This interaction has been described in a number of other reports.[1,3,4,6–10,13] One study showed that chloramphenicol more than doubled the half-life of phenytoin.[1]

(b) Serum chloramphenicol levels reduced or increased

A child on a six-week course of chloramphenicol (100 mg/kg/day intravenously in four divided doses) showed a reduction in peak and trough serum levels of 46 and 74% respectively within two days of beginning additional treatment with phenytoin (4 mg/kg/day). Levels were further reduced by 63 and 87% respectively when additionally treated with phenobarbitone (4 mg/kg/day).[11]

In contrast, six children (aged 1 month to 12 years) developed raised chloramphenicol levels into the toxic range while concurrently receiving phenytoin.[12]

Mechanisms

It seems probable that chloramphenicol, a known enzyme inhibitor, depresses the liver enzymes concerned with the metabolism of phenytoin, thereby reducing its rate of clearance from the body.[5] The changes in the pharmacokinetics of chloramphenicol in children is not understood.

Importance and management

The rise in serum phenytoin levels (a) in adults is well-documented and clinically important. A two- to four-fold rise can occur within a few days of beginning concurrent treatment. Concurrent use should be avoided unless the effects can be closely monitored and appropriate phenytoin dosages reduction made as necessary. The general clinical importance of the changes in serum chloramphenicol levels in children (b) is uncertain, but the effects of concurrent use should certainly be monitored. More study is needed. It seems very doubtful if enough chloramphenicol is absorbed from eye-drop solutions or ointments for an interaction to occur, but this needs confirmation.

References

1 Christensen LK and Skovsted L. Inhibition of drug metabolism by chloramphenicol. Lancet (1969) ii, 1397.

2 Ballek RE, Reidenberg MM amd Orr L. Inhibition of DPH metabolism by chloramphenicol. Lancet (1973) i, 150.

3 Houghton GW, Richens A. Inhibition of phenytoin metabolism by other drugs used in epilepsy. Int J Clin Pharmacol (1975) 12, 210.

4 Rose JQ, Choi HK, Schentag JJ, Kinkel WR, Jusko WJ. Intoxication caused by interaction of chloramphenicol and phenytoin. J Amer Med Ass (1977) 237, 2630.

5 Dixon RL and Fouts JR. Inhibition of microsomal drug metabolism pathway by chloramphenicol. Biochem Pharmacol (1962) 11, 715.

6 Koup JR, Gibaldi M, McNamara P, Hilligoss DM, Colburn WA, Bruck E. Interaction of chloramphenicol with phenytoin and phenobarbital. Clin Pharmacol Ther (1978) 24, 571.

7 Vincent FM, Mills L and Sullivan JK. Chloramphenicol-induced phenytoin intoxication. Ann Neurol (1978) 3, 469.

8 Harper JM, Yost RL, Stewart RB, Ciezkowski J. Phenytoin-chloramphenicol interaction. Drug Intell Clin Pharm (1979) 13, 425.

9 Greenlaw CW. Chloramphenicol-phenytoin drug interaction. Drug Intell Clin Pharm (1979) 13, 609.

10 Saltiel MS, Stephens NM. Phenytoin-chloramphenicol interaction. Drug Intell Clin Pharm (1980) 14, 221.

11 Powell DA, Nahata M, Durrell DC, Glazer JP, Hilty MD. Interactions among chloramphenicol, phenytoin and phenobarbitone in a pediatric patient. J Pediat (1981) 98, 1001.

12 Karasinski K, Kusmiesz H, Nelson JD. Pharmacological interactions among chloramphenicol, phenytoin and phenobarbital. Pediatr Infect Dis (1982) 1, 232–5.

13 Cosh DG, Rowett DS, Lee PC, McCarthy PJ. Case report-phenytoin therapy complicated by concurrent chloramphenicol and enteral nutrition. Aust J Hosp Pharm (1987) 17, 51–3.

Phenytoin + Chlorpheniramine

Abstract/Summary

Phenytoin intoxication in two patients has been attributed to the concurrent use of chlorpheniramine.

Clinical evidence, mechanism, importance and management

A week or so after starting to take chlorpheniramine (12 mg daily), a woman on phenytoin and phenobarbitone developed phenytoin intoxication with serum phenytoin levels of about 65 μg/ml. The toxic symptoms disappeared and phenytoin levels fell when the chlorpheniramine was withdrawn.[1] Another woman on anticonvulsants, including phenytoin, developed slight grimacing of the face and involuntary jaw movements (but no speech slurring, ataxia or nystagmus) within 12 days of starting to take 12–16 mg chlorpheniramine daily. Her serum phenytoin levels had risen to 30 μg/ml but they fell when the chlorpheniramine was withdrawn.[2] The reason for these reactions is not clear but it has been suggested that chlorpheniramine may have inhibited the metabolism of phenytoin by the liver. These are isolated cases so there would seem to be no good reason for avoiding concurrent use in all patients, but it would be reasonable to monitor the effects. There seem to be no reports of interactions between phenytoin and other antihistamines.

References

1 Pugh RNH, Geddes AM, Yeoman WB. Interaction of phenytoin with chlorpheniramine. Br J clin Pharmac (1975) 2, 173.
2 Ahmad S, Laidlaw J, Houghton GW, Richens A. Involuntary movements caused by phenytoin intoxication in epileptic patients. J Neurol Neurosurg Psychiat (1975) 38, 225.

Phenytoin + Cholestyramine or Colestipol

Abstract/Summary

Neither cholestyramine nor colestipol affect the absorption of phenytoin from the gut.

Clinical evidence, mechanism, importance and management

Neither cholestyramine (5 g) nor colestipol (10 g) had a significant effect on the absorption of a single 500 mg dose of phenytoin in six normal subjects.[1] Another study in six normal subjects found that 4 g cholestyramine four times daily had no significant effect on the extent of the absorption of 400 mg phenytoin, although it was absorbed a little more rapidly.[2] No special precautions would seem to be necessary if either of these drugs and phenytoin is taken concurrently.

References

1 Callaghan JT, Tsuru M, Holtzman JL and Hunningshake DB. Effect of cholestyramine and colestipol on the absorption of phenytoin. Eur J Clin Pharmacol (1983) 24, 675–8.
2 Barzaghi N, Monteleone M, Amione C, Lecchini S, Perucca E, Frigo GM. Lack of effect of cholestyramine on phenytoin bioavailability. J Clin Pharmacol (1988) 28, 1112–4.

Phenytoin + Cimetidine, Famotidine and Ranitidine

Abstract/Summary

Phenytoin serum levels are raised by the use of cimetidine. Toxicity may occur if the phenytoin dosage is not reduced appropriately. Very rarely bone marrow depression develops with concurrent use. Neither ranitidine nor famotidine normally interact with phenytoin, but they appear to do so on rare occasions.

Clinical evidence

(a) Phenytoin + Cimetidine

Nine patients showed a 60% rise (from 5.7 to 9.1 μg/ml) in serum phenytoin levels after taking cimetidine (1 g daily) for 3 weeks. The serum phenytoin fell to its former levels within 2 weeks of withdrawing the cimetidine.[1,2,5,6]

This interaction has been described in many reports and studies involving numerous patients and subjects.[3,4,8,9,11–15,23] Phenytoin toxicity developed in some individuals. The extent of the rise is very variable (13–33% over six days in one report[3] and 22–280% over 2 weeks in another[10]). Severe and life-threatening agranulocytosis in two patients[2,7] and thrombocytopenia in five others[19,20] have been attributed to concurrent use.

(b) Phenytoin + Famotidine or Ranitidine

Studies in four patients given ranitidine for 2 weeks[17] found that no interaction occurred, and a study in 10 subjects given famotidine demonstrated that the phenytoin pharmacokinetics remained unaltered.[16,18] However a single case report describes phenytoin intoxication and a doubled serum level (from 18 to 33 μg/ml) in a patient when given famotidine.[21] Another patient showed a 40% increase in serum phenytoin levels over a month when treated with 300 mg ranitidine daily.[22]

Mechanism

Cimetidine is a potent enzyme inhibitor which depresses the activity of the liver enzymes concerned with the metabolism of phenytoin, thus allowing it to accumulate in the body and, in some instances, to reach toxic concentrations. Neither famotidine nor ranitidine normally affect these enzymes. Cimetidine may also possibly delay the dissolution of phenytoin in tablet form by raising the gastric pH.[23] Agranulocytosis and thrombocytopenia are relatively rare manifestations of bone marrow depression caused by these drugs

Importance and management

The phenytoin-cimetidine interaction is well documented and clinically important. It is not possible to identify individuals who will show the greatest response, but those with serum levels at the top end of the therapeutic range are most at risk. Cimetidine should not be given to patients taking phenytoin unless the serum levels can be monitored and suitable dosage reductions made if necessary. Ranitidine and famotidine normally do not interact like cimetidine, but the isolated cases cited show that monitoring is advisable even with these H$_2$-blockers.

References

1 Neuvonen PJ, Ritta A, Tokola R, Kaste M. Cimetidine-phenytoin interaction: effect of serum phenytoin concentration and antipyrine test in man. Nauyn-Schmied Arch Pharmacol (1980) 313 (Suppl) R60.
2 Sazie E, Jaffe JP. Severe granulocytopenia with cimetidine and phenytoin. Ann Intern Med (1980) 93, 151.
3 Hetzel DJ, Bochner F, Hallpike JF, Shearman DJC and Hann CS. Cimetidine interaction with phenytoin. Brit Med J (1981) 282, 1512.
4 Algozzine GJ, Steward RB, Springer PK. Decreased clearance of phenytoin with cimetidine. Ann Intern Med (1981) 95, 244.
5 Neuvonen PJ, Tokola R, Kaste M. Cimetidine interaction with phenytoin. Brit Med J (1981) 283, 501.
6 Ibid. Cimetidine-phenytoin interaction: effect on serum phenytoin concentration and antipyrine test. Eur J Clin Pharmacol (1981) 21, 215–20.
7 Al-Kawas FH, Lenes BA, Sacher RA. Cimetidine and agranulocytosis. Ann Intern Med (1979) 90, 992–3.
8 Bartle WK, Walker SE, Shapero I. Effect of cimetidine on phenytoin metabolism. Clin Pharm Ther (1982) 31, 202.
9 Bartle WK, Walker SE, Shapero I. Dose-dependent effect of cimetidine on phenytoin kinetics. Clin Pharmacol Ther (1983) 33, 649–55.
10 Watts RW, Hetzel DJ, and Bochner F. Lack of interaction between ranitidine and phenytoin. Brit J clin Pharmac (1983) 15, 499–500.
11 Phillips P, Hansky J. Phenytoin toxicity secondary to cimetidine administration. Med J Aust (1984) 141, 602.
12 Griffin JW, May JR, DiPiro JT. Drug interactions: theory versus practice. Amer J Med (1984) 77 (Suppl 5B) 85–9.
13 Frigo GM, Lecchini S, Caravaggi M, Gatti G, Tonini M, D'Angelo L, Perucca E, Crema A. Reduction of phenytoin clearance caused by cimetidine. Europ J Clin Pharmacol (1983) 25, 135–7.
14 Salem RB, Breland BD, Mishra SK, Jordan JE. Effect of cimetidine on phenytoin serum levels. Epilepsia (1983) 24, 284–8.
15 Iteogu MO, Murphy JE, Shleifer N, Davis R. Effect of cimetidine on single-dose phenytoin kinetics. Clin Pharm (1983) 2, 302–3.
16 Sambol NC, Upton RA, Chremos AN, Lin ET, Williams RL. A comparison of the influence of famotidine and cimetidine on phenytoin elimination and hepatic blood flow. Br J clin Pharmac (1989) 27, 83–7.
17 Hetzel DJ, Watts RW, Bochner F, Shearman. Ranitidine, unlike cimetidine, does not interact with phenytoin. Aust NZ J Med (1983) 13, 324.
18 Sambol NC, Upton RA, Chremos AN, Lin E, Gee W, Williams RL. Influence of famotidine and cimetidine on the disposition of phenytoin and indocyanine green. Clin Pharmacol Ther (1986) 39, 225.
19 Wong YY, Lichtor T, Brown FD. Severe thrombocytopenia associated with phenytoin and cimetidine therapy. Surg Neurol (1985) 23, 169–72.
20 Yue CP, Mann KS, Chan KH. Severe thrombocytopenia due to combined cimetidine and phenytoin therapy. Neurosurgery (1987) 20, 963–5.
21 Shinn AF. Unrecognized drug interactions with famotidine and nizatidine. Arch intern Med (1991) 151, 810–4.
22 Bramhall D, Levine M. Possible interaction of ranitidine with phenytoin. Drug Intell Clin Pharm (1988) 22, 979–80.
23 Hsieh Y-Y, Huang J-D, Lai M-L, Lin M-S, Liu R-T, Wan E C-J. The complexity of cimetidine-phenytoin interaction. J Formosan Med Assoc (1986) 85, 395–402.

Phenytoin + Cloxacillin

Abstract/Summary

A marked reduction in serum phenytoin levels in one patient has been attributed to the concurrent use of cloxacillin.

Clinical evidence, mechanism, importance and management

An epileptic woman taking 400 mg phenytoin daily, hospitalized for second degree burns sustained during a generalized seizure, showed an '...astonishing drop...' in serum phenytoin levels (from 21.8 to 3.5 µg/ml) which was attributed to the concurrent use of cloxacillin, 0.5 g 6-hourly. Serum phenytoin values within the original range and using the original dosage were only satisfactorily restored when the cloxacillin was withdrawn. The authors of the report advise a 'watchful awareness' if both drugs are used.[1] This seems to be the only report of an adverse interaction between phenytoin and a penicillin. Its incidence and general importance would seem to be very small if viewed against the very wide-spread use of the pencillins.

Reference

1 Fincham RW, Wiley DE, Schottelius DD. Use of phenytoin levels in a case of status epilepticus. Neurology (1976) 26, 879.

Phenytoin + Diazoxide

Abstract/Summary

Four children showed very marked reductions in serum phenytoin levels when diazoxide was given and seizure control was lost in one case. There is some evidence that the effects of diazoxide may also be reduced.

Clinical evidence

Two children receiving 17 and 30 mg/kg/day phenytoin respectively failed to achieve therapeutic phenytoin serum levels when given diazoxide. When the diazoxide was withdrawn, satisfactory serum phenytoin levels were achieved with dosages of only 6.6 and 10 mg/kg/day. When diazoxide was restarted experimentally in one child, the serum phenytoin fell to undetectable levels over 3 days and seizures occurred.[1,2] Two other reports describe this interaction.[3,5] In addition it appears that the effects of the diazoxide can also be reduced.[3,4]

Mechanism

What is known[1-3] suggests that diazoxide increases the metabolism and the clearance of phenytoin from the body. The half-life of diazoxide is reduced by phenytoin.[4]

Importance and management

Information is limited to these reports concerning children, but the interaction would appear to be established. Monitor the effects of concurrent use, being alert for the need to increase the phenytoin dosage. The clinical importance of the reduced diazoxide effects is uncertain.

References

1 Roe TF, Podosin RL and Blaskovics ME. Drug interaction. Diazoxide and diphenylhydantoin. Pediatr Res (1975) 9, 285.
2 Roe TF, Podison RL and Blascovics ME. Drug Interaction. Diazoxide and diphenylhydantoin. J Pediatr (1975) 87, 480.
3 Petro DJ, Vannucci RC, Kulin HE. Diazoxide-diphenylhydantoin interaction. J Pediatr (1976) 89, 331.
4 Pruitt AW, Dayton PG, Patterson JH. Disposition of diazoxide in children. Clin Pharmacol Ther (1973) 14, 73.
5 Turck D, Largilliere C, Depuis B, Farriaux JP. Interaction entre le diazoxide et la phenytoine. Presse Med (1986) 15, 31.

Phenytoin + Dichloralphenazone

Abstract/Summary

Serum phenytoin levels may be reduced by the concurrent use of dichloralphenazone. Some loss in seizure control is possible.

Clinical evidence, mechanism, importance and management

After taking 1 g dichloralphenazone each night for 13 nights the total body clearance of phenytoin (single dose given intravenously) in five normal subjects was doubled.[1] The phenazone component of dichloralphenazone is a known enzyme-inducer and the increased clearance of phenytoin may be due to an enhancement of its metabolism. There seem to be no reports of adverse effects in patients given both drugs so that the clinical importance of this interaction is uncertain, but it would seem prudent to watch for falling serum phenytoin levels if dichloralphenazone is added to established treatment with phenytoin.

Reference

1 Riddell JG, Salem SAM and McDevitt DG. Interaction between phenytoin and dichloralphenazone. Br J clin Pharmacol (1980) 9, 118P.

Phenytoin + Felbamate

Abstract/Summary

Felbamate increases serum phenytoin levels. Toxicity may occur in some individuals if the dosage is not reduced. Felbamate serum levels are reduced but the importance of this is uncertain.

Clinical evidence

A very brief report about four patients, associated later with a study in five normal subjects, found that felbamate increases serum phenytoin levels. After a 20% reduction in the phenytoin dosage before the felbamate was given (30–54.9 mg/kg/day), one subject needed a slight increase in dosage, whereas two others needed a further reduction in phenytoin dosage.[1] Other studies in patients and normal subjects clearly showed that felbamate increases serum phenytoin levels.[4,5] Another report says that felbamate clearance is reduced if the dosage of phenytoin is reduced.[3]

Mechanism

Uncertain but felbamate probably inhibits the metabolism of the phenytoin, thereby reducing its loss from the body and increasing its serum levels,[1,2] whereas phenytoin induces felbamate metabolism, thereby increasing its clearance (about 20%).[3]

Importance and management

Established interactions. Anticipate the need to reduce the phenytoin dosage if felbamate is added to avoid toxicity, and to increase it if felbamate is withdrawn. An initial reduction of 20% was tried in the study cited.[1] The importance of the reduced felbamate levels is uncertain.

References

1 Fuerst RH, Graves NM, Leppik IE, Remmel RP, Rosenfeld WE, Sierzant TL. A preliminary report on alteration of carbamazepine and phenytoin metabolism by felbamate. Drug Intell Clin Pharm (1986) 20, 465–6.
2 Fuerst RH, Graves NM, Leppik IE, Brundage RC, Holmes GB, Remmel RP. Felbamate increases phenytoin but decreases carbamazepine concentrations. Epilepsia (1988) 29, 488–91.
3 Wagner ML, Graves NM, Marienau K, Holmes GB, Remmel RP, Leppik IE. Discontinuation of phenytoin and carbamazepine in patients receiving felbamate. Epilepsia (1991) 32, 398–406.
4 Sachedo R, Sachedo S, Wagner M, Reitz J, Schumaker RC, Perhach JL, Ward DL. Steady-state pharmacokinetics of felbamate (Felbatol) when coadministered with phenytoin. Epilepsia (1992) 33, Suppl 3, 84.
5 Sachedo R, Wagner M, Sachedo S, Schumaker RC, Perhach JL, Ward DL. Steady-state pharmacokinetics of phenytoin when coadministered with felbamate (Felbatol). Epilepsia (1992) 33, Suppl 3, 84.

Phenytoin + Fluconazole

Abstract/Summary

Phenytoin serum levels can rise rapidly if fluconazole is given. Toxicity will develop unless the phenytoin dosage is reduced appropriately. Ketoconazole levels may also possibly be reduced.

Clinical evidence

10 subjects on 200 mg phenytoin daily for three days and 200 mg fluconazole for 14 days were compared with 10 other subjects not given fluconazole. The phenytoin AUC_{0-24} (area under the curve over 24 h) was raised by 75%, and the trough phenytoin serum levels by 128%. Phenytoin appeared not to affect fluconazole trough serum levels.[1,5]

A patient on 300 mg phenytoin daily developed signs of toxicity (dizziness, nystagmus, ataxia) within two days of starting to take 400 mg fluconazole daily. His serum phenytoin levels had risen from a range of 30–40 μmol/l to 140 μmol/l. Serum levels fell and the toxicity rapidly disappeared when the phenytoin dosage was reduced.[2] At least four other cases of phenytoin toxicity caused by fluconazole have been documented.[3,4,9] A study in man found that 400 mg fluconazole daily for 6 days raised the AUC of a single dose of phenytoin by a third.[6,8] An undetailed report also suggests that phenytoin reduces fluconazole levels in some patients.[7]

Mechanism

Not established. A reduction in the metabolism and clearance of the phenytoin by the fluconazole is a probable explanation.[1,2] It is suggested that fluconazole causes a dose related inhibition of the human cytochrome P-450 system.[2]

Importance and management

Information is limited but the interaction(s) would appear to be established. Monitor serum phenytoin levels closely during concurrent use, and reduce the dosage to prevent toxicity. In the case report cited above[2] a reduction from 300 to 200 mg phenytoin daily controlled this interaction. Also be alert for any evidence of reduced fluconazole effects.

References

1 Blum RA, Wilton JH, Hilligoss DM, Gardner MJ, Chin EB, Schentag JJ. Effect of fluconazole on the disposition of phenytoin. Clin Pharmacol Ther (1990) 47, 182.
2 Mitchell AS, Holland JT. Fluconazole and phenytoin: a predictable interaction. Br Med J (1989) 298, 1315.
3 Howittt KM, Oziemski MA. Phenytoin toxicity induced by fluconazole. Med J Aust (1989) 151, 603–4.
4 Wooller HO (Pfizer). Personal communication quoted in reference 3.
5 Blum RA, Wilton JH, Hilligoss DM, Gardner MJ, Henry EB, Harrison NJ, Schentag JJ. Effect of fluconazole on the disposition of phenytoin. Clin Pharmacol Ther (1991) 49, 420–5.
6 Touchette MA, Chandrasekar PH, Millad MA, Edwards DJ. Differential effects of ketoconazole and fluconazole on phenytoin and testosterone concentrations in man. Pharmacotherapy (1991) 11, 275.
7 Tett S, Carey D, Lee H-S. Drug interactions with fluconazole. Med J Aust (1992) 156, 365.
8 Touchette MA, Chandrasekar PH, Millad MA, Edwards DJ. Contrasting effects of ketoconazole and fluconazole on phenytoin and testosterone disposition in man. Br J clin Pharmac (1992) 34, 75–8.
9 Sugar AM. Quoted as Personnal Communication by Grant SM, Clissold SP. Fluconazole. A review of its pharmacodynamic and pharmcokinetic properties, and therapeutic potential in superficial and system mycoses. Drugs (1990) 39, 877–916.

Phenytoin + Food

Abstract/Summary

The absorption of phenytoin can be affected some foods. A very marked reduction in phenytoin absorption has been described when given with enteral feeds (e.g. *Fortison*, *Isocal*, *Osmolite*) administered by nasogastric tube.

Clinical evidence

(a) Phenytoin + Food eaten normally

A study showed that serum drug levels were low when the phenytoin was disguised in vanilla pudding and given to mentally retarded children, but were doubled when mixed with apple sauce. Three out of 10 patients developed serum phenytoin levels within the toxic range.[5] An epileptic showed a marked fall in his serum phenytoin levels accompanied by an increased seizure frequency when the phenytoin was given at bedtime with a food supplement (*Ensure*).[10] Another patient showed reduced phenytoin serum levels when given phenytoin as an oral suspension and oral *Fresubin* liquid food concentrate.[18] Absorption of phenytoin as the acid in a micronized form (*Fentoin*, ACO, Sweden) may be increased by 27% and peak serum levels can average 40% higher when given with food.[2] One single dose study found that when taken with a meal the total absorption of phenytoin was was not affected, although it was slightly delayed.[1]

(b) Phenytoin + Food by nasogastric tube

A patient on 300 mg phenytoin daily who was being fed with *Fortison* through a nasogastric tube achieved a phenytoin serum level of only 1.0 mg/l until the phenytoin was given diluted in water and separated from the food by 2 h. Using this method and with an increase in the dose to 420 mg daily a serum level of 6 mg/l was achieved.[6] This report describes a similar reaction in another patient.[6]

A study in 20 patients and five normal subjects found that a 73–75% reduction in phenytoin absorption occurred when given by nasogastric tube with an enteral food product (*Isocal*).[3] Other reports describe the same interaction in patients given *Osmolite*, *Fortison* or other enteral foods.[4,7,8,12–14,16,17]

Mechanism

Not fully resolved. Phenytoin can bind to some food substances.[9,11] It can also become bound to the nasogastric tubing[15] and may also be poorly absorbed if the tubing empties into the duodenum rather than the stomach.[15]

Importance and management

(a) Phenytoin is often taken with water or food to reduce gastric irritation. This normally appears not to have a marked effect on absorption but the studies cited above show that some formulations and some foods can interact. If there are problems with the control of convulsions or evidence of toxicity, review how and when the patient is taking the phenytoin.

(b) The interaction between phenytoin and enteral foods given by nasogastric tube is well established and clinically important. The markedly reduced bioavailability has been successfully managed by giving the phenytoin diluted in water 2 h after stopping the feed, flushing with 60 ml of water, and waiting another 2 h before restarting the feed.[3,6,12] Some increase in the phenytoin dosage may also be needed. However one limited study failed to confirm that this method is successful. Monitor concurrent use closely.

References

1 Kennedy MC, Wade DN. The effect of food on the absorption of phenytoin. Aust NZ J Med (1982) 12, 258–61.
2 Melander A, Brante G, Johansson O, Wahlin-Boll E. Influence of food on the absorption of phenytoin in man. Eur J Clin Pharmacol (1979) 15, 269.
3 Bauer LA. Interference of oral phenytoin absorption by continuous nasogastric feedings. Neurology (1982) 32, 570–2.
4 Hatton RC. Dietary interaction with phenytoin. Clin Pharm (1984) 3, 110–1.
5 Jann MW, Bean J, Fidone G. Interaction of dietary pudding with phenytoin. Pediatrics (1986) 78, 952–3.
6 Summers VM, Grant R. Nasogastric feeding and phenytoin interaction. Pharm J (1989) 243, 181.
7 Weinryb J, Cogen R. Interaction of nasogastric phenytoin and enteral feeding solution. J Amer Geriatr Soc (1989) 37, 195–6.
8 Pearce GA. Apparent inhibition of phenytoin absorption by an enteral nutrient formula. Aust J Hosp Pharm (1988) 18, 289–92.
9 Millar SW, Strom JG. Stability of phenytoin in three enteral nutrient formulas. Am J Hosp Pharm (1988) 45, 2529–32.
10 Longe RL and Smith OB. Phenytoin interaction with an oral feeding results in loss of seizure control. J Amer Geriatr Soc (1988) 36, 542–4.
11 Hooks MA, Longe RL and Taylor AT. Recovery of phenytoin from an enteral nutrient formula. Am J Hosp Pharm (1986) 43, 685.
12 Summers VM, Grant R. Nasogastric feeding and phenytoin interaction. Pharm J (1989) 243, 181.
13 Worden JP, Wood CA, Workman CH. Phenytoin and nasogastric feedings. Neurology (1984) 34, 132.
14 Fitzsimmons WE, Garnett WR, Kreuger KA. Phenytoin and enteral feeding. Drug Intell Clin Pharm (1988) 22, 920.
15 Fleishner D, Sheth N, Kou JH. Phenytoin interaction with enteral feedings administered through nasogastric tubes. J Parenteral Enteral Nutr (1990) 14, 513–6.
16 Ozuna J, Friel P. Effect of enteral tube feeding on serum phenytoin levels. J Neurosurg Nursing (1984) 16, 289–91.
17 Maynard GA, Jones KM, Guidry JR. Phenytoin absorption from tube feedings. Arch intern Med (1987) 147, 1821.
18 Taylor DM, Massey CA, Willson WG, Dhillon S. Lowered serum phenytoin concentrations during therapy with liquid food concentrates. Ann Pharmacother (1993) 27, 369.

Phenytoin + Hypoglycaemic agents

Abstract/Summary

Large and toxic doses of phenytoin have been observed to cause hyperglycaemia, but normal therapeutic doses do not usually affect the control of diabetes. Two isolated cases of phenytoin intoxication have been attributed to the use of tolazamide and tolbutamide.

Clinical evidence

(a) The effect of phenytoin on the response to hypoglycaemic agents

Phenytoin has been shown in a number of reports[1–4,7,8] to raise the blood sugar levels of both diabetics and non-diabetics, but in virtually all the cases on record the phenytoin dosage was large or even in the toxic range, and there is no evidence that a hyperglycaemic response to usual doses of phenytoin is normally large enough to interfere with the control of diabetes either with diet alone or with conventional hypoglycaemic agents. In a single case involving hyperglycaemia in which both insulin and phenytoin were used, the situation was complicated by the use of other drugs and by kidney impairment.[2]

(b) The effect of hypoglycaemic agents on the response to phenytoin

17 patients on phenytoin (100–400 mg daily) who were given tolbutamide (500 mg three times a day) showed a transient rise in the amount of non-protein-bound phenytoin, but no signs of intoxication appeared.[11] A man given phenytoin and tolazamide developed phenytoin toxicity which disappeared when the tolazamide was replaced by insulin.[10] A woman previously successfully treated with phenytoin and tolbutamide developed intoxication on a later occasion when again given tolbutamide.[13]

Mechanisms

Studies in animals and man[5,6,9] suggest that phenytoin-induced hyperglycaemia occurs because the release of insulin from the pancreas is impaired. This implies that no interaction is possible without functional pancreatic tissue. Just why the phenytoin/tolazamide and phenytoin/tolbutamide interactions occurred is uncertain,[12] but it is possible that they compete for metabolism by the same cytochrome (P-4502C9).[14]

Importance and management

The weight of evidence shows that no interaction of clinical importance normally occurs between phenytoin and the hypoglycaemic agents. No special precautions seem normally to be necessary. There appear to be only two unexplained cases on record of a sulphonylurea-phenytoin interaction.

References

1 Klein JP. Diphenylhydantoin intoxication associated with hyperglycaemia. J Paediatr (1966) 69, 463.
2 Goldberg EM, Sanbar SS. Hyperglycaemic, non-ketotic coma following administration of Dilantin (diphenylhydantoin). Diabetes (1969) 18, 101.
3 Peters BH, Samaan NA. Hyperglycaemia with relative hypoinsulinaemia in diphenylhydantoin intoxication. N Engl J Med (1969) 281, 91.
4 Millichap JG. Hyperglycaemic effect of diphenylhydantoin. N Engl J Med (1969) 281, 447.
5 Kizer JS, Cordon-Vargas M, Brendel K, Bressler R. The in vitro inhibition of insulin secretion by diphenylhydantoin. J Clin Invest (1970) 49, 1942.
6 Levin SR, Booker J, Smith DF, Grodsky M. Inhibition of insulin secretion by diphenylhydantoin in the isolated perfused pancreas. J Clin Endocrinol Metab(1970) 30, 400.
7 Farfiss BL and Lutcher CL. Diphenylhydantoin-induced hyperglycaemia and impaired insulin release. Diabetes (1971) 46, 563.
8 Treasure T, Toseland PA. Hyperglycaemia due to phenytoin toxicity. Arch Dis Child (1971) 46, 563.
9 Malherbe C, Burrill KC, Levin SR, Karam JH, Forsham PH. Effect of diphenylhydantoin on insulin secretion in man. N Engl J Med (1972) 286, 339.
10 Pannekoek JH (1969) cited in 11.
11 Wesseling H, Mols-Thurkow I. Diphenylhydantoin (DPH) and tolbutamide in man. Eur J clin Pharmacol (1975) 8, 75.
12 Wesseling H, Mols-Thurkow I, Mulder GJ. Effect of sulphonylureas (tolazamide, tolbutamide and chlorpropamide) on the metabolism of diphenylhydantoin in the rat. Biochem Pharmacol (1973) 22, 3033.
13 Beech E, Mathur SV, Harrold BP. Phenytoin toxicity produced by tolbutamide. Br Med J (1988) 297, 1613–4.
14 Tasseaneeyakul W, Veronese ME, Birkett DJ, Doecke CJ, McManus ME, Sansom LN, Miners JO. Co-regulation of phenytoin and tolbutamide metabolism in humans. Br J clin Pharmac (1992) 34, 494–8.

Phenytoin + Influenza vaccines

Abstract/Summary

Influenza vaccine is reported to increase, decrease or to have no effect on the serum levels of phenytoin. The efficacy of the vaccine remains unchanged.

Clinical evidence

(a) Phenytoin serum levels increased

Eight epileptic children on phenytoin showed an approximately 50% increase in their serum phenytoin levels (from 9.5 to 15.16 µg/ml) 7 days after being given 0.5 ml influenza virus vaccine, USP, types A and B, whole virus (Squibb). Four patients in a group cited below[2] whose phenytoin levels were unchanged after immunization, showed serum phenytoin increases ranging from 46 to 170% over weeks 4–17 after being immunized with 0.5 ml inactivated whole-virion trivalent vaccine.[2] Rises in serum phenyton levels in three patients, temporarily related to influenza vaccination, are briefly described in another report.[5]

(b) Phenytoin serum levels decreased

Within four days of receiving 0.5 ml subviron, trivalent influenza vaccine the serum phenytoin levels of seven patients were reduced 11–14%.[1]

(c) Phenytoin serum levels unchanged

A study on 16 patients given 0.5 ml inactivated whole-virion trivalent influenza vaccine showed that 7 and 14 days later their mean serum phenytoin levels were not significantly altered.[2] The efficacy of influenza vaccine is reported to be unchanged by phenytoin.[3]

Mechanism

Where an interaction occurs it is suggested that it may be due to the inhibitory effect of the vaccine on the liver enzymes concerned with the metabolism of the phenytoin, resulting in a reduced clearance from the body.[4]

Importance and management

The outcome of immunization with influenza vaccine is uncertain. Concurrent use need not be avoided but it would be prudent to monitor the effects closely.

References

1 Sawchuk RJ, Rector TS, Fordice JJ, Leppik IE. Case report. Effect of influenza vaccination on plasma phenytoin concentrations. Ther Drug Monit (1979) 1, 285–8.
2 Levine M, Jones MW, Gribble M. Increased serum phenytoin concentration following influenza vaccination. Clin Pharm (1984) 3, 505–9.
3 Levine M, Beattie BL, McLean DM, Corman D. Phenytoin therapy and immune response to influenza vaccine. Clin Pharm (1985) 4, 191–4.
4 Jann MW, Fidone GS. Effect of influenza vaccine on serum anticonvulsant concentrations. Clin Pharm (1986) 5, 817–20.
5 Mooradian AD, Hernandez L, Tamai IC, Marshall C. Variability of serum phenytoin concentrations in nursing home patients. Arch Intern Med (1989) 149, 890–2.

Phenytoin + Isoniazid

Abstract/Summary

Phenytoin serum levels can be raised by the concurrent use of isoniazid. Those who are 'slow metabolizers' of isoniazid (10–25%) may develop phenytoin intoxication if the dosage of phenytoin is not reduced appropriately.

Clinical evidence

A study in 32 patients on phenytoin (300 mg daily) showed that, within a week of starting to take isoniazid (300 mg daily) and para-aminosalicylic acid (15 g daily), six of them had phenytoin levels almost 5 µg/ml higher than the rest of the group, and on the following days when levels climbed above 20 µg/ml the typical signs of phenytoin toxicity were seen. All six had unusually high serum isoniazid serum levels.[1,2]

Rises in serum phenytoin levels and toxicity induced by the concurrent use of isoniazid has been described in numerous other reports involving large numbers of patients, one of which describes a fatality.[3-14] It occurs in those who are 'slow metabolizers (acetylators)' of isoniazid (see 'Mechanism' below) and the incidence is between 10 and 25%.

Mechanism

Isoniazid inhibits the liver microsomal enzymes which metabolize phenytoin, as a result the phenytoin accumulates and its serum levels rise.[1,2] Only those who are 'slow metabolizers (acetylators)' of isoniazid (this is genetically determined) attain blood levels of isoniazid which are sufficiently high to cause extensive inhibition of the phenytoin metabolism, whereas the 'fast metabolizers' remove the isoniazid too quickly for this to occur. Thus some individuals will show a rapid rise in phenytoin levels which eventually reaches toxic concentrations, whereas others will show only a relatively slow and unimportant rise to a plateau within, or only slightly above the therapeutic range.

Importance and management

A well-documented, well-established, clinically important and potentially serious interaction. About 50% of the population are slow or relatively slow metabolizers of isoniazid, but not all of them develop serum phenytoin levels in the toxic range (20 µg/ml plus). The reports indicate that somewhere between 10 and 25% are at risk.[1-4,10] This adverse interaction may take only a few days to develop fully in some patients, but several weeks in others so that concurrent use should be very closely monitored, making suitable dosage reductions as necessary. One patient is reported to have had better seizure control with fewer side-effects while taking both drugs than with phenytoin alone.[15] See also 'Phenytoin + Rifampicin', and 'Phenytoin + Isoniazid/Rifampicin'.

References

1 Kutt H, Brennan R, Dehejia H, Verebeley K. Diphenylhydantoin intoxication. A complication of isoniazid therapy. Amer Rev Resp Dis (1970) 101, 377.

2 Brennan RW, Dehejia H, Kutt H, Verebelely K, McDowell F. Diphenylhydantoin intoxication attendant to slow inactivation of isoniazid. Neurology (1970) 20, 687.

3 Murray FJ, Outbreak of unexpected reactions among epileptics taking isoniazid. Amer Rev Resp Dis (1962) 86, 729.

4 Kutt H, Winters W, McDowell FH. Depression of parahydroxylation of diphenylhydantoin by antituberculosis chemotherapy. Neurol (1966) 16, 594.

5 Manigand G, Thieblot Ph and Deparis M. Accidents de la diphenylhydantoine induits par les traitements antituberculeux. Presse Med (1971) 79, 815.

6 Beauvais P, Mercier D, Hanoteau J, Brissand H-E. Intoxication a la diphenylhydantoine induite par l'isoniazide. Arch Franc Ped (1973) 30, 541.

7 Johnson J. Epanutin and isoniazid interaction. Br Med J (1975) 1, 152.

8 Johnson J, Freeman HL. Death due to isoniazid (INH) and phenytoin. Br J Psychiatr (1975) 129, 511.

9 Geering JM, Ruch W, Dettli L. Diphenylhydantoin-Intoxikation durch

Diphenylhydantoin-Isoniazid Interaktion. Schweiz med Wsch (1974) 104, 1224.

10 Miller RR, Porter J, Greenblatt DJ. Clinical importance of the interaction of phenytoin and isoniazid. A report from the Boston Collaborative Drug Surveillance Program. Chest (1979) 75, 356.

11 Witmer DR, Ritschel WA. Phenytoin-isoniazid interaction: a kinetic approach to management. Drug Intell Clin Pharm (1984) 18, 483–6.

12 Perucca E, Richens A. Anticonvulsant drug interactions. In: Tyrer J (ed) The treatment of epilepsy. MTP Lancaster. (1980) pp 95–128.

13 Sandyk R. Phenytoin toxicity induced by antituberculous drugs. S Afr Med J (1982) 61, 382.

14 Yew WW, Lau KS, Ling MHM. Phenytoin toxicity in a patient with isoniazid-induced hepatitis. Tubercle (1991) 72, 309–10.

15 Thulasimnay M, Kela AK. Improvement of psychomotor epilepsy due to interaction of phenytoin-isoniazid. Tubercle (1984) 65, 229–30.

Phenytoin + Loxapine

Abstract/Summary

A single case report describes depressed serum phenytoin levels during concurrent treatment with loxapine.

Clinical evidence

The serum phenytoin levels of an epileptic patient were depressed by the concurrent use of loxapine, and showed a marked rise when it was withdrawn.[1] The general importance of this is uncertain, but it would now seem prudent to monitor the effects in any patient, particularly as loxapine can lower the convulsive threshold. More study is needed.

Reference

1 Ryan GM, Matthews PA. Phenytoin metabolism stimulated by loxapine. Drug Intell Clin Pharm (1977) 11, 428.

Phenytoin + Methylphenidate

Abstract/Summary

Raised serum phenytoin levels and phenytoin toxicity have been seen in three patients when given methylphenidate, but it is an uncommon reaction. One of the patients also showed raised serum primidone and phenobarbitone levels.

Clinical evidence

A hyperkinetic epileptic boy of five taking 8.9 mg/kg phenytoin and 17.7 mg/kg primidone daily, developed ataxia without nystagmus when additionally treated with 20–40 mg methylphenidate daily. Serum levels of the anticonvulsants were found to be at toxic concentrations and only began to fall when the methylphenidate dosage was reduced.[1]

A further case of phenytoin intoxication occurred in another child when given methylphenidate,[5] but only one other case was seen in other clinical studies and observations on three subjects,[2] 11 patients,[3] and over 100 other patients.[4] A patient who demonstrated phenytoin intoxication on one occasion when given methylphenidate later failed to do so.[2]

Mechanism

Not fully understood. The suggestion is that methylphenidate acts as an enzyme inhibitor, slowing the metabolism of the phenytoin by the liver and leading to its accumulation in those few individuals whose drug metabolizing system is virtually saturated by large doses of phenytoin.

Importance and management

An established but uncommon interaction. Concurrent use need not be avoided but be alert for any evidence of phenytoin intoxication, particularly if the dosage is high.

References

1 Garrettson KJ, Perel JM, Dayton PG. Methylphenidate interaction with both anticonvulsants and ethyl biscoumacetate. A new action of methylphenidate. J Amer Med Ass (1969) 207, 2053.
2 Mirkin BL and Wright F. Drug interactions: effect of methylphenidate on the disposition of diphenylhydantoin in man. Neurology (1971) 21, 1123.
3 Kupferberg HJ, Jeffery W, Hunningshake DB. Effect of methylphenidate on plasma anticonvulsant levels. Clin Pharmacol Ther (1972) 13, 201.
4 Oettinger L. Interaction of methylphenidate and diphenylhydantoin. Drug Ther (1976) 5, 107.
5 Ghofrani M. Possible phenytoin-methylphenidate interaction. Dev Med Child Neurol (1988) 30, 267–8.

Phenytoin + Metronidazole

Abstract/Summary

A small and usually clinically unimportant rise in serum phenytoin levels may occur if metronidazole is used concurrently although a few patients have developed toxic levels.

Clinical evidence, mechanism, importance and management

A pharmacokinetic study[1] in normal subjects found that metronidazole (750 mg daily) increased the half-life of a single 300 mg intravenous dose of phenytoin by 44% (from 16 to 23 h) and reduced the clearance by 14.75%. In another study in normal subjects the pharmacokinetics of a single 300 mg oral dose of phenytoin were unaffected by 800 mg metronidazole daily for 5 days.[2] An anecdotal report describes '...several patients...' who developed toxic phenytoin serum levels when given metronidazole.[3] The reason for these discordant reports is not clear, but if and when metronidazole affects serum phenytoin levels the rise seems to be relatively small and usually of minimal clinical importance except possibly in those whose levels are already high and close to the toxic threshold. Monitor the outcome. More study is needed.

References

1 Blyden GT, Scavone JM, Greenblatt DJ. Metronidazole impairs clearance of phenytoin but not of alprazolam or lorazepam. Clin Pharmacol Ther (1988) 28, 240–5.
2 Jensen JC, Gugler R. Interaction between metronidazole and drugs eliminated by oxidative metabolism. Clin PharmacolTher (1985) 37, 407–10.
3 Picard EH. Side effects of metronidazole. Mayo Clin Proc (1983) 58, 401.

Phenytoin + Miconazole

Abstract/Summary

Two reports describe phenytoin intoxication in two patients when concurrently treated with miconazole

Clinical evidence, mechanism, importance and management

An epileptic man,[1] well controlled on phenytoin, developed signs of intoxication within a day of starting treatment with intravenous miconazole (500 mg eight-hourly) and flucytosine. After a week of concurrent treatment his serum phenytoin levels had climbed by 50% (from 29 to 43 µg/ml). He had some signs of very mild phenytoin intoxication even before the antifungal treatment was started. Another patient became intoxicated (nystagmus, ataxia) within 5 days of starting to take 500 mg miconazole daily. His serum phenytoin climbed to 41 ug/ml.[2] A probable explanation is that the miconazole can depress the metabolism and clearance of the phenytoin by the liver, resulting in its accumulation in the body. Evidence for this interaction seems to be limited to these reports, even so it would be prudent to avoid concurrent use unless serum phenytoin levels can be monitored and appropriate reductions made in the phenytoin dosage if necessary. The interaction apparently develops very rapidly.

References

1 Rolan PE, Somogyi AA, Drew MJR, Cobain WG, South D, Bochner F. Phenytoin intoxication during parenteral treatment with miconazole. Brit Med J (1983) 287, 1760.
2 Loupi E, Descotes J, Lery N, Evereux J Cl. Interactions medicamenteuses et miconazole. A propos de 10 observations. Therapie (1982) 37, 437–41.

Phenytoin + Nitrofurantoin

Abstract/Summary

An isolated report describes a reduction in serum phenytoin levels and poor seizure control in a patient when given nitrofurantoin.

Clinical evidence, mechanism, importance and management

A patient with seizures due to a brain tumour was treated with 300 mg phenytoin daily. He had a seizure within a day of starting additional treatment with 200 mg nitrofurantoin for a urinary tract infection and his serum phenytoin levels were found to be modestly reduced (from 36 to 30 µmol/l). They continued to fall to 25 µmol/l despite an increase in the phenytoin dosage to 350 and then 400 mg daily. When the nitrofurantoin was stopped he was restabilized on his original dosage of phenytoin. The reasons are not understood but, on the basis of a noted rise in serum gamma GT levels during the use of the nitrofurantoin, the authors speculate that it increased the metabolism of the phenytoin by the liver.[1] The general importance of this interaction is uncertain but it would now seem prudent to monitor concurrent use in any patient.

Reference

1 Heipertz R, Pilz H. Interaction of nitrofurantoin with diphenylhydantoin. J Neurol (1978) 218, 297–301.

Phenytoin + Omeprazole

Abstract/Summary

A study in patients found that 20 mg omeprazole daily did not affect the serum levels of phenytoin, whereas earlier studies in normal subjects suggested that phenytoin levels might be raised by 40 mg omeprazole daily.

Clinical evidence

20 mg omeprazole daily for 3 weeks caused no changes in the mean steady-state serum phenytoin levels in eight patients.[3] Four patients had unchanged levels, two had falls and two had rises, but none of them was adversely affected by the omeprazole treatment.[3]

A double-blind cross-over study in 10 normal subjects found that after taking 40 mg omeprazole daily for nine days the AUC (area under the curve) of a single 300 mg dose of phenytoin was increased by 25% (from 122 to 151 µg/ml/h) and the half-life was increased by 45% (from 17.9 to 25.9 h).[1] In another study the clearance of a 250 mg IV dose of phenytoin was reduced by 15% (from 0.025 to 0.021 l/h/kg) by 40 mg omeprazole given for 8 days.[2]

Mechanism

Not understood. A possible explanation is that if the dosage of omeprazole is high enough, it may possibly reduce the metabolism of phenytoin, thereby reducing its loss from the body.

Importance and management

Information is very limited but it seems that 20 mg omprazole daily does not affect serum phenytoin levels, whereas 40 mg daily may possibly do so. Until more is known it would be prudent to monitor concurrent use whatever the dosage.

References

1 Prichard PJ, Walt RP, Kitchingman GK, Somerville KW, Langman MJS, Williams J, Richens A. Oral phenytoin pharmacokinetics during omeprazole therapy. Br J clin Pharmac (1987) 24, 534–5.
2 Gugler R, Jensen JC. Omeprazole inhibits oxidative drug metabolism. Gastroenterology (1985) 89, 1235–41.
3 Andersson T, Lagerström P-O, Unge P. A study of the interaction between omeprazole and phenytoin in epileptic patients. Ther Drug Monit (1990) 12, 329–33.

Phenytoin + Pheneturide

Abstract/Summary

Phenytoin serum levels can be increased by about 50% if pheneturide is used concurrently.

Clinical evidence, mechanism, importance and management

The half-life of phenytoin was prolonged from 32 to 47 h by pheneturide in nine patients. Mean serum levels were raised about 50% (from 35 to 53 uM) but fell rapidly when the pheneturide was withdrawn.[1] This study confirms a previous report of this interaction.[2] The reason for this reaction is uncertain, but since the two drugs have a similar structure it is possible that they compete for the same metabolizing enzymes in the liver, thereby resulting, at least initially, in a reduction in the metabolism of the phenytoin. If concurrent use is undertaken the outcome should be well monitored. Reduce the phenytoin dosage as necessary.

References

1 Houghton GW, Richens A. Inhibition of phenytoin metabolism by other drugs used in epilepsy. Int J Clin Pharmacol (1975) 12, 210.
2 Hulsman JW, van Heycop Ten Ham MW and van Zijl CHW. Influence of ethylphenacemide on serum levels of other anticonvulsant drugs. Epilepsia (1970) 11, 207.

Phenytoin + Phenothiazines

Abstract/Summary

The serum levels of phenytoin can be raised or lowered by the use of chlorpromazine, thioridazine or prochlorperazine.

Clinical evidence

The reports are inconsistent. A patient on phenytoin, primidone and sulthiame showed a doubling in his serum phenytoin levels (from 7 to 15 μg/ml) after taking 50 mg chlorpromazine daily for a month. Four other patients on 50–100 mg chlorpromazine showed no interaction.[1] In another report[2] one out of three patients showed a fall in serum phenytoin levels when given chlorpromazine, and a fall is described in a further report.[5] Yet another report[3] states (without giving details) that in rare instances chlorpromazine and prochlorperazine have been noted to impair phenytoin metabolism. One out of six patients on phenytoin, phenobarbitone and thioridazine showed a marked rise in serum phenytoin levels, whereas four others showed a fall.[2] Phenytoin intoxication has also been described in two patients on thioridazine.[4] A retrospective study on 27 patients on phenytoin showed that four had an increase, two had a decrease and the rest demonstrated no changes in phenytoin serum levels when given thioridazine.[6] Another retrospective study of 28 patients also found no evidence that thioridazine increased the risk of toxicity in patients on phenytoin.[7] A further study found no changes in serum phenytoin or thioridazine levels in patients given both drugs, but serum mesoridazine (active metabolite of thioridazine) levels were reduced.[8]

Mechanism

Uncertain, but it may be related to changes in the metabolism of the phenytoin caused by the phenothiazines.

Importance and management

A confusing situation. The concurrent use of phenytoin and the phenothiazines cited need not be avoided, but it would be prudent to watch for any signs of changes in serum phenytoin levels which would affect anticonvulsant control. Whether other phenothiazines interact similarly is uncertain.

References

1 Houghton GW, Richens A. Inhibition of phenytoin metabolism by other drugs used in epilepsy. Int J clin Pharmacol (1975) 12, 210.
2 Siris JH, Pippenger CE, Werner WL and Masland RL. Anticonvulsant drug-serum levels in psychiatric patients with seizure disorders. Effects of certain psychotropic drugs. NY State J Med (1974) 74, 1554.
3 Kutt H, McDowell F. Management of epilepsy with diphenylhydantoin sodium. Dosage regulation for problem patients. J Amer Med Ass (1968) 203, 969.
4 Vincent FM. Phenothiazine-induced phenytoin intoxication. Ann Int Med (1980) 93, 56.
5 Haidukewych D, Rodin EA. Effect of phenothiazines on serum antiepileptic drug concentrations in psychiatric patients with seizure disorder. Ther Drug Monit (1985) 7, 401.
6 Sands CD, Robinson JD, Salem RB, Stewart RB, Muniz C. Effect of thioridazine on phenytoin serum concentration: a retrospective study. Drug Intell Clin Pharm (1987) 21, 267–72.
7 Gotz VP, Yost RL, Lamadrid ME, Buchanan CD. Evaluation of a potential interaction: thioridazine-phenytoin — negative findings. Hospital Pharmacy (1984) 19, 555–7.
8 Linnoila M, Viukari M, Vaisanen K, Auvinen J. Effect of anticonvulsants

on plasma haloperidol and thioridazine levels. Am J Psychiatry (1980) 137, 819–21.

Phenytoin + Phenylbutazone, Oxyphenbutazone

Abstract/Summary

Phenytoin serum levels can be increased by phenylbutazone. Intoxication may occur if the phenytoin dosage is not reduced appropriately. It seems likely that oxyphenybutazone will interact similarly.

Clinical evidence

Six epileptic patients on phenytoin (200–250 mg daily) given 300 mg phenylbutazone daily showed a mean fall in their phenytoin serum levels from 15 to 13 μg/ml over the first three days, after which the levels climbed steadily to 19 μg/ml over the next 11 days. One patient developed signs of toxicity. His levels of free phenytoin more than doubled.[1]

Mechanism

The predominant effect of phenylbutazone seems to be the inhibition of the enzymes concerned with the metabolism of phenytoin (half-life increased from 13.7 to 22 h[3]), leading to its accumulation in the body and a rise in its serum levels. The initial transient fall may possibly be related in some way to the displacement by the phenylbutazone of the phenytoin from its plasma protein binding sites.[2]

Importance and management

An established interaction, although the documentation is very limited. Patients on both drugs should be monitored and suitable phenytoin dosage reductions made where necessary to ensure that intoxication does not occur. There is no direct evidence that oxyphenbutazone interacts like phenylbutazone, but since it is the main metabolic product of phenylbutazone in the body and has been shown to prolong the half-life of phenytoin[4] it would be expected to interact similarly.

References

1 Neuvonen PJ, Lehtovaara R, Bardy A, Elomaa E. Antipyretic analgesics in patients on anti-epileptic drug therapy. Eur J Clin Pharmacol (1979) 15, 263.
2 Lunde PKM. Plasma protein binding of diphenylhydantoin in man: interaction with other drugs and the effect of temperature and plasma dilution. Clin Pharmacol Ther (1970) 11, 846.
3 Andreasen PB, Froland A, Skovsted L, Andersen SA, Haugue M. Diphenylhydantoin half-life in man and its inhibition by phenylbutazone: the role of genetic factors. Acta Med Scand (1973) 193, 561.
4 Soda DM, Levy G. Inhibition of drug metabolism by hydroxylated metabolites: cross-inhibition and specificity. J Pharm Sci (1975) 64, 1928.

Phenytoin + Phenyramidol

Abstract/Summary

Serum phenytoin levels can be markedly increased (as much as threefold) by the concurrent use of phenyramidol. Phenytoin toxicity may occur unless the phenytoin dosage is reduced appropriately.

Clinical evidence, mechanism, importance and management

The observation that poorly controlled epileptics taking phenytoin improved when given phenyramidol prompted more detailed study. Five subjects given phenytoin (100 mg three times daily) doubled their serum phenytoin levels (from 6.6 to 12.0 µg/ml) after taking 1200 mg phenyramidol daily for 6 days.[1] The evidence suggests that phenyramidol inhibits the liver microsomal enzymes concerned with the metabolism of the phenytoin, thereby prolonging its stay in the body (phenytoin half-life increased from 26 to 55 h).[1]

Information seems to be limited to this study, but interaction would seem to be established. The incidence is uncertain, but all five subjects demonstrated rises in serum levels ranging from about 40 to 200%.[1] Phenytoin serum levels should be closely monitored if phenyramidol is given concurrently, and the phenytoin dosage reduced appropriately to ensure that intoxication does not occur.

Reference

1 Solomon HM, Schrogie JJ. The effect of phenyramidol on the metabolism of diphenylhydantoin. Clin Pharmacol Ther (1967) 8, 554–6.

Phenytoin + Rifampicin (Rifampin), Rifampicin/Clofazimine, Rifampicin/Isoniazid

Abstract/Summary

Serum phenytoin levels are markedly reduced by the concurrent use of rifampicin. If isoniazid is also given, serum phenytoin levels may also fall in patients who are fast acetylators of isoniazid, but may rise in those who are slow acetylators. Clofazimine may also reduce serum phenytoin levels.

Clinical evidence

(a) Phenytoin + Rifampicin

Studies in six patients showed that the clearance of phenytoin (100 mg given intravenously) doubled (from 46.7 to 97.8 ml/min) after taking 450 mg rifampicin daily for 2 weeks[1] A man on phenytoin needed a dosage reduction to keep his serum phenytoin levels within the therapeutic range when his treatment with rifampicin came to an end.[2]

(b) Phenytoin + Rifampicin/Clofazimine

A man with AIDS taking a number of drugs (rifampicin, clofazimine, ciprofloxacin, ethambutol, clarithromycin, diphenoxylate, bismuth, ocreotide, co-trimoxazole, amphotericin, 5-flurocytosine, amikacin, zalcitabine) was additionally given phenytoin to control a right-sided seizure disorder. Despite taking 1600 mg daily, his trough phenytoin plasma levels remained less than 0.25 µg/dl until the rifampicin was withdrawn, when they rose to 5 µg/ml. When the clofazimine was withdrawn the levels rose to 10 µg/ml.[4]

(c) Phenytoin + Rifampicin/Isoniazid

A patient on 300 mg phenytoin daily developed progressive drowsiness (a sign of phenytoin toxicity) during the first week of starting treatment with isoniazid, rifampicin and ethambutol. His serum phenytoin levels climbed to 46.1 mg/l. He slowly recovered when the phenytoin was stopped. He was later stabilized on only 200 mg phenytoin daily. He proved to be a slow acetylator of isoniazid.[3] Later another patient on 300 mg phenytoin daily was also started on isoniazid, rifampicin and ethambutol but, in anticipation of the response seen in the previous patient, his phenytoin dosage was reduced to 200 mg daily. Within three days he developed seizures because his serum phenytoin levels had fallen to only 8 mg/l. He needed a daily dosage of 400 mg phenytoin to keep the serum levels within the therapeutic range. He was a fast acetylator of isoniazid.[3]

The clearance of phenytoin also doubled in 14 patients given 450 mg rifampicin, 300 mg isoniazid and 1200 mg ethambutol daily for 2 weeks. No further changes occurred in the kinetics of phenytoin after three months antitubercular treatment.[1] These patients were apparently fast acetylators of isoniazid.

Mechanism

Rifampicin (a known potent liver enzyme-inducing agent) increases the metabolism and clearance of the phenytoin from the body so that a larger dose is needed to maintain adequate serum levels. If isoniazid is also given, its enzyme inhibitory effects may oppose the effects of rifampicin in those who are slow acetylators of isoniazid (ie because the isoniazid accumulates in the body), but in those who are fast acetylators, the isoniazid will be cleared too quickly for it effectively to oppose the rifampicin effects. The interaction involving clofazimine is not understood.

Importance and management

Direct information seems to be limited to these reports, but the interactions appear to be of clinical importance. Monitor the serum phenytoin levels and increase the dosage appropriately if rifampicin alone is started. Reduce the dosage if the rifampicin is stopped. If both rifampicin and isoniazid are given, the outcome will depend on the isoniazid acetylator status of the patient. Those who are fast acetylators will probably need an increased phenytoin dosage. Those who are slow acetylators will probably need a smaller phenytoin dosage if toxicity is to be avoided. It is clearly important to know the acetylator status of the patient on phenytoin before giving isoniazid and rifampicin together so that the likely outcome, and the appropriate measures, can be chosen. Information about clofazimine seems to be limited to one report. Monitor concurrent use, anticipating the need to increase the phenytoin dosage.

References

1 Kay L, Kampmann JP, Svendsen TL, Vergman B, Hansen JEM, Skovsted L and Kristensen M. Influence of rifampicin and isoniazid on the kinetics of phenytoin. Br J clin Pharmac (1985) 20, 323–6.
2 Abajo FJ. Phenytoin interaction with rifampicin. Br Med J (1988) 297, 1048.
3 O'Reilly D, Basran GS, Hourihan B, Macfarlane JT. Interaction between phenytoin and antituberculous drugs. Thorax (1987) 42, 736.
4 Cone LA, Woodard DR, Simmons JC, Sonnensheim MA. Drug interaction in patients with AIDS. Clin Infect Dis (1992) 15, 1066–8.

Phenytoin + *Shankhapushpi* (SRC)

Abstract/Summary

Two case reports, assocated with animal studies, indicate that an anticonvulsant Ayurvedic herbal preparation — SRC (*Shankhapushpi*) — can markedly reduce serum phenytoin levels, leading to an increased seizure frequency if the phenytoin dosage is not raised.

Clinical evidence

An epileptic man on phenobarbitone (120 mg daily) and phenytoin (500 mg daily) developed an increased seizure frequency after starting additional treatment with SRC three times a day. His serum phenytoin levels were found to have fallen from 18.2 to 9.3 µg/ml whereas his phenobarbitone levels were little changed (from 10.2 to 9.7 µg/ml). When the SRC was stopped both the phenobarbitone and phenytoin serum levels climbed to 15.7 and 30.3 µg/ml respectively. A boy of 10 also developed an increased fit-frequency, associated with a fall in serum phenytoin levels (approximately halved), when given SRC. His phenytoin dosage had been reduced at the same time from 175 to 150 mg daily.[1–3,6]

Subsequent studies in rats showed that SRC approximately halves the serum levels of phenytoin.[2,3,6]

Mechanism

Not understood. There is some evidence from animal studies that SRC may affect the pharmacokinetics of the phenytoin and possibly its pharmacodynamics as well,[2,3] thereby reducing its anticonvulsant activity. It is also suggested that one of the ingredients of SRC may have some convulsant activity.[3]

Importance and management

Information about this interaction appears to be limited to these reports.[1–3,6] SRC is given because it has some anticonvulsant activity (demonstrated in animal studies[1]), but there is little point in combining it with phenytoin if the outcome is a fall in serum phenytoin levels, accompanied by an increase in fit-frequency. For this reason concurrent use should be avoided. SRC (*Shankhapushpi*) is a syrup containing in each 15 ml dose the leaves of *convolvulus pluricaulis* (2 g), the rhizome of *nardostachys jatamansi* (0.5 g), the whole plant of *centella asiatica* (0.25 g), nepeta hindostana (0.25 g) and nepeta elliptica (0.25 g), and the leaves and flowers of *onosma bracteatum* (0.10 g).[3] The first three of these plants appear to contain compounds with anticonvulsant activity.[4,5]

References

1 Kshirsagar N A, Chandra R S, Dandekar U P, Dalvi S S, Sharma A V, Joshi M V, Gokhale P C, Shah P U. Investigation of a novel clinically important interaction between phenytoin and Ayurvedic preparation. Eur J Pharmacol (1990) 183, 519. (Abstract).
2 Kshirsagar N A, Personnal communication 1991.
3 Dandekar U P, Chandra R S, Dalvi S S, Joshi M V, Gokhale P C, Sharma A V, Shah P U, Kshirsagar N A. Analysis of a novel clinically important interaction between phenytoin and an Ayurvedic preparation. J Ethnopharmacology (1992) 35, 285–8.
4 Sharma V N, Barar F S K, Khanna N K, Mahawar M M. Some pharmacological actions of *convolvulus pluricaulis chois* — an indigenous herb. Indian J Med Res (1965) 53, 871.
5 Arora R B. In: Nardostachys jatamansi: a chemical, pharmacological and clinical appraisal. Pharmacological actions of Jatamansi. Indian Council of Medical Research Publications, Delhi (1965), 136.
6 Kshirsagar NA, Dalvi SS, Joshi MV, Sharma SS, Sani HM, Shah PU, Chandra RS. Phenytoin and ayurvedic preparation — clinically important interaction in epileptic patients. J Assoc Phys India (1992) 40, 354–5.

Phenytoin + Sodium valproate

Abstract/Summary

Concurrent use is common and usually uneventful. Initially total serum phenytoin levels may fall but this is offset by a rise in the levels of free (and active) phenytoin which may very occasionally cause some toxicity. After continued use the serum phenytoin levels rise once again. There is also some very limited evidence that concurrent use possibly increases the incidence of sodium valproate hepatotoxicity

Clinical evidence

A number of reports clearly show that total serum phenytoin levels fall during early concurrent use while the concentrations of free phenytoin rise.[7–12] In one of them it was noted that within 4–7 days the total serum phenytoin levels had fallen from 19.4 to 14.6 µg/ml.[7] A study extending over a year on eight patients taking phenytoin and sodium valproate showed that by the end of 10 weeks the serum phenytoin levels of six of them had fallen by as much as 50%, but had returned to their original levels by the end of the year.[1] Similar results were found in another study.[13] The occasional patient may show signs of phenytoin toxicity during this period and the dosage may need to be reduced.[2] Delerium was seen in one patient on sodium valproate when given phenytoin.[10] Sodium valproate levels are reduced by the presence of phenytoin.[3,4] Very occasionally (and inexplicably) the fit-frequency has increased in patients on phenytoin given sodium valproate. Epidemiological studies suggest that polytherapy with enzyme inducers such as phenytoin increases the incidence of sodium valproate induced hepatotoxicity[14] whereas monotherapy reduces it,[15] so that concurrent use apparently carries some small risk.

Mechanism

The initial fall in serum phenytoin levels appears to result from the displacement of phenytoin by the sodium valproate from its protein binding sites (the extent being subject to diurnal variation[5]).[7-12] This allows more of the unbound drug to be exposed to metabolism by the liver and the total phenytoin levels fall. After several weeks the metabolism of the phenytoin is inhibited by the valproate and its levels rise.[8,11] Phenytoin reduces sodium valproate levels, probably because it increases its metabolism by the liver.[3] Because phenytoin is an enzyme inducer it may also possibly increase the formation of a minor but heptatotoxic metabolite of sodium valproate (2-propyl-4-pentenoic acid or 4-ene-VPA).[16.]

Importance and management

An extremely well-documented interaction (only a selection of the references being listed here). Concurrent use is common and usually advantageous, the adverse effects of the interactions between the drugs usually being of only minor practical importance, however the effects should be monitored. A few patients may experience mild and transient toxicity if sodium valproate is started, but most patients on phenytoin do not need a dosage change. During the first few weeks total serum phenytoin levels may fall by 20–50%, but usually no increase in the dosage is needed because it is balanced by an increase in the levels of free (active) phenytoin levels. In the period which then follows, the phenytoin levels may rise again 40–50%. Saliva sampling which measures free phenytoin is more reliable in this situation than total serum levels.[6] When monitoring concurrent use it is important to understand fully the implications of changes in 'total' and 'free' or 'unbound' serum phenytoin concentrations. A useful nomogram has been designed for predicting unbound phenytoin concentrations during concurrent use.[17] Also bear in mind the evidence that the incidence of sodium valproate induced liver toxicity may be increased.

References

1 Vakil SD, Critchley EMR, Philips JC, Haydock D, Cocks A, Dyer T. The effect of sodium valproate (Epilim) on phenytoin and phenobarbitone blood levels. In 'Clinical and Pharmacological Aspects of Sodium Valproate (Epilim) in the Treatment of Epilepsy'. Proceedings of a symposium held at Nottingham University, September 1975, MCS Consultants, England, p 75.

2 Haigh D, Forsythe WI. The treatment of childhood epilepsy with sodium valproate. Dev Med Child Neurol (1975) 17, 743–8.

3 Rambeck B, May T. Serum concentrations of valproic acid: influence of dose and co-medication. Ther Drug Monit (1985) 7, 387–90.

4 Sackellares JC, Sato S, Dreifuss FE, Penry JK. Reduction of steady-state valproate levels by other antiepileptic drugs. Epilepsia (1981) 22, 437–41.

5 Riva R, Albani F, Contin M, Perucca E, Ambrosetto G, Gobbi G, Santucci M, Procaccianti G, Baruzzi A. Time-dependent interaction between phenytoin and valproic acid. Neurology (1985) 35, 510–15.

6 Knott C, Hamshaw-Thomas A, Reynolds F. Phenytoin-valproate interaction: importance of saliva monitoring in epilepsy. Br Med J (1982) 284, 13–16.

7 Mattson RH, Cramer JA, Williamson PD, Novelly RA. Valproic acid in epilepsy: clinical and pharmacological effects. Ann Neurol (1978) 3, 20–5.

8 Perucca E, Hebdige S, Frigo GM, Gatti G, Lecchini S, Crema A. Interaction between phenytoin and valproic acid: plasma protein binding and metabolic effects. Clin Pharmacol Ther (1980) 28, 779–89.

9 Tsanaclis LM, Allen J, Perucca E, Routledge PA, Richens A. Effect of valproate on free plasma phenytoin concentrations. Br J clin Pharmac (1984) 18, 17–20.

10 Tollefson GD. Delerium induced by the competitive interaction between phenytoin and dipropylacetate. J Clin Psychopharmacol (1981) 1, 154–8.

11 Bruni J, Gallo JM, Lee CS, Pershalski RJ, Wilder BJ. Interactions of valproic acid with phenytoin. Neurology (1980) 30, 1233–6.

12 Friel PN, Leal KW, Wilensky AJ. Valproic acid-phenytoin interaction. Ther Drug Monit (1979) 1, 243–8.

13 Bruni J, Wilder BJ, Willmore LJ and Barbour B. Valproic acid and plasma levels of phenytoin. Neurology (1979) 29, 904–5.

14 Dreifuss FE, Santilli N, Langer DH, Sweeney KP, Moline KA, Menander KB. Valproic acid fatalities: a retrospective review. Neurology (1987) 37, 379–85.

15 Dreifuss FE, Langer DH, Moline KA, Maxwell DE. Valproic acid hepatic fatalities. II. US experience since 1984. (1989) 39, 201–7.

16 Levy RH, Rettenmeier AW, Anderson GD, Wilensky AJ, Friel PN, Bailiie TA, Acheampong A, Tor J, Guyot M, Poiseau P. Effects of polytherapy with phenytoin, carbamazepine, and stiripentol on formation of 4-ene-valproate, a hepatotoxic metabolite of valproic acid. Clin Pharmacol Ther (1990) 48, 225–35.

17 May TW, Rambeck B, Nothebaum N. Nomogram for the prediction of unbound phenytoin concentrations in patients on a combined treatment of phenytoin and valproic acid. Eur Neurol (1991) 31, 57–60.

Phenytoin + Sucralfate

Abstract/Summary

The absorption of phenytoin can be reduced about 7–20% by the concurrent use of sucralfate. There is indirect evidence that the interaction can be avoided by giving the phenytoin 2 h after the sucralfate.

Clinical Evidence

In a double-blind cross-over study with eight normal subjects, the concurrent administration of 1 g sucralfate was found to reduce the absorption of a single 300 mg dose of phenytoin by 20%, measured over a 48 h period.[1] Peak serum phenytoin levels were also reduced, but this was said not to be statistically significant. Another study demonstrated an absorption reduction of 7.7–9.5%.[2] A similar interaction has been demonstrated in dogs.[3]

Mechanism

Uncertain.

Importance and management

Information is limited, but this interaction would appear to be established. The reduction in absorption is small, but it might be enough to reduce the steady-state serum concentrations of phenytoin in some patients to levels where seizure control is lost. Concurrent use should be monitored. A study in dogs[2] showed that no change in absorption occurred if the phenytoin was given 2 h after the sucralfate, so it seems possible that the same precaution might prevent this interaction in man.

References

1 Smart HL, Somerville KW, Williams J, Richens A, Langman MJS. The effects of sucralfate upon phenytoin absorption in man. Br J clin Pharmac (1985) 20, 238–40.
2 Hall TG, Cuddy PG, Glass CJ, Melethil S. Effect of sucralfate on phenytoin bioavailability. Drug Intell Clin Pharm (1986) 20, 607–11.
3 Lacz JP, Groschang AG, Giesing DH, Browne RK. The effect of sucralfate on drug absorption in dogs. Gastroenterology (1982) 82, 1108.

Phenytoin + Sulphinpyrazone

Abstract/Summary

Some limited evidence indicates that phenytoin serum levels may be markedly increased by the concurrent use of sulphinpyrazone. Toxicity may possibly occur unless the phenytoin dosage is reduced appropriately.

Clinical evidence

The serum phenytoin levels of two out of five patients on phenytoin (250–350 mg daily) were doubled (from approximately 10 to 20 µg/ml) within 11 days of starting to take 800 mg sulphinpyrazone daily. One of the remaining patients showed a small increase and the other two no changes at all. When the sulphinpyrazone was withdrawn, the serum phenytoin concentrations fell to their former levels.[1] A clinical study in patients showed that 800 mg sulphinpyrazone daily for a week increased the phenytoin half-life from 10 to 16.5 h and reduced the metabolic clearance from 59 to 32 ml/min.[2]

Mechanism

Uncertain. It seems probable that sulphinpyrazone inhibits the metabolism of the phenytoin by the liver, thereby allowing it to accumulate in the body and leading to a rise in its serum levels. Displacement of phenytoin from its plasma protein binding sites may also have some part to play.

Importance and management

Information seems to be limited to just two reports (one is an abstract and the other an indirect reference) which await confirmation. A similar interaction is reported with phenylbutazone with which sulphinpyrazone has a very close chemical relationship. Thus what is known suggests that concurrent use should be monitored and suitable phenytoin dosage reductions made where necessary. The incidence is uncertain, but two out of the five patients studied[1] are reported to have demonstrated this interaction. More study is needed.

References

1 Hansen JM, Busk G, Niemi G, Haase NJ, Lumholtz B, Skovsted L and Kampmann JP. Inhibition of phenytoin metabolism by sulphinpyrazone. In: Turner P, Padgham C (eds). Abstracts of the world conference on clinical pharmacology and therapeutics. London. (Macmillan, London) (1980) Abstract 584.
2 Simonsen K, Busk G, Niemi G, Haase HNJ, Lumholtz B, Skovsted L, Kampmann JP, Hansen JM. Influence of sulphinpyrazone on the metabolism of antipyrine, phenytoin and tolbutamide. Clin Pharmacol Ther (1982) in press. Quoted thus by Pedersen AK, Kacobsen P, Kampmann JP, Hansen JM. Clinical pharmacokinetics and potentially important drug interactions of sulphinpyrazone. Clin Pharmacokinet (1982) 7, 42–56.

Phenytoin + Sulphonamides

Abstract/Summary

Phenytoin serum levels can be raised by the concurrent use of co-trimoxazole, sulphamethizole, sulphamethoxazole, sulphaphenazole and trimethoprim. Phenytoin intoxication may develop. Sulphadimethoxine, sulphamethoxypyridazine, sulphamethoxydiazine and sulphafurazole (sulfisoxazole) are reported not to interact.

Clinical evidence

(a) Phenytoin + Co-trimoxazole (sulphamethoxazole + trimethoprim)

A patient on 400 mg phenytoin daily developed intoxication (ataxia, nystagmus, loss of balance) within two weeks of starting to take 960 mg co-trimoxazole twice daily. His serum levels were found to have climbed to 152 µmol/l (normal range 40–80 µmol/l).[6] A child developed phenytoin intoxication within 48 h of starting co-trimoxazole. She was also taking sulthiame.[7] A clinical study showed that co-trimoxazole and trimethoprim can increase the phenytoin half-life by 30 and 51% respectively, and decrease the mean metabolic clearance by 27–30%.[5] Sulphamethoxazole alone had only a small effect.

(b) Phenytoin + sulphamethizole

The development of phenytoin intoxication in a patient given sulphamethizole prompted a study of this interaction in eight patients. After 7 days' treatment with sulphamethizole (1 g four times daily) the phenytoin half-life had lengthened from 11.3 to 20.5 h. Three out of four patients showed rises in serum phenytoin levels from 22 to 33, from 19 to 23 and from 4 to 7 µg/ml respectively. The fourth patient was not affected.[1,2] Another single-dose study showed that the half-life of phenytoin was similarly increased and the mean metabolic clearance reduced by 36%.[5]

(c) Phenytoin + Sulphaphenazole or Sulphadiazine

After taking 2 g sulphaphenazole (13 patients) or 4 g sulphadiazine (eight patients) daily for a week, the half-life of single IV doses of phenytoin were found to have increased by 237 and 80% respectively. The mean metabolic clearance decreased by 67 and 45% respectively.[5]

(d) Phenytoin + Other sulphonamides

Sulphadimethoxine, sulphamethoxypyridazine, sulphamethoxydiazine and sulphafurazole (sulfisoxazole) have been found not to interact with phenytoin significantly.[2,4,7]

Mechanism

The sulphonamides which interact appear to do so by inhibiting the metabolism of the phenytoin by the liver, resulting in its accumulation in the body. This would also seem to be true for trimethoprim.[3]

Importance and management

The documentation seems to be limited to the reports cited, but the interaction is established. Co-trimoxazole, sulphamethizole, sulphadiazine, sulphaphenazole and trimethoprim can increase serum phenytoin levels. It probably occurs in most patients but the small number of adverse reaction reports suggests that the risk of intoxication is small. It is clearly most likely in those with serum phenytoin levels at the top end of the range. If concurrent use is thought appropriate, the serum phenytoin levels should be closely monitored and the phenytoin dosage reduced if necessary. Alternatively use a non-interacting sulphonamide (see (d) above). There seems to be no information about other sulphonamides but it would be prudent to be alert for this interaction if any is given with phenytoin.

References

1 Lumholtz B, Siersbaek-Nielsen K, Skovsted L, Kampmann J, Hansen JM. Sulfamethizole-induced inhibition of diphenylhydantoin, tolbutamide and warfarin metabolism. Clin Pharmacol Ther (1975) 17, 731.
2 Siersbaek-Nielsen K, Hansen M, Skovsted L, Lumholtz B, Kampmann J. Sulphamethizole-induced inhibition of diphenylhydantoin and tolbutamide metabolism in man. Clin Pharmacol Ther (1973) 14, 148.

3 Hansen JM, Siersbaek-Nielsen K, Skovsted L, Kampmann JP, Lumholtz B. Potentiation of warfarin by co-trimoxazole. Br Med J (1975) 1, 684.
4 Hansen JM, Kristensen M, Skovsted L and Christensen LK. Dicoumarol-induced diphenylhydantoin intoxication. Lancet (1966) ii, 265.
5 Hansen JM, Kampmann JP, Siersbaek-Nielsen K, Lumholtz B, Arroe M, Abildgaard U, Skovsted L. The effect of different sulphonamides on phenytoin metabolism in man. Acta Med Scand (1979) Suppl, 624, 106.
6 Wilcox JB. Phenytoin intoxication and co-trimoxazole. NZ Med J (1981) 96, 235–6.
7 Gillman MA, Sandyk R. Phenytoin intoxication and co-trimoxazole. Ann Intern Med (1985) 102, 559.

Phenytoin + Sulthiame

Abstract/Summary

Serum phenytoin levels can be approximately doubled by the concurrent use of sulthiame. Phenytoin intoxication may occur unless suitable phenytoin dosage reductions are made.

Clinical evidence

The serum phenytoin levels of six out of seven epileptic patients approximately doubled within 5–25 days of starting to take 400 mg sulthiame daily. All experienced an increase in side-effects and definite phenytoin intoxication occurred in two of them. Phenytoin serum levels fell when the sulthiame was withdrawn.[1] All of the patients were also taking phenobarbitone (phenobarbital) and greater variations in serum phenobarbitone were seen, but this was not clinically important.[1]

A number of other reports confirm this interaction,[2–8] some of which describe the development of phenytoin intoxication.

Mechanism

The evidence suggests that sulthiame interferes with the metabolism of the phenytoin by the liver, leading to its accumulation in the body. In one study the phenytoin half-life almost doubled (from 28 to 52 h) during treatment with sulthiame.

Importance and management

A reasonably well-documented, established and clinically important interaction. The incidence seems to be high. If sulthiame is added to established treatment with phenytoin, increases in serum phenytoin levels of up to 75% may be expected.[3,7] Phenytoin serum levels should be closely monitored and appropriate dosage reductions made to prevent the development of intoxication. The changes in phenobarbitone (phenobarbital) levels appear to be unimportant.

References

1 Olesen OV, Jensen ON, Drug-interaction between sulthiame (Ospolot) and phenytoin in the treatment of epilepsy. Dan Med Bull (1969) 16, 154.
2 Houghton GW, Richens A. Inhibition of phenytoin metabolism by sulthiame. Br J Pharmac (1973) 49, 157P.
3 Houghton GW, Richens A. Inhibition of phenytoin metabolism by sulthiame in epileptic patients. Br J clin Pharmac (1974) 1, 59.

4 Richens A, Houghton GW. Phenytoin intoxication caused by sulthiame. Lancet (1973) ii, 1442.

5 Houghton GW, Richens A. Inhibition of phenytoin metabolism by other drugs during epilepsy. Int J Clin Pharmacol (1975) 12, 210.

6 Frantzen E, Hansen JM, Hansen OE, Kristensen M. Phenytoin (Dilantin) intoxication. Acta Neurol Scandinav (1967) 43, 440.

7 Houghton GW, Richens A. Phenytoin intoxication induced by sulthiame in epileptic patients. J Neurol Neurosurg Psychiat (1974) 37, 275.

8 Hansen JM, Kristensen L and Skovsted L. Sulthiame (Ospolot) as inhibitor of diphenylhydantoin metabolism. Epilepsia (1968) 9, 17.

Phenytoin + Theophylline

Abstract/Summary

The serum levels of each drug and their therapeutic effects can be markedly reduced by the presence of the other. Dosage increases may be needed to maintain adequate concentrations. Separating the oral dosage by 1–2 h can minimize the effects of theophylline on phenytoin.

Clinical evidence

(a) Reduced phenytoin serum levels

The seizure frequency of an epileptic woman on phenytoin (400 mg daily) increased when she was given intravenous and later oral theophylline. Her serum phenytoin levels had more than halved (from 15.7 to 5–8 µg/ml). An increase in the phenytoin dosage to 600 mg daily raised her serum phenytoin levels to only 7–11 µg/ml until the drugs were given 1–2 h apart. The patient then developed phenytoin intoxication with a serum level of 33 µg/ml. A subsequent study in four normal subjects confirmed that separating the dosages raised the serum levels of both drugs.[1]

A study on 14 subjects showed that, after two weeks of concurrent use, withdrawal of the theophylline resulted in a 40% rise in the mean serum phenytoin levels of five of the subjects and a mean rise of 30% in the total group.[2]

(b) Reduced theophylline serum levels

The observation that a patient on phenytoin needed an increase in the dosage of theophylline prompted a study in 10 normal subjects. After taking phenytoin for 10 days (serum levels 10–20 µg/ml) the clearance of theophylline was increased by 73%, and both the area under the time-concentration curve and the half-life were reduced about 50%.[3] A study in six normal subjects showed that after taking 300 mg phenytoin daily for 3 weeks the mean clearance of theophylline was increased by 45% (range 31–65%).[4] Other reports on individual asthmatic patients and normal subjects have shown that phenytoin can cause a two- to three-fold increase in the clearance of theophylline.[5,6,9,10] Another study[8] and a case report[11] show that the effects of phenytoin (and phenobarbitone) on theophylline can be additive with the effects of smoking.

Mechanisms

(a) Uncertain. The evidence suggests that theophylline inhibits the absorption of phenytoin from the gut. (b) It seems probable that the phenytoin, a known enzyme-inducing agent, increases the metabolism of the theophylline by the liver, thereby hastening its clearance from the body.

Importance and management

These mutual interactions are established and of clinical importance. Patients given both drugs should be monitored to confirm that therapy remains effective. Ideally the serum levels should be measured to confirm that they remain within the therapeutic range. Dosage increases of up to 50% or more may be required.[7] Separating the oral dosages by 1–2 h apparently minimizes the effects of theophylline on phenytoin.

References

1 Fincham RW, Schottelius DD, Wyatt R, Hendeles L and Weinberger M. Phenytoin-theophylline interaction: a case report. In Advances in Epileptology. Xth Epilepsy Int Symp. Wada JA, Perry JK (eds) Raven Press, NY (1980) p 505.

2 Taylor JW, Hendeles L, Weinberger M, Lyon LW, Wyatt R, Riegelman S. The interaction of phenytoin and theophylline. Drug Intell Clin Pharm (1980) 14, 638.

3 Marquis J-F, Carruthers SG, Spense JD, Brownstone YS, Toogood JH. Phenytoin-theophylline interaction. N Engl J Med (1982) 307, 1189–90.

4 Miller M, Cosgriff J, Kwong T, Morken DA. Influence of phenytoin on theophylline clearance. Clin Pharmacol Ther (1984) 35, 656–9.

5 Sklar SJ, Wagner JC. Enhanced theophylline clearance secondary to phenytoin therapy. Drug Intell Clin Pharm (1985) 19, 34–6.

6 Reed RC, Schwartz HJ. Phenytoin-theophylline-quinidine interaction. N Engl J Med (1983) 308, 724–5.

7 Slugg PH, Pippenger CE. Theophylline and its interactions. Cleve Clin Q (1985) 52, 417–24.

8 Crowley JJ, Cusack BJ, Jue SG, Koup JR, Vestal RE. Cigarette smoking and theophylline metabolism: effects of phenytoin. Clin Pharmacol Ther (1987) 42, 334–40.

9 Landsberg K, Shalansky S. Interaction between phenytoin and theophylline. Can J Hosp Pharm (1988) 41, 31–2.

10 Adebayo GI. Interaction between phenytoin and theophylline in healthy volunteers. Clin Exp Pharmacol Physiol (1988) 15, 883–7.

11 Nicholson JP, Basile SA, Cury JD. Massive theophylline dosing in a heavy smoker receiving both phenytoin and phenobarbital. Ann Pharmacother (1992) 26, 334–6.

Phenytoin + Tienilic acid (Ticrynafen)

Abstract/Summary

Phenytoin intoxication occurred in two patients when they were additionally treated with tienilic acid.

Clinical evidence, mechanism

An epileptic patient, well controlled on phenobarbitone and phenytoin for 6 years, developed various adverse effects within three weeks of starting to take tienilic acid (250 mg daily) and, despite a reduction in the phenytoin dosage from 300 mg to

100 mg daily, developed clear signs of phenytoin intoxication a week later. His serum phenytoin levels had increased threefold (to 30.2 μg/ml). Three weeks after stopping the tienilic acid, his serum phenytoin levels had fallen again, and all adverse symptoms had disappeared at the end of a further 3 weeks.[1] Phenytoin intoxication is described elsewhere in another patient treated with tienilic acid.[2]

Mechanism

Not understood. Tienilic acid is highly protein bound and may displace phenytoin from its binding sites, but it seems more likely that the interaction results from its inhibition of the metabolism of the phenytoin which allows it to accumulate in the body.

Importance and management

Although information seems to be limited to only two patients, concurrent use should be avoided unless the serum phenytoin levels can be monitored and suitable downward adjustments made if necessary. More study is needed. Tienilic acid has been withdrawn in some countries because it can cause serious liver damage.

References

1 Ahmad S. Ticrynafen-induced phenytoin toxicity: an interaction. J Roy Soc Med (1981) 74, 162.
2 Weber KT, Fisherman AP. In 'A new class of diuretics with uricosuric activity'. Postgrad Med Comm (1979) pp 57–63.

Phenytoin + Trazodone

Abstract/Summary

A single case report describes phenytoin intoxication in a patient when concurrently treated with trazodone.

Clinical evidence, mechanism, importance and management

A patient taking 300 mg phenytoin daily developed signs of phenytoin intoxication after taking 500 mg trazodone daily for six weeks. His serum phenytoin levels had risen from 17.5 to 46 μg/ml.[1] Therapeutic phenytoin serum levels were restored by reducing the phenytoin dosage to 200 mg daily and the trazodone to 400 mg daily. The reasons for this apparent interaction are not understood. Concurrent use need not be avoided but patients should be monitored if given both drugs.

Reference

1 Dorn JM. A case of phenytoin toxicity possibly precipitated by trazodone. J Clin Psychiatry (1986) 47, 89–90.

Phenytoin + Tricyclic antidepressants

Abstract/Summary

Some very limited evidence suggests that imipramine can raise serum phenytoin levels but nortriptyline and amitriptyline appear not to do so. Phenytoin possibly reduces serum desipramine levels. The tricyclics also lower the convulsive threshold.

Clinical evidence

(a) Serum phenytoin levels increased or unchanged

The serum phenytoin levels of two patients rose over a three-month period when concurrently treated with imipramine, 75 mg daily. One of them showed an increase from 30 to 60 μmol/l and developed mild intoxication. These signs disappeared and the phenytoin serum levels of both patients fell when the imipramine was withdrawn. One of them was also taking nitrazepam and clonazepam, and the other sodium valproate and carbamazepine.[1]

Other studies have shown that nortriptyline, 75 mg daily, had a small but non-significant effect on the serum phenytoin levels of five patients,[2] and that amitriptyline had no effect on the elimination of phenytoin in three subjects.[3]

(b) Serum tricyclic antidepressant levels reduced

A report describes two patients who had low serum desipramine levels, despite taking standard dosages, while concurrently taking phenytoin.[5]

Mechanisms

One suggestion is that imipramine inhibits the metabolism of the phenytoin by the liver which results in its accumulation in the body. The reduced desipramine levels may be a result of enzyme induction by the phenytoin.

Importance and management

The documentation is very limited indeed and none of these interactions is adequately established. The tricyclic antidepressants as a group lower the seizure threshold[4] which raises the question of the advisability of giving them to epileptic patients. If concurrent use is undertaken the effects should be very well monitored.

References

1 Perucca E, Richens A. Interaction between phenytoin and imipramine. Br J clin Pharmac (1977) 4, 485.
2 Houghton GW, Richens A. Inhibition of phenytoin metabolism by other drugs used in epilepsy. Int J clin Pharmacol (1975) 12, 210.
3 Pond SM, Graham GG, Birkett DJ, Wade DN. Effects of tricyclic antidepressants on drug metabolism. Clin Pharmacol Ther (1975) 18, 191.

4 Dallos V, Heathfield K. Iatrogenic epilpesy due to antidepressant drugs. Brit Med J (1969) 4, 80.
5 Fogel BS, Haltzman S. Desipramine and phenytoin: a potential drug interaction of relevance. J Clin Psychiatry (1987) 48, 387–8.

Phenytoin + Zidovudine

Abstract/Summary

Although zidovudine does not alter the pharmacokinetics of phenytoin, there is preliminary evidence that an adverse response may sometimes occur.

Clinical evidence, mechanism, importance and management

Although there are said to have been 13 cases of a possible interaction between zidovudine and phenytoin,[1]12 asymptomatic HIV positive patients showed no significant changes in the pharmacokinetics of phenytoin (300 mg orally) while taking 200 mg ziodovudine every 4 h.[1] Until the situation is more clearly defined it would be prudent to monitor concurrent use.

References

1 Sarver P, Lampkin TA, Dukes GE, Messenheimer JA, Kirby MG, Dalton MJ, Hak JL. Effect of zidovudine on the pharmacokinetic disposition of phenytoin in HIV positive asymptomatic patients. Pharmacotherapy (1991) 11, 108–9.

Primidone + Barbiturates

Abstract/Summary

Elevated serum phenobarbitone (phenobarbital) levels may develop if primidone and phenobarbitone are given concurrently.

Clinical evidence, mechanism, importance and management

Primidone is substantially converted into phenobarbitone within the body. For example, a group of patients taking primidone without phenobarbitone developed serum primidone levels of 9 µg/ml and serum phenobarbitone levels of 31 µg/ml.[1] If phenobarbitone is given at the same time the serum levels may become excessive. This effect may be possibly exacerbated if phenytoin is also being given. If concurrent use is undertaken be particularly alert for any evidence of phenobarbitone intoxication.

Reference

1 Booker HE, Hosokowa K, Burdette RD. A clinical study of serum primidone levels. Epilepsia (1970) 11, 395.

Primidone + Carbamazepine, Clonazepam or Clorazepate

Abstract/Summary

Carbamazepine is reported to reduce, whereas clonazepam is reported to raise serum primidone levels. Clorazepate with primidone may possibly cause personality changes.

Clinical evidence, mechanism, importance and management

An extremely brief report on 155 epileptic children indicated that the serum levels of primidone may be reduced by carbamazepine but no details were given.[1] The same report stated that in children aged 3–15 the concurrent use of clonazepam increased the concentrations of primidone to toxic levels.[1] Another report suggested that the concurrent use of primidone and clorazepate may have been responsible for the development of irritability, aggression and depression in a group of patients.[2] None of these effects appears to be well documented or confirmed but some caution would seem appropriate during concurrent use.

References

1 Windorfer A, Sauer W. Drug interactions during anticonvulsant therapy in childhood: diphenylhydantoin, primidone, phenobarbitone, clonazepam, nitrazepam, carbamazepine and dipropylacetate. Neuropadiatrie (1977) 8, 29.
2 Feldman RG. Clorazepate in temporal lobe epilepsy. J Am Med Ass (1976) 236, 2603.

Primidone + Isoniazid

Abstract/Summary

A single case report describes elevated serum primidone levels and reduced phenobarbitone levels during concurrent treatment with primidone and isoniazid.

Clinical evidence, mechanism, importance and management

A patient on primidone showed raised serum primidone levels and reduced serum phenobarbitone levels due, it was demonstrated, to the concurrent use of isoniazid which inhibited the metabolism of the primidone by the liver. The half-life of primidone rose from 8.7 to 14 h while taking isoniazid and steady-state primidone levels rose by 83%. The importance of this interaction is uncertain but prescribers should be aware that it can occur if concurrent treatment is undertaken.[1]

Reference

1 Sutton G, Kupferberg HJ. Isoniazid as an inhibitor of primidone metabolism. Neurology (1975) 25, 1179.

Primidone + Phenytoin

Abstract/Summary

Serum phenobarbitone levels are increased in patients on primidone when concurrently treated with phenytoin. This is normally an advantageous interaction, but phenobarbitone intoxication occurs occasionally.

Clinical evidence

A study in 44 epileptic patients taking primidone and phenytoin showed that their serum phenobarbitone:primidone ratio was high (4.35) compared with 15 other patients (1.05) who were only taking primidone.[1] Similar results are described in other studies.[2–4,7,8] A few patients may develop intoxication.[6,7]

Mechanism

Phenytoin increases the metabolic conversion of primidone to phenobarbitone while possibly depressing the subsequent metabolic destruction of the phenobarbitone. The net effect is a rise in phenobarbitone levels.[5]

Importance and management

Well documented. Concurrent use is common. This is normally an advantageous interaction since a metabolic product of primidone is phenobarbitone which is itself an active anticonvulsant. However it should be borne in mind that phenobarbitone serum levels can sometimes reach toxic concentrations,[6] even if only a small dose of phenobarbitone is added.[1]

References

1 Fincham RW, Schottelius DD, Sahs AL. The influence of diphenylhydantoin on primidone metabolism. Arch Neurol (1974) 30, 259.
2 Fincham RW, Schottelius DD, Sahs AL. The influence of diphenylhydantoin on primidone metabolism. Trans Am Neurol Ass (1973) 98, 197.
3 Schmidt D. The effect of phenytoin and ethosuximide on primidone metabolism in patients with epilepsy. J Neurol (1975) 209, 115.
4 Reynolds EH, Fenton G, Fenwick P, Johnson AL and Laundy M. Interaction of phenytoin and primidone. Br Med J (1975) 2, 594.
5 Porro MG, Kupferberg HJ, Porter RJ, Theodore WH, Newmark ME. Phenytoin: an inhibitor and inducer of primidone metabolism in an epileptic patient. Br J clin Pharmac (1982) 14, 294–7.
6 Galdames P, Ortizo M, Saavedra S, Aguilera O. Interaccion fenitoina-primidona: intoxicacion por fenobarbital, en un adulto tratado con ambas drogas. Rev Med Chile (1980) 108, 716.
7 Gallagher BB, Baumel IP, Mattson RH, Woodbury SG. Primidone, diphenylhydantoin and phenobarbital. Aspects of acute and chronic toxicity. Neurology (1973) 23, 145–9.
8 Callaghan N, Feeley M, Duggan F, O'Callaghan M, Seldrup J. The effect of

anticonvulsant drugs which induce liver microsomal enzymes on derived and ingested phenobarbitone levels. Acta Neurol Scan (1977) 56, 1–6.

Primidone + Sodium valproate

Abstract/Summary

Increases in serum primidone and phenobarbitone levels due to sodium valproate have been reported. The reports are inconsistent.

Clinical evidence

(a) Increased serum primidone levels

The serum primidone levels of seven children taking 10–18 mg/kg daily were seen to have risen by a factor of 2–3 when sodium valproate (dosage not stated) was given concurrently. After 1–3 months the effect of the sodium valproate had almost disappeared in three of the patients but persisted in one. The effects on the other three are not recorded.[1] This interaction is described in other reports: ataxia, drowsiness and marked sedation were seen.[2–5]

(b) Reduced serum primidone levels or no changes

Five patients failed to show any significant changes in serum primidone or phenobarbitone levels when concurrently treated with sodium valproate,[6] whereas another study in two patients found a reduction in serum primidone levels of 24 and 42% respectively when treated with sodium valproate.[7] A retrospective study of 100 epileptic adults and children found no changes in primidone levels, but serum phenobarbitone levels were significantly increased.[8]

Mechanism

Not understood. One suggestion is that the sodium valproate initially slows or blocks the metabolism of the primidone, but later this effect is lost.[1]

Importance and management

There seems to be no consistency about the response of patients to concurrent use. More study is needed. If concurrent use is undertaken, the outcome should be well monitored. Be alert for any signs of primidone or phenobarbitone intoxication.

References

1 Windorfer A, Sauer W, Gadeke R. Elevation of diphenylhydantoin and primidone serum concentrations by addition of dipropylacetate, a new anticonvulsant drug. Acta Paediatr Scand (1975) 64, 771.
2 Wilder BJ, Willmore LJ, Bruni J, Villarreal HJ. Valproic acid: interaction with other anticonvulsant drugs. Neurology (1978) 28, 892.
3 Haigh D, Forsythe WI. The treatment of childhood epilepsy with sodium valproate. Dev Med Child Neurol (1975) 17, 743.

4 Richens A, Ahmad S. Controlled trial of sodium valproate in severe epilepsy. Br Med J (1975) 3, 255.

5 Volzke E, Doose H. Dipropylacetate (Depakine, Ergenyl) in the treatment of epilepsy. Epilepsia (1973) 14, 185.

6 Bruni J. Valproic acid and plasma levels of primidone and derived phenobarbital. Can J Neurol Sci (1981) 8, 91.

7 Varma R, Michos GA, Varma RS, Hoshino AY. Clinical trials of Depakene (valproic acid) coadministered with other anticonvulsants in epileptic patients. Res Comm Psychol Psychiat Behav (1980) 5, 265.

8 Yukawa E, Higuchi S, Aoyama T. The effect of concurrent administration of sodium valproate on serum levels of primidone and its metabolite phenobarbital. J Clin Pharmacy Ther (1989) 14, 387–92.

Semisodium valproate + Fluoxetine

Abstract/Summary

An isolated report describes a 50% rise in serum valproic acid levels in a patient taking semisodium valproate when given fluoxetine.

Clinical evidence, mechanism, importance and management

A mentally retarded patient with an atypical bipolar disorder on 3 g semisodium valproate (divalproex sodium) daily showed a rise in serum valproic acid levels from 93.5 to 152 mg/l within 2 weeks of starting to take 20 mg fluoxetine daily. The valproate dosage was reduced to 2.25 g daily and two weeks later the serum valproic acid levels had fallen to 113 mg/l. No adverse effects were seen.[1] The reason for this response and its clinical importance are unknown.

Reference

1 Sovner R, Davis JM. A potential drug interaction between fluoxetine and valproic acid. J Clin Psychopharmacol (1991) 11, 389.

Sodium valproate + Antacids

Abstract/Summary

The absorption of sodium valproate is slightly increased by *Maalox* (aluminium-magnesium hydroxide) but not by magnesium trisilicate or calcium carbonate suspension.

Clinical evidence, mechanism, importance and management

The AUC (area under the curve) of a single dose of sodium valproate (given 1 h after breakfast) was increased by 12% (range 3–28%) in normal subjects given 62 ml *Maalox* 1h and 3 h after breakfast and at bedtime. Neither magnesium trisilicate suspension (*Trisogel*) nor calcium carbonate suspension (*Titralac*) had a significant effect on absorption.[1] No special precautions would seem necessary during concurrent use.

Reference

1 May CA, Garnett WR, Small RE, Pellock JM. Effects of three antacids on the bioavailability of valproic acid. Clin Pharm (1982) 1, 244–7.

Sodium valproate + Aspirin, Naproxen

Abstract/Summary

Sodium valproate toxicity developed in three patients when given large and repeated doses of aspirin. Naproxen appears not to interact.

Clinical evidence

A girl of 17 taking 21 mg/kg sodium valproate daily was prescribed 18 mg/kg of aspirin daily for lupus arthritis. Within a few days she developed a disabling tremor which disappeared when the aspirin was stopped. Total serum valproate levels were not significantly changed, but the free fraction fell from 24 to 14% when the aspirin was withdrawn. Similar toxic reactions (tremor, nystagmus, drowsiness, ataxia) were seen in two children of six and four given 12–20 mg/kg aspirin 4-hourly while taking sodium valproate (25–48 mg/kg daily).[1]

A study in six normal subjects found that 500 mg naproxen moderately displaces sodium valproate from its protein binding sites, but not enough to have any clinical relevance.[2,4]

Mechanism

Aspirin displaces sodium valproate from its protein binding sites[2] and also decreases its metabolism by the liver[3] so that the levels of free (and pharmacologically active) sodium valproate rise. This would be expected to increase both the therapeutic and toxic effects of the sodium valproate.

Importance and management

Direct information seems to be limited to the studies cited. It would be prudent to avoid giving repeated doses of aspirin to patients taking sodium valproate, unless the response can be monitored and the dosage adjusted appropriately, but the occasional single dose probably does not matter. More study is needed. No clinically important interaction occurs between sodium valproate and naproxen.

References

1 Goulden KJ, Dooley JM, Camfield PR, Fraser AD. Clinical valproate toxicity induced by acetylsalicylic acid. Neurology (1987) 37, 1392–4.

2 Orr JM, Abbott FS, Farrell K, Ferguson S, Sheppard I, Godolphin W. Interaction between valproic acid in epileptic children: serum protein binding and metabolic effects. Clin Pharmacol Ther (1982) 31, 642–9.

3 Abbott FS, Kassam J, Orr JM, Farrell K. The effect of aspirin on valproic acid metabolism. Clin Pharmacol Ther (1986) 40, 94–100.

4 Grimaldi R, Lecchini S, Crema F, Perucca E. In vivo plasma protein binding interaction between valproic acid and naproxen. Eur J Drug Metab Pharmacokinet (1984) 9, 359–63,

Sodium valproate + Benzodiazepines

Abstract/Summary

The concurrent use of sodium valproate and clonazepam may cause an increase in side-effects but some patients are benefitted. Diazepam serum levels may be raised by sodium valproate.

Clinical evidence, mechanism, importance and management

A study in epileptic children and adolescents showed that the addition of clonazepam increased the unwanted effects (drowsiness, absence status) in nine out of the 12 patients. The authors suggested that this combination should be avoided.[1] However it has been pointed out in a very brief letter that neither affects the the serum concentrations of the other drug and that '...it would be improper to conclude that clonazepam and valproic acid should never be given together in patients with absence seizures since some patients with refractory absence seizures have an excellent response to this combination of drugs.'[3] Enhanced sedation has been briefly described during the concurrent use of sodium valproate and other unnamed benzodiazepines.[2] Sodium valproate can also increase the serum levels of diazepam but the importance of this is uncertain.[4]

References

1 Jeavons PM, Clark JE, Mahashwari MC. Treatment of generalized epilepsies of childhood and adolescence with sodium valproate ('Epilim'). Dev Med Child Neurol (1977) 19, 9.
2 Volzke E, Doose H. Dipropylacetate (Depakine, Ergenyl) in the treatment of epilepsy. Epilepsia (1973) 14, 185.
3 Browne TR. Interaction between clonazepam and sodium valproate. N Engl J Med (1979) 300, 678.
4 Dhillon SA, Richens A. Valproic acid and diazepam interaction in vivo. Br J Clin Pharmacol (1982) 13, 553.

Sodium valproate + Chlorpromazine

Abstract/Summary

Sodium valproate serum levels are slightly raised in patients given chlorpromazine, but this appears to be of minimal clinical importance. An isolated report describes severe hepatotoxicity with concurrent use.

Clinical evidence, mechanism, importance and management

The sodium valproate steady-state trough serum levels of six patients taking 400 mg daily rose by 22% when given 100–300 mg chlorpromazine daily. The half-life increased by 14% and the clearance fell by 13% (possibly due to some reduction in the metabolism by the liver)[1]. This interaction would normally seem to be of minimal importance, however severe heptatoxicity occurred in another patient when given both drugs.[2]

Concurrent use should be monitored.

References

1 Ishizaki T, Chiba K, Saito M, Kobayashi K, Iizuka R. The effects of neuroleptics (haloperidol and chlorpromazine) on the pharmacokinetics of valproic acid in schizophrenic patients. J Clin Psychopharmacol (1984) 4, 254–61.
2 Bach N, Thung SN, Schaffner F, Tobias H. Exaggerated cholestasis and hepatic fibrosis following simultaneous administration of chlorpromazine and sodium valproate. Dig Dis Sci (1989) 34, 1303–7.

Sodium valproate + Cimetidine or Ranitidine

Abstract/Summary

Ranitidine does not interact with sodium valproate, and cimetidine interacts only minimally.

Clinical evidence, mechanism, importance and management

The clearance of sodium valproate was reduced in six patients to a small extent (2–17%) by cimetidine, but not by ranitidine.[1] It seems doubtful if the sodium valproate-cimetidine interaction is of clinical importance.

Reference

1 Webster LK, Mihaly GW, Jones DB, Smallwood RA, Phillips JA, Vajda FJ. Effect of cimetidine and ranitidine on carbamazepine and sodium valproate pharmacokinetics. Eur J Clin Pharmacol (1984) 27, 341–3.

Sodium valproate + Felbamate

Abstract/Summary

Felbamate can raise sodium valproate serum levels

Clinical evidence, mechanism, importance and management

The steady-state sodium valproate levels in eight epileptics were raised 28% (from 66.9 to 85.4 µg/ml) by 1200 mg felbamate daily, and by 54% (from 66.9 to 103.0 µg/ml) by 2400 mg daily.[1] The reasons are not understood. It may be necessary to reduce the sodium valproate dosage to avoid toxicity if felbamate is given. More study is needed to establish the clinical importance of this interaction.

Reference

1 Wagner ML, Graves NM, Leppik IE, Remmel RP, Ward DL, Shumaker RC. The effect of felbamate on valproate disposition. Epilepsia (1991) 32, Suppl 3, 15.

Sodium valproate + Isoniazid

Abstract/Summary

An isolated report describes the development of raised serum sodium valproate levels and toxicity in a child when concurrently treated with isoniazid.

Clinical evidence, mechanism, importance and management

A girl of 5 with left partial seizures, successfully controlled on 600 mg sodium valproate daily and clonazepam for 7 months, developed signs of sodium valproate toxicity (drowsiness, asthenia) shortly after starting to take 200 mg isoniazid daily (because of a positive tuberculin reaction). Her serum valproate levels were found to have risen (121–139 mg.l^{-1}; normal therapeutic range 50–100 mg.l^{-1}). Over the next few months various changes were made in her treatment, the most significant being a 62% reduction in the dosage of sodium valproate to maintain satisfactory therapeutic levels. Later when the isoniazid was stopped, her valproate levels fell below therapeutic levels and seizures re-occurred. It was then found necessary to increase the valproate to its former dosage. The suggested explanation is that the isoniazid inhibited the metabolism (oxidation) of the sodium valproate by the liver so that it accumulated and, in effect, became an overdose. The child was found to be a very slow acetylator of isoniazid which made the interaction more likely to occur.[1]

The general importance of this interaction is uncertain, but it would clearly be prudent to monitor sodium valproate levels closely if isoniazid is added, reducing the dosage where necessary.

Reference

1 Jonville AP, Gauchez AS, Autret E, Billard C, Barbier P, Nsabiyumva F, Breteau M. Interaction between isoniazid and valproate: a case of valproate overdosage. Eur J Clin Pharmacol (1991) 40, 197–8.

Chapter 8
Antihypertensive Drug Interactions

Hypertension (elevated blood pressure) can be controlled by the use of a very wide spectrum of drugs acting either centrally within the brain or peripherally. The drugs dealt with in this chapter include the centrally acting drugs (clonidine, methyldopa), adrenergic neurone blockers (guanethidine), vasodilators (alpha-1 blockers such as prazosin, indoramin and others whose mode of action is uncertain—e.g. hydralazine, diazoxide), angiotensin-converting enzyme (ACE) inhibitors and diuretics. The beta-blockers, calcium channel blockers, and pargyline (MAOI) are dealt with in separate chapters. Table 8.1 lists the drugs dealt with in this chapter and some of their proprietary names. Where these drugs are the affecting agent rather than the drug affected, the interactions are described elsewhere. The index must be consulted for a full listing of all the interactions.

Table 8.1 Antihypertensive drugs

Non-proprietary names	Proprietary names
ACE inhibitors	
Benazepril	
Captopril	*Acepril, Alopresin, Capoten, Captolane, Cesplon, Cor Tensobon, Dilabar, Garranil, Loprin, Lopril, Tensoprel*
Cilazapril	
Enalapril	*Converten, Enapren, Innovace, Naprilene, Pres, Reniten, Vasotec, Xanef*
Lisinopril	*Carace, Zestril*
Quinapril	
Pentopril	
Ramipril	
Trandolapril	*Gopten*
Adrenergic neurone blockers	
Bethanidine	*Bendogen, Esbatal, Batel, Benzoxine, Betaling, Eusmanid, Hypersin, Regulin*
Guanadrel	*Hylorel*
Guanethidine	*Ganda, Ismelin(e), Antipres, Dopom, Ipotidina, Normoten, Solo-ethidine, Visutensil*
Guanfacine	*Entulic, Estulic, Tenex*
Guanoclor	*Vatensol*
Guanoxan	*Envacar*
Alpha-blocking agents	
Bunazosin	
Doxazosin	
Indoramin	*Baratol, Indorene, Wydora*
Phenoxybenzamine	*Dibenyline, Dibenzyline, Dibenzyran*
Phentolamine	*Rogitine, Regitine*

Continued on page 351

Table 8.1 (Continued)

Non-proprietary names	Proprietary names
Prazosin	*Hypovase, Duramipress, Eurex, Hexapress, Perpress, Pratsiol*
Terazosin	
Trimazosin	

Calcium channel blockers

See Chapter 11

Centrally-acting agents

Clonidine	*Catapres(s)(an), Clonilou, Clonistada, Drylon, Ipotensium, Tensinova, Tenso-Timelets*
Debrisoquine	*Declinax, Equitonil*
Methyldopa	*Aldomet, Dopamet, Hydromet, Alphamex, Dimal, Elanpres, Equibar, Grospisk, Hyperpax, Hypodopa, Medomet, Medopren, Methoplain, Novomedopa, Sembrina, Sinepress*
Moxonidine	
Rilmenidine	

Directly-acting vasodilators

Diazoxide	*Eudemine, Hyperstat, Hypertonalum, Proglicem, Proglycem*
Hydralazine	*Apresolin(e), Alphapress, Aprelazine) Dralzine, Hydrapres, Hyperazin, Hyperex, Hyperphen, Ipolina, Rolazine, Supres, Vasodur*
Minoxidil	*Loniten, Regaine, Alopepil, Alostil, Minodyl, Rogaine*
Tolazoline	

Diuretics (see also Table 14.2 in Chapter 14)

Potassium depleters
Azosemide
Bumetanide
Chlorthalidone
Ethacrynic acid
Frusemide (furosemide)
Piretanide
Thiazides

Potassium-sparers
Amiloride
Azolimine
Canrenoate potassium
Spironolactone
Triamterene

Rauwolfia alkaloids

Reserpine

Serotonin Blockers

Ketanserin
Sufrexal

ACE inhibitors + Allopurinol

Abstract/Summary

Three cases of serious Stevens-Johnson syndrome (one fatal) and two cases of hypersensitivity have been attributed to the concurrent use of captopril and allopurinol.

Clinical evidence

An elderly man with hypertension, chronic renal failure and mild polyarthritis on multiple drug treatment which included captopril (50 mg daily) and diuretics developed fatal Stevens-Johnson syndrome within five weeks of starting to take 200 mg allopurinol daily.[1] Two other patients similarly treated developed the syndrome 3–5 weeks after allopurinol was added to their treatment with captopril.[1] A later report describes fever, arthralgia and myalgia in a man similarly treated. He improved when the captopril was withdrawn.[2] Exfoliatory facial dermatitis was seen in another patient with renal failure.[3]

Mechanism

Not understood. It is uncertain whether this is an interaction because allopurinol alone can cause severe hypersensivity reactions, particularly in the presence of renal failure and the use of diuretics. Captopril is also capable of inducing a hypersensitivity reaction.

Importance and management

This interaction is not clearly established. All that can be constructively said is that patients on both drugs should be very closely monitored for any signs of hypersensitivity and, if necessary, the drugs should be withdrawn at once.

References

1 Pennell DJ, Nunan TO, O'Doherty MJ, Croft DN. Fatal Stevens-Johnson syndrome in a patient on captopril and allopurinol. Lancet (1984) i, 463.
2 Samanta A, Burden AC. Fever, myalgia and arthralgia in a patient on captopril and allopurinol. Lancet (1984) i, 679.
3 Beeley L, Daly M, Stewart P. Bulletin W Midlands Centre for Adverse Drug Reaction Reporting (1987) 24, 9.

ACE-inhibitors + Alpha blockers

Abstract/Summary

Severe first-dose hypotension occurred in a patient on enalapril when given bunazosin. Additive hypotensive effects occur in normal subjects.

Clinical evidence

Prompted by the observation of a patient on enalapril who experienced severe first-dose hypotension when given bunazosin, a study of this interaction was made in six normal subjects. When given 10 mg enalapril or 2 mg bunazosin, their systolic/diastolic pressures over 6 h were reduced by 9.5/6.7 mmHg. When given the enalapril followed by the bunazosin an hour later, the pressure falls were 27/28 mmHg. Even with a much smaller dose of enalapril (2.5 mg) the fall when given both drugs was 19/22 mmHg.[1]

Mechanism

Additive hypotensive effects.

Importance and management

Direct information is limited to this study but acute hypotension (dizziness, fainting) sometimes occurs unpredictably with the first dose of other alpha-blockers and this can be exacerbated if the patient is given or is already taking a beta-blocker or a calcium channel blocker (see 'Prazosin + Beta-blockers', and 'Prazosin + Calcium Channel blockers'). It would therefore seem prudent to apply the same precautions, namely to give test doses of these drugs and monitor the effects. Giving the drugs at bedtime has been suggested because the acute hypotensive reaction appears to be short-lived. Other alpha blockers (doxazosin, prazosin, terazosin, trimazosin) and ACE inhibitors probably behave similarly. More study is needed.

Reference

1 Baba T, Tomiyama T, Takebe K. Enhancement by an ACE inhibitor of first-dose hypotension caused by an alpha$_1$-blocker. N Eng J Med (1990) 322, 1237.

ACE inhibitors + Antacids

Abstract/Summary

Antacids have been found to reduce the absorption of captopril and fosinopril by about one-third.

Clinical evidence, mechanism, importance and management

An antacid containing aluminium hydroxide, magnesium carbonate and magnesium hydroxide reduced the bioavailability of 50 mg captopril in 10 normal subjects by about a third.[1] Another study found that *Mylanta* (aluminium and magnesium hydroxides) similarly reduced the bioavailability of fosinopril by about a third.[2] The mechanism of this interaction and its clinical significance is uncertain but be alert for evidence of reduced effects if antacids are used concurrently. More study is needed.

Reference

1 Mantyla R, Mannisto PT, Vuorela A, Sundberg S, Ottoila P. Impairment of captopril bioavailability by concomitant food and antacid intake. Int J Clin Pharmacol Ther Toxicol (1984) 22, 626–9.
2 Moore L, Kramer A, Swites B, Kramer P, Tu J. Effect of cimetidine and antacid on the kinetics of the active diacid of fosinopril in healthy subjects. J Clin Pharmacol (1988) 28, 946–59.

ACE inhibitors + Azathioprine

Abstract/Summary

The concurrent use of captopril and azathioprine occasionally results in leucopenia.

Clinical evidence, mechanism, importance and management

Both captopril and azathioprine given alone can cause bone marrow depression which results in a fall in the white cell count. Sometimes these effects appear to be additive when both drugs are given. A patient whose white cell count fell sharply when treated with captopril and azathioprine together, showed no leucopenia when given each drug separately.[1] Another patient, previously treated with azathioprine, developed leucopenia when later given captopril.[2] Other patients have similarly shown leucopenia when given both drugs, in one case only occurring when rechallenged with captopril alone.[3,4] As the development of this interaction is not predictable, it would be prudent to monitor the white cell count during concurrent or sequential use. There seems to be nothing documented about other ACE inhibitors.

References

1 Kirchetz EF, Grone HJ, Rieger J, Holscher M, Scheler F. Successful low dose captopril rechallenge following drug induced leucopenia. Lancet (1981) i, 1363.
2 Case DB, Whitman HH, Laragh JH, Spiera H. Successful low dose captopril rechallenge following drug induced leucopenia. Lancet (1981) i, 1362–3.
3 Elijovisch F, Krakoff OR. Captopril associated with granulocytopenia in hypertension after renal transplant. Lancet (1980), i, 927–8.
4 Edwards CRW, Drury P, Penketh A, Damnlinji SA. Successful reintroduction of captopril after neutropenia. Lancet (1981) i, 723.

ACE inhibitors + Capsaicin

Abstract/Summary

An isolated report describes cough in a woman taking an ACE inhibitor each time she used a topical cream containing capsaicin.

Clinical evidence, mechanism, importance and management

A woman of 53 who had been maintained on an un-named ACE inhibitor for several years, complained of cough each time she applied *Axsain*, a cream containing 0.075% capsaicin, to her lower extremities.[1] It would appear that some of the absorbed capsaicin had a distant effect on the lungs. Pretreatment with an ACE inhibitor is know to enhance the cough caused by inhaled capsaicin. The general clinical importance of this reaction is not known.

Reference

1 Hakas JF. Topical capsaicin induces cough in patient receiving ACE inhibitor. Ann Allergy (1990) 65, 322–3.

ACE inhibitors + Diuretics

Abstract/Summary

Captopril combined with diuretics can be safe and effective but (a) a few patients may feel dizzy or lightheaded within an hour of taking the first dose, and acute hypotension can occur. (b) Hyperkalaemia is possible if potassium-sparing diuretics (e.g. amiloride, spironolactone, triamterene) and/or potassium supplements are used. (c) Hypokalaemia may occur if potassium-depleting diuretics (frusemide, ethacrynic acid, etc.) are used. (d) Severe renal deterioration and failure has been seen in patients with renal arterial stenosis.

Clinical evidence, mechanism, importance and management

(a) High doses, hypovolaemia, sodium depletion

Normally concurrent use is safe and effective but hypotensive symptoms such as dizziness and lightheadedness occasionally occur, particularly in those on high diuretic doses, within an hour or so of taking the first dose of captopril. For example, severe hypotension is very briefly described in a patient given captopril and *Moduretic* (amiloride + chlorothiazide).[17] Those most at risk appear to be patients with hypovolaemia and sodium depletion caused by the use of a diuretic. The effects should be closely monitored. A case of renal failure has been described in a patient with congestive heart failure when treated with captopril and metolazone.[7] Another patient with congestive heart failure developed non-oliguric renal failure while on enalapril and frusemide which resolved when the sodium balance was restored.[18]

(b) Potassium-sparing diuretics and/or potassium supplements

Five patients on potassium-sparing diuretics (not named) and/or potassium supplements showed a serum potassium level increase from 3.88 to 4.84 mmol/l when concurrently treated with captopril. Serum potassium levels climbed out of the normal clinical range in three of the patients, but no signs or symptoms of hyperkalaemia occurred.[6] Hyperkalaemia is said to have occurred in a patient given *Dyazide* (hydrochlorothiazide + triamterene) and captopril.[13] Increased serum potassium levels have been seen with captopril alone so it would seem that the effects are additive. Potassium-sparing diuretics such as amiloride, spironolactone or triamterene and/or potassium supplements should not be given with captopril unless the serum potassium levels can be closely monitored. It may be necessary to reduce the dosages or withdraw one of the drugs. However a comparative study has shown that enalapril added to frusemide and amiloride did not affect serum potassium levels, and no differences were seen when compared with patients taking frusemide and amiloride alone.[10]

(c) Potassium-depleting diuretics

Although ACE inhibitors can maintain body potassium, the concurrent use of potassium-depleting diuretics can result in hypokalaemia.[13,16] A patient developed hypokalaemia over a two-month period (a fall from 4.9 to 3.4 mmol/l) accompanied by acute pulmonary oedema, ventricular tachycardia and multifocal premature beats when given on captopril, frusemide, amiodarone and isosorbide dinitrate.[9] Another patient on captopril, frusemide, flecainide, digoxin and allopurinol also developed hypokalaemia (a fall from 4.2 to 3.1 mmol/l) and cardiac arrhythmias despite a potassium supplement.[9] Four other cases of hypokalaemia have been briefly reported elsewhere in elderly patients given captopril and frusemide.[13] The authors of this report[9] and another[16] advise regular monitoring of the serum potassium levels if patients are treated with ACE inhibitors and diuretics of this kind (i.e. frusemide, bumetanide, ethacrynic acid, etc.).

One study says that captopril does not affect the diuretic effects of frusemide,[11] however another found that during the first collecting period captopril reduced the diuretic response to 50% and the natriuretic response to nearly 30%, but neither enalapril nor ramipril significantly affect the diuretic effects of frusemide.[12] Another study also confirmed that the diuresis of frusemide was reduced by captopril.[14] No adverse effects on blood pressure and diuresis appear to occur if frusemide and benazepril are given together.[15]

(d) Renal arterial stenosis

Six studies describe renal deterioration or failure (rises in blood urea and serum creatinine levels) in patients with renal arterial stenosis given captopril or enalapril with frusemide, bendrofluazide, hydrochlorothiazide-amiloride, chlorthalidone or spironolactone.[1-5,8] In one study there was evidence that captopril caused no renal deterioration except when combined with the diuretic. Stopping or starting the diuretic initiated or reversed the deterioration. The reasons are not understood.[5] The outcome of using this drug combination should be very closely monitored in patients with renal arterial stenosis. Withdrawal of the diuretic and a reduction in the dosage of the captopril may be needed.

References

1 Curtis JJ, Luke RG, Whelchel JD, Dietheim AG, Jones P, Dunstan HP. Inhibition of angiotensin-converting enzyme in renal transplant recipients with hypertension. N Engl J Med (1983) 308, 377–81.

2 Silas JH, Klenza Z, Solomon SA, Bone MJ. Captopril induced reversible renal failure: a marker of renal stenosis affecting a solitary kidney. Br Med J (1983) 286, 1702–3.

3 Hricik DE, Browning PJ, Kopelman R, Goorno WE, Madia NE, Dzau VJ. Captopril-induced functional renal insufficiency in patients with bilateral renal artery stenosis. N Engl J Med (1983) 308, 373–6.

4 Watson ML, Bell GM, Muir AL, Buist TAS, Kellett RJ, Padfield PL. Captopril/diuretic combinations in severe renovascular disease: a cautionary note. Lancet (1983) ii, 404–5.

5 Hoefnagels WHL, Strijk SP, Thien T. Reversible renal failure following treatment with captopril and diuretics in patients with renovascular hypertension. Neth J Med (1984) 27, 269–74.

6 Burnakis TG, Mioduch HJ. Combined therapy with captopril and potassium supplementation. A potential for hyperkalaemia. Arch Intern Med (1984) 144, 2371–2.

7 Hogg KJ, Hillis WS. Captopril/metolazone induced renal failure. Lancet (1986) i, 501–2.

8 O'Donnell D. Renal failure due to enalapril and captopril in bilateral artery stenosis: greater awareness needed. Med J Aust (1988) 148, 525–7.

9 Begg EJ. Dosing regimens of captopril and enalapril in elderly patients and those with renal insufficiency. NZ Med J (1987) 100, 695.

10 Radley AS, Fitzpatrick RW. An evaluation of the potential interaction between enalapril and amiloride. J Clin Pharmacy Ther (1987) 12, 319–23.

11 Fujimura A, Shimokawa Y, Ebihara A. Influence of captopril on urinary excretion of furosemide in hypertensive subjects. J Clin Pharmacol (1990) 30, 538–42.

12 Toussaint C, Masselink A, Gentges A, Wambach G, Bönner G. Interference of different ACE-inhibitors with the diuretic action of furosemide and hydrochlorothiazide. Klin Wschschr (1989) 67, 1138–46.

13 Manchon ND, Bercoff E, Lemarchand P, Chassagne P, Senant J, Bourreille J. Fréquence et gravité des interactions médicamenteuses dan une population âgée: étude prospective concernant 63 malades. Rev Med Interne (1989) 10, 521–5.

14 Sommers De K, Meyer EC, Moncrieff J. Acute interaction of furosemide and captopril in healthy salt-replete man. SA Tydskr Wet (1991) 87, 375–7.

15 De Lepeleire I, Van Hecken A, Verbesselt R, Kaiser G, Barner A, Holmes I, De Schepper PJ. Interaction between furosemide and the converting enzyme inhibitor benazepril in healthy volunteers. Eur J clin Pharmacol (1988) 34, 465–8.

16 D'Costa DF, Basu SK, Gunasekera NPR. ACE inhibitors and diuretics causing hypokalaemia. BJCP (1990) 44, 26–7.

17 Beeley L, Stewart P. Bulletin of W Midlands Centre for Adverse Drug Reaction Reporting (1987) 25, 8.

18 Funck-Brentano C, Chatellier G, Alexandre J-M. Reversible renal failure after combined treatment with analapril and frusemide in a patient with congestive heart failure. Br Heart J (1986) 55, 596–8.

ACE inhibitors + Haemodialysis membranes

Abstract/Summary, clinical evidence, mechanism, importance and management

An anaphylactoid reaction (facial swelling, flushing, hypotension and dyspnoea) can occur in patients on ACE inhibitors within a few minutes of starting haemodialysis using high flux polyacrylonitrile membranes ('*AN69 Hospal*'). The reasons are not known.[1] Use an alternative membrane or an alternative hypotensive agent.

Reference

1 Anon. Anaphylactoid reactions to high-flux polyacrylonitrile membranes in combination with ACE inhibitors. CSM Current Problems Series (1992) 33, 2.

ACE inhibitors + Miscellaneous drugs

Abstract/Summary

No clinically important adverse interactions have been seen between captopril, enalapril, fosinopril, quinapril or pentopril and cimetidine; between cilazapril, quinapril and propranolol; between captopril and probenecid or procainamide; between lisinopril and nifedipine, or between ramipril and felodipine.

Clinical evidence, mechanism, importance and management

Cimetidine in normal subjects does not appear to alter the pharmacokinetics or pharmacological effects of captopril[1] or enalapril,[11] nor the pharmacokinetics of quinapril[4] or fosinopril.[10] Cimetidine can reduce the clearance of pentopril by 11–14% and pentopril can reduce the clearance of cimetidine by 21%,[5] but it seems doubtful if either of these two effects is clinically important. The pharmacokinetics of captopril and procainamide are unaffected by concurrent use.[2] Steady-state levels of captopril are only slightly increased by the use of probenecid but no interaction of clinical importance seems to occur.[3] No evidence of either a pharmacokinetic or pharmacodynamic interaction was seen in 12 normal subjects given single doses of nifedipine (20 mg) and lisinopril (20 mg).[6] No pharmacokinetic interaction was found to occur between ramipril and felodipine, but some increased hypotensive effects were seen.[13] 80 mg propranolol three times daily was found not to affect the pharmacokinetics of a single 20 mg dose of quinapril in 10 normal subjects.[7,8] No adverse interaction occurs between cilazapril and propranolol but the reductions in blood pressure are more pronounced and long-lasting.[9,12]

References

1 Richer C, Bah M, Cadilhalez C, Giudicelli JF. Cimetidine does not alter free unchanged captopril pharmacokinetics and biological effects in healthy volunteers. J Pharmacol (Paris) (1986) 17, 338–42.
2 Sugerman AA, McKown J. Lack of kinetic interaction of captopril (CP) and procainamide (PA) in healthy subjects. J Clin Pharmacol (1985) 25, 455–74.
3 Singhvi SM, Duchin KL, Willard DA, McKinstry DN, Migdalof BH. Renal handling of captopril: effect of probenecid. Clin Pharmacol Ther (1982) 32, 182–9.
4 Ferry JJ, Cetnarowski AB, Sedman AJ, Thomas RW, Horvath AM. Multiple-dose cimetidine administration does not influence the single-dose pharmacokinetics of quinapril and its active metabolite (CI-928). J Clin Pharmacol (1988) 28, 48–51.
5 Kochak GM, Rakhit A, Thompson TN, Hurley ME. Pentopril–cimetidine interaction caused by a reduction in hepatic blood flow. J Clin Pharmacol (1988) 28, 222–7.
6 Lees KR, Reid JL. Lisinopril and nifedipine: no acute interaction in normotensives. Br J clin Pharmac (1988) 25, 307–13.

7 Horvath AM, Blake DS, Ferry JJ, Colburn WA. Propranolol does not influence quinapril pharmacokinetics in healthy volunteers. J Clin Pharmacol (1987) 27, 719.
8 Horvath AM, Pilon D, Caille G, Colburn WA, Ferry JJ, Frank GJ, Lacasse Y, Olson SC. Multiple dose propranolol does not influence the single dose pharmacokinetics of quinapril and its active metabolite (quinaprilat). Biopharm Drug Disp (1990) 11, 191–6.
9 Belz GG, Essig J, Kleinbloesem CH, Hoogkamer JFW, Wiegand UW, Wellstein A. Interactions between cilazapril and propranolol in man; plasma drug concentrations, hormone and enzyme responses, haemodynamics, agonist dose-effect curves and baroreceptor reflex. Br J clin Pharmac (1988) 26, 547–56.
10 Moore L, Kramer A, Swites B, Kramer P, Tu J. Effect of cimetidine and antacid on the kinetics of the active diacid of fosinopril in healthy subjects. J Clin Pharmacol (1988) 28, 946–59.
11 Ishizaki T, Baba T, Murabayashi S, Kubota K, Hara K, Kuromoto F. Effect of cimetidine on the pharmacokinetics and pharmacodynamics of enalapril in normal volunteers. J Cardiovasc Pharmacol (1988) 12, 512–9.
12 Belz GG, Essig J, Erb K, Breithaupt K, Hoogkamer JFW, Kneer J, Kleinbloesem CH. Pharmacokinetic and pharmacodynamic interactions between the ACE inhibitor cilazapril and beta-adrenceptor antagonist propranolol in healthy subjects and in hypertensive patients. Br J clin Pharmac (1989) 27, 317–22S.
13 Bainbridge AD et al. A study of the acute pharmacodynamic interaction of ramipril and felodipine in normotensive subjects. Br J clin Pharmac (1991) 31, 148.

ACE inhibitors + Non-steroidal anti-inflammatory drugs (NSAIDs)

Abstract/Summary

The antihypertensive effects of captopril can be reduced or abolished by indomethacin, ibuprofen and aspirin, whereas sulindac only has a very small effect. Indomethacin modestly reduces the antihypertensive effects of perindopril, and interacts to some extent with lisinopril and possibly enalapril. Lornoxicam (chlortenoxicam) causes a small rise in diastolic pressures in those on enalapril.

Clinical evidence

(a) Captopril + Aspirin

Eight patients with essential hypertension showed a 20 mmHg fall in diastolic blood pressure when given single 25–100 mg doses of captopril. The diastolic blood pressures of four of them rose by an average of 7 mmHg when additionally given 600 mg aspirin six-hourly for 24 h.[1] The same interaction has been mentioned in another report.[4]

(b) Captopril + Indomethacin or Ibuprofen

Five patients with essential hypertension demonstrated a fall in blood pressure from 178/116 to 132/92 mmHg when given 100–200 mg captopril twice daily. The addition of 50 mg indomethacin twice daily caused a blood pressure rise to 144/103 mmHg.[2] This same interaction has been described in patients with hypertension and in normal subjects given indomethacin in doses ranging from 50 to 250 mg.[3–8,14,16,18,21] One of these studies found that 50 mg captopril lowered the mean blood pressure of eight normal subjects when lying from 85 to 74 mmHg. The addition of either 50 mg indomethacin or 800 mg ibuprofen caused the blood pressure to rise to 84 mmHg.[7] A case report describes abolition of the hypertensive effects of captopril by ibuprofen in an elderly man.[20]

(c) Captopril + Sulindac

In the study detailed above[2] it was also found that 200 mg sulindac twice daily given to patients taking captopril caused only a small rise in blood pressure: from 132/92 to 137/95 mmHg.[2]

(d) Enalapril + Indomethacin, Lornoxicam, Sulindac

Indomethacin (100 mg daily) caused a small rise in blood pressure (from 134/89 to 143/93 mmHg) in 29 hypertensives taking 40 mg enalapril daily, whereas sulindac (400 mg daily) had little or no effect.[9] Another study found a rise from 155/91 to 179/100 mmHg in patients on enalapril 1 h after being given 50 mg indomethacin.[17] A further study found SBP/DBP rises of 11/6–12/7 mmHg due to 100 mg indomethacin daily in those on 5–20 mg enalapril daily.[22] However other studies found no significant interaction between indomethacin and enalapril.[10,13,14] 8 mg Lornoxicam was found to have no effect on the systolic blood pressures of hypertensive patients on enalapril, but a small rise in diastolic pressures (from 88.2 to 93.3 mmHg) occurred after 2 h.[17]

(e) Lisinopril + Indomethacin

Indomethacin was found to have little effect on the hypotensive effects of lisinopril in one study[11] whereas another found a SBP/DBP rises of 15/10–18/7 mmHg.[22]

(f) Pentopril + Indomethacin

No change in the disposition of pentopril occurs if indomethacin is used, but the effects on blood pressure do not seem to have been assessed.[12]

(g) Perindopril + Indomethacin

The antihypertensive effects of perindopril (4–8 mg daily) were found to be reduced 30% by 100 mg indomethacin daily.[19]

Mechanism

The antihypertensive effects of some ACE inhibitors can be interfered with by drugs which block prostaglandin synthesis. One study found that captopril and ibuprofen had opposing effects on sodium and water handling by the kidney.[15]

Importance and management

The captopril-indomethacin interaction is well established. The incidence is reported to be high (nine out of 10 in one study[1]). Not enough is known about the captopril-ibuprofen interaction for its incidence to be known, whereas half of the patients showed an effect with aspirin.[1] Occasional doses of aspirin or ibuprofen probably do not matter, but if aspirin, ibuprofen or indomethacin are used regularly the blood pressure should be monitored. Raise the captopril dosage if necessary. It seems possible that this interaction may occur with some other NSAIDs but information so far is lacking. Sulindac appears not to interact significantly.

Information about enalapril with indomethacin is inconsistent so that the effects should be monitored. Lornoxicam has a small effect and the effects on lisinopril of indomethacin should be monitored. Information about pentopril is very limited but the effects of indomethacin on perindopril should also be monitored.

References

1 Moore TJ, Crantz FR, Hollenberg NK, Koletsky RJ, Leboff MS, Swartz SL, Levine L, Podolsky S, Dluhy RG, Williams GH. Contribution of prostaglandins to the antihypertensive action of captopril in essential hypertension. Hypertension (1981) 3, 168–73.

2 Salvetti A, Pedrinelli R, Magagna A, Ugenti P. Differential effects of selective and non-selective prostaglandin-synthesis inhibition on the pharmacological responses to captopril in patients with essential hypertension. Clin Sci (1982) 63, 261S–263S.

3 Silberbauer K, Stanek B, Templ H. Acute hypotensive effect of captopril in man modified by prostaglandin synthesis inhibition. Br J Clin Pharmacol (1982) 14, 87–93S.

4 Swartz SL and Williams GH. Angiotensin-converting enzyme inhibition and prostaglandins. Am J Cardiol (1982) 49, 1405–9.

5 Witzgall H, Hirsch F, Schere B, Weber PC. Acute haemodynamic and hormonal effects of captopril are diminished by indomethacin. Clin Sci (1982) 62, 611–5.

6 Dzau VJ, Packer M, Lilly LS, Swartz SL, Hollenberg NK, Williams GH. Prostaglandins in severe congestive heart failure. Relation to activation of the renin-angiotensin system and hyponatremia. N Engl J Med (1984) 310, 347–52.

7 Goldstone R, Martin K, Zipser R, Horton R. Evidence for a dual action of converting enzyme inhibitor on blood pressure in normal man. Prostaglandins (1981) 22, 587–98.

8 Ogihara T, Maruyama A, Hata T, Mikami H, Nakamaru M, Naka T, Ohde H, Kumahara Y. Hormonal responses to long term converting enzyme inhibition in hypertensive patients. Clin Pharmacol Ther (1981) 30, 328–35.

9 Oparil S, Horton R, Wilkins LH, Irvin J, Hammett DK, Dustan HP. Antihypertensive effect of enalapril (MK-421) in low renin essential hypertension: role of vasodilatory prostaglandins. Clin Res (1983) 31, 538A.

10 Oparil S, Horton R, Wilkins LH, Irvin J, Hammett DK. Antihypertensive effect of enalapril in essential hypertension: role of prostacyclin. Am J Med Sci (1987) 294, 395–402.

11 Shae W, Shapiro D, Antonello J, Cressman M, Vlasses P, Oparil S. Indomethacin does not blunt the antihypertensive effect of lisinopril. Clin Pharmacol Ther (1987) 41, 219.

12 Lin S, Rahkit A, Redalieu E, Hurley M, Garg D, Weidler D. Effect of indomethacin on the disposition of pentopril in man. J Clin Pharmacol (1986) 26, 546.

13 Salvetti A, Abdel-Haq B, Magagna A, Pedrinelli R. Indomethacin reduces the antihypertensive action of enalapril. Clin and Exp Theory and Practice (1987) A9 (2 and 3) 559–67.

14 Koopmans PP, Van Megen T, Thien T, Gribnau FWJ. The interaction

between indomethacin and captopril or enalapril in healthy volunteers. J Intern Med (1989) 226, 139–42.

15 Allon M, Pasque CB, Rodriguez M. Interaction of captopril and ibuprofen on glomerular and tubular function in humans. Am J Physiol (1990) 259, F233–8.

16 Fujita T, Yamashita N, Yamashita K. Effect of indomethacin on antihypertensive actions of captopril in hypertensive patients. Clin Exptl Hypertension (1981) 3, 939–52.

17 Waldern RJ, Owens CWI, Graham BR, Snape A, Nutt J, Prichard BNC. NSAIDs and the control of hypertension: pilot study. Br J clin Pharmacol (1991) 33, 241P.

18 Iniesta AR, de Léon N, Serna JCM. Bloqueo de la acción antihipertensiva del captoprilo por indometacina. Medicina Clinica (1991) 11, 438.

19 Abdel-Haq B, Magagna A, Favilla S, Salvetti A. Hemodynamic and humoral interaction between perindopril and indomethacin in essential hypertensive patients. J Cardiovasc Pharmacol (1991) 18 (Suppl 7) S33–6.

20 Espino DV, Lancaster MC. Neutralization of the effects of captopril by the use of ibuprofen in an elderly man. J Am Board Fam Pract (1992) 5, 319–21.

21 Sanchez FM, Martinez JCA, Nieto MJA. Interacción entre captorpil e indometacina. An Med Intern (Madrid) (1992) 9, 74.

22 Duffin D, Leahey W, Brennan G, Johnston GD. The effects of indomethacin on the antihypertensive responses to enalapril and lisinopril. Br J clin Pharmac (1992) 34, 456P.

ACE inhibitors + Other antihypertensives

Abstract/Summary, clinical evidence, mechanism, importance and management

There is some evidence that the effects of captopril may be delayed when patients are switched from clonidine.[1] The hypotensive effects of captopril and either minoxidil or sodium nitroprusside appear to be additive and it may be necessary to reduce the dosages to avoid excessive hypotension.[2,3]

References

1 Grone H-J, Kirchertz EJ, Rieger J. Mogliche Komplikationenen und Probleme der Captopriltherapie bei Hypertonikern mit ausgepraten Gefasschaden. Therapiewoche (1981) 31, 5280–7.

2 Jennings GL, Gelman JS, Stockigt JR, Korner PI. Accentuated hypotensive effect of sodium nitroprusside in man after captopril. Clin Sci (1981) 61, 521–6.

3 Traub YM, Levey BA. Combined treatment with minoxidil and captopril in refractory hypertension. Arch Intern Med (1983) 143, 1142–4.

ACE-inhibitors + Pergolide

Abstract/Summary

An isolated report describes severe hypotension in a patient on lisinopril when given pergolide.

Clinical evidence, mechanism, importance and management

A man successfully treated for hypertension with 10 mg lisinopril four times daily experienced a severe hypotensive reaction within four hours of taking a single 0.05 mg dose of pergolide for periodic leg movements during sleep. He needed hospitalization and treatment with intravenous fluids. It is not clear whether this patient was extremely sensitive to the pergolide or whether what occurred was due to an interaction, but it would now seem prudent to monitor the concurrent of pergolide and ACE inhibitors, or other antihypertensives. The authors of this report suggest that the initial dose of pergolide should be 0.025 mg.[1]

Reference

1 Kando JC, Keck PE, Wood PA. Pergolide-induced hypotension. DICP Ann Pharmacotherapy (1990) 24, 543.

ACE Inhibitors + Rifampicin

Abstract/Summary

Two reports describe a rise in blood pressure in a two hypertensive patients attributed to an interaction between enalapril and rifampicin.

Clinical evidence, mechanism, importance and management

A man with a prosthetic aortic valve and essential hypertension was treated with warfarin, enalapril, acebutolol, bendrofluazide, dipyridamole, metoclopramide and *Gaviscon*. When he became pyrexic (38°) because of a probable *Brucella abortus* infection, he was additionally started on streptomycin, oxytetracycline and rifampicin, whereupon his blood pressure rose over the next 5–6 days from 164/104 to 180/115 mmHg. It was suspected that an interaction with the rifampicin was possibly responsible. Subsequent studies showed that after stopping and then restarting the rifampicin, the AUC_{0-7} (area under the concentration-time curve over 7 h) of enalaprilat, the active metabolite of the enalapril, was reduced by 31%. The mechanism of this interaction is not clear because the rifampicin is a potent liver enzyme inducing agent which might have been expected to cause the production of more, rather than less, enalaprilat from enalapril, however the authors postulate that the rifampicin might have increased the loss of the enalaprilat in the urine.[1] There is also the hint of this interaction in another report.[2]

The general importance of this interaction is uncertain, but it would now seem prudent to monitor the effects of concurrent use. There seems to be nothing reported about any of the other ACE inhibitors.

Reference

1 Kandiah D, Penny W J, Fraser A G, Lewis M J. A possible drug interaction between rifampicin and enalapril. Eur J Clin Pharmacol (1988) 35, 431–2.

2 Tada Y, Tsuda Y, Otsuka T, Nagasawa K, Kimura H, Kusaba T, Sakata T. Case report: nifedipine-rifampicin interaction attenuates the effect on blood pressure in a patient with essential hypertension. Am J Med Sci (1992) 303, 25–7.

ACE inhibitors + Stable plasma protein solution (SPPS)

Abstract/Summary

Acute hypotension has been seen in patients taking enalapril when rapidly infused with a stable plasma protein solution.

Clinical evidence

A patient on enalapril (10 mg in the morning) underwent surgery for groin lymph node resection under spinal and general anaesthesia. When rapidly infused with 500 ml stable plasma protein solution (SPPS), the pulse rose to 90–100 bpm and systolic blood pressure fell from 100 to 60 mmHg and a red flush was noted on all exposed skin. The blood pressure was controlled with metaraminol (4.5 mg over 10 min) at 90–95 mmHg. When the SPPS was finished, the blood pressure and pulse rate spontaneously restabilized.[1]

Two very similar cases involving patients on enalapril when given SPPS have been recorded.[2,3]

Mechanism

Not fully established, but it is believed that SPPS contains low levels of pre-kallikrein activator which stimulates the production of bradykinin and other kinases which can cause vasodilatation and hypotension. Normally they are destroyed by kininase II (ACE), but with the ACE inhibited by the enalapril, their inactivation appear to be delayed so that their hypotensive effects are exaggerated and prolonged.[4]

Importance and management

An established interaction of clinical importance. The authors of one report suggest that if rapid expansion of intravascular volume is needed in patients taking ACE inhibitors, an artificial colloid might be a safer choice than SPPS.[1] There appear to be no reports about other ACE inhibitors but they would be expected to interact similarly.

Reference

1 McKenzie AJ. Possible interaction between SPPS and enalapril. Anaesth Intens Care (1990) 18, 127–31.
2 Young K. Enalapril and SPPS. Anesth Intens Care (1990) 18, 583.
3 Young K. Hypotension from the interaction of ACE inhibitors with stable plasma protein solution. Anaesth (1993) 48, 356.
4 Bonner G, Preis S, Schunk U, Toussaint C, Kaufman W. Haemodynamic effects of bradykinin on systemic and pulmonary circulation in healthy and hypertensive patients. J Cardiovasc Pharmacol (1990) 15, S46–56.

Acetazolamide + Beta-blockers

Abstract/Summary

The concurrent use of acetazolamide and timolol eye-drops resulted in severe mixed acidosis in a patient with chronic obstructive lung disease.

Clinical evidence, mechanism, importance and management

An elderly man with severe chronic obstructive lung disease was given 750 mg acetazolamide daily orally and 0.5% timolol maleate eye-drops, one drop in each eye twice daily, as operative premedication to reduce ocular hypertension before surgery for glaucoma. Five days later a progressive worsening of dyspnoea was seen and he was found to have a severe mixed acidosis.[1] The reason seems to have been the additive effects of acetazolamide which blocked the excretion of hydrogen ions in the kidney, and the bronchoconstrictor effects of the timolol which was sufficiently absorbed systemically to exacerbate the airway obstruction in this patient and thereby reduced the respiration. This isolated case emphasizes the potential risks of using beta-blockers in patients with obstructive lung disease and of concurrent use with acetazolamide even if kidney function is normal.

Reference

1 Boada JE, Estopa R, Izquierdo J, Dorca J, Manresa F. Severe mixed acidosis by combined therapy with acetazolamide and timolol eye drops. Eur J Resp Dis (1986) 68, 226–8.

Alpha blockers + Calcium channel blockers

Abstract/Summary

The blood pressure may fall sharply if calcium channel blockers are given to patients already taking prazosin. Only administer together if the response can be closely monitored. No such adverse effect seems to occur with doxazosin and nifedipine.

Clinical evidence

(a) Doxazosin + Nifedipine

No serious adverse events or postural symptoms were seen in 12 normal subjects given 20 mg nifedipine twice daily for 10 days, to which was added 2 mg doxazosin once daily for 10 days. No pharmacokinetic interactions were found. There was a tendency for the hypotensive effects to be greater than with either drug alone.[4]

(b) Prazosin + Nifedipine

Two patients with severe hypertension given prazosin (2–5 mg) experienced a sharp fall in blood pressure shortly after being given nifedipine sublingually. One of them had a fall in standing blood pressure from 200/120 to 88/48 mmHg about 20 min after being given a total of 15 mg nifedipine. He complained of dizziness. Eight other patients with hypertension given prazosin showed falls in blood pressure 20 min after nifedipine from 198/108 to 173/96 mmHg when lying and from 192/114 to 168/97 mmHg when standing.[1]

(c) Prazosin + Verapamil

A study in eight normal subjects given single 1 mg doses of prazosin showed that the average serum prazosin levels were raised 86% (from 5.2 to 9.6 ng/ml) when given with 160 mg verapamil, and the prazosin AUC (area under the curve) increased by 62%. The standing blood pressure fell from 114/82 to 99/81 mmHg after the prazosin and after both drugs to 89/60 mmHg at 4 h.[2]

Mechanism

It would seem to be that the vasodilatory effects of prazosin and the calcium channel blockers can be additive. The increase in serum prazosin levels resulting from the interaction with verapamil is possibly because the metabolism of the prazosin by the liver is reduced.[3]

Importance and management

The prazosin/nifedipine and prazosin/verapamil interactions would appear to be established and of clinical importance although the documentation is limited. Marked additive hypotensive effects can occur. It has been suggested that concurrent use should only be undertaken if the effects can be closely monitored.[1] When nifedipine is added to prazosin treatment, a 5 mg test dose of nifedipine should be given with the patient lying down. If the patient is already taking nifedipine, a test dose of 0.5 mg prazosin should be given.[1] The same precautions would also seem applicable with verapamil or any other calcium channel blocker. No adverse effects of this kind were seen in the trial with doxazosin and nifedipine.

References

1 Jee LD and Opie LH. Acute hypotensive response to nifedipine added to prazosin in treatment of hypertension. Br Med J (1983) 287, 1514.
2 Pasanisi F, Meredith PA, Elliott HL and Reid JL. Verapamil and prazosin: pharmacodynamic and pharmacokinetic interactions in normal man. Br J clin Pharmac (1984) 18, 290P.
3 Meredith PA, Elliott HL, Pasanisi F, Reid JL. Prazosin and verapamil: a pharmacokinetic and pharmacodynamic interaction. Br J clin Pharmac (1986) 21, 85P.
4 Donnelly R, Elliott HL, Meredith PA, Howie CA, Reid JL. The pharmacodynamics and pharmacokinetics of the combination of nifedipine and doxazosin. Eur J Clin Pharmacol (1993) 44, 279–82.

Amiloride + Cimetidine

Abstract/Summary

Cimetidine does not alter serum amiloride levels or its diuretic effects but amiloride can cause some reduction in the cimetidine levels.

Clinical evidence, mechanism, importance and management

A study in eight normal subjects given 5 mg amiloride daily found that the concurrent use of 400 mg cimetidine twice daily for 12 days reduced the renal clearance of amiloride by 17% (from 358 to 299 ml/min) and the urinary excretion of amiloride from 65 to 53% of the administered dose. The amiloride also reduced the excretion of the cimetidine from 43 to 32% of the dose and the AUC was reduced by 14%.[1] No changes in the diuretic effects (urinary volume, Na^+ or K^+ excretion) occurred. It seems that each drug reduces the gastrointestinal absorption of the other drug by as yet unidentified mechanisms. The overall serum levels of the amiloride remain unchanged because the reduced absorption is offset by a reduction in its renal excretion.

These mutual interactions seem to be clinically unimportant but confirmation from studies in patients is needed.

Reference

1 Somogyi AA, Hovens CM, Muirhead MR, Bochner F. Renal tubular secretion of amiloride and its inhibition by cimetidine in humans and in an animal model. Drug Metab Disp (1989) 17, 190–6.

Antihypertensives + Alcohol

Abstract/Summary

Chronic moderate to heavy drinking raises the blood pressure and reduces to some extent the effectiveness of antihypertensive drugs. A few patients may experience postural hypotension, dizziness and fainting shortly after having a drink.

Clinical evidence, mechanisms, importance and management

(a) Hypertensive reaction

A study in 44 men with essential hypertension, treated with diuretics, beta-blockers, verapamil, prazosin, captopril or methyldopa and who were moderate to heavy drinkers, showed that when they reduced their drinking over a 6-week period from an average of 450 ml ethanol weekly (about six drinks daily) to 64 ml ethanol weekly, their average blood pressure fell by 5.0/3.0 mmHg.[1] The reasons are uncertain. These findings are consistent with those of other studies.[2,3] It seems likely that this effect will occur with any antihypertensive. Patients with hypertension should be encouraged to reduce their intake of alcohol. It may then become possible to reduce the dosage of the antihypertensive.

(b) Hypotensive reaction

A few patients taking some antihypertensives feel dizzy, begin to 'black out' or faint if they stand up quickly or after exercise. This orthostatic and exertional hypotension may be exaggerated in some patients shortly after drinking alcohol because it causes vasodilatation and can lower the output of the heart (noted in patients with various types of heart disease[4,5,6]). Patients just beginning hypertensive treatment should be warned.

References

1 Puddey IB, Beilin LJ and Vandongen R. Regular alcohol use raises blood pressure in treated hypertensive subjects. A randomized controlled trial. Lancet (1987) i, 647–51.
2 Potter JF, Beevers DG. Pressor effect of alcohol in hypertension. Lancet (1984) i, 119–22.
3 Puddey IB, Beilin LJ, Vandongen R, Rouse IL and Rogers P. Evidence for a direct effect of alcohol on blood pressure in normotensive men - a randomized controlled trial. Hypertension (1985) 7, 707–13.
4 Gould L, Zahir M, DeMartino A, Gomerbrecht RF. Cardiac effects of a cocktail. J Amer Med Ass (1971) 218, 1799.
5 Conway N. Haemodynamic effects of ethyl alcohol in patients with coronary heart disease. Brit Heart J (1968) 30, 638.
6 Noble EP, Parker E, Alkana R, Cohen H, Birch H. Propranolol-ethanol interaction in man. Fed Proc (1973) 32, 724.

Antihypertensives + Bupropion, Mianserin or Maprotiline

Abstract/Summary, clinical evidence, mechanism, importance and management

Mianserin does not affect the control of blood pressure with propranolol, hydralazine, clonidine, guanethidine, bethanidine[1,2,3,6] or methyldopa.[4,6] Bupropion and maprotiline do not reduce the antihypertensive effects of clonidine.[5,7]

References

1 Burgess CD, Turner P, Wadsworth J. Cardiovascular responses to mianserin hydrochloride: a comparison with tricyclic antidepressant drugs. Br J clin Pharmac (1978) 5, 215.
2 Coppen A, Ghose K, Swade C, Wood K. Effect of mianserin hydrochloride on peripheral uptake mechanisms for noradrenaline and 5-hydroxytryptamine in man. Br J clin Pharmac (1978) 5, 135.
3 Elliott HL, Mc Lean K, Reid JL and Sumner DJ. Pharmacodynamic studies on mianserin and its interaction with clonidine. Br J clin Pharmac (1981) 11, 122P.
4 Elliott HL, Whiting B, Reid JL. Assessment of the interaction between mianserin and centrally-acting antihypertensive drugs. Br J clin Pharmac (1983) 15, 323–8S.
5 Gundert-Remy U, Amann E, Hildbrandt R, Weber E. Lack of interaction between the tetracyclic antidepressant maprotiline and the centrally

acting antihypertensive drug clonidine. Eur J Clin Pharmacol (1983) 25, 595–9.

6 Elliot HL, McLean K, Sumner DJ, Reid JL. Absence of effect of mianserin on the actions of clonidine or methyldopa in hypertensive patients. Eur J Clin Pharmacol (1983) 24, 15–19.
7 Cubeddu LX, Cloutier G, Gross K, Grippo PA-CR, Tanner L, Lerea L, Shakarjian M, Knowlton G, Harden TK, Arendshorst W, Rogers JF. Bupropion does not antagonize cardiovascular actions of clonidine in normal subjects and spontaneously hypertensive rats. Clin Pharmacol Ther (1984) 35, 576–84.

Antihypertensives + Fenfluramine

Abstract/Summary

Fenfluramine can cause a small but clinically unimportant increase in the blood pressure lowering effects of antihypertensive agents.

Clinical evidence, mechanism, importance and management

Fenfluramine has some hypotensive activity, but in a number of trials with considerable numbers of obese hypertensive patients given 60 mg fenfluramine daily, the changes in blood pressure in those taking beta-blockers, bethanidine, debrisoquine, guanethidine, methyldopa, reserpine or diuretics were small and, in the context of adverse interactions, of little or no clinical importance.[1-3]

References

1 Waal-Manning J, Simpson FO. Fenfluramine in obese patients on various antihypertensive drugs. Double-blind controlled trial. Lancet (1969) ii, 1392.
2 Simpson FO, Waal-Manning J. Use of fenfluramine in obese patients on antihypertensive therapy. S Afr Med J (1971) 45 (Suppl), 47.
3 General Practitioner Clinical Trials. Hypotensive effect of fenfluramine in the treatment of obesity. Practitioner (1971) 207, 101.

Antihypertensives + Food

Abstract/Summary

The ingestion of food has little or no effect on the absorption of spironolactone, captopril, cilazapril, enalapril, pentopril or possibly perinodopril but it reduces the bioavailability of hydralazine. Hypertension has been seen in negroes after eating large amounts of pork.

Clinical evidence, mechanism, importance and management

Some early studies suggested that food reduced the bioavailability of captopril and delayed its antihypertensive effects,[1,2] but long-term work has shown that the absorption and bioavailability are not significantly changed.[5,6] Other studies show that food has little or no effect on either enalapril,[3] cilazapril[12] or pentopril,[4] but the situation with perindopril is not clear.[10,11] A single dose study suggested that food reduces the bioavailability of perindopril.[11] A study in subjects given 100 mg spironolactone showed that food did not affect steady-state levels, blood pressure or heart rate. This supports the recommendation that it should be taken with breakfast to avoid gastric irritation.[7] Food can markedly reduce the bioavailability and peak serum levels of hydralazine.[13,14] Studies in negroes in southern USA have shown that those who eat extremely large amounts of pork can experience unpleasant symptoms including dizziness, nausea, vomiting, headache, diarrhoea, blurred vision, fainting, scotoma, lacrimation and general malaise.[8] Two members of one family experienced very marked hypertension and one of them died after eating a considerable amount of pork.[9] Salt pork possibly represents an additional problem. This is not, strictly speaking, an interaction, but rather an undesirable reaction in those under treatment for hypertension or cardiac failure. Whether it is confined to negroes is uncertain. More study is needed.

References

1 Mantyla R, Mannisto PT, Vuorela A, Sundberg S, Ottoila P. Impairment of captopril bioavailability by concomitant food and antacid intake. Int J Clin Pharmacol Ther Toxicol (1984) 22, 626–9

2 Singhvi SM, McKinstry DN, Shaw JM, Willard DA, Migdalof BH. Effect of food on the bioavailability of captopril in healthy subjects. J Clin Pharmacol (1982) 22, 135–40.

3 Swanson BN, Vlasses PH, Ferguson RK, Bergquist PA, Till AE, Irvin JD, Harris K. Influence of food on the bioavailability of enalapril. J Pharm Sci (1984) 73, 1655–7.

4 Rahkhit A, Hurley ME, Redalieu E, Kochak G, Tipnis V, Coleman J, Rommel A. Effect of food on the bioavailability of pentopril, an angiotensin-converting enzyme inhibitor, in healthy subjects. J Clin Pharmacol (1985) 25, 424–8.

5 Ohman KP, Kagedal B, Larsson R, Karlberg BE. Pharmacokinetics of captopril and its effect on blood pressure during acute and chronic administration and in relation to food intake. J Cardiovasc Pharmacol (1985) 7, S20–4.

6 Salvetti A, Pedrinelli R, Magagna A, Abdel-Haq B, Graziadei L. Influence of food on acute and chronic effects of capropril in essential hypertensive patients. J Cardiovasc Pharmacol (1985) 7, S25–9.

7 Thulin T, Wahlin-Boll E, Liedholm H, Lindholm L and Melander A. Influence of food intake on antihypertensive drugs: spironolactone. Drug-Nutrient Interactions (1983) 2, 169–73.

8 Burch GE, Phillips JH, Wood W. The high-pork diet of the Negro of the Southern United States (Editorial). Arch Intern Med (1957) 100, 859.

9 Burch GE. Pork and hypertension. Am Heart J (1973) 86, 713.

10 Funck-Brentano C, Lecocq B, Jaillon P, Devissaguet M. Effects of food on the pharmacokinetics and ACE-inhibition of perindopril in healthy volunteers. Excerpta Medica Int Congr Series (1989) 839, 277–80.

11 Lecocq B, Funck-Brentano C, Lecocq V, Ferry A, Gardin M-E, Devissaguet M, Jaillon P. Influence of food on the pharmacokinetics of perindopril and the time course of angiotensin-converting enzyme inhbition in serum. Clin Pharmacol Ther (1990) 47, 397–402.

12 Massarella JW, DeFeo TM, Brown AN, Lin A, Wills RJ. The influence of food on the pharmacokinetics and ACE inhibition of cilazpril. Br J clin Pharmac (1989) 27, 205–9S.

13 Jackson SHD, Shepherd AMM, Ludden TM, Jamieson MJ, Woodworth J, Rogers D, Ludden LK, Muir KT. Effect of food on oral bioavailability of apresoline and controlled release hydralazine in hypertensive patients. J Cardiovasc Pharmacol (1990) 16, 624–8.

14 Semple HA, Koo W, TAm YK, Ngo LY, Coutts RT. Interactions between hydralazine and oral nutrients in humans. Ther Drug Monit (1991) 13, 304–8.

Antihypertensives + Phenothiazines

Abstract/Summary

The hypotensive side-effects of the phenothiazines may increase the effects of some antihypertensive agents and patients may feel faint if they stand up quickly. Guanethidine-like drugs are the probable exception because their effects are opposed by the phenothiazines. An isolated report describes hypertension in a patient given methyldopa and trifluoperazine.

Clinical evidence, mechanism, importance and management

Some of the phenothiazines such as chlorpromazine cause postural hypotension so that patients feel faint and dizzy if they stand up quickly. It is particularly marked with methotrimeprazine. This reaction may be exaggerated in the presence of an antihypertensive agent and may prove to be problematical. For example, a patient experienced dizziness and hypotension (systolic pressure of 70 mmHg) a little over an hour after being given 100 mg chlorpromazine, 0.1 mg clonidine and 40 mg frusemide.[2] Another patient experienced fainting and marked orthostatic hypotension (blood pressure 66/48 mmHg) when given 6.25 mg captopril twice daily and 200 mg chlorpromazine three times daily. He had had no problems while taking chlorpromazine, nadolol, prazosin and hydrochlorothiazide.[4] A patient on chlorpromazine and given nifedipine showed marked hypotension during surgery which was controlled with noradrenaline.[5] There is also an isolated and unexplained case on record of a psychotic patient on fluphenazine decanoate who began to demonstrate delerium, agitation disorientation, short-term memory loss, confusion and clouded consciousness within 10 days of starting to take 0.2 mg clonidine daily. These symptoms disappeared when the clonidine was stopped and returned when the clonidine was re-started.[3] An isolated report describes a paradoxical rise in blood pressure in a patient with systemic lupus erythematosus and renal disease when treated with methyldopa and trifluoperazine. The suggested explanation is that the phenothiazine blocked the uptake of the 'false transmitter' (alpha-methyl noradrenaline) produced during therapy with methyldopa.[1]

These reports emphasise the need to monitor the reaction of patients on antihypertensives, particularly during the first period of treatment with chlorpromazine or other phenothiazines. Dosage adjustment may be necessary. Guanethidine-like drugs behave differently because their antihypertensive actions can be opposed to some extent by the phenothiazines (see 'Guanethidine and related drugs + Phenothiazines').

References

1 Westhervelt FB, Atuk NO. Methyldopa-induced hypertension. J Amer Med Ass (1974) 227, 557.

2 Fruncillo RJ, Gibbons WJ, Vlasses PH, Ferguson RK. Severe hypotension associated with concurrent clonidine and antipsychotic medication. Am J Psychiatry (1985) 142, 274.

3 Allen RM, Flemenbaum A. Delirium associated with combined sulphenazine-clonidine therapy. J Clin Psychiatry (1979) 236, 55.

4 White WB. Hypotension with postural syncope secondary to the combination of chlorpromazine and captopril. Arch Intern Med (1986) 146, 1833–4.

5 Stuart-Taylor ME, Crosse MM. A plea for noradrenaline. Anaesthesia (1989) 44, 916–7.

Antihypertensives + Phenylpropanolamine

Abstract/Summary

A sustained-release preparation of phenylpropanolamine and brompheniramine was found to cause a minor and clinically insignificant rise in the blood pressures of patients with drug-controlled hypertension.

Clinical evidence, mechanism, importance and management

A randomized double-blind crossover study in 13 patients with hypertension controlled with un-named diuretics (7), ACE-inhibitors (6), beta-blockers (5), calcium channel blockers (1) and a centrally acting alpha-agonist (1) found that a single dose of *Dimetapp Extentabs* (75 mg phenylpropanolamine + 12 mg brompheniramine) caused only a minor systolic/diastolic blood pressure rise (+ 1.7/ + 0.9 mmHg) over 4 h.[1] This sustained release preparation in this dosage has therefore no clinically important effect on the blood pressure, but (as the authors point out) these results do not necessarily apply to different doses and immediate-release preparations.

Reference

1 Petrulis AS, Imperiale TF, Speroff T. The acute effect of phenylpropanolamine and brompheniramine on blood pressure in controlled hypertension. J Gen Intern Med (1991) 6, 503–6.

Antihypertensives + Pyrazolone compounds

Abstract/Summary

Phenylbutazone and kebuzone reduce the antihypertensive effects of guanethidine and chlorothiazide. This would be expected to occur with other antihypertensive agents.

Clinical evidence, mechanism, importance and management

15 patients on 75 mg guanethidine daily showed a mean blood pressure rise of 13 mmHg (from 123 to 136 mmHg, i.e. diastolic + one-third pulse pressure) when concurrently treated with 750 mg phenylbutazone or kebuzone daily.[1] A similar rise in pressure was seen in 20 other patients taking 50 mg hydrochlorothiazide daily when given phenylbutazone.[1] These rises represent an approximately two-thirds reduction in the antihypertensive effects of guanethidine and hydrochlorothiazide. The mechanism of this interaction is uncertain but it is probably due to salt and water retention by these pyrazolone compounds. Direct evidence of this interaction seems to be limited to this report but it is in line with what is known about these anti-inflammatory compounds. Patients taking any antihypertensive agent should be monitored if phenylbutazone, kebuzone or oxyphenbutazone are given concurrently. A number of other NSAIDs do not interact like this.

Reference

1 Polak F. Die hemmende Wirkung von Phenylbutazon auf die durch einige Antihypertonika hervorgerufene Blutdrucksenkung bei Hypertonikern. Zsch inn Med (1976) 22, 375.

Antihypertensives + Salbutamol (Albuterol)

Abstract/Summary

Severe hypotension attributed to the use of a salbutamol infusion in the presence of methyldopa has been reported.

Clinical evidence, mechanism, importance and management

The manufacturers of salbutamol issued a general warning in 1979 about the concurrent use of salbutamol infusion with either methyldopa or any other drug with an acute hypotensive effect.[1] Three reports had been received of acute hypotension following the use of salbutamol infusion to postpone delivery in premature labour in women already taking 2–2.5 g methyldopa daily for the hypertension of pregnancy.[1] The suggested reason is that it results from peripheral vasodilation due to stimulation of the beta-receptors by the salbutamol. There is as yet nothing to suggest that salbutamol given orally will interact similarly.

Reference

1 Allen and Hanbury Ltd. Letter, 16th February 1979.

Clonidine + Beta-Blockers

Abstract/Summary

Concurrent use can be therapeutically valuable, but a sharp and serious rise in blood pressure ('rebound hypertension') can follow sudden withdrawal of the clonidine which may be worsened by the presence of a beta-blocker. Isolated cases of marked bradycardia and hypotension have been seen with clonidine and esmolol. There are also two reports describing abolition by the beta-blockers of the hypotensive effects of clonidine and even hypertension.

Clinical evidence

(a) Exacerbation of the clonidine-withdrawal hypertensive rebound

A woman with a blood pressure of 180/140 mmHg was treated with clonidine and timolol. When the clonidine was stopped in error, she developed a violent throbbing headache and became progressively confused, ataxic and semicomatose during which she also had a grand mal convulsion. Her blood pressure was found to have risen to 300 + /185 mmHg.[3]

A number of other reports describe similar cases of hypertensive rebound (a sudden and serious rise in blood pressure) within 24 and 72 h of stopping the clonidine, apparently worsened by the presence of propranolol[5–8,10] or timolol.[3] The symptoms resemble those of phaeochromocytoma and include tremor, apprehension, flushing, nausea, vomiting, severe headache and a serious rise in blood pressure. One patient died from a cerebellar haemorrhage.[8]

(b) Bradycardia and hypotension

A man of 80 anaesthetised with thiopentone and diamorphine, with oxygen, nitrous oxide, enflurane and atracurium was given 50 µg clonidine to control hypertension. 15 min later he became tachycardic with rates up to 170 beats/min. 75 mg esmolol was given by slow infusion, whereupon his heart rate fell to 20. He responded to 1.2 mg atropine, 1 mg adrenaline and 10 ml calcium chloride with a stable heart rate of 110 beats per min.[13] Another report describes marked hypotension in another patient on clonidine when given esmolol during surgery. This responded well to 10 mg ephedrine.[14]

(c) Antagonism of the hypotensive effects

When sotalol in daily doses of 160 mg was given to 10 hypertensive patients taking 0.45 mg clonidine daily, the fall in blood pressure caused by the clonidine was abolished in six of the patients. Two of the other patients had blood pressures which were lower than with either drug alone, and the remaining two patients were unresponsive to treatment.[1]

Two cases of hypertension involving clonidine with propranolol have also been described.[2]

Mechanism

The normal additive hypotensive effects of these drugs result from the two acting in concert at different but complementary sites in the cardiovascular system. Just why antagonism sometimes occurs is unexplained. The reliability of one of the reports[1] has been questioned. The hypertensive rebound following clonidine withdrawal is thought to be due to an increase in the levels of circulating catecholamines. With the beta (vasodilator) effects blocked by a beta-blocker, the alpha (vasoconstrictor) effects of the catecholamines are unopposed and the hypertension is further exaggerated.

Importance and management

The rebound hypertension following clonidine withdrawal, seriously worsened by the presence of a beta-blocker, is well established. Control this adverse effect by stopping the beta-blocker several days before the clonidine is gradually withdrawn.[4] A successful alternative is to replace the clonidine and the beta-blocker with labetalol[9] which is both an alpha- and a beta-blocker. If this is done, the blood catecholamine levels still rise markedly (× 20) and the patient may experience tremor, nausea, apprehension and palpitations, but no serious blood pressure rise or headaches occur.[9] The dosage of labetalol (800–1200 mg) will need to be titrated for the patient, with regular checks on the blood pressure over 2–3 days. If a hypertensive episode develops, control it with an alpha-blocking agent such as phentolamine (5 mg IV).[5] Diazoxide is effective[3,8] and oral nifedipine has been used for other hypertensive situations. Re-introduction of the clonidine, given orally or intravenously, should also stabilize the situation. It is clearly important to emphasize to patients taking clonidine and beta-blockers that they must keep taking their drugs.

What are the advantages and disadvantages of combined treatment? Patients given clonidine and either propranolol[11] or atenolol[12] (non-selective blockers) showed additive hypotensive effects and smaller doses of clonidine could be used which decreased its troublesome side-effects (sedation and dry mouth). In contrast, with nadolol[12] (cardio-selective) the blood pressure reductions were the same as with either drug alone. The weight of evidence is that adverse reactions (abolition of the blood pressure lowering effects or even hypertension) are rare.[1,2] The authors of one of these reports suggest that clonidine and propranolol should not be used together in cases of refractory hypertension.[2]

References

1 Saarimaa H. Combination of clonidine and sotalol in hypertension. Br Med J (1976) 1, 810.
2 Warren SE, Ebert E, Swerdlin A-H, Steinerger SM, Stone R. Clonidine and propranolol paradoxical hypertension. Arch Intern Med (1979) 139, 252–3.
3 Bailey RR, Neale TJ. Rapid clonidine withdrawal with blood pressure overshoot exaggerated by beta-blockade. Br Med J (1976) 1, 942.
4 Harris AL. Clonidine withdrawal and beta-blockade. Lancet (1976) i, 596.
5 Bruce DL, Croley TF, Less JS. Preoperative clonidine withdrawal syndrome. Anesthesiology (1979) 51, 90–2.
6 Cairns SA, Marshall AJ. Clonidine withdrawal. Lancet (1976) i, 368.
7 Strauss FG, Franklin SS, Lewin AJ, Maxwell MH. Withdrawal of hypertensive therapy. (1977) J Amer Med Ass. 238, 1734–6.
8 Vernon C, Sakula A. Fatal rebound hypertension after abrupt withdrawal of clonidine and propanolol. Br J Clin Pract (1979) 33, 112.
9 Rosenthal T, Rabinowitz B, Boichis H, Elazar E, Brauner A, Neufeld A. Use of labetalol in hypertensive patients during discontinuation of clonidine therapy. Eur J Clin Pharmacol (1981) 20, 237–40.
10 Reid JL, Wing LMH, Dargie HJ, Hamilton CA, Davies DS, Dollery CT. Clonidine withdrawal in hypertension. Changes in blood pressure and plasma and urinary noradrenaline. Lancet (1977) i, 1171–4.

11 Lilja M, Jounela AJ, Juustila H, Mattila MJ. Interaction of clonidine and beta-blockers. Acta Med Scand (1980) 207, 173–6.

12 Fogari R, Corradi L. Interaction of clonidine and beta blocking agents in the treatment of essential hypertension. In 'Low dose oral and transdermal therapy of hypertension' (Proceedings of Conference 1984), edited by Weber MA, Drayer JIM and Kolloch R. Springer-Verlag, 1985, pp. 118–21.

13 Perks D, Fisher GC. Esmolol and clonidine — a possible interaction. Anaesthesia (1992) 47, 533–4.

14 Kanitz DD, Ebert TJ, Kampine JP. Introperative use of bolus doses of esmolol to treat tachcardia. J Clin Anesthesiol (1990) 2, 238–42.

Clonidine or Apomorphine + Contraceptives, oral

Abstract/Summary

The sedative effects of clonidine are increased by the concurrent use of the pill, but those of apomorphine are decreased.

Clinical evidence, mechanism, importance and management

An experimental study[1] on alpha-2-receptors in a group of women showed that the sedative effects of clonidine and of apomorphine were increased and decreased respectively while taking an oral contraceptive (ethinyloestradiol 30 µg, levonorgestrel 150 or 250 µg). The clinical importance of this is uncertain.

Reference

1 Chalmers JS, Fulli-Lemaire I .Cowen PJ. Effects of the contraceptive pill on sedative responses to clonidine and apomorphine in normal women. Psych Med (1985) 15, 363–7.

Clonidine + Prazosin

Abstract/Summary

There is some evidence that prazosin may possibly reduce the antihypertensive effects of clonidine whereas other evidence suggests that this does not occur.

Clinical evidence

A study in 18 patients with essential hypertension showed that the hypotensive effects of an intravenous dose of clonidine were reduced by the presence of prazosin.[1] A later crossover study by the same group with 17 patients with essential hypertension (mean blood pressures 170/103 mmHg) found that 0.3 mg clonidine for 3 days reduced pressures to132/85 mmHg, whereas 6 mg prazosin daily for 3 days reduced the pressures to 160/99 mmHg. However when given together the pressures were only reduced to 158/97 mmHg.[5] Other studies failed to find this effect.[2–4] In the presence of prazosin the rebound hypertension following clonidine withdrawal is only moderate

(a rise from 145/85 to 169/104 mmHg).[4] More work is needed to establish what happens with certainty but it seems possible that concurrent use may not always be favourable. Monitor the effects.

References

1 Kapocsi J, Farsang C, Vizi ES. Prazosin partly blocks clonidine-induced hypotension in patients with essential hypertension. Eur J Clin Pharmacol (1987) 32, 331–4.

2 Kuokkanen K, Mattila MJ. Antihypertensive effects of prazosin in combination with methyldopa, clonidine or propanolol. Ann Clin Res (1979) 11, 18–24.

3 Stokes GS, Gain JM, Mahoney JE, Raaftos J, Steward JH. Long term use of prazosin in combination or alone for treating hypertension. Med J Aust (1977) 2 (Suppl) 13–16.

4 Andrejak M, Fievet P, Makdassi R, Conroy E, de Fremont JF, Coevoet B, Fournier A. Lack of antagonism in the antihypertensive effects of clonidine and prazosin in man. Clin Sci (1981) 61, 453–5S.

5 Farsang C, Varga K, Kaposcsi J. Prazosin-clonidine and prazosin-guanfacine interactions in hypertension. Pharmacol Res Comm (1988) 20, Suppl 1, 85–6.

Clonidine + Rifampicin (Rifampin)

Abstract/Summary

Rifampicin does not interact with clonidine

Clinical evidence, mechanism, importance and management

600 mg rifampicin twice daily for seven days had no effect on the elimination kinetics of clonidine nor on the pulse rates or blood pressures of six normal subjects taking 0.4 mg clonidine daily.[1] No special precautions would seem necessary.

Reference

1 Affrime MB, Lowenthal DT, Rufo M. Failure of rifampicin to induce the metabolism of clonidine in normal volunteers. Drug Intell Clin Pharm (1981) 15, 964–6.

Clonidine + Tricyclic antidepressants

Abstract/Summary

Clomipramine, desipramine and imipramine reduce or abolish the antihypertensive effects of clonidine. Other tricyclics are expected to behave similarly. A hypertensive crisis developed in a woman on clonidine when given imipramine, and severe pain in a man on amitriptyline and diamorphine when given clonidine intrathecally.

Clinical evidence

Four out of five hypertensive patients on 600–1800 µg clonidine daily (with chlorthalidone or hydrochlorothiazide) showed blood pressure rises averaging 22/15 mmHg when lying and 12/10 mmHg when standing after taking 75 mg desipramine daily for two weeks.[2]

This interaction has been seen in other patients taking clomipramine, desipramine and imipramine.[1,2,3,10-12,14] The antihypertensive effects of clonidine were reduced about 50% in six patients given desipramine,[10] and by 40–50% in eight normal subjects given 75 mg imipramine and single 300 μg doses of clonidine.[9] A man on 800 μg clonidine daily showed a blood pressure rise from 150/90 to 220/130 mmHg within four days of starting 75 mg clomipramine daily.[11]

An elderly woman on 200 μg clonidine daily developed severe frontal headache, dizziness, chest and neck pain and tachycardia (120 bpm) with hypertension (230/140–130 mmHg) on the second day of taking 50 mg imipramine for incontinence.[4] The effects of the withdrawal of clonidine from another elderly patient may also have been made worse by the presence of amitriptyline.[5] A man with severe pain, well controlled with amitriptyline, sodium valproate and intrathecal boluses of diamorphine, experienced severe pain within 5 min of an intrathecal test dose of 75 g clonidine.[13]

Mechanism

Not understood. One idea is that the tricyclics block the uptake of clonidine into neurones within the brain.[6] Another is that the tricyclics desensitize alpha-2-receptors.

Importance and management

The clonidine-tricyclics interaction is established and clinically important. The incidence is uncertain but it is not seen in all patients.[2] Avoid concurrent use unless the effects can be monitored. Increasing the dosage of clonidine may possibly be effective. 'Titration' of the clonidine dosage was apparently done successfully in 10 out of 11 hypertensive patients already on amitriptyline or imipramine.[7] Only clomipramine, desipramine and imipramine have been implicated so far, but other tricyclics would be expected to behave similarly (seen in animals with amitriptyline, nortriptyline and protriptyline[8]). Alternative antidepressants which do not interact with clonidine are maprotiline, mianserin and bupropion (see appropriate synopsis).

References

1 Conolly ME, Paterson JW, Dollery CT. In 'Catapres in Hypertension', Conolly ME (ed), Butterworths, London (1969) p 167.

2 Briant RH, Reid JL and Dollery CT. Interaction between clonidine and desipramine in man. Br Med J (1973) 1, 522.

3 Coffler DE. Antipsychotic drug interaction. Drug Intell Clin Pharm (1976) 10, 114.

4 Hui KK. Hypertensive crisis induced by interaction of clonidine with imipramine. J Amer Ger Soc (1983) 31, 164–5.

5 Stiff JL and Harris DB. Clonidine withdrawal complicated by amitriptyline therapy. Anesthesiology (1983) 59, 73–4.

6 van Spanning HW and van Zwieten PA. The interference of tricyclic antidepressants with the central hypotensive effect of clonidine. Eur J Pharmacol (1973) 24, 402.

7 Raftos J, Bauer GE, Lewis RG, Stokes GS, Mitchell AS, Young AA, Maclachalan I. Clonidine in the treatment of severe hypertension. Med J Aust (1973) 1, 786–93.

8 van Zwieten PA. Interaction between centrally active hypotensive drugs and tricyclic antidepressants. Arch Int Pharmacodyn Ther (1975) 214, 12.

9 Cubeddu LX, Cloutier G, Gross K, Grippo PA-CR, Tanner L, Lerea L, Shakarjian M, Knowlton G, Harden TK, Arendshorst W, Rogers JF. Bupropion does not antagonize cardiovascular actions of clonidine in normal subjects and spontaneously hypertensive rats. Clin Pharmacol Ther (1984) 35, 576–84.

10 Checkley SA, Slade AP, Shur E, Dawling S. A pilot study on the mechanism of action of desipramine. Br J Psychol (1981) 138, 248–51.

11 Andrejak M, Fournier A, Hardin JM, Coevoet B, Lambrey G, De Fremont JF, Quichaud J. Suppression de l'effet antihypertenseur de la clonidine par la prise simultanee d'un antidepresseur tricyclique. Nouv Presse med (1977) 6, 2603.

12 Lacomblez L, Warot D, Bouche P, Derousesne C. Suppression de l'effet antihypertenseur de la clonidine par la clomipramine. Rev Med Interne (1988) 9, 291–3.

13 Hardy PA, Wells JC. Pain after spinal intrathecal clonidine. An adverse interaction with tricyclic antidepressants? Anaesthesia (1988) 43, 1026–7.

14 Manchon ND, Bercoff E, Lemarchand P, Chassagne P, Senant J, Bourreille J. Fréquence et gravité des interactions médicamenteuses dan une population âgée: étude prospective concernant 63 malades. Rev Med Interne (1989) 10, 521–5.

Diazoxide + Hypoglycaemic agents and Hypotensive agents

Abstract/Summary

(a) Severe hypotension, in some cases fatal, has followed the administration of diazoxide before or after hydralazine. (b) Excessive hyperglycaemia is possible if diazoxide is given with other drugs with hyperglycaemic activity (e.g. the thiazides, clorpromazine).

Diazoxide has two main effects and two main therapeutic uses: it lowers blood pressure and is used to control severe hypertension, and it raises blood sugar levels and is used for intractable hypoglycaemia. If other drugs are used which either increase or oppose either of these two effects (antihypertensives, diuretics, hypo- or hyperglycaemics) the sum of the responses should be monitored and controlled to ensure that an overall balance is maintained, bearing in mind that some of these other drugs may also have dual activity. The hypotensive and hyperglycaemic effects of diazoxide may represent an unwanted side-effect when the other therapeutic use is being exploited.

(a) Diazoxide + Hydralazine

Clinical evidence

A previously normotensive 25-year old woman had a blood pressure of 250/150 mmHg during the 34th week of pregnancy which failed to respond to magnesium sulphate given intravenously. It fell transiently to 170/120 mmHg when given 15 mg hydralazine. One hour later intravenous diazoxide, 5 mg/kg resulted in a blood pressure fall to 60/0 mmHg. Despite large doses of noradrenaline, the hypotension persisted and the woman died.[1]

Other cases of severe hypotension are described in other studies and reports.[1-8] In some instances the patients had also had other antihypertensive agents such as methyldopa[3,4] or reserpine.[8] At least three of the cases had a fatal outcome.[8]

Mechanism

Not fully understood. The hypotensive effects (vasodilatory) of the two drugs are additive, and it would seem that in some instances the limit of the normal compensatory responses of the cardiovascular system to maintain an adequate blood pressure is reached.

Importance and management

An established, adequately documented and clinically important interaction. Concurrent use should be extremely cautious and thoroughly monitored. The authors of one of the reports cited[1] warn that '...diazoxide should be administered with caution to patients being concurrently treated with other potential vasodilatory or catechol-amine depleting agents.' The concurrent use of diazoxide and beta-blockers seems to be safe and effective (see 'Beta-blockers + Hydralazine').

(b) Diazoxide + Chlorpromazine and Bendrofluazide

Clinical evidence, mechanism, importance and management

An isolated report[8] describes a child on long-term treatment for hypoglycaemia with diazoxide, 8 mg/kg, and bendrofluazide, 1.25 mg daily, who developed a diabetic precoma and severe hyperglycaemia after a single 30 mg dose of chlorpromazine. The reason is not understood but one idea is that all three drugs had additive hyperglycaemic effects. Enhanced hyperglycaemia has been seen in other patients given diazoxide and trichlormethiazide.[9] Caution is clearly needed to ensure that the hyperglycaemic effects do not become excessive.

References

1 Henrich WL, Cronin R, Miller PD, Anderson RJ. Hypotensive sequelae of diazoxide and hydralazine therapy. J Am Med Ass (1977) 237, 264–5.
2 Miller WE, Gifford RW, Humphrey DC, Vidt DG. Management of severe hypertension with intravenous injections of diazoxide. Am J Cardiol (1969) 24, 870–5.
3 Kumar GK, Pastoor FC, Robayo JR, Razzaque MA. Side effects of diazoxide. J Am Med Ass (1973) 225, 275–6.
4 Tansey WA, Williams EG, Landerman RH, Schwartz MJ. Diazoxide. J Am Med Ass (1973) 225, 749.
5 Saker BM, Mathew TH, Eremin J, Kincaid-Smith P. Diazoxide in the treatment of the acute hypertensive emergency. Med J Aust (1968) 1, 592–3.
6 Finnerty FA. Hypertensive encephalopathy. Am J Med (1972) 52, 672–8.
7 Davey M, Moodley J, Soutter P. Adverse effects of a combination of diazoxide and hydralazine therapy. SA Med J (1981) 59, 496.
8 Aynsley-Green A, Illig R. Enhancement by chlorpromazine of hyperglycaemic action of diazoxide. Lancet (1975) ii, 658.
9 Seltzer HS, Allen EW. Hyperglycaemia and inhibition of insulin secretion

during administration of diazoxide and trichlormethiazide in man. Diabetes (1969) 18, 19.

Diuretics (potassium-sparing) + Potassium supplements and salt substitutes

Abstract/Summary

The concurrent use of potassium-sparing diuretics (spironolactone, triamterene, amiloride) and potassium supplements can result in severe and even life-threatening hyperkalaemia unless potassium levels are well monitored and controlled. Potassium-containing salt substitutes can be equally hazardous.

Clinical evidence

One study found that hyperkalaemia developed in 5.7% patients on spironolactone alone and 15.4% in those also taking a potassium supplement. The incidence rose to 42% in those with azotemia given spironolactone and a potassium supplement.[1] A retrospective survey of another group of patients on spironolactone found that half of them developed hyperkalaemia when given potassium chloride supplements.[2] The pacemaker of a patient failed because of hyperkalaemia caused by the concurrent use of *Dyazide* (triamterene + hydrochlorothiazide) and '*Slow-K*'.[3] Three patients on spironolactone became hyperkalaemic[4,5] because they took potassium-containing salt substitutes ('*No Salt*' in one case[4]). Two developed heart arrhythmias.[5]

Mechanism

The effects of these potassium conserving diuretics and the potassium supplements are additive, resulting in hyperkalaemia.

Importance and management

The interaction with spironolactone is well established, well documented and of clinical importance. Triamterene and amiloride would be expected to behave similarly. Avoid potassium supplements in patients on potassium-sparing diuretics except in cases of marked potassium depletion and where the effects can be closely monitored. Warn patients about the risks of salt substitutes containing potassium which may increase the potassium intake by 50–60 mEq daily.[5] The signs and symptoms of hyperkalaemia include muscular weakness, fatigue, parasthesia, flaccid paralysis of the extremities, bradycardia, shock and ECG abnormalities which may develop slowly and insidiously.

References

1 Greenblatt DJ, Koch-Weser J. Adverse reactions to spironolactone. A report from the Boston Collaborative Drug Surveillance Program. Clin Pharmacol Ther (1973) 14, 136–7.
2 Simborg DN. Medication prescribing on a university medical service - the

incidence of drug combinations with potential adverse interactions. Johns Hopkins Med J (1976) 139, 23.

3 O'Reilly MV, Murnaghan DP, Williams MB. Transvenous pacemaker failure induced by hyperkalemia. J Amer Med Ass (1974) 228, 336–7.

4 McCaughan D. Hazards of non-prescription potassium supplements. Lancet (1984) i, 513–14.

5 Yap V, Patel A, Thomsen J. Hyperkalemia with cardiac arrhythmia. Induction by salt substitutes, spironolactone and azotemia. J Am Med Ass (1976) 236, 2775.

Diuretics + Trimethoprim

Abstract/Summary

Excessively low serum sodium levels have been seen a few patients taking thiazide diuretics when given trimethoprim or co-trimoxazole.

Clinical evidence

A 75-year-old woman with multiple medical conditions and taking methyldopa, thyroxine and *Moduretic* (hydrochlorothiazide + amiloride) developed nausea and anorexia and was found to have hyponatremia (107 mmol/l) within four days of starting to take trimethoprim. The problem resolved when the *Moduretic* and trimethoprim were stopped. She was later discharged on methyldopa, thyroxine and *Moduretic*. When rechallenged four months later with trimethoprim in the absence of *Moduretic* no hyponatraemia occurred, but it developed rapidly when the *Moduretic* restarted.[1] The authors of this report say that they have seen several other patients who developed hyponatraemia within 4–12 days of taking trimethoprim or co-trimoxazole (sulphamethoxazole + trimethoprim), all of whom were elderly and all but one was taking a diuretic.[1]

Two other patients are described in another report who developed hyponatraemia when co-trimoxazole was added to treatment with *Moduret* (hydrochlorothiazide + amiloride) or hydrochlorothiazide/triamterene.[2]

Mechanism

Both the thiazides and trimethoprim can cause sodium loss and in these cases their additive effects were enough to cause extreme hyponatraemia.

Importance and management

Information is limited but it would seem prudent to be on the alert for any signs of hyponatremia (nausea, anorexia, etc.) in any patient in this category while taking these drugs.

References

1 Eastall R, Edmonds CJ. Hyponatraemia associated with trimethoprim and a diuretic. Br Med J (1984) 289, 1658–9.

2 Hart TL, Johnston LJ, Edmonds MW, Brownscombe L. Hyponatremia secondary to thiazide-trimethoprim interaction. Can J Hosp Pharm (1989) 42, 243–6.

Frusemide (Furosemide) + Chloral hydrate

Abstract/Summary

The intravenous injection of frusemide after treatment with chloral occasionally causes sweating, hot flushes, a variable blood pressure, tachycardia and uneasiness.

Clinical evidence

Six patients in a coronary care unit given an intravenous bolus of 40–120 mg frusemide and who had had chloral hydrate during the previous 24 h developed sweating, hot flushes, variable blood pressure, tachycardia and uneasiness. The reaction was immediate and lasted about 15 min. No special treatment was given.[1] A retrospective study of hospital records revealed that out of 43 patients who had had both drugs, one patient developed this reaction and two others may have done so.[2] The interaction has also been described in an 8-year-old boy.[3]

Mechanism

Not understood. One suggestion is that frusemide displaces trichloroacetic acid (the metabolite of chloral) from its protein binding sites, which in its turn displaces thyroxine or alters the serum pH so that the levels of free thyroxine rise.[1] There is no experimental confirmation of this idea.

Importance and management

An established interaction, but information is limited to three reports. The incidence is uncertain but probably low. Concurrent use need not be avoided, but it would be prudent to given intravenous frusemide cautiously if chloral has been given recently. It seems possible that variants of chloral hydrate (dichloralphenazone, petrichloral, chloral betaine) might interact similarly. There is no evidence that frusemide given orally or chloral given to patients already on frusemide initiates this reaction.[2]

References

1 Malach M, Berman N. Furosemide and chloral hydrate. Adverse drug interaction. J Amer Med Ass (1975) 232, 638.

2 Pevonka MP, Yost RL, Marks RG, Howell WS, Steward RB. Interaction of chloral hydrate and furosemide. A controlled retrospective study. Drug Intell Clin Pharm (1977) 11, 332.

3 Dean RP, Rudinsky BF, Kelleher MD. Interaction of chloral hydrate and intravenous furosemide in a child. Clin Pharm (1991) 10, 385–7.

Frusemide (Furosemide) + Cholestyramine or Colestipol

Abstract/Summary

Cholestyramine and colestipol markedly reduce the absorption and diuretic effects of frusemide. Giving the frusemide 2–3 h before either of these other drugs should minimize the effects of this interaction.

Clinical evidence

8 g cholestyramine reduced the absorption of a single 40 mg dose of frusemide in six normal subjects by 95%. The 4 h diuretic response was reduced by 76% (from 1510 to 350 ml). 10 g colestipol reduced the frusemide absorption by 80% and the 4 h diuretic response by 60% (from 1510 to 630 ml).[1]

Mechanism

Both cholestyramine and colestipol are anionic exchange resins which can bind frusemide within the gut, thereby by reducing its absorption and its effects.

Importance and management

An established interaction, although direct evidence seems to be limited to this study. The absorption of frusemide is relatively rapid so that giving it 2–3 h before either the cholestyramine or colestipol should be an effective way of overcoming this interaction. This needs confirmation.

Reference

1 Neuvonen P J, Kivistö K, Hirvisalo E L. Effects of resins and activated charcoal on the absorption of digoxin, carbamazepine and frusemide. Br J clin Pharmac (1988) 25, 229–33. s20

Frusemide (Furosemide) + Clofibrate

Abstract/Summary

Additional treatment with clofibrate in patients with nephrotic syndrome already receiving frusemide has led to marked diuresis and muscular symptoms.

Clinical evidence, mechanism, importance and management

Six patients with hypoalbuminaemia and hyperlipoprotein-aemia secondary to nephrotic syndrome, receiving 80–500 mg frusemide daily, developed muscle pain, low lumbar backache, stiffness and general malaise with pronounced diuresis within three days of receiving additional treatment with 1–2 g clofibrate daily.[1]

Mechanism

Not understood. The marked diuresis may have been due to competition and displacement of the frusemide by the clofibrate from its plasma protein binding sites. Clofibrate occasionally causes a muscular syndrome which could have been exacerbated by (a) the urinary loss of Na^+ and K^+ and (b) the increase in the half-life of clofibrate (from 12 to 36 h).

Importance and management

The clinical documentation seems to be limited to this report. The authors of this report suggest that serum proteins and renal function should be checked before giving clofibrate. If serum albumins are low, the total daily dosage of clofibrate should not exceed 0.5 g for each 1 g per 100 ml of the albumin concentration. More study is needed.

Reference

1 Bridgeman JF, Rosen SM, Thorp JM. Complications during clofibrate treatment of nephrotic syndrome hyperlipoproteinaemia. Lancet (1972) ii, 506.

Frusemide (Furosemide) + Food

Abstract/Summary

Food reduces the bioavailability of frusemide and its diuretic effects.

Clinical evidence

10 normal subjects were given 40 mg frusemide at 8.00 am with and without breakfast (milk, roll, cheese, butter, egg). The food reduced the peak serum levels by 55% (from 933 to 423 ng/ml) and the bioavailability was reduced approximately 30%.[1] The results were almost identical in five other subjects given a heavy meal (avacado with cream, fish, potatoes, fruit salad).[1] The diuresis over 10 h was reduced by 21% (from 2072 to 1640 ml) and over 24 h by 15% (from 2668 to 2270 ml).[1] When these figures were compared with urinary output of other subjects who were not given frusemide, the increased amount of urine when the frusemide was given without breakfast was about 600 ml whereas the increase was only 200 ml when given with breakfast, representing an approximately two-thirds reduction. Another study also found a reduction in the urinary recovery of frusemide.[2]

Mechanism

Not understood.

Importance and management

Information is limited. The authors of the first study cited say that frusemide should not be given with food. A two-thirds reduction is very considerable.

References

1 Beerman B, Midskov C. Reduced bioavailability and effect of furosemide given with food. Eur J Clin Pharmacol (1986) 29, 725–7.
2 Manarlund MM, Paalzow LK and Odlind B. Pharmacokinetics of furosemide in man after intravenous and oral administration. Application of moment analysis. Eur J Clin Pharmacol (1984) 26, 197–207.

Frusemide (Furosemide), Bumetanide or Torasemide + Indomethacin and other NSAIDs

Abstract/Summary

The antihypertensive and diuretic effects of frusemide can be reduced or even abolished by the concurrent use of indomethacin. Diclofenac, diflunisal, flurbiprofen, lornoxicam, naproxen, piroxicam and tolfenamic acid also appear to interact similarly although much less information is available. Azapropazone, dipyrone, flupirtine, ibuprofen, ketoprofen, pirprofen, mofebutazone, oxindanac, sulindac and tenoxicam may possibly not interact at all or may do so to a much lesser extent. Bumetanide and torasemide appear to behave like frusemide.

Clinical evidence

(a) Bumetanide + Aspirin, Indomethacin

640 mg aspirin four times daily reduced the 24 h urinary output in response to 1 mg bumetanide in eight normal subjects by 18%.[34] Indomethacin also reduces the diuretic effects of bumetanide.[4]

(b) Frusemide + Azapropazone

10 normal subjects showed no change in their urinary excretion caused by frusemide (40 mg daily) when they were concurrently given azapropazone (1200 mg daily). The frusemide did not antagonize the uricosuric effects of the azapropazone.[21]

(c) Frusemide + Diclofenac

A study in patients with heart failure and cirrhosis showed that 150 mg diclofenac daily reduced the frusemide-induced excretion of sodium by 38%, but the excretion of potassium was unaltered.[19]

(d) Frusemide + Diflunisal

A study in 12 normal subjects showed that 500 mg diflunisal twice daily interacted with frusemide like indomethacin: sodium excretion was reduced 59% but potassium excretion remained unchanged.[17] In patients with heart failure and cirrhosis treated with frusemide, 500–700 mg diflunisal daily decreased the sodium excretion by 36% and the potassium

excretion by 47%.[19] However another study failed to find an interaction.[22]

(e) Frusemide + Dipyrone (metamizole)

A study in 9 normal subjects found that while taking 3 g dipyrone daily for three days, the clearance of 20 mg frusemide IV was reduced (from 175 to 141 ml/min) but the diuretic effects of the frusemide were unchanged.[26]

(f) Frusemide + Flurbiprofen

A study in seven normal subjects showed that the increase in renal osmolal clearance of a standard water load, in response to 40 mg frusemide given orally or intravenously, fell from 105 to 19% and from 140 to 70% respectively following concurrent treatment with 100 mg flurbiprofen.[6] A single dose study in normal subjects showed that 100 mg flubiprofen reduced by 10% the urinary volume and sodium and potassium excretion following 80 mg frusemide orally.[7]

(g) Frusemide + Flupirtine

A study in normal subjects found that a single 200 mg dose of flupirtine did not affect the overall frusemide diuresis, but it was slightly delayed.[28]

(h) Frusemide + Ibuprofen

An elderly man with cardiac failure treated with digoxin, isosorbide and 80 mg frusemide daily, developed congestive heart failure with ascites when given 1200 mg ibuprofen daily. His serum urea and creatinine levels climbed and no diuresis occurred even when the frusemide dosage was doubled. Two days after withdrawing the ibuprofen, brisk diuresis took place, renal function returned to normal and his condition improved steadily.[5] Another elderly patient similarly showed a poor response to frusemide (and later to metolazone as well) until ibuprofen (600 mg four times daily) and at least two aspirin daily were stopped.[24] This was due to hyponatraemic hypovolaemia.

(i) Frusemide or Bumetanide + Indomethacin

A study in four normal subjects and six patients with essential hypertension showed that frusemide alone (240 mg daily) reduced the mean blood pressure by 13 mmHg, but when given with indomethacin (200 mg daily) the blood pressures returned to virtually pretreatment levels. Moreover the normal urinary sodium loss induced by the frusemide was significantly reduced.[1] A study in normal subjects and patients with congestive heart failure given frusemide showed that 100 mg indomethacin reduced the urinary output by 53% and also reduced the excretion of Na^+, K^+ and Cl^- by 64%, 48% and 62% respectively.[8] Another study found a 20–30% reduction in urinary output.[3] 100 mg indomethacin was also found to reduce the bumetanide-induced output of urine, Na^+ and Cl^-

(but not K^+) by about 25%.[10,13] There are other reports confirming the interaction between frusemide or bumetanide and indomethacin, some of which are detailed clinical studies whereas others describe individual patients who have developed cardiac failure as a result of this interaction.[2,11,12,15,16,34] An early study in normal subjects suggested that torasemide was not affected by indomethacin,[30] but on the basis of later work the same workers now say that pathological factors in patients may allow the same interaction to occur.[31]

(j) Frusemide + Ketoprofen

A study in 12 normal subjects given 40 mg frusemide found that 100 mg ketoprofen reduced the 6 h urine output by 67 ml, and the 24 h output by 651 ml on the first day of treatment. However no significant differences were seen after 5 days treatment.[29]

(k) Frusemide + Lornoxicam

A study in 12 normal subjects found that 4 mg lornoxicam signficantly antagonized the diuretic and natriuretic effects of frusemide.[33]

(l) Frusemide + Mofebutazone

A study in 10 normal subjects showed that 600 mg mofebutazone had no effect on the diuretic effects of 40 mg furosemide. The urinary volume and excretion of sodium, potassium and chloride were unchanged.[18]

(m) Frusemide + Naproxen

Two elderly women with congestive heart failure failed to respond to treatment with frusemide and digoxin until the naproxen they were taking was withdrawn.[5] A single dose study in patients with cardiac failure showed that the volume of urine excreted in response to frusemide was reduced about 50% by naproxen.[3]

(n) Frusemide + Oxindanac

A study in eight subjects found that 300 mg oxindanac twice daily did not affect the natriuresis of 40 mg frusemide twice daily.[32]

(o) Frusemide + Piroxicam

A 96-year-old woman with congestive heart failure failed to respond adequately to frusemide until the dosage of piroxicam she was taking was reduced from 20 to 10 mg daily.[23]

(p) Frusemide + Pirprofen

A study of eight patients showed that 800 mg pirprofen did not significantly affect the diuresis induced by frusemide or the urinary excretion of sodium.[20]

(q) Frusemide or Bumetanide + Sulindac or Tolfenamic acid

A study in eight normal subjects showed that tolfenamic acid (300 mg) reduced the diuretic response (volume, sodium, potassium and chloride) to a single 1 mg dose of bumetanide by 34% at 2 h, whereas the effects of 300 mg sulindac were smaller and not statistically significant.[14] Another study showed that in patients with cirrhosis and ascites that 150 mg sulindac reduced the diuretic effects (volume, sodium, potassium) of 80 mg frusemide given IV by 75%, 84% and 42% respectively.[9]

(r) Frusemide + Tenoxicam

A study in 12 patients showed that 20–40 mg tenoxicam daily had no significant effect on the urinary excretion of sodium or chloride due to 40 mg frusemide, and blood pressure, heart rate and body weight also were not affected.[25]

Mechanism

Uncertain and complex. It seems almost certain that a number of different mechanisms come into play. One possible mechanism is concerned with the synthesis of renal prostaglandins which occurs when the loop diuretics cause sodium excretion. If this synthesis is blocked by drugs such as the NSAIDs, then renal blood flow and diuresis will be altered.[27] Indomethacin is a non-specific inhibitor of cyclo-oxygenase, whereas sulindac selectively inhibits cyclo-oxygenase outside the kidney which might explain why it interacts to a lesser extent.

Importance and management

The frusemide-indomethacin interaction is very well documented and of clinical importance, whereas far less is known about the interactions with other NSAIDs. Concurrent use often need not be avoided but the effects should be checked and the frusemide dosage raised as necessary. Patients at greatest risk are likely to be the elderly with cirrhosis, cardiac failure and/or renal insufficiency. Some of the data comes from studies in normal subjects rather than patients so that the total picture is still far from clear. Diclofenac, diflunisal, flurbiprofen, ketoprofen, naproxen, piroxicam and tolfenamic acid are known to interact in some individuals, but not necessarily to the same extent as indomethacin. If raising the diuretic dosage is ineffective, another NSAID such as azapropazone, dipyrone, flupirtine, ibuprofen, oxindanac, pirprofen, sulindac or tenoxicam may prove not to interact significantly (this is not necessarily true for patients with cirrhosis and ascites[9]). Not every NSAID seems to have been investigated but be alert for this interaction with any of them. Phenylbutazone and oxyphenbutazone would be expected to interact because they cause sodium retention and oedema. Much less is known about bumetanide, and even less about torasemide, but the evidence suggests that they interact like frusemide with indomethacin. It would therefore seem prudent to be alert for interactions with any of the NSAID's with which frusemide interacts. More study is needed.

References

1 Patal RV, Moorkerjee BK, Bentzel CJ, Hysert PE, Babej M, Lee JB. Antagonism of the effects of frusemide by indomethacin in normal and hypertensive man. Prostaglandins (1975) 10, 649.

2 Allan SG, Knox J, Kerr F. Interaction between diuretics and indomethacin. Br Med J (1981) 283, 1611.

3 Faunch R. Non-steroidal anti-inflammatory drugs and frusemide-induced diuresis. Br Med J (1981) 283, 988.

4 Aggernaes KH. Indometacinehaemning of bumetaniddiurese. Ugeskr Laeg (1980) 142, 691.

5 Laiwah ACY and Mactier RA. Antagonistic effect of non-steroidal anti-inflammatory drugs on frusemide-induced diuresis in cardiac failure. Br Med J (1981) 283, 714.

6 Rawles JM. Antagonism between non-steroidal anti-inflammatory drugs and diuretics. Scott Med J (1982) 27, 37–40.

7 Symmons D, Kendall MJ. Non-steroidal anti-inflammatory drugs and frusemide-induced diuresis. Br Med J (1981) 283, 989.

8 Sorgel F, Koob R, Gluth WP, Kruger B, Lang E. The interaction of indomethacin and furosemide in patients with congestive heart failure. Clin Pharmacol Ther (1985) 37, 231.

9 Kronborg I, Daskalopuolos D, Katkov W, Zipser RD. The influence of sulindac and indomethacin on renal function and furosemide-induced diuresis in patients with cirrhosis and ascites. Clin Res (1984) 32, 14A.

10 Brater C, Chennavasin P. Indomethacin and the response to bumetanide. Clin Pharmacol Ther (1980) 27, 421–5.

11 Ahmad S. Indomethacin-bumetanide interaction: an alert. Am J Cardiol (1984) 54, 246–7.

12 Poe TE, Scott RB, Keith JF. Interaction of indomethacin with furosemide. J Fam Pract (1983) 16, 610–16.

13 Brater DC, Fox WR, Chennavasin P. Interaction studies with bumetanide and furosemide. Effects of probenecid and of indomethacin on response to bumetanide in man. J Clin Pharmacol (1981) 21, 647–53.

14 Pentikainen PJ, Tokola O, Vapaatalo H. Non-steroidal anti-inflammatory drugs and bumetanide response in man. Comparison of tolfenamic acid and sulindac. Clin Pharmacol Ther (1986) 39, 219.

15 Ritland S. Alvorlig interaksjon mellom indometacin og furosemid. Tidsskr Nor Laegeforen (1983) 103, 2003.

16 Nordrehaug JE. Alvorlig interaksjon mellom indometacin og furosemid. Tisskr Nor Laegeforen (1983) 103, 1680–1.

17 Favre L, Glasson PH, Riondel A, Vallotton MB. Interaction of diuretics and non-steroidal anti-inflammatory drugs in man. Clin Sci (1983) 64, 407–15.

18 Matthei U, Grabensee B, Loew D. The interaction of mofebutazone and furosemide. Curr Med Res Op (1987) 10, 638–44.

19 Jean G, Meregalli G, Vasiloco M, Silvani A, Scapiaticci R, Della Ventura GF, Baiocchi C, Thiella G. Interazioni tra terapia diuretica e farmaci antiinfiammatori nonsteroidei. Clin Ter (1983) 105, 471–5.

20 Sorgel F, Hemmerlein M, Lang E. Wirkung von Pirprofen und Indometacin auf die Effekte von Oxprenolon und Furosemid. Arzneim Forsch/Drug Res (1984) 34, 1330–2.

21 Williamson PJ, Enen MD, Roberts CJC. A study of the potential interactions between azapropazone and frusemide in man. Br J clin Pharmac (1984) 18, 619–23.

22 Tobert JA, Ostazewski T, Reger B, Mesinger MAP and Cook TJ. Diflunisal-furosemide interaction. Clin Pharmacol Ther (1980) 27, 290.

23 Baker DE. Piroxicam-furosemide interaction. Drug Intell Clin Pharm (1988) 22, 505–6.

24 Goodenough GK, Lutz LJ. Hyponatremic hypervolemia caused by a drug-drug interaction mistaken for syndrome of inappropriate ADH. J Amer Geriatr Soc (1988) 36, 285–6.

25 Hartmann D, Kleinbloesem CH, Lucker PW, Vetter G. Study on the possible interaction between tenoxicam and furosemide. Arzneim-Forsch/Drug Res (1987) 37, 1072–6.

26 Rosenkranz B, Lehr K-H, Mackert G, Seyberth HW. Metamizole-furosemide interaction study in healthy volunteers. Eur J Clin Pharmacol (1992) 42, 593–8.

27 Passmore AP, Copeland S, Johnston CD. The effects of ibuprofen and indomethacin on renal function in the presence and absence of frusemide in healthy volunteers on a restricted sodium diet. Br J clin Pharmac (1990) 29, 311–9.

28 Johnston A, Warrington SJ, Turner P, Riethmuller-Winzen H. Comparison of flupirtine and indomethacin on frusemide-induced diuresis. Postgrad Med J (1987) 63, 959–61.

29 Li Kam Wa TC, Lawson M, Jackson SHD, Hitoglou-Makedou A, Turner P. Interaction of ketoprofen and frusemide in man. Postgrad Med J (1991) 67, 655–8.

30 Van Ganse E, Douchamps J, Deger F, Staroukine M, Verniory A, Herchuelz A. Failure of indomethacin to impair the diuretic and natriuretic effects of the loop diuretic torasemide in healthy volunteers. Eur J Clin Pharmacol (1986) 31, 43–7.

31 Herschuelz A, Derenne F, Deger F, Juvent M, van Ganse E. Staroutkine M, Verniory A, Boeynaems AM, Douchamps J. Interaction between non-steroidal anti-inflammatory drugs and loop diuretics: modulation by sodium balance. J Pharmacol Exptl Ther (1989) 248, 1175–81.

32 Tamm C, Favre L, Spence S, Pfister S, Vallotton MB. Interaction of oxindanac and frusemide in man. Eur J Clin Pharmacol (1989) 37, 17–21.

33 Ravic M, Johnston A, Turner P. clinical pharmacological studies of some possible interactions of lornoxicam with other drugs. Postgrad Med J (1990) 66, Suppl 4, S30–4.

34 Kaufman J, Hamburger R, Matheson J, Flamenbaum W. Bumetanide-induced diuresis and natriuresis: effect of prostaglandin synthetase inhibition. J Clin Pharmacol (1981) 21, 663–7.

Frusemide (Furosemide) + Phenytoin

Abstract/Summary

The diuretic effects of frusemide can be reduced as much as 50% if phenytoin is used concurrently.

Clinical evidence

The observation that dependent oedema in a group of epileptics was higher than expected, and the response to diuretic treatment seemed to be reduced, prompted further study. 30 patients taking 200–400 mg phenytoin daily with 60–180 mg phenobarbitone produced a maximal diuresis in reponse to 20 or 40 mg frusemide after 3–4 h instead of the usual 2 h, and the total diuresis was reduced 68 and 51% respectively. When given 20 mg frusemide intravenously the total diuresis was reduced 50%. Some of the patients were also taking carbamazepine, pheneturide, ethosuximide, diazepam or chlordiazepoxide.[1] Another study in five normal subjects given 300 mg phenytoin daily for 10 days showed that the maximal serum frusemide levels when given 20 mg frusemide, orally or intravenously, were reduced by 50%.[2]

Mechanism

Not fully understood. One suggestion is that the phenytoin causes changes in the jejunal Na$^+$ pump activity which reduces the absorption of the frusemide, but this is not the whole story because an interaction also occurs when frusemide is given intravenously.[3] Another suggestion is that the phenytoin generates a 'liquid membrane' which blocks the transport of the frusemide to its active site.[4]

Importance and management

Information is limited but the interaction is established. A reduced diuretic response should be expected in the presence of phenytoin. A dosage increase may be needed.

References

1 Ahmad S. Renal insensitivity to frusemide caused by chronic anticonvulsant therapy. Br Med J (1974) 3, 657.
2 Fine A, Henderson JS, Morgan DR, Tilstone WJ. Malabsorption of frusemide caused by phenytoin. Br Med J (1977) 2, 1061.
3 Noach EL, Rees H and de Wolff PA. Effects of diphenylhydantoin (DPH) on absorptive processes in the rat jejunum. Arch Int Pharmacodyn Ther (1973) 206, 392.
4 Srivastava RC, Bhise SB, Sood R, Rao MNA. On the reduced furosemide response in the presence of diphenylhydantoin. Colloids and Surfaces (1986) 19, 83–8.

Frusemide (Furosemide) or Bumetanide + Probenecid

Abstract/Summary

Probenecid can reduce the urinary loss of sodium caused by frusemide but it appears not to affect bumetanide.

Clinical evidence, mechanism, importance and management

(a) Frusemide

Concurrent use has been closely studied to sort out renal pharmacological mechanisms. One study in patients given 40 mg frusemide daily found that the addition of 0.5 g probenecid twice daily for three days reduced their urinary excretion of sodium by almost 40% (from 56.7 to 35.9 mmol daily).[5] Other studies have also found some changes in diuresis (a fall in some studies, a rise in others).[1-4] The clinical importance of these interactions is uncertain.

(b) Bumetanide

A study in eight normal subjects showed that 1 g probenecid did not affect their response to 0.5–1.0 mg bumetanide.[6] Another study reported a fall in natriuresis and in the clearance of bumetanide, but of minimal clinical importance.[7]

References

1 Brater DC. Effects of probenecid on furosemide response. Clin Pharmacol Ther (1978) 24, 548.
2 Homeida M, Roberts C, Branch RA. Influence of probenecid and spironolactone on furosemide kinetics and dynamics in man. Clin Pharmacol Ther (1977) 22, 402.
3 Honari J, Blair AD, Cutler RE. Effects of probenecid on furosemide kinetics and natriuresis in man. Clin Pharmacol Ther (1977) 22, 395.
4 Smith DE, Gee WL, Brater DC, Lin ET, Benet LZ. Preliminary evaluation

of furosemide-probenecid interaction in humans. J Pharm Sci (1980) 69, 571–5.
5 Hsieh Y-Y, Hsieh B-S, Lien W-P and Wu T-L. Probenecid interferes with the natriuretic action of furosemide. J Cardiovasc Pharmacol (1987) 10, 530–4.
6 Brater DC, Chennavasin P. Effect of probenecid on response to bumetanide in man. J Clin Pharmacol (1981) 21, 311–15.
7 Lant AF. Effects of bumetanide on cation and anion transport. Postgrad Med J (1975) 51 (Suppl 6) 35.

Guanethidine and related drugs + Haloperidol or Thiothixene

Abstract/Summary

The antihypertensive effects of guanethidine can be reduced by the concurrent use of haloperidol or thiothixene.

Clinical evidence

Three hypertensive patients taking 60–150 mg guanethidine daily showed rises in their blood pressures when haloperidol (6–9 mg daily) was added: from 132/95 to 149/99 mmHg in the first patient; from 125/84 to 148/100 mmHg in the second; and from 138/91 to 154/100 mmHg in the third. One of the patients later tested with 60 mg thiothixene daily showed a rise from 126/87 to 156/110 mmHg.[1] These results have been reported elsewhere.[2,3]

Mechanism

Haloperidol and thiothixene prevent the entry of guanethidine into the adrenergic neurones of the sympathetic nervous system so that its blood pressure lowering effects are reduced or lost. This is essentially the same mechanism of interaction as that seen with the tricyclic antidepressants and chlorpromazine.

Importance and management

Information seems to be limited to this report, but it is supported by the well-documented pharmacology of these drugs. It appears to be clinically important. If haloperidol or thiothixene are given to patients on guanethidine, monitor their blood pressures and raise the guanethidine dosage as necessary.[3] There is no direct evidence of an interaction between guanethidine or related drugs and other butyrophenones or thioxanthenes but it would be prudent to adopt the same precautions.

References

1 Janowsky DS, El-Yousef MK, Davis JM, Fann WE, Oates JA. Guanethidine antagonism by antipsychotic drugs. J Tenn State Med Ass (1972) 65, 620.
2 Davis JM. Psychopharmacology in the aged. Use of psychotropic drugs in geriatric patients. J Geriatric Psychiatry (1974) 7, 145.
3 Janowsky DS, El-Yousef MK, Davis JM, Fann WE. Antagonism of guanethidine by chlorpromazine. Am J Psychiatry (1973) 130, 808.

Guanethidine and related drugs + Levodopa

Abstract/Summary

When additionally given levodopa it was possible to reduce the dosage of guanethidine in one patient, and another was able to stop using a diuretic.

Clinical evidence, mechanism, importance and management

A brief report describes a patient on guanethidine and a diuretic who, when given levodopa (dose not stated but said to be within the ordinary therapeutic range) required a reduction in his daily dose of guanethidine from 60 to 20 mg. Another patient similarly treated was able to discontinue the diuretic.[1] The suggested reason is that the hypotensive side-effects of the levodopa are additive with the effects of the guanethidine. Direct information seems to be limited to this report but it would be a wise precaution to confirm that excessive hypotension does not develop if levodopa is added to treatment with guanethidine or guanethidine-like drugs.

Reference

1 Hunter KR, Stern GM, Laurence DR. Use of levodopa with other drugs. Lancet (1970) ii, 1283.

Guanethidine and related drugs + Monoamine oxidase inhibitors (MAOIs)

Abstract/Summary

The antihypertensive effects of guanethidine can be reduced by nialamide

Clinical evidence, mechanism, importance and management

Four out of five hypertensive patients on guanethidine (25–35 mg daily) showed a blood pressure rise from 140/85 to 165/100 mmHg 6 h after being given a single 50 mg dose of nialamide.[1] The reason is not understood but one idea is that MAOIs possibly oppose the guanethidine-induced loss of noradrenaline from sympathetic neurones. Direct information seems to be limited to this single dose study so that the outcome of long-term use is uncertain, but it would be prudent to monitor the effects if any MAOI is given to patients taking any guanethidine-like drug.

Reference

1 Gulati OD, Dave BT, Gokhale SD, Shah KM. Antagonism of adrenergic neuron blockade in hypertensive subjects. Clin Pharmacol Ther (1966) 7, 510.

Guanethidine and related drugs + Phenothiazines

Abstract/Summary

Large doses of chlorpromazine may reduce or even abolish the antihypertensive effects of guanethidine although in some patients the inherent hypotensive effects of the chlorpromazine may possibly predominate.

Clinical evidence

Two severely hypertensive patients, well controlled on 80 mg guanethidine daily, were additionally given 200–300 mg chlorpromazine. The diastolic blood pressure of one rose over 10 days from 94 to 112 mmHg and continued to climb to 116 mmHg even when the chlorpromazine was withdrawn. The diastolic pressure of the other rose from 105 to 127 mmHg, and then on to 150 mmHg even after the chlorpromazine had been withdrawn.[1] Other reports similarly describe marked rises in blood pressure in patients on guanethidine when given chlorpromazine (100–400 mg daily).[2–4]

Mechanism

Chlorpromazine prevents the entry of guanethidine into the adrenergic neurones of the sympathetic nervous system so that its blood pressure lowering effects are lost. This is essentially the same mechanism of interaction as that seen with the tricyclic antidepressants.

Importance and management

Direct information is very limited but the interaction is established and can be clinically important. It may take several days to develop. Not all patients may react to the same extent.[2,6] Monitor concurrent use and raise the guanethidine dosage if necessary. It is uncertain how much chlorpromazine is needed before a significant effect occurs but the smallest dose of chlorpromazine used in the documented studies was 100 mg with 90 mg guanethidine which raised the blood pressure from 113/82 to 153/105 mmHg. The inherent hypotensive effects of the chlorpromazine may possibly reduce the effects of this interaction. Other guanethidine-like antihypertensives (bethanidine, debrisoquine, guanoclor, etc.) would be expected to interact similarly but nobody seems to have checked on the effects of phenothiazines other than chlorpromazine. The effects should be monitored. Molindone is reported not to interact.[5]

References

1 Fann WE, Janowsky DS, Davis JM, Oates JA. Chlorpromazine reversal of the antihypertensive action of guanethidine. Lancet (1971) ii, 436.

2 Janowsky DS, El-Yousef MK, Davis JM, Fann WE, Oates JA. Guanethidine antagonism by antipsychotic drugs. J Tenn State Med Ass (1972) 65, 620.

3 Janowsky DS, El-Yousef MK, Davis JM, Fann WE. Antagonism of guanethidine by chlorpromazine. Am J Psychiatry (1973) 130, 808.

4 Davis JM. Psychopharmacology in the aged. Use of psychotropic drugs in geriatric patients. J Geriatric Psychiatry (1974) 7, 145.

5 Simpson LL. Combined use of molindone and guanethidine in patients with schizophrenia and hypertension. Am J Psychiatry (1979) 136, 1410.

6 Tuck D, Hamberger B, Sjoqvist F. Drug interactions: effect of chlorpromazine on the uptake of monoamines into adrenergic neurones in man. Lancet (1972) ii, 492.

Guanethidine and related drugs + Pizotifen

Abstract/Summary

An isolated report describes the abolition of the antihypertensive effects of debrisoquine by pizotifen.

Clinical evidence, mechanism, importance and management

A man with severe focal glomerulonephritis and hypertension, well controlled on debrisoquine, 30 mg daily, timolol 10 mg and frusemide 40 mg eight-hourly, was additionally given pizotifen (*Sandomigran*) as a prophylactic for migraine. Over the next few weeks his blood pressure climbed from 130/90 to 195/145 mmHg. It was found impossible to lower the pressure with either diazoxide or prazosin, but within 48 h of withdrawing the pizotifen the pressure had fallen to 105/82 mmHg and later stabilized at 140/90 mmHg.[1] The reason is not known but Sandoz, the manufacturers of pizotifen, suggest that as it is structurally similar to the tricyclic antidepressants, it may possibly oppose the actions of debrisoquine in a similar way by blocking the entry of the antihypertensive into the adrenergic neurones of the sympathetic nervous system.[1] Information is limited to this report but it would be wise to check for this interaction in any patient on debrisoquine or any other guanethidine-like hypertensive if pizotifen is given.

Reference

1 Bailey RR. Antagonism of debrisoquine sulphate by pizotifen (*Sandomigran*). NZ Med J (1976) 1, 449.

Guanethidine and Related drugs + Sympathomimetic amines (directly-acting)

Abstract/Summary

The pressor effects of noradrenaline (norepinephrine, levarterenol), phenylephrine, metaraminol and similar drugs can be increased two- to four-fold in the presence of guanethidine and related drugs (bethanidine, debrisoquine, guanadrel,

etc.). The mydriatic effects are similarly enhanced and prolonged.

Clinical evidence

(a) Pressor responses

A study in six normal subjects, given 200 mg guanethidine on the first day of study and 100 mg daily for the next two days, showed that their pressor responses (one third pulse pressure + diastolic pressure) when infused with noradrenaline in a range of doses were enhanced two-and-a-half to four times. Moreover cardiac arrhythmias appeared at lower doses of noradrenaline and with greater frequency than in the absence of guanethidine, and were more serious in nature.[1] There are reports of this enhanced pressor response involving debrisoquine with phenylephrine,[3,4] (even when given orally[9]), with bretylium and noradrenaline,[5] and guanethidine with metaraminol.[2] In the latter instance, 10 mg metaraminol given intravenously rapidly caused a blood pressure rise to 220/130 mmHg accompanied by severe headache and extreme angina. An increased blood pressure (from 165/92 to 210/120 mmHg) was also seen in a patient on guanethidine who, prior to surgery, was treated with phenylephrine eye drops.[10]

(b) Mydriatic responses

The mydriasis due to phenylephrine administered as a 10% eyedrop solution was observed to be prolonged for up to 10 h in a patient concurrently receiving guanethidine for hypertension.[6] This enhanced mydriatic response has been described in other studies involving guanethidine with adrenaline, phenylephrine or methoxamine;[7] and debrisoquine with phenylephrine[9] or ephedrine.[7]

Mechanism

If sympathetic nerves are cut surgically, the receptors which they normally stimulate become hypersensitive. By preventing the release of noradrenaline (norepinephrine) from adrenergic neurones, guanethidine and other adrenergic neurone blockers cause a temporary 'drug-induced sympathectomy' which is also accompanied by hypersensitivity of the receptors. Hence the increased response to the stimulation of the receptors by directly acting sympathomimetics.

Importance and management

An established, well-documented and potentially serious interaction. Since the pressor effects are grossly exaggerated, dosages of directly-acting sympathomimetics (alpha-agonists) should be reduced appropriately. The pressor effects of noradrenaline (norepinephrine) are increased two- to four-fold, and of phenylephrine twofold. In addition it should be remembered that the incidence and severity of heart arrhythmias is increased.[1,4] Considerable care is required. Direct evidence seems to be limited to noradrenaline, phenylephrine and metaraminol, but dopamine and methoxamine possess direct sympathomimetic activity and may be expected to interact similarly. No interaction would be expected with the beta-agonist drugs used for the treatment of asthma (such as terbutaline, salbutamol). Bethanidine and other guanethidine-like drugs (guanoclor, guanoxan, guanadrel, etc.) are also expected to behave like guanethidine. If as a result of this interaction the blood pressure becomes grossly elevated, it can be controlled by the administration of an alpha-adrenergic blocker such as phentolamine.[3,9] 10 mg oral nifedipine with water may also be effective. Phenylephrine is contained in a number of over-the-counter cough and cold preparations, a few of which contain up to 10 mg in a dose. This dose is only likely to cause a moderate blood pressure rise, compared with the marked rise seen in subjects on debrisoquine given 0.75 mg/kg (roughly 45 mg in a 10-stone individual).[4,8] However this requires confirmation. An exaggerated pressor response is clearly much more potentially serious than enhanced and prolonged mydriasis, but the latter is also possible and undesirable. It can occur whether or not the guanethidine-like drug has been given systemically or topically. The same precautions apply about using smaller amounts of the sympathomimetic drugs.

References

1 Mulheims GH, Entrup RW, Palewonsky D, Mierzwiak DS. Increased sensitivity of the heart to catecholamine-induced arrhythmias following guanethidine. Clin Pharmacol Ther (1965) 6,757.

2 Stevens FRT. A danger of sympathomimetic drugs. Med J Aust (1966) 2, 576.

3 Aminu J, D'Mello A, Vere DW. Interaction between debrisoquine and phenylephrine. Lancet (1970) ii, 935.

4 Allum W, Aminu J, Bloomfield TH, Davies C, Scales AH, Vere DW. Interaction between debrisoquine and phenylephrine in man. Brit J Pharmacol (1973) 47, 675P.

5 Laurence DR, Nagle RE. The interaction of bretylium with pressor agents. Lancet (1961) i, 593.

6 Cooper B. Neo-synephrine (10%) eye drops. Med J Aust (1968) 55,420.

7 Sneddon JM, TurnerP. The interactions of local guanethidine: tolerance and effects on adrenergic nerve function and response to sympathomimetic amines. Brit J Pharmacol (1962) 19, 13.

8 Boura ALA and Green AF. Comparison of bretylium and guanethidine; tolerance and effects on adrenergic nerve function and responses to sympathomimetic amines. Br J Pharmac (1962) 19, 13–41.

9 Allum W, Aminu J, Bloomfield TH, Davies C, Scales AH, Vere DW. Interaction between debrisoquine and phenylephrine in man. Br J Clin Pharmac (1974) 1, 51.

10 Kim JM, Stevenson CE, Matthewson HS. Hypertensive reactions to phenylephrine eyedrops in patients with sympathetic denervation. Am J Ophthalmol (1978) 85, 862–8.

Guanethidine and related drugs + Sympathomimetic amines (indirectly acting) and related drugs

Abstract/Summary

The antihypertensive effects of guanethidine-like drugs (bethanidine, debrisoquine, guanoclor, etc.) can be reduced or abolished by the concurrent use of indirectly-acting sympathomimetics and related drugs which are contained in cough, cold and influenza remedies or are used as appetite suppressants (amphetamines, ephedrine, pseudoephedrine, phenylpropranolamine, mazindol, methylphenidate, etc.). The blood pressure may even rise higher than before treatment with the antihypertensive.

Clinical evidence

When 16 hypertensive patients on 25–35 mg guanethidine daily were additionally given dextroamphetamine (10 mg orally), ephedrine (90 mg orally), methamphetamine (30 mg IM) or methylphenidate (20 mg orally), the effects of the guanethidine were completely abolished and in some instances the blood pressures rose higher than before treatment with the guanethidine.[1] Other reports describe the same interaction between guanethidine and dextroamphetamine[6] or methamphetamine;[5] bethanidine and phenylpropanolamine[2] or mazindol;[13] bretylium and amphetamine;[3] debrisoquine and mazindol;[14] and an unnamed adrenergic blocker and ephedrine.[4]

Mechanism

Indirectly-acting sympathomimetic amines not only prevent guanethidine-like drugs from entering the adrenergic neurones of the sympathetic nervous system, but they can also displace the antihypertensive drug already there.[10] As a result the blood pressure lowering effects are lost. In addition these amines release noradrenaline from the neurones which raises the blood pressure. Thus the antihypertensive effects are not only opposed, but the pressure may even be raised higher than before treatment.[7-12] Mazindol is related to the tricyclic antidepressants and probably interacts solely by blocking the entry of the guanethidine-like drugs into adrenergic neurones.

Importance and management

Well documented, well established and clinically important interactions. Patients taking guanethidine and related drugs (bretylium, bethanidine, debrisoquine, guanoclor, guanacline, guanadrel, etc.) should avoid indirectly-acting sympathomimetics (named above). Warn them against the temptation to use proprietary over-the-counter nasal decongestants containing any of these amines to relieve the nasal stuffiness commonly associated with the use of guanethidine and related drugs. The same precautions apply to the sympathomimetics used as appetite suppressants. However diethylpropion appears not to interact with guanethidine or bethanidine.[15] Not every guanethidine-like antihypertensive-sympathomimetic combination has been investigated in man, but from their well-understood pharmacology they are expected to behave similarly.

References

1 Gulati OD, Dave BT, Gokhale SD, Shah KM. Antagonism of adrenergic neurone blockade in hypertensive subjects. Clin Pharmacol Ther (1966) 7, 510.

2 Misage JR, McDonald RH. Antagonism of hypotensive action of bethanidine by 'common cold' remedy. Br Med J (1970) 2, 347.

3 Wilson R, Long C. Action of bretylium antagonized by amphetamine. Lancet (1960) ii, 262.

4 Starr KJ, Petrie JC. Drug interactions in patients on long-term oral anticoagulant and antihypertensive adrenergic neurone-blocking drugs. Br Med J (1972) 2, 133.

5 Laurence DR, Rosenheim ML. Ciba Foundation Symposium on adrenergic mechanisms. London (1960) p 201.

6 Ober KF, Wang RIH. Drug interactions with guanethidine. Clin Pharmacol Ther (1973) 14, 190.

7 Day MD, Rand MJ. Antagonism of guanethidine and bretylium by various agents. Lancet (1962) i, 1282.

8 Day MD, Rand MJ. Evidence for a competitive antagonism of guanethidine by dexamphetamine. Br J Pharmacol (1963) 20, 17.

9 Day MD. Effect of sympathomimetic amines on the blocking action of guanethidine, bretylium and xylocholine. Br J Pharmacol (1962) 18, 421.

10 Feagin OT, Morgan DH, Oates JA, Shand DG. The mechanism of the reversal of the effect of guanethidine by amphetamines in cat and man. Br J Pharmacol (1970) 39, 253.

11 Starke K. Interactions of guanethidine and indirectly-acting sympathomimetic amines. Arch Int Pharmacodyn Ther (1972) 195, 309.

12 Boura ALA and Green AF. Comparison of bretylium and guanethidine: tolerance and effects on adrenergic nerve function and responses to sympathomimetic amines. Br J Pharmacol (1962) 19, 13–41.

13 Boakes AJ. Antagonism of bethanidine by mazindol. Br J clin Pharmacol (1977) 4, 486.

14 Parker J. Wander Pharmaceuticals, England. Personal communication (1976).

15 Seedat YK, Roddy J. Diethylpropion hydrochloride (Tenuate, Dospin) in the treatment of obese hypertensive patients. S Afr med J (1974) 48, 569.

Guanethidine and related drugs + Tricyclic antidepressants

Abstract/Summary

The antihypertensive effects of guanethidine, bethanidine, bretylium and debrisoquine are reduced or abolished by the concurrent use of tricyclic antidepressants such as amitriptyline, desipramine, imipramine, nortriptyline and protriptyline. Doxepin in doses of more than 200–250 mg daily interacts similarly, but in smaller doses appears not to do so. Maprotiline only interacts in a few individuals.

Clinical evidence

Five hypertensive patients, controlled on 50–150 mg guanethidine daily, showed a blood pressure rise of 27 mmHg (diastolic pressure + one-third pulse pressure) when given 50–75 mg desipramine or 20 mg proptriptyline daily for 1–9 days. The full antihypertensive effects of the guanethidine were not re-established until five days after the antidepressants were withdrawn.[1] The same interaction has been described in other reports between guanethidine and desipramine,[2,3] imipramine,[4,5] amitriptyline,[6–8] protriptyline[3] and nortriptyline;[17] between bethanidine and desipramine,[1–3,9] imipramine,[8,10] amitriptyline,[10,20] and nortriptyline;[10,20] between debrisoquine and desipramine[3] and amitriptyline;[8,10] and between bethanidine and maprotiline in one out of six patients,[11] and in one other patient.[8] In some cases the interaction develops rapidly and fully within a few hours and lasts for many days (e.g. two 25 mg doses of imipramine — less than a day's dosage —

completely abolished the effects of bethanidine for an entire week[2]), whereas the interaction with guanethidine may take several days to develop fully. Tricyclic antidepressants have also been deliberately used to return the blood pressure to normal in patients taking bretylium, without reducing its antiarrhythmic efficacy.[21]

Mechanism

The guanethidine-like drugs exert their hypotensive actions firstly by entering the adrenergic nerve endings associated with blood vessels using the noradrenaline (norepinephrine) uptake mechanism. The tricyclics successfully compete for the same mechanism so that the antihypertensives fail to reach their site of action and, as a result, the blood pressure rises once again.[19] The differences in the rate of development, duration and extent of the interactions reflect the differences between the various guanethidine-like drugs and the various tricyclics, as well as individual differences between patients.

Importance and management

A very well documented and well established interaction of clinical importance. Not every combination of guanethidine-like drug and tricyclic antidepressant has been studied but all are expected to interact similarly. Concurrent use should be avoided unless the effects are very closely monitored and the interaction balanced by raising the dosage of the antihypertensive. Alternative and probably better solutions are as follows:

(a) Choose a different antidepressant

Maprotiline only appears to interact in a few patients[8,11] (no interaction was seen in two patients on guanethidine and one on debrisoquine)[8] but there seems to be no way of predicting the outcome. Doxepin does not interact until doses of about 200–250 mg daily are used, but with 300 mg or more daily it interacts to the same extent as other tricyclics.[9,12–16,22] Mianserin is reported not to interact (see 'Antihypertensives + Bupropion, Mianserin or Maprotiline') and theoretically iprindole does not do so, but this needs confirmation.

(b) Choose a different antihypertensive

Clonidine should be avoided because it interacts similarly (see 'Clonidine + Tricyclic antidepressants'). Depression is also associated with methyldopa and the rauwolfia alkaloids which makes them unsuitable, but beta-blockers[18] and ACE-inhibitors appear not to be affected.

References

1 Mitchell JR, Arias L and Oates JA. Antagonism of the antihypertensive actions of guanethidine sulfate by desipramine hydrochloride. J Am Med Ass (1967) 202, 973.

2 Oates JA, Mitchell JR, Feagin OT, Kaufmann JS, Shand DG. Distribution of guanidium antihypertensives-mechanism of their selective action. Ann NY Acad Sci (1971) 197, 302.

3 Mitchell JR, Cavanaugh JH, Arias L and Oates JA. Guanethidine and

related agents. III. Antagonism by drugs which inhibit the norepinephrine pump in man. J Clin Invest (1970) 49, 1596.

4 Leishmann AWD, Matthews HL and Smith AJ. Antagonism of guanethidine by imipramine. Lancet (1963) i, 112.

5 Boston Collaborative Drug Surveillance Program. Adverse reactions to the tricyclic antidepressant drugs. Lancet (1972) i, 529.

6 Meyer JF, McAllister CK, Godlberg LI. Insidious and prolonged antagonism of guanethidine by amitriptyline. J Am Med Ass (1970) 213, 1487.

7 Ober KF, Wang RIH. Drug interactions with guanethidine. Clin Pharmacol Ther (1973) 14, 190.

8 Smith AZJ and Bant WP. Interactions between post-ganglionic sympathetic blocking drugs and antidepressants. J Int Med Res (1975) 3, (Suppl 2) 55.

9 Oates JA, Fann WE, Cavanaugh JH. Effect of doxepin on the norepinephrine pump. A preliminary report. Psychosomatics (1969) 10 (Suppl), 12.

10 Skinner C, Coull DC, Johnston AW. Antagonism of the hypotensive action of bethanidine and debrisoquine by tricyclic antidepressants. Lancet (1969) ii, 564.

11 Briant RH, George CF. The assessment of potential drug interaction with a new tricyclic antidepressant drug. Br J clin Pharmac (1974) 1, 113.

12 Fann WE, Cavanaugh JH, Kaufmann JS, Griffith JD, Davis JM, Janowsky DS, Oates JA. Doxepin: effects on transport of biogenic amines in man. Psychopharmacologica (1971) 22, 111.

13 Gerson IM, Friedman R, Unterberg H. Non-antagonism of anti-adrenergic agents by dibenzoxepine (preliminary report). Dis Nerv Syst (1970) 31, 780.

14 Ayd FJ. Long-term administration of doxepin (Sinequan). Dis Nerv Syst (1971) 32, 617.

15 Ayd FJ. Doxepin with other drugs. South med J (1973) 66, 465.

16 Ayd FJ. Maintenance doxepin (Sinequan) therapy for depressive illness. Dis Nerv Syst (1975) 36, 109.

17 McQueen EG. New Zealand Committee on Adverse Reactions: Ninth Annual Report 1974. NZ Med J (1974) 80, 305.

18 Cocco G, Ague C. Interactions between cardioactive drugs and antidepressants. Eur J Clin Pharmacol (1977) 11, 389.

19 Cairncross KD. On the peripheral pharmacology of amitriptyline. Arch Int Pharmacodyn (1965) 154, 438.

20 La Corte WStJ, Ryan JR, McMahon FG, Jain AK, Ginzler F, Duncan W, Morley E. Titrating nortriptyline with bethanidine to eliminate the hypotensive effects in normal males. Clin Pharmacol Ther (1982) 31, 241.

21 Woosley RL, Stots B, Keele MD, Roden DM, Nies AM, Oates JA. Pharmacological reversal of hypotensive effect cnmplicating antiarrhythmic therapy with bretylium. Clin Pharmacol Ther (1982) 32, 313–21.

22 Poe TE, Edwards JL, Taylor RB. Hypertensive crisis possibly due to drug interaction. Postgrad Med (1979) 66, 235–7.

Guanethidine and related drugs + Tyramine-rich foods

Abstract/Summary

One study found no interaction between debrisoquine and tyramine, but a single case report describes a serious hypertensive reaction in a patient who ate 50 g Gruyére cheese.

Clinical evidence

(a) No interaction

A study in four hypertensive patients taking 40–60 mg debrisoquine daily showed that when they were given oral doses of tyramine in water only a moderate and unimportant increase in their sensitivity occurred. Intestinal MAO-activity remained unchanged.[1]

(b) Hypertensive reaction

A hypertensive woman, treated for a week with doses of debrisoquine progressively increased to 70 mg daily, was given 50 g Gruyére cheese to eat. Within 5 min her blood pressure had risen from 135/85 mmHg to 170/90 mmHg, and by the end of an hour it had climbed to 195/165 mmHg. It fell to 160/95 mmHg when 2 mg phentolamine was given, but rose again to 200/110 mmHg during the next hour.[2]

Mechanism

Not understood. Debrisoquine has some MAO-inhibitory activity but (unlike the antidepressant MAO-inhibitors) it appears not to affect the MAO in the gut wall so that tyramine is metabolized normally.[1,3] For a detailed account of the MAO-tyramine interaction see 'MAO Inhibitors + Tyramine-rich foods'. In the isolated case cited it may have been that the cheese contained particularly large amounts of tyramine which were absorbed through the mucosal lining of the mouth while being chewed. If this is what happened, the tyramine by-passed the liver and was able to release the noradrenaline from the adrenergic sympathetic neurones resulting in a rise in blood pressure.

Importance and management

Information seems to be limited to the reports cited. The absence of other reports of a hypertensive reaction would seem to be a measure of its rarity. Prescribers may feel it prudent to warn their patients about tyramine-rich foods. A list of these is to be found in the synopsis 'MAO Inhibitors + Tyramine-rich foods'. No interaction would be expected with the other guanethidine-like drugs.

References

1 Pettinger WA, Korn A, Spiegel H, Solomon HM, Pocelinko R, Abrams WB. Debrisoquin, a selective inhibitor of intraneuronal monoamine oxidase in man. Clin Pharmacol Ther (1969) 10, 667.

2 Amery A, Deloof W. Cheese reaction during debrisoquine treatment. Lancet (1970) ii, 613.

3 Pettinger WA, Horst WD. Quantifying metabolic effects of antihypertensive and other drugs at the sympathetic neuron level: clinical and basic correlations. Ann NY Acad Sci (1971) 179, 310.

Guanfacine + Tricyclic antidepressants

Abstract/Summary

A single report describes a reduced antihypertensive response to guanfacine in a patient given amitriptyline and later imipramine.

Clinical evidence

A woman of 38 with hypertension, well controlled with 2 mg

guanfacine daily, showed a rise in her blood pressure from 138/89 mmHg to 150/100 mmHg after taking 75 mg amitriptyline daily for 7–14 days. The pressure fell again when the amitriptyline was stopped. A month later her blood pressure rose to 142/98 mmg Hg after taking 50 mg imipramine daily for two days, and fell again when it was stopped.[1]

Mechanism

Uncertain. A possible reason is, that like clonidine (another alpha-2 agonist), the uptake of guanfacine into neurones within the brain is blocked by tricyclic antidepressants, thereby reducing its effects.

Importance and management

Direct information is limited to this report, but it is supported by animal studies[2] and consistent with the way another alpha-2 agonist (clonidine) interacts with tricyclic antidepressants (see 'Clonidine + Tricyclic antidepressants'). Be alert for this interaction in any patient given guanfacine and any tricyclic antidepressant. Guanabenz is another alpha-2 agonist which might interact similarly, but as yet there is no direct clinical evidence that it does so.

References

1 Buckley M and Feeley J. Antagonism of antihypertensive effect of guanfacine by tricyclic antidepressants. Lancet (1991) 337, 1173–4.
2 Ohkubo K, Suzuki K, Oguma T, Otorii T. Central hypotensive effects of guanfacine in anaesthetised rabbits. Nippon Yakarigaku Zasshi (1982) 79, 263–74.

Hydralazine + Indomethacin or Diclofenac

Abstract/Summary

It is uncertain whether indomethacin does or does not reduce or abolish the hypotensive effects of hydralazine, whereas diclofenac appears to oppose dihydralazine.

Clinical evidence, mechanism, importance and management

After taking 200 mg indomethacin, the hypotensive response to 0.15 mg/kg hydralazine given intravenously to normal subjects was abolished, and the subjects only responded when given another dose 30 min later.[1] In contrast another study, also in normal subjects, found that 100 mg indomethacin did not affect the hypotensive response to 0.2 mg/kg hydralazine given intravenously.[2] Thus it is not clear if indomethacin interacts with hydralazine given intravenously, and equally uncertain if an interaction occurs when hydralazine is given orally. On the other hand a study in four hypertensive subjects found that the actions of dihydralazine (hypotensive, urinary excretion, heart

rate, sodium clearance) are reduced by diclofenac.[3] Concurrent use should be monitored.

References

1 Cinquegrani MP, Liang C-s. Indomethacin attenuates the hypotensive action of hydralazine. Clin Pharmacol Ther (1986) 39, 564–70.
2 Jackson SHD and Pickles H. Indomethacin does not attenuate the effects of hydralazine in normal subjects. Eur J Clin Pharmacol (1983) 25, 303–5.
3 Reimann IW, Ratge D, Wisser H, Frohlich JC. Are prostaglandins involved in the antihypertensive effect of dihydralazine? Clin Sci (1981) 61, 319–21S.

Indoramin + Alcohol

Abstract/Summary

The serum levels of both indoramin and alcohol may be raised by concurrent use. The increased drowsiness may possibly increase the risk of driving.

Clinical evidence

A double-blind study in 10 normal subjects given 50 mg indoramin and 0.5 g/kg alcohol in 600 ml alcohol-free lager showed that the AUC (area under the curve) of the indoramin was increased by 25% and the peak levels raised by 58%. When given alcohol intravenously (0.175 mg/kg) the indoramin caused a 26% rise in blood alcohol levels during the first hour-and-a-quarter after dosing. Both alcohol and indoramin caused sedation[1,2]

Mechanism

Uncertain. Increased absorption of the indoramin from the gut or reduced liver metabolism may be responsible for the raised indoramin serum levels.

Importance and management

Information is limited but the interactions appear to be established. The clinical importance of the raised serum indoramin and alcohol levels is uncertain, however since indoramin sometimes causes drowsiness when it is first given, there is the possibility that alertness will be reduced which could increase the risks of driving or handling other machinery. Patients should be warned. More study is needed.

References

1 Abrams SML, Pierce DM, Franklin RA, Johnston A, Marrott PK, Cory EP, Turner P. Effect of ethanol on indoramin pharmacokinetics. Br J clin Pharmac (1984) 18, 294P.
2 Abrams SM, Pierce DM, Johnston A, Hedges A, Franklin RA, Turner P. Pharmacokinetic interaction between indoramin and ethanol. Hum Toxicol (1989) 8, 237–41.

Ketanserin + Beta-blockers

Abstract/Summary

The pharmacokinetics of neither drug appears to be affected by the presence of the other but additive hypotensive effects may occur. Very marked and acute hypotension has been seen in two patients on atenolol when first given ketanserin.

Clinical evidence, mechanism, importance and management

A study in six patients and two normal subjects given ketanserin (40 mg thrice daily for three weeks) showed that the concurrent use of propranolol (80 mg twice daily for six days) did not significantly alter the steady-state serum levels of ketanserin.[1] Another study on normal subjects, using single doses of both drugs, showed that the pharmacokinetics of neither drug was affected by the presence of the other.[3] The hypotensive effects of the ketanserin were slightly increased by the propranolol in the study already cited[1] and additive hypotensive effects were seen in a study in patients with essential hypertension.[2] Acute hypotension is reported to have occurred in two patients taking atenolol within an hour of additionally being given a 40 mg oral dose of ketanserin. One of them briefly lost consciousness.[4] Concurrent use can be valuable and uneventful but a few patients may experience marked hypotensive effects when first given ketanserin. Patients should be warned. Information about other beta-blockers seems not to be available.

References

1 Trenk D, Luh A, Radkow N, Jahnchen E. Lack of effect of propranolol on the steady-state plasma levels of ketanserin. Arzneim-Forsch/Drug Res (1985) 35, 1286–8.
2 Hedner T, Persson B. Antihypertensive properties of ketanserin in combination with beta-adrenergic blocking agents. J Cardiovasc Pharmac (1985) 7 (Suppl 7) S161–3.
3 Williams FM, Leeser JE, Rawlins MD. Pharmacodynamics and pharmacokinetics of single doses of ketanserin and propranolol alone and in combination in healthy volunteers. Br J clin Pharmac (1986) 22, 301–8.
4 Waller PC, Cameron HA, Ramsey LE. Profound hypotension after the first dose of ketanserin. Postgrad Med J (1987) 63, 305–7.

Ketanserin + Diuretics

Abstract/Summary

Sudden deaths, probably from heart rhythym abnormalities, are markedly increased in patients taking potassium-losing diuretics if they are concurrently treated with high doses of ketanserin. Potassium-sparing diuretics do not appear to interact in this way and no interaction seems to occur with low doses of ketanserin.

Clinical evidence, mechanism, importance and management

A large multi-national study[1]involving 3899 patients found that a harmful and potentially fatal interaction could occur in those given ketanserin (40 mg three times daily) and potassium-losing diuretics. 35 of 249 patients on both drugs died (16 suddenly) compared with only 15 of 260 (five suddenly) taking a placebo and potassium-losing diuretics. No significant increase in the number of deaths occurred in those on ketanserin and potassium-sparing diuretics.

The reason for the deaths seems to be that the ketanserin accentuates and exaggerates the harmful effects of the potassium-losing diuretics on the heart which can worsen arrhythmias. It was found that the corrected QT interval of the heart was prolonged as follows: ketanserin alone (18 ms), ketanserin + potassium-sparing diuretics (24 ms), ketanserin + potassium-losing diuretics (30 ms). In some individuals this can apparently have a fatal outcome. A later study on 33 patients using a smaller dose of ketanserin (20 mg twice daily) with potassium-losing diuretics (frusemide, thiazides) found no evidence that this dose prolonged the QT_c interval.[2] The pharmacokinetics of ketanserin are not altered by single doses of hydrochlorothiazide.[3] Potassium-losing diuretics (thiazides, frusemide, etc.) with relatively high doses of ketanserin (40 mg three times daily) should be avoided but lower doses seem to be safe. Potassium-sparing diuretics (amiloride, triamterene, etc.) also seem to be safe even with the higher dose of ketanserin.

Reference

1 Prevention of Atherosclerotic Complications with Ketanserin Trial Group. Prevention of atherosclerotic complications: controlled trial of ketanserin. Br Med J (1989) 298, 424–30.
2 Van Gool R, Symoens J. Ketanserin in combination with diuretics: effect on QT_c interval. Eur Heart J (1990) 11, (Suppl) 57.
3 Botha JH, McFadyen ML, Leary WPP, Janssen M. No effect of single-dose hydrochlorothiazide on the pharmacokinetics of single-dose ketanserin. Curr Ther Res (1991) 49, 225–30.

Ketanserin + Miscellaneous drugs

Abstract/Summary

Ketanserin should not be given with certain antiarrhythmics, naftidrofuryl or tricyclic antidepressants because of the risk of potentially serious heart disturbances. Drowsiness and dizziness are common side-effects which may possibly be additive with the effects of other CNS depressants.

Clinical evidence, mechanism, importance and management

Ketanserin has weak class-III antiarrhythmic activity and can prolong the QT_c interval. For safety reasons it has therefore been advised that it should be avoided in patients with existing QT_c prolongation, atrioventricular of sinoauricular block of higher degree, or severe bradycardia (<50 beats/min).[1] For the same reason the concurrent use of drugs which affect repolarization (antiarrhythmics of classes Ia, Ic, III) or those which cause conduction disturbances (naftidrofuryl, tricyclic antidepressants) should be avoided.[1] Dizziness and drowsiness are common side-effects and therefore it seems likely that these will be additive with other CNS depressants and alcohol which may possibly make driving more hazardous. This needs confirmation.

Reference

1 Distler A. Clinical aspects during therapy with the serotonin antagonist ketanserin. Clin Physiol Biochem (1990) 8 (suppl 3) 64–80.

Ketanserin + Nifedipine

Abstract/Summary

A few elderly patients given ketanserin and nifedipine may experience an increase in heart arrhythmias.

Clinical evidence, mechanism, importance and management

A study in 20 normal subjects aged 60 or more, with normal or slightly raised blood pressures, found that the concurrent use of ketanserin and nifedipine for a week did not, on average, affect their blood pressures, heart rates, or the QT intervals, but two of the subjects monitored over 24 h showed a marked increase in the frequency of ectopic beats, couplets and ventricular tachycardia.[1] The reasons are not understood. The authors of this study say that their findings do not exclude the possibility that the combined use of these two drugs might therefore increase arrhythmia in some elderly patients.[1] Concurrent use in the elderly should be monitored.

Reference

1 Alberio L, Beretta-Piccoli C, Tanzi F, Koch P, Zehender M. Kardiale Interaktionen zwischen Ketanserin und dem Calcium-Antagonisten Nifedipin. Schweiz Med Wochenschr (1992) 122, 1723–7.

Methyldopa + Barbiturates

Abstract/Summary

The effects of methyldopa are not altered by the use of phenobarbitone.

Clinical evidence, mechanism, importance and management

Indirect evidence from one study in man suggested that phenobarbitone could reduce methyldopa levels,[1] but later work

which directly measured the blood levels of methyldopa failed to find any evidence of an interaction.[2]

References

1 Kaldor A, Juvancz P, Demeczky M, Sebestynen and Palotas J. Enhancement of methyldopa metabolism with barbiturate. Br Med J (1971) 3, 518.
2 Kristensen M, Jorgensen M, Hansen T. Plasma concentration of alphamethyldopa and its main metabolite, methyldopa-O-sulphate, during long term treatment with alphamethyldopa with special reference to possible interaction with other drugs given simultaneously. Clin Pharmacol Ther (1973) 14, 139.

Methyldopa + Cephalosporins

Abstract/Summary

Two reports describe the development of pustular eruptions in two women taking methyldopa when they were given cephradine or cefazolin.

Clinical evidence, mechanism, importance and management

A black woman aged 74 on methyldopa and insulin developed pruritis on her arms and legs within 2 h of starting to take cephradine. Over the next two days fever and a widespread pustular eruption developed.[1] Another black woman of 65 on methyldopa and frusemide experienced severe pruritis within 8 h of starting to take 1 g cefazolin sodium every 12 h. Over the next two days superficial and coalescing pustules appeared on her trunk, arms and legs.[2] The reasons are not understood. There seem to be no other reports of this reaction. The concurrent use of methyldopa may possibly have been purely coincidental.

References

1 Kalb RE, Grossman ME. Pustular eruption following administration of cephradine. Cutis (1986) 38, 58–60.
2 Stough D, Guin JD, Baker GF, Haynie L. Pustular eruptions following administration of cefazolin: a possible interaction with methyldopa. J Amer Acad Dermatol (1987) 16, 1051–2.

Methyldopa + Disulfiram

Abstract/Summary

An isolated report describes a patient whose hypertension failed to respond to methyldopa in the presence of disulfiram.

Clinical evidence, mechanism, importance and management

The hypertension of an alcoholic patient on disulfiram failed to respond to moderate to high doses of intravenous methyldopa, but did so when given oral low dose clonidine. The postulated reason is that disulfiram blocks the activity of dopamine beta-hydroxylase, the enzyme responsible for the conversion of the methyldopa to its active form.[1] The general importance of this alleged interaction is uncertain.

Reference

1 McCord RW, LaCorte WS. Hypertension refactory to methyldopa in a disulfiram-treated patient. Clin Res (1984) 32, 923A.

Methyldopa + Haloperidol

Abstract/Summary

Three cases of dementia have been attributed to the use of methyldopa and haloperidol, but concurrent use without serious problems has also been described.

Clinical evidence

Two patients on long term treatment with methyldopa (1–1.5 g daily) without problems developed a dementia syndrome (mental retardation, loss of memory, disorientation, etc.) within three days of starting to take 6–8 mg haloperidol daily. The symptoms cleared within 72 h of withdrawing the haloperidol.[1] Another patient treated with these drugs showed severe irritability and aggressive behaviour.[3]

Mechanism

Not understood. Among the side-effects of methyldopa relevant to this interaction are sedation, depression and dementia; and of haloperidol, drowsiness, dizziness and depression.

Importance and management

These three cases must be viewed alongside another report of a 4-week trial in 10 schizophrenics given 500 mg methyldopa and 10 mg haloperidol daily. Among the important side-effects were somnolence (eight patients) and dizziness (six patients) but no serious interaction of the kind described above.[2] Concurrent use need not be avoided but it would be prudent to be on the alert for the development of adverse effects.

References

1 Thornton WE. Dementia induced by methyldopa with haloperidol. N Engl J Med (1976) 243, 1222.
2 Chouinard G, Pinard G, Serrano M, Tetreault L. Potentiation of haloperidol by alpha-methyldopa in the treatment of schizophrenic patients. Curr Ther Res (1973) 15, 473.
3 Nadel I, Wallach M. Drug interaction between haloperidol and methyldopa. Br J Psychiatry (1979) 135, 484.

Methyldopa + Iron salts

Abstract/Summary

The antihypertensive effects of methyldopa can be reduced by the concurrent use of ferrous sulphate. Ferrous gluconate appears to interact similarly.

Clinical evidence

Arising out of a metabolic study of the interaction between methyldopa and ferrous sulphate, five hypertensive patients who had been taking 500–1500 mg methyldopa daily for more than a year were additionally given 325 mg ferrous sulphate three times daily. After 2 weeks the blood pressures of all of them had risen. The systolic pressures of three of them had risen by more than 15 mmHg. Four had diastolic pressure rises, two of them exceeding 10 mmHg.[1] Reductions of 88% and 79% in the renal excretion of unmetabolized methyldopa were seen when methyldopa was given with ferrous sulphate and ferrous gluconate respectively.[1] Another study found that if the ferrous sulphate is given at the same time, or 1 h or 2 h before the methyldopa, the bioavailability is reduced 83%, 55% and 42% respectively.[2]

Mechanism

Uncertain. One suggestion is that the iron chelates or complexes with the methyldopa in the gut, thereby reducing its absorption (reduced 50%).[1,3] The increase in the metabolic sulphonation of the methyldopa also seems to have a part to play.

Importance and management

Information is limited and this interaction is as yet unconfirmed but it appears to be clinically important. Monitor the effects of concurrent use and increase the methyldopa dosage as necessary. Separating the dosages by up to 2 h apparently only partially reduces the effects of this interaction. Ferrous gluconate appears to interact like ferrous sulphate.

References

1 Campbell N, Paddock V, Sundaram R. Alteration of methyldopa absorption, metabolism, and blood pressure control caused by ferrous sulphate and ferrous gluconate. Clin Pharmacol Ther (1988) 43, 381–6.
2 Campbell NRC, Hasinoff BB. Iron supplements: a common cause of drug interactions. Br J clin Pharmac (1991) 31, 251–55.
3 Campbell NRC, Campbell RRA, Hasinoff BB. Ferrous sulfate reduces methyldopa absorption: methyldopa: iron complex formation as a likely mechanism. Clin Invest Med (1990) 13, 329–32.

Methyldopa + Oxazepam

Abstract/Summary

A single case report suggests that blood pressure control in essential hypertension with methyldopa may possibly be made more difficult in the presence of oxazepam.

Clinical evidence, mechanism, importance and management

It was found difficult to establish good blood pressure control in a 54-year-old woman with insomnia and essential hypertension even when given 750 mg methyldopa daily and a thiazide diuretic. She was also a moderate drinker. Within a week of stopping 60 mg oxazepam nightly, she developed grand mal convulsions and hypertension (190/90 mmHg standing, 240/140 mmHg lying) but was eventually discharged, and remained very well controlled, on atenolol and prazosin. The authors of this report suggest that short-acting benzodiazepines such as oxazepam, plus alcohol, may possibly exacerbate essential hypertension and its management.[1] The general importance of this possible interaction is not established.

Reference

1 Stokes GS. Can short-acting benzodiazepines exacerbate essential hypertension? Cardiovasc Rev Rep (1989) 10, 60–1.

Methyldopa + Phenoxybenzamine

Abstract/Summary

An isolated case report describes total urinary incontinence in a patient treated with methyldopa and phenoxybenzamine after bilateral lumbar sympathectomy.

Clinical evidence, mechanism, importance and management

A woman who had previously had bilateral lumbar sympathectomy for Reynauds disease developed total urinary incontinence when given 500–1500 mg methyldopa and 12.5 mg phenoxybenzamine daily, but not with either drug alone. This would seem to be the outcome of the additive effects of the sympathectomy and the two drugs on the sympathetic control of the bladder sphincters.[1] Stress incontinence has previously been described with these drugs. The general importance of this interaction is probably small.

Reference

1 Fernandez PG, Shani S, Galway BA, Granter S, McDonald J. Urinary incontinence due to interaction of phenoxybenzamine and alpha-methyldopa. Can Med Ass J (1981) 124, 174.

Methyldopa + Sympathomimetics (indirectly-acting)

Abstract/Summary

Indirectly-acting sympathomimetics might be expected to cause a blood pressure rise in patients taking methyldopa, and an isolated case report describes such a reaction in a patient taking methyldopa and oxprenolol when he took a decongestant containing phenylpropanolamine, but in practice this interaction normally seems to be of little or no general practical importance. The mydriatic effects of ephedrine are reported to be depressed by methyldopa.

Clinical evidence, mechanism, importance and management

Studies in man have shown that after taking 2–3 g methyldopa daily, the pressor (rise in blood pressure) effects of tyramine were doubled.[1] In another study the pressor rise was 50/16 mmHg compared with 18/10 before methyldopa treatment.[2] A man with renal hypertension, whose blood pressure was well controlled with 500 mg methyldopa and 480 mg oxprenolol daily, showed a rise in blood pressure from about 120–140/70–80 mmHg to 200/150 mmHg within two days of starting to take two tablets of Triogesic (phenylpropanolamine 12.5 mg and paracetamol 500 mg) three times a day. His blood pressure fell when the Triogesic was withdrawn.[4] The reason for this is uncertain. One suggestion is that the methyldopa causes the replacement of noradrenaline (epinephrine) at adrenergic nerve endings by methyl-noradrenaline which has weaker pressor (alpha) activity but greater vasodilator (beta) activity. With the vasodilator activity blocked by the oxprenolol, the vasoconstrictor activity (pressor) of the phenylpropanolamine would be unopposed and exaggerated. Despite the information derived from the studies outlined above[1,2] and the single report cited, there seems to be nothing else in the literature to suggest that indirectly-acting sympathomimetics normally cause an adverse reaction (rise in blood pressure) with methyldopa. More study is needed. One report states that the normal mydriatic effects of ephedrine are depressed by methyldopa.[3]

References

1 Pettinger W, Horwitz D, Spector S, Sjoerdsma A. Enhancement by methyldopa of tyramine sensitivity in man. Nature (1963) 200, 1107.

2 Dollery CT, Harrington M, Hodge JV. Haemodynamic studies with methyldopa: effect on cardiac output and response to pressor amines. Br Heart J (1963) 25, 670.

3 Sneddon JM, Turner P. Ephedrine mydriasis in hypertension and the response to treatment. Clin Pharmacol Ther (1969) 10, 64.

4 McLaren EH. Severe hypertension produced by interaction of phenylpropanolamine with methyldopa and oxprenolol. Br Med J (1976) 3, 283.

Methyldopa + Tricyclic antidepressants

Abstract/Summary

The antihypertensive effects of methyldopa are not normally adversely affected by the concurrent use of desipramine but an isolated report describes hypertension, tachycardia, tremor and agitation in man on methyldopa when additionally treated with amitriptyline.

Clinical evidence

A hypertensive man, controlled on 700 mg methyldopa daily with a diuretic, experienced tremor, agitation, tachycardia (148 beats/min) and hypertension (a rise from 120–150/80–90 mmHg to 170/110 mmHg) within 10 days of starting to take 75 mg amitriptyline daily. A week after stopping the amitriptyline his pulse rate was 100 and his blood pressure 160/90 mmHg.[1] In contrast, a double-blind cross-over study in five volunteers (one with mild hypertension) found that 75 mg desipramine daily for three days had no significant effect on the hypotensive effects of single 750 mg doses of methyldopa.[5] Another study in three hypertensive patients on methyldopa (2.5–3.0 g daily) found that when given 75 mg desipramine daily for 5–6 days, the blood pressure (diastolic + one-third pulse pressure) fell by 5 mmHg.[2]

Mechanism

Not understood. Antagonism of the antihypertensive actions of methyldopa by tricyclic antidepressants is seen in animals and it seems to occur within the brain, possibly within the rhombencephalon.[3,4]

Importance and management

Normally no adverse interaction occurs, nevertheless it would seem prudent to monitor the effects of concurrent use if amitriptyline or any other tricyclic antidepressant is given to patients on methyldopa. Methyldopa sometimes induces depression so that it may not be the best choice of antihypertensive in depressed patients.

References

1 White AG. Methyldopa and amitriptyline. Lancet (1965) ii, 441.
2 Mitchell JR, Cavanaugh JH, Arias L and Oates JA. Guanethidine and related agents. III. Antagonism by drugs which inhibit the norepinephrine pump in man. J Clin Invest (1970) 49, 1596.
3 Van Spanning HW and van Zwieten PA. The interaction between alpha-methyldopa and tricyclic antidepressants. Int J Clin Pharmacol (1975) 11, 65.
4 Van Zwieten PA. Interaction between centrally acting hypotensive drugs and tricyclic antidepressants. Arch Int Pharmacodyn Ther (1975) 214, 12.
5 Reid JL, Porsius AJ, Zambulis C, Polak G, Hamilton CA, Dean CR. The effects of desmethylimipramine on the pharmacological actions of alpha-methyldopa in man. Eur J Clin Pharmacol (1979) 16, 75.

Piretanide + Miscellaneous drugs

Abstract/Summary

The urinary excretion of sodium due to piretanide is reduced by probenecid and indomethacin, but not by piroxicam.

Clinical evidence, mechanism, importance and management

A comparative study into the pharmacological mechanisms underlying the way drugs interfere with the actions of loop diuretics found that 1 g probenecid, 50 mg indomethacin and 20 mg piroxicam reduced the peak fractional excretion of sodium due to piretanide (6 mg orally) by 65%, 35% and 0% respectively.[1] Another study confirmed that probenecid reduces the natriuretic effects of piretanide.[2] The clinical importance of these changes was not studied, but it would now seem prudent to check the effectiveness of piretanide in the presence of either probenecid or indomethacin.

Reference

1 Dixey JJ, Noormohamed FH, Pawa JS, Lant AF, Brewerton DA. The influence of nonsteroidal anti-inflammatory drugs and probenecid on the renal response to and kinetics of piretanide in man. Clin Pharmacol Ther (1988) 44, 531–9.
2 Noormohamed FQ, Lant AF. Analysis of the natriuretic action of a loop diuretic, piretanide, in man. Br J clin Pharmac (1991) 31, 463–9.

Prazosin + Beta-blockers

Abstract/Summary

Prazosin causes some patients to faint when they first start treatment. It is more likely to occur if the patient is already taking a beta-blocker.

Clinical evidence

Some patients experience acute postural hypotension, tachycardia and palpitations when they begin to take prazosin. A few even collapse in a sudden faint within 30–90 min and this can be exacerbated if they are already taking beta-blockers. Three out of six hypertensive patients on 0.8 mg alprenolol daily experienced this 'first dose' hypotensive reaction when given 0.5 mg prazosin. Other patients already taking prazosin showed no unusual fall in blood pressure when given the first of several doses of alprenolol.[1] The severity and the duration of this 'first dose' response was also found to be increased in normal subjects taking propranolol or primidolol when they were given prazosin.[2] The pharmacokinetics of prazosin are not affected by either atenolol[1] or propranolol.[3]

Mechanism

The normal cardiovascular response (increased heart output and rate) which should follow the first dose hypotensive reaction to prazosin is apparently compromised by the presence of a beta-blocker. The problem is usually only short-lasting because, within hours or days, some physiological compensation occurs which allows the blood pressure to be lowered without falling precipitously.

Importance and management

An established interaction. It has been recommended that those already on beta-blockers should begin with less than 0.5 mg prazosin.[1] They should also be told what may happen and what to do. Giving the first dose just before going to bed is a sensible precaution. No particular precautions seem necessary in patients already taking prazosin who are additionally given beta-blockers.

References

1 Seideman P, Grahnen A, Haglund K, Lindstrom B and von Bah C. Prazosin first dose phenomenon during combined treatment with a beta-adrenoceptor in hypertensive patients. Br J clin Pharmacol (1982) 13, 865–70.
2 Elliott HL, McLean K, Sumner DJ, Meredith PA, Reid JL. Immediate cardiovascular reponses to oral prazosin-effects of beta-blockers. Clin Pharmacol Ther (1981) 29, 303–9.
3 Rubin P, Jackson G, Blaschke T. Studies on the clinical pharmacology of prazosin. II: The influence of indomethacin and of propranolol on the action and the disposition of prazosin. Br J clin Pharmacol (1980) 10, 33–9.

Rauwolfia alkaloids + Tricyclic antidepressants

Abstract/Summary

The rauwolfia alkaloids cause depression and are not usually used in patients needing treatment for depression, but there are a few reports of their successful use in some resistant forms of depression when combined with the tricyclic antidepressants.

Clinical evidence, mechanism, importance and management

Depression and sedation are among the very well-recognized side-effects of rauwolfia treatment. For example, out of a total of 270 patients given treatment for hypertension with rauwolfia, 23% developed depressive episodes within seven months of starting treatment.[1] Animals treated with reserpine have been widely used by pharmacologists as experimental models of depression when testing the effectiveness of new compounds with potential antidepressant activity. The rauwolfia alkaloids cause adrenergic (noradrenaline-releasing) and serotoninergic (5-HT-releasing) neurones to become depleted of their normal stores of neurotransmitter, the result being that very reduced amounts are available for release by nerve impulses. Because of

this action at adrenergic sympathetic nerve endings the blood pressure falls. The brain possesses both types of neurone and failure in transmission is believed to be responsible for the sedation and depression which can occur. However one study describes 14 out of 15 patients with endogenous depression resistant to imipramine who responded well when given up to 300 mg imipramine and 7.5–10.0 mg reserpine daily after an initial manic response.[2] Other reports describe the use of reserpine with desipramine[3,5] and imipramine[4] although the authors of the latter question the advantages claimed by other workers. However, in general, concurrent use should be avoided. Only in well-controlled situations and with patients unresponsive to other forms of treatment should this combination be used.

References

1 Bolte E, Marc-Aurele J, Brouillet J, Beauregard P, Verdy M, Genest J. Mental depressive episodes during rauwolfia therapy for arterial hypertension with special reference to dosage. Can Med Ass J (1959) 80, 291.
2 Haskovec L and Rysanek K. The action of reserpine in imipramine-resistant depressive patients. A clinical and biochemical study. Psychopharmacologica (1967) 11, 18.
3 Poldinger W. Combined administration of desipramine and reserpine or tetrabenazine in depressed patients. Psychopharmacologia (1963) 4, 308.
4 Carney MWP, Thakurdas H, Sebastian J. Effects of imipramine and reserpine in depression. Psychopharmacologia (1969) 14, 349.
5 Amsterdam JD, Berwish N. Treatment of refractory depression with combination reserpine and tricyclic antidepressant therapy. J Clin Psychopharmacol (1987) 7, 238–42.

Spironolactone + Aspirin and Salicylates

Abstract/Summary

The antihypertensive effects of spironolactone are unaffected by the concurrent use of aspirin in patients with hypertension, although there is evidence that the spironolactone-induced loss of sodium in the urine is reduced in normal subjects.

Clinical evidence

(a) Effects in hypertensive patients

Five patients with low-renin essential hypertension, well-controlled for four months or more with 100–300 mg spironolactone daily, were examined in a double blind crossover trial. Daily doses of aspirin of 2.4 to 4.8 g given over six-week periods had no effect on blood pressure, serum electrolytes, body weight, urea nitrogen or plasma renin activity.[4]

(b) Effects in normal subjects

A six-week crossover study in 10 normal subjects given single 25, 50 and 100 mg doses of spironolactone showed that 600 mg of aspirin reduced the urinary excretion of electrolyte. The effectiveness of the spironolactone was reduced 70%, and the overnight sodium excretion reduced by a third in seven of

10 subjects given 25 mg spironolactone daily and a single 600 mg dose of aspirin.[1] Reductions in sodium excretion are described in other studies.[2,3] In one of these the sodium excretion was completely abolished when aspirin was given one-and-a-half hours after the spironolactone, but only partially reduced when administered in the reverse order.[3]

Mechanism

Uncertain. There is evidence that the active secretion of canrenone (the active metabolite of spironolactone) is blocked by aspirin, but the significance of this is not entirely clear.[2]

Importance and management

An adequately but not extensively documented interaction. Despite the results of the studies in normal subjects, the study in hypertensive patients shows that the blood pressure lowering effects of spironolactone are not affected by aspirin. Concurrent use need not be avoided, but it would be prudent nonetheless to monitor the response to confirm that no adverse interaction is taking place.

References

1 Tweedale MG, Ogilvie RI. Antagonism of spironolactone-induced natriuresis by aspirin in man. N Engl J Med (1973) 289, 198.
2 Ramsay LE, Harrison IR, Shelton JR, Vose CW. Influence of acetylsalicylic acid on the renal handling of a spironolactone metabolite in healthy subjects. Eur J clin Pharmacol (1976) 10, 43.
3 Elliott HC. Reduced adrenocortical steroid excretion rates in man following aspirin administration. Metabolism (1962) 11, 1015.
4 Hollifield JW. Failure of aspirin to antagonize the antihypertensive effect of spironolactone in low-renin hypertension. South Med J (1976) 69, 1034.

Spironolactone + Dextropropoxyphene

Abstract/Summary

A single case report describes the development of gynecomastia and a rash in a man on spironolactone when he was given dextropropoxyphene.

Clinical evidence, mechanism, importance and management

A patient who had been taking spironolactone uneventfully for four years developed swollen and tender breasts and a rash on his chest and neck a fortnight after starting to take *Darvon*, a compound preparation containing dextropropoxyphene, aspirin, phenacetin and caffeine. The problem disappeared when both drugs were withdrawn but the rash reappeared when the *Darvon* alone was given. It disappeared again when it was withdrawn. No problems occurred when the spironolactone was given alone, but both the rash and the gynecomastia recurred when the *Darvon* was added.[1] The reasons for this reaction are not understood. Gynecomastia is a known side-

effect of spironolactone (incidence 1.2%). The authors of this report reasonably surmise that the dextropropoxyphene component of *Darvon* was responsible in some way. Concurrent use need not be avoided but prescribers should be aware of this case.

Reference

1 Licata AA, Bartter FC. Spironolactone-induced gynecomastia related to allergic reaction to 'darvon compound'. Lancet (1976) ii, 905.

Terazosin + Calcium channel blockers

Abstract/Summary

The antihypertensive effects of terazosin and verapamil are additive. Early in treatment some patients may experience faintness when they stand up.

Clinical evidence, mechanism, importance and management

A three week study in 24 hypertensive patients found that when 120 mg verapamil daily was added to treatment with 1-5 mg terazosin, the peak serum levels and the AUC of the terazosin were increased 24–25%.[1] A related study by the same group confirmed that concurrent use increased the antihypertensive effects and found that orthostasis was more common when the verapamil was first added to terazosin.[2] In addition to the warning and advice about 'first dose collapse' with terazosin ('take it at bedtime'), patients should be told that early in treatment they may also feel faint and dizzy when they stand up.

References

1 Varghese A, Lenz M, Locke C, Granneman R. Laddue A. Pool J, Piwinski S, Taylor A. Combined terazosin and verapamil therapy in essential hypertension: pharmacokinetic interactions. Clin Pharmacol Ther (1991) 49, 130.
2 Lenz M, Varghese A, Pool J, Laddu A, Johnston W, Piwinski S, Taylor A. Combined terazosin and verapamil therapy in essential hypertension: hemodynamic interactions. Clin Pharmacol Ther (1991) 49, 146.

Thiazides + Cholestyramine or Colestipol

Abstract/Summary

The absorption of hydrochlorothiazide from the gut can be reduced by a third if colestipol is given concurrently, and two-thirds by cholestyramine. The diuretic effects are reduced accordingly. Separating the dosages of the thiazide and the cholestyramine by 4 h can reduce but not totally overcome the effects of this interaction.

Clinical evidence

The blood levels of the hydrochlorothiazide were reduced to about one-third in six subjects taking 8 g cholestyramine 2 min before and 6 and 12 h after a single 75 mg oral dose. Total urinary excretion fell to 15%. In a parallel study with 10 mg colestipol, the blood levels of the thiazide fell to about two-thirds and the total urinary excretion fell to 57%.[1] A further study showed that giving the cholestyramine 4 h after the hydrochlorothiazide reduced the effects of the interaction but the absorption was still reduced by a third.[3] Another study demonstrated a 42% reduction when using chlorothiazide and colestipol.[2]

Mechanism

Hydrochlorothiazide becomes bound to these non-absorbable anionic exchange resins within the gut, and less is available for absorption.

Importance and management

Established interactions of clinical importance. The best dosing schedule would appear to be to give the hydrochorothiazide 4 h before the cholestyramine to minimize mixing in the gut. Even so a one-third reduction in thiazide absorption occurs.[3] The optimum time-interval with colestipol has not been investigated but it would be reasonable to take similar precautions. Information about other thiazides is lacking although it seems likely that they will interact similarly.

References

1 Hunningshake DB, King S, La Croix K. The effect of cholestyramine and colestipol on the absorption of hydrochlorothiazide. Int J Clin Pharmacol Ther Toxicol (1982) 20, 151–4.
2 Kauffmann RE, Azarnoff DL. Effect of colestipol on gastrointestinal absorption of chlorothiazide in man. Clin Pharmacol Ther (1973) 14, 886.
3 Hunningshake DB, Hibbard DM. Influence of time intervals for cholestyramine dosing on the absorption of hydrochlorothiazide. Clin Pharmacol Ther (1986) 39, 329–34.

Thiazides + Indomethacin and other NSAIDs

Abstract/Summary

The antihypertensive effects of the thiazides can be reduced to some extent by indomethacin, but it appears to be of only moderate clinical importance and may possibly only be a transient interaction. Ibuprofen appears to interact to a lesser extent or not at all. No adverse interaction appears to occur with diclofenac, diflunisal, naproxen or sulindac.

Clinical evidence

(a) Thiazides + Indomethacin

A double-blind controlled trial in seven patients with hypertension on 5–10 mg bendrofluazide or amiloride 5 mg + hydrochlorothiazide 50 mg, found that additional treatment with 100 mg indomethacin daily for 3 weeks raised their systolic/diastolic blood pressures by 13/9 mmHg when lying and by 16/9 mmHg when standing. Body weight increased by 1.1 kg.[1] A later study found a 6/3 mmHg blood pressure rise in patients given indomethacin for 2 weeks which had gone after 4 weeks.[7] Only a 5/1 mmHg blood pressure rise was seen in another study in hypertensive patients on hydrochlorothiazide given 100 mg indomethacin daily,[4] whereas no significant changes in blood pressure were seen in healthy subjects.[3] 100 mg indomethacin was found to reduce the urinary excretion of sodium and chloride caused by bemetizide by 47 and 44% respectively in normal subjects,[5] but it had no effect on the sodium excretion caused by hydrochlorothiazide.[2] Indomethacin does not affect the pharmacokinetics of hydrochlorothiazide.[2,3]

(b) Thiazides + Other NSAIDs

375 mg diflunisal twice daily caused the plasma levels of hydrochlorothiazide to rise by 25–30%, but this appears to be clinically unimportant.[8,9] Diflunisal also has uricosuric activity which counteracts the uric acid retention which occurs with hydrochlorothiazide. Diclofenac, sulindac and naproxen do not reduce either the hypotensive or diuretic effects of hydrochlorothiazide, and may even slightly enhance the antihypertensive effects.[4,6,7,10] Another study found that diclofenac and sulindac do not affect blood pressures controlled with *Moduretic* (hydrochlorothiazide + amiloride) and beta-blockers.[15] Ibuprofen (1200 mg daily) caused a small rise in systolic but not in diastolic pressures in one study,[10] but not in another involving bendrofluazide.[11] Another study found that 1200 mg ibuprofen daily had no effect on blood pressures controlled by triameterene-hydrochlorothiazide, although one patient showed a marked fall in kidney function.[14] 3200 mg ibuprofen daily for a week had little effect on blood pressures controlled with hydrochlorothiazide in yet another study.[13] Both ibuprofen and diclofenac can cause a weight rise.[10]

Mechanism

Not understood. Since the prostaglandins have a role to play in kidney function, drugs such as the NSAIDs which inhibit their synthesis might be expected to have some effect on the actions of diuretics whose effects also depend on the activity of the prostaglandins. A study in rats suggested that indomethacin may oppose the thiazides by reducing chloride delivery to the site of thiazide action in the distal tubule.[12]

Importance and management

The thiazide-indomethacin interaction is well documented although the findings are not entirely consistent. It seems to be of only moderate clinical importance but the effects of concurrent use should be monitored and the thiazide dosage modified if necessary. Ibuprofen interacts to a lesser extent or not at all, and no adverse interaction appears to occur with diclofenac, naproxen, sulindac or diflunisal. The uricosuric effects of diflunisal may be usefully exploited to counteract the uric acid retention which occurs with hydrochlorothiazide. The effects of other NSAIDs do not seem to have been studied.

References

1 Watkins J, Abbott EC, Hensby CN, Webster J, Dollery CT. Attenuation of hypotensive effect of propranolol and thiazide diuretics by indomethacin. Br Med J (1980) 281, 702–5.
2 Williams RL, Davies RO, Berman RS, Holmes GI, Huber P, Gee WL, Lin ET, Benet LZ. Hydrochlorothiazide pharmacokinetics and pharmacologic effect: the influence of indomethacin. J Clin Pharmacol (1982) 22, 32–41.
3 Koopmans PP, Wim GPM, Tan Y, van Ginneken CAM and Gribnau FWJ. Effects of indomethacin and sulindac on hydrochlorothiazide kinetics. Clin Pharmacol Ther (1985) 37, 625–8.
4 Koopmans PP, Thien Th, Thomas CMG, van den Berg RJ, Gribnau FWJ. The effects of sulindac and indomethacin on the antihypertensive and diuretic action of hydrochlorothiazide in patients with mild to moderate essential hypertension. Br J clin Pharmac (1986) 21, 417–23.
5 Dusing R, Nicolas V, Glatte B, Glanzer K, Kipnowski J, Kramer HJ. Interaction of bemetizide and indomethacin in the kidney. Br J clin Pharmac (1983) 16, 377–84.
6 Steiness E, Waldorff S. Different interactions of indomethacin and sulindac with thiazides in hypertension. Br Med J (1982) 285, 1702–3.
7 Koopmans PP, Thien Th and Gribnau FWJ. Influence of non-steroidal anti-inflammatory drugs on diuretic treatment of mild to moderate essential hypertension. Br Med J (1984) 289, 1492–4.
8 Tempero KF, Cirillo VJ, Steelman SL. Diflunisal: a review of the pharmacokinetic and pharmacodynamic properties, drug interactions and special tolerability studies in humans. Br J clin Pharmac (1977) 4, 31S.
9 Tempero KF, Cirillo VJ, Steelman SL, Besselaar GH, Smit Sibinga CTh, De Schepper P, Tjandramaga TB, Dresse A, Gribnau FWJ. Special studies on diflunisal, a novel salicylate. Clin Res (1975) 23, 224A.
10 Koopmans PP, Thien Th and Gribnau FWJ. The influence of ibuprofen, dicolfenac and sulindac on the blood pressure lowering effect of hydrochlorothiazide. Eur J Clin Pharmacol (1987) 31, 553–7.
11 Davies JG, Rawlins DC, Busson M. Effect of ibuprofen on blood pressure control by propranolol and bendrofluazide. J Int Med Res (1988) 16, 173–81.
12 Kirchner KA, Brandon S, Mueller RA, Smith MJ, Bower JD. Mechanism of attenutated hydrochlorothiazide response during indomethacin administration. Kidney Int (1987) 31, 1097–1103.
13 Wright JT, McKenney JM, Lehany AM, Bryan DL, Cooper LW and Lambert CM. The effect of high-dose short-term ibuprofen on antihypertensive control with hydrochlorothiazide. Clin Pharmacol Ther (1989) 46, 440–4.
14 Gehr TWB, Sica DA, Steiger BW, Marshall C. Interaction of triamterene-hydrochlorothiazide and ibuprofen. Clin Pharmacol Ther (1990) 47, 200.
15 Stokes GS, Brooks PM, Johnson HJ, Monaghan JC, Okoro EO, Kelly D. The effects of sulindac and diclofenac in essential hypertension controlled by treatment with a beta-blocker and/or diuretic. Clin Exp Hyper Theory Prac (1991) A13, 1169–78.

Thiazides + Propantheline

Abstract/Summary

Propantheline can substantially increase the absorption of hydrochlorothiazide from the gut.

Clinical evidence, mechanism, importance and management

The absorption of hydrochlorothiazide in six normal subjects was delayed but substantially increased (+ 40%) by the concurrent use of 60 mg propantheline, due, it is suggested, to a slower delivery of the drug to its areas of absorption.[1] The clinical importance of this is uncertain, but some increase in the diuretic effects would be expected.

Reference

1 Beerman B, Groschinsky-Grind M. Enhancement of the gastrointestinal absorption of hydrochlorothiazide by propantheline. Eur J Clin Pharmacol (1978) 13, 385.

Tolazoline + H$_2$-blockers

Abstract/Summary

Cimetidine and ranitidine can reduce or abolish the effects of tolazoline when used as a pulmonary vasodilator in children.

Clinical evidence

A newborn infant with persistent foetal circulation was given a continuous infusion of tolazoline to reduce pulmonary hypertension. The oxygenation improved but gastrointestinal bleeding occurred. When cimetidine was given, the condition of the child deteriorated with a decrease in in oxygen saturation and arterial Po_2 values.[1] This report is similar to another in which the fall in pulmonary arterial pressure in a child due to tolazoline was reversed when cimetidine was given for acute gastrointestinal haemorrhage.[3] Another study found that ranitidine (3 mg/kg IV) abolished the fall in pulmonary and systemic vascular resistance in 12 children who had been treated with tolazoline (1–2 mg/kg) as a pulmonary vasodilator.[2]

Mechanism

Tolazoline dilates the pulmonary vascular system by stimulating both H$_1$ and H$_2$ receptors. Cimetidine and ranitidine block H$_2$ receptors so that at least part of the tolazoline effects are abolished. It has been suggested that this interaction is confined to children.[3]

Importance and management

An established interaction. Cimetidine and ranitidine are not suitable agents against the gastrointestinal side-effects of tolazoline in children. Other H$_2$-blockers would be expected to behave similarly. Antacids have been used, and omeprazole is a possible alternative but this needs confirmation.

References

1 Roll C, Hanssler L. Interaction of tolazoline and cimetidine in persistent fetal circulation of the newborn infant. Montasschrift Kinderheilkunde (1993) 141, 297–9.

2 Bush A. Busst CM, Knight WB, Shinebourne EA. Cardiovascular effects of tolazoline and ranitidine. Arch Dis Child (1987) 62, 241–6.

3 Jones ODH, Shore DF, Rigby ML. The use of tolazoline hydrochloride as a pulmonary vasodilator in potentially fatal episodes of pulmonary vasoconstriction after cardiac surgery in children. Circulation (1981) 64 (Suppl II) 134–9.

Trandolapril + Miscellaneous drugs

Abstract/Summary

Trandolapril appears not to interact adversely with nifedipine, frusemide, digoxin, warfarin, or in diabetic patients. Based on the way other ACE-inhibitors behave, the makers of trandolapril advise caution with diuretics, potassium supplements, lithium, some neuroleptics and antidepressants.

Clinical evidence, mechanism, importance and management

Knoll, the makers of trandolapril say that 'no significant interactions between trandolapril and nifedipine, frusmide, or digoxin have been found, and trandolapril does not alter the anticoagulant activity of warfarin.'[5] This is based on the results of a series of unpublished studies.[1–4] Other studies (also quoted by the makers) identified no problems when trandolapril was given to diabetic patients and others with glucose intolerance, but as a precaution they recommend monitoring blood glucose levels.[5,6]

In their datasheet the makers point out the risks of hyperkalaemia if trandolapril is given with potassium-sparing diuretics (amiloride, spironolactone, triamterene) or potassium supplements, particularly in renal failure. They also point out the risks of initial excessive hypotension if trandolapril is given to patients already taking diuretics, of orthostatic hypotension in those taking neuroleptics or tricyclic antidepressants, and possible changes in serum lithium levels. These warnings are based, not unreasonably, on the adverse reactions seen with other ACE-inhibitors, but not apparently on direct observations with trandolapril.[7] See also other ACE-inhibitors.

References

1 Patat A, Granier J Surjus A et al. study of the potential pharmacokinetic interaction of digoxin and trandolapril at steady state. RU internal report F/87/570/24, 1989.

2 Meyer BH, Muller FO, Lenfant B et al. Pharmacokinetic interaction study between trandolapril and furosemide. RU internal report, ZA/89/570/43. 1990.

3 Patat A, Granier J, Tremablay D et al. Investigation into possible pharmacokinetic and pharmacodynamic interaction between nifedipine (sustained release form) and trandolapril administered in a single dose to healthy volunteers. RU internal report 90/2183/CN, 1991.

4 Meyer BH, Muller Fo, Du P, Heyns A et al. Interaction between warfarin and trandolapril. RU internal report, ZA/88/570/28, 1989.

5 New Horizons in Antihypertensive therapy. Gopten'a8 Trandolapril. Knoll AG 1992.

6 Bauduceau B, Vaur L, Chemama L et al. Effect of trandolapril on glucose tolerance and microalbuminaria in diabetic hypertensive patients. In Abstract 14th Scientific Meeting of the International Society of Hypertension, Madrid, 1992, 183.

7 Das S (Knoll Ltd). Personal communication, 1993.

Triamterene + Cimetidine or Ranitidine

Abstract/Summary

Ranitidine reduces the absorption and the diuretic effects of triamterene but the clinical importance of this is uncertain. Cimetidine appears not to interact with triamterene significantly.

Clinical evidence

(a) Cimetidine

A study in six normal subjects given 100 mg triamterene daily for four days showed that although 800 mg cimetidine daily increased the triamterene AUC by 22%, reduced its metabolism (hydroxylation) by 32% and its renal clearance by 28% as well as its absorption, the loss of sodium in the urine was not significantly changed nor were its potassium-sparing effects altered.[2]

(b) Ranitidine

A study in eight normal subjects showed that taking 300 mg ranitidine daily for four days approximately halved the absorption of triamterene, 100 mg daily (as measured by its renal clearance). Its metabolism was also reduced, the total effect being a 24% reduction in the AUC. As a result of the reduced serum triamterene levels the urinary sodium loss was reduced to some extent but potassium excretion remained unchanged.[1]

Mechanism

These changes are due to reduced triamterene absorption from the gut and reduced liver metabolism and renal excretion caused by the these H_2-blockers.

Importance and management

Information about the triamterene-ranitidine interaction is limited and the clinical importance remains uncertain. Nobody seems to have measured whether this interaction significantly reduces the diuretic effects of triamterene in patients. The outcome of concurrent use should therefore be monitored.

Cimetidine also interacts with triamterene but this appears to be clinically unimportant because its diuretic effects are minimally changed.[2] No dosage changes are likely to be necessary.

References

1 Muirhead M, Bochner F, Somogyi A. Pharmacokinetic drug interactions between triamterene and ranitidine in humans: alterations in renal and hepatic clearances and gastrointestinal absorption. J Pharmacol exp Ther (1988) 244, 734–9.
2 Muirhead MR, Somoygi AA, Rolan PE, Bochner F. Effect of cimetidine on renal and hepatic drugs elimination: studies with triamterene. Clin Pharmacol Ther (1986) 40, 400–7.

Triamterene + Indomethacin

Abstract/Summary

Concurrent use may rapidly lead to acute renal failure.

Clinical evidence

A study in four normal subjects showed that the concurrent use of indomethacin (150 mg daily) and triameterene (200 mg daily) over a 3-day period reduced the creatinine clearance of two of them by 62 and 72% respectively. Kidney function returned to normal after a month. Indomethacin alone caused an average 10% fall in creatinine clearance, but triamterene alone caused no consistent change in kidney function. No adverse reactions were seen in 18 other subjects treated in the same way with indomethacin and three other diuretics (frusemide, chlorothiazide, spironolactone).[1,2] Five patients have been described who rapidly developed acute renal failure after receiving indomethacin and triamterene either concurrently or sequentially.[3–6]

Mechanism

Uncertain. One suggestion is that triamterene causes renal ischaemia for which the kidney compensates by increasing prostaglandin (PGE_2) production, thereby preserving renal blood flow. Indomethacin opposes this by inhibiting prostaglandin synthesis, so that the damaging effects of triamterene on the kidney continue unchecked.

Importance and management

Information is limited to these reports, but the interaction is established. The incidence is uncertain but it occurred in two of the four subjects in the study cited.[1,2] Since acute renal failure can apparently develop unpredictably and very rapidly it would seem prudent to avoid concurrent use.

References

1 Favre L, Glasson P, Vallotton MB. Reversible acute renal failure from combined triamterene and indomethacin. A study in healthy subjects. Ann Intern Med (1982) 96, 317–20.
2 Favre L, Glasson PH, Riondel A, Vallotton MB. Interaction of diuretics and non-steroidal anti-inflammatory drugs in man. Clin Sci (1983) 64, 407–15.
3 McCarthy JT, Torres VE, Romero JC, Wochos DN, Velosa JA. Acute intrinsic renal failure induced by indomethacin: role of prostaglandin synthetase inhibition. Mayo Clin Proc (1982) 57, 289–96.
4 McCarthy JT. Drug induced renal failure. Mayo Clin Proc (1982) 57, 463.
5 Weinberg MS, Quigg RJ, Salant DJ, Bernard DB. Anuric renal failure precipitated by indomethacin and triamterene. Nephron (1985) 40, 216–18.
6 Mathews A, Baillie FR. Acute renal failure and hyperkalaemia associated with triamterene and indomethacin. Vet Hum Toxicol (1986) 28, 224–5.

Chapter 9
Antiparkinsonian Drug Interactions

The drugs in this chapter are classified together because their major therapeutic application is in the treatment of Parkinson's disease. This disease is named after Dr James Parkinson who a century-and-a-half ago described the four mains signs of the disease, namely muscle rigidity, tremor, muscular weakness and hypokinesia. Similar symptoms may also be displayed as the unwanted side-effects of therapy with certain drugs.

The basic cause of the disease lies in the basal ganglia of the brain, particularly the corpus striatum and the substantia nigra, where the normal balance between dopaminergic nerve fibres (those which use dopamine as the chemical transmitter) and the cholinergic nerve fibres (acetylcholine as the transmitter) is lost because the dopaminergic fibres degenerate. As a result the cholinergic fibres come to be in dominant control. Much of the treatment of Parkinson's disease is based on an attempt to redress the balance, either by limiting the activity of the cholinergic fibres with anticholinergic (atropine-like) drugs, and/or by 'topping up' the dopaminergic system with dopamine in the form of levodopa, or with other agents such as amantadine or bromocriptine which increase dopaminergic activity in the brain. Dopamine cannot penetrate the blood-brain barrier so that its precursor, dopa, is given instead. These days it is common to include with dopa an enzyme-inhibitor such as carbidopa (in *Sinemet*) or benserazide (in *Madopar*) which prevents the 'wasteful' enzymic metabolism of the levodopa outside the brain and thereby allows the use of lower oral doses which have fewer side-effects.

In addition to the interactions discussed in this chapter, some of the drugs are involved in interactions described elsewhere. Consult the index for a full listing.

Table 9.1 Antiparkinsonian drugs

Non-proprietary names	Proprietary names
Anticholinergics	
Benazpryzine	*Brizin*
Benzhexol (trihexiphenidyl)	*Antispas, Aparkane, Apo-Trihex, Artane, Artilan, Bentex, Novoheidyl, Paralest, Pargitan, Parkinane Retard, Peragit, Tremin, Trixyl*
Benztropine	*Bensylate, Cogentin(e)(ol)*
Biperiden	*Akineton, Akinophyl, Tasmolin*
Bornaprine	*Sormodren*
Caramiphen	*Rescaps-d, Tuss-ade, Tuss-ornade*
Chlorphenoxamine	*Clorevan, Phenoxene, Systral(leten)*
Cycrimine	*Pagitan(e)*
Dexetimide	*Tremblex*
Diethazine	

continued on p. 391

Table 9.1 (*Continued*)

Non-proprietary names	Proprietary names
Ethopropazine (profenamine)	*Lysivane, Parkin, Parsidol, Parsitan, Parsotil*
Ethylbenztropine	*Ponalid* *PKM*

Ethylbenzhydramine

Mazaticol	*Pentona*
Methixene	*Methyloxan, Tremaril, Tremarit, Tremonil, Tremoquil, Trest*
Orphenadrine (mephenamine)	*Biophen, Brocadispal, Distalene, Euflex, Lysantin, Mefeamina, Myotrol, Norflex, Orpadrex, Orphenate, Tega-flex, X-otag*
Piroheptine	*Trimol*
Procyclidine	*Arpicolin, Kemadrin(e), Kemadren, Osnervan Procyclid*
Tigloidine	*Mepidium*
Tropatepine	*Lepticur*

Other drugs possessing anticholinergic (antimuscarinic) activity are listed in Table 9.2

Amantadine	*Amantan, Amazolon, Antadine, Aontenton, Mantadan(e), Mantadix, PK-Merz, Solu-Contenon, Symmetrel, Trivaline, Virofal, Virosol*
Bromocriptine	*Bagren, Lactismine, Parlodel, Pravidel*
Levodopa (L-Dopa)	*Bendopa, Berkdopa, Brocadopa, Cidandopa, Dopaidan, Dopaken, Dopalfher, Dopar, Doparkine, Doparl, Dopasol, Dopaston, Dopastral, Eldopal, Eldopa, Eldopatec, Larodopa, Levopa, Syndopa, Veldopa*
Levodopa + benserazide	*Madopar*
Levodopa + carbidopa	*Sinemet*
Pergolide	
Piribedil	*Circularina, Trivastal, Trivastan*

Amantadine + Co-trimoxazole

Abstract/Summary

An elderly patient on amantadine developed acute mental confusion when given co-trimoxazole (sulphamethoxazole + trimethoprim).

Clinical evidence, mechanism, importance and management

An 84-year-old man with Parkinson's disease, chronic obstructive pulmonary disease and chronic atrial fibrillation, was treated with 100 mg amantadine twice daily and digoxin for at least two years. Within 72 h of starting co-trimoxazole (*Septra DS*) twice daily for bronchitis he became mentally confused, incoherent and combative. He also showed cogwheel rigidity and a resting tremor. Within 24 h of stopping the amantadine and co-trimoxazole, the patient's mental status returned to normal.[1] The reasons for this reaction are not understood but, on the basis of animal studies, the authors suggest that the trimethoprim component of the co-trimoxazole may have competed with the amantadine for renal secretion, resulting in an accumulation of amantadine with its toxic effects.[1] In fact both drugs can cause some mental confusion. This interaction is more likely in the elderly because ageing results in a decrease in the clearance of these and many other drugs.

The general importance of this interaction is uncertain, but it would now seem prudent to monitor the effects of concurrent use in any patient, particularly the elderly.

Reference

1 Speeg KV, Leighton JA, Maldonoado AL. Case report: toxic delerium in a patient taking amantadine and trimethoprim-sulfamethoxazole. Am J Med Sci (1989) 298, 410–12.

Amantadine + Miscellaneous drugs

Abstract/Summary

The use of amantadine in patients taking amphetamines, other CNS stimulants, or having treatment with other drugs for epilepsy, gastrointestinal ulceration, Parkinson's disease or congestive heart failure may cause problems.

Clinical evidence, mechanism, importance and management

Geigy, the manufacturers of amantadine, say that although adverse interactions have not been reported, they recommend that amantadine should be given with caution if amphetamines or other CNS stimulants are being used. They advise that amantadine is not given to those who are subject to convulsions or with a history of gastric ulceration. They also warn that amantadine can aggravate the CNS, gastro-intestinal and other side-effects of drugs used in the treatment of Parkinson's disease (anticholinergics, levodopa).[1] Amantadine sometimes causes peripheral oedema which may possibly have an adverse effect on the control of congestive heart failure.

Reference

1 ABPI Data Sheet Compendium 1991–2. Datapharm Publications, London (1991).

Amantadine + Thiazides

Abstract/Summary

Concurrent use can be successful and uneventful but two patients have been described who developed amantadine toxicity when given hydrochlorothiazide-triamterene or cyclopenthiazide-K.

Clinical evidence

A patient developed signs of amantadine toxicity (ataxia, agitation, hallucinations) within a week of additionally starting treatment with two tablets of *Dyazide* (hydrochlorothiazide-triamterene) daily. The symptoms rapidly disappeared when all the drugs were withdrawn. In a later study this patient showed a 50% rise in amantadine serum levels (from 156 to 243 ng/ml) after taking the diuretic for 7 days.[1] Another very brief report describes confusion and hallucinations in a patient given amantadine and cyclopenthiazide K.[2] In contrast, the successful and apparently uneventful concurrent use of amantadine and diuretics (named as a thiazide in one of them)[3] has also been described.[3,4]

Mechanism

Uncertain. Amantadine is largely excreted unchanged in the urine and it seems probable that these diuretics reduce the renal clearance.[1]

Importance and management

Information about an adverse interaction appears to be limited to these two reports. Its incidence is uncertain. There seems to be little reason for avoiding concurrent use, but the effects should be well monitored.

References

1 Wilson TW, Rajput AH. Amantadine-*Dyazide* interaction. Can Med Ass J (1983) 129, 974–5.
2 New Zealand Committee on Adverse Drug Reactions. 11th year. April 1975-March 1976. Serial no 5476.
3 Birdwood GFB, Gilder SSB, Wink CAS (eds). Parkinson's Disease. A new approach to treatment. Int Clin Symp Report on Symmetrel in Parkinsonism. London June 1971. Academic Press (1971) p 66.

4 Parkes JD, Marsden CD, Price P. Amantadine-induced heart failure. Lancet (1977) i, 904.

Anticholinergics + Anticholinergics

Abstract/Summary

Additive anticholinergic effects, both peripheral and central, can develop if drugs with anticholinergic effects are used together. The outcome may be harmful.

Clinical evidence, mechanism, importance and management

The anticholinergic (antimuscarinic) effects of some drugs are exploited therapeutically. These include atropine, and drugs such as benzhexol and benztropine which are used for the control of Parkinsonian symptoms. Other drugs with a broader spectrum of activity may also possess some anticholinergic properties as an unwanted side-effect which may be troublesome but often not serious. They can however be worsened and possibly made clinically important if another drug with similar properties is added.

The easily recognized and common peripheral anticholinergic effects are blurred vision, dry mouth, constipation, difficulty in urination, reduced sweating, tachycardia and possibly exacerbation of narrow angle glaucoma. Central effects include confusion, disorientation, visual hallucinations, agitation, irritability, delerium, memory problems, belligerence and even assaultiveness. Problems are most likely to arise with patients with particular physical conditions such as glaucoma (drainage worsened), prostatic hypertrophy (urination made even more difficult) or constipation. Table 9.2 lists some of the drugs with anticholinergic effects which may be expected to be additive if used together, but apart from some reports describing life-threatening reactions (see 'Neuroleptics Butyrophenones, Phenothiazines, Thioxanthenes + Anticholinergics') there are very few reports describing this simple additive interaction, probably because the outcome is so obvious. Many of these interactions, unlike virtually all of the other interactions described in this book, are therefore 'theoretical' but their probability is high.

Some drugs with minimal anticholinergic properties may sometimes cause difficulties if given with another anticholinergic: a patient on isopropamide iodide (an anticholinergic antispasmodic) only developed urinary retention needing catheterization when additionally given 75 mg trazodone daily, but not with either drug alone.[1] Trazodone is usually regarded as having little or no anticholinergic effects.

If the central anticholinergic syndrome caused by the use of anticholinergic drugs is not clearly recognized for what it is, there is the possibility that neuroleptic (antipsychotic) agents may additionally be prescribed. Many of these drugs also have anticholinergic side-effects so that matters are simply made worse. If the patient then demonstrates dystonias, akathisia, tremor and rigidity it is possible that even more anticholinergic agents may be added to control the extrapyramidal effects,

Table 9.2 Drugs with Anticholinergic effects (main or side-effects)

Drug group	Individual drugs
Antiarrhythmics	Disopyramide, propafenone
Antiemetics	Cyclizine, dimenhydrinate, meclizine, hyoscine (scopolamine)
Antihistamines	Brompheniramine, chlorpheniramine, cyproheptadine, diphenhydramine, hydroxyzine, triprolidine
Antiparkinson agents (anticholinergics) see Table 9.1	
Antispasmodics	Atropine, belladonna, dicyclomine, flavoxate, hyoscine (scopolamine), isopropamide, oxybutynin, propantheline
Antiulcer drugs	Pirenzepine
Cycloplegic mydriatics	Atropine, homatropine, hyoscine (scopolamine), cyclopentolate, tropicamide
Muscle relaxants	Baclofen, cyclobenzaprine, orphenadrine
Neuroleptics	Chlorpromazine, chlorprothixene, clozapine, loxapine, perphenazine, pimozide, mesoridazine, trifluoperazine, thioridazine
Peripheral vasodilator	Papaverine
Tricyclic and related antidepressants	Amitriptyline, amoxapine, clomipramine, desipramine, doxepin, imipramine, maprotiline, protripytline, nortriptyline, trimipramine

After Barkin RL, Stein ZLG. South Med J (1989) 82, 1547.

which merely adds to the continuing downward spiral of drug-induced problems.

In addition to the obvious and very well recognized drugs with anticholinergic effects, a study of the 25 drugs most commonly prescribed for the elderly was able to identify detectable anticholinergic activity (using an anticholinergic radioreceptor assay) in 14 of them, 10 of which (ranitidine, codeine, dipyridamole, warfarin, isosorbide, theophylline, nifedipine, digoxin, lanoxin and prednisolone) have been shown to cause significant impairment in tests of memory and attention in the elderly.[2] Thus the problem may not necessarily be confined to those drugs which most obviously have anticholinergic properties, but also with these are not normally thought of as possessing these properties. See also 'Neuroleptus + Anticholinergus' in Chapter 19.

References

1 Chan CH, Ruskiewicz RJ. Anticholinergic side-effects of trazodone combined with another pharmacological agent. Am J Psychiatry (1990) 147, 533.

2 Tune L, Carr S, Hoag E, Cooper T. Anticholinergic effects of drugs commonly prescribed for the elderly: potential means for assessing risk of delerium. Am J Psychiatry (1992) 149, 1393–4.

Anticholinergics + Betel nuts

Abstract/Summary

The control of the extrapyramidal (parkinsonian) side-effects of fluphenazine and flupenthixol with procyclidine was lost in two patients when they began to chew betel nuts.

Clinical evidence

An Indian patient on depot fluphenazine (50 mg every three weeks) for schizophrenia, and mild parkinsonian tremor controlled with procyclidine (5 mg twice daily), developed marked rigidity, bradykinesia and jaw tremor when he began to chew betel nuts. The symptoms were so severe he could barely speak. When he stopped chewing the nuts his stiffness and abnormal movements disappeared. Another patient on flupenthixol developed marked stiffness, tremor and akathisia, despite taking up to 20 mg procyclidine daily, when he began to chew betel nuts. The symptoms vanished within four days of stopping the nuts.[1]

Mechanism

Betel nuts contain arecoline which mimics the actions of acetylcholine. It seems that the arecoline opposed the actions of the anticholinergic procyclidine which was being used to control the extrapyramidal side-effects of the two neuroleptics, thereby allowing these side-effects to emerge.

Importance and management

Direct information seems to be limited to this report but the interaction would seem to be established and clinically important. Patients taking anticholinergic drugs for the control of drug-induced extrapyramidal (Parkinson-like) symptoms or Parkinson's disease should avoid betel nuts. The authors of this report suggest that a dental inspection for the characteristic red stains of the betel may possibly provide a simple explanation for the sudden and otherwise mysterious deterioration in the symptoms of patients from Asia and the East Indies.

Reference

1 Deahl M. Betel nut-induced extrapyramidal syndrome: an unusual drug interaction. Movement Disorders (1989) 4, 330–3.

Antiparkinsonian agents + Fluoxetine

Abstract/Summary

Preliminary evidence suggests that fluoxetine can cause extrapyramidal side-effects and may therefore be unsuitable for patients being treated for Parkinson's disease.

Clinical evidence, mechanism, importance and management

5 patients developed extrapyramidal side-effects (clumsiness, shuffling gait, mask-like look of the face) when treated with 20 mg fluoxetine daily.[1] Extrapyramidal effects were seen in another patient taking haloperidol and fluoxetine,[2] and generalized muscle stiffness in another.[3] One of the reports[1] also says that deterioration of parkinsonian patients has been seen in other patients given serotonin reuptake inhibitors. The reasons are not known, however the indications are that fluoxetine should possibly not be used in patients treated for parkinsonism. More study is needed.

References

1 Bouchard RH, Pourcher E, Vincent P. Fluoxetine and extrapyramidal side-effects. Am J Psychiatry (1989) 146, 1352–3.
2 Tate JL. Extrapyramidal symptoms in a patient taking haloperidol and fluoxetine. Am J Psychiatry (1989) 146, 399–400.
3 Brod TM. Fluoxetine and extrapyramidal side-effects. Am J Psychiatry (1989) 146, 1353.

Bromocriptine + Alcohol

Abstract/Summary

There is some very limited evidence that the adverse effects of bromocriptine may possibly be increased by alcohol.

Clinical evidence, mechanism, importance and management

Intolerance to alcohol has been briefly mentioned in a report about patients taking bromocriptine for acromegaly.[1] In another report two patients with high prolactin levels are said to have developed the side-effects of bromocriptine even in low doses while continuing to drink.[2] When they abstained, the frequency and the severity of the side-effects fell, even with higher doses of bromocriptine. This, it is suggested, may be due to some alcohol-induced increase in the sensitivity of dopamine receptors.[1] No other reports of this interaction have been traced.[3] There would seem to be little reason, on the basis of this extremely sparse evidence, to tell all patients on bromocriptine not to drink, but it would be reasonable to warn them to avoid alcohol if side-effects develop.

References

1 Wass JAH, Thorner MO, Morris DV, Rees LH, Mason AE, Besser EM. Long-term treatment of acromegaly with bromocriptine. Br Med J (1977) 1, 875.
2 Ayres J, Maisey MN. Alcohol increases bromocriptine side-effects. N Engl J Med (1980) 302, 806.
3 Hunt M (Sandoz). Personal communication (1990).

Bromocriptine + Griseofulvin

Abstract/Summary

Evidence from a single case where bromocriptine was being used for acromegaly suggests that its effects can be opposed by griseofulvin.

Clinical evidence, mechanism, importance and management

The effects of bromocriptine, used for the treatment of acromegaly, were blocked when a patient was given griseofulvin for the treatment of a mycotic infection.[1] The mechanism of this interaction and its general importance are unknown, but prescribers should be aware of it when treating patients with bromocriptine.

Reference

1 Schwinn G, Dirks H, McIntosh C, Kobberling J. Metabolic and clinical studies in patients with acromegaly treated with bromocriptine over 22 months. Eur J Clin Invest (1977) 7, 101.

Bromocriptine + Macrolide antibiotics

Abstract/Summary

Bromocriptine toxicity occurred in an elderly man when given josamycin. Another study found that erythromycin causes an increase in serum bromocriptine levels.

Clinical evidence

(a) Erythromycin

A study in five normal subjects found that 250 mg erythromycin estolate four times daily for four days caused a marked change in the pharmacokinetics of a single 5 mg oral dose of bromocriptine. The clearance of the bromocriptine was decreased by 70.6%, the peak serum levels were raised by 460% and the AUC was increased by 268%.[2,3]

Another report describes two women on levodopa and bromocriptine for parkinsonism which was better controlled when erythromycin was added. Bromocriptine serum levels were found to be 40–50% higher.[4]

(b) Josamycin

An elderly man with Parkinson's disease, well-controlled for 10 months on daily treatment with levodopa (and benserazide) 200 mg, bromocriptine 70 mg and domperidone 60 mg, was additionally given 2 g josamycin daily for a respiratory infection. Shortly after the first dose he became drowsy with visual hallucinations, and began to show involuntary movements of his limbs similar to the dystonic and dyskinetic movements seen in choreo-athetosis. These adverse effects (interpreted as bromocriptine toxicity) disappeared within a few days of withdrawing the antibiotic.[1]

Mechanism

Not understood. One suggestion is that these macrolide antibiotics inhibits the metabolism of the bromocriptine by the liver, thereby reducing its loss from the body and raising its serum levels.[1]

Importance and management

Information seems to be limited to these reports. Concurrent use should be well monitored if either of these macrolide antibiotics is added to bromocriptine treatment. Moderately increased bromocriptine levels may be therapeutically advantageous, but grossly elevated levels can be toxic. There seems to be no direct evidence about any other macrolides, but some of them certainly inhibit liver metabolism and can raise the serum levels of other drugs.

References

1 Montastruc JL, Rascol A. Traitement de la maladie de Parkinson par doses elevees de bromocriptine. Interaction possible avec josamycine. La Presse Med (1984) 13, 2267–8.
2 Nelson MV, Berchou RC, Kareti D, LeWitt PA. Pharmacokinetic evaluation of erythromycin and caffeine administered with bromocriptine in normal subjects. Clin Pharmacol Ther (1990), 47,166.
3 Nelson MV, Berchou RC, Kareti D, LeWitt PA. Pharmacokinetic evaluation of erythromycin and caffeine administered with bromocriptine. Clin Pharmacol Ther (1990) 47, 694–7.
4 Sibley WA, Laguna JF. Enhancement of bromocriptine clinical effect and plasma levels with erythromycin. Excerpta Medica (1981) 548, 329–30.

Bromocriptine + Sympathomimetics

Abstract/Summary

Two young healthy women with severe headache, apparently due to bromocriptine taken for milk-suppression, developed worsening headache and hypertension with serious cardiac arrhythmias or seizures with cerebral vasospasm when additionally given isometheptene or phenylpropanolamine.

Clinical evidence, mechanism, importance and management

Two women normal healthy women who had given birth 3–4 days previously developed severe headaches while taking bromocriptine (2.5 mg twice daily) for milk suppression. After additionally taking three one-hourly 65 mg doses of isomethepetene mucate (a sympathomimetic), the headache of one of them markedly worsened, and hypertension with life-threatening ventricular tachycardia and cardiac dysfunction developed. The other developed seizures and cerebral vasospasm after taking two 75 mg doses of phenylpropanolamine.[1] The reasons are not understood but cases of hypertension, stroke and seizures have been seen with bromocriptine alone and it is suggested that in these two cases the additional use of the sympathomimetics exacerbated the adverse effects of the bromocriptine.[1] Information is limited but it would now seem prudent to withdraw the bromocriptine if severe headache develops, and take particular care with drugs which can raise the blood pressure.

Reference

1 Kulig K, Moore LL, Kirk M, Smith D, Stallworth J, Rumack B. Bromocriptine-associated headache: possible life-threatening sympathomimetic interaction. Obst Gynecol (1991) 78, 941–3.

Levodopa + Antacids

Abstract/Summary

Antacids appear not to interact significantly with levodopa, except possibly with one slow-release preparation, the bioavailability of which is reduced.

Clinical evidence, mechanism, importance and management

Levodopa can be metabolized in the stomach so that, in theory at least, antacids which increase gastric emptying might decrease this 'wasteful' metabolism and increase the amounts available for absorption. This would seem to be confirmed by one study which found that an aluminium-magnesium hydroxide antacid raised peak serum levodopa levels and they occurred sooner.[2,3] However no interaction was seen when magaldrate was used,[4] nor in a study in 15 parkinsonian patients taking bromocriptine, levodopa and carbidopa who were given six 30 ml doses of aluminium hydroxide (*Mylanta*) daily. No effect was seen on the fluctuations in response to levodopa which normally occur.[1] However in another study using *Madopar* HBS, a sustained release preparation of levodopa and benserazide, the concurrent use of an un-named antacid reduced the bioavailability by about one third.[5] The overall picture is that concurrent use need not be avoided, but the outcome should be monitored.

References

1 Lau E, Waterman K, Glover R, Schulzer M, Calne DB. Effect of antacid on levodopa therapy. Clin Neuropharmacol (1986) 9, 477–9.
2 Rivera-Calimlim L, Dujovne CA, Morgan JO, Lasagna L, Bianchine JR. Absorption and metabolism of L-dopa by the human stomach. Eur J Clin Invest (1971) 1, 313.
3 Pocelinko GBT, Solomon HM. The effect of an antacid on the absorption and metabolism of levodopa. Clin Pharmacol Ther (1972) 13, 149.
4 Leon AS, Spiegel HE. The effect of antacid administration on the absorption and metabolism of levodopa. J Clin Pharmacol (1972) 12, 263.
5 Malcolm SL, Allen JG, Bird H, Quinn NP, Marion MH, Marsden CD. Single dose pharmacokinetics of *Madopar* HBS in patients and effect of food and antacid on the absorption of Madopa HBS in volunteers. Eur Neurol (1987) 27, 28–35.

Levodopa + Anticholinergics

Abstract/Summary

Although anticholinergic drugs are very widely used in conjunction with levodopa, they may reduce the absorption of levodopa and reduce its therapeutic effects to some extent.

Clinical evidence

A study in six normal subjects and six patients with Parkinson's disease showed that the administration of benzhexol (trihexyphenidyl) lowered the peak serum levels and reduced the absorption of levodopa in about half of the subjects by an average of 16–20%.[1]

A patient who needed 7 g levodopa daily while taking homatropine developed levodopa toxicity when the homatropine was withdrawn, and he was subsequently restabilized on 4 g levodopa daily.[2] This interaction is described in another report.[3]

Mechanism

Anticholinergics delay gastric emptying which gives the gastric mucosa more time to metabolize the levodopa 'wastefully' so that less is available for absorption in the small intestine.[4]

Importance and management

Anticholinergics are almost certainly the most commonly co-administered drugs with levodopa (one study suggests that the incidence may be as much as 50%[1]). Prescribers should be alert for evidence of a reduced levodopa response if anticholinergics are added, or for levodopa toxicity if they are withdrawn.

References

1 Algeri S, Cerletti C, Curcio M, Morselli PL, Bonollo L, Buniva M, Minazzi M, Minoli G. Effect of anticholinergic drugs on gastrointestinal absorption of L-dopa in rats and man. Eur J Pharmacol (1976) 35, 293.
2 Fermaglich J, O'Doherty DS. Effect of gastric motility on levodopa. Dis Nerv Syst (1972) 33, 624.
3 Birket-Smith E. Abnormal involuntary movements in relation to anti-

cholinergics and levodopa therapy. Acta Neurol Scand (1975) 52, 158.

4 Rivera-Calimlim L, Morgan JP, Dujovne CA, Bianchine JR, Lasagna L. L-dopa absorption and metabolism by the human stomach. J Clin Invest (1970) 49, 79.

Levodopa + Benzodiazepines

Abstract/Summary

The therapeutic effects of levodopa can be reduced or abolished in some patients by the concurrent use of chlordiazepoxide, diazepam or nitrazepam.

Clinical evidence

Eight patients on levodopa were concurrently treated with various benzodiazepines, mostly in unstated doses but said to be within the normal therapeutic range. No adverse interaction occurred in three given chlordiazepoxide or one given oxazepam, but a dramatic deterioration in the control of parkinsonism was seen in a man given 5 mg diazepam twice daily, from which he spontaneously recovered. Two out of three given nitrazepam also showed marked deterioration but failed to react in the same way when rechallenged with nitrazepam in three further tests.[1] There are other reports of a loss in the control of the parkinsonism in nine patients given chlordiazepoxide[2-6] and three patients given diazepam.[5] However another report says that diazepam and especially flurazepam are valuable for sleep induction and maintenance in patients on levodopa.[7]

Mechanism

Not understood.

Importance and management

Established and clinically important interactions but the incidence is uncertain. Apparently it only affects some patients. Concurrent use need not be avoided but monitor the outcome closely for any sign of deterioration in the control of the parkinsonism. Information about other benzodiazepines is lacking but it would seem reasonable to apply the same precautions. 75 mg hydroxyzine daily was found to be a non-interacting substitute for chlordiazepoxide in one patient.[6]

References

1 Hunter KR, Stern GM, Laurence DR. Use of levodopa with other drugs. Lancet (1970) ii, 1283.
2 Mackie L. Drug antagonism. Br Med J (1971) 2, 651.
3 Schwartz GA, Fahn S. Newer medical treatments in parkinsonism. Med Clin N Amer (1970) 54, 773.
4 Brogden RN, Speight TM, Avery GS. Levodopa: a review of its pharmacological properties and therapeutic use with particular reference to Parkinsonism. Drugs (1971) 2, 262.
5 Wodak J, Gilligan BS, Veale JL, Dowty BJ. Review of 12 months' treatment

with L-dopa in Parkinson's disease with remarks on usual side-effects. Med J Aust (1972) 2, 1277.
6 Yosselson-Superstine S, Lipman AG. Chlordiazepoxide interaction with levodopa. Ann Intern Med (1982) 96, 259.
7 Kales A, Ansel RD, Markham CH, Scharf MB, Tan T-L. Sleep in patients with Parkinson's disease and normal subjects prior to and following levodopa administration. Clin Pharmacol Ther (1971) 12, 397–406.

Levodopa + Beta-blockers

Abstract/Summary

Concurrent use normally appears to be favourable, but the long-term effects of the elevated growth hormone levels are uncertain.

Clinical evidence, mechanism, importance and management

Most of the effects of combined use seem to be favourable. Dopamine derived from levodopa stimulates beta-receptors in the heart which can cause heart arrhythmias. These receptors are blocked by propranolol.[1] An enhancement of the effects of levodopa and a reduction in tremor in some[2] but not all patients[3,5] have been described. However there is evidence that growth hormone levels are substantially raised,[4] but to what extent this might prove to be an adverse response during long-term treatment appears not to have been assessed.

References

1 Goldberg LI, Whitsett TL. Cardiovascular effects of levodopa. Clin Pharmacol Ther (1971) 12, 376.
2 Kissel P, Tridon P, Andre JM. Levodopa-propranolol therapy in parkinsonian tremor. Lancet (1974) ii, 403.
3 Sandler M, Fellows LE, Calne DB, Findley LJ. Oxprenolol and levodopa in parkinsonian patients. Lancet (1975) i, 168.
4 Camanni F, Massara F. Enhancement of levodopa-induced growth hormone stimulation by propranolol. Lancet (1974) i, 942.
5 Marsden CD, Parkes JD, Rees JE. Propranolol in Parkinson's disease. Lancet (1974) ii, 410.

Levodopa or Piribedil + Clonidine

Abstract/Summary

Clonidine is reported to oppose the effects of levodopa or piribedil used to control Parkinson's disease.

Clinical evidence

A study in seven patients (five taking piribedil and two taking levodopa with benserazide) found that concurrent treatment with 1.5 mg clonidine daily for 10–24 days caused a worsening of the symptoms of Parkinson's disease (an exacerbation of rigidity and akinesia). The concurrent use of anticholinergic drugs reduced the effects of this interaction.[1]

Another report on 10 hypertensive and three normotensive

patients with Parkinson's disease, some of them taking levodopa and some of them not, claimed that concurrent treatment with clonidine did not affect the control of the parkinsonism, although two patients stopped taking the clonidine because of an increase in tremor and gait disturbance.[2]

Mechanism

Not understood. A suggestion is that the clonidine opposes the antiparkinson effects by stimulating alpha-receptors in the brain. Another idea is that the clonidine directly stimulates post-synaptic dopaminergic receptors.

Importance and management

Information seems to be limited to these reports. Be alert for a reduction in the control of the Parkinson's disease during concurrent use. The effects of this interaction appear to be reduced if anticholinergic drugs are also being used.

References

1 Shoulson I, Chase TN. Clonidine and the antiparkinsonian response to L-dopa or piribedil. Neuropharmacology (1976) 15, 25–7.
2 Tarsy D, Parkes JD, Marsden CD. Clonidine in Parkinson's disease. Arch Neurol (1975) 32, 134–6.

Levodopa + Dacarbazine

Abstract/Summary

An isolated report describes a reduction in the effects of levodopa caused by dacarbazine.

Clinical evidence, mechanism, importance and management

A patient who had been treated surgically for melanoma in 1973 continued to have dacarbazine treatment (200 mg IV daily) for sporadic positive melanuria. He developed Parkinson's disease in 1978 for which levodopa was started in 1985, but he complained that its effects were reduced each time he was treated with dacarbazine: his daily living Schwab and England activities score fell by as much as 25%. A subsequent double-blind study on the patient confirmed that this was so using a modified Columbia Score.[1] The reasons are not understood but since the serum dopamine levels remained unchanged it is suggested that competition between the two drugs at the blood-brain barrier may be the explanation.[1] Be alert for the need to increase the levodopa dosage if dacarbazine is used concurrently.

Reference

1 Merello M, Esteguy M, Perazzo F, Leiguarda R. Impaired levodopa

response in Parkinson's Disease during melanoma therapy. Clin Neuropharmacol ((1992) 15, 69–74.

Levodopa or Bromocriptine + Domperidone

Abstract/Summary

Domperidone can be used to prevent nausea and vomiting caused by levodopa or bromocriptine used for parkinsonism, but it seems possible that it will oppose the effects of bromocriptine when used to reduce prolactin levels.

Clinical evidence, mechanism, importance and management

Domperidone is a dopamine antagonist, similar to metoclopramide, which can be used to control the nausea and vomiting associated with the treatment of parkinson's disease with levodopa or bromocriptine. It acts on the dopamine receptors in the stomach wall and normally appears not to oppose the effects of levodopa within the brain because it does not readily cross the blood-brain barrier, although some extrapyramidal symptoms have been observed. It may even slightly increase the bioavailability and effects of levodopa.[1] Domperidone raises prolactin levels, sometimes causing galactorrhoea,[2,4,5] gynecomastia or mastalgia,[3,4] and may therefore be inappropriate for patients being treated with bromocriptine to reduce prolactin levels. This needs confirmation.

References

1 Shindler JS, Finnerty GT, Towlson K, Dolan AL, Davies CL, Parkes JD. Domperidone and levodopa in Parkinson's disease. Br J clin Pharmac (1984) 18, 959–62.
2 Cann PA, Read NW, Holdsworth CD. Galactorrhoea as a side-effect of domperidone. Br Med J (1983) 286, 1395–6.
3 Van der Steen M, Du Caju MVL, Van Acker KJ. Gynecomastia in a male infant given domperidone. Lancet (1982) 2, 884–5.
4 Cann PA, Read NW, Holdsworth CD. Oral domperidone: double blind comparison with placebo in irritable bowel syndrome. Gut (1983) 24. 1135–40.
5 Moriga M. A multicentre Double-blind study of domperidone and metoclopramide in the symptomatic control of dyspepsia. Roy Soc Med Int Congr Symp Ser (1981) 36, 77–9.

Levodopa + Ferrous sulphate

Abstract/Summary

Ferrous sulphate can reduce the bioavailability of levodopa and carbidopa, and may possibly reduce their control of parkinson's disease.

Clinical evidence

A study in 9 patients with parkinson's disease showed that a single 325 mg dose of ferrous sulphate reduced the AUC (area under the curve) of levodopa by 30% and of carbidopa by more than 75%. Some, but not all, of the patients showed showed some worsening in the control of their disease.[3]

In a previous study eight normal subjects were given a single 250 mg dose of levodopa, with and without a single 325 mg dose of ferrous sulphate, and the serum levodopa levels were measured for the following 6 h. Peak serum levodopa levels were reduced by 55% (from 3.6 to 1.6 nmol/l) and the AUC was reduced by 51% (from 257 to 125 nmol.min/ml). Those subjects who had the highest peak levels and greatest absorption showed the greatest reductions when given ferrous sulphate.[1]

This interaction has also been demonstrated in animal experiments.[2]

Mechanism

Ferrous iron rapidly oxidizes to ferric iron at the pH values found in the gastro-intestinal tract which then binds strongly to carbidopa and levodopa to form chelation complexes which are poorly absorbed.[1,4]

Importance and management

Information appears to be limited to these studies. The importance of this interaction in patients taking both drugs chronically awaits further study, but the extent of the reductions in absorption (30%) and the hint of worsening control[3] suggests that this interaction may be of clinical importance. Be alert for any evidence of this. Increasing the levodopa or carbidopa dosage or separating the adminstration of the iron as much as possible may prove to be effective. More study is needed.

References

1 Campbell NRC, Hasinoff B. Ferrous sulfate reduces levodopa bio-availability: chelation as a possible mechanism. Clin Pharmacol Ther (1989) 45, 220–5.
2 Campbell RRA, Hasinoff B, Chernenko G, Barrowman J, Campbell NRC. The effect of ferrous sulfate and pH on L-dopa absorption. Can J Physiol Pharmacol (1990) 68, 603–7.
3 Campbell NRC, Rankine D, Goodridge AE, Hasinoff BB, Kara M. Sinemet-ferrous sulphate interaction in patients with Parkinson's disease. Br J clin Pharmac (1990) 30, 599–605.
4 Greene RJ, Hall AD, Hider RC. The interaction of orally administered iron with levodopa and methyldopa. J Pharm Pharmacol (1990) 42, 502–4.

Levodopa + Food

Abstract/Summary

The fluctuations in response to levodopa experienced by some patients may be due to timing of meals and the kind of diet, particularly the protein content, both of which can reduce the effects of levodopa.

Clinical evidence

(a) Changes in absorption

A study in patients with Parkinson's disease treated with levodopa showed that if taken with a meal, the mean absorption of the levodopa from the gut and the peak plasma levels were reduced by 27 and 29% respectively, and the peak serum level was delayed by 34 min.[1] Another study showed that peak serum levodopa levels were reduced if taken with food rather than when fasting.[2] A study in normal subjects found that a low protein meal caused a small reduction in absorption.[6]

(b) Changes in response

A study showed that glycine and lysine given to four patients receiving levodopa as a constant IV infusion had no effect, but phenylalanine, leucine and isoleucine reduced the clinical response although the serum levodopa levels remained unchanged.[1] Other studies have shown that a high daily intake of protein reduces the effects of levodopa, compared with the situation when the intake of protein is low.[3,4,5]

Mechanism

(a) Meals which delay gastric emptying allow the levodopa to be exposed to 'wasteful' metabolism in the gut which reduces the amount available for absorption. In addition (b) some large neutral amino acids arising from the digestion of proteins can compete with levodopa for transport into the brain so that the therapeutic response may be reduced, whereas other amino acids do not have this effect.[1,4,6]

Importance and management

An established interaction, but unpredictable. Since the fluctuations in the response of patients to levodopa may be influenced by what is eaten, and when, a change in the pattern of drug and food administration on a trial-and-error basis may be helpful. Multiple small doses of levodopa and distributing the intake of proteins may also iron out the effects of these interactions. Diets which conform to the recommended daily allowance of protein (0.8 g/kg body weight) are reported to eliminate this adverse drug-food interaction.[4]

References

1 Anon. Timing of meals may affect clinical response to levodopa. Am Pharm (1985) 25, 34–5.
2 Morgan JP, Bianchine JR, Spiegel HE, Nutley NJ, Rivera-Calimlim L, Hersey RM. Metabolism of levodopa in patients with Parkinson's disease. Arch Neurol (1971) 25, 39–44.
3 Gillespie NG, Mena I, Cotzias GC. Diets affecting treatment of parkinsonism with levodopa. J Am Diet Ass (1973) 62, 525–8.
4 Juncos JL, Fabbrini G, Mouradian MM, Serrati C, Chase TN. Dietary influences on the antiparkinsonian response to levodopa. Arch Neurol (1987) 44, 1003–5.
5 Carter JH, Nutt JG, Woodward WR, Hatcher LF, Trotman TL. Amount

and distribution of dietary protein affects clinical response to levodopa in Parkinson's disease. Neurology (1989) 39, 552–6.

6 Robertson DRC, Higginson I, Macklin BS, Renwick AG, Waller DG, George CF. The influence of protein containing meals on the pharmacokinetics of levodopa in healthy volunteers. Br J clin Pharmac (1991) 31, 413–7.

Levodopa + Methionine

Abstract/Summary

The effects of levodopa can be reduced by methionine.

Clinical evidence

14 patients with Parkinson's disease and treated with levodopa were given a low-methionine diet for a period of eight days. Five out of seven then given 4.5 g methionine daily showed a definite worsening of the symptoms (gait, tremor, rigidity, etc) which ceased when the methionine was withdrawn. Three out of seven given a placebo showed some subjective improvement.[1] This report confirms the results of a previous study.[2]

Mechanism

Uncertain. One idea is that the methionine competes with the levodopa for active transport into the brain so that its effects are reduced.

Importance and management

Information is very limited but it indicates that large doses of methionine should be avoided in patients being treated with levodopa.

References

1 Pearce LA, Waterbury LD. L-methionine: a possible levodopa antagonist. Neurology (Minneap) (1974) 24, 640.
2 Pearce LA, Waterbury LD. L-methionine: a possible levodopa antagonist. Neurology (Minneap) (1971) 21, 410.

Levodopa + Methyldopa

Abstract/Summary

Methyldopa can increase the effects of levodopa and permit a reduction in the dosage in some patients, but it can also worsen dyskinesias in others. A small increase in the hypotensive actions of methyldopa may also occur.

Clinical evidence

(a) Effects on the response to levodopa

A double-blind cross-over trial in 10 patients with Parkinson's disease who had been taking levodopa for 12–40 months, showed that the optimum daily dose of levodopa, 5.5 g, fell by 78% when using the highest doses of methyldopa studied (1920 mg daily) and by 50% with 800 mg methyldopa daily.[1] A one-third[2] and a two-thirds[3] reduction in the levodopa dosage during concurrent treatment with methyldopa have been described in other reports. Another report states that the control of Parkinson's disease in some patients improved during concurrent use, but worsened the dyskinesias in others.[9] Methyldopa on its own can cause a reversible parkinsonian-like syndrome.[6–8]

(b) Effects on the response to methyldopa

A study in 18 patients with Parkinson's disease showed that levodopa and methyldopa taken together lowered the blood pressure in doses which, when given singly, did not alter the pressure. Daily doses of 1–2.5 g levodopa with 500 mg methyldopa caused a 12/6 mm Hg fall in blood pressure. No change in the control of the Parkinson's disease was seen, but the study lasted only a few days.[4]

Mechanism

Not understood. (a) One idea is that the methyldopa inhibits the enzymic destruction of levodopa outside the brain so that more is available to exert its therapeutic effects. Another is that a false neurotransmitter produced from methyldopa opposes the effects of levodopa. (b) The increased hypotension may simply be due to the additive effects of the two drugs.

Importance and management

Well documented, but the picture presented is a little confusing. Concurrent use need not be avoided but the outcome should be well monitored. The use of methyldopa may allow a reduction in the dosage of the levodopa (the reports cited[1–3] quote figures of between 30 and 78%) and enhance the control of Parkinson's disease, but it should also be borne in mind that in some patients the control may be worsened. The increased hypotensive effects seem to be small but they too should be checked.

References

1 Fermaglich J, Chase TN. Methyldopa or methyldopa hydrazine as levodopa synergists. Lancet (1973) i, 1261.
2 Mones KJ. Evaluation of alpha-methyldopa and alpha-methyldopa hydrazine with L-dopa therapy. NY State J Med (1974) 74, 47.
3 Fermaglich J, O'Doherty DS. Second generation of l-dopa therapy. Neurology (1971) 21, 408.
4 Gibberd FB, Small E. Interaction between levodopa and methyldopa. Br Med J (1973) 2, 90.

5 Smith SE. The pharmacological actions of 3.4-dihydroxy-phenyl-alpha-methylalanine (alpha-methyldopa), an inhibitor of 5-hydroxytryptophan decarboxylase. Br J Pharmacol (1960) 15, 319.

6 Groden BM. Parkinsonism occurring with methyldopa treatment. Br Med J (1963) 2, 1001.

7 Peaston MJT. Parkinsonism associated with alpha-methyldopa therapy. Br Med J (1964) 2, 168.

8 Strang RR. Parkinsonism occurring during methyldopa therapy. Can Med Ass J (1966) 95, 928.

9 Sweet RD, Lee JE, McDowell FH. Methyldopa as an adjunct to levodopa treatment of Parkinson's disease. Clin Pharmacol Ther (1972) 13, 23–7.

Levodopa + Metoclopramide

Abstract/Summary

Some of the effects of levodopa are increased by metoclopramide and other effects are opposed. The outcome of concurrent use is uncertain.

Clinical evidence, mechanism, importance and management

Metoclopramide is a dopamine antagonist and occasionally it causes extrapyramidal disturbances (parkinson-like symptoms) especially in children.[1] On the other hand metoclopramide opposes the effects of levodopa on stomach emptying which can result in an increase in the bioavailability of levodopa.[2,3] The outcome of these two opposite effects (reduced effects and increased bioavailability) is uncertain, but it would be prudent to monitor concurrent use. There seem to be no clinical reports describing an adverse interaction.

References

1 Castells-Van Daele M, Jaeken J, Van der Schueren P. Dystonic reactions in children caused by metoclopramide. Arch Dis Child (1970) 45, 130–3.

2 Berkowitz DM, McCallum RW. Interaction of levodopa and metoclopramide on gastric emptying. Clin Pharmacol Ther (1980) 27, 415–20.

3 Mearrick PT et al. Metoclopramide, gastric emptying and L-dopa absorption. Aust NZ J Med (1974) 4, 144.

Levodopa or Whole broad beans + Monoamine oxidase inhibitors (MAOIs)

Abstract/Summary

A rapid, serious and potentially life-threatening hypertensive reaction can occur in patients on MAOIs if they are concurrently given levodopa or if they eat whole broad beans which contain dopa. An interaction with compound levodopa preparations containing carbidopa or benserazide (*Sinemet, Madopar*) is unlikely. Selegiline (*Deprenyl*) and moclobemide do not interact adversely with levodopa.

Clinical evidence

(a) Levodopa + Monoamine oxidase inhibitor

A patient who had been taking phenelzine daily for 10 days was given 50 mg levodopa by mouth. Within an hour his blood pressure had risen from 135/90 to about 190/130 mm Hg, and despite the IV injection of 5 mg phentolamine it continued to rise over the next 10 min to 200/135 mm Hg, before falling in response to a further 4 mg injection of phentolamine. Next day the experiment was repeated with 25 mg levopa but no blood pressure changes were seen. Three weeks after withdrawal of the phenelzine even 500 mg levodopa had no effect on the blood pressure.[1]

Similar cases of severe hypertension, accompanied in most instances by flushing, throbbing and pounding in the head, neck and chest, and lightheadedness have been described in other case reports and studies involving the concurrent use of levodopa with pargyline,[2] nialamide,[3,4] tranylcypromine,[4,5,7] phenelzine[6,14] and isocarboxazid.[12]

(b) Whole broad beans + Monoamine oxidase inhibitor

A similar hypertensive reaction can occur in patients taking MAOI who have eaten WHOLE cooked broad beans (*Vicia faba* L), that is to say the beans with pods, the latter normally containing dopa.[10] The reports involve pargyline[8] and phenelzine.[9]

Mechanism

Not fully understood. Levodopa is enzymically converted in the body, firstly to dopamine and then to noradrenaline (norepinephrine), both of which are normally under enzymic attack by monoamine oxidase. But in the presence of a monoamine oxidase inhibitor this attack is suppressed which means that the total levels of dopamine and noradrenaline are increased. Precisely how this then leads to a sharp rise in blood pressure is not clear, but either dopamine or noradrenaline, or both, directly or indirectly stimulate the alpha-receptors of the cardiovascular system.

Importance and management

A well documented, serious and potentially life-threatening interaction. Patients should not be given levodopa during treatment with any of the older MAOI cited here, whether used for depression or hypertension, and for a period of 2–3 weeks after their withdrawal. The same precautions apply to the eating of WHOLE cooked broad beans, the dopa being in the pods but not in the beans. If accidental ingestion occurs the hypertensive reaction can be controlled by the IV injection of an alpha-blocker such as phentolamine, or by chewing and swallowing with water the contents of a 10 mg nifedipine capsule. This interaction is inhibited in man by the presence of dopa decarboxylase inhibitors[5] such as carbidopa (in *Sinemet*) and benserazide (in *Madopar*) so that a serious interaction is unlikely to occur with these preparations, even so the makers continue to list the MAOI among their contraindications.

Selegiline (*Deprenyl*) which is an inhibitor of MAO-B does not interact adversely with levodopa and is sometimes used as an adjunct.[11,13] The makers say that if selegiline is given with maximal doses of levodopa, involuntary movements and agitation may occur, but these will disappear if the levodopa dosage is reduced (about 30% is suggested). No adverse interaction appears to occur between levodopa and moclobemide.[15]

References

1 Hunter KR, Boakes AJ, Laurence DR, Stern GM. Monoamine oxidase inhibitors and L-dopa. Br Med J (1970) 3, 388.
2 Hodge JV. Use of monoamine oxidase inhibitors. Lancet (1965) i, 764.
3 Friend DG, Bell WR, Kline NS. The action of L-dihydroxyphenylalanine in patients receiving nialamide. Clin Pharmacol Ther (1965) 6, 363.
4 Horowitz D, Goldberg LI, Sjoerdsma A. Increased blood pressure responses to dopamine and norepinephrine produced by monoamine oxidase inhibitors in man. J Lab Clin Med (1960) 56, 747.
5 Teychenne PF, Calne DB, Lewis PJ, Findley LJ. Interactions of levodopa with inhibitors of monoamine oxidase and L-aromatic amino acid decarboxylase. Clin Pharmacol Ther (1975) 18, 273.
6 Schildkraut JJ, Klerman G, Friend I, Greenblatt M. Biochemical and pressor effects of oral D,L-dihydroxyphenylalanine in patients pretreated with antidepressant drugs. Ann NY Acad Sci (1963) 107, 1005.
7 Sharpe J, Marquez-Julio A, Ashby P. Idiopathic orthostatic hypotension treated with levodopa and MAO inhibitor: a preliminary report. Can Med Ass J (1972) 107, 296.
8 Hodge JV, Nye ER, Emerson GW. Monoamine oxidase inhibitors, broad beans and hypertension. Lancet (1964) i, 1108.
9 Bromley DJ. Monoamine oxidase inhibitors. Lancet (1964) i, 1181.
10 McQueen EG. Interactions with monoamine oxidase inhibitors. Br Med J (1975) 3, 101.
11 Birkmayer W, Riederer P, Ambrozi I, Youdim MBH. Implications of combined treatment with 'Madopar' and L-deprenil in Parkinson's disease. Lancet (1977) i, 439.
12 Birkmayer W, Hornykiewicz O. Archiv fur Psychiatrie und der Nervenkrankheiten vereinigt mit Zeitschrift fur die gesamte Neurologie und Psychiatrie (1962) 203, 560. Quoted in ref 1.
13 Elsworth JD, Glover V, Reynolds GP, Sandler M, Lees AJ, Phuapradit P, Shaw KM, Stern GM, Kumar P. *Deprenyl* administration in man: a selective monoamine oxidase B inhibitor without a 'cheese effect'. Psychopharmacology (1978) 57, 33.
14 Kassirer JP, Kopleman RI. A modern medical Descartes. Hosp Prac (1987) September 15th, 17–25.
15 Dingemanse J. An update of recent moclobemide interaction data. Int Clin Psychopharmacol (1993) 7, 67–80.

Levodopa + Papaverine

Abstract/Summary

There are case reports of a deterioration in the control of parkinsonism in patients treated with levodopa when given papaverine, but a controlled trial failed to confirm this interaction.

Clinical evidence

(a) Reduced levodopa effects

A woman with long-standing parkinsonism, well controlled on levodopa and later levodopa with benserazide, began to show a steady worsening of her parkinsonism within a week of additionally starting 100 mg papaverine daily. The deterioration continued until the papaverine was withdrawn. The normal response to levodopa returned within a week. Four other patients showed a similar response.[1]

Two other similar cases have been described in another report.[2]

(b) No change in levodopa effects

A double-blind cross-over trial was carried out on nine patients with parkinsonism being treated with levodopa (range 100–750 mg daily) plus a decarboxylase inhibitor. Two of them were also taking bromocriptine (40 mg daily) and two benzhexol (15 mg daily). No changes in the control of their disease were seen when they were concurrently treated with 150 mg papaverine hydrochloride daily for 3 weeks.[5]

Mechanism

Not understood. One suggestion is that papaverine blocks the dopamine receptors in the striatum of the brain, thereby inhibiting the effects of the levodopa.[1,3] Another is that papaverine may have a reserpine-like action on the vesicles of adrenergic neurones.[1,4]

Importance and management

Direct information seems to be limited to the reports cited. Concurrent use can apparently be uneventful, however in the light of the reports of adverse interactions it would be prudent to monitor the outcome closely. Carefully controlled trials can provide a good picture of the general situation, but may not necessarily pick out the occasional patient who may be affected by an interaction.

References

1 Duvoisin RC. Antagonism of levodopa by papaverine. J Amer Med Ass (1975) 231, 845.
2 Posner DM. Antagonism of levodopa by papaverine. J Amer Med Ass (1975) 233, 768.
3 *Gonzalez-Vegas JA.* Antagonism of dopamine-mediated inhibition in the nigro-striatal pathgay: a mode of action of some catatonia-inducing drugs. Brain Res (1974) 80, 219.
4 Cebeddu LX, Weiner JA. Relationship between a granular effect and exocytic release of norepinephrine by nerve stimulation. Pharmacologist (1974) 16, 190.
5 Montastruc JL, Rascol O, Belin J, Ane M, Rascol A. Does papaverine interact with levodopa in Parkinson's disease? Ann Neurol (1987) 22, 558–9.

Levodopa + Phenothiazines or Butyrophenones

Abstract/Summary

Phenothiazines and butyrophenones can oppose the effects of levodopa. The antipsychotic effects and extrapyramidal side-effects of the phenothiazines can be opposed by levodopa.

Interaction, mechanism, importance and management

Phenothiazines (eg chlorpromazine) and butyrophenones (eg haloperidol, droperidol) block the dopamine receptors in the brain and can therefore upset the balance between cholinergic and dopaminergic components within the corpus striatum and substantia nigra. As a consequence they may not only induce the development of extrapyramidal (parkinson-like) symptoms, but they can aggravate parkinsonism and antagonize the effects of levodopa used in its treatment.[1-3] Antiemetics such as prochlorperazine[1,2] and trifluoperazine[2] can behave in this way. For this reason drugs of this kind are generally regarded as contraindicated in patients under treatment for Parkinson's disease, or they are only to be used with great caution in carefully controlled conditions. Non-phenothiazine antiemetics which do not antagonize the effects of levodopa include cyclizine (*Marzine*) and diphenidol (*Vontrol*).

The extrapyramidal symptoms which frequently occur with the phenothiazines have been treated with varying degrees of success with levodopa, but the levodopa may also antagonize the antipsychotic effects of the phenothiazines.[4,5]

References

1 Duvoisin R.C. Diphenidol for levodopa-induced nausea and vomiting. J Amer Med Ass (1972) 221, 1408.
2 Campbell JB. Long-term treatment of Parkinson's disease with levodopa. Neurology (1970) 20 (December Suppl), 18.
3 Klawans HL, Weiner WJ. Attempted use of haloperidol in the treatment of L-dopa induced dyskinesias. J Neurol Neurosurg Psychiatry (1974) 37, 427–30.
4 Yaryura-Tobias JA. Action of L-dopa in drug-induced extrapyramidalism. Dis Nerv Syst (1970) 1, 60.
5 Hunter KR, Stern GM, Laurence DR. Use of levodopa and other drugs. Lancet (1970) ii, 1283.

Levodopa + Phenylbutazone

Abstract/Summary

A single case report describes antagonism of the effects of levodopa by phenylbutazone.

Interaction, mechanism, importance and management

A patient who was very sensitive to levodopa found that only by taking frequent small doses (0.125 g) was he able to prevent the involuntary movements of his tongue, jaw, neck and limbs. If these developed he was able to suppress them with phenylbutazone, but this also lessened the beneficial effect.[1] The reason is not understood. This interaction has not been confirmed by anyone else and its general importance is not known, but prescribers should be aware of this isolated case.

Reference

1 Wodak J, Gilligan BS, Veale JL, Dowty BJ. Review of 12 months treatment with L-dopa in Parkinson's disease, with remarks on unusual side-effects. Med J Aust (1972) 2, 1277–82.

Levodopa + Phenytoin

Abstract/Summary

The therapeutic effects of levodopa can be reduced or abolished by the concurrent use of phenytoin.

Clinical evidence, mechanism, importance and management

In a study on five patients treated with levodopa (630–4600 mg plus 150–225 mg carbidopa daily) for Parkinson's disease, it was found that when they were additionally given phenytoin (100–500 mg daily) for 5–19 days the levodopa dyskinesias were relieved but the beneficial effects of the levodopa were also reduced or abolished. The patients became slow, rigidity re-emerged and some of them became unable to get out of a chair. Within two weeks of stopping the phenytoin, their parkinsonism was again well controlled by the levodopa.[1] The mechanism of this interaction is not understood. Information seems to be limited to this study, nevertheless it would seem prudent to avoid giving phenytoin to patients already taking levodopa. If both drugs are used it may be necessary to increase the dosage of the levodopa.

Reference

1 Mendez JS, Cotzias GC, Mena I, Papavasiliou PS. Diphenylhydantoin blocking of levodopa effects. Arch Neurol (1975) 32, 44.

Levodopa + Piperidine

Abstract/Summary

Piperidine hydrochloride opposes both the dyskinesia associated with the use of levodopa and the beneficial effects of levodopa.

Clinical evidence, mechanism, importance and management

A study on 11 patients with Parkinson's diseases and levodopa-induced dyskinesia showed that piperidine hydrochloride, in daily doses of 700–6300 mg over periods of 10–33 days, diminished the dyskinesia, but it also opposed the effects of the levodopa so that the parkinsonian symptoms re-emerged.[1] This is probably because piperidine has cholinergic effects which upset the cholinergic/dopaminergic balance for which the levodopa had originally been given. This was essentially an experimental study undertaken in the hope that piperidine might prove to be beneficial. It would seem that there is no therapeutic value in the concurrent use of these drugs.

Reference

1 Tolosa ES, Cotzias GC, Papavasilou PS, Lazarus CB. Antagonism by piperidine of levodopa effects in Parkinson's disease. Neurology (1977) 27, 875.

Levodopa + Pyridoxine (Vitamin B6)

Abstract/Summary

The effects of levodopa are reduced or abolished by the concurrent use of pyridoxine, but no adverse interaction occurs with levodopa-carbidopa or levodopa-benserazide preparations (e.g. *Sinemet, Madopar*).

Clinical evidence

(a) Levodopa + Pyridoxine

A study in 25 patients being treated with levodopa showed that if they were given high doses of pyridoxine (750–1000 mg daily) the effects of the levodopa were completely abolished within 3–4 days, and some reduction in the effects were evident within 24 h. Daily doses of 50–100 mg also reduced or abolished the effects of levodopa, and an increase in the signs and symptoms of parkinsonism occurred in eight out of 10 patients taking only 5–10 mg pyridoxine daily.[1]

The antagonism of the effects of levodopa by pyridoxine has been described in numerous other reports.[2–11]

(b) Levodopa-carbidopa + Pyridoxine

A study on six chronic levodopa-treated patients with Parkinson's disease showed that when given 250 mg levodopa with 50 mg pyridoxine their mean levodopa plasma levels fell by 70% (from 356 to 109 ng/ml). With levodopa-carbidopa their mean plasma levels rose almost three-fold (to 845 ng/ml) and with 50 mg pyridoxine as well a further slight increase occurred (to 891 ng/ml), although the plasma-integrated area fell 22% from that obtained with levodopa-carbidopa.[11]

The absence of an interaction is confirmed in another report.[12]

Mechanism

The conversion of levodopa to dopamine within the body requires the presence of pyridoxal-5-phosphate (derived from pyridoxine) as a co-factor. When dietary amounts of pyridoxine are high, the 'wasteful' metabolism of levodopa outside the brain is increased so that less is available for entry into the CNS and its effects are reduced accordingly. Pyridoxine may also alter levodopa metabolism by Schiff-base formation. However in the presence of dopa-decarboxylase inhibitors such as carbidopa or benserazide, this 'wasteful' metabolism of levodopa is reduced and much larger amounts are available for entry into the CNS, even if quite small doses are given. So even in the presence of large amounts of pyridoxine, the peripheral metabolism remains unaffected and the serum levels of levodopa are virtually unaltered.

Importance and management

A clinically important, well documented and well established. Doses of pyridoxine as low as 5 mg daily can reduce the effects of levodopa and should be avoided. Warn patients about the self-administration of proprietary pyridoxine-containing preparations. Martindale's Extra Pharmacopoeia lists numerous over-the-counter preparations containing varying amounts of pyridoxine (ranging from 0.1 to 25 mg in each tablet or capsule) many of which could undoubtedly interact to a significant extent. Some breakfast cereals are fortified with pyridoxine and other vitamins, but the amounts are usually too small to matter. For example, a normal serving of *Kellogg's Corn Flakes* or *Rice Krispies* (UK preparations) contains only about 0.6 mg pyridoxine, and a whole 500 g packet contains only 9 mg. There is no good clinical evidence to suggest that a low-pyridoxine diet is desirable, and indeed it may be harmful since the normal dietary requirements are about 2 mg daily. The problem of this interaction can be totally solved by using levodopa-carbidopa or levodopa-benserazide preparations (e.g. *Sinemet* or *Madopar*) which are unaffected by pyridoxine.

References

1 Duvoisin RC, Yahr MD, Cote LD. Pyridoxine reversal of L-dopa effects in parkinsonism. Trans Amer Neurol Ass (1969) 94, 81.
2 O'Reilly S. Pyridoxine reversal of L-dopa effects in parkinsonism. Trans Amer Neurol Ass (1969) 94, 81.
3 Markham CH. Pyridoxine reversal of L-dopa effects in parkinsonism. Trans Amer Neurol Ass (1969) 94, 81.
4 Schwab RS. Pyridoxine reversal of L-dopa effects in parkinsonism. Trans Amer Neurol Ass (1969) 94, 81.
5 Celesia GG, Barr AN. Psychosis and other psychiatriac manifestations of levodopa therapy. Arch Neurol (1970) 23, 193.
6 Carter AB. Pyridoxine and parkinsonism. Br Med J (1973) 4, 236.
7 Cotzias GC, Papavasiliou PS. Blocking the negative effects of pyridoxine on patients receiving levodopa. J Amer Med Ass (1971) 215, 1504.
8 Leon AS, Spiegel HE, Thomas G, Abrams WB. Pyridoxine antagonism of levodopa in parkinsonism. J Amer Med Ass (1971) 218, 1924.
9 Hildick-Smith M. Pyridoxine in parkinsonism. Lancet (1973) ii, 1029.

10 Yahr MD, Duvoisin RC. Pyridoxine and levodopa in the treatment of parkinsonism. J Amer Med Ass (1972) 220, 861.

11 Mars H. Levodopa, carbidopa and pyridoxine in Parkinson's disease: metabolic interactions. Arch Neurol (1974) 30, 444.

12 Papavasiliou PS, Cotzias GC, Duby SE, Steck AJ, Fehling C, Bell MA. Levodopa in parkinsonism: potentiation of central effects with a peripheral inhibitor. N Engl J Med (1972) 286, 8–14.

Levodopa + Rauwolfia alkaloids

Abstract/Summary

The effects of levodopa are opposed by the concurrent use of rauwolfia alkaloids such as reserpine.

Clinical evidence, mechanism, importance and management

Reserpine and other rauwolfia alkaloids deplete the brain of monoamines, including dopamine, thereby reducing their effects.[1] This opposes the actions of administered levodopa. There are sound pharmacological reasons for believing that this is an interaction of clinical importance, and a reduction in the antiparkinsonian activity of levodopa by reserpine has been observed.[2] The rauwolfia alkaloids should be avoided in patients with Parkinson's disease, whether or not they are taking levodopa.

References

1 Bianchine JR, Sunyapridakul L. Interactions between levodopa and other drugs: significance in the treatment of Parkinson's disease. Drugs (1973) 6, 364.

2 Yahr MD. Personal communication (1977).

Levodopa + Spiramycin

Abstract/Summary

The serum levels of levodopa are reduced by the concurrent use of spiramycin, thereby reducing its therapeutic effects.

Clinical evidence

The observation of a patient with Parkinson's disease on levodopa/carbidopa (*Sinemet*) who became less well-controlled when treated with spiramycin, prompted further study in seven normal subjects given 250 mg levodopa + 25 mg carbidopa. After taking 1 g spiramycin twice daily for 3 days, the AUC (area under the curve) of the levodopa fell to 43% (from 253809 to 109558 ng/ml/min) while maximum serum levels fell from 2161 to 1679 ng/ml (not significant). The serum levels of the carbidopa were barely detectable (an AUC fall from 27706 to 1059 ng/ml/min).[1]

Mechanism

Not fully established. In some way the spiramycin markedly reduces the absorption of the carbidopa, possibly by forming a non-absorbable complex in the gut or by accelerating its transit through the gut. As a result, not enough carbidopa is absorbed to inhibit the 'wasteful' metabolism of the levodopa within the body so that the effects of the levodopa are reduced.[1]

Importance and management

Information is very limited but the interaction appears to be established and of clinical importance. If spiramycin is given, anticipate the need to increase the dosage of the levodopa/carbidopa preparation (approximately double the dose). It is not known whether other macrolide antibiotics behave in a similar way, or whether spiramcyin affects levodopa/benserazide preparations. More study is needed.

Reference

1 Brion N, Kollenbach K, Marion MH, Grégoire A, Adveneir C, Pays M. Effect of a macrolide (spiramycin) on the pharmacokinetics of L-dopa and carbidopa in healthy volunteers. Clin Neuropharmacol (1992) 15, 229–35.

Levodopa + Tricyclic antidepressants

Abstract/Summary

Concurrent use is usually uneventful although a small reduction in the effects of levodopa may occur. Two unexplained hypertensive crises have also occurred when both drugs were used.

Clinical evidence

(a) Reduced levodopa effects

A study in man showed that the concurrent use of imipramine, 100 mg daily for three days, reduced the absorption of a single 500 mg dose of levodopa. Peak serum concentrations of levodopa were reduced about 50% although the 24-hr cumulative excretion was not significantly different from the control.[1]

(b) Hypertensive crises

A hypertensive crisis (blood pressure 210/110 mmHg) associated with agitation, tremor and generalized rigidity developed in a woman taking six tablets of *Sinemet* (levodopa 100 mg + 10 mg carbidopa) when she started to take 25 mg imipramine three times a day. It occurred again when she was later accidentally given the same dosage of amitriptyline.[5]

A similar hypertensive reaction (a rise from 190/110 to 270/140 mmHg) occurred over 36 h in another woman taking amitriptyline when given half a tablet of *Sinemet* and 10 mg metoclopramide three times a day.[2]

Mechanisms

(a) The tricyclics have anticholinergic activity which slows gastric emptying, and this allows more time for the gastric mucosa to metabolize the levodopa 'wastefully', thereby reducing the amount available for entry into the brain. (b) The hypertensive reactions are not understood.

Importance and management

Information seems to be limited to these reports. Concurrent use is normally successful and uneventful[3,4,6] but it would be prudent to check that the effects of the levodopa are not undesirably reduced. Also be alert for the possibility of a hypertensive reaction which resolves if the tricyclic antidepressant is withdrawn.

References

1 Morgan JP, Rivera-Calimlim L, Messiha F, Sandaresan PR, Trabert N. Imipramine-mediated interference with levodopa absorption from the gastrointestinal tract in man. Neurology (1975) 25, 1029.
2 Rampton DS. Hypertensive crisis in a patient given *Sinemet*, metoclopramide and amitriptyline. Br Med J (1977) 3, 607.
3 Yahr MD. The treatment of Parkinsonism-Current concepts. Med Clin N Amer (1972) 56, 1377.
4 Calne DB, Reid JL. Antiparkinsonian drugs: pharmacological and therapeutic aspects. Drugs (1972) 4, 49.
5 Edwards M. Adverse interaction of levodopa with tricyclic antidepressants. The Practitioner (1982) 226, 1448.
6 van Wiegeren A, Wright J. Observations on patients with Parkinson's disease treated with L-dopa. Trial and evaluation of L-dopa therapy. SA Med J (1972) 46, 1262.

Levodopa + L-tryptophan

Abstract/Summary

L-tryptophan can reduce levodopa blood levels.

Clinical evidence, mechanism, importance and management

The blood levels of dopa were markedly reduced in normal healthy subjects when 0.5 g levodopa was taken with 1.0 g L-tryptophan. The reasons are not understood. The clinical importance of this was not assessed. L-Tryptophan has been withdrawn in the USA and UK because of a possible association with the development of a serious eosinophilia-myalgia syndrome.

Reference

1 Weitbrecht W-U, Weigel K. Der Einfluss von L-Tryptophan auf die L-Dopa Resorption. Dtsch med Wschr (1976) 101, 20–2.

Chapter 10
Beta-Blocker Drug Interactions

The adreno-receptors of the sympathetic nervous system are of two main types, namely alpha and beta. The beta-adrenoreceptor blocking drugs (better known as the beta-blockers) are sufficiently selective to block only the beta-receptors and this property is therapeutically exploited to reduce, for example, the normal sympathetic stimulation of the heart. The activity of the heart in response to stress and exercise is reduced, its consumption of oxygen is diminished, and in this way the angina of effort can be treated. Beta-blockers given orally can also be used in the treatment of cardiac arrhythmias, hypertension, and in the form of eye-drops for glaucoma and ocular hypertension.

Some of the beta-blockers are sufficiently selective to show that all beta-receptors are not identical but can be further subdivided into two groups, beta-1 and beta-2. The former are found in the heart and the latter in the bronchi. Since one of the unwanted side-effects of generalized beta-blockade can be the loss of the normal noradrenaline-stimulated bronchodilation (leading to bronchospasm), there was clear therapeutic advantage in the development of the cardioselective beta-1 blocking drugs (e.g. practolol, metoprolol) which leave the beta-2 receptors virtually unaffected. These cardioselective beta-blockers are therefore particularly valuable in patients such as asthmatics where bronchospasm is clearly unacceptable, although it should be emphasised that the selectivity is not absolute because a few asthmatics even develop bronchospasm with these

Table 10.1 Cardioselective beta-blockers (beta-1 receptors only)

Non-proprietary names	Proprietary names
Acebutolol	*Acecor, Alol, Diasectral, Molson, Neptal, Prent, Rhodiasectral, Secadrex, Sectral, Westfalin*
Atenolol	*Atenol, Beta-Adalat, Blokium, Ibinolo, Kalten, Myocord, Neatenol, Prenormine, Seles beta, Telvodin, Tenif, Tenoret(ic), Tenormin(e), Vericordin*
Betaxolol	*Betoptic, Betoptima, Kerlone*
Bevantolol	
Bisoprolol	*Concor, Detensiel, Emcor, Monocor*
Celiprolol	*Selectol*
Cycloprolol (Cicloprolol)	
Esmolol	*Brevibloc*
Metoprolol	*Beloc, Beprolo, Betaloc, Co-betaloc, Lopres(s)or, Metoros, Novometoros, Prelis, Selokeen, Selo-Zok*
Practolol	*Dalzic, Eraldin*
Talinolol	

drugs. Tables 10.1 and 10.2 list most of the beta-blockers currently available.

In addition to the interactions with the beta-blockers detailed in this chapter, there are others discussed elsewhere. See the Index for a full listing.

Table 10.2 Non-selective beta-blockers (block beta-1 and beta-2 receptors)

Non-proprietary names	Proprietary names
Alprenolol	*Apllobal, Aptin(e), Aptol, Gubernal, Regletin, Sinalol, Vasoton*
Befunolol	*Bentos, Glauconex*
Bopindolol	*Sandonorm*
Bucindolol	
Bufetolol	*Adobiol*
Bufuralol	
Bunitrolol	*Stresson*
Bupranolol	*Betadran, Betadrenol, Looser, Monobeltin, Ophtorenin, Panimit*
Butofilolol	*Cafide*
Carazolol	*Conducton*
Carteolol	*Arteolol, Arteoptic, Carteol, Cartol, Endak, Mikelan, Teoptic*
Dilevalol	
Indenolol	*Pulsan, Securpres*
Levobunolol	*Betagan, Vistagan*
Moprolol	*Levotensin, Omeral*
Mepindolol	*Betagon, Corindolan, Mepicor*
Metipranolol	*Betamann, Betanol, Beta-ophthiole, Disorat, Glauline, Turoptin*
Nadolol	*Corgard, Corgaretic, Solgol*
Nifenalol	*Impeasel, Inpea*
Oxprenolol	*Apsolox, Captol, Laracor, Lo-Tone, Oxanol, Slow-Pren, Trasicor, Trasidex*
Penbutolol	*Betapressin(e), Blocotin, Ipobab, Lasiprersin, Levatol*
Pindolol	*Barbloc, Betadren, Carvicken, Decreten, Dubapindol, Hexapindol, Pectobloc, Pinbetol, Viskaldix, Viskeen, Visken(e)*
Propranolol	*Angilol, Apsolol, Avlocardyl, Bedranol, Beprane, Berkolol, Beta-neg, Betaryl, Beta-Tablinen, Beta-Timeleds, Blocardyl, Cartdinol, Cardispare, Caridolol, Deralin, Detensol, Dociton, Efekotolol, Elbrol, Euprovasin, Frekven, Herzul, Inderal(ici), Indobloc, Kemi, Noloten, Novopranol, Pranolol, Prano-puren, Prolol, Pronovan, Propabbloc, Propalong, Propayerst, Propranur, Pur-bloka, Pylapron, Rexigen, Sagittol, Sumial, Tensiflex, Tesnol*
Sotalol	*Beta-cardone, Betades, Sotacor, Sotalex, Sotapor*
Tertatolol	*Artex*
Timolol	*Betim, Blocadren, Blocanol, Cusimolol, Oftan-timolol, Proflax, Temserin, Tenopt, Timacor, Timoptic, Timoptol*

Table 10.3 Drugs with both alpha and beta-blocking activity

Non-proprietary names	Proprietary names
Carvedilol	
Labetolol	Abetol, Alfabetal, Amipress, Ipolab, Labrocol, Lolum, Mitalolo, Normodyne, Presdate, Pressalolo, Trandate
Medraxolol	

Beta-blockers + Alcohol

Abstract/Summary

The effects of metoprolol and atenolol are not changed by the concurrent use of alcohol, nor does propranolol change the effects of alcohol.

Clinical evidence, mechanism, importance and management

No significant changes in blood pressures or pulse rates or in the pharmacokinetics of single doses of 100 mg of atenolol or metoprolol occurred in eight subjects 6 h after drinking the equivalent of 200 ml absolute alcohol.[1] The performance of a number of psychomotor tests was unaltered in 12 subjects by 160 mg propranolol when given with 50 ml/70 kg body weight of alcohol,[2] although some effect on divided attention was seen in another study.[3] There do not seem to be any strong reasons for avoiding concurrent use, however your attention is drawn to the synopsis, 'Antihypertensives + Alcohol'.

References

1 Kirch W, Spahn H, Hutt HJ, Ohnhaus EE, Mutschler E. Interaction between alcohol and metoprolol or atenolol in social drinking. Drugs (1983) 25 (Suppl 2) 152.
2 Lindenschmidt R, Brown D, Cerimele B, Walle T, Forney RB. Combined effects of propranolol and ethanol on human psychomotor performance. Toxicol Appl Pharmacol (1983) 67, 117–21.
3 Noble EP, Parker E, Alkana R, Cohen H, Birch H. Propranolol-ethanol interaction in man. Fed Proc (1973) 32, 724.

Beta-blockers + Allopurinol

Abstract/Summary, clinical evidence, mechanism, importance and management.

Allopurinol does not affect the pharmacokinetics of atenolol.[1]

References

1 Schafer-Korting M, Kirch W, Axthelm T, Kohler H, Mutschler E. Atenolol interaction with aspirin, allopurinol, and ampicillin. Clin Pharmacol Ther (1983) 33, 283–8.

Beta-blockers + Antacids

Abstract/Summary

Although some antacids and antidiarrhoeals may cause a modest reduction in the absorption of propranolol, atenolol and other beta-blockers, and possibly an increase in the absorption of metoprolol, the clinical importance of these interactions is probably minimal.

Clinical evidence

(a) Propranolol + aluminium hydroxide

30 ml aluminium hydroxide gel affected neither the plasma concentrations nor the increases in heart rates caused by exercise in six subjects given 40 mg propranolol.[1]

In contrast, another study in five subjects found that 30 ml aluminium hydroxide gel given with single 80 mg doses of propranolol reduced the plasma propranolol levels and the AUC (area under the curve) by almost 60%.[2] Animal studies have shown that bismuth subsalicylate, kaolin-pectin and magnesium trisilicate can also reduce the absorption of propranolol.[5,6]

(b) Atenolol or metoprolol + aluminium hydroxide or calcium gluconate/carbonate

5.6 g aluminium hydroxide given to six subjects caused an insignificant fall (20%) in plasma atenolol levels, after a single 100 mg dose. Six hypertensive subjects, given 500 mg calcium as the lactate, gluconate or carbonate, showed a reduction in the absorption of atenolol after a single 100 mg dose. The half-life was prolonged but the beta-blocking effects were not significantly changed.[3]

Another study showed that an aluminium and magnesium-containing antacid reduced the bioavailability of atenolol 37% but increased that of metoprolol by 25%.[4]

(c) Indenolol + aluminium/magnesium hydroxide/ simethicone or kaolin/pectin

A study in rats showed that when given indenolol with either *Simeco* or Kaopectate, the 6 h AUC (area under the curve) were reduced 15 and 30% respectively.[7]

Mechanism

Uncertain. The reduction in absorption could possibly be related to a delay in gastric emptying caused by the antacid, or to some complexation between the two drugs in the gut which reduces absorption.

Importance and management

The documentation is limited and in some instances somewhat contradictory. It is also largely confined to single dose or animal studies which may not be clinically relevant. Some changes in absorption may possibly occur but nobody seems to have shown that it has a significant effect on the therapeutic effectiveness of the beta-blockers. Nevertheless it might be prudent to be on the alert for any changes in the response to beta-blockers during concurrent use. Separating the dosages would seem a simple way of avoiding any problems. There seems to be no information about other beta-blockers and antacids.

References

1 Hong CY, Hu SC, Lin SJ, Chiang BN. Lack of influence of aluminium hydroxide on the bioavailability and beta-adrenoceptor blocking activity of propranolol. Int J Clin Pharmacol Ther Toxicol (1985) 23, 244–46.
2 Dobbs JH, Skoutakis VA, Acchardio SR, Dobbs BR. Effects of aluminium hydroxide on the absorption of propranolol. Curr Ther Res (1977) 21, 887.
3 Kirch W, Schafer-Korting M, Axthelm T, Kohler H, Mutschle E. Interaction of furosemide and calcium and aluminium salts. Clin Pharmacol Ther (1981) 30, 429–35.
4 Regardh CG, Lundborg P, Persson BA. The effect of antacid, metoclopramide and propantheline on the bioavailability of metoprolol and atenolol. Biopharm Drug Dispos (1981) 2, 79–87.
5 Moustafa MA, Gouda MW, Tariq M. Decreased bioavailability of propranolol due to interactions with adsorbent antacids and antidiarrhoeal mixtures. Int J Pharmaceutics (1986) 30, 225–8.
6 McElnay JC, D'Arcy PF, Leonard JK. The effect of activated dimethicone, other antacid constituents, and kaolin on the absorption of propranolol. Experentia (1982) 38, 605–7.
7 Tariq M, Babhair SA. Effect of antacid and antidiarrhoeal drugs on the bioavailability of indenolol. IRCS Med Sci (1984) 12, 87–8.

Beta-blockers + Anticholinesterases

Abstract/Summary

Normally no adverse reaction occurs, but a small number of reports describe marked bradycardia and hypotension during the recovery period from anaesthesia and neuromuscular blockade in patients on beta-blockers when given anticholinesterase drugs. Myasthenic symptoms have occurred in a few patients given practolol, propranolol or oxprenolol.

Clinical evidence

A patient on nadolol, recovering from surgery during which succinylcholine had been used for tracheal intubation and pancuronium for general muscular relaxation, developed prolonged bradycardia (32–36 bpm) and hypotension (systolic pressure 60–70 torr) when neostigmine and atropine were given to reverse the neuromuscular blockade.[1] Another patient on propranolol and anaesthetized with N_2O/O_2 and alcuronium also developed severe bradycardia (a fall from 65 to 40 bpm) and hypotension (systolic pressure 70 mmHg) when given physostigmine.[2] Prolonged bradycardia and hypotension were seen in an elderly woman on atenolol when given neostigmine and atropine for the reversal of muscle relaxation at the end of general anaesthesia.[6] Other reports similarly describe this effect when neostigmine was used.[3–5]

These reports contrast with a study in eight hypertensive patients taking beta-blockers (atenolol or propranolol) who showed no significant changes in heart rates when given pyridostigmine (30 mg three times daily for 2 days) and no adverse reactions.[8]

Four patients developed myasthenic symptoms when treated with beta-blockers (two on propranolol, one on oxprenolol and the other on practolol). Two of them were effectively treated with pyridostigmine.[7]

Mechanism

It would appear that the heart-slowing effects of the beta-blockers and the acetylcholine-like effects of these anticholinesterase drugs can be additive. In the instances cited, these were inadequately controlled by the use of atropine. The reason for the myasthenic symptoms is not understood.

Importance and management

The information available indicates that marked adverse reactions are uncommon, but concurrent use should be well monitored to ensure that the occasional problem is dealt with promptly.

References

1 Seidl DC, Martin DE. Prolonged bradycardia after neostigmine administration in a patient taking nadolol. Anesth Analg (1984) 63, 365–7.
2 Baraka A, Dajani A. Severe bradycardia following physostigmine in the presence of beta-adrenergic blockade. Middle Eastern J Anaesthesiology (1984) 7, 291–3.
3 Sprague DH. Severe bradycardia after neostigmine in a patient taking propranolol to control paroxsymal atrial tachycardia. Anesthesiology (1975) 42, 208–10.
4 Wagner DL, Moorthy SS, Stoertling RK. Administration of anticholinesterase drugs in the presence of beta-blockade. Anesth Analg (1982) 61, 153–4.
5 Prys-Roberts C. Cardiovascular responses to anaesthesia and surgery in patients receiving beta-receptor antagonists. In 'Beta-blockade and Anaesthesia', Poppers PJ, van Dijk B and van Elzakker AHM. (eds). Rijswijk, Netherlands: Astra Pharmaceutica (1980) 164–70.
6 Eldor J, Hoffmann B, Davidson JT. Prolonged bradycardia and hypotension after neostigmine administration in a patient receiving atenolol. Anaesthesia (1987) 42, 1294–7.
7 Herishanu Y, Rosenberg P. Beta-blockers and myasthenia gravis. Ann Intern Med (1975) 83, 834–5.
8 Arad M, Roth A, Zelinger J, Zivner Z, Rabinowitz B, Atsmon J. Safety of pyridostigmine in hypertensive patients receiving beta blockers. Am J Cardiol (1992) 69, 518–22.

Beta-blockers + Barbiturates

Abstract/Summary

The serum levels and the effects of those beta-blockers which are mainly removed from the body by liver metabolism (e.g. propranolol, alprenolol, metoprolol, etc.) are reduced by the concurrent use of barbiturates. Alprenolol concentrations are halved, but the others are possibly not affected as much. Beta-blockers which are mainly lost unchanged in the urine (e.g. atenolol, sotalol, nadolol, etc.) are not affected by the barbiturates.

Clinical evidence

100 mg pentobarbitone for 10 days at bedtime reduced the serum alprenolol levels (400 mg twice daily) of six hypertensive patients by 59%. Mean pulse rates at rest rose by 6% (from 67 to 75 bpm) and blood pressures rose 8–9% (from 138/93 to

143/97 mm Hg). In a further study on the same patients, resting pulse rates rose from 70 to 74 bpm, and blood pressures rose from 134/89 to 145/97 mm Hg within 4–5 days of starting the barbiturate, and fell once again within 8–9 days of stopping.[6]

These results confirm previous studies by the same authors and others. Pentobarbitone was found to cause a 40% reduction in serum alprenolol levels after a single 200 mg dose of alprenolol. There was also a 20% reduction in the effects of the beta-blocker on the heart rate during exercise.[2] The AUC (area under curve) of alprenolol was reduced by about 80% after 100 mg pentobarbitone daily for 10–14 days.[1] Other studies have shown that 100 mg pentobarbitone for 10 days reduced the AUC of metoprolol by 32% (eight normal subjects),[3] and 100 mg phenobarbitone daily for seven days reduced the AUC of timolol by 24% (12 normal subjects).[4] Phenobarbitone also seems to increase the clearance of propranolol, but not sotalol.[5]

Mechanism

Barbiturates are potent liver enzyme inducing agents which can increase the metabolism and clearance of other drugs from the body. Beta-blockers which are removed from the body principally by liver metabolism (e.g. alprenolol, propranolol, metoprolol, timolol, etc.) can therefore be cleared more quickly in the presence of a barbiturate, whereas other beta-blockers which are lost mainly unchanged in the urine (e.g. sotalol) are not affected.

Importance and management

The alprenolol-pentobarbitone interaction is well documented and likely to be of clinical importance when the beta-blocker is being used to treat hypertension, and possibly angina. Since blood levels are roughly halved, it seems reasonable to expect that the dosage will need to be doubled to accommodate this interaction. This needs confirmation. Other barbiturates would be expected to do the same. A reduced response is likely with any of the beta-blockers which are extensively metabolized (e.g. propranolol, metoprolol, alprenolol, timolol, etc.), but the effects on the AUC's of metoprolol and timolol are less than with alprenolol (32%, 24% and 80% respectively) so that the dosage increases which are needed may proportionately less. Detailed information about the clinical importance of this interaction with propranolol and other beta-blockers is lacking. The interaction can almost certainly be avoided by using one of the beta-blockers which are primarily lost unchanged in the urine (e.g. atenolol, sotalol, nadolol, etc.).

References

1 Alvan G, Piafsky K, Lind M, von Bah C. Effect of pentobarbital on the disposition of alprenolol. Clin Pharmacol Ther (1977) 22, 316.
2 Collste P, Seideman P, Borg K-O, Haglund K, von Bah C. Influence of pentobarbital on effects and plasma levels of alprenolol and 4-hydroxy-alprenolol. Clin Pharmacol Ther (1979) 25, 423–7.
3 Haglund K, Seiderman P, Collste P, Borg K-O, von Bah C. Influence of pentobarbital on metoprolol plasma levels. Clin Pharmacol Ther (1979) 26, 326.
4 Mantyla R, Mannisto P, Nykanen S, Kopenen A, Lamminsivu U. Pharmacokinetic interactions of timolol with vasodilating drugs, food and phenobarbitone in healthy volunteers. Eur J Clin Pharmacol (1983) 24, 227–30.
5 Sotaniemi EA, Anttila M, Pelkonen RO, Jarvensivu P, Sundquist H. Plasma clearance of propranolol and sotalol and hepatic drug-metabolizing activity. Clin Pharmacol Ther (1979) 26, 153–161.
6 Seideman P, Borg K-O, Haglund K, von Bah C. Decreased plasma concentrations and clinical effects of alprenolol during combined treatment with pentobarbitone in hypertension. Br J clin Pharmac (1987) 23, 267–71.

Beta-blockers + Calcium channel blockers

Abstract/Summary

The concurrent use of the beta-blockers and calcium channel blockers cited below (felodipine, isradipine, lacipine, nimodipine, nisoldipine) appears to be useful and safe, but adverse effects, some quite serious, can occur with some drug combinations (see other synopses about beta-blockers + diltiazem, nicardipine, nifedipine, verapamil.) Changes in the pharmacokinetics of the beta-blockers may also occur.

Clinical evidence

(a) Felodipine

A double-blind crossover study in eight normal subjects showed that, over a five-day period, metoprolol (100 mg twice daily) did not affect the pharmacokinetics of felodipine (10 mg twice daily). On the other hand the bioavailability of metoprolol was increased by 30% and its peak serum levels by 38%.[1] Another study in 10 normal subjects given 10 mg felodipine with either 100 mg metoprolol, 5 mg pindolol, 80 mg propranolol or 10 mg timolol found no changes in heart rate, PR interval or blood pressure which might be considered to be harmful to patients with hypertension or angina,[2] however seven of the ten reported some increase in adverse reactions.

(b) Isradipine

A study in 24 subjects found that the concurrent use of 80 mg propranolol and 10mg isradipine daily caused some modest changes in the pharmacokinetics both drugs (peak propranolol serum levels + 17%, peak isradipine serum levels – 18%), but the AUCs were unaltered.[4] A previous study by some of the same authors found an increase in the propranolol AUC (+ 22%), a reduction in the isradipine AUC (– 18%) and a 59% increase in the peak propranolol levels.[6]

(c) Lacidipine

Single dose studies in 24 normal subjects found that 160 mg propranolol reduced the peak serum levels and AUC of lacidipine (4 mg) by 38 and 42% respectively, while the peak serum levels of the propranolol were increased by 35 and 26% respectively. There was a modest additive reduction (4–6 mm Hg) in blood pressures, and heart rates were reduced by 5 bpm. No significant adverse effects were seen.[7]

(d) Nimodipine

30 mg nimodipine three times daily for four days in 12 normal subjects had no significant effect on the changes in heart rate, blood pressure or cardiac output due to either 40 mg propranolol or 25 mg atenolol three times daily, or on their pharmacokinetics.[8]

(e) Nisoldipine

Two studies[3,5] in 12 and 8 subjects found that single 20 mg oral doses of nisoldipine with 40–160 mg propranolol increased the propranolol AUC by 30–43% and the peak propranolol levels by 50–68%. With 100 mg atenolol the maximum serum level was increased by 20%. In one study both the fall in blood pressure the extent of beta-blockade were increased.

Mechanisms

Not understood. Where pharmacokinetic changes are seen, a possible reason is that the metabolism of the beta-blockers is changed by changes in blood flow through the liver.

Importance and management

The concurrent use of beta-blockers and calcium channel blockers is common and normally valuable but not always entirely free of problems. Serious cardiodepression has been seen in a few patients on beta-blockers given nifedipine, diltiazem and particularly verapamil (see 'Beta-blockers + Diltiazem', 'Beta-blockers + Nifedipine', 'Beta-blockers + Verapamil'). Against this background it would seem prudent to monitor concurrent use for any evidence of undesirable cardiodepression.

References

1 Smith SR, Wilkins MR, Jack DB, Kendall MJ, Laugher S. Pharmacokinetic interactions between felodipine and metoprolol. Eur J Clin Pharmacol (1987) 31, 575–8.
2 Carruthers SG, Bailey DG. Tolerance and cardiovascular effects of single dose felodipine/beta-blocker combinations in healthy subjects. J Cardiovasc Pharmacol (1987) 10 (Suppl 1) S169–77.
3 Levine MAH, Ogilvie RI, Leenen FHH. Pharmacokinetic and pharmacodynamic interactions between nisoldipine and propranolol. Clin Pharmacol Ther (1988) 43, 39–48.
4 Schran HF, Shepherd AM, Choc MM, Gonasun LM, Brodie CL. The effect of concomitant administration of isradipine and propranolol on their steady-state bioavailability. Pharmacologist (1989) 31, 153.
5 Elliott HL, Meredith PA, McNally C, Reid JL. The interactions between nisoldipine and two beta-adrenoceptor antagonists — atenolol and propranolol. Br J clin Pharmac (1991) 32, 379–85.
6 Shepherd AMM, Brodie CL, Carrillo DW, Kwan CM. Pharmacokinetic interactions between isradipine and propranolol. Clin Pharmacol Ther (1988) 43,194.

7 Hall ST, Hardin SM, Hassani H, Keene ON, Pellegatti M. The pharmacokinetic and pharmacodynamic interaction between lacidipine and propranolol in healthy volunteers. J Cardiovasc Pharmacol (1991) 18, Suppl 11) S13–17.
8 Horstmann R, Weber H, Wingender W, Ramsch K-O, Kühlmann J. Does nimodipine interaction with beta adrenergic blocking agents ? Eur J Clin Pharmacol (1989) 36, A258.

Beta-blockers + Cholestyramine or Colestipol

Abstract/Summary

Although both cholestyramine and colestipol can reduce the absorption of propranolol to some extent, this does not seem to reduce its effects.

Clinical evidence

(a) Cholestyramine

When single 120 mg doses of propranolol and 8 g doses of cholestyramine were taken together by six normal subjects, peak propranolol serum levels were reduced by almost 25% and the AUC (area under the curve) was reduced 13%. An additional dose of cholestyramine 12 h before the propanolol reduced the AUC by 43%. No changes in blood pressures or pulse rates were seen.[2] A study on five patients with type II hyperlipidaemia on 160 mg propranolol daily demonstrated no significant changes in blood levels of propranolol after being given a single (unstated) dose of cholestyramine.[1]

(b) Colestipol

When single 120 mg doses of propranolol and 10 mg doses of colestipol were taken together by six normal subjects, the peak serum propranolol levels were raised. But they were decreased if an additional 10 mg dose of colestipol was taken 12 h before the propranolol, and the AUC was reduced by about 30%. No changes in blood pressure or pulse rates were seen.[2]

Mechanism

Uncertain. It seems probable that both the cholestyramine and colestipol can bind to the propranolol in the gut, thereby reducing its absorption.

Importance and management

Information is limited. Even though both cholestyramine and colestipol can apparently reduce the absorption of propranolol, no changes in its pharmacological effects were reported[2] which suggests that the interaction is clinically unimportant. There is no obvious reason for avoiding concurrent use. There seems to be no information about other beta-blockers.

References

1 Schwartz DE, Schaeffer E, Brewer HB, Franciosa JA. Bioavailability of propranolol following administration of cholestyramine. Clin Pharmacol Ther (1982) 31, 268.

2 Hibbard DM, Peters JR, Hunningshake DB. Effects of cholestyramine and colestipol on the plasma concentrations of propranolol. Br J clin Pharmac (1984) 18, 337–42.

Beta-blockers + Cimetidine

Abstract/Summary

The blood levels of beta-blockers which are extensively metabolized by the liver (e.g. metoprolol, propranolol) can be doubled by the concurrent use of cimetidine, but normally this appears to be clinically unimportant. No important interaction normally seems to occur with other beta-blockers. An isolated report describes profound bradycardia (heart rate 36 beats/min) in a patient given atenolol and cimetidine. Marked postural hypotension occurred in another patient on labetalol and cimetidine, and an irregular heart beat in yet another taking metoprolol and cimetidine.

Clinical evidence

(a) Propranolol

12 normal subjects were given 1.2 g cimetidine daily for a week. From day 3 onwards they were also given two 80 mg daily doses of propranolol, morning and evening, until the end of the week. The mean steady-state blood levels of propranolol were raised 57%, the AUC increased 47% and the half-life was prolonged by 17%, but heart rates remained unchanged.[1]

A number of other single-dose and steady-state studies confirm that cimetidine can cause marked rises (up to 100%) in blood levels of propranolol[2] but no changes occur in either resting or exercised heart rates,[3–7] nor in blood pressures.[5,7] In contrast, one study showed a reduction in pulse rates.[16] One patient given 1 g cimetidine daily for six weeks showed an approximately threefold increase in serum propranolol level (AUC + 340%) when given a single 80 mg dose of propranolol.[11]

(b) Atenolol, Betaxolol, Dilevalol, Nadolol, Penbutolol or Pindolol

A report describes a patient taking atenolol for angina who developed profound sinus bradycardia (36 beats/min) and hypotension when additionally treated with cimetidine.[11,12] The original report does not specifically name atenolol, but it is identified elsewhere in a letter.[12] In contrast, well-controlled studies in other subjects have shown that cimetidine does not normally significantly alter blood levels of atenolol,[6,8–10] nor does it affect heart rates whether resting or exercised.[9,10] Blood levels and the pharmacokinetics of betaxolol[21] and nadolol[5] are similarly unaffected. Dilevalol, pindolol and penbutolol plasma levels are modestly raised or unaffected, while exercise-induced heart rates and other effects of the beta-blockers are not changed.[17,19,22,24]

(c) Metoprolol

A study in six normal subjects given 100 mg metoprolol daily for a week found that the concurrent use of 1 g cimetidine daily increased the peak plasma levels by 70% and the AUC rose by 61%, but there were no changes in resting or exercised heart rates, nor in blood pressures.[6] Some other studies confirm that cimetidine increases metoprolol serum levels[8,13,14,20,23] whereas another did not.[9] No changes in exercised heart rates were seen.[14,20,23] One patient complained of a 'very irregular heart beat' while taking both drugs, but it was much less marked when he took the two drugs separated as much as possible.[25]

(d) Labetalol (an alpha- and beta-blocker)

A study in three normal subjects showed that the bioavailability of labetalol was increased about 80% after 4 days treatment with cimetidine (1 g daily).[15] One subject in a related study developed postural hypotension (70/40 mm Hg), felt light-headed and almost fainted on standing.[18]

Mechanism

The blood levels of beta-blockers extensively metabolized by liver (propranolol, metoprolol and penbutolol) are increased because cimetidine reduces their metabolism, both by inhibiting the activity of the liver enzymes and by reducing the flow of blood to the liver.[6,17] Those beta-blockers which are not metabolized to a significant extent (atenolol, nadolol) are not affected because they are largely excreted unchanged in the urine.[5,10] Pindolol[17] falls between these two groups of drugs.

Importance and management

The concurrent use of beta-blockers and cimetidine has been well studied yet, despite the very considerable rises in blood levels which can occur with some beta-blockers, the effects of these interactions normally appear — perhaps surprisingly — to be clinically unimportant. Concurrent use is common but only one case of profound bradycardia involving atenolol appears to have been reported (see case cited above). Marked hypotension also seems to be rare. Combined use need not be avoided, however it has been suggested that patients with impaired liver function who are given beta-blockers which are extensively metabolized (metoprolol, propranolol, etc.) might possibly develop grossly elevated blood levels which could cause adverse effects. This needs confirmation.

References

1 Donn KH, Powell JR, Rogers JF, Eshelman FN. The influence of H_2-receptor antagonists on steady-state concentrations of propranolol and 4-hydroxypropranolol. J Clin Pharmacol (1984) 24, 500–8.

2 Kirch W, Kohler H, Spahn H, Mutschler I. Interaction of cimetidine with metoprolol, propranolol or atenolol. Lancet (1981) ii, 531

3 Reimann IW, Klotz U, Frohlich JC. Effects of cimetidine and ranitidine on steady-state propranolol kinetics and dynamics. Clin Pharmacol Ther (1982) 32, 749–57.

4 Reimann IW, Klotz U, Siems B, Frohlich JC. Cimetidine increases steady-state plasma levels of propranolol. Br J clin Pharmac (1981) 12, 785–90.

5 Duchin KL, Stern MA, Willard DA, McKinstry DN. Comparison of kinetic interactions of nadolol and propranolol with cimetidine. Am Heart J (1984) 108, 1084–6.

6 Kirch W, Spahn H, Kohler H, Mutschler E. Accumulation and adverse effects of metoprolol and propranolol after concurrent administration of cimetidine. Arch Toxicol (1983) Suppl 6, 379–83.

7 Markiewicz A, Hartleb M, Lelek A, Boldys H, Nowak A. The effect of treatment with cimetidine and ranitidine on bioavailability of, and circulatory response to, propranolol. Zbl Pharm (1984) 123, 516–8.

8 Kirch W, Spahn H, Kohler H, Mutschler E. Interaction of metoprolol, propranolol and atenolol with cimetidine. Clin Sci (1982) 63, 451s-53s.

9 Houtzagers JJR, Streurman O, Regardh CG. The effect of pretreatment with cimetidine on the bioavailability and disposition of atenolol and metoprolol. Br J clin Pharmac (1982) 14, 67–72.

10 Ellis ME, Hussain M, Webb AK, Barker NP, Fitzsimons TJ. The effect of cimetidine on the relative cardioselectivity of atenolol and metoprolol in asthmatic patients. Br J clin Pharmac (1984) 17, 59S–64S.

11 Donovan MA, Heagerty AM, Patel L, Castleden M, Pohl JEF. Cimetidine and bioavailability of propranolol. Lancet (1981) i, 164.

12 Rowley-Jones D, Flind AC. Drug interactions with cimetidine. Pharm J (1981) 283, 659.

13 Kendall MJ, Laugher SJ, Wilkins MR. Ranitidine, cimetidine and metoprolol. Gastroenterol (1986) 90, 1490.

14 Kirch W, Ramsch K, Janisch HD, Ohnhaus EE. The influence of two histamine H$_2$-receptor anagonists, cimetidine and ranitidine, on plasma levels and clinical effect of nifedipine and metoprolol. Arch toxicol (1984) Suppl 7, 256–9.

15 Daneshmend TK, Roberts CJC. Cimetidine and bioavailability of labetalol. Lancet (1981), i, 505.

16 Feeley J, Wilkinson GR, Wood AJJ. Reduction in liver blood flow and propranolol metabolism by cimetidine. N Engl J Med (1981) 304, 692–5.

17 Spahn H, Kirch W, Mutschler E. The interaction of cimetidine with metoprolol, atenolol, propranolol, pindolol and penbutolol. Br J clin Pharmac (1983) 15, 500–1.

18 Daneshmend TK, Roberts CJC. The effects of enzyme induction and enzyme inhibition on labetalol pharmacokinetics. Br J clin Pharmac (1984) 18, 393–400.

19 Spahn H, Kirch W, Hajdu P, Mutschler E, Ohnhaus EL. Penbutolol pharmacokinetics: the influence of concomitant administration of cimetidine. Eur J Clin Pharmacol (1986) 29, 555–60.

20 Toon S, Davidson EM, Garstang FM, Batra H, Bowers RJ, Rowland M. The racemic metoprolol H$_2$-antagonist interaction. Clin Pharmacol Ther (1988) 43, 283–9.

21 Rey E, Jammet P, d'Athis P, de Lauture D, Christoforov B, Weber S, Olive G. Effect of cimetidine on the pharmacokinetics of the new beta-blocker betaxolol. Arzneim-Forsch./Drug Res (1987) 37, 953–6.

22 Tenero DM, Bottorff MB, Given ED, Kramer WG, Affrime MB, Patrick JE, Lalonde RL. Pharmacokinetics and pharmacodynamics of dilevalol. Clin Pharmacol Ther (1989) 46, 648–56.

23 Chellingsworth MC, Laugher S, Akhlaghi S, Jack DB, Kendall MJ. The effects of ranitidine and cimetidine on the pharmacokinetics and pharmacodynamics of metoprolol. Aliment Pharmacol Therap (1988) 2, 521–7.

24 Somogyi AA, Bochner F, Sallustio BC. Stereoselective inhibition of pindolol renal clearance by cimetidine in humans. Clin Pharmacol Ther (1992) 51, 379–87.

25 Anon. Adverse Drug Reactions Advisory Committee. Seven case studies. Med J Aust (1982) 2, 190–1.

Beta-blockers + Cimetidine + Phenylephrine

Abstract/Summary

A patient undergoing surgery had a low blood pressure probably resulting from an exaggeration of the effects of labetalol due to an interaction with cimetidine. Bronchospasm occurred later, probably as a result of the combined actions of labetalol and phenylephrine.

Clinical evidence, mechanism, importance and management

An elderly asthmatic patient, treated with nitrates and labetalol (650 mg) for unstable angina and hypertension before surgery for double aortocoronary vein grafting, was given cimetidine (400 mg) as part of his premedication. During the surgery, hypotension (40–45 mm Hg) occurred despite phenylephrine 14 mg. This was followed during rewarming by a rise in pressure to 150 mm Hg and, on cessation of bypass, protracted bronchospasm was seen.[1] The possible reasons are that the cimetidine reduced the metabolism and clearance of the labetalol (see 'Beta-blockers + Cimetidine'). The increase in its alpha-blocking (vasodilating) effects opposed the alpha-stimulating (vasoconstrictor) effects of the phenylephrine so that the blood pressure was low. Later the beta-blocking effects of the labetalol and the alpha-stimulating effects of the phenylephrine combined to cause bronchospasm. The authors of the report point out that higher doses of phenylephrine may be needed in the presence of labetalol, but that this may carry an increased risk of bronchospasm in asthmatic patients.

Reference

1 Durant PAC, Joucken K. Bronchospasm and hypotension during cardiopulmonary bypass after preoperative cimetidine and labetalol therapy. Br J Anaesth (1984) 56, 917–20.

Beta-blockers + Ciprofloxacin

Abstract/Summary

Ciprofloxacin reduces the loss of metoprolol from the body but this is probably clinically unimportant.

Clinical evidence, mechanism, importance and management

Pretreatment with five 12-hourly 500 mg doses of ciprofloxacin increased the AUC of (+) metoprolol in seven subjects by 54% and reduced it clearance by 38.5%. The AUC of (–) metoprolol was increased by 29% and the clearance reduced by 12%.[1] The reason appears to be that the ciprofloxacin inhibits the activity of the P-450 isozymes concerned with the metabolism and clearance of these metoprolol isomers from the body. Beta-blocker AUC changes of this size, or even more, with other enzyme inhibiting drugs have proved not to be clinically important, and it seems probable that this will be the case with ciprofloxacin, but this needs confirmation. There appears to be no information about interactions between other beta-blockers and other quinolone antibiotics.

Reference

1 Waite NM, Rutledge DR, Warbasse LH, Edwards DJ. Disposition of the (+) and (−) isomers of metoprolol following ciprofloxacin treatment. Pharmacotherapy (1990) 10, 236.

Beta-blockers + Contraceptives (oral)

Abstract/Summary

The blood levels of metoprolol are increased in women taking oral contraceptives, but the clinical importance is uncertain.

Clinical evidence, mechanism, importance and management

The peak serum levels and the AUC of a single 100 mg dose of metoprolol were increased by 36 and 70% respectively in 12 women on low-dose combined oral contraceptives when compared with a similar group not taking the pill.[1] It seems likely that this is because the pill inhibits the metabolism of the metoprolol. The clinical effects of interaction seem not to have been studied, but changes of this size caused by interactions of other drugs with beta-blockers do not usually have clinically important effects. Beta-blockers such as propranolol which are metabolized similarly are possibly affected in the same way, but not those which are largely excreted unchanged in the urine (e.g. atenolol).

Reference

1 Kendall MJ, Quarterman CP, Jack DB, Beeley L. Metoprolol pharmacokinetics and the oral contraceptive pill. Br J clin Pharmacol (1982) 14, 120–2.

Beta-blockers + Dextromoramide

Abstract/Summary

Two patients developed marked bradycardia and severe hypotension when given propranolol and dextromoramide following the induction of anaesthesia.

Clinical evidence, mechanism, importance and management

Two women about to undergo partial thyroidectomy were given 30 mg propranolol and dextromoramide (1.25 and 4 mg respectively) by injection during the pre-operative period following the induction of anaesthesia with a barbiturate. Each developed marked bradycardia and severe hypotension which responded rapidly to the intravenous injection of atropine.[1] The reasons for this response are not understood.

Reference

1 Cabanne F, Wilkening M, Caillard B, Foissac JC, Aupecle P. Interferences medicamenteuses induites par l'association propranolol-dextromoramide. Anesth Anal Rean (1973) 30, 369–75.

Beta-blockers + Dextropropoxyphene

Abstract/Summary

A single dose study has shown that the bioavailability of metoprolol is markedly increased, and of propranolol to a lesser extent, by the concurrent use of dextropropoxyphene. There seem to be no reports of adverse reactions when both drugs are used.

Clinical evidence, mechanism, importance and management

A single dose study in normal subjects showed that after taking dextropropoxyphene for a day (dose not stated) the bioavailability of metoprolol (100 mg orally) was increased almost fourfold and the total body clearance was reduced 18%. The bioavailability of propranolol (40 mg orally) was increased by about 70%.[1] The probable reason is that the dextropropoxyphene inhibits the metabolism of these beta-blockers by the liver so that they are cleared from the body more slowly. From this it would be expected that the effects of these beta-blockers would be markedly increased, but there seems to be no other evidence that concurrent use presents any problems. Nevertheless it would seem prudent to monitor the effects of giving both drugs. No interaction would be expected with those beta-blockers which, unlike metoprolol and propranolol, are largely excreted unchanged in the urine (e.g. nadolol, sotalol, atenolol, etc.)

Reference

1 Lundborg P, Regard CG. The effect of propoxyphene pretreatment on the disposition of metoprolol and propranolol. Clin Pharmacol Ther (1981) 29, 263–4.

Beta-blockers + Diltiazem

Abstract/Summary

Concurrent use is normally safe and uneventful but a few patients with pre-existing ventricular failure or conduction abnormalities may develop serious and potentially life-threatening bradycardia. **Diltiazem increases the serum levels of propranolol and metoprolol, but not those of atenolol.**

Clinical evidence

The concurrent use of beta-blockers and diltiazem is common, appears to be valuable and is normally without major problems,[1-4] but adverse effects have also been described:

Ten patients were admitted to an intensive coronary care unit during one year with severe bradycardia (heart rates of 24–44 bpm). All were relatively elderly and presented with lethargy, dizziness, syncope, chest pain, and (in one case) pulmonary oedema. The ECG abnormalities were localised in the sinus node, the primary rhythm disorders being junctional escape rhythm, sinus bradycardia and sinus pause. They were taking diltiazem (90–360 mg daily) with propranolol (30–120 mg daily), atenolol (50–100 mg daily) or pindolol (90 mg daily). The rhythm abnormalities resolved within 24 h of withdrawing the drugs.[8]

Symptomatic and severe bradycardia of this kind has been described in over 20 other patients involving diltiazem and atenolol,[15] metoprolol,[15,16] propranolol,[6-12,15,16] sotalol or pindolol.[5] Profound bradycardia and unconsciousness occurred in a 68-year-old woman, taking 320 mg sotalol daily for supraventricular tachycardia and ventricular premature beats, two days after starting to take 60 mg diltiazem three times a day. Her pulse rate fell to 15 bpm and her blood pressure was unrecordable. Another woman of 77 on 30 mg pindolol three times daily became cold and dizzy 2 h after taking a first 60 mg dose of diltiazem. Her pulse rate fell to 25 bpm and systolic blood pressure to 70 mm Hg.[5]

Diltiazem increases the AUC (area under the curve) of propranolol and metoprolol by 48 and 33% respectively, and the maximal serum concentrations by 45 and 71%, but atenolol is not significantly affected.[13] Another study found a 24–25% reduction in propranolol clearance.[14]

Mechanism

The heart slowing effects of the beta-blockers can be additive with the effects of the delay in conduction through the atrioventricular node caused by the diltiazem.[13] This advantageously increases the antianginal effects in most patients, but in a few these effects may exacerabate the effects of their existing cardiac abnormalities. Diltiazem apparently also inhibits the metabolism of propranolol and metoprolol (thereby increasing its effects), but not atenolol.

Importance and management

Concurrent use is unquestionably valuable and uneventful in many patients, but severe adverse effects develop in a few. This is well established. A not dissimilar adverse interaction can occur with verapamil (see 'Beta-blockers + Verapamil'). On the basis of six reports, the incidence of symptomatic bradyarrhythmia seems to be about 10–15%.[8] It can occur with different beta-blockers, even with very low doses, and any time from

within a few hours of starting treatment up to 2 years.[8] The main risk factors seem to be ventricular dysfunction or antecedent sinoatrial or AV nodal conduction abnormalities.[8] Patients with normal ventricular function and no evidence of conduction abnormalities seem not to be at risk. Concurrent use should be very well monitored for evidence of adverse effects.

References

1 Tilmant PY, Lablanche JM, Thieuleux FA, Dupuis BA, Bertrand ME. Detrimental effect of propranolol in patients with coronary arterial spasm countered by combination with diltiazem. Am J Cardiol (1983) 52, 230–33.
2 Rocha P, Baron B, Delestrain A, Pathe M, Cazor J-L, Kahn J-C. Hemodynamic effects of intravenous diltiazem in patients treated chronically with propranolol. Am Heart J (1986) 111, 62.
3 Humen DP, O'Brien P, Puves P, Johnson D, Kostuk WJ. Effort angina with adequate beta-receptor blockade: comparison with diltiazem alone and in combination. J Am Coll Cardiol (1986) 7, 329–35.
4 Kostuk WJ, Plugfelder P. Comparative effects of calcium entry blocking drugs, beta-blocking drugs and their combination in patients with chronic stable angina. Circulation (1987) 75, (Suppl V), 114–21.
5 Hassell AB, Creamer JE. Profound bradycardia after the addition of diltiazem to a beta-blocker. Br Med J (1989) 298, 675.
6 O'Hara MJ, Khurmi NS, Bowles MJ, Raftery BB. Diltiazem and propranolol combination for the treatment of chronic stable angina pectoris. Clin Cardiol (1987) 10, 115–23.
7 Sagie A, Strasberg B, Kusnieck J, Sclarovsky S. Symptomatic bradycardia induced by the combination of oral diltiazem and beta blockers. Clin Cardiol (1991) 14, 314–6.
8 Hung J, Lamb I, Connolly SJ, Jutzy KR, Goris ML, Schroder JS. The effect of diltiazem and propranolol alone and in combination on exercise performance on left ventricular function in patients with stable effort angina: a double blind randomized placebo controlled study. Circulation (1983) 68, 560.
9 Strauss WE, Parisi AF. Superiority of combined diltiazem and propranolol therapy for angina pectoris. Circulation (1985) 71, 951.
10 Kenny J, Bergman DG, Kerkez S, Jewitt DE. Beneficial effects of diltiazem combined with beta blockade in angina pectoris. Eur Heart J (1985) 6, 418.
11 Hossack KF. Conduction abnormalities due to diltiazem. N Eng J Med (1982) 307, 953.
12 Ishikawa T, Imamura T, Korwaya Y, Tanaka K. Atrioventricular dissociation and sinus arrest induced by oral diltiazem. N Eng J Med (1983) 309, 1124.
13 Tateishi T, Nakashima H, Shitou T, Kumagain Y, Ohashi K, Hosada S, Ebihara A. Effect of diltiazem on the pharmacokinetics of propranolol, metoprolol and atenolol. Eur J Clin Pharmacol (1989) 36, 67–70.
14 Hung BA, Bottorff MB, Herring VL, Self TH, Lalonde RL. Effects of calcium channel blockers on the pharmacokinetics of propranolol stereoisomers. Clin Pharmacol Ther (1990) 47, 584–91.
15 Yust I, Hoffman M, Aronson RJ. Life-threatening bradycardic reactions due to beta blocker-diltiazem interactions. Isr J med Sci (1992) 28, 292–4.
16 Lan Cheong Wah LSH, Robinet G, Guiavarc'h M, Garo B, Boles JM. États de choc au cours de l'association diltiazem-β-bloquant. Rev Med Interne (1992) 13, 80–1.

Beta-blockers + Enprostil

Abstract/Summary

Enprostil is reported not to interact with propranolol.

Clinical evidence, mechanism, importance and management

A double-blind crossover study in nine healthy subjects showed that after taking 70 g enprostil twice daily for 6 days the elimination of propranolol given orally or intravenously was not affected (whereas it was affected by cimetidine).[1] No special precautions seem necessary during concurrent use. Direct information about other beta-blockers is lacking, but it seems likely that they will behave similarly.

Reference

1 Reilly CS, Biollaz J, Koshakji RP, Wood AJJ. Enprostil, in contrast to cimetidine, does not inhibit propranolol metabolism. Clin Pharmacol Ther (1986) 40, 37–41.

Beta-blockers + Ergotamine, Dihydroergotamine or Methysergide

Abstract/Summary

The concurrent use of beta-blockers and ergotamine for the treatment of migraine is usually safe and effective, but three cases of severe peripheral vasoconstriction and one of hypertension have been described. There is also an isolated case of exacerbated migraine.

Clinical evidence

A man with recurrent migraine headaches, reasonably well-controlled over a 6-year period with two daily suppositories of *Cafergot* (ergotamine tartrate 2 g, caffeine 100 mg, butalbital 100 mg, belladonna leaf alkaloids 250 g) developed progressively painful and purple feet a short while after additionally starting to take 30 mg propranolol daily. When he eventually resumed taking the *Cafergot* alone there was no further evidence of peripheral vasoconstriction.[1]

A similar situation occurred in a woman taking oxprenolol and ergotamine tartrate (dosages unknown) for some considerable time, as well as a number of other drugs.[4] Another report describes a similar reaction in a man after taking 3 mg methysergide and 120 mg propranolol daily for two weeks.[4] It was necessary to amputate both his legs below the knee because of gangrene. A woman on propranolol for migraine became hypertensive (BP 180/120 mm Hg) with a crushing substernal pain immediately after being given oxygen, 5 mg compazine and 0.75 mg dihydroergotamine (IV). She recovered uneventfully. She was later found to be hyperthyroidic.[5]

The exacerbation of migraine has also been described in a single patient.[2]

These reports contrast with another stating that concurrent use in 50 patients was both effective and uneventful.[3]

Mechanism

Uncertain. One suggestion is that additive vasoconstriction occurs.[1,4] Ergot causes vasoconstriction. The beta-blockers do the same by blocking the normal (beta-2-stimulated) sympathetic vasodilatation. The beta-blockers also reduce blood flow by reducing cardiac output. Severe vasoconstriction with ergot compounds alone is not unknown.

Importance and management

Concurrent use is usually safe and effective, and there are only five reports of adverse interactions. However it would clearly be prudent to be on the alert for any signs of an adverse response.

References

1 Baumrucker JF. Drug interaction propranolol and cafergot. N Engl J Med (1973) 288, 916.
2 Blank NK, Rieder MJ. Paradoxical response to propranolol in migraine. Lancet (1973) ii, 1336.
3 Diamond S. Propranolol and ergotamine tartrate (cont.) N Engl J Med (1973) 289, 159.
4 Venter CP, Joubert PH, Buys AC. Severe peripheral ischaemia during concomitant use of beta-blockers and ergot alkaloids. Brit Med J (1984) 2, 289.
5 Gandy W. Dihydroergotamine interaction with propranolol. Ann Emerg Med (1990) 19, 221.

Beta-blockers + Erythromycin or Neomycin

Abstract/Summary

Erythromycin and neomycin can increase the serum concentrations of nadolol, but the clinical importance of this is not known.

Clinical evidence, mechanism, importance and management

In eight normal subjects given either 0.5 g neomycin or 0.5 g erythromycin, four times a day for two days, the peak serum nadolol concentration after a single 80 mg oral dose more than doubled (from 146 to 397 ng/ml). The AUC stayed the same but its half-life fell from 17.3 to 11.6 h.[1] The reasons are not understood. More study is needed to find out whether this interaction is of clinical importance. The effects of concurrent use should be monitored. No information seems to be available about other beta-blockers.

Reference

1 du Souich P, Caille G, Larochelle P. Enhancement of nadolol elimination by activated charcoal and antibiotics. Clin Pharmacol Ther (1983) 33, 585–90.

Beta-blockers + Etintidine

Abstract/Summary

The serum levels of propranolol can be markedly increased by etintidine.

Clinical evidence

400 mg etintidine twice daily for four days increased the AUC (area under the curve) of a single 40 mg oral dose of propranolol in 12 normal subjects by almost 300% (from 146 to 573 ng.h/ml). The elimination half-life and peak serum concentrations doubled and the clearance fell from 102 to 41 l/h.[1]

Mechanism

The most likely explanation is that etintidine, which is a chemical analogue of cimetidine, can (like cimetidine) inhibit the metabolism of the propranolol by the liver, thereby reducing its loss from the body.

Importance and management

Direct information seems to be limited to this single dose study. Its clinical importance is uncertain but the changes seen are so large that increased propranolol effects would be expected. Monitor the effects if etintidine is added or withdrawn. Ranitidine is a non-interacting alternative (see 'Beta-blockers + Ranitidine'). The beta-blockers which interact with cimetidine (see 'Beta-blockers + Cimetidine') would also be expected to interact with etintidine. Thus metoprolol, penbutolol and labetolol are metabolized like propranolol and would be expected to interact similarly, but not nadolol or atenolol.

Reference

1 Huang S-M, Weintraub HS, Marriott TB, Marinan B, Abels R. Etintidine-propranolol interaction study in humans. J Pharmacokinet Biopharm (1987) 15, 557–67.

Beta-blockers + Famotidine

Abstract/Summary

Famotidine does not interact with beta-blockers

Clinical evidence, mechanism, importance and management

A survey of 15 patients taking beta-blockers (acebutolol, atenolol, betaxolol, nadolol, pindolol, propranolol or sotalol) for 6–8 weeks found no evidence of changes in their response (increased antihypertensive effects or enhanced bradycardia) while concurrently taking 40 mg famotidine daily.[1] No interaction would be expected and no special precautions would seem necessary if famotidine is taken with these or any other beta-blocker.

Reference

1 Chichmanian RM, Mignot G, Spreux A, Jean-Girard C, Hofliger P. Tolérance de la famotidine. Étude due réseau médecins sentinelles en pharmacovigilance. Therapie (1992) 47, 239–43.

Beta-blockers + Flecainide

Abstract/Summary

There is some limited evidence that combined use may possibly cause excessive cardiac depression.

Clinical evidence, mechanism, importance and management

A study on cardiac function and drug clearance in 10 normal subjects found that the AUCs of propranolol and flecainide were increased 20–30% when given together, and they had some additive negative inotropic effects on the heart.[1] There is a report of a patient developed bradycardia and fatal atrioventricular conduction block after sotalol was added to flecainide.[2] Careful monitoring has therefore been recommended if beta-blockers are added to therapy with other antiarrhythmic agents. Serious cardiac depression has been seen following the concurrent use of flecainide and other drugs with negative inotropic effects (e.g. verapamil). See Index.

References

1 Holtzman JL, Kvam DC, Berry DA, Mottonen L, Borrell G, Harrison LI, Conard GJ. The pharmacodynamic and pharmacokinetic interaction of flecainide acetate with propranolol: effects on cardiac function and drug clearance. Eur J Clin Pharmacol (1987) 33, 97–9.
2 Warren R, Vohra J, Hunt D, Hamer A. Serious interactions of sotalol with amiodarone and flecainide. Med J Aust (1990) 152, 277.

Beta-blockers + Fluoxetine

Abstract/Summary

An isolated report describes lethargy and profound bradycardia in a man on metoprolol shortly after starting to take fluoxetine.

Clinical evidence, mechanism, importance and management

100 mg metoprolol daily improved the angina of a man who

had had a coronary artery bypass 4 years earlier. A month later he was given 20 mg fluoxetine daily for depression. Within two days he complained of profound lethargy, and his resting heart rate was found to have fallen from 64 to 37 beats per minute. The fluoxetine was withdrawn, whereupon his heart rate returned to 64 within 5 days. The metoprolol was replaced by 80 mg sotalol twice daily without problems.[1]

Mechanism

Not only can fluoxetine alone can cause bradycardia, it also probably inhibits the oxidative metabolism of the metoprolol (mediated by cytochrome P-450 CYP2D6) so that it accumulates, the result being that its effects are increased (bradycardia being one of them).[1]

Importance and management

Direct information seems to be limited to this report. Its general importance is uncertain because other SSRIs such as fluvoxamine can cause a very marked rise in serum propranolol levels, apparently without causing problems (see 'Fluvoxamine + Miscellaneous drugs'). It is suggested this interaction can be avoided by giving water soluble beta-blockers such as atenolol or sotalol.[1]

References

1 Walley T, Pirmohamed M, Proudlove C, Maxwell D. Interaction of metoprolol and fluoxetine. Lancet (1993) 341, 967–8.

Beta-blockers + Food

Abstract/Summary

Food can increase, decrease or not affect the bioavailability of beta-blockers, but none of the changes has been shown to be of importance.

Clinical evidence, mechanism, importance and management

Food increases the bioavailability of propranolol and metoprolol by 30–80%,[1–3] and of labetalol by about 40%[4] by changing the extent of their metabolism during their first pass through the liver. Food has very little effect on the absorption of oxprenolol[5,6] or pindolol,[8] whereas the bioavailability of atenolol is reduced about 20%.[7] None of these changes has been shown to be of clinical importance, and it is not clear whether it matters if patients take these drugs in a regular pattern in relation to meals.

References

1 Melander A, Danielson K, Schersten B, Wahlin E. Enhancement of the bioavailability of propranolol and metoprolol by food. Clin Pharmacol Ther (1977) 22, 108–12.

2 Liedholm H, Melander A. Concomitant food intake can increase the bioavailability of propranolol by transient inhibition of its presystemic primary conjugation. Clin Pharmacol Ther (1986) 40, 29–36.
3 McLean AJ, Isbister C, Bobik A, Dudley F. Reduction of first-pass hepatic clearance of propranolol by food. Clin Pharmacol Ther (1981) 30, 31–4.
4 Daneshmend TK, Roberts CJC. The influence of food on the oral and intravenous pharmacokinetics of a high clearance drug: a study with labetalol. Br J Clin Pharmacol (1982) 14, 73–8.
5 Dawes CP, Kendall MJ, Welling PG. Bioavailability of conventional and slow-release oxprenolol in fasted and non-fasted individuals. Br J clin Pharmac (1979) 7, 299–302.
6 John VA, Smith SE. Influence of food intake on plasma oxprenolol concentrations following oral administration of conventional and Oros preparations. Br J clin Pharmac (1985) 19, 191–5S.
7 Melander A, Stenberg P, Liedholm H, Schersten B, Wahlin-Boll E. Food-induced reduction in bioavailability of atenolol. Eur J Clin Pharmacol (1979) 16, 327–30.
8 Kiger JL, Lavene D, Guillaume MF, Guerret M, Longchampt J. The effect of food and clopamide on the absorption of pindolol in man. Int J Clin Pharmacol (1976) 13, 228–32.

Beta-blockers + Halofenate

Abstract/Summary

The serum levels and the therapeutic effects of propranolol can be reduced by the concurrent use of halofenate.

Clinical evidence

In a cross-over study four healthy subjects were given 1 g halofenate or a placebo daily for 21 days. During the last two days they were given either 80 or 160 mg of propranolol. Their steady-state plasma levels of propranolol were reduced by 74 and 81% respectively. The reduction in the beta-blocking effects were checked using isoprenaline and the cardiac response correlated with the reduction in beta-blockade in three of the four subjects.[1]

Mechanism

Unknown. One idea is that the halofenate increases the metabolism and clearance of the propranolol from the body.[1]

Importance and management

Information seems to be confined to this study, but this interaction would seem to be established.[1] Such a large reduction in serum propranolol levels would be expected to cause a reduction in the control of hypertension and angina but this needs confirmation. If both drugs are given, the response should be monitored, anticipating the need to increase the propranolol dosage. If the mechanism of interaction suggested above is true, then an interaction with other beta-blockers which are extensively metabolized (e.g. alprenolol, metoprolol, timolol) also seems a possibility.

References

1 Huffman DH, Azarnoff DL, Shoeman DW, Dujorne CA. The interaction between halofenate and propranolol. Clin Pharmacol Ther (1976) 19, 807.

Beta-blockers + Haloperidol

Abstract/Summary

An isolated case report describes severe hypotension and cardiopulmonary arrest in a woman on three occasions shortly after being given haloperidol and propranolol.

Clinical evidence, importance and management

A middle-aged woman with schizophrenia and hypertension experienced three episodes of severe hypotension within 30–120 min of being given propranolol (40–80 mg) and haloperidol (10 mg).[1] On two of the occasions cardiopulmonary arrest took place. She fainted each time, became cyanotic, had no palpable pulses and showed severe hypotension, but rapidly responded to cardiopulmonary resuscitation. She suffered no adverse consequences. The reasons for this reaction are not understood, but one suggestion[1] is that this patient was unduly sensitive to the additive relaxant effect of both drugs on peripheral blood vessels.

This seems to be the only case of this interaction on record. Bearing in mind the wide-spread use of propranolol, other beta-blockers and haloperidol, this interaction is obviously rare. There would seem to be little reason for avoiding concurrent use.

Reference

1 Alexander HE, McCarty K, Giffen MB. Hypotension and cardiopulmonary arrest associated with concurrent haloperidol and propranolol therapy. J Amer Med Ass (1984) 252, 87–8.

Beta-blockers + Hydralazine

Abstract/Summary

Concurrent use is not uncommon in the treatment of hypertension. Serum levels of propranolol and other extensively metabolized beta-blockers (metoprolol, oxprenolol) are increased but no adverse effects seem to have been reported.

Clinical evidence

(a) Effect of hydralazine on beta-blockers

25 and 50 mg hydralazine increased the AUC (area under the curve) of single 40 mg doses of propranolol in five normal subjects by 60% and 110%, and raised the peak serum levels by 144 and 240% respectively.[1]

Other studies confirm that hydralazine increases the bioavailability of propranolol by 31–57%,[3] of oxprenolol by 41%,[4] of metoprolol by 30%[2] and 38%[5], but not acebutolol or nadolol.[2] The increased levels of oxprenolol[4] did not significantly reduce either diastolic or systolic blood pressures.

(b) Effect of beta-blockers on hydralazine

Oxprenolol was found not to have a significant effect on the pharmacokinetics of hydralazine.[4]

Mechanism

Originally it was believed[3] that hydralazine inhibited the liver enzymes concerned with the metabolism of propranolol (and other extensively metabolized beta-blockers such as metoprolol), thereby increasing their bioavailability, but more recent evidence suggests that the hydralazine reduces metabolism by reducing the blood flow into the liver.[1] Beta-blockers which are not extensively metabolized (nadolol, acebutolol, etc.) would not be expected to be affected because they are largely excreted unchanged in the urine.

Importance and management

Moderately well-documented and established interactions, but the increased beta-blocker serum levels appears to be advantageous rather than adverse. Concurrent use is common and usually valuable in the treatment of hypertension. No particular precautions seem to be necessary but the outcome should be monitored.

References

1 Schnek DW, Vary JE. Mechanism by which hydralazine increases propranolol bioavailability. Clin Pharmacol Ther (1984) 35, 447–53.
2 Jack DB, Kendall MJ, Dean S, Laugher SJ, Zaman R, Tenneson ME. The effect of hydralazine on the pharmacokinetics of three different beta-adrenoceptor antagonists: metoprolol, nadolol and acebutolol. Biopharm Drug Dispos (1982) 3, 47–54.
3 McLean AJ, Skews H, Bobik A, Dudley FJ. Interaction between oral propranolol and hydralazine. Clin Pharmacol Ther (1980) 27, 726–32.
4 Hawksworth GM, Dart AM, Chiang K, Parry K, Petrie JC. Effect of oxprenolol on the pharmacokinetics and pharmacodynamics of hydralazine. Drugs (1983) 25 (Suppl 2) 136–40.
5 Lindeberg S, Holm B, Lundborg P, Regårdh CG, Sandström B. The effect of hydralazine on steady-state plasma concentrations of metoprolol in pregnant hypertensive women. Eur J Clin Pharmacol (1988) 35, 131–5.

Beta-blockers + Indomethacin and other NSAIDs

Abstract/Summary

Indomethacin reduces the antihypertensive effects of the beta-blockers. This interaction can be accommodated either by raising the dosage of the beta-blocker or by using a non-interacting NSAID. Piroxicam interacts similarly while normally diclofenac, imidazole salicylate, isoxicam, naproxen, oxaprozin, pirprofen and sulindac do not interact. Isolated cases have been reported with naproxen and ibuprofen. The situation with aspirin is uncertain. Indomethacin has also been reported to cause a marked hypertensive response in women with eclampsia. Indomethacin and sulindac reduce the effects of labetalol to some extent.

Clinical evidence

(a) Beta-blockers + Aspirin and other salicylates

A study in 11 patients taking a number of antihypertensives which included propranolol and pindolol showed that 1950 mg aspirin daily did not affect the control of their blood pressure.[12] In contrast another study found that aspirin reduced the hypotensive effects of pindolol and propranolol,[19] whereas it is reported not to affect the control of hypertension by metipranolol.[25] Sodium salicylate was found to affect neither the pharmacokinetics of alprenolol nor its effects on heart rate and blood pressure during exercise.[18] Another study in six normal subjects showed that aspirin did not affect the kinetics of atenolol.[17] Imidazole salicylate does not affect the blood pressure control of patients treated with atenolol.[21]

(b) Beta-blockers + Diclofenac

Studies in patients taking atenolol, metoprolol, propranolol and pindolol, with and with hydrochlorothiazide/amiloride, found that 50 mg diclofenac three times daily had no effect on the control of blood pressure.[27]

(c) Beta-blockers + Ibuprofen

The antihypertensive effects of pindolol and possibly metoprolol were antagonized by the concurrent use of ibuprofen in two patients,[14] but no changes in the control of blood pressure with propranolol were seen in another study.[16]

(d) Beta-blockers + Indomethacin

The diastolic blood pressures of seven hypertensive patients treated with pindolol (15 mg daily) or propranolol (80–160 mg daily) rose from 82 to 96 mm Hg when they were also given indomethacin, 100 mg daily, over a 10 day period. Changes in systolic pressures were not statistically significant.[1]

In other studies 100 mg indomethacin raised systolic/diastolic blood pressures of patients on propranolol by 14/5 mm Hg when lying and 16/9 mm Hg when standing.[2] This interaction has also been seen in other patients on metipranolol,[25] propranolol,[4] oxprenolol[3,5] and atenolol.[9,10] Two women with eclampsia treated with pindolol and propranolol became markedly hypertensive (rises from 135/85 to 240/140 mm Hg, and from 130/70 to 230/130 mm Hg) within 4–5 days of being given indomethacin because of premature contractions.[22]

(e) Beta-blockers + Isoxicam

A study in 10 normal subjects showed that 200 mg isoxicam daily did not alter the effects of propranolol on either blood pressure or heart rate.[15]

(f) Beta-blockers + Naproxen or pirprofen

A study in hypertensive patients treated with timolol, hydrochlorothiazide and amiloride showed that 500 mg naproxen daily caused an insignificant rise in blood pressures,[7] but three cases of poor blood pressure control attributed to the use of naproxen have been described. Another study found that naproxen caused no changes in hypertension controlled with propranolol,[20] although one patient in another report showed a marked rise in blood pressure.[29] Yet another found that 500 mg naproxen twice daily caused an average 4 mm Hg rise in diastolic blood pressures of patients on atenolol.[23] Pirprofen in daily doses of 800 mg was found not to affect the antihypertensive effects of oxprenolol.[5]

(g) Beta-blockers + Oxaprozin

A study in 32 hypertensive arthritic patients found that 1200 mg oxaprozin daily for four weeks did not affect the antihypertensive effects of metoprolol (100 mg twice daily).[26]

(h) Beta-blockers + Piroxicam

An extensive study[11] found that about a quarter of the patients given 20 mg piroxicam daily and propranolol developed diastolic pressure rises of 10 mmHg or more when lying or standing.[11] Increases in both systolic and diastolic pressures (+ 8.1/5.2 mmHg lying and + 8.5/8.9 mmHg standing) were seen in another study.[13] In contrast, patients taking propranolol and piroxicam for 4 weeks (doses not stated) showed systolic/diastolic blood pressure rises of 5.8/2.4 mmHg when lying and 0.5/3.5 mm Hg when standing,[8] but these were said not to be statistically significant. No significant rises were seen in another study in patients given timolol and 20 mg piroxicam daily.[7]

(i) Beta-blockers + Sulindac

400 mg sulindac had little or no effect on the control of hypertension in patients taking atenolol, metoprolol, propranolol, pindolol[27] or timolol,[7] with hydrochlorothiazide and amiloride. No statistically significant rises in blood pressure occurred in other patients on propranolol[11] or atenolol[23,27] given 400 mg sulindac daily. No change in the hypertensive response to propranolol was seen in other studies.[13,20] In contrast, another study claimed that patients given propranolol and sulindac for four weeks (doses not stated) showed systolic/diastolic blood pressure rises of 4.8/10.3 mmHg and 2.4/7.1 mmHg when standing or lying,[8] but these were said not to be statistically significant.[4]

(j) Labetalol + Naproxen, sulindac

A crossover study in 26 hypertensive patients given labetalol found that 50 mg indomethacin twice daily or 200 mg sulindac twice daily for 7 days raised the mean systolic blood pressure by

6 mmHg when sitting, and by 9–14 mmHg when standing. Diastolic pressures while taking indomethacin were raised about 2 mmHg, but sulindac had no effect.[24]

Mechanism

Indomethacin alone can raise blood pressure (13 hypertensive patients given 150 mg indomethacin daily for 3 days showed a mean systolic blood pressure rise from 118 to 131 mmHg).[6] One suggested reason is that it inhibits the synthesis and release into the circulation of two prostaglandins (PGA and PGE) from the kidney medulla which have a potent dilating effect on peripheral arterioles throughout the body. In their absence the blood pressure rises. Thus the hypotensive actions of the beta-blockers are opposed by the hypertensive actions of indomethacin. This mechanism has been questioned and it is possible that other physiological and pharmacological mechanisms have a part to play.[28,30] It seems likely that NSAIDs which behave like indomethacin interact by similar mechanisms.

Importance and management

Some of the beta-blocker/NSAID interactions have been well studied and are of clinical importance but others are not. The concurrent use of beta-blockers and indomethacin need not be avoided (except in patients with eclampsia) but anticipate the need to increase the dosage of the beta-blocker. Alternatively exchange the indomethacin for a non-interacting NSAID. Piroxicam interacts similarly while normally diclofenac, imidazole salicylate, isoxicam, naproxen, oxaprozin, pirprofen and sulindac only interact minimally or not at all. The situation with aspirin is unresolved. Because the occasional patient may show a marked interaction even with NSAID's which normally do not interact (e.g. naproxen, ibuprofen), it would be prudent to monitor the effects when any NSAID is given. Direct information about other NSAID's seems not to be available. Many of the antihypertensive agents appear to be affected by this interaction so that exchanging one for another may not avoid the problem. Monitor the effects of any NSAID with labetalol and raise the dosage if necessary.

References

1 Durao V, Prata MM, Goncalves LMP. Modification of antihypertensive effects of beta-adrenoceptor blocking agents by inhibition of endogenous prostaglandin synthesis. Lancet (1977) ii, 1005–7.

2 Watkins J, Abbott EC, Hensby CN, Webster J, Dollery CT. Attenuation of hypotensive effects of propranolol and thiazide diuretics by indomethacin. Br Med J (1980) 281, 702–5.

3 Salvetti A, Arzillis F, Pedrinelli R, Beggi P, Motolese M. Interaction between oxprenolol and indomethacin on blood pressure in essential hypertensive patients. Eur J Clin Pharmacol (1982) 22, 197–201.

4 Lopez-Overjero JA, Weber MA, Drayer JIM, Sealey JE, Laragh JH. Effects of indomethacin alone and during diuretic or beta-adrenoceptor blockade therapy on blood pressure and the renin system in essential hypertension. Clin Sci Mol Med (1978) 55, 203–5s.

5 Sorgel F, Hemmerlein M, Lang E. Wirkung von Pirprofen und Indometacin auf die Effekte von Oxprenolol und Furosemid. Arneim-Forsch./Drug Res (1984) 34, 1330–2.

6 Barrientos A, Alcazar V, Ruilope L, Jarillo D, Rodicio JL. Indomethacin and beta-blockers in hypertension. Lancet (1978) i, 277.

7 Wong DG, Spence JD, Lamki L, Freeman D, McDonald JWD. Effect of non-steroidal anti-inflammatory drugs on control of hypertension by beta-blockers and diuretics. Lancet (1986) i, 997–1001.

8 Alvarez CR, Baez MA, Weidler DJ. Effect of sulindac and piroxicam adminstration on the antihypertensive effect of propranolol. J Clin Pharmacol (1986) 26, 544.

9 Ylitalo P, Pitkajavvi T, Pyykonen M-L, Nurmi A-K, Seppala E, Vapaatal H. Inhibition of prostaglandin synthesis by indomethacin interacts with the antihypertensive effect of atenolol. Clin Pharmacol Ther (1985) 38, 443–9.

10 Salvetti A, Pedrinelli R, Alberci A, Magagna A, Abdel-Haq B. The influence of indomethacin and sulindac on some pharmacological actions of atenolol in hypertensive patients. Br J clin Pharmacol (1984) 17, 108–11S.

11 Ebel DL, Rhymer AR, Stahl E. Effect of sulindac, piroxicam and placebo on the hypotensive effect of propranolol in patients with mild to moderate essential hypertension. Adv Ther (1985) 2, 131–42.

12 Mills EH, Whitworth JA, Andrews J, Kincaid-Smith P. Non-steroidal anti-inflammatory drugs and blood pressure. Aust NZ J Med (1982) 12, 478–82.

13 Pugliese F, Simonetti BM, Cinotte GA, Ciabattoni G, Catella F, Vastano S, Ghidini Ottonelli A, Pierucci A. Differential interaction of piroxicam and sulindac with the anti-hypertensive effect of propranolol. Eur J Clin Invest (1984) 14, 54.

14 Reid ALA. Antihypertensive effect of thiazides. Med J Aust (1981) 2, 109–10.

15 Staiger J, Gharieb AK, Keul J. Zur interaktion von Betablockern (Propranolol) und Antirheumatika (Isoxicam). Herz/Krauslauf (1983) 15, 141–3.

16 Davies JG, Rawlins DC, Busson M. Effect of ibuprofen on blood pressure control by propranolol and bendrofluazide. J Int Med Res (1988) 16, 173–81.

17 Schafer-Korting M, Kirch W, Axthelm T, Kohler H, Mutschler E. Atenolol interaction with aspirin, allopurinol, and ampicillin. Clin Pharmacol Ther (1983) 33, 283–8.

18 Johnsson G, Regardh CG, Solvell L. Lack of biological interaction of alprenolol and salicylate in man. Eur J clin Pharmacol (1973) 6, 9–14.

19 Sziegoleit W, Rausch J, Polak G, Gyorgy M, Dekov E, Bekes M. Influence of acetylsalicylic acid on acute circulatory effects of the beta-blocking agents pindolol and propranolol in humans. Int J Clin Pharmac Ther Tox (1982) 20, 423–30.

20 Schuna AA, Vejraska BD, Hiatt JG, Kochar M, Day R, Goodfriend TL. Lack of interaction between sulindac or naproxen and propranolol in hypertensive patients. J Clin Pharmacol (1989) 29, 524–8.

21 Abdel-Haq B, Magagna A, Avilla S, Salvetti A. The interference of indomethacin and of imidazole salicylate on blood pressure control of essential hypertensive patients treated with atenolol. Int J Clin Pharmacol Ther Toxicol (1987) 25, 598–600.

22 Schoenfeld A, Freedman S, Hod M, Ovadia Y. Antagonism of antihypertensive drug therapy in pregnancy by indomethacin? Am J Obst Gynecol (1989) 161, 1204–5.

23 Abate MA, Layne RD, Neeley JL, D'Alessandri R. Effect of naproxen and sulindac on blood pressure response to atenolol. DICP Ann Pharmacotherapy (1990) 24, 810–3.

24 Abate MA, Neeley JL, Layne RD, D'Alessandri R. Interaction of indomethacin and sulindac with labetalol. Br J clin Pharmacol (1991) 31, 363–6.

25 Macek K, Jurin I. Effects of indomethacine and aspirin on the antihypertensive action of metipranolol — a clinical study. Eur J Pharmacol (1990) 183, 839–40.

26 Halabi A, Linde M, Zeidler H, König J, Kirch W. Double-blind study on the interaction of oxaprozin with metoprolol in hypertensives. Cardiovasc Drug Ther (1989) 3, 441–3.

27 Stokes GS, Brooks PM, Johnson HJ, Monaghan JC, Okoro EO, Kelly D. The effects of sulindac and diclofenac in essential hypertension controlled by treatment with a beta-blocker and/or diuretic. Clin Exp Hyper Theory Prac (1991) A13, 1169–78. also Johnson H. Personnal Communication 1992.

28 Frölich JC, Whorten AR, Walker L, Smigel M, Oates JA, France R, Hollifield JW, Data JL, Gerber JG, Nies AS, Williams W, Robertson GL. Renal prostaglandins: regional differences in synthesis and role in renin release and ADH action. 7th Int Congr Nephrol, Montreal (1978). 108–114.

29 Anon. Adverse Drug Reactions Advisory Committee. Seven case studies. Med J Aust (1982) 2, 190–1.
30 Walker LA, Frölich JC. Renal prostaglandins and leukotrienes. Rev Physiol Biochem Pharmacol (1987) 107, 2–50.

Beta-blockers + Misoprostol

Abstract/Summary

Misoprostol does not interact significantly with propranolol.

Clinical evidence, mechanism, importance and management

400 µg misoprostol twice daily had no significant effect on the pharmacokinetics of a single dose of propranolol, nor on its steady state (80 mg twice daily) in 12 normal subjects.[1] This study did not confirm earlier observations by the same authors that misoprostol increased propranolol serum levels.[2] No special precautions would seem necessary during concurrent use.

References

1 Bennett PN, Fenn GC, Notarianni LJ, Lee CE. Misoprostol does not alter the pharmacokinetics of propranolol. Postgrad Med J (1991) 67, 455–7.
2 Bennett PN, Fenn GC, Notarianni LJ. Potential drug interactions with misoprostol: effects on the pharmacokinetics of antipyrine and propranolol. Postgrad Med J (1988) 64, (Suppl 1) 21–4.

Beta-blockers + Morphine

Abstract/Summary

Morphine can raise the serum levels of esmolol. The fatal dose of morphine is markedly reduced in animals by propranolol, but whether this also occurs in man is uncertain.

Clinical evidence, mechanism, importance and management

After being given an injection of 3 mg morphine the steady-state levels of esmolol (an infusion of 300 g/kg/min over 4 h) in 10 normal men were generally higher, but were only statistically significantly higher (by 46%) in two of the subjects. The pharmacokinetics of morphine were unchanged.[1] This interaction should be borne in mind if both drugs are given. There seems to be no information about other interactions with other beta-blockers. Studies in animals have shown that the fatal dose of morphine is reduced 2–7-fold in mice[2] and 15–16-fold in rats[3] by propranolol. The same interaction has also been seen in dogs.[3] So far there seems to be no confirmation that this occurs in man with propranolol or any other beta-blocker but it would seem prudent to use this drug combination cautiously until more is known.

References

1 Lowenthal DT, Porter RS, Saris SD, Bies CM, Slegowski MB, Staudacher A. Clinical pharmacology, pharmacodynamics and interactions of esmolol. Am J Cardiol (1985) 56, 14–18F.
2 Murmann W, Almirante L, Saccani-Guelfi M. Effects of hexobarbital, ether, morphine and urethane upon the acute toxicity of propranolol and D-(-)-INPEA. J Pharm Pharmacol (1966) 18, 692–4.
3 Davis WM, Hatoum NS. Possible toxic interaction of propranolol and narcotic analgesics. Drug Intell Clin Pharm (1981) 15, 290.

Beta-blockers + Nicardipine

Abstract/Summary

No important interaction appears to occur between atenolol or propranolol and nicardipine in healthy subjects but the response in patients should be checked.

Clinical evidence, mechanism, importance and management

A study in 12 normal subjects given 80 mg propranolol and 30 mg nicardipine daily for 6 days showed that no changes in the pharmacokinetics of either drug occurred.[1] This contrasts with two single dose studies which found that 30 mg nicardipine increased the AUC of a single 80 mg dose of propranolol by 47%,[3] and of an 80 mg sustained release formulation by 17%.[4] Another study found that nicardipine does not affect the pharmacokinetics or pharmacodynamics of atenolol in normal subjects.[2] However some patients have shown adverse effects (hypotension, heart failure) when beta-blockers and other calcium channel blockers were used together (see 'Beta-blockers + Nifedipine', 'Beta-blockers + Verapamil') so that the outcome of using beta-blockers and nicardipine should be well monitored.

Reference

1 Macdonald FC, Dow RJ, Wilson RAG, Yee KF, Finlayson J. A study to determine potential interactions between nicardipine and propranolol in healthy volunteers. Br J clin Pharmac (1987), 23, 626–7P.
2 Vercruysse I, Schoors DF, Musch G, Massart DL, Dupont AG. Nicardipine does not influence the pharmacokinetics and pharmacodynamics of atenolol. Br J clin Pharmac (1990) 30, 499–500.
3 Schoors DF, Vercruysse I, Musch G, Massart DL, Dupont AG. Influence of nicardipine on the pharmacokinetics and pharmacodyanics of propranolol in healthy volunteers. Br J clin Pharmac (1990) 29, 497–501.
4 Vercruysse I, Schoors DF, Massart DL, Dupont AG. Influence of nicardipine on the pharmacokinetics of sustained release propranolol in healthy volunteers. Br J clin Pharmac (1992) 34, 445P.

Beta-blockers + Nifedipine

Abstract/Summary

Concurrent use is common in the treatment of hypertension and angina, and usually both beneficial and uneventful, but a few cases of excessive hypotension and heart failure have been reported.

Clinical evidence

Some reports indicate that nifedipine interacts with beta-blockers such as atenolol, betaxolol, celiprolol, propranolol and metoprolol to affect their pharmacokinetics or pharmacodynamics, whereas others have found little or no interaction. Concurrent use normally appears to be useful and there is usually no evidence of haemodynamic deterioration,[5-7,9-13] however there are a few reports of adverse effects:

Two patients with angina under treatment with beta-blockers (alprenolol, propranolol) developed heart failure when additionally given 10 mg nifedipine three times a day. The signs of heart failure disappeared when the nifedipine was withdrawn.[1] One out of 15 patients with hypertension and exertional angina developed hypotension when given 10 mg nifedipine twice daily in addition to treatment with atenolol (50–100 mg), prazosin (9 mg) and diuretics. The situation was controlled by withdrawing the nifedipine.[2] Severe and prolonged hypotension developed in a patient treated with propranolol and nifedipine which may have been a factor which led to fatal myocardial infarction.[3] Cardiac failure is also described in another patient on atenolol when additionally given nifedipine.[4]

Mechanism

Nifedipine depresses the contractility of the heart muscle. This is counteracted by a sympathetic reflex increase in heart rate due to a nifedipine-induced peripheral vasodilation so that the ventricular output stays the same or is even improved. The presence of a beta-blocker may oppose this to some extent by slowing the heart rate which allows the negative inotropic effects of nifedipine to go unchecked.

Importance and management

The concurrent use of beta-blockers and nifedipine in the treatment of hypertension and angina pectoria is normally beneficial, safe and uneventful. A number of clinical studies confirm the value of this combination, however the existence of a handful of reports of adverse reactions emphasizes the need for some care during combined use. Patients should be monitored for any signs of excessive hypotension or cardiac depression. Those likely to be particularly at risk are patients with impairment of left ventricular function[8] and/or those taking beta-blockers in high dosage.

References

1 Anastassiades CJ. Nifedipine and beta-blocker drugs. Br Med J (1980) 281, 1251.
2 Opie LH, White DA. Adverse interaction between nifedipine and beta-blockade. Br Med J (1980) 281, 1462.
3 Staffurth JS, Emery P. Adverse interaction between nifedipine and beta-blockade. Br Med J (1981) 282, 225.
4 Robson RH, Vishwanath MC. Nifedipine and beta-blockade as a cause of cardiac failure. Br Med J (1982) 284, 104.
5 Gangji D, Juvent M, Niset G, Wathieu M, Degreve M, Bellens R, Poortmans J, Degre S, Fitzsimons TJ, Herchuelz A. Study of the influence of nifedipine on the pharmacokinetics and pharmacodynamics of propranolol, metoprolol and atenolol. Br J clin Pharmac (1984) 17, 29–35S.
6 Kendall MJ, Jack DB, Laugher SJ, Lobo J, Smith R. Lack of a pharmacokinetic interaction between nifedipine and the beta-adrenoceptor blockers metoprolol and atenolol. Br J clin Pharmac (1984) 18, 331–5.
7 Rowland E, Razis P, Sugrue D, Krikler DM. Acute and chronic haemodynamic and electrophysiological effects of nifedipine in patients receiving atenolol. Br Heart J (1983) 50, 383–9.
8 Brooks N, Cattell M, Pigeon J, Balcon R. Unpredictable response to nifedipine in severe cardiac failure. Br Med J (1980) 281, 1324.
9 Elkayam U, Roth A, Weber L, Kulick D, Kawanishi D, McKay C, Rahimtoola SH. Effects of nifedipine on hemodynamic and cardiac function in patients with left ventricular ejection fraction already treated with propranolol. Am J Cardiol (1986) 58, 536–40.
10 Vineneux Ph, Canal M, Domart Y, Roux A, Cascio B, Orofiamma B, Larribaud J, Flouvat B, Carbon C. Pharmacokinetic and pharmacodynamic interactions between nifedipine and propranolol or betaxolol. Int J Clin Pharmacol Ther Toxicol (1986) 24, 153–8.
11 Rosenkranz B, Ledermann H, Frolich JC. Interaction between nifedipine and atenolol: pharmacokinetics and pharmacodynamics in normotensive volunteers. J Cardiovasc Pharmacol (1986) 8, 943–9.
12 Vetrovec GW, Parker VE. Nifedipine, beta-blocker interaction: effect on left ventricular function. Clin Res (1984) 32, 833A.
13 Silke B, Verma SP, Guy S. Hemodynamic interactions of a new beta blocker, celiprolol, with nifedipine in angina pectoris. Cardiovasc Drug Ther (1991) 5, 681–8.

Beta-blockers + Nizatidine

Abstract/Summary

The heart-slowing effects of atenolol are increased by nizatidine.

Clinical evidence, mechanism, importance and management

A study in 12 normal subjects found that 3 h after taking 100 mg atenolol their resting heart rates fell by 10.6 beat per minute (from 63.7 to to 53.1 bpm). A further fall by 6.0 bpm occurred when additionally given 300 mg nizatidine.[1] It seems probable that nizatidine will have the same effects in the presence of other beta-blockers. The clinical significance of these effects is uncertain, but it could possibly be important in elderly patients. More study is needed.

Reference

1 Halabi A, Kirch W. Negative chronotropic effect of nizatidine. Gut (1991) 32, 630–4.

Beta-blockers + Omeprazole

Abstract/Summary

Omeprazole does not interact with metoprolol or propranolol.

Clinical evidence, mechanism, importance and management

20 mg omeprazole daily for eight days in eight normal subjects had no effect on the steady-state serum levels of propranolol (160 mg daily), nor on its clinical effects (resting and exercised heart rates, blood pressure).[1] Another study found that 40 mg omeprazole daily for eight days had no effect on the steady-state serum levels of metoprolol (100 mg daily).[2] No special precautions are needed.

References

1 Henry D, Brent P, Whyte I, Mihaly G, Devenish-Meares S. Propranolol steady-state pharmacokinetics are unaltered by omeprazole. Eur J Clin Pharmacol (1987) 33, 369–73.
2 Andreasson T, Lundborg P, Regårdh CG. Lack of effect of omeprazole treatment on steady-state plasma levels of metoprolol. Eur J Clin Pharmacol (1991) 40, 61–5.

Beta-blockers + Penicillins

Abstract/Summary

Serum atenolol levels are halved by the concurrent use of 1 g doses of ampicillin. The clinical importance of this is uncertain, but possibly not large. No important interaction occurs if the ampicillin is given in divided doses.

Clinical evidence

A study in six normal subjects found that when 100 mg atenolol was given with 1 g ampicillin daily for 6 days, the mean steady-state serum atenolol levels were reduced by 52% (from 199 to 95 ng/ml).[1] The AUC was also reduced by 52%. The blood pressure lowering effects of atenolol at rest were not affected by the presence of ampicillin, but after exercise a small rise in systolic pressures occurred. The effects of atenolol on heart rate during exercise were diminished (from 24% to 11% at 12 h).[1]

Another study showed that when 50 mg atenolol and 1 g ampicillin were given concurrently by mouth, the AUC was reduced by 51.5%, whereas when the ampicillin was given as four 250 mg doses over 24 h, the AUC was only reduced by 18.2%.[1]

Mechanism

Uncertain. Ampicillin apparently affects the absorption of the atenolol.

Importance and management

An established interaction although information is limited. If the minimal effects on blood pressure and heart rate can be taken as a measure, it would appear to be of only moderate or minor clinical importance. It is not clear therefore why the authors of the paper cited[1] say that the atenolol dosage may need to be doubled to achieve the desired antihypertensive effect, and are adamant that doubling the dosage is necessary in the treatment of angina. The second study[2] showed that if the ampicillin is given divided into four 250 mg doses instead of as a single 1 g dose, the effects of the interaction are almost certainly trivial. If a large dose of ampicillin is needed, it has been suggested that the atenolol is given first.[2] Information about other beta-blockers is lacking, although it seems possible that other penicillins will interact like ampicillin.

References

1 Schafer-Korting M, Kirch W, Axthelm T, Kohler H, Mutschler E. Atenolol interaction with aspirin, allopurinol, and ampicillin. Clin Pharmacol Ther (1983) 33, 283–8.
2 McLean AJ, Tonkin A, McCarthy P, Harrison P. Dose-dependence of atenolol-ampicillin interaction. Br J Clin Pharmac (1984) 18, 969–71.

Beta-blockers + Phenothiazines

Abstract/Summary

The concurrent use of chlorpromazine and propranolol can result in a marked rise in the serum levels of both drugs. Excessive hypotension has been seen. Two patients showed 3–5-fold increases in serum thioridazine levels when given propranolol.

Clinical evidence

(a) Serum propranolol or pindolol levels raised

The mean steady-state propranolol levels (80 mg eight-hourly) of four normal subjects and one patient were raised 70% (from 41.5 to 70.2 ng/ml) when additionally given 50 mg chlorpromazine eight-hourly.[1] The increase was considerable in some subjects but barely detectable in others. Another subject on propranolol climbed out of bed after the first dose of chlorpromazine and promptly fainted. He was found to have a pulse rate of 35–40 per min and a blood pressure of 70/0 mmHg. He rapidly recovered with a pulse rate of 85 and blood pressure of 120/70 when given 3 mg atropine.[1]

Another case of hypotension during the concurrent use of chlorpromazine and sotalol has been reported.[2] Thioridazine also increases serum pindolol levels.[9]

(b) Serum chlorpromazine levels raised

Propranolol (mean dose 8.1 mg/kg) increased the serum chlorpromazine levels of seven schizophrenics taking 6.7 mg/kg three times daily by 100–500%, and raised the plasma levels of the active metabolites of chlorpromazine by 50–100%.[4] The same or similar work by the same authors is described elsewhere.[5] One of the patients was withdrawn from the study because he suffered a cardiovascular collapse while taking both drugs.[5] It has been suggested that the value of propranolol in the treatment of schizophrenia probably results from the rise in serum chlorpromazine levels.[5,6]

A schizophrenic patient taking chlorpromazine and thiothixene experienced delerium, grand mal seizures and skin photosensitivity, attributed to a rise in serum levels of the neuroleptic drugs after additionally being given propranolol.[7]

(c) Serum thioridazine levels raised

Two patients stabilized on 600 or 800 mg daily showed rises in serum thioridazine levels from 0.3 to 1.6, and from 0.4 to 1.5 g/ml respectively when concurrently treated over 26–40 days with propranolol given in increasing doses up to a total of 800 mg daily. No thioridazine toxicity was seen although serum levels had risen into the toxic range.[8] Another study confirmed that thioridazine levels rise markedly.[10] Pindolol also increases serum thioridazine levels by up to 50%.[9]

Mechanism

Pharmacokinetic evidence[1] and animal studies[3] suggest that propranolol and chlorpromazine mutually inhibit the liver metabolism of the other drug so that both accumulate within the body. The hypotensive episodes reported[1,2,5] are presumably due to the additive hypotensive effects of both drugs. The mechanism of the propranolol-thioridazine interaction is not understood.

Importance and management

The propranolol-chlorpromazine interaction appears to be established although information is limited. Concurrent use should be well monitored and the dosages reduced if necessary. The same precautions apply with propranolol and thioridazine.[8] There seems to be no information about any other beta-blocker/phenothiazine interactions, but if the mechanism of interaction suggested above is true, it seems possible that other beta-blockers which are mainly cleared from the body by liver metabolism (e.g. alprenolol, metoprolol) might interact similarly with chlorpromazine, whereas those mainly cleared unchanged in the urine (e.g. atenolol, nadolol) are less likely to do so.

References

1 Vestal RE, Kornhauser DM, Hollifield JW, Shand DG. Inhibition of propranolol metabolism by chlorpromazine. Clin Pharmacol Ther (1979) 25, 19.
2 Baker L, Barcai A, Kaye R, Haque N. Beta-adrenergic blockade and juvenile diabetes: acute studies and long-term therapeutic trial. J Pediat (1969) 75, 19.
3 Shand DG, Oates JA. The metabolism of propranolol by rat liver microsomes and its inhibition by phenothiazine and tricyclic antidepressants. Biochem Pharmacol (1971) 20, 1720.
4 Peet M, Middlemiss DN, Yates RA. Pharmacokinetic interaction between propranolol and chlorpromazine in schizophrenic patients. Lancet (1980) ii, 978.
5 Peet M, Middlemiss DN, Yates RA. Propranolol in schizophrenia, II. Clinical and biochemical aspects of combining propranolol with chlorpromazine. Br J Psychiat (1981) 138, 112.
6 Lindstrom IH, Persson E. Propranolol in chronic schizophrenia: a controlled study in neuroleptic treated patients. Br J Psychiat (1980) 137, 126.
7 Miller FA, Rampling D. Adverse effects of combined propranolol and chlorpromazine therapy. Am J Psychiat (1982) 139, 1198–9.
8 Silver JM, Yudofsky SC, Kogan M, Katz BL. Elevation of thioridazine plasma levels by propranolol. Am J Psychiatry (1986) 143, 1290–2.
9 Greendyke RM, Gulya A. Effect of pindolol administration on serum levels of thioridazine, haloperidol and phenobarbital. J Clin Psychiatry (1988) 49, 105–7.
10 Greendyke RM, Kanter DR. Plasma propranolol levels and their effect on plasma thioridazine and haloperidol concentrations. J Clin Psychopharmacol (1987) 7, 178–82.

Beta-blockers + Propafenone

Abstract/Summary

Serum metoprolol and propranolol levels can be markedly raised (2–5-fold) by the concurrent use of propafenone. Toxicity may develop.

Clinical evidence

Four patients with ventricular arrhythmias showed a 2–5 fold rise in steady-state serum metoprolol levels (150–200 mg daily) when given 150 mg propafenone three times daily. One of them developed distressing nightmares and the other had acute left ventricular failure with pulmonary oedema and haemoptysis which disappeared when the metoprolol dosage was reduced or stopped. Single dose studies in normal subjects found a two-fold decrease in the clearance of metoprolol and a 20% reduction in the heart rate increase due to exercise at 90 min. Serum propafenone levels in four other patients were found to be unaffected by metoprolol.[1]

A patient developed neurotoxicity (vivid nightmares, fatigue, headache, etc) when given 100 mg metoprolol daily which worsened while it was being withdrawn and replaced by 300 mg propafenone.[3]

225 mg propafenone daily more than doubled the steady-state propranolol levels (50 mg 8-hourly) of 12 subjects. The beta-blocking effects were only modestly increased. The propafenone pharmacokinetics remained unchanged.[2]

Mechanism

Uncertain, but it is suggested that the propafenone reduces the metabolism of the metoprolol and propranolol by the liver, thereby reducing their clearance and raising serum levels.[1,2]

Importance and management

Information is limited but the interaction would seem to be established. Concurrent use need not be avoided but anticipate the need to reduce the dosage of metoprolol and propranolol. Monitor closely because some patients may experience adverse effects. If the suggested mechanism of interaction is correct it is possible that other beta-blockers which undergo liver metabolism will interact similarly but not those largely excreted unchanged in the urine (e.g. atenolol, nadolol). This needs confirmation.

References

1 Wagner F, Kalusche D, Trenk D, Jahnchen E, Roskamm H. Drug interaction between propafenone and metoprolol. Br J clin Pharmac (1987) 24, 213–20.

2 Kowey PR, Kirsen EB, Fu C-HJ, Mason WD. Interaction between propranolol and propafenone in healthy volunteers. J Clin Pharmacol (1989) 29, 512–17.

3 Ahmad S. Metoprolol-induced delerium perpetuated by propafenone. Am Fam Phys (1991) 44, 1142–3.

Beta-blockers + Ranitidine

Abstract/Summary

Ranitidine does not alter the steady-state plasma levels of atenolol, metoprolol, propranolol or teratolol and their therapeutic effects remain unchanged.

Clinical evidence

300 mg ranitidine daily for six days given to five normal subjects did not affect their steady-state plasma levels of propranolol (160 mg daily), nor were their exercise-induced heart rates or blood pressures affected.[1] Similarly no changes in plasma propranolol levels, pulse rates or blood pressures were seen in other studies.[2–6]

Another study on 12 normal subjects found that the serum levels of metoprolol (100 mg daily) were unaffected by 300 mg ranitidine daily for seven days.[7] Some studies confirm these findings,[8,9,13,15] but other single doses studies report increases in serum metoprolol levels and AUC's (+50%) by ranitidine.[10–12] No changes in exercise-induced heart rates were found.[8,13,15] No changes in the pharmacokinetics of atenolol or teratolol by ranitidine were reported in two other studies.[10,14] A further study found that ranitidine raised peak serum metoprolol levels by 30%.[16]

Mechanism

The rises in metoprolol serum levels caused by ranitidine in the single dose studies are not understood.[10–12,16]

Importance and management

The possible effects of ranitidine on the serum levels and effects of propranolol and metoprolol have been well studied, but less is known about atenolol and teratolol. No clinically important interactions have been seen. There is nothing to suggest that the concurrent use of ranitidine and any beta-blocker should be avoided, nor that there is any need to take particular precautions.

References

1 Reimann IW, Klotz U, Frohlich JC. Effects of cimetidine and ranitidine on steady-state propranolol kinetics and dynamics. Clin Pharmacol Ther (1982) 32, 749–57.

2 Donn KH, Powell JR, Rogers JF, Eshelman FN. The influence of H_2-receptor antagonists on steady-state concentrations of propranolol and 4-hydroxypropranolol. J Clin Pharmacol (1984) 24, 500–8.

3 Markiewicz A, Hartler M, Lelek H, Boldys H, Nowak A. The effect of treatment with cimetidine and ranitidine on bioavailability of, and circulatory response to, propranolol. Zbl Pharm (1984) 123, 516–18.

4 Heagerty AM, Castleden CM, Patel L. Failure of ranitidine to interact with propranolol. Br Med J (1982) 284, 1304.

5 Heagerty AM, Donovan MA, Castleden CM, Pohl JEF, Patel L. The influence of histamine (H_2) antagonists on propranolol pharmacokinetics. Int J clin Pharmac Res (1986) 2, 203–5.

6 Patel L, Weerasuriya K. The effect of cimetidine and ranitidine on propranolol clearance. Br J Clin Pharmac (1983) 15, 152P.

7 Toon S, Batra HK, Garstang FM, Rowland M. Comparative effects of ranitidine and cimetidine on metoprolol in man. Br J Pharmacol (1987). Abstract presented to the British Pharmacological Society meeting, September 1986.

8 Kelly JG, Salem SAM, Kinney CD, Shanks RG, McDevitt DG. Effects of ranitidine on the disposition of metoprolol. Br J clin Pharmac (1985) 19, 219–24.

9 Kendall MJ, Laugher SJ, Wilkins MR. Ranitidine, cimetidine and metoprolol-a pharmacokinetic interaction study. Gastroenterol (1986) 90, 1490.

10 Spahn H, Mutschler E, Kirch W, Ohnhaus EE, Janisch HD. Influence of ranitidine on plasma metoprolol and atenolol concentrations. Br Med J (1983) 286, 1546–7.

11 Kelly JG, Shanks RG, McDevitt DG. Influence of ranitidine on plasma metoprolol concentrations. Br Med J (1983) 287, 1218–19.

12 Kirch W, Ramsch K, Janisch HD, Ohnhaus EE. The influence of two histamine H_2-receptor antagonists, cimetidine and ranitidine, on the plasma levels and clinical effect of nifedipine and metoprolol. Arch Toxicol (1984) 7, 256–9.

13 Tom S, Davidson EM, Garstang FM, Batra H, Bowers RJ, Rowland M. The racemic metoprolol H_2-antagonist interaction. Clin Pharmacol Ther (1988) 43, 283–9.

14 Kirch W, Milferstädt S, Halabi A,Rocher I, Efthymiopoulos C, Jung L. Interaction of teratolol with rifampicin and ranitidine pharmacokinetics and antihypertensive activity. Cardiovasc Drug Ther (1990) 4, 487–92.

15 Chellingsworth MC, Laugher S, Akhlaghi S, Jack DB, Kendall MJ. The effects of ranitidine and cimetidine on the pharmacokinetics and pharmacodynamics of metoprolol. Aliment Pharmacol Therap (1988) 2, 521–7.

16 Mutschler E, Spahn H, Kirch W. The interaction between H_2-receptor antagonists and beta-adrenoceptor blockers. Br J Clin Pharmac (1984) 17, 51–7S.

Beta-blockers + Rifampicin (Rifampin)

Abstract/Summary

Rifampicin increases the loss of bisoprolol, propranolol, metoprolol and teratolol from the body and reduces their serum levels. The extent to which this reduces the therapeutic response to these beta-blockers is uncertain, but it is probably small.

Clinical evidence

600 mg rifampicin daily for three weeks increased the oral clearance of propranolol in six normal subjects from 35.7 to 96.1 ml min^{-1} kg^{-1}. Increasing the dose of rifampicin to 900 or 1200 mg daily did not increase the clearance. Four weeks after withdrawing the rifampicin the blood levels of propranolol had returned to normal.[1]

A similar interaction occurs with metoprolol: 600 mg rifampicin daily for 15 days reduced the peak serum metoprolol levels (after single 100 mg doses) of 10 normal subjects by 33% and the AUC by 40%.[2] Another study showed that the AUC of bisoprolol was reduced by 34% in subjects given 600 mg rifampicin daily.[3] A further study found that 600 mg rifampicin for a week increased the clearance of teratolol almost threefold (from 89 to 241 ml/min) and reduced the half-life from 9 to 3.4 h. A slight reduction in the effects of teratolol on blood pressure was seen and heart rates were raised from 68 to 74 bpm.[4]

Mechanism

Rifampicin is a potent liver enzyme inducing agent which increases the metabolism and loss of the these beta-blockers from the body.

Importance and management

These interactions are established. Their Clinical importance is uncertain but probably small,[4] nevertheless concurrent use should be monitored. Increase the dosage of the beta-blocker if there is any evidence that the therapeutic response is inadequate. Only those beta-blockers which undergo extensive liver metabolism would be expected to be affected by rifampicin (e.g. propranolol, metoprolol, alprenolol, etc.), unlike those mainly lost unchanged in the urine (atenolol, nadolol, etc.).

References

1 Herman RJ, Nakamura K, Wilkinson GR, Wood AJJ. Induction of propranolol metabolism by rifampicin. Br J Clin Pharmac (1983) 16, 565–9.
2 Bennett PN, John VA, Whitmarsh VB. Effects of rifampicin on metoprolol and antipyrine kinetics. Br J Clin Pharmac (1982) 13, 387.
3 Kirch W, Rose I, Klingmann I, Pabst J, Ohnhaus EE. Interaction of bisoprolol with cimetidine and rifampicin. Eur J Clin Pharmacol (1986) 31, 59–62.
4 Kirch W, Milferstädt S, Halabi A, Rocher I, Efthymiopoulos C, Jung L. Interaction of teratolol with rifampicin and ranitidine pharmacokinetics and antihypertensive activity. Cardiovasc Drug Ther (1990) 4, 487–92.

Beta-blockers + Sulphasalazine

Abstract/Summary

Sulphasalazine markedly reduces the absorption of talinolol.

Clinical evidence, mechanism, importance and management

The AUC_{0-4} (area under the curve over four hours) of 50 mg talinolol in eight subjects was reduced to 9% (from 958 to 84 ng/ml/h) when simultaneously given with 4 g sulphasalazine. The maximum serum levels were also markedly reduced: from 112 to 23 ng.ml^{-1} in three subjects, and to undetectable levels in the other five.[1]

Mechanism

Not known. It is suggested that the talinolol is adsorbed onto the sulphasalazine, thereby preventing its absorption.[1] Sulphasalazine also reduces the absorption of digoxin, folic acid and iron.

Importance and management

Information is limited to this study but it would appear to be an established and probably Clinically important interaction. The efficacy of the talinolol would be expected to be markedly reduced, but nobody yet seems to have checked on this. If the mechanism suggested by the authors is true, their advice to separate the dosages by 2–3 h should minimize this interaction.[1] More study is needed to confirm how effective this is, and whether other beta blockers behave similarly.

Reference

1 Terhaag B, Palm U, Sahre H, Richter K, Oertel R. Interaction of talinolol and sulfasalazine in the human gastrointestinal tract. Eur J Clin Pharmacol (1992) 42, 461–2.

Beta-blockers + Sulphinpyrazone

Abstract/Summary

The antihypertensive effects of oxprenolol can be reduced or abolished by the concurrent use of sulphinpyrazone.

Clinical evidence

10 hypertensive patients were given 80 mg oxprenolol twice daily, as a result of which their mean supine blood pressures were reduced from 161/101 to 149/96 mmHg, and their heart rates fell from 72 to 66 beats per min. When additionally given 400 mg sulphinpyrazone twice daily, their blood pressures climbed again to approximately their former levels. Heart rates remained unaffected.[1] Cardiac workload (Systolic blood pressure × heart rate) was only slightly increased (+ 8%).

Mechanism

Not understood. One idea is that the sulphinpyrazone inhibits the production of prostaglandins by the kidney which have vasodilatory (antihypertensive) activity. This would oppose the actions of the oxprenolol. Another idea is that the sulphinpyrazone increases the metabolism of the oxprenolol, thereby increasing its loss from the body and reducing its effects.

Importance and management

Information seems to be limited to this study. If sulphinpyrazone is given to patients taking oxprenolol for hypertension, the effects should be monitored. It seems likely that this interaction could be accommodated by raising the dosage of the oxprenolol. The effects of this interaction on cardiac workload appear to be minimal but it would still be prudent to monitor concurrent use if oxprenolol is used for angina. It is not known whether other beta-blockers interact similarly but it would seem wise at the moment to assume that they do.

Reference

1 Ferrara LA, Mancini M, Marotta T, Pasanisi F, Fasano ML. Interference by sulphinpyrazone with the antihypertensive effects of oxprenolol. Eur J Clin Pharmacol (1986) 29, 717–19.

Beta-blockers + Sympathomimetics, directly-acting

Abstract/Summary

(i) Effects on blood pressure and heart rate

The pressor effects of adrenaline (epinephrine) can be markedly increased in patients taking non-selective beta-blockers such as propranolol. A severe and potentially life-threatening hypertensive reaction and/or marked bradycardia can develop. An isolated report describes a fatal hypertensive reaction with propranolol and phenylephrine but concurrent use normally seems to be uneventful.

(ii) Effects on bronchi

Non-selective beta-blockers (e.g. propranolol) should not be used in asthmatic subjects because they may cause serious bronchoconstriction. Even cardio-selective blockers can sometimes cause problems. No adverse interaction normally occurs during the concurrent use of sympathomimetic brochodilators (e.g. isoprenaline, isoproterenol etc) and cardio-selective beta-blockers (e.g. metoprolol).

(iii) Anaphylaxis

The incidence of anaphylaxis is possibly increased by the beta-blockers, and patients may be resistant to treatment with adrenaline (epinephrine) or other sympathomimetics.

Clinical evidence

(i) Effects on blood pressure and heart rate

(a) Propranolol + Adrenaline (epinephrine) or levonordefrin

Five normal subjects and four patients with hyperthyroidism showed a small increase in heart rate but little change in blood pressure after the subcutaneous injection of 0.4 mg adrenaline. After pre-treatment with 40 mg propranolol the same dose of adrenaline caused a 20–40 mmHg rise in blood pressure and a fall in heart rate of 23–36 beats per minute.[1]

Six patients on 20–80 mg propranolol daily and undergoing plastic surgery experienced marked hypertensive reactions (blood pressures in the range 190/110 to 260/150 mmHg) and bradycardia when their eyelids and/or faces were infiltrated with 8–40 ml of local anaesthetic solutions of lignocaine (lidocaine) containing 1:100,000 or 1:200,000 adrenaline (epinephrine). Cardiac arrest occurred in one patient.[7]

Similar marked increases in blood pressure,[2–5,10,11,20,22,27] associated with marked bradycardia, sometimes severe, have been described in other reports involving propranolol. In contrast only a small blood pressure rise was seen in a comparative study with metoprolol.[4] This was confirmed in another study in which patients given identical infusions of adrenaline (epinephrine) developed a hypertensive-bradycardial reaction while taking propranolol but not while taking metoprolol.[8] A hypertensive reaction has also been seen in a patient on propranolol when given an injection of 2% mepivacaine with 1:20,000 levonordefrin.[21]

(b) Propranolol + Phenylephrine

A woman on 30 mg propranolol four times daily for hypertension was given one drop of a 10% phenylephrine hydrochloride solution in each eye during an ophthalmic examination. 45 min later she complained of a sudden and sharp bi-temporal pain and shortly afterwards became unconscious. She later died of an intracerebral haemorrhage due to the rupture of a berry aneurysm. She had had a similar dose of phenylephrine on a previous occasion in the absence of propranolol without any problems.[9] No change in blood pressure was seen in another study in subjects taking metoprolol who were administered 0.5–4.0 mg doses of phenylephrine intranasally[6] or in 12 hypertensive patients on propranolol or metoprolol when given intravenous infusions of phenylephrine.[11]

Mechanism

Adrenaline stimulates alpha- and beta-receptors of the cardiovascular system, the former results in vasoconstriction and the latter in both vasodilatation and stimulation of the heart. The net result is usually a modest increase in heart rate and a small rise in blood pressure. If however the beta-receptors are blocked, the unopposed alpha vasoconstriction causes a marked rise in blood pressure, followed by bradycardia due to the unopposed increase in reflex vagal tone. Cardioselective beta-blockers have a much smaller effect on the beta-2 receptors in the blood vessels and therefore the effects of any interaction is relatively small. Phenylephrine is largely an alpha-stimulator.

Importance and management

The propranolol-adrenaline (epinephrine) interaction is established. It may be serious and potentially life-threatening, depending on the dosage of adrenaline (epinephrine) used.

Marked and serious blood pressure rises and severe bradycardia have occurred in patients given 300–400 µg adrenaline subcutaneously[1,9] or 80–400 µg by infiltration of skin and eyelids during plastic surgery. 15 µg given intravascularly can cause an almost 40% fall in heart-rate.[27] Patients on non-selective beta-blockers such as propranolol should only be administered adrenaline in very reduced dosages because of the marked bradycardia and hypertension which can occur. A less marked effect is likely with the selective beta-blockers such as metoprolol.[4] A list of the different types of beta-blockers is given in the introduction to this chapter. Local anaesthetics used in dental surgery usually contain very low concentrations (e.g. 5–20 µg/ml, i.e. 1 in 200,000–1 in 50,000) and only small volumes are usually given, so that an undesirable interaction is unlikely.

No interaction between phenylephrine and the beta-blockers would be expected. Apart from the single unexplained case cited above,[9] the literature would appear to be silent. Concurrent use normally appears to be Clinically unimportant,[6,11] particularly bearing in mind the widespread use of the beta-blockers and the ready availability of phenylephrine in the form of over-the-counter cough-and-cold remedies and nasal decongestants.

Acute hypertensive episodes can be controlled with chlorpromazine given in 1 mg increments, or phentolamine, both of which are alpha-blockers. Intravenous hydralazine, 20 mg in 250 ml saline, administered at 40 drops per min for 10–20 min has been used successfully[7]. Nifedipine has also been used;[20] chewing and swallowing the contents of a capsule with water can be very effective.

(ii) Effects on bronchi

(a) Cardio-selective beta-blockers + Beta-agonist bronchodilators

The cardio-selective beta-blockers would not be expected to affect the beta-receptors in the bronchi, but an increasing number of reports indicate that bronchospasm can sometimes occur following their use by asthmatics, particularly if high doses are used (see also 'Antiasthmatics + Beta-blockers'.)

No adverse interaction normally occurs between beta-agonist sympathomimetic bronchodilators and these beta-blockers. A study in 29 patients with chronic bronchial asthma on 200 mg practolol daily found that the effects of terbutaline, 15 mg daily, were unaltered and no subjective or objective worsening of the asthmatic symptoms was seen.[14] Similar results have been described in other studies with celiprolol, metoprolol[12,13] or practolol[12] with isoprenaline (isoproterenol); atenolol, celiprolol or metoprolol with terbutaline;[17,31] or atenolol and celiprolol with salbutamol (albuterol).[23,29,30]

(b) Non-selective beta-blockers + Beta-agonist bronchodilators

Non-selective beta-blockers (e.g. propranolol and oxprenolol) are contraindicated in asthmatic subjects because they can cause bronchospasm, reduce lung ventilation and may possibly precipitate a severe asthmatic attack in some subjects. Fatalities have occurred.[24] They block the normal dilation of the bronchi which is under the control of the sympathetic nervous system.[12,13] They also oppose the effects of bronchodilators such as salbutamol (albuterol).[23] Even eye drops containing the non-selective beta-blockers timolol[15,28] and metipranolol[26] have been reported to precipitate asthmatic attacks.

Mechanism

Non-selective beta-blockers, intended for their actions on the heart, also block the beta-receptors in the bronchi so that the normal brochodilation which is under the control of the sympathetic nervous system is reduced or abolished. As a result the brochoconstriction of asthma can be made worse. Cardioselective beta-blockers on the other hand preferentially block beta-1 receptors in the heart, leaving the beta-2 receptors largely unaffected, so that beta-2 stimulating bronchodilators such as isoprenaline, terbutaline, etc. continue to have their bronchodilator effects.

Importance and management

Well established. Avoid non-selective beta-blockers in asthmatics and those with chronic obstructive airways disease (COPD), (ie those already likely to be taking beta-agonist bronchodilators) whether given orally or in eye-drops because serious and life-threatening bronchospasm may occur. The cardioselective beta-blockers are generally safer but not entirely free from risk in some patients, particularly in high dosage. Celiprolol (a selective blocker) appears to be exceptional in causing bronchodilatation in asthmatics and not bronchconstriction, but some caution is still necessary.[29] The cardioselective and non-selective beta-blockers are listed in tables 10.1–10.3 while the the beta-agonist bronchodilators are listed in table 22.1.

(iii) Anaphylaxis: resistance to treatment

Clinical evidence, mechanism, importance and management

A patient who suffered an anaphylactic reaction after receiving an allergy injection was resistant to the bronchodilatory effects of adrenaline (epinephrine) because she was taking propranolol.[15] Resistance to treatment in patients on beta-blockers has been described in a number of reports.[16] It may be necessary to use much larger doses of adrenaline (epinephrine) or other sympathomimetics to overcome the resistance. An 80-fold increase in the IV dose of isoprenaline (isoproterenol) has even been suggested.[18] It has also been proposed that the incidence of anaphylactic reactions may be increased in those on beta-blockers,[18,19] one idea being that the adrenoceptors concerned with suppressing the release of the mediators of anaphylaxis may be blocked by either beta-1 or beta-2 antagonists.[18] However one study failed to find any evidence to support this idea.[25]

References

1 Varma DR, Sharma KK, Arora RC. Response to adrenaline and propranolol in hyperthyroidism. Lancet (1976), 1, 260.

2 Kram J, Bourne HR, Melmon KL, Malbach H. Propranolol. Ann Int Med (1974) 80, 282.

3 Harris WS, Schoenfeld CD, Brooks RH, Weissler AM. Effect of beta adrenergic blockade on the hemodynamic responses to epinephrine. Amer J Cardiol (1966) 17, 484.

4 van Herwaarden CLA. Effects of adrenaline during treatment with propranolol and metoprolol. Br Med J (1977) 2, 1029.

5 Berchtold P, Bessman AN. Propranolol. Ann Int Med (1974) 80, 119.

6 Myers MG, Iazetta JJ. Intranasally administered phenylephrine and blood pressure. Can Med Ass J (1982) 127, 365–8.

7 Foster CA, Aston SJ. Propranolol-epinephrine interaction: a potential disaster. Plastic Surg and Reconstr Surg (1983) 72, July, 74–8.

8 Houben H, Thien T, Laor VA. Effect of low-dose epinephrine infusion on hemodynamics after selective and non-selective beta-blockade in hypertension. Clin Pharmacol Ther (1982) 31, 685.

9 Cass E, Kadar D, Stein HA. Hazards of phenylephrine topical medication in persons taking propranolol. Can Med Ass J (1979) 120, 1261–2.

10 Hansbrough JF, Near A. Propranolol-epinephrine antagonism with hypertension and stroke. Ann InternMed (1980) 92, 717.

11 Myers MG. Beta-adrenoceptor antagonism and pressor response to phenylephrine. Clin Pharmacol Ther (1984) 36, 57–63.

12 Thringer G, Svedmyr N. Interaction of orally administered metoprolol, practolol and propranolol with isoprenaline in asthmatics. Eur J Clin Pharmacol (1976) 10, 163.

13 Johnsson G, Svedmyr N, Thurnier G. Effects of intravenous propranolol and metoprolol and their interaction with isoprenaline on pulmonary function, heart rate and blood pressure in asthmatics. Eur J Clin Pharmacol (1975) 8, 175.

14 Fromgren H, Eriksson NE. Effects of practolol in combination with terbutaline in the treatment of hypertension and arrhythmias in asthmatic patients. Scand J Resp Dis (1975) 56, 217.

15 Charan NB, Lakshminarayan S. Pulmonary effects of topical timolol. Arch Intern Med (1980) 120, 843.

16 Newman BR, Schultz LK. Epinephrine-resistant anaphylaxis in a patient taking propranolol hydrochloride. Ann Allergy (1981) 47, 35.

17 Lofdahl C-G, Svedmyr N. Cardioselectivity of atenolol and metoprolol. A study in asthmatic patients. Eur J Resp Dis (1981) 62, 396–404.

18 Toogood JH. Beta-blocker therapy and the risk of anaphylaxis. Canad Med Ass J (1987) 136, 929–33.

19 Berkelman RL, Finton RJ, Elsea W. Beta-adrenergic antagonists and fatal anaphylactic reactions to oral penicillin. Ann Intern Med (1986) 104, 143.

20 Whelan TV. Propranolol, epinephrine and accelerated hypertension during hemodialysis. Ann Intern Med (1987) 106, 327.

21 Mito RS, Yagiela JA. Hypertensive response to levonordefrin in a patient receiving propranolol: report of a case. J Am Dent Ass (1988) 116, 55–7.

22 Gandy W. Severe epinephrine-propranolol interaction. Ann Emerg Med (1989) 18, 98–9.

23 Fogari R, Zoppi A, Tettamanti F, Poletti L, Rizzardi G, Fiocchi G. Comparative effects of celiprolol, propranolol, oxprenolol, and atenolol on respiratory function in hypertensive patients with chronic obstructive lung disease. Cardiovasc Drugs Ther (1990) 4, 1145–50.

24 Anon. Beta-blocker caused death of asthmatic. Pharm J (1991) 246, 185.

25 Hepner MJ, Ownby DR, Anderson JA, Rowe MS, Sears-Ewald D, Brown EB. Risk of systemic reactions in patients taking beta-blocker drugs receiving allergen immunotherapy injections. J Allergy Clin Immunol (1990) 86, 407–11.

26 Vinti H, Chichmanaian RM, Fournier JP, Pesce A, Taillan B, Fuzibet JG, Cassuto JP, Dujardin P. Accidents systémiques des bêta-bloquants en collyres. A propos de six observations. Rev Med Interne (1989) 10, 41–4.

27 Mackie K, Lam A. Epinephrine-containing test dose during beta-blockade. J Clin Monit (1991) 7, 213–6.

28 Jones FL, Ekberg NL. Exacerbation of obstructive airway disease by timolol. J Amer Med Ass (1980) 244, 2730.

29 Pujet JC, Dubreuill C, Fluery B, Provendier O, Abella ML. Effects of celiprolol, a cardioselective beta-blocker, on respiratory function in asthmatic patients. Eur Resp J (1992) 5, 196–200.

30 Doshan HD, Rosenthal RR, Brown R, Slutsky A, Applin WJ, Caruso FS. Celiprolol, atenolol and propranolol: a comparison of pulmonary effects in

asthmatic patients. J Cardiovasc Pharmacol (1986) 8, Suppl 4) S105–8.

31 Matthys H, Doshan HD, Rühle K-H, Applin WJ, Braig H, Pohl M. Bronchosparing properties of celiprolol, a new beta-1, alpha-2 blocker, in propranolol-sensitive asthmatic patients. J Cardiovasc Pharmacol (1986) 8, Suppl 4, S40–2.

Beta-blockers + Sympathomimetics, Indirectly-acting

Abstract/Summary

A small but probably Clinically unimportant rise in blood pressure may occur in patients on beta-blockers who take phenylpropanolamine. A marked rise has been seen in one patient also taking methyldopa.

Clinical evidence, mechanism, importance and management

A study in seven hypertensive patients controlled with beta-blockers (five on atenolol, and the other two on metoprolol or propranolol) found that single 25 mg doses of rapid-release phenylpropanolamine (*Super Odrinex*) increased peak systolic/diastolic blood pressures by 8.0/4.9 mmHg on average over a 6 h period.[1] Another study found that *Dimetapp Extentabs* (75 mg phenylpropanolamine + 12 mg brompheniramine) given to five hypertensive patients on un-named beta-blockers caused systolic/diastolic blood pressure rises of 1.7/0.9 mmHg over a 4 h period.[2] These rises in blood pressure are small and relatively short-lived, and probably of little Clinical importance, but they may possibly mislead the interpretation of blood pressure measurements. See also 'Methyldopa + Sympathomimetics (indirectly-acting)'

References

1 O'Connell MB, Gross CR. The effect of single-dose phenylpropanolamine on blood pressure in patients with hypertension controlled by beta blockers. Pharmacotherapy (1990) 10, 85–91.

2 Petrulis AS, Imperiale TF, Speroff T. The acute effect of phenylpropanolamine and brompheniramine on blood pressure in controlled hypertension. J Gen Intern Med (1991) 6, 503–6.

Beta-blockers + Thallium scans

Abstract/Summary

Beta-blockers may falsify the results of stress thallium scans used for the diagnosis of coronary heart disease.

Clinical evidence, mechanism, importance and management

A comparative study in patients, given 201-thallous chloride during exercise for the diagnosis of coronary heart disease, showed that there was a marked reduction in the sensitivity to stress thallium scans in those on beta-blockers when compared with other patients not taking beta-blockers. The suggestion was made that consideration should be given to discontinuing beta-blockers before evaluating these patients.[1] Strictly speaking this is not an interaction in the usual sense of the word.

Reference

1 Henkin RE, Chang W, Provus R. The effect of beta-blockers on thallium scans. J Nucl Med (1982) 23, P35.

Beta-blockers + Tobacco smoking and/or Coffee and Tea drinking

Abstract/Summary

The beta-blockers reduce the heart rate and the blood pressure. These therapeutically useful effects are exploited in the treatment of angina and hypertension but are reduced to some extent if patients smoke. Drinking tea or coffee may have the same but smaller effect. Some increase in the dosage of the beta-blocker may be necessary.

Clinical evidence

(a) Beta-blockers + Tobacco smoking

A double blind study in 10 smokers with angina pectoris, taking daily doses of either 240 mg propranolol, 100 mg atenolol or a placebo, found that smoking reduced their plasma propranolol levels by 25%. Plasma atenolol levels were not significantly altered. Both of the beta-blockers reduced heart rates at rest and when exercised, but the reductions were less when they smoked (rises of 8–14%).[1]

Other studies found that serum propranolol levels were 200% higher in non-smokers[2] and that smoking reduced propranolol levels.[2,3] In addition to these pharmacokinetic effects, smoking can abolish the beneficial effects of propanolol on ST segment depression in patients with angina.[6]

(b) Beta-blockers + Caffeine

Two 150 mg cups of coffee (made from 24 g coffee) increased the blood pressures of 12 normal subjects while taking 240 mg propranolol, 300 mg metoprolol or a placebo. Systolic/diastolic blood pressure rises were + 7%/ + 22% (propranolol), + 7%/ + 19% (metoprolol) and + 4%/ + 16% mmHg (placebo). The beta-blockers and placebo were given in divided doses over 15 hours before the test.[4]

(c) Beta-blockers + Tobacco smoking + Caffeine

Eight patients with mild hypertension taking daily doses of 160 mg propranolol, 160 mg oxprenolol or 100 mg atenolol over a 6 week period were additionally tested with two tipped cigarettes and coffee (200 mg caffeine). Their mean systolic/diastolic blood pressure rises over the following 2 h were 8.5/8/0 mmHg (propranolol), 12.1/9.1 mmHg (oxprenolol) and 5.2/4.4 mmHg (atenolol).[5]

Mechanism

Smoking on its own increases the heart rate, the blood presure and the severity of myocardial ischaemia (oxygen starvation of the heart muscle).[6] These actions oppose and may even totally abolish the beneficial actions of the beta-blockers. In addition, smoking stimulates the liver enzymes concerned with the metabolism of some beta-blockers (eg propranolol, metoprolol) so that their serum levels and their effects are reduced. Smoking also reduces the oxygen-carrying capacity of the blood which may also be significant in those with angina. Caffeine on its own causes the release into the blood of catecholamines, such as adrenaline, which could account for the increases in heart rate and blood pressure which are seen.[5] The blood pressure rise may be exaggerated in the presence of beta-blockers which block vasodilatation, leaving the alpha (vasoconstrictor) effects of adrenaline unopposed. This too opposes the actions of the beta-blockers.

Importance and management

These interactions are established. Smoking tobacco and (to a very much lesser extent) drinking tea or coffee oppose the effects of the beta-blockers in the treatment of angina or hypertension. Patients should be encouraged to stop smoking because, quite apart from its other toxic effects, it aggravates myocardial ischaemia, increases heart rates and can change satisfactorily controlled blood pressures into those which are not. If this encouragement is unsuccessful it may be necessary to raise the dosages of the beta-blockers. The effects of atenolol (a selective beta-1 blocker) are opposed less than those of propranolol,[5] and it seems possible that this will also be true for other beta-blockers which are largely cleared unchanged in the urine (eg nadolol, pindolol etc). The effects of the caffeine in tea, coffee, *Coca-Cola*, etc. are quite small and there seems to be no strong reason to forbid them, but the excessive consumption of large amounts may not be a good idea, particularly in those who also smoke.

References

1 Fox K, Deansfield J, Krikler S, Ribeiro P, Wright C. The interaction of cigarette smoking and beta-adrenoceptor blockade. Br J Clin Pharmac (1984) 17, 92–93S.

2 Vestal RE, Wood AJJ, Branch RA, Shand DG, Wilkinson GR. Effects of age and cigarette smoking on propranolol disposition. Clin Pharmacol Ther (1979) 26, 8–15.

3 Gardner MJ, Cady WJ, Ong YS. Effect of smoking on the elimination of propranolol hydrochloride. Int J Clin Pharmacol Ther Toxicol (1980) 18, 421–4.

4 Smits P, Hoffmann H, Thien T, Houben H, van't Laar A. Hemodynamic and humoral effects of coffee after beta-selective and nonselective beta-blockade. Clin Pharmacol Ther (1983) 34, 153–8.

5 Freestone S, Ramsey LE. Effect of beta-blockade on the pressor response to coffee plus smoking in patients with mild hypertension. Drugs (1983) 25 (Suppl 2), 141–5.

6 Fox KM, Jonathan A, Williams H, Selwyn A. Interaction between cigarettes and propranolol in the treatment of angina pectoris. Br Med J (1980) 3, 191–3.

Beta-blockers + Verapamil

Abstract/Summary

Although beta-blockers and verapamil have been used together very successfully and uneventfully, serious cardiodepression (bradycardia, asystole, sinus arrest) sometimes occurs and it has been suggested that the combination should only be given to those who can initially be closely supervised. An adverse interaction can occur even with beta-blockers given as eye drops (e.g. timolol).

Clinical evidence

(a) Adverse interactions

Forty out of 50 patients on 100 mg atenolol and 360 mg verapamil daily experienced a reduction in anginal episodes over a mean period of 10 months while taking both drugs. 16 needed a reduced dosage or withdrawal. Three had bradyarrhythmias (drugs withdrawn) and seven experienced dyspnoea (four withdrawals and three dosage reductions) presumed to be secondary to left ventricular failure. Other complications were tiredness (two patients), postural hypotension (one patient) and dizziness (one patient), all of which were dealt with by reducing the dosage.[15]

In another study[16] on 15 patients given atenolol and verapamil, four experienced profound lethargy, one had left ventricular failure and four had bradyarrhythmias. Other reports describe cardiac failure, sinus arrest,[6,20] ventricular asystole,[1,16] heart block,[12] hypotension,[13,19] and bradycardia[11,13,16,19,24] in patients on atenolol,[6,20,24] practolol,[1,2] metoprolol,[8,11,13] propranolol[3,5,7,9,10,19,21,24] or pindolol[8] and verapamil. In two cases the patients were using timolol in the form of eye drops.[16-18]

(b) Pharmacokinetic interactions

When verapamil was added to metoprolol, its AUC (area under the curve) in 10 patients was increased by 33% and the peak serum levels were raised 41%.[13] Pulse rates and blood pressures were also less than with metoprolol alone. The pharmacokinetics of atenolol were not altered by verapamil in a study on a single patient,[14] nor were the mean values changed in another in 10 patients although individual patients showed AUC increases of more than 100%.[22] Verapamil was found in another study to reduce the clearance of propanolol by 26–32%.[23]

Mechanism

Both drugs have negative inotropic (cardiac depressant) effects on the heart which can be additive (see the mechanism of interaction suggested for Beta-blockers + Nifedipine). Given together they can cause marked bradycardia and may even depress the contraction of the ventricle completely. Verapamil can also raise the serum levels of the beta-blockers which are extensively metabolized in the liver by inhibiting their metabolism (e.g. metoprolol, propranolol).

Importance and management

Well-documented and well-established interactions. Although concurrent use can be uneventful and successful, the reports cited here amply demonstrate that it may not always be safe, the difficulty being to identify the patients most at risk. The makers list the following among their contraindications and warnings with verapamil alone: hypotension associated with cardiogenic shock, marked bradycardia, uncompensated heart failure, second or third degree atrioventricular block and sick sinus syndrome.[4] These and high doses of either drug are likely predisposing factors. The BNF says that oral concurrent use should only be contemplated if myocardial function is well preserved. There is also a note saying that verapamil should not be injected in patients recently given beta-blockers because of the risks. If the verapamil injection is given first, wait 30 min before giving a beta-blocker, but the safety of this too is open to doubt.[25]

It has been advised that the initiation of treatment should be restricted to hospital practice where the dose of each drug can be carefully titrated and the patient closely supervised, particularly during the first few days when adverse effects are most likely to develop.[15,16,24] If adverse haemodynamic effects occur, the drug dosage should be reduced or withdrawn.[11] One method is to give 50 mg atenolol and 240 mg verapamil daily. If after two weeks no adverse effects develop and the symptoms persist, the verapamil dosage is raised to 360 mg.[15] Beta-blockers which are extensively metabolized (eg metoprolol, propranolol) may possibly carry some additional risk because the verapamil raises the serum levels.[14]

References

1 Boothby CB, Garrard CS, Pickering D. Verapamil in cardiac arrhythmias. Br Med J (1972) 2, 349.

2 Seabia-Gomes R, Richards A, Sutton R. Hemodynamic effects of verapamil and practolol. Eur J Cardiol (1976) 4, 79.

3 Livesley B, Catley PF, Campbell RC, Oram S. Double-blind evaluation of verapamil, propranolol, and isosorbide dinitrate against a placebo in the treatment of angina pectoris. Br Med J (1973) 1, 375.

4 ABPI Data Sheet Compendium. Datapharm Publications Ltd (1985) p1.

5 Ljungstrom A, Aberg H. Interaktion mellan betareceptorblockerare och verapamil. Lalartidingen (1973) 70, 3548.

6 McQueen EG. New Zealand Committee on Adverse Reactions: 14th Annual Report 1979. NZ Med J (1980) 91, 226.

7 McAllister RG, Todd GD, Slack JD, Shearer ME, Hobbs PJ. Hemodynamic and pharmacokinetic aspects of the interaction between propranolol and verapamil. Clin Res (1981) 29, 755A.

8 Wayne VS, Harper RW, Laufer E, Federman J, Anderson ST, Pitt A. Adverse interaction between beta-adrenergic blocking drugs and verapamil--report of 3 cases. Aust NZ J Med (1982) 12, 285–9.

9 Balasubramian V, Bowles M, Davies AB, Raferty EB. Combined treatment with verapamil and propranolol in chronic stable angina. Br Heart J (1981) 45, 349–50.

10 Leon MB, Rosing DR, Bonow RO, Epsteind SE. Clinical efficacy of verapamil alone and combined with propranolol in treating patients with chronic stable angina pectoris. Circulation (1980) 62, (Suppl III) 87.

11 Eisenberg JNH, Oakley GDG. Probable adverse interaction between oral metoprolol and verapamil. Postgrad Med J (1984) 60, 705–6.

12 Hutchison SJ, Lorimer AR, Lakhdar A, McAlpine SG. Beta-blockers and verapamil: a cautionary tale. Br Med J (1984) 289, 659–60.

13 Keech AC, Harper RW, Harrison PM, Pitt A, McLean AJ. Pharmacokinetic interaction between oral metoprolol and verapamil for angina pectoris. Am J Cardiol (1986) 58, 551–2.

14 McLean AJ, Knight R, Harrison PM, Harper RW. Clearance-based oral drug interaction between verapamil and metoprolol and comparison with atenolol. Am J Cardiol (1985) 55, (13 part 1), 1628–9.

15 McCourty JC, Silas JH. Beta-blockers and verapamil: a cautionary tale. Br Med J (1984) 289, 1624.

16 Findlay I, McInnes GT, Dargie HJ. Beta-blockers and verapamil: a cautionary tale. Br Med J (1984) 289, 1074.

17 Sinclair NI, Benzie JL. Timolol eye drops and verapamil – a dangerous combination. Med J Aust (1983) 1, 548.

18 Pringle SD, MacEwen CJ. Severe bradycardia due to interaction of timolol eye drops and verapamil. Br Med J (1987) 294, 155–6.

19 Zatuchini J. Bradycardia and hypotension after propranolol HCl and verapamil. Heart and Lung (1985) 14, 94–5.

20 Misra M, Thakur R, Bhandari K. Sinus arrest caused by atenolol-verapamil combination. Clin Cardiol (1987) 10, 365–7.

21 Ruboldt Z, Bakovic Z, Bagatin J. Opasna kardiodepresivna interakcija izmedu verapamila i propranolola. Lijnecniki Vjesnki (1979) 101, 430–2.

22 Keech AC, Harper RW, Harrison PM, Pitt A, McLean AJ. Extent and pharmacokinetic mechanisms of oral atenolol-verapamil interaction in man. Eur J Clin Pharmacol (1988) 35, 363–6.

23 Hung BA, Bottorff MB, Herring VL, Self TH, Lalonde RL. Effects of calcium channel blockers on the pharmacokinetics of propranolol stereo-isomers. Clin Pharmacol Ther (1990) 47, 584–91.

24 McCourty JC, Silas JH, Tucker GT, Lennard MS. The effect of combined therapy on the pharmacokinetics and pharmacodynamics of verapamil and propranolol in patients with angina pectoris. Br J Clin Pharmac (1988) 25, 349–57.

25 Prasad AB (ed.) British National Formulary (1992) 24, 70.

Beta-blockers + X-Ray contrast media

Abstract/Summary

Severe hypotension has been seen in two patients taking beta-blockers when given sodium meglumine diatrizoate as a contrast agent.

Clinical evidence, mechanism, importance and management

Two patients, one taking nadolol and the other propranolol, developed severe hypotensive reactions when given sodium meglumine diatrizoate as a contrast agent for X-ray urography. Both patients developed slowly progressive erythema on the face and arms followed by tachycardia and a weak pulse. Each was treated with subcutaneous adrenaline and hydrocortisone, and placed in the Trendelenburg position. It is suggested that the reaction was due to the release of histamine by the contrast medium, the ability of the body to cope with the hypotension being compromised by the beta-blockade.[1]

Reference

1 Hamilton G. Severe adverse reactions to urography in patients taking beta-adrenergic blocking agents. Can Med Ass J(1985) 133, 122.

Chapter 11
Calcium Channel Blocker Drug Interactions

This chapter is concerned with those interactions where the activity of the calcium channel blockers (sometimes called calcium antagonists) is changed by the presence of another drug. The table below lists all the calcium channel blockers whose interactions are described in this book, but not all are necessarily dealt with in this chapter because, where the calcium channel blocker is the affecting agent, the relevant synopsis is categorized under the heading of the drug affected. The index should be consulted for a full listing.

The calcium channel blockers have an increasingly wide application and are used for paroxysmal supraventricular tachycardia and angina, arrhythmias, hypertension, congestive heart failure, pulmonary disorders, gastrointestinal disorders and migraine headaches.

Table 11.1 Calcium channel blockers

Non-proprietary names	Proprietary names
Amlodipine	
Bepridil	*Bepadil, Cordium, Cruor, Vascor*
Darodipine	
Diltiazem	*Cardizem*
Felodipine	
Gallopamil	*Procorum*
Isradipine	
Lacidipine	
Nicardipine	*Angioflebil, Cardene, Dagan, Flusemide, Lecibral, Lincil, Loxen, Nerdipina, Nicardal, Nicodel, Perdipina, Perdipine, Ranvil, Vasodin, Vasonase, Vastrasin*
Nifedipine	*Adalat(e), Anifed, Aprical, Citilat, Coral, Cordicant, Cordilan, Corotrend, Dilcor, Duranifin, Fedipina, Hinoxon, Nifecor, Nifedicor, Nifedin, Nifedipat, Nifelat, Nifeniastron, Nife-Puren, Nifical, Pidilat, Procardia, Tibricol*
Nimodipine	
Nisoldipine	
Nitrendipine	*Bayotensin, Baypress*
Prenylamine	*Angormin, Angoran, Bismetin, Carditin-same, Crespasin, Daxauten, Epocol, Eucardion, Herzcon, Hostagina, Incoran, Lactamine, Nyuple, Onlemin,Piboril, Reocorin, Sedolatan, Segontin(e), Synadrin, Wasangor*
Tiapamil	
Verapamil	*Azupamil, Berkatens, Calan, Cardiagutt, Cardibeletin, Cardimil, Cavartil, Coridilox, Durasoptin, Geangin, Hexasoptin, Isoptin(e/o), Manidon, Praecicor, Securon, Univer, Vasolan, Verakard, Veraloc, Veramex, Veramil, Veroptinstada.*

Calcium channel blockers + Aspirin

Abstract/Summary

The antiplatelet effects of the calcium channel blockers may be increased by the concurrent use of aspirin. Abnormal bruising has been seen.

Clinical evidence, mechanism, importance and management

It is recognized that calcium channel blockers such as vera-pamil, nifedipine and diltiazem can inhibit platelet aggregation because they interfere with the movement of calcium ions through cell membranes. These effects may be additive with those of other antiplatelet drugs. One report describes abnormal bruising and prolonged bleeding times in a patient taking 240 mg verapamil daily while taking two 325 mg aspirin tablets several times a week for headaches. The bruising ceased when the aspirin was stopped.[1] A healthy volunteer taking the same dose of verapamil observed the appearance of new petechiae when also taking aspirin.[1] Concurrent use need not be avoided unless the outcome is clearly adverse.

Reference

1 Ring ME, Martin GV, Fenster PE. Clinically significant antiplatelet effects of calcium-channel blockers. J Clin Pharmacol (1986) 26, 719–20.

Calcium channel blockers + Bupivacaine

Abstract/Summary

On theoretical grounds the potentially serious cardiac depressant effects of IV bupivacaine may be enhanced in patients taking calcium channel blockers.

Clinical evidence, mechanism, importance and management

A number of factors (e.g. hypoxia, hyperkalaemia, acidosis, pregnancy and age)[1] can enhance the myocardial depression of IV bupivacaine, and studies in dogs have now confirmed the suspicion that calcium channel blockers such as nifedipine[1] and verapamil[2] can do the same. Elderly patients with impaired cardiovascular function on calcium channel blockers would therefore appear to be at considerable risk if bupivacaine is accidentally given intravenously during regional anaesthesia.

References

1 Howie MB, Mortimer W, Candler EM, McSweeney TD, Frolicher DA. Does nifedipine enhance the cardiovascular depressive effects of bupivacaine ? Regional Anesth (1989) 14, 19–25.

2 Liu P, Feldman HS, Covino BM. Acute cardiovascular toxicity of intravenous amide local anesthetics in anesthetized dogs. Anesth Analg (1982) 61,134–8.

Calcium channel blockers + Calcium channel blockers

Abstract/Summary

Blood levels of nifedipine are increased by diltiazem and blood pressure is reduced accordingly. This is claimed to be an advantageous interaction.

Clinical evidence

Pretreatment of six normal subjects with 30 mg or 90 mg of diltiazem three times daily for three days was found to increase the AUC (area under the concentration-time curve) of single 20 mg doses of nifedipine two- and threefold respectively. With the placebo the AUC was 637 ng.h.ml^{-1}; with 30 mg diltiazem 1365 ng.h.ml^{-1} and with 90 mg diltiazem 2005 ng.h.ml^{-1}.[1,3] Similar results are reported elsewhere.[2] An isolated report attributes complete or partial intestinal occlusion in a patient on diltiazem when nifedipine was added on three occasions.[3]

Mechanism

A reduction in the metabolism of the nifedipine by the diltiazem is suggested.[1] Additive relaxant effects on smooth muscle is suggested for the case of intestinal occulsion.[4]

Importance and management

Information is very limited but the authors of these reports suggest that the effects of concurrent use are usually beneficial rather than adverse, and that the dosage of the nifedipine can be reduced. Fewer side-effects and better compliance are predicted.[3]

References

1 Tateishi T, Ohashi K, Toyosaki N, Hosada S, Sugimoto K, Kumagai Y, Kotegawa T, Ebihara A, Toyo-oka T. The effect of diltiazem on plasma nifedipine concentration in human volunteers. Jap Circ J (1987) 51, 921.

2 Ohashi K, Tateishi T, Sudo T, Sakamoto K, Toyosaki N, Hosoda S, Toyo-oka T, Sugimoto K, Kumagai Y, Ebihara A. Effects of diltiazem on the pharmacokinetics of nifedipine. J Cardiovasc Pharmacol (1990) 15, 96–101.

3 Tateishi T, Ohashi K, Sudo T, Sakamoto K, Toyosaki N, Hosada S, Toyo-oka T, Kumagai Y, Sugimoto K, Fujimura A, Ebihara A. Dose dependent effect of diltiazem on the pharmacokinetics of nifedipine. J Clin Pharmacol (1989) 29, 994–7.

4 Lamaison D, Abrieu V, Fialip J, Dumas R, Andronikoff M, Lavarenne J. Occlusion intestinale aiguë et antagonistes calciques. Therapie (1989) 44, 201–2

Calcium channel blockers + Calcium salts

Abstract/Summary

The concurrent use of verapamil and intravenous calcium salts can be therapeutically useful, but an isolated report describes antagonism of the antiarrhythmic effects of verapamil due to the use of calcium adipate and calciferol.

Clinical evidence, mechanism, importance and management

Verapamil alone is effective in treating atrial fibrillation and supraventricular arrhythmias, and if preceded by an intravenous infusion of calcium gluconate or chloride, its hypotensive and possible negative inotropic effects are reduced or prevented without compromising its antiarrhythmic effects.[1-5] Concurrent use is therefore normally valuable but an isolated report describes an adverse response:

An elderly woman, successfully treated for over a year with verapamil, re-developed atrial fibrillation within a week of starting to take 1.2 g calcium adipate and 3000 IU calciferol daily for diffuse osteoporosis. Her serum calcium levels had risen from 2.45 to 2.7 mmol/l. Normal sinus rhythm was restored by giving 500 ml saline and repeated doses of 20 mg frusemide and 5 mg verapamil by injection.[6] Verapamil acts by inhibiting the passage of calcium ions into cardiac muscle cells and it would appear that in this case the increased concentration of calcium ions outside the cells opposed the effects of the verapamil.

The general importance of this isolated case is uncertain, but it would clearly be prudent to monitor concurrent use for any signs of reduced verapamil effects.

References

1 Roguin N, Shapir Y, Blazer S, Zeltzer M, Berant M. The use of calcium gluconate prior to verapamil in infants with paroxysmal supraventricular tachycardia. Clin Cardiol (1984) 7, 613–6.
2 Salerno DM, Anderson B, Sharkey PJ, Iber C. Intravenous verapamil for treatment of multifocal atrial tachcardia with and without calcium pretreatment. Ann Intern Med (1987) 107, 623–8.
3 Haft JI, Habbab MA. Treatment of atrial arrhythmias. Effectiveness of verapamil when preceded by calcium infusion. Arch Intern Med (1986) 146, 1085–9.
4 Schoen MD, Parker RB, Hoon TJ, Hariman RJ, Bauman JL, Beckman KJ. Evaluation of the pharmacokinetics and electrocardiographic effects of intravenous verapamil with intravenous calcium chloride pretreatment in normal subjects. Amer J Cardiol (1991) 67, 300–4.
5 Weiss AT, Lewis BS, Halon DA, Hasin Y, Gotsman MS. The use of calcium with verapamil in the management of supraventricular tachyarrhythmias. Int J Cardiol (1983) 4, 275–84.
6 Bar-Or D, Yoel G. Calcium and calciferol antagonize effect of verapamil in atrial fibrillation. Brit Med J (1981) 282, 1585.

Calcium channel blockers + Clonidine, Indomethacin, Spironolactone

Abstract/Summary

Indomethacin appears not to reduce the hypotensive effects of nicardipine or felodipine, whereas clonidine has a small additive hypotensive effect. The situation with nifedipine and indomethacin is uncertain. Spironolactone does not interact adversely with felodipine.

Clinical evidence, mechanism, importance and management

A study in a total of 21 patients with mild to moderate essential hypertension, given 20 mg nifedipine twice daily, showed that 100 mg indomethacin daily for a week did not significantly change the hypotensive effects of the nifedipine,[1] whereas 250 g clonidine daily for a week increased the hypotensive effects by about 5 mmHg (mean blood pressure).[1] In contrast, another study in eight hypertensive patients treated with 15–40 mg nifedipine daily found that 100 mg indomethacin daily raised the mean arterial pressure of five of them by 17–20 mm Hg.[5] Two other studies in normal subjects found that indomethacin does not affect the blood pressure lowering effects of felodipine[2] or nicardipine.[3] 50 mg spironolactone was found not to affect the pharmacokinetics or felodipine or its clinical effects.[4]

No special precautions seem to be necessary if any of these drugs is given with the calcium channel blockers cited, the exception being nifedipine and indomethacin. Their concurrent use should be monitored for any evidence of a reduced hypotensive response.

References

1 Slavetti A, Pedrinelli R, Magagna A, Stornello M, Scapellato L. Calcium antagonists: interactions in hypertension. Am J Nephrol (1986) 6 (Suppl 1) 95–99.
2 Hardy BG, Bartle WR, Myers M, Bailey DG, Edgar B. Effect of indomethacin on the pharmacokinetics and pharmacodynamics of felodipine. Br J Clin Pharmac (1988) 26, 557–62.
3 Debbas NPG, Raoof NT, Al Gassab HK, Jackson SHD, Turner P. Does indomethacin antagonize the effects of nicardipine? Acta Pharmacol Toxicol (1986) 59, Suppl V, 181.
4 Janzon K, Edgar B. Lundborg P, Regardh CG. The influence of cimetidine and spironolactone on the pharmacokinetics and haemodynamic effects of felodipine in healthy subjects. Acta Pharmacol Toxicol (1986) 59, Suppl 4, 98.
5 Thatte UM, Shah SJ, Salvi SS, Suraokar S, Temulkar P, Anklesaria P, Kshirsager NA. Acute drug interaction between indomethacin and nifedipine in hypertensive patients. J Ass Phys India (1988) 36, 695–8.

Calcium channel blockers + Co-trimoxazole

Abstract/Summary

Co-trimoxazole normally appears not to interact with nifedipine, but adverse effects (leg cramps, facial flushing) have been reported in one patient.

Clinical evidence, mechanism, importance and management

The observation of a patient on nifedipine who developed leg cramps and facial flushing (evidence of raised serum nifedipine levels) when treated with co-trimoxazole, prompted further study of this possible interaction in 9 normal subjects. After taking 960 mg co-trimoxazole twice daily for 3 days the pharmacokinetics of single 20 mg doses of nifedipine and blood pressures in these subjects were found to be unchanged.[1] No special precautions would therefore normally seem to be necessary but monitor the outcome of concurrent use.

Reference

1 Edwards C, Monkman S, Cholerton S, Rawlins MD, Idle JR, Ferner RE. Lack of effect of co-trimoxazole on the pharmacokinetics and pharmacodynamics of nifedipine. Br J Clin Pharmac (1990) 30, 889–91.

Calcium channel blockers + Dantrolene

Abstract/Summary

An isolated report describes acute hyperkalaemia and cardiovascular collapse when dantrolene was given in the presence of verapamil, but not nifedipine.

Clinical evidence, mechanism, importance and management

A 90-year-old man with coronary artery disease taking 80 mg verapamil three times daily, with a history of malignant hyperthermia and undergoing surgery, showed marked myocardial depression and hyperkalaemia (7.1 mmol/l) within 2 h of being given dantrolene intravenously.[1] Six months later similar preoperative and intraoperative procedures were undertaken uneventfully when the verapamil was replaced by nifedipine. Hyperkalaemia and cardiovascular collapse have been seen in pigs and dogs given dantrolene and verapamil or diltiazem, but not with nifedipine.[2–6]

These observations would seem to link with a report of three patients taking verapamil who developed hypotension and sinus bradycardia, all of whom were noted to be hyperkalaemic. In two cases their severe left ventricular dysfunction reversed when they were given intravenous calcium.[6] Studies in dogs confirmed that hyperkalaemia reduced myocardial contractility in the presence of verapamil, and this was reversed by calcium.[6]

The overall picture is that hyperkalaemia can apparently increase the myocardial depression caused by verapamil, and it seems possible that drugs other than dantrolene which can raise blood potassium levels may be among the factors which may predispose patients to severe left ventricular dysfunction. More study is needed.

References

1 Rubin AS, Zablocki AD. Hyperkalaemia, verapamil and dantrolene. Anesthesiology (1987) 66, 246–9.
2 Lynch C, Durbin CG, Fisher NA, Veselis RA, Althaus JS. Effects of dantrolene and verapamil on atrioventricular conduction and cardiovascular performance in dogs. Anesth Analg (1986) 65, 252–8.
3 San Juan AC, Port JD, Wong KC. Hyperkalaemia after dantrolene administration in dogs. Anesth Analg (1986) 65, S131.
4 Saltzman LS, Kates RA, Corke BC, Norfleet EA, Heath KR. Hyperkalaemia and cardiovascular collapse after verapamil and dantrolene administration in swine. Anesth Analg (1984) 63, 473–8.
5 Saltzman LS, Kates RA, Norfleet EA, Corke BC, Heath KR. Hemodynamic interactions of diltiazem-dantrolene and nifedipine and nifedipine-dantrolene. Anaesthesiology (1984) 61, A11.
6 Jolly SR, Keaton N, Movahed A, Rose GC, Reeves WC. Effect of hyperkalaemia on experimental myocardial depression by verapamil. Am Heart J (1991) 121, 517–23.

Calcium channel blockers + Diclofenac or Naproxen

Abstract/Summary

Diclofenac reduces serum verapamil levels, but naproxen appears not to interact.

Clinical evidence, mechanism, importance and management

A study in 25 hypertensive subjects taking 240 mg slow-release verapamil daily found that the concurrent use of 75 mg diclofenac twice daily reduced the AUC (area under the concentration-time curve) by 26% (from 3207 to 2389 ng/ml h), whereas 375 mg naproxen twice daily had no effect.[1] The reasons are not understood. Whether this interaction with diclofenac has a clinically important effect on treatment with verapamil appears not to have been assessed, but be alert for any signs of a reduced response to verapamil.

Reference

1 Peterson C, Basch C, Cohen A. Differential effects of naproxen and diclofenac on verapamil pharmacokinetics. Clin Pharmacol Ther (1990) 49, 129.

Calcium channel blockers + Erythromycin

Abstract/Summary

An isolated report describes increased felodipine effects and toxicity in a patient when erythromycin was added.

Clinical evidence, mechanism, importance and management

A hypertensive woman on 10 mg felodipine daily developed tachycardia, flushing and massive ankle oedema within 2–3 days of starting to take 250 mg erythromycin twice daily. Her blood pressure had fallen from 120/90 to 110/70 mmHg. She fully recovered within a few days stopping the erythromycin. The suggested explanation is that the metabolism of the felodipine was inhibited by the erythromycin resulting in a marked increase in its effects.[1] The general importance of this interaction is not known, but it would now seem prudent to monitor the effect is erythromycin is added to felodipine in any patient. There seem to be no reports of interactions between any of the other calcium channel blockers and macrolide antibiotics.

Reference

1 Liedholm H, Nordin G. Erythromycin-felodipine interaction. DICP Ann Pharmacotherapy (1991) 25, 1007–8.

Calcium channel blockers + Fluoxetine

Abstract/Summary

Two patients on verapamil and one on nifedipine developed what seem to be increased side-effects (oedema, headaches, nausea, flushing) attributable to the concurrent use of fluoxetine.

Clinical evidence, mechanism, importance and management

A woman on 240 mg verapamil daily developed oedema of the feet and ankles and neck vein distention within six weeks of starting 20 mg fluoxetine daily. The oedema resolved within 2–3 weeks of reducing the verapamil dosage to 120 mg daily.[1] Another patient taking 240 mg verapamil daily for the prophylaxis of migraine developed morning headaches (believed by the patient not to be migraine) within a week of increasing his fluoxetine dosage from 20 to 40 mg daily. The headaches stopped when the verapamil dosage was reduced and then stopped. Yet another patient on 60 mg nifedipine daily developed nausea and flushing following the addition of 20 mg fluoxetine every other day. The adverse effects gradually disappeared over the next 2–3 weeks when the fluoxetine dosage was halved.

The development of these common calcium channel blocker side-effects (oedema, headaches, nausea, flushing) appeared to be related to the use of fluoxetine. The author of the report suggests that the fluoxetine may have reduced the metabolism of the calcium channel blockers by the liver, thereby increasing their effects. Although information is as yet very limited, it would seem reasonable to monitor concurrent use, being alert for the need to reduce the drug dosages. More study is needed.

Reference

1 Sternbach H. Fluoxetine-associated potentiation of calcium-channel blockers. J Clin Psychopharmacol (1991) 11, 390.

Calcium channel blockers + Food

Abstract/Summary

Food appears not to have an important effect on the absorption of bepridil, nifedipine nor verapamil in a sustained-release formulation. Grapefruit juice very markedly increases the bioavailability of felodipine, nifedipine and nitrendipine, but only the side-effects of felodipine appear to be increased.

Clinical evidence, mechanism, importance and management

(a) Food

The absorption of two 200 mg capsules of bepridil in 15 normal subjects was delayed by food (peak serum times prolonged from 2.6 to 3.8 h) but the amount absorbed was unchanged.[1] It seems likely that steady-state levels will be unaffected by food. Some single dose studies suggested that food might delay the absorption of nifedipine and reduce its peak levels,[2–4] but a multiple dose study found that food does not have an important effect on the steady-state levels.[5] No significant effects on the absorption of verapamil from a multiparticulate sustained release preparation were seen when given with food.[8]

(b) Fruit juices

A study in six men with borderline hypertension found that the mean bioavailability of a 5 mg dose of felodipine was almost three-fold greater when taken with 250 ml double strength grape fruit juice ('*Old South*') than when taken with either water or orange juice. The AUC was increased by 284% (range 164–469%). The pharmacological effects were also increased. Diastolic blood pressures fell by 20% (compared with 11% with water) and the heart rates rose by 22% (compared with 9% with water) when the blood concentrations of felodipine were at their highest. Side effects such as headaches, facial flushing and lightheadedness were also increased.[6] This confirmed the results of a previous study.[11] Another study found that 200 ml single-strength grapefruit juice also tripled the bioavailability of felodipine.[7,12] In a related study in six normal men, the mean bioavailabity of 10 mg nifedipine was increased 134% (range 108–169%) by grapefruit juice,[6] and a further study found that the bioavailability of 20 mg nitrendipine was increased 106% by grapefruit juice,[9] but no adverse haemodynamic effects were seen. Suggested reasons for these increases in bioavailability are that the flavenoid[6] or sesquiterpenoid[10] components of the fruit juice inhibit the activity of cytochrome P450 in the liver so that the metabolism of these calcium channel blockers is reduced, thereby increasing their effects.

The clinical importance of these findings is uncertain, but it would be worth checking the diet of any patient who complains of increased side-effects with any of these drugs.

References

1 Easterling DE, Stellar SM, Nayak RK, Desiraju RK. The effect of food on the bioavailability of bepridil. J Clin Pharmacol (1984) 24, 416.
2 Ochs HR, Ramsch KD, Verburg-Ochs B, Greenblatt DJ, Gerloff J. Nifedipine: kinetics and dynamics after a single oral dose. Klin Wsch(1984) 62, 427–9.
3 Reitberg DP, Love SJ, Quercia GT, Zinny MA. Effect of food on nifedipine pharmacokinetics. Clin Pharmacol Ther (1987) 42, 72–5.
4 Challenor VF, Waller DG, Gruchy BS, Renwick AG, George CF. Food and nifedipine pharmacokinetics. Br J clin Pharmac (1987) 23, 248–9.
5 Rimoy GH, Idle JR, Bhaskar NK, Rubin PC. The influence of food on the pharmacokinetics of 'biphasic' nifedipine at steady state in normal subjects. Br J clin Pharmac (1989) 28, 612–5.
6 Bailey DG, Spence JD, Munoz C, Arnold JMO. Interaction of citrus juices with felodipine and nifedipine. Lancet (1990) 337, 268–9.
7 Edgar B, Bailey DG, Bergstrand R, Johnsson G, Lurje L. Formulation dependent interaction between felodipine and grapefruit juice. Clin Pharmacol Ther (1990) 47, 181.
8 Devane JG, Kelly JG. Effect of food on the bioavailability of a multiparticulate sustained-release verapamil formulation. Advances in Therapy (1991) 8, 48–53.
9 Soons PA, Vogels BAPM, Roosemalen MCM, Schoemaker HC, Uchida E, Edgar B, Lundahl J, Cohen AF, Breimer DD. Grapefruit juice and cimetidine inhibit stereoselective metabolism of nitrendipine in humans. Clin Pharmacol Ther (1991) 50, 394–403.
10 Chayen R, Rosenthal T. Interaction of citrus juices with felodipine and nifedipine. Lancet (1991) 337, 854.
11 Bailey DG, Spence JD, Edgar B, Bayliff CD, Arnold JMO. Ethanol enhances the hemodynamic effects of felodipine. Clin Invest Med (1989) 12, 357–62.
12 Edgar B, Bailey D, Bergstrand R, Johnsson G, Regårdh CG. Acute effects of drinking grapefruit juice on the pharmacokinetics and dynamics on felodipine — and its potential clinical relevance. Eur J Clin Pharmacol (1992) 42, 313–7.

Calcium channel blockers + H$_2$-blockers

Abstract/Summary

The serum levels of diltiazem and nifedipine are increased by cimetidine and it may possibly be necessary to reduce the dosages. Serum felodipine, nimodipine, nisoldipine and nitrendipine levels are also increased but this seems to be clinically unimportant. It is uncertain whether cimetidine interacts significantly with verapamil. Ranitidine appears to interact only minimally with calcium channel blockers but famotidine may possibly reduce heart activity undesirably.

Clinical evidence

(a) Diltiazem

1200 mg cimetidine daily for a week increased the AUC of a single 60 mg oral dose of diltiazem in six normal subjects by 50% (from 14637 to 22435 ng min/ml) and peak serum levels by 57% (from 46.4 to 73.1 ng/ml). 300 mg ranitidine daily for a week increased the AUC by 15% (statistically insignificant).[11] Serum diltiazem increases of 40% and AUC increases of 25–50% were seen in another study using cimetidine.[12]

(b) Felodipine

1 g cimetidine daily increased the AUC of 10 mg felodipine in 12 subjects by 56%, and raised the peak serum level by 54%. There was short lasting effect on their heart rates but the clinical effects were minimal.[28]

(c) Nifedipine

1 g cimetidine daily for a week increased the AUC of a single 40 mg oral doze of nifedipine by about 60% and increased maximum serum levels by about 80% (from 46.1 to 87.7 ng/ml). 300 mg ranitidine daily for a week caused a non-significant rise of about 25% in maximum nifedipine serum levels and AUC. Seven hypertensive patients showed a fall in mean blood pressure from 127 to 109 mmHg after taking 40 mg nifedipine daily for 4 weeks, and a further fall to 95 mmHg after additionally taking 1 g cimetidine daily for two weeks. When they took 300 mg ranitidine instead, there was a non-significant fall to 103 mmHg.[1,2,17]

Other studies clearly confirm that cimetidine causes a very significant rise in serum nifedipine levels and an increase in its effects, whereas ranitidine interacts only minimally.[3–6,19,20,23]

(d) Nifedipine, Nicardipine

A study found no pharmacokinetic interaction between nifedipine and famotidine, but the famotidine reversed the effects of nifedipine on systolic time intervals and significantly reduced the stroke volume and cardiac output.[18,22,25] No adverse interaction was seen in 24 patients given nifedipine, nicardipine or diltiazem with famotidine for 6–8 weeks.[27]

(e) Nimodipine, Nisoldipine, Nitrendipine

Seven days treatment with 1 g cimetidine daily increased the bioavailability of 30 mg nimodipine three times daily in eight subjects by 75%, but the haemodynamic effects were unchanged. Ranitidine did not interact.[29] A study in eight normal subjects showed that after taking 1200 mg cimetidine for a day the bioavailability of a single 10 mg dose of nisoldipine was increased by about 50%, but the haemodynamic effects of the nisoldipine were unaltered.[13] 200 mg cimetidine was found to increase the bioavailability of nitrenidipine by 154% but the haemodynamic effects were unchanged.[24] Another study showed that ranitidine increased the AUC of a single oral dose of nitrendipine by about 50% and decreased its clearance, but no changes in the haemodynamic measurements (systolic time intervals, impedance cardiography).[14] Two further studies, including one of the same authors confirmed that a pharmacokinetic interaction (AUC + 89%) occurs but it appears to be clinically unimportant.[26,30]

(f) Verapamil

A study in eight normal subjects showed that after taking 300 mg cimetidine six-hourly for eight days no changes occurred in the pharmacokinetics of a single 10 mg intravenous dose of verapamil, but the bioavailability of a 120 mg oral dose increased from 26 to 49%. A small insignificant change in clearance occurred but no change in AUC. The changes in the PR interval caused by the verapamil were unaltered in the presence of cimetidine.[10]

Another study found that 1200 mg cimetidine daily for five days reduced the clearance of verapamil by 21% and increased its elimination half-life by 50%.[7] 800 mg cimetidine daily for a week increased its bioavailability from 35 to 42% and its clearance fell from 45.9 to 33.2 ml/min/kg in another study.[21] Yet another found a small increase in the bioavailability of both enantiomers of verapamil.[8] In contrast, other studies found that the pharmacokinetics of verapamil were unaffected by cimetidine.[6,7,9]

Mechanism

It is believed that cimetidine increases nifedipine levels by inhibiting its oxidative metabolism by the liver. Like ranitidine it may also increase the bioavailability of nifedipine by lowering gastric acidity.[4] The mechanisms of the other interactions are probably similar.

Importance and management

The diltiazem-cimetidine and nifedipine-cimetidine interactions are established. Concurrent use need not be avoided but the increase in the calcium channel blocker effects should be taken into account. It has been suggested that the dosage of diltiazem should be reduced by 30–35%[15] and of nifedipine by 40%.[15,16] The evidence available suggests that although cimetidine increases the serum levels of felodipine, nimodipine, nisoldipine and nitrendipine, the haemodynamic changes are unimportant. This needs confirmation. The verapamil-cimetidine interaction is not well established, but monitor the effects until more is known.

Ranitidine does not to interact significantly with diltiazem, nimodipine or nifedipine and is possibly a non-interacting alternative for cimetidine with other calcium channel blockers.

Famotidine does not have a pharmacokinetic interaction with nifedipine, but its negative inotropic effects may possibly be undesirable in the elderly or those with heart failure.[18,22,25] and therefore some care may be needed.

References

1 Kirch W, Janisch HD, Heidemann H, Ramsch K, Ohnhaus EE. Einfluss von Cimetidin und Rantidin auf Pharmakokinetik und antihypertensiven Effekt von Nifedipin. Dtsch Med Wsch (1983) 108, 1757–61.
2 Kirch W, Ramsch K, Janisch HD, Ohnhaus EE. The influence of two histamine H₂-receptor antagonists, cimetidine and ranitidine, on the plasma levels and clinical effect of nifedipine and metoprolol. Arch Toxicol (1984) Suppl 7, 256–9.
3 Smith SR, Kendall MJ, Lobo J, Beerahee A, Jack DB, Wilkins MR. Ranitidine and cimetidine: drug interactions with single dose and steady-state nifedipine administration. Br J Clin Pharmac (1987) 23, 311–5.
4 Adams LJ, Antonow DR, McClain CJ, McAllister R. Effect of ranitidine on bioavailability of nifedipine. Gastroenterology (1986) 90, 1320.
5 Kirch W, Ohnhaus EE, Hoensch H, Janisch HD. Ranitidine increases bioavailability of nifedipine. Clin Pharmacol Ther (1985) 37, 204.
6 Abernethy DR, Schwartz JB, Todd EL. Lack of interaction between verapamil and cimetidine. Clin Pharmacol Ther (1985) 38, 342–9.
7 Loi C-M, Rollins DE, Dukes GE, Peat MA. Effect of cimetidine on verapamil disposition. Clin Pharmacol Ther (1985) 37, 654–7.
8 Mikus G, Kroemer HK, Klotz U, Eichelbaum M. Stereochemical considerations of the cimetidine-verapamil interaction. Clin Pharmacol Ther (1988) 43, 134.
9 Wing LMH, Miners JO, Lillywhite KJ. Verapamil disposition-effects of sulphinpyrazone and cimetidine. Br J Clin Pharmac (1985) 19, 385–91.
10 Smith MS, Benyunes MC, Bjornsson TD, Shand DG, Pritchett MD. Influence of cimetidine on verapamil kinetics and dynamics. Clin Pharmacol Ther (1984) 36, 551–4.
11 Winship LC, McKenney JM, Wright JT, Wood JH, Goodman RP. The effect of ranitidine and cimetidine on single-dose diltiazem pharmacokinetics. Pharmacotherapy (1985) 5, 16–9.
12 Mazhar M, Popat KD, Sanders C. Effect of cimetidine on diltiazem blood levels. Clin Res (1984) 32, 741A.
13 Van Harten J, van Brummelen P, Lodewijks M Th M, Danhof M, Breimer DD. Pharmacokinetics and hemodynamic effects of nisoldipine and its interaction with cimetidine. Clin Pharmacol Ther (1988) 43, 332–41.
14 Kirch W, Nahoui R, Ohnhaus EE. Ranitidine:nitrendipine interaction. Clin Pharmacol Ther (1988) 43, 149.
15 Piepho RW, Culbertson VL, Rhodes RS. Drug interactions with the calcium entry blockers. Circulation (1987) 75 (Suppl V) V-181–94.
16 Piepho RW. Individualization of calcium-entry blocker dosage for systemic hypertension. Am J Cardiol (1985) 56, 105H.
17 Kirch W, Hoensch H, Ohnhaus EE. Ranitidin-Nifedipin-Interaktion. Dtsch med Wsch (1984) 109, 1223.
18 Halabi A, Ohnhaus EE, Kirch W. Influence of famotidine on non-invasive haemodynamic parameters and nifedipine plasma levels. Eur J Clin Invest (1988) 18, A23.
19 Schwartz JB, Upton RA, Lin ET, Williams RL, Benet LZ. Effect of cimetidine or ranitidine administration on nifedipine pharmacokinetics and pharmacodynamics. Clin Pharmacol Ther (1988) 43, 673–80.
20 Renwick AG, Le Vie J, Challenor VF, Waller DG, Gruchy B, George CF. Factors affecting the pharmacokinetics of nifedipine. Eur J Clin Pharmacol (1987) 32, 351–55.
21 Mikus G, Stuber H. Influence of cimetidine treatment on the physiological disposition of verapamil. Naunyn-Schmied Arch Pharmacol (1987) 335, Suppl R106.
22 Kirch W, Halabi A, Linde M, Ohnhaus EE. Negativ-inotrope Wirkung von Famotidin. Schweiz med Wschr (1988) 118, 1912–4.
23 Khan A, Langley SJ, Mullins FPG, Dixon JS, Toon S. The pharmacokinetics and pharmacodynamics of nifedipine at steady state during concomitant administration of cimetidine or high dose ranitidine. Br J Clin Pharmac (1991) 32, 519–22.
24 Soons PA, Vogels BAPM, Roosemalen MCM, Schoemaker HC, Uchida E, Edgar B, Lundahl J, Cohen AF, Breimer DD. Grapefruit juice and cimetidine inhibit stereoselective metabolism of nitrendipine in humans. Clin Pharmacol Ther (1991) 50, 394–403.
25 Kirch W, Halabi A. Linde M, Santos SR, Ohnhaus EE. Negative effects of famotidine on cardiac performance assessed by noninvasive heodynamic measurements. Gastroenterology (1989) 96, 1386–92.
26 Halabi A, Nahoui R, Kirch W. Influence of ranitidine on kinetics of nitrendipine and on noninvasive hemodynamic parameters. Ther Drug Monit (1990) 12, 303–4.

27 Chichmanian RM, Mignot G, Spreux A, Jean-Girard C, Hofliger P. Tolérance de la famotidine. Étude due réseau médecins sentinelles en pharmacovigilance. Therapie (1992) 47, 239–43.
28 Janzon K, Edgar B, Lundborg P, Regårdh CG. The influence of cimetidine and spironolactone on the pharmacokinetics and haemodynamic effects of felodipine in healthy subjects. Acta Pharmacol Toxicol (1986) 59, Suppl 4, 98.
29 Mück W, Wingender W, Seiberling M, Woelke E, Rämsch K-D, Kuhlmann J. Influence of the H_2-receptors antagonists cimetidine and ranitidine on the pharmacokinetics of nimodipine in healthy volunteers. Eur J Clin Pharmacol (1992) 42, 325–8.
30 Santos SR, Storpirtis S, Moreira-Filho L, Donzella H, Kirch W. Ranitidine increases the bioavailability of nitrendipine in patients with arterial hypertension. Brazilian J Med Biol Res (1992) 25, 337–47.

Calcium channel blockers + Local anaesthetics

Abstract/Summary

Severe hypotension and bradycardia have been seen in patients taking verapamil after epidural anaesthesia with bupivacaine, but not with lignocaine (lidocaine).

Clinical evidence

Four patients on long-term verapamil treatment developed severe hypotension (systolic pressures as low as 60 mmHg) and bradycardia (48 bpm) after epidural block with bupivacaine (0.5% with adrenaline). This was totally resistant to atropine and ephedrine, and responded only to calcium gluconate or chloride. No such interaction was seen in a similar group of patients when epidural lignocaine was used.[1]

Animal experiments have shown that the presence of verapamil increases the toxicity of lignocaine, and increases toxicity of bupivacaine even more.[2]

Mechanism

Not understood.

Importance and management

Information seems to be limited to these studies involving verapamil. In the absence of more information it would be prudent to assume that other calcium channel blockers may possibly behave similarly. Lignocaine would appear to be preferable to bupivacaine for epidural blockade. Intravenous calcium effectively controls the hypotension and bradycardia produced by verapamil.[3]

References

1 Collier C. Verapamil and epidural bupivacaine. Anaesth Intens Care (1985) 13, 101.
2 Tallman RD, Rosenblatt RM, Weaver JM, Wang Y. Verapamil increases the toxicity of local anaesthetics. J Clin Pharmacol (1988) 28, 317–21.
3 Coaldrake LA. Verapamil overdose. Anaesth Intens Care (1984) 12, 174–5.

Calcium channel blockers + Magnesium salts

Abstract/Summary

A pregnant woman with premature uterine contractions developed muscle weakness and paralysis when given nifedipine and magnesium sulphate concurrently.

Clinical evidence, mechanism, importance and management

A pregnant woman at 32 weeks' gestation was effectively treated for premature uterine contractions with nifedipine, 60 mg orally over 3 h, and later 20 mg over 8 h. 12 h later when contractions began again she was given 500 mg magnesium sulphate intravenously. She developed jerky movements of the extremities, complained of difficulty in swallowing, paradoxical respirations and an inability to lift her head from the pillow. The magnesium was stopped and the muscle weakness disappeared over the next 25 min.[1] The reasons for this reaction are not fully understood. Magnesium ions have neuromuscular blocking activity on skeletal muscle, and both agents can affect the intracellular flow of calcium ions in both skeletal and smooth muscle. Although information seems to be limited to this report, the authors recommend that both drugs should not be used together for tocolysis.

Reference

1 Snyder SW, Cardwell MS. Neuromuscular blockade with magnesium sulphate and nifedipine. Am J Obst Gynecol (1989) 161, 35–6.

Calcium channel blockers + Miscellaneous drugs

Abstract/Summary

The concurrent use of prenylamine and other drugs with negative inotropic effects such as beta-blockers and quinidine, procainamide, amiodarone or lignocaine should be avoided because of the risk of the development of torsades de pointes.

Clinical evidence, mechanism, importance and management

The manufacturers of prenylamine say that prenylamine should not be given with negative inotropic drugs such as beta-blockers, quinidine, procainamide, amiodarone or lignocaine because there is the risk of the development of torsades de pointes associated with a prolongation of the Q-T interval. Other risk factors are hypokalaemia[5] and conduction disorders.[5] The recommendation is based on reports of atypical ventricular tachycardia (AVT or torsades de pointes) occurring in patients taking prenylamine and propranolol,[1,2] sotalol[3] and other beta-blockers or quinidine-like compounds such as lignocaine (lidocaine).[6,7] The extent of the risk seems not to have been measured but there is evidence that some of these drugs (propranolol, acebutalol, atenolol, oxprenolol, sotalol) have been used concurrently without problems although the Q-T interval was observed to be prolonged.[4]

References

1 Evans TR and Krikler DM. Drug-aggravated sinoatrial block. Proc Roy Soc Med (1975) 68, 808–9.
2 Puritz R, Henderson MA, Baker SN, Chamberlain DA. Ventricular arrhythmias caused by prenylamine. Br Med J (1977) 2, 608–9.
3 Kontopoulos A, Filindris A, Manoudis F, Metaxas P. Sotalol-induced torsades de pointes. Postgrad Med J (1981) 57, 321–3.
4 Oakley D, Jennings K, Puritz R, Krikler D, Chamberlain D. The effect of prenylamine on the QT interval of the resting electrocardiogram in patients with angina pectoris. Postgrad Med J (1980) 56, 753–6.
5 Warembourg H, Pauchant M, Ducloux G, Delbecque M, Vermeersch M, Tonnel-Levy M. Les torsades de pointe. A propos de 30 observations. Lille med (1974) 19, 1–11.
6 Grenadier E, Alpan G, Keidar S, Palant A. Atrio-ventricular block after administation of lignocaine in patients treated with prenylamine. Postgrad Med J (1982) 58, 175–7.
7 Cantle J (Hoechst UK Ltd). Personal communication (1981).

Calcium channel blockers + Omeprazole

Abstract/Summary

The loss from the body of both nifedipine and omeprazole is modestly reduced by concurrent use, but this seems unlikely to be of clinical importance.

Clinical evidence, mechanism, importance and management

After taking 20 mg omeprazole daily for 7 days the clearance of nifedipine in 10 normal subjects was reduced 21% (from 75 to 59.4 L/h). The same subjects showed a 14% reduction (from 24.9 to 28.8 L/h) in the clearance of a 40 mg IV dose of omeprazole after 5 days treatment with 10 mg nifedipine three times daily.[1] In a related study the same group of workers found that 20 mg omeprazole increased the AUC of nifedipine by 26%, but no changes in blood pressure or heart rates were seen.[2] None of these changes is large and they are unlikely to be of clinical importance. This needs confirmation.

Reference

1 Danhof M, Soons PA, van den Berg G, Van Brummelen P, Jansen JBMJ. Interactions between nifedipine and omeprazole. Eur J Clin Pharmacol (1989) 36 (Suppl) A258.
2 Soons PA, van den Berg G, Danhof M, van Brummelen P, Jansen JBMJ, Lamers CBHWL, Breimer DD. Influence of single- and multiple-dose omeprazole treatment on nifedipine pharmacokinetics and effects in healthy subjects. Eur J Clin Pharmacol (1992) 42, 319–24.

Calcium channel blockers + Rifampicin (Rifampin)

Abstract/Summary

Verapamil serum levels are markedly reduced by the concurrent use of rifampicin and may become therapeutically ineffective unless the dosage is raised appropriately. This also appears to be true for diltiazem. Three reports describe reduced serum nifedipine levels and reduced antianginal and antihypertensive effects in three patients when given rifampicin.

Clinical evidence

(a) Diltiazem

A study in six extensive and six poor metabolizers found that the peak serum level following a single 120 mg oral dose of diltiazem alone was 186 ng/ml, but after taking 600 mg rifampicin daily for eight days maximum serum diltiazem levels were only 5–8 ng/ml.[8]

(b) Nifedipine and Nisoldipine

A hypertensive woman well controlled on nifedipine (40 mg twice daily) showed a blood presssure rise from 140–160/80–90 mmHg to 200/110 mmHg within two weeks of starting to take antitubercular treatment which included 450 mg rifampicin daily. When the rifampicin was stopped and then restarted, the blood pressure fell and then rose again. The peak nifedipine serum levels and the AUC fell to about 40% while taking the rifampicin.[6] There was also some extremely limited evidence that nisoldipine and enalapril were also ineffective in reducing blood pressure while taking rifampicin.[6]

Reduced nifedipine levels (peak levels and AUCs roughly halved) and an increase in anginal attacks were seen a patient when given rifampicin,[5] and another showed a loss of blood pressure control when given rifampicin.[7]

(c) Verapamil

The observation of a patient whose hypertension was not reduced by verapamil while on antitubercular drugs, prompted a study in four other patients.[1] No verapamil could be detected in the plasma of three of them similarly treated for tuberculosis (rifampicin 450–600 mg daily; isoniazid 5 mg/kg daily; ethambutol 15 mg/kg daily) after receiving a single 40 mg dose of verapamil. A maximum of 20 ng/ml was found in the fourth patient. Six other subjects not taking antitubercular drugs had a maximum verapamil serum concentration of 35 ng/ml after being given a single 40 mg dose.

Similar results are reported in another study.[3] Supraventricular tachycardia was inadequately controlled in a patient taking 600 mg rifampicin and 300 mg isoniazid, despite the administration of 480 mg verapamil every 6 h.[2] Substitution of the rifampicin by ethambutol resulted in a four-fold rise in serum verapamil levels. A later study in six normal subjects showed that after taking rifampicin for two weeks the oral bioavailability of verapamil was reduced from 26 to 2%, and the effects of verapamil on the ECG were abolished.[4]

Mechanism

The most likely explanation is that the rifampicin (known to be a potent liver enzyme inducing agent) increases the metabolism of the diltiazem, verapamil and nifedipine by the liver, thereby increasing their clearance from the body.

Importance and management

Established interactions but the documentation is very limited. Monitor the effects closely if diltiazem, verapamil or nifedipine and rifampicin are given concurrently, anticipating the need to make a marked increase in the dosage of the calcium channel blocker. Ethambutol is a non-interacting alternative antitubercular. There seems to be no information about other calcium channel blockers.

References

1 Rahn KH, Mooy K, Bohm R, van den Vet, A. Reduction of bioavailability of verapamil by rifampin. N Eng J Med (1985) 312, 920–21.
2 Barbarash RA. Verapamil-rifampin interaction. Drug Intell Clin Pharm (1985) 19, 559–60.
3 Mooy J, Bohm R, van Baak M, Kemenade J, v d Vet A, Rahn RH. The influence of antituberculosis drugs on the plasma level of verapamil. Eur J Clin Pharmacol (1987) 32, 107–9.
4 Barbarash RA, Bauman JL, Fischer JH, Kondos G, Batenhorst RL. Near total reduction in verapamil bioavailability by rifampin: electrocardiographic correlates. J Amer Coll Cardiol (1988) 11, 205A.
5 Tsuchihashi K, Fukami K, Kishimoto H, Sumiyoshi T, Haze K, Saito M, Hiramori K. A case of variant angina exacerbated by administration of rifampicin. Heart Vessels (1987) 3, 214–7.
6 Tada Y, Tsuda Y, Otsuka T, Nagasawa K, Kimura H, Kusaba T, Sakata T. Case report: nifedipine-rifampicin interaction attenuates the effect on blood pressure in a patient with essential hypertension. Am J Med Sci (1992) 303, 25–7.
7 Takasugi T. A case of hypertension suggesting nifedipine and rifampicin drug interaction. Igaku To Yakugaku (1989) 22, 132–5.
8 Drda KD, Bastian TL, Self TH, Lawson J, Lanman RC, Burlew BS, Lalonde RL. Effects of debrisoquine hydroxylation phenotype and enzyme induction with rifampin on diltiazem pharmacokinetics and pharmacodynamics. Pharmacotherapy (1991) 11, 278.

Calcium channel blockers + Sulphinpyrazone

Abstract/Summary

The clearance of verapamil is markedly increased by sulphinpyrazone.

Clinical evidence, mechanism, importance and management

A study in eight normal subjects showed that after taking 800 mg sulphinpyrazone daily for a week, the clearance of a single oral dose of verapamil was increased about threefold (from 4.27 to 13.77 l/h/kg), possibly due to an increase in its liver metabolism.[1] The clinical importance of this is uncertain, but be alert for reduced verapamil effects. It seems probable that the dosage may need to be increased.

Reference

1 Wing LMH, Miners JO, Lillywhite KJ. Verapamil disposition-effects of sulphinpyrazone and cimetidine. Br J Clin Pharmac (1985) 19, 385–91.

Calcium channel blockers + Vancomycin

Abstract/Summary

An isolated case report suggests that the hypotensive effects of the rapid infusion of vancomycin may occur more readily in those who are already vasodilated with nifedipine.

Clinical evidence, mechanism, importance and management

A man with severe systemic sclerosis was hospitalized for Raynaud's phenomenon and dental extraction. After being started on 40 mg nifedipine daily, he was given intravenous vancomycin (1 g in 200 ml 5% dextrose) over 30 min. After 20 min he experienced a severe headache and was found to have a marked macular erythema on the upper trunk, head, neck and arms. His blood pressure fell to 100/60 mmHg and his pulse rate was 90. He recovered spontaneously.[1] The suggested reason is that the vasodilatory effects of the nifedipine were additive with those of the vancomycin (known to cause hypotension and erythema if infused quickly). The authors of this report suggest that vasodilators should be discontinued several days before giving vancomycin, and the blood pressure should be well monitored during infusion.

Reference

1 Daly BM, Sharkey I. Nifedipine and vancomycin-associated red man syndrome. Drug Intell Clin Pharm (1986) 20, 986.

Calcium channel blockers + X-ray contrast media

Abstract/Summary

The hypotensive effects of an intravenous bolus of ionic X-ray contrast medium can be increased by the presence of calcium channel blockers (diltiazem, nifedipine, verapamil, etc.). No interaction or only a small interaction appears to occur with non-ionic contrast media. A case report describes serious ventricular tachycardia in a patient on prenylamine when given sodium iothalamate.

Clinical evidence, mechanism, importance and management

(a) Hypotensive effects increased

It is well recognized that ionic X-ray contrast media used for ventriculography reduce the systemic blood pressure due to peripheral vasodilation. They also have a direct depressant effect on the heart muscle. A comparative study of the haemodynamic response of 65 patients showed that the hypotensive effect of a bolus dose of an ionic agent (0.5 ml/kg diatrizoate meglumine and diatrizoate sodium with edetate sodium or disodium) was increased by the concurrent use of nifedipine or diltiazem: it occurred earlier (3.1 s instead of 12.9 s), was more profound (a fall in systolic pressure of 48.4 instead of 36.9 mm Hg) and more prolonged (62s instead of 36s).[1] A similar interaction was seen in dogs given verapamil.[2] No interaction or only a minimal interaction was seen in the patients and dogs when non-ionic contrast media (iopamidol or iohexol) were used instead.[1,2] Concurrent use should be undertaken with care.

(b) Ventricular arrhythmia precipitated

An elderly man who had been taking 60 mg prenylamine and 10 mg nifedipine three times a day for two years experienced cardiorespiratory arrest a few seconds after a bolus intravenous injection of 80 ml sodium iothalamate 70% (Contray 420), and a further arrest 90 seconds later. On the second occasion the rhythm was identified as ventricular tachycardia, converted to sinus rhythm by a 100 Joule DC shock.[3] The reason is thought to be the additive effects of the prenylamine and sodium iothalamate both of which can prolong the QT_c (corrected QT interval of the heart) which predisposes the development of serious ventricular arrhythmias. Concurrent use should be avoided or undertaken with great care. The manufacturers of sodium iothalamate also advise the avoidance of hypokalaemia and of drugs such as procainamide and quinidine which also tend to prolong the QTC interval.

References

1 Morris DL, Wisneski JA, Gertz EW, Wexman M, Axelrod R, Langberg JJ. Potentiation by nifedipine and diltiazem of the hypotensive response after contrast angiography. J Am Coll Cardiol (1985) 6, 785–91.

2 Higgins CB, Kuber M, Slutsky RA. Interaction between verapamil and contrast media in coronary arteriography: comparison of standard ionic and new non-ionic media. Circulation (1983) 68, 628–35.

3 Duncan JS, Ramsay LE. Ventricular tachycardia precipitated by sodium iothalamate (Contray 420) injection during prenylamine treatment: a predictable adverse drug interaction. Postgrad Med J (1985) 61, 415–7.

Chapter 12
Oral Contraceptive and Related Sex-Hormone Drug Interactions

The oral contraceptives are of two main types: (i) the combined oestrogen-progestogen fixed dose preparations, and the combined sequential preparations with the doses of each steroid varied throughout the cycle; (ii) the progestogen-only preparations. The oestrogens commonly used are ethinyloestradiol in doses of 20–50 g, or mestranol in doses of 50–100 g. The progestogens are either those derived from 19-norethisterone (e.g. norethynodrel, ethynodiol acetate, norgestrel, norethisterone, lynoestrenol) or more uncommonly from 17 alpha-hydroxyprogesterone (e.g. megestrol) in doses ranging from about 0.25–5.0 mg. There are now very many different oral contraceptive preparations available throughout the world but most seem to be variants on these two broad themes.

The combined and sequential preparations are taken for 20–21 days, followed by a period of seven days during which withdrawal bleeding occurs. Some of them include six or seven tablets of lactose to be taken at this time so that the daily habit of taking a tablet is not broken. These contraceptives act in several ways: the oestrogenic component suppresses ovulation while the progestogen acts to change the endometrial structure so that even if conception were to occur, implantation would be unlikely. In addition the cervical mucus becomes unusually viscous which inhibits the free movement of the sperm.

The progestogen-only or 'mini-pills' are taken continuously. They do not inhibit ovulation but probably act by increasing the viscosity of the cervical mucus so that movement of the sperm is retarded. They may also cause changes in the endometrium which inhibit successful implantation.

Almost all of the interactions described here in this chapter and elsewhere in this book involve the combined oral contraceptives. Very little seems to be known about the interactions with the progestogen-only contraceptives. One should not therefore uncritically assume that interactions known to occur with the former type of contraceptive also occur with the latter, but there may possibly be some overlap. Much more study is needed to define the situation more clearly.

Gestrinone + Miscellaneous drugs

Abstract/Summary

The makers say that gestrinone should not be used with oral contraceptives and that rifampicin and antiepileptic drugs may reduce its effects. An isolated report describes bleeding in a woman on warfarin given gestrinone.

Clinical evidence, mechanism, importance and management

Although gestrinone can inhibit ovulation, it is not sufficiently reliable to be used as a contraceptive. The makers emphasise the importance of using a barrier method instead of oral contraception while on gestrinone because they say that not only are the effects of gestrinone possibly modified by oral contraceptives, but its use in pregnancy is totally contra-indicated.[1]

The makers also suggest that rifampicin and anticonvulsants (not named, but by implication phenytoin, phenobarbitone and carbamazepine) can accelerate the metabolism of gestrinone thereby reducing its effects,[1] but so far there appear to be no reports that this actually occurs.[3] An isolated report briefly describes an increased INR with vaginal bleeding and multiple bruising in a woman on warfarin and gestrinone.[2] Good monitoring is advisable if any of these drugs is given concurrently, with dosage adjustments where it becomes clearly necessary.

References

1 Dimetriose (Gestrinone). Roussel laboratories. ABPI Datasheet Compendium 1991–2, 1307.
2 Beeley L, Cunningham H, Carmichael A, Brennan A. Bulletin of the W. Midlands Centre for Adverse Drug Reporting (1992) 35, 13.
3 Roberts G (Rousell Labs). Personnal Communication 1992.

Oestrogens (Estrogens) + Phenothiazines

Abstract/Summary

Oestrogens can increase the serum levels of butaperazine.

Clinical evidence, mechanism, importance and management

When a dystonic reaction to a single dose of prochlorperazine was seen in a pregnant woman (presumed to be due to increased serum butaperazine levels resulting from the high oestrogen levels), a further study was undertaken in four postmenopausal schizophrenic women. While taking 1.25 mg conjugated oestrogens (*Premarin*) daily, their serum butaperazine levels in response to two 40 mg doses daily were increased by 48% (from 231 to 343 ng/ml) and the AUC (area under the curve) was increased by 92%.[1] The reasons are not understood but increased absorption or reduced liver metabolism are suggested.[1] The general clinical importance of these findings is not known. There seem to be no other reports of adverse reactions but it would be prudent to monitor concurrent use. There seems to be no information about other phenothiazines or the effects of the oestrogens contained in oral contraceptives.

Reference

1 El-Yousef MK, Manier DH. Estrogen effects on phenothiazine derivative blood levels. J Amer Med Ass (1974) 228, 827–8.

Oral contraceptives + Alcohol

Abstract/Summary

The detrimental effects of alcohol may be reduced to some extent in women on oral contraceptives, but blood alcohol levels are possibly unaltered.

Clinical evidence

A controlled study in 54 women showed that those on oral contraceptives (30, 35 or 50 µg oestrogen) tolerated the effects of alcohol better than those not taking oral contraceptives (as measured by a reaction-time test and a bead-threading test), but their blood-alcohol levels and its rate of clearance were unchanged.[1] Two other studies suggest that blood alcohol levels may be reduced in those taking oral contraceptives.[2,3] The authors of the report cited[1] say that they do not recommend women on oral contraceptives to drink more than usual. No special precautions would seem to be necessary.

References

1 Hobbes J, Boutagy J, Shenfield GM. Interactions between ethanol and oral contraceptive steroids. Clin Pharmacol Ther (1985) 38, 371–80.
2 Jones MK, Jones BM. Ethanol metabolism in women taking oral contraceptives. Alcoholism (1984) 8, 24–8.
3 Zeiner AR, Kegg PS. Effects of sex steroids on ethanol pharmacokinetics and autonomic reactivity. Prog Biochem Pharmacol (1981) 18, 130–42.

Oral contraceptives + Antacids

Abstract/Summary

Despite *in vitro* evidence that magnesium trisilicate might possibly reduce the effects and the reliability of the oral contraceptives, other evidence from human studies suggests that concurrent use is safe.

Clinical evidence, mechanism, importance and management

Although *in vitro* studies[1] have clearly shown that 0.5 and 1.0% suspensions of magnesium trisilicate in water adsorb 50–90% of ethisterone, mestranol and norethisterone, a single-dose study[2] in 12 women given a single pill (30 μg ethinyloestradiol and either norethisterone acetate 1 mg or levenorgestrel 150 μg) with a single tablet containing magnesium trisilicate (0.5 g) and aluminium hydroxide (0.25 g), showed that the bioavailability of the contraceptive remained unchanged. This is in line with common experience. Nor does there appear to be an important interaction with any other antacid or adsorbent. No special precautions seem to be necessary.

References

1 Khalil SAH. The *in vitro* uptake of some oral contraceptive steroids by magnesium trisilicate. J Pharm Pharmac (1976) 28, (Suppl). 47P.
2 Joshi JV, Sankolli GM, Shah RS, Joshi UM. Antacid does not reduce the bioavailability of oral contraceptive steroids in women. Int J Clin Pharmac Ther Toxicol (1986) 24, 192–5.

Oral contraceptives + Anti-asthmatic preparations

Abstract/Summary

No recorded interactions, but asthma is included by some manufacturers of oral contraceptives among their 'special precautions' because the asthmatic condition may be worsened. Sometimes it may be improved.

Clinical evidence, mechanism, importance and management

There have been instances in which women have developed allergic conditions such as rhinitis, atopic eczema, urticaria or asthma while taking oral contraceptives.[1–3] In contrast there are other instances where pre-existing asthma and other allergic conditions have improved.[2] For this reason it has been claimed that '... it is always worth while giving an oral contraceptive a trial for patients with any of these complaints [eczema, asthma, vasomotor rhinitis, migraine] as there is an even chance that she will be improved; if the condition is aggravated, it will return to its previous state as soon as the medication is stopped.[1]

References

1 Mears E. Oral contraceptives. Lancet (1964) i, 980.
2 Falliers CJ. Oral contraceptives and allergy. Lancet (1974) ii, 515.
3 Horan JD, Lederman JJ. Possible asthmogenic effect of oral contraceptives. Can Med Ass J (1968) 99, 130.

Oral contraceptives + Antibiotics and Anti-infective agents

Abstract/Summary

Failure of oral contraceptives to prevent pregnancy has been attributed to the concurrent use of a tetracycline (doxycycline, lymecycline, oxytetracycline, minocycline, tetracycline) in almost 30 cases. One or two cases of failure have been reported with each of the following: chloramphenicol, cephalexin, cephalexin with clindamycin, dapsone, erythromycin, isoniazid, spiramycin, nitrofurantoin with sulphafurazole (sulfisoxazole) sulphamethoxypyridazine, sulphonamides, trimethoprim and metronidazole. The risk of contraceptive failure appears to be very low.

Clinical evidence

(a) Tetracyclines

A woman on *Microgynon 30* (ethinyloestradiol + D-norgestrel) became pregnant, the evidence indicating that she had conceived while taking a course of tetracycline (500 mg 6-hourly for three days and then 250 mg 6-hourly for 2 days) or in the week following. There was no evidence of either nausea or vomiting which might have been an alternative explanation for the contraceptive failure.[1] A case of break-through bleeding and another pregnancy attributed to the concurrent use of tetracycline are also described in this report.[1,2]

The Committee on the Safety of Medicines (CSM) in the UK has reports of 12 cases of contraceptive failure with tetracyclines (tetracycline, oxytetracycline).[3,9] Another survey describes six failures due to doxycycline, lymecycline or minocycline,[8] and a further two cases involving tetracycline are described elsewhere by the same author.[16] Two others describe three failures with tetracycline.[10,19] Further reports describe other failures attributed to oxytetracycline and minocycline,[11,17] and intermenstrual bleeding due to doxycycline and oxytetracyline.[12] See also 'Tetracyclines + Ethinyloestradiol' for reports of facial pigmentation due to minocycline and ethinyloestradiol.

(b) Chloramphenicol, Cephalexin/clindamycin, Dapsone, Erythromycin, Isoniazid, Nitrofurantoin, Para-Aminosalicylic acid, Spiramycin, Streptomycin, Sulphonamides and Trimethoprim

Two women on oral contraceptives are briefly reported to have shown break-through bleeding and to have become pregnant. One was taking chloramphenicol and the other sulphamethoxypyridazine.[4,5] One or two cases of failure have been attributed to concurrent treatment with each of the following: chloramphenicol, cephalexin, cephalexin/clindamycin, dapsone, erythromycin, isoniazid, nitrofurantoin, spiramycin, sulphafurazole (sulfisoxazole), sulphonamides, and trimethoprim.[3,9,10,18,19] Break-through bleeding due to erythromycin, clindamycin and chloramphenicol has also been described.[12] The CSM also has on record five cases implicating co-trimoxazole in contraceptive failure — see 'Contraceptives, oral + Co-trimoxazole'. No evidence of ovulation or of changes in serum contraceptive steroid levels was seen in a study of eight women treated with triple antitubercular therapy (para-aminosalicyclic acid, isoniazid, streptomycin).[15]

(c) Metronidazole

Three out of 25 women on oral contraceptives ovulated while taking metronidazole, but no cases of pregnancy were reported.[6] Pregnancy occurred in another woman on metronidazole, but she was also taking doxycycline.[8] Another study found no evidence that metronidazole affected the reliability of the combined oral contraceptives,[7] yet the CSM has three cases of pregnancy on their records attributed to an interaction with metronidazole.[9] Another occurs in a further report.[10]

Mechanism

Not understood. Suppression of intestinal bacteria which results in a fall in contraceptive serum levels is one suggested explanation (see 'Mechanism' in the synopsis dealing with 'Oral contraceptives + Penicillins'), but two studies failed to find evidence that this actually occurs.[13,14]

Importance and management

The cases cited here appear to be the sum of the reports involving these drugs. The incidence would seem to be very low indeed, although one study suggested that the risk of contraceptive failure is increased six-fold by antibiotics.[11] The majority of women appear not to be at risk, but there is as yet no way as yet of predicting who is likely to be affected. The precautions suggested for 'Oral contraceptives + Penicillins' should be followed.

References

1 Bacon JF, Shenfield GM. Pregnancy attributable to interaction between tetracycline and oral contraceptives. Br Med J (1980) 1, 293.
2 Lesqueux A. Grossesse sous contraceptif oral apres prise de tetracycline. Louvain Med (1980) 99, 413.
3 Back DJ, Breckenridge AM, Crawford FE, MacIver M, Orme LE, Rowe PH. Interindividual variation and drug interactions with hormonal steroids. Drugs (1981) 21, 46.
4 Hempel E, Bohm W, Carol W, Klinger G. Medikamentose Enzyminduktion und hormonal Kontrazeption. Zbl Gynak (1973) 95, 1451.
5 Hempel E. Personal communication (1975).
6 Joshi JV, Gupta KC, Joshi UM, Krishna U, Saxena BN. Interactions of oral contraceptives with other drugs and nutrition. Contracep Delivery Syst (1982) 3, 60.
7 Viswanathan MK, Govindarajulu P. Metronidazole therapy on the efficacy of oral contraceptive steroid pills. J Reprod Biol Comp Endocrinol (1985) 5, 69–72.
8 Sparrow MJ. Pill method failures. NZ J Med (1987) 100, 102–5.
9 Back DJ, Grimmer FM, Orme L'E, Proudlove C, Mann RD, Breckenridge AM. Evaluation of Committee on Safety of Medicines yellow card reports on oral contraceptive-drug interactions with anticonvulsants and antibiotics. Br J clin Pharmac (1988) 25, 527–32.
10 Kovacs GT, Riddoch G, Duncombe P, Welberry L, Chick P, Weisberg E, Leavesley GM, Baker G. Inadvertent pregnancies in oral contraceptive users. Med J Aust (1989) 150, 549–51.
11 Hughes BR, Cunliffe WJ. Interactions between the oral contraceptive pill and antibiotics. Br J Dermatol (1990) 122, 717.
12 Hetényi G. Possible interactions between antibiotics and oral contraceptives. Ther Hung (1989) 37, 86–9.
13 Murphy AA, Zacur HA, Charache P, Burkman RT. The effect of tetracycline on levels of oral contraceptives. Am J Obst Gynecol (1991) 164, 28–33.
14 Neeley JL, Abate M, Swinker M, D'Angio R. The effect of doxycycline on serum levels of ethinyl estradiol, norethindrone, and endogenous progesterone. Obstet Gynecol (1991) 77, 416–20.
15 Joshi JV, Joshi UM, Sankolli GM, Gupta K, Rao AP, Hazari K, Sheth UK, Saxena BN. A study of interaction of low-dose combination oral contraceptive with antitubercular drugs. Contraception (1980) 21, 617–29.
16 Sparrow MJ. Pregnancies in reliable pill takers. NZ Med J (1989) 102, 575–7.
17 De Groot AC, Eshuis H, Stricker BHC. Inefficacy of oral contraception during use of minocycline, Ned T Geneeskd (1990) 134, 1227–9.
18 Pedretti E, Brunenghi GM, Morali GC. Interazione tra antibiotici e contraccettivi orali: la spiramicina. Quad Clin Obstet Ginecol (1991) 46, 153–4.
19 DeSano EA, Hurley SC. Possible interactions of antihistamines and antibiotics with oral contraceptive effectiveness. Fertil Steril (1982) 37, 853–4.

Oral contraceptives + Anticonvulsants

Abstract/Summary

Oral contraceptives are unreliable during concurrent treatment with phenytoin, primidone, barbiturates, carbamazepine or oxcarbazepine. Intermediate break-through bleeding and spotting can take place and pregnancies have occurred. The failure of contraceptive implants has also been reported. Seizure control may sometimes be disturbed. Sodium valproate and lamotrigine appear not to interact with the oral contraceptives.

Clinical evidence

(a) Contraceptive failure

An epileptic woman taking 200 mg phenytoin and 50 mg sulthiame daily (with ferrous gluconate and folic acid) became pregnant despite the regular use of an oral contraceptive containing 0.05 mg ethinyloestradiol and 3 mg norethisterone acetate.[1]

Since this first report[1] in 1972, at least 29 pregnancies have been reported in the literature in epileptic women taking a range of oral contraceptives and anticonvulsants which have included either phenytoin, a barbiturate or primidone.[2–6,10,11,15,25,28,34] Carbamazepine has also been clearly implicated[13,25–9] and possibly ethosuximide.[26] In addition the Committee on the Safety of Medicines in the UK has received another 43 reports[12,26] making a total of more than 70 cases in the 1968–92 period. It is also reported that subdermal contraceptive implants containing levonorgestrel (*Norplant*) failed to prevent pregnancy in three women taking phenytoin.[21,22] There is also good clinical evidence that oxcarbazepine may interact similarly but so far no cases of pregnancy have been reported.[35,36] In addition to these interactions, a report describes a menopausal woman on replacement treatment with conjugated oestrogens (*Premarin*), 1.25 mg daily, which became inadequate when she began to take 300 mg phenytoin daily.[16]

(b) Disturbance of seizure control

Epilepsy is included by most oral contraceptive manufacturers among the 'special precautions' to be observed because seizure control may sometimes be made worse, but it also may remain unaltered or even improve. For example, an epileptic woman under treatment with phenytoin and phenobarbitone became much worse while taking *Lyndiol* but improved when *Gynovlar* and later *Ovulen* were substituted.[7] Another report describes 20 epileptics on a variety of anticonvulsants whose condition was unaltered by *Norinyl-1*.[8] A woman on phenytoin and phenobarbitone was completely fit-free until she discontinued the oral contraceptive (un-named) she had been taking.[9]

Mechanism

The likeliest explanation is that these anticonvulsants act as potent liver enzyme inducing agents which increase the metabolism and clearance of the contraceptives from the body, thereby reducing their effects, and in some instances allowing ovulation to occur. A study using single doses of *Eugynon 50* in epileptic patients found that phenytoin (200–300 mg daily) or carbamazepine (300–600 mg daily) almost halved the AUC of the ethinyloestradiol and levonorgestrel.[30,31] Changes in seizure control have been attributed to changes in fluid retention which can influence seizure frequency.[7,8]

Importance and management

These are important interactions. Contraceptive failure in the presence of phenobarbitone, phenytoin, primidone and carbamazepine is well established. It also seems likely with oxcarbazepine, but is uncertain with ethosuximide. The incidence is unknown. It may be quite small (a failure-rate of 3.1 per 100 woman years is reported[24]). On the other hand the incidence of spotting and break-through bleeding is high.[17–19] One study reported it in seven out of eleven patients on phenobarbitone, one out of two on phenytoin, and four out of six on carbamazepine.[17] Another reported a 60% incidence in adolescents taking un-named anticonvulsants.[18] The unsolved problem is the identification of those whose menstrual cycles are sufficiently disturbed to allow pregnancy to take place.

Several practical solutions have been proposed to increase the contraceptive reliability and reduce the unpleasant break-through bleeding: (a) Raise the ethinyloestradiol dosage (or its equivalent). Use contraceptives containing 50 μg ethinyloestradiol.[12,13,17] If break-through bleeding still occurs, give in addition a preparation containing 30 or even 50 μg ethinyloestradiol.[12,14] Reliable contraception in most patients is said to be achievable with 80–100 μg ethinyloestradiol daily,[17, 30–32] although the advisability of giving such large doses has been

questioned.[23] (b) Use a non-interacting anticonvulsant: neither sodium valproate[17,20] nor lamotrigine[33] normally appear to interact with the oral contraceptives. (c) Use a barrier contraceptive method routinely while taking any of these interacting anticonvulsants. If anticonvulsants are used short-term, the Family Planning Association in the UK recommend that additional precautions are used for at least seven days after stopping the anticonvulsants, and if the seven days run beyond the end of a packet, the new packet should be started without a break, omitting any of the inactive tablets. Allow 4–8 weeks for the liver metabolism to recover following withdrawal of long-term anticonvulsants. It is also important to be on the alert for changes in seizure control if the interacting anticonvulsants are used.

References

1 Kenyon IE. Unplanned pregnancy in an epileptic. Br Med J (1972) 1, 686.
2 Hempel von E, Bohm W, Carol W, Klinger G. Medikamentose Enzyminduktion und hormonale Kontrazeption. Zbl Gynak (1973) 95, 1451–7.
3 Janz D, Schmidt D. Anti-epileptic drugs and failure of oral contraceptives. Lancet (1974) i, 1113.
4 Janz D, Schmidt D. Anti-epileptic drugs and the safety of oral contraceptives. Paper delivered to the German Section of the International League against Epilepsy. Berlin, 1st September 1974.
5 Belaisch J, Driguez P, Janaud A. Influence de certains medicaments due l'action des pilules contraceptives. Nouv Presse Med (1976) 5, 1645.
6 Gagnaire JC, Tchertchian J, Revol A, Rochet Y. Grossesses sous contraceptifs oraux chez les patientes recevant des barbituriques. Nouv Presse Med (1975) 4, 3008.
7 McArthur J. Notes and comments. Oral contraceptives and epilepsy. Br Med J (1967) 3, 162.
8 Espir M, Wallace ME, Lawson JP. Epilepsy and oral contraception. Br Med J (1969) 1, 294.
9 Copeman H. Oral contraceptives. Med J Aust (1963) 2, 969.
10 Back DJ, Orme ML'E. Drug interactions with oral contraceptive steroids. Prescribers Journal (1977) 17, 137.
11 Coulam CB, Annegers JF. Do anticonvulsants reduce the efficacy of oral contraceptives ? Epilepsia (1979) 20, 519.
12 Editorial. Drug interaction with oral contraceptive steroids. Br Med J (1980) 3, 93.
13 Hempel E, Klinger W. Drug stimulated biotransformation of hormonal contraceptive steroids. Clinical implications. Drugs (1976) 12, 442.
14 Back DJ, Bates M, Bowden A, Breckenridge AM, Hall MJ, Jones H, MacIver M, Orme M, Perucca E, Richens A, Rowe PH, Smith E. The interaction of phenobarbital and other anticonvulsants with oral contraceptive steroid therapy. Contraception (1980) 22, 495.
15 Fanoe E. P-pillesvigt-antagelig pa grund af interaktion me fenemal. Ugeskr Laege (1977) 139, 1485.
16 Notelovitz M, Tjapkes A, Ware M. Interaction between estrogen and Dilantin in a menopausal woman. N Engl J Med (1981) 304, 788.
17 Sonnen AEH. Sodium valproate and the pill. In 'Advances in Epileptology', XIIIth Epilepsy Int Symp. Akimoto H, Kazamatsuri H, Seino M, Ward A (Eds). Raven Press, NY (1982) 4229–32.
18 Diamond MP, Thompson JM. Oral contraceptive use in epileptic adolescents. J Adolesc Health Care (1981) 2, 82.
19 Diamond MP, Greene JW, Thompson JM, VanHooydonk JE, Wentz AC. Interaction of anticonvulsants and oral contraceptives in epileptic adolescents. Contraception (1985) 31, 623–32.
20 Crawford P, Chadwick D, Cleland P, Tjia J, Cowie A, Back DJ, Orme ML'E. Sodium valproate and oral contraceptive steroids. Brit J Clin Pharmacol (1985) 20, 288P.
21 Odlind V, Olsson S-E. Enhanced metabolism of levonorgestrel during phenytoin treatment in a woman with *Norplant* implants. Contraception (1986) 33, 257–61.
22 Haukkamaa M. Contraception by *Norplant* subdermal capsules is not reliable in epileptic patients on anticonvulsant treatment. Contraception (1986) 33, 559–65.
23 Elkington KW. Use of oral contraceptives by women with epilepsy. J Amer Med Ass (1986) 256, 2961.

24 Kay CR. Progestogen and arterial disease. Evidence from the Royal college of General Practitioners study. Am J Obst Gynecol (1982) 142, 762–6.

25 Sparrow MJ. Pill method failures. NZ J Med (1987) 100, 102–5.

26 Back DJ, Grimmer FM, Orme L'E, Proudlove C, Mann RD, Breckenridge AM. Evaluation of Committee on Safety of Medicines yellow card reports on oral contraceptive-drug interactions with anticonvulsants and antibiotics. Br J clin Pharmac (1988) 25, 527–32.

27 Beeley L, Magee P, Hickey FM. Bulletin of the West Midlands Centre for Adverse Drug Reaction Reporting (1989) 28, 21.

28 Kovacs GT, Riddoch G, Duncombe P, Welberry L, Chick P, Weisberg E, Leavesley GM, Baker G. Inadvertent pregnancies in oral contraceptive users. Med J Aust (1989) 150, 549–51.

29 Rapport DJ, Calabrese JR. Interactions between carbamazepine and birth control pills. Psychosomatics (1989) 30, 462–3.

30 Orme M, Back DJ, Chadwich DJ, Crawford P, Martin C, Tjia J. The interaction of phenytoin and carbamazepine with oral contraceptive steroids. Eur J Pharmacol (1990) 183, 1029.

31 Crawford P, Chadwick DJ, Martin C, Tjia J, Back DJ, Orme M. The interaction of phenytoin and carbamazepine with combined oral contraceptive steroids. Br J clin Pharmac (1990) 30, 892–6.

32 Orme M, Back DJ. Oral contraceptive steroids — pharmacological issues of interest to the prescribing physician. Advances in Contraception (1991) 7, 325–31.

33 Holdich T, Whiteman P, Orme M, Back D, Ward S. Effect of lamotrigine on the pharmacology of the combined oral contraceptive pill. Epilepsia (1991) 32, Suppl 1, 96.

34 van der Graaf WT, van Loon AJ, Postmus PE, Sleijfer DT. Twee patienten met hersenmetastasen die zwanger werden tijdens fenytoinegebruik. Ned-Tijdschr-Geneeskd (1992) 136, 2236–8.

35 Klosterkov Jensen P, Saano V, Haring P, Svenstrup B, Menge GP. Possible interaction between oxcarbazepine and an oral contraceptive. Epilepsia (1992) 33, 1149–52.

36 Sonnen AEH. Oxcarbazepine and oral contraceptives. Acta Neurol Scand (1990) 82 (Suppl 133) 37.

Oral contraceptives + Antihypertensive agents

Abstract/Summary

The hypertension caused by the oral contraceptives is frequently resistant to antihypertensive therapy with guanethidine or methyldopa.

Clinical evidence, mechanism, importance and management

Virtually all women who take oestrogen-containing oral contraceptives show some rise in blood pressure. One study[1] on 83 women showed that the average rise in systolic/diastolic pressures was 9.2/5.0 mmHg, and that it was about twice as likely to occur as in those not on the pill. There are many reports confirming this response but, despite extensive work, the reason for it is not understood although much of the work has centred around the increases seen in the activity of the renin-angiotensin system. Once the contraceptive is withdrawn, the blood pressure usually returns to its former levels.[2]

Attempts to control gross rises in pressure using guanethidine or methyldopa have been unsatisfactory[3–5] and one report[3] states that '...concurrent medication with guanethidine and oral contraceptives made satisfactory control of hypertension difficult or impossible.' It seems therefore that hypertension associated with, or exacerbated by, the use of oral contraceptives may not respond to drugs whose major actions are at adrenergic neurones.

References

1 Weir RJ, Briggs E, Mack A, Naismith L, Taylor L, Wilson E. Blood pressure in women taking oral contraceptives. Br Med J (1974) 1, 533.

2 Editorial (Anon.) Hypertension and oral contraceptives. Br Med J (1978) 1, 1570.

3 Clezy TM. Oral contraceptives and hypertension: the effect of guanethidine. Med J Aust (1970) 1, 638.

4 Wallace MR. Oral contraceptives and severe hypertension. Aust NZ J Med (1971) 1, 49.

5 Woods JW. Oral contraceptives and hypertension. Lancet (1967) iii, 653.

Oral contraceptives + Antimalarial drugs

Abstract/Summary

Chloroquine and primaquine do not reduce the serum levels of the combined oral contraceptives nor do they seem to affect their reliability. Chloroquine and quinine serum levels remain unchanged during concurrent use and their efficacy appears to be unaltered. Oral contraceptives appear not to affect the treatment of falciparum malaria with mefloquine.

Clinical evidence, mechanism, importance and management

(a) Effect of chloroquine and primaquine on oral contraceptives

A pharmacokinetic study[1] in two groups of women (12 and 7) on low-dose oral contraceptives (ethinyloestradiol + norethisterone) showed that the prophylactic use of chloroquine phosphate, 500 mg once a week for four weeks, caused a small increase in blood levels of the oestrogen (AUC + 15%), but there was nothing to suggest that the normal effects of the contraceptives were changed in any way. Chloroquine blood levels remained unaltered. Another study[2] in six women given a single dose of *Microgynon* (ethinyloestradiol + levonorgestrel) confirmed that neither chloroquine (300 mg) nor primaquine (45 mg) had a significant effect on the pharmacokinetics of either the oestrogen or the progestogen. Further confirmation of the absence of an interaction comes from studies in rhesus monkeys infected with malaria in which it was shown that the efficacy of chlorquine was not altered by the use of either *Norinyl* or *Ovral-28*.[3]

(b) Effect of oral contraceptives on mefloquine

A study in 12 Thai women with falciparum malaria found that their response (parasite and fever clearance) to treatment with mefloquine was not affected by the concurrent use of oral contraceptives. However the half-life and residence time of mefloquine were found to be shorter than in six normal healthy Thai women taking oral contraceptives.[4] There would seem to be no reason for avoiding concurrent use.

(c) Effect of oral contraceptives on quinine

A controlled study in Thai women showed that the pharmacokinetics of single 600 mg doses of quinine in seven women taking oral contraceptives were not significantly different from those in seven other women not taking contraceptives. The contraceptives were *Microgynon 30, Eugynon, Eugynon ED, Noriday* and *Triquilar*. There seem to be no reports that quinine affects the reliability of the oral contraceptives and there would seem to be no reason for avoiding concurrent use.[5]

References

1 Gupta KC, Joshi JV, Desai NK, Sankolli GM, Chowdhary VN, Joshi UM, Chitalange S, Satoskar RS. Kinetics of chloroquine and contraceptive steroids in oral contraceptive users during concurrent chloroquine prophylaxis. Indian J Med Res (1984) 80, 658–662.
2 Back DJ, Breckenridge AM, Grimmer SFM, Orme MLE, Purba HS. Pharmacokinetics of oral contraceptive steroids following the administration of the antimalarial drugs primaquine and chloroquine. Contraception (1984) 30, 289–295.
3 Dutta GP, Puri SK, Kamboj KK, Srivastava SK, Kamboj VP. Interactions between oral contraceptives and malaria infections in rhesus monkeys. Bull WHO (1984) 62, 931–9.
4 Karbwang J, Looareesuwan S, Back DJ, Migasana S, Bunnag D, Breckenridge AM. Effect of oral contraceptive steroids on the clinical cause of malaria infection and on the pharmacokinetics of mefloquine in Thai women. Bull WHO (1988) 66, 763–7.
5 Wanwimolruk S, Kaewvichit S, Tanthayaphinant O, Suwannarach C, Oranratnachai A. Lack of effect of oral contraceptive use on the pharmacokinetics of quinine. Br J clin Pharmac (1990) 31,179–81.

Oral contraceptives + Antischistosomal drugs

Abstract/Summary

Early schistosomiasis and the use of praziquantel or metriphonate do not appear to have any effect on the oral contraceptives.

Clinical evidence, mechanism, importance and management

Women with advanced schistosomal infections which affect the liver are not given oral contraceptives because their impaired liver function can affect the metabolism of drugs, but there seems to be no reason for withholding these contraceptives from those with only urinary or intestinal infections.[1,2] A study in 25 women with early active schistosomiasis (*S. haematobium* or *S. mansoni*) showed that neither the disease itself nor the concurrent use of antischistosomal drugs (a single 40 mg/kg dose of praziquantel, or metriphonate in three doses of 10 mg/kg at fortnightly intervals) had any effect on their serum oral contraceptive steroid levels when given *Ovral* (50 ug ethinyloestradiol + 500 ug levonorgestrel).[3]

References

1 Shaaban MM, Hammad WA, Fathalla MF, Ghaneimah SA, El-Sharkawy MM, Salim TH, Liaso WC, Smith SC. Effects of oral contraception on liver function tests and serum protein in women with active schistosomiasis. Contraception (1982) 26, 65–74.
2 El-Raghy I, Back DJ, Osman F, Nafeh MA, Orme ML'E. The pharmacokinetics of antipyrine in patients with graded severity of schistosomiasis. Br J Clin Pharmac (1985) 20, 313–6.
3 El-Raghy I, Back DJ, Osman F, Orme ML'E, Fathalla M. Contraceptive steroid concentrations in woman with early active schistosomias: lack of effect of antischistosomal drugs. Contraception (1986) 33, 373–7.

Oral contraceptives + Cimetidine or Ranitidine

Abstract/Summary

Cimetidine, but not ranitidine, raises endogenous serum oestradiol levels but whether it raises serum contraceptive steroid levels is uncertain.

Clinical evidence, mechanism, importance and management

800 mg cimetidine twice daily for 2 weeks was found to increase the serum oestradiol (endogenous) levels of nine men by about 20%, due apparently to the well-recognised inhibitory effects of cimetidine on the metabolism of oestradiol (2-hydroxylation) by the liver. 400 mg twice daily for a week had the same effect in another six men,[1] but ranitidine, 150 mg twice daily, was found not to raise serum oestradiol levels. These raised levels are a possible explanation of the signs and symptoms of oestrogen excess (gynecomastia, sexual dysfunction) which sometimes occurs in men after taking cimetidine for some time. Whether cimetidine has the same effect on administered oestradiol or other oestrogens (in oral contraceptives for instance) is uncertain but the possibility of increased effects should be borne in mind during concurrent use. There is no evidence that this is a clinically important interaction.

Reference

1 Galbraith RA, Michnovicz JJ. Effects of cimetidine on the oxidative metabolism of estradiol. N Eng J Med (1989) 321, 269–74.

Oral contraceptives + Ciprofloxacin

Abstract/Summary

Ciprofloxacin appears unlikely to affect the reliability of the combined oral contraceptives.

Clinical evidence, mechanism, importance and management

No significant changes in gonadotropin (LH, FSH) or oestradiol levels occurred in 10 healthy women on oral contraceptives (ethinyloestradiol + desogestrel, gestodene or levonogestrel) while also taking 500 mg ciprofloxacin twice daily for seven days, starting on the first day of contraceptive intake. No break-through bleeding occurred. It was concluded that no adverse interaction occurs.[1] It should however be pointed out that some other antibiotics have similarly been shown not to interact in trials, but rare cases of failure have nevertheless occurred in the population at large (none so far with any of the quinolones). Another quinolone, temafloxacin (now withdrawn) has also been shown not to interact with oral contraceptives.[2]

Reference

1 Maggiolo F, Puricelli G, Dottorini M, Caprioli S, Bianchi W, Suter F. The effect of ciprofloxacin on oral contraceptive steroid treatments. Drugs Exptl Clin Res (1991) XVII, 451–4.
2 Back DJ, Tija J, Martin C, Millar E, Mant T, Morrison P, Orme M. The lack of interaction between temafloxacin and combined oral contraceptives. Contraception (1991) 43, 317–23.

Oral contraceptives + Clarithromycin, Roxithromycin

Abstract/Summary

Clarithromycin and roxithromycin appear unlikely to cause oral contraceptive failure.

Clinical evidence and mechanism

(a) Oral Contraceptives + Clarithromycin

10 women on combined oral contraceptives (*Microgynon, Ovranette, Marvelon*) showed a very slight (but not statistically significant) rise in serum ethinyloestradiol levels while also taking 250 mg clarithromycin twice daily for seven days. No changes in levonorgestrel levels occurred in those taking *Microgynon* or *Ovranette*, but levels of the active metabolite of desogestrel were increased in those on *Marvelon*. Progesterone levels remained suppressed and FSH and LH levels were reduced. There was no evidence that clarithromycin reduced the effectiveness of these oral contraceptives, and some evidence (reduced levels of FSH and LH) that it actually increases their efficacy.[1]

(b) Oral Contraceptives + Roxithromycin

While taking 150 mg roxithromycin twice daily, the anti-ovulatory effects of a low dose triphasic oral contraceptive remained unchanged during one cycle in 21 normal women. As a contrast, during another cycle while taking 300 mg rifampicin daily instead (known to reduce the effects of the oral contraceptives), 11 of the 21 women ovulated (52%). Ovulation was detected by measuring serum progesterone levels on day 21 (a value of above 10 nmol/l being considered indicative), and confirmed by sonography of the ovaries on day 13.[2,3]

Importance and management

Information seems to be limited to these studies, on the basis of which the authors concluded that these antibiotics are unlikely to cause oral contraceptive failure in most women. However it should be pointed out that even though contraceptive failure with other antibiotics (eg ampicillin) has similarly not been demonstrated in clinical studies, yet failure has nevertheless occurred in a very few other individuals. See 'Oral contraceptives + Antibiotics' and Anti-infectives, and 'Oral contraceptives + Penicillins'.

References

1 Back DJ, Tija J, Martin C, Millar E, Salmon P, Orme M. The interaction between clarithromycin and combined oral-contraceptive steroids. J Pharm Med (1991) 2, 81–7.
2 Meyer BH, Muller FO, Wessels P. Lack of interaction between roxithromycin and an oral contraceptive. Eur J Pharmacol (1990) 183, 1031–2.
3 Meyer BH, Muller FO, Wessels P, Maree J. A model to detect interactions between roxithromycin and oral contraceptives. Clin Pharmacol Ther (1990) 47, 671–4.

Oral contraceptives + Co-trimoxazole

Abstract/Summary

A human study has shown that co-trimoxazole (sulphamethoxazole + trimethoprim) would be expected to increase the effectiveness of the oral contraceptives, yet there are 15 cases on record of contraceptive failure attributed to the concurrent use of co-trimoxazole.

Clinical evidence

A study in nine women taking a triphasic contraceptive (*Trinordiol*) containing ethinyloestradiol and levonorgestrel showed that while taking two tablets of co-trimoxazole daily (320 mg trimethoprim + 1600 mg sulphamethoxazole in each tablet) their blood levels of ethinyloestradiol rose 30–50% (from 29.3 to 38.2 ng/ml at 12 h and from 18.9 to 27.8 ng/ml at 24 h). Levonorgestrel levels remained unaltered.[1]

In contrast, the Committee on the Safety of Medicines in the UK has on its records five cases of oral contraceptive failure attributed to the use of co-trimoxazole,[2,4] and another is reported elsewhere.[5] Three other surveys describe a total of nine other cases of contraceptive failure while taking co-trimoxazole or trimethoprim.[3,6,7]

Mechanism

The rise in ethinyloestradiol levels[1] is probably due to inhibition by the sulphamethoxazole of the liver enzymes concerned with the metabolism and clearance of the oestrogen from the body. It is not clear why co-trimoxazole should sometimes paradoxically seem to be the cause of contraceptive failure.

Importance and management

The picture is confusing and contradictory. The authors of the study cited[1] say that '... the effects of contraceptive steroid preparations are enhanced rather than reduced by co-trimoxazole; and it is unlikely that clinical problems will arise in women taking long-term oral contraceptive steroids who are given short courses of co-trimoxazole.' This study appears to have been carefully carried out and well controlled, whereas the CSM and other reports are simply uncontrolled individual case reports. However some risk, however small, seems to exist and the precautions suggested for 'Oral contraceptives + Penicillins' would seem to be appropriate.

References

1　Grimmer SFM, Allen WL, Back DJ, Breckenridge AM, Orme M,and Tjia T. The effect of co-trimoxazole on oral contraceptive steroids in women. Contraception (1983) 28, 53–9.
2　Back DJ, Breckenridge AM, Crawford FE, MacIver M, Orme ML'E, Rowe PH. Interindividual variation and drug interactions with hormonal steroid contraceptives. Drugs (1981) 21, 46–61.
3　Sparrow MJ. Pill method failures. NZ Med J (1987) 100, 102–5.
4　Back DJ, Grimmer FM, Orme L'E, Proudlove C, Mann RD, Breckenridge AM. Evaluation of Committee on Safety of Medicines yellow card reports on oral contraceptive-drug interactions with anticonvulsants and antibiotics. Br J clin Pharmac (1988) 25, 527–32.
5　Beeley L, Magee P, Hickey FM. Bull W Midl Centre for Adverse Drug Reaction Reporting (1989) 28, 32.
6　Kovacs GT, Riddoch G, Duncombe P, Welberry L, Chick P, Weisberg E, Leavesley GM, Baker G. Inadvertent pregnancies in oral contraceptive users. Med J Aust (1989) 150, 549–51.
7　Sparrow MJ. Pregnancies in reliable pill takers. NZ Med J (1989) 102, 575–7.

Oral contraceptives + Danazol

Abstract/Summary

The makers of danazol say that concurrent use should be avoided because of a theoretical risk that the effects of both drugs might be altered or reduced.

Clinical evidence, mechanism, importance and management

Danazol can inhibit ovulation, apparently by depressing the LH surge which precedes and triggers ovulation, but in daily doses of 200 mg or more its side-effects are too unacceptable for it to be used routinely as an oral contraceptive, and at lower doses it is too unreliable.[1–3] Despite this ability to prevent conception, the makers of danazol advise against the concurrent use of oral contraceptives and suggest that non-hormonal contraceptive methods should be used instead. They say that there is a theoretical risk that danazol and the oral contraceptives might possibly compete for the same oestrogen, progestogen and androgen receptors, thereby altering the effects of both drugs.[4] However as yet there appears to be no direct evidence that this actually happens.

References

1　Greenblatt R B, Oettinger M, Borenstein R, Bohler C S-S. Influence of danazol (100 mg) on conception and contraception. J Reprod Med (1974) 13, 201–3.
2　Colle M L, Greenblatt R B. Contraceptive properties of danazol. J Reprod Med (1976) 17, 98–102.
3　Lauerson N H, Wilson K H. The effect of danazol in the treatment of chronic cystic mastitis. Obstet Gynecol (1976) 48, 93–8.
4　Sterling-Winthrop, Personnal communication 1990.

Oral contraceptives + Enprostil

Abstract/Summary

Enprostil appears not to interact with the oral contraceptives.

Clinical evidence, mechanism, importance and management

A double-blind cross-over study on 22 normal women taking *Norinyl®* 1 + 35 (norethindrone 1 mg + ethinyloestradiol 0.035 mg) showed that the concurrent use of 35 µg enprostil for seven days had no significant effect on the pharmacokinetics of either of the contraceptive steroids. The bioavailability of the oral contraceptives remained unaltered.[1]

Reference

1　Winters L, Wilberg C. Enprostil, a synthetic prostaglandin E_2 analog does not affect oral contraceptive bioavailability. Gastroenterology (1988) 94, A500. Also published in Curr Ther Res (1988) 44, 46–50.

Oral contraceptives + Fluconazole

Abstract/Summary

Two pregnancies and six cases of intermenstrual bleeding have been described in women using oral contraceptives, attributed to the use of fluconazole. This interaction (if such it is) is rare.

Clinical evidence

Two pregnancies have been reported, despite the use of oral contraceptives, attributed to an interaction with single 150 mg doses of fluconazole. Intermenstrual bleeding has also been described in six other women on oral contraceptives when given a single 150 mg dose of fluconazole. No withdrawal bleeding was reported in one other patient.[1,2]

In contrast a study in 10 women taking combined oral contraceptives found no evidence that a single 50 mg dose of fluconazole or 50 mg fluconazole daily for 10 days had significant effects on the pharmacokinetics of an oral contraceptive (30 μg ethinyloestradiol and 150μg leveonorgestrel).[3] Two other studies in women taking oral contraceptives found no clinically significant changes in their endocrinological profiles while taking 50 mg fluconazole daily.[5,6] During clinical trials in which single 150 mg doses of fluconazole were used by over 700 women taking oral contraceptives, no evidence of an interaction was seen.[4]

Mechanism

Not understood. Unlike ketoconazole, fluconazole appears to have little effect on liver enzyme activity (P450-cytochrome mediated reactions).

Importance and management

The weight of evidence suggests that contraceptive failure is unlikely if low-dose fluconazole (50 mg) is given. The contraceptive failures and intermenstrual bleeding cited here have only been attributed to the use of higher dose fluconazole (150 mg) and then only in a very small number of patients. The ultracautious might therefore consider advising the additional use of a barrier method of contraception if pregnancy is to be avoided more certainly. More study is needed.

References

1 Pfizer Ltd. Summary of unpublished reports: Female reproductive disorders possibly associated with Diflucan. Data on file (Ref DIFLU:diflu41.1) (1990).
2 Bulletin of West Midlands Centre for Adverse Drug Reaction Reporting. January (1990), 30.
3 Pfizer Ltd. An open study to examine the effect of fluconazole on the metabolism of an oral contraceptive in healthy female volunteers. Unpublished data on file (ref 29/VG) (1990).
4 Dodd GJ (Pfizer Ltd). Personal communication (1990).
5 Devenport MH, Crook D, Wynn V, Lees LJ. Metabolic effects of low-dose fluconazole in healthy female users and non-users of oral contraceptives. Br J clin Pharmac (1989) 27, 851–9.
6 Lazar JD, Wilner KD. Drug interactions with fluconazole. Rev Infect Dis (1990) 12, Suppl 3, S327–33.

Oral contraceptives + Griseofulvin

Abstract/Summary

The effects of the oral contraceptives may possibly be disturbed (either intermenstrual bleeding or amenorrhoea) if griseofulvin is taken concurrently. A woman taking an oral contraceptive became pregnant while taking griseofulvin and two others on oral contraceptives became pregnant while taking griseofulvin and a sulphonamide.

Clinical evidence

15 out of 22 women experienced transient intermenstrual bleeding and five had amenorrhoea during the first or second cycle after starting to take griseofulvin (0.5–1.0 g daily). Four of the 22 (two with intermenstrual bleeding and two with amenorrhoea) developed their original reactions when re-challenged with griseofulvin. Two other women on the pill are reported to have become pregnant while taking griseofulvin and a sulphonamide (co-trimoxazole in one instance and an unknown sulphonamide in the other)[1].

Oligomenorrhoea and irregular menses have been described in a woman on an oral contraceptive when given griseofulvin (250–500 mg daily). When the oral contraceptive was substituted by another with 57% more oestrogen, the menstrual flow became normal again.[2] Break-through bleeding has also been seen in three other women on the pill given griseofulvin[3] and one case of contraceptive failure has been reported.[4]

Mechanism

Not understood. Griseofulvin may possibly stimulate the activity of the liver enzymes concerned with the metabolism of the contraceptive steroids, thereby reducing their effects. This might explain the cases of break-through bleeding, but not those involving oligomenorrhoea and amenorrhoea. Contraceptive failure attributed to co-trimoxazole has also been reported (see 'Oral contraceptives + Co-trimoxazole').

Importance and management

Information about this interaction is very limited.[1-4] The risk of total contraceptive failure is uncertain but probably very small. It would now seem prudent for prescribers to warn women on oral contraceptives who are given griseofulvin that menstrual disturbances may possibly be signs of contraceptive unreliability, and that additional contraceptive precautions should be taken. For maximal contraceptive protection a barrier method should be used routinely while taking griseofulvin and for at least seven days afterwards. The Family Planning Association in the UK recommend that if the seven days run beyond the end of a packet, the new packet should be started without a break, omitting any of the inactive tablets.

References

1 Van Dijke CPH, Weber JCP. Interaction between oral contraceptives and griseofulvin. Br Med J (1984) 288, 1125–6.
2 McDaniel PA, Caldroney RD. Oral contraceptives and griseofulvin interaction. Drug Intell Clin Pharm (1986) 20, 384.
3 Beeley L, Stewart P. Bulletin of the West Midlands Centre for Adverse Drug Reaction Reporting. (1987) 25, 23.
4 Back DJ, Grimmer FM, Orme L'E, Proudlove C, Mann RD, Breckenridge AM. Evaluation of Committee on Safety of Medicines yellow card reports on oral contraceptive-drug interactions with anticonvulsants and antibiotics. Br J clin Pharmac (1988) 25, 527–32.

Oral contraceptives + Ketoconazole

Abstract/Summary

Ketoconazole can reduce the effectiveness of the oral contraceptives and cause intermenstrual bleeding. So far no pregnancies have been reported.

Clinical evidence, mechanism, importance and management

Seven out of 147 women taking low dose oral contraceptives (*Ovidon*, *Rigevidon*, *Anteovin*) experienced break-through bleeding or spotting within 2–5 days of starting a five-day course of ketoconazole, 400 mg daily. No pregnancies occurred.[1] The reason for this reaction is not understood. Its incidence is low (about 5%), its general importance is uncertain and information seems to be limited to this single report, however intermenstrual bleeding is a sign of a decrease in the effectiveness of the oral contraceptives so that the precautions suggested when taking antibiotics such as the penicillins (use an additional barrier contraceptive) might be a wise precaution if pregnancy is be avoided with certainty (see 'Oral contraceptives + Penicillins').

Reference

1 Kovacs L, Somos P, Hamori M. Examination of the potential interaction between ketoconazole (Nizoral) and oral contraceptives with special regard to products of low hormone content (*Rigevidon*, *Anteovin*). Ther Hung (1986) 34, 167.

Oral contraceptives + Penicillins

Abstract/Summary

Very infrequently and unpredictably the penicillins can cause the combined oral contraceptives to fail. Rare failures of the progestogen-only oral contraceptives have also been attributed to the use of a penicillin, but cause-and-effect has not been established.

Clinical evidence

A woman is reported to have had two unwanted pregnancies while taking *Minovlar* (ethinyloestradiol + norethisterone). She had also been treated with wide-spectrum antibiotics, particularly ampicillin. Another woman on *Minovlar* for five years, with no history of break-through bleeding, lost a quantity of blood similar to a normal period loss within a day of starting to take ampicillin, one capsule four times a day. There was no evidence of diarrhoea or vomiting in either case.[1,2]

The British Committee on the Safety of Medicines (CSM) in the UK has on record 32 further cases of contraceptive failure over the 1968–84 period attributed to penicillin antibiotics: ampicillin, ampicillin with either fusidic acid, tetracycline or flucloxacillin; amoxycillin, talampicillin, phenoxymethyl-penicillin (one also with oxytetracycline) and 'penicillin'.[8,13] Another survey describes contraceptive failures due to amoxycillin (16 cases), flucloxacillin, phenoxymethylpenicillin, pivampicillin (five cases) and amoxycillin with phenoxymethylpenicillin (two cases).[12] Two other reports describe a total of 26 cases with amoxycillin and six cases with 'penicillin'.[14,16] Further cases attributed to oxacillin and Triplopen (benethamine, procaine and benzyl penicillins) are reported elsewhere.[9,11]

Mechanism

Not understood. The oestrogen component of the contraceptive is cycled in the entero-hepatic shunt (i.e. it is repeatedly secreted in the bile as steroid sulphate and glucuronide conjugates which are then hydrolysed by the gut bacteria before reabsorption). One idea is that if these bacteria are decimated by the use of an antibiotic, the steroid conjugates fail to undergo bacterial hydrolysis and are very poorly reabsorbed, resulting in lower-than-normal concentrations of circulating oestrogen in a very small number of women and in an inadequate suppression of ovulation.[7] However, although the penicillins reduce urinary oestriol secretion in pregnant women,[3–5] no marked changes in serum oestrogen[6,8,19] or progestogen[17] levels in women on contraceptives have been found in formal studies. The progestogens do not take part in the entero-hepatic shunt.

Importance and management

An established but controversial interaction. The incidence is unknown but it is probably very low indeed. Despite the very wide use of both the oral contraceptives and the penicillins, relatively speaking there are few reports of contraceptive failure. Most women do not appear to be at risk, but as yet there seems to be no way of identifying the few who are likely to be affected. Spotting and break-through bleeding are possible signs of diminished contraceptive effectiveness. For maximal protection a barrier contraceptive method should be used routinely while taking a short course of a penicillin, and for at least seven days afterwards.[18] The Family Planning Association in the UK recommend that if the seven days run beyond the end of a packet, the new packet should be started without a break, omitting any of the inactive tablets. It has been suggested that those on long-term antibiotics for acne need only take extra precautions for the first two weeks because, after that, the gut flora becomes resistant to the antibiotic,[10] but this was not apparently borne out in the case of a woman on long-term minocycline who became pregnant.[15] Four contraceptive failures attributed to a progestogen-only contraceptive/pencillin interaction occur in the CSM records, but no definite link has been established.

References

1 Dossetor EJ. Drug interactions with oral contraceptives. Br Med J (1975) 4, 467.
2 Dossetor EJ. Personal communication (1976).

3 Willman K, Pulkkinen MO. Reduced maternal plasma and urinary oestriol during ampicillin treatment. Amer J Obstet Gyn (1971) 109, 893.

4 Tikkanen MJ, Aldercreutz H, Pulkinnen MO. Effect of antibiotics on oestrogen metabolism. Br Med J (1973) 1, 369.

5 Pulkinnen MO, Willeman K. Maternal oestrogen levels during penicillin treatment. Br Med J (1971) 4, 48.

6 Friedman CJ, Huneke AL, Kim MH, Powell J. The effect of ampicillin on oral contraceptive effectiveness. Obst Gynec (1980) 55, 33.

7 Back DJ, Breckenridge AM, Crawford FE, MacIver M, Orme L and Rowe PH. Interindividual variation and drug interactions with hormonal steroid contraceptives. Drugs (1981) 21, 46.

8 Back DJ, Breckenridge AM, MacIver M, Orme M, Rowe PH, Staiger Ch, Thomas E, Tjia A. The effect of ampicillin on oral contraceptive steroids in women. Br J Clin Pharmac (1982) 14, 43–8.

9 Silber TJ. Apparent oral contraceptive failure associated with antibiotic administration. J Adolesc Health Care (1983) 4, 287–9.

10 Szarewski A, Guillebaud J. Hormonal contraception. In 'Update Postgraduate Centre Series. Contraception', McFadzean W (ed). Update-Siebert Publications, Guildford (1988) p 9–18.

11 Bainton R. Interaction between antibiotic therapy and contraceptive medication. Oral Surgery, Oral Medicine, Oral Pathology (1986) 61, 453–5.

12 Sparrow MJ. Pill method failures. NZ Med J (1987) 100, 102–5.

13 Back DJ, Grimmer FM, Orme L'E, Proudlove C, Mann RD, Breckenridge AM. Evaluation of Committee on Safety of Medicines yellow card reports on oral contraceptive-drug interactions with anticonvulsants and antibiotics. Br J Clin Pharmac (1988) 25, 527–32.

14 Kovacs GT, Riddoch G, Duncombe P, Welberry L, Chick P, Weisberg E, Leavesley GM, Baker G. Inadvertent pregnancies in oral contraceptive users. Med J Aust (1989) 150, 549–51.

15 Hughes BR, Cunliffe WJ. Interactions between the oral contraceptive pill and antibiotics. Br J Dermatol (1990) 122, 717.

16 Sparrow MJ. Pregnancies in reliable pill takers. NZ Med J (1989) 102, 575–7.

17 Joshi JV, Sankoli KT, Mandlekar A, Joshi UM, Gupta K, Krishna U, Virkar KD, Sheth UK, Saxena BN. Interaction of an oral contraceptive with metronidazole and ampicillin therapy. J Steroid Biochem (1978) 9, 862.

18 Orme M, Back DJ. Oral contraceptive steroids — pharmacological issues of interest to the prescribing physician. Advances in Contraception (1991) 7, 325–31.

19 Philipson A. Plasma and urine levels produced by an oral dose of ampicillin 0.5 g administered to women taking oral contraceptives. Acta Obstet Gynecol Scand (1979) 58, 69–71.

Oral contraceptives + Pethidine (Meperidine)

Abstract/Summary

Oral contraceptives do not appear to interact with pethidine (meperidine).

Clinical evidence, mechanism, importance and management

One early study suggested that women on oral contraceptives excreted more unchanged pethidine in the urine than a control group not taking contraceptives who were found to excrete more of the demethylated metabolite.[1] However a later, well controlled, comparative study in 24 normal subjects (eight women taking 0.5 mg norgestrel + 0.05 mg ethinyloestradiol, and eight women and eight men not taking contraceptives) found no differences between the serum levels or excretion patterns of the three groups.[2] There would seem to be no reason for avoiding concurrent use.

References

1 Crawford JS, Rudofsky S. Some alterations in the pattern of drug metabolism associated with pregnancy, oral contraceptives and the newly-born. Br J Anaesth (1966) 38, 446.

2 Stambaugh JE, Wainer IW. Drug interactions I: meperidine and combination oral contraceptives. J Clin Pharmacol (1975) 15, 46–51.

Oral contraceptives + Retinoids

Abstract/Summary

There seems to be no evidence that the reliability of the combined oral contraceptives is affected by acitretin or isotretinoin. Any changes in the effects of the progestogen-only contraceptives caused by acitretin seem to be clinically unimportant.

Clinical evidence, mechanism, importance and management

(a) Oral contraceptives + acitretin

Eight women on combined oral contraceptives (*Stediril, Minidiril, Adepal*) and one on a progestogen-only contraceptive (*Microval*) were given 25–40 mg acitretin daily for at least two cycles. No changes in progesterone levels were seen in those taking the combined contraceptives, but the patient taking the progestogen-only contraceptive (0.03 mg levonorgestrel) showed a significant increase in progesterone levels after 3 cycles with acitretin. Plasma progesterone levels rose from 2.15 ng/ml before taking the acitretin to 3.87–13.46 ng/ml with acitretin. This rise in progesterone levels was taken as evidence that a corpus luteum had developed and hence that ovulation had occurred.[1]

Direct information seems to be limited to this report,[1] however no special precautions would seem to be necessary if acitretin is taken by women on either type of contraceptive. (however see the note at the end of (b)) Acitretin appears to have no effect on the anti-ovulatory effects of the combined contraceptives, and since the progestogen-only contraceptives are believed act primarily by altering the cervical mucous so that it become a sperm barrier, it probably does not matter whether acitretin allows ovulation to occur or not while taking this type of oral contraceptive. There seems to be no evidence in the literature that either acitretin (the main metabolite of etretinate) or etretinate itself has ever been responsible for oral contraceptive failure.

(b) Oral contraceptives + isotretinoin

A study in nine women on a combined oral contraceptive showed that the plasma concentrations of ethinyloestradiol and levonorgestrel were not significantly changed by the use of 0.5 mg/kg isotretinoin for severe pustular acne.[2] The authors concluded that oral contraceptives remain reliable during concurrent use, and they say that it seems unlikely that an interaction would occur with 1.0 mg/kg which is the dose commonly recommended in the USA.

It should however be emphasised that women who have used these retinoids should avoid becoming pregnant because of the risk of teratogenicity. The current recommendation is that pregnancy should be avoided for two years after these retinoids are stopped.

References

1 Berbis Ph, Bun H, Geiger J M, Rognin C, Durand A, Serradimigni A, Hartmann D, Privat Y. Acitretin (RO10–1670) and oral contraceptives: interaction study. Arch Dermatol Res (1988) 280, 388–9.
2 Orme M, Back DJ, Shaw MA, Allen WL, Tjia J, Cunliffe WJ, Jones DH. Isotretinoin and contraception. Lancet (1984) ii, 752–3

Oral contraceptives + Rifampicin (Rifampin)

Abstract/Summary

Oral contraceptives are very unreliable during concurrent treatment with rifampicin. Intermediate break-through bleeding and spotting commonly occur and conception may not be prevented.

Clinical evidence

62 out of 88 women on oral contraceptives are described in a report as having developed menstrual cycle disorders of various kinds when treated with rifampicin. Five pregnancies in women taking both drugs are also mentioned.[1,2]

Beginning with the first report[3] in 1971, a very marked increase in the frequency of intermenstrual break-through bleeding has been described in women on oral contraceptives when given rifampicin. Other reports have confirmed this interaction and at least 15 pregnancies have been reported.[4–8,14] One study found that 11 out of 21 women (52%) on a triphasic oral contraceptive ovulated while taking 300 mg rifampicin daily.[15,16] In another study, two out of seven on low dose oral contraceptives ovulated while taking rifampicin.[17] Contraceptive failure in a woman given rifampicin, streptomycin and isoniazid has also been described.[13]

Mechanism

600 mg rifampicin daily for only six days increases the hydroxylation of ethinyloestradiol fourfold[9,10] and reduces serum norethisterone levels significantly.[12] Mestranol is probably similarly affected.[11] As a result of this enzyme induction the reduced steroid levels may be insufficient to prevent the reestablishment of a normal menstrual cycle with ovulation, which would explain the break-through bleeding and pregnancies which can occur. The trend towards low-dose oestrogen contraceptives has possibly increased its likelihood.

Importance and management

The oestrogen/progestogen + rifampicin interaction is well documented and established. Menstrual cycle disturbances of 50–70%[1,2,15] and an ovulation rate of 52%[15,16] clearly indicate that women on these contraceptives should use an alternative or additional form of contraception if pregnancy is to be avoided with certainty while on rifampicin, and for 4–8 weeks after its withdrawal[18] (a UK Family Planning Association recommendation). No failures due to rifampicin have been reported with the progestogen-only contraceptives, but their reliability in the presence of rifampicin is doubtful.[12]

References

1 Reimers D, Nocke-Finck L, Breuer H. Rifampicin causes a lowering in efficacy of oral contraceptives by influencing oestrogen excretion. Reports on Rifampicin: XII International Tuberculosis Conference, Tokyo, September 1974.
2 Reimers D, Nocke-Finck L, Breuer H. Rifampicin, 'pill' do not go well together. J Amer Med Ass (1974) 227, 608.
3 Reimers D, Jezek A. Rifampicin und andere Antituberkulotika bei gleichzeitiger oraler Kontrazeption. Prax Pneumol (1971) 25, 255.
4 Kropp R. Rifampicin und Ovulationshemmer. Prax Pneumol (1974) 28, 270.
5 Bessot J-C, Vandevenne A, Petitjean R, Burghard G. Effets opposes de la rifampicine et de l'isoniazide sur le metabolisme des contraceptifs oraux? Nouv Presse med (1977) 6, 1568.
6 Hirsch A. Pilules endormies. Nouv Presse Med (1973) 2, 2957.
7 Piguet B, Muglioni JF, Chaline G. Contraception orale et rifampicine. Nouv Presse med (1975) 4, 115.
8 Skolnik JL, Stoler BS, Katz DB, Anderson WH. Rifampicin, oral contraceptives and pregnancy. J Amer Med Ass (1976) 236, 1382.
9 Bolt HM, Kappus H, Bolt M. Rifampicin and oral contraception. Lancet (1974) i, 1280.
10 Bolt HM, Kappus H, Bolt M. Effect of rifampicin treatment on the metabolism of oestradiol and 17 alpha-ethinyloestradiol by human liver microsomes. Europ J Clin Pharmacol (1975) 8, 301.
11 Bolt HM, Bolt WH. Pharmacokinetics of mestranol in man in relation to its oestrogenic activity. Europ J Clin Pharmacol (1974) 7, 295.
12 Back DJ, Breckenridge AM, Crawford F, MacIver M, Orme ML'E, Park BK, Rowe PH, Smith E. The effect of rifampicin on norethisterone pharmacokinetics. Europ J Clin Pharmacol (1974) 7, 193.
13 Back DJ, Breckenridge AM, Crawford FE, MacIver M, Orme L'E, Rowe P. Interindividual variation and drug interactions with hormonal steroid contraceptives. Drugs (1981) 21, 46.
14 Gupta KC, Ali MY. Failure of oral contraceptive with rifampicin. Med J Zambia (1980/81) 15, 23.
15 Meyer B H, Muller F O, Wessels P. Lack of interaction between roxithromycin and an oral contraceptive. Eur J Pharmacol (1990) 183, 1031–2.
16 Meyer BH, Muller FO, Wessels P, Maree J. A model to detect interactions between roxithromycin and oral contraceptives. Clin Pharmacol Ther (1990) 47, 671–4.
17 Joshi JV, Joshi UM, Sankolli GM, Gupta K, Rao AP, Hazari K, Sheth UK, Saxena BN. A study of interaction of low-dose combination oral contraceptive with antitubercular drugs. Contraception (1980) 21, 617–29.
18 Orme M, Back DJ. Oral contraceptive steroids — pharmacological issues of interest to the prescribing physician. Advances in Contraception (1991) 7, 325–31.

Contraceptives, oral + SCH 39304

Abstract/Summary

Preliminary evidence suggests that SCH 39304 is unlikely to affect the reliability of the combined oral contraceptives.

Clinical evidence, mechanism, importance and management

A study in 15 women found that a single 400 mg oral dose of SCH 39304 (a triazole antifungal) on day 7 of the cycle did not interfere with the inhibitory action of a low dose combined oral contraceptive, as judged from the serum progesterone values.[1] This antifungal seems unlikely to affect the reliability of the oral contraceptives in most women, however it must be pointed out that other antifungals and antibiotics which have failed to show evidence of an interaction during clinical trials, have nevertheless been implicated (though rarely) in oral contraceptive failures. More study is needed.

Reference

1 Lunell N-O, Pschera H, Zador G, Carlström K. Evaluation of the possible interaction of the antifungal triazole SCH 39304 with oral contraceptives in normal healthy women. Gynecol Obstet Invest (1991) 32, 91–7.

Oral contraceptives + Tobacco smoking

Abstract/Summary

The risk of thromboembolic disease in women on oral contraceptives is increased if they smoke.

Clinical evidence, mechanism, importance and management

A study in women in the 40–41 age group on oral contraceptives who smoked showed that they had a lower level of high-density lipoprotein in their serum than women who neither smoked nor took the pill.[1] The significance of this finding is that low levels are a major risk factor in the development of coronary heart disease and related thrombotic diseases. This is borne out by epidemiological studies which show that the incidence of thromboembolic diseases in women on the pill increases both with age and if the subjects smoke.[2,3] For example, one study found a relative risk ('rate ratio') of non-fatal myocardial infarction in women on the pill of 4.5 in non-smokers and 39 for heavy smokers.[4] Another study found a relative risk of subarachnoid haemorrhage in women on the pill of 6.5 for non-smokers and 22.0 for smokers.[5] Just another good reason why smoking should be discouraged.

References

1 Arntzenius AC, van Gent CM, van der Voort H, Stegerhoek C, Styblo K. Reduced high-density lipoprotein in women aged 40–41 using oral contraceptives. Lancet (1978) i, 1221.

2 Fredriksen H, Ravenholt RT. Thromboembolism, oral contraceptives and cigarettes. Public Health Rep (1970) 85, 197.

3 Collaborative Group for the study of stroke in young women. J Amer Med Ass (1975) 231, 718.

4 Shapiro S, Slone D, Rosenberg L. Oral contraceptive use in relation to myocardial infarction. Lancet (1979) 1, 743–7.

5 Petitti DB, Wingard J. use of oral contraceptives, cigarette smoking and risk of subarachnoid hemorrhage. Lancet (1978) 2, 234–6.

Oral contraceptives + Triacetyloleandomycin

Abstract/Summary

Severe pruritis and jaundice have been observed in women taking oral contraceptives shortly after starting treatment with triacetyloleandomycin.

Clinical evidence

A report describes 10 cases of cholestatic jaundice and pruritis in women taking oral contraceptives and triacetyloleandomycin. All had been using the contraceptive for 7–48 months and were given the antibiotic in 250 or 500 mg doses four times a day. The pruritis was intense, lasting 2–24 days, and preceded the jaundice which, in eight of the patients, persisted for over a month.[1]

There are numerous other reports of this adverse reaction,[2-13] one of which describes 24 cases.[5,6] The adverse reactions (fatigue, anorexia, severe itching, jaundice) can begin very rapidly, sometimes within two days, and may last up to 14 weeks.[13]

Mechanism

Uncertain. Hepatotoxicity has been associated with the use of both types of drug, but it is not common. The reaction suggests that their damaging effects on the liver may be additive or supra-additive.

Importance and management

A well established, well documented and clinically important interaction. The incidence is unknown. Concurrent use should be avoided.

References

1 Miguet JP, Monange C, Vuitton D, Allemand H, Hirsch JP, Carayon P, Gisselbrecht H. Ictere cholestatique survenu apres administration de triacetyloleandomycine: interference avec les contraceptifs oraux? Dix observations. Nouv Presse med (1978)7, 4304.

2 Perol R, Hincky J, Desnos M. Hepatites cholestatiques lors de la prise de troleandomycine chez deux femmes prenant des estrogenes. Nouv Presse med (1978) 7, 4302.

3 Goldfain D,Cauveinc L, Guillan J, Verudron J. Ictere cholestatique chez des femmes prenant simultanement de triacetyloleandomycine et des contraceptifs oraux. Nouv Presse med (1979) 8, 1099.

4 Rollux R, Plottin F, Mingat J, Bessard G. Ictere apres association estroprogestatif-troleandomycine. Trois observations. Nouv Presse med (1979) 8, 1694.

5 Miguet J-P, Vuitton D, Pessayre D, Allemand H, Metreau J-M, Poupon R, Capron JP, Blanc F. Jaundice from troleandomycin and oral contraceptives. Ann Intern Med (1980) 92, 434.

6 Miguet JP, Vuitton D, Allemand H, Pessayre D, Monange C, Hirsch J-P, Metreau J-M, Poupon R, Capron J-P and Blanc F. Une epidemie d'icteres due a l'association troleandomycine-contraceptifs oraux. Gastroenterol Clin Biol (1980) 4, 420.

7 Haber I, Hubens H. Cholestatic jaundice after triacetyloleandomycin and oral contraceptives. Acta Gastro-Enterol Belg (1980) 43, 475.

8 Claudel S, Euvrard P, Bory R, Chaivallon A, Paliard P. Cholestase intrahepatique apres association triacetyloleandomycine-estroprogestatif. Nouv Presse med (1979) 8, 1182.

9 Descotes J, Evreux J Cl, Fouatier N, Gaumer R, Girard D, Savoye B, Trois nouvelles observations d'ictere apres estroprogestatifs et troleandomycine. Nouv Presse med (1979) 8, 1182.

10 Anon. Levertoxiciteit van troleandomycine en oestrogen. Fol Pharmaceutica (Brussels) (1979) 6, 64.

11 Dellas JA, Hugues FC, Roussel G, Marche J. Contraception orale et troleandomycine. Un nouveau cas d'ictere. Therapie (1982) 37, 443–6.

12 Girard D, Pillon M, Bal A, Petigny A, Savoye B. Hepatite au decours d'un traitement au TAO chez les jeunes femmes sous oestro-progestatifs. LL M Medecine Sud Est (1980) 16, 2335–44.

13 Fevery J, Van Steenbergen W, Desmet V, Deruyttiere M, De Groote J. Severe intraheptic cholestasis due to the combined intake of oral contraceptives and triacetyloleandomycin. Acta Clin Belg (1983) 38, 242–5.

Oral contraceptives + Vitamins

Abstract/Summary

The oral contraceptives are reported to raise serum levels of vitamin A, and lower levels of ascorbic acid, cyanocobalamin, folic acid and pyridoxine. Ascorbic acid can raise serum ethinyloestradiol levels and pyridoxine may relieve depression in women on oral contraceptives, but the general clinical importance of concurrent treatment with these vitamins is uncertain.

Clinical evidence, mechanism, importance and management

There is evidence that the use of oral contraceptives can cause a biochemical deficiency of several vitamins, but clinical deficiency does not necessarily manifest itself. Serum levels of cyanocobalamin can be lowered,[1] folate deficiency with anaemia can occur,[2,3] and reduced levels of ascorbic acid[3-5] and pyridoxine[6,7] have been described. Treatment of pyridoxine deficiency has been shown to improve the mood of depressed women on oral contraceptives.[11] Raised levels of vitamin A has also been reported.[8] These changes in vitamin requirements induced by the oral contraceptives are reviewed in detail elsewhere.[9]

A study has shown that 1 g ascorbic acid can substantially raise serum ethinyloestradiol levels (+48% measured at 24 h) in women taking oral contraceptives,[14] and a single case report describes a woman on *Logynon* who experienced heavy breakthrough bleeding within 2–3 days of stopping her self-administered 1 g daily dose of ascorbic acid.[14] Another, paradoxically, attributes contraceptive failure to ascorbic acid and multivitamins.[15]

Routine prophylactic treatment with vitamins in women on oral contraceptives has been advised by some,[10] but questioned by others[12,13] because an increased intake of some vitamins in some circumstances may be harmful. For example, in areas of the world where protein malnutrition is rife, a pyridoxine supplement might lead to an undesirable increase in amino-acid catabolism in those on a low daily intake of protein.[12] One author's comment on the indiscriminate supplementation of the diet with multivitamin preparations in women on oral contraceptives is that it can hardly be justified.[13]

References

1 Wertalik LF, Metz EN, LoBuglio AF, Balcerzak SP. Decreased serum B$_{12}$ levels with oral contraceptive use. J Amer Med Ass (1972) 221, 1371.

2 Streiff RR. Folate deficiency and oral contraceptives. Ibid (1970) 214, 214.

3 Meguid MM, Loebl WY. Megaloblastic anaemia associated with the oral contraceptive pill. Postgrad Med J (1974) 60, 470.

4 Harris AB, Pillay M, Hussein S. Vitamins and oral contraceptives. Lancet (1975) ii, 82.

5 Briggs M, Briggs M. Vitamin C requirements and oral contraceptives. Nature (1972) 238, 277.

6 Bennick HJTC, Schreurs WHP. Disturbance of tryptophan metabolism and its correction during hormonal contraception. Contraception (1972) 9, 347.

7 Doberenz AR, van Miller JP, Green JR, Beaton JR. Vitamin B6 depletion in women using oral contraceptives as determined by erythrocyte glutamic-pyruvic transaminase activities. Proc Soc Exp Biol Med (1971) 137, 1100.

8 Wild J, Schorah CJ, Smithells RW. Vitamin A, pregnancy and oral contraceptives. Br Med J (1974) 1, 57.

9 Larsson-Cohn U. Oral contraceptives and vitamins. A review. Amer J Obst Gynec (1975) 121, 84.

10 Briggs M, Briggs M. Oral contraceptives and vitamin requirements. Med J Aust (1975) 1, 407.

11 Adams PW, Wynn V, Seed M, Foklhard J. Vitamin B6, depression and oral contraception. Lancet (1974) ii, 515.

12 Adams PW, Wynn V, Rose DP, Folkhard J, Seed M, Strong R. Effect of pyridoxine hydrochloride (vitamin B6) upon depression associated with oral contraception. Lancet (1973) i, 897.

13 Back DJ, Breckenridge AM, MacIver M, Orme ML'E, Purba H, Rowe PH. Interaction of ethinyloestradiol with ascorbic acid in man. Br Med J (1981) 282, 1516.

14 Morris JC, Beeley L, Ballantine N. Interaction of ethinyloestradiol with ascorbic acid in man. Br Med J (1981) 283, 503.

15 DeSano EA, Hurley SC. Possible interactions of antihistamines and antibiotics with oral contraceptive effectiveness. Fertil Steril (1982) 37, 853–4.

Intrauterine contraceptive devices (IUDs) + Anti-inflammatory agents

Abstract/Summary

There is some evidence that the very occasional failure of an IUD to prevent pregnancy may have been due to the concurrent use of a steroidal or non-steroidal anti-inflammatory agent.

Clinical evidence, mechanism, importance and management.

Two women out of a total of about 1000 fitted with *Multiload 250* (an IUD) became pregnant. One had taken aspirin, and the other mefenamic acid during the month when conception occurred. Another woman using a *Lippes* C conceived during the month when she took *Veganin* (aspirin, codeine, paracetamol).[1] Four women have been described who, despite being fitted with IUDs, became pregnant.[2,5] Two were taking corticosteroids regularly and the other two often took aspirin for migraine. Unwanted pregnancies have also been reported elsewhere in women with IUDs treated with corticosteroids.[3,4]

The evidence for this possible interaction is very slim and inconclusive, but the suggestion that drugs which affect prostaglandins might possibly affect the actions of the IUDs bears further investigation.

References

1 Dossetor J. Personal communication (1983).
2 Buhler M, Papiernik E. Successive pregnancies in women fitted with intrauterine devices who take anti-inflammatory drugs. Lancet (1983) 1, 483.
3 Inkeles DM, Hansen RI. Unexpected pregnancy in women using an intrauterine device and receiving steroid therapy. Ann Ophthalmol (1982) 14, 975.
4 Zerner J, Miller AB, Festino MJ. Failure of an intrauterine device concurrent with administration of corticosteroids. Fertil Steril (1976) 27, 1467.
5 Papiernik R, Rozenbaum H, Amblard P, Dephot N, de Mouzon J. Intrauterine device failure: relation with drug use. Eur J Obst Gyn Rep Biol (1989) 32, 205–12.

Medroxyprogesterone or Megestrol + Aminoglutethimide

Abstract/Summary

Aminoglutethimide markedly reduces the serum levels of medroxyprogesterone and megestrol. The dosage may need to be doubled to accommodate this interaction.

Clinical evidence

(a) Medroxyprogesterone + Aminoglutethimide

The concurrent use of aminoglutethimide (500–1000 mg daily) halved the plasma levels of the medroxyprogesterone (1500 mg daily) in six postmenopausal women with breast cancer.[1]

Another study in six postmenopausal women found that 1000 mg aminoglutethimide daily reduced medroxyprogestone levels by 63% (from 70 to 26 ng/ml) and of megestrol by 78% (from 177 to 38 ng/ml).[2] In another study on six women with advanced breast cancer, it was found that as the dosage of aminoglutethimide was gradually reduced and finally withdrawn, so the serum levels of medroxyprogesterone steadily climbed, although the dose remained constant.[3]

(b) Megestrol + Aminoglutethimide

1000 mg aminoglutethimide daily reduced serum megestrol levels in six postmenopausal women by 78% (from 177 to 38 ng/ml).[2]

Mechanism

The most likely reason is that the aminoglutethimide acts as an enzyme inducing agent, increasing the metabolism of the progestins, thereby increasing their loss from the body.

Importance and management

Both interactions appear to be established and of clinical importance. A 50% reduction in the serum levels of medroxyprogesterone and megestrol should be expected during concurrent use. The authors of one report[3] say that to achieve adequate serum medroxyprogesterone acetate levels (> 100 ng/ml) a daily dose of 800 mg is necessary in the presence of 125 or 250 mg aminoglutethimide twice daily. This is double the usual recommended dose of 400 mg daily.

References

1 Van Deijk WA, Blijhan GH, Mellink WAM, Meulenberg PMM. Influence of aminoglutethimide on plasma levels of medroxyprogesterone acetate: its correlation with serum cortisol. Cancer Treat Rep (1985) 69, 85–90.
2 Lundgren S, Lønning PE, Aakvaag A, Kvinnsland S. Influence of aminoglutethimide on the metabolism of medroxyprogesterone acetate and megestrol acetate in postmenopausal women with advanced breast cancer. Cancer Chemother Pharmacol (1990) 27, 101–5.
3 Halpenny O, Bye A, Cranny A, Feely J, Daly PA. Influence of aminoglutethimide on plasma levels of medroxyprogesterone acetate. Med Oncol & Tumour Pharmacother (1990) 7, 241–7.

Chapter 13
Cytotoxic Drug Interactions

The cytotoxic drugs (antineoplastics, cytostatics) are used in the treatment of malignant disease in conjunction with radiotherapy, surgery and immunosuppressants such as the corticosteroids and lymphocytic antisera. They also find application in the treatment rheumatoid arthritis, of skin conditions such as psoriasis, and a few are used with other immunosuppressant drugs (cyclosporin, corticosteroids) to prevent transplant rejection. These other immunosuppressant drugs are dealt with in Chapter 16.

Of all the drugs discussed in this book, the cytotoxic drugs are amongst the most toxic and have a low therapeutic index. This means that a quite small increase in their activity can lead to the development of serious and life-threatening toxicity. A list of the cytotoxic agents which are featured appears in Table 13.1. Unlike most of the other interaction synopses in this book, some of the information on the cytotoxic drugs is derived from animal experiments and still requires confirmation in man. The reason for including this data is that the drugs in this group generally do not lend themselves readily to the kind of clinical studies which can be undertaken with other drugs, and there would seem to be justification in this instance for including indirect evidence. The aim is not to make definite predictions, but to warn users of the interaction possibilities.

Table 13.1 Cytotoxic drugs

Non-proprietary names	Proprietary names
Aclarubicin (aclacinomycin A)	*Aclacin*
Actinomycin (dactinomycin)	*Cosmegen, Lyovac*
Altretamine (hexamethylmelamine)	*Hexastat, Hexinawas*
Aminoglutethimide	*Cytraden, Orimeten, Orimeten*
Azathioprine	*Azamune, Azanin, Azapress, Imuran, Imurek, Imurel, Thioprine*
Bleomycin	*Blenoxane, Bleo-oil, Bleo-s, Blocamicina, Verbublen*
Carmofur	*Mifurol, Yamaful*
Carmustine (BCNU)	*Becenun, BiCNU, Carmubris, Citrumon*
Chlorambucil	*Leukeran, Linfolysin*
Chlorozotocin	
Cis-platin (CPDD)	*Cisplatyl, Citoplatino, Neoplatin, Placis, Platamine, Platiblastin, Platinex,Platinol, Platistin, Platosin*
Colaspase (asparaginase)	*Crasnitin(e), Elspar, Erwinase, Kidrolase, Leucogen, Leunase, Laspar*
Cyclophosphamide	*Carloxan, Cycloblastin, Cyclostin(e), Cytoxan, Endoxan(a), Enduxan, Genoxal, Neosar, Procytox, Sendoxan*
Cytarabine (cytosine arabinoside)	*Alexan, Arabitin, Aracytin(e), Erpalfa, Iretin*

continued on p. 463

Table 13.1 *(Continued)*

Non-proprietary names	Proprietary names
Dacarbazine	*DTIC-Dome*
Daunorubicin (daunomycin, rubidomycin)	*Cerubidin(e), Daunoblastin(a)*
Doxorubicin (adriamycin)	*Adriacin, Adriblastina, Farmiblastina*
Estramustine	
Etoposide	*Etopol, Vepesid*
Fluorouracil (5-FU)	*Adrucil, Arumel, Effluderm, Efudex, Efudix, Fluoroplex, Fluoroblastin(e), Timazin*
Hydroxyurea	*Hydrea, Litalir, Onco-Carbide*
Ifosfamide	*Holoxan, Mitoxana, Tronoxal*
Lomustine (CCNU)	*Belustine, Cecenu, CeeNU, CiNU, Lucostrine*
Melphalan	*Alkeran(a)*
Mercaptopurine	*Ismipur, Purinethol*
Methotrexate (amethopterin)	*Emtexate, Emthexat(e), Farmotrex, Folex, Ledertrexate, Maxtrex, Methotrexat, Metotraxato, Metrexan, Mexate, Tremetex*
Meturedepa	*Turloc*
Misonidazole	
Mitomycin (mitomycin C)	*Ametycine, Mitomycine-C, Mutamycin*
Mithramycin (plicamycin)	*Mithracin*
Mitotane	*Lysodren*
Mustine (methchlormethamine, Nitrogen mustard)	*Caryolysine, Cloramin, Mustargen*
Procarbazine	*Matulane, Natulan(ar)*
Streptozocin (streptozotocin)	*Zanosar*
Tamoxifen	*Istubol, Kessar, Noltam, Nolvadex, Tamaxin, Tamofen, Tamoxasta, Zitazonium*
Teniposide	
Thioguanine	*Lanvis*
Thiotepa	*Ledertepa, Onco-Tiotepa, Tifosyl*
Vinblastine	*Velban, Velbe*
Vincristine	*Kyocristine, Onconvin, Pericristine*
Vindesine	*Eldesine, Enison*

Aclarubicin and Cytotoxic drugs

Abstract/Summary

The bone marrow depressant effects of aclarubicin can be increased by previous treatment with nitrosoureas or mitomycin.

Clinical evidence, mechanism, importance and management

Myelosuppression is among the adverse effects of aclarubicin (aclacinomycin A). The makers warn that the concurrent use of other drugs with similar myelosuppressant actions may be expected to have additive effects and dosage reductions should be considered.[3] Prior treatment with nitrosoureas (not specifically named) or mitomycin has been shown to increase the severity of the myelosuppression.[1,2]

References

1 Van Echo DA, Whitacre MY, Aisner J, Applefeld MM, Wiernik PH. Phase I trial of aclacinomycin A. Cancer Treat Rep(1982) 66, 1127–32.
2 Bedikian AY, Karlin D, Stoehlein J, Valdivieso M, Korinek J, Bodey G. Phase II evaluation of aclacinomycin A (ACM-A, NSC 208734) in patients with metastatic colorectal cancer. Am J Clin Oncol (CCT) (1983) 6, 187–190.
3 Aclacin (aclarubicin hydrochloride) data sheet. Lundbeck (Feb 1990).

Altretamine (Hexamethylmelamine) + Antidepressants

Abstract/Summary

Severe orthostatic hypotension has been described in patients concurrently treated with altretamine and either phenelzine, amitriptyline or imipramine.

Clinical evidence, mechanism, importance and management

Five patients experienced very severe (described by the authors as potentially life-threatening) orthostatic hypotension when concurrently treated with altretamine (150–250 mg/m^2) and either phenelzine (60 mg), amitriptyline (50–150 mg) or imipramine (50 mg).[1] They experienced incapacitating dizziness, severe lightheadedness and/or fainting within a few days of taking both drugs concurrently. Standing blood pressures as low as 50/30 and 60/40 mm Hg were recorded. The reasons are not known. One of the patients had no problems when imipramine was replaced by nortriptyline (50 mg). The incidence of this interaction is unknown but it is clear that the concurrent use of these drugs should be closely monitored.

Reference

1 Bruckner HW, Schleifer SJ. Orthostatic hypotension as a complication of

hexamethylmelamine antidepressant interaction. Cancer Treat Rep (1983) 67, 516.

Aminoglutethimide + Bendroflumethiazide

Abstract/Summary

A single case report describes the severe loss of sodium in a patient after 10 months treatment with both drugs.

Clinical evidence, mechanism, importance and management

A woman who for several years had been taking four tablets daily of bendroflumethiazide (2.5 mg) and potassium chloride (578 mg) for hypertension and mild cardiac incompensation, was additionally treated with aminoglutethimide, 1 g daily, and hydrocortisone, 60 mg daily, for breast cancer. After 10 months' treatment she was hospitalized with severe hyponatremia due, apparently, to the combined inhibitory effects of the aminoglutethimide on aldosterone production (which normally retains sodium in the body) and the diuretic. The serum sodium levels were subsequently kept normal by the addition of fludrocortisone (0.1 mg daily).[1]

Reference

1 Bork E, Hansen M. Severe hyponatremia following simultaneous administration of aminoglutethimide and diuretics. Cancer Treat Rep (1986) 70, 689–90.

Azathioprine/Mercaptopurine + Allopurinol

Abstract/Summary

The effects of azathioprine and mercaptopurine are markedly increased by the concurrent use of allopurinol. The dosage of the cytotoxic drug should be reduced to a third or a quarter if toxicity is to be avoided. No interaction possibly occurs if these cytotoxic drugs are given intravenously. This needs confirmation.

Clinical evidence

(a) Azathioprine + Allopurinol

A patient on 300 mg allopurinol daily for gout was additionally given 100 mg azathioprine daily to treat autoimmune haemolytic anaemia. Within 10 weeks his platelet count fell from 236 to 45 x 10^9 /L, his white cell count fell from 9.4 to 0.8 x 10^9/L and his haemoglobin concentration fell from 115 to 53 g/L.[9]

A number of other reports similarly describe reversible bone marrow damage associated with anaemia, leucocytopenia and thrombocytopenia in patients when concurrently treated with azathioprine and allopurinol.[3-6,9-13] At least 13 cases have been reported. One fatality has been described.[11]

(b) Mercaptopurine + Allopurinol

Seven patients with chronic granulocytic leukaemia, treated with 50 mg mercaptopurine daily, showed a fall in granulocyte counts equivalent to four or five times the dose of mercaptopurine when additonally given 400 mg allopurinol daily.[1]

Profound pancytopenia developed in three children under treatment with mercaptopurine 2.5 mg/kg/day and allopurinol 10 mg/kg/day, but when the mercaptopurine dosage was halved no untoward effects were seen.[2] A pharmacokinetic study found that allopurinol caused a five-fold increase in peak plasma mercaptopurine concentrations and AUC when the mercaptopurine was given orally. The bioavailability increased from 12 to 59%.[7] This did not occur when the mercaptopurine was given intravenously.[7,8] Leucopenia and thrombocytopenia occurred in another patient given both drugs.[14]

Mechanism

Azathioprine is firstly metabolized in the liver to mercaptopurine and then enzymatically oxidized in the liver and intestinal wall by xanthine oxidase to an inactive compound (6-thiouric acid) which is excreted. Allopurinol inhibits this latter enzyme (inhibition of first-pass metabolism) so that the mercaptopurine accumulates, blood levels rise and its toxic effects develop (leucopenia, thrombocytopenia etc). In effect the patient suffers a gross overdose.

Importance and management

A well documented, well established, clinically important and potentially life-threatening interaction. The dosages of azathioprine and mercaptopurine should be reduced to about a third or a quarter when given orally to prevent the development of toxicity. On the basis of two studies[7,8] it would seem that this precaution may not be necessary if mercaptopurine is given intravenously, even so very close monitoring is advised with any route of administration.

References

1 Rundles RW, Wyngaarden JB, Hitchings GH, Elion GB, Silberman HR. Effects of xanthine oxidase inhibitor on thiopurine metabolism, hyperuricaemia and gout. Trans Assoc Am Phys (1963) 76, 126.

2 Levine AS, Sharpt HL, Mitchell J, Krivit W, Nesbit M. Combination therapy with 6-mercaptopurine (NSC-755) and allopurinol (NSC 1390) during induction and maintenance of remission of acute leukaemia in children. Cancer Chemother Rep (1969) 53, 53.

3 Glogner P, Heni N. Panzytopenie nach kombinationsbehandlung mit allopurinol und azathioprin. Med Welt (1976) 27, 1545.

4 Brooks RJ, Dorr RT, Durie BGM. Interaction of allopurinol with 6-mercaptopurine and azathioprine. Biomedicine (1982) 36, 217–22.

5 Klugkist H, Lincke HO. Panzytopenie unter Behandlung mit Azathioprin durch Interaktion mit Allopurinol bei Myasthenia gravis. Akt Neurol (1987) 14, 165–7.

6 Zazgornik J, Kopsa H, Schmidt P, Pils P, Kuschan K, Deutch E. Increased danger of bone marrow damage in simultaneous azathioprine-allopurinol therapy. Int J Clin Pharmacol Ther Toxicol (1981) 19, 96.

7 Zimm S, Collins JM, O'Neill D, Chabner BA, Poplak DG. Inhibition of first-pass metabolism in cancer chemotherapy: interaction of 6-mercaptopurine and allopurinol. Clin Pharmacol Ther (1983) 34, 810–17.

8 Coffey JJ, White CA, Lesk AB, Rogers WI, Serpick AA. The effect of allopurinol on the pharmacokinetics of 6-mercaptopurine in cancer patients. Cancer Res (1972) 32, 1283–9.

9 Boyd IW. Allopurinol-azathioprine interaction. J Intern Med (1991) 229, 386.

10 Raman GV, Sharman VL, Lee HA. Azathioprine and allopurinol: a potentially dangerous combination. J Intern Med (1990) 228, 69–71.

11 Adverse Drug Reactions Advisory Committee. Allopurinol and azathioprine. Fatal interaction. Med J Aust (1980) 2, 130.

12 Adverse Drug Reactions Advisory Committee. A reminder — the allopurinol azathioprine interactions. Australian Adverse Drug Reactions Bulletin. February 1985.

13 Garcia-Ortiz RE, De Los Angeles Rdriguez M. Pancytopenia associated with the interaction of allopurinol and azathioprine. J Pharm Technol (1991) 7, 224–6.

14 Berns A, Rubenfelds, Rymzo WI, and Calabro JJ. Hazard of combining allopurinol and thiopurine. N Engl J Med (1972) 286, 730–1.

Azathioprine/Mercaptopurine + Co-Trimoxazole or Trimethoprim

Abstract/Summary

The risk of potentially life-threatening haematological toxicity may be increased in renal transplant patients taking azathioprine if they are treated with co-trimoxazole or trimethoprim, particularly if given for extended periods. The same interaction would be expected with mercaptopurine.

Clinical evidence

The observation that haematological toxicity often seemed to occur in renal transplant patients given azathioprine and co-trimoxazole, prompted a retrospective survey of the records of 40 patients. It was found that there was no difference in the incidence of thrombocytopenia and neutropenia in those given azathioprine alone or with co-trimoxazole (160–20 mg trimethoprim + 800–1600 mg sulphamethoxazole daily) for a short time (6–16 days), but a significant increase occurred in the incidence and duration of these cytopenias if both drugs were given together for 22 days or more.[1]

A marked fall in white cell counts in renal transplant recipients during concurrent treatment with either co-trimoxazole (described as frequent) or trimethoprim (three cases) has been reported elsewhere.[2] In one case the fall occurred within five days and was treated by temporarily withdrawing the azathioprine and reducing the trimethoprim dosage from 300 to 100 mg daily.[2]

Mechanism

Not understood. It seems possible that the bone marrow depressant effects of all three drugs may be additive. In addition, impaired renal function may allow co-trimoxazole levels to become elevated, and haemodialysis may deplete folate levels which could exacerbate the anti-folate effects of the co-trimoxazole.

Importance and management

Information appears to be limited to the studies cited, but the interaction would seem to be established. The use of co-trimoxazole or trimethoprim in renal transplant patients may clearly be hazardous and potentially life-threatening. An as yet untested suggestion by the authors of the first study[1] is that folinic acid might be an effective treatment for bone marrow suppression without affecting the antimicrobial effects of the co-trimoxazole. A similar interaction would be expected with mercaptopurine. More study is needed.

References

1 Bradley PP, Warfen GD, Maxwell JG, Rothstein G. Neutropenia and thrombocytopenia in renal allograft recipients treated with trimethoprim-sulfamethoxazole. Ann Intern Med (1980) 93, 560.
2 Bailey RR. Leukopenia due to a trimethoprim-azathioprine interaction. NZ Med J (1984) 97, 739.

Azathioprine/Mercaptopurine + Doxorubicin (Adriamycin)

Abstract/Summary

The heptatoxicity of mercaptopurine and probably azathioprine can be increased by doxorubicin.

Clinical evidence, mechanism, importance and management

Liver damage induced by treatment with mercaptopurine was increased in 11 patients by the concurrent use of doxorubicin.[1] Since azathioprine is converted to mercaptopurine within the body, it would seem probable that increased hepatotoxicity will also be seen with this drug and doxorubicin.

Reference

1 Minow RA, Stern MH, Casey JH. Clinico-pathological correlation of liver damage in patients treated with 6-mercaptopurine. Cancer (1976) 38, 1524.

Bleomycin + Cisplatin

Abstract/Summary

Cisplatin can increase the pulmonary toxicity of bleomycin by reducing its renal excretion. Raynaud's phenomenon and arterial thrombosis have also been described.

Clinical evidence

30 patients with cervix carcinoma were given bleomycin followed by cisplatin intramuscularly every 12 h for four days. Another 15 patients with germ cell tumours were given bleomycin and then cisplatin by continuous infusion over 72 h. Nine of the patients with normal renal function and no previous pulmonary disease developed serious pulmonary toxicity and six died from respiratory failure.[7]

A study in 18 patients given both drugs for the treatment of disseminated testicular non-seminoma found that the cisplatin-induced reduction in renal function was paralleled by an increase in bleomycin-induced pulmonary toxicity. Two patients developed pneumonitis.[2]

A man with unrecognized acute renal failure due to cisplatin treatment died from pulmonary toxicity when he was given bleomycin.[4] A study in patients showed that the total clearance of bleomycin was halved (from 39 to 18 ml/min/m²) when concurrently treated with cisplatin in doses exceeding 300 mg/m² and the renal clearance in one patient fell from 30 to 8.2 ml/min/m². There was no evidence of severe bleomycin toxicity in these patients.[1] Renal dysfunction alone has also been reported in some instances to cause bleomycin toxicity.[3] Another report describes arterial thrombosis associated with pathological vascular changes arteries in a man treated with both drugs,[5] and Raynaud's phenomena is reported to occur in up to 41% of patients treated.[6]

Mechanism

Excretion by the kidney accounts for almost half of the total body clearance of bleomycin. Cisplatin is nephrotoxic and reduces the glomerular filtration rate so that the clearance of the bleomycin is reduced. The accumulating bleomycin apparently causes the pulmonary toxicity.

Importance and management

Pulmonary toxicity with bleomycin is an established reaction with a potentially serious, sometimes fatal, outcome. Concurrent use should be very closely monitored and renal function checked. One of the problems is that levels of creatinine may not accurately indicate the extent of renal damage, both during and after cisplatin treatment. The renal toxicity of cisplatin may also not develop gradually. Other toxic effects on the vascular system can also occur. One group of authors strongly advise that the bleomycin should, wherever possible, be given before the cisplatin to prevent accumulation of bleomycin in the plasma.[7]

References

1 Yee GC, Crom WR, Champion JE, Brodeur GM, Evans WE. Cisplatin-induced changes in bleomycin elimination. Cancer Treat Rep (1983) 67, 587–9.
2 van Barneveld PWC, Sleijfer D Th, van der Mark Th W, Mulder NH, Donker AJM, Meijer S, Schraffordt Koops H, Sluiter HJ, Peset R. Influence of platinum-induced pulmonary toxicity in patients with disseminated testicular carcinoma. Oncology (1984) 41, 4–7.

3 Perry DJ, Weiss RB, Taylor HG. Enhanced bleomycin toxicity during acute renal failure. Cancer Treat Rep (1982) 66, 592–3.

4 Bennett WM, Pastore L, Houghton DC. Fatal pulmonary toxicity in cis-platin-induced renal failure. Cancer Treat Rep (1980) 64, 921–4.

5 Garstin IWH, Cooper GG, Hood JM. Arterial thrombosis after treatment with bleomycin and cisplatin. Br Med J (1990) 300, 1018.

6 Vogelzang NJ, Bosi GJ, Johnson K, Kennedy BJ, Raynaud's phenomenon : a common toxicity after combination chemotherapy for testicular cancer. Ann Intern Med (1981) 95, 288–92.

7 Rabinowits M, Souhami L, Gil RA, Andrade CAV, Paiva HC. Increased pulmonary toxicity with bleomycin and cisplatin chemotherapy combinations. Am J Clin Oncol (1990) 13, 132–8.

Bleomycin + Oxygen

Abstract/Summary

Serious and potentially fatal pulmonary toxicity can develop in patients treated with bleomycin who are exposed to conventional oxygen concentrations during anaesthesia.

Clinical evidence

Five patients under treatment with bleomycin, exposed to oxygen concentrations of 39% during and immediately following anaesthesia, developed a severe respiratory distress syndrome and died. Bleomycin-induced pneumonitis and lung fibrosis were diagnosed at post-mortem. Another group of 12 matched patients who underwent the same procedures but with lower oxygen concentrations (22–25%) recovered uneventfully.[1]

Another comparative study similarly demonstrated that adult respiratory distress syndrome (ARDS) in patients on bleomycin was reduced by the use of lower oxygen concentrations (22–30%).[3] Bleomycin-induced pulmonary toxicity in man apparently related to oxygen concentrations has been described in other reports,[2,4,10,12,13] and has also been demonstrated in mice,[5] rats[6] and hamsters.[7] Other reports however found no obvious increase in pulmonary complications in patients on bleomycin exposed to oxygen in concentrations above 30%.[8,9]

Mechanism

Not understood. One suggestion is that bleomycin-injured lung tissue is less able to scavenge free oxygen radicals which may be present and damage occurs as a result.[2]

Importance and management

An established, well-documented, serious and potentially fatal interaction. It is advised that any patient on bleomycin undergoing general anaesthesia should have their inspired oxygen concentrations limited to less than 30% and the fluid replacement should be carefully monitored to minimize the crystalloid load. This is clearly very effective because having used these precautions Dr Goldiner writes that '...since ...1978 we have operated on more than 700 bleomycin treated patients....we

have seen no postoperative pulmonary failure in this group of patients.'[11] It has also been suggested that reduced oxygen levels should be continued during the recovery period and at any time during hospitalization.[2] If an oxygen concentration equal or greater than 30% has to be used, short term prophylactic corticosteroid administration should be considered. Intravenous corticosteroids should be given at once if bleomycin toxicity is suspected.[2]

References

1 Goldiner PL, Carlon CG, Cvitkovic E, Schweizer O, Howland WS. Factors influencing postoperative morbidity and mortality in patients treated with bleomycin. Br Med J (1978) 1, 1664.

2 Gilson AJ, Sahn SA. Reactivation of bleomycin lung toxicity following oxygen administration. A second response to corticosteroids. Chest (1985) 88, 304–6.

3 El-Baz N, Ivankovich AD, Faber LP, Logas WG. The incidence of bleomycin lung toxicity after anesthesia for pulmonary lung resection: a comparison between HFV and IPPV. Anesthesiology (1984) 61, A107.

4 Cersosimo RJ, Matthews SJ, Hong WK. Bleomycin pneumonitis potentiated by oxygen administration. Drug Intell Clin Pharm (1985) 19, 921–3.

5 Toledo CH, Ross WE, Block ER. Potentiation of bleomycin toxicity by oxygen. Cancer Treat Rep (1982) 66, 359–62.

6 Berend N. The effect of bleomycin and oxygen on rat lung. Pathology (1984) 16, 136–9.

7 Rinaldo J, Goldstein RH, Snider GL. Modification of oxygen toxicity after lung injury by bleomycin in hamsters. Am Rev Resp Dis (1982) 126, 1030–3.

8 Douglas MJ, Coppin CML. Bleomycin and subsequent anesthesia: a retrospective study at Vancouver General Hospital. Can Anaesth Soc J (1980) 27, 449–52.

9 Mandelbaum I, Williams SD, Einhorn LH. Aggressive surgical management of testicular carcinoma metastatic to lungs and mediastinum. Ann Thorac Surg (1980) 30, 224–9.

10 Hulbert JC, Grossman JE, Cummings KB. Risk factors of anesthesia and surgery in bleomycin-treated patients. J Urol (1983) 130, 163–4.

11 Goldiner PL. Editorial comment. J Urol (1983) 130, 164.

12 Allen SC, Riddell GS, Butchart EG. Bleomycin therapy and anaesthesia. The possible hazards of oxygen administration to patients after treatment with bleomycin. Anesthesia (1981) 36, 60–3.

13 Donohue JP, Rowland RG. Complications of retroperitoneal lymph node dissection. J Urol (1981) 125, 338–40.

Bleomycin + Various cytotoxic regimens

Abstract/Summary

There is evidence that the concurrent use of other cytotoxic drugs can increase the occurrence of bleomycin-induced pulmonary reactions.

Clinical evidence, mechanism, importance and management

18% (15 of 83) of the patients treated for non-Hodgkin's lymphomas with bleomycin (mean total dose 36 units) in conjunction with other cytotoxic drugs (M-Bacod, methotrexate, bleomycin, doxorubicin, cyclophosphamide, vincristine, dexamethasone), developed acute but completely reversible pulmonary reactions.[1] This is high compared with the 3–10%

incidence reported in those receiving bleomycin alone. Patients should be closely monitored. See also 'Bleomycin + Cisplatin.'

Reference

1 Bauer KA, Skarin AT, Balikina JP, Garnick MB, Rosenthal DS, Canellos GP. Pulmonary complications associated with combination chemotherapy program containing bleomycin. Am J Med (1983) 74, 557–63.

Carmofur + Alcohol

Abstract/Summary

A disulfiram-like reaction occurred in a patient on carmofur when given coeliac plexus blockade with alcohol.

Clinical evidence, mechanism, importance and management

A man with pancreatic carcinoma treated with 500 mg carmofur daily for 25 days experienced a disulfiram-like reaction (facial flushing, diaphoresis, hypotension — BP 60/30 mm Hg, and tachycardia — 128 bpm) within 30 min of being given coeliac plexus alcohol blockade for pain relief. Blood acetaldehyde levels were found to have risen sharply supporting the belief that the underlying mechanism is similar to the disulfiram-alcohol interaction (see 'Alcohol + Disulfiram'). It is suggested that alcohol blockade should be avoided for seven days after treatment with carmofur.[1]

Reference

1 Noda J, Umeda S, Mori K, Fukunaga T, Mizoi Y. Disulfiram-like reaction associated with carmofur after celiac plexus alcohol block. Anesthesiology (1987) 76, 908.

Carmustine (BCNU) + Cimetidine

Abstract/Summary

The bone marrow depressant effects of carmustine can be increased by the concurrent use of cimetidine. The fall in neutrophil and thrombocyte counts may become serious.

Clinical evidence

Six out of eight patients treated with carmustine, 80 mg/m^2 daily, for three days, cimetidine, 300 mg six-hourly, and steroids demonstrated marked leucopenia and thrombocytopenia after the first administrations. Biopsy confirmed the marked decrease in granulocytic elements. In comparison only six out of 40 patients treated similarly but without cimetidine showed comparable white cell and platelet depression.[1]

This increased myelotoxicity with marked falls in neutrophil counts has been described in another report.[2]

Mechanism

Cimetidine alone occasionally causes a marked fall in neutrophil numbers[3] and in some way, as yet not understood, it can augment the bone marrow depressant effects of carmustine.

Importance and management

Information appears to be limited to the reports cited, but it seems to be an established reaction. Patients given both drugs should be closely monitored for changes in neutrophil and platelet counts because the neutropenia may be life-threatening.

References

1 Selker RG, Moore P, LoDolce D. Bone-marrow depression with cimetidine plus carmustine. N Engl J Med (1978) 299, 834.
2 Volkin A, Shadduck RK, Winkelstein A, Zeigler ZR, Selker G. Potentiation of carmustine-cranial irradiation-induced myelosuppression by cimetidine. Arch Intern Med (1982) 142, 243–5.
3 Klotz S, Kay B. Cimetidine and agranulocytosis. Ann Intern Med (1978) 88, 579.

Cisplatin + Aminoglycoside antibiotics

Abstract/Summary

Acute and possibly life-threatening renal failure can occur in patients treated concurrently with cisplatin and aminoglycoside antibiotics such as gentamicin and tobramycin.

Clinical evidence

Four patients treated with cisplatin in dosages ranging from low to very high (eight doses of 0.5 to 5 mg/kg) and who were subsequently given gentamicin/cephalothin developed acute and fatal renal failure. Autopsy revealed extensive renal tubular necrosis.[1]

Two similar cases of severe renal toxicity attributed to the concurrent use of cisplatin with gentamicin/cephalothin are described elsewhere.[2,3] A very marked reduction in kidney function (as measured by a fall in creatinine clearance) has been described in three patients on cisplatin when they were subsequently treated with gentamicin or tobramycin.[5] A comparative study on 17 patients on cisplatin and gentamicin confirmed that the incidence of nephrotoxicity was increased by concurrent use, but the renal insufficiency was described as usually mild and not clinically significant.[4] There is also evidence from studies in children to show that the half-life of gentamicin is approximately doubled by the presence of cisplatin,[6] and aminoglycosides increase the risk of nephrotoxicity.[9] Both cisplatin and the aminoglycosides can cause the excessive loss of magnesium and combined use increases this loss.[7,9]

Mechanism

Cisplatin is nephrotoxic and it would appear that its damaging effects on the kidney are additive with the nephrotoxic and possibly the ototoxic effects of the aminoglycoside antibiotics. Enhanced renal toxicity and ototoxicity have been reported in guinea pigs concurrently treated with cisplatin and kanamycin.[8] The magnesium-losing effects of both also seem to be additive.

Importance and management

An established and potentially serious interaction. It has been recommended that these antibiotics should only be given with caution, or probably not at all, to patients under treatment with cisplatin,[1,2] although one report describing the use of gentamicin without cephalothin claims that concurrent use can be relatively safe.[4] There is some evidence that previous treatment with cisplatin can delay the clearance of the aminoglycosides.[10] Sequential use should therefore be well monitored and the magnesium status checked.

References

1 Gonzalez-Vitale JC, Hayes DM, Cvitkovic E, Sternberg SS. Acute renal failure after cis-Dichlorodiammineplatinum (II) and gentamicin-cephalothin therapies. Cancer Treat Rep (1978) 62, 693.

2 Salem PA, Jabboury KW, Khalil MF. Severe nephrotoxicity: a probable complication of cis-dichorodiammineplatinum (II) and cephalothin-gentamicin therapy. Oncology (1982) 39, 31–2.

3 Leite JBF, De Campelo Gentil F, Burchenal J, Marques A, Teixeira MIC, Abrao FA. Insuficienza renal aguda apos o uso de cis-diamino-dicloroplatina, gentamicina e cefalosporina. Rev Paul Med (1981) 97, 75–7.

4 Haas A, Anderson L, Lad T. The influence of aminoglycosides on the nephrotoxicity of cis-Diamminedichloroplatinum in cancer patients. J Infect Dis (1983) 147, 363.

5 Dentino M, Luft FC, Yum MN, Williams SD, Eihorn LH. Long term effect of cis-diamminedichloride platinum (CDDP) on renal functions and structure in man. Cancer (1978) 41, 1274–81.

6 Stewart CF, Christensen ML, Crom WR, Evans WE. The effect of cisplatin therapy on gentamicin pharmacokinetics. Drug Intell Clin Pharm (1984) 18, 512.

7 Flombaum CD. Hypomagnesiemia associated with cisplatin combination chemotherapy. Arch Intern Med (1984) 144, 2336–7.

8 Schweitzer VG, Hawkins JE, Lilly DJ, Litterst CJ, Abrams G, Davis JA, Christy M. Ototoxic and nephrotoxic effects of combined treatment with cis-diamminedichloroplatinum and kanamycin in the guinea pig. Otolaryngol (1984) 92, 38–49.

9 Pearson ADJ, Kohli M, Scott GW, Craft AW. Toxicity of high dose cisplatinum in children — the additive role of aminoglycosides. Proc Am Ass Cancer Res (1987) 28, 221.

10 Christensen ML, Stewart CF, Crom WR. Evaluation of aminoglycoside disposition in patients previously treated with cisplatin. Ther Drug Monit (1989) 11, 631–6.

Cisplatin + Antihypertensive agents

Abstract/Summary

A single report describes the development of kidney failure in a patient whose cisplatin-induced hypertension was treated with frusemide, hydralazine, diazoxide and propranolol.

Clinical evidence, mechanism, importance and management

Three hours after receiving cisplatin intravenously (70 mg/m² body surface area) a patient experienced severe nausea and vomiting and his blood pressure rose from 150/90 to 248/140 mm Hg. This was treated with frusemide (40 mg IV), hydralazine (10 mg IM), diazoxide (300 mg IV) and propranolol (40 mg orally for two days). Nine days later the patient showed evidence of renal failure which resolved within three weeks. The patient was subsequently similarly treated on two occasions with cisplatin and again developed hypertension, but no treatment was given and there was no evidence of kidney dysfunction.[1] The reasons for the kidney failure are not known, but studies in dogs[2] and rats[3] indicate that kidney damage may possibly be related to the concentrations of cisplatin and that frusemide can increase cisplatin levels in the kidney.

Information seems to be limited to the reports cited and its general clinical importance is uncertain, however the authors of the clinical report '...advise caution in treating hypertension or altering in any way renal hemodynamics in a patient receiving cisplatin.'[1]

References

1 Markman M, Trump DL. Nephrotoxicity with cisplatin and antihypertensive medications. Ann Intern Med (1982) 96, 257.

2 Cvitkovic E, Spauldind J, Bethune V. Improvement of cis-dichloro-diammineplatinum (NSC 119875): therapeutic index in an animal model. Cancer (1977) 39, 1357–61.

3 Pera MF, Zook BC, Harder HC. Effects of mannitol or furosemide diuresis on the nephrotoxicity and physiological disposition of cis-dichlor-diammineplatinum (II) in rats. Cancer Res (1979) 39, 1269–79.

Cisplatin + Ethacrynic acid

Abstract/Summary

Animal studies show that the damaging effects of cisplatin on the ear can be markedly increased by the concurrent use of ethacrynic acid. It seems possible that this could also occur in man.

Clinical evidence, mechanism, importance and management

Both cisplatin and ethacrynic acid given alone can be ototoxic in man. A study[1] carried out on guinea pigs showed that when cisplatin (7 mg/kg) or ethacrynic acid (50 mg/kg) were given alone their ototoxic effects were reversible, but when given together the damaging effects on the ear were '...profound, and prolonged, if not permanent.' Although this adverse interaction has not yet been reported in man, in the light of this study and what is already known about the ototoxicity of these two drugs in man, it seems possible that this may be a clinically important interaction. Audiometric tests should be carried out if these drugs are used concurrently.

Reference

1 Komune S, Snow JB. Potentiating effects of cisplatin and ethacrynic acid in ototoxicity. Arch Otolaryngol (1981) 107, 594–7.

Cisplatin + Methotrexate

Abstract/Summary

The risk of fatal methotrexate toxicity appears to be markedly increased by previous treatment with cisplatin.

Clinical evidence, mechanism, importance and management

Six out of 106 patients died with clinical signs of methotrexate toxicity 6–13 days after receiving 20–50 mg/m^2 in the absence of the usual signs of renal dysfunction and despite having previously been treated with methotrexate without serious toxicity. All had had prior treatment with cisplatin. Four of the patients were regarded as good-risk.[1] A study in children and adolescents suggested that the cumulative dose of cisplatin received appears to increase the risk of methotrexate toxicity.[2] Another study indicated that the sequential use of cisplatin and high-dose methotrexate was nephrotoxic and decreased the amount of methotrexate which could be given.[3] A report on 14 patients on high dose methotrexate indicated that prior treatment with one course of cisplatin sharply increased their serum levels of methotrexate, and after two courses the increase was even more marked (an eightfold rise).[4]

The picture is not totally clear but it seems possible that prior treatment with cisplatin causes kidney damage which may not necessarily be detectable with the usual creatinine clearance tests. The effect is to cause a marked reduction in the clearance of the methotrexate. The serum methotrexate levels of these patients should be closely monitored so that any delay in its clearance is detected early and appropriate measures taken.[2]

References

1 Haim N, Kedar A, Robinson E. Methotrexate-related deaths in patients previously treated with cis-diamminedichloride platinum. Cancer Chemother Pharmacol (1984) 13, 223–5.
2 Crom WR, Pratt CB, Green AA, Champion JE, Crom DB, Stewart CF, Evans WE. The effect of prior cisplatin therapy on the pharmacokinetics of high-dose methotrexate. J Clin Oncol (1984) 2, 655–61.
3 Pitman SW, Mino DR, Papac R. Sequential methotrexate-leucovorin (MTX-LCV) and cis-platinum (CDDP) in head and neck cancer. Proc AACR/ASCO (1979) 21, 166.
4 Crom WR, Teresi ME, Meyer WH, Green AA, Evans WE. The intrapatient effect of cisplatin therapy on the pharmacokinetics of high-dose methotrexate. Drug Intell Clin Pharm (1985) 19, 467.

Cisplatin + Probenecid

Abstract/Summary

On the basis of studies on animals it is uncertain whether the nephrotoxicity of cisplatin is increased or reduced by probenecid.

Clinical evidence, mechanism, importance and management

One study[1] in rats showed that probenecid could reduce cisplatin-induced nephrotoxicity, but other studies[2] found the complete opposite. The combination of cisplatin and probenecid was decidedly more toxic than cisplatin alone. Until this interaction has been more thoroughly studied this drug combination should be used with great care.

References

1 Ross DA, Gale GR. Reduction of renal toxicity of cis-dichloro-diammineplatinum (II) by probenecid. Cancer Treat Rep (1979) 63, 781–7.
2 Daley-Yates PT, McBrien DCH. Enhancement of cisplatin nephrotoxicity by probenecid. Cancer Treat Rep (1984) 68, 445–6.

Cyclophosphamide + Allopurinol

Abstract/Summary

There is evidence that the incidence of serious bone marrow depression caused by cyclophosphamide can by markedly increased by the concurrent use of allopurinol, but this was not confirmed in one study.

Clinical evidence

A retrospective epidemiological survey of patients in four hospitals who, over a four-year period, had been treated with cyclophosphamide showed that the incidence of serious bone marrow depression was 57.7% in 26 patients who had also received allopurinol, and 18.8% in 32 patients who had not. A threefold difference.[1]

A study in nine patients with malignant disease and two normal subjects showed that while taking 200 mg allopurinol daily the concentration of the cytotoxic metabolites of cyclophosphamide increased by an average of 37.5% (range – 1.5 to + 109%).[2] Agranulocytosis has been reported in another patient.[5] However another study,[4] designed as a follow-up to the study cited above[1] involving cytotoxic regimens which contained cyclophosphamide, failed to confirm that allopurinol increased the toxicity in patients with Hodgkin's or non-Hodgkin's lymphoma.

Mechanism

Not fully resolved. Cyclophosphamide itself is inactive, but it is converted in the liver into metabolites which are cytotoxic. Allopurinol possibly increases the activity of the liver enzymes concerned with the production of these metabolites.[2] Another idea is that it inhibits their loss from the kidneys.[2] Since the toxicity is related to the concentration of the metabolites,[3] the increased incidence of bone marrow depression is explained.

Importance and management

This interaction is not established with any certainty. The authors of the survey[1] cited write that '...there seem to be good grounds for re-evaluating the routine practice of administering allopurinol [with cyclophosphamide] prophylactically.' This does not forbid concurrent use, but introduces a strong note of caution.

References

1 Boston Collaborative Drug Surveillance Programme. Allopurinol and cytotoxic drugs. Interaction in relation to bone marrow depression. J Amer Med Ass (1974) 227, 1036.
2 Witten J, Fredericksen PL, Mouridsen HT. The pharmacokinetics of cyclophosphamide in man after treatment with allopurinol. Acta pharmacol et toxicol (1980) 46, 392.
3 Mouridsen HT, Witten J, Fredericksen PL,Hulsbaek I. Studies on the correlation between rate of biotransformation and haematological toxicity of cyclophosphamide. Acta pharmacol et toxicol (1978) 42, 81.
4 Stolbach L, Begg C, Bennett JM, Silverstein M, Falkson G, Harris DT, Glick J. Evaluation of bone marrow toxic reaction in patients treated with allopurinol. J Amer Med Ass (1982) 247, 334–6.
5 Beeley L, Daly M, Steward P. Bulletin of the W Midlands Centre for Adverse Drug Reaction Reporting (1987) 24, 26.

Cyclophophamide + Azathioprine

Abstract/Summary

A report describes liver damage in four patients given cyclophosphamide who had previously been treated with azathioprine.

Clinical evidence, mechanism, importance and management

Four patients (two with systemic lupus erythematosus, one with Sjogren's syndrome, and one with Wegeners granulomatosis) developed liver injury when given cyclosphosphamide. All had previously been treated with azathioprine. Three of them showed liver cell necrosis. Liver biopsy showed cytolytic necrosis of perihepatic venous hepatocytes. Two of them had had cyclophosphamide previously without apparent liver damage.[1] The relationship between the sequential use of these drugs is not established but these cases draw attention to the possibility of this adverse effect in other patients.

Reference

1 Shaunak S, Munro JM, Weinbren K, Walport MJ, Cox TM. Cyclophosphamide-induced liver necrosis: a possible interaction with azathioprine. Quart J Med (1988) New Series 76, 252, 309–17.

Cyclophosphamide + Barbiturates

Abstract/Summary

Despite some animal data, the evidence from studies in man suggests that neither the toxicity nor the therapeutic effects of cyclophosphamide are significantly affected by the concurrent use of the barbiturates.

Clinical evidence, mechanism, importance and management

There is evidence from a number of animal studies that the barbiturates and other potent liver enzyme-inducing agents can affect the activity of cyclophosphamide,[1,2] but studies undertaken in man indicate that although some changes in the pharmacokinetics of cyclophosphamide occur, neither the toxicity nor the therapeutic effects of cyclophosphamide are significantly altered.[3–5] No special precautions seem to be necessary.

References

1 Donelli MG, Colombo T, Garattini S. Effect of cyclophosphamide on the activity and distribution of pentobarbital in rats. Biochem Pharmacol (1973) 22, 2609.
2 Alberts DS, Van Daalen Wetters T. The effect of phenobarbital on cyclophosphamide antitumour activity. Cancer Res (1976) 36, 2785.
3 Bagley CM, Bostick FW, De Vita VT. Clinical pharmacology of cyclophosphamide. Cancer Res (1973) 33, 226.
4 Jao JY, Jusko WJ, Cohen JL. Phenobarbital effects on cyclophosphamide pharmacokinetics in man. Cancer Res (1972) 32, 2761.
5 Mellet LB. Chemistry and metabolism of cyclophosphamide: in Vancil (Ed) 'Immunosuppressive Properties of Cyclophosphamide', Mead Johnson and Co, Indiana. (1971) pp6–34.

Cyclophosphamide + Benzodiazepines

Abstract/Summary

Animal studies suggest that the benzodiazepines may possibly increase the toxicity of cyclophosphamide.

Clinical evidence, mechanism, importance and management

Studies in mice found that 3 days' treatment with benzodiazepines (chlordiazepoxide, diazepam, oxazepam) increased the lethality of the cyclophosphamide (without improving its effectiveness against Ehrlich solid tumour).[1] This may be due, it is suggested, to the induction of the liver enzymes concerned with the metabolism of cyclophosphamide to its active cytotoxic products. The importance of this possible interaction in man is uncertain, but the possibility should be borne in mind during concurrent use.

Reference

1 Sasaki K-I, Furusawa S, Takayanagi G. Effects of chlordiazepoxide, diazepam and oxazepam on the antitumour activity, the lethality and the blood levels of active metabolites of cyclophosphamide and cyclophosphamide oxidase activity in mice. J Pharm Dyn (1983) 6, 767–72.

Cyclophosphamide + Chloramphenicol

Abstract/Summary

Some limited evidence suggests that chloramphenicol may reduce the production of the therapeutically active metabolites of cyclophosphamide, thereby reducing its activity.

Clinical evidence, mechanism, importance and management

Cyclophosphamide itself is inactive, but after administration it is metabolized within the body to active alkylating metabolites. Animal studies[1] have shown that pretreatment with chloramphenicol reduces the activity (lethality) of cyclophosphamide because, it is believed, the antibiotic inhibits its conversion to these active metabolites. Studies[2] in four patients showed that 2 g chloramphenicol daily for 12 days prolonged the mean half-life of cyclophosphamide from 7.5 to 11.5 h and the production of the active metabolites fell. So it seems possible that a reduction in the activity of cyclophosphamide may also occur in man, but the extent to which this affects treatment with cyclophosphamide is uncertain. Concurrent use need not be avoided, but be on the watch for evidence of a reduced response. More study is needed.

References

1 Dixon RL. Effect of chloramphenicol on the metabolism and lethality of cyclophosphamide in rats. Proc Soc Exp Biol Med (1968) 127, 1151–5.
2 Faber OK, Mouridson HT, Skovsted L. The effect of chloramphenicol and sulphaphenazole on the biotransformation of cyclophosphamide in man. Br J Clin Pharmac (1975) 2, 281–5.

Cyclophosphamide + Corticosteroids

Abstract/Summary

There is evidence that single doses of prednisone can reduce the activity of cyclophosphamide, but longer term treatment may increase its activity.

Clinical evidence and mechanism

Cyclophosphamide itself is inactive, but after administration it is metabolized in the body to active metabolites. Single doses of prednisone have been shown to inhibit the activation of cyclophosphamide in man[1] (and animals[2]), probably due to competition for the drug-metabolizing enzymes in the liver. Longer-term treatment on the other hand (50 mg daily for 1–2 weeks) has been shown in man to have the opposite effect and increases the rate of activation of the cyclophosphamide, probably due to the induction of the liver enzymes.

Importance and management

The documentation is very limited and the interaction is poorly established, but changes in the activity of the cyclophosphamide should be watched for during concurrent use. Whether other corticosteroids behave in the same way as prednisone is uncertain. More study is needed.

References

1 Faber OK, Mouridsen HT. Cyclophosphamide activation and corticosteroids. N Engl J Med (1974) 291, 211.
2 Sladek NE. Therapeutic efficacy of cyclophosphamide as a function of inhibition of its metabolism. Cancer Res (1972) 32, 1848.

Cyclophosphamide + Dapsone

Abstract/Summary

Some extremely limited evidence suggests that dapsone might be capable of reducing the activity of cyclophosphamide.

Clinical evidence, mechanism, importance and management

An unexplained and undetailed report has described patients with leprosy on dapsone and cyclophosphamide who showed inhibition of the leucopenia normally associated with cyclophosphamide treatment.[1] Whether this indicates a reduction in the effects of cyclophosphamide is uncertain, but it would seem prudent to be on the alert for signs of a depressed therapeutic response to cyclophosphamide during concurrent treatment. More study is needed.

Reference

1 Quoted by Warren RD, Bender RA. Drug interactions with antineoplastic agents. Cancer Treat Rep (1977) 61, 1231.

Cyclophosphamide + Doxorubicin (Adriamycin)

Abstract/Summary

A single case report suggests that the damaging effects of cyclophosphamide and doxorubicin on the bladder may be additive.

Clinical evidence, mechanism, importance and management

A woman was treated with cyclophosphamide (100–150 mg daily orally) for three years for the treatment of breast cancer. The cyclophosphamide was withdrawn and replaced by doxorubicin (30 mg weekly IV). After five doses she developed a severe haemorrhagic cystitis, and bladder biopsy showed that the cyclophosphamide had caused chronic subclinical bladder damage which apparently was further damaged by the doxorubicin. The authors recommend that patients given doxorubicin should be carefully examined for microscopic haematuria, particularly if they have previously had cyclophosphamide or pelvic irradiation.[1]

Reference

1 Ershler WB, Gilchrist KW, Citrin DL. Adriamycin enhancement of cyclophosphamide-induced bladder injury. J Urol (1980) 123, 121–2.

Cyclophosphamide + Indomethacin

Abstract/Summary

A single case report describes acute water intoxication in a patient taking indomethacin when given low dose intravenous cyclophosphamide.

Clinical evidence, mechanism, importance and management

A patient with multiple myelomatosis and adequate renal function on 50 mg indomethacin 8-hourly, developed acute water intoxication and salt retention after being given a single bolus IV injection of 500 mg cyclophosphamide (10 mg/kg). The reasons are not understood, but it is suggested that it was due to the additive or synergistic effects of the two drugs. Indomethacin inhibits the production of the renal vasodilatory prostaglandins (PgE_2, PgI_2) which affect the renal blood flow and also inhibit salt and water reabsorption by the kidney. The cyclosphophamide produces metabolites which have antidiuretic effects.

The general importance of this case is uncertain, but the authors of the report suggest caution if both drugs are used.

Reference

1 Webberley M J, Murray J A. Life-threatening acute hyponatremia induced by low dose cyclophosphamide and indomethacin. Postgrad Med J (1989) 65, 950–2.

Cyclophosphamide or Mustine + Morphine or Pethidine

Abstract/Summary

Animal studies indicate that the toxicity of cyclophosphamide and mustine is increased by morphine or pethidine.

Clinical evidence, mechanism, importance and management

Studies in mice[1] have shown that morphine in doses of 5–25 mg/kg increases sublethal doses of cyclophosphamide (300 mg/kg) and mustine (5 mg/kg) into maximally lethal doses. The effect of pethidine (meperidine) was less marked. This work suggests that there may be a need to re-evaluate the concurrent use of these drugs in man.

Reference

1 Akintonwa A. Potentiation of nitrogen mustard toxicity by narcotic analgesic. Clin Toxicol (1981) 18, 451–8.

Cyclophosphamide + Ranitidine

Abstract/Summary

Ranitidine appears not to increase the bone marrow toxicity of cyclophosphamide.

Clinical evidence, mechanism, importance and management

A study in seven cancer patients found that although 300 mg oral ranitidine daily signficantly prolonged the half-life and increased the AUC (area under the curve) of cyclosphosphamide (600 mg/m^2 cyclophosphamide given intravenously), it did not significantly affect the AUCs of the two major oncolytic metabolites of cyclophosphamide nor did it affect its bone marrow toxicity (leucopenia, granulocyopenia).

The authors of the study conclude that ranitidine can safely be given with cyclosphosphamide.[1]

Reference

1 Alberts DS, Mason-Liddil N, Plezia PM, Roe DJ, Dorr RT, Struck RF, Phillips JG. Lack of ranitidine effects on bone cyclophosphamide bone marrow toxicity or metabolism: a placebo-controlled clinical trial. J Nat Cancer Inst (1991) 83, 1739–43.

Cyclophosphamide + Sulphaphenazole

Abstract/Summary

Some very limited evidence suggests that sulphaphenazole may increase or decrease the activity of cyclophosphamide, but the clinical importance of this is uncertain.

Clinical evidence, mechanism, importance and management

A study[1] in seven subjects on a 50 g dose of cyclophosphamide given 2 g sulphaphenazole daily for 9–14 days showed that the half-life of the cyclophosphamide was unchanged in three, longer in two and shorter in the remaining two. The reasons are not clear. Whether this has any practical importance or not is uncertain, but it would seem prudent to be on the watch for changes in the response to cyclophosphamide if sulphaphenazole is given concurrently. More study is needed. Information about other sulphonamides appears to be lacking.

Reference

1 Faber OK, Mouridsen HT, Skovsted L. The effect of chloramphenicol and sulphaphenazole on the biotransformation of cyclophosphamide in man. Br J Clin Pharmac (1975) 2, 281.

Cytotoxics + Calcium channel blockers

Abstract/Summary

Verapamil can increase the efficacy of doxorubicin both in tissue culture systems and in patients. It raises serum doxorubicin levels. The absorption of verapamil can be reduced by COPP and VAC cytotoxic drug regimens.

Clinical evidence, mechanism, importance and management

(a) The effect of calcium channel blockers on cytotoxics

The efficacy of doxorubicin can be increased by verapamil and nicardipine in doxorubicin-resistant tissue culture systems[1] and its pharmacokinetics can also be changed by verapamil. A study[2] in five patients with small cell lung cancer given doxorubicin, vincristine and cyclophosphamide showed that when given verapamil (240–480 mg daily) the AUC of the doxorubicin was doubled, peak serum levels were raised and the clearance was reduced. No increased toxicity was seen in this study or in two others,[3,4] but be alert for this possibility if drugs are used.

effect of cytotoxics on calcium channel blockers

In nine patients with a variety of malignant diseases showed that treatment with cytotoxic drugs reduced the absorption of 160 mg verapamil given orally. The AUC in eight patients was reduced by 40% (range 7–58%). One patient showed a 26% increase. Five patients received a modified COPP regimen (cyclophosphamide, onconvin, procarbazine, prednisone) and four VAC (vindesine, adriamycin, cisplatin).[5] It is believed that these cytotoxics damage the lining of the upper part of the small intestine which impairs the absorption of verapamil. Patients should be monitored for signs of a reduced response to verapamil during concurrent treatment.

References

1 Ramu A, Spanier R, Rahamimoff H, Fuks Z. Restoration of doxorubicin responsiveness in doxorubicin-resistant P388 murine leukaemia cells. Br J Cancer (1984) 50, 501–7.

2 Kerr DJ, Graham J, Cummings J, Morrison JG, Thompson GG, Brodie MJ, Kaye SB. The effect of verapamil on the pharmacokinetics of adriamycin. Cancer Chemother Pharmacol (1986) 18, 32.

3 Ozols RF, Rogan AM, Hamilton TC, Klecker R, Young RC. Verapamil plus adriamycin in refractory ovarian cancer: design of a clinical trial on basis of reversal of adriamycin resistance in human ovarian cancer cell lines. AACR (1986) Abstract 1186.

4 Presant CA, Kennedy P, Wiseman C, Gala K, Wyres M. Verapamil plus adriamycin — a phase I-II clinical study. Proc Am Soc Clin Oncol (1984) 3, 1–124.

5 Kuhlmann J, Woodcock B, Wilke J, Rietbrock N. Verapamil plasma concentrations during treatment with cytostatic drugs. J Cardiovasc Pharmacol (1985) 7, 1003–6.

Cytotoxics + Food

Abstract/Summary

The absorption of melphalan can be reduced by food, but etoposide is unaffected. Low dose methotrexate appears not to be significantly affected by food.

Clinical evidence, mechanism, importance and management

(a) Etoposide

The plasma etoposide concentrations of 11 patients with extensive small cell lung carcinoma given 100 mg oral doses were unaffected when taken with breakfast (milk, cornflakes, sugar, egg, sausage, bread, margarine, marmalade, coffee or tea). Also no changes were seen when the etoposide was taken with cyclophosphamide (100 mg/m²), methotrexate (12.5 mg/m²) or procarbazine (60 mg/m²) given orally.[3]

(b) Melphalan

A study in five patients with multiple myeloma showed that the half-life of melphalan (5mg/m²) was unaffected when taken with a standardized breakfast, but the area under the curve was reduced to an average of 43% (range 0–78%). In one patient no melphalan was detectable when given with food.[2]

(c) Methotrexate

The peak serum methotrexate levels (measured at 1.5 h) of 10 children with lymphoblastic leukemia, following an oral dose (15 mg/m^2) were reduced about 40% when taken with a milky meal (milk, cornflakes, sugar, white bread and butter). The area under the 4 h concentration/time curve was reduced about 25%. A smaller reduction was seen after a 'citrus meal' (orange juice, fresh orange, white bread, butter and jam).[1] However a four-hour study is too short to assess the extent of the total absorption. Another study in 16 other children given 8–22.7 mg/m^2 methotrexate found that peak levels were lower if given before a meal, but the AUC was unaffected.[4] Yet another study in 12 healthy subjects found that a high fat-content breakfast delayed the absorption of methotrexate (7.5 mg orally) by about 30 min but the extent of the absorption was unchanged.[5]

References

1 Pinkerton CR, Welshman SG, Glasgow JFT, Bridges JM. Can food influence the absorption of methotrexate in children with acute lymphoblastic leukaemia? Lancet (1980) 2, 944–5.
2 Kotasek D, Dale BM, Morris RG, Reece PA, Sage RE. Food reduces melphalan absorption. Aust NZ J Med (1985) 15 (Suppl 1) 120.
3 Harvey VJ, Slevin ML, Joel SP, Johnston A, Wrigley PFM. The effect of food and concurrent chemotherapy on the bioavailability of oral etoposide. Br J Cancer (1985) 52, 363–7.
4 Mandat F, Awidi A, Shaheen O, Ottman S, Al-Turk W. Effects of food and gender on the pharmacokinetics of methorexate in children. Res Commun Chem Pathol Pharmacol (1987) 55, 279–82.
5 Kozloski GD, De Vito JM, Kisicki JC, Johnson JB. The effect of food on the absorption of methotrexate sodium tablets in healthy volunteers. Arth Rheum (1992) 35, 761–4.

Cytotoxics + Gentamicin

Abstract/Summary

There is evidence that the use of gentamicin with daunorubicin, thioguanine and cytarabine may cause hypomagnesaemia.

Clinical evidence, mechanism, importance and management

The observation of hypomagnesaemia in two patients given gentamicin (with lincomycin or mezlocillin) during induction therapy for non-lymphoblastic leukaemia prompted further study in another nine patients. They were all treated with the same cytotoxic regimen: daunorubicin 50 mg/m^2 IV day 1, thioguanine 100 mg/m^2 twice daily orally on days 1–5, and cytarabine 100 mg/m^2 twice daily IV on days 1–5. Six out of 11 patients demonstrated hypomagnesaemia.[1] The reasons are not known but suggestions include a direct nephrotoxic action of the cytotoxic drugs, or the cytotoxics may sensitize the kidneys to the actions of gentamicin. Concurrent use should be well monitored.

Reference

1 Davey P, Gozzard D, Goodall M, Leyland MJ. Hypomagnesaemia: an underdiagnosed interaction between gentamicin and cytotoxic chemotherapy for acute non-lymphoblastic leukaemia. J Antimicrob Chemother (1985) 15, 623–8.

Cytotoxics + Ondansetron

Abstract/Summary

Cisplatin and 5-fluorouracil do not affect the pharmacokinetics of ondansetron, but ondansetron appears to increase the nephrotoxicity of zeniplatin. Dexamethasone can be safely given with ondansetron.

Clinical evidence, mechanism, importance and management

No significant changes in the pharmacokinetics of ondansetron occurred in 20 cancer patients on cisplatin (20–40 mg/m^2) and/or 5-fluorouracil (1 g/m^2) for five days but the clearance was lower than in normal subjects.[1] Preliminary data indicate that ondansetron can be safely combined with dexamethasone to increase the antiemetic effects.[2]

A phase II trial of zeniplatin in 308 patients found that nephrotoxicity occurred in 22 of them (7%). 32 of the 308 had been given ondansetron hydrochloride alone or with dexamethasone as antiemetic treatment, and 14 of the 32 (ie 44%) developed nephrotoxicity of varying severity. Only 8 of the other patients (3%) who had not had ondansetron developed nephrotoxicity.[3] The reasons for this increased nephrotoxicity are not known but these preliminary observations suggest that concurrent use should be undertaken with caution.

References

1 Hsyu P-H, Bozigian HP, Pritchard JF, Kernodle A, Panella J, Hansen LA, Griffin RH. Effect of chemotherapy on the pharmacokinetics of oral ondansetron. Pharm Res (1991) 8 (Suppl 10) S-257.
2 Kris MG. Rationale for combination antiemetic therapy and strategies for the use of ondansetron in combination. Semin Oncol (1992) 19 (Suppl 10) 61–6.
3 Aamdal S. Can ondansetron hydrochloride (Zofran®) enhance the nephrotoxic potential of other drugs ? Ann Oncol (1992) 3, 774.

Cytotoxics + Propofol

Abstract/Summary

Severe pain may occur in patients given intravenous propofol who have previously had intravenous chemotherapy.

Clinical evidence, mechanism, importance and management

A girl of 15 with acute lymphoblastic leukaemia who been

treated with several injections of cyclophosphamide, methotrexate and vincristine during the previous 6 months, was cannulated in her hand and infused with *Plasmlyte B*. An injection of 60 μg fentanyl was painful and 20 mg lignocaine helped, but 20 mg (2 ml) propofol caused extreme pain and a further 20 mg lignocaine was given. The whole hand became blue and congested, and blood began to move backwards up the drip tubing. The venous congestion gradually subsided over the next 15 min.[1] This case is similar to another in which severe pain after iv administration of propofol with lignocaine occurred in a patient on chemotherapy.[2] The authors of the first report cited[1] recommend that propofol should be avoided in patients who have recently had intravenous chemotherapeutic agents.[1]

References

1 Butt AD, James MFM. Venospasm due to propofol. SAMT (1990) 77, 168.
2 Whitlock JC, Nicol ME, Pattison J. Painful injection of propofol. Anaesthesia (1989) 44, 618.

Cytotoxics + Vaccines

Abstract/Summary

The immune response of the body is suppressed by cytotoxic drugs. The effectiveness of the vaccine may be poor and generalized infection may occur in patients immunized with live vaccines.

Clinical evidence, mechanism, importance and management

Since the cytotoxic drugs are immunosuppressants, the response of the body to immunization is reduced. A study[1] in 53 patients with Hodgkins disease showed that chemotherapy reduced the antibody response 60% when measured three weeks after immunization with a pneumococcal vaccine. The patients were treated with mustine, vincristine, prednisone and procarbazine. A few of them also had bleomycin, vinblastine or cyclophosphamide. Subtotal radiotherapy reduced the response a further 15%. The response to influenza immunization in children with various malignancies was also found to be markedly suppressed by chemotherapy. The cytotoxic drugs used were mercaptopurine, methotrexate, vincristine and prednisone. Some of them were also treated with vincristine, actinomycin and cyclophosphamide.[2] Only nine out of 17 children with leukaemia and other malignant diseases treated with methotrexate, cyclosphosphamide, mercaptopurine and prednisone developed a significant response to immunization with inactivated measles vaccine.[5]

Immunization with live vaccines may result in a potentially life-threatening infection. For example, a woman who was under treatment with 15 mg methotrexate daily for psoriasis and who was vaccinated against smallpox, developed a generalized vaccinial infection.[3] Studies in animals given smallpox vaccine confirmed that they were more susceptible to infection if treated with methotrexate, mercaptopurine or cyclophosphamide.[4]

Smallpox is no longer a problem, but other live vaccines such as rubella, measles, mumps and others continue to be used. Extreme care should therefore be exercised in immunizing patients with live vaccines who are receiving cytotoxics or other immunosuppressive treatment (see also 'Corticosteroids + Live Vaccines').

References

1 Siber GR, Weitzman SA, Aisenberg AC, Weinstein HJ, Schiffman A. Impaired antibody response to pneumococcal vaccine after treatment for Hodgkins disease. N Engl J Med (1978) 299, 442–8.
2 Gross PA, Lee H, Wolff JA, Hall CB, Minnefore AB, Lazicki ME. Influenza immunization in immunosuppressed children. J Pediatr (1978) 92, 30–5.
3 Allison J. Methotrexate and smallpox vaccination. Lancet (1968) ii, 1250.
4 Rosenbaum EH, Cohen RA, Glatstein HR. Vaccination of a patient receiving immunosuppresive therapy for lymphosarcoma. J Amer Med Ass (1966) 198, 737.
5 Stiehm ER, ABlin A, Kushner JH, Zoger S. Measles vaccination in patients on immunosuppressive drugs. Amer J Dis Child (1966) 111, 191–4.

Doxorubicin (Adriamycin) + Actinomycin + Plicamycin (Mithramycin)

Abstract/Summary

A case of fatal cardiomyopathy attributed to the concurrent use of doxorubicin (adriamycin), actinomycin-D and plicamycin (mithramycin) has been described.

Clinical evidence, mechanism, importance and management

A patient developed fatal cardiomyopathy apparently due to the use of doxorubicin, actinomycin-D and plicamycin. The general importance of this is uncertain, but it would seem prudent to be on the alert for changes in cardiac function in patients treated with these drugs.[1]

Reference

1 Kushner JP, Hansen VL, Hammar SP. Cardiomyopathy after widely separated courses of adriamycin exacerbated by actinomycin-D and mithramycin. Cancer (1975) 36, 1577.

Doxorubicin (Adriamycin) + Barbiturates

Abstract/Summary

The effects of doxorubicin may be reduced by the concurrent use of barbiturates.

Clinical evidence, mechanism, importance and management

A comparative study in patients treated with doxorubicin showed that those concurrently taking barbiturates had a plasma clearance which was 50% higher than those who were not (318 compared with 202 ml/min).[1] This clinical study confirms previous studies in mice.[2] A possible explanation is that the barbiturate increases the metabolism of the doxorubicin. It seems likely that the dosage of doxorubicin will need to be increased in barbiturate-treated patients to achieve maximal therapeutic effects.

References

1 Riggs CE, Engel S, Wesley M, Wiernik PH, Bachur NR. Doxorubicin pharmacokinetics, prochlorperazine and barbiturate effects. Clin Pharmacol Ther (1982) 31, 263.
2 Reich SD, Bachur NR. Alterations in adriamycin efficacy by phenobarbital. Cancer (1976) 36, 3803.

Doxorubicin (Adriamycin) + Beta-blockers

Abstract/Summary

Animal data suggest that additive cardiotoxicity may occur with doxorubicin and propranolol. This awaits clinical confirmation.

Clinical evidence, mechanism, importance and management

A very well recognized problem with doxorubicin is its cardiotoxicity and cardiomyopathy. Studies in mice[1] showed that mortality was significantly increased when doxorubicin (18 and 23 mg/kg) and propranolol (1 and 10 mg/kg) were given concurrently, possibly because both drugs can inhibit the activity of two cardiac CoQ_{10} enzymes (succinoxidase, NADH oxidase) which are essential for mitochondrial respiration. There is no clinical confirmation of this interaction in man, but the authors of this animal study suggest that concurrent use may be contraindicated.

Reference

1 Choe JY, Combs AB, Folkers K. Potentiation of the toxicity of adriamycin by propranolol. Res Comm Chem Pathol Pharmacol (1978) 21, 577.

Doxorubicin (Adriamycin) + Cyclosporin(e)

Abstract/Summary

An isolated report describes severe neurotoxicity and coma in a patient previously on cyclosporin when given doxorubicin.

Clinical evidence, mechanism, importance and management

A cardiac transplant patient was treated with cyclosporin (2 mg/kg daily) for 22 months. The cyclosporin was stopped and he was given 60 mg doxorubicin, 2 mg vincristine, 600 mg cyclophosphamide and 80 mg prednisone to treat Burkitt's lymphoma stage IVB. 8 h later he developed disturbances of consciousness which lead to stage I coma from which he spontaneously recovered 12 h later. A week later a similar course of chemotherapy was started. 10–15 min later he lost consciousness and generalized tonic clonic seizures progressively developed. He died eight days later without recovering from the coma. On the basis of later studies in animals the authors of this report suggest that the cyclosporin may have affected the blood-brain barrier, thereby allowing the diffusion of the doxorubicin into the brain where it has neurotoxic effects. They suggest that whatever the mechanism of this interaction, caution should be exercised in giving doxorubicin to cancer patients on cyclosporin.[1]

Reference

1 Barbui T, Rambaldi A, Parenzan L, Zucchelli M, Perico N, Remuzzi G. Neurological symptoms and coma associated with doxorubicin administration during chronic cyclosporin therapy. Lancet (1992) 339, 1421.

Estramustine + Food or milk

Abstract/Summary

The absorption of estramustine is reduced by milk and foods containing calcium.

Clinical evidence

A randomized three-way crossover study in six patients with prostatic cancer showed that the absorption of single doses of the disodium salt, equivalent to 140 mg of estramustine, were reduced to 41% when taken with 200 ml milk, and to 67% when taken with a standardized breakfast (2 pieces of white bread with margarine, ham, tomato, marmalade and water). Peak serum estramustine levels were reduced to 32 and 57% respectively.[1]

Mechanism

In vitro studies suggest that estramustine combines with calcium ions in milk and food to form a poorly-soluble complex which is not as well absorbed as the parent compound.[1]

Importance and management

An established interaction although the information is limited. The authors suggest that estramustine should be taken at a set time in relation to food intake, and not with milk, calcium-containing milk products (eg yoghourt) or food if maximal absorption is to be achieved. If the suggested mechanism of interaction is correct, estramustine should also not be taken with calcium-containing drugs (eg some antacids).

Reference

1 Gunnarsson P O, Davidsson T, Andersson S-B, Backman C, Johansson S-Å. Impairment of estamustine phosphate absorption by concurrent intake of milk and food. Eur J Clin Pharmacol (1990) 38, 189–93.

Etoposide + Anticonvulsants

Abstract/Summary, clinical evidence, mechanism, importance and management

A preliminary study found that the clearance of etoposide (doses 320–500 mmg/m²) was increased 170% in five paediatric patients with cancer taking phenobarbitone or phenytoin (doses not stated).[1] Be alert for the need to give larger doses of etoposide if these anticonvulsants are used.

Reference

1 Rodman JH, Murry DJ, Madden T, Santana VM. Pharmacokinetics of high doses of etoposide and the influence of anticonvulsants in pediatric cancer patients. Clin Pharmacol Ther (1992) 51, 156.

Etoposide + Cisplatin

Abstract/Summary

The clearance of etoposide is reduced by cisplatin given acutely but not when given chronically.

Clinical evidence, mechanism, importance and management

A study in 17 children with neuroblastoma found that when cisplatin (90 mg/m² iv) was given acutely, the clearance of etoposide (780 mg/m²) fell and the serum levels rose. But when the cisplatin was given chronically, it had no effect on the clearance of etoposide.[1] The reasons are not understood. The clinical importance of these findings is uncertain.

Reference

1 McLeod HL, Santana VM, Bowman LC, Furman WL, Relling MV. Etoposide pharmacokinetic are influenced by acute but not by chronic cisplatin exposure. Proc Amer Ass Cancer Res (1992) 33, 531.

Etoposide + Cyclosporin(e)

Abstract/Summary

High dose cyclosporin markedly raises etoposide serum levels and increases the suppression of white blood cell production. Severe toxiicity has been reported in one patient.

Clinical evidence

A comparative study in 16 patients with multidrug resistance and advanced cancer given 20 paired courses of etoposide alone or with cyclosporin found that cyclosporin concentrations of either more or less than 2000 ng/ml increased the etoposide AUC by 80% or 50% respectively, decreased the total clearance by 38% or 28%, increased its half-life by 108 or 40%, reduced the leucocyte count nadir by − 64 or − 37% and altered the volume of distribution at steady state by 46 and 1.4%.[1] The patients were given 150–200 mg/m² etoposide for 3 consecutive days as a 2-hr IV infusion and cyclosporin as a 3-day continuous infusion in doses ranging from 5–21 mg/kg/day.[1]

The leukaemic cells in the bone marrow of a patient with acute T-lymphocyte leukaemia were totally cleared with cyclosporin (8.3 mg/kg orally twice daily) and etoposide (100–300 mg daily for 2–5 days), but the side-effects were severe (mental confusion, renal and hepatic toxicity). The patient died from respiratory failure.[2]

Mechanism

It is suggested that the cyclosporin decreases the metabolism of the etoposide (by inhibiting its cytochrome P-450 mediated metabolism and inhibiting P-glycoprotein mediated efflux from the hepatocyte) as well as inhibiting some unknown non-renal clearance mechanism.[1] The total effect is to cause the retention of etoposide in the body, thereby increasing its effects.

Importance and management

An established interaction. The authors of report cited advise an etoposide dosage reduction of 50% if used with high-dose cyclosporin in patients with normal kidney and liver function.[1] More study is needed to find out the possible effects of low-dose cyclosporin.

References

1 Lum BL, Kaubisch S, Yahanda AM, Adler KM, Jew L, Ehsan MN, Brophy NA, Halsey J, Gosland MP, Sikic BI. Alteration of etoposide pharmacokinetics and pharmacodynamics by cyclosporine in a phase I trial to modulate multidrug resistance. J Clin Oncol (1992) 10, 1635–42.
2 Kloke O, Isieka R. Interaction of cyclosporin A, antineoplastic agents. Klin Wsch (1985) 63, 1081–2.

5-Fluorouracil + Aminoglycosides

Abstract/Summary

Neomycin can delay the gastrointestinal absorption of 5-fluorouracil, but the clinical importance of this is uncertain.

Clinical evidence, mechanism, importance and management

Some preliminary information from a study in 12 patients under treatment for adenocarcinoma showed that treatment with oral neomycin (2 g daily for a week) delayed the absorption of 5-fluorouracil, but the effects were generally too small to reduce the therapeutic response, except possibly in one patient.[1] It seems probable that this interaction occurs because neomycin can induce a malabsorbtion syndrome. If neomycin, paromomycin or kanamycin are used in patients on 5-fluorouracil, the possibility of this interaction should be borne in mind.

Reference

1 Bruckner HW, Creasey WA. The administration of 5-fluorouracil by mouth. Cancer (1974) 33, 14.

5-Fluorouracil + Cimetidine

Abstract/Summary

Serum 5-fluorouracil levels are increased about 75% by the concurrent use of cimetidine for a month.

Clinical evidence

A study in six patients with carcinoma under treatment with 5-fluorouracil (15 mg/kg daily for five days, repeated every 4 weeks) showed that treatment with 1 g cimetidine daily for 4 weeks increased peak plasma 5-FU concentrations by 74% and the AUC by 72% when given orally. When given intravenously the AUC was increased by 27%. The total body clearance was reduced by 28%.[1] The pharmacokinetics of 5-FU were unaltered by the use of cimetidine for only a week.

Mechanism

Uncertain. It is probably a combination of a reduction in the metabolism of the 5-FU caused by the cimetidine (a well-known enzyme inhibitor) and a reduction in blood flow through the liver.

Importance and management

Direct information appears to be limited to this study, but the interaction would seem to be established. Concurrent treatment should be undertaken with particular care because of the risks of 5-FU overdosage. A reduction in the dosage may be necessary.

Reference

1 Harvey VJ, Slevin ML, Dilloway MR, Clark PI, Johnston A, Lant AF. The influence of cimetidine on the pharmacokinetics of 5-fluorouracil. Br J clin Pharmac (1984) 18, 421–30.

5-Fluorouracil + Cisplatin

Abstract/Summary

The addition of low-dose cisplatin to fluorouracil infusion markedly increases the toxicity. Cardiotoxicity may possibly be increased with higher doses of methotrexate.

Clinical evidence, mechanism, importance and management

The addition of weekly low-dose cisplatin ($20\ mg/m^2$) to continuous ambulatory fluorouracil infusions ($300\ mg/m^2/day$) considerably increased the toxicity (nausea, vomiting, anorexia, diarrhoea, stomatitis, myelosuppression) of 18 patients with advanced cancers. More than half developed multiple toxicities, and severe toxicity occurred in two-thirds. Leucopenia occurred in 28% given both drugs whereas it is virtually nonexistent with 5-FU alone. 55% of patients on 5-FU alone had toxicity requiring treatment interruption or dose reduction. This rose to 94% when given both drugs.[1] In another study of 80 patients with carcinoma of the head, neck, oesophagus and stomach it was found that concurrent use increased the cardiotoxicity (chest pain, ST-T wave changes, arrhythmias) by 15%.[2] Concurrent use clearly needs careful evaluation.

References

1 Jeske J, Hansen RM, Libnoch JA, Anderson T. 5-Fluorouracil infusion and low-dose weekly cisplatin: an analysis of increased toxicity. Am J Clin Oncol (CCT) (1990) 13, 485–8.
2 Jeremic B, Jevremovic S, Djuric L, Mijatoivic L. Cardiotoxicity during chemotherapy treatment with 5-flurouracil and cisplatin. J Chemotherapy (1990) 2, 264–7.

5-Fluorouracil + Metronidazole or Misonidazole

Abstract/Summary

The toxicity of 5-fluorouracil, but not its efficacy, is increased by metronidazole. Its toxicity is also increased by misonidazole.

Clinical evidence

27 patients with metastatic colorectal cancer were given 750 mg/m² metronidazole IV 1 h before 600 mg/m² 5-fluorouracil IV five days per week for four weeks. The 5-FU toxicity was markedly increased: granulocytopenia occurred in 74%, anaemia in 41%, stomatitis and oral ulceration in 34%, nausea and vomiting in 48% and thrombocyopenia in 19%. A pharmacokinetic study in ten patients showed that the metronidazole reduced the clearance of the 5-FU by 27% over the five day period and increased the AUC. *In vitro* studies with human colon cancer cells failed to show any increased efficacy.[1]

Studies using another nitroimidazole, misonidazole, in patients with colorectal cancer also found an increased incidence and severity of gastrointestinal toxicity with concurrent use,[2,3] a slightly increased incidence of leucopenia[2] and a reduction in the clearance.[3]

Mechanism

Metronidazole reduces the clearance of 5-FU, thereby increasing its toxic effects.

Importance and management

Information is limited but the 5-FU/metrondiazole interaction apppears to be established. The toxicity of 5-FU is increased without an increase in its therapeutic efficacy. The authors of the report do not recommend use of this drug combination.[1] Be aware that misonidazole can apparently behave similarly.

References

1 Bardakji Z, Jolivet J, Langelier Y, Besner J-G, Ayoub J. 5-fluorouracil-metronidazole combination therapy in metastatic colorectal cancer. Cancer Chemother Pharmacol (1986) 18, 140–44.
2 Spooner D, Bugden RD, Reckham MJ, Wist EA. The combination of 5-flurouracil with misonidazole in patients with advanced colorectal cancer. Int J RAdiat Oncol Biol Phys (1982) 8, 387.
3 McDermott BJ, van den Berg HW, Martin WMC, Murphy RF. Pharmacokinetic rationale for the interaction of 5-fluorouracil and misonidazole in humans. Br J Cancer (1983) 48, 705.

5-Fluorouracil + Miscellaneous drugs

Abstract/Summary

The toxicity and effects of 5-fluorouracil appear to be unaffected by the drugs listed below (antihistamines, phenothiazines etc).

Clinical evidence, mechanism, importance and management

A study in 250 patients given 5-fluorouracil for the treatment of gastrointestinal cancer found that the following drugs did not cause any significant increase in its toxicity or decrease its therapeutic effects when compared with a placebo: chlorprothixene, cinnarizine, pipamazine, prochlorperazine, sodium pentobarbitone (pentobarbital), thiethlperazine, thiopropazate, trimethobenzamide.[1] No special precautions would seem necessary.

Reference

1 Meertal CG, Reitemeier RJ, Hahn RG. Effect of concomitant drug treatment on toxic and therapeutic activity of 5-fluorouracil (5-FU, NSC-19893). Cancer Chemother Rep (1972) 56, 245–7.

Hydroxyurea + CNS depressants

Abstract/Summary

Increased CNS depression may occur.

Clinical evidence, mechanism, importance and management

Hydroxyurea has CNS-depressant effects and can cause drowsiness. This may be expected to be increased by other drugs which can also cause drowsiness (e.g. alcohol, antiemetics, antihistamines, barbiturates, cough and cold remedies, phenothiazines, narcotic analgesics, tranquillizers, some tricyclic antidepressants, etc.)

Ifosfamide + Barbiturates

Abstract/Summary

Encephalopathy developed in a girl on phenobarbitone when given a single first dose of ifosfamide/mesna.

Clinical evidence

A 15-year-old girl who had been taking phenobarbitone for epilepsy since infancy developed confusion and gradually became unconscious 6 h after being given a first dose of ifosfamide for metastatic rhabdomyosarcoma. She was treated with ifosfamide (3 g/m²), mesna (3.6 g/m²) vincristine (2 mg) and actinomycin D (1000 μg). An ECG revealed signs of severe diffuse encephalopathy. She remained unconscious for 24 h but was asymptomatic after 48 h.

Mechanism

Encephalopathy due to ifosfamide has been seen in other patients and apparently results from the alteration in the balance of dechloroethylation of ifosfamide and the clearance of chloracetaldehyde.[2–4] The doses used were greater than in the case cited (<3.5 g/m² daily) and repeated. The reason for the encephalopathy in this case is not understood but the authors of the report suggest that the enzyme induction caused by the phenobarbitone might have resulted in increased activation of the single dose of ifosfamide, resulting in increased toxicity. The vincristine may also have had additive effects.[1]

Importance and management

The relationship between this encephalopathy and the use of phenobarbitone is not established, but this case serves to emphasize the need for particular caution and good monitoring if concurrent use is undertaken. More study is needed.

References

1 Ghosn M, Carde P, Leclerq B, Flamant F, Friedman S, Droz JP, Hayat M. Ifosfamide/mesna related encephalopathy: a case report with a possible role of phenobarbital in enhancing neurotoxicity. Bull Cancer (1988) 75, 391–2.
2 Cantwell BMJ, Harris AL. Ifosfamide/mesna and encephalopathy. Lancet (1985) i, 752.
3 Goren MP, Wright RK, Pratd CB, Pell FR. Dechloroethylation of ifosfamide and neurotoxicity. Lancet (1986) ii, 1219–20.
4 Salloum E, Flamant F, Ghosn M, Taleb N, Akatcherian C. Irreversible encephalopathy with ifosfamide/mesna. J Clin Oncol (1987) 5, 1303–4.

Ifosfamide + Cisplatin

Abstract/Summary

Ifosfamide toxicity is more common in those who have had prior treatment with cisplatin. Ifosfamide increases the hearing loss due to cisplatin.

Clinical evidence

A comparative study in 36 children with malignant solid tumours on a range of drugs including some known to be potentially nephrotoxic (high dose methotrexate, aminoglycosides, cyclophosphamide), indicated that previous treatment with cisplatin increased their susceptibility to ifosfamide toxicity (neurotoxicity, severe leucopenia or acute tubular damage).[1]

This confirms other studies in which pretreatment with cisplatin appeared to increase the nephrotoxicity of ifosfamide,[2,3] but not another study which suggested that no such interaction occurs.[4] A further comparative study found that when ifosfamide was added to cisplatin, the hearing loss caused by cisplatin was exacerbated.[5]

Mechanism

It is thought that prior treatment with cisplatin damages the kidney tubules so that the clearance of the ifosfamide metabolites from the body is reduced and their toxic effects are thereby increased. Damaged kidney tubules may also be less capable of converting mesna to its active kidney-protecting form. The increase in the hearing loss is not understood.

Importance and management

These interactions appear to be established. The authors of the paper cited[1] point out that the majority of patients who develop toxicity have persistently high urinary NAG concentrations, even though serum creatinine levels remain within the acceptable range for ifosfamide treatment. They suggest that evidence of subclinical tubular damage should be sought for by monitoring the excretion of urinary NAG. The authors of the report about hearing loss advise that serial audiograms are given to patients treated with both drugs.[5]

References

1 Goren MP, Wright RK, Pratt CB, Horowitz ME, Dodge RK, Viar MJ, Kovnar EH. Potentiation of ifosfamide neurotoxicity, hematoxicity, and tubular nephrotoxicity by prior cis-diamminedichloroplatinum(II) therapy. Cancer Res (1987) 47, 1457–60.
2 Wheeler BM, Loehrer PJ, Williams SD, Einhorn LH. Ifosfamide in refractory male germ cell tumors. J Clin Oncol (1986) 4, 28–34.
3 Niederle N, Scheulen ME, Cremer M, Schutte J, Schmidt CG, Seeber S. Ifosfamide in combination chemotherapy for sarcomas and testicular carcinomas. Cancer Treat Rev (1983) 10 (Suppl A) 129–35.
4 Hacke M, Schmoll H-J, Alt JM, Bauman K, Stolte H. Nephrotoxicity of cis-diamminedichloroplatinum with or without ifosfamide in cancer treatment. Clin Physiol Biochem (1983) 1, 17–26.
5 Meyer WH, Ayers D, McHaney VA, Roberson P, Pratt CB. Ifosfamide and exacerbation of cisplatin-induced hearing loss. Lancet (1993) 341, 754–5.

Lomustine (CCNU) + Theophylline

Abstract/Summary

A single case report describes thrombocytopenia and bleeding attributed to the concurrent use of lomustine and theophylline.

Clinical evidence, mechanism, importance and management

An asthmatic woman taking theophylline and under treatment for medulloblastoma with lomustine, prednisone and vincristine, developed severe nose bleeding and thrombocytopenia three weeks after the third cycle of chemotherapy.[1] This was attributed to the concurrent use of the lomustine and theophylline. It is suggested that the theophylline inhibited the activity of phosphodiesterase within the blood platelets, thereby increasing cyclic AMP levels and disrupting normal platelet function. This theory seems to be supported by an experimental study.[2] What is known is far too limited to act as more than a warning of the possibility of increased thrombopathia and myelotoxicity during the concurrent use of theophylline and lomustine.

References

1 Zeltzer PM, Feig SA. Theophylline-induced lomustine toxicity. Lancet (1979) ii, 960.
2 DeWys WD, Bathina S. Synergistic anti-tumour effect of cyclic AMP elevation (induced by theophylline) and cytotoxic drug treatment. Proc Am Assoc Cancer Res (1978) 19, 104.

Melphalan + Cimetidine

Abstract/Summary

Cimetidine reduces the bioavailability of melphalan.

Clinical evidence, mechanism, importance and management

A study in eight patients with multiple myeloma or monoclonal gammopathy showed that pretreatment with 1 g cimetidine daily for six days reduced the bioavailability of a 10 mg oral dose of melphalan by 30%.[1] The melphalan half-life was reduced from 1.94 to 1.57 h. The reasons for this reaction and its clinical importance await assessment.

Reference

1 Sviland L, Robinson A, Proctor SJ, Bateman DN. Interaction of cimetidine with oral melphalan. Cancer Chemother Pharmacol (1987) 20, 173–5.

Melphalan + Interferon

Abstract/Summary

Interferon modestly increases the loss of melphalan, but melphalan cytoxicity is possibly increased because of the interferon-induced fever.

Clinical evidence, mechanism, importance and management

The AUC (area under the curve) of melphalan (0.25 mg.kg) in 10 myeloma patients was reduced by 13% when given 5 h after the administration of human interferon alfa (7 x 10^6 IU/m^2) due to the fever caused by the interferon.[1] The clinical importance of this is uncertain but the authors of the report suggest that despite this small loss the cytotoxicity of the melphalan is increased by the fever. More study is needed.

Reference

1 Ehrsson H, Eksborg S, Wallin I, Österborg A, Mellstedt H. Oral melphalan pharmacokinetics: influence of interferon-induced fever. Clin Pharmacol Ther (1990) 47, 86–90.

Mercaptopurine + Food

Abstract/Summary

Food reduces and delays the absorption of mercaptopurine.

Clinical evidence

A study in 17 children with acute lymphoblastic leukaemia showed that the absorption of 6-mercaptopurine (75 mg/m^2) was markedly reduced if given 15 min after a standard breakfast (250 ml of milk and 50 g biscuits) compared with the situation when fasting. The area under the time-concentration curve (AUC) was reduced by 26% (from 143 to 105 μM min). The maximum serum concentration was reduced 36% (from 0.98 to 0.63 μM) and delayed from 1.2 to 2.3 h.[1] Some individuals showed more marked effects than others. One subject showed a 2.6-fold decrease in AUC and a sixfold decrease in maximum serum levels.[1]

This study confirms the findings of another study on two patients.[2]

Mechanism

Not understood. Delayed gastric emptying is a suggested reason.[1]

Importance and management

The documentation is small but this interaction appears to be established and of clinical importance. Mercaptopurine should be taken while fasting to optimize its absorption.

References

1 Riccardi R, Balis FM, Ferrara P, Lasorella A, Poplak DG, Mastrangelo R. Influence of food intake on bioavailability of oral 6-mercaptopurine in children with acute lymphoblastic leukaemia. Paed Haematol Oncol (1986) 3, 319–24.
2 Burton NK, Aherne GW, Marks VA. Novel method for the quantitation of 6-mercaptopurine in human plasma using high-peformance liquid chromatography with fluorescent detection. J Chromatogr (1984) 309, 409–14.

Methotrexate + Alcohol

Abstract/Summary

There is some inconclusive evidence that the consumption of alcohol may increase the risk of methotrexate-induced hepatic cirrhosis and fibrosis.

Clinical evidence, mechanism, importance and management

It has been claimed that alcohol can increase the hepatotoxic effects of methotrexate.[2] Two studies indicate that this may be so, in one of which three out of five patients with methotrexate-induced cirrhosis were reported to have taken alcohol concurrently,[1,3] but the evidence is by no means conclusive and no direct causal relationship has been established. The manufacturers of methotrexate (Lederle) advise the avoidance of drugs, including alcohol, which have hepatotoxic potentialities.

References

1 Tobias H, Auerbach R. Hepatotoxicity of long-term methotrexate therapy. Arch Intern Med (1973) 132, 391.

2 Pai SH, Werthamer S, Zak FG. Severe liver damage caused by treatment of psoriasis with methotrexate. NY State J Med (1973) 73, 2585.

3 Almeyda J, Barnardo D, Baker H. Drug reactions XV. Methotrexate, psoriasis and the liver. Br J Dermatol (1971) 85, 302–5.

Methotrexate + Amiodarone

Abstract/Summary

An isolated case report tentatively attributes the development of methotrexate toxicity to additional treatment with amiodarone.

Clinical evidence, mechanism, importance and management

An elderly woman, effectively treated for two years with methotrexate for psoriasis, developed ulceration of the psoriatic plaques within two weeks of starting treatment with amiodarone. The reason is not understood. A modest increase in her dosage of frusemide is a suggested contributory factor because it might have interfered with the excretion of the methotrexate.[1]

Reference

1 Reynolds NJ, Jones SK, Crossley J, Harman RRM. Methotrexate induced skin necrosis: a drug interaction with amiodarone? Br Med J (1989) 299, 980–1.

Methotrexate + Aminoglycoside Antibiotics

Abstract/Summary

There is evidence that the gastrointestinal absorption of methotrexate can be reduced by paromomycin, neomycin and possibly other oral aminoglycosides, but increased by kanamycin.

Clinical evidence

A study in 10 patients with small cell bronchogenic carcinoma treated with methotrexate found that when additionally given a range of oral antibiotics (paromomycin, vancomycin, polymyxin B, nystatin) the gastrointestinal absorption of the methotrexate was reduced by over one third (from 69 to 44%).[1] The paromomycin was believed to have been responsible. In another study the concurrent use of neomycin (500 mg four times a day for three days) reduced the methotrexate area under the curve and the 72-hour culmulative excretion by 50%.[2] In contrast, the same report suggests that kanamycin can increase the absorption of methotrexate, but no details are given.

Mechanism

Paromomycin[3] and neomycin, in common with other oral aminoglycosides, can cause a malabsorption syndrome which reduces drug absorption. Kanamycin may possibly be different because it causes less malabsorption. It also reduces the activity of the gut flora which metabolize methotrexate so that more is available for absorption.

Importance and management

The documentation of these interactions is sparse, but it would seem prudent to be on the alert for a reduction in the response to methotrexate if patients are given oral aminoglycosides such as paromomycin or neomycin. An increased response may possibly occur with kanamycin. No interaction would be expected if the aminoglycosides are given parenterally.

References

1 Cohen MH, Creaven PJ, Fossieck BE, Johnston AV, Williams CL. Effect of oral prophylactic broad spectrum nonabsorbable antibiotics on the gastrointestinal absorption of nutrients and methotrexate in small cell bronchogenic carcinoma patients. Cancer (1976) 38, 1556.

2 Shen DD, Azarnoff D. Clinical pharmacokinetics of methotrexate. Clin Pharmacokinetics (1978) 3, 1–13.

3 Keusch GT, Troneale FJ, Buchanan RD. Malabsorption due to paromomycin. Arch Intern Med (1970) 125, 273.

Methotrexate + Ascorbic Acid (Vitamin C)

Abstract/Summary

The urinary excretion of methotrexate is not significantly changed by the concurrent ingestion of large amounts of vitamin C (1–3 g daily) and it may possibly relieve the nausea of chemotherapy.

Clinical evidence, mechanism, importance and management

A patient with breast cancer, treated with methotrexate and cyclophosphamide, and who was also taking propranolol, amitriptyline, perphenazine and prochlorperazine said that the nausea caused by the cytotoxic therapy was relieved by large daily doses of vitamin C. A study on this patient showed that the concurrent ingestion of 1–3 g vitamin C daily had little effect on the excretion of methotrexate in the urine.[1]

Reference

1 Sketris IS, Farmer PS, Fraser A. Effect of vitamin C on the excretion of methotrexate. Cancer Treat Rep (1984) 68, 446–7.

Methotrexate + Barbiturates

Abstract/Summary

Animal studies suggest that phenobarbitone may possibly enhance the alopecia caused by methotrexate.

Clinical evidence, mechanism, importance and management

A study in rats showed that severe alopecia could be induced by the concurrent use of methotrexate and phenobarbitone in dosages which when given alone failed to cause any hair loss.[1] Whether this occurs in man is uncertain.

Reference

1 Basu TK, Williams DC, Raven RW. Methotrexate and alopecia. Lancet (1973) ii, 331.

Methotrexate + Chloramphenicol, PAS, Sodium Salicylate, Sulphamethoxypyridazine, Tetracycline, Tolbutamide

Abstract/Summary

Animal studies suggested that the toxicity of methotrexate might be increased by the use of these drugs, but confirmation of this in man has only been seen with the salicylates, sulphonamides and tetracycline.

Clinical evidence, mechanism, importance and management

Some lists, reviews and books on interactions say that the drugs listed above interact with methotrexate, apparently based largely on a study in which male mice were treated for five days with each of four doses of methotrexate (1.53–12.25 mg/kg IV) and immediately afterwards with non-toxic intraperitoneal doses of the drugs listed. These drugs '...appeared to be capable of decreasing the lethal dose and/or decreasing the median survival time of the mice.'[1] That is to say, the toxicity of the methotrexate was increased. The reasons are not understood, but it is suggested that displacement of the methotrexate from its plasma protein binding sites could result in a rise in the levels of unbound and active methotrexate, and in the case of sodium salicylate to a decrease in renal clearance.

These animal studies were done in 1968. Since then the clinical importance of the interaction with salicylates has been confirmed, there are three cases involving another sulphonamide (sulphamethoxazole in the form of co-trimoxazole) and there is an isolated case report of an interaction with tetracycline (see appropriate synopsis), but there appears to be no direct clinical evidence of interactions between methotrexate and any of the other drugs. The results of animal experiments cannot be applied directly and uncritically to man and it now seems probable that some of these suggested or alleged interactions are more theoretical than real.

Reference

1 Dixon RL. The interaction between various drugs and methotrexate. Toxicol Appl Pharmacol (1968) 12, 308.

Methotrexate + Cholestyramine

Abstract/Summary

The serum methotrexate levels of two patients (methotrexate given by infusion) were markedly reduced by the concurrent use of cholestyramine.

Clinical evidence

A girl of 11 with osteosarcoma who developed colitis when treated with high dose intravenous methotrexate, was subsequently treated with 2 g cholestyramine six hourly from 6 to 48 h after the methotrexate. Serum methotrexate concentrations at 24 h were approximately halved. A marked fall in serum methotrexate levels were seen in another patient similarly treated.[1]

Mechanism

Methotrexate (whether given orally or by infusion) takes part in the entero-hepatic cycle, that is to say it is excreted into the gut in the bile and re-absorbed further along the gut. If cholestyramine is given orally, it can bind strongly to the methotrexate[1] in the gut, thereby preventing its reabsorbtion and, as a result, the serum levels fall.

Importance and management

The documentation seems to be limited to this study.[1] In this instance the cholestyramine was deliberately used to reduce serum methotrexate levels, but in some circumstances it might represent an unwanted interaction. Since methotrexate is excreted into the gut in the bile, separating the oral dosages of the cholestyramine and methotrexate may not necessarily prevent their coming into contact and interacting together. Monitor concurrent use and make any dosage adjustments as necessary.

Reference

1 Erttmann R, Landbeck G. Effect of oral cholestyramine on the elimination of high-dose methotrexate. J Cancer Res Clin Oncol (1985) 110, 48.

Methotrexate + Corticosteroids

Abstract/Summary

Methotrexate may have a 'steroid-sparing' effect, but there is evidence that the toxicity of methotrexate is increased. The efficacy of methotrexate may also possibly be reduced by hydrocortisone with cephalothin.

Clinical evidence

(a) Steroid-sparing effect

Methotrexate and the corticosteroids have been used together successfully, for example in the treatment of psoriatic arthritis, where a 50% reduction in the corticosteroid dosage was possible,[2,3] and in steroid-dependent asthmatics where 30–38% reductions in prednisone doses were achieved.[6,7] However one study found no evidence of a steroid-sparing effect with prednisone.[8]

(b) Increased methotrexate effects, toxicity

Two patients being treated for psoriasis with methotrexate (5 mg daily for 5–7 days) and on long-term corticosteroid therapy died apparently from severe bone marrow depression. One was also on chloramphenicol.[1] Another patient taking 30 mg prednisone daily for psoriasis and who was given 50 mg, 100 mg and 150 mg methotrexate by injection at 10-day intervals, developed severe leucopenia and thrombocytopenia.[2] Yet another patient, debilitated from arthritis and prolonged corticosteroid therapy, died of generalized systemic moniliasis after two doses of methotrexate. She had no haematological abnormalities.[4] There is some evidence that low-dose prednisolone (15 mg daily) given long term (but not short term) can reduce the clearance of methotrexate and increase its serum levels.[9]

(c) Reduced methotrexate effects with cephalothin/ hydrocortisone

In vitro experiments with blast cells from seven patients with acute myelogenous leukaemia indicated that the intracellular uptake of methotrexate is reduced by the presence of cephalothin (21μg/ml) and hydrocortisone (20μg/ml) which are normal achievable clinical serum concentrations.[5]

Mechanisms

Not understood. The 'steroid sparing' effect is possibly the result of a reduction in the steroid metabolism due to the methotrexate.[6]

Importance and management

These interactions between methotrexate and the corticoster-oids are not well documented nor well established, but there is sufficient evidence to suggest that particular care should be exercised during concurrent use to confirm that the clinical outcome is, as intended, advantageous. Be alert for any evidence of methotrexate toxicity.

References

1 Haim S, Alrey G. Methotrexate in psoriasis. Lancet (1967) i, 1156.
2 Black RL, O'Brien WM, Van Scott EJ, Auerbach R, Eisen AZ, Bunim JJ. Methotrexate therapy in psoriatic arthritis. J Amer Med Ass (1964) 189, 743.
3 Schewach-Millet M, Ziprkowski L. Methotrexate in psoriasis. Br J Derm (1968) 80, 535.
4 Roenigk HH, Fowler-Bergfeld W, Curtis GH. Methotrexate for psoriasis in weekly oral doses. Arch Derm (1969) 99, 86.
5 Bender AR, Bleyer WA, Frisby SA, Oliverio VJ. Alterations in methotrex-ate uptake in human leukaemia cells by other agents. Cancer Res (1975) 35, 1305–8.
6 Sockin SM, Ostro MG, Goldman MA, Bloch KJ. The effect of methotrexate on plasma prednislone levels in steroid dependent asthmatics. J Allergy Clin Immunol (1992) 89, 286.
7 Sorkness CA, Joseph J, Busse WW, Bush RK. The effect of oral methotrex-ate discontinuation in corticosteroid-dependent adult asthma. J Allergy Clin Immunol (1992) 89, 286.
8 Caldwell EJ, Vogel BM, Dziodzio JT, Bagwell S. The effects of methotrexate on prednisone dosing in steroid-dependent asthma. Am Rev Resp Dis (1992) 145, A420.
9 Lafforgue P, Monjanel-Mouterde S, Durand A, Catalin J, Acquaviva PC. Is there an interaction between low doses of corticosteroids and methotrex-ate in patients with rheumatoid arthritis ? A pharmacokinetic study in 33 patients. J Rheumatol (1993) 20, 263–7.

Methotrexate + Co-trimoxazole or Trimethoprim

Abstract/Summary

Ten cases of severe bone marrow depression have been reported, two of them fatal, caused by the concurrent use of methotrexate and co-trimoxazole (sulphamethoxazole + trimethoprim) or trimethoprim. There is good evidence that co-trimoxazole increases the effective concentrations of metho-trexate.

Clinical evidence

A 61-year-old patient with rheumatoid arthritis, taking 7.5 mg methotrexate daily, developed generalized bone marrow hy-poplasia over 2 months after a 10-day course of treatment with co-trimoxazole for a urinary tract infection. She had taken a total of 775 mg methotrexate when the hypoplasia appeared.[1]

Nine other cases of severe bone marrow depression, two of them fatal, have been described in patients on methotrexate when given co-trimoxazole or trimethoprim concurrently or sequentially.[2,3,7–9,11,12,14] Skin ulceration and marked pancy-topenia occurred in a woman on methotrexate and naproxen when given trimethoprim.[6] Life-threatening complications (no details given) are said to have occurred in two patients on methotrexate given un-named sulphonamides.[13]

Mechanism

Uncertain. One mechanism seems to be that the co-trimoxazole causes an almost 30% increase in 'free' concentrations of methotrexate while the renal clearance is more than halved.[10] This is calculated to increase the exposure to methotrexate by 66%.[10] Both drugs can also suppress the activity of dihydrofolate reductase and it seems possible that the methotrexate and co-trimoxazole can act additively to produce folate deficiency, which could lead to some of the bone marrow changes seen. Another sulphonamide, sulphafurazole (sulfisoxazole),[5] has been found to cause a small reduction in the clearance of methotrexate by kidneys. However one study in children with acute lymphoblastic leukaemia found that the concurrent use of co-trimoxazole had no effect on the pharmacokinetics of methotrexate.[4]

Importance and management

Information seems to be limited to the reports cited but the interaction is established. Concurrent use should probably be avoided. If these drugs are given either concurrently or sequentially, the haematological picture should be very closely monitored because the outcome can be life-threatening. One of the studies cited suggested that concurrent use may cause a mean 66% increase in the exposure to methotrexate.[10]

References

1 Thomas MH, Gutterman LA. Methotrexate toxicity in a patient receiving trimethoprim-sulfamethoxazole. J Rheumatol (1986) 13, 440–1.
2 Dan M, Shapira I. Possible role of methotrexate in trimethoprim-sulphamethoxazole-induced acute megaloblastic anemia. Isr J Med Sci (1984) 20, 262–3.
3 Kobrinsky NL, Ramsay NKC. Acute megaloblastic anaemia induced by high dose trimethoprim-sulfamethoxazole. Ann Intern Med (1981) 94, 780–1.
4 Beach BJ, Woods WG, Howell SB. Influence of cotrimoxazole on methotrexate pharmacokinetics in children with acute lymphoblastic leukaemia. Am J Pediatr Hematol Oncol (1981) 3, 115–9.
5 Liegler DG, Henderson ES, Hahn MA, Oliverio VT. The effect of organic acids on renal clearance of methotrexate in man. Clin Pharmacol Ther (1969) 10, 849–57.
6 Ng HWK, MacFarlane AW, Graham RM, Verbov JL. Near fatal drug interactions with methotrexate given for psoriasis. Br Med J (1987) 295, 752–3.
7 Therenet JP, Ristori JM, Cure H, Mizony MH, Bussiere JL. Pancytopenie au cours du traitement d'une polyarthrite rheumatoide par methotrexate apres administration de trimethoprime-sulphamethoxazole. La Presse Med (1987) 16, 1487.
8 Groenendal H, Rampen FHJ. Methotrexate and trimethoprim-sulphamethoxazole — a potentially hazardous combination. Clin Exp Dermatol (1990) 15, 358–60.
9 Maricic M, Davis M, Gall EP. Megaloblastic pancytopenia in a patient receiving concurrent methotrexate and trimethoprim-sulphamethoxazole treatment. Arth Rheum (1986) 29, 133–5.
10 Ferrazzini G, Klein J, Sulh H, Chung D, Griesbrecht E, Koren G. Interaction between trimethoprim-sulfamethoxazole and methotrexate in children with leukaemia. J Pediatr (1990) 117, 823–6.
11 Jeurissen ME, Boerbooms AM, van de Putte LB. Pancytopenia and methotrexate with trimethoprim-sulfamethoxazole. Ann Intern Med (1989) 111, 261.
12 Liddle BJ, Marsden JR. Drug interactions with methotrexate. Br J Dermatol (1989) 120, 582.
13 Zachariae H. Methotrexate and non-steroidal anti-inflammatory drugs. Br J Dermatol (1992) 126, 95.
14 Govert JA, Patton S, Fine RL. Pancytopenia from using trimethoprim and methotrexate. Ann Intern Med (1992) 117, 877–8.

Methotrexate + Diuretics

Abstract/Summary

There is some unconfirmed evidence that bone marrow suppression may possibly be increased by concurrent use.

Clinical evidence, mechanism, importance and management

A study in nine patients showed that neither frusemide nor hydroflumethiazide had any effect on the clearance of methotrexate in the urine.[1] However a study in women with breast cancer and under treatment with methotrexate, cyclophosphamide and 5-fluorouracil found that the concurrent use of a thiazide diuretic appeared to increase the myelosuppressant effects.[2] It is uncertain which of the cytotoxic drugs was responsible. Concurrent use should clearly be undertaken with caution.

References

1 Krisensen LO, Weismann K, Hutters L. Renal function and the rate of disappearance of methotrexate from serum. Eur J Clin Pharmacol (1975) 8, 439–44.
2 Orr LE. Potentiation of myelosuppression from cancer chemotherapy and thiazide diuretics. Drug Intell Clin Pharm (1981) 15, 967.

Methotrexate + 5-Fluorouracil (5-FU)

Abstract/Summary

Two patients on low dose methotrexate had a toxic skin reaction when they started to use a cream containg 5-FU. *In vitro* and animal data also suggest that the cytotoxic effects of methotrexate and 5-fluorouracil may possibly be reduced by concurrent use, but this has yet to be confirmed in man.

Evidence, mechanism, importance and management

(a) Methotrexate + Topical 5-FU

Two patients with rheumatoid arthritis on low dose methotrexate (7.5–12.5 mg weekly) for 6–14 months were given 2% fluorouracil cream topically for actinic keratosis. Within 2–3 days both patients developed erythema, blister formation and necrosis. The cream was stopped and the the lesions healed over the next 2–3 weeks.[7] It would seem that concurrent use should be avoided.

(b) Methotrexate + Systemic 5-FU

5-FU and another compound, 5-fluorodeoxyuridine (FldUrd), are metabolized in the body to a third compound, FldUrd monophosphate which is the active cytotoxic agent. This acts by inhibiting an enzyme (thymidilate synthetase) which takes part in the biosynthesis of DNA so that DNA production is reduced. In this way 5-FU and FldUrd impair tumour growth.[4,5] Tests on tumour cells in culture indicate that methotrexate interferes with and reduces the activity of FldUrd.[1] *In vitro* studies in the L1210 cells system, Friend leukaemia system and in human bone marrow have similarly shown that in the presence of methotrexate the activity of 5-FU is also suppressed.[2] The likely reason is that the methotrexate inhibits a co-factor (5,10,methylenetetrahydrofolic acid) which is required by the FldUrd in order to allow it to bind to thymidilate synthetase. Thus the activity of the FldUrd is weakened (and by implication 5-FU as well) which would explain the antagonistic effects of methotrexate.

One cannot uncritically extrapolate tissue culture or animal experiments to man, moreover there is already considerable debate about the time-scheduling of administration[3] and whether combinations of methotrexate and 5-FU are antagonistic or even additive.[6,8] However the evidence (if it does nothing else) emphasises that these two drugs should not be given concurrently without a full awareness that they may possibly be less effective than each drug given alone.

References

1 Maugh TH. Cancer chemotherapy: an unexpected drug interaction. Science (1976) 194, 310.
2 Waxman S, Bruckner H. Antitumour drug interactions: additional data. Science (1976) 194, 672.
3 Bertino J, Sawicki WL, Lindquist CA, Gupta VS. Schedule-dependent antitumour effects of methotrexate and 5-fluorouracil. Cancer Res (1977) 37, 327.
4 Tattersall MNH, Jackson RC, Connors TA, Harrap KR. Combination chemotherapy: the interaction of methotrexate and 5-fluorouracil. Eur J Cancer (1973) 9, 733.
5 Waxman S, Rubinoff M, Greenspan E, Bruckner H. Interaction of methotrexate (MTX) and 5-fluorouracil (5-FU): effect on de novo DNA synthesis. Proc Am Assoc Cancer Res (1976) 17, 157.
6 Brown I, Ward HWC. Therapeutic consequences of antitumour drug interactions: methotrexate and 5-fluorouracil in the chemotherapy of C3H mice with transplanted mammary adenocarcinoma. Cancer Letters (1978) 5, 291.
7 Blackburn WD, Alarcón GS. Toxic response to topical fluorouracil in two rheumatoid arthritis patients receiving low dose weekly methotrexate. Arth Rheum (1990) 33, 303–4.
8 Bertino JR. Modulation of fluorouracil by methotrexate. J Clin Oncol (1991) 9, 1511–12.

Methotrexate + Folinic Acid (Leucovorin)

Abstract/Summary

Folinic acid opposes both the adverse and beneficial effects of methotrexate in the treatment of cancer and rheumatoid arthritis.

Clinical evidence, mechanism, importance and management

Folinic acid (leucovorin) is frequently used an antidote to high dose methotrexate in cancer therapy because it competes for entry into cells, and repletes the pools of tetrahydrofolate within cells (the so-called leucovorin rescue). However a study in 7 patients found that it also antagonizes the effects of low dose methotrexate (7.5 – 12.0 mg weekly) given for rheumatoid arthritis. Calcium folinate (45 mg weekly) taken 4–6 h after the methotrexate was successful in causing the nausea associated with methotrexate to disappear, but at the same time the disease worsened in all of the patients (subjective clinical assessment, Ritchie articular index, grip strength, ESR, C-reactive protein).[1] Concurrent use should therefore be closely evaluated.

Reference

1 Tishler M, Caspi D, Fishel B, Yaron M. The effects of leucovorin (folinic acid) on methotrexate therapy in rheumatoid arthritis patients. Arth Rheum (1988) 31, 906–8.

Methotrexate + Nitrous Oxide

Abstract/Summary

Methotrexate-induced stomatitis and other toxic effects may possibly be increased by the use of nitrous oxide.

Clinical evidence, mechanism, importance and management

Studies in which intravenous methotrexate, cyclophosphamide and 5-fluorouracil were used after mastectomy suggested that the stomatitis which can develop may be caused by a toxic interaction between methotroxate and nitrous oxide used during anaesthesia. A possible reason is that the effects of methotrexate on tetrahydrofolate metabolism are increased by nitrous oxide. It was found that the incidence of stomatitis, severe leucopenia, thrombocytopenia, and of severe systemic and local infections could be reduced by giving calcium folinate (leucovorin), intravenous hydration and withdrawal of the drugs where necessary.[1]

Reference

1 Goldhirsch A, Gelber RD, Tattersall MNH, Rudenstam C-M, Cavalli F. Methotrexate/nitrous oxide toxic interaction in perioperative chemotherapy for early breast cancer. Lancet (1987) ii, 151.

Methotrexate + Non-Steroidal Anti-Inflammatory Drugs (NSAIDs)

Abstract/Summary

Increased methotrexate toxicity, sometimes life-threatening, has been seen in few patients concurrently treated with NSAID's (amidopyrine, aspirin, azapropazone, choline magnesium trisalicylate, diclofenac, dipyrone, flurbiprofen, ibuprofen, indomethacin, naproxen, phenylbutazone, sodium salicylate and tolmetin) whereas other patients have been treated uneventfully. The development of toxicity may possibly be related to the methotrexate dosage. The risk appears to be lowest in those taking low-dose methotrexate for rheumatoid arthritis.

Clinical evidence

(a) Methotrexate + Aspirin and other salicylates

Lethal pancytopenia in two patients given methotrexate and aspirin prompted a retrospective survey of the records of other patients treated with intra-arterial infusions of methotrexate (50 mg daily for 10 days) for epidermoid carcinoma of the oral cavity. Six out of seven who developed a rapid and serious pancytopenia were found to have had aspirin or other salicylates.[1] Similar results were found in studies on mice.[1]

There are other case reports[2,3] of methotrexate toxicity in patients taking salicylates but whether a causal relationship exists is uncertain. A study in eight patients with rheumatoid arthritis found that 975 mg aspirin daily increased the AUC of a single 10 mg bolus of methotrexate by 28%. The methotrexate clearance was reduced.[19] Another study in four patients found that the renal clearance of methotrexate was reduced by 35% when given an infusion of sodium salicylate (2 g initially, then 33 mg/min).[6] Two further studies found that choline magnesium trisalicylate reduced the clearance (compared with paracetamol — acetaminophen) by 24–41%, and increased the unbound fraction by 28%.[24,29] It has been suggested that pneumonitis in patients on low-dose methotrexate may have resulted from the concurrent use of 4–5 g aspirin daily.[6]

(b) Methotrexate + Amidopyrine

Megaloblastic pancytopenia occurred in a woman with rheumatoid arthritis given methotrexate (15 mg weekly) and amidopyrine (1.0–1.5 g daily).[22]

(c) Methotrexate + Azapropazone

A woman given methotrexate (25 mg weekly for four years) for psoriasis showed acute toxicity (oral and genital ulceration, bone marrow failure) shortly after starting to take azapropazone (1.2 g daily). She was also taking 300 mg aspirin daily.[5] Life-threatening bone marrow suppression occurred in another woman similarly treated within 2 weeks of starting azapropazone.[21]

(d) Methotrexate + Dipyrone

A study in a patient with osteosarcoma showed that 4 g dipyrone daily more than doubled the methotrexate AUC (from 636 to 1476 μmol.h.l^{-1}) during the first cycle of high dose methotrexate treatment.[27]

(e) Methotrexate + Etodolac

A pharmacokinetic study in patients with rheumatoid arthritis found that 600 mg etodolac daily did not affect the AUC of methotrexate, but duration of exposure was lengthened (half-life increased from 10.3 to 14.2 h). The clinical significance of this was not assessed.[30]

(f) Methotrexate + Flurbiprofen

An elderly woman who had been taking 2.5 mg methotrexate three times a week for 3 years for rheumatoid arthritis developed haematemesis, neutropenia and thrombocytopenia (diagnosed as methotrexate toxicity) within 1–2 weeks of starting to take 100 gm flurbiprofen daily.[31]

(g) Methotrexate + Ibuprofen

A patient on methotrexate who was given ibuprofen required leucovorin rescue because the clearance of methotrexate had fallen by two-thirds.[12] Another patient had severe methotrexate-induced kidney toxicity and delayed excretion of methotrexate while taking 400 mg ibuprofen 4-hourly.[18] A study in seven patients found that the clearance of methotrexate (7.5–15 mg orally) was halved by ibuprofen (40 mg.kg/day) when compared with paracetamol (acetaminophen).[24] In a related study the clearance was reduced by 40%.[29]

(h) Methotrexate + Indomethacin

Two patients on sequential intermediate dose methotrexate and 5-fluorouracil who were concurrently taking indomethacin (75–100 mg daily) died from acute drug toxicity which the authors of the report attributed to indomethacin-associated renal failure.[7]

Another case of acute renal failure has been described,[10] and toxicity has been seen in a patient given methotrexate and indomethacin,[8] but not in four other patients on methotrexate given either paracetamol (acetaminophen) or indomethacin.[3] An elderly woman died after a single 10 mg IM dose of methotrexate while taking 50 mg indomethacin daily rectally and 100 mg diclofenac daily intravenously.[25] A child of 9 months on methotrexate showed an AUC increase of 140% when given indomethacin and aspirin.[15]

(i) Methotrexate + Ketoprofen or diclofenac

A retrospective study[8] of 118 cycles of high-dose methotrexate treatment in 36 patients showed that four out the nine patients who developed severe methotrexate toxicity (800–8300 mg/m^2; mean 3200 mg/m^2) had also taken ketoprofen (150–200 mg daily for 2–15 days). Three of them died. A marked and prolonged rise in serum methotrexate levels were observed. Another patient who showed toxicity had also been given diclofenac (150 mg in one day). See also (h) above.

(j) Methotrexate + Naproxen

A woman died of gross methotrexate toxicity apparently exacerbated by the concurrent use of naproxen.[11] Two children aged 1 and 2 showed increases in the AUC of methotrexate of 22% and 71% when given naproxen with aspirin or indomethacin respectively.[15] Five patients on low-dose methotrexate (7.5 — 12.5 mg weekly) for psoriasis or rheumatoid arthritis developed neutropenias. Three of them died.[26] However a study in patients with rheumatoid arthritis with normal renal function found that no toxicity was caused by 500 mg naproxen twice daily with 15 mg methotrexate given orally or intravenously, nor was the methotrexate clearance altered.[20] Another study found that the clearance was decreased 22%.[24,29]

(k) Methotrexate + Phenylbutazone

Two patients on methotrexate for psoriasis developed methotrexate toxicity and skin ulceration shortly after starting to take phenylbutazone (200–600 mg daily). One of them died from septicaemia following bone marrow depression.[9]

(l) Methotrexate + Tolmetin

Three children aged 6 months, 6 months and 2 years showed increases in the AUC of methotrexate of 42%, and 18%, 25% respectively when given tolmetin alone, and in the last two cases tolmetin with aspirin.[15]

Mechanisms

Methotrexate is largely cleared unchanged from the body by renal excretion. The NSAIDs as a group inhibit the synthesis of the prostaglandins (PGE$_2$) resulting in a fall in renal perfusion which would lead to a rise in serum methotrexate levels, accompanied by increased toxicity. In addition, salicylates and phenylbutazone competitively inhibit the tubular secretion of methotrexate which would further reduce its clearance.[4] Phenylbutazone and indomethacin can also cause renal failure which would allow the methotrexate to accumulate. Both phenylbutazone, amidopyrine and methotrexate cause bone marrow depression which could be additive. Protein binding displacement of the major extracellular metabolite of methotrexate (7-hydroxy-methotrexate) has also been suggested as a possible additional mechanism because it is highly bound to plasma proteins.[14] There is also some evidence that this metabolite is cleared more slowly in the presence of NSAID's.[16]

Importance and management

None of these interactions is very well documented, but the overall picture seems to be that the risks are greatest with high-dose methotrexate and in patients with impaired kidney function, but less in patients given low doses and with normal kidney function.

The evidence so far suggests that aspirin and possibly some other salicylates should be avoided. Remind patients of the many over-the-counter preparations which contain aspirin. The authors of the report cited[1] above state that ketoprofen should not be given at the same time as methotrexate, but it may be safe to give it 12–24 h after high dose methotrexate because 50% of the methotrexate is excreted by the kidneys within 6–12 h. This was tried in two patients without ill-effects.

The evidence about amidopyrine, azapropazone, choline magnesium trisalicylate, diclofenac, dipyrone, etodolac, flurbiprofen, ibuprofen, naproxen, indomethacin, phenylbutazone and tolmetin is much thinner, and there appears to be no direct evidence against any other NSAID, nevertheless it seems that many of them can impair the renal clearance of methotrexate to some extent, quite apart from any other toxic effects they may have. If concurrent use is thought appropriate, it should be closely monitored (see the measures suggested below). The use of amidopyrine and dipyrone is to be discouraged because even on their own they can cause agranulocytosis.

The incidence of serious reactions seems to be very much lower with low-dose methotrexate. A study of 87 patients on long-term treatment with methotrexate (mean weekly dose 8.19 mg), most of whom were also taking unspecified NSAIDs, found that the majority (72%) experienced no untoward effects and in the rest they were only relatively mild.[13] Concurrent use in more than 450 patients with psoriatic arthritis or rheumatoid arthritis 'without clinical problems due to interactions (with NSAIDs)..' is briefly described in another report.[28] Other studies have found no changes in the pharmacokinetics of methotrexate in patients with rheumatoid arthritis taking NSAIDs (flurbiprofen, ibuprofen, indomethacin, diclofenac, diflunisal, naproxen, sulindac).[17,20,23] Concurrent use in these circumstances may therefore possibly be quite uneventful. However one study suggests that even with low dose therapy it would be reasonable to do white cell and platelet counts twice weekly for two weeks, and regularly thereafter if interacting NSAIDs are given, especially in the elderly or those with high creatinine levels. Folinic acid rescue therapy should be available.[26]

References

1 Zuik M, Mandel MA. Methotrexate-salicylate interaction: a clinical and experimental study. Surg For (1975) 26, 567.

2 Dubin HV, Harrell RE. Liver disease associated with methotrexate treatment of psoriatic patients. Arch Dermatol (1970) 102, 498–503.

3 Baker H. Intermittent high dose oral methotrexate therapy in psoriasis. Br J Derm (1970) 82, 65.

4 Liegler DG, Henderson ES, Hahn MA, Oliverio VT. The effect of organic acids on renal clearance of methotrexate in man. Clin Pharmacol Ther (1969) 10, 849–57.

5 Daly HM, Scott GL, Boyle J, Roberts CJC. Methotrexate toxicity precipitated by azapropazone. Br J Dermatol (1986) 114, 733–35.

6 Maier WP, Leon-Perez R, Miller SB. Pneumonitis during low-dose methotrexate therapy. Arch Intern Med (1986) 146, 602–3.

7 Ellison NM, Servi RJ. Acute renal failure and death following sequential intermediate-dose methotrexate and 5-FU: a possible adverse effect due to concomitant indomethacin administration. Cancer Treat Rep (1985) 69, 342–3.

8 Thyss A, Milano G, Kubar J, Namer M, Schneider M. Clinical and pharmacokinetic evidence of a life-threatening interaction between methotrexate and ketoprofen. Lancet (1986) i, 256–8.

9 Adams JD, Hunter GA. Drug interaction in psoriasis. Aust J Derm (1976) 17, 39.

10 Maiche AG. Acute renal failure due to concomitant action of methotrexate and indomethacin. Lancet (1986) i, 1390.

11 Singh RR, Malaviya AN, Pandey JN, Guleria JS. Fatal interaction between methorexate and naproxen. Lancet (1986) i, 1390.

12 Bloom EJ, Ignoffo RJ, Reis CA, Cadman E. Delayed clearance (CL) of methotrexate (MTX) associated with antibiotics and antiinflammatory agents (abstract). Clin Res (1986) 34, 560A.

13 Wilke WS, Calabrese LH, Segal AM. Incidence of untoward reactions in patients with rhematoid arthritis treated with methotrexate. Arthritis Rheum (1983) 26 (Suppl) S56.

14 Slordal L, Sager G, Aarbakke J. Pharmacokinetic interactions with methotrexate: is 7-hydroxy-methotrexate the culprit? Lancet (1988) i, 591–2.

15 Dupuis LL, Koren G, Shore A, Silverman ED, Laxer RM. Methotrexate-nonsteroidal antiinflammatory drug interaction in children with arthritis. J Rheumatol (1990) 17, 1469–73.

16 Furst DE, Herman RA, Koehnke R, Erickson N,. Hash L, Riggs CE, Porras A, Veng-Pedersen P. Effect of aspirin and sulindac on methotrexate clearance. J Pharm Sci (1990) 79, 782–6.

17 Ahern M, Booth J, Loxton A, McCarthy P, Meffin P, Kevat S. Methotrexate kinetics in rheumatoid arthritis: is there an interaction with nonsteroidal antiinflammatory drugs ? J Rheumatol (1988) 15, 1356–60.

18 Cassano WF. Serious methotrexate toxicity caused by interaction with ibuprofen. Am J Ped Hematol/Oncol (1989) 11, 481–2.

19 Stewart CF, Fleming RA, Magneson P, Germain B, Evans WE. Effect of aspirin on the disposition of methotrexate in patients with rheumatoid arthritis. Clin Pharmacol Ther (1990) 47, 139.

20 Stewart CF, Fleming RA, Arkin CR, Evans WE. Coadministration of naproxen and low-dose methotrexate in patients with rheumatoid arthritis. Clin Pharmacol Ther (1990) 47, 540–6.

21 Burton JL. Drug interactions with methotrexate. Br J Dermatol (1991) 124, 300–1.

22 Noskov SM. Megaloblastic pancytopenia in a female patient with rheumatoid arthritis given methotrexate and amidopyrine. Terapeuticheskiy Arkhiv (1990) 62, 122–3.

23 Skeith KJ, Russell AS, Jamali F, Coates J, Friedman H. Lack of significant interaction between low dose methotrexate and ibuprofen or flurbiprofen in patients with arthritis. J Rheumatol (1990) 17, 1008–10.

24 Tracy TS, Jones DR, Hall SD, Brater DC, Bradley JD. The effect of NSAIDs on methotrexate disposition in patients with rheumatoid arthritis. Clin Pharmacol Ther (1990) 47, 138.

25 Gabrielli A, Leoni P, Danieli G. Methotrexate and non-steroidal anti-inflammatory drugs. Br Med J (1987) 294, 776.

26 Mayall B, Poggi G, Parkin JD. Neutropenia due to low-dose methotrexate therapy for psoriasis and rheumatoid arthritis may be fatal. Med J Aust (1991) 155, 480–4.

27 Hernández de la Figuera y Gómez T, Torres NVJ. Ronchera Oms CL, Ordovás Baines JP. Interacción farmacocinetica entre metotrexato a altas dosis y dipirona. Rev Farmacol Clin Exp (1989) 6, 77–81.

28 Zachariae H. Methotrexate and non-steroidal anti-inflammatory drugs. Br J Dermatol (1992) 126, 95.

29 Tracy TS, Krohn K, Jones DR, Bradley JD, Hall SD, Brater DC. The effects of salicylate, ibuprofen and naproxen on the disposition of methotrexate in patients with rheumatoid arthritis. Eur J Clin Pharmacol (1992) 42, 121–5.

30 Anaya J-M, Fabre D, Bressolle F, Alrice R, Dropsy R, Sany J. Effects of etodolac on methotrexate pharmacokinetics in rheumatoid arthitis patients. Arth Rheum (1992) 35, S343.

31 Frenia ML, Long KS. Methotrexate and non-steroidal antiinflammatory drug interactions. Ann Pharmacother (1992) 26, 234–7.

Methotrexate + Penicillins

Abstract/Summary

The loss of methotrexate from the body can be markedly reduced by the concurrent use of penicillins. There is a considerable risk of methotrexate toxicity. Deaths have occurred.

Clinical evidence

Four patients treated with methotrexate showed a marked reduction in its clearance when concurrently treated with different penicillins: with penicillin a 35% reduction; with piperacillin 66%; with ticarcillin 40%; and with dicloxacillin and indomethacin 93%. Prolonged use of leucovorin rescue was necessary. They were given the methotrexate as an intravenous bolus (15–60 mg/m^2) and then 15–60 mg by infusion over 36 h.[1]

A patient under treatment with 50 mg methotrexate (weekly, given intravenously) diethylstilboestrol, prednisone and frusemide, developed severe methotrexate toxicity within a week of starting to take 250 mg penicillin every other day.[2] Increased methotrexate plasma levels and decreased excretion, attributed to the use of 30 mg carbenicillin daily, and necessitating an increase in the folinic acid dosage, is described in another patient.[3] A marked reduction in methotrexate clearance was seen in patient when concurrently treated with mezlocillin (330 mg/kg daily) accompanied by increased gastrointestinal toxicity.[4] Five patients on low dose methotrexate (7.5–12.5 mg weekly) for psoriasis or rheumatoid arthritis developed neutropenia and thrombocytopenia when treated with penicillins (piperacillin, amoxycillin, flucloxacillin, benzylpenicillin). Three died and the other two were extensively hospitalized.[5]

Mechanism

It is thought that weak acids such as the penicillins can successfully compete with methotrexate in the kidney tubules for excretion so that the methotrexate is retained, thereby increasing its effects and its toxicity.

Importance and management

An established interaction. Considerable care and good monitoring is needed if penicillins are given. Recommendations include twice weekly platelet and white cell counts for two weeks initially, determination of methotrexate levels if toxicity is suspected and treatment for sepsis if necessary.[5] Folinic acid rescue should be available.[5] The author of one report advises avoidance.[1]

References

1 Bloom EJ, Ignoffo RJ, Reis CA, Cadman E. Delayed clearance (CL) of methotrexate (MTX) associated with antibiotics and anti-inflammatory agents. Clin Res (1986) 34, 560A.

2 Nierenberg DW, Mamelok RD. Toxic reaction to methotrexate in a patient receiving penicillin and furosemide: a possible interaction. Arch Dermatol (1983) 119, 449–50.

3 Gibson DL, Bleyer AW, Savitch JL. Carbenicillin potentiation of methotrexate plasma concentration during high dose methotrexate therapy. Am Soc Hosp Pharm. Mid year clinical meeting abstracts, New Orleans, Dec 6–10 (1981) p 111.

4 Dean R, Nachman J, Lorenzana AN. Possible methotrexate-mezlocillin interaction. Am J Ped Hematol/Oncol (1992) 14, 88–92.

5 Mayall B, Poggi G, Parkin JD. Neutropenia due to low-dose methotrexate therapy for psoriasis and rheumatoid arthritis may be fatal. Med J Aust (1991) 155, 480–4.

Methotrexate + Pristinamycin

Abstract/Summary

An isolated report describes severe methotrexate toxicity in a patient when treated with pristinamycin.

Clinical evidence

A boy of 13 with acute lymphoblastic leukaemia had a relapse and began a series of regimes with methotrexate in combination with other cytotoxics including dexamethasone, mercaptopurine, vincristine, cytarabine and asparaginase, thioguanine and ifosfamide. During a late cycle during which he was also taking 2 g pristinamycin daily for a staphylococcal infection, the clearance of the methotrexate became markedly increased (half-life prolonged from the usual 6 h to 203 h). He developed severe methotrexate toxicity (oral mucositis, anusitis, balanitis, neutropenia and thrombocyopenia) and was given leucovorin rescue and haemodialysis.[1]

Mechanism

Not understood, but on the basis of experimental evidence the authors of the report excluded the possibilities of kidney impairment or reduction by the pristinamycin of liver metabolism.[1]

Importance and management

This appears to be the first and only report of an interaction between methotrexate and a macrolide antibiotic. Its general importance is unknown but the authors strongly advise the avoidance of pristinamycin in patients treated with methotrexate, and caution with other macrolides.[1]

Reference

1 Thyss A, Milano G, Renée N, Cassuto-Viguier E, Jambou P, Soler C. Severe interaction between methotrexate and a macrolide-like antibiotic. J Natl Cancer Inst (1993) 85, 582–3.

Methotrexate + Probenecid

Abstract/Summary

Serum methotrexate levels are markedly increased (3–4-fold) by the concurrent use of probenecid. The dosage of methotrexate may need to be reduced to avoid the development of toxicity.

Clinical evidence

The concurrent use of probenecid (500–1000 mg) and methotrexate (200 mg/m^2 intravenous bolus injection) resulted in serum methotrexate levels in four patients which were four times higher at 24 h than in four others who had not received probenecid (0.4 compared with 0.09 mg/l).[1]

In another study on four other patients the methotrexate serum levels were raised threefold at 24 h when probenecid was given concurrently.[2] Severe and life-threating pancytopenia occurred in a woman taking low dose methotrexate (7.5 mg weekly) for rheumatoid arthritis when given probenecid. She also had renal insufficiency, hypoalbinaemia and was using salicylates.[7]

Mechanism

Studies in rats have shown that probenecid inhibits the excretion of methotrexate by the kidney and in the bile. A similar effect on renal excretion has been seen in monkeys.[3,4] This is also probably the mechanism in man. Changes in the protein binding of methotrexate may have some part to play.[5] The increased methotrexate levels increase the risk of serious bone marrow depression.

Importance and management

An established and clinically important interaction. A marked increase in methotrexate toxicity can occur, apparently even with low doses if other risk factors are present.[7] The dosage of the methotrexate may need to be reduced. Some evidence from animal studies suggests that despite the rise in methotrexate levels caused by the probenecid, the clinically useful cytotoxic (antitumour) effects of the methotrexate may actually be reduced by the presence of probenecid.[6]

References

1 Aherne GW, Piall E, Marks V, Mould G, White WF. Prolongation and enhancement of serum methotrexate concentrations by probenecid. Brit Med J (1978) 1, 1097–99.

2 Howell SB, Olshen RA, Rice JA. Effect of probenecid on cerebrospinal fluid methotrexate kinetics. Clin Pharmacol Ther (1979) 26, 641–6.

3 Bourke RS, Chhada G, Bremer A, Watanabe O, Tower DB. Inhibition of renal tubular transport of methotrexate by probenecid. Cancer Res (1975) 35, 110–6.

4 Kates RE, Tozer TN, Sorby DL. Increased methotrexate toxicity due to concurrent probenecid administration. Biochem Pharmacol (1976) 25, 1485–8.

5 Paxton JW. Interaction of probenecid with the protein binding of metho-trexate. Pharmacology (1984) 28, 86–9.

6 Gangji D, Ross WE, Bleyer WA, Poplak DG, Glaubiger DL. Probenecid inhibition of methotrexate toxicity in mouse L1210 leukaemia cells. Cancer Treat Rep (1984) 68, 521–5.

7 Basin KS, Escalante A, Beardmore TD. Severe pancytopenia in a patient taking low dose methotrexate and probenecid. J Rheumatol (1991) 18, 609–10

Methotrexate + Retinoids

Abstract/Summary

Although concurrent use can be successful, the incidence of severe liver toxicity appears to be considerably increased. The serum levels of methotrexate may possibly be increased to some extent by etretinate.

Clinical evidence

A study in a man with chronic discoid psoriasis who was being treated weekly with methotrexate (infusion of 10 mg over 48 h) found that when given 30 mg (0.05 mg/kg) etretinate daily his serum methotrexate levels were almost doubled. Concentra-tions at 12 and 24 h during the infusion were 0.11 mmol/l, compared with 0.07 and 0.05 mmol/l before the etretinate.[1]

A later pharmacokinetic study in six psoriatic patients found that etretinate increased the maximum serum levels of metho-trexate by 27%.[8] Other reports describe severe toxic hepatitis in other patients when these drugs were used concurrently.[2,3,7] It may take several months to develop.[7] Signs of liver toxicity were seen in two out of ten patients in one clinic given both drugs,[8] but none in another 531 patients given methotrexate alone or in 110 patients given etretinate alone.[2]

Mechanism

Not understood. The increased incidence of toxic hepatitis may possibly be related to the increased methotrexate serum levels.

Importance and management

Although both drugs have apparently been used concurrently with success for psoriasis, pityriasis rubra pilaris and Reiter's disease,[4–6] the risk of severe drug-induced hepatitis seems to be very considerably increased. One author says that he has decided not to use this combination in future.[2] Concurrent use should clearly be undertaken with great care.

References

1 Harrison PV, Peat M, James R, Orrell D. Methotrexate and retinoids in combination for psoriasis. Lancet (1987) i, 512.

2 Zachariae H. Danger of methotrexate/etretinate combination therapy. Lancet (1988) i, 422.

3 Zachariae H. Methotrexate and etretinate as concurrent therapies in the treatment of psoriasis. Arch Dermatol (1984) 120, 155.

4 van der Veen E, Ellis C, Cambell J. Methotrexate and etretinate as

concurrent therapies in severe psoriasis. Arch Dermatol (1982) 118, 660.

5 Adams J. Concurrent methotrexate and etretinate therapy for psoriasis. Arch Dermatol (1983) 119, 793.

6 Rosenbaum M, Roenigk H. Treatment of generalised pustular psoriasis with etretinate (RO-10–9359) and methotrexate. J Am Acad Dermatol (1984) 10, 357–61.

7 Beck H-I, Foged EK. Toxic hepatitis due to combination therapy with methotrexate and etretinate in psoriasis. Dermatologica (1983) 166, 94–6.

8 Larsen FG, Nielsen-Kudsk F, Jakobsen P, Schroder H, Kradballe K. Interaction of etretinate with methotrexate pharmacokinetics in psoriatic patients. J Clin Pharmacol (1990) 30, 802–7.

Methotrexate + Tetracycline

Abstract/Summary

An isolated case report describes the development of meth-otrexate toxicity in a patient when additionally given tetra-cycline.

Clinical evidence, mechanism, importance and management

A man being successfully and uneventfully treated for psoriasis with methotrexate (25 mg weekly) was additionally started on 2 g tetracycline daily for a mycoplasmal infection. Within five days he developed recurrent fever, ulcerative stomatitis and diarrhoea, and he was found to have a white cell count of 1000 and a platelet count of 30 000 — all signs of methotrexate toxicity. The problem resolved when the methotrexate was withdrawn, but the psoriasis returned.[1] This interaction has also been observed in mice.[2] It may possibly be due to displace-ment of the methotrexate from its binding sites.

This appears to be the only clinical report of this interaction on record. Concurrent treatment should be well monitored.

References

1 Turck M. Successful psoriasis treatment then sudden 'cytotoxicity'. Hosp Pract (1984) 19, 175–6.

2 Dixon RL. The interaction between various drugs and methotrexate. Toxicol Appl Pharmacol (1968) 12, 308.

Methotrexate + Urinary Alkalinizers

Abstract/Summary

Alkalinization increases the solubility of the methotrexate in the urine but also increases its excretion.

Clinical evidence, mechanism, importance and management

Methotrexate is much more soluble in alkaline than in acid fluids. For this reason urinary alkalinizers (and ample fluids) have been given to patients on high dose methotrexate therapy to prevent the precipitation of methotrexate in the kidney tubules which would cause damage. However alkalinization also increases the loss of methotrexate in the urine because at high pH values more of the drug exists in the ionized form which is not readily reabsorbed by the tubules. This increased loss was clearly shown in a very large number of patients (69–75) in whom alkalinization of the urine (pH7+) with sodium bicarbonate and hydration reduced the serum methotrexate concentrations at 24 h by 40%, at 48 h by 73% and at 72 h by 77%.[1] In this instance the interaction was being exploited therapeutically to avoid toxicity. This interaction has also been shown by others.[2] Its possible consequences should be recognized if concurrent use is undertaken.

References

1 Nirenberg A, Mosende C, Mehta BM, Gisolfi AL and Rosen G. High dose methotrexate with citrovorum factor rescue: predictive value of serum methotrexate concentrations and corrective measures to avert toxicity. Cancer Treat Rep (1977) 61, 779–83.
2 Sand TE, Jacobsen S. Effect of urine pH and flow on renal clearance of methotrexate. Eur J Clin Pharmacol (1981) 19, 453–6.

Misonidazole + Cimetidine

Abstract/Summary

There is evidence that cimetidine does not interact with misonidazole.

Clinical evidence, mechanism, importance and management

Cimetidine increases the half-life and area under the curve of misonidazole in mice,[2] but 1 g cimetidine daily given to six normal human subjects for nine days had no effect on the pharmacokinetics of misonidazole.[1] Even so it would be prudent to monitor the effects to confirm that cimetidine used for longer periods does not interact.

References

1 Workman P, Donaldson J, Smith NC. Effects of cimetidine, antipyrine and pregnenolone carbonitrile on misonidazole pharmacokinetics. Cancer Treat Rep (1983) 67, 723–5.
2 Begg EJ, Williams KM, Wade DN, O'Shea KF. No significant effect of cimetidine on the pharmacokinetics of misonidazole in man. Br J clin Pharmac (1983) 15, 575–6.

Misonidazole + Miscellaneous Drugs

Abstract/Summary

Phenytoin, phenobarbitone and dexamethasone increase the clearance of misonidazole from the body. Dexamethasone appears to reduce the neurotoxicity of misonidazole without reducing its radiosensitizing effects, but this does not seem to be true for phenytoin and phenobarbitone. Metoclopramide does not interact with misonidazole.

Clinical evidence, mechanism, importance and management

A study in patients suggests that the use of corticosteroids confers some protection against the peripheral neuropathy which can occur with misonidazole,[3] a possible explanation being provided by another study which showed that dexamethasone increased the clearance of misonidazole and reduced the plasma area under the curve.[6]

A study in normal subjects showed that after taking phenytoin (300 mg daily for a week) or phenobarbitone (200 mg daily for a week) the half-life of misonidazole was decreased by 27 and 23% respectively. The clearance increased by 42 and 31%.[1] This confirms previous human studies in which phenytoin shortened the misonidazole half-life by 31%[2] and 30–40%.[4] Both phenytoin and phenobarbitone were found to reduce plasma misonidazole concentrations.[3] It seems probable that this interaction results from an increase in the metabolism of the misonidazole caused by these two enzyme-inducing drugs. Whether concurrent use helps to reduce the neurotoxicity of misonidazole is uncertain although this was not apparent in two studies.[3,5] Peak plasma concentrations of misonidazole are not affected so that its radiosensitizing effects may not be reduced.[1]

A study in six normal subjects indicates that metoclopramide has no significant effect on the pharmacokinetics of misonidazole.[7]

References

1 Williams K, Begg E, Wade D, O'Shea K. Effects of phenytoin, phenobarbital and ascorbic acid on misonidazole elimination. Clin Pharmacol Ther (1983) 33, 314–21.
2 Workman P, Bleehen NM, Wiltshire CR. Phenytoin shortens the half-life of the hypoxic cell radiosensitizer misonidazole in man: implications for possible reduced toxicity. Br J Cancer (1980) 41, 302–4.
3 Walker MD, Strike TA. Misonidazole peripheral neuropathy. Its relationship to plasma concentration and other drugs. Cancer Clin Trials (1980) 3, 105–9.
4 Moore JL, Paterson ICM, Dawes PJD K, Henk JM. Misonidazole in patients receiving radical radiotherapy: pharmacokinetic effects of phenytoin tumor response and neurotoxicity. Int J Radiation Oncology Biol Phys (1982) 8, 361–4.
5 Jones DH, Bleehen NM, Workman P, Smith NC. The role of microsomal enzyme inducers in the reduction of misonidazole neurotoxicity. Br J Radiol (1983) 56, 865–70.
6 Jones DH, Bleehen P, Workman P, Walton MI. The role of dexamethasone in the modification of misonidazole pharmacokinetics. Br J Cancer (1983) 48, 553–7.
7 Williams KM, Begg EJ, Wade DN, O'Shea K. No significant effect of metoclopramide on misonidazole elimination in man. Br J clin Pharmac (1983) 15, 390–1.

Mitomycin + Chlorozotocin

Abstract/Summary

Pneumonitis developed in a patient concurrently treated with mitomycin and chlorozotocin.

Clinical evidence, mechanism, importance and management

A woman with pancreatic cancer developed acute interstitial pneumonitis (characterized by increasing dyspnoea and a dry cough) after receiving modest doses of mitomycin and chlorozotocin in combination with 5-fluorouracil and doxorubicin (FAM-chlorozotocin). Mitomycin and chlorozotocin rarely cause lung damage at low doses and it is concluded that when given concurrently they may act synergistically or additively to cause lung damage. The problem responded rapidly to treatment with prednisone.[1]

Reference

1 Godert JJ, Smith FP, Tsou E, Weiss RB. Combination chemotherapy pneumonitis: a case report of possible synergistic toxicity. Med Paed Oncol (1983) 11, 116–18.

Mitomycin + Frusemide (Furosemide)

Abstract/Summary

Frusemide does not interact with mitomycin C.

Clinical evidence, mechanism, importance and management

A study in five patients with advanced solid tumours treated with mitomycin C ($10 \, mg/m^2$) showed that frusemide given as a 40 mg IV bolus either 120 or 200 min after the mitomycin had no effect on its pharmacokinetics.[1]

Reference

1 Verweij J, Kerpel-Fronius S, Stuurman M, de Vries J, Pinedo HM. Absence of interaction between furosemide and mitomycin C. Cancer Chemother Pharmacol (1987) 19, 84–6.

Mitotane + Spironolactone

Abstract/Summary

An isolated report describes the abolition of the effects of mitotane in Cushing's disease by spironolactone.

Clinical evidence, mechanism, importance and management

A woman with Cushing's disease under treatment with chlorpropamide, digoxin, frusemide was given 200 mg spironolactone daily to control hypokalaemia. She was additionally treated for five months with 3 g mitotane daily to control the elevated cortisol levels but without effect.[1] When an interaction was suspected (on the basis of animal studies[2]) it was decided to withdraw the spironolactone, whereupon severe nausea and profuse diarrhoea developed with 24–48 hr, suggesting mitotane toxicity. This subsided and then redeveloped when the mitotane was stopped and then restarted a week later. The mechanism of this apparent interaction is not understood. It would seem that mitotane can become ineffective in the management of Cushing's syndrome in the presence of spironolactone. More confirmatory study is needed.

References

1 Wortsman J, Soler NG. Mitotane. Spironolactone antagonism in Cushing's syndrome. J Amer Med Ass (1977) 238, 2527.
2 Menard RH, Culter GB, Rifka SM et al. Spironolactone and adrenal cytochrome P-450; inhibition of o.p'DDD (mitotane) induced adrenal atrophy and necrosis. Read before the 59th Annual Meeting of the Endocrine Society, Chicago, June 10th, 1977. Quoted in ref 1.

Procarbazine + Miscellaneous drugs

Abstract/Summary

The effects of drugs which can cause CNS depression or lower blood pressure may possibly be increased by the presence of procarbazine.

Clinical evidence, mechanisms, importance and management

Procarbazine can cause CNS depression ranging from mild drowsiness to profound stupor. The incidence is variously reported as being 31%, 14% and 8%.[1-3] Additive CNS depression may therefore be expected if other drugs possessing CNS-depressant activity are given concurrently.

Orthostatic hypotension has been described in four out of 48 patients on procarbazine.[3] Elsewhere a patient with hypertension and Hodgkin's disease has been reported whose blood pressure returned to normal when treated with procarbazine.[4] Additive hypotensive effects may therefore be seen with the concurrent use of antihypertensive drugs.

An isolated report describes an acute dystonic reaction (difficulty in speaking or moving, intermittent contractions of muscles on the left side of the neck) in a patient on procarbazine when given prochlorperazine.[5]

References

1 Brunner KW, Young CW. A methylhydrazine derivative in Hodgkin's

disease and other malignant neoplasms: therapeutic and toxic effects studies in 51 patients. Ann Intern Med (1965) 63, 69.

2 Stolinsky DC, Solomon J, Pugh RP, Jacobs EM, Irwin LE, Wood DA, Steinfeld JL and Bateman JR. Clinical experience with procarbazine in Hodgkin's disease, reticulum cell sarcoma and lymphosarcoma. Cancer (1970) 26, 984.

3 Samuels ML, Leary WB, Alexanian R, Howe CD, Frei E. Clinical trials with N-isopropyl-alpha-(2-methylhydrazino)-p-toluamide hydrochloride in malignant lymphoma and other disseminated neoplasia. Cancer (1967) 20. 1187.

4 Frei E. Quoted as a personal communication by De Vita VT, Hahn MA, Oliverio VT in Monoamine oxidase inhibition by a new carcinostatic agent, N-isopropyl-alpha-(2-methylhydrazino)-p-toluamide (MIH). Proc Soc Exp Biol Med (1965) 120, 561.

5 Poster DS. Procarbazine-prochlorperazine interaction: an underreported phenomenon. J Med (1978) 9, 519–24.

Procarbazine + Mustine (Mechlorethamine, Nitrogen Mustard)

Abstract/Summary

A report on two patients suggests that the concurrent use of high doses of procarbazine with mustine may result in neurological toxicity.

Clinical evidence, mechanism, importance and management

Two patients with acute myelogenous leukaemia admitted to hospital for marrow transplantation and who were given high doses of procarbazine (12.5/15 mg/kg) and mustine (0.75/1.0 mg/kg) on the same day became lethargic, somnolent and disorientated for about a week. Although no interaction has been proved, the authors suggest that the mustine may have enhanced the neurotoxic effects of the procarbazine, and advise that it would be prudent to avoid high-dose administration of these drugs on the same day.[1]

Reference

1 Weiss GB, Weiden PL, Thomas ED. Central nervous system disturbances after combined administration of procarbazine and mechlorethamine. Cancer Treat Rep (1977) 61, 1713.

Procarbazine + Tyramine-Containing Foods and Sympathomimetic Amines

Abstract/Summary

It seems doubtful whether the weak MAO-inhibitory properties of procarbazine can normally cause a hypertensive reaction with tyramine or other sympathomimetic amines. An itching skin reaction attributed to an interaction with cheese has been described in one patient.

Clinical evidence, mechanism, importance and management

The manufacturers of procarbazine state that it '... is a weak MAO inhibitor and therefore interactions with certain foodstuffs and drugs, although very rare, must be borne in mind.' This is apparently based on the results of animal experiments which show that the monoamine oxidase inhibitory properties of procarbazine are weaker than pheniprazine.[1] There seem to be no formal reports of a hypertensive reaction in patients on procarbazine who have eaten tyramine-containing foods (e.g. cheese) or after using indirectly-acting sympathomimetic amines (e.g. phenylpropanolamine, amphetamines, etc.). The only account I have been able to trace is purely anecdotal and unconfirmed: '...I recall one patient who described vividly reactions to wine and chicken livers which had occurred while he was taking MOPP chemotherapy several years earlier. Since he had not been forewarned, the reactions had been a frightening experience.'[3] An itching skin eruption observed after the ingestion of cheese has been attributed to the MAO-inhibitory properties of procarbazine.[2]

A practical way of dealing with this interaction problem has been suggested by a practitioner in an Oncology unit:[3] patients on procarbazine should ideally be given a list of the potentially interacting foodstuffs (see 'Tyramine-rich foods + MAOI'), with a warning about the nature of the possible reaction but also with the advice that it very rarely occurs. The foods may continue to be eaten, but patients should start with small quantities to ensure that they still agree with them. Those taking MOPP should also be told that any reaction is most likely to occur during the second week while on a 14 day treatment with procarbazine, and during the week following when not taking it.

References

1 De Vita VT, Hahn MA, Oliverio VT. Monoamine oxidase inhibition by a new carciostatic agents. N-isopropyl-alpha(2-methylhydrazino)-p-toluamide (MIH). Proc Soc Exp Biol Med (NY) (1965) 120, 561.

2 Cooper IA, Madigan RC, Motteran R, Maritz JS, Turner C. Combination chemotherapy (MOPP) in the management of advanced Hodgkin's disease. A progress report on 55 patients. Med J Aust (1972) 1, 41.

3 Maxwell MB. Re-examining the dietary restrictions with procarbazine (an MAOI). Cancer Nursing (1980) December, 451–7.

Streptozocin + Phenytoin

Abstract/Summary

A single case report indicates that phenytoin can reduce or abolish the cytotoxic effects of streptozocin (streptozotocin).

Clinical evidence, mechanism, importance and management

A patient with an organic hypoglycaemic syndrome, due to a metastatic apud cell carcinoma of the pancreas, and who was treated with 2 g streptozocin daily for four days together with 400 mg phenytoin, failed to show the expected response until the phenytoin was withdrawn.[1] It would seem that the phenytoin protected the beta-cells of the pancreas from the cytotoxic effects of the streptozocin by some mechanism as yet unknown. Although this is an isolated case report its authors recommend that concurrent use should be avoided.

Reference

1 Koranyi L and Gero L. Influence of diphenylhydantoin on the effect of streptozotocin. Brit Med J (1979) 1, 127.

Tamoxifen + Aminoglutethimide

Abstract/Summary

Aminoglutethimide markedly increases the loss of tamoxifen from the body and reduces its serum levels.

Clinical evidence, mechanism, importance and management

A study in six menopausal women with breast cancer, treated with 80–320 mg tamoxifen daily, found that when also given 1 g aminoglutethimide daily for 6 weeks the serum levels of tamoxifen and most of its metabolites were markedly reduced. The clearance of the tamoxifen was increased 222% (from 189 to 608 ml/min) and the tamoxifen AUC was reduced by 75% (range 56–80%).[1] The probable reason is that aminoglutethimide is an enzyme inducing agent which increases the metabolism of the tamoxifen by the liver, thereby increasing its loss from the body. Tamoxifen appears not to affect the pharmacokinetics of aminoglutethimide.[1]

The authors of this report say that their findings may explain why combined use appears to be no more effective than tamoxifen on its own. They suggest that serum tamoxifen levels should be monitored and the dosage possibly increased to compensate for this interaction. More study is needed.

Reference

1 Lien EA, Anker G, Lonning PE, Solheim E, Ueland PM. Decreased serum concentrations of tamoxifen and its metabolites induced by aminoglutethimide. Cancer Res (1990) 50, 5851–7.

Tamoxifen + Medroxyprogesterone acetate

Abstract/Summary

Medroxyprogesterone affects the metabolism of tamoxifen but the clinical importance of this is uncertain.

Clinical evidence, mechanism, importance and management

The addition of 500 mg medroxyprogesterone acetate twice daily only slightly reduced the tamoxifen serum levels over a six month period in 20 women with breast cancer given 20 mg tamoxifen twice daily, but considerably reduced the levels of the desmethyl metabolite of tamoxifen, presumably because of some effect on the metabolism of the tamoxifen by the liver.[1] The clinical importance of this interaction awaits assessment.

Reference

1 Reid AD, Horobin JM, Newman EL, Preece PE. Tamoxifen metabolism is altered by simultaneous administration of medroxyprogesterone acetate in breast cancer patients. Breast Cancer Res Treat (1992) 22, 153–6.

Teniposide + Anticonvulsants

Abstract/Summary

Carbamazepine, phenytoin and phenobarbitone markedly increase the clearance of teniposide. A reduction in its cytotoxic effects may occur.

Clinical evidence, mechanism, importance and management

A study in 6 children with acute lymphocytic leukaemia found that the clearance of teniposide was increased two-threefold (from 13 to 33 ml/min/m²) while taking phenytoin or phenobarbitone concurrently.[1,2] Another patient showed a twofold increase in teniposide clearance when treated with carbamazepine.[2] The most probable reason is that these anticonvulsants are potent liver enzyme inducing agents which increase the metabolism of teniposide by the liver, thereby increasing its loss from the body. A previous study found that the oncolytic response to teniposide was reduced in those showing an increased teniposide clearance.[1] The authors of these two reports conclude that increased dosages of teniposide will be needed in the presence of these anticonvulsants to achieve a systemic exposure to the drug comparable to that in their absence.

Reference

1 Baker DK, Rodman JH, Pui CH, Rivera GK, Evans WE. Anticonvulsants increase clearance of teniposide. Clin Pharmacol Ther (1991) 49,195.
2 Baker DK, Relling MV, Pui C-H, Christensen ML, Evans WE, Rodman JH. Increased teniposide clearance with concomitant anticonvulsant therapy. J Clin Oncol (1992) 10, 311–5.

Vinblastine + Bleomycin + Cisplatin

Abstract/Summary

This drug combination appears to cause serious life-threatening cardiovascular toxicity.

Clinical evidence, mechanism, importance and management

A report describes five patients (aged 23, 24, 33, 42 and 58) under treatment for germ cell tumours who died from acute life-threatening vascular events (myocardial infarction, rectal infarction, cerebrovascular accident) following VBP therapy (vinblastine, bleomycin, cisplatin). A survey of the literature by the authors of this paper revealed 14 other cases of both acute and long-term cardiovascular problems (myocardial infarction, coronary heart disease, cerebrovascular accident) in patients given VBP therapy.[1] Reynaud's phenomenon is common (37%) in those treated with vinblastine and bleomycin or VBP and there is evidence that blood vessels are pathologically altered.[2] This drug combination is very effective in the treatment of testicular carcinoma but its potential toxicity is clearly very serious.[1,2]

References

1 Samuels BL, Vogelzang NJ, Kennedy BJ. Severe vascular toxicity associated with vinblastine, bleomycin and cisplatin chemotherapy. Cancer Chemother Pharmacol (1987) 19, 253–6.
2 Vogelzang NJ, Bosl GJ, Johnson K, Kennedy BJ. Raynaud's phenomenon: a common toxicity after combination chemotherapy for testicular cancer. Ann intern Med (1981) 95, 288–92.

Vinca Alkaloids + Mitomycin

Abstract/Summary

Vinblastine and vindesine can increase the pulmonary toxicity of mitomycin. Severe and life-threatening bronchospasm has been described.

Clinical evidence, mechanism, importance and management

There are now several reports describing an increase in lung disease in patients treated with mitomycin and vinca alkaloids. Diffuse lung damage characterized by interstitial infiltrates and pleural effusions resulting in respiratory distress and cough have been described after treatment with vinblastine.[1-3] Severe and life-threatening bronchospasm has also been described when vindesine sulphate was given after treatment with mitomycin.[4] The potential hazards of combining these drugs should be recognized.

References

1 Konits PH, Aisner J, Sutherland JC, Wiernik PH. Possible pulmonary toxicity secondary to vinblastine. Cancer (1982) 50, 2771–4.
2 Gunstream SR, Seidenfeld JJ, Sobonya RE, McMahon LJ. Mitomycin-associated lung disease. Cancer Treat Rep (1983) 67, 301–4.
3 Ozols RF, Hogan WM, Ostchega T, Young RC. MVP (mitomycin, vinblastine, progesterone): a second-line regimen in ovarian cancer with a high incidence of pulmonary toxicity. Cancer Treat Rep (1983) 67, 721–2.
4 Dyke RW. Acute bronchospasm after a vinca alkaloid in patients previously treated with mitomycin. N Engl J Med (1984) 310, 389.

Vincristine + Colaspase, Isoniazid and Pyridoxine

Abstract/Summary

Some limited evidence suggests that vincristine neurotoxicity may possibly be increased by the concurrent use of these drugs.

Clinical evidence, mechanism, importance and management

Severe neurotoxicity has been described in three patients who were under treatment with vincristine. One of them was also taking colaspase and the other two were concurrently receiving isoniazid and pyridoxine.[1] A definite link between the use of these drugs and this serious toxicity has not been established, but the evidence suggests that particular care should be exercised if given concurrently.

Reference

1 Hildebrand J, Kenis Y. Vincristine neurotoxicity. N Engl J Med (1972) 287, 517.

Chapter 14
Digitalis Glycoside Drug Interactions

Plant extracts containing cardiac glycosides have been in use for thousands of years. The ancient Egyptians were familar with squill, as were the Romans who used it as a heart tonic and diuretic. The foxglove was mentioned in the writings of Welsh physicians in the thirteenth century and features in *An Account of the Foxglove and some of its Medical Uses*, published by William Withering in 1785, in which he described its application in the treatment of 'dropsy' or the oedema which results from heart failure.

The most commonly used cardiac glycosides are those obtained from the members of the foxglove family, *Digitalis purpurea* and *Digitalis lanata*. The leaves of these two plants are the source of a number of purified glycosides (digoxin, digitoxin, gitoxin, lanatoside C and others), of gitalin (an amorphous mixture largely composed of digitoxin and digoxin), and of powdered whole leaf digitalis. Occasionally ouabain or strophanthin (also of plant origin) are used for particular situations, while for a number of years the Russians have exploited cardiac glycosides from lily of the valley. All of these cardiac glycosides have similar actions, but they differ in their potency and in their rates of elimination from the body, and this determines how much is given and how often. Table 14.1 lists many of the cardiac glycosides in use.

Digitalization

The cardiac glycosides have two main actions and two main applications: for the treatment of cardiac arrhythmias and fibrillation, and to a much lesser extent these days, for congestive heart failure. Because the most commonly used glycosides are derived from digitalis, the achievement of the desired therapeutic serum concentration of any cardiac glycoside is usually referred to as 'digitalization'. The digitalis glycosides are said to have a 'positive inotropic effect' on the heart muscle, meaning that the force of contraction of the heart muscle is increased.

It is usual to start treatment with a large 'loading dose' so that the therapeutic concentrations are achieved reasonably quickly, but once this has been reached the amount is reduced to a maintenance dose which is intended to keep a nice balance between drug intake and drug loss. This has to be done carefully because there is a relatively narrow gap between serum concentrations which are therapeutic and those which are toxic. Normal therapeutic levels are about one third of those which are fatal, and serious toxic arrhythmias begin at about two thirds of the fatal levels. If a patient is over-digitalized, signs of intoxication will occur: firstly loss of appetite, followed by nausea and vomiting. Visual disturbances may also be experienced, headache, drowsiness, occasionally diarrhoea, and the pulse rate can fall as low as 40 beats per min. Death can take place from cardiac arrhythmias which are associated with total AV block. Patients under treatment for cardiac arrhythmias can therefore demonstrate arrhythmias when they are both under- as well as over-digitalized, which may complicate the decision to increase or reduce the dosage.

Interactions of the cardiac glycosides

The pharmacological actions of these glycosides are very similar, but their rates and degree of absorption, metabolism and clearance are different and this determines the dosages used. For example, the half-life of digoxin is 30–40 h compared with 4–6 days for digitoxin, and this is reflected in their daily maintenance doses of 0.125–0.5 mg and 0.15 mg respectively. It is therefore most important not to

Table 14.1 Cardiac glycosides

Non-proprietary names	Proprietary names
Acetyldigitoxin	*Acetil Digitoxina, Acylanid(e)*
Acetyldigoxin	*Agolanid, Allocor, Cardioreg, Cedigocin(a)(e), Cedigossina, Ceverin, Decardil, Digisistabil, Digostada, Digostab, Dioxanin, Kardiamed, Lanadigin, Longidox, Novodigal, Sandolanid, Stillacor*
Acetylstrophanthidin	
Convallaria	
Cymarin	*Alvonal MR*
Delanoside	*Cedilanid, Desace, Desaci*
Digitalin	
Digitalis leaf	
Prepared digitalis	*Augentonicum, Digifortis, Digiglusin, Digiplex, Digitalysat, Pil-digis*
Digitoxin	*Asthensilo, Coramedan, Crystodigin, Digicor, Digilong, Digimed, Digimerck, Digipural, Digitalina-Bescansa, -Mialhe, -Nativelle, Digitasid, Digitox, Digitoxina Simes, Digitoxine, Digitrin, Ditaven, Mono-Glycocard, Purodigin, Tardigal*
Digoxin	*Allocor, Cardigox(in), Cardioreg, Cardiox, Coragoxine, Digacin, Digazolan, Digivern, Digomal, Dixina, Eudigox, Lanacordin, Lanacrist, Lanorale, Lanoxicaps, Lanoxin(e), Lenoxin, Natigoxin, Novodigal, Prodigox, Purgoxin*
Gitalin	*Cistaloxine, Formigitalin, Gitalide, Gitaligin, Verodigeno*
Gitoformate	*Dynocard, Formiloxine*
Lanatoside C	*Cedilanid(e), Celenat(e), Dilanosid-C, Lanatosid, Lanimerck, Lanocide*
Medigoxin	*Cardiolan, Lanirapid, Lanitop, Metidi, Miopat*
Meproscillarin	*Clift*
Ouabain (Stophanthin-G)	*g-Strofantin, Ouabaine Aguettant, Arnaud, Purostrophan, Strodival, Strophoperm*
Pengitoxin	*Carnacid-Cor, Cordoval*
Proscillaridin	*Caradrin, Proscillan, Sandoscill, Stelarid, Sucblorin, Talucard, Talusin, Tradenal, Urgilan, Wirnesin*
Strophanthin-K	*Estrofosid, Kombetin, Myokombin, Strofopan, Strophosid, Trauphantin*

extrapolate an interaction seen with one glycoside and apply it uncritically to any other. Because the therapeutic ratio of the cardiac glycosides is low, a quite small change in serum levels may lead to inadequate digitalization or to toxicity. For this reason interactions which have a relatively modest effect on serum levels may sometimes have serious consequences.

Digitalis glycosides + ACE inhibitors

Abstract/Summary

Some studies have found that serum digoxin levels rise by about 20–25% if captopril is used concurrently, but others have found no significant changes. No interaction has been seen with enalapril, lisinopril, ramipril or spirapril. It has been suggested that an interaction with any ACE inhibitor is only likely to occur in those patients who have pre-existing renal impairment. Digitoxin and captopril appear not to interact.

Clinical evidence

(a) Digoxin + Captopril

The serum digoxin levels of 20 patients with severe chronic congestive heart failure rose by 26% (from 1.38 to 1.74 nmol/l) while taking captopril (averaging 93.7 mg daily). Three of them had serum digoxin levels above the therapeutic range (2.6 nmol/l) but no toxicity was seen. All had impaired renal function and were being treated with diuretics.[1] A later study by the same workers showed that captopril increased serum digoxin levels by about 21%.[6]

Another controlled study in 31 patients with stable congestive heart failure, given 25 mg captopril three times daily, found no significant changes in serum digoxin levels over a 6-month period.[7] Two other studies in normal subjects and patients with congestive heart failure found no evidence of an interaction.[9,10]

(b) Digoxin + Enalapril, Lisinopril, Ramipril or Spirapril

20 mg enalapril daily for 30 days had no significant effect on the pharmacokinetics of digoxin (0.25 mg daily) in seven patients with congestive heart failure.[4] 5 mg lisinopril daily for 4 weeks had no significant effect on the serum digoxin levels of another 14 patients.[2] This confirms the findings of two single dose studies.[3,8] 5 mg ramipril daily for 14 days had no effect on the serum digoxin levels of 12 normal subjects.[5] 12–48 mg spirapril daily did not significantly affect the pharmacokinetics nor the steady-state serum levels of digoxin in 15 normal subjects on 0.5 mg digoxin.[11]

(c) Digitoxin + Captopril

A study in 12 normal subjects given 0.07 mg digitoxin daily for up to 58 days found no evidence that the addition of 25 mg captopril daily had a relevant effect on the pharmacokinetics of digitoxin, or its effects on the heart.[12]

Mechanism

Not fully understood. It has been suggested that an interaction is only likely to occur in those who have renal impairment. The glomerular filtration rate of these patients may be maintained by the vasoconstrictor action of angiotensin II on the postglomer-ular blood vessels, which would be impaired by ACE inhibition. As a result some of the loss of digoxin through the tubules is reduced.[9]

Importance and management

Information about the digoxin/ACE inhibitor interactions is limited. It has been suggested that no interaction is likely in patients with normal renal function, and that serum digoxin monitoring is only needed in those who have a high risk of reversible ACE inhibitor induced renal failure (e.g. patients with congestive heart failure during chronic diuretic treatment, with bilateral renal artery stenosis or unilateral renal artery stenosis in a solitary kidney).[9] It seems that in these patients their serum digoxin levels may rise modestly (20–25%). The critical factor seems to be not the particular ACE inhibitor used but the existence of abnormal renal function. This needs confirmation.

No interaction apparently occurs between digitoxin and captopril in normal subjects, but this needs confirmation in patients.

References

1 Cleland JGF, Dargie HJ, Hodsman GP, Robertson IS, Ball SG. Interaction of digoxin and captopril. Br J clin Pharmac (1984) 17, 214P.

2 Vandenburg MJ, Kelly JG, Wiseman HT, Mannering D, Long C, Glover DR. The effect of lisinopril on digoxin pharmacokinetics in patients with congestive heart failure. Br J clin Pharmac (1988) 21, 657P.

3 Morris FP, Tamrazian S, Marks C, Kelly J, Stephens JD, Vandenberg MJ. An acute pharmacokinetic study of the potential interaction of lisinopril and digoxin in normal volunteers. Br J clin Pharmac (1985) 20, 281–2P.

4 Douste-Blazy Ph, Blanc M, Montastruc JL, Conte D, Cotonat J, Galinier F. Is there any interaction between digoxin and enalapril? Br J clin Pharmac (1986) 22, 752.

5 Doering W, Maass L, Irmisch R, Konig E. Pharmacokinetic interaction study with ramipril and digoxin in healthy volunteers. Am J Cardiol (1987) 59, 60–4D.

6 Cleland JGF, Dargie HJ, Pettigrew A, Gillen C, Robertson JLS. The effects of captopril on serum digoxin and urinary urea and digoxin clearances in patients with congestive heart failure. Amer Heart J (1986) 112, 130–5.

7 Magelli C, Bassein L, Ribani MA, Liberatore S, Ambrosioni E, Magnani B. Lack of effect of captopril on serum digoxin in congestive heart failure. Eur J Clin Pharmacol (1989) 36, 99–100.

8 Vandenburg MJ, Morris F, Marks C, Kelly JG, Dews IM, Stephens JD. A study of the potential pharmacokinetic interaction of lisinopril and digoxin in normal volunteers. Xenobiotica (1988) 18, 1179–84.

9 Rossi GP, Semplicini A, Bongiovi S, Mozzato MG, Paleari CD, Pessina AC. Effect of acute captopril administration on digoxin pharmacokinetics in normal subjects. Curr Ther Res (1989) 46, 439–44.

10 Miyakawa T, Shionoiri H, Takasaki I, Kobayashi K, Ishii M. The effect of captopril on pharmacokinetics of digoxin in patients with mild congestive heart failure. J Cardiovasc Pharmacol (1991) 17, 576–80.

11 Johnson BF, Wilson J, Johnson J, Flemming J. Digoxin pharmacokinetics and spirapril, a new Ace inhibitor. J Clin Pharmacol (1991) 31, 527–30.

12 de Mey C, Elich D, Schroeter V, Butzer R, Belz GG. Captopril does not interact with the pharmacodynamics and pharmacokinetics of digitoxin in healthy man. Eur J Clin Pharmacol (1992) 43, 445–7.

Digitalis glycosides + Acipimox

Abstract/Summary

Acipimox does not interact with digoxin.

Clinical evidence, mechanism, importance and management

150 mg acipimox three times daily for a week had no significant effect on the serum digoxin levels, clinical condition, ECGs, plasma urea or electrolyte levels of six elderly patients.[1,2] No special precautions during concurrent use would seem necessary.

Reference

1 Chijioke PC, Pearson RM, Johnston A, Blackett A. Effect of acipimox on plasma digoxin levels in elderly patient volunteers. Br J clin Pharmac (1987) 25, 102–3P.
2 Chijioke CP, Pearson RM, Benedetti S. Lack of acipimox-digoxin interaction in patient volunteers. Hum Exp Toxicol (1992)11, 357–9.

Digitalis glycosides + Allopurinol

Abstract/Summary

Allopurinol has been shown not to affect serum digoxin levels.

Clinical evidence, mechanism, importance and management

No significant changes in the serum digoxin levels of five normal subjects occurred over a 7-day period while taking 300 mg allopurinol daily.[1] No special precautions would appear to be necessary.

Reference

1 Havelund T, Abildtrup N, Birkebaek N, Breddam E, Rosager AM. Allopurinols effekt pa koncentrationen af digoksin i serum. Ugeskr Laeger (1984) 146, 1209–11.

Digitalis glycosides + Amiloride

Abstract/Summary

Amiloride has little effect on blood digoxin levels in normal subjects, but it reduces the contractility of the heart. In patients with renal impairment it possibly raises serum digoxin levels.

Clinical evidence, mechanism, importance and management

Amiloride (10 mg daily for 8 days) virtually doubled the renal clearance of digoxin (from 1.3 to 2.4 ml/kg/min) in six normal subjects, but almost blocked the extra-renal clearance (from 2.1 to 0.2 ml/kg/min). The balance of the two effects was to cause a small fall in total body clearance and a small rise in serum digoxin levels.[1] The positive inotropic effects of digoxin were reduced, but whether this is clinically important or not is

uncertain. Studies in patients with congestive heart failure are needed. Patients with poor kidney function would be expected to show a rise in digoxin levels but the clinical importance of this also awaits confirmation. The effects of concurrent use should be well monitored.

Reference

1 Waldorff S, Hansten PB, Kjaergard H, Buch J, Egeblad H, Steiness E. Amiloride-induced changes in digoxin dynamics and kinetics: abolition of digoxin-induced inotropism with amiloride. Clin Pharmacol Ther (1980) 30, 1981.

Digitalis glycosides + Aminoglutethimide

Abstract/Summary

The clearance of digitoxin is markedly increased by the concurrent use of aminoglutethimide and a reduction in its effects would be expected.

Clinical evidence, mechanism, importance and management

The clearance of digitoxin was increased by 109% in six patients while receiving aminoglutethimide, 250 mg four times a day.[1] The likely reason is that the aminoglutethimide increases the metabolism of the digitoxin by the liver. This would be expected to be clinically important, but it appears not to have been assessed. Check that patients do not become underdigitalized during concurrent treatment. No interaction would be expected with digoxin because it is largely excreted unchanged in the urine and therefore metabolism by the liver has little part to play in its clearance.

Reference

1 Lonning PE, Kvinnsland S, Bakke OM. Effect of aminoglutethimide on antipyrine, theophylline and digitoxin disposition in breast cancer. Clin Pharmacol Ther (1984) 36, 796–802.

Digitalis glycosides + Aminoglycoside antibiotics

Abstract/Summary

Blood levels of digoxin can be reduced by the concurrent use of neomycin

Clinical evidence

Neomycin (1–3 g orally) was found to depress and delay the absorption of digoxin by the gut in normal sujbects.[1,2] The AUC (area under the curve) was reduced as much as 50%. Absorption was affected even when the neomycin was given 3–6 h before the digoxin. The probable reason is that neomycin can cause a general but reversible malabsorption syndrome which affects the absorption of several drugs. The extent of this is probably offset in some patients because the neomycin also depresses the destruction of the digoxin by the bacteria in the gut.[3] Information is limited but it appears to be an established interaction. Patients on digoxin should be monitored for reduced effects if neomycin is given and suitable dosage adjustments made if necessary. Separating the dosages of the two drugs does not prevent this interaction. Kanamycin and paromomycin possibly interact similarly, but this requires confirmation. There seems to be no information about other aminoglycosides.

References

1 Lindenbaum J, Maulitz RM, Saha JR, Butler VP. Impairment of digoxin absorption by neomycin. Clin Res (1972) 20, 410.
2 Lindenbaum J, Maulitz RM, Butler V. Inhibition of digoxin absorption by neomycin. Gastroenterology (1976) 71, 399.
3 Lindenbaum J, Tse-Eng D, Butler BV, Rund DG. Urinary excretion of reduced metabolites of digoxin. Amer J Med (1981) 71, 67.

Digitalis glycosides + (Para) – Aminosalicylic acid (PAS)

Abstract/Summary

Blood levels of digoxin in normal subjects are reduced to a small extent by p-aminosalicyclic acid, but the importance of this in patients is uncertain.

Clinical evidence, mechanism, importance and management

10 normal subjects showed a 20% reduction in the absorption of a single 0.75 mg dose of digoxin (using urinary excretion as a measure) when concurrently treated with 8 g p-aminosalicylic acid (PAS) daily for 2 weeks.[1] This seems to be just another aspect of the general malabsorption caused by aminosalicylic acid. The importance of this interaction in patients is not known (it is probably small) but it would be prudent to monitor concurrent use.

Reference

1 Brown DD, Juhl RP, Warner SL. Decreased bioavailability of digoxin due to hypocholesterolemic interventions. Circulation (1978) 58, 164.

Digitalis glycosides + Amiodarone

Abstract/Summary

Blood levels of digoxin can be approximately doubled by the concurrent use of amiodarone. Some individuals may show even greater increases. Digitalis intoxication will occur if the dosage of digoxin is not reduced appropriately.

Clinical evidence

The observation[1] that patients on digoxin developed intoxication and unexpectedly high digoxin blood levels when given amiodarone prompted study of this interaction. Seven patients on constant daily doses of digoxin for 14 days showed a mean rise in serum digoxin levels of 69% (from 1.17 to 1.98 µg/ml) when given 600 mg amiodarone daily. Two other patients similarly treated also showed this interaction.[1]

Numerous studies in large numbers of patients have confirmed this interaction, with reported increases in serum digoxin levels of 75%,[9] 90%,[7] 95%[11] and 104%.[12] The occasional patient may show three- to four-fold increases, whereas others may show little or no change.[7,14] Children seem particularly sensitive with two- to three-fold rises, and even as much as eight-fold.[13] Other reports confirm that the digoxin levels are markedly increased or roughly doubled, and intoxication can occur.[4–6,8,14,15,19,20,22] In contrast, one group of workers state that they observed no change in serum digoxin levels in five patients given amiodarone.[2,3] There is also some evidence that in the treatment of resistant atrial tachyarrhythmias the risk of arrhythmias may be increased by concurrent use.[23]

Mechanism

Not fully understood. Amiodarone reduces both the renal and non-renal excretion of digoxin,[10] and amiodarone-induced changes in thyroid function may also have some part to play in this interaction.[18] Displacement of digoxin from its binding sites has been suggested.[16,17] One study suggests that increased absorption from the gut is responsible.[21]

Importance and management

A well-documented and well-established interaction of considerable clinical importance. It occurs in most patients. It is clearly evident after a few days and develops over the course of 1–4 weeks.[11] If no account is taken of this interaction the patient may develop digitalis intoxication. Reduce the digoxin dosage by a third to a half when amiodarone is added[1,9,8,21] with further adjustment of the dosage after a week or two, and possibly a month or more, as necessary.[8] Children may show much larger rises in digoxin levels than adults so that particular care is needed. Amiodarone is lost from the body very slowly so that the effects of this interaction will persist for several weeks after its withdrawal.[22]

References

1 Moysey JO, Jaggarao NSV, Grundy EN, Chamberlain DA. Amiodarone increases plasma digoxin concentrations. Br Med J (1981) 282, 272.

2 Achilli A, Serra N. Amiodarone increases plasma digoxin concentrations. Br Med J (1981) 282, 1630.

3 Achilli A, Giacci M, Capezzuto A, de Luca F, Guerra R, Serra N. Interazione digossina-chinida e digossina-amiodarone. G Ital Cardiol (1981) 11, 918–25.

4 Nademanee K, Kannan R, Hendrikson JA, Burbham M, Kay I, Singh BN. Amiodarone digoxin interaction during treatment of resistant cardiac arrhythmias. Am J Cardiol (1982) 49, 1026.

5 McQueen EG. New Zealand Committee on Adverse Drug Reactions. 17th Annual Report 1982. NZ J Med (1983) 96, 95–9.

6 McGovern B, Garan H, Kelly E, Ruskin JN. Adverse reactions during treatment with amiodarone hydrochloride. Br Med J (1983) 287, 175–80.

7 Oetgen WJ, Sobol SM, Tri TB, Heydorn WH, Davia JE, Rakita L. Amiodarone-digoxin interaction. Clinical and experimental observations. Chest (1984) 86, 75–9.

8 Marcus FI, Fenster PE. Drug therapy. Digoxin interactions with other cardiac drugs. J Cardiovasc Med (1983) 8, 25–8.

9 Fornaro G, Rossi P, Padrini R, Piovan D, Ferrari M, Fortina A, Tomassini G, Aquili C. Ricerca farmacologico-clinica sull'interazione digitale-amiodarone in pazienti cardiopatici con insufficiencza cardiaca di vario grado. G Ital Cardiol (1984) 14, 990–8.

10 Fenster PE, White NW, Hanson CD. Pharmacokinetic evaluation of the digoxin-amiodarone interaction. J Amer Coll Cardiol (1985) 5, 108–12.

11 Vitale P, Jacono A, *Gonzales* y Reyero E, Zeuli L. Effect of amiodarone on serum digoxin levels in patients with atrial fibrillation. Clin Trial J (1984) 21, 199–206.

12 Nademanee K, Kannan R, Hendrickson J, Ookhtens M, Kay I, Singh BN. Amiodarone-digoxin interaction: clinical significance, time course of development, potential pharmacokinetic mechanisms and therapeutic implications. J Amer Coll Cardiol (1984) 4, 111–16.

13 Koren G, Hesslein PS, MacLeod SM. Digoxin toxicity associated with amiodarone therapy in children. J Pediatr (1984) 104, 467–70.

14 Nager F, Nager G. Interaktion zwischen Amiodaron und Digoxin. Schweiz med Wsch (1983) 113, 1727–30.

15 Strocchi E, Malini PL, Graziani A, Ambrosioni E, Magnani B. L'interazione tra digossina e amiodarone. G Ital Cardiol (1984) 14, 12–15.

16 Douste-Blazy Ph, Montastruc JL, Bonnet B, Auriol P, Conte D, Bernadet P. Influence of amiodarone on plasma and urine digoxin concentrations. Lancet (1984) i, 905.

17 Mingardi G. Amiodarone and plasma digoxin levels. Lancet (1984) i, 1238.

18 Ben-Chetrit E, Ackerman Z, Eliakim M. Case-report: Amiodarone-associated hypothyroidism-a possible cause of digoxin intoxication. Amer J Med Sci (1985) 289, 114–16.

19 Robinson KC, Walker S, Johnston A, Mulrow JP, McKenna WJ, Holt DW. The digoxin-amiodarone interaction. Circulation (1986) 74, II-225.

20 Johnston A, Walker S, Robinson KC, McKenna WJ, Holt DW. The digoxin-amiodarone interaction. Br J clin Pharmac (1987) 24, 253P.

21 Santostasi G, Fantin M, Marango I, Gaion RM, Basadonna O, Dalla-Volta S. Effects of amiodarone on oral and intravenous digoxin kinetics in healthy subjects. J Cardiovasc Pharmacol (1987) 9, 385–90.

22 Robinson K, Johnston A, Walker S, Mulrow JP, McKenna WJ, Holt DW. The digoxin-amiodarone interaction. Cardiovasc Drugs Therapy (1989) 3, 25–28.

23 Bajaj BP, Baig MW, Perrins EJ. Amiodarone-induced torsades de pointes: the possible facilitatory role of digoxin. Int J Cardiol (1991) 33, 335–8.

Digitalis glycosides + Amphotericin

Abstract/Summary

Amphotericin causes potassium loss which could lead to the development of digitalis toxicity.

Clinical evidence, mechanism, importance and management

Among the well-recognized adverse effects of amphotericin treatment is increased potassium loss.[1–3] The hypokalaemia can be severe. Although there seem to be no reports of adverse interactions, it would be logical to expect that digitalis toxicity could develop in patients given both drugs if the potassium levels were allowed to fall unchecked. Concurrent treatment should be well monitored and any potassium deficiency made good. Amiloride has been successfully used to counteract the potassium loss caused by amphotericin.[4]

References

1 Holeman CW, Einstein H. The toxic effects of amphotericin B in man. Californ Med (1963) 99, 290.

2 Butler WT, Bennett JE, Hill GJ, Szwed CF, Cotlove E. Electrocardiographic and electrolyte abnormalities caused by amphotericin B in dog and man. Proc Soc Exp Biol Med (1964) 116, 857.

3 Miller RP, Bates JH. Amphotericin B toxicity. A follow-up report of 53 patients. Ann Intern Med (1969) 71, 1089.

4 Smith SR, Galloway MJ, Reilly JT, Davies JM. Amiloride prevents amphotericin B related hypokalaemia in neutropenic patients. Clin Pathol (1988) 41, 494–7.

Digitalis glycosides + Antacids

Abstract/Summary

Although the bioavailability of digoxin is reduced by some antacids, the clinical importance of this is uncertain. It may be advisable to separate the dosages by 1–2 h to avoid admixture in the gut. This is effective with digitoxin.

Clinical evidence

(a) Digoxin

(i) Evidence of an interaction with digoxin

A study in 10 normal subjects given 0.75 mg digoxin (*Lanoxin*) with 60 ml of either 4% aluminium hydroxide gel, 8% magnesium hydroxide gel or magnesium trisilicate showed that the cumulative 6-day urinary excretion expressed as a percentage of the original dose was as follows: control 40%; aluminium hydroxide 31%; magnesium hydroxide 27%.[1]

Other studies describe reductions in digoxin absorption of 11% with aluminium hydroxide, 15% with bismuth carbonate and light magnesium carbonate, and 99.5% with magnesium trisilicate.[2] *In vitro* studies with digitoxin suggest that it may possibly interact similarly,[3] but lanatoside C probably does not.[4]

(ii) Evidence of no interaction

A study on four patients chronically treated with 250–500 µg digoxin daily showed that concurrent treatment with either 10 ml aluminium hydroxide mixture BP or magnesium trisilicate mixture BP, three times a day, did not reduce the bioavailability of the digoxin and none of the patients showed any reduction in the control of their symptoms.[5]

Other bioavailability studies failed to show a significant interaction between digoxin (in capsule but not tablet form)[7] or beta-acetyldigoxin[6] and magnesium-aluminium hydroxide.

(b) Digitoxin: Evidence of no interaction

A study in 10 patients with heart failure showed that their steady-state serum digitoxin levels were slightly but not significantly raised (from 13.6 to 15.1 ng/ml) while taking 20 ml aluminium-magnesium hydroxide gel three or four times a day, separated from the digitoxin dosage by at least 1–2 h.[8]

Mechanism

Not established. One suggestion is that the digoxin can become adsorbed onto the antacids and therefore unavailable for absorption.[1,3]

Importance and management

The digoxin-antacid interactions are moderately well documented but their clinical importance is not established. Watch for any evidence of a reduced response to digoxin if given concurrently. Raise the digoxin dosage if necessary. Alternatively, separate the dosages by 1–2 h to minimize admixture in the gut. This is effective with digitoxin and many other drugs which interact within the gut.

References

1 Brown DD, Juhl RP, Lewis K, Schrott M, Bartels B. Decreased bioavailability of digoxin due to antacids and kaolin-pectin. N Engl J Med (1976) 295, 1034.
2 McElnay JC, Harron DWG, D'Arcy PF, Eagle MRG. Interaction of digoxin with antacid constituents. Br Med J (1978) i, 1554.
3 Khalil SAH. The uptake of digoxin and digitoxin by some antacids. J Pharm Pharmac (1974) 26, 961.
4 Aldous S, Thomas R. Absorption and metabolism of lanatoside. Clin Pharmacol Ther (1977) 21, 647.
5 Cooke J, Smith JA. Absence of interaction of digoxin with antacids under clinical conditions. Br Med J (1978) 2, 1166.
6 Bonelli J, Hruby K, Magometschigg D, Hitzenberger G, Kaik G. The bioavailability of beta-acetyldigoxin alone and combined with aluminium hydroxide and magnesium hydroxide. Int J Clin Pharmacol (1977) 15, 337.
7 Allen MD, Greenblatt DJ, Harmatz JS, Smith TW. Effect of magnesium-aluminium hydroxide and kaolin-pectin on the absorption of digoxin from tablets and capsules. J Clin Pharmacol (1981) 21, 26.
8 Kuhlmann J. Plasmaspiegel und renale Elimination von Digitoxin bei Langzeittherapie mit Aluminium-Magnesium-Hydroxide-Gel. Dtsch med Wsch (1984) 109, 59–61.

Digitalis glycosides + Aspirin

Abstract/Summary

Aspirin does not interact with digoxin.

Clinical evidence, mechanism, importance and management

Although aspirin can double the serum concentrations of digoxin in dogs, a study in eight normal subjects demonstrated no interaction, even when taking high doses (975 mg three times a day).[1] This finding is in line with common experience.

Reference

1 Fenster PE, Comess KA, Hanson CD, Finley PR. Kinetics of digoxin-aspirin combination. Clin Pharmacol Ther (1982) 32, 428–30.

Digitalis glycosides + Azapropazone

Abstract/Summary

Azapropazone appears not to interact with digitoxin in most patients, but the occasional patient may possibly show a small rise in serum levels. The importance of this is uncertain.

Clinical evidence, mechanism, importance and management

900 mg azapropazone daily did not significantly alter the mean half-life of a single intravenous dose of digitoxin or the AUC in eight arthritic patients, although two of them showed individual half-life increases of almost a third and a half.[1] This suggests that concurrent use is normally likely to be uneventful, but the possibility of an interaction in the occasional patient cannot be dismissed. Information about digoxin appears to be lacking.

Reference

1 Faust-Tinnefeldt G, Gilfrich HJ. Digitoxin-Kinetik und der antirheumatischer Therapie mit Azapropazon. Arzneim-Forsch./Drug Res (1977) 27, 2009.

Digitalis glycosides + Barbiturates

Abstract/Summary

Blood levels of digitoxin can be halved by the concurrent use of phenobarbitone. Its effects may be expected to be reduced accordingly.

Clinical evidence

After taking 180 mg phenobarbitone daily for 12 weeks, the steady-state serum digitoxin levels in a group of patients (0.1 mg daily) fell by 50%.[1]

In associated studies the half-life of digitoxin decreased from eight to five days during phenobarbitone treatment.[1,2] In another study[1] the rate of conversion of digitoxin to digoxin in one patient increased from 4% to 27% while taking 96 mg phenobarbitone daily for 13 days.

In contrast, a study in 10 normal subjects given digitoxin (0.4 mg), digoxin (1 mg) or acetyldigitoxin (0.8 mg) daily failed to find changes in the serum concentrations of any of these glycosides while concurrently taking 100 mg phenobarbitone daily for 7–9 days.[4]

Mechanism

Phenobarbitone and other barbiturates are well known as potent liver enzyme inducing agents which, it would seem, can increase the metabolism and conversion of digitoxin to digoxin.[1–3] The failure of one study to demonstrate this interaction may possibly have been because the barbiturate was taken for a relatively short time.[4]

Importance and management

An established interaction, although its clinical importance is somewhat uncertain because there seem to be few reports of the effects of concurrent use or of problems in practice. Nevertheless, patients taking both drugs should be monitored for expected underdigitalization and the dosage of digitoxin increased if necessary. The result of this interaction is an increase in the levels of digoxin, but as its duration of action is considerably shorter than digitoxin, a much larger dose is needed to achieve the same degree of digitalization. Thus an increased conversion of digitoxin to digoxin means a reduction in the total activity of the two glycosides. It seems likely that digoxin itself will not be affected by the barbiturates because it is largely excreted unchanged in the urine. Other barbiturates would be expected to behave like phenobarbitone.

References

1 Jelliffe RW, Blankenhorn DH. Effect of phenobarbital on digitoxin metabolism. Clin Res (1966) 14, 160.
2 Solomon HM, Reich S, Gaul Z, Pocelinko R, Abrams WB. Induction of the metabolism of digitoxin in man by phenobarbital. Clin Res (1971) 19, 356.
3 Solomon HM, Abrams WB. Interactions between digitoxin and other drugs in man. Amer Heart J (1972) 83, 277.
4 Kaldor A, Somogyi GY, Debreczeni LA, Gachalyi B. Interaction of heart glycosides and phenobarbital. Int J Clin Pharmacol (1975) 12, 403.

Digitalis glycosides + Benoxaprofen

Abstract/Summary

Benoxaprofen does not interact with digoxin

Clinical evidence, mechanism, importance and management

Over a 4-week period the concurrent use of benoxaprofen, 600 mg daily, had no effect on the serum digoxin levels of 12 patients with rheumatic disease.[1] Benoxaprofen has been withdrawn from general use in most countries because of its adverse side-effects.

Reference

1 Zoller B, Engel HJ, Faust-Tinnefeldt G, Geissler HE, Gilfrich HJ, Zimmer M. An interaction study between benoxaprofen and digoxin. Eur J Rheumatol Inflamm (1982) 5, 82–6.

Digitalis glycosides + Benzodiazepines

Abstract/Summary

An isolated case report describes digoxin intoxication in a patient when given alprazolam, but a later trial in normal subjects failed to confirm this interaction. A reduction in the urinary clearance of digoxin has been described during the use of diazepam, but no interaction seems to occur with metaclazepam.

Clinical evidence

(a) Alprazolam

An elderly woman on maprotiline, isosorbide dinitrate, frusemide, potassium chloride, and with a serum digoxin concentration of 1.6–1.8 ng/ml, was additionally given 1 mg alprazolam daily. During the second week she began to demonstrate signs of digitalis intoxication and on admission to hospital her serum digoxin levels were found to have risen about 300% (to 4.3 ng/ml). The apparent oral clearance had fallen from 126.3 to 49.8 l/day.[1] However a two-way crossover study in eight normal subjects found no changes in the clearance of digoxin while taking 1.5 mg alprazolam daily.[3]

(b) Diazepam, Metaclazepam

The observation[2] that three patients showed raised digoxin levels while taking diazepam prompted a further study in seven normal subjects. After taking 5 mg diazepam with a single 0.5 mg dose of digoxin, and another 5 mg diazepam 12 h later, all of them were said to have a 'substantial reduction in urinary excretion' and five of them showed a 'modest increase in the digoxin half-life'. No further details were given.[2] No statistically significant interaction was seen in nine patients on digoxin (β-acetyldigoxin) when given metaclazepam.[4]

Mechanism

Uncertain. The suggestion is that diazepam may possibly alter the extent of the protein binding of digoxin within the plasma, which may have some influence on the renal tubular excretion.[2] The reason for the digoxin-alprazolam interaction in the patient described is not understood.

Importance and management

The adverse interaction with alprazolam cited above is an isolated report and it was not confirmed by a later study. Both digoxin and the benzodiazepines have been used for a very considerable time and these reports appear to be among the few on record. There would therefore seem to be no good reason for avoiding concurrent use but the effects should be monitored. More study is needed.

References

1 Tollefson G, Lesar T, Grothe D, Garvey M. Alprazolam-related digoxin toxicity. Am J Psychiatry (1984) 141, 1612–14.
2 Castillo-Ferrando JR, Garcia M, Carmona J. Digoxin levels and diazepam. Lancet (1980) ii, 368.
3 Ochs HR, Greenblatt DJ, Verburg-Ochs B. Effect of alprazolam on digoxin kinetics and creatinine clearance. Clin Pharmacol Ther (1985) 38, 595–8.
4 Völker D, Müller R, Günther C, Bode R. Digoxin-Plasmaspiegel während der Behandlung mit Metaclazepam. Arzneim-Forsch/Drug Res (1988) 88, 923–5.

Digitalis glycosides + Beta-blockers

Abstract/Summary

Concurrent use is common and often efficacious, but controversial. Excessive and potentially fatal bradycardia can occur if beta-blockers are used to control digitalis-induced arrhythmias unless appropriate precautions are taken.

Clinical evidence, mechanism, importance and management

Digitalis glycosides and beta-blockers are commonly used together, but such use is controversial. Some claim that it is beneficial[2] whereas others say that it is not.[1]

Cardiac arrhythmias and cardiac flutter which can occur in digitalis intoxication can be controlled with propranolol, but under these circumstances patients appear to be particularly sensitive to the actions of propranolol and show marked bradycardia.[3] There have been fatalities. It has been suggested that if propranolol is used in this situation, it would be wise to give the patient a test dose of 5 mg or less before giving the full dose, or to combine the full dose with a protective dose of atropine.[4] Atropine can be used in this way because it blocks the normal parasympathetic (heart slowing) activity which, if not adequately balanced by sympathetic (heart accelerating) activity, results in further bradycardia. Marked bradycardia (35–50 bpm) was seen in a very elderly patient on digoxin while using timolol eye drops.[11]

The pharmacokinetics of digoxin has been shown to be unaffected by the concurrent use of acebutolol,[5] cycloprolol (cicloprolol),[12] epanolol,[8] esmolol[6] or sotalol.[10] Sotalol is also reported to be well tolerated in patients on digoxin.[10] The pharmacodynamics of digoxin are also unaffected by esmolol and epanolol[8] and no significant changes in heart rate or blood pressure occur,[6,7] whereas cycloprolol has a positive inotropic effect.[12] A single dose study in normal subjects given 25 mg carvedilol (a vasodilator beta-blocker) found that maximal serum levels of digoxin (0.5 mg dose) were increased by 0.97 ng/ml (+60%) and the AUC by approximately 20%, but the authors of the study say that the clinical effects are likely to be small, although they advise monitoring. No interaction was seen when the carvedilol was given intravenously,[9] and no significant pharmacokinetic interaction was found in another study of carvedilol with digitoxin.[13]

References

1 O'Reilly M, Goldberg E, Chaithiraphan S. Propranolol and digitalis. Lancet (1974) i, 138.
2 Crawford MH, LeWinter M, Karliner JS, O'Rourke RA. Propranolol and digitalis. Lancet (1974) i, 458.
3 Turner JRB. Propranolol in the treatment of digitalis-induced and digitalis resistant tachycardias. Amer J Cardiol (1966) 18, 450.
4 Watt DAL. Sensitivity to propranolol after digoxin intoxication. Br J Med (1968) 3, 413.
5 Ryan JR. Clinical pharmacology of acebutolol. Am Heart J (1985) 109, 1131–6.
6 Lowenthal DT, Porter RS, Conry K, Bies C, Laddu A, Turlapaty P, Hulse JD. Digoxin-esmolol drug interaction. Clin Pharmacol Ther (1985) 37, 209.
7 Lowenthal DT, Porter RS, Achari R, Turlapaty P, Laddu AR, Matier WL. Esmolol-digoxin drug interaction. J Clin Pharmacol (1987) 27, 561–6.
8 Lefebvre RA, Bogaert MG, Duprez D. Investigation of possible pharmacokinetic and pharmacodynamic interactions between epanolol and digoxin. Eur J Clin Pharmacol (1990) 38, 505–7.
9 De Mey C, Brendel E, Enterling D. Carvedilol increases the systemic bioavailability of oral digoxin. Br J clin Pharmac (1990) 29, 486–90.
10 Singh S, Saini RK, DiMarco J, Kluger J, Gold R, Chen Y. Efficacy and safety of sotalol in digitalized patients with chronic atrial fibrillation. Am J Cardiol (1991) 68, 1227–30.
11 Rynne MV. Timolol toxicity: ophthalmic medication complicating systemic disease. J Maine Med Ass (1980) 71, 82.
12 Weber S, Kahan A, Pinquier JL, Julien J, Rosenzweig P, Bianchetti G, Morselli PL, Dessaut O, De Lauture D, Strauch G. Pharmacodynamic without pharmacokinetic interaction between cicloprolol, a partial β_1-adrenoceptor agonist, and digoxin in healthy subjects. Br J Clin Pharmac (1990) 30, 411–6.
13 Caspary S, Merz P-G, Brei R, Harder S. Interaction profile of carvedilol: investigations with digitoxin and phenprocoumon. Int J Clin Pharmacol Ther Toxicol (1992) 30, 537–8.

Digitalis glycosides + Calcium channel blockers

Abstract/Summary

Concurrent use can be valuable, but tiapamil may cause an approximately 50% and bepridil a 33% rise in serum digoxin levels which may possibly cause toxicity if the digoxin dosage is not reduced. Felodipine, gallopamil, nicardipine and nisoldipine cause small but normally clinically unimportant increases (about 15%), while amlodipine, isradipine and nimodipine appear not to affect serum digoxin levels. The situation with nitrendipine is uncertain but it possibly only causes a small rise. The interactions of digoxin with diltiazem, nifedipine and verapamil are dealt with individually elsewhere.

Clinical evidence

(a) Digoxin + Amlodipine

5 mg amlodipine had no significant effect on the serum digoxin levels or its renal clearance in 21 normal subjects given 0.375 mg daily.[6,17]

(b) Digoxin + bepridil

300 mg bepridil daily for a week raised the serum digoxin levels of 12 normal subjects on 0.375 mg daily by 34% (from 0.93 to 1.25 ng/ml).[1] Five of them experienced mild headache, nausea and dizziness for 1–3 days shortly after concurrent use started. The heart-slowing effects of the two were found to be additive, while the negative inotropic effects of the bepridil and the positive inotropism of the increased serum digoxin levels were almost balanced.[7,8]

In another study on 23 subjects given 0.25 mg digoxin and 300 mg bepridil daily for 14 days, peak serum digoxin levels rose by 48% (from 1.49 to 2.2 ng/ml) and the AUC rose by 21% (from 18.7 to 22.6 ng/h/ml).[9]

(c) Digoxin + Felodipine

10 mg felodipine twice daily for eight weeks raised the serum digoxin levels of 23 patients by a clinically non-significant amount (+15%).[20] 14 similar patients on 10 mg felodipine daily for a week (plain or slow-release preparations) also had no significant changes in digoxin levels.[13] A third study found that digoxin levels were transiently raised about 40% 1 h after intake.[21]

(d) Digoxin + Gallopamil

150 mg gallopamil daily for 2 weeks raised the serum digoxin levels of 12 normal subjects on 0.375 mg daily by 16% (from 0.57 to 0.67 ng/ml).[10]

(e) Digoxin + Isradipine

Isradipine (5–15 mg daily) for 10 days did not interact significantly in 24 normal subjects given digoxin by infusion.[5] Another 19 normal subjects on 15 mg isradipine daily for seven days similarly showed no changes in steady-state serum digoxin levels or in its absorption.[15]

(f) Digoxin + Nicardipine

The serum digoxin levels of 10 patients on 0.13–0.25 mg daily increased by 15% (said not to be statistically significant) when given 20 mg nicardipine three times a day for 14 days.[11] Another 20 patients with congestive heart failure also had no significant changes in steady-state serum digoxin levels (doses 0.25 − 0.5 mg daily) while taking 30 mg nicardipine three times daily for 5 days.[19]

(g) Digoxin + Nimodipine

30 mg nisoldipine twice daily caused no change in the pharmacokinetics or haemodynamic effects of digoxin in 12 normal subjects.[16]

(h) Digoxin + Nisoldipine

20 mg nisoldipine daily increased serum trough digoxin levels of 10 patients with heart failure by about 15%.[4,12,14] 10 mg nisoldipine twice daily caused no changes in the pharmacokinetics or haemodynamic effects of digoxin in eight normal subjects.[16]

(i) Digoxin + Nitrendipine

A study in eight normal subjects who had been taking 0.5 mg digoxin daily for 2 weeks showed that the concurrent use of 10 mg nitrendipine daily caused a slight but insignificant rise in plasma digoxin levels. 20 mg nitrendipine daily increased the digoxin AUC by 15% (from 9.7 to 11.2 ng/ml) and maximum plasma digoxin levels rose from 1.34 to 2.10 ng/ml. Clearance fell by 13% (from 315.1 to 274.5 ml/min). One subject dropped out of the study because of dizziness, nausea, palpitation, insomnia and nervousness.[1–3]

Another study found that plasma digoxin levels were approximately doubled when nitrendipine was given,[12] but two others in 12 normal subjects and eight patients found that 20 mg nitrendipine twice daily caused no change in the pharmacokinetics or haemodynamic effects of digoxin.[16,18]

(j) Digoxin + Tiapamil

Eight patients on digoxin who were given tiapamil (200 mg three times a day) for 14 days showed an approximately mean 50% rise in serum digoxin levels. No signs of digitalis toxicity occurred.[11]

Mechanism

Where an interaction occurs it is probably due to changes in the renal excretion of the digoxin.

Importance and management

Information about the effects of concurrent use is limited but it can apparently be therapeutically valuable. Monitor the effects of bepridil or tiapamil to ensure that digoxin serum levels do not rise excessively. Reduce the digoxin dosage as necessary. The other calcium channel blockers listed here (felodipine, gallopamil, nicardipine, nisoldipine) either cause only minimal increases which are unlikely to be clinically important in most patients, or do not interact at all (amlodipine, isradipine, nimodipine). The situation with nitrendipine needs clarification. The interactions of digoxin with diltiazem, nifedipine and verapamil are detailed in individual synopses.

References

1 Kirch W, Logemann C, Heidemann H, Santos SR, Ohnhaus EE. Effect of two different doses of nitrendipine on steady-state plasma digoxin levels and systolic time intervals. Eur J Clin Pharmacol (1986) 31, 391–5.
2 Kirch W, Logemann C, Santos SR, Ohnhaus EE. Influence of different doses of nitrendipine on digoxin plasma concentrations. Br J clin Pharmacol (1986) 23, 111–2P.
3 Kirch W, Logemann C, Santos SR, Ohnhaus EE. Nitrendipine increases digoxin plasma levels dose dependently. J Clin Pharmacol (1986) 26, 553.
4 Kirch W, Stenzel J, Dylewicz P, Hutt HJ, Santos SR, Ohnhaus EE. Influence of nisoldipine on haemodynamic effects and plasma levels of digoxin. Br J clin Pharmac (1986) 22, 155–9.
5 Johnson BF, Wilson J, Marwaha R, Hoch K, Johnson J. The comparative effects of verapamil and a new dihydropyridine calcium channel blocker on digoxin pharmacokinetics. Clin Pharmacol Ther (1987) 42, 66–7.
6 Schwartz JB. Amlodipine does not affect serum digoxin concentrations or renal clearance. Clin Res (1987) 35, 380A.
7 Belz GG, Wistuba S, Matthews JH. Digoxin and bepridil: pharmacokinetic and pharmacodynamic interactions. Clin Pharmacol Ther (1986) 39, 65–71.
8 Fenzl E, Toburen D, Wistuba S, Stern HC, Belz GG. Pharmacodynamic interactions between digoxin and bepridil. J Mol Cell Cardiol (1984) 16, (Suppl 3, no. 12).
9 Doose DR, Wallen S, Nayak RK, Minn FL. Pharmacokinetic interaction of bepridil and digoxin in steady-state. Clin Pharmacol Ther (1987) 42, 204.
10 Belz GG, Doering W, Munkes R, Matthews J. Interaction between digoxin and calcium antagonists and antiarrhythmic drugs. Clin Pharmacol Ther (1983) 33, 410–17.
11 Lessem J, Bellinetto A. Interaction between digoxin and the calcium antagonists nicardipine and tiapamil. Clin Therapeutics (1983) 5, 595–602.
12 Kirch W, Hutt HJ, Heidemann H, Ramsch K, Janisch HD, Ohnhaus EE. Drug interactions with nitrendipine. J Cardiovasc Pharmacol (1984) 6, S982–5.
13 Kirch W, Laskowski M, Ohnhaus EE. The felodipine/digoxin interaction. A placebo-controlled study in patients with heart failure. Br J clin Pharmac (1988) 26, 644P.
14 Kirch W, Stenzel J, Santos SR, Ohnhaus EE. Nisoldipine, a new calcium channel antagonist, elevates plasma levels of digoxin. Arch Toxicol (1987) Suppl, 11, 310–12.
15 Rodin SM, Johnson BF, Wilson J, Ritchie P, Johnson J. Comparative effects of verapamil and isradipine on steady-state digoxin levels. Clin Pharmacol Ther (1988) 43, 668–72.
16 Ziegler R, Horstmann R, Wingender W, Kuhlmann J. Do dihydropyridines influence pharmacokinetic and hemodynamic parameters of digoxin? J Clin Pharmacol (1987) 27, 712.
17 Schwartz JB. Effects of amlodipine on steady-state digoxin concentrations and renal digoxin clearance. J Cardiovasc Pharmacol (1988) 12, 1–5.
18 Debbas NMG, Johnston A, Jackson SHD, Banim SO, Camm AJ, Turner P. The effect of nitrendipine on predose digoxin serum concentration. Br J clin Pharmac (1988) 19, 151P.
19 Debruyne D, Commeau Ph, Grollier G, Huret B, Scanu P, Moulin M. Nicardipine does not significantly affect serum digoxin concentrations at the steady-state of patients with congestive heart failure. Int J Clin Pharm Res (1989) IX, 15–19.
20 Dunselman PHJM, Scaf AHJ, Kuntze CEE, Lie KI, Wessling H. Digoxin-felodipine interaction in patients with congestive heart failure. Eur J Clin Pharmacol (1988) 35, 461–5.
21 Rehnqvist N, Billing E, Moberg L, Lundman T, Olsson G. Pharmacokinetics of felodipine and effect on digoxin plasma levels in patients with heart failure. Drugs (1987) 34, (Suppl 3) 33–42.

Digitalis glycosides + Calcium preparations

Abstract/Summary

The effects of digitalis can be increased by increases in blood calcium levels, and the administration of intravenous calcium may result in the development of potentially life-threatening digitalis-induced heart arrhythmias.

Clinical evidence

Two patients developed heart arrhythmias and died after being given digitalis intramuscularly and either calcium chloride or gluconate intravenously. No absolutely certain causative relationship was established.[1]

There is other evidence that increases or decreases in blood calcium levels can increase or decrease respectively the effects of digitalis. A patient with congestive heart failure and atrial fibrillation was resistant to the actions of digoxin in the usual therapeutic range (1.5–3.0 ng/ml) until his serum calcium levels were raised from 6.7 to about 8.5 mg% by the administration of calcium and oral vitamin D.[2] Disodium edetate[3–5] and sodium and potassium citrate[6] which lower ionic blood calcium levels have been used successfully in the treatment of digitalis intoxication.

Mechanism

The actions of the cardiac glycosides (even now not fully understood) are closely tied up with movement of calcium ions into heart muscle cells. Increased concentrations of calcium outside these cells increase the inflow of calcium and this enhances the activity of the glycosides. This can lead to effective over-digitalization and even potentially life-threatening arrhythmias.

Importance and management

The report cited[1] (published in 1936) seems to be the only direct clinical evidence of a serious adverse interaction, although there is plenty of less direct evidence that an interaction is possible. Intravenous calcium should be avoided in patients on cardiac glycosides. If that is not possible, it has been suggested[7] that it should be given slowly or only in small amounts in order to avoid transient serum calcium levels higher than 15 mmol/l.

References

1 Bower JO, Mengle HAK. The additive effects of calcium and digitalis. A warning with a report of two deaths. J Amer Med Ass (1936) 106, 1151.
2 Chopra D, Janson P, Sawin CT. Insensitivity to digoxin associated with hypocalcaemia. N Engl J Med (1977) 296, 917.
3 Jick S, Karsh R. The effect of calcium chelation on cardiac arrhythmias and conduction disturbances. Amer J Cardiol (1959) 43, 287.
4 Szekely P, Wynne NA. Effects of calcium chelation on digitalis induced cardiac arrhythmias. Br Heart J (1963) 25, 589.

5 Rosenbaum JL, Mason D, Seven M. The effect of disodium EDTA on digitalis intoxication. Amer J Med Sci (1960) 240, 77.

6 Barbieri FF, Gold H, Lang TW, Bernstein H, Corday E. Sodium and potassium citrate salts for the treatment of digitalis toxicity. Amer J Cardiol (1964) 14, 650.

7 Nola GT, Pope S, Harrison DC. Assessment of the synergistic relationship between serum calcium and digitalis. Amer Heart J (1970) 79, 499.

Digitalis glycosides + Carbamazepine

Abstract/Summary, clinical evidence, importance and management

Bradycardia seen in patients on digitalis and carbamazepine was tentatively attributed to their concurrent use[1], but as yet this has not been confirmed by other observations. No special precautions seem to be necessary.

Reference

1 Killian JM, Fromm GH. Carbamazepine in the treatment of neuralgia. Use and side-effects. Arch Neurol (1968) 19, 129.

Digitalis glycosides + Carbenoxolone

Abstract/Summary

Carbenoxolone can raise blood pressure, cause fluid retention and reduce serum potassium levels. It is generally regarded as contraindicated in those using digitalis for congestive heart failure.

Clinical evidence, mechanism, importance and management

The side-effects of carbenoxolone treatment include an increase in blood pressure (both systolic and diastolic), fluid retention and reduced serum potassium levels. The incidence of these side-effects is said in some reports to be as high as 50%. Others quote lower figures, nevertheless it is clear that they are not an uncommon occurrence. Hypertension and fluid retention occur early in carbenoxolone treatment, whereas the hypokalaemia develops later and may occur in the absence of the other two side-effects.[1–4] The hypokalaemia may be exacerbated if thiazide diuretics are used to control the fluid retention without the use of suitable potassium supplements. For example, severe hypokalaemia has been described in a patient taking carbenoxolone and chlorthalidone without potassium supplementation.[5] For all these reasons carbenoxolone is unsuitable for patients with congestive heart failure, or those taking digitalis glycosides unless measures to avoid hypokalaemia are taken.

References

1 Geismar P, Mosebech J, Myren J. A double-blind study of the effect of carbenoxolone sodium in the treatment of gastric ulcer. Scand J Gastroenterol (1973) 8, 251.

2 Turpie AGG, Thomson TJ. Carbenoxolone sodium in the treatment of gastric ulcer with special reference to side-effects. Gut (1965) 6, 591.

3 Langman MJS, Knapp DR, Wakley E. Treatment of chronic gastric ulcer with carbenoxolone and gefarnate; a comparative trial. Br Med J (1973) 3, 84.

4 Davies GJ, Rhodes J, Calcraft BJ. Complications of carbenoxolone therapy. Br Med J (1974) 3, 400.

5 Descamps C. Rhabdomyocysis and acute tubular necrosis associated with carbenoxolone and diuretic treatment. Br Med J (1977) 1, 272.

Digitalis glycosides + Cholestyramine

Abstract/Summary

The blood levels of both digoxin and digitoxin can be reduced by the concurrent use of cholestyramine, but the clinical importance of this is uncertain. Minimize the possible effects of this interaction by giving the cholestyramine not less than one-and-a-half hours after the cardiac glycoside.

Clinical evidence

(a) Digitalis glycoside serum levels unaffected

10 patients on long-term treatment with either digoxin (0.125–0.25 mg daily) or digitoxin (0.1–0.2 mg daily) were concurrently treated for a year with 12 g cholestyramine or a placebo taken 1.5 h after the digitalis. Their serum digitalis levels were not significantly altered by the cholestyramine.[6]

The half-life of digitoxin is reported to have remained unchanged when cholestyramine was used.[10]

(b) Digitalis glycoside serum levels reduced

A study carried out with 12 subjects given 0.75 mg digoxin showed that the cumulative 6-day recovery of the digoxin from the urine was reduced almost 20% (from 40.5 to 33.1%) when 4 g cholestyramine was given concurrently.[1]

Other reports describe a fall in serum digoxin levels during the concurrent use of cholestyramine[2,9,11] and an increase in the loss of digoxin and its metabolites in the faeces during concurrent long-term use.[3] A reduction by cholestyramine of the half-life of digitoxin of 35 to 40% has been described.[4,5,8]

Mechanism

Not totally understood. Cholestyramine appears to bind with digitoxin in the gut, thereby reducing its bioavailability and interfering with the enterohepatic cycle so that its half-life is shortened. Just how digoxin interacts is uncertain.[3]

Importance and management

The overall picture is far from clear. Some interaction seems possible but the extent to which it impairs the treatment of patients on these glycosides is uncertain. Be alert for any evidence of under-digitalization if digoxin or, more particularly,

digitoxin are given with cholestyramine. Give the cholestyramine not less than 1.5–2 h after the digitalis to minimize
the possibility of an interaction.[6] An alternative is to use
beta-methyldigoxin which one study suggests may be minimally affected by cholestyramine.[7] Another study showed that
giving digoxin as a solution in a capsule reduced the effects of
this interaction.[11]

References

1 Brown DD, Juhl RP, Warner SL. Decreased bioavailability of digoxin
  produced by dietary fibre and cholestyramine. Amer J Cardiol (1977) 39,
  297.
2 Smith TW. New approaches to the management of digitalis intoxication.
  In 'Symposium on Digitalis' Glydendal Norsk Forlag, Oslo (1977) 39, 312.
3 Hall WH, Shappell SD, Doherty JE. Effect of cholestyramine on digoxin
  absorption and excretion in man. Amer J Cardiol (1977) 39, 213.
4 Caldwell JH, Greenberger NJ. Cholestyramine enhances digitalis excretion
  and protects against lethal intoxication. Clin Invest (1970) 49, 16a.
5 Caldwell JH, Bush CA, Greenberger NJ. Interruption of the enterohepatic
  circulation of digitoxin by cholestyramine. J Clin Invest (1971) 50, 2638.
6 Bazzano G, Bazzano GS. Effects of digitalis binding resins on cardiac
  glycoside plasma levels. Clin Res (1972) 20, 24.
7 Hahn K-J, Weber E. Effect of cholestyramine on absorption of drugs. In
  'Frontiers of Internal Medicine' 12th Int Cong Int Med, Tel Aviv 1974.
  Karger, Basel (1975) p. 409.
8 Carruthers SG, Dujovne CA. Cholestyramine and spironolactone and their
  combination in digitoxin elimination. Clin Pharmacol Ther (1980) 27,
  184.
9 Brown DD, Juhl RP, Warner SL. Decreased bioavailability of digoxin due
  to hypocholesterolemic interventions. Circulation (1978) 58, 164.
10 Pabst J, Leopold D, Schad W, Meub R. Bioavailability of digitoxin during
  chronic administration and influence of food and cholestyramine on the
  bioavailability after a single dose. Nauyenschmiedbergs Arch Pharmacol
  (1979) 307, R70.
11 Brown DD, Schmidt J, Long RA, Hull JH. A steady-state evaluation of the
  effects of propanthenline bromide and cholestyramine on the bioavailability of digoxin when administered as tablets or capsules. J Clin Pharmacol
  (1985) 25, 360–4.

Digitalis glycosides + Cibenzolone

Abstract/Summary

Cibenzoline does not interact with digoxin.

Clinical evidence, mechanism, importance and management

A study in 12 normal subjects taking 0.25–0.375 mg digoxin
daily showed that the concurrent use of 160 mg cibenzoline
twice daily for seven days had no effect on the pharmacokinetics of the digoxin.[1]

Reference

1 Khoo K-C, Givens SV, Parsonnet M, Massarella JW. Effect of oral cibenzoline on steady-state concentrations in healthy volunteers. J Clin Pharmacol (1988) 28, 29–35.

Digitalis glycosides + Cicletanine

Abstract/Summary

Cicletanine appears not to affect serum digoxin levels.

Clinical evidence, mechanism, importance and management

Single 50 mg and 100 mg doses of cicletanine were found to
have no effect on the serum digoxin levels of six patients
stabilized on long term treatment (0.125–0.25 mg digoxin
daily).[1] This absence of an interaction needs further confirmation.

Reference

1 Clement DL, Teirlynck O, Belpaire F. Lack of effect of cicletanine on
  plasma digoxin levels. Int J Clin Pharm Res (1988) VIII, 9–11.

Digitalis glycosides + Cimetidine, Ranitidine

Abstract/Summary

Changes in serum digoxin levels, both rises and falls, have
been seen in patients given cimetidine, but these do not appear
to be of clinical importance. Ranitidine appears not to interact.

Clinical evidence, mechanism, importance and management

While taking 600–1200 mg cimetidine daily the steady-state
serum digoxin levels of 11 patients with congestive heart failure
fell on average by 25% (from 2.0 to 1.5 ng/ml), but none of
them showed any ECG changes or signs that their condition
had worsened.[1] Four other patients with stable congestive
heart failure showed no significant changes in the pharmacokinetics of digoxin (0.125–0.25 mg daily) when treated with
1200 mg cimetidine daily.[6] Three single dose studies on 11 and
eight normal subjects respectively and six patients with duodenal ulcers[5] found that cimetidine (600–1200 mg) had no
significant effect on the absorption[2] or the kinetics[3,5] of digoxin.
Another study found a small increase in digoxin levels in
normal subjects, but only a small statistically insignificant rise
(0.02 ng/ml) in the steady-state levels of 11 patients given
1600 mg cimetidine daily.[4] Six patients with chronic congestive
heart failure given beta-methyldigoxin showed no changes in
their serum digoxin levels when concurrently treated with
150 mg ranitidine twice daily for a week.[7]

No interaction of clinical importance with either of these
H_2-blockers has been established and no special precautions
would seem to be necessary.

References

1 Fraley DS, Britton HL, Schwinghammer TL, Kalla R. Effect of cimetidine on steady-state serum digoxin concentrations. Clin Pharm (1983) 2, 163–5.

2 Ochs HR, Gugler R, Guthoff T, Greenblatt DJ. Effect of cimetidine on digoxin kinetics and creatinine clearance. Amer Heart J (1984) 107, 170–2.

3 Jordaens L, Hoegaerts J, Belpaire F. Non-interaction of cimetidine with digoxin absorption. Acta Clin Belg (1981) 36, 109.

4 Crome P, Curl B, Holt D, Volans GN, Bennett PN, Cole DS. Digoxin and cimetidine: investigation of the potential for a drug interaction. Human Toxicol (1985) 4, 391–9.

5 Garty M, Perry G, Shmueli H, Illfield D, Boner G, Pitlik S, Rosenfeld J. Effect of cimetidine on digoxin disposition in peptic ulcer patients. Eur J Clin Pharmacol (1986) 30, 489–91.

6 Mouser B, Nykamp D, Murphy JE, Krissman PH. Effect of cimetidine on oral digoxin absorption. DICP Ann Pharmacother (1990) 24, 286–8.

7 Enomoto N, KUrasawa T, Ichikawa M, Shimuzu T, Matsuyama T, Sakai K, Shimamura K, Oda M. Lack of interaction of beta-methyldigoxin with ranitidine in patients with chronic congestive heart failure. Eur J Clin Pharmacol (1992) 43, 205–6.

Digitalis glycosides + Cisapride

Abstract/Summary

Cisapride causes a small but probably clinically unimportant fall in the absorption of digoxin.

Clinical evidence, mechanism, importance and management

10 mg cisapride three times a day reduced the digoxin AUC (area under the curve) and the peak serum concentrations by 12–13% in six normal subjects taking 0.75–1.0 mg daily.[1] This is probably too small normally to be of much, if any, clinical importance. This needs confirmation.

Reference

1 Kirch W, Janisch HD, Santos SR, Duhrsen U, Dylewicz P, Ohnhaus EE. Effect of cisapride and metoclopramide on digoxin bioavailability. Eur J Drug Metab Pharmacokinet (1986) 11, 249–50.

Digitalis glycosides + Clovoxamine or Fluvoxamine

Abstract/Summary

Neither clovoxamine nor fluvoxamine appear to interact with digoxin.

Clinical evidence, mechanism, importance and management

After taking 150 mg clovoxamine or 100 mg fluvoxamine daily for 15 days, the pharmacokinetics (distribution, elimination and clearance) of a single intravenous dose of 1.25 mg digoxin were unchanged in eight normal subjects.[1] It seems unlikely therefore that either of these drugs will affect the steady-state serum levels of digoxin in patients, but this needs confirmation.

Reference

1 Ochs HR, Greenblatt DJ, Verburg-Ochs B, Labedski L. Chronic treatment with fluvoxamine, clovoxamine and placebo: interaction with digoxin and effects on sleep and alertness. J Clin Pharmacol (1989) 29, 91–95.

Digitalis glycosides + Colestipol

Abstract/Summary

Colestipol appears not to interfere with the absorption of either digoxin or digitoxin if it is given at least 1.5 h after the glycoside. It can be used to reduce serum digitoxin or digoxin levels if intoxication occurs.

Clinical evidence

(a) Digitoxin and Digoxin levels reduced in intoxication

Four patients intoxicated with digitoxin were given 10 g colestipol at once and 5 g every 6–8 h to reduce their digitoxin serum levels. The average digitoxin half-life fell to 2.75 days compared with an untreated control patient in whom the digitoxin half-life was 9.3 days. Another patient intoxicated with digoxin was similarly treated. His digoxin half-life was 16 h compared with 1.8–2.0 days in two other control patients.[2]

(b) Digitoxin and Digoxin levels unaffected

10 patients on long-term treatment with either digoxin (0.125–0.25 mg daily) or digitoxin (0.1–0.2 mg daily) were concurrently treated for a year with 15 g colestipol daily or a placebo, taken 1.5 h after the digitalis. Their serum digitalis levels were not significantly altered by the colestipol.[3]

A comparative study in 11 patients with serum digitoxin levels above the therapeutic range (40 ng/ml) showed that giving 5 g colestipol four times daily before meals and stopping the digitoxin immediately did not affect the digitoxin half-life (6.3 days) when compared with 11 other patients not given colestipol (6.8 days).[1]

Mechanism

Colestipol is an ion-exchange resin which can bind to digitalis glycosides.[2] It can apparently interfere with the entero-hepatic circulation and increase the loss during intoxication.

Importance and management

This interaction is neither well established nor apparently of great clinical importance. Giving either digoxin or digitoxin followed by the colestipol at least 1.5 h later appears to avoid any possible interaction in the gut.[3] In cases of intoxication it may possibly reduce serum digitalis levels because under these circumstances the excretion of digitalis in the bile increases and more becomes available for binding in the gut.[3]

References

1 Van Bever RJ, Duchateau AMJ A, Pluym BFM, Merkus FWHM. The effect of colestipol on digitoxin serum levels. Arzneimittel Forsch (1976) 26, 1891–3.

2 Bazzano G, Bazzano GS. Digitalis intoxication. Treatment with a new steroid-binding resin. J Amer Med Ass (1972) 220, 828.

3 Bazzano G, Bazzano GS. Effect of digitalis-binding resins on cardiac glycosides plasma levels. Clin Res (1972) 20, 24.

Digitalis glycosides + Cyclosporin(e)

Abstract/Summary

A report describes kidney dysfunction and marked rises in serum digoxin levels in patients concurrently treated with cyclosporin.

Clinical evidence

Four patients on digoxin developed kidney dysfunction and elevated serum digoxin levels when given cyclosporin before receiving heart transplants. Two of them on 0.375 mg digoxin daily showed four-fold rises (from 1.5 to 5.7 nmol/l, and 2.6 to 10.6 nmol/l respectively) within 2–3 days of starting to take 400 mg cyclosporin twice daily. Marked rises in creatinine levels occurred (a reflection of kidney dysfunction). A subsequent study on four other patients given both drugs found that serum creatinine levels rose sharply and in two of them plasma digoxin clearances fell by 58 and 47%.[1] The apparent volume of distribution of the digoxin also decreased markedly. This interaction has been studied in a further seven patients by the same group of authors.[2,3]

Mechanism

Not fully understood. Cyclosporin appears to reduce the renal excretion of digoxin.[2]

Importance and management

Information seems to be limited to the studies cited. If concurrent use is thought appropriate, the effects should be very closely monitored and the digoxin dosage should be substantially lowered if necessary.

Reference

1 Dorian P, Cardella C, Strauss M, David T, East S, Ogilvie R. Cyclosporine nephrotoxicity and cyclosporine-digoxin interaction prior to heart transplantation. Transplant Proc (1987) 19, 1825–7.

2 Robieux LC, Dorian P, Klein J, Cheung D, Ogilvie R, Koren G. The effect of cardiac transplantation and cyclosporin therapy on digoxin pharmacokinetics. Clin Pharmacol Ther (1991) 49, 129.

3 Robieux LC, Dorian P, Klein J, Chung D, Zborowska-Sluis D, Ogilvie R, Koren G. The effects of cardiac transplantation and cyclosporine therapy on digoxin pharmacokinetics. J Clin Pharmacol (1992) 32, 338–43.

Digitalis glycosides + Cytotoxic (Antineoplastic) agents

Abstract/Summary

Treatment with radiation and/or cytotoxic agents can damage the lining of the intestine so that digoxin is much less readily absorbed when given in tablet form. This can be overcome by giving the digoxin in liquid or liquid-in-capsule form, or by substituting digitoxin.

Clinical evidence

A study in 13 patients with various forms of neoplastic disease showed that radiation therapy and/or various high dose cytotoxic regimens (including carmustine (BCNU), cyclophosphamide, melphalan, cytarabine and methotrexate) reduced the absorption of digoxin from tablets (*Lanoxin*) by almost 46%, but the reduction was not significant (15%) when the digoxin was given in capsule form (*Lanoxicaps*).[4]

Other studies in patients confirm that a 50% reduction in serum digoxin levels (using beta-acetyldigoxin) occurred while using drug regimens of cyclophosphamide, onconvin, procarbazine and prednisone (COPP); cyclophosphamide, onconvin and prednisone (COP); cyclophosphamide, onconvin, cytarabine and prednisone (COAP); and adriamycin, bleomycin and prednisone (ABP). These effects disappeared about a week after withdrawal.[2] Radiation has a smaller effect.[3] Digitoxin absorption is not affected.[5]

Mechanism

The reduced absorption is thought to result from damage to the intestinal epithelium caused by the cytotoxic agents.[1]

Importance and management

The interaction appears to be established. Patients on digoxin and receiving treatment with cytotoxic drugs should be monitored for signs of under-digitalization. The problem can be overcome by replacing digoxin tablets with digoxin in liquid form or in solution inside a capsule. The effects of the interaction are short-lived so that a downward readjustment may be necessary about a week after treatment is withdrawn. An alternative is to use digitoxin which is not affected.

References

1 Jusko WB, Conti DR, Molson A, Kuritzky P, Giller J, Schultz. Digoxin

absorption from tablets and elixir: the effect of radiation-induced malabsorption. J Amer Med Ass (1974) 230, 1554–5

2 Kuhlmann J, Zilly W, Wilke J. Effects of cytostatic drugs on plasma levels and renal excretion of beta-acetyldigoxin. Clin Pharmacol Ther (1981) 30, 518–27.

3 Sokol GH, Greenblatt DJ, Lloyd BL, Georgotas A, Allen MD, Harmatz JS, Smith TW, Shader RI. Effect of abdominal radiation therapy on drug absorption in humans. J Clin Pharmacol (1978) 18, 388–96.

4 Bjornsson TD, Huang AT, Roth P, Jacob SS, Christenson R. Effects of high-dose cancer chemotherapy on the absorption of digoxin in two different formulations. Clin Pharmacol Ther (1986) 39, 25–8.

5 Kuhlmann J, Wilke J, Rietbrock N. Cytostatic drugs are without significant effect on digitoxin plasma level and renal excretion. Clin Pharmacol Ther (1982) 32, 646–51.

Digitalis glycosides + Dietary fibre (bran) and Laxatives

Abstract/Summary

Bisacodyl reduces serum digoxin levels to a small extent. Large amounts of dietary fibre, guar gum and neither of two bulk-forming laxatives containing isphagula (psyllium) appear to have a significant effect on the absorption of digoxin from the gut.

Clinical evidence

(a) Digoxin + Bisacodyl

Bisacodyl reduced the mean serum digoxin levels of 11 subjects by about 12%. When the bisacodyl was taken 2 h before the digoxin, serum digoxin levels were slightly raised, but not to a statistically significant extent.[10]

(b) Digoxin + Fibre (bran)

The serum digoxin levels of 12 patients (0.125–0.25 mg daily taken 15–30 min before breakfast) were unchanged over a 10 day period while on a diet supplemented each day with 22 g dietary fibre. The fibre was given in this way to simulate the conditions which might be encountered clinically (for example to reduce the symptoms of diverticular disease).[1]

7.5 g wheat bran twice daily caused a small reduction (10%) in serum digoxin levels of 16 geriatric patients after 2 weeks, but no significant change after 4 weeks.[7] 11 g bran fibre caused a 6–7% reduction in the absorption and the steady-state serum levels of digoxin in 16 normal subjects.[9] The cumulative urinary recovery of single oral doses of digoxin in normal subjects was reduced almost 20% by 5 g and 15 g fibre respectively, whereas a normal amount of fibre (0.75 g) had no effect.[2,3]

(c) Digoxin + Guar gum

5 g guar gum (*Guarem*, 95% guar gum) reduced the peak serum levels of a single 0.25 mg oral dose of digoxin by 21% and the AUC_{0-6h} was reduced by 16% in 10 normal subjects, but the amount excreted in the urine over 24 h was only minimally reduced.[11] 18 g guar gum with a test meal did not affect steady-state serum digoxin levels in 10 normal subjects on 0.5 mg digoxin daily for 3 days.[12]

(d) Digoxin + Ispaghula (psyllium)

An ispaghula formulation (*Vi-Siblin S*) was found to have no significant effect on serum digoxin levels of 16 geriatric patients.[7] The same lack of effect was seen in another study in 15 patients given 3.6 g psyllium (*Metamucil*) three times a day.[8]

Mechanism

Not established. Bisacodyl possibly increases the absorption of digoxin from the gut. Digoxin can bind to some extent to fibre within the gut[5] and *in vitro* studies show that the cellulose component is probably responsible.[4] However other *in vitro* studies (with bran, pectin, sodium pectinate, xylan and carboxymethylcellulose) have shown that most of the binding is reversible.[6]

Importance and management

Information seems to be limited to these reports. The reduction in serum digoxin levels caused by bisacodyl is small, probably of little clinical importance, and apparently preventable by giving the bisacodyl 2 h before the digoxin. Neither dietary fibre (bran), guar gum nor the two bulk-forming laxatives (*Vi-Siblin*, *Metamucil*) have a clinically important effect on serum digoxin levels. No special precautions would appear to be necessary.

References

1 Woods MN, Ingelfinger JA. Lack of effect of bran on digoxin absorption. Clin Pharmacol Ther (1979) 26, 21.

2 Brown DD, Juhl RP, Warner SL. Decreased bioavailability of digoxin produced by dietary fibre and cholestyramine. Amer J Cardiol (1977) 39, 297.

3 Brown DD, Juhl RP, Warner SL. Decreased bioavailability of digoxin due to hypocholesterolemic interventions. Circulation (1978) 58, 164.

4 Spector R, Vernick R, Lorenzo AV. Effects of pressure on the plasma binding of digoxin and ouabain in an ultrafiltration apparatus. Biochem Pharmacol (1973) 22, 2485.

5 Floyd RA, Greenberg WM, Caldwell C. In vitro interaction between digoxin and bran. Presented at the 12th Annual ASHP Midyear Clinical Meeting, Atlanta, Georgia, December 1977.

6 Hamamura J, Burros BC, Clemens RA, Smith CH. Dietary fiber and digoxin. Fed Proc (1985) 44, 759.

7 Nordstrom M, Melander A, Robertsson E, Steen B. Influence of wheat bran and of a bulk-forming isphaghula cathartic on the bioavailability of digoxin in geriatric in-patients. Drug-Nutrient Interactions (1987) 5, 67–9.

8 Walan A, Bergdahl B, Skoog M-L. Study of digoxin bioavailability during treatment with a bulk forming laxative (*Metamucil*). Scand J Gastroenterol (1977) 12 (Suppl 45), 111.

9 Johnson BF, Rodin SM, Hoch K, Shekar V. The effect of dietary fiber on the bioavailability of digoxin in capsules. J Clin Pharmacol (1987) 27, 487–90.

10 Wang D-J, Chu K-M, Chen J-D. Drug interaction between digoxin and bisacodyl. J Formosan Med Assoc (1990) 89, 913–9.

11 Huupponen R, Seppälä P, Iisalo E. Effect of guar gum, a fibre preparation,

on digoxin and penicillin absorption in man. Eur J Clin Pharmacol (1984) 26, 279–81.
12 Lembcke B, Häsler K, Kramer P, Caspary WF, Creuzfeldt W. Plasma digoxin concentrations during administration of dietary fibre (guar gum) in man. Z Gastroenterologie (1982) 20, 164–7.

Digitalis glycosides + Diltiazem

Abstract/Summary

Serum digoxin levels are reported in a number of studies to be unchanged by the concurrent use of diltiazem, but others describe increases ranging from 20 to 85%. An approximately 20% rise in serum digitoxin levels has also been described.

Clinical evidence

(a) Digoxin

(i) Evidence of no interaction

120 or 240 mg diltiazem daily had no significant effect on the serum digoxin levels of nine patients treated chronically for heart disease with 0.25 mg daily.[1] Other studies in 12 patients,[3] and nine, five, seven and eight normal subjects[2,7,8,13,14] given 120–360 mg diltiazem daily confirmed the absence of an interaction.

(ii) Evidence of an interaction

A study in 17 Japanese patients, some with rheumatic valvular disease, and taking either digoxin or medigoxin found that 180 mg diltiazem daily for two weeks increased their serum digoxin levels measured at 24 h by 36 and 51% respectively.[6] Other studies in European and American patients have shown rises of 20–85% in plasma digoxin levels while taking diltiazem.[4,9,10,12,15–18]

(b) Digitoxin

Five out of 10 patients on digitoxin showed a 6–31% (mean 21%) rise in serum digitoxin levels while taking 180 mg diltiazem daily for 4–6 weeks.[11]

Mechanism

Uncertain. Falls in total digoxin clearance of about 25% have been described.[5,10]

Importance and management

A thoroughly investigated interaction but there is no clear explanation for the inconsistent results. All patients on digoxin given diltiazem should be well monitored for signs of over-digitalization and dosage reductions should be made if neces-

sary. Those most at risk are patients with digoxin levels near the top end of the range. Similar precautions would appear to be necessary with digitoxin, although the documentation of this interaction is very limited.

References

1 Elkayam U, Parikh K, Torkan B, Weber L, Cohen JL, Rahimtoola SH. Effect of diltiazem on renal clearance and serum concentration of digoxin in patients with cardiac disease. Am J Cardiol (1985) 55, 1393–5.
2 Boden WE, More G, Sharma S, Bough EW, Korr KS, Shulman RS, Does high-dose diltiazem increase serum digoxin levels? J Am Coll Cardiol (1985) 5, 419.
3 Schrager BR, Pina I, Frangi M, Applewhite S, Sequeira R, Chahine RA. Diltiazem, digoxin interaction? Circulation (1983) 68, Suppl III-368.
4 Gallet M, Aupetit JF, Manchon M, Manchon J, Lopez M, Leizorovicz A. Effet du diltiazem sur la concentration serique de digoxine. La Presse Med (1984) 13, 2455–6.
5 Yoshida A, Fujita M, Kurosawa N, Nioka M, Shichinohe T, Asrakawa M, Fukuda R, Owada E, Ito K. Effects of diltiazem on plasma level and urinary excretion of digoxin in healthy subjects. Clin Pharmacol Ther (1984) 35, 681–5.
6 Oyama Y, Fujii S, Kanda K, Akino E, Kawasaki H, Nagata M, Goto K. Digoxin-diltiazem interaction. Am J Cardiol (1984) 53, 1480–1.
7 Beltrami TR, May JJ, Bertino JS. Lack of effects of diltiazem on digoxin pharmacokinetics. J Clin Pharmacol (1985) 25, 390–392.
8 Young PM, Boden WE, More G. Lack of effect of high dose diltiazem on serum digoxin levels. Clin Pharmacol Ther (1985) 37, 239.
9 Kuhlmann J St M, Frank KH. Effects of nifedipine and diltiazem on the pharmacokinetics of digoxin. Naunyn-Schmiedberg Arch Pharmacol (1983) 324 (Suppl) R81.
10 Rameis H, Magometschnigg D, Ganzinger U. The diltiazem-digoxin interaction. Clin Pharmacol Ther (1984) 36, 183–9.
11 Kuhlmann J. Effects of verapamil, diltiazem, and nifedipine on plasma levels and renal excretion of digitoxin. Clin Pharmacol Ther (1985) 38, 667–73.
12 North DS, Mattern AL, Hiser WW. The influence of diltiazem hydrochloride on trough serum digoxin levels. Drug Intell Clin Pharm (1986) 20, 500–3.
13 Boden WE, More G, Sharma S, Bough EW, Korr KS, Young PM, Shulman RS. No increase in serum digoxin concentrations with high dose diltiazem. Am J Med (1986) 81, 425–8.
14 Jones WN, Kern KB, Rindone JP, Mayersohn M, Bliss M, Goldman S. Digoxin-diltiazem interaction: a pharmacokinetic evaluation. Eur J Clin Pharmacol (1986) 31, 351–3.
15 Gallet M, Aupetit JF, Lopez M, Manchon J, Lestaevel M, Lefrancois JJ. Interaction diltiazem-digoxine. Evolution de la digoxinemie et de parametres electocardiographique chez le sujet sain. Arch Mal Coeur (1986) 79, 1216–20.
16 Andrejak M, Hary L, Andrjak M-Th, Lesbre J Ph. Diltiazem increases steady state digoxin serum levels in patients with cardiac disease. J Clin Pharmacol (1987) 27, 967–70.
17 Larman RC. A pharmacokinetic evaluation of the digoxin-diltiazem interaction. J Pharm Sci (1987) 76, S79.
18 King T, Mallet L. Diltiazem-digoxin interaction in an elderly woman: a case report. J Geriat Drug Ther (1991) 5, 79–83.

Digitalis glycosides + Disopyramide or Procainamide

Abstract/Summary

Neither disopyramide nor procainamide normally cause a significant change in serum digoxin levels. A single report describes intoxication in a patient on digitoxin and disopyramide.

Clinical evidence, mechanism, importance and management

(a) Disopyramide

A number of studies have clearly shown that disopyramide causes only a very small increase or no increase at all in the serum concentrations of digoxin.[1-5,7] A small but insignificant reduction in systolic time intervals has been seen[6] but the weight of evidence suggests that no adverse interaction occurs if these drugs are used together. However, a very brief report describes intoxication and serious arrhythmia in one patient given digitoxin and disopyramide.[9]

(b) Procainamide

A study in 26 patients who had been taking digoxin for at least seven days showed that while taking procainamide the serum digoxin levels remained unaltered.[2,8] No special precautions seem necessary.

References

1 Doering W. Digoxin-quinidine interaction. N Engl J Med (1979) 301, 400–5.
2 Leahey EB, Reiffel JA, Giardina E-G, Bigger JT. The effect of quinidine and other oral antiarrhythmic drugs on serum digoxin: a prospective study. Ann Intern Med (1980) 92, 605–8.
3 Manolas EG, Hunt D, Sloman G. Effects of quinidine and disopyramide on serum digoxin concentrations. Aust NZ J Med (1980) 10, 426–9.
4 Wellens HJ, Gorgels AP, Braat SJ, Vanagt EJ, Phaf B. Effect of oral disopyramide on serum digoxin levels. A prospective study. Am Heart J (1980) 100, 934–5.
5 Risler T, Burk M, Peters U, Grabensee B, Seipel L. On the interaction between digoxin and disopyramide. Clin Pharmacol Ther (1983) 34, 176–80.
6 Elliott HL, Kelman AW, Sumner DJ, Bryson SM, Campbell BC, Hillis WS, Whiting B. Pharmacodynamic and pharmacokinetic evaluation of the interaction between digoxin and disopyramide. Br J Clin Pharmac (1982) 14, 141P.
7 Garcia-Barreto D, Groning E, Gonzalez-Gomera A, Perez A, Hernandez-Canero A, Toruncha A. Enhancement of the antiarrhythmic action of disopyramide by digoxin. J Cardiovasc Pharmacol (1981) 3, 1236–42.
8 Leahey EB, Giardina EGV, Reiffel JA, Bigger JT. Serum digoxin concentrations during administration of oral antiarrhythmic drugs. Clin Res (1986) 25, 602A.
9 Manchon ND, Bercoff E, Lemarchand P, Chassagne P, Senant J, Bourreille J. Fréquence et gravité des interactions médicamenteuses dans une population âgée: étude prospective concernant 63 malades. Rev Med Interne (1989) 10, 521–5.

Digitalis glycosides + Diuretics, Potassium depleting

Abstract/Summary

It is generally believed, but not unequivocally established, that the potassium loss caused by these diuretics increases the toxicity of the digitalis glycosides. It is common practice to give these diuretics with potassium supplements or potassium-sparing diuretics.

Clinical evidence

(a) Evidence of an interaction

A comparative study[1] of the medical records of 418 patients on digitalis over the 1950–52 period, and of 679 patients over the period 1964–66, showed that the incidence of digitalis toxicity had more than doubled. 8.6% of the earlier group showed toxicity (58% on diuretics, mainly of the organomercurial type) compared with 17.17% of the latter group (81% taking diuretics, mainly the chlorothiazides, frusemide, ethacrynic acid, chlorthalidone), the conclusion being that the increased toxicity was related to the increased usage of potassium-depleting diuretics.

A retrospective study[2] of another large number of patients on digoxin showed that almost one in five had some toxic reactions attributable to the use of the glycoside. Of these, 16% had demonstrable hypokalaemia (less than 3.5 mmol/l). Almost half of the patients who showed toxicity were taking potassium-depleting diuretics, notably hydrochlorothiazide or frusemide. Similar results were found in other studies[3-9] on a considerable number of patients. There are other reports not listed here. In addition there is also some evidence that frusemide may raise serum digoxin levels.[13]

(b) Evidence of no interaction

A retrospective study of 191 patients who developed digitalis toxicity showed that the likelihood of its development in those with potassium levels below 3.5 mmol/l was no greater than those with normal potassium levels.[10]

Table 14.2 Potassium-depleting diuretics

Carbonic anhydrase inhibitors	Acetazolamide, dichlorphenamide, disulphamide, ethoxzolamide, methazolamide
Loop diuretics	Azosemide, ethacrynic acid, etolozin, frusemide, bumetanide, mefruside, muzolimine, piretanide, torasemide
Organomercurials	Chlormerodrin, meraluride, mercaptomerin
Thiazides and related diuretics	Althiazide, ambuside, bemetizide, bendrofluazide, benzthiazide, benzylhydrochlorothiazide, buthiazide, chlorothiazide, chlorthalidone, clopamide, clorexolone, cyclopenthiazide, cyclothiazide, epithiazide, ethiazide, fenquizone, hydrobentizide, hydrochlorothiazide, hydroflumethiazide, indapamide, mebutizide, mefruside, methylclothiazide, meticrane, metolazone, polythiazide, quinethazone, teclothiazide, trichlormethiazide, xipamide

Two other studies on a total of almost 200 patients failed to detect any association between the development of digitalis toxicity and the use of diuretics or changes in potassium levels.[11,12] A study in 10 normal subjects found that 10 mg torasemide daily had no significant effect on the pharmacokinetics of digoxin[14]

Mechanism

Not fully understood. The cardiac glycosides inhibit sodium-potassium ATP-ase which is concerned with the transport of sodium and potassium ions across the membranes of the myocardial cells, and this is associated with an increase in the availability of calcium ions concerned with the contraction of the cells. Potassium loss caused by these diuretics exacerbates the potassium loss from the myocardial cells, thereby increasing the activity and the toxicity of the digitalis. Some loss of magnesium may also have a part to play. The mechanism of this interaction is still being debated.

Importance and management

A direct link between the use of these diuretics and the development of digitalis toxicity is not established beyond doubt, but current thinking favours the belief that concurrent use can result in digitalis intoxication. Because it is only a short step from effective therapy with digitalis to a state of intoxication, those given potassium-depleting diuretics should be well monitored for signs of toxicity. Ideally serum potassium (normal range 3.8 to 5.0 mmol/l) and magnesium levels should be monitored. One of the problems is that serum potassium levels and body stores of potassium are not uniformly correlated. If necessary potassium supplements should be given. It may be possible to do this with foods which are high in potassium but low in sodium (citrus fruits, bananas, peaches, dates, wheat germ, potatoes). An alternative is to use a potassium-sparing diuretic such as triamterene or spironolactone.

References

1 Jorgenson AW, Sorensen OH. Digitalis intoxication: a comparative study on the incidence of digitalis intoxication during the periods 1950–1952 and 1964–1966. Acta Med Scand (1970) 188, 179.
2 Shapiro S, Slone D, Lewis GP, Jick H. The epidemiology of digoxin. A study in three Boston Hospitals. J Chron Dis (1969) 22, 361.
3 Tawakkol AA, Nutter DO, Massumi RA. A prospective study of digitalis toxicity in a large city hospital. Med Ann D C (1967) 36, 402.
4 Soffer A. The changing clinical picture of digitalis intoxication. Arch Int Med (1961) 107, 681.
5 Rodensky PL, Wasserman F. Observation on digitalis intoxication. Arch Int Med (1961) 108, 171.
6 Steiness E, Olesen KH. Cardiac arrhythmias induced by hypokalaemia and potassium loss during maintenance digoxin therapy. Br Heart J (1976) 38, 167.
7 Binnion PE. Hypokalaemia and digoxin-induced arrhythmias. Lancet (1975) i, 343.
8 Poole-Wilson PA, Hall R, Cameron IR. Hypokalaemia, digitalis and arrhythmias. Lancet (1975) i, 575.
9 Shapiro W, Taubert K. Hypokalaemia and digoxin induced arrhythmias. Lancet (1975) ii, 604.
10 Ogilvie RI, Ruedy J. An educational program in digitalis therapy. J Amer Med Ass (1972) 222, 50.
11 Smith TW, Haber E. Digoxin intoxication: the relationship of clinical presentation to serum digoxin concentration. J Clin Invest (1970) 49, 2377.
12 Beller GA, Smith TW, Abelmann WH, Haber E, Hood WB. Digitalis intoxication: a prospective clinical study with serum level correlations. N Engl J Med (1971) 284, 989.
13 Tsutsumi E, Fujiki H, Takeda H, Fukushima H. Effect of furosemide on serum clearance and renal excretion of digoxin. J Clin Pharmacol (1979) 19, 200.
14 Krämer BK, Ress KM, von Möllendorff E, Piesche L, Achhammer I, Müller GA, Risler T. Influence of torasemide on serum level and renal elimination of digoxin in healthy volunteers. Progr Pharmacol & Clin Pharmacol (1990) 8, 39–46.

Digitalis glycosides + Edrophonium

Abstract/Summary

Excessive bradycardia and AV-block may occur in patients on digitalis glycosides given edrophonium.

Clinical evidence, mechanism, importance and management

The rapid IV injection of 10 mg edrophonium has proved to be useful in the differentiation of cardiac arrhythmias, but it has been recommended that it should not be given to patients with auricular flutter or tachycardia who are taking digitalis glycosides because of the risk of producing AV-block due to the additive heart slowing effects.[1] This recommendation is reinforced by the case of an elderly woman who developed bradycardia, AV block and asystole following concurrent use.[2]

References

1 Reddy RCV, Gould L, Gomprecht RF. Use of edrophonium (Tensilon) in the evaluation of cardiac arrhythmias. Amer Heart J (1971) 82, 742.
2 Gould L, Zahir M, Gomprecht RF. Cardiac arrest during edrophonium administration. Amer Heart J (1971) 81, 437.

Digitalis glycosides + Encainide

Abstract/Summary

Digoxin and encainide do not interact adversely.

Clinical evidence, mechanism, importance and management

No significant changes occurred in serum digoxin levels of 17 patients when concurrently taking 100–200 mg encainide daily. A further study in 10 patients with severe congestive heart failure confirmed these findings. The efficacy of neither drug was changed.[1] No special precautions seem to be necessary.

Reference

1 Quart BD, Gallo DG, Sami MH, Wood AJJ. Drug interaction studies and encainide use in renal and hepatic impairment. Am J Cardiol (1986) 58, 104–13C.

Digitalis glycosides + Enoximone

Abstract/Summary

Enoximone does not affect the serum levels of either digoxin or digitoxin.

Clinical evidence, mechanism, importance and management

A study in 23 patients on long-term treatment with digitalis glycosides (18 on digoxin and five on digitoxin) showed that the concurrent use of enoximone, 100 mg three times daily for a week, had no significant effect on the serum levels of either of these glycosides.[1,2] Cardiac function was improved. No special precautions seem necessary.

References

1 Glauner T, Winkelmann FHB, Dieterich HA, Trenk D, Jähnchen E. Lack of effect of enoximone on steady-state plasma concentrations of digoxin and digitoxin. Eur Heart J (1988) 9 (Suppl 1) 151.
2 Trenk D, Hertrich F, Winkelmann B, Glauner T, Dieterich HA, Jähnchen E. Lack of effect of enoximone on the pharmacokinetics of digoxin in patients with congestive heart failure. J Clin Pharmacol (1990) 30, 235–40.

Digitalis glycosides + Erythromycin, Tetracycline or other antibiotics

Abstract/Summary

Blood digoxin levels may be approximately doubled in about 10% of patients treated with erythromycin. Digitalis intoxication has been seen. A smaller increase may occur with tetracycline. No interaction normally occurs with cefazolin or rokitamycin. No important interaction occurs between ampicillin and digitoxin.

Clinical evidence

(a) Erythromycin

An elderly woman with a prosthetic heart valve was under treatment for left ventricular dysfunction with warfarin, frusemide, hydralazine, isosorbide and digoxin, to which was added erythromycin. Four days later her serum digoxin levels were found to have risen to 2.6 ng/ml from a normal steady-state range of 1.4–1.7 ng/ml, and she showed evidence of digitalis intoxication.[1]

This report is in line with a previous report describing two patients on 0.5 mg digoxin daily whose serum digoxin levels roughly doubled after five days of erythromycin (1–2 g daily).[2] A patient on digoxin developed signs of toxicity (nausea, vomiting, cardiac arrhythmias) within four days of starting to take 500 mg erythromycin three times daily. Her serum digoxin levels were elevated. This patient recalled having similar problems during a previous course of erythromycin.[7] Another patient given 250 mg erythromycin 6-hourly similarly showed elevated serum digoxin levels within six days.[8]

(b) Other antibiotics

2 g tetracycline daily has been responsible for a 30% rise in serum digoxin levels over five days in one patient. A marked fall in the excretion of digoxin metabolites from the gut (see Mechanism) in the presence of erythromycin and tetracycline is confirmed in another brief report, but not with cefazolin and only occasionally with penicillin.[4] A later report found that ampicillin did not have a significant effect on digitoxin serum levels.[6] Rokitamycin also does not interact.[5]

Mechanism

About 10% of patients on oral digoxin excrete it in substantial amounts in the faeces and urine as inactive metabolites (digoxin reduction products or DRPs). This metabolism seems to be the responsibility of the gut flora, in particular *Eubacterium lentum*, which is anaerobic and gram positive.[2,3,8] In the presence of antibiotics which decimate these organisms, much more digoxin is available for absorption which results in a marked rise in serum levels. At the same time the inactive metabolies derived from the gut disappear.[3]

Importance and management

The digoxin/erythromycin and /tetracycline interactions are not strongly established. Only a small proportion of patients (about 10%) is likely to be at risk, the difficulty being that it is usually not known if a particular patient falls into this 'excretor' category or not (see 'Mechanism'). Monitor patients for signs of increased digoxin effects if they are given antibiotics which reduce the activity of the gut flora, reducing the digoxin dosage as necessary. There is unconfirmed evidence that it does not occur with cefazolin, only occasionally with penicillin,[4] and no changes in digoxin levels occur if rokitamycin is given.[5] Ampicillin does not interact significantly with digitoxin.[6]

References

1 Friedman HS, Bonventre MV. Erythromycin-induced digoxin toxicity. Chest (1982) 82, 202.
2 Lindenbaum J, Rund DG, Butler VP, Tse-Eng D, Saha JR. Inactivation of digoxin by the gut flora: reversal of antibiotic therapy. N Engl J Med (1981) 305, 789–94.

3 Lindenbaum J, Tse-Eng D, Butler VP, Rund DG. Urinary excretion of reduced metabolites of digoxin. Am J Med (1981) 71,67.
4 Dobkin JF, Saha JR, Butler VP, Lindenbaum J. Effects of antibiotic therapy on digoxin metabolism. Clin Res (1982) 30,517A.
5 Ishioka T. Effect of a new macrolide antibiotic 3'-O-propionyl-leucomycin A5 (Rotikamycin) on serum concentrations of theophylline and digoxin in the elderly. Acta Therapeutica (1987) 13,17–23.
6 Lucena MI, Moreno A, Fernandez MC, Garcia-Morillas M, Andrade R. Digitoxin elimination in healthy subjects taking ampicillin. Int J Clin Pharm Res (1987) VII, 33–7.
7 Maxwell DL, Gilmour-White SK, Hall MR. Digoxin toxicity due to interaction of digoxin with erythromycin. Br Med J (1989) 298, 572.
8 Morton MR, Cooper JW. Erythromycin-induced digoxin toxicity. DICP Ann Pharmacotherapy (1989) 23, 668–70.

Digitalis Glycosides + Fenoldopam

Abstract/Summary

Fenoldopam appears to cause a small and clinically unimportant reduction in serum digoxin levels in most patients, but more marked changes may occur in a few individuals.

Clinical evidence, mechanism, importance and management

Ten patients with congestive heart failure on chronic digoxin treatment (doses not stated) were additionally given 100 mg fenoldopam three times daily for 9 days. The mean AUC and steady-state digoxin levels were reduced about 20%. The steady-state serum levels of two patients fell by 48% (from 1.36 to 0.71 ng/ml) and 68% (from 1.36 to 0.71 ng/ml), and rose by 45% (from 1.03 to 1.49 ng/ml) in another.[1] Most patients appear therefore not to show marked changes in serum digoxin levels, but a few individuals may possibly need some dosage adjustment. Monitor the effects of concurrent use.

Reference

1 Strocchi E, Tartagni F, Malini PL, Valtancoli G, Ambrosioni E, Pasinelli F, Riva E, Fuccella LM. Interaction study of fenoldopam-digoxin in congestive heart failure. Eur J Clin Pharmacol (1989) 37, 395–7.

Digitalis Glycosides + Flecainide

Abstract/Summary

Serum digoxin levels are unaltered or only modestly increased by the use of flecainide, but this is not likely to be important in most patients.

Clinical evidence

While taking 100–200 mg flecainide twice daily for 7 days the serum digoxin levels of five patients with congestive heart failure remained unaltered. The same result was seen in four patients over a 4-week period.[3]

In contrast, a study in 15 normal subjects showed that while taking 200 mg flecainide twice daily, their serum digoxin levels measured just before and 6 h after taking their daily dose of digoxin (0.25 mg) rose by 24% and 13% respectively.[1] The changes observed in vital signs were not clinically significant. In a single dose study the steady-state digoxin levels were predicted to rise about 15% while taking 200 mg flecainide twice daily.[2]

Mechanism

Uncertain. It is suggested that any changes may be due to alterations in the volume of distribution.[2]

Importance and management

Documentation is limited but what is known suggests that either no interaction occurs, or any changes are small and unlikely to be clinically important in most patients. However the authors of one of the reports[1] suggest that patients with high drug levels, atrioventricular nodal dysfunction, or both, should be monitored during concurrent treatment.

References

1 Weeks CE, Conard GJ, Kvam DC, Fox JM, Chang SF, Paone RP, Lewis GP. The effect of flecainide acetate, a new antiarrhythmic, on plasma digoxin levels. J Clin Pharmacol (1986) 26, 27–31.
2 Tjandramaga TB, Verbesselt R, van Hecken A, Mullie A, De Schepper PJ. Oral digoxin pharmacokinetics during multiple-dose flecainide treatment. Arch Int Pharmacodyn (1982) 260, 302–3.
3 McQuinn RL, Kvam DC, Parrish SL, Fox TL, Miller AM, Franciosa JA. Digoxin levels in patients with congestive heart failure are not altered by flecainide. Clin Pharmacol Ther (1988) 44, 150.

Digitalis Glycosides + Guanethidine and Related Drugs

Abstract/Summary

Guanadrel does not affect the pharmacokinetics of digoxin.

Clinical evidence, mechanism, importance and management

No change in the pharmacokinetics of a single intravenous dose of digoxin occurred in 13 normal subjects after taking 10 mg guanadrel sulphate orally every 12 h for 3 days. One subject experienced a 10 min. episode of asymptomatic second degree heart block (Wenckebach) 3 h after the dose of digoxin, the reason for which was not clear.[1] There seem to be no reports of adverse interactions between the digitalis glycosides and any of the guanethidine-like antihypertensive drugs.

Reference

1 Wright CE, Andreadis NA. Digoxin pharmacokinetics when administered concurrently with guanadrel sulfate. Drug Intell Clin Pharm (1986) 20, 465.

Digitalis Glycosides + Hydroxychloroquine and Chloroquine

Abstract/Summary

The blood levels of digoxin were found to be markedly increased (+ 70%) in two elderly patients while they were treated with hydroxychloroquine. A similar increase has been seen with chloroquine in dogs.

Clinical evidence, mechanism, importance and management

Two women of 65 and 68 who had been taking digoxin (0.25 mg daily) for 2–3 years for heart arrhythmias were concurrently treated with hydroxychloroquine (0.25 g twice daily) for rheumatoid arthritis. When the hydroxychloroquine was withdrawn the serum digoxin levels of both women fell by 70–75% (from 3.0 to 0.7 nmol/l and from 3.1 to 0.9 nmol/l respectively). Neither showed any evidence of intoxication during concurrent use, and one of them claimed that the regularity of her heart rhythm had been improved.[1] The reason for this apparent interaction is not understood. It would now seem prudent to check on the effects of adding or withdrawing hydroxychloroquine in any patient on digoxin. No interaction between digoxin and chloroquine has been described in man, but increases (+ 77%) in peak serum digoxin levels have been seen in dogs.[2]

References

1 Leden I. Digoxin-hydroxychloroquine interaction? Acta Med Scand (1982) 211, 411–12.
2 McElnay JC, Sidahmed AM, D'Arcy PF, McQuale RD. Chloroquine-digoxin interaction. Int J Pharmaceut (1985) 26, 267–74.

Digitalis Glycosides + Fenbufen, Ibuprofen, Ketoprofen

Abstract/Summary

One study found that ibuprofen raised serum digoxin levels. Another found no evidence of an interaction. The outcome of concurrent use remains uncertain. Fenbufen causes a slight increase in serum digoxin levels but ketoprofen has no effect.

Clinical evidence, mechanism, importance and management

The serum digoxin levels of 12 patients are reported to have risen by about 60% after being treated with 1600 mg ibuprofen daily for a week, but after a month of concurrent treatment they had fallen to their former levels.[1] The reason is not understood. This interaction is not well established because half of the patients were not satisfactorily compliant. Another study found that 1800 mg ibuprofen daily for 10 days had no effect on steady-state serum levels of eight patients.[2] However until the situation has been further investigated it would seem reasonable to monitor patients for changes in the effects of digoxin if ibuprofen is started or stopped.

900 mg fenbufen daily was found to cause a slight and unimportant rise in the serum levels of patients on maintenance digoxin,[3] and 50 mg ketoprofen four times daily for 4 days had no effect on the serum digoxin levels of 12 patients.[4] No special precautions seem necessary.

References

1 Quattrocchi FP, Robinson JD, Curry RW, Grieco ML and Schulman SG. The effect of ibuprofen on serum digoxin concentrations. Drug Intell Clin Pharm (1983) 17, 286.
2 Jorgensen HK, Christensen HR, Kampmann JP. Interaction between digoxin and indomethacin or ibuprofen. Br J Clin Pharmac (1991) 31, 108–110.
3 Dunky A, Eberi R. Anti-inflammatory effects of a new anti-rheumatic drug fenbufen in rheumatoid arthritis. XIV Int Congr Rheumatology, June 26- July 1 (1977), Abstract No 379.
4 Lewis GR, Jacobs SG, Vavra I. Effect of ketoprofen on serum digoxin concentrations. Curr Ther Res (1985) 38, 494–9.

Digitalis Glycosides + Indomethacin

Abstract/Summary

Serum digoxin levels in premature and full-term infants and adult patients can be raised up to 40% by the use of indomethacin. Toxicity can occur if the digoxin dosage is not reduced appropriately.

Clinical evidence

(a) Premature and full-term infants

A study in 11 preterm babies (25–33 weeks) given digoxin showed that when 4 days later they were given indomethacin (mean total dose of 0.32 mg/kg) for the treatment of patient ductus arteriosus, their mean serum digoxin levels rose on average by 40%. The digoxin was stopped in five of them because serum concentrations were potentially toxic.[1]

This confirms the observation of digitalis toxicity in three other preterm babies when treated similarly,[2] and of toxic serum digoxin concentrations in another.[3] A further report describes very high levels (8.2 ng/ml) without toxicity in a full-term neonate.[7]

(b) Adults

50 mg indomethacin daily for 10 days increased steady-state serum digoxin levels of 10 adults patients by about 40% (from 0.73 to 1.02 nmol l^{-1}), with a range of 0–100%.[6] This contrasts with the results of a single dose study in six normal adult subjects[4] and another study in six normal adult subjects who had digoxin by infusion over 4 h,[5] both of which suggested that no interaction occurs.

Mechanism

Uncertain. Indomethacin probably reduces the clearance of digoxin by the kidney, thereby allowing it to accumulate in the body.[1,3] The digoxin half-life can be doubled.[1]

Importance and management

Documentation is limited but the interaction appears to be established. It has been suggested that the digoxin dosage should be halved if indomethacin is given to preterm or full-term infants and the serum digoxin levels and urinary output monitored. The same precautions would also seem appropriate for adults. More study is needed.

References

1 Koren G, Zarfin Y, Perlman M, MacLeod SM. Effects of indomethacin on digoxin pharmacokinetics in preterm babies. Ped Pharmacol (1984) 4, 25–30.
2 Mayes LC and Boerth RC. Digoxin-indomethacin interaction. Pediatric Res (1980) 14, 469.
3 Schimmel MS, Inwood RL, Eidelman AI, Eilath U. Toxic digitalis levels associated with indomethacin therapy in a neonate. Clin Pediatr (1980) 19, 768–9.
4 Finch MB, Johnston GD, Kelly JG, McDevitt DG. Pharmacokinetics of digoxin alone and in the presence of indomethacin therapy. Br J Clin Pharmac (1984) 17, 353–5.
5 Sziegoleit W, Weimss M, Fah A, Forster W. Are serum levels and cardiac effects of digoxin influenced by indomethacin? Pharmazie (1986) 41, 340.
6 Jorgensen HK, Christensen HR, Kampmann JP. Interaction between digoxin and indomethacin or ibuprofen. Br J clin Pharmac (1991) 31, 108–110.
7 Haig GM, Brookfield EG. Increase in serum digoxin concentrations after indomethacin therapy in a full-term neonate. Pharmacotherapy (1992) 12, 334–6.

Digitalis Glycosides + Isoxicam and Piroxicam

Abstract/Summary

Isoxicam and piroxicam do not interact with digoxin.

Clinical evidence, mechanism, importance and management

200 mg isoxicam daily did not affect the steady-state serum levels of 12 normal subjects taking beta-acetyldigoxin.[1] This confirms the findings of a previous study.[2] 10 patients taking digoxin for mild cardiac failure similarly demonstrated that 10 or 20 mg piroxicam daily for 15 days had no effect on steady-state digoxin levels, nor were consistent effects seen on the pharmacokinetics of digoxin.[3] No special precautions would seem necessary.

References

1 Zoller B, Engel HJ, Faust-Tinnefeldt G, Gilfrich HJ, Zimmer M. Untersuchungen zur Wechselwirkung von Isoxicam und Digoxin. Z. Rheumatol (1984) 43, 182–4.
2 Chlud K. Zur Frage der Interaktionen in der Rheumatherapie: Untersuchungen von Isoxicam und Glibenclamid bei Diabeten mit rheumatischen Enkrankungen. Tempo Medical (1983) 12A, 15–18.
3 Rau R. Interaction study of piroxicam with digoxin. In 'Piroxicam: A New Non-steroidal Anti-inflammatory Agent.' Proc IXth Eur Cong Rheumatol, Wiesbaden, September 1979, pp 41–6. Academy Professional Information Services, NY.

Digitalis glycosides + Itraconazole

Abstract/Summary

Itraconazole can cause a marked increase in serum digoxin levels. Toxicity may occur unless the dosage is suitably reduced.

Clinical evidence

A man of 68 on 0.5 mg digoxin daily and ibuprofen developed nausea and fatigue (interpreted later as digoxin toxicity) after starting 400 mg itraconazole daily for an infected elbow. The symptoms disappeared when both the itraconazole and ibuprofen were stopped, but returned when the itraconazole was restarted. After 7 days use his heart rate had fallen from 60 to 40 bpm and his digoxin level had doubled (from 1.6 to 3.2 ng/ml). He was later restabilized on a quarter of the digoxin dosage (0.125 mg daily) with serum digoxin levels in the range 0.8–1.8 ng/ml while taking the same dose of itraconazole.[1]

Two other patients developed digoxin toxicity after taking itraconazole for nine days.[2–4] The serum digoxin levels of one them had roughly doubled and she was restabilized on a quarter of her previous digoxin dosage.[2] The other was restabilized on a 40% dosage.[3,4] The last report briefly quotes six other cases of this interaction.[3,4]

Mechanism

Not understood. Decreased digoxin clearance has been suggested.[4]

Importance and management

In established interaction but of uncertain incidence. Monitor the effects if itraconazole is started or stopped, anticipating the need to adjust the digoxin dosage. Two of the patients cited above were restabilized on a 25% digoxin dosage[1,2] and another on about one-third while taking itraconazole.[3,4]

References

1 Rex J. Itraconazole-digoxin interaction. Ann Intern Med (1992) 116, 525.
2 Kauffman CA, Bagnasco FA. Digoxin toxicity associated with itraconazole therapy. Clin Infect Dis (1992) 15, 886–7.
3 Sachs MK, Green PJ. Itraconazole-digoxin interaction. Janssen Pharmaceuticals, Report N80541.
4 Sachs MK, Blanchard LM, Green PJ. Interaction of itraconazole and digoxin. Clin Infect Dis (1993) 16, 400–3.

Digitalis Glycosides + Kaolin-pectin

Abstract/Summary

Serum digoxin levels can be reduced by kaolin-pectin, but the reduction is small and probably of minimal clinical importance. The interaction can be avoided by taking the two drugs 2 h apart, or by giving the digoxin in liquid or capsule form.

Clinical evidence

The concurrent use of kaolin-pectin suspension and digoxin reduced the peak serum digoxin levels of seven patients by 36%, while the area under the 24 h concentration/time curve was reduced by 15%. When two doses of kaolin-pectin were taken, one 2 h before and the other 2 h after the digoxin, no significant changes were seen.[1]

Single dose studies have found 42% and 62% reductions in the bioavailability of digoxin caused by kaolin-pectin.[2,3] Another study showed an interaction with digoxin tablets but not with digoxin capsules.[4]

Mechanism

Not understood. The digoxin may possibly become adsorbed onto the kaolin so that less is available for absorption. Another possibility is that the kaolin reduces the motility of the gut which normally increases mixing and brings the digoxin into contact with the absorbing surface.

Importance and management

Steady-state studies reflect the every-day situation much more closely than single dose studies, and the one cited above[1] indicates that the total reduction in digoxin absorption is small (15%). This is unlikely to be of clinical importance, however the interaction can be avoided by separating the dosages (in any order) by 2 h or by giving the digoxin in capsule or liquid form.

References

1 Albert KS, Elliott WJ, Abbott RD, Gilbertson TJ, Data JL. Influence of

kaolin-pectin on steady-state digoxin levels. J Clin Pharmacol (1981) 21, 449–55.
2 Brown DD, Juhl RP, Lewis K, Schrott M, Bartels B. Decreased bioavailability of digoxin due to antacids and kaolin-pectin. N Engl J Med (1976) 295, 1034.
3 Albert KS, Ayres JW, Disanto AR, Weidler DJ, Sakmar E, Hallmark MR, Stoll RG, Desante KA, Wagner JG. Influence of kaolin-pectin suspension on digoxin bioavailability. J Pharm Sci (1978) 67, 1582.
4 Allen MD, Greenblatt DJ, Harmatz JS, Smith TW. Effect of magnesium aluminium hydroxide and kaolin-pectin on absorption of digoxin from tablets and capsules. J Clin Pharmacol (1981) 21, 26.

Digitalis Glycosides + Ketanserin

Abstract/Summary

Experimental evidence suggests that ketanserin is unlikely to affect the serum levels of either digoxin or digitoxin.

Clinical evidence, mechanism, importance and management

80 mg ketanserin daily did not cause significant changes in the pharmacokinetics of single doses of either digoxin or digitoxin in 10 normal subjects, and it is concluded that ketanserin is unlikely to alter serum concentrations of either glycoside during clinical use.[1]

Reference

1 Ochs HR, Verburg-Ochs B, Holler M, Greenblatt DJ. Effect of ketanserin on the kinetics of digoxin and digitoxin. J Cardiovasc Pharmacol (1985) 7, 205–7.

Digitalis Glycosides + Lithium

Abstract/Summary

No pharmacokinetic interaction occurs between digoxin and lithium but the addition of digoxin to lithium possibly has a detrimental short-term effect on the control of mania. An isolated report describes severe bradycardia in one patient given both drugs.

Clinical evidence, mechanism, importance and management

A study in six normal subjects taking lithium carbonate (mean steady-state serum levels 0.76 mmol/l, range 0.4–1.0 mmol/l) showed that the pharmacokinetics of digoxin given intravenously were unchanged, and no significant effects on sodium pump activity or electrolyte concentrations were found.[1] However an experimental seven day study in patients with manic-depressive psychoses found that there was a greater improvement in those given lithium + placebo than those given lithium + digoxin. This may be a reflection of changes in Na-K ATP-ase.[2] An isolated report describes tremor, confusion and severe nodal bradycardia in a patient given both drugs. The bradycardia worsened (30 bpm) even after both drugs were stopped.[3] The clinical significance of all of these findings is uncertain. More study is needed.

References

1 Cooper SJ, Kelly JG, Johnston GD, Copeland S, King DJ, McDevitt DG. Pharmacodynamics and pharmacokinetics of digoxin in the presence of lithium. Br J Clin Pharmac (1984) 18, 21–5.
2 Chambers CA, Smith AHW, Naylor GJ. The effect of digoxin on the response to lithium therapy in mania. Psychological Med (1982) 12, 57–60.
3 Winters WD, Ralph DD. Digoxin-lithium drug interaction. Clin Toxicol (1977) 10, 487–8.

Digitalis glycosides + Lomoparan

Abstract/Summary

Digoxin and lomoparan appear not to interact together adversely.

Clinical evidence, mechanism, importance and management

Lomoparan (bolus injection of 3250 anti-Xa units) caused a small decrease in the AUC and serum levels of digoxin (0.25 mg daily for 8 days), and a small increase in the clearance of plasma anti-Xa activity in six subjects,[1] nevertheless none of these changes appears to be clinically important. More confirmatory study of this is needed.

Reference

1 de Boer A, Stiekema JCJ, Danhof M, Moolenaar AJ, Breimer DD. Interaction of ORG 10172, a low molecular weight heparinoid, and digoxin in healthy volunteers. Eur J Clin Pharmacol (1991) 41, 245–50.

Digitalis Glycosides + Methyldopa

Abstract/Summary

Methyldopa does not affect serum digoxin levels, but marked bradycardia has been seen in two elderly women when given both drugs.

Clinical evidence

(a) Serum digoxin levels unchanged

250 mg methyldopa daily had no effect on their steady-state serum digoxin levels of eight normal subjects taking 0.25 mg daily.[1]

(b) Bradycardia

Two elderly women with hypertension and left ventricular failure developed marked bradycardia when given digoxin and methyldopa (375 or 750 mg daily) but not with digoxin alone. Average and minimum heart rates of 50 and 32, and 48 and 38 beats per min respectively were recorded. They were subsequently discharged on digoxin and hydralazine with heart rates within the normal range.[2]

Mechanism

Uncertain. Both digoxin and methyldopa can cause some bradycardia[3] but these effects seem to have been more than simply the sum of the two.

Importance and management

Information is limited but it would seem that concurrent use need not be avoided, but monitor the effects for any evidence of excessive heart slowing.

References

1 May CA, Vlasses PH, Rocci ML, Rotmensch HH, Swanson BN, Tannenbaum RP, Ferguson RK, Abrams WB. Methyldopa does not alter the disposition of digoxin. J Clin Pharmacol (1984) 24, 386–9.
2 Davis JC, Reiffel JA, Bigger JT. Sinus node dysfunction caused by methyldopa and digoxin. J Amer Med Ass (1981) 245, 1241.
3 Lund-Johansen P. Hemodynamic changes on long term alpha-methyldopa therapy of essential hypertension. Acta Med Scand (1972) 192, 221.

Digitalis Glycosides + Metoclopramide

Abstract/Summary

The serum levels of digoxin may be reduced by about a third if metoclopramide and slowly dissolving forms of digoxin are given concurrently. No interaction is likely with digoxin in liquid form or in fast dissolving preparations.

Clinical evidence

A study on 11 patients on a slowly dissolving digoxin formulation found that metoclopramide (10 mg three times a day for 10 days) reduced the serum digoxin levels by 36% (from 0.72 to 0.46 ng/ml).[1] The digoxin concentrations rose to their former levels when the metoclopramide was withdrawn.

Another study in normal subjects found a 19% reduction in AUC and a 27% reduction in peak serum digoxin levels while taking digoxin in an un-named formulation.[6] Yet another study clearly showed that an interaction occurred between metoclopramide and digoxin tablets but not in capsule form.[7]

Mechanism

It would seem[3-5] that the metoclopramide increases the motility of the gut to such an extent that full dissolution and absorption of the digoxin is unfinished by the time it is lost in the faeces. Another idea[2] is that the metoclopramide stimulates the excretion of digoxin in the bile.

Importance and management

Information is very limited, but the interaction seems to be established. It is not likely to occur with solid form, fast-dissolving digoxin preparations or digoxin in liquid form, but only those preparations which are slowly dissolving. A reduction in digoxin levels of a third could result in underdigitalization. There is no information about digitoxin.

References

1 Manninen V, Apajalahti A, Melin J, Kavesoja M. Altered absorption of digoxin in patients given propantheline and metoclopramide. Lancet (1973) i, 398.
2 Thompson WG. Altered absorption of digoxin in patients given propantheline and metoclopramide. Lancet (1973) i, 783.
3 Manninen V, Apajalahti A, Simonen H, Reissell P. Effect of propantheline and metoclopramide on the absorption of digoxin. Lancet (1973) i, 1118.
4 Medin S, Nyberg L. Effect of propantheline and metoclopramide on the absorption of digoxin. Lancet (1973) i, 1393.
5 Fraser EJ, Leach RH, Poston JW, Bold AM, Culank LS and Lipede AB. Dissolution rates and bioavailability of digoxin tablets. Lancet (1973) i, 1393.
6 Kirch W, Janisch HD, Santos SR, Duhrsen U, Dylewicz P, Ohnhaus EE. Effect of cisapride and metoclopramide on digoxin bioavailability. Eur J Drug Metab Pharmacokinet (1986) 11, 249–50.
7 Johnson BF, Bustrack JA, Urbach DR, Hull JH, Marawaha R. Effect of metoclopramide on digoxin absorption from tablets and capsules. Clin Pharmacol Ther (1984) 36, 724–30.

Digitalis Glycosides + Mexiletine

Abstract/Summary

Serum digoxin levels are not significantly altered by mexiletine.

Clinical evidence, mechanism, importance and management

The steady-state serum digoxin levels of 10 normal subjects on 0.25 mg daily were slightly but not significantly altered while concurrently taking 600 mg mexiletine daily for 4 days (a fall from 0.32 to 0.27 ng/ml).[1,2] When the mexiletine was given with 30 ml of an aluminium magnesium hydroxide antacid the digoxin AUC was approximately halved (from a range of 4.1–15.6 to 2.6–8.5 ng/ml h). This is in line with other studies showing that antacids can reduce serum digoxin levels (see 'Digitalis Glycosides + Antacids'). The serum mexiletine levels were not significantly altered by the antacid. Another study on nine patients confirmed that mexiletine does not significantly affect serum digoxin levels.[3]

References

1 Affrime MB, Lowenthal DT, Saris S. Drug interaction study of oral mexiletine and digoxin. Drug Intell Clin Pharm (1982) 16, 469.
2 Saris SD, Lowenthal DT, Affrime MB. Steady-state digoxin concentration during oral mexiletine administration. Ther Res (1983) 34, 662–66.
3 Leahey EB, Reiffel JA, Giardina E-GV and Bigger T. The effect of quinidine and other oral antiarrhythmic drugs on serum digoxin. Ann Intern Med (1980) 92, 605–8.

Digitalis glycosides + Moricizine (Ethmozine)

Abstract/Summary

Serum digoxin levels are not significantly increased by the concurrent use of moricizine in patients with normal renal function, however some adverse conduction effects have been seen.

Clinical evidence

13 patients on digoxin (0.125–0.25 mg daily) showed a non-significant rise in their serum digoxin levels of 10–15% when concurrently treated with moricizine (10 mg/kg) for 2 weeks. Nine patients concurrently treated for 1–6 months showed no significant changes in their serum digoxin levels.[1]

No changes in the pharmacokinetics of digoxin were seen in a single dose study of digoxin and moricizine in nine normal subjects[2] nor in another study in patients over a 13-day period, however heart arrhythmias (AV junctional rhythm and heart block) were seen which disappeared when the moricizine was stopped.[3] Concurrent use can cause a significant increase in the PR interval.[5]

Importance and management

Although no clinically important changes in serum digoxin levels appear to occur during concurrent use, the occurrence of arrhythmias in a few patients indicates that good monitoring is advisable. It has been pointed out that the additive effects of both drugs on intranodal and intraventricular conduction may be excessive in some patients with heart disease.[4] More study is needed.

References

1 Kennedy HL, Sprague MK, Redd RM, Wiens RD, Blum RI, Buckingham TA. Serum digoxin concentrations during ethmozine anti-arrhythmic therapy. Am Heart J (1986) 111, 667–72.
2 MacFarland RT, Moeller VR, Pieniaszek HJ, Whitney CC, Marcus FI. Assessment of the potential pharmacokinetic interaction between digoxin and ethmozine. J Clin Pharmacol (1985) 25, 138–43.
3 Antman EM, Arnold JM, Friedman PL, White H, Bosak M, Smith TW. Drug interactions with cardiac glycosides: evaluation of a possible digoxin-ethmozine pharmacokinetic interaction. J Cardiovasc Pharmacol (1987) 9, 622–7.
4 Quoted as data on file, Du Pont Pharmaceuticals in reference 5.
5 Siddoway LA, Schwartz SL, Barbey JT, Woosley RL. Clinical Pharmacokinetics of moricizine. Am J Cardiol (1990) 65, 21–25D.

Digitalis glycosides + Moxonidine

Abstract/Summary

Moxonidine and digoxin appear not to interact together.

Clinical evidence, mechanism, importance and management

No interaction was found in 15 normal subjects taking 0.2 mg moxonidine twice daily and, after a 0.4 mg loading dose, 0.2 mg digoxin daily for at least 5 days. The pharmacokinetics of neither drug was changed to a clinically significant extent under steady-state conditions. No special precautions would seem necessary during concurrent use.[1]

Reference

1 Pabst G, Weimann H-J, Weber W. Lack of pharmacokinetic interactions between moxonidine and digoxin. Clin Pharmacokinet (1992) 23, 477–81.

Digitalis glycosides + Neuromuscular blockers

Abstract/Summary

Serious cardiac arrhythmias can develop in patients receiving digitalis glycosides who are given suxamethonium (succinylcholine) or pancuronium.

Clinical evidence

Eight out of 17 digitalized patients (anaesthetized with sodium thiamylal and then maintained with nitrous oxide and oxygen) developed serious ventricular arrhythmias following the intravenous injection of 40–100 mg suxamethonium. Three of the others had immediate and definite ST/T wave changes, and the remaining six showed frequent multifocal premature ventricular contractions.[1]

There are other reports of this interaction.[2,3] Another report describes sinus tachycardia and atrial flutter in six out of 18 patients on digoxin when given pancuronium.[4] In contrast, five out of eight patients with ventricular arrhythmias returned to normal rhythm when given 15–30 mg tubocurarine, and one patient returned to a regular nodal rhythm from ventricular tachycardia.[1]

Mechanism

Not understood. One possibility is that the suxamethonium may cause the rapid removal of potassium from the myocardial cells. Another idea is that it affects catecholamine-releasing cholinergic receptors.

Importance and management

Information is limited but the interaction appears to be established. Suxamethonium should be avoided, or used with great caution, in patients taking digitalis glycosides. Similar caution would seem appropriate with pancuronium.

References

1 Dowdy EG, Fabian LW. Ventricular arrhythmias induced by succinylcholine in digitalized patients. A preliminary report. Anesth Analg (1963) 42, 501.
2 Perez HR. Cardiac arrhythmia after succinylcholine. Anesth Analg (1970) 49, 33.
3 Smith RB, Petrusack J. Succinylcholine, digitalis and hypercalcaemia; a case report. Anesth Analg (1972) 51, 202.
4 Bartolone RS, Rao TLK. Dysrhythmia following muscle relaxant administration in patients receiving digitalis. Anesthesiology (1983) 58, 567.

Digitalis glycosides + Nifedipine

Abstract/Summary

Serum digoxin levels are normally unchanged or only modestly increased by the concurrent use of nifedipine. One unexplained and conflicting study indicated that a 45% rise could occur. Digitoxin appears not to interact.

Clinical evidence

(a) Digoxin

(i) Serum digoxin levels unchanged

Studies on 14 patients,[4] 10 patients[7,11] and 28 subjects[5,6,15] showed that serum digoxin levels were not significantly altered while taking 30–60 mg nifedipine daily. Similarly no significant changes in the pharmacokinetics of digoxin were found in six patients[8] or eight subjects[9] on 60–90 mg nifedipine daily when given a single intravenous dose of digoxin. No changes in the pharmacokinetics of nifedipine were seen.[8]

(ii) Serum digoxin levels increased

30 mg nifedipine increased the serum digoxin levels of 12 normal subjects taking 0.375 mg daily by 45% (from 0.505 to 0.734 ng/ml) over 14 days.[1]

20 mg nifedipine daily increased the steady-state serum digoxin levels of nine patients by 15% (from 0.87 to 1.04 ng/ml).[2] A 15% increase was also seen in a study[3,16] in seven subjects given 15–60 mg nifedipine daily.

(b) Digitoxin

A study in eight and 10 normal subjects showed that 40–60 mg nifedipine daily had no significant effect on their steady-state serum digitoxin levels over a 6-week period.[17]

Mechanism

Not understood. Changes and lack of changes in both renal and non-renal excretion of digoxin have been reported.

Importance and management

The digoxin-nifedipine interaction is well documented but the findings are inconsistent. The weight of evidence appears to be that serum digoxin levels are normally unchanged or only very moderately increased by nifedipine. Concurrent use appears normally to be safe and effective,[10,12,13] but it would clearly be prudent to monitor the response. One report suggests that nifedipine has some attenuating effect on the digoxin-induced inotropism.[14] Another points out that under some circumstances (renal insufficiency or pre-existing digoxin overdosage) some risk of an undesirable interaction still exists.[3] Nifedipine appears not to interact with digitoxin significantly.

References

1 Belz GG, Doering W, Munkes R, Matthews J. Interaction between digoxin and calcium antagonists and antiarrhythmic drugs. Clin Pharmacol Ther (1983) 33, 410–17.
2 Kleinbloesem CH, van Brummelen P, Hillers J, Moolenaar AJ, Breimer DD. Interaction between digoxin and nifedipine at steady state in patients with atrial fibrillation. Ther Drug Monit (1985) 7, 372–6.
3 Kirch W, Hutt HJ, Dylewicz P, Graf KJ, Ohnhaus EE. Dose-dependence of the nifedipine-digoxin interaction? Clin Pharmacol Ther (1986) 39, 35–9.
4 Schwartz JB, Raizner A, Akers S. The effect of nifedipine on serum digoxin concentrations in patients. Am Heart J (1984) 107, 669–73.
5 Schwartz JB, Migliore PJ. Nifedipine does not alter digoxin level or clearance. J Am Coll Cardiol (1984) 3, 478.
6 Schwartz JB, Migliore PJ. Effect of nifedipine on serum digoxin concentration and renal clearance. Clin Pharmacol Ther (1984) 36, 19–24.
7 Kuhlmann J, Marcin S, Frank KH. Effects of nifedipine and diltiazem on the pharmacokinetics of digoxin. Naunyn-Schmied Arch Pharmacol (1983) 324 (Suppl) R81.
8 Garty M, Shamir E, Ilfield D, Pilik S, Rosenfeld JB. Non-interaction of digoxin and nifedipine in cardiac patients. J Clin Pharmacol (1986) 26, 304–5.
9 Koren G, Zylber-Katz E, Granit L and Levy M. Pharmacokinetic studies of nifedipine and digoxin co-administration. Int J Clin Pharmacol Ther Toxicol (1986) 24, 39–42.
10 Pedersen KE, Dorph-Pedersen A, Hvidt S, Klitgaard NA, Kjaer K, Nielsen-Kudsk F. Effect of nifedipine on digoxin kinetics in healthy subjects. Clin Pharmacol Ther (1982) 32, 562–5.
11 Kuhlmann J. Effects of nifedipine and diltiazem on levels and renal excretion of beta-acetyldigoxin. Clin Pharmacol Ther (1985) 37, 150–6.
12 Belz GG, Aust PE, Munkes R. Digoxin concentrations and nifedipine. Lancet (1981) i, 844.
13 Cantelli I, Pavesi PC, Parchi C, Naccarella F, Bracchetti D. Acute hemodynamic effects of combined therapy with digoxin and nifedipine in patients with chronic heart failure. Am Heart J (1983) 106, 308–15
14 Hansen PB, Buch J, Rasmussen OO, Waldorff S, Steiness E. Influence of atenolol and nifedipine on digoxin-induced inotropism in humans. Br J Clin Pharmacol (1984) 18, 817–22.
15 Pedersen KE, Madsen JL, Klitgaard NA, Kjoer K, Hvidt S. Non-interaction between nifedipine and digoxin. Dan Med Bull (1986) 33, 109–10.
16 Hutt HJ, Kirch W, Dylewicz P, Ohnhaus EE. Dose-dependence of the nifedipine/digoxin interaction? Arch Toxicol (1986) Suppl 9, 209–12.
17 Kuhlmann J. Effects of quinidine, verapamil and nifedipine on the pharmacokinetics and pharmacodynamics of digitoxin during steady-state conditions. Arzneim-Forsch/Drug Res (1987) 37, 545–8.

Digitalis glycosides + Penicillamine

Abstract/Summary

Serum digoxin levels can be reduced by the concurrent use of penicillamine.

Clinical evidence

While taking 1 g penicillamine daily 2 h after taking digoxin orally, the serum digoxin levels of 10 patients measured 2, 4 and 6 h later were reduced by 13, 20 and 39% respectively. In 10 other patients similarly treated but given digoxin intravenously, the serum digoxin levels measured 4 and 6 h later were reduced by 23 and 64% respectively.[1]

This interaction is reported by the same authors to occur in children.[2]

Mechanism

Unknown.

Importance and management

Information seems to be limited to the reports cited. Patients on digoxin should be checked for signs of under-digitalization if penicillamine is added. Information about digitoxin appears to be lacking.

References

1 Moezzi B, Fatourechi V, Khozain R, Eslami B. The effect of penicillamine on serum digoxin levels. Jpn Heart J (1978) 19, 366–70.
2 Moezzi B, Khozain R, Pooymeh F, Shakibi JG. Reversal of digoxin-induced changes in erythrocyte electrolyte concentrations by penicillamine in children. Jpn Heart J (1980) 21, 335–9.

Digitalis glycosides + Phenylbutazone

Abstract/Summary

Serum digitoxin levels can be approximately halved by the concurrent use of phenylbutazone.

Clinical evidence

On two occasions when concurrently taking 200 or 400 mg phenylbutazone daily, the serum digitoxin levels of six patients taking 0.1 mg daily were approximately halved within 8–10 days. They returned to their former values within roughly the same period of time following the phenylbutazone withdrawal.[1]

A similar response has been described elsewhere in one patient.[2]

Mechanism

Not understood, One suggestion is that the phenylbutazone increases the rate of metabolism of the digitoxin by the liver.[1]

Importance and management

Information is limited but the interaction appears to be established. The dosage of digitoxin will need to be increased to avoid under-digitalization if phenylbutazone is added to established treatment. Phenylbutazone may be inappropriate for some patients because it can cause sodium retention and oedema. There seems to be nothing documented about other digitalis glycosides and phenylbutazone.

References

1 Wirth KE. Arzneimittelinteraktionen bei der Anwendung herzwirksamer Glykoside. Med Welt (1981) 32, 234.
2 Solomon HM, Reich S, Spirt N, Abrams WB. Interactions between digitoxin and other drugs *in vitro* and in vivo. Ann NY Acad Sci (1971) 179, 362.

Digitalis glycosides + Phenytoin

Abstract/Summary

Phenytoin is of proven value in the treatment of digitalis-induced heart arrhythmias but sudden cardiac arrest has been reported. Phenytoin reduces serum digoxin levels and a marked fall in serum digitoxin levels has also been seen. There is a single case report of marked bradycardia.

Clinical evidence

(a) Bradycardia and cardiac arrest

A patient with digitalis-induced heart arrhythmias died following the intravenous injection of phenytoin.[1] Sudden cardiac arrest has also been seen in dogs.[5] Marked bradycardia (34 bpm) and complete heart block has been described in a mongol patient taking 0.25 mg digoxin daily for mitral insufficiency when he was given 200 mg phenytoin daily.[7]

(b) Reduced serum digoxin levels

A study in six normal subjects showed that after taking 400 mg phenytoin daily for a week the half-life of digoxin was reduced by 30% (from 33.9 to 23.7 h) and the AUC by 23% (from 31.6 to 24.4 ng/ml/h). Total clearance increased by 27% (from 258.6 to 328.3 ml/min).[8]

(c) Reduced serum digitoxin levels

The serum digitoxin levels of a man were observed to fall on three occasions when he was concurrently treated with pheny-toin. On the third occasion while taking 0.2 mg digitoxin daily, the addition of 900 mg phenytoin daily caused a 60% fall (from 25 to 10 µg/ml) over a 7–10 day period.[6]

Mechanisms

Phenytoin has a stabilizing effect on the responsiveness of the myocardial cells to stimulation so that the toxic threshold at which arrhythmias occurs is raised. But the heart-slowing effects of the digitalis are not opposed and the lethal dose is unaltered, so that the cardiac arrest would appear to be the result of the excessive bradycardia. It seems possible that the fall in serum digitoxin levels may have been due to a phenytoin-induced increase in the metabolism of the digitoxin by the liver. The reduction in serum digoxin levels by phenytoin is not understood.

Importance and management

The value of phenytoin in the treatment of digitalis-induced arrhythmias is well established.[2–5] The authors of one report[5] warn that phenytoin should not be used in patients with a high degree of heart block or marked bradycardia because of the risk that cardiac arrest may occur. This is confirmed by the reports cited.[1,5,7] Information about the effects of phenytoin on serum digitoxin seems to be confined to these single reports, but it would now be prudent to check that patients on digoxin or digitoxin who are subsequently given phenytoin do not become under-digitalized.

References

1 Zoneraich S, Zoneraich O, Siegel J. Sudden death following intravenous sodium diphenylhydantoin. Am Heart J (1976) 91, 375.
2 Helfant RH, Seuffert GW, Patton RD, Stein E, Damato AN. The clinical use of diphenylhydantoin (Dilantin) in the treatment and prevention of cardiac arrhythmias. Am Heart J (1969) 77, 315.
3 Lang TW, Bernstein H, Barbieri F, Gold H, Corday E. Digitalis toxicity. Treatment with diphenylhydantoin. Arch Intern Med (1965) 116, 573.
4 Karliner JS. Intravenous diphenylhydantoin sodium (Dilantin) in cardiac arrhythmias. Dis Chest (1967) 51, 256.
5 Rosen MR, Lisak R, Rubin IL. Diphenylhydantoin in cardiac arrhythmias. Am J Cardiol (1967) 20, 674.
6 Solomon HM, Reich S, Spirt N, Abrams WB. Interactions between digitoxin and other drugs *in vitro* and in vivo. Ann NY Acad Sci (1971) 179, 362.
7 Vlukari NMA and Aho K. Digoxin-phenytoin interaction. Br Med J (1970) 2, 51.
8 Rameis H. On the interaction between phenytoin and digoxin. Eur J Clin Pharmacol (1985) 292, 49–53.

Digitalis glycosides + Pinaverium bromide

Abstract/Summary

Serum digoxin levels are not affected by the concurrent use of pinaverium bromide in patients taking either beta-acetyl or beta-methyl digoxin.

Clinical evidence, mechanism, importance and management

A double-blind study[1] on 25 patients, taking either beta-acetyldigoxin or beta-methyl digoxin for congestive heart failure, found that pinaverium bromide (50 mg three times a day) for 12 days had no significant effect on their serum digoxin levels. No special precautions seem necessary.

Reference

1 Weitzel O, Seidel G, Engelbert S, Berksoy M, Eberhardt G, Bode R. Investigation of possible interaction between pinaverium bromide and digoxin. Curr Med Res Op (1983) 8, 600–2.

Digitalis glycosides + Prazosin

Abstract/Summary

A rapid and marked rise in serum digoxin levels occurs if prazosin is given.

Clinical evidence

A study in 20 patients with steady-state serum digoxin levels of 0.30–1.80 ng/ml found that when given 5 mg prazosin for a day their serum plasma digoxin rose by 43% (to 1.34 ng/ml), and after three days by 60% (to 1.51 ng/ml). Three days after the prazosin was stopped the serum digoxin levels had fallen to their previous values.[1] The reason for this response is not understood. Serum digoxin levels should be closely monitored and appropriate dosage reductions made if prazosin is added. More study is needed.

Reference

1 Copur S, Tokgozoglu L, Oto A, Oram E, Ugurlu S. Effects of oral prazosin on total plasma digoxin levels. Fundam Clin Pharmacol (1988) 2, 13–17.

Digitalis glycosides + Probenecid

Abstract/Summary

Probenecid has no clinically significant effects on serum digoxin levels.

Clinical evidence, mechanism, importance and management

A study[1] over a 16 day period on two normal subjects taking 0.25 mg digoxin daily showed that while concurrently taking two daily doses of *ColBenemid* (probenecid 500 mg + colchicine 0.5 mg) for three days their serum digoxin levels were slightly but not significantly raised (from 0.67 to 0.70 ng/ml, and from 0.60 to 0.67 ng/ml respectively). Another study in six normal subjects found that 2 g probenecid daily for 8 days had no significant effect on the pharmacokinetics of digoxin.[2] No special precautions would seem necessary during concurrent use.

Reference

1 Jaillon P, Weissenburger J, Cheymol G, Graves P, Marcus F. Les effets de probenecide sur la concentration plasmatique a l'equilibre de digoxine. Thérapie (1980) 35, 635.
2 Hedman A, Angelin B, Arvidsson A, Dahlqvist R. No effect of probenecid on the renal and biliary clearances of digoxin in man. Br J Clin Pharmac (1991) 32, 63–7.

Digitalis glycosides + Propafenone

Abstract/Summary

Propafenone can increase serum digoxin levels by 30–90% or even more. A digoxin dosage reduction may be necessary.

Clinical evidence

900 mg propafenone daily for three days increased the mean serum digoxin levels of five patients (taking 0.125–0.25 mg daily) by 83%. Three of them continued to take both drugs for six months and showed a 63% rise. No digitalis toxicity was seen.[3]

600 mg propafenone daily increased the serum digoxin levels of nine other patients by 90% (from 0.97 to 1.54 ng/ml) and two of them showed symptoms of intoxication (nausea, vomiting).[6,7] Another found a steady-state level increase of 28%.[5] Three children showed rises in serum digoxin levels of 112–254% over 3–24 days when given 250–500 mg/m^2 propafenone daily.[9] 450 mg propafenone daily increased the mean serum digoxin levels of 12 normal subjects by about 35% (from 0.58 to 0.78 ng/ml), and the cardiac effects were increased accordingly.[1,2] A pharmacokinetic study found a 24 h AUC increase of about 25%.[4]

Mechanism

Not understood. One suggestion is that propafenone increases the bioavailability of the digoxin.[4] Another is that the volume of distribution and non-renal clearance of digoxin are changed by the propafenone.[8]

Importance and management

An established interaction of clinical importance. Monitor the effects of concurrent use and reduce the digoxin dosage appropriately in order to avoid toxicity. Most patients appear to be affected[6] and dosage reductions in the range 13–79% were found necessary in one of the studies cited.[6,7] The data available suggests that the extent of the rise may possibly depend on the dose of propafenone used.[8]

References

1 Belz GG, Matthews J, Doering W, Belz G. Digoxin-antiarrhythmics: pharmacodynamic and pharmacokinetic studies with quinidine, propafenone and verapamil. Clin Pharmacol Ther (1982) 31, 202.

2 Belz GG, Doering W, Munkes R, Matthews J. Interaction between digoxin and calcium antagonists and antiarrhythmic drugs. Clin Pharmacol Ther (1983) 33, 410–17.

3 Salerno DM, Granrud G, Sharkey P, Asinger R, Hodges M. A controlled trial of propafenone for treatment of frequent and repetitive ventricular premature complexes. Am J Cardiol (1984) 53, 77–83.

4 Cardaioli P, Compostella L, De Domenico R, Papalia D, Zeppellini R, Libardoni M, Pulido E, Cucchini F. Influenza del propafenone sulla farmococinetica della digossina somministrata per via orale: studio su volontari sani. G Ital Cardiol (1986) 16, 237–40.

5 Nolan PE, Marcus FI, Erstad BL, Hoyer GK, Furman C, Kirsten EB. Pharmacokinetic interaction between propafenone and digoxin. J Amer Coll Cardiol (1988) 11, 168A.

6 Calvo MV, Martin-Suarez A, Avila MC, Luengo CM. Interaccion digoxina-propafenona. Medicina Clinica (1987) 89, 171–2.

7 Calvo MV, Martin-Suarez A, Luengo CM, Avila C, Cascon M, Hurle AD-G. Interaction between digoxin and propafenone. Ther Drug Monit (1989) 11, 10–15.

8 Nolan PE, Marcus FI, Erstad BL, Hoyer GK, Furman C, Kirsten E. Effects of coadministration of propafenone on the pharmacokinetics of digoxin in healthy subjects. J Clin Pharmacol (1989) 29, 46–52.

9 Zalzstein E, Koren G, Bryson SM, Freedom RM. Interaction between digoxin and propafenone in children. J Pediatr (1990) 116, 310–2.

Digitalis glycosides + Propantheline

Abstract/Summary

Serum digoxin levels may be increased by a third or more if propantheline and slowly-dissolving forms of digoxin are given concurrently. No interaction is likely with digoxin given as a liquid or in soft-gelatine capsules or in the form of fast-dissolving tablets such as *Lanoxin*.

Clinical evidence

The serum digoxin levels of nine out of 13 patients rose by 30% (from 1.02 to 1.33 ng/ml) while taking a slowly dissolving formulation of digoxin with 15 mg propantheline daily for 10 days. Serum levels stayed the same in three patients and fell slightly in one. An associated study in four normal subjects given digoxin in liquid form, with and without propantheline, found that serum digoxin levels were higher than those when given digoxin in tablet form, and they remained unaffected by propantheline.[1]

Another study by the same workers showed that propantheline only increased digoxin serum levels (by 40%) with slowly dissolving formulations, but not with fast dissolving preparations.[2] Increased bioavailability of digoxin in capsule form when propantheline is given is confirmed by another study.[4]

Mechanism

Propantheline is an anticholinergic agent which reduces gut motility. This allows the slowly-dissolving formulations of digoxin more time to pass into solution so that more is available

for absorption. Propantheline may also reduce the excretion of digoxin in the bile.[3]

Importance and management

An established interaction, but only of importance if slowly-dissolving digoxin formulations are used. No interaction is likely with liquid or soft gelatine capsule forms of digoxin, or with fast-dissolving tablets such as *Lanoxin* which fulfill BP or USP standards. With slowly dissolving forms of digoxin it may be necessary to reduce the digoxin dosage. No interaction seems likely with digitoxin because it is better absorbed from the gut than digoxin, but this requires confirmation.

References

1 Manninen V, Apajalahti A, Melin J, Kavesoja M. Altered absorption of digoxin in patients given propantheline and metoclopramide. Lancet (1973) i, 398.

2 Manninen V, Apajalahti A, Simonen H, Reissel P. Effect of propantheline and metoclopramide on absorption of digoxin. Lancet (1973) i, 1118.

3 Thompson WG. Altered absorption of digoxin in patients given propantheline and metoclopramide. Lancet (1973) i, 783.

4 Brown DD, Schmidt J, Long RA, Hull JH. A steady-state evaluation of the effects of propantheline bromide and cholestyramine on the bioavailability of digoxin when administered as tablets or capsules. J Clin Pharmacol (1985) 25, 360–4.

Digitalis glycosides + Prostaglandins

Abstract/Summary

Neither enprostil, iloprost nor rioprostil interact significantly with digoxin.

Clinical evidence, mechanism, importance and management

35 μg enprostil daily for 6 days in 12 normal subjects had no effect on the pharmacokinetics of digoxin (0.25 mg daily). No clinically significant ECG abnormalities were seen.[1,3] 600 mg rioprostil daily in nine normal subjects decreased the rate of absorption of digoxin but not its extent. Steady-state digoxin levels were not significantly changed.[2] The digoxin pharmacokinetics of 12 patients showed no significant changes when treated for 20 days with 6-hour infusions of iloprost (2 ng/kg/min), although the digoxin absorption was delayed by an hour.[4,5] No special precautions would seem to be necessary with any of these prostaglandins.

References

1 Winters L, Windle S, Cohen A, Wolbach R. Enprostil does not interact with steady state digoxin. Gastroenterology (1988) 94, A500.

2 Demol P, Wingender W, Weihrauch TR, Kuhlmann J. Effect of rioprostil, a synthetic prostaglandin E1 on the bioavailability of digoxin. Gastroenterology (1988) 92, 1368.

3 Cohen A, Winters L. Enprostil leaves steady state digoxin pharmacokinetics unaltered. Curr Ther Res (1988) 44, 541–6.

4 Cabane J, Penin I, Bouslama K, Benchouieb A, Giral Ph, Picard O, Wattiaux MJ, Cheymol G, Souvignet G, Imbert JC. Traitement par iloprost des ischémies critiques des membres inférieurs associées à une insuffisiance cardiaque. Therapie (1991) 46, 235–40.

5 Penin E, Cheymol G, Bouslama K, Benchouieb A, Cabane J, Souvignet G. No pharmacokinetic interaction between iloprost and digoxin. Eur J Clin Pharmacol (1991) 41, 505–6.

Digitalis glycosides + Quinidine

Abstract/Summary

The serum levels of digoxin in most patients are doubled within five days if quinidine is added. The digoxin dosage will need to be halved if intoxication is to be avoided. Digitoxin levels are also increased but it occurs more slowly and the extent may be less.

Clinical evidence

(a) Digoxin + Quinidine

Arising out of the observation that quinidine appeared to increase serum digoxin levels, a retrospective study of patient records revealed that 25 out 27 patients on digoxin had shown a significant rise (from 1.4 to 3.2 ng/ml) in serum digoxin levels when given quinidine. 16 showed typical signs of intoxication (nausea, vomiting, anorexia) which resolved in 10 of them when the digoxin dosage was reduced or withdrawn, and in five when the quinidine was reduced.[1]

This is one of the first reports published in 1978 (two other groups independently reported it the same year[2,6]) which clearly describe this interaction, although hints of its existence can be found in papers published over the previous 50 years. Since then very considerable numbers of research reports, both retrospective and prospective, and case studies on very considerable numbers of patients have confirmed and established the extent (a 100% increase in serum digoxin levels) and incidence (+ 90%) of this interaction beyond doubt. I have on file almost 150 reports and reviews, only a selection of which are listed here for economy of space. Two reviews published in 1982 and 1983 contain extensive and valuable bibliographies.[13,16]

(b) Digitoxin + Quinidine

The steady-state serum digitoxin levels of eight normal subjects rose by 45% (from 13.6 to 19.7 ng/ml) over 32 days while taking 750 mg quinidine daily.[17]

Another study over only 10 days found a 31% increase in serum digitoxin levels,[18] whereas yet another found a 115% increase.[19] A study in five subjects found that quinidine reduced the total body clearance of digitoxin by 63% and the serum digitoxin levels were raised.[7]

Mechanisms

Quinidine reduces the renal excretion of digoxin by 40–50%,

and it also appears to have some effects on non-renal clearance which includes an approximately 50% reduction in its excretion in the bile.[14] It displaces digoxin from tissue binding sites and significant changes in the volume of distribution occur. There is also some limited evidence that changes in the rate and extent of absorption of digoxin from the gut may have a small part to play.[9] Digoxin also appears to cause a small reduction in the renal clearance of quinidine.[15] Quinidine appears to increase digitoxin serum levels by reducing the non-renal clearance.

Importance and management

The digoxin-quinidine interaction is overwhelming well-documented, well-established and of clinical importance. Since serum digoxin levels are usually roughly doubled (up to a five-fold increases have been seen[8]) and most (90% +) patients are affected, digitalis toxicity will develop unless the dosage of digoxin is reduced appropriately (approximately halved).[1,3,4,8] A suggested rule-of-thumb is that if serum digoxin levels are no greater than 0.9 ng/ml the addition of quinidine is unlikely to cause cardiotoxic digoxin levels (if serum potassium levels are normal) whereas with levels of 1.0 ng/ml or more, toxic concentrations may develop.[12] Monitor the effects and readjust the dosage as necessary. Significant effects occur within a day of taking the quinidine and reach a maximum after about 3–6 days (quicker or slower in some patients), but it will only stabilize when the quinidine has reached steady-state and that depends on whether a loading dose is given. The effects are to some extent dose-related but the correlation is not good: less than 400–500 mg quinidine daily have minimal effects, and increasing doses up to 1200 mg having greater effects.[3,5] About five days are needed after withdrawing the quinidine before serum digoxin levels fall to their former levels. It has been recommended that patients with chronic renal failure should have their digoxin dosage reduced to a half or a third.[10,11,20] An appropriate upward readjustment will be necessary if the quinidine is subsequently withdrawn.

Far less is known about the digitoxin-quinidine interaction but the same precautions should be taken. It develops much more slowly.

Alternative non-interacting antiarrhythmics include disopyramide, mexiletine, procainamide and possibly flecainide.

References

1 Leahey EB, Reiffel JA, Drusin RE, Heisenbuttel RH, Lovejoy WP, Bigger JT. Interaction between quinidine and digoxin. J Amer Med Ass (1978) 240, 533.

2 Ejvinsson G. Effect of quinidine on plasma concentrations of digoxin. Br Med J (1978) 1, 279.

3 Doering W. Quinidine-digoxin interaction: pharmacokinetics, underlying mechanism and clinical implications. N Engl J Med (1979) 301, 400–4.

4 Leahey EB, Reiffel JA, Heissenbuttel RH, Drusin RE, Lovejoy WP, Bigger JT. Enhanced cardiac effect of digoxin during quinidine treatment. Arch Intern Med (1979) 139, 519–21.

5 Fenster PE, Powell JR, Hager WD, Graves PE, Conrad K, Goldman S. Onset and dose dependence of digoxin-quinidine interaction. Amer J Cardiol (1980) 45, 413.

6 Reid PR, Meek AG. Digoxin-quinidine interaction. Johns Hopkins Med J (1979) 145, 227–9.

7 Garty M, Sood P, Rollins DE. Digitoxin elimination reduced during quinidine therapy. Ann Intern Med (1981) 94, 35–7.

8 Bigger JT, Leahey EB. Quinidine and digoxin. An important interaction. Drugs (1982) 24, 229–39.

9 Pedersen KE, Christiansen BD, Klitgaard NA, Nielsen-Kudsk F. Effect of quinidine on digoxin bioavailability. Eur J Clin Pharmacol (1983) 24, 41–7.

10 Fichtl B, Doering W, Seidel H. The quinidine-digoxin interaction in patients with impaired renal function. Int J Clin Pharmacol Ther Toxicol (1983) 21, 229–33.

11 Fenster PE, Hager WD, Perrier D, Powell JR, Graves PE, Michael UF. Digoxin-quinidine interaction in patients with chronic renal failure. Circulation (1982) 66, 1277–80.

12 Friedman HS, Chen T-S. Use of control steady-state digoxin levels for predicting serum digoxin concentration after quinidine administration. Am Heart J (1983) 104, 72–6.

13 Bigger JT, Leahey EB. Quinidine and digoxin. An important drug interaction. Drugs (1982) 24, 229–39.

14 Schenck-Gustafsson K, Angelin B, Hedman A, Arvidsson A, Dahlqvist R. Quinidine-induced reduction of the biliar excretion of digoxin in patients. Circulation (1985) 72, Suppl III-19.

15 Rameis H. Quinidine-digoxin interaction: are the pharmacokinetics of both drugs altered? Int J Clin Pharmacol Ther Toxicol (1985) 23, 145–53.

16 Fichtl B, Doering W. The quinidine-digoxin interaction in perspective. Clin Pharmacokinet (1983) 8, 137–54.

17 Kuhlmann J, Dohrmann M, Marcin S. Effects of quinidine on pharmacokinetics and pharmacodynamics of digitoxin achieving steady-state conditions. Clin Pharmacol Ther (1986) 39, 288–94.

18 Peters U, Risler T, Graben see B, Falkstein U, Kroukou J. Interaktion von Chinidin und Digitoxin beim Menschen. Dtsch Med Wsch (1980) 105, 438–42.

19 Kreutz G, Keller F, Gast D, Prokein E. Digitoxin-quinidine interaction achieving steady-state conditions for both drugs. Naunyn-Schmied Arch Toxicol (1982) 319, R82.

20 Woodcock BG, Rietbrock N. Digitalis-quinidine interactions. TIPS (1982) 3, 118–22.

Digitalis + Quinidine + Pentobarbitone

Abstract/Summary

Digitalis toxicity arising from the digoxin-quinidine interaction only manifested itself in an elderly woman when the enzyme-inducing effects of pentobarbitone were removed.

Clinical evidence, mechanism, importance and management

A woman in her nineties who had been taking 100 mg pentobarbitone at bedtime for at least a year was given digoxin and quinidine to control paroxysmal atrial fibrillation. Her serum quinidine levels remained below the therapeutic range and its half-life was unusually short (1.6 h compared with the normal 10 h) until the pentobarbitone was withdrawn, whereupon both the quinidine and the digoxin levels rose, accompanied by signs of digoxin toxicity.[1] It seems that the pentobarbitone (an enzyme-inducer) kept the quinidine levels depressed by allowing rapid liver metabolism, as a result of which the normal digoxin-quinidine interaction was minimal. Once the enzyme-inducing agent was withdrawn, the quinidine serum levels climbed and the digoxin-quinidine interaction (see 'Digitalis Glycosides + Quinidine') which results in elevated digoxin levels was able to manifest itself fully. An interaction involving the interplay of three drugs like this is fairly unusual.

Reference

1 Chapron DJ, Mumford D, Pitegoff GJ. Apparent quinidine-induced digoxin toxicity after withdrawal of pentobarbital. A case of sequential drug interactions. Arch Int Med (1979) 139, 363.

Digitalis glycosides + Quinine

Abstract/Summary

Some but not all patients may show a marked rise (+ 60%) in serum digoxin levels if given quinine.

Clinical evidence

The steady-state digoxin levels of four normal subjects on 0.25 mg daily rose by 63% (from 0.63 to 1.03 nmol/l) after taking 300 mg quinine four times daily for a day. After taking the quinine for a further three days the digoxin levels rose another 11% (to 1.10 nmol/l). Digoxin renal clearance fell by 20% (from 2.32 to 1.86 ml/min/kg).[1]

250 mg quinine daily for seven days given to seven normal subjects increased their mean serum digoxin levels by 25% (from 0.64 to 0.80 ng/ml). When given 750 mg daily there was a further 8% rise. Considerable individual differences were seen, one subject demonstrating a 92% rise.[4] In contrast, 17 patients given 750 mg quinine daily showed only a small and statistically insignificant rise in serum digoxin levels (from 0.80 to 0.91 ng/ml). Serum levels were virtually unaltered in 11 patients, decreased in two and markedly increased (amount not stated) in four.[3] Another study found that quinine reduced the total body clearance of digoxin by 26%.[2]

Mechanism

Not fully understood. Unlike quinidine, a reduction in non-renal clearance is apparently largely responsible for the rise in serum digoxin levels.[2,4,5] This is possibly due to changes in digoxin metabolism or in its biliary excretion.[2,5]

Importance and management

An established interaction of clinical importance but only moderately documented compared with digoxin/quinidine. Monitor the effects of concurrent use and reduce the digoxin dosage where necessary. Some patients may show a substantial increase in serum digoxin levels whereas others will show only small or moderate rise. There appear to be no case reports of digoxin intoxication because of concurrent use.

References

1 Aronson JK, Carver JG. Interaction of digoxin with quinine. Lancet (1981) i, 1418.
2 Wandell M, Powell JR, Hager WD, Fenster PE, Graves PE, Conrad KA, Goldman S. Effect of quinine on digoxin kinetics. Clin Pharmacol Ther (1980) 28, 425–30.
3 Doering W. Is there a clinically relevant interaction between quinine and digoxin in human beings? Am J Cardiol (1981) 48, 975–6.
4 Pedersen KE, Madsen JL, Klitgaard NA, Kjaer K, Hvidt S. Effect of quinine on plasma digoxin concentration and renal digoxin clearance. Acta Med Scand (1985) 218, 229–32.
5 Hedman A, Angelin B, Arvidsson A, Dahlqvist R, Nilsson B. Interactions in the renal and biliary elimination of digoxin: stereoselective difference between quinine and quinidine. Clin Pharmacol Ther (1990) 47, 20–6.

Digitalis glycosides + Rauwolfia Alkaloids

Abstract/Summary

Concurrent use is not uncommon and usually uneventful, but the incidence of arrhythmias appears to be increased, particularly in those with atrial fibrillation. Excessive bradycardia and hypotension have also been described.

Clinical evidence

(a) Increased cardiac arrhythmias

Three patients on digoxin and either reserpine or whole root *Rauwolfia serpentina* developed arrhythmias: atrial tachycardia with 4:1 Wenckebach irregular block; ventricular bigeminy and tachycardia; and atrial fibrillation. A large number of other patients received both drugs without problems.[1]

The incidence of premature ventricular systoles was roughly doubled (seven out of 15) in patients taking both drugs compared with a similar group taking only rauwolfia.[2] Reserpine reduced the tolerated dose of acetyl strophanthidin in 15 patients with congestive heart failure; eight out of nine with atrial fibrillation showed advanced toxic rhythms during acute digitalization compared with only one who responded in this way without reserpine.[3]

(b) Excessive bradycardia and syncope

A man on digoxin (0.25 and 0.375 mg alternate days) and reserpine (0.25 mg daily) developed a very slow heart rate, sinus bradycardia and carotid sinus supersensitivity. He was hospitalized because of syncope which remitted when the reserpine was withdrawn.[4]

Mechanism

Not understood. A possible explanation is that the rauwolfia alkaloids deplete the sympathetic nerve supply (i.e. accelerator) to the heart of its neurotransmitter which allows the parasympathetic vagal supply (i.e. heart slowing) to have full rein. Digitalis also causes heart slowing, so that the total additive bradycardia becomes excessive. In this situation the rate could become so slow that ectopic foci which would normally be swamped by a faster, more normal beat, begin to fire, leading to the development of arrhythmias. Syncope could also result from the combination of bradycardia and the hypotensive effects of reserpine elsewhere in the cardiovascular system.

Importance and management

Concurrent use is not unusual, but some caution is advisable. One group of authors who, despite having described the adverse reactions cited above,[1] conclude that '...time has proven the safety of the combination.' However they continue with the proviso that '...the development of arrhythmias must be anticipated and appropriate steps taken at their appearance...'. Particular risk of arrhythmias seems to occur with patients with atrial fibrillation (eight out of nine in the report cited[3]), and with digitalized patients given reserpine parenterally because of the sudden release of catecholamines which takes place.[4]

References

1 Dick HLH, McCawley EL and Fisher WA. Reserpine-digitalis toxicity. Arch Intern Med (1962) 109, 49.
2 Schreader CJ, Etzel MM. Premature ventricular contractions due to rauwolfia therapy. J Amer Med Ass (1956) 162, 1256.
3 Lown B, Ehrlich L, Lipschultz B, Blake J. Effect of digitalis in patients receiving reserpine. Circulation (1961) 24, 1185.
4 Bigger JT, Strauss HC. Digitalis toxicity: drug interactions prompting toxicity and the management of toxicity. Seminars in Drug Treatment (1972) 2, 147.

Digitalis glycosides + Rifampicin (Rifampin)

Abstract/Summary

The serum levels of digitoxin can be halved by the concurrent use of rifampicin. Digoxin serum levels may be similarly affected in patients with kidney failure, but it is unlikely to occur in those with normal kidney function.

Clinical evidence

(a) Digitoxin

A comparative study[1] on 21 tuberculous patients and 19 normal subjects taking 0.1 mg digitoxin daily showed that the serum digitoxin levels of the patients on rifampicin were approximately 50% of those not on rifampicin (18.4 compared with 39.1 ng/ml). The half-life of digitoxin was found to be reduced by the rifampicin from 8.2 to 4.5 days.

There are case reports confirming that rifampicin can markedly reduce serum digitoxin levels.[2,4]

(b) Digoxin

A woman, hospitalized for endocarditis and under treatment with digoxin (0.25–0.375 mg daily), frusemide, aspirin, isosorbide and potassium chloride, showed a marked fall (about 80%) in her serum digoxin levels when given 600 mg rifampicin daily. The serum digoxin climbed to its former levels when the rifampicin was withdrawn.[3] She had only moderate renal impairment (serum creatinine 2.5 mg/dl).

Another report describes two patients on renal dialysis whose digoxin dosage needed to be doubled while taking rifampicin, and similarly reduced when the rifampicin was withdrawn.[5] This confirms an earlier report.[7]

Mechanism

Rifampicin is a potent liver enzyme inducing agent which can increase the normal metabolism of digitoxin (and reduce its half-life[1,6]) thereby hastening its clearance. Digoxin on the other hand is largely excreted unchanged in the urine, so that a similar increase in its metabolism would not be expected to increase its clearance except in patients with poor kidney function. However the case cited[3] would suggest that non-renal clearance may sometimes account for a considerable amount of the total body clearance.

Importance and management

The digitoxin/rifampicin interaction is established and clinically important. Under-digitalization may occur unless the digitoxin dosage is increased appropriately (approximately doubled). An interaction of the same magnitude can occur with digoxin in patients with renal failure,[5] and sometimes in those with only moderate renal impairment,[3] but a digoxin/rifampicin interaction is unlikely in patients with normal kidney function in whom most of the digoxin is eliminated unchanged in the urine.

References

1 Peters U, Hausmen T-U and Gross-Brockhoff F. Einfluss von Tuberkulostatika auf die Pharmakokinetik des Digitoxins. Deut Med Wchsch (1974) 99, 2381.

2 Boman G, Eliasson K, Odarcederlof I. Acute cardiac failure during treatment with digitoxin an interaction with rifampicin. Br J clin Pharmacol (1980) 10, 89.

3 Bussey HI, Merritt GJ, Hill EG. The influence of rifampin on quinidine and digoxin. Arch Intern Med (1984) 144, 1021–3.

4 Poor DM, Self TH, Davis HL. Interaction of rifampin and digitoxin. Arch Intern Med (1983) 143, 599.

5 Gault H, Longerich L, Dawe M, Fine A. Digoxin-rifampin interaction. Clin Pharmacol Ther (1984) 35, 750–4.

6 Zilly W, Breimer DD, Richter E. Pharmacokinetic interactions with rifampicin. Clin Pharmacokinetics (1977) 2, 61.

7 Novi C, Bissoli F, Simonati V, Volpini T, Baroli A, Vignati G. Rifampin and digoxin: possible drug interaction in a dialysis patient. J Amer Med Ass (1980) 244, 2522–3.

Digitalis glycosides + Ro 405967

Abstract/Summary

Ro 405967, a new calcium channel blocker, increases serum digoxin levels.

Clinical evidence, mechanism, importance and management

42 normal subjects on 0.375 mg digoxin daily showed the following mean maximum increases in serum digoxin levels when given Ro 405967 for a week: 50 mg daily (+24%), 100 mg and 150 mg daily (+43%). The AUCs, ECGs and other haemodynamic measurements were also changed in a dose-dependent manner.[1] If and when this drug is used clinically, the precautions suggested for verapamil would seem to be appropriate (see index). Ro 405967 is a calcium channel blocker similar to verapamil.

Reference

1 Kirch W, Mescneder A. Dose dependence of the calcium antagonist/digoxin interaction. Clin Pharmacol Ther (1993) 53, 164.

Digitalis glycosides + Spironolactone

Abstract/Summary

The available evidence suggests that serum digoxin levels may be increased 25% by spironolactone, but as spironolactone or its metabolite can interfere with some digoxin assay methods, the evaluation of this interaction is difficult. The effects of digitoxin are reported to be both increased and decreased by spironolactone.

Clinical evidence

(a) Digoxin

The serum digoxin levels of nine patients were increased about 20% (from 0.85 to 1.0 ng/ml) when given 200 mg spironolactone daily. One patient showed a 3–4-fold rise.[1]

The clearance of digoxin in four patients and four subjects after single 0.75 mg intravenous doses was reduced about 25% following five days treatment with 200 mg spironolactone daily.[2] A marked fall in serum digoxin was reported in an elderly patient when spironolactone was withdrawn[6] but the accuracy of the assay method used is uncertain. One study found that no clinically important reduction in digoxin clearance occurred when *Aldactazide* (spironolactone-hydrochlothiazide) was used.[5]

(b) Digitoxin

A study[3] in six normal subjects who had been taking 0.1 or 0.15 mg digitoxin daily for 30 days showed that the concurrent use of 300 mg spironolactone daily increased the digitoxin half-life by a third (from 141 to 192 h).

Other studies however found that the digitoxin half-life was reduced (from 256 to 204 h).[4]

Mechanism

Not fully understood. Spironolactone inhibits the excretion of digoxin by the kidney (by 13%) but not its biliary clearance,[8] and probably causes a reduction in the volume of distribution.

Importance and management

The digoxin/spironolactone interaction appears to be established. What is known suggests a rise of about 25% in serum digoxin levels, although much greater increases can apparently occur.[1] Monitor concurrent use carefully for signs of over-digitalization. The reports cited here appear to be reliable, but the total picture of this interaction is confused by a number of other reports (not cited) of doubtful reliability. The problem is that spironolactone or its metabolite, canrenone, interfere with some assay methods (eg radioimmunoassay with Gamma Coat[125] I, and Abbott TDX fluorescence polarization immunoassay).[7] This means that monitoring is difficult unless the digoxin assay method is known to be reliable. The situation with digitoxin is even more confusing because the reports are contradictory. Concurrent use should be monitored, but the effects are uncertain.

References

1 Steiness E. Renal tubular secretion of digoxin. Circulation (1974) 50. 103.
2 Waldorff S, Andersen JD, Heeboll-Nielsen N, Nielsen OG, Moltke E, Steiness E. Spironolactone-induced changes in digoxin kinetics. Clin Pharmacol Ther (1978) 24, 162.
3 Carruthers SG, Dujovne CA. Cholestyramine and spironolactone and their combination in digitoxin elimination. Clin Pharmacol Ther (1980) 27, 184.
4 Wirth KE, Frohlich JC, Hollifield JW, Falkner FC, Sweetman BS, Oates JA. Metabolism of digitoxin in man and its modification by spironolactone. Europ J Clin Pharmacol (1976) 9, 345.
5 Finnegan TP, Spence JD, Cape R. Potassium-sparing diuretics: interaction with digoxin in elderly men. J Amer Ger Soc (1984) 32, 129–31.
6 Paladino JA, Davidson KH, McCall BB. Influence of spironolactone on serum digoxin concentration. J Amer Med Ass (1984) 251, 470–1.
7 Foukaridis GN. Influence of spironolactone and its metabolite canrenone on serum digoxin assays. Ther Drug Monit (1990) 12, 82–4.
8 Hedman A, Anglein B, Arvidsson A, Dahlqvist R. Digoxin-interactions in man: spironolactone reduces renal but not biliary digoxin clearance. Eur J Clin Pharmacol (1992) 42, 481–5.

Digitalis glycosides + Sucralfate

Abstract/Summary

Sucralfate caused only a small reduction (19%) in the absorption of digoxin in normal subjects, but an isolated report describes a marked reduction in one patient.

Clinical evidence

1 g sucralfate four times daily for 2 days given to 12 normal subjects had no effect on most of the pharmacokinetic parameters of single 0.75 mg doses of digoxin, except that the AUC was reduced by 19% (from 41.85 to 39.47 ng/ml/h) and the amount eliminated in the urine was reduced by 12%. It was also absorbed faster.[1] No interaction occurred when the digoxin was given 2 h before the sucralfate.[1] One elderly patient is reported to have had subtherapeutic serum digoxin levels while taking sucralfate, even though the dosages were separated by 2 h.[2]

Mechanism

Uncertain. One possibility is that the digoxin and sucralfate bind together in the gut which reduces the digoxin absorption.

Importance and management

Information is limited to the reports cited. Give the digoxin 2 h before the sucralfate to reduce admixture in the gut, and be alert for any evidence of reduced digoxin effects. More study is needed.

References

1 Giesing DH, Lamman RC, Dimmitt DC, Runser DJ. Lack of effect of sucralfate on digoxin pharmacokinetics. Gastroenterology (1983) 84, 1165.
2 Rey AM, Gums JG. Altered absorption of digoxin, sustained-release quinidine, and warfarin with sucralfate absorption. DICP Ann Pharmacotherapy (1991) 25, 745–6.

Digitalis glycosides + Sulphasalazine

Abstract/Summary

Serum digoxin levels can be reduced by the concurrent use of sulphasalazine.

Clinical evidence, mechanism, importance and management

The observation that a patient taking 8 g sulphasalazine daily had low serum digoxin levels, prompted a cross-over study in 10 normal subjects given 0.5 mg digoxin alone and later after

6 days' treatment with 2–6 g sulphasalazine daily. Digoxin absorption was reduced, ranging from 50% to virtually nothing, depending on the dosage of sulphasalazine used.[1] Serum digoxin levels were depressed accordingly.[1] The reasons are not understood. This seems to be the only report of this interaction, but it appears to be established. Concurrent use need not be avoided, but serum digoxin levels should be monitored and/or the patient checked for signs of under-digitalization. In one patient examined, separating the dosages appeared not to prevent this interaction.

Reference

1 Juhl RP, Summers RW, Guillory JK, Blaug SM, Cheng FH, Brown DD. Effect of sulfasalazine on digoxin availability. Clin Pharmacol Ther (1976) 20, 387.

Digitalis glycosides + Sympathomimetics (beta-agonists)

Abstract/Summary

Salbutamol (albuterol) causes a small reduction in serum digoxin levels.

Clinical evidence, mechanism, importance and management

A study[1] in 10 normal subjects who had taken 0.5 mg digoxin daily for 10 days found that 3 h after taking 3–4 mg salbutamol (albuterol) orally their serum digoxin levels had fallen by 0.3 nmol/l and their serum potassium levels by 0.58 mmol/l. A follow-up study suggested that the digoxin distribution to skeletal muscle may have been increased.[2] Terbutaline alone as well as with frusemide also causes a fall in serum potassium levels (see 'Terbutaline + Diuretics') which may possibly affect the response of patients to digoxin. The clinical importance of these changes is uncertain.

Reference

1 Edner M, Jogestrand T. Oral salbutamol decreases serum digoxin concentration. Eur J Clin Pharmacol (1990) 38, 195–7.
2 Edner M, Jogestrand T, Dahlqvist R. Effect of salbutamol on digoxin pharmacokinetics. Eur J Clin Pharmacol (1992) 42, 197–201.

Digitalis glycosides + Thyroid hormones and antithyroid drugs

Abstract/Summary

There is some indirect evidence that thyrotoxic patients may need a reduced digitalis dosage if treated with anti-thyroid drugs, and hypothyroidic patients may need more digitalis if started on thyroid hormones.

Clinical evidence, mechanism, importance and management

The clinical effectiveness of digitalis treatment is influenced by the thyroid status of the patient. Based on dose, hyperthyroidic patients have lower serum digoxin concentrations than euthyroid (normal) individuals, and hypothyroidic patients have higher serum digoxin concentrations.[1,3] Thyrotoxic patients are also insensitive to the chronotropic effects of digitalis.[2] The reasons are not understood, although there is evidence that in some patients the glomerular filtration rate is changed by the thyroid status.

In practical terms it seems probable that as the thyroid status is returned to normal by the use of drugs (antithyroid drugs or thyroid hormones), the dosage of the digitalis glycosides may need to be adjusted accordingly. Hyperthyroidic patients may need a reduced digitalis dosage whereas hypothyroidic patients may need an increase. There seems to be little or nothing in the literature to suggest that this is normally an important interaction, but be alert for the possibility of changed digitalis requirements during treatment. Strictly speaking this is a drug-disease not a drug-drug interaction.

References

1 Lawrence JR, Sumner DJ, Kalk WJ, Ratcliffe WA, Whiting B, Gray K, Lindsay M. Digoxin kinetics in patients with thyroid dysfunction. Clin Pharmacol Ther (1977) 22, 7–13.
2 Huffman DH, Klaassen CD, Hartman CR. Digoxin in hyperthyroidism. Clin Pharmacol Ther (1977) 22, 533–8.
3 Croxson MS, Ibbertson HK. Serum digoxin in patients with thyroid disease. Br Med J (1975) 3, 566–8.

Digitalis glycosides + Tiaprofenic Acid

Abstract/Summary

Serum digoxin levels are slightly but not significantly increased by the concurrent use of tiaprofenic acid.

Clinical evidence, mechanism, importance and management

600 mg tiaprofenic acid daily for 10 days caused a non-significant rise (from 0.97 to 1.12 ng/ml, i.e. about 15%) in serum digoxin levels of 12 normal subjects.[1] No particular precautions would seem to be necessary.

Reference

1 Doering Von W, Isbary J. Der Einfluss von Tiaprofensäure auf die Digoxin-Konzentration im Serum. Arzneim-Forsch/Drug Res (1983) 33, 167–8.

Digitalis glycosides + Ticlopidine

Abstract/Summary

Ticlopidine causes a small reduction in serum digoxin levels.

Clinical evidence, mechanism, importance and management

Ticlopidine, 250 mg twice daily for 10 days, reduced the peak serum digoxin concentrations in 15 normal subjects on 0.125–0.5 mg daily by 11% and the AUC by 9%.[1] These reductions are small and unlikely to be of clinical importance.

Reference

1 Vargas R, Reitman M, Teitelbaum P, Ryan JR, McMahon FG, Jain AK, Ryan M, Regel G. Study of the effect of ticlopidine (T) on digoxin (D) blood levels. Clin Pharmacol Ther (1988) 43, 146.

Digitalis glycosides + Trapidil

Abstract/Summary

Trapidil does not alter serum digoxin levels.

Clinical evidence, mechanism, importance and management

Trapidil (400 mg daily) for 8 days had no effect on the steady-state serum digoxin levels of 10 normal subjects taking digoxin (0.375 mg daily). It was noted that trapidil opposed the negative chronotropic effect of digoxin to a small extent.[1] No special precautions would seem necessary.

Reference

1 Sziegoleit W, Weiss M, Fah A, Scharfe S. Trapidil does not affect serum levels and cardiotonic action of digoxin in healthy humans. Jap Circ J (1987) 51, 1305–9.

Digitalis glycosides + Trazodone

Abstract/Summary

A rise in serum digoxin levels, accompanied by intoxication in one instance, has been seen in two patients on digoxin when treated with trazodone.

Clinical evidence, mechanism, importance and management

An elderly woman stabilized on digoxin (and also taking quinidine, clonidine and a triamterene-hydrochlorthiazide diuretic) complained of nausea and vomiting within a fortnight of starting to take trazodone (50–300 mg daily for 11 days). Her serum digoxin levels had risen more than threefold (from 0.8 to 2.8 ng/ml). The digoxin was stopped and then restarted at half the original dosage which maintained therapeutic levels.[1] The patient had poor renal function, but this did not change significantly during this incident. Another case has been reported.[2]

Even though direct information seems to be limited to these two reports, and a study in dogs failed to confirm this interaction,[3] it would now seem prudent to monitor the effects of concurrent use.

References

1 Rauch PK, Jenike MA. Digoxin toxicity possibly precipitated by trazodone. Psychosomatics (1984) 25, 334–5.
2 Knapp JE. Mead Johnson Pharmaceutical Newsletter, 1983.
3 Dec GW, Jenike MA, Stern TA. Trazodone-digoxin interaction in an animal model. J Clin Psychopharmacol (1984) 4, 153–5.

Digitalis glycosides + Trimethoprim

Abstract/Summary

Serum digoxin levels can be increased about 25% or more by trimethoprim but some individuals may show a much greater rise.

Clinical evidence

After taking 400 mg trimethoprim daily for 14 days the mean serum digoxin levels in nine patients had risen by an average of 22% (from 1.17 to 1.50 nmol/l). One patient showed a 75% rise. When the trimethoprim was withdrawn, the serum digoxin levels fell once again.[1,2]

Mechanism

It is suggested that the trimethoprim reduces the renal excretion of digoxin and may also reduce the liver metabolism as well.[1,2]

Importance and management

Information seems to be limited to the reports cited, but the interaction appears to be established. More study is needed to confirm the observations. Normally the serum digoxin rise is modest, but monitor the effects because some individuals can apparently experience a marked rise. Reduce the digoxin dosage if necessary. Trimethoprim is contained in co-trimoxazole, but the dosage is relatively small (80 mg per tablet) so that it is uncertain therefore whether co-trimoxazole will also interact.

References

1 Kastrup J, Bartram R, Petersen P, Hansen JM. Trimethoprims indvirkning pa serum-digoksin og serum-kreatinin. Ugeskr Laeger (1983) 145, 2286–8.
2 Petersen P, Kastrup J, Bartram R, Hansen JM. Digoxin-trimethoprim interaction. Acta Med Scand (1985) 217, 423–7.

Digitalis glycosides + Urapidil

Abstract/Summary

Urapidil appears not to interact adversely with digoxin.

Clinical evidence, mechanism, importance and management

Four days treatment with 60 mg urapidil twice daily for 4 days had no significant effects on serum digoxin levels of 12 normal subjects. Blood pressures and pulse rates were not significantly changed.[1] No special precautions seem necessary.

Reference

1 Solleder P, Haerlin R, Wurst W, Klingmann I, Mosberg H. Effect of urapidil on steady-state serum digoxin concentration in healthy subjects. Eur J Clin Pharmacol (1989) 37, 193–4.

Digitalis glycosides + Vasodilators

Abstract/Summary

A reduction in serum digoxin levels can occur during the concurrent use of sodium nitroprusside or hydralazine, but the importance of this is as yet uncertain.

Clinical evidence, mechanism, importance and management

An experimental study[1] on eight patients with congestive heart failure showed that when they were given either sodium nitroprusside by infusion (7–425 μg/min) or hydralazine by injection (5 mg every 10–20 min), their total renal digoxin clearance went up by 50% and their serum digoxin levels fell by 20% and 11% respectively. It is not known whether these changes would be sustained during chronic concurrent treatment, or the extent to which the digoxin dosage might need to be increased. More study is needed to find out if this interaction is of practical importance.

Reference

1 Cogan JJ, Humphreys MH, Carlson CJ, Benowitz NL and Rapaport E. Acute vasodilator therapy increases renal clearance of digoxin in patients with congestive heart failure. Circulation (1981) 64, 973–6.

Digitalis glycosides + Verapamil

Abstract/Summary

Serum digoxin levels are increased about 40% by the concurrent use of 160 mg verapamil daily, and about 70% by 240 mg verapamil or more daily. Digoxin toxicity may develop if the dosage is not reduced. Deaths have occurred. A rise of about 35% occurs with digitoxin.

Clinical evidence

(a) Digoxin

After 2 weeks treatment with 240 mg verapamil daily the mean serum digoxin levels of 29 patients with chronic atrial fibrillation had risen by 72%. It was seen in most patients. Most (90%) of this rise occurred within the first 7 days. The rise was less with a smaller dose of verapamil (160 mg). Some of the patients showed signs of digoxin toxicity.[1]

Reports on nine and 12 normal subjects,[8,9] and on 41 and six and seven patients[3,6,24] describe rises in serum digoxin levels of 44%, 53%, 69%, 70% and 96% (range 44–147%) when given 240–360 mg verapamil daily. A 40% rise was seen with 160 mg verapamil daily.[14] Similar rises are reported elsewhere.[12–15] An approximately 50% rise was seen in chronic haemodialysis patients given 120–240 mg verapamil daily.[23] Nine normal subjects on digoxin showed a 53% rise while taking 240 mg verapamil daily for a fortnight which increased to a total of 155% when additionally given 480 mg quinidine daily.[8] Toxicity[20] and a fatality[2] occurred in patients whose digoxin levels became markedly increased by verapamil. Both asystole and sinus arrest have been described.[16,21] A single dose study indicated that cirrhosis magnifies the extent of this interaction.[22]

(b) Digitoxin

Eight out of 10 patients showed a mean 35% rise (range 14–97%) in serum digitoxin levels over a 4–6 week period while taking 240 mg verapamil daily. Two patients showed no changes, and no changes in the pharmacokinetics of a single dose digitoxin were found in three normal subjects.[18,19]

Mechanism

The rise in serum digoxin levels is due to reductions in renal and especially extra-renal (biliary) clearance; a diminution in the volume of distribution also takes place.[3,4,7,12,14,24] Impaired extra-renal excretion is suggested as the reason for the rise in serum digitoxin levels.[18]

Importance and management

The digoxin/verapamil interaction is well documented and well established. It occurs in most patients.[11,12] Serum digoxin levels should be well monitored and downward dosage adjustments made to avoid digoxin toxicity (deaths have occurred[2]). A 33–50% dosage reduction has been recommended.[10,17] The interaction develops within 2–7 days, approaching or reaching a maximum within 14 days or so.[1,6] The magnitude of the rise is dose-dependent[5] with a significant increase if the verapamil dosage is increased from 160 to 240 mg daily,[1] but with no further increase if the dose is raised any higher.[9] The mean response to 160 mg daily is about 40%, and with 240 mg verapamil or more it is about 60–80%, but the response is variable. Some patients may show rises of up to 150% while others show only a modest increase. One study found that serum digoxin levels which had risen by 60% within a week had fallen to about 30% 5 weeks later.[12] Regular monitoring and dosage adjustments would seem to be necessary.

The documentation of the digitoxin/verapamil interaction is limited, but the interaction appears to be established. The incidence was 80% in the study cited.[18] Downward dosage adjustment may be necessary, particularly in some patients. Serum digitoxin levels rise less than digoxin levels and more slowly so that they are easier to control. It has been suggested therefore that digitoxin is a valuable alternative to digoxin in this situation.[18] For alternative non-interacting calcium-channel blockers see 'Digitalis + Calcium channel blockers' and 'Digitalis + Nifedipine'.

References

1 Klein HO, Lang R, Weiss E, Segni ED, Libhaber C, Guerrero J, Kaplinsky E. The influence of verapamil on serum digoxin concentrations. Circulation (1982) 65, 998–1003.

2 Zatuchni J. Verapamil-digoxin interaction. Am Heart J (1984) 108, 412–3.

3 Klein HO, Lang R, Di Segni E, Kaplinsky E. Verapamil-digoxin interaction. N Engl J Med (1980) 303, 160.

4 Pedersen KE, Dorph-Pedersen A, Hvidt S, Litgaard NA, Nielsen-Kudsk F. Digoxin-verapamil interaction. Clin Pharmacol Ther (1981) 30, 311.

5 Schwartz JB, Keefe D, Kates RE, Kirsten E, Harrison DC. Acute and chronic pharmacodynamic interaction of verapamil and digoxin in atrial fibrillation. Circulation (1982) 65, 1163.

6 Merola P, Badin A, Paleari DC, De Petris A, Maragno I. Influenza del verapamile sui livelli plasmatici di digossina nell'uomo. Cardiologia (1984) 27, 683–7.

7 Pedersen KE et al. Digoxin-verapamil interaction. Acta Med Scand (1982) 211 (Suppl 655) 37.

8 Doering W. Effect of co-administration of verapamil and quinidine on serum digoxin concentration. Eur J Clin Pharmacol (1983) 25, 517–21.

9 Belz GG, Doering W, Munkes R, Matthews J. Interaction between digoxin and calcium antagonists and antiarrhythmic drugs. Clin Pharmacol Ther (1983) 33, 410–17.

10 Marcus FI. Pharmacokinetic interactions between digoxin and other drugs. J Amer Coll Cardiol (1985) 5, 82–90A.

11 Belz GG, Aust PE, Munkes R. Digoxin plasma concentrations and nifedipine. Lancet (1981) i, 844.

12 Pedersen KE, Dorph-Pedersen A, Hvidt S, Klitgaard NA, Pedersen KK. The long term effect of verapamil on plasma digoxin concentrations and renal digoxin clearance in healthy subjects. Eur J Clin Pharmacol (1982) 22, 123–7.

13 Klein HO, Saba K, Lang R, Di Segni E, Sareli P, David D, Kaplinsky E. Oral verapamil versus digoxin in the management of chronic atrial fibrillation. Chest (1980) 78, 524.

14 Lang R, Klein HO, Saba K, Weiss E, Libhaber C, Kaplinsky E. Effect of verapamil on digoxin blood levels and clearance. Chest (1980) 78, 525.

15 Schwartz JB, Keefe D, Kates RE, Harrison DC. Verapamil and digoxin. Another drug-drug interaction. Clin Res (1981) 29, 501A.

16 Kounis NG. Asystole after verapamil and digoxin. Brit J Clin Prac (1980) 34, 57.

17 Klein HO, Kaplinsky E. Verapamil and digoxin: their respective effects on atrial fibrillation and their interaction. Am J Cardiol (1982) 50, 894–902.

18 Kuhlmann J, Marcin S. Effects of verapamil on pharmacokinetics and pharmacodynamics of digitoxin in patients. Am Heart J (1985) 110, 1245–50.

19 Kuhlmann J. Effects of verapamil, diltiazem, and nifedipine on plasma levels and renal excretion of digitoxin. Clin Pharmacol Ther (1985) 38, 667–73.

20 Gordon M, Goldenberg LMC. Clinical digoxin toxicity in the aged in association with co-administered verapamil. A report of two cases and a review of the literature. J Am Geriatr Soc (1986) 34, 659–62.

21 Kounis NG, Mallioris C. Interactions with cardioactive drugs. Br J Clin Prac (1986) 40, 537–8.

22 Maragno I, Gianotti C, Tropeano PF, Rodighiero V, Gaion RM, Paleari C, Prandoni R, Menozzi L. Verapamil-induced changes in digoxin kinetics in cirrhosis. Eur J Clin Pharmacol (1987) 32, 309–11.

23 Rendtorff C, Johannessen AC, Halck S, Klitgaard NA. Verapamil-digoxin interaction in chronic hemodialysis patients. Sand J Urol Nephrol (1990) 24, 137–9.

24 Hedman A, Angelin B, Arvidsson A, Beck O, Dahlqvist R, Nilsson B, Olsson M, Schenck-Gustafsson K. Digoxin-verapamil interaction: reduction of biliary but not renal digoxin clearance. Clin Pharmacol Ther (1991) 49, 256–62.

Chapter 15
Hypoglycaemic Agent Drug Interactions

The hypoglycaemic agents are used to control diabetes mellitus, a disease in which there is total or partial failure of the beta-cells within the pancreas to secrete into the circulation enough insulin, one of the hormones concerned with the handling of glucose. In some cases there is evidence to show that the disease results from the presence of factors which oppose the activity of insulin.

With insufficient insulin, the body tissues are unable to take up and utilize the glucose which is in circulation in the blood. Because of this, the glucose which is derived largely from the digestion of food and which would normally be removed and stored in tissues throughout the body, accumulates and boosts the glucose in the blood to such grossly elevated proportions that the kidney is unable to cope with such a load and glucose appears in the urine. Raised blood sugar levels (hyperglycaemia) with glucose and ketone bodies in the urine (glycosuria and ketonuria) are among the manifestations of a serious disturbance in the metabolic chemistry of the body which, if untreated, can lead on to the development of diabetic coma and death.

There are two main types of diabetes: one develops early in life and occurs when the ability of the pancreas suddenly, and often almost totally, fails to produce insulin. The first is called Type I, Juvenile or insulin-dependent diabetes (IDDM). The other form of diabetes is the maturity-onset type and is most often seen in those over 40. This occurs when the pancreas gradually loses the ability to produce insulin over a period of months or years. It is often associated with being over-weight and can sometimes be satisfactorily controlled simply by losing weight and adhering to an appropriate diet. Its alternative names are Type II or non-insulin dependent diabetes mellitus (NIDDM).

The modes of action of the hypoglycaemic agents

Insulin

Insulin extracted from the pancreatic tissue of pigs and cattle is so similar to human insulin that it can be used as a replacement. Human insulin is also increasingly being used because it can now be made by micro-organisms which have been modified by genetic engineering. It is given, not by mouth, but by injection in order to bypass the enzymes of the gut which would digest and destroy it like any other protein. There are now many formulations of insulin, some of them designed to delay absorption from the subcutaneous or intramuscular tissue into which the injection is made so that repeated daily injections can be avoided, but all of them sooner or later release insulin into the circulation where it acts to replace or top-up the insulin from the human pancreas.

Sulphonylurea and biguanide oral hypoglycaemic agents

The sulphonylurea and other sulphonamide-related compounds such as chlorpropamide and tolbutamide were the first synthetic compounds used in medicine as hypoglycaemic agents which had the advantage of being given by mouth. Among their actions they stimulate the remaining beta-cells of the pancreas to grow and secrete insulin which, with a restricted diet, controls blood sugar levels and permits normal metabolism to occur. Clearly they can only be effective in those diabetics whose pancreas still has the capacity to produce some insulin, so their use is confined to the maturity-onset, Type II, non-insulin dependent diabetics.

Table 15.1 Hypoglycaemic agents

Approved or generic names	Proprietary names
Biguanides	
Buformin	*Diabrin, Silubin Retard, Sindiatil*
Metformin	*Diabex, Diaberit, Diabetosan, Diabexyl, Glufagos, Glucadal, Glucophage, Islotin, Metiguanide, Orabet, Stagid, Mellitin*
Phenformin	*Cronoformin, DBI, Diabenide, Dibotin, Dipar, Glucopostin, Insoral (also used for carbutamide), Meltrol*
Sulph(f)onylureas	
Acetohexamide	*Dimelor, Dymelor, Gamadiabet, Metaglucina, Ordimel*
Carbutamide (glybutamide)	*Biouren, Carbutil, Diabetin, Diabetoplex, Diabutan, Dia-Tablinen, Dibefanil, Dicarbul, Glucidoral, Glucofren, Insoral (see also phenformin), Invenol, Nadisan*
Chlorpropamide	*Bioglumin, Clordiabet, Clordiasan, Cloro-Hipoglucina, Diabet, Glucosulfina, Catanil, Diabetasi, Diabexan, Diatron, Gliconorm, Melisar, Normoglig, Chloromide, Chloronase, Diabenal, Diabetal, Diabinese, Diabines, Diabetoral, Diabinese, Glymese, Insulase, Melitase, Mellinese, Nogluc, Novopropamide, Promide*
Glibenclamide (glyburide)	*Adiab, Calabren, Daonil, DiaBeta, Euglucan, Euglucon, Gilemal, Libanil, Malix, Glidiabet, Glucolon, Gliben, Micronase*
Glibornuride	*Glutril, Giltrim, Gluborid, Glutrid*
Gliclazide	*Diamicron, Dramion*
Glipizide	*Glibenese, Glucutrol, Minodiab, Minidiab*
Gliquidone	*Glurenorm, Glurenor*
Glisoxepide	*Glisepin, Glucoben, Pro-Diaban*
Glybuzole	*Gludease*
Glycopyramide	*Deamelin-S*
Glycyclamide	*Diaborate*
Metahexamide	*Isodiane*
Tolazamide	*Diabewas, Norglycin, Ronase, Tolinase, Tolamide*
Tolbutamide	*Aglicem, Aglycid, Arcosal, Artosin, Chembutamide, Diaben, Diabeton, Diasulfon, Dolipol, Fordex, Glyconon, Guabeta N, Insilange-D, Mellitol, Metilato, Mobenol, Neo-Insoral, Nigloid, Neo-Dibetic, Novobutamide, Oramide, Oribetic, Orinase, Pramidex, Proinsul, Rastinon, Tolbutone*
Sulph(f)onamide-related compounds	
Gliflumide	
Glymidine (glycodiazine)	*Glyconormal, Gondafon, Lycanol, Redul*
Enzyme inhibitor	
Acarbose	*Glucobay*

The mode of action of the other synthetic oral hypoglycaemic agents, the biguanides such as metformin, is obscure, but they do not stimulate the pancreas like the sulphonylureas to release insulin, but appear to facilitate the uptake and utilization of glucose by the cells in some way. Their use is restricted to maturity-onset diabetics because they are not effective unless insulin is also present.

Other oral hypoglycaemic agents

Acarbose has recently been introduced and acts against alphaglucosidases and specifically against sucrase in the gut to delay the digestion and absorption of monosaccharides from starch and sucrose. Outside orthodox Western medicine, there are herbal preparations which are used to treat diabetes and which can be given by mouth. Blueberries were traditionally used by the Alpine peasants, and bitter gourd or karela (*Momordica charantia*) is an established part of herbal treatment in the Indian subcontinent and elswhere. The Chinese herbals also contain remedies for diabetes. As yet it is not known how these herbal remedies act and their efficacy awaits formal clinical evaluation.

Interactions

The commonest interactions are those which result in a rise or fall in blood glucose levels, thereby disturbing the control of diabetes. These are detailed in this chapter. Other interactions where the hypoglycaemic agent is the affecting agent are described elsewhere. A full listing is to be found in the Index.

Acarbose + Miscellaneous drugs

Abstract/Summary

Neomycin may increase the gastrointestinal side-effects of acarbose, and cholestyramine may possibly increase its effects. Charcoal and digestive enzyme preparations are expected to reduce its effects.

Clinical evidence, mechanism, importance and management

(a) Neomycin

Neomycin (1 g three times daily) increased the unpleasant gastrointestinal side-effects (flatulence, cramps and diarrhoea) of acarbose (200 mg three times daily) in seven normal subjects.[1]

(b) Cholestyramine

4 g cholestyramine daily for 6 days given to eight normal subjects taking 100 mg acarbose three times daily increased the reduction in postprandial insulin levels due to acarbose.[2] The mean serum insulin levels fell from 318 to 246 μUm^{-1} while taking both drugs, but showed a 'rebound' rise to 417μUm^{-1} when both were stopped.[2] The clinical importance of this in diabetics is uncertain.

(c) Digestive enzyme preparations

The makers of acarbose reasonably suggest the avoidance of intestinal adsorbents (e.g. charcoal) or digestive enzyme preparations because these would be expected to reduce and oppose the effects of acarbose,[3] but this is based on theoretical considerations.[2]

References

1 Lembke B, Caspary WF, Fölsch UR, Creutzfeldt W. Influence of neomycin on postprandial metabolic changes and side-effects of an alpha-glucosidehydrolase inhibitor (BAY g 5421). I Effects on intestinal hydrogen gas production and flatulence. In Frontiers of Hormone Research, vol 7. The Entero-Insular Axis. Satellite Symposium to Xth IDF-Meeting, September 7–8, Göttingen 1979, p 294–5.
2 Gillespie H. (Bayer) Personnal Communication, June, July 1993.
3 Glucobay (Acarbose) Datasheet 1993.

Hypoglycaemic agents + ACE inhibitors

Abstract/Summary

Concurrent use normally appears to be uneventful but marked hypoglycaemia has been seen in a few diabetics taking insulin or sulphonylureas when treated with captopril or enalapril.

Clinical evidence

(a) Evidence of hypoglycaemia

Two diabetics on glibenclamide and metformin developed marked hypoglycaemia (2.2 and 2.9 mmol/l) within 24–48 h of starting to take captopril.[6] Two other stable patients on glibenclamide experienced hypoglycaemic episodes almost immediately after starting to take enalapril or captopril. One of them was restabilized on half the dose of glibenclamide while continuing to take enalapril.[7] Three unexplained cases of hypoglycaemia in diabetics given captopril are briefly reported elsewhere.[1] Two diabetics experienced recurrent hypoglycaemia when treated with enalapril. The insulin requirements of one of them fell, and the sulphonylurea was withdrawn from the other.[2] There are nine other cases of hypoglycaemia in diabetics taking unspecified sulphonylureas while concurrently taking ACE inhibitors (five on captopril and four on enalapril) in the records of the Centre Régionaux de Pharmacovigilance in France, recorded over the 1985–90 period.[9] Hypoglycaemia has also been seen in diabetics on insulin when given captopril (but see (b) below).[1]

(b) Evidence of no interaction

A study, prompted by three unexplained cases of hypoglycaemia in insulin-dependent diabetics on captopril, failed to find any evidence of an interaction.[1] Further studies in diabetics (on insulin or sulphonylureas and/or metformin) given enalapril (20–40 mg daily) or captopril (37.5–100 mg daily)[3,4] also failed to find any evidence of an adverse interaction. Another study found that the control of diabetes was improved by enalapril.[8]

Mechanism

Uncertain. An increase in glucose utilization and increased insulin sensitivity has been suggested.[9]

Importance and management

Established interactions but the incidence appears to be very low. Just why it only affects a few individuals is not understood. Concurrent use need not be avoided but it would be prudent to warn patients on insulin or oral hypoglycaemic agents who are starting ACE inhibitors that excessive hypoglycaemia occurs very occasionally and unpredictably. A false positive urine ketone test can also occur with captopril when using the alkaline-nitroprusside test (*Keto-diastix*, Ames).[5]

References

1 Ferriere M, Lachkar H, Richard J-L, Bringer J, Orsetti A, Mirouze J. Captopril and insulin sensitivity. Ann Intern Med (1985) 102, 134–5.
2 McMurray J, Fraser DM. Captopril, enalapril and blood glucose. Lancet (1986) i, 1035.

3 Passa Ph, Marre M, Leblanc H. Enalapril, captopril and blood glucose. Lancet (1986) i, 1447.

4 Geissler C, Horton T. Captopril and blood glucose. Lancet (1986) ii, 461.

5 Warren SE. False-positive urine ketone test with captopril. N Engl J Med (1980) 303, 1003–4.

6 Rett K, Wicklmayr M, Dietz GJ. Hypoglycemia in hypertensive diabetic patients treated with sulfonylureas, biguanides and captopril. N Engl J Med (1988) 319, 1609.

7 Arsuz-Pacheco C, Ramirez LC, Rios JM, Raskin P, Hypoglycaemia induced by angiotensin-converting enzyme inhibitors in patients with non-insulin-dependent diabetes receiving sulfonylurea therapy. Am J Med (1990) 89, 811–3.

8 Whitcroft IA, Thomas JM, Rawsthorne A, Wilkinson N, Thompson H. Effects of alpha and beta adrenoceptor blocking drugs and ACE inhibitors on long term glucose and lipid control in hypertensive non-insulin dependent diabetics. Horm Metab Res Suppl (1990) 22,42–46.

9 Girardin E, Vial T, Pham E, Evreux J-C. Hypoglycémies induites par les sulfamides hypoglycémiants. Ann Med Interne (1992) 143, 11–17.

Hypoglycaemic agents + Alcohol

Abstract/Summary

Diabetics controlled on insulin or oral hypoglycaemic agents or diet alone need not abstain from alcohol, but they should only drink in moderation and accompanied by food. Alcohol makes the signs of hypoglycaemia less clear and delayed hypoglycaemia can occur. The CNS depressant effects of alcohol plus hypoglycaemia can make driving or the operation of dangerous machinery much more hazardous. A flushing reaction is common in patients on chlorpropamide who drink, but is rare with other sulphonylureas. Alcoholic patients may require above-average doses of tolbutamide.

Clinical evidence

(a) Hypoglycaemic agents in general + Alcohol

The blood glucose levels of diabetics may be reduced or may remain unchanged by alcohol. In one study, two out of seven diabetics using insulin became severely hypoglycaemic after drinking the equivalent of about three measures of spirits.[2] In a hospital study over a three-year period, five insulin-dependent diabetics were hospitalized with severe hypoglycaemia after going on the binge. Two of them died without recovery from the initial coma and the other three suffered permanent damage to the nervous system.[3] In another study it was found that alcohol was involved in 4% of hypoglycaemic episodes requiring hospitalization.[4] In contrast to these alcohol-induced hypoglycaemic episodes, it was found in two other studies[5,6] that pure alcohol and dry wine had little effect on blood glucose levels. An extensive study found that alcohol causes some deterioration in the metabolic control of elderly non-insulin dependent diabetics (increased lipolysis, raised triglyceride levels, ketogenesis).[31]

(b) Sulphonylureas + Alcohol

About one third of those on chlorpropamide who drink alcohol, even in quite small amounts, experience a warm, tingling or burning sensation of the face, and sometimes the neck and arms as well. It may also involve the conjunctivae. This can begin within 5–20 min. of drinking, reaching a peak within 30–40 min, and may persist for 1–2 h. Very occasionally headache occurs, and lightheadedness, palpitations, wheezing and breathlessness have also been experienced.[11]

This flushing reaction has been described in numerous reports (far too many to list here) involving large numbers of patients on chlorpropamide. These reports have been extensively reviewed.[7–10] A similar reaction can occur, but only very rarely, with other sulphonylureas (gliclazide,[32] glipizide,[11] glibenclamide,[11,12] tolbutamide,[13–15] tolazamide[16]). A comparative study showed that the mean half-life of tolbutamide in alcoholics was reduced about a third (from 384 to 232 min).[17] Alcohol is also reported to prolong but not increase the hypoglycaemic effects of glipizide.[30]

(c) Biguanides + Alcohol

A controlled study in five ketosis-resistant type II diabetics taking 50–100 mg phenformin daily showed that the equivalent of 3 oz whisky markedly raised their blood lactate and lactate-pyruvate levels. Two of them attained blood-lactate levels of more than 50 mg%, and one of these patients had previously experienced nausea, weakness and malaise while taking phenformin and alcohol.[18] The ingestion of alcohol is described in other reports as having preceded the onset of phenformin-induced lactic-acidosis[19–23] or a rise in blood lactate levels. Some patients have complained that alcohol tastes metallic. Phenformin has been withdrawn because of the high incidence of lactic acidosis.

Mechanism

The exacerbation of hypoglycaemia by alcohol is not fully understood, however it is known that if hypoglycaemia occurs when liver glycogen stores are low, the liver turns to the formation of new glucose from amino acids (neoglucogenesis) which is released into the circulation. This neoglucogenesis is inhibited by the presence of alcohol so that the fall in blood glucose levels may not be prevented and a full-scale hypoglycaemic episode can result. The chlorpropamide-alcohol flush (CPAF) reaction, although extensively studied, is by no means fully understood. It seems to be related to the disulfiram-alcohol reaction and is accompanied by a rise in blood-acetaldehyde levels (see 'Alcohol + Disulfiram'). It also appears to be genetically determined[11] and may involve both the prostaglandins and the endogenous opioids.[24] The decreased half-life of tolbutamide in alcoholics is probably due to the inducing effects of alcohol on liver microsomal enzymes.[17,25,26]

The reasons for the raised blood lactate levels seen during the concurrent use of phenformin and alcohol are not clear, but one suggestion is that it may possibly be related to the competitive demands for NAD by the reactions which convert alcohol to acetaldehyde, and lactate to pyruvate.[18]

Importance and management

The documentation of the hypoglycaemic agent-alcohol interactions is surprisingly patchy (with the exception of chlorpropamide and alcohol) but they are of recognized clinical importance. The following contains the main recommendations of The British Diabetic Association based on a review of what is currently known.[1]

General comments

Most diabetics need not avoid alcohol totally, but they are advised not to exceed three drinks daily, and the fewer the drinks the better. 'A drink' is defined as either half a pint (300 ml) beer, a single measure of spirits (one-sixth of a gill or 25 ml) or one small glass of sherry or wine. Drinks with a high carbohydrate content (sweet sherries, sweet wines and most liqueurs) should be avoided. Diabetics should not drink on an empty stomach but should avoid the simultaneous use of readily absorbed carbohydrates, and they should know that the warning signs of hypoglycaemia may possibly be obscured by the effects of the alcohol. Particular care is needed if they intend to drive or handle dangerous machinery because the CNS depressant effects of alcohol plus hypoglycaemia can be particularly hazardous. Warn them of the risks of hypoglycaemia occurring several hours after drinking. Those with peripheral neuropathy should be told that alcohol may aggravate the condition and they should not have more than one drink daily. Provided drinking is restricted as suggested and drinks containing a lot of carbohydrate are avoided, there is no need to include the drink in the dietary allowance. However diabetics on a weight-reducing diet should not exceed one drink daily and should include it in their daily calorie allowance.

Additional comments about the oral hypoglycaemic agents

The chlorpropamide-alcohol interaction (flushing reaction) is very well documented, but of minimal importance. It is a nuisance and may be socially embarrassing but normally requires no treatment. Patients should be warned. The incidence is said to lie between 13 and 33%[27,28] although one study claims that it may be as low as 4%.[29] Since it can be provoked by quite small amounts of alcohol (half a glass of sherry or wine) it is virtually impossible for sensitive patients to avoid it if they drink. Most manufacturers give a warning about the possibility of this reaction with other sulphonylureas, but it is very rarely seen and can therefore almost always be avoided by exchanging chlorpropamide for another sulphonylurea. Alcoholic subjects may need above-average doses of tolbutamide.

Metformin does not carry the same risk of lactic acidosis seen with phenformin (now withdrawn), and in the paper[1] prepared for and approved by the British Diabetic Association it is suggested that one or two drinks a day are unlikely to be harmful, however it should not be given to alcoholic patients because of the possibility of liver damage.

References

1 Connor H, Marks V. Alcohol and diabetes. A position paper prepared by the Nutrition Subcommittee of the British Diabetic Association's Medical Advisory Committee and approved by the Executive Council of the British Diabetic Association. Human Nutr: Appl Nutr (1985) 39A, 393–9.

2 Walsh CH, O'Sullivan DJ. Effect of moderate alcohol intake on control of diabetes. Diabetes (1974) 23, 440–2.

3 Arky RA, Veverbrandts E, Abramson EA. Irreversible hypoglycaemia. J Amer Med Ass (1968) 206, 575–8.

4 Potter J, Clarke P, Gale EAM, Dave SH, Tattersall RB. Insulin induced hypoglycaemia in an accident and emergency department: the tip of an iceberg? Br Med J (1982) 285, 1180–2.

5 McMonagle J, Felig P. Effects of ethanol ingestion on glucose tolerance and insulin secretion in normal and diabetic subjects. Metabolism (1975) 24, 625–32.

6 Lolli G, Balboni C, Ballatore C. Wine in the diets of diabetic patients. QJ Stud Alcohol (1963) 24, 412–6.

7 Johnston C, Wiles PG, Pyke DA. Chlorpropamide-alcohol flush: the case in favour. Diabetologia (1984) 26, 1–5.

8 Hillson RM, Hockaday TDR. Chlorpropamide-alcohol flush: a critical appraisal. Diabetologia (1984) 26, 6–11.

9 Waldhausl W. To flush or not to flush? Comments on the chlorpropamide-alcohol flush. Diabetologia (1984) 26, 12–14.

10 Groop L, Eriksson CJP, Huupponen R, Ylikahri R, Pelkonen R. Roles of chlorpropamide, alcohol and acetaldehyde in determining the chlorpropamide-alcohol flush. Diabetologia (1984) 26, 34–38.

11 Leslie RDG and Pyke DA. Chlorpropamide-alcohol flushing: a dominantly inherited trait associated with diabetes. Br Med J (1978) 2, 1519.

12 Stowers JM. Alcohol and glibenclamide. Br Med J (1971) 3, 533.

13 Doger H. Experience with the tolbutamide treatment of 500 cases of diabetes on an ambulatory basis. Ann NY Acad Sci (1957) 71, 275.

14 Signorelli S. Tolerance for alcohol in patients on chlorpropamide. Ann NY Acad Sci (1959) 74, 900.

15 Buttner H. Athanolunvertraglichkeit beim Menschen nach Sulfonylharnstoffen. Dtsch Arch Klin Med (1961) 207, 1.

16 McKendry JBR and Gfeller KF. Clinical experience with the oral antidiabetic compound tolazamide. Can Med Ass J (1967) 96, 531.

17 Carulli N, Manenti F, Gallo M, Salvioli GF. Alcohol-drugs interaction in man: alcohol and tolbutamide. Eur J clin Invest (1971) 1, 421.

18 Johnson HK, Waterhouse C. Relationship of alcohol and hyperlactatemia in diabetic subjects treated with phenformin. Am J Med (1968) 45, 98.

19 Davidson MB, Bozarth WR, Challoner DR, Goodner CJ. Phenformin hypoglycaemia and lactic acidosis. Report of an attempted suicide. N Engl J Med (1966) 275, 886.

20 Gottlieb A, Duberstein J, Geller A. Phenformin acidosis. N Engl J Med (1962) 267, 806.

21 Maclachlan MJ, Rodman GP. Effects of food, fast and alcohol on serum uric acid and acute attacks of gout. Am J Med (1967) 42, 38.

22 Dubas TC, Johnson WJ. Metformin-induced lactic acidosis: potentiation by ethanol. Res Comm Chem Pathol Pharmacol (1981) 33, 21.

23 Schaffalitzky de Muckadell OB, Koster A, Jensen SL. Fenformin-alkohol interaktion. Ugeskr Laeg (1973) 135, 925.

24 Johnston C, Wiles PG, Medbak S, Bowcock S, Cooke ED, Pyke DA, Rees LH. The role of endogenous opioids in the chlorpropamide alcohol flush. Clin Endocrinol (1984) 21, 489–97.

25 Kater RMH, Roggin G, Tobon F, Zieve P, Iber FL. Increased rate of clearance of drugs from the circulation of alcoholics. Amer J Med Sci (1969) 258, 35.

26 Kater RMH, Tobon F, Iber FL. Increased rate of tolbutamide metabolism in alcoholic patients. J Amer Med Ass (1969) 207, 363.

27 Fitzgerald MG, Gaddie R, Malins JM, O'Sullivan DJ. Alcohol sensitivity in diabetics receiving chlorpropamide. Diabetes (1962) 11, 40.

28 Daeppen JP, Hofstetter JR, Curchod B, Saudan Y. Traitment oral du diabete par un nouvel hypoglycemiant, le P 607 ou Diabinese. Schweiz med Woch (1959) 89, 817.

29 De Silva NE, Tunbridge WMG and Alberti KGMM. Low incidence of chlorpropamide-alcohol flushing in diet-treated, non-insulin-dependent diabetics. Lancet (1981) i, 128–31.

30 Hartling SG, Faber OK, Wegmann M-L, Wahlin-Boll E, Melander A. Interaction of ethanol and glipizide in humans. Diabetes Care (1987) 10, 683–6.

31 Ben G, Gnudi L, Maran A, Gigante A, Duner E, Iori E, Tiengo A, Avogaro A. Effects of chronic alcohol intake on carbohydrate and lipid metabolism in subjects with type II (non-insulin dependent) diabetes. Amer J Med (1991) 90, 70–6.
32 Conget JI, Vendrell J, Esmatjes E, Halperin I. Gliclazide alcohol flush. Diabetes Care (1989) 12, 44.

Hypoglycaemic agents + Allopurinol

Abstract/Summary

An increase in the half-life of chlorpropamide, and a decrease in the half-life of tolbutamide during treatment with allopurinol have been described, but the effect of these changes on the hypoglycaemic response of patients is uncertain. Marked hypoglycaemia and coma occurred in one patient on gliclazide.

Clinical evidence

(a) Chlorpropamide + Allopurinol

A brief report describes seven patients given chlorpropamide and allopurinol concurrently. The half-life of chlorpropamide in one patient with gout but normal renal function exceeded 200 h (normal 36 h) after taking allopurinol for 10 days. In two others the half-life was extended to 44 and 55 h respectively. The other three patients were given allopurinol for only 1 or 2 days and the half-life of chlorpropamide remained unaltered.[1]

(b) Gliclazide + Allopurinol

Severe hypoglycaemia (1.6 mmol/L) and coma occurred in a patient taking gliclazide and allopurinol, possibly exacerbated by renal insufficiency.[4] Hypoglycaemia has been seen in another patient taking both drugs, but enalapril and ranitidine were also involved.[4]

(b) Tolbutamide + Allopurinol

Fifteen days treatment with allopurinol (2.5 mg/kg twice daily) reduced the half-life of intravenous tolbutamide in 10 normal subjects by 25% (from 360 to 267 m).[2,3]

Mechanism

Not understood. In the case of chlorpropamide it has been suggested that it possibly involves some competition for renal tubular mechanisms.[1]

Importance and management

Information is very limited. Only gliclazide has been implicated in severe hypoglycaemia and there seem to be no reports of either grossly enhanced hypoglycaemia with chlorpropamide, or reduced hypoglycaemia with tolbutamide. More study is needed to find out whether any of these interactions has general clinical importance, but in the meantime patients should be given an appropriate warning if allopurinol is added. Information about other hypoglycaemic agents seems to be lacking.

References

1 Petitpierre B, Perrin L, Rudhardt M, Herrera A, Fabre J. Behaviour of chlorpropamide in renal insufficiency and under the effects of associated drug therapy. Int J clin Pharmacol (1972) 6, 120.
2 Gentile S, Porcellini M, Loguercio C, Foglia F, Coltorti M. Modificazione della depurazione plasmatica di tolbutamide e rifampicina-SV indotte del trattamento con allopurinolo in volontari sono. Il Progresso Medico (Roma) (1979) 35, 637.
3 Gentile S, Porcellini M, Foglia F, Loguercio C, Coltorti M. Influenza di allopurinolo sull'emivita plasmatica di tolbutamide e rifampicina-SV in soggetti sono. Boll Soc Ital Sper (1979) 55, 345.
4 Girardin E, Vial T, Pham E, Evreux J-C. Hypoglycémies induites par les sulfamides hypoglycémiants. Ann Med Interne (1992) 143, 11–17.

Hypoglycaemic agents + Amiloride

Abstract/Summary

There is some limited evidence that diabetic patients may possibly be predisposed to the development of amiloride-induced hyperkalaemia.

Clinical evidence, mechanism, importance and management

Two cases of hyperkalaemia (6.5 mEq/l or more) occurred in four hypertensive diabetic patients treated with amiloride. One of them died.[1] Another diabetic on glibenclamide and metformin developed progressive muscular paralysis and difficulty in breathing within a week of starting to take *Moduretic* (amiloride/hydrochlorothiazide).[2]

It is suggested that diabetics may have some electrolyte abnormality which predisposes them to hyperkalaemia during the use of potassium-retaining diuretics. Merck Sharp and Dohme who make amiloride say that the renal status of diabetics should be determined before giving amiloride, and that the diuretic should be discontinued for at least 3 days before giving glucose tolerance tests. However there is also evidence that concurrent use can be uneventful.[1] Strictly speaking this is not an interaction but an adverse response to amiloride in patients who need hypoglycaemic agents.

References

1 Lowenthal DT, Gould A, Shirk J, Mazzella J, Affrine MB, Walker F, Onesti G. Effects of amiloride on oral glucose loading, serum potassium, renin, and aldosterone in diet-controlled diabetics. Clin Pharmacol Ther (1980) 27, 661.
2 Freeman SJ, Fale AD. Muscular paralysis and ventilatory failure caused by hyperkalaemia. Br J Anaesth (1993) 70, 226–7.

Hypoglycaemic agents + Anabolic steroids

Abstract/Summary

Nandrolone (norandrostenolone), methandienone (methandrostenolone), testosterone and stanozolol can enhance the blood sugar reducing effects of insulin. The dosage of the hypoglycaemic agent may need to be lowered.

Clinical evidence

In a study in 54 diabetics under treatment with 25 mg nandrolone (norandrostenolone) phenylpropionate given weekly or 50 mg decanoate given 3-weekly, it was found necessary to reduce the insulin dosage by an average of 36% (reduction range of 4 to 56 U).[1]

Other reports similarly describe this response in diabetics treated with insulin and nandrolone,[2,3] methandienone (methandrostenolone),[4] testosterone propionate[7] or stanozolol.[6] A reduction in blood sugar levels has also been seen in normal subjects given testosterone propionate.[5] No changes were seen when ethyloestrenol was used.[1,2]

Mechanism

Uncertain.

Importance and management

An established interaction. The total picture is incomplete because not all of the anabolic steroids appear to have been studied and they may not necessarily behave identically. A fall in the dosage requirements of insulin (an 'insulin-sparing' effect) may be expected in many patients with the steroids cited. An average reduction of a third is reported.[1] Whether this is also true with every anabolic steroid appears not to have been documented.

References

1 Houtsmuller AJ. The therapeutic applications of anabolic steroids in ophthalmology: biochemical results. Acta Endocrinol (1961) 39 (Suppl 63) 154.
2 Dardenne U. The therapeutic applications of anabolic steroids in ophthalmology. Acta Endocrinol (1961) 39 (Suppl 63) 143–53.
3 Weissel W. Anaboles Hormon bei malignem oder kompliziertem Diabetes mellitus. Wien Klin Wsch (1962) 74, 234.
4 Landon J, Wqnl V, Samois E, Bilkus D. The effect of anabolic steroids on blood sugar and plasma insulin levels in man. Metabolism (1963) 12, 924–5.
5 Talaat M, Habib YA, Habib M. The effect of testosterone on the carbohydrate metabolism in normal subjects. Arch Int pharmacodyn (1957) 61, 215–26.
6 Pergola F. El estanozolol, nuevo anabolico. La Prensa Med Argent (1962) 49, 274–90.
7 Veil WH, Lipprocs O. 'Unspezifische' wirkungen der Mannlichen keimdrucenhormone. Klin Wchnsch (1938) 19, 655–8.

Hypoglycaemic agents + Anaesthetics

Abstract/Summary

Halothane and thiopentone-nitrous oxide appear to have relatively unimportant effects on blood sugar and insulin levels. A change from oral antidiabetic treatment to insulin may be advisable if the surgical procedures are very extensive.

Clinical evidence

The Table 15.2 summarizes the findings of 10 studies carried out on a large number of patients.

Mechanism

Extremely complex and by no means fully understood.

Importance and management

Among the work summarized in the table, halothane[2] or nitrous oxide-thiopentone[1] have been recommended as anaesthetics for diabetics because they neither increase the blood sugar or growth hormone levels significantly nor do they decrease insulin levels. A change from oral hypoglycaemics to insulin before anaesthesia has been a not uncommon practice, but it would seem that there is now an increasing tendency to leave the patient's antidiabetic treatment unchanged,[9,10] although one recommendation is that those undergoing extensive and prolonged procedures should be switched to insulin.[11]

References

1 Yoshimura N, Kodama K, Yoshitake J. Carbohydrate metabolism and insulin release during ether and halothane anaesthesia. Br J Anaesth (1971) 43, 1022.
2 Oyama T, Takasawa T. Effect of halothane anaesthesia and surgery on human growth hormone and insulin levels in plasma. Br J Anaesth (1971) 43, 573.
3 Merin RG, Samuelson PN, Schalch DS. Major inhalation anaesthetics and carbohydrate metabolism. Anaesth Analg (Curr Res) (1971) 50, 625.
4 Allison SP, Tomblin PJ, Chamberlain MJ. Some effects of anaesthesia and surgery on carbohydrate and fat metabolism. Br J Anaesth (1969) 41, 588.
5 Oyama T, Takiguchi M, Kudo T. Metabolic effects of anaesthesia: effect of thiopentone-nitrous oxide anesthesia on human growth hormone and insulin levels in plasma. Can Anaesth Soc J (1971) 18, 442.
6 Oyama T, Takiguchi M. Effects of neuroleptanaesthesia on plasma levels of growth hormone and insulin. Br J Anesth (1970) 42, 1105.
7 Oyama T, Takasawa T. Effects of diethyl ether anaesthesia and surgery on carbohydrate and fat metabolism in man. Can Anaesth Soc J (1971) 18, 51.
8 Oyama T, Takasawa T. Effect of methoxyflurane anaesthesia and surgery on human growth hormone and insulin levels in plasma. Can Anaesth Soc J (1970) 17, 347.
9 Hagan JJ, Kendall CHG. Insulin and oral antidiabetic drugs. Int Anesthesiol Clinics (1975) 13, 127.
10 Fletcher J, Langman MJS and Kelloch TD. Effects of surgery on blood sugar levels in diabetes mellitus. Lancet (1965) 22, 52.
11 Stehling L. Clinical Anaesthesia: Pharmacology of adjuvant drugs. Philadelphia (1973) vol 10, 219.

Table 15.2 The effects of anaesthetics on blood sugar & insulin levels (after Hagan & Kendall[9])

Anaesthetic	Patient nos	Glucose load	Insulin levels (μU/ml)		Glucose levels (mg%)		References
			Before	After	Before	After	
Ether-N$_2$O	10	—	16	25 at 30' 28 at 60'	83	118 at 60'	1
Ether-N$_2$O	19	—	38	30 at 60' 30 at 45'	85	124 at 45'	7
Halothane-N$_2$O	8	—	17	14 at 60'	80	88 at 60'	1
Halothane-N$_2$O	20	—	11	10 at 45'	83	93 at 45'	2
Halothane-N$_2$O	5	—	16	15 at 30'	78	102 at 30'	3
Halothane-N$_2$O	4	—	18	14 at 20'	84	94 at 20'	4
Thiopentone-N$_2$O	20	—	12	12 at 45'	92	135 at 45'	5
Methoxyflur.-N$_2$O	5	—	8	8 at 30'	84	103 at 30'	3
Methoxyflur.-N$_2$O	20	—	23	19 at 45'	99	108 at 45'	8
Droperidol-N$_2$O	25	+	16	24 at 45'	102	169 at 30'	6

Hypoglycaemic agents + Antacids

Abstract/Summary

Magnesium hydroxide increases the bioavailability of tolbutamide, chlorpropamide, and some formulations of glibenclamide. Sodium bicarbonate increases the bioavailability of glipizide, but there appear to be no reports of adverse responses in diabetic patients as a result of any of these interactions.

Clinical evidence

(a) Chlorpropamide + Magnesium hydroxide

850 mg magnesium hydroxide increased the rate of absorption of 250 mg chlorpropamide in normal subjects, but the insulin and glucose responses were unaffected.[4]

(b) Glibenclamide + Magnesium hydroxide and Aluminium hydroxide

A single dose study in normal subjects found that magnesium hydroxide had little effect on the rate or extent of absorption of a micronized glibenclamide preparation (*Semi-Euglucon*), but it caused a a three-fold increase in the peak serum concentration and the bioavailability of a non-micronised preparation (*Gilemid*).[3] Aluminium hydroxide appeared to have no effect. *Maalox* (magnesium and aluminium hydroxides) increases the AUC of a formulation of glibenclamide by a third, and its maximal serum level by 50%.[2]

(c) Glipizide + Sodium bicarbonate

Sodium bicarbonate significantly increases the absorption of glipizide and enhances its effects to some extent, but the total absorption is unaltered.[1]

(d) Tolbutamide + Magnesium hydroxide

850 mg magnesium hydroxide increased the 0–1 h and 0–2 h tolbutamide AUCs (area under the curve) by five-fold and 2.5-fold respectively in normal subjects given a single 500 mg dose, but the total AUC was unaffected. The maximum insulin response was increased four-fold and occurred about an hour earlier, and the glucose responses were also greater and earlier.[4]

Mechanism

Uncertain. The small increase in gastric pH caused by these antacids possibly increases the solubility of these sulphonylureas and therefore increases their absorption.

Importance and management

Although these interactions certainly occur in normal subjects, their clinical importance in diabetics is uncertain. There do not appear to be any reports of any adverse interactions, nevertheless be alert for any evidence of changes in diabetic control in patients given sulphonylureas and antacids, in particular with tolbutamide and magnesium hydroxide where some transient hypoglycaemia might occur. Separating the dosages as much as possible would probably minimize any effects.

References

1 Kivistö KT, Neuvonen PJ. Enhancement of absorption and effect of glipizide by magnesium hydroxide. Clin Pharmacol Ther (1991) 49, 39–43.

2 Zuccaro P, Pacifici R, Pichini S, Avico U, Federzoni G, Pini LA, Sternieri E. Influence of antacids on the bioavailability of glibenclamide. Drugs Exptl Clin Res (1989) XV, 165–9.

3 Neuvonen PJ, Kivisto KT. The effects of magensium hydroxide on the absorption and efficacy of two glibenclamide preparations. Br J Clin Pharmac (1991) 32, 215–20.

4 Kivistö KT, Neuvonen PJ. Effect of magnesium hydroxide on the absorption and efficacy of tolbutamide and chlorpropamide. Eur J Clin Pharmacol (1992) 42, 675–80.

Hypoglycaemic agents + Anticoagulants

Abstract/Summary

Dicoumarol and tolbutamide mutually interact. This can result in increased hypoglycaemia (possibly coma) and increased anticoagulant effects (possibly bleeding). Dicoumarol can also increase the hypoglycaemic effects of chlorpropamide and this has also been seen in one patient given acenocoumarol (nicoumalone). Three reports describe increased warfarin effects in two patients given glibenclamide and another given tolbutamide. The effects of phenprocoumon are reduced by metformin but bleeding was seen in another patient on warfarin given phenformin. Other anticoagulants and hypoglycaemic agents seem not to interact together.

Clinical evidence

Effect of anticoagulants on hypoglycaemic agents:

(a) Tolbutamide + Dicoumarol or Phenindione

Dicoumarol can increase the serum levels of tolbutamide, prolong its half-life (more than three-fold), and reduce blood sugar levels in both diabetics[1] and normal subjects.[1,2] The hypoglycaemic effects are increased. This may become excessive in a few patients and coma has been described.[1,3,6,8] Phenindione does not affect the half-life of tolbutamide.[1]

(b) Chlorpropamide + Dicoumarol or Nicoumalone (Acenocoumarol)

The observation of severe hypoglycaemia in a patient on chlorpropamide while taking dicoumarol prompted further study in three other patients and two non-diabetics. Dicoumarol doubled the serum chlorpropamide levels within 3–4 days and the half-life was more than doubled.[9] A woman with normal kidney function showed an increase in the half-life of chlorpropamide to 88 h (normally about 36 h) when treated with nicoumalone.[13]

(c) Glibenclamide, Glibornuride, Glymidine, Tolbutamide + Phenprocoumon

Phenprocoumon has been found to cause a slight increase in the half-life of glibornuride,[11] but the pharmacokinetics of glibenclamide[12] and the hypoglycaemic effects of tolbutamide remained unchanged. The half-life of glymidine is increased.

Effect of hypoglycaemic agents on anticoagulants:

(a) Dicoumarol + Tolbutamide

Two patients on dicoumarol showed marked increases in prothrombin times (a rise from 33 to 60 s) within two days of starting tolbutamide but no bleeding occurred. Increases were seen in three other patients.[5] Another patient on dicoumarol showed a similar increase in his prothrombin time and bled (haematuria, purpura) within five days of starting tolbutamide.[6] The half-life of dicoumarol was approximately halved in two out of four normal subjects given tolbutamide, but the hypoprothrombinaemic effects were unchanged.[14] A retrospective study on 15 patients treated concurrently found no evidence that the anticoagulant effects of the dicoumarol were altered by tolbutamide but the form of the study may possibly have obscured evidence of an interaction.[7] No change in overall anticoagulant control was seen in another study.[4]

(b) Phenprocoumon and Warfarin + Metformin

The observation that a woman diabetic needed more phenprocoumon while taking metformin prompted further study in 13 diabetics. It was found that those taking 1.0–4.0 g metformin daily were less well anticoagulated than those taking only 0.4–1.0 g, even though the phenprocoumon dosage of the former was slightly higher.[1] The half-life of phenprocoumon is reduced about a third (from 123 to 85 h) while taking 1700 mg metformin daily.[17]

Haematuria occurred in a patient on warfarin three months after concurrent treatment with phenformin was started. Her prothrombin values were normal.[16] The phenformin may have increased fibrinolysis to the point where it was additive with the effects of the warfarin.

(c) Other Anticoagulants + Hypoglycaemic agents

Treatment of diabetic patients and normal subjects for a week with glibenclamide, glibornuride, tolbutamide or insulin had no effect on the plasma levels or half-life of single doses of phenprocoumon.[10] A retrospective study of 24 patients given dicoumarol and 54 given warfarin suggested that insulin did not alter their anticoagulant effects; similarly tolbutamide is said not to have altered the anticoagulant effects of warfarin taken by 42 patients.[7] However what is not clear is whether this study would have revealed an interaction because the patients were already taking the hypoglycaemic agent and would have been routinely stabilized on the anticoagulant. Three isolated reports describe increased warfarin effects (serious in one instance) in two patient given glibenclamide,[15,18] and another given tolbutamide.[19]

Mechanisms

Dicoumarol appears to increase the effects of tolbutamide by inhibiting its metabolism by the liver.[1,2] This may also be true for chlorpropamide.[9] The increase in the anticoagulant effects of dicoumarol by tolbutamide may in part be due to a plasma protein binding interaction. In the case of phenprocoumon there seem to be several different mutually opposing processes going on which cancel each other out and produce a 'silent' interaction.[4] Metformin possibly reduces the effects of phenprocoumon by altering blood flow to the liver and interfering with the enterohepatic circulation. There is no clear explanation for most of these interactions.

Importance and management

Information is patchy and very incomplete. Dicoumarol with tolbutamide has been most thoroughly investigated and the interactions are clinically important. Increased hypoglycaemic effects may be expected if dicoumarol is given to patients taking tolbutamide and there is a risk of coma. If tolbutamide is given to those taking dicoumarol an increase in prothrombin times and possibly bleeding will occur. Avoid concurrent use unless the outcome can be well monitored and dosage adjustments made. The same precautions should be taken with dicoumarol and chlorpropamide, but what is known is limited to one study.[9] Some caution is appropriate with nicoumalone (acenocoumarol) and chlorpropamide, and warfarin with glibenclamide or tolbutamide although information seems to be limited to isolated observations.[13,17,19] A small increase in the dosage of phenprocoumon may be necessary if metformin is given. There appears to be no other information about interactions between other hypoglycaemic agents and anticoagulants but monitoring is advisable.

The 'Clinical Evidence' section lists those which seem to be free from interactions: tolbutamide + phenindione; glibornuride + phenprocoumon; dicoumarol or warfarin + tolbutamide; phenprocoumon + glibenclamide, glibornuride, tolbutamide or insulin; warfarin + tolbutamide. Warfarin and phenprocoumon seem to be safer than dicoumarol, nevertheless be alert for any evidence of changes in the anticoagulant or hypoglycaemic effects if either is given with any hypoglycaemic agent.

References

1 Kristensen M, Hansen JM. Potentiation of the tolbutamide effect by dicoumarol. Diabetes (1967) 16, 211–14.
2 Solomon HM, Schrogie JJ. Effect of phenyramidol and bishydroxycoumarin on the metabolism of tolbutamide in human subjects. Metabolism (1967) 16, 1029–33.
3 Spurney OM, Wolf JW, Devins GS. Protracted tolbutamide-induced hypoglycaemia. Arch Intern med (1965) 115, 53.
4 Jahnchen E, Meinertz T, Gilfrich H-J and Groth U. Pharmacokinetic analysis of the interaction between dicoumarol and tolbutamide in man. Eur J Clin Pharmacol (1976) 10, 349–56.
5 Chaplin H, Cassell M. Studies on the possible relationship of tolbutamide to dicoumarol in anticoagulant therapy. Am J Med Sci (1958) 235, 706–15.
6 Schwartz JF. Tolbutamide-induced hypoglycaemia in Parkinson's disease. A case report. J Amer Med Ass (1961) 176, 106–9.
7 Poucher RL and Vecchio TJ. Absence of tolbutamide effect on anticoagulant therapy. J Amer Med Ass (1966) 197, 1069–70.
8 Fontana G, Addavil F, Peta G. Su di uno casa di coma ipoglicemico in corso di terapie con tolbutamide e dicumarolici. G Clin Med (1968) 49, 849.

9 Kristensen M, Hansen JM. Accumulation of chlorpropamide caused by dicoumarol. Acta Med Scand (1968) 183, 83–6.
10 Heine P, Kewitz H, Wiegboldt K-A. The influence of hypoglycaemic sulphonylureas on elimination and efficacy of phenprocoumon following a single oral dose in diabetic patients. Eur J Clin Pharmacol (1976) 10, 31–6.
11 Eckhardt W, Rudolph R, Sauer H, Schuber WR, Undeutsch D. Zur pharmacologischen Interferenz von Glibornurid mit Sulfaphenazol, Phenylbutazon und phenprocoumon beim Menschen. Arzneim-Forsch (1972) 22, 2212.
12 Schulz E, Schmidt FH. Uber den Einfluss von Sulphaphenazol, Phenylbutazon und Phenprocumarol auf die Elimination von Glibenclamid beim Menschen. Vern Dtsch Ges Inn Med (1970) 76, 435.
13 Petitpierrre B, Perrin L, Rudhardt M, Herrera A, Fabre J. Behaviour of chlorpropamide in renal insufficiency and under the effect of associated drug therapy. Int J Clin Pharmacol (1972) 6, 120.
14 Jahnchen E, Gilfrich HJ, Groth U, Meinertz T. Pharmacokinetic analysis of the dicoumarol-tolbutamide interaction in man. Naunyn-Schmied Arch Pharmacol (1975) 287 (Suppl) R88.
15 Beeley L, Stewart P, Hickey FM. Bull W Midlands Centre for Adverse Drug Reaction Reporting. (1988) 26, 27.
16 Hamblin TJ. Interaction between warfarin and phenformin. Lancet (1971) ii, 1323.
17 Ohnhaus EE, Berger W, Duckert F, Oesch F. The influence of dimethylbiguanide on phenprocoumon elimination and its mode of action. Klin Wchsch (1983) 61, 851–8.
18 Jassal SV. Drug points. Br Med J (1991) 303, 789
19 Beeley L, Magee P, Hickey FN. Bulletin of the West Midlands Centre for Adverse Drug Reaction Reporting (1990) 30, 32.

Hypoglycaemic agents + Azapropazone

Abstract/Summary

Two case reports and a study in three normal subjects show that azapropazone can increase the effects of tolbutamide and cause severe hypoglycaemia.

Clinical evidence

A diabetic woman, well controlled for 3 years on 500 mg tolbutamide daily, became confused and semi-comatose four days after starting to take 900 mg azapropazone daily. She complained of having felt agitated since starting the azapropazone so that it was withdrawn on suspicion of causing hypoglycaemia. Later that evening she became semi-comatose and was found to have a plasma glucose level of 2.0 mmol/l.[1] A subsequent study in three normal subjects found that the same dosage of azapropazone increased the serum half-life of tolbutamide three-fold (from 7.7 to 25.2 h) and reduced its clearance accordingly.[1]

Acute hypoglycaemia occurred in a patient on tolbutamide 5.5 h after taking a single 600 mg dose of azapropazone.[2]

Mechanism

The clinical study suggests that azapropazone can inhibit the liver enzymes concerned with the metabolism of the tolbutamide, thereby prolonging its stay in the body and increasing its effects.[1] The rapidity of the second case suggests that displacement from plasma protein binding may also occur.[2]

Importance and management

The cases cited and the associated clinical study appear to be all that is on record about this interaction so far. It would be prudent to avoid concurrent use. Information about other sulphonylurea hypoglycaemic agents seems to be lacking.

References

1 Andreasen PB, Simonsen K, Brocks K, Dimo B, Bouchelouche P. Hypoglycaemia induced by azapropazone-tolbutamide. Br J Clin Pharmac (1980) 12, 581.
2 Waller DG, Waller D. Hypoglycaemia due to azapropazone-tolbutamide interaction. Brit J Rheumatol (1984) 23, 24–5.

Hypoglycaemic agents + Barbiturates

Abstract/Summary

The hypoglycaemic effects of glymidine are reported not to be affected by phenobarbitone. There appear to be no reports of adverse hypoglycaemic agent/barbiturate interactions.

Clinical evidence, mechanism, importance and management

A study in man showed that the hypoglycaemic effects of glymidine were unaffected by the concurrent use of phenobarbitone.[1] There seems to be nothing in the literature to suggest that an adverse interaction takes place between any of the hypoglycaemic agents and barbiturates. No special precautions would appear necessary.

Reference

1 Gerhards E, Kolb KH, Schulz PE. Uber 2-Benzolsulfonylamino- 5-(beta-methoxy-athoxy)-pyrimidin (Glycodiazin). V. In vitro- und in vivo-Versuche zum Einfluss von Phenylathylbarbitursaure (Luminal) auf en Stoffwechsel und die blutzuckersendkende Wirkung des Glycodiazins. Naunyn-Schmied Arch Pharmak u exp Path (1966) 255, 200.

Hypoglycaemic agents + Benzodiazepines

Abstract/Summary

No adverse interaction normally occurs between these drugs but an isolated case of hyperglycaemia has been seen in an insulin-treated diabetic associated with the use of chlordiazepoxide.

Clinical evidence, mechanism, importance and management

A woman with maturity-onset diabetes of 27 years' duration,

controlled on 45 U isophane insulin suspension daily, showed a fasting blood sugar rise from 200 to 400 mg/100 ml during a three-week period while taking 40 mg chlordiazepoxide daily. Four other diabetics, two controlled on diet alone and the other two on tolbutamide, showed no changes in blood sugar levels while taking chlordiazepoxide.[1] No change in the half-life of chlorpropamide is reported to have occurred in another study when diazepam was used concurrently.[2] There seems to be nothing in the literature to suggest that an adverse interaction normally takes place between the hypoglycaemic agents and the benzodiazepines. No special precautions would normally appear to be necessary.

References

1 Zumoff B, Hellman L. Aggravation of diabetic hyperglycemia by chlordiazepoxide. J Amer Med Ass (1977) 237, 1960.
2 Petitpierre B, Perrin L, Rudhardt M, Herrera A, Fabre J. Behaviour of chlorpropamide in renal insufficiency and under the effect of associated drug therapy. Int J Clin Pharmacol (1972) 6, 120.

Hypoglycaemic agents + Beta-blockers

Abstract/Summary

In diabetics using insulin, the normal recovery reaction (blood sugar rise) if hypoglycaemia occurs may be impaired to some extent by propranolol, but serious and severe hypoglycaemia and hypertension has only been seen in a few patients. Other beta-blockers normally interact to a lesser extent or not at all. The hypoglycaemic effects of the sulphonylureas may possibly be reduced by the beta-blockers. Whether insulin, the sulphonylureas or the biguanides is given, be aware that some of the familiar warning signs of hypoglycaemia (tachycardia, tremor) may not occur, although sweating may be increased.

Clinical evidence

(A) Insulin + Beta-blockers in Insulin-dependent, Type I diabetics

(i) Hypoglycaemia

Although propranolol has occasionally been associated with spontaneous episodes of hypoglycaemia in non-diabetics,[1] and a number of studies in patients[4] and normal subjects[5-8] have shown that propranolol impairs the normal blood sugar rebound which should follow if blood sugar levels fall, there appear to be few reports of severe hypoglycaemia or coma in diabetics on insulin given propranolol. Marked hypoglycaemia and/or coma occurred in five diabetic patients on insulin due to the use of propranolol,[1-3] pindolol,[3] and timolol eye-drops.[13] Other contributory factors (fasting, haemodialysis, etc.) probably had some part to play.[3] Metoprolol interacts like propranolol but to a lesser extent,[5,7,20] whereas the other beta-blockers examined (acebutalol,[4,7] alprenolol[9], atenolol,[10,12] oxprenolol,[20] penbutolol,[8] pindolol[11]) were found to interact minimally or not at all. The situation with pindolol is therefore not clear. Propranolol (a vasoconstrictor) has also been found to reduce the rate of absorption of subcutaneous insulin by almost 50%, but the importance of this is uncertain.[26]

(ii) Hypertension

Marked increases in blood pressure (systolic and diastolic) and bradycardia may develop if hypoglycaemia occurs in diabetics on insulin and beta-blockers.[15] Systolic/diastolic pressure rises of + 38.8/ + 14.3 mmHg with propranolol, + 27.9/0 mmHg with atenolol and + 15.6/-9.2 mmHg with placebo were seen in one study in insulin-treated diabetics.[16] In another study rises of + 27/ + 14 mmHg were seen with alprenolol, but no rise with metoprolol.[17] A report describes a pressure rise to 258/144 mmHg in a patient within two days of starting propranolol.[2] Another patient on metoprolol experienced a rise from 190/96 to 230/112 mmHg during a hypoglycaemic episode.[16]

(B) Oral hypoglycaemic agents + Beta-blockers in non-insulin dependent, Type II, maturity-onset diabetics

(i) Hyperglycaemia, hypoglycaemia or no interaction

The sulphonylurea-induced insulin-release from the pancreas can be inhibited by beta-blockers so that the hypoglycaemic effects are opposed to some extent. The effects of glibenclamide,[22] chlorpropamide[18] and tolbutamide[19] have been shown to be inhibited by propranolol. Acebutalol affects glibenclamide about the same as propranolol but has fewer unwanted haemodynamic effects[22] and has no effect on tolbutamide.[23] Two isolated cases of hypoglycaemia have been seen with acebutolol, in one patient taking gliclazide and the other taking chlorpropamide.[27] One study failed to find an interaction between tolbutamide and either propranolol or metoprolol,[21,24] and another found no interaction between betaxolol and glibenclamide or metformin.[25] An isolated report describes hyperosmolar non-ketotic coma in a patient on tolbutamide and propranolol.[14]

Mechanism

Among other mechanisms, the normal physiological response to a fall in blood sugar levels is the mobilization of glucose from the liver under the stimulation of adrenaline (epinephrine) from the adrenals. This sugar mobilization is blocked by non-selective beta-blockers (such as propranolol) so that recovery from hypoglycaemia is delayed and may even proceed into a full-scale episode in a hypoglycaemia-prone diabetic. Normally the adrenaline would also increase the heart rate, but with the beta-receptors in the heart already blocked this fails to occur. A rise in blood pressure occurs because the stimulant effects of adrenaline on the beta-2 receptors (vasodilation) are blocked leaving the alpha (vasoconstriction) effects unopposed. Non-selective beta-blockers can also block beta-2 receptors in the pancreas concerned with insulin-release, so that the effects of the sulphonylureas may be blocked.

Importance and management

Extremely well-studied interactions. Concurrent use can be uneventful but there are some risks. The overall picture is as follows:

(A) Diabetics on insulin may have (i) a prolonged or delayed recovery response to hypoglycaemia while on beta-blockers, but very severe hypoglycaemia and/or coma is rare. (ii) If hypoglycaemia occurs it may be accompanied by a sharp rise in blood pressure. The risk is greatest with propranolol and possibly other non-selective blockers and least with the cardio-selective blockers (e.g. atenolol, metoprolol, etc.). Monitor the effects of concurrent use well, avoid the non-selective blockers, and check for any evidence that the insulin dosage needs some adjustment. Warn all patients that some of the normal pre-monitory signs of 'going hypo' may not appear, in particular tachycardia and tremors, whereas the hunger, irritability and nausea signs may be unaffected and sweating may even be increased.

(B) Diabetics taking oral sulphonylureas rarely seem to have serious hypoglycaemic episodes caused by beta-blockers, and any reductions in the hypoglycaemic effects of the sulphonylureas normally appear to be of little clinical importance. The selective beta-blockers are probably safer than the non-selective, however always monitor concurrent use to confirm that diabetic control is well maintained (increase the dosage if necessary), and warn all patients (as above) that some of the premonitory signs of hypoglycaemia may not occur.

(C) One experimental study indicated no interaction between betaxolol and metformin, but direct information about other biguanides seems to be lacking. However warn patients on biguanides that the premonitory signs of hypoglycaemia may possibly be obscured.

There is also a hint from one report that the peripheral vasoconstrictive effects of non-selective beta-blockers and the poor peripheral circulation in diabetics could be additive.[2] Another good reason for avoiding this type of beta-blocker in diabetics.

References

1 Kotler MN, Berman L and Rubenstein AH. Hypoglycaemia precipitated by propranolol. Br Med J (1966) 1, 1389.
2 McMurty RJ. Propranolol, hypoglycemia, and hypertensive crisis. Ann Intern Med (1974) 80, 669–70.
3 Samii K, Ciancioni C, Rottembourg J, Bisseliches F, Jacobs C. Severe hypoglycaemia due to beta-blocking drugs in haemodialysis patients. Lancet (1976) i, 545–6.
4 Deacon SP, Karunanayake A, Barnett D. Acebutalol, atenolol, and pro-pranolol and metabolic response to acute hypoglycaemia in diabetics. Br Med J (1977) 2, 1255–7.
5 Davidson NM, Corrall RJM and Shaw TRD. Observations in man of hypoglycaemia during selective and non-selective beta-blockade. Scott Med J (1976) 22, 69–72.
6 Abramson EA, Arky RA, Woeber KA. Effects of propranolol on the hormonal and metabolic responses to insulin-induced hypoglycaemia. Lancet (1966) i, 1386–9.
7 Newman RJ. Comparison of propranolol, metoprolol and acebutalol on insulin-induced hypoglycaemia. Br Med J (1976) 2, 447–9.
8 Sharma SD, Vakil BJ, Samuel MR et al. Comparison of penbutolol and propranolol during insulin-induced hypoglycaemia. Curr Ther Res (1979) 26, 252–9.

9 Eisalo A, Heino A, Munter J. The effect of alprenolol in elderly patients with raised blood pressure. Acta Med Scand (1974) Suppl, 554, 32–31.

10 Deacon SP, and Barnett D. Comparison of atenolol and propranolol during insulin-induced hypoglycaemia. Br Med J (1976) 2, 272–3.

11 Patsch W, Patsch JR, Sailer S. Untersuchung zur Wirkung von Pindolol auf Kohlehydrat- und Fettstoffwechsel bei Diabetes Mellitus. Int J Clin Pharmacol Biopharm (1977) 15, 394–6.

12 Waal-Manning HJ. Atenolol and three non-selective beta-blockers in hypertension. Clin Pharmacol Ther (1979) 25, 8–18.

13 Angelo-Nielsen K. Timolol topically and diabetes mellitus. J Amer Med Ass (1980) 244, 2263.

14 Podolsky S, Pattavina CG. Hyperosmolar non-ketotic diabetic coma. A complication of propranolol therapy. Metabolism (1973) 22, 685–93.

15 Shepherd AMM, Lin M-S and Keeton TK. Hypoglycaemia-induced hypertension in a diabetic patient on metoprolol. Ann Intern Med (1981) 94, 357–8.

16 Ryan JR, Lacorte W, Jain A, McMahon FG. Response of diabetics treated with atenolol or propranolol to insulin-induced hypoglycaemia. Drugs (1983) 25 (Suppl) 256–7.

17 Ostman J, Arner P, Haglund K, Juhlin-Dannfelt A, Nowak J, Wennlund A. Effect of metoprolol and alprenolol on the metabolic, hormonal and haemodynamic response to insulin-induced hypoglycaemia in hypertensive, insulin-dependent diabetics. Acta Med Scand (1982) 211, 381–8.

18 Holt RJ, Gaskins JD. Hyperglycaemia associated with propranolol and chlorpropamide administration. Drug Intell Clin Pharm (1981) 15, 599–600.

19 Massara F, Stumia E, Camanni E, Mollnatti GM. Depressed tolbutamide-induced insulin response in subjects treated with propranolol. Diabetalogia (1971) 7, 287–9.

20 Vibert GC, Stimmler M, Kein H. The effect of oxprenolol and metoprolol on the hypoglycaemic response to insulin in normals and insulin-dependent diabetics. Diabetalogia (1978) 15, 278.

21 Groop L, Totterman KJ, Harna K, Gordin A. Influence of beta-blocking drugs on glucose metabolism in patients with non-insulin dependent diabetes. Acta Med Scand (1982) 211, 7–12.

22 Zaman R, Kendall MJ, Biggs PI. The effect of acebutalol and propranolol on the hypoglycaemic action of glibenclamide. Br J Clin Pharmac (1982) 13, 507–12.

23 Ryan JR. Clinical pharmacology of acebutalol. Amer Heart J (1985) 109, 1131–6.

24 Totterman KJ, Groop LC. No effect of propranolol and metoprolol on the tolbutamide-stimulated insulin-secretion in hypertensive diabetic and non-diabetic patients. Ann Clin Res (1982) 14, 190–3.

25 Sinclair AJ, Davies JB, Warrington SJ. Betaxolol and glucose-insulin relationships: studies in normal subjects taking glibenclamide or metformin. Br J clin Pharmac (1990) 30, 699–702.

26 Veenstra J, van der Hulst JP, Wildenborg IH, Njoo SF, Verdegaal WP, Silberbusch J. Effect of antihypertensive drugs on insulin absorption. Diabetes Care (1991) 14, 1089–92.

27 Girardin E, Vial T, Pham E, Evreux J-C. Hypoglycémies induites par les sulfamides hypoglycémiants. Ann Med Interne (1992) 143, 11–17.

Hypoglycaemic agents + Calcium channel blockers

Abstract/Summary

Calcium channel blockers are known to have effects on insulin secretion and glucose regulation but significant disturbances in the control of diabetes are uncommon. A report describes a patient whose diabetes worsened and who needed more insulin when treated with diltiazem. Another patient needed a 30% increase in insulin while taking nifedipine, and hypoglycaemia occurred in a patient taking gliclazide and nicardipine.

Clinical evidence

(a) Diltiazem

An insulin-dependent diabetic developed worsening and intractable hyperglycaemia (mean serum glucose levels above 13 mmol) when given 90 mg diltiazem 6-hourly. Her insulin requirements dropped when the diltiazem was withdrawn. When restarted on 30 mg diltiazem 6-hourly her blood sugar levels were still high, but she needed less insulin than when taking the higher diltiazem dosage.[14]

A study in normal subjects showed that 60 mg diltiazem three times daily had no effect on the secretion of insulin or glucagon, or on plasma glucose levels.[12]

(b) Nifedipine, nicardipine and nitrendipine

A study in 20 non-insulin dependent diabetics (five on metformin and 15 diet-controlled) showed that neither nifedipine (10 mg 8-hourly) nor nicardipine (30 mg 8-hourly) for 4 weeks had any effect on glucose tolerance tests and no effect on the control of the diabetes, but significant reductions in blood pressures occurred (4–7 mmHg diastolic and systolic).[1] Another study on eight non-diabetics and 8 diabetics (three on chlorpropamide, one on glipizide and four on diet alone) showed that the use of 30 mg nifedipine daily for a month did not significantly alter their glucose tolerance tests.[2] No important changes occurred in seven diabetic patients taking glibenclamide when chronically treated for 12–75 weeks with 20–60 mg nifedipine daily.[8] Another study on six diabetics showed that single 20 mg doses of nifedipine had no effect on the pharmacokinetics or actions of glipizide (5–20 mg daily).[7] This confirms other studies with nifedipine[3] and nicardipine.[4] 30 mg nitrendipine daily over a 5-year period is reported to have had no adverse effect on the control of diabetes in 14 elderly patients using insulin or oral hypoglycaemic agents.[16] There are however other reports of a deterioration in glucose tolerance during the use of nifedipine,[5,6] and the need to increase insulin dosage by 30%.[15] One study found that 10 mg nifedipine increased the rate of absorption of subcutaneous insulin by about 50%.[17] An isolated case of hypoglycaemia has been described in a patient on gliclazide when treated with nicardipine.[18]

(c) Verapamil

A study in 23 Type II diabetics, seven of whom were taking glibenclamide, showed that verapamil improved the oral glucose tolerance test but did not increase the hypoglycaemic effects of the glibenclamide.[9] Two studies in Type II diabetics found that verapamil improved glucose tolerance tests,[10,11] but no alterations in the hypoglycaemic effects of glibenclamide were found in another study.[10] A study in normal subjects found that verapamil raised serum glibenclamide levels but plasma glucose levels were unchanged.[13]

Mechanism

The changes which occur are not fully understood. Suggestions include inhibition of insulin secretion by the calcium channel blockers and inhibition of glucagon secretion by glucose; changes in glucose uptake by liver and other cells; blood glucose rises following catecholamine release after vasodilation, and changes in glucose metabolism.

Importance and management

Very extensively studied, but many of the reports describe single-dose studies or multiple dose studies in normal subjects (only a few are cited here) which give no clear picture of what may be expected in diabetic patients. Those studies which have concentrated on diabetics indicate that the control of the diabetes is not usually adversely affected by concurrent use although isolated cases with diltiazem, nicardipine and nifedipine have been reported.[13,15,18] No particular precautions normally seem to be necessary, nevertheless be alert for any signs of a worsening control of the diabetes. More study in diabetics is needed.

References

1 Collins WCJ, Cullen MJ, Feeley J. Calcium channel blocker drugs and diabetic control. Clin Pharmacol Ther (1987) 42, 420–3.

2 Donnelly T, Harrower ADB. Effect of nifedipine on glucose tolerance and insulin secretion in diabetic and non-diabetic patients. Curr Ther Res Opin (1980) 6, 690–3.

3 Abadia E, Passa PH. Diabetogenic effects of nifedipine. Br Med J (1984) 289, 438.

4 Sakta S, Miura K. Effect of nicardipine in a hypertensive patient with diabetes mellitus. Clin Therap (1984) 6, 600–2.

5 Guigliano D, Torella R, Cacciapuoti F, Gentile S, Kerza M, Varricchio M. Impairment of insulin secretion in man by nifedipine. Eur J Clin Pharmacol (1980) 18, 395–8.

6 Bhatnagar SK, Amin MMA and Al-Yusuf AR. Diabetogenic effects of nifedipine. Br Med J (1984) 289, 19.

7 Connacher AA, El Debani AH, Stevenson IH. A study of the influence of nifedipine on the disposition and hypoglycaemic action of glipizide. Brit J clin Pharmac (1986) 22, 240 P.

8 Kantatsuna T, Nakano K, Mori H, Kano Y, Nishioka H, Kajiyama S, Kitagawa Y, Yoshida T, Kondo M, Nakamura N, Aochi O. Effects of nifedipine on insulin secretion and glucose metabolism in rats and hypertensive type two (non-insulin dependent) diabetes. Arzneim Forsch (1985) 35, 514.

9 Rojdmark S, Andersson DEH. Influence of verapamil on human glucose tolerance. Am J Cardiol (1986) 57, 39–43D.

10 Rojdmark S, Andersson DEH. Influence of verapamil on glucose tolerance. Acta Med Scand (1984) Suppl 681, 37–42.

11 Andersson DEH and Rojdmark S. Improvement of glucose tolerance by verapamil in patients with non-insulin-dependent diabetes mellitus. Acta Med Scand (1981) 210, 27–33.

12 Segrestaa JM, Caulin C, Dahan R, Houlbert D, Thiercelin JF, Herman P, Sauvanet JP. Effect of diltiazem on plasma glucose, insulin and glucagon during an oral glucose tolerance test in healthy volunteers. Eur J clin Pharmacol (1984) 26, 481–3.

13 Semple CG, Omile C, Buchanan KD, Beastall GH, Paterson KR. Effect of oral verapamil on glibenclamide stimulated insulin secretion. Br J clin Pharmac (1986) 22, 187–90.

14 Pershadsingh HA, Grant N, McDonald JM. Association of diltiazem therapy with increased insulin resistance in a patient with type one diabetes mellitus. J Am Med Ass (1987) 257, 930–1.

15 Heyman SN, Heyman A, Halperin I. Diabetogenic effect of nifedipine.

DICP Ann Pharmacother (1989) 23, 236–7.

16 Trost BN, Weidmann P. 5 years of antihypertensive monotherapy with the calcium antagonist nitrendipine do not alter carbohydrate homeostasis in diabetic patients. Diabetes Res Clin Prac (1988) 5 (Suppl 1) S511.

17 Veenstra J, van der Hulst JP, Wildenborg IH, Njoo SF, Verdegaal WP, Silberbusch J. Effect of anthypertensive drugs on insulin absorption. Diabetes Care (1991) 14, 1089–92.

18 Girardin E, Vial T, Pham E, Evreux J-C. Hypoglycémies induites par les sulfamides hypoglycémiants. Ann Med Interne (1992) 143, 11–17.

Hypoglycaemic agents + Chloramphenicol

Abstract/Summary

The hypoglycaemic effects of tolbutamide and chlorpropamide can be increased by the concurrent use of chloramphenicol. Acute hypoglycaemia can occur.

Clinical evidence

While taking 2 g chloramphenicol daily, a man was additionally started on a course of 2 g tolbutamide daily. Three days later he had a typical hypoglycaemic collapse and was found to have serum tolbutamide levels 3–4-fold higher than expected.[1]

Studies in diabetics have shown that 2 g daily doses of chloramphenicol can approximately double the half-lives of tolbutamide[2] and chlorpropamide,[3] and double the serum levels of tolbutamide.[3] Other studies using 1 g daily doses of chloramphenicol similarly showed that serum levels of tolbutamide could be doubled, and blood sugar levels reduced 25–30%.[4,5] Hypoglycaemia, acute in one case, developed in two other patients on tolbutamide given chloramphenicol.[6,7]

Mechanism

Chloramphenicol inhibits the liver enzymes concerned with the metabolism of tolbutamide, and probably chlorpropamide as well, leading to their accumulation in the body. This is reflected in prolonged half-lives, reduced blood sugar levels and occasionally acute hypoglycaemia.[1–6]

Importance and management

The tolbutamide/chloramphenicol interaction is well-established and of clinical importance. The incidence is uncertain, but an increased hypoglycaemic response should be expected if both drugs are given. The chlorpropamide/chloramphenicol interaction is less well documented. The dosage of both sulphonylureas should be reduced appropriately. Some patients may show a particularly exaggerated response. The manufacturers of other sulphonylureas often list chloramphenicol as an interacting drug, based on its interactions with tolbutamide and chlorpropamide, but direct information of an interaction appears not to be available. No interaction would be expected with chloramphenicol eye drops because the systemic absorption is likely to be small. This needs confirmation.

References

1 Hansen JM, Kristensen M. Tolbutamide in the treatment of Parkinson's disease. Dan Med Bull (1965) 12, 181.

2 Christensen LK and Skovsted L. Inhibition of drug metabolism by chloramphenicol. Lancet (1969) ii, 1397.

3 Petitpierre B, Perrin L, Rudhardt M, Herrera A, Fabre J. Behaviour of chlorpropamide in renal insufficiency and under associated drug therapy. Int J Clin Pharmacol (1972) 6, 120.

4 Brunova E, Slabachova Z, Platilova H. Influencing the effect of dirastan (tolbutamide). Simultaneous administration of chloramphenicol in patients with diabetes and bacterial urinary tract inflammation. Cas Lek ces (1974) 113, 72.

5 Brunova E, Slabachova Z, Platilova H, Pavlik F, Grafnetterova J, Dvoracek K. Interaction of tolbutamide and chloramphenicol in diabetic patients. Int J Clin Pharmacol (1977) 15, 7.

6 Ziegelasch H-J. Extreme Hypoglykamie unter kombinierter Behandlung mit Tolbutamid, n-1-Butylbiguanidhydrochlorid und Chloramphenikol. Z Gesamte inn Med (1972) 27, 63.

7 Soeldner JS, Steinke J. Hypoglycemia in tolbutamide-treated diabetes. J Amer Med Ass (1965) 193, 398–9.

Hypoglycaemic agents + Chlorpromazine

Abstract/Summary

Chlorpromazine can raise blood sugar levels, particularly in daily doses of 100 mg or more, and disturb the control of diabetes. It may be necessary to increase the dosage of the hypoglycaemic agent.

Clinical evidence

A long-term study over the period 1955–1966 on a large number of women treated for a year or more with chlorpromazine in daily doses of 100 mg or more, showed that about 25% developed hyperglycaemia accompanied by glycosuria, compared with only about 9% in the control group who were not taking phenothazines of any kind. Of those given chlorpromazine, about a quarter showed complete remission of the symptoms when the chlorpromazine was withdrawn or the dosage reduced.[2]

There are numerous other reports of this response.[1,3–12,14,15] A single report is out of step in claiming that chlorpromazine has no effect at all on blood sugar levels.[13] Chlorpromazine in doses of less than 100 mg daily (50–70 mg) does not affect blood sugar levels significantly.[15]

Mechanism

It seems that chlorpromazine can inhibit the release of insulin, and possibly cause adrenaline (epinephrine) release from the adrenals, both of which could result in a rise in blood sugar levels.

Importance and management

A well-documented and long-established reaction first recog-
nized in the early 1950s. The incidence is about 25% with daily doses of chlorpromazine of 100 mg or more. Increases in the dosage requirements of the hypoglycaemic agent should be anticipated during concurrent use. Smaller daily doses (50–70 mg) do not apparently cause hyperglycaemia. There seems to be no clinical evidence that other phenothiazines significantly disturb blood sugar levels in diabetics.

References

1 Hiles BH. Hyperglycaemia and glycosuria following chlorpromazine therapy. J Amer Med Ass (1956) 162, 1651.

2 Thonnard-Neumann E. Phenothiazines and diabetes in hospitalized women. Am J Psychiat (1968) 124, 978.

3 Dobkin A, Lamoreux R, Gilbert RGB. Some studies with largactil. Can Med Ass J (1954) 2, 565.

4 Lancaster NP, Jones DH. Chlorpromazine and insulin in psychiatry. Br Med J (1954) 2, 565.

5 Glacobini F, Lassenius B. Chlorpromazine therapy in psychiatric practice: secondary effects and complications. Nord Med (1954) 52, 1693.

6 Moyer J, Kinross-Wright V, Finney RM. Chlorpromazine as a therapeutic agent in clinical medicine. Arch Int Med (1955) 95, 202.

7 Celice J, Porcher P, Plas S. Action de la chlorpromazine sur la vesicule biliare et le clon droit. Therapie (1955) 10, 30.

8 Charatan F, Bartlett N. The effect of chlorpromazine ('Largactil') on glucose tolerance. J Ment Sci (1955) 101, 351.

9 Cooperberg AA, Eidlow S. Haemolytic anaemia, jaundice and diabetes mellitus following chlorpromazine therapy. Can Med Ass J (1956) 75, 746.

10 Blair D, Brady DM. Recent advances in the treatment of schizophrenia: group training and tranquillizers. J Ment Sci (1958) 104. 625.

11 Amidsen A. Diabetes mellitus as a side-effect of treatment with tricyclic neuroleptics. Acta Psychiat Scand (1964) 40 (Suppl 180) 411.

12 Arneson G. Phenothiazine derivatives and glucose metabolism. J Neuropsychiatr (1964) 5, 181.

13 Schwarz L and Munoz R. Blood sugar levels in patients treated with chlorpromazine. Amer J Psychiat (1968) 125, 253.

14 Korenyl C, Lowenstein B. Chlorpromazine induced diabetes. Dis Ner Syst (1971) 32, 777.

15 Erle G, Basso M, Federspil G, Sicolo N, Scandellari C. Effect of chlorpromazine on blood glucose and plasma insulin in man. Eur J Clin Pharmacol (1977) 11, 15.

Hypoglycaemic agents + Cholestyramine

Abstract/Summary

There is evidence that the absorption of glipizide may be reduced about a third if taken at the same time as cholestyramine. Tolbutamide is reported not to interact.

Clinical evidence

8 g cholestyramine in 150 ml water reduced the absorption of a single 5 mg dose of glipizide in six normal subjects by 29%. One subject had a 41% reduction. Peak serum levels were reduced by 33%. The AUC (area under the curve over 10 hr) was used to measure absorption.[1]

A single dose study indicated that cholestyramine does not reduce the amount of tolbutamide absorbed, although the rate may be changed.[2]

Mechanism

Cholestyramine is an anion-exchange resin, intended to bind to bile acids within the gut, but it can also bind with some acidic drugs thereby reducing the amount available for absorption.

Importance and management

Information about glipizide is limited to this single dose study so that the clinical importance of the interaction awaits further study, but it would now seem prudent to monitor the effects of concurrent use in patients. It has been suggested[1] that the glipizide should be taken 1–2 h before the cholestyramine to minimize admixture in the gut, but this may only be partially effective because it is believed that glipizide undergoes some entero-hepatic circulation (ie after absorption it is re-excreted in the bile). The effect of cholestyramine on other sulphonylureas is uncertain, with the exception of tolbutamide which is reported not to interact.

References

1 Kivisto K T, Neuvonen P J. The effect of cholestyramine and activated charcoal on glipizide absorption. Br J Clin Pharmac (1990) 30, 733–6.

2 Hunninghake D B, Pollack E W. Effect of bile acid sequestering agents on the absorption of aspirin, tolbutamide and warfarin. Fed Proc (1977) 35, 996.

Hypoglycaemic agents + Cibenzoline (Cifenline)

Abstract/Summary

Hypoglycaemia has been seen in a few patients while taking cibenzoline alone, and in one case with gliclazide. The risk factors appear to be age, renal insufficiency and high dosage.

Clinical evidence, mechanism, importance and management

For reasons which are not understood, cibenzoline occasionally and unpredictably causes hypoglycaemia which may be severe. Marked hypoglycaemia was first seen in an 67-year-old patient when given cibenzoline.[1] Since then 20 other cases have been described in elderly patients with renal insufficiency and taking large doses.[2] Hypoglycaemia also occurred in a patient of 61 with renal insufficiency taking gliclazide.[3] The reasons are not understood. This appears to be a drug-disease rather than a drug–drug interaction and diabetic patients do not seem to be more at risk than non-diabetics, but good monitoring is advisable if cibenzoline is given.

References

1 Hilleman DE, Mohiuddin SM, Ahmed IS, Dahl JM. Cibenzoline induced hypoglycemia. Drug Intell Clin Pharm (1987) 21, 38–40.

2 Houdent C, Noblet C, Vandoren C, Levesque H, Morin C, Moore N, Courtois H, Wolf LM. Hypoglycémia induite par la cibenzoline chez le sujet âgè. Rev Med Interne (1991) 12, 143–5.

3 Girardin E, Vial T, Pham E, Evreux J-C. Hypoglycémies induites par les sulfamides hypoglycémiants. Ann Med Interne (1992) 143, 11–17.

Hypoglycaemic agents + Cimetidine or Ranitidine

Abstract/Summary

Isolated cases of hypoglycaemia have been seen with gliclazide/cimetidine and glibenclamide/ranitidine, but marked changes in the control of diabetes in patients on most sulphonylureas when given either cimetidine or ranitidine seem to be unusual. A possible exception is glipizide with cimetidine. Cimetidine appears to reduce the clearance of metformin.

Clinical evidence

(A) Studies in diabetic patients given sulphonylureas

(a) Gliclazide, glibenclamide

An elderly diabetic taking 160 mg gliclazide daily developed very low blood sugar levels (1 mmol/l) after starting treatment with 800 mg cimetidine daily.[7] Marked hypoglycaemia was seen in a patient on glibenclamide when treated with ranitidine,[10] and another report briefly describes hypoglycaemia in two patients given cimetidine, and two others given ranitidine, while taking un-named sulphonylureas.[14]

(b) Glipizide

Non-insulin dependent diabetics were given 400 mg cimetidine 1 h before taking a dose of glipizide (average 5.7 mg dose) and then 3 h later they were given a standard meal with 200 mg of cimetidine. The expected rise in blood sugar levels after the meal was reduced by 40% and in some of the patients it fell to less than 3 mmol/l.[6,15] Two studies in non-insulin dependent diabetics found that 300 mg ranitidine had no significant effects on the pharmacokinetics or the effects of glipizide, except that the absorption was delayed,[8,13] whereas a later study by the same group of workers found that the expected rise in blood sugar levels after a meal was reduced by 25%.[15]

(B) Studies in normal subjects given sulphonylureas

The pharmacokinetics of the tolbutamide (250 mg daily for 4 days) were not significantly changed in seven subjects when given 800 mg cimetidine daily for a further 4 days.[3] Other studies also found no interaction between tolbutamide[2,12] or chlorpropamide[4] and cimetidine, or tolbutamide and ranitidine,[4] and the hypoglycaemic activities of tolbutamide, chlorpropamide, glibenclamide and glipizide remained unaltered.[5] In contrast, in another study the AUC of tolbutamide was found to be increased by 20% and the elimination half-life decreased by 17% by 1200 mg cimetidine, but plasma glucose levels were not significantly changed. Ranitidine had no effect.[1] Yet another study reported that the hypoglycaemic effects of glibenclamide were reduced by cimetidine and ranitidine.[9]

(C) Study in normal subjects given a biguanide

800 mg cimetidine daily was found to reduce the renal clearance of metformin in seven normal subjects by 27% and increase the AUC by 50%.[11]

Mechanism

If an interaction occurs[1] it may be because the cimetidine inhibits the metabolism of the sulphonylurea by the liver, thereby increasing its effects. Cimetidine appears to inhibit the excretion of metformin by the kidneys.[11]

Importance and management

Information is limited and difficult to assess because of the differences between the sulphonylureas and between normal subjects and diabetics, but all the evidence cited here, as well as the relative paucity of adverse reports, suggests that most diabetics do not experience any marked changes in their diabetic control if given cimetidine. However warn them that rarely and unpredicably hypoglycaemia occurs. The dosage of metformin may need to be reduced if cimetidine is used, bearing in mind the possibility of lactic acidosis if levels become too high. Ranitidine normally appears not to interact.

References

1 Case EW, Rogers JF, Powell JR. Inhibition of tolbutamide elimination by cimetidine but not ranitidine. J Clin Pharmacol (1986) 26, 372–7.
2 Dey NG, Castleden CM, Ward J, Cornhill J, McBurney A. The effect of cimetidine on tolbutamide kinetics. Br J Clin Pharmacol (1983) 16, 438–440.
3 Stockley C, Keal J, Rolan P, Bochner F, Somogyi A. Lack of inhibition of tolbutamide hydroxylation by cimetidine in man. Eur J Clin Pharmacol (1986) 31, 235–7.
4 Shah GF, Ghandi TP, Patel PR, Patel MR, Gilbert RN, Shridhar PA. Tolbutamide and chlorpropamide kinetics in the presence of cimetidine in human volunteers. Indian Drugs (1985) 22, 455–8.
5 Shah GF, Ghandi TP, Patel PR, Patel MR, Gilbert RN, Shridhar PA. The effect of cimetidine on the hypoglycaemic activity of four commonly used sulphonylurea drugs. Indian Drugs (1985) 22, 570–2.
6 Feeley J, Peden N. Enhancement of sulphonylurea-induced hypoglycaemia with cimetidine. Br J Clin Pharmacol (1983) 15, 607.
7 Archambeaud-Mouveroux F, Nouaille Y, Nadalon S, Treves R, Merles L. Interaction between gliclazide and cimetidine. Eur J Clin Pharmacol (1987) 31, 631.
8 MacWalter RS, El Debani AH, Feeley J, Stevenson IH. Potentiation by ranitidine of the hypoglycaemic response to glipizide in diabetic patients. Br J Clin Pharmac (1985) 21, 121–2P.
9 Kubacka RT, Antal EJ, Juhl RP. The paradoxical effects of cimetidine and ranitidine on glibenclamide pharmacokinetics and pharmacodynamics. Br J Clin Pharmac (1987) 23, 743–51.
10 Leek K, Mize R, Lowenstein SR. Glyburide-induced hypoglycaemia and ranitidine. Ann Intern Med (1987) 107, 261–2.
11 Somogyi A, Stockley C, Keal J, Rolan P, Bochner F. Reduction of

metformin renal tubular secretion by cimetidine in man. Br J Clin Pharmac (1987) 23, 545–51.
12 Adebayo GI, Coker HAB. Lack of efficacy of cimetidine and ranitidine as inhibitors of tolbutamide metabolism. Eur J Clin Pharmacol (1988) 34, 653–6.
13 Stevenson IH, El Debani AH, MacWalter RS. Glipizide pharmacokinetics and effect in diabetic patients given ranitidine. Acta Pharmacol Toxicol (1986) 59, Suppl 4, 97.
14 Girardin E, Vial T, Pham E, Evreux J-C. Hypoglycémies induites par les sulfamides hypoglycémiants. Ann Med Interne (1992) 143, 11–17.
15 Feeley J, Collins WCJ, Cullen M, El Debani AH, Macwalter RS, Peden NR, Stevenson IH. Potentiation of the hypoglycaemic response to glipizide in diabetic patients by histamine H2-receptor antagonists. Br J Clin Pharmac (1993) 35, 321–3.

Hypoglycaemic agents + Clofibrate

Abstract/Summary

(a) The effects of the sulphonylurea hypoglycaemic agents can be enhanced by clofibrate in some patients, possibly advantageously in those with poorly controlled diabetes. A reduction in the dosage of the hypoglycaemic agent may be necessary. (b) The antidiuretic effects of clofibrate in the treatment of diabetes insipidus are opposed by glibenclamide, and the diuretic effects of glibenclamide are opposed by carbamazepine and desmopressin.

Clinical evidence

(a) Increased hypoglycaemic effects

Over a 5 day period while taking 2 g clofibrate daily, the control of the diabetes was improved in six out of 13 maturity-onset diabetics on various sulphonylureas (not named). Hypoglycaemia (blood glucose levels of 30–40 mg per 100 ml) was seen in four patients.[1]

Other studies confirm that some, but not all, patients show a fall in blood glucose levels while taking clofibrate and the control of the diabetes can improve.[2,3,4–6,8–11] One study showed that the clofibrate increased the half-life of chlorpropamide from 38 to 47 h.[1]

(b) Reduced antidiuretic effects

Clofibrate reduced the volume of urine excreted by 11 patients with pituitary diabetes insipidus, but when given with glibenclamide the volume increased once again. For example, one patient without treatment excreted 5.8 litre urine daily, but only 2.3 litre while taking 2 g clofibrate, whereas with glibenclamide and clofibrate he excreted 3.61 litre daily. The action of glibenclamide was also found to be inhibited by carbamazepine and desmopressin (DDAVP).[12]

Mechanism

(a) Not understood. Among the suggestions are the displacement of the sulphonylureas from their plasma protein binding sites,[5] alterations in their renal excretion,[1] and a decrease in insulin resistance.[4,7] Clofibrate has also been shown to have a hypoglycaemic action of its own which improves the glucose tolerance of diabetics.[11] It seems possible that any or all of these mechanisms might contribute towards the enhanced hypoglycaemia which is seen. (b) Not understood.

Importance and management

(a) The sulphonylurea-clofibrate interaction is established and well documented. The incidence is uncertain, but what is known suggests that between about a third and a half may be affected. Concurrent use need not be avoided, but patients should be monitored for excessive hypoglycaemia (reported with ciprofibrate, an analogue of clofibrate, and an un-named sulphonylurea[13]). Reduce the dosage of the hypoglycaemic agent if necessary. (b) Information about reduced diuretic effects is limited. It would seem prudent to avoid the concurrent use of drugs with actions which are antagonistic rather than additive.

References

1 Petitpierre B, Perrin L, Rudhardt M, Herrera A, Fabre J. Behaviour of chlorpropamide in renal insufficiency and under the effect of associated drug therapy. Int J Clin Pharmacol (1972) 6, 120.
2 Jain AK, Ryan JR, McMahon FG. Potentiation of hypoglycaemic effect of sulphonylureas by halofenate. N Engl J Med (1975) 293, 1283–6.
3 Daubresse J-C, Luyckx AS, Lefebrve P. Potentiation of hypoglycaemic effect of sulphonylureas by clofibrate. N Engl J Med (1976) 294, 613.
4 Ferrari C, Frezzati S, Testori GP, Bertazzoni A. Potentiation of hypoglycaemic response to intravenous tolbutamide by clofibrate. N Engl J Med (1976) 294, 1184.
5 Jain AK, Ryan JR, McMahon FG. Potentiation of hypoglycaemic effect of sulphonylureas by clofibrate. N Engl J Med (1976) 294, 613.
6 Daubresse J-C, Daigneux D, Bruwler M, Luyckx A, Lefebvre PJ. Clofibrate and diabetes control in patients treated with oral hypoglycaemic agents. Br J Clin Pharmac (1979) 7, 599.
7 Ferrari C, Frezzati S, Romussi M, Bertazzoni A, Testori GP, Antonini S, Paracchi A. Effect of short-term clofibrate administration on glucose tolerance and insulin secretion in patients with chemical diabetes or hypertriglyceridaemia. Metabolism (1977) 26, 129.
8 Miller RD. Atromid in the treatment of post-climacteric diabetes. J Atheroscler Res (1963) 3, 694.
9 Csogor SI, Bornemisza P. The effect of clofibrate (Atromid) on intravenous tolbutamide, oral and intravenous glucose tolerance tests. Clin Trials J (1977) 14, 15.
10 Herriott SC, Percy-Robb IW, Strong JA, Thompson CG. The effect of Atromid on serum cholesterol and glucose tolerance in diabetes mellitus. J Atheroscler Res (1963) 3, 679.
11 Barnett D, Craig JG, Robinson DS, Rogers MP. Effect of clofibrate on glucose tolerance in maturity-onset diabetics. Br J Clin Pharmac (1977) 4, 455.
12 Rado JP, Szende L, Marosi J, Juhos E, Sawinsky I, Tako J. Inhibition of the diuretic action of glibenclamide by clofibrate, carbamazepine and 1-deamino-8-D-arginine-vasopressin (DDAVP) in patients with pituitary diabetes insipidus. Acta diabet lat (1974) 11, 179.
13 Girardin E, Vial T, Pham E, Evreux J-C. Hypoglycémies induites par les sulfamides hypoglycémiants. Ann Med Interne (1992) 143, 11–17.

Hypoglycaemic agents + Clonidine

Abstract/Summary

There is evidence that clonidine may possibly suppress the signs and symptoms of hypoglycaemia in diabetic patients

Clinical evidence, mechanism, importance and management

Studies in normal subjects and patients with hypertension found that their normal response to hypoglycaemia (tachycardia, palpitations, perspiration) caused by a dose of insulin was markedly reduced when they were taking 0.45–0.9 mg clonidine daily.[1,2] The reason is that clonidine depresses the output of the catecholamines (adrenaline, noradrenaline) which are secreted in an effort to raise blood sugar levels and which are also responsible for these signs. It seems possible that clonidine will similarly suppress the signs and symptoms of hypoglycaemia which can occur in diabetics, but this appears not to have been reported. Nevertheless diabetic patients should be warned.

References

1 Hedeland H, Dymling J-F and Hokfelt A. The effect of insulin induced hypoglycaemia on plasma renin activity and urinary catecholamines before and following clonidine (Catapresan) in man. Acta Endocrinol (1972) 71, 321–33.
2 Hedeland H, Dymling J-F and Hokfelt A. Pharmacological inhibition of adrenaline secretion following insulin-induced hypoglycaemia in man: the effect of Catapresan. Acta Endocrinol (1971) 67, 97–103.

Hypoglycaemic agents + Contraceptives (oral)

Abstract/Summary

Some diabetics may require small increases or decreases in their dosage of hypoglycaemic agent while taking oral contraceptives, but it is unusual for the control of diabetes to be seriously disturbed.

Clinical evidence

More than half of a group of 30 menopausal diabetics showed abnormal tolerance when given an oral contraceptive (norethynodrel 5 mg + mestranol 0.075 mg) but the changes in their requirements of insulin or oral hypoglycaemic agent were '...few, scattered and slight in magnitude.'[1]

34% of a group[2] of 179 diabetic women needed an increase in insulin and 7% a decrease when given a variety of oral contraceptives, whereas in another group of 38 insulin dependent diabetics it was found that progestogen-only and combined oral contraceptives had little effect on the control of diabetes.[8] Another report[3] about women on *Orthonovin* (norethisterone + mestranol) stated that no insulin changes were necessary. In contrast there are a few scattered reports of individual diabetics who experienced a marked disturbance of their diabetic control when given an oral contraceptive.[4–6]

Mechanism

Not understood. Many mechanisms have been considered including changes in cortisol secretion, alterations in tissue glucose utilization, production of excesssive amounts of growth hormone, alterations in liver function, and others.[7]

Importance and management

Moderately well documented. Concurrent use need not be avoided, but because some patients need a small adjustment in their dosage of hypoglycaemic agent (increases or decreases) and because very occasionally serious disturbances occur, the diabetic response should be monitored.

References

1 Cochran B, Pote WWH. C-19 nor-steroid effects on plasma lipid and diabetic control of postmenopausal women. Diabetes (1963) 12, 366.

2 Zeller WJ, Brehm H, Schoffling K, Melzer H. Vertraglichkeit von hormonalen Ovulationshemmern bei Diabetikerinnen. Arzneim-Forsch (1974) 24, 351.

3 Tyler ET, Olsen HJ, Gotlib M, Levin M, Behne D. Long term usage of norethindrone with mestranol preparations in the control of human fertility. Clin Med (1964) 71, 997.

4 Kopera H, Dukes NG, Ijzerman GL. Critical evaluation of clinical data on *Lyndiol*. Int J Fertil (1964) 9, 69.

5 Peterson WF, Stell MW, Coyne RY. Analysis of the effect of ovulatory suppressants on glucose tolerance. Amer J Obst Gyn (1966) 95, 484.

6 Reder JA, Tulgan H. Impairment of diabetic control by norethynodrel with mestranol. NY State J Med (1967) 67, 1073.

7 Spellacy WN. A review of carbohydrate metabolism and the oral contraceptives. Amer J Obst Gynecol (1969) 104, 448.

8 Radberg T, Gustafson A, Skryten A, Karlsson K. Oral contraception in diabetic women. Diabetes control, serum and high density lipoprotein lipids during low-dose progestogen, combined oestrogen/progestogen and non-hormonal contraception. Acta Endocrinol (1981) 98, 246–51.

Hypoglycaemic agents + Corticosteroids

Abstract/Summary

The blood sugar lowering effects of the hypoglycaemic agents are opposed by the concurrent use of corticosteroids with glucocorticoid (hyperglycaemic) activity. It may be necessary to raise the dosage of the hypoglycaemic agent appropriately.

Clinical evidence, mechanism, importance and management

Corticosteroids with glucocorticoid activity can raise blood sugar levels and induce diabetes.[1] This can oppose the blood sugar lowering effects of the hypoglycaemic agents used in the treatment of diabetes mellitus. For example, a disturbance of the control of diabetes is very briefly described in a patient treated with insulin and hydrocortisone.[4] A study in five diabetics showed that a single 200 mg dose of cortisone modified their glucose tolerance curves while taking an unstated amount of chlorpropamide. The blood glucose levels of four of them rose (three showed an initial fall), whereas in a previous test with chlorpropamide alone the blood sugar levels of four of them had fallen.[2] This almost certainly reflects a direct antagonism between the pharmacological effects of the two drugs, and this would seem to be confirmed by a study in normal subjects which showed that another glucocorticoid, prednisone, had no significant effect on the metabolism or clearance of tolbutamide.[3]

There are very few studies of this interaction, probably because the hyperglycaemic activity of the corticosteroids has been known for such a long time that the outcome of concurrent use is self-evident. The effects of corticosteroid treatment in diabetics (using insulin or oral hypoglycaemic agents) should be closely monitored and the dosage of the hyperglycaemic agent raised as necessary. Hypoglycaemic agents are sometimes deliberately given to non-diabetic patients taking corticosteroids to reduce blood sugar levels.

References

1 David DS, Cheigh JS, Braun DW, Fotino M, Stenzel KH, Rubin AL. HLA-A28 and steroid-induced diabetes in renal transplant patients. J Amer Med Ass (1980) 423, 532–3.

2 Danowski TS, Mateer FM, Moses C. Cortisone enhancement of peripheral utilization of glucose and the effects of chlorpropamide. Ann NY Acad Sci (1959) 74, 988.

3 Breimer DD, Zilly W, Richter E. Influence of corticosteroids on hexobarbital and tolbutamide disposition. Clin Pharmacol Ther (1978) 24, 208.

4 Manchon ND, Bercoff E, Lemarchand P, Chassagne P, Senant J, Bourreille J. Fréquence et gravité des interactions médicamenteuses dan une population âgée: étude prospective concernant 63 malades. Rev Med Interne (1989) 10, 521–5.

Hypoglycaemic agents + Cytotoxics

Abstract/Summary

Colaspase (L-asparaginase) sometimes induces diabetes mellitus. Changes in the hypoglycaemic agent dosage requirements seems a possibility in some diabetic patients. There is also evidence that the control of diabetes can also be severely disturbed in patients given cyclophosphamide.

Clinical evidence and mechanisms

(a) Colaspase (L-asparaginase)

Three patients with acute lymphocytic leukaemia developed diabetes after treatment with colaspase (asparaginase): two of them two and 4 days after a single dose of colaspase, and another patient 2 days after the fourth dose. Plasma insulin was undetectable. A normal insulin reponse returned in one patient after 23 days, whereas the other two showed a suboptimal reponse two weeks and nine months afterwards.[1] In another study, five out of 39 patients developed hyperglycaemia and glycosuria after treatment with colaspase.[2] The reasons are not understood but suggestions include inhibition of insulin synthesis,[5] direct damage to the Islets of Langerhans,[1] and reduced insulin binding.[5]

(b) Cyclophosphamide

Acute hypoglycaemia has been described in two diabetic patients under treatment with insulin and carbutamide who were concurrently treated with cyclophosphamide.[3] Three cases of diabetes, apparently induced by the use of cyclophosphamide, have also been reported.[4] The reasons are not understood.

Importance and management

Strictly speaking none of these reactions is probably an interaction, but they serve to underline the importance of monitoring the diabetic control of patients receiving either colaspase or cyclophosphamide.

References

1 Gailani S, Nussbaum A, Takao O, Freeman A. Diabetes in patients treated with asparaginase. Clin Pharmacol Ther (1971) 12, 487.
2 Ohnuma T, Holland JF, Freeman A, Sinks L. Biochemical and pharmacological studies with asparaginase in man. Cancer Res (1970) 30, 2297.
3 Kruger H-U. Blutzuckersenkende Wirkung von Cyclophosphamid bei Diabetikern. Med Klin (1966) 61, 1462.
4 Pengelly CR. Diabetes mellitus and cyclophosphamide. Br Med J (1965) 1, 1312.
5 Burghen G, Pui C-H, Yasuda K, Kitabchi AE. Decreased insulin binding and production: probable mechanism for hyperglycaemia due to therapy with prednisone (PRED) and l-asparaginase (ASP). Ped Res (1981) 15, 626.

Hypoglycaemic agents + Danazol

Abstract/Summary

On theoretical grounds danazol would be expected to oppose the effects of hypoglycaemic agents, but the practical clinical importance of this is uncertain.

Clinical evidence, mechanism, importance and management

Danazol can disturb glucose metabolism. A study in 14 non-diabetic subjects showed that 3 months treatment with 600 mg danazol daily caused a mild but definite deterioration in glucose tolerance, associated with high insulin levels. Insulin resistance was also seen in five subjects on danazol when given intravenous tolbutamide.[1] Another study in nine non-diabetic women found that 600 mg danazol daily raised insulin levels in response to glucose or IV tolbutamide. This was attributed to the effects of danazol on the beta-cells of the pancreas.[2] However the authors of another study in nine non-diabetic women attributed the mild deterioration in glucose tolerance and the marked increase in the insulin response to the androgenic properties of the danazol.[3] Danazol can displace testosterone from sex hormone binding globulin sites.

For these reasons the makers of danazol advise caution if danazol is given to diabetic patients. Danazol would be expected to oppose the actions of hypoglycaemic agents to some extent, but nobody seems to have checked to see whether this is clinically important or not.

References

1 Wynn V. Metabolic effects of danazol. J Int Med Res (1977) 5, Suppl 3, 25–35.
2 Goettenberg N, Schlienger J L, Becmeur F, Dellenbach P. Traitement de l'endométriose pelvienne par le danazol. Incidence sur le métabolisme glucidique. Nouv Presse Méd (1982) 11, 3703–6.
3 Vaughan-Williams C A, Shalet S M. Glucose tolerance and insulin resistance after danazol treatment. J Obstet Gynaecol (1989) 9, 229–32.

Hypoglycaemic agents + Dextropropoxyphene

Abstract/Summary

Dextropropoxyphene does not interact with tolbutamide. Hypoglycaemia was seen in a patient on an unnamed sulphonylurea and dextroproproxyphene-paracetamol.

Clinical evidence, mechanism, importance and management

After taking 65 mg dextropropoxyphene eight-hourly for four days the clearance of tolbutamide (500 mg given IV) in six normal subjects was not affected.[1] An isolated case of hypoglycaemia has been reported with an un-named sulphonylurea and dextropropoxyphene/paracetamol.[2] There would seem to be little reason for avoiding concurrent use or for taking particular precautions.

Reference

1 Robson RA, Miners JO, Whitehead AG, Birkett DJ. Specificity of the inhibitory effect of dextropropoxyphene on oxidative drug metabolism in man: effects on theophylline and tolbutamide disposition. Br J Clin Pharmac (1987) 23, 772–5.
2 Girardin E, Vial T, Pham E, Evreux J-C. Hypoglycémies induites par les sulfamides hypoglycémiants. Ann Med Interne (1992) 143, 11–17.

Hypoglycaemic agents + Disopyramide

Abstract/Summary

Disopyramide occasionally causes hypoglycaemia which may be severe.

Clinical evidence, mechanism, importance and management

For reasons which are not understood disopyramide occasionally and unpredictably causes hypoglycaemia which may be severe.[1-5] Impaired renal function and impaired cardiac function may be predisposing factors. The makers of disopyramide advise close monitoring of blood glucose levels and withdrawal of disopyramide if problems arise.[6] This is not simply a problem for diabetics, but certainly within the context of diabetes the hypoglycaemic effects of disopyramide may possibly cause particular difficulties. Concurrent use should be well monitored.

References

1 Goldberg IJ, Brown LK, Rayfield EJ. Disopyramide (Norpace-induced hypoglycaemia. Am J Med (1980) 69, 463–6.
2 Quevdeo SF, Kraus DS, Chazan JA, Crosafulli FS, Kahn CB. Fasting hypoglycaemia secondary to disopyramide therapy. Report of two cases. J Amer Med Ass (1981) 245, 2424.
3 Strathman I, Schubert EN, Cohen A, Nitzberg DM. Hypoglycemia in patients receiving disopyramide phosphate. Drug Intell Clin Pharm (1983) 17, 635–8.
4 Semel JD, Wortham E, Karl DM. Fasting hypoglycaemia associated with disopyramide. Am Heart J (1983) 106, 1160–1.
5 Seriès C. Hypoglycémie induite ou favorisée par le disopyramide. Rev Med Interne (1988) 9, 528–9.
6 Rhythmodan (Roussel Labs). Drug Datasheet Compendium (1992–3) 1311.

Hypoglycaemic agents + Disulfiram

Abstract/Summary

Disulfiram does not interact with tolbutamide and there appears to be no evidence that it interacts with any other hypoglycaemic agent.

Clinical evidence, mechanism, importance and management

Studies on 10 normal subjects showed that disulfiram (first day 400 mg three times; second day 400 mg; third and fourth days 200 mg) had no significant effect on the half-life or clearance of tolbutamide given intravenously.[1] No special precautions seem to be necessary.

Reference

1 Svendsen TL, Kristensen MB, Hansen JM, Skovsted L. The influence of disulfiram on the half-life and metabolic clearance rate of diphenylhydantoin and tolbutamide in man. Eur J Clin Pharmacol (1976) 9, 439.

Hypoglycaemic agents + Erythromycin

Abstract/Summary

An isolated report describes severe liver damage with prolonged cholestasis in a patient on chlorpropamide after concurrent treatment with erythromycin. An isolated case of hypoglycaemia has been described in another patient on glibenclamide when given erythromycin.

Clinical evidence, mechanism, importance and management

A man with Type II diabetes was treated with phenformin for 10 years. Four months after the phenformin was replaced by chlorpropamide, he was treated with 1 g erythromycin ethylsuccinate daily for 3 weeks for a respiratory infection. Two weeks later he complained of increasing fatigue and fever. A short episode of pruriginous skin rash was followed by the appearance of dark urine, jaundice and hepatomegaly. The picture over the next two years was that of profound cholestasis, complicated by steatorrhoea and marked hyperlipidaemia with disappearance of interlobular bile ducts. He died of ischemic cardiomyopathy.[1] The reasons for this serious reaction are not understood, but the authors point out that liver damage occurs in a very small number of patients given sulphonylureas, such as chlorpropamide, which in this instance, appears to have been markedly increased by the erythromycin.[1] No general conclusions can be drawn from this unusual case about the advisability of concurrent use.

An isolated case of hypoglycaemia occurred in a patient given glibenclamide and erythromycin,[2] but an earlier single-dose study in 12 non-insulin dependent diabetics found that erythromycin had little effect on glibenclamide pharmacokinetics or on its hypoglycaemic effects.[3] Nevertheless concurrent use should be monitored.

References

1 Geubel AP, Nakad A, Rahier J, Dive C. Prolonged cholestasis and disappearance of interlobular bile ducts following chlorpropamide and erythromycin ethylsuccinate. Case of drug interaction? Liver (1988) 8, 350–3.
2 Girardin E, Vial T, Pham E, Evreux J-C. Hypoglycémies induites par les sulfamides hypoglycémiants. Ann Med Interne (1992) 143, 11–17.
3 Fleishaker JC, Phillips JP. Evaluation of a potential interaction between erythromycin and glyburide in diabetic volunteers. J Clin Pharmacol (1991) 31, 259–62.

Hypoglycaemic agents + Ethacrynic acid

Abstract/Summary

Ethacrynic acid can raise blood sugar levels in diabetics which opposes to some extent the effects of the hypoglycaemic agents. The clinical importance of this seems to be small.

Clinical evidence and mechanism

A double-blind study on 24 hypertensive patients, one third of whom were diabetics, showed that daily treatment with 200 mg ethacrynic acid over a 6-week period impaired their glucose tolerance and raised the blood sugar levels of those who were diabetic to the same extent as those taking hydrochlorothiazide.[1] In another study[2] no changes in carbohydrate metabolism was seen in six diabetics given 150 mg ethacrynic acid daily for a week. The reasons are not understood.

Importance and management

Information is very limited indeed. Some impairment of the glucose tolerance may possibly occur, but there seems to be a singular lack of evidence in the literature to show that normally ethacrynic acid has much effect on the control of diabetes in most patients. Nevertheless it would be prudent to monitor the effects of concurrent use.

References

1 Russell RP, Lindeman RD, Prescott LF. Metabolic and hypotensive effects of ethacrynic acid. Comparative study with hydrochlorothiazide. J Amer Med Ass (1968) 205, 81.

2 Dige-Petersen H. Ethacrynic acid and carbohydrate metabolism. Nord Med (1966) 75, 123–5.

Hypoglycaemic agents + Fenfluramine

Abstract/Summary

Fenfluramine has inherent hypoglycaemic activity which can add to, or in some instances replace, the effects of conventional hypoglycaemic agents.

Clinical evidence, mechanism, importance and management

A study in a group of obese maturity-onset diabetics who were given either fenfluramine (initially 40 mg daily increased over four weeks to 160 mg) or a placebo showed that four of the six were better controlled than when previously taking a biguanide hypoglycaemic agent.[1] The hypoglycaemic effects of fenfluramine are described elsewhere.[2,4] It seems that fenfluramine increases the uptake of glucose into skeletal muscle, thereby lowering blood glucose levels.[3,4]

This is a well established and, on the whole, an advantageous rather than an adverse reaction, but it would be prudent to check on the extent of the response if fenfluramine is added or withdrawn from the treatment being received by diabetics.

References

1 Jackson WPU. Fenfluramine trials in a diabetic clinic. S Afr med J (1971) 45, (Suppl), 29.

2 Turtle JR, Burgess JA. Hypoglycaemic effect of fenfluramine in diabetes mellitus. Diabetes (1973) 22, 858.

3 Kirby MJ, Turner P. Effect of amphetamine, fenfluramine and norfenfluramine on glucose uptake into human isolated skeletal muscle. Br J Clin Pharmac (1974) 1, 340P.

4 Dykes JRW. The effect of a low-calorie diet with and without fenfluramine, and fenfluramine alone on the glucose tolerance and insulin secretion of overweight non-diabetics. Postgrad med J (1973) 49, 314.

Hypoglycaemic agents + Fibrates (Bezafibrate, Ciprofibrate, Fenofibrate, Gemfibrozil)

Abstract/Summary

A small improvement in the control of diabetes may possibly occur, but excessive hypoglycaemia has been seen in a few patients on sulphonylurea hypoglycaemic agents when given these fibrates. See also 'Hypoglycaemic agents + Clofibrate'.

Clinical evidence, mechanism, importance and management

A study in diabetic patients on insulin (1), acetohexamide (4), chlorpropamide (6) or glipizide (1) found that the control of their diabetes was not impaired and even slightly improved when concurrently treated with gemfibrozil (800 mg daily initially, reduced later to 400–600 mg daily).[1] A later study found that a slight increase in the oral hypoglycaemic agent dosage was needed.[2] A single report describes hypoglycaemia in a diabetic on glibenclamide (glyburide) when started on 1200 mg gemfibrozil daily. The glibenclamide dosage was accordingly reduced from 5 to 1.25 mg daily with satisfactory diabetic control. When the gemfibrozil was later stopped and restarted, the dosage of the glibenclamide had to be increased and then again reduced.[3]

The French Centres Régionaux de Pharmacovigiliance recorded a number of cases of hypoglycaemia during the period 1985–90 in patients on unnamed sulphonylureas when given fibrates (1 with bezafibrate, 3 with ciprofibrate, 3 with fenofibrate).[4]

There would seem to be no strong reason for avoiding the concurrent use of hypoglycaemic agents and fibrates, but patients should be warned that excessive hypoglycaemia occurs occasionally and unpredictably.

References

1 De Salcedo I, Gorringe JAL, Silva JL and Santos JA. Gemfibrozil in a group of diabetics. Proc Roy Soc Med (1976) 69, Suppl 2, 64–70.

2 Kontinnen A, Kuisma I, Ralli R, Pohjola S, Ojala K. The effect of gemfibrozil on serum lipids in diabetic patients. Ann Clin Res (1979) 11, 240–5.

3 Ahmad S. Gemfibrozil: interaction with glyburide. South Med J (1991) 84, 102.

4 Girardin E, Vial T, Pham E, Evreux J-C. Hypoglycémies induites par les sulfamides hypoglycémiants. Ann Med Interne (1992) 143, 11–17.

Hypoglycaemic agents + Fluconazole

Abstract/Summary

An isolated report describes a hypoglycaemic coma in a patient on glipizide when given fluconazole. Fluconazole raises serum tolbutamide levels in normal subjects.

Clinical evidence

(a) Glipizide

A diabetic on glipizide, 2.5 mg three times daily, developed a hypoglycaemic coma within 4 days of starting to take 200 mg fluconazole daily. Her blood sugar levels had fallen to less than 1 g/l. She rapidly recovered when given glucose.[2]

(b) Tolbutamide

After taking 100 mg fluconazole daily for 6 days and then for a further 7 days, the AUCs of single 500 mg doses of tolbutamide in 13 normal subjects were increased by 47 and 52% respectively and the peak serum levels were raised. The half-life of the tolbutamide was increased about 40%. Blood glucose levels remained unaltered and none of the subjects showed any evidence of hypoglycaemia. [1]

Mechanism

Not understood.

Importance and management

Neither of these two interactions is well documented nor well established. Their general importance is uncertain because the interaction with glipizide involves only one patient and the study with tolbutamide was in normal healthy subjects. However if fluconazole is given to diabetics on either of these hypoglycaemic agents, warn them to be alert for any evidence of increased hypoglycaemia.

References

1 Lazar D J, Wilner K D. Drug interactions with fluconazole. Rev Infect Dis (1990) 12 (Suppl 3) S327–333.
2 Fournier JP, Schneider S, Martinez P, Mahagne MH, Haffner M, Thiercelin D, Chichmanain GM, Bertrand F. Coma hypoglycémique chez une patients traitée par glipizide et fluconazole: une possible interaction? Therapie (1992) 47, 446–7.

Hypoglycaemic agents + Frusemide

Abstract/Summary

The control of diabetes is not usually disturbed by the concurrent use of frusemide, although there are a few reports showing that it can sometimes raise blood sugar levels.

Clinical evidence, mechanism, importance and management

Although frusemide can elevate blood sugar levels[1] (but to a much lesser extent than the thiazide diuretics), worsen glucose tolerance tests[5] and occasionally cause glycosuria and even acute diabetes in individual patients,[2] the general picture is that the control of diabetes is not usually affected by the use of frusemide.[3] It has been described as the 'diuretic of choice for the diabetic patient.'[4] Even so, prescribers should be aware of its hyperglycaemic potentialities.

References

1 Hutcheon DE, Leonard G. Diuretic and antihypertensive action of frusemide. J Clin Pharmac (1967) 7, 26.
2 Toivnonen S, Mustala O. Diabetogenic action of frusemide. Br Med J (1966) 1, 920.
3 Bencomo L, Fyvolent J, Kahana S, Kahana L. Clinical experience with a new diuretic, furosemide. Curr Ther Res (1965) 7, 339.
4 Malins JM. Diuretics in diabetes mellitus. Practitioner (1968) 201, 529.
5 Breckenridge A, Welborn TA, Dollery CT, Frazer R. Glucose tolerance in hypertensive patients on long-term diuretic therapy. Lancet (1967) i, 61–4.

Hypoglycaemic agents + Guanethidine and Related drugs

Abstract/Summary

Guanethidine has hypoglycaemic activity which may possibly add to the effects of conventional hypoglycaemic agents. Soluble insulin may also exaggerate the hypotensive effects of debrisoquine.

Clinical evidence and mechanism

(a) Hypoglycaemia increased

A diabetic needed an insulin increase from 70 to 94 units daily when guanethidine was withdrawn.[1] A later study on three maturity-onset diabetics showed that guanethidine in daily doses of 50–90 mg caused a significant improvement in their glucose tolerance.[2] Other reports also describe the hypoglycaemic effects of guanethidine in man.[3,4] A suggested reason is that guanethidine can impair the homeostatic mechanism concerned with raising blood sugar levels by affecting the release of catecholamines. The balance of the system thus impaired tends to be tipped in favour of a reduced blood sugar level, resulting in a reduction in hypoglycaemic agent needs.

(b) Hypotension increased

An insulin-dependent man taking debrisoquine (20 mg twice daily) developed severe postural hypotension within an hour of using a short-acting insulin (28 units soluble insulin + 20 units isophane insulin). He became dizzy and was found to have a standing blood pressure of 97/72 mmHg. The postural fall in systolic pressure was 65 mmHg. He had no evidence of hypoglycaemia and no hypotension when using 48 units of isophane insulin.[4] Insulin can cause hypotension but this is only seen in those with an impaired reflex control of blood pressure.[5]

Importance and management

Information about the guanethidine-insulin interaction is limited, the case cited being the only one describing an adverse response. Check on the dosage requirements of the hypoglycaemic agent if guanethidine or related drugs (bethanidine, guanadrel, debrisoquine, etc.) are started or stopped. Also check patients given debrisoquine and insulin, particularly if they are taking vasodilators, to ensure that excessive hypotension does not develop.

References

1 Gupta KK, Lillicrap CA. Guanethidine and diabetes. Br Med J (1968) 2, 697.
2 Gupta KK. The antidiabetic action of guanethidine. Postgrad Med J (1969) 45, 455.
3 Kansal PC, Buse J, Durling FC. Effect of guanethidine and reserpine on glucose tolerance. Curr Ther Res (1971) 13, 517.
4 Woeber KA, Arky R, Braverman LE. Reversal by guanethidine of abnormal oral glucose tolerance in thyrotoxicosis. Lancet (1966) i, 895.
5 Hume L. Potentiation of hypotensive effect of debrisoquine by insulin. Diabetic Medicine (1985) 2, 390–1.

Hypoglycaemic agents + Guar gum or Glucomannan

Abstract/Summary

Guar gum appears not to affect the absorption of glipizide nor one formulation of glibenclamide, but glucomannan appears to reduce the absorption of glibenclamide.

Clinical evidence, mechanism, importance and management

(a) Guar gum

5 g guar gum alone or taken 30 min. later with breakfast did not significantly affect the absorption of a single 2.5 mg dose of glipizide in 10 normal subjects.[1] Guar gum was found to reduce the absorption of glibenclamide in one formulation (*Semi-Euglucon*) but not another newer formulation (*Semi-Euglucon-N*),[2] possibly because the latter preparation is more rapidly and completely absorbed. There seems to be nothing documented about any of the other sulphonylureas.

(b) Glucomannan

3.9 g glucomannan markedly reduced the serum levels of glibenclamide in nine normal subjects after taking a single 2.5 mg dose. Four samples taken over the period 30–150 min. showed reductions in the serum levels of glibenclamide by about 50%.[3] The extent to which affects the control of diabetes in patients appears not to have been studied.

References

1 Huupponen R, Karhuvaara S, Seppälä P. Effect of guar gum on glipizide absorption in man. Eur J Clin Pharmacol (1985) 28, 717–9.
2 Neugebauer G, Akpan W, Abshagen U. Interaktion von Guar mit Glibenclamid und Bezafibrat. Beitr Infusionther Klin Ernähr (1983) 12, 40–7.
3 Shima K, Tanaka A, Ikegami H, Tabata M, Sawazaki N, Kumahara Y. Effect of dietary fiber, glucomannan, on absorption of sulfonylurea in man. Hormon metabol Res (1983) 15, 1–3.

Hypoglycaemic agents + Halofenate

Abstract/Summary

Halofenate can raise sulphonylurea serum levels and enhance the blood sugar lowering effects of chlorpropamide, tolbutamide, tolazamide and phenformin in some patients.

Clinical evidence

A double-blind trial over 48 weeks on diabetics with type IV hyperlipoproteinaemia found that halofenate (0.5 to 1.5 g) enhanced the effects of the sulphonylureas and biguanides in some patients. The dosages were reduced as follows: chlorpropamide 80% (four patients), tolazamide 46% (four patients), phenformin 33% (five patients) but no change was needed in two patients taking insulin. Some of the patients taking the sulphonylureas were also given phenformin. A study in 12 normal subjects also showed that halofenate increased serum tolbutamide levels and decreased blood sugar levels.[1]

Similar results have been described in other studies.[2,3] One of them found that 0.5–1.0 g halofenate daily improved diabetic control in four patients, two of whom showed rises in chlorpropamide serum levels of 25–35%.[3]

Mechanism

Not understood. One suggestion is that the halofenate displaces the sulphonylureas from their protein binding sites in the plasma, thereby increasing the biological activity.[1] As a full explanation this seems unlikely because the full effects take up to a month to develop.

Importance and management

An established interaction. Concurrent use need not be avoided. The dosage of the hypoglycaemic agent can be reduced with full control of the diabetes, but the interaction may take 2–4 weeks to develop fully. Not all patients may show this interaction.[1,2] Excessive hypoglycaemia has not been reported, but the possibility should be borne in mind. Information about other hypoglycaemic agents appears to be lacking.

References

1 Jain AK, Ryan JR, McMahon FG. Potentiation of hypoglycaemic effect of sulphonylureas by halofenate. N Engl J Med (1975) 293, 1283–6.
2 Kudzma DJ, Friedenberg SJ. Potentiation of hypoglycaemic effect of chlorpropamide and phenformin by halofenate. Diabetes (1977) 26, 291.
3 Kohl EA, Persellin S, Friedberg SJ. Halofenate-chlorpropamide combined regimen in the treatment of maturity onset diabetes mellitus. Clin Res (1979) 27, 790A.

Hypoglycaemic agents + Heparin

Abstract/Summary

Two reports describe hypoglycaemia in a diabetic on glipizide and another on glibenclamide, both attributed to concurrent treatment with heparin.

Clinical evidence, mechanism, importance and management

A diabetic, treated for 6 months with glipizide with fair control, experienced recurring episodes of hypoglycaemia over a period of 4 days after taking a single 5 mg dose of glipizide while hospitalized for the treatment of peripheral vascular disease. It was suggested that this might possibly have been due to an interaction with subcutaneous heparin calcium (5000 U every 12 h) which, it is postulated, might have displaced the glipizide from its protein binding sites.[1] The patient was also treated with diamorphine. Another very brief report describes hypoglycaemia in a patient treated with glibenclamide and heparin.[2] Concurrent use should be monitored.

References

1 McKillop G, Fallon M, Slater SD. Possible interaction between heparin and a sulphonylurea: a cause of prolonged hypoglycaemia? Brit Med J (1986) 293, 1073.
2 Beeley L, Daly M, Stewart P. Bulletin of the West Midlands Centre for Adverse Drug Reaction Reporting. (1987) 24, 24.

Hypoglycaemic agents + Isoniazid

Abstract/Summary

Some reports state that isoniazid can raise blood sugar levels in diabetics, whereas one describes a fall. The outcome of con-current use is uncertain. The dosage of the hypoglycaemic agent may possibly need to be adjusted to control the diabetes adequately.

Clinical evidence

A study on six diabetics taking insulin showed that while taking 250–400 mg isoniazid daily their fasting blood sugar levels were raised 40% (from an average of 255 to 357 mg%), and their glucose tolerance curves rose and returned to normal levels more slowly. After 6 days treatment the average rise was only 20%. Two other patients needed an increased dosage of insulin while taking 200 mg isoniazid daily, but a reduction when the isoniazid was withdrawn.[1]

Another report describes glycosuria and the development of frank diabetes in three out of 50 patients given 300 mg isoniazid daily,[2] and hyperglycaemia has been seen in cases of isoniazid poisoning.[3]

In contrast, a study in six out of eight diabetics[4] showed that isoniazid can have a hypoglycaemic effect. A 500 mg dose of isoniazid caused an 18% (range 5–34%) reduction in blood sugar levels after 4 h; 3 mg tolbutamide caused a 28% (19–43%) reduction, and together they caused a 35% (17–57%) reduction. One patient however showed a 10% increase after isoniazid, a 41% decrease after tolbutamide, and a 30% decrease after taking both. The other diabetic responded to neither drug.

Mechanism

Not understood.

Importance and management

The major documentation for these reactions dates back to the 1950s, since when the literature has been virtually (and perhaps significantly?) silent. The outcome of concurrent use is therefore somewhat uncertain. Nevertheless it would be prudent for diabetics given isoniazid to be monitored for changes in the control of the diabetes. Appropriate dosage adjustments (up or down?) of the hypoglycaemic agent should be made where necessary.

References

1 Luntz GRWN and Smith SG. Effect of isoniazid on carbohydrate metabolism in controls and diabetics. Br Med J (1953) 1, 296.
2 Dickson I. Glycosuria and diabetes mellitus following INAH therapy. Med J Aust (1962) 49, 325.
3 Tovarys A, Siler Z. Diabetic syndrome and intoxication with INH. Prakt Lekar (1968) 48, 286; quoted in Int Pharm Abs (1968) 5, 286.
4 Seggara FO, Sherman DS, Charif BS. Experiences with tolbutamide and chlorpropamide in tuberculous diabetic patients. Ann NY Acad Sci (1959) 74, 656.

Hypoglycaemic agents + Karela

Abstract/Summary

The hypoglycaemic effects of chlorpropamide can be increased by the concurrent use of karela (*Momordica charantia*).

Clinical evidence, mechanism, importance and management

Karela (also known as bitter gourd, bitter melon, balsam pear, cundeamor) is the fruit of *Momordica charantia* which is indigenous to Asia and South America. It is used to flavour foods such as curries, and also used as a herbal medicine, both fresh and dried, for the treatment of diabetes mellitus. It contains a hypoglycaemic peptide, polypeptide-p,[2] which produces a significant improvement in glucose tolerance in non-insulin-dependent diabetics[1,4,5]

A report of a diabetic who was poorly controlled on diet and chlorpropamide, but much better controlled when she also ate karela, provides evidence that the hypoglycaemic effects of karela and conventional oral hypoglycaemic agents can be additive.[3] What is not clear is whether excessive hypoglycaemia might occur in diabetics taking conventional hypoglycaemic agents, if they were additionally to begin to take karela as a food or as a herbal medicine. Karela is now available in both forms in the UK and elsewhere, and prescribers should therefore be aware that Asian patients may possibly be using karela as well as more orthodox drugs to control their diabetes.

References

1 Leatherdale BA, Panesar K, Singh G, Atkins TW, Bailey J, Bignell AH. Improvement in glucose tolerance due to *Momordica charantia* (karela). Br Med J (1981) 282, 1823–4.
2 Khanna P, Jain SC, Panaqariya A, Dixit VP. Hypoglycaemic activity of polypeptide-p from a plant source. J Nat Prod (1981) 44, 648–55.
3 Aslam M, Stockley I H. Interaction between curry ingredient (karela) and drug (chlorpropamide). Lancet (1979) 1, 607.
4 Welihinda J, Karunanayake EH, Sheriff MHR, Jaysinghe KSA . Effect of *Momordica Charantia* on the glucose tolerance in maturity onset diabetes. J Ethnopharmacology (1986) 17, 277–82.
5 Akhtar S. Trial of *Momordica Charantia* Linn (Karela) powder in patients with maturity-onset diabetes. JPMA (1982) 32, 106–7.

Hypoglycaemic agents + Ketotifen

Abstract/Summary

Concurrent use appears to be well tolerated, but a fall in the number of blood platelets has been seen in one study in patients on biguanides while taking ketotifen. The clinical importance of this is uncertain.

Clinical evidence, mechanism, importance and management

A study in 30 hospitalized diabetics (10 on diet alone, 10 on unnamed sulphonylureas, 10 on unnamed biguanides) found that the concurrent use of ketotifen for 14 days was generally well tolerated. However those on biguanides showed a significant decrease in platelet counts and three showed a marked fall on day 14 to slightly below $100 \times 19^9/l$ which returned to normal after a few days.[1] This finding underlies the precaution issued by the makers of ketotifen (Sandoz) that the combination '...should be avoided until this phenomenon has been satisfactorily explained.' However no other studies appear to have confirmed the fall in thrombocyte count so that its importance still remains uncertain.[2]

References

1 Dolecek R. Ketotifen in the treatment of diabetics with various allergic conditions. Pharmatherapeutica (1981) 2, 568–74.
2 Sandoz. Personnal communication (1991).

Hypoglycaemic agents + Lithium carbonate

Abstract/Summary

Lithium carbonate can raise blood sugar levels and in some instances cause the development of diabetes mellitus, but there is little or no evidence that its use normally disturbs the control of diabetes significantly.

Clinical evidence, mechanism, importance and management

A study in 10 psychiatric patients showed that when treated with lithium carbonate for 2 weeks their blood glucose levels were raised and their glucose tolerance tests impaired.[1] Other reports describe the development of hyperglycaemia and frank diabetes mellitus in patients treated with lithium carbonate.[2–4]

Although there appear to be no reports of disturbed diabetic control in diabetics treated with lithium carbonate (any marked effect might be expected to have been reported by now), it would seem prudent to monitor the response if lithium is added to the treatment being received by diabetic patients.

References

1 Shopsin B, Stern S, Gershon S. Altered carbohydrate metabolism during treatment with lithium carbonate. Arch Gen Psychiat (1972) 26, 566–71.
2 Craig J, Abu-Saleh M, Smith B, Evans I. Diabetes mellitus in patients on lithium. Lancet (1977) ii, 1028.
3 Johnstone BB. Diabetes mellitus in patients on lithium. Lancet (1977) ii, 935.
4 Martinez-Maldone M, Terrell J. Lithium carbonate-induced nephrogenic diabetes insipidus and glucose intolerance. Arch Intern Med (1973) 132, 881–4.

Hypoglycaemic agents + Lovastatin

Abstract/Summary

Lovastatin does not affect serum chlorpropamide levels and the control of diabetes is unchanged.

Clinical evidence, mechanism, importance and management

A study in seven non-insulin dependent diabetic patients on chlorpropamide and with hypercholesterolaemia showed that lovastatin (20 mg twice daily for 6 weeks) reduced low-density lipoprotein cholesterol by 28%, total cholesterol by 24% and apolipoprotein B by 24%. Chlorpropamide and lovastatin serum levels were unchanged, and diabetic control unaltered.[1] There would seem to be no reason for avoiding concurrent use.

Reference

1 Johnson B F, LaBelle P, Wilson J, Allan J, Zupkis R V, Ronca P D. Effects of lovastatin in diabetic patients treated with chlorpropamide. Clin Pharmacol Ther (1990) 48, 467–72.

Hypoglycaemic agents + Methysergide

Abstract/Summary

A preliminary study indicates that methysergide may enhance the activity of tolbutamide.

Clinical evidence, mechanism, importance and management

A study of eight maturity-onset diabetics showed that two days' pretreatment with methysergide (2 mg 6-hourly) increased the amount of insulin secreted in response to 1 g tolbutamide given intravenously by almost 40%.[1] Whether in practice the addition or withdrawal of methysergide adversely affects the control of diabetes is uncertain, but prescribers should be aware of this reaction.

Reference

1 Baldridge JA, Quickel KE, Feldman JM, Lebovitz HE. Potentiation of tolbutamide-mediated insulin release in adult onset diabetics by methysergide maleate. Diabetes (1974) 23, 21.

Hypoglycaemic agents + Metolazone

Abstract/Summary

An isolated report describes severe hypoglycaemia in a patient on glibenclamide shortly after starting treatment with metolazone.

Clinical evidence, mechanism, importance and management

A diabetic man, stabilized on glibenclamide and hospitalized for congestive heart failure, became clinically hypoglycaemic (blood glucose levels unmeasurable by Labstix) within 40 h of starting 5 mg metolazone daily. He was treated with IV glucose. Although both glibenclamide and metolazone were stopped, he had four further hypoglycaemic episodes over the next 30 h.[1] The reasons are not understood. *In vitro* studies failed to find any evidence that metolazone displaces glibenclamide from its protein binding sites which might possibly have provided some explanation for what happened.[1] The general importance of this apparent interaction is not clear, but until more is known it would seem prudent to monitor the effects of concurrent use. More study is needed.

References

1 George S, McBurney A, Cole A. Possible protein binding displacement interaction between glibenclamide and metolazone. Eur J Clin Pharmacol (1990) 38, 93–5.

Hypoglycaemic agents + Mianserin

Abstract/Summary

The control of diabetes appears to be unaffected by the use of mianserin.

Clinical evidence, mechanism, importance and management

Although there is some evidence of a change in glucose metabolism during treatment with mianserin,[1,2,4] the alteration failed to affect the control of diabetes in 10 patients under study and there appear to be no reports of adverse effects caused by concurrent use.[3]

References

1 Fell PJ, Quantock DC and van der Burg WJ. The human pharmacology of GB94--a new psychotropic agent. Eur J Clin Pharmac (1973) 5, 166.
2 Peet M, Behagel H. Mianserin: a decade of scientific development. Br J Clin Pharmac (1978) 5, 5S.
3 Weinges A. Unpublished data quoted in ref. 2.
4 Moonie J. Unpublished data quoted by Brogden RN, Heel RC, Speight TM, Avery GS. Mianserin: a review of its pharmacological properties and therapeutic efficacy in depressive illness. Drugs (1978) 16, 273.

Hypoglycaemic agents + Miconazole

Abstract/Summary

Hypoglycaemia has been seen in diabetics taking tolbutamide, glibenclamide or gliclazide when they were concurrently treated with miconazole.

Clinical evidence, mechanism, importance and management

A diabetic patient taking tolbutamide was hospitalized with severe hypoglycaemia about 10 days after starting to take miconazole.[1] In 1983 the French Commission Nationale de Pharmacovigilance reported six cases of hypoglycaemia in diabetics on sulphonylureas within 2–6 days of beginning treatment with miconazole (five with gliclazide and one with glibenclamide).[1] The same organisation report a further nine cases in the 1986–1990 period but individual sulphonylureas were not named.[3] Three other cases (two on gliclazide and one on glibenclamide) are reported elsewhere in patients given miconazole (250–1250 mg daily).[2]

Mechanism

Not understood. It is thought that the miconazole inhibits the metabolism of the sulphonylureas by the liver, causing them to accumulate and thereby increasing their effects.[3]

Importance and management

An established and clinically important interaction but the incidence is uncertain, probably small. Concurrent use should be monitored and the dosage of the sulphonylurea reduced as necessary. Patients should be warned. Information about other sulphonylureas not cited is lacking but it seems possible that they may interact similarly.

References

1 Meurice JC, Lecomte P, Renard JP, Girard JJ. Interaction miconazole et sulfamides hypoglycemiants. La Presse Medicale. (1983) 12, 1670.
2 Loupi E, Descotes J, Lery N, Evreux JCl. Interactions medicamenteuses et miconazole. A propos de 10 observations. Therapie (1982) 37, 437–41.
3 Girardin E, Vial T, Pham E, Evreux J-C. Hypoglycémies induites par les sulfamides hypoglycémiants. Ann Med Interne (1992) 143, 11–17.

Hypoglycaemic agents + Monoamine oxidase inhibitors (MAOI)

Abstract/Summary

The hypoglycaemic effects of insulin and the oral hypoglycaemic agents can be increased by the concurrent use of the MAOI. This may improve the control of blood sugar levels in most diabetics, but in a few it may cause undesirable hypoglycaemia. This can be controlled by reducing the dosage of the hypoglycaemic agent. Moclobemide appears not to interact.

Clinical evidence

A woman diabetic, stabilized on insulin-zinc suspension, exhibited hypoglycaemic sopors and postural syncope when treated with 15–25 mg mebanazine daily. She required a 30% reduc-

tion in the dosage of insulin (from 48 to 35 units daily) to achieve restabilization. Her insulin requirements rose once again when the mebanazine was withdrawn.[1]

Other reports on diabetics showed that the concurrent use of mebanazine increased the hypoglycaemic activity of insulin, tolbutamide and chlorpropamide, and improved the control of their diabetes.[2–5] No clinically relevant interaction is reported to occur between glibenclamide and moclobemide.[9] A study in normal subjects on 2.5 mg glibenaclamide daily found that 200 mg moclobemide three times daily for a week had no effect on glucose or insulin concentrations after oral glucose tolerance tests.[10] Clinical trials in eight diabetics taking glibenclamide, gliclazide, metformin and chlorpropamide also found that moclobemide had no effect on blood gluocose levels or any other evidence of an interaction.

Mechanism

Not fully understood. A reduction in blood sugar levels has been demonstrated in man in the absence of conventional hypoglycaemic agents with mebanazine,[3] iproniazid,[6] isocarboxazid,[7] and phenelzine,[3] possibly due to some direct action by the MAOI on the pancreas which causes the release of insulin.[8] It would seem that this can be additive with the effects of the conventional hypoglycaemics.

Importance and management

An established interaction of only moderate clinical importance. It can benefit the control of diabetes in many patients, but some individuals may need a reduction in their hypoglycaemic agent dosage to avoid excessive hypoglycaemia. The effects of concurrent use should be monitored. Only a few MAOI-hypoglycaemic agent combinations appear to have been examined, but this interaction would seem possible with any of them. This requires confirmation.

Reference

1 Cooper AJ, Keddie KMG. Hypotensive collapse and hypoglycaemia after mebanazine-a monoamine oxidase inhibitor. Lancet (1964) i, 1133.
2 Wickstrom L and Pettersson K. Treatment of diabetics with monoamine oxidase inhibitors. Lancet (1964) ii, 995.
3 Adnitt PI. Hypoglycaemic actions of monoamine oxidase inhibitors (MAOI's). Diabetes (1968) 17, 628.
4 Cooper AJ. The action of mebanazine, a monoamine oxidase inhibitor antidepressant drug in diabetes-part II. Int J Neuropsychiatry (1966) 2, 342.
5 Adnitt PI, Oleesky S, Schneiden H. The hypoglycaemic action of monoamine oxidase inhibitors (MAOI's). Diabetologia (1968) 4, 379.
6 Weiss J, Weiss S, Weiss B. Effects of iproniazid and similar compounds on the gastrointestinal tract. Ann NY Acad Sci (1959) 80, 854.
7 Van Praag HM, Leijnse B. The influence of some antidepressives of the hydrazine type on the glucose metabolism in depressed patients. Clin Chim Acta (1963) 8, 466.
8 Bressler R, Vargas-Cordon M, Lebovitz HE. Tranylcypromine: a potent insulin secretagogue and hypoglycaemic agent. Diabetes (1968) 17, 617.
9 Zimmer R, Gieschke R, Fischbach R, Gasic S. Interaction studies with moclobemide. Acta Psychiatr Scand (1990) Suppl 360, 84–6.
10 Amrein R, Güntert TW, Dingemanse J, Lorscheid T, Stabl M, Schmid-Burgk W. Interactions of moclobemide with concomitantly administered

medication: evidence from pharmacological and clinical studies. Psychopharmacology (1992) 106, S24–31.

Hypoglycaemic agents + Naftidrofuryl oxalate

Abstract/Summary, clinical evidence, mechanism, importance and management

There are two very brief reports describing severe hypoglycaemia during the concurrent use of glibenclamide and naftidrofuryl oxalate, possibly due to an interaction.[1] No details are given.

Reference

1 Beeley L, Magee P, Hickey FN. Bulletin of the West Midlands Centre for Adverse Drug Reaction Reporting (1990) 30, 17.

Hypoglycaemic agents + Non-steroidal anti-inflammatory drugs (NSAIDs)

Abstract/Summary

No adverse interactions normally occur between chlorpropamide or tolbutamide and ibuprofen; glibenclamide and acemetacin, diclofenac, tenoxicam or tolmetin; glipizide or tolbutamide and indoprofen; glibornuride and tenoxicam; or between tolbutamide and diflunisal, naproxen or sulindac. There are isolated case reports of hypoglycaemia in patients given fenclofenac with chlorpropamide and metformin, and glibenclamide with diflunisal. Another describes loss of diabetic control attributed to indomethacin. Indobufen increases the effects of glipizide, and piroxicam increases the effects of glibenclamide. See the Index for interactions with azapropazone, phenylbutazone, oxyphenbutazone and the salicylates.

Clinical evidence

(a) Chlorpropamide or Tolbutamide + Ibuprofen

1200 mg ibuprofen had no significant effect on the blood sugar levels of diabetic patients taking 62.5–375 mg chlorpropamide daily.[7] In other patients on tolbutamide it was found that ibuprofen lowered fasting blood sugar levels, but not below the normal lower limits.[8]

(b) Chlorpropamide + Fenclofenac or Flurbiprofen

A woman diabetic, well controlled on 500 mg chlorpropamide and 850 mg metformin daily, developed hypoglycaemia within two days of exchanging flurbiprofen + indomethacin for 1200 mg fenclofenac daily. The hypoglycaemic agents were withdrawn the next day, but later in the evening she went into a hypoglycaemic coma. The reasons for this are not understood.[5] However another isolated report briefly describes loss of diabetic control with chlorpropamide possibly due to indomethacin.[16]

(c) Glibenclamide + Acemetacin, Diclofenac, Diflunisal, Tenoxicam or Tolmetin

The blood sugar levels of 12 glibenclamide-treated diabetics with rheumatic diseases remained unchanged when they were concurrently treated with 150 mg diclofenac daily for 4 days,[2] but an isolated case of hypoglycaemia has been reported with diflunisal.[17] No changes were seen in the blood sugar levels of 40 other diabetics on glibenclamide given 1200 mg tolmetin daily for 5 days.[6] No changes in the control of diabetes was seen in 20 patients on glibenclamide when concurrently treated with 60 mg acemetacin three times daily.[12] 20 mg tenoxicam daily was found not to affect the glycoregulation of 12 normal subjects given 2.5 mg glibenclamide daily.[13] Normal subjects and diabetics showed an increased hypoglycaemic response to glibenclamide (blood sugar levels down 13–15%) when additionally given 10 mg piroxicam.[18]

(d) Glibornuride + Tenoxicam

A study in normal subjects found that tenoxicam did not affect the pharmacokinetics of glibornuride nor the responses of plasma insulin and blood glucose to glibornuride.[14]

(e) Glipizide + Indobufen

Six normal subjects showed a rise in serum glipizide levels when treated with 200 mg indobufen for 15 days and blood sugar levels were lowered.[11]

(f) Glipizide or Tolbutamide + Indoprofen

No important changes in blood sugar levels occurred in 24 diabetic patients on tolbutamide or glipizide when given 600 mg indoprofen daily for 5 days.[10] A single dose study showed that although 200 mg indoprofen lowered the plasma levels of 5 mg glipizide, the blood sugar levels remained unaffected.[9]

(g) Tolbutamide + Diflunisal, Naproxen or Sulindac

A brief report states that no changes in serum tolbutamide or in fasting blood glucose levels were seen in diabetics given 375 mg diflunisal twice daily.[3,4] 12 maturity-onset tolbutamide-treated diabetics demonstrated no changes in tolbutamide half-life, serum levels, time-to-peak or AUC when given 400 mg sulindac daily. An unimportant reduction in fasting blood sugar levels was seen.[1] Naproxen (375 mg 12-hourly) had no effect on the pharmacokinetics or pharmacological effects of tolbutamide when given to 10 maturity onset diabetics over 3 days.[15]

Importance and management

The reports briefly quoted here indicate that no adverse interaction normally occurs between the oral hypoglycaemic agents and the NSAIDs cited. The general quietness in the literature would seem to add confirmation, but some caution is needed with fenclofenac and indobufen. In contrast, adverse interactions can certainly occur between hypoglycaemic agents and azapropazone, phenylbutazone, oxyphenbutazone and salicylates, details of which are given in the appropriate synopses. See Index.

References

1 Ryan JR, Jain MD, McMahon FG, Vargas R. On the question of an interaction between sulindac and tolbutamide in the treatment of diabetes. Clin Pharmacol Ther (1976) 21, 231.

2 Chlud K, von. Untersuchungen zur Wechselwirkung von Diclofenac und Glibenclamid. Zeit Rheumatologie (1976) 35, 377.

3 Tempero KF, Cirillo VJ, Steelman SL. Diflunisal: a review of the pharmacokinetic and pharmacodynamic properties, drug interactions, and special tolerability studies in human. Br J Clin Pharmac (1977) 4, 31S.

4 McMahon FG, Ryan JR. Unpublished observations quoted in ref. 3.

5 Allen PA, Taylor RT. Fenclofenac and thyroid function tests. Brit Med J (1980) 281, 1642.

6 Chlud K, Kaik B. Clinical studies of the interaction between tolmetin and glibenclamide. J Clin Pharmacol (1977) 15, 409.

7 Shah SJ, Bhandarkar SD, Satoskar RS. Drug interaction between chlorpropamide and non-steroidal anti-inflammatory drugs, ibuprofen and phenylbutazone. Int J Clin Pharmacol Ther Toxicol (1984) 22, 470–2.

8 Andersen LA. Ibuprofen and tolbutamide drug interaction study. Br J Clin Pract (1980) 34 (Suppl 6) 10.

9 Melander A, Wahlin-Boll E. Interaction of glipizide and indoprofen. Eur J Rheum Inflamm (1981) 4, 22–5.

10 Pedrazzi F, Bommartini F, Freddo J, Emanueli A. A study of the possible interaction of indoprofen with hypoglycemic sulphonylureas in diabetic patients. Eur J Rheum Inflamm (1981) 4, 26–31.

11 Elvander-Stahl E, Melander A, Wahlin-Boll E. Indobufen interacts with the sulphonylurea, glipizide, but not with the beta-adrenergic receptor antagonists, propranolol and atenolol. Br J Clin Pharmac (1984) 18, 773–8.

12 Haupt E, Hoppe FK, Rechziegler H, Zundorf P. Zur Frage der Interaktionen von nichtsteroidalen Antirheumatika mit oralen Antidiabetika: Acemetacin--Glibenclamid. Z. Rheumatol (1987) 46, 170–3.

13 Hartmann D, Korn A, Komjati M, Heinz G, Haefelfinger P, Defoin R, Waldhäusl WK. Lack of effect of tenoxicam on dynamic response to concurrent oral doses of glucose and glibenclamide. Br J Clin Pharmac (1990) 30, 245–52.

14 Stoeckel K, Trueb V, Dubach UC, Heintz RC, Ascalone V, Forgo I, Hennes U. lack of effect of tenoxicam on glibornuride kinetics and response. Br J Clin Pharmac (1985) 19, 249–54.

15 Whiting B, Williams RL, Lorenzi M, Varady JC, Robins DS. Effect of naproxen on glucose metabolism and tolbutamide kinetics and dynamics in maturity onset diabetics. Br J Clin Pharmac (1981) 11, 295–302.

16 Beeley L, Beadle F, Elliott D. Bulletin W Midlands Centre for Adverse Drug Reactions Reporting (1985) 21, 19.

17 Girardin E, Vial T, Pham E, Evreux J-C. Hypoglycémies induites par les sulfamides hypoglycémiants. Ann Med Interne (1992) 143, 11–17.

18 Diwan PV, Sastry MSP, Satyanarayana NV. Potentiation of hypoglycaemic response of glibenclamide by piroxicam in rats and humans. Ind J Exp Biol (1992) 30, 317–9.

Hypoglycaemic agents + Phenylbutazone or Oxyphenbutazone

Abstract/Summary

The hypoglycaemic effects of tolbutamide, acetohexamide, chlorpropamide, carbutamide, glymidine and glibenclamide can be increased by the concurrent use of phenylbutazone. Severe hypoglycaemia has occurred in a few patients. Oxyphenbutazone may be expected to behave similarly.

Clinical evidence

A diabetic man under treatment with tolbutamide experienced an acute hypoglycaemic episode 4 days after beginning to take 200 mg phenylbutazone three times a day, although there was no change in his diet or in the dosage of tolbutamide. He was able to control the hypoglycaemia by eating a large bar of chocolate.[1]

There are numerous other case reports and studies of this interaction involving phenylbutazone with tolbutamide,[2,4,5,8,10,11,17,21] carbutamide,[3] acetohexamide,[6] chlorpropamide,[11,20] glibenclamide,[12] and glymidine,[18,19] some of which describe acute hypoglycaemic episodes.[2,5,6,10] There is a report suggesting that the glibornuride-phenylbutazone may not be clinically important.[7] Oxyphenbutazone has been shown to interact with glymidine[13] and tolbutamide.[15,16] In contrast to these reports, a single study describes a paradoxical rise in blood sugar levels in three negro patients while receiving tolbutamide and phenylbutazone.[14] In addition to these reports there is some evidence that tolbutamide increases the metabolism of phenylbutazone by 42%,[21] but the extent to which this affects its therapeutic effects is uncertain.

Mechanism

Not fully resolved. Some evidence shows that phenylbutazone can inhibit the renal excretion of glibenclamide,[12] tolbutamide,[8] and the active metabolite of acetohexamide[6] so that they are retained in the body longer and their hypoglycaemic effects are increased and prolonged. It has also been shown that phenylbutazone can inhibit the metabolism of the sulphonylureas[15,21] as well as causing their displacement from protein binding sites.[9]

Importance and management

Well-documented and potentially clinically important interactions. Blood sugar levels may be lowered, but the number of reports of acute hypoglycaemic episodes seems to be small. Concurrent use should therefore be well monitored. A reduction in the dosage of the sulphonylurea may be necessary if excessive hypoglycaemia is to be avoided. Not all sulphonylureas have been shown to interact (glibornuride probably does not do so) but it would be prudent to assume that they all interact until the contrary is proved. Oxyphenbutazone may be expected to interact similarly (it is the metabolite of phenylbutazone).

References

1 Mahfouz M, Abdel-Maguid R, El-Dakhakhny M. Potentiation of the hypoglycaemic action of tolbutamide by different drugs. Arzneim-Forsch (1970) 20, 120.

2 Dalgas M, Christiansen I, Kjerulf K. Fenylbutazoninduceret hypoglykaemitilfaelde hos klorpropamidbehandlet diabetiker. Ugeskr Laeg (1965) 127, 834.

3 Kaindl F, Kretschy A, Puxkandl H, Wutte J. Zur steigerung des Wirkundseffektes peroraler Antidiabetika durch Pyrazolonderivate. Wien Klin Wcsch (1961) 73, 79.

4 Gulbrandsen R. Okt tolbutamid-effekt ved hjelp av fenylbutazon? Tidskr Norsk Laeg (1959) 79, 1127.

5 Tannenbaum H, Anderson LG and Soeldner JS. Phenylbutazone-tolbutamide drug interaction. N Engl J Med (1974) 290, 344.

6 Field JB, Ohata M, Boyle C, Remer A. Potentiation of acetohexamide hypoglycaemia by phenylbutazone. N Engl J Med (1967) 277, 889.

7 Eckhardt W, Rudolph R, Sauer H, Schubert WR, Undeutsch D. Zur pharmackologischen Interferenz von Glibornurid mit Sulfaphenazol, Phenylbutazon und Phenprocoumon beim Menschen. Arzneim-Forsch (1972) 22, 2212.

8 Ober K-F. Mechanism of interaction of tolbutamide and phenylbutazone in diabetic patients. Europ J Clin Pharmacol (1974) 7, 291.

9 Hellman B. Potentiating effects of drugs on the binding of glibenclamide to pancreatic beta cells. Metabolism (1974) 23, 839.

10 Dent LA and Jue SG. Tolbutamide + phenylbutazone: a dangerous and predictable interaction. Drug Intell Clin Pharm (1976) 10, 711.

11 Schulz E. Severe hypoglycaemic reactions after tolbutamide, carbutamide and chlorpropamide. Arch Klin Med (1968) 214, 135.

12 Schulz E, Koch K, Schmidt FH. Ursachen der Potenzierung der hypoglykamischen Wirkung von Sulfonylharnstoffderivaten durch Medikamente. II. Pharmakokinetik und Metabolismus von Glibenclamid (HN 419) in Gegenwart von Phenylbutazon. Eur J Clin Pharmacol (1971) 4, 32.

13 Held H, Scheible G, von Olderhausen HF. Uber Stoffwechsel under Interferenz von Arzneimittelen bei Gesunden und Leberkranken. Kongress fur Innere Medizin (Wiesbaden) (1970) 76, 1153.

14 Owasu SK, Ocran K. Paradoxical behaviour of phenylbutazone in African diabetics. Lancet (1972) i, 440.

15 Pond SM, Birkett J, Wade DN. Mechanisms of inhibition of tolbutamide metabolism: phenylbutazone, oxyphenbutazone, sulfafenazole. Clin Pharmacol Ther (1977) 22, 573.

16 Kristensen M, Christensen LK. Modificazioni dell'effeto ipoglicemizzante del farmaci ipoglicemizzanti indotte da altri farmaci. Acta diabet lat (Milan) (1969) six (Suppl 1) 116.

17 Christensen LK, Hansen JM, Kristensen M. Sulphaphenazole-induced hypoglycaemic attacks in tolbutamide-treated diabetics. Lancet (1963) ii, 1298.

18 Held H, Kaminski B and von Olderhausen HF. Die beeinflussung der Elimination von Glycodiazin durch Leber und Nierenfunktionsstorungen und durch eine Behandlung mit Phenylbutazon, Phenprocoumarol und Doxycyclin. Diabetologia (1970) 6, 386.

19 Held von H, Scheible G. Interaktion von Phenylbutazon und Oxyphenbutazon mit glymidine. Arzneim-Forschd/Drug Res. (1981) 31, 1036–8.

20 Shah SJ, Bhandarkar SD, Satoskar RS. Drug interaction between chlorpropamide and non-steroidal anti-inflammatory drugs, ibuprofen and phenylbutazone. Int J Clin Pharmacol Ther Toxicol (1984) 22, 470–2.

21 Szita M, Gacháalyi B, Tornyossy M, Kálsor A. Interaction of phenylbutazone and tolbutamide in man. Int J Clin Pharmacol Ther Toxicol (1980) 18, 378–80.

Hypoglycaemic agents + Phenylephrine

Abstract/Summary

Insulin-dependent diabetics can develop elevated blood pressures if treated with phenylephrine eye-drops.

Clinical evidence, mechanism, importance and management

A comparative study of 14 insulin-dependent diabetics who over a period of 2 h before ocular surgery were given phenylephrine eye-drops (a total of four doses of one or two drops of 10%), showed that they demonstrated an average blood pressure rise of 34/17 mmHg, whereas another 176 non-diabetic patients similarly treated showed no increases in blood pressure.[1] The reason for this pressor reaction is not understood but clearly enough phenylephrine was absorbed systemically to stimulate the adrenoceptors of the sympathetic system which innervates the cardiovascular system. The authors of this report say that they readily controlled these hypertensive reactions with halothane and by neuroleptanalgesia accompanying regional block with anaesthesia standby. Strictly speaking this is not a drug interaction, but a drug-disease reaction. The mydriatic dosage of phenylephrine should be reduced in insulin-dependent diabetics but whether this is also true for non insulin-dependent diabetics is uncertain.

Reference

1 Kim JM, Stevenson CE, Mathewson HS. Hypertensive reactions to phenylephrine eyedrops in patients with sympathetic denervation. Am J Ophthalmol (1978) 85, 862–8.

Hypoglycaemic agents + Phenyramidol

Abstract/Summary

The hypoglycaemic effects of tolbutamide are increased by phenyramidol but the clinical importance of this is uncertain.

Clinical evidence, mechanism, importance and management

The half-life of tolbutamide was increased from 7 to 18 h and serum tolbutamide levels raised in three normal subjects after taking 1200 mg phenyramidol daily for 4 days because (so it is suggested) the phenyramidol inhibits the metabolism of the tolbutamide by the liver, thereby prolonging its stay in the body.[1] A reduction in the dosage of tolbutamide may be necessary to avoid excessive hypoglycaemia, but this requires confirmation. Information about other sulphonylureas is lacking.

Reference

1 Solomon HM, Schrogie JJ. Effect of phenyramidol and bishydroxycoumarin on the metabolism of tolbutamide in human subjects. Metabolism (1967) 16, 1029.

Hypoglycaemic agents + Probenecid

Abstract/Summary

The clearance of chlorpropamide from the body is prolonged by probenecid, but the clinical importance of this is uncertain.

Clinical evidence, mechanism, importance and management

A study in six patients given single oral doses of chlorpropamide showed that the concurrent use of probenecid (1–2 g daily) increased its half-life from about 36 to 50 h.[1] It seems that the probenecid reduces the renal excretion of chlorpropamide. Another report claimed that the half-life of tolbutamide was also prolonged by probenecid,[2] but this was not confirmed by another properly controlled study.[3]

Information is very limited but it may possibly be necessary to reduce the dosage of the chlorpropamide in the presence of probenecid. Information about other sulphonylureas (with the exception of tolbutamide) appears to be lacking.

References

1 Petitpierre B, Perrin L, Rudhardt M, Herrera A, Fabre J. Behaviour of chlorpropamide in renal insufficiency and under the effect of associated drug therapy. Int J Clin Pharmacol (1972) 6, 120.
2 Stowers JM, Mahler RF, Hunter RB. Pharmacology and mode of action of the sulphonylureas in man. Lancet (1958) i, 278.
3 Brook R, Schrogie JJ, Solomon HM. Failure of probenecid to inhibit the rate of metabolism of tolbutamide in man. Clin Pharmacol Ther (1968) 9, 314.

Hypoglycaemic agents + Quinine or Quinidine

Abstract/Summary

Patients with falciparum malaria who are treated with quinine or quinidine may show very severe hypoglycaemia. The impact of this on the control of diabetes has yet to be determined. Quinine very occasionally causes hypoglycaemia in non-diabetics.

Clinical evidence, mechanism, importance and management

Patients with severe faciparum malaria who are treated with quinine may develop severe and life-threatening hypoglycaemia.[1,2] The reasons are not fully understood but it seems that in these patients the quinine causes the release of large amounts of insulin from the pancreas, possibly associated with an increase in the sensitivity to insulin as the malaria improves,[4] although other factors may also be involved. Quinidine has been shown to have a similar effect.[3] Whether these changes can also occur in patients with malaria and diabetes, despite their pancreatic beta cell impairment, seems not to have been studied, but any interpretation of disturbances in the control of the diabetes should take into account these possible effects of quinine or quinidine. Chloroquine, amodiaquine, mefloquine and halofantrine do not apparently stimulate the release of insulin.[3]

Quinine has also been responsible for hypoglycaemia in non-diabetic patients, one of whom was taking 325 mg four times daily for leg muscle cramps.[5] Two other non-diabetic patients, one with congestive heart failure and the other with terminal cancer, similarly developed hypoglycaemia when given quinine for leg cramps.

References

1 White NJ, Warrell DA, Chanthavanich P, Looareesuwan S, Warrell MJ, Krishna S, Williamson DH, Turner RC. Severe hypoglycaemia and hyperinsulinemia in falciparum malaria. N Engl J Med (1983) 309, 61–6.
2 Looareesuwan S, Phillips RE, White NJ, Kietinun S, Karbwang J, Rackow C, Turner RC, Warrell DA. Quinine and severe falciparum malaria in late pregnancy. Lancet (1985) ii, 4–8.
3 Phillips RE, Looaressuwan S, White NJ, Chanthavanich P, Karbwang J, Supanaranond W, Turner RC, Warrell DA. Hypoglycaemia and antimalarial drugs: quinidine and release of insulin. Br Med J (1986) 292, 1319–21.
4 Davis TME, Pukrittayakamee S, Supanaranond W, Looareesuwan S, Krishna S, Nagachinta B, Turner RC, White NJ. Glucose metabolism in quinine-treated patients with uncomplicated falciparum malaria. Clin Endocrinol (1990) 33, 739–49.
5 Limburg PJ, Katz H, Grant CS, Service FJ. Quinine-induced hypoglycaemia. Ann Intern Med (1993) 119, 218
6 Harats N, Ackerman Z, Shalit M. Quinine-related hypoglycemia. N Engl J Med (1984) 310, 1331.
7 Jones RG, Sue-Ling HM, Kear C, Wiles PG, Quirke P. Severe symptomatic hypoglycemia due to quinine therapy. J Roy Soc Med (1986) 79, 426–8.

Hypoglycaemic agents + Rifampicin (Rifampin)

Abstract/Summary

Rifampicin reduces the serum levels of tolbutamide, glycodiazine, chlorpropamide (single case) and glibenclamide (single case). A reduction in the hypoglycaemic effects of these sulphonylureas would be expected.

Clinical evidence

After 4 weeks' treatment with rifampicin the half-life of tolbutamide in nine patients with tuberculosis was reduced by 43%, and the serum concentrations measured at 6 h were halved compared with other patients not taking rifampicin.[1]

Similar results have been found in other studies in patients with cirrhosis or cholestasis,[2] in normal subjects[3] and in other patients.[6] The half-life of glymidine in man is also approximately halved by the concurrent use of rifampicin.[4] A single case report describes a diabetic man who needed an increase in his daily dosage of chlorpropamide from 250 to 400 mg daily when he was given 600 mg rifampicin daily, and a reduction 12 months later when the rifampicin was withdrawn.[5] Another diabetic showed a marked rise in serum glibenclamide levels (trough levels from 40 to 200 ng/ml) when rifampicin was stopped, but no hypoglycaemia occurred.[7]

Mechanism

Rifampicin is a potent inducer of the liver microsomal enzymes concerned with the metabolism of tolbutamide and other drugs, which hastens their clearance from the body, thereby reducing their effects.[1-3]

Importance and management

The tolbutamide-rifampicin interaction is established. Patients taking tolbutamide may need an increase in the dosage while taking rifampicin (possibly roughly doubled, but this needs confirmation). This also seems possibly to be true for glymidine, glibenclamide and chlorpropamide, but the documentation about these three drugs is very limited indeed. Information about other hypoglycaemic agents does not seem to be available.

References

1 Syvalahti EKG, Pihlajamaki KK, Ilsalo EJ. Rifampicin and drug metabolism. Lancet (1974) i, 232.
2 Zilly W, Breimer DD, Richter E. Stimulation of drug metabolism by rifampicin in patients with cirrhosis or cholestasis measured by increased hexobarbital and tolbutamide clearance. Eur J Clin Pharmacol (1977) 11, 287.
3 Zilly W, Breimer DD, Richter E. Induction of drug metabolism in man after rifampicin treatment measured by hexobarbital and tolbutamide clearance. Eur J Clin Pharmacol (1975) 9, 219.
4 Held HK, Schoene B, Laar HJ, Fleischmann R. Die Aktivat der Benzepyrenhydroxylaze im Leberpunktat des Menschen in vitro und ihre Beziehung zur Eliminations-geschwindigkeit von Glycodiazin in vivo. Verhandhlungen der Deutschen Gesellschaft fur Innere Medizin (1974) 80, 501.
5 Self TH, Morris T. Interaction of rifampin and chlorpropamide. Chest (1980) 77, 800-1.
6 Syvalahti E, Pihlajamki K, Iisalo E. Effect of tuberculostatic agents on the response of serum growth hormone and immunoreactive insulin to intravenous tolbutamide, and on the half-life of tolbutamide. Int J Clin Pharmacol (1976) 13, 83-9.
7 Self TH, Tsiu SJ, Fowler JW. Interaction of rifampin and glyburide. Chest (1989) 96, 1443-4.

Hypoglycaemic agents + Salicylates

Abstract/Summary

Aspirin and other salicylates can lower blood sugar levels, but small analgesic doses do not normally have an adverse effect on patients taking hypoglycaemic agents. Some reduction in the dosage of the hypoglycaemic agent may be appropriate if large doses of salicylate are used.

Clinical evidence

(a) Insulin

12 juvenile diabetics treated with insulin showed a reduction in blood glucose levels averaging 15% (from 188 to 159 mg%) when additionally given either 1200 mg daily doses of aspirin (patients under 60 lb) or 2400 mg (patients over 60 lb) daily for a week. No significant changes in insulin requirements were necessary.[1]

Eight patients on 12–48 U insulin zinc suspension daily required no insulin when treated for 2–3 weeks with aspirin in doses large enough to give blood concentrations of 350–450 mg/ml. Six other patients were able to reduce their insulin requirements by about a half (from 22–112 to 10–72 U).[5]

(b) Chlorpropamide

A study in five normal subjects showed that the blood glucose lowering effects of chlorpropamide and sodium salicylate were additive; a further study on six subjects showed that 100 mg chlorpropamide with 1.5 g sodium salicylate lowered blood sugar levels the same amount as either 200 mg chlorpropamide or 3 g sodium salicylate.[6]

The blood glucose levels of a patient on 500 mg chlorpropamide daily were lowered about two-thirds by aspirin in doses sufficient to give serum salicylate levels of 26 mg%.[2]

Mechanism

It has been known for over 100 years that aspirin and salicylates have hypoglycaemic properties and in relatively large doses can be used on their own in the treatment of diabetes.[3,4,8,9] The simplest explanation for this interaction is that the blood sugar lowering effects are additive,[6] but there is some evidence that other mechanisms may some into play.[10] In addition aspirin can raise serum chlorpropamide levels so that its effects are increased, possibly by interfering with renal tubular excretion.[2]

Importance and management

An established interaction but of limited importance. Considering the extremely wide use of aspirin it might reasonably be expected that any generally serious interaction would have come to light by now. The data available, coupled with the common experence of diabetics,[7] is that excessive and unwanted hypoglycaemia is very unlikely with small analgesic doses. Some downward readjustment of the dosage of the hypoglycaemic agent may be appropriate if large doses of salicylates are used. Information about other hypoglycaemic agents and salicylates appears to be lacking, but they may be expected to behave similarly

References

1 Kay R, Athreya BH, Kunzman EE, Baker L. Antipyretics in patients with juvenile diabetes mellitus. Amer J Dis Child (1966) 112, 52.
2 Stowers JM, Constable LW and Hunter RB. A clinical and pharmacological comparison of chlorpropamide and other sulfonylureas. Ann NY Acad Sci (1959) 74, 689.
3 Gilgore SG, Rupp JJ. The long-term response of diabetes mellitus to salicylate therapy. Report of a case. J Amer Med Ass (1962) 180, 65.
4 Reid J, Macdougall AI, Andrews MM. Aspirin and diabetes mellitus. Br Med J (1957) 2, 1071.
5 Reid J, Lightbody TD. The insulin equivalence of salicylate. Br Med J (1959) 1, 897.
6 Richardson T, Foster J, Mawer GE. Enhancement by sodium salicylate of the blood glucose lowering effect of chlorpropamide--drug interaction or summation of similar effects? Br J Clin Pharmac (1986) 22, 43–48.
7 Logie AW, Galloway DB, Petrie JC. Drug interactions and long-term diabetic treatment. Br J Clin Pharmac (1976) 3, 1027–32.
8 Ebstein W. Zur Therapie des Diabetes mellitus, insbesondere über die Anwendung des Salizylsaüren Natrons bei demselben. Berl klin Wschr (1876) 13, 337.
9 Bartels K. Über die therapeutische Verwertung der Salizylsäure und ihres Nastronsalzes in der Inneren Medizin. Dtsch Med Wschr (1878) 4, 423.
10 Catteneo AG, Caviezel F, Pozza G. Pharmacological interaction between tolbutamide and acetylsalicylic acid: study on insulin secretion in man. Int J Clin Pharmacol Ther Toxicol (1990) 28, 229–34.

Hypoglycaemic agents + Sucralfate

Abstract/Summary

Sucralfate appears not to interact significantly with chlorpropamide.

Clinical evidence, mechanism, importance and management

A two-way cross-over study in 12 normal subjects showed that 1 g sucralfate four times a day 1 h before meals had no effect on the pharmacokinetics of a single 250 mg dose of chlorpropamide, except for a small but statistically significant change in the zero to infinity AUC.[1] This seems unlikely to be clinically important, but it needs confirmation. There seems to be no information about the effects of sucralfate on other hypoglycaemic agents.

Reference

1 Letendre PW, Carlson JD, Siefert RD, Dietz AJ, Dimmit D. Effect of sucralfate on the absorption and pharmacokinetics of chlorpropamide. J Clin Pharmacol (1986) 26, 622–5.

Hypoglycaemic agents + Sugar-containing pharmaceuticals

Abstract/Summary

Some pharmaceutical preparations such as cough linctuses, liquid antibiotics, bulk laxatives and others can contain significant amounts of sugar. Diabetics should be warned.

Clinical evidence, mechanism, importance and management

Many pharmaceuticals contain sugar in considerable amounts. Some liquid oral antibiotic preparations may contain up to 70% sucrose (e.g. *Broxil*, 7 g/10 ml, *Erythroped* Pi, 6.8 g/10 ml) and the sugar-content of many elixirs and linctuses (e.g. *Phensedyl*, 3.36 g per 5 ml dose) also may be high. The extent to which the administration of preparations like these will affect the control of diabetes clearly depends upon the amounts ingested, but the problem is by no means merely theoretical. One report[1] describes a significant loss of control in a woman diabetic with diverticulitis when she was prescribed a psyllium effervescent powder (*Metamucil* instant-mix) which contains sugar. The range of other sugar-containing preparations is far too extensive to be listed here, but diabetics should be made aware that sugar is present in a variety of pharmaceuticals in unsuspected guises and disguises. Unfortunately package labels are not always as informative as they might be. The National Pharmaceutical Association has published two very useful lists[2,3] of the sugar content of prescribed and over-the-counter medicines available in the UK, one of them drawn up in collaboration with the British Diabetic Association.[3] Another valuable list appeared in the Pharmaceutical Journal.[4]

References

1 Catellani J, Collins RJ. Drug labelling. Lancet (1978) ii, 98.
2 The NPA notes for proprietors. Sugar content of medicines. Published by the National Pharmaceutical Association, Mallinson House, 40–42 St Peters Street, St Albans, Herts, England. December (1986).
3 Carbohydrate content of proprietary medicines available without prescription. Published by the National Pharmaceutical Association (address above) and the British Diabetic Association, 10 Queen Anne St, London W1M 0BD. April (1987).
4 Greenwood J. Sugar content of liquid prescription medicines. Pharm J (1989) 243, 553–7.

Hypoglycaemic agents + Sulphinpyrazone

Abstract/Summary

Sulphinpyrazone has no effect on the insulin requirements of diabetics, nor does it affect the control of patients taking glibenclamide. There is good evidence that excessive hypoglycaemia might occur with tolbutamide, but as yet there appear to be no case reports of this interaction, nor of any adverse interactions with other hypoglycaemic agents.

Clinical evidence

(a) Insulin + Sulphinpyrazone

A double blind study, extending over 12 months, on 41 adult diabetics showed that the daily administration of 600–800 mg sulphinpyrazone had no clinically significant effects on their insulin requirements.[1]

(b) Glibenclamide + Sulphinpyrazone

A study of 19 Type II diabetics taking glibenclamide showed that 800 mg sulphinpyrazone daily did not affect the control of their diabetes.[3]

(c) Tolbutamide + Sulphinpyrazone

A detailed study of the pharmacokinetics of tolbutamide in six normal subjects showed that after taking 200 mg sulphinpyrazone every 6 h for a week, the half-life of tolbutamide was almost doubled (from 7.3 to 13.2 h) and the plasma clearance reduced by 40%.[2]

Mechanism

The available evidence suggests that the tolbutamide/sulphinpyrazone interaction occurs because the sulphinpyrazone inhibits the metabolism of tolbutamide by the liver.[2]

Importance and management

Information about the tolbutamide/sulphinpyrazone interaction appears to be limited to the report cited. So far there appear to be no reports of adverse interactions in patients, but what is known suggests that excessive hypoglycaemia could occur if the dosage of tolbutamide is not reduced. Such an interaction has been described with phenylbutazone with which sulphinpyrazone has a close structural similarity (see appropriate synopsis). There seems to be nothing documented about any other clinically important hypoglycaemic agent/sulphinpyrazone interaction.

References

1 Pannebakker MAG, den Ottolander JH and ten Pas, JG. Insulin requirements in diabetic patients treated with sulphinpyrazone. J Int Med Res (1979) 7, 328.
2 Miners JO, Foenander T, Wanwimolruk S, Gallus AS, Birkett DJ. The effect of sulphinpyrazone on oxidative drug metabolism in man: inhibition of tolbutamide elimination. Eur J Clin Pharmacol (1982) 22, 321.
3 Kritz H, Najemnik C, Irsigler K. Interaktionsstudie mit Sulfinpyrazon (Anduran) und Glibenclamid (Euglucon) bei Typ-II-Diabetikern. Wien Med Wschr (1983) 133, 237–43.

Hypoglycaemic agents + Sulphonamides

Abstract/Summary

The hypoglycaemic effects of chlorpropamide, glibenclamide, glibornuride, gliclazide and tolbutamide can be increased by some sulphonamides and acute hypoglycaemia sometimes occurs. Some sulphonylurea/sulphonamide pairs do not interact. There appear to be no reports of adverse insulin/sulphonamide interactions.

Clinical evidence

The Table 15.3 summarizes the information I have been able to trace on the hypoglycaemic agent/sulphonamide interactions.

Mechanism

Not fully understood. The sulphonamides may inhibit the metabolism of the sulphonylureas so that they accumulate in the body. In this way their serum levels and effects are

Table 15.3 Hypoglycaemic agent/Sulphonamide interactions

Drugs	Information documented	Refs
Chlorpropamide		
+ sulphafurazole (sulfisoxazole)	1 case of acute hypoglycaemia	7
+ sulphamethizole	1 case of acute hypoglycaemia	8
+ co-trimoxazole	2 cases of acute hypoglycaemia	9,14
Glibenclamide		
+ co-trimoxazole	11% incidence of hypoglycaemia	15
	8 cases of hypoglycaemia	19, 20
	Stated to be no pharmacokinetic interaction	17
Glibornuride		
+ sulphaphenazole	Stated to be no interaction	10
Gliclazide		
+ co-trimoxazole	4 cases of acute hypoglycaemia	20
Glipizide		
+ co-trimoxazole	1 case of acute hypoglycaemia	18
Tolbutamide		
+ co-trimoxazole	Clearance reduced 25%, half-life increased 30%	16
+ sulphafurazole (sulfisoxazole)	3 cases of severe hypoglycaemia	1,2
	2 reports state no interaction	6, 11
+ sulphamethizole	Half-life of tolbutamide increased 60%. Metabolic clearance reduced 40%	3, 4
+ sulphaphenazole	1 case of severe hypoglycaemia	5, 11
	Half-life of tolbutamide increased ×4–6	
+ sulphadiazine	Half-life of tolbutamide increased 50%	5
+ sulphadimethoxine	Stated to be no interaction	6
+ sulphamethoxy-pyridazine	Stated to be no interaction	6
+ sulphamethoxazole	Clearance reduced 14%, half-life increased 20%	16
Unnamed sulphonylurea		
+ co-trimoxazole	1 case of acute hypoglycaemia	13

enhanced.[3,5,6,12] There is also evidence that the sulphonamides can displace the sulphonylureas from their protein binding sites. Hypoglycaemia induced by sulphonamides, in the absence of a hypoglycaemic agent, and sometimes associated with renal failure has been described.

Importance and management

Established interactions of clinical importance, but of uncertain incidence. Serious interactions seem uncommon. Firm predictions cannot be made about what will, or what will not, interact in individual patients, nor how clinically important the reaction may prove to be, but table 15.2 can be used as a broad guide. Warn diabetics when first given a sulphonamide that increased hypoglycaemia, sometimes excessive, has been seen to occur. There appear to be no reports of adverse interactions in patients given insulin and a sulphonamide.

References

1 Soeldner JS, Steinke J. Hypoglycaemia in tolbutamide-treated diabetes. J Amer Med Ass (1965) 193, 148.
2 Robinson DS. The application of basic principles of drug interaction to clinical practice. J Urology (1975) 113, 100.
3 Lumholtz B, Siersbaek-Nielsen K, Skovsted L, Kampmann J, Hansen JM. Sulphamethizole-induced inhibition of diphenylhydantoin, tolbutamide, and warfarin metabolism. Clin Pharmacol Ther (1975) 17, 731.
4 Siersbaek-Nielsen K, Hansen JM, Skovsted L, Lumholtz B, Kampmann J. Sulphamethizole-induced inhibition of diphenylhydantoin and tolbutamide metabolism in man. Clin Pharmacol Ther (1973) 14, 148.
5 Kristensen M, Christensen LK. Drug induced changes of blood glucose lowering effect of oral hypoglycaemic agents. Acta diabet lat (1969) 6 (Suppl 1) 116.
6 Christensen IK, Hansen JM, Kristensen M. Sulphaphenazole-induced hypoglycaemic attacks in tolbutamide-treated diabetics. Lancet (1963) ii, 1298.
7 Tucker HSG and Hirsch JI. Sulphonamide-sulphonylurea interaction. N Eng J Med (1972) 286, 110.
8 Dall JLC, Conway H, McAlpine SG. Hypoglycaemia due to chlorpropamide. Scot Med J (1967) 12, 403.
9 Ek I. Langvarigt klorpropamidutlost hypoglykemitillstand Lakemedelsinteraktion? Lakartidningen (1974) 71, 2597.
10 Eckhardt W, Rudolph R, Sauer H, Schubert WR, Undeutsch D. Zur pharmakologischen Interferenz von Glibornurid mit Sulfaphenazol, Phenylbutazon und Phenprocoumon beim Menschen. Artzneim-Forsch (1972) 22, 2212.
11 Dubach UC, Buckert A, Raaflaub J. Einfluss von Sulfonamiden auf die blutzuckersenkende Wirkung oraler Antidiabetica. Schweiz med Wsch (1966) 96, 1483.
12 Hellman B. Potentiating effects of drugs on the binding of glibenclamide to pancreatic beta cells. Metabolism (1974) 23, 839.
13 Baciewicz AM, Swafford WB. Hypoglycaemia induced by the interaction of chlorpropamide and co-trimoxazole. Drug Intell Clin Pharm (1984) 181, 3093–3110.
14 Mihac M, Mautner LS, Feness JZ, Grant K. Effect of trimethoprim-sulphamethoxazole on blood insulin and glucose concentrations of diabetics. Can Med Assoc J (1975), 112, 80s.
15 Sjoberg S, Widholm BE, Gunnarsson R, Emilsson H, Thunberg E, Christenson I, Ostman J. No evidence for pharmacokinetic interaction between glibenclamide and trimethoprim-sulfametoxazole. Diabetes Res Clin Prac (1985) (Suppl 1) S 522.
16 Wing LMH and Miners JO. Co-trimoxazole as an inhibitor of oxidative drug metabolism effects of trimethoprim and sulfamethoxazole separately and combined on tolbutamide disposition. Br J Clin Pharmacol (1985) 20, 482–5.
17 Sjoberg S, Wiholm BE, Gunnarsson R, Emilsson H, Thunberg E, Christenson I, Ostman J. Lack of pharmacokinetic interaction between glibenclamide and trimethoprim-sulphamethoxazole. Diabet Med (1987) 4, 245–7.
18 Johnson JF, Dobmeier ME. Symptomatic hypoglycemia secondary to a glipizide-trimethoprim/sulfamethoxazole drug interaction. DICP Ann Pharmacotherapy (1990)24, 250–1.
19 Asplund K, Wiholm BE, Lithner F. Glibenclamide-associated hypoglycemia: a report on 57 cases. Diabetologia (1983) 24, 412–7.
20 Girardin E, Vial T, Pham E, Evreux J-C. Hypoglycémies induites par les sulfamides hypoglycémiants. Ann Med Interne (1992) 143, 11–17.

Hypoglycaemic agents + Tetracyclines

Abstract/Summary

A few scattered reports indicate that the hypoglycaemic effects of insulin and the sulphonylureas may sometimes be increased by oxytetracycline, and limited evidence suggests that this may also occur with doxycycline.

Clinical evidence

(a) Insulin or Sulphonylureas + Tetracyclines

A poorly controlled diabetic needed a marked reduction in his insulin dosage (from 104 to 62 units daily) in order to control the hypoglycaemia which developed when also given 250 mg oxytetracyline four times a day. This reaction was also seen in another patient.[1]

Marked hypoglycaemia occurred in an elderly patient on tolbutamide when given oxytetracycline,[2] and the hypoglycaemic effects of oxytetracycline have also been demonstrated in dogs.[2] Another study in diabetic subjects similarly showed that oxytetracycline can reduce blood sugar levels.[11] A very brief report describes hypoglycaemia in a patient on insulin when given doxycycline.[3] The half-life of glymidine in man has been shown to be prolonged from 4.6 to 7.6 h by doxycycline,[4] whereas a brief comment in another report suggests that demeclocycline may not affect chlorpropamide.[5]

(b) Biguanides + Tetracyclines

There are now at least six cases on record of lactic-acidosis in patients on phenformin which was apparently precipitated by the concurrent use of tetracycline.[6-10]

Mechanisms

Not understood.

Importance and management

Information about the interaction between the sulphonylureas or insulin and the tetracyclines is very limited indeed. Concurrent use need not be avoided but be alert for any signs of hypoglycaemia, particularly with oxytetracycline and doxycycline. Reduce the dosage of the hypoglycaemic agent if necessary. Phenformin has been withdrawn because of the high incidence of lactic acidosis but there is nothing to suggest that there is an increased risk if tetracyclines are given with metformin.

References

1 Miller JB. Hypoglycaemic effect of oxytetracycline. Brit Med J (1966) 2, 1007.
2 Hiatt N, Bonorris G. Insulin response in pancreatectomised dogs treated with oxytetracycline. Diabetes (1970) 19, 307–10.
3 New Zealand Committee on Adverse Drug Reactions. Ninth Annual Report. NZ Dent J (1975) 71, 28.
4 Held H, Kaminski B and von Olderhausen HF. Die beeinflussung der Elimination von Glycodiazin durch Leber- und Nierenfunctionssorungen und durch eine Behandlung mit Phenylbutazon, Phenprocoumarol und Doxycyclin. Diabetologica (1970) 6, 386.
5 Petitpierre B, Perrin L, Rudhardt M, Herrera A, Fabre J. Behaviour of chlorpropamide in renal insufficiency and under the effect of associated drug therapy. Int J Clin Pharmacol (1972) 6, 120.
6 Aro A, Korhonen T, Halinen M. Phenformin-induced lactic acidosis precipitated by tetracycline. Lancet (1978) 1, 673.
7 Tashima CK. Phenformin, tetracycline and lactic acidosis. Brit Med J (1971) 4, 557.
8 Blumenthal SA, Streeten DHP. Phenformin-related lactic acidosis in a 30-year old man. Ann Intern Med (1976) 84, 55.
9 Korhonen T, Idanpaan-Heikkila JE, Aro A. Unpublished data quoted in reference 6.
10 Philips PJ, Pain RW. Phenformin, tetracycline and lactic acidosis. Ann Intern Med (1977) 86, 111.
11 Sen S, Mukerjee AB. Hypoglycaemic action of oxytetracycline. A preliminary study. J Indian Med Ass (1969) 52, 366–9.

Hypoglycaemic agents + Thiazides, Chlorthalidone or related diuretics

Abstract/Summary

(a) By raising blood sugar levels, the thiazide diuretics, chlorthalidone and other related diuretics can reduce the effects of the hypoglycaemic agents and impair the control of diabetes. Some, but by no means all, patients will require a modest increase in the dosage of their hypoglycaemic agent. (b) Hyponatraemia also occurs occasionally.

Clinical evidence

(a) Reduced hypoglycaemic effects

Chlorothiazide, the first of the thiazide diuretics, was found within a year of its introduction in 1958 to have hyperglycaemic effects.[1] Since then a very large number of reports have described this same effect with other thiazides, the precipitation of diabetes in prediabetics, and the disturbance of blood sugar control in diabetics. One example from many:

A long-term study on 53 diabetics showed that treatment with chlorothiazide (0.5 or 1 g daily) or trichlormethiazole (4 or 8 mg daily) caused a mean rise in blood sugar levels from 120 to 140 mg%. Only seven patients needed a change in their treatment: four required more of their oral agent, two an increase in insulin, and one was transferred from tolbutamide to insulin. The oral agents used included tolbutamide, chlor-

propamide, acetohexamide and phenformin.[2]

A rise in blood sugar levels has been observed with bendrofluazide,[10] benzthiazide,[3] hydrochlorothiazide,[5] dihydroflumethiazide,[5] and chlorthalidone.[6]

(b) Hyponatraemia

A hospital report describes eight cases of low serum sodium concentrations observed over a 5-year period in patients taking chlorpropamide and *Moduretic* (hydrochlothiazide 50 mg + amiloride 5 mg).[11]

Mechanisms

(a) Not understood. One study suggested that the hyperglycaemia is due to some inhibition of insulin release by the pancreas.[9] Another is that the peripheral action of insulin is affected in some way.[8] There is also evidence that it may be related in part to potassium depletion. (b) The hyponatraemia appears to be due to the additive sodium-losing effects of the chlorpropamide, thiazide and amiloride.

Importance and management

(a) The reduction in hypoglycaemia is extremely well-documented but of only moderate practical importance. A full list of references is not given here to save space. The report of the study cited above[2] stated that '...it is not of serious degree... and in no patient was a dramatic deterioration of diabetic control observed.' The incidence is said to lie between 10 and 30%.[2,4] Concurrent use need not be avoided but the outcome should be monitored. There is evidence that the full effects may take many months to develop in some patients.[10] Most patients respond to a modest increase in the dosage of the hypoglycaemic agent, or to a change from an oral drug to insulin. The adverse hyperglycaemic effects can also be reversed significantly by the use of potassium supplements.[7]

In addition to the thiazides already named, the interaction may be expected to occur with the other thiazides in common use (cyclopenthiazide, cyclothiazide, methyclothiazide, polythiazide) and possibly related diuretics such as clopamide, clorexolone, metolazone, quinethazone etc. This requires confirmation. However see also Hypoglycaemics + Metolazone.

(b) Hyponatraemia seems to be uncommon but be aware that it can occur during concurrent use.

References

1 Wilkins RW. New drugs for the treatment of hypertension. Ann Intern Med (1959) 50,1.
2 Kansal PC, Buse J, Buse MG. Thiazide diuretics and control of diabetes mellitus. S Med J (1969) 62,1374.
3 Runyan JW. Influence of thiazide diuretics on carbohydrate metabolism in patients with mild diabetes. N Eng J Med (1961) 267,541.
4 Wolff FW, Parmley WW, White KW, Okun RJ. Drug-induced diabetes. Diabetogenic activity of long-term administration of benzothiadiazines. J Amer Med Ass (1963) 185,568.
5 Goldner MG, Zarowitz H, Akgun S. Hyperglycaemia and glycosuria due to

thiazide derivatives administered in diabetes mellitus. N Eng J Med (1960) 262,403.

6 Carliner NH, Schelling J-L, Russell RP, Okun R, Davis M. Thiazide- and phthalimidine-induced hyperglycaemia in hypertensive patients. J Amer Med Ass (1965) 191, 535.

7 Rapoport MI, Hurd HF. Thiazide-induced glucose intolerance treated with potassium. Arch Intern Med (1964) 113, 405.

8 Remenchik AP, Hoover C, Talso PJ. Insulin secretion by hypersensitive patients receiving hydroclorothiazide. J Amer Med Ass (1970) 212, 869.

9 Fajans SS, Floyd JC, Knopf RF, Rull J, Guntsche EM, Conn JW. Benzothiazide suppression of insulin release from normal and abnormal islet tissue in man. J Clin Invest (1966) 45, 481.

10 Lewis PJ, Kohner EM, Petrie A, Dollery CT. Deterioration of glucose tolerance in hypertensive patients on prolonged diuretic treatment. Lancet (1976) 1, 564–6.

11 Zalin AM, Hutchinson CE, Jong M, Matthews K. Hyponatraemia during treatment with chlorpropamide and *Moduretic* (amiloride plus hydrochlorothiazide). Br Med J (1984) 289, 659.

Hypoglycaemic agents + Tobacco smoking

Abstract/Summary

Diabetics who smoke need more insulin than those who do not.

Clinical evidence, mechanism, importance and management

Two studies[1,2] carried out on large numbers of insulin-dependent smokers showed that on average they needed 15–20% more insulin than non-smokers, and up to 30% more if they smoked heavily. This is apparently because smoking causes a significant rise (40–120%) in the levels of the hormones which oppose the actions of insulin.[3] A consequence of this interaction is that diabetics who give up smoking may need a downward adjustment of their insulin dosage.

References

1 Klemp P, Staberg B, Madsbad S, Kolendorf K. Smoking reduces insulin absorption from subcutaneous tissue. Brit Med J (1982) 284, 237.

2 Madsbad S, McNair P, Christensen MS, Christiansen C, Faber OK, Binder C, Transbol I. Influence of smoking on insulin requirement and metabolic status in diabetes mellitus. Diabetes Care (1980) 3, 41–3.

3 Helve E, Yki-Jarvinen H, Koivisto VA. Smoking and insulin sensitivity in type I diabetes. Diabetes Res Clin Prac (1985) (Suppl 1) S 232.

Hypoglycaemic agents + Tricyclic antidepressants

Abstract/Summary

Three isolated reports describe hypoglycaemia in three patients, one on tolazamide and the other on chlorpropamide shortly after starting treatment with doxepin and nortriptyline respectively, and the last on insulin when given amitriptyline.

Clinical evidence, mechanism, importance and management

A patient on tolazamide became hypoglycaemic 11 days after starting to take 75 mg doxepin daily; another on chlorpropamide developed marked hypoglycaemia three days after starting 125 mg nortriptyline daily;[2] a further patient on insulin developed violent and agitated behaviour (but no adrenergic symptoms) and hypoglycaemia when she started to take 25 mg amitriptyline at bedtime.[3] The reasons are not understood. An earlier study suggested that no interaction was likely: four patients given nine days' treatment with 25 mg amitriptyline daily showed no change in the half-life of a single 500 mg dose of tolbutamide.[1]

Apart from these cases the literature seems to be silent about interactions between these hypoglyaemics and the tricyclic antidepressants. Bearing in mind the length of time these groups of drugs have been available, the risk of a clinically important interaction would seem to be small, nevertheless be alert for any evidence of increased hypoglycaemia if both are given. The patient on doxepin was eventually stabilized on a daily dose of tolazamide which was only 10% of that used before the doxepin was given.[2]

References

1 Pond SM, Graham GG, Birkett DJ, Wade DN. Effects of tricyclic antidepressants on drug metabolism. Clin Pharmacol Ther (1975) 18, 191.

2 True BL, Perry PJ, Burns EA. Profound hypoglycemia with the addition of a tricyclic antidepressant to maintenance sulfonylurea therapy. Am J Psychiatry (1987) 144, 1220–1.

3 Sherman KE, Bornemann M. Amitriptyline and asymptomatic hypoglycaemia. Ann Intern Med (1988) 109, 683–4.

Hypoglycaemic agents + Urinary alkalinizers and acidifiers

Abstract/Summary

On theoretical grounds the response to chlorpropamide may be decreased if the urine is made alkaline, and increased if urine is acidified, but so far no adverse interactions appear to have been reported.

Clinical evidence, mechanism, importance and management

A study in six normal subjects given 250 mg oral doses of chlorpropamide showed that when their urinary pH was raised from 7.1 to 8.2 with sodium bicarbonate, the half-life of the chlorpropamide was reduced from 50 to 13 h, and the 72 h clearance was increased four-fold. In contrast, when their urinary pH was lowered from 5.5 to 4.7 with ammonium chloride, the chlorpropamide half-life was increased from 50 to 69 h and the 72 h urinary clearance was decreased to one-twentieth.[1] Another study showed that the renal clearance was almost 100 times greater at pH 7 than at pH 5.[2] The reasons are that changes in urinary pH affect the ionization of the chlorpropamide, and this affects the ability of the kidney to reabsorb it from the kidney filtrate (see more details of this interaction mechanism in the introductory chapter.)

There appear to be no reports of adverse interactions between chlorpropamide and drugs which can alter urinary pH, but prescribers should be aware of the possibilities: a reduced response if the pH is raised significantly (e.g. with sodium bicarbonate, acetazolamide, some antacids); an increased response if the pH is made more acid than usual (e.g. with ammonium chloride).

References

1 Neuvonen PJ, Karkkainen S. Effects of charcoal, sodium bicarbonate and ammonium chloride on chlorpropamide kinetics. Clin Pharmacol Ther (1983) 33, 386–393.

2 Neuvonen PJ, Karkkainen S, Lehtovaara R. Pharmacokinetics of chlorpropamide in epileptic patients: effects of enzyme induction and urine pH on chlorpropamide elimination. Eur J Clin Pharmacol (1987) 32, 297–301.

Hypoglycaemic agents + Vinpocetine

Abstract/Summary

Vinpocetine does not interact with glibenclamide.

Clinical evidence, mechanism, importance and management

A study in 18 elderly patients with Type II diabetes, under treatment with glibenclamide, and symptoms of dementia showed that 4 day's treatment with 10 mg vinpocetine, three times daily, did not affect either the pharmacokinetics of the glibenclamide or the control of blood glucose levels.[1] There would seem to be no reason for avoiding concurrent use. There seems to be no information about the effects of vinpocetine on other hypoglycaemic agents.

Reference

1 Grandt R, Braun W, Schulz H-U, Lührmann B, Frercks H-J. Glibenclamide steady-state plasma levels during concomitant vinpocetine administration in type II diabetic patients. Arzneim Forsch/Drug Res (1989) 39, 1451–4.

Chapter 16
Immunosuppressant Drug Interactions

The immunosuppressant drugs dealt with in this chapter are the corticosteroids and cyclosporin. Other drugs which are also used for immunosuppression (e.g. azathioprine and methotrexate) are to be found in Chapter 13 which deals with the cytotoxic drugs. When any of these drugs acts as the interacting agent the relevant synopsis is categorized in the chapter dealing with the drug whose effects are changed. A list of the agents which are featured here appears in Table 16.1.

Table 16.1

Non-proprietary names	Proprietary names
Cyclosporin A (Cyclosporin(e))	*Sandimunn*
Corticosteroids	
Cloprednol	
Dexamethasone	
Hydrocortisone (cortisol)	
Fludrocortisone	
Methylprednisolone	
Prednisolone	
Prednisone	
Tacrolimus (FK-506)	
OKT3 (Murine monoclonal antibody)	

Corticosteroids + Aminoglutethimide

Abstract/Summary

The effects of dexamethasone but not hydrocortisone can be reduced or abolished by the concurrent use of aminoglutethimide.

Clinical evidence

When given 500–750 mg aminoglutethimide daily the half-life of dexamethasone (1 mg daily) in six patients was reduced from 264 to 120 min. In another 22 patients it was found that increasing the dexamethasone dosage to 1.5–3.0 mg daily compensated for the increased dexamethasone metabolism and complete adrenal suppression was achieved over a prolonged period.[1]

A patient, dependent on dexamethasone due to brain oedema caused by a tumour, deteriorated rapidly with headache and lethargy when additionally treated with aminoglutethimide. The problem was solved by withdrawing the aminoglutethimide and temporarily increasing the dexamethasone dosage.[2]

Mechanism

Aminoglutethimide is an enzyme inducing agent and it seems probable that it interacts by increasing the metabolism and clearance of the steroids by the liver, thereby reducing their effects.[4]

Importance and management

Information is limited but the interaction appears to be established. The reduction in the serum corticosteroid levels can be enough to reduce or even abolish intended adrenal suppression[1] or to cause loss of control of a disease condition.[2] The former situation has been successfully accommodated by increasing the dosage of the corticosteroid or by increasing the dosage of both.[1] An alternative is to use hydrocortisone which appears not to be affected by aminoglutethimide.[3] A standard fixed dose regimen of 1 g aminoglutethimide and 40 mg hydrocortisone daily has been shown to block adrenal steroid synthesis effectively without the 'adrenal escape phenomenon'.[3]

References

1 Santen RJ, Lipton A, Kendall J. Successful medical adrenalectomy with aminoglutethimide. Role of altered drug metabolism. J Amer Med Ass (1974) 230, 1661–5.
2 Halpern J, Catane R, Baerwald H. A call for caution in the use of aminoglutethimide: negative interactions with dexamethasone and beta blocker treatment. Journal of Medicine (1984) 15, 59–63.
3 Santen RJ, Wells SA, Runic S, Gupta C, Kendall J, Ruby EB, Samojlik E. Adrenal suppression with aminoglutethimide. I. Differential effects of aminoglutethimide on glucocorticoid metabolism as a rationale for the use of hydrocortisone. J Clin Endocrinol Metab (1977) 45, 469–79.
4 Santen RJ, Brodie AMH. Suppression of oestrogen production as treatment of breast carcinoma: pharmacological and clinical studies with aromatase inhibitors. Clinics in Oncology (1982) 1, 77–130.

Corticosteroids + Antacids

Abstract/Summary

The absorption of prednisone can be reduced by large but not small doses of aluminium and magnesium hydroxide antacids. Prednisolone probably behaves similarly. Dexamethasone absorption is reduced by magnesium trisilicate. Phosphate-depletion caused by antacids can confuse the diagnostic picture.

Clinical evidence

(a) Prednisone or Prednisolone

20 ml *Gastrogel* (aluminium hydroxide, magnesium hydroxide and trisilicate) had no significant effect on serum levels, half-life or prednisone AUCs (10 or 20 mg doses) in five patients and two normal subjects.[1]

Other studies in eight normal subjects given 20 mg doses of prednisolone showed that 30 ml Magnesium Trisilicate Mixture BP or *Aludrox* (aluminium hydroxide gel) caused small but not statistically significant changes in peak prednisolone levels and absorption, however one subject given magnesium trisilicate had considerably reduced levels.[2] Aluminium phosphate has also been found not to affect prednisolone absorption.[6,7] In contrast, another study in normal subjects and patients given 60 ml of *Aldrox* or *Melox* (both containing aluminium hydroxide and magnesium hydroxide) found that the bioavailability of 10 mg prednisone was reduced on average by 30%, and even 40% in some individuals.[5]

(b) Dexamethasone

5 g magnesium trisilicate in 100 ml of water considerably reduced the bioavailability of single 1 mg oral doses of dexamethasone given to six subjects. Using the urinary excretion of 11-hydroxycorticosteroids as a measure, the reduction was about 75%.[4]

Mechanism

The reduction in dexamethasone absorption is attributed to adsorption onto the surface of the magnesium trisilicate.[4,8]

Importance and management

Information seems to be limited to these studies. The indication is that large doses of some antacids can reduce bioavailability, but small doses do not. More study is needed to confirm this. Concurrent use should be monitored to confirm that the therapeutic response is adequate. Also be alert for evidence of a phosphate-depletion syndrome which can mimic steroid-induced side-effects and confuse the diagnostic picture.[3] This has been reported in a prednisolone-dependent asthmatic man given *Maalox* and *Mylanta*, both of which are phosphate-binding antacids.[1]

References

1 Tanner AR, Caffin JA, Halliday JW, Powell LW. Concurrent administration of antacids and prednisone: effect on serum levels of prednisolone. Br J Clin Pharmac (1979) 7, 397.
2 Lee DAH, Taylor GM, Walker JG, James VHT. The effect of concurrent administration of antacids on prednisolone absorption. Br J Clin Pharmac (1979) 8, 92.
3 Goodman M, Solomons CC, Miller PD. Distinction between the common symptoms of the phosphate-depletion syndrome and glucocorticoid-induced disease. Am J Med (1978) 65, 868.
4 Naggar VF, Khalil SA, Gouda MW. Effect of concomitant administration of magnesium trisilicate on GI absorption of dexamethasone in humans. J Pharm Sci (1978) 67, 1029.
5 Uribe M, Casian C, Rojas S, Sierra JG, Go VLW, Munoz RM, Gil S. Decreased bioavailability of prednisone due to antacids in patients with chronic active liver disease and in healthy subjects. Gastroenterology (1981) 80, 661.
6 Albin H, Vincon G, Demotes-Mainard F, Begaud B, Bedjauoi A. Effects of aluminium phosphate on bioavailability of cimetidine and prednisolone. Eur J Clin Pharmacol (1984) 26, 271–3.
7 Albin H, Vincon G, Pehourcq F, Lecorre C, Fleury B, Conri C. Influence d'un anti-acide sur la biodisponibilite de la prednisolone. Therapie (1983) 38, 61–5.
8 Prakash A, Verma RK. In vitro adsorption of dexamethasone and betamethasone on antacids. Ind J Pharm Sci (1984) Jan-Feb, 55–6.

Corticosteroids + Anti-infective agents

Abstract/Summary

Because the corticosteroids can suppress the normal responses of the body to attack by micro-organisms, it is important to ensure that any anti-infective 'cover' is sufficient to prevent local or even generalized and potentially life-threatening infections.

Clinical evidence

A patient with severe cystic acne vulgaris given low dose oral tetracyline, 500 mg daily, and betamethasone, 2 mg daily, for seven months became toxaemic and pyrexic with severe acne and cellulitis of the face due to the emergence of a gram-negative organism not susceptible to the antibiotic.[1] A child with *Tinea corporis* developed a permanently scarred knee when treated with a cream containing 1% clotrimazole and 0.05% betamethasone diproprionate.[2]

Mechanism

The corticosteroids reduce inflammation, impair antibody formation and, if given systemically, cause adrenal suppression. This increases the susceptibility of the body to infection. In both of the cases cited the infections were insufficiently con-trolled by the anti-infective agents during this immunosuppression.

Importance and management

Not, strictly speaking, interactions, but the cases cited amply illustrate the importance of monitoring concurrent use. The author of one of the reports points out that '...it appears that if oral corticoids or combined therapy are ever warranted, they should be very carefully policed because of the risk of turning a benign disease into one that is potentially fatal.'[1]

Reference

1 Paver K. Complications from combined oral tetracycline and oral corticoid therapy on acne vulgaris. Med J Aust (1970) 1, 509.
2 Reynolds RD, Boiko S, Lucky AW. Exacerbation of tinea corporis during treatment with 1% clotrimazole/0.05% betamethasone diproprionate (Lotrisone) Am J Dis Child (1991) 145, 1224–5.

Corticosteroids + Barbiturates

Abstract/Summary

The therapeutic effects of systemically administered corticosteroids (dexamethasone, hydrocortisone, methylprednisolone, prednisone and prednisolone) are decreased by the concurrent use of phenobarbitone (phenobarbital) because the loss of these corticosteroids from the body is increased. An increase in the corticosteroid dosage may be needed. Other barbiturates probably interact similarly.

Clinical evidence

(a) Asthmatic patients on prednisone, Prednisolone, Methylprednisolone

Three prednisone-dependent patients with bronchial asthma taking 10–40 mg prednisone daily showed a marked worsening of their symptoms within a few days of starting to take 120 mg phenobarbitone daily. There was a deterioration in their pulmonary function tests (FEV1, degree of bronchospasm) and a rise in eosinophil counts, all of which improved when the phenobarbitone was stopped. The prednisone clearance increased while taking the phenobarbitone.[1]

Phenobarbitone increased the clearance of prednisolone in asthmatic children by 41% and of methylprednisolone by 209%.[8] In contrast, the prednisone requirements of other children were unaltered while taking a compound preparation containing 24 mg phenobarbitone daily.[3]

(b) Kidney transplant patients on prednisone

The survival of kidney transplants in a group of 75 children being given azathioprine and prednisone as immunosuppressants was reduced in those given anticonvulsant treatment with

60–120 mg phenobarbitone daily. Two of the 11 epileptic children were also taking 100 mg phenytoin daily.[4]

(c) Patients with rheumatoid arthritis on prednisolone

Nine patients with rheumatoid arthritis on 8–15 mg prednisolone daily showed strong evidence of clinical deterioration (worsening joint tenderness, pain, morning stiffness, fall in grip strength) when treated with phenobarbitone for 2 weeks (plasma concentrations 0–2 mg%). The prednisolone half-life fell by 25%.[6]

Mechanism

Phenobarbitone is a recognized potent liver enzyme inducing agent which increases the metabolism and loss from the body of administered corticosteroids, thereby reducing their effects. Pharmacokinetic studies in man have shown that phenobarbitone reduces the half-lives of these corticosteroids and increases their clearances by 10–209%.[1,5,8]

Importance and management

Well-documented and well-established interactions of clinical importance. Concurrent use need not be avoided but the outcome should be well monitored and the corticosteroid dosage increased as necessary. Dexamethasone,[1] hydrocortisone,[2] methylprednisolone,[5,8] prednisone[1,4] and prednisolone[6,8] are all known to be affected. Prednisone and prednisolone appear to be less affected than methylprednisolone and may be preferred.[8] Be alert for the same interaction with other corticosteroids and other barbiturates (which also are enzyme-inducing agents) although direct evidence seems to be lacking. The dexamethasone adrenal suppression test may be expected to be unreliable in those taking phenobarbitone, however 50 mg hydrocortisone instead of dexamethasone can give reliable results in the presence of phenytoin[7] (another potent enzyme inducer) and might also be considered for those on barbiturates (see 'Corticosteroids + Phenytoin').

References

1 Brooks SM, Werk EE, Ackerman SJ, Sullivan I, Thrasher K. Adverse effects of phenobarbital on corticosteroid metabolism in patients with bronchial asthma. N Engl J Med (1972) 286, 1125.
2 Burstein S, Klaiber EL. Phenobarbital-induced increase in 6-beta-hydroxycortisol excretion: clue to its significance in human urine. J Clin Endocrinol Metab (1965) 25, 293.
3 Falliers CJ. Corticosteroids and phenobarbital in asthma. N Engl J Med (1972) 287, 201.
4 Wassner SJ, Pennisi AJ, Malekzadeh MH, Fine RN. The adverse effect of anticonvulsant therapy on renal allograft survival. J Pediat (1976) 88, 134.
5 Stjernholm MR, Katz FH. Effects of diphenylhydantoin, phenobarbital and diazepam on the metabolism of methylprednisolone and its sodium succinate. J Clin Endocrinol Metab (1975) 41, 887.
6 Brooks PM, Buchanan WW, Grove M, Downie WW. Effects of enzyme induction on metabolism of prednisolone. Clinical and laboratory study. Ann Rheum Dis (1975) 35, 339.
7 Meikle AW, Stanchfield JB, West CD, Tyler FH. Hydrocortisone suppression test for Cushings syndrome: therapy with anticonvulsants. Arch Intern Med (1974) 134, 1068.
8 Bartoszek M, Brenner AM, Szefler SJ. Prednisolone and methylprednisolone kinetics in children receiving anticonvulsant therapy. Clin Pharmacol Ther (1987) 42, 424–32.

Corticosteroids + Beta-blockers

Abstract/Summary

An isolated report describes hyperkalaemia in a man attributed to the concurrent use of timolol eye drops and prednisone.

Clinical evidence, mechanism, importance and management

A patient with radiation pneumonitis and glaucoma treated with timolol eye drops (two drops 0.5% daily) developed severe hyperkalaemia shortly after starting 60 mg prednisone daily. His serum potassium levels fell when the timolol was stopped, and rose when it was restarted. Other possible contributory factors included a history of obstructive liver disease and the use of heparin.[1] This appears to be a rare and unusual case.

Reference

1 Swenson ER. Severe hyperkalaemia as a complication of timolol, a topically applied beta-adrenergic antagonist. Arch Intern Med (1986) 146, 1220–1.

Corticosteroids + Caffeine

Abstract/Summary

The results of the dexamethasone suppression test can be falsified by the ingestion of substantial amounts of caffeine.

Clinical evidence, mechanism, importance and management

A study in 22 normal subjects and six depressed patients showed that when they were given a single 480 mg dose of caffeine at 2.0 pm following a single 1 mg dose of dexamethasone at 11.0 am, cortisol levels taken at 4.0 pm were increased from 2.3 to 5.3 g/dl, but at 8.0 am they were unaffected.[1] Thus the equivalent of about 4–5 cups of coffee might effectively falsify the results of the dexamethasone suppression test.

Reference

1 Unde TW, Bieren LM, Post RM. Caffeine-induced escape from dexamethasone suppression. Arch Gen Psychiatry (1985) 42, 737–8.

Corticosteroids + Carbamazepine

Abstract/Summary

The loss of dexamethasone, methylprednisolone and prednisolone from the body is increased in patients taking carbamazepine and a dosage increase will be needed. The results of the dexamethasone suppression test may be invalid.

Clinical evidence

A study in eight patients on long-term treatment with carbamazepine showed that the elimination half-life of prednisolone was 27% shorter (1.98 compared with 2.73 h) and the clearance was 42% higher (4.2 versus 2.96 ml/min/kg) than in nine normal subjects.[1]

A study in asthmatic children found that carbamazepine increased the clearance of prednisolone by 97% and of methylprednisolone by 342%.[4] A study in eight normal subjects found that while taking 800 mg carbamazepine daily the dosage of dexamethasone needed to suppress cortisol secretion (as part of the dexamethasone adrenal suppression test) was increased 2–4-fold.[2] A further study found that it took 2–13 days for false-positive results to occur and 3–12 days to recover when the carbamazepine was stopped.[3]

Mechanism

The almost certain reason is that the carbamazepine stimulates the liver enzymes to metabolize the corticosteroids much faster.

Importance and management

Information is limited but the interaction appears to be established. Patients taking carbamazepine will need increased doses of dexamethasone, methylprednisolone or prednisolone. Prednisolone is less affected than methylprednisolone and is probably preferred. The same interaction seems likely with other corticosteroids but more study is needed to confirm this.

References

1 Olivesi A. Modified elimination of prednisolone in epileptic patients on carbmazepine monotherapy, and in women using low-dose oral contraceptives. Biomed and Pharmacother (1986) 40, 301–8.
2 Kobberling J, v zur Muhlen A. The influence of diphenylhydantoin and carbamazepine on the circadian rhythm of free urinary corticoids and on the suppressibility of the basal and the 'impulsive' activity of dexamethasone. Acta Endocrinol (1973) 72, 303–18.
3 Privitera MR, Greden JF, Gardner RW, Ritchie JC, Carroll BJ. Interference by carbamazepine with the dexamethasone suppression test. Biol Psychiat (1982) 17, 611–20.
4 Bartoszek M, Brenner AM, Szefler SJ. Prednisolone and methylprednisolone kinetics in children receiving anticonvulsant therapy. Clin Pharmacol Ther (1987) 42, 424–32.

Corticosteroids + Carbimazole or Methimazole

Abstract/Summary

The loss of prednisolone from the body is increased by the use of carbimazole or methimazole. Its dosage may therefore need to be increased.

Clinical evidence

A comparative study was made of (a) eight women taking thyroxine and under treatment with 2.5 mg methimazole or 5 mg carbimazole daily for Grave's ophthalmology, (b) six women on thyroxine who had had subtotal thyroidectomy, and (c) six other normal women. All were euthyroid. It was found that the clearance of 0.54 mg/kg iv prednisolone in those taking the methimazole or carbimazole was much greater than in the other two groups (0.37, 0.24 and 0.20 l/h.kg respectively). After 6 h the plasma prednisolone levels in methimazole/carbimazole groups were only about 10% of those in the normal women and none was detectable after 8 h, whereas total and unbound prednisolone levels were much higher and measurable over the 10 hour study period in the two control groups. In another group of previously hyperthyroidic patients, now euthyroid because of carbimazole treatment, the total prednisolone clearance was 0.40 l/h.[1]

Mechanism

Not established. It seems possible that the methimazole and carbimazole increase the metabolism of the prednisolone by the liver microsomal enzymes, thereby increasing its loss from the body.

Importance and management

Direct information seems to be limited to this study although the authors point out that there is a clinical impression that higher doses of prednisolone are needed in patients with Grave's disease. Be alert for the need to use higher doses of prednisolone in patients taking either methimazole or carbimazole.

Reference

1 Legler UF. Impairment of prednisolone disposition in patients with Graves disease taking methimazole. J Clin Endocrinol Metab (1988) 66, 221–3.

Corticosteroids + Cholestyramine

Abstract/Summary

Cholestyramine reduces the absorption of hydrocortisone from the gut. Its effects are expected to be reduced.

Clinical evidence

4 g cholestyramine reduced the AUC of 50 mg oral hydrocortisone (cortisol) in 10 normal subjects from 103.5 to 58.9 μmol.min.l.$^{-1}$ Peak levels were lower and were reached about 50 min. later.[1] Two of the subjects were given both 4 g and 8 g cholestyramine. Their AUCs were reduced by 47 and 97%, and by 59 and 86% respectively.[1]

Mechanism

It seems that the hydrocortisone becomes bound to the cholestyramine in the gut, thereby reducing its absorption.

Importance and management

Direct information is limited to this study. It seems almost certain that the hydrocortisone effects will be reduced but this need confirmation. Separate the administration of the two drugs as much as possible to minimize admixture in the gut. The authors of the report warn that this may not necessarily avoid this interaction because their data show that the cholestyramine may remain in the gut for a considerable time.[1] Monitor the effects and increase the hydrocortisone dosage if necessary. Information about other corticosteroids is lacking but be alert for this interaction with any of them if given orally.

Reference

1 Johansson C, Adamsson U, Stierner U, Lindsten T. Interaction of cholestyramine on the uptake of hydrocortisone in the gastrointestinal tract. Acta Med Scand (1978) 204, 509–12.

Corticosteroids + Cimetidine, Ranitidine

Abstract/Summary

Cimetidine does not interact with prednisolone, prednisone or dexamethasone, nor ranitidine with prednisone.

Clinical evidence, mechanism, importance and management

Prednisone is a pro-drug which must be converted to prednisolone within the body to become active. A double-blind cross-over study in nine normal subjects showed that after taking either cimetidine (300 mg 6-hourly) or ranitidine (150 mg twice daily) for 4 days the pharmacokinetics of the prednisolone after a single 40 mg oral dose of prednisone were little changed.[1] Another double-blind cross-over study also showed that 1 g cimetidine daily only caused minor changes in plasma prednisolone levels following the administration of 10 mg of enteric-coated prednisolone.[2] Yet another study found that seven days' treatment with 1200 mg cimetidine daily had no effect on the pharmacokinetics of a single 8 mg IV dose of dexamethasone sodium phosphate.[3] There would seem to be no reason for avoiding concurrent use. Information about other corticosteroids appears to be lacking.

References

1 Sirgo MA, Rocci ML, Ferguson RK, Eshleman FN, Vlasses PH. Effects of cimetidine and ranitidine on the conversion of prednisone to prednisolone. Clin Pharmacol Ther (1985) 37, 534–8.
2 Morrison PJ, Rogers HJ, Bradbrook ID, Parsons C. Concurrent administration of cimetidine and enteric-coated prednisolone: effect on plasma levels of prednisolone. Br J Clin Pharmac (1980) 10, 87.
3 Peden NR, Rewhorn I, Champion MC, Mussani R, Ooi TC. Cortisol and dexamethasone elimination during treatment with cimetidine. Br J Clin Pharmac (1984) 18, 101–3.

Corticosteroids + Contraceptives (oral)

Abstract/Summary

The serum levels of prednisone, prednisolone, cloprednol and possibly other corticosteroids are considerably increased in those taking oral contraceptives. Both the therapeutic and toxic effects may be expected to be increased accordingly. Fluocortolone is not affected.

Clinical evidence

A comparative pharmacokinetic study on six women showed that, while taking an oral contraceptive, the plasma clearance of a single dose of prednisolone was decreased by a factor of 2.5, the area under the plasma concentration time curve was increased by 6, and the half-life increased by 2.5.[1]

This is in broad agreement with the results of other studies,[2,3,5–8,11] in one of which[2] the plasma clearance of prednisolone was roughly halved and the area under the plasma concentration time curve approximately doubled in eight women taking an oral contraceptive. A marked increase in plasma cloprednol levels has also been reported.[9] In another study in women with skin diseases, the use of oestrogens (chlorotrianisene or hexestrol) markedly increased the anti-inflammatory effects of prednisone or hydrocortisone given by mouth[4] and increased the concentration of serum corticosteroids by a factor of 3.

In contrast, a study in seven women showed that the pharmacokinetics of fluocortolone were unaffected by the concurrent use of oral contraceptives.[10]

Mechanism

Not understood. The possibilities include a change in the metabolism of the corticosteroids, or in their binding to serum proteins.[6]

Importance and management

An established interaction. Concurrent use should be monitored. Both the therapeutic and the toxic effects of the corticosteroids would be expected to be increased but there seem to be no clinical reports of adverse reactions. A dosage reduction may be necessary to avoid corticosteroid overdosage. Only prednisone, prednisolone, cloprednol and hydrocortisone have been reported to interact but other corticosteroids possibly behave similarly, the exception being fluocortolone.

References

1 Legler UF, Benet LZ. Marked alterations in prednisolone elimination for women taking oral contraceptives. Clin Pharmacol Ther (1982) 31, 243.

2 Boekenoogen SJ, Szefler SJ, and Jusko WJ. Prednisolone disposition and protein binding in oral contraceptive users. J Clin Endocrinol Metab (1983) 56, 702–9.

3 Kozower M, Veatch L, Kaplan MM. Decreased clearance of prednisolone, a factor in the development of corticosteroid side-effects. J Clin Endocrinol Metab (1974) 38, 407–12.

4 Spangler AS, Antoniades HN, Sotman SL, Inderbitizin TM. Enhancement of the anti-inflammatory action of hydrocortisone by estrogen. J Clin Endocrinol Metab (1969) 29, 650–5.

5 Legler UF, Benet LZ. Marked alterations in dose-dependent prednisolone kinetics in women taking oral contraceptives. Clin Pharmacol Ther (1986) 39, 425–9.

6 Frey BM, Schaad HJ, Frey FL. Pharmacokinetic interaction of contraceptive steroids with prednisone and prednisolone. Eur J Clin Pharmacol (1984) 26, 505–11.

7 Meffin PJ, Wing LMH, Sallustio BC, Brooks PM. Alterations in prednisolone disposition as a result of oral contraceptive use and dose. Br J Clin Pharmacol (1984) 17, 655–64.

8 Olivesi A. Modified elimination of prednisolone in epileptic patients on carbamazepine monotherapy, and in women using low-dose oral contraceptives. Biomed Pharmacother (1986) 40, 301–8.

9 Legler UF. Altered cloprednol disposition in oral contraceptive users. Clin Pharmacol Ther (1987) 41, 237.

10 Legler UF. Lack of impairment of fluocortolone disposition in oral contraceptive users. Eur J Clin Pharmacol (1988) 35, 101–3.

11 Legler UF, Benet LZ. Veränderungen der Prednisolonkinetik in Frauen, die orale Kontrazeptiva einnehmen. Hoppe-Seylers Zeitschrift fur Physiologische Chemie (1983) 364, 348.

Corticosteroids + Diuretics, Potassium-losing

Abstract/Summary

Since both of these groups of drugs cause potassium to be lost from the body, severe potassium depletion may occur during concurrent use. The intake of potassium may need to be increased to balance this loss.

Clinical evidence, mechanism, importance and management

Some corticosteroids and some diuretics can cause a significant loss of potassium from the body. An exaggeration of the loss would therefore be expected if taken together and severe potassium depletion is possible (eg seen with hydrocortisone and frusemide[1]) but there seem to be no formal clinical studies describing the extent of the depletion. The effects should be monitored and the intake of potassium increased as necessary to balance this loss.

The corticosteroids which cause the greatest potassium loss are those which are naturally occurring. These include cortisone and hydrocortisone. Fludrocortisone also causes potassium loss. Corticotrophin (ACTH) which is a pituitary hormone and tetracosactrin (a synthetic polypeptide) stimulate corticosteroid secretion by the adrenal cortex and can thereby indirectly cause potassium loss. The synthetic corticosteroids (glucocorticoids) have a much less marked potassium-losing effect and are less likely to cause problems. These include prednisone, prednisolone, dexamethasone, betamethasone and triamcinolone.

The potassium-losing diuretics include bumetanide, frusemide, ethacrynic acid, piretanide, the thiazides and related diuretics (e.g. bendrofluazide, benzthiazide, chlorothiazide, clopamide, cyclopenthiazide, hydrochlorothiazide, hydroflumethiazide, indapamide, mefruside, methyclothiazide, metolazone, polythiazide, xipamide).

Reference

1 Manchon ND, Bercoff E, Lemarchand P, Chassagne P, Senant J, Bourreille J. Fréquence et gravité des interactions médicamenteuses dans une population âgée: étude prospective concernant 63 malades. Rev Med Interne (1989) 10, 521–5.

Corticosteroids + Ephedrine and Theophylline

Abstract/Summary

Ephedrine increases the loss of dexamethasone from the body, but theophylline appears not to interact.

Clinical evidence, mechanism, importance and management

Nine asthmatic patients showed a 40% increase in the clearance of the dexamethasone when concurrently given 100 mg ephedrine daily for 3 weeks and a similar reduction in its half-life.[1] This would be expected to reduce the overall control of asthma, but this requires confirmation. Be alert for any evidence that the dexamethasone effects are reduced if both drugs are used. It is not clear whether other corticosteroids behave similarly. Theophylline appeared not to interact.[1]

Reference

1 Brooks SM, Sholiton LJ, Werk EE, Altenau P. The effects of ephedrine and theophylline on dexamethasone metabolism in bronchial asthma. J Clin Pharmacol (1977) 17, 308.

Corticosteroids + Glycyrrhizin

Abstract/Summary

Glycyrrhizin can reduce the clearance of prednisolone from the body.

Clinical evidence, mechanism, importance and management

A study in six subjects found that after taking four 50 mg oral doses of glycyrrhizin 8-hourly followed by a bolus injection of 0.096 mg/kg prednisolone hemisuccinate, the AUC of total prednisolone was increased by 50% (from 591 to 882 µg.h/l) and of free prednisolone by 55% (from 117 to 182 µg.h/l).[1] This confirms the findings of two previous studies in which the glycyrrhizin was given by intravenous infusion.[2,3] The probable reason is that the glycyrrhizin inhibits the metabolism of the prednisolone by the liver so that it is cleared by the body more slowly. In one of the studies it was also found that glycyrrhizin increased the effects of prednisolone in some patients with rheumatoid arthritis and polyarteritis nodosa.

The clinical importance of these observations is uncertain, but increased effects can be beneficial and in excess can be toxic. Concurrent use should be well monitored. More study is needed.

References

1 Chen M-F, Shimada F, Kato H, Yano S, Kanaok M. Effect of oral administration of glycyrrhizin on the pharmacokinetics of prednisolone. Endocrinol Japon (1991) 38, 167–74.
2 Chen M-F, Shimada F, Kato H, Yano S, Kanaok M. Effect of glycyrrhizin on the pharmacokinetics of prednisolone following low dosage of prednisolone hemisuccinate. Endocrinol Japon (1990) 37, 331–41.
3 Ojima M, Itoh N, Satoh K, Fukuchi S. The effects of glycyrrhizin preparations on patients with difficult in release of steroids treatment. Minophagen Med Rev (1987) Suppl 17, 120–5.

Corticosteroids + Ketoconazole

Abstract/Summary

Ketoconazole reduces the metabolism and loss of methylprednisolone from the body. The corticosteroid dosage should be reduced. The situation with prednisone and prednisolone is uncertain.

Clinical evidence

(a) Methylprednisolone

A study in six normal subjects showed that 200 mg ketoconazole daily for six days increased the mean AUC of a single 20 mg dose of methylprednisolone by 135% and decreased the clearance by 60%. The 24 h cortisol AUC was reduced by 44%.[1]

These findings are confirmed by another study by the same group of workers.[2]

(b) Prednisone and Prednisolone

A study in 10 normal subjects found that 200 mg ketoconazole daily for 6–7 days caused a 50% rise in the total and unbound prednisolone serum levels following oral prednisone or intravenous prednisolone.[3] In contrast, two other studies failed to find any effect of 200 mg ketoconazole for 6 days on either the pharmacokinetics or the pharmacodynamics of prednisolone, as measured by the suppressive effects on serum cortisol, blood basophil and helper T lymphocyte values of prednisolone.[4,5]

Mechanism

Ketoconazole inhibits cytochrome P-450 dependent enzymes in the liver so that the metabolism of some corticosteroids and endogenous cortisol is reduced, thereby reducing their loss from the body and increasing their effects.

Importance and management

The methylprednisolone/ketoconazole appears to be established and clinically important. A 50% reduction in the corticosteroid dosage is recommended in one study.[2] It has been pointed out that increased corticosteroid serum levels have an increased immunosuppressive effect which may be undesirable in those with a fungal infection needing treatment with ketoconazole.[3] The situation with prednisone and prednisolone is as yet uncertain.[6,7] More study is needed to clarify the situation.

References

1 Glynn AM, Slaughter RL, Brass C, D'Ambrosio R, Jusko WJ. Effects of ketoconazole on methylprednisolone pharmacokinetics and cortisol secretion. Clin Pharmacol Ther (1986) 39, 654–9.
2 Kandrotas RJ, Slaughter RL, Brass C, Jusko WJ. Ketoconazole effects on methylprednisolone disposition and their joint suppression of endogenous cortisol. Clin Pharmacol Ther (1987) 42, 465–70.
3 Zurcher RM, Frey BM, Frey FJ. Impact of ketoconazole on the metabolism of prednisolone. Clin Pharmacol Ther (1989) 45, 366–72.
4 Yamashita SK, Ludwig EA, Middleton E, Jusko WJ. Lack of pharmacokinetic and pharmacodynamic interactions between ketoconazole and prednisolone. Clin Pharmacol Ther (1991) 49, 558–70.
5 Ludwig EA, Slaughter RL, Savilwala M, Brass C, Jusko WJ. Steroid-specific effects of ketoconazole on prednisolone disposition: unaltered prednisolone elimination. Drug Intell Clin Pharm (1989) 23, 858–61.
6 Jusko WJ. Ketoconazole effects on corticosteroid disposition. Clin Pharmacol Ther (1990) 47, 418–9.
7 Zurcher RM, Frey BM, Frey FJ. Ketoconazole effects on corticosteroid disposition. Clin Pharmacol Ther (1990) 47, 419–20.

Corticosteroids + Macrolide antibiotics

Abstract/Summary

Triacetyloleandomycin and, to a lesser extent, erythromycin can reduce the loss of methylprednisolone from the body, thereby increasing both its therapeutic and toxic effects. Prednisolone appears not to be affected except in those taking enzyme-inducing agents such as phenytoin and phenobarbitone. Other corticosteroids are probably not affected.

Clinical evidence

(a) Methylprednisolone + Erythromycin

A study in nine adolescents aged 9–18 with asthma showed that after taking 250 mg erythromycin four times a day for a week, the clearance of methylprednisolone was decreased by 46% (range 28–61%) and the half-life was increased by 51% (from 2.34 to 3.45 h).[4]

(b) Methylprednisolone and Prednisolone + Triacetyloleandomycin

A pharmacokinetic study in four children and six adult steroid-dependent asthmatics found that one week's treatment with 14 mg/kg triacetyloleandomycin daily increased the half-life of methylprednisolone by 90% (from 2.46 to 4.63 h) and reduced the total body clearance by 44% (from 406 to 146 ml/min/1.73 m²). All 10 showed cushingoid symptoms (cushingoid facies and weight gain) which resolved when the methylprednisolone dosage was reduced, without any loss in the control of the asthma.[1]

A later study by the same group of workers confirmed these findings but they also found that prednisolone clearance was not affected except in those who were also taking phenytoin or phenobarbitone which are enzyme inducers.[2,3]

A number of other reports confirm that triacetyloleandomycin can act as a 'steroid-sparing' agent.[5–12] One of them reported a 50% reduction in steroid clearance.[7] However a case report suggests that the risk of disseminated varicella infection may possibly be increased by concurrent use.[8]

Mechanism

What is known suggests that these macrolide antibiotics inhibit the metabolism of methylprednisolone, thereby reducing its loss from the body and increasing its effects. The volume of distribution is also decreased.[1–4]

Importance and management

Information about the erythromycin/methylprednisolone interaction is much more limited than with triacetyloleandomycin/methylprednisolone, but both appear to be established and of clinical importance. This 'steroid-sparing' effect should be taken into account during concurrent use and appropriate dosage reductions made to avoid the development of corticosteroid overdosage side-effects. The authors of one study suggest that this reduction should be '...empirical and based primarily on clinical symptomatology.'[1] Another group found that a 68% reduction in methylprednisolone dosage was possible within two weeks,[10] and yet another group found that a four- to

five-fold reduction was possible.[11] Triacetyloleandomycin appears to have a larger effect than erythromycin.

Prednisolone seems not to interact with triacetyloleandomycin and is a non-interacting alternative except in those taking enzyme-inducing drugs (e.g. phenytoin, phenobarbitone). The general silence in the literature suggests that these macrolide antibiotics do not interact with other corticosteroids but be on the alert for any changes until this is confirmed. There also seems to be no information about other macrolide antibiotics.

References

1 Szefler SJ, Rose JQ, Ellis EF, Spector SL, Green AW, Jusko WJ. The effect of troleandomycin on methylprednisolone elimination. J Allergy Clin Immunol (1980) 66, 447–51.

2 Szefler SJ, Ellis EF, Brenner M, Rose JQ, Spector SL, Yurchak A, Andrews F, Jusko WJ. Steroid-specific and anticonvulsant interaction aspects of triacetyloleandomycin-steroid therapy. J Allergy Clin Immunol (1982) 69, 455–60.

3 Szefler SJ, Brenner M, Jusko WJ, Spector SL, Flesher KA, Ellis EF. Dose- and time-related effects of troleandomycin on methylprednisolone elimination. Clin Pharmacol Ther (1982) 32, 166–171.

4 Laforce CF, Szefler SJ, Miller MF, Ebling W, Brenner M. Inhibition of methylprednisolone elimination in the presence of erythromycin. J Allergy Clin Immunol (1983) 72, 34–9.

5 Fox JL. Infectious asthma treated with triacetyloleandomycin. Penn Med J (1961) 64, 634–5.

6 Itkin IH, Menzel M. The use of macrolide antibiotic substances in the treatment of asthma. J Allergy (1970) 45, 146–62.

7 Ball BD, Hill M, Brenner M, Sanks R, Szefler SJ. Critical assessment of troleandomycin in severe steroid-requiring asthmatic children. Ann Allergy (1988) 60, 155.

8 Lantner R, Rockoff JB, DeMasi J, Boran-Ragotzy R, Middleton E. Fatal varicella in a corticosteroid-dependent asthmatic receiving troleandomycin. Allergy Pro (1990) 11, 83–7.

9 Eitches RW, Rachelefsky GS, Katz RM, Mendoza GR, Siegel SC. Methylprednisolone and troleandomycin in treatment of steroid-dependent asthmatic children. Am J Dis Child (1985) 139, 264–8.

10 Wald JA, Friedman BF, Farr RS. An improved protocol for the use of troleandomycin (TAO) in the treatment of steroid-requiring asthma. J Allergy Clin Immunol (1986) 78, 36–43.

11 Zeiger RS, Schatz M, Sperling W, Simon RA, Stevenson DD. Efficacy of troleandomycin in outpatients with severe, corticosteroid-dependent asthma. J Allergy Clin Immunol (1980) 66, 438–46.

12 Kamada AK, Hill MR, Brenner AM, Szefler SJ. Glucocorticoid reduction with troleandomycin in chronic, severe asthmatic children: implication for future trials and clinical application. J All Clin Immunol (1992) 89, 285.

Corticosteroids + Non-steroidal anti-inflammatory drugs (NSAIDs)

Abstract/Summary

Concurrent use increases the incidence of gastro-intestinal bleeding and probably ulceration. Indomethacin and naproxen can have a 'steroid sparing' effect.

Clinical evidence, mechanism, importance and management

(a) Gastrointestinal bleeding and ulceration

A retrospective study of more than 20 000 patients who had

had corticosteroids found that the incidence of upper gastrointestinal bleeding was no greater than in the control group who had not had corticosteroids (95 compared with 91), however the risk of bleeding was increased if the patients were also taking aspirin or other non-steroidal anti-inflammatory drugs.[1] This is consistent with the results of another study on patients taking prednisone and indomethacin,[2] and gives support to the widely held belief that concurrent use of the NSAIDs (well-known as gastric irritants) can cause bleeding and ulceration. Concurrent use should be very well monitored. See also 'Aspirin and Salicylates + Corticosteroids'.

(b) Steroid-sparing effect

A study in 11 patients with stable rheumatoid disease on regular corticosteroid therapy showed that when given either 75 mg indomethacin or 250 mg naproxen twice daily for two weeks the total serum levels of a single 7.5 mg dose of prednisolone remained unchanged but the amount of unbound (free) prednisolone increased by 30–60%.[3] The probable reason is that these NSAIDs displace administered and endogenous corticosteroids from their plasma protein binding sites. It should therefore be possible to reduce the corticosteroid dosage while maintaining the therapeutic effects. One study found that the dosage of paramethasone could be reduced by almost 60% when naproxen was given.[4]

References

1 Carson JL, Strom BL, Schinnar R, Sim E, Maislin G, Morse ML. Do corticosteroids really cause upper GI bleeding? Clin Res (1987) 35, 340A.
2 Emmanuel JH, Montgomery RD. Gastric ulcer and anti-arthritic drugs. Postgrad Med J (1971) 47, 227.
3 Rae SA, Williams IA, English J, Baylis EM. Alteration of plasma prednisolone levels by indomethacin and naproxen. Br J Clin Pharmac (1982) 14, 459–61.
4 Flores JJB, Rojas SV. Naproxen: corticosteroid-sparing effect in rheumatoid arthritis. J Clin Pharmacol (1975) 15, 373–7.

Corticosteroids + Omeprazole

Abstract/Summary

An isolated report describes a reduction in the effects of prednisone in a patient when treated with omeprazole.

Clinical evidence, mechanism, importance and management

A man suffering from bullous pemphigoid was given prednisone (1 mg/kg daily), and a week later was additionally started on ranitidine (200 mg daily) for a gastric ulcer. Four weeks later when the skin lesions were well controlled, it was decided to replace the ranitidine with 40 mg omeprazole daily. Within 4 days the skin lesions began progressively to worsen, although the prednisone dosage remained unchanged, until after 3 weeks it was decided to stop the omeprazole and restart

the ranitidine because an adverse interaction between the prednisone and the omeprazole was suspected. Within about a week, the skin condition had begun to improve.[1] The suggested explanation is that the omeprazole inhibited the liver enzyme (11β-hydroxylase) which normally converts prednisone into its active form (prednisolone) so that in effect the pemphigoid became inadequately treated.[1]

This is the first and, so far, the only report of this interaction. Its general importance is unknown but it would now be prudent to be on the alert if these drugs are given concurrently. More study is needed.

Reference

1 Joly P, Chosidow O, Laurent-Puig P, Delchier J-C, Roujeau J-C, Revuz J. Possible interaction prednisone-oméprazole dans la pemphigoïde bulleuse. Gastroenterol Clin Biol (1990) 14, 682–3.

Corticosteroids + Phenytoin

Abstract/Summary

(a) The therapeutic effects of dexamethasone, prednisone, prednisolone, methylprednisolone (probably other glucocorticoids) and fludrocortisone can be markedly reduced by the concurrent use of phenytoin. (b) The results of the dexamethasone adrenal suppression test may prove to be unreliable, and (c) serum phenytoin levels may be changed by dexamethasone.

Clinical evidence

(a) Reduced corticosteroid levels

A comparative pharmacokinetic study in six neurological or neurosurgical patients taking dexamethasone (orally) and phenytoin showed that the average amount of dexamethasone which reached the general circulation was a quarter of that observed in nine other patients taking only dexamethasone (mean oral bioavailability fractions of 0.21 and 0.84 respectively).[1]

Other patients have been described who needed increased doses of dexamethasone while taking phenytoin.[2] The fludrocortisone dosages of two patients required marked increases (four-fold in one patient and 10–20 times in the other) while taking phenytoin.[17] Renal allograft survival is decreased in patients on prednisone taking phenytoin due (it is believed) to reduced immunosuppressant effects.[8] The effects of phenytoin on the half-lives and clearance rates of other corticosteroids are shown in Table 16.2.

(b) Interference with the dexamethasone adrenal suppression test

A study on seven patients showed that while taking 300–400 mg phenytoin daily their plasma cortisol levels were only

Table 16.2 A comparison of the effects of phenytoin on the kinetics of different glucocorticoids (after Petereit and colleagues[3])

Corticosteroid	Daily dosage of phenytoin (mg)	Half-life without phenytoin (min)	Decreased half life with phenytoin (%)	Increased mean clearance rate with phenytoin (%)	Reference
Hydrocortisone	300–400	60–90	– 15	+ 25	11
Methylprednisolone	300	165	– 56	+ 130	12
Prednisone	Prednisolone is the biologically active metabolite of prednisone so that the values for prednisone and prednisolone should be similar.				13
Prednisolone	300	190–240	– 45	+ 77	7,8
Dexamethasone	300	250	– 51	+ 140	14,15

reduced by dexamethasone from 22 to 19 µg% compared with a reduction from 18 to 4 µg% in the absence of phenytoin.[4]

Other studies confirm that plasma cortisol and urinary 17-hydroxycorticosteroid levels are suppressed far less than might be expected with small doses of dexamethasone (0.5 mg 6-hourly for eight doses), but with larger doses (2.0 mg 6-hourly for eight doses) suppression was normal.[5]

(c) Serum phenytoin levels increased or decreased

A post-traumatic epilepsy prophylaxis study showed that the serum phenytoin levels in those taking dexamethasone (16–150 mg: mean 63.6 mg) was 40% higher than those on phenytoin alone (17.7 compared with 12.5 g/ml). The phenytoin was given as a loading dose of 11 mg/kg IV and then 13 mg/kg IM.[6]

A retrospective study of 40 patient records indicated that dexamethasone reduced serum phenytoin levels. The serum phenytoin levels of six patients on fixed doses of phenytoin were halved by the presence of dexamethasone.[7] Another patient needed a large dose of phenytoin (>10 mg/kg) while taking dexamethasone. He showed an almost 300% rise in serum phenytoin levels when dexamethasone was stopped.[19]

Mechanism

Phenytoin is a potent liver enzyme inducing agent which increases the metabolism of the corticosteroids so that they are cleared from the body more quickly, reducing both their therapeutic and adrenal suppressant effects

Importance and management

(a) The fall in serum corticosteroid levels is established and of clinical importance where treatment depends upon transport by the circulation (e.g. in immunosuppression), but it seems unlikely to affect the response to steroids administered topically or by inhalation, intra-articular injection or enema.[3] The interaction can be accommodated in several ways: (i) Increase the corticosteroid dosage proportionately to the increase in clearance (see Table 16.2). With prednisolone an average increase of 100% (range 58–260% in five individuals) proved effective.[3] A four-fold increase may be necessary with dexamethasone,[1] and much greater increases have been required with fludrocortisone.[17] (ii) Exchange the corticosteroid

for another which is less affected (see Table 16.2). A switch from dexamethasone to equivalent doses of methylprednisolone has been reported to be effective[9] but another report found that methylprednisolone was affected more than prednisolone.[18] In another case the exchange of 16 mg dexamethasone daily for 100 mg prednisone was successful.[10] (iii) Exchange the phenytoin for another anticonvulsant: Barbiturates, and to some extent primidone[16] and carbamazepine, are also enzyme-inducing agents, but sodium valproate is a successful non-interacting alternative.[2]

(b) The effects on the dexamethasone adrenal suppression test can apparently be accommodated by using larger than usual doses of dexamethasone (2 mg every 6 h for eight doses)[5] or by using an overnight test using 50 mg hydrocortisone.[9]

(c) The reports on the changes in serum phenytoin levels are inconsistent (rises and falls). The effects of concurrent use should be monitored.

References

1 Chalk JB, Ridgeway K, Brophy TrO'R, Yelland JDN and Eadie MJ. Phenytoin impairs the bioavailability of dexamethasone in neurological and neurosurgical patients. J Neurol Neurosurg Psychiatry (1984) 47, 1087–90.

2 McLelland J, Jack W. Phenytoin/dexamethasone interaction: a clinical problem. Lancet (1978) i, 1096.

3 Petereit LB, Meikle AW. Effectiveness of prednisolone during phenytoin therapy. Clin Pharmacol Ther (1977) 22, 912.

4 Werk EE, Choi Y, Sholiton L, Olinger C, Haque N. Interference in the effect of dexamethasone by diphenylhydantoin. N Engl J Med (1969) 281, 32.

5 Jubiz W, Meikle AW, Levinson RA, Mizutani S, West CD, Tyler FH. Effect of diphenylhydantoin on the metabolism of dexamethasone. N Engl J Med (1970) 283, 11.

6 Lawson LA, Blouin RA, Smith RB, Rapp RP, Young AB. Phenytoin-dexamethasone interaction: a previously unreported observation. Surg Neurol (1981) 16, 23.

7 Wong DD, Longenecker RG, Liepman M, Baker S, LaVergne M. Phenytoin-dexamethasone: a possible drug-drug interaction. J Amer Med Ass (1985) 254, 2062–3.

8 Wassner SJ, Pennisi AJ, Malekzadeh MH, Fine RN. The adverse effect of anticonvulsant therapy on renal allograft survival. J Pediat (1976) 88, 134–7.

9 Meikle AW, Stanchfield JB, West CD, Tyler FH. Hydrocortisone suppression test for Cushing syndrome: therapy with anticonvulsants. Arch Intern Med (1974) 134, 1068.

10 Boyland JJ, Owen DS, Chin JB. Phenytoin interference with dexamethasone. J Amer Med Ass (1976) 235, 802.

11 Choi Y, Thrasher K, Werk EE, Sholiton LJ, Ollinger C. Effect of diphenylhydantoin on cortisol kinetics in humans. J Pharmacol Exp Ther (1971) 176, 27.

12 Stjernholm MR, Katz FH. Effects of diphenylhydantoin, phenobarbitone

and diazepam on the metabolism of methylprednisolone and its hemisuccinate. J Clin Endocrinol Metab (1975) 41, 887.

13 Meikle AW. Weed JA, Tyler FH. Kinetics and interconversion of prednisolone and prednisone studies with new radio-immunoassays. J Clin Endocrinol Metab (1975) 41, 717.

14 Brooks SM, Werk EE, Ackerman S, Sullivan I, Thrasher K. Adverse effects of phenobarbital on corticosteroid metabolism in patients with bronchial asthmas. N Engl J Med (1972) 286, 1125.

15 Haque N, Thrasher K, Werk EE, Knowles HC, Sholiton LJ. Studies of dexamethasone metabolism in man. Effect of diphenylhydantoin. J Clin Endocrinol Metab (1972) 34, 44.

16 Hancock KW, Levell MJ. Primidone/dexamethasone interaction. Lancet (1978) i, 97.

17 Keilholz U, Guthrie GP. Case report: adverse effect of phenytoin on mineralocorticoid replacement with fludrocortisone in adrenal insufficiency. Amer J Med Sci (1986) 291, 280–3.

18 Bartoszek M, Brenner AM, Szefler SJ. Prednisolone and methylprednisolone kinetics in children receiving anticonvulsant therapy. Clin Pharmacol Ther (1987) 42, 424–32.

19 Lackner TE. Interaction of dexamethasone with phenytoin. Pharmacotherapy (1991) 11, 344–7.

Corticosteroids + Primidone

Abstract/Summary

A case report describes a reduction in the effects of dexamethasone due to the concurrent use of primidone. Primidone may also possibly invalidate the results of the dexamethasone adrenal suppression tests.

Clinical evidence, mechanism, importance and management

Direct evidence of an interaction seems to be limited to a letter describing a reduction in the effects of dexamethasone in a woman with congenital adrenal hyperplasia when treated with primidone for petit mal.[1] The probable reason for this reaction is that primidone is metabolized to phenobarbitone which is a potent liver enzyme inducing agent. This would be expected to increase the metabolism of the dexamethasone by the liver, thereby hastening its loss from the body and reducing its effects. For the same reason the results of the dexamethasone adrenal suppression test should be viewed with caution in patients taking primidone. See also 'Corticosteroids + Barbiturates'.

Reference

1 Hancock KW, Leveli A. Primidone/dexamethasone interaction. Lancet (1978) ii, 97.

Corticosteroids + Rifampicin (Rifampin)

Abstract/Summary

The effects of the corticosteroids can be markedly reduced by the concurrent use of rifampicin.

Clinical evidence

A child with nephrotic syndrome on prednisolone, accidentally given BCG vaccine, was treated with rifampicin and isoniazid to prevent possible dissemination of the vaccine. When the nephrotic condition failed to respond, the prednisolone dosage was raised from 2 to 3 mg/kg daily without any evidence of corticosteroid overdosage. Later when the rifampicin and isoniazid were withdrawn, remission of the nephrotic condition was achieved with the original dosage of prednisolone.[3]

A number of other reports describe a reduction in the response to corticosteroids (prednisone, prednisolone, methylprednisolone) in patients when given rifampicin, including a number who had had renal transplants.[2–5,7,8,11] A patient with Addison's disease stabilized on cortisone and fludrocortisol showed typical signs of corticosteroid overdosage when the rifampicin he was taking was replaced by ethambutol.[1] A pharmacokinetic study in patients with TB showed that the AUC of prednisolone was reduced 66% by rifampicin.[7] Another study found a 48% reduction and a decrease in the elimination half-life from 3.72 to 2.11 h.[9]

Mechanism

Rifampicin is a potent liver enzyme inducing agent which increases the metabolism of the corticosteroids by the liver,[4,6] thereby increasing their loss from the body and reducing their effects.

Importance and management

An established, well documented and clinically important interaction. The need to increase the dosage of cortisone, hydrocortisone, fludrocortisone, prednisone, prednisolone and methylprednisolone should be expected if rifampicin is given. A number of workers suggest that as a first approximation the dosage should be increased 2–3-fold, and reduced proportionately if the rifampicin is withdrawn.[4,7,9,10] There seems to be no direct information about other corticosteroids but be on the alert for them to be similarly affected.

References

1 Edwards OM, Courtnay-Evans RJ, Galley JM, Hunter J, Tait AD. Changes in cortisol metabolism following rifampicin therapy. Lancet (1974) ii, 549.

2 Hendrickse W, McKiernan J, Pickup M, Lowe J. Rifampicin-induced non-responsiveness to corticosteroid treatment in nephrotic syndrome. Br Med J (1979) 1, 306.

3 Van Marle W, Woods KL, Beeley L. Concurrent steroid and rifampicin therapy. Br Med J (1979) 1, 1020.

4 Buffington GA, Dominguez JH, Piering WF, Hebert LA, Kaufmaln HM, Lemann J. Interactiol of rifampin and glucocorticoids. J Amer Med Ass (1976) 236, 1958.

5 Mendez-Picon G, Murai M, Pierce JC. Tuberculosis in transplant patients: two possible cases of rifampin renal toxicity. Read before the 8th Annual Meeting of the American Society of Nephrology, Washington 1975.

6 Sotaniemi EA, Medzihradsky F, Eliasson G. Glutaric acid as an indicator of use of enzyme-inducing drugs. Clin Pharmacol Ther (1974) 15, 417.

7 McAllister WAC, Thompson PJ, Al-Habet SM, Rogers HJ. Rifampicin reduces effectiveness and bioavailability of prednisolone. Br Med J (1983) 286, 923–5.

8 Powell-Jackson A, Gray BJ, Heaton RW, Costello JF, Williams R, English J. Adverse effect of rifampicin administration on steroid-dependent asthma. Am Rev Resp Dis (1983) 128, 307–10.

9 Bergram H, Refvan OK. Altered prednisolone pharmacokinetics in patients treated with rifampicin. Acta Med Scand (1983) 213, 339–43.

10 Lofdahl C-G, Mellstrand T, Svedmyr N, Wahlen P. Increased metabolism of prednisolone and rifampicin after rifampicin treatment. Am Rev Resp Dis (1984) 129, A201.

11 Bitaudeau Ph, Clement S, Chartier JPh, Papapietro PM, Bonnafoux A, Arnaud M, Treves R, Desproges-Gotteron R. Interaction rifampicine-prednisolone. A propos de deux cas au cours d'une maladie de Horton. Rev Rhumatisme (1989) 56, 87–8.

Corticosteroids + Sucralfate

Abstract/Summary

Sucralfate appears not to interact with prednisone.

Clinical evidence, mechanism, importance and management

1 g sucralfate every 6 h had no effect on the pharmacokinetics of single 20 mg doses of prednisone in 12 normal subjects, except that the peak serum levels were delayed by about three-quarters of an hour when given at the same time, but not when the sucralfate was given 2 h after the prednisone.[1] No particular precautions are likely to be needed in patients given both drugs. Information about other corticosteroids is lacking.

Reference

1 Gambertoglio JG, Romac DR, Yong C-L, Birnbaum J, Lizak P, Amend WJ C. Lack of effect of sucralfate on prednisone bioavailability. Amer J Gastroenterology (1987) 82, 42–5.

Corticosteroids + Live vaccines

Abstract/Summary

Patients who are immunized with live virus vaccines while receiving immunosuppressive doses of corticosteroids may develop generalized, possibly life-threatening, infections

Clinical evidence, mechanism, importance and management

The administration of the corticosteroids can reduce the number of circulating lymphocytes and suppress the normal immune response so that concurrent immunization with live vaccines can lead to generalized infection. It is suggested that prednisone in doses greater than 10–15 mg daily will suppress the immune response, whereas 40–60 mg doses on alternate days probably do not.[4] However a patient with lymphosarcoma and hypogammaglobulinaemia, taking 15 mg prednisone daily, developed a generalized vaccinial infection when she was vaccinated.[1] A fatal vaccinial infection developed in another patient treated with cortisone.[2] This type of problem can be controlled with immunoglobulin to give cover against a general infection while immunity develops, and this has been successfully used in steroid-dependent patients needing smallpox vaccination.[3]

Smallpox vaccination is no longer necessary but other live attenuated vaccines (measles, mumps, rubella, poliomyelitis, BCG) are still used and the principles relevant for smallpox are probably generally applicable, but no studies seem to have been done to establish what is safe.[4] These are some of the published warnings: '...extreme caution must be observed in administering live virus vaccine to any patient receiving steroid therapy...' and '...it seems unwise to administer live virus vaccines to any person receiving steroids for a systemic effect in any dosage.'[4] Problems with topical or inhaled steroids in normal dosages seem unlikely because the amounts absorbed are relatively small,[4] however this needs confirmation.

References

1 Rosenbaum EH, Cohen RA, Glatstein HR. Vaccination of a patient receiving immunosuppressive therapy for lymphosarcoma. J Amer Med Ass (1966) 198, 737–40.

2 Olansky S, Smith JG, Hansen OC E. Fatal vaccinia associated with cortisone therapy. J Amer Med Ass (1956) 162, 887–8.

3 Joseph MR. Vaccination of patients on steroid therapy. Med J Aust (1974) 2, 181.

4 Shapiro L. Questions and Answers. Live virus vaccine and corticosteroid therapy. J Amer Med Ass (1981) 246, 2075–6. Answered by Fauci AS, Bellanti JA, Polk IJ, Cherry JD.

Cyclosporin + ACE inhibitors

Abstract/Summary

Acute kidney failure developed in two kidney transplant patients on cyclosporin when given enalapril. Oliguria was seen in another patient when given captopril.

Clinical evidence, mechanism, importance and management

Two patients with kidney transplants on cyclosporin developed acute renal failure 10–42 days after starting to take 5–10 mg enalapril daily. Recovery was complete when the enalapril was stopped in one of the patients, and when both were stopped in the other. The latter had no problems when the cyclosporin was restarted. Both recovered renal function after 10–30 days. Two other patients appeared to tolerate concurrent use well. The reasons for these reactions are not understood. Neither had any previous evidence of transplant artery stenosis or chronic rejection which are conditions known to predispose to renal failure during ACE inhibitor treatment.[1] Transient oliguria was seen in another patient given cyclosporin and captopril.[2] Considerable care and good monitoring is clearly needed if ACE inhibitors and cyclosporin are used. More study is needed.

References

1 Murray BM, Venuto RC, Kohli R, Cunningham EE. Enalapril-associated renal failure in renal transplants: possible role of cyclosporine. Am J Kid Dis (1990) XVI, 66–9.
2 Cockburn I, (Sandoz, Basel). Cyclosporin A: a clinical evaluation of drug interactions. Transplantation Proc (1986) 18, (Suppl 5) 50–5.

Cyclosporin(e) + Alcohol

Abstract/Summary

An isolated report describes a marked increase in serum cyclosporin levels in a patient when he went on the binge, but a subsequent study found that moderate single doses of alcohol in other patients had no such effect.

Clinical evidence, mechanism, importance and management

Prompted by the case of a renal transplant patient whose serum cyclosporin levels doubled (from 101 to 205 ng/ml) and remained high for about four days after going on a 2-day binge, a study was undertaken in eight other patients with kidney transplants. No changes in serum cyclosporin or creatinine levels were seen in these patients when they drank 50 ml of 100% alcohol (equivalent to 4 oz of whisky).[4] Alcoholic patients with liver transplants and on cyclosporin have been reported to have a much higher rate of alcohol abstinence than other alcoholics,[1,2] but a subsequent study failed to find any evidence that this was due to the development of a disulfiram-like reaction which would make drinking unpleasant,[3] and there was no suggestion in the report cited above that such a reaction ever occurs.[4] The authors of this study say that they currently advise their patients to avoid heavy drinking but that an occasional drink probably does not affect cyclosporin levels.[4]

References

1 Starzl E, Van Thiel D, Tzakis AG. Orthoptic liver transplantation for alcoholic cirrhosis. J Amer Med Ass (1988) 260, 2542.
2 Orrego H, Blendis LM, Blake J E, Kapur BM, Israel Y. Reliability of assessment of alcohol intake based on personal interviews in a liver clinic. Lancet (1979) 2, 1354.
3 Giles HG, Orrego H, Sandrin S, Saldivia V. The influence of cyclosporine on abstinence from alcohol in transplant patients. Transplantation (1990) 49, 1201–2.
4 Paul MD, Parfrey PS, Smart M, Gault H. The effect of ethanol on serum cyclosporine A levels in renal transplant patients. Am J Kidney Dis (1987) X, 133–5.

Cyclosporin(e) + Aminoglycoside antibiotics

Abstract/Summary

Both animal and human studies indicate that kidney toxicity may be increased by concurrent use of cyclosporin and ami-

kacin, gentamicin, tobramycin, framycetin or possibly other aminoglycosides.

Clinical evidence, mechanism, importance and management

A comparative study in patients given 30 mg gentamicin with lincomycin just prior to transplantation found that the concurrent use of cyclosporin increased the incidence of nephrotoxicity from 5% to 67%.[1] When ampicillin, ceftazidime and lincomycin were used instead the incidence of nephrotoxicity was 10%.[1] Three other reports describe increased nephrotoxicity associated with the concurrent use of cyclosporin and gentamicin,[6] tobramycin[2,3] or framycetin.[2] This interaction has also been well demonstrated in animals.[4,5] Another report describes damaged renal function in a patient on cyclosporin with minocycline and amikacin.[7] All of these studies indicate that the aminoglycosides and cyclosporin can have additive nephrotoxic effects and should therefore be avoided or only used with great caution.

References

1 Termeer A, Hoitsma AJ, Koene RAP. Severe nephrotoxicity caused by the combined use of gentamicin and cyclosporine in renal allograft recipients. Transplantation (1986) 42, 220–1.
2 Hows JM, Chipping PM, Fairhead S, Smith J, Baughan A, Gordon-Smith EC. Nephrotoxicity in bone marrow transplant recipients treated with cyclosporin A. Br J Haematol (1983) 54, 69–78.
3 Hows JM, Palmer S, Want S, Dearden C, Gordon-Smith EC. Serum levels of cyclosporin A and nephrotoxicity in bone marrow transplant patients. Lancet (1981) ii, 145–6.
4 Whiting PH, Simpson JG. The enhancement of cyclosporin A-induced nephrotoxicity by gentamicin. Biochem Pharmacol (1983) 32, 2025–8.
5 Ryffel B, Muller AM, Mihatsch MJ. Experimental cyclosporine nephrotoxicity: risk of concomitant chemotherapy. Clin Nephrol (1986) 25, Suppl 1, S121–5.
6 Morales JM, Andres A, Prieto C, Rolon JAD, Rodicio JL. Reversible acute renal toxicity by toxic synergic effect between gentamicin and cyclosporine. Clin Nephrol (1988) 29, 272.
7 Thaler F, Gotainer B, Teodori G, Dubois C, Loirat Ph. Mediastinitis due to Nocardia asteroides after cardiac transplantation. Intensive Care Med (1992) 18, 127–8.

Cyclosporin(e) + Amiodarone

Abstract/Summary

Cyclosporin serum levels can be increased by amiodarone. Cyclosporin dosage reductions are needed to avoid nephrotoxicity.

Clinical evidence

Eight patients with heart transplants and three with heart-lung transplants on cyclosporin were given amiodarone for atrial flutter or fibrillation. Despite a 13–14% reduction in the cyclosporin dosage, the cyclosporin serum levels rose by 9%, serum creatinine levels rose by 38% (from 157 to 216 µmol/l), and blood urea nitrogen rose by 30%.[3] In a previous report by some of the same authors one patient is said to have shown a 50% decrease in the clearance of cyclosporin when given amiodarone.[2]

Eight patients with heart transplants were effectively treated with amiodarone for atrial flutter and/or atrial fibrillation, but they also showed a 31% rise in serum cyclosporin levels (from 248 to 325 ng/ml) despite a 44% reduction in the cyclosporin dosage (from 6.2 to 3.5 mg/kg/day). Serum creatinine levels rose from 158 to 219.[1]

Mechanism

Uncertain. A reduction in the metabolism of the cyclosporin by the amiodarone has been suggested.[2]

Importance and management

An established and clinically important interaction. Concurrent use need not be avoided but close monitoring and cyclosporin dosage reductions are needed to minimize the potential nephrotoxicity.

References

1 Mamprin F, Mullins P, Graham T, Kendall S, Biocine B, Large S, Wallwork J, Schofield P. Amiodarone-cyclosporine interaction in cardiac transplantation. Am Heart J (1992) 123, 1725–6.
2 Nicolau DP, Uber WE, Crumbley AJ, Strange C. Amiodarone-cyclosporine interaction in a heart transplant patient. J Heart Lung Transplant (1992) 11, 564–8.
3 Egami J, Mullins PA, Mamprin F, Chauhan A, Large SR, Wallwork J, Schofield PM. Increase in cyclosporin levels due to amiodarone therapy after heart and heart-lung transplantation. J Am Coll Cardiol (1993) 21, 141A.

Cyclosporin(e) + Amphotericin (B)

Abstract/Summary

The risk of kidney toxicity is increased if cyclosporin and amphotericin are used concurrently.

Clinical evidence

A comparative study in 47 patients with bone marrow transplants found that the concurrent use of amphotericin B increased the incidence of kidney toxicity. Out of a total of 10 patients who had had both drugs, five doubled and three tripled their serum creatinine levels within 5 days. In contrast only eight out of 21 (38%) on cyclosporin alone and three out of 16 (19%) on methotrexate and amphotericin B doubled their serum creatinine within 14–30 and 5 days respectively.[1]

Another study in patients on cyclosporin with bone marrow transplants found that amphotericin B contributed significantly to renal failure. It can apparently develop even after the amphotericin has been withdrawn.[2] Marked nephrotoxicity is described in one patient in another report.[3]

Mechanism

Not understood. Simple additive kidney damaging effects is one possible explanation.

Importance and management

An established and clinically important interaction. The authors of one report say that 'if amphotericin must be given, witholding cyclosporine until the serum level is less than about 150 ng/ml may be a means of decreasing renal toxicity without losing the immunosuppressive effect.[1]

References

1 Kennedy MS, Deeg HJ, Siegel M, Crowley JJ, Storb R, Thomas ED. Acute renal toxicity with combined use of amphotericin B and cyclosporine after bone marrow transplantation. Transplantation (1983) 35, 211–15.
2 Tutschka PJ, Beschorner WE, Hess AD, Santos GW. Cyclosporin-A to prevent graft-versus-host-disease: a pilot study in 22 patients receiving allogeneic marrow transplants. Blood (1983) 61, 318–25.
3 Conti DJ, Tolkoff-Rubin NE, Baker GP, Doran M, Cosinin AB, Delmonico F, Auchincloss H, Russell PS, Rubin RH. Successful treatment of invasive fungal infection with fluconazole in organ transplant recipients, Transplantation (1989) 48, 692–4.

Cyclosporin(e) + Anticoagulants

Abstract/Summary

The cyclosporin levels of a patient fell when given warfarin. When the cyclosporin dosage was raised an increase in the warfarin dosage was needed. Another report describes a rise in serum cyclosporin levels when an un-named anticoagulant was given. Yet another describes increased nicoumalone effects while receiving cyclosporin.

Clinical evidence, mechanism, importance and management

A man with erythrocyte aplasia effectively treated with cyclosporin for 18 months, relapsed within a week of starting warfarin. His cyclosporin levels had fallen from a range of 300–350 to 170 ng/ml. He responded well when the cyclosporin dosage was increased from 3 to 7 mg/kg daily, but his prothrombin activity rose from 17% of control to 64% and he needed an increase in the warfarin dosage to achieve satisfactory anticoagulation. The patient was also taking phenobarbitone.[1] Another patient on nicoumalone (acenocoumarol) showed the opposite effect. His anticoagulant dosage needed to be approximately halved when he was started on cyclosporin following a kidney transplant.[3] The reasons are not understood. Another report briefly says that serum cyclosporin levels rose in a patient when given a warfarin derivative.[2]

These reports serve to emphasize the need to monitor concurrent use. The outcome is clearly uncertain.

References

1 Snyder DS. Interaction between cyclosporine and warfarin. Ann Intern Med (1988) 108, 311.

2 Cockburn I (Sandoz, Basel). Cyclosporin A: a clinical evaluation of drug interactions. Transplantation Proc (1986) 18, (Suppl 5) 50–5.

3 Campistol JM, Maragall D, Andreu J. Interaction between cyclosporin A and sintrom. Nephron (1989) 53, 291–2

Cyclosporin(e) + Anticonvulsants

Abstract/Summary

Serum cyclosporin levels are markedly reduced by the concurrent use of carbamazepine, phenobarbitone and phenytoin. The dosage of cyclosporin may need to be increased 2–3-fold to maintain adequate immunosuppression. Sodium valproate appears not to affect cyclosporin levels but it may sometimes possibly damage renal grafts and cause liver damage.

Clinical evidence

(a) Cyclosporin + Carbamazepine

The cyclosporin serum levels of a kidney transplant patient fell from 346 to 64 ng/ml within 3 days of starting to take 200 mg carbamazepine three times daily. A week later serum levels were down to 37 ng/ml. They rose again when the carbamazepine was stopped but fell once more when it was restarted. The cyclosporin dosage was increased to keep the levels within the therapeutic range.[3]

Four other patients have shown this interaction.[4,14,17] One needed her cyclosporin dosage to be doubled in order to maintain adequate serum levels while taking 800 mg carbamazepine daily.[4] When the carbamazepine was replaced by sodium valproate in three patients, the cyclosporin dosages became normal again.[4,14]

(b) Cyclosporin + Phenobarbitone

A 4-year-old child on phenobarbitone (50 mg twice daily) with a bone marrow transplant had serum cyclosporin levels of less than 60 ng/ml even after raising the dosage to 18 mg/kg daily. When the phenobarbitone dosage was halved and later halved again the trough serum cyclosporin levels rose to 205 ng/ml.[5]

A threefold increase in cyclosporin clearance was seen in another child with a kidney transplant while on phenobarbitone (12.6 compared with 3.8 ml/min/kg).[6] Reductions in cyclosporin levels due to phenobarbitone have been described in other patients.[8,12,16,18,20]

(c) Cyclosporin + Phenytoin

The observation of five patients on cyclosporin who needed dosage increases while taking phenytoin prompted a further study in six normal subjects. It was found that while taking 300 or 400 mg phenytoin daily the maximal serum cyclosporin levels and the AUC following a single 15 mg/kg dose were reduced by 37% (from 1325 to 831 g/l) and 47% (10.4 to 5.5 mg l^{-1} h) respectively.[1,13]

Another report by the same authors describes six patients whose serum cyclosporin levels were more than halved while treated with phenytoin (750–1000 mg daily orally and intravenously) despite an almost twofold increase in the cyclosporin dosage. It persisted for about a week after the phenytoin was stopped.[2] Two four-fold increases in cyclosporin dosages were needed in nine heart transplant patients when given phenytoin,[9] and increases were also needed in an 11-year-old boy with a bone marrow transplant.[10] Another study found reduced serum cyclosporin levels (136 compared with 182 ng/ml) in 13 patients on phenytoin despite doses which were more than double those of other patients not taking phenytoin.[19] 1.55 mg/kg/day increases in cyclosporin dosages were found necessary in other patients taking phenytoin.[20]

Mechanisms

Not fully resolved. It is thought that phenytoin,[1,2] carbamazepine[3] and phenobarbitone[5,12] increase the metabolism of the cyclosporin by the liver (hepatic P450 oxygenase system) thereby increasing its loss from the body and lowering the serum levels accordingly. Phenytoin also possibly reduces the absorption of the cyclosporin.[7]

Importance and management

None of these interactions is extensively documented but all appear to be established and of clinical importance. Serum cyclosporin levels should be well monitored if carbamazepine, phenobarbitone or phenytoin are given concurrently and the cyclosporin dosage increased appropriately (by a factor of two or even more). The effects of the interaction may persist for a week or more after the anticonvulsant is withdrawn. Sodium valproate seems to be a non-interacting anticonvulsant,[4,11,18] however it may not always be without problems because interstitial nephritis was suspected in one patient with a renal graft[8] and fatal valproate-induced hepatotoxicty occurred in another.[15]

References

1 Freeman DJ, Laupacis A, Keown PA, Stiller CR, Carruthers SG. Evaluation of cyclosporin-phenytoin interaction with observations on cyclosporin metabolites. Br J Clin Pharmac (1984) 18, 887–93.

2 Keown PA, Laupacis A, Carruthers G, Stawecki M, Koegler J, McKenzie FN, Wall W, Stiller CR. Interaction between phenytoin and cyclosporine following organ transplantation. Transplantation (1984) 38, 304–6.

3 Lele P, Peterson P, Yang S, Jarell B, Burke JF. Cyclosporine and tegretol — another drug interaction. Kidney Int (1985) 27, 344.

4 Hillebrand G, Castro LA, van Scheidt W, Beukelmann D, Land W, Schmidt D. Valproate for epilepsy in renal transplant recipients receiving cyclosporine. Transplantation (1987) 43, 915–16.

5 Carstensen H, Jacobsen N, Dieperink H. Interaction between cyclosporin A and phenobarbitone. Br J Clin Pharmac (1986) 21, 550–1.

6 Burckart GJ, Venkataramanan R, Starz T, Ptachcinski J, Gartner JC,

Rosenthal T. Cyclosporine clearance in children following organ transplantation. J Clin Pharmacol (1984) 24, 412.

7 Rowland M, Gupta SK. Cyclosporin-phenytoin interaction: re-evaluation using metabolite data. Br J Clin Pharmac (1987) 24, 329–34.

8 Kramer G, Dillmann U, Tettenborn B. Cyclosporine-phenobarbital interaction. Epilepsia (1989) 30, 701.

9 Grigg-Damberger MM, Costanzo-Nordin R, Kelly MA, Bahamon-Dussan JE, Silver M, Zucker MJ, Celesia GG. Phenytoin may compromise efficacy of cyclosporine immunosuppresion in cardiac transplant patients. Epilepsia (1988) 29, 693.

10 Schmidt H, Naumann R, Jaschonek K, Einsele H, Dopfer R, Ehninger G. Drug interaction between cyclosporin and phenytoin in allogeneic bone marrow transplantation. Bone Marrow Transplantation (1989) 4, 212–13.

11 Noguchi M, Kiuchi C, Akiyama H, Sakamaki H, Onozawa Y. Interaction between cyclosporin A, anticonvulsants. Bone Marrow Transplant (1992) 9, 391.

12 Beierle FA, Bailey L. Cyclosporine metabolism impeded/blocked by co-administration of phenobarbitol. Clin Chem (1989) 35, 1160.

13 Freeman DJ, Laupacis A, Keown P, Stiller C, Carruthers G. The effects of agents that alter drug metabolizing enzyme activity on the pharmacokinetics of cyclosporin. Ann Roy Coll Phys Can (1984) 17, 301.

14 Schofield OMV, Camp RDR, Levene GM. Cyclosporin A in psoriasis: interaction with carbamazepine. Br J Dermatol (1990) 122, 425–6.

15 Fischmann MA, Hull D, Bartus SA, Schweizer RT. Valproate for epilepsy in renal transplant recipients receiving cyclosporine. Transplantation (1989) 48, 542.

16 Wideman CA. Pharmacokinetic monitoring of cyclosporine. Transplant Proc (1983) XV, Suppl 1, 3168–75.

17 Alvarez JS, Del Castillo JAC, Ortiz MJA. Effect of carbamazepine on ciclosporin blood level. Nephron (1991) 58, 235–6.

18 Matsuura T, Akiyama T, Kurita T. Interaction between phenobarbital and ciclosporin following renal transplantation: a case report. Hinyokika Kiyo (1990) 36, 447–50.

19 Schweitzer EJ, Canafax DM, Gillingham KJ, Najarian JS, Matas AJ. Phenytoin administration in kidney recipients on CSA immunosuppression. J Am Soc Nephrol (1991) 2, 816.

20 Castelao AM. Cyclosporine A – drug interactions. In Sunshine I (Ed.) Recent developments in therapeutic drug monitoring and clinical toxicology. 2nd Int Conf Therapeutic Drug Monitoring Toxicology, Barcelona, Spain, (1992) 203–9.

Cyclosporin(e) + Benzodiazepines

Abstract/Summary

Cyclosporin and midazolam appear not to interact.

Clinical evidence, mechanism, importance and management

On the basis of an experimental study in nine patients it was concluded that the dosage of midazolam needs no adjustment in those on cyclosporin. Midazolam also appears to have no effect on cyclosporin.[1]

Reference

1 Li G, Treiber G, Meinshausen J, Wolf J, Werringloer J, Klotz U. Is cyclosporin A an inhibitor of drug metabolism ? Br J Clin Pharmac (1990) 30, 71–7.

Cyclosporin(e) + Busulphan and Cyclophosphamide

Abstract/Summary

The development of seizures in patients with bone marrow transplants on cyclosporin has been attributed to previous treatment with busulphan and cyclophosphamide.

Clinical evidence, mechanism, importance and management

Five of 182 patients receiving allogenic bone marrow transplants developed seizures within 22–61 days of starting cyclosporin and methylprednisolone. All of them had had 16 mg/kg busulphan and 120 mg/kg cyclophosphamide as preparative therapy without radiation.[1] Magnetic resonance imaging showed brain abnormalities which resolved a few days after the cyclosporin was withdrawn. The reasons are not understood, nor is the association between the use of the preparative drugs, the cyclosporine and the development of the seizure clearly established. The authors of the report recommend that if seizures develop the cyclosporine should be stopped and anticonvulsants started.

Reference

1 Ghany AM, Tutschaka PJ, McGhee RB, Avalos BR, Cunningham I, Kapoor N, Copelan EA. Cyclosporine-associated seizures in bone marrow transplant recipients given busulfan and cyclophosphamide preparative therapy. Transplantation (1991) 52, 310–5.

Cyclosporin(e) + Calcium channel blockers

Abstract/Summary

Diltiazem, nicardipine and verapamil raise serum cyclosporin levels but also appear to possess both kidney-tissue protective and increased immunosuppressive effects which can improve the viability of transplanted kidneys. Isradipine, nifedipine and nitrendipine normally appear not to raise serum cyclosporin levels, but rises and falls have been seen in a few patients on nifedipine. The interaction of diltiazem with cyclosporin has been exploited to save costs.

Clinical evidence

(a) Cyclosporin + Diltiazem

65 kidney transplant patients on cyclosporin and diltiazem needed less cyclosporin than 63 control patients not given diltiazem (7.3 compared with 9 mg/kg/day). There were considerable individual differences.[18]

Other studies clearly confirm that diltiazem can raise cyclosporin serum levels.[26,28,31,33,34,36-9,47] In some cases the serum cyclosporin levels were not only controlled by reducing the cyclosporin dosage by about one-third but it appeared that diltiazem had a kidney protective role (reduced nephrotoxicity, fewer rejection episodes and haemodialyses).[5,6,7,17,26,37-9,48] See also cost-saving under 'Importance and management' below.

(b) Cyclosporin + Felodipine

A single 10 mg dose of felodipine in cyclosporin treated kidney transplant patients was found to have beneficial effects on blood pressure, renal haemodynamics, renal tubular sodium and water handling. The effects of long-term use were not studied.[49]

(c) Cyclosporin + Isradipine

12 kidney transplant patient showed no changes in cyclosporin levels over 4 weeks while taking up to 2.5 mg isradipine twice daily.[42] Two other studies in seven and six kidney transplant patients confirmed the absence of an interaction.[43,51]

(d) Cyclosporin + Nicardipine

20 mg nicardipine three times a day in nine patients raised their serum cyclosporin levels by 110% (from 226 to 430 ng/ml-range 24 to 341%). Their serum creatinine levels rose from 135 to 147 µmol/l.[3] Other studies have found increases in serum cyclosporin levels, in some cases as much as 2-3-fold, when nicardipine was given.[10,14,23,24,30,50]

(e) Cyclosporin + Nifedipine

Five of nine patients who showed an interaction with nicardipine (see above) showed no interaction when given nifedipine.[3] No changes in cyclosporin levels were seen in other studies.[17,25,28,29,32,40] but raised[37,47] and reduced levels[27] have been reported in others. Two studies found that nifedipine appeared to protect patients against the nephrotoxicity of cyclosporin,[8,45] however there is some evidence that the side-effects of nifedipine (flushing, rash)[16] and gingival overgrowth may be increased.[52]

(f) Cyclosporin + Nitrendipine

20 mg nitrendipine daily for three weeks had no significant effect on serum cyclosporin levels of 16 kidney transplant patients.[35]

(g) Cyclosporin + Verapamil

22 kidney transplant patients on cyclosporin and verapamil had serum cyclosporin levels which were 50-70% higher than in 18 other patients not given verapamil although the dosages were the same. Serum creatinine levels were lower. Moreover only three of the 22 had rejection episodes within four weeks compared with 10 out of 18 not given verapamil.[21]

Other studies have demonstrated that 120-320 mg verapamil daily can increase, or double or even triple serum cyclosporin levels in individual patients with kidney or heart transplants.[4,9,11,13,22,26,28,32]

Mechanism

The increased cyclosporin levels are largely due to inhibition by the calcium channel blockers of its metabolism by the liver. The reduced loss results in a serum level rise. Diltiazem also appears to reduce ischaemia-induced tubular necrosis.[44]

Importance and management

The interactions of cyclosporin with diltiazem, nicardipine or verapamil are established and relatively well documented. Concurrent use need not be avoided but cyclosporin levels should be well monitored and dosage reductions made as necessary. Even though cyclosporin serum levels are increased, these calcium channel blockers appear to have both a kidney-protective effect and to improve immunosuppression. One study noted that '...calcium channel blockers lead to an alteration of the cyclosporin pharmacokinetics by increasing cyclosporin blood levels...this interference, however, is of no harm to the patient, since no change in kidney function was observed despite drastic elevation of cyclosporin levels.'[19] With diltiazem and verapamil the cyclosporin dosage can apparently be reduced by about 25-50%, but possibly larger reductions with nicardipine. One study found that the costs of cyclosporin for heart transplant patients could be reduced by using 30 mg diltiazem three times daily initially, increasing to 60 mg three times daily at 1 month: a 32% saving in year 1 and 43% in the ensuing years.[31] Others estimate an annual 1991 cost saving of $1700 (Can.) and $2000 (US) per patient using 60-360 mg diltiazem daily.[33,41,46]

The situation with nifedipine is not totally clear (no effect, decreases or increases) but it appears to have a kidney-protective effect.[40] So too does felodipine. Isradipine and nitrendipine appear to be non-interacting alternatives. More study is needed to find out what happens with other calcium channel blockers.

References

1 Pochet JM, Pirson Y. Cyclosporin-diltiazem interaction. Lancet (1986) i, 979.
2 Grino JM, Sabate I, Castelao AM, Alsina J. Influence of diltiazem on cyclosporin clearance. Lancet (1986) i, 1387.
3 Bourbigot B, Guiserix J, Airiau J, Bressollette L, Morin JF, Cledes J. Nicardipine increases cyclosporin blood levels. Lancet (1986) i, 1447.
4 Lindholm A, Henricsson S. Verapamil inhibits cyclosporin metabolism. Lancet (1987) 1, 1262-3
5 Neumayer H-H, Wagner K. Diltiazem and economic use of cyclosporin. Lancet (1986) ii, 523.
6 Wagner K, Albrecht S, Neumayer H-H. Prevention of delayed graft function in cadaveric kidney transplantation by a calcium antagonist. Preliminary results of two prospective randomized trials. Transplant Proc (1986) 18, 510-15.

7 Wagner K, Albrecht S, Neumayer H-H. Prevention of delayed graft function by a calcium antagonist- a randomized trial in renal graft recipients on cyclosporin A. Transplant Proc (1986) 18, 1269–71.

8 Feehally J, Walls J, Mistry N, Horsburgh T, Taylor J, Veitch PS, Bell PRF. Does nifedipine ameliorate cyclosporin A nephrotoxicity ? Br Med J (1987) 295, 310.

9 Hampton EM, Stewart CF, Herrod HG, Valenski WR. Augmentation of in vitro immunosuppressive effects of cyclosporin by verapamil. Clin Pharmacol Ther (1987) 41, 169.

10 Cantarovich M, Hiesse C, Lockiec F, Charpentier B, Fries D. Confirmation of the interaction between cyclosporine and the calcium channel blocker nicardipine in renal transplant patients. Clin Nephrol (1987) 28, 190–3.

11 Robson RA, Fraenkel M, Barratt LJ, Birkett DJ. Cyclosporin-verapamil interaction. Br J Clin Pharmac (1988) 25, 402–3.

12 Brockmoller J, Wagner K, Neumayer HH, Heinemeyer G. Interaction of ciclosporine and diltiazem. Naunyn-Schmied Arch Pharmakol (1988) 337, Suppl R126.

13 Angermann CE, Spes CH, Anthuber M, Kemkes BM, Theisen K. Verapamil increases cyclosporin-A blood trough levels in cardiac recipients. J Amer Coll Cardiol (1988) 11, 206A.

14 Kessler M, Renoult E, Jonon B, Vigneron T, Huu C, Netter P. Interaction ciclosporine-nicardipine chez le transplante renal. Therapie (1987) 42, 273–5.

15 Kunzerdorf G, Walz G, Neumayer H-H, Wagner K, Keller F, Offermann G. Einfluss von Diltiazem auf die Ciclosporin-Blutspiegel. Klin Wschr (1987) 65, 1101–3.

16 McFadden JP, Pontin JE, Powles AV, Fry L, Idle JR. Cyclosporin decreases nifedipine metabolism. Br Med J (1989) 299, 1224.

17 Wagner K, Philipp TH, Heinemeyer G, Brockmuller F, Roots I, Neumayer HH. Interaction of cyclosporin and calcium antagonists. Transplant Proc (1989) 21, 1453–6.

18 Kohlhaw K, Wonigeit K, Frei U, Oldhafer K, Neumann K, Pichlmayr R. Effect of calcium channel blocker diltiazem on cyclosporin A blood levels and dose requirements. Transplant Proc (1988) XX Suppl 2, 572–4.

19 Wagner K, Henkel M, Heinemeyer G, Neumayer H-H. Interaction of calcium blockers and cyclosporine. Transplant Proc (1988) XX, Suppl 2, 561–8.

20 Sabate I, Grino JM, Castelao AM, Huguet J, Seron D, Blanco A. Cyclosporin-diltiazem interaction: comparison of cyclosporin levels measured with two monoclonal antibodies. Transplant Proc (1989) 21, 1460–1.

21 Dawidson I, Rooth P, Fry WR, Sandor Z, Willms C, Coorpender L, Alway C, Reisch J. Prevention of acute cyclosporin induced renal blood flow inhibition and improved immunosuppression with verapamil. Transplantation (1989) 48, 575–80.

22 Sabate I, Grino JM, Castelao AM, Ortola J. Evaluation of cyclosporin-verapamil interaction, with observations on parent cyclosporin and metabolites. Clin Chem (1989) 34, 2151–2.

23 Deray G, Aupeptit B, Martinez F, Baumelou A, Worcel A, Benhmikda M, Lagrand JC, Jacobs C. Cyclosporin-nicardipine interaction. Am J Nephrol (1989) 9, 349.

24 Kessler M, Netter P, Renoult E, Jonon B, Mur JM, Trechot P, Dousset B. Influence of nicardipine on renal function and plasma cyclosporin in renal transplant patients. Eur J Clin Pharmacol (1989) 36, 637–8.

25 McNally P, Mistry N, Idle J, Walls J, Freehally J. Calcium channel blockers and cyclosporin metabolism. Transplantation (1989) 48, 1071.

26 Ki Chul Choi, Young Joon Kang, Shin Kon Kim, Soo Bang Ryu. Effects of the calcium channel blocker diltiazem on the blood and serum levels of cyclosporin A. Chonnam J Med Sci (1989) 2, 131–6.

27 Howard RL, Shapiro JI, Babcock S, Chan L. The effect of clacium channel blockers on the cyclosporine dose requirment in renal transplant recipients. Renal Failure (1990) 12, 89–92.

28 Campistol JM, Oppenheimer F, Vilardell J, Ricart MJ, Alcaraz A, Ponz E, Andreu J. Interaction between ciclosporin and diltiazem in renal transplant patients. Nephron (1991) 57, 241–2.

29 Rossi SJ, Harlharan S, Schroeder TJ, First MR. Cyclosporine dosing and blood levels in renal transplants receiving Procardia XL. Clin Pharmacol Ther (1993) 53, 238.

30 Todd P, Garioch JJ, Rademaker M, Thomson J. Nicardipine interacts with cyclosporin. Br J Dermatol (1989) 121, 820.

31 Valantine H, Keogh A, McIntosh N, Hunt S, Oyer P, Schroeder J. Cost containment. Coadministration of diltiazem with cyclosporine following cardiac transplant. J Heart Transplant (1990) 9, 68.

32 Ogborn MR, Crocker JFS, Grimm PC. Nifedipine, verapamil and cyclosporin A pharmacokinetics in children. Pediatr Nephrol (1989) 3, 314–6.

33 Bourge RC, Kirklin JK, Naftel DC, Figg WD, White-Williams C, Ketchum C. Diltiazem-cyclosporine interaction in cardiac transplant recipients: impact on cyclosporine dose and medication costs. Am J Med (1991) 90, 402–4.

34 Maddux MS, Veremis SA, Bauma WD, Pollak R. Significant drug interactions with cyclosporine. Hospital Therapy (1987) 12, 56–70.

35 Copur MS, Tasdmir I, Turgan C, Yasavul Ü, Caglar S. Effects of nitrendipine on blood pressure and blood ciclosporin A level in patients with posttransplant hypertension. Nephron (1989) 52, 227–30.

36 Brockmöller J, Neumayer H-H, Wagner K, Weber W, Heinemeyer G, Kewitz H, Roots I. Pharmacokinetic interaction between cyclosporin and ditliazem. Eur J Clin Pharmacol (1990) 38, 237–42.

37 Diaz C, Gillum DM. Interaction of ditliazem and nifedipine with cyclosporine in renal transplant recipients. Kidney Int (1989) 35, 513.

38 Wagner K, Albrecht S, Neumayer H-M. Prevention of posttransplant acute tubular necrosis by the calcium antagonist diltiazem: a propective randomized study. Am J Nephrol (1987) 7, 287–91.

39 McCauley J, Ptachcinski RJ, Shapiro R. The cyclosporine-sparing effects of diltiazem in renal transplantation. Transplant Proc (1989) 21, 3955–7.

40 Propper DJ, Whiting PH, Power DA, Edward N, Catto GRD. The effect of nifedipine on graft function in renal allograft recipients treated with cyclosporin A. Clin Nephrol (1989) 32, 62–7.

41 Moody HR, Bickell-Feist L, Friesen I, Huizinga R, Halloran PF. Benefits of cyclosporine dose reduction using diltiazem. Clin Invest Med (1991) 14, Suppl A, A142.

42 Endresen L, Bergan S, Holdaas H, Pran T, Singing-Larsen B, Berg KJ. Lack of effect of the calcium antagonist isradipine on cyclosporin pharmacokinetics in renal transplant patients. Ther Drug Monit (1991) 13, 490–5.

43 Martinez F, Pirson Y, Wallemacq P, van Ypersele de Strihou C. No clinically significant interaction between ciclosporin and isradipine. Nephron (1991) 59, 658–9.

44 Oppenheimer F, Alcaraz A, Manalich M, Ricart MJ, Vilardell J, Campistol JM, Andreu J, Talbot-Wright R, Fernandez-Cruz L. Influence of the calcium blocker diltiazem on the prevention of acute renal failure after renal transplantation. Transplant Proc (1992) 24, 50–1.

45 Morales JM, Andrés A, Alvarez C, Prieto C, Ortuno B, Paternina ER, Poblete GH, Praga M, Ruilope LM, Rodicio JL. Calcium channel blockers and early cyclosporin nephrotoxicity after renal transplantation: a prospective randomized study. Transplant Proc (1990) 22, 1733–5.

46 Smith CL, Hampton EM, Pederson JA, Pennington LR, Bourne DWA. Influence of diltiazem on the pharmacokinetics and dose/cost relationships of cyclosporin in renal transplant patients. J Am Soc Nephrol (1991) 2, 816.

47 Castelao AM. Cyclosporine A — drug interactions. In Sunshine I (Ed.) Recent developments in therapeutic drug monitoring and clinical toxicology. 2nd Int Conf Therapeutic Drug Monitoring Toxicology, Barcelona, Spain,(1992) 203–9.

48 Neumayer H-H, Kunzendorf U, Schreiber M. Protective effects of calcium antagonists in human renal transplantation. Kidney Int (1992) 41, Suppl 36, S87–93.

49 Pedersen EB, Sorensen SS, Eiskjoer H, Skovbon H, Thomsen K. Interaction between cyclosporine and felodipine in renal transplant recipients. Kidney Int (1992) 41, Suppl 36, S82–6.

50 Bouquet S, Chapelle G, Barrier L, Boutaud Ph, Menu P, Courtois PH. Interactions ciclosporine-nicardipine chez un transplanté cardiaque, adaption poslogique. J Pharm Clin (1992) 11, 59.

51 Vernillet L, Bourbigot B, Codet JP, Le Saux L, Moal MC, Morin JF. Lack of effect of isradipine on cyclosporin pharmacokinetics. Fund Clin Pharmacol (1992) 6, 367–74.

52 Thomason JM, Seymour RA, Rice N. The prevalence and severity of cyclosporin and nifedipine-induced gingival overgrowth. J Clin Peridont (1993) 20, 37–40.

Cyclosporin + Cephalosporins

Abstract/Summary

Two patients developed elevated cyclosporin serum levels when given ceftriaxone. Ceftazidime possibly interacts similarly.

Clinical evidence, mechanism, importance and management

Two kidney transplant patients showed marked rises (2–4 fold) in cyclosporin levels within 2–3 days of starting 1 g ceftriaxone twice daily. Levels fell when the antibiotic was stopped. The reason is uncertain but the suggestion is that ceftriaxone possibly inhibits the metabolism of the cyclosporin by the liver.[1] Ceftazidime has also been implicated in an increase in serum cyclosporin levels.[2] Information about both of these cephalosporins is very limited but it would clearly be prudent to monitor cyclosporin levels closely if either is given.

References

1 Alvarez JS, Del Castillo JAS, Ortiz MJA. Interaction between ciclosporin and ceftriaxone. Nephron (1991) 59, 681–2.
2 Cockburn I. Cyclosporin A: a clinical evaluation of drug interactions. Transplantation Proc (1986) 18, (Suppl 5), 50–5.

Cyclosporin(e) + Cholestyramine and Food

Abstract/Summary

Cholestyramine, different drinks and food can have a marked effect (increases and decreases) on the absorption of cyclosporin.

Clinical evidence, mechanism, importance and management

Four transplant patients on cyclosporin and prednisolone given cholestyramine for a week had only a very small average change (+6%) in the AUC of the cyclosporin, but one patient had a 55% increase and another a 23% decrease.[1] Patients taking cyclosporin with milk had a 39% higher AUC after food and 23% higher when fasting compared with others taking cyclosporin with orange juice.[1] Food more than doubled the AUC of cyclosporin (bioavailability increased from 20.7 to 53%) and almost tripled its maximal serum levels (from 783 to 2062 ng/ml).[3] Another study in 18 patients with kidney transplants found that when the cyclosporin was mixed with 240 ml chocolate milk and taken with a standard hospital breakfast, peak cyclosporin levels rose by 30% (from 1120 to 1465 ng/ml), trough serum levels rose by 21% (from 228 to 267 ng/ml), and the AUC rose 60.6% (from 7881 to 11430 ng/h/ml). Very considerable individual variations occurred.[2] 11 of 13 kidney

transplant patients showed a mean 32% rise in trough serum cyclosporin levels while taking 8 ounces of grapefruit juice for a week. The levels decreased again in 10 of 11 when the juice was stopped (two patients failed to complete the study).[4]

All of these studies suggest that some cost savings might be achieved with patients if the cyclosporin were to be taken with certain foods and/or drinks. More study is needed.

References

1 Keogh A, Day R, Critchley L, Duggin G, Baron D. The effect of food and cholestyramine on the absorption of cyclosporine in cardiac transplant patients. Transplant Proc (1988) 20, 27–30.
2 Ptachcinski RJ, Venkataaramanan R, Rosenthal JT, Burckart GJ, Taylor RJ, Hakala TR. The effect of food on cyclosporin absorption. Transplantation (1985) 40, 174–6.
3 Gupta SK, Benet LZ. Food increases the bioavailability of cyclosporin in healthy volunteers. Clin Pharmacol Ther (1989) 45,148.
4 Edwards DJ, Ducharme MP, Provenzano R, Dehoorne-Smith M. Effect of grapefruit juice on blood concentrations of cyclosporine. Clin Pharmacol Ther (1993) 53, 237.

Cyclosporin(e) + Cimetidine, Famotidine and Ranitidine

Abstract/Summary

An uncertain situation: some reports say that cimetidine and ranitidine do not affect serum cyclosporin levels whereas others say that cimetidine and ranitidine raise serum cyclosporin levels. Rises in serum creatinine levels (interpreted as a deterioration in kidney function) have been seen in some studies with cimetidine and ranitidine, but not others. Cases of thrombocytopenia and hepatotoxicity have also occurred. Famotidine is reported not to interact.

Clinical evidence

(a) Cimetidine, Ranitidine

Cimetidine or ranitidine increased the mean serum creatinine levels in seven kidney transplant patients on cyclosporin by 62% (from 2.28 to 3.22 mg/dl). All of them showed a rise, whereas only two out of five other patients with heart transplants showed a serum creatinine level rise when given either cimetidine or ranitidine, nevertheless the mean rise was 37% (from 1.72 to 2.36 mg/dl). No changes in serum cyclosporin levels were seen.[1]

Raised serum cyclosporin levels have been seen in eight liver transplant patients,[10,15] and in another patient when treated with cimetidine and metronidazole.[6] Elsewhere cimetidine is stated not to affect the pharmacokinetics of cyclosporin in normal subjects.[7] A study in five liver transplant patients found that cimetidine transiently raised peak cyclosporin levels but no changes in trough cyclosporin levels were seen after 4 h, and the conclusion was reached that it was safe to use cimetidine over at least a 4-week period.[14]

Three further reports claim that ranitidine does not alter serum cyclosporin levels[4,11,13] nor the creatinine or inulin clearance,[11] but another claims a decrease in cyclosporin levels in two patients when ranitidine was stopped.[15] A report describes thrombocytopenia in a man with a kidney transplant on cyclosporin when given ranitidine.[2] Another patient experienced hepatotoxicity while taking cyclosporin when given ranitidine.[3]

(b) Famotidine

Famotidine is reported not to affect serum cyclosporin levels.[8,16]

Mechanisms

Not understood. In a study in which azathioprine and prednisone were used for immunosuppression in patients with kidney transplants, no changes in serum creatinine levels were found when cimetidine was used for 6 weeks.[5] This possibly suggests that the rise in serum creatinine levels described in the studies cited results from a cyclosporin/H_2-antagonist interaction.

Importance and management

Information about cimetidine and ranitidine is limited and the results are confusing. The practical solution is to monitor serum cyclosporin levels, and be alert for any evidence of kidney function deterioration if cimetidine or ranitidine are used. One report puts forward the idea that any rises in serum creatinine levels are not a reflection of increased nephrotoxicity, but occur simply because these H_2-blockers compete with creatinine for secretion by the kidney tubules.[9] This needs confirmation. Another suggestion is that any interaction possibly depends on how much cyclosporin is being used.[12] More study is needed to clarify the situation. Famotidine is reported not to interact.

References

1 Jarowenko MV, Van Buren CT, Kramer WG, Lorber MI, Flechner SM, Kahan BD. Ranitidine, cimetidine and the cyclosporin-treated recipient. Transplantation (1986) 42, 311–12.
2 Bailey RR, Walker RJ, Swainson CP. Some new problems with cyclosporin A ? NZ Med J (1985) 98, 915–6.
3 Hiesse C, Cantarovich M, Santelli C, Francais P, Charpentier B, Fries D. Ranitidine heptatotoxicity in renal transplant patient. Lancet (1985) i, 1280.
4 Zazgornik J, Schindler J, Gremmel F, Balcke P, Kopsoa H, Derfler K, Minar E. Ranitidine does not influence the blood cyclosporin levels in renal transplant patients (RTP). Kidney Int (1985) 28, 410.
5 Garvin PJ, Carney K, Castenada M, Codd JE. Peptic ulcer disease following transplantation: the role of cimetidine. Am J Surg (1982) 114, 545.
6 Zylber-Katz E, Rubinger D, Berlatsky Y. Cyclosporine interactions with metronidazole and cimetidine. Drug Intell Clin Pharm (1988) 22, 504.
7 Freeman DJ, Laupacis A, Keown P, Stiller C, Carruthers G. The effect of agents that alter drug metabolyzing enzyme activity on the pharmacokinetics of cyclosporin. Ann Roy Coll Phys Surg Can (1984) 17, 301.
8 Von Schütz A, Kemkes BM. Ciclosporinspiegel unter Gabe von Famotidin. Fortschr Med (1990) 23, 457–8.
9 Pachon J, Lorber MI, Bia MJ. Effects of H_2-receptor antagonists on renal function in cyclosporine-treated renal transplant patients. Transplantation (1989) 47, 254–9.
10 Puff MR, Carey WD, Pippenger CE, Vogt DP. Cimetidine alters cyclosporin A metabolism in liver transplantation patients. Gastroenterol (1989), 96, A647.
11 Jadoul M, Hené RJ. Ranitidine and the cyclosporine treated recipient. Transplantation (1989) 48, 359.
12 Kahan BD, Jarawenko MV. Reply to ref 11. Transplantation (1989) 48, 359.
13 Popovic J, Cameron JS. Effects of ranitidine on renal function in transplant recipients. Nephrol Dial Transplant (1990) 5, 980–1.
14 Puff MR, Carey WD. The effect of cimetidine on cyclosporine A levels in liver transplant recipients: a preliminary report. Am J Gastroenterol (1992) 87, 287–91.
15 Castelao AM. Cyclosporine A — drug interactions. In Sunshine I (Ed.) Recent developments in therapeutic drug monitoring and clinical toxicology. 2nd Int Conf Therapeutic Drug Monitoring Toxicology, Barcelona, Spain,(1992) 203–9.
16 Morel D, Bannwarth B, Vincon G, Penouil F, Elouaerr-Blanc L, Aparicio M, Potaux L. Effect of famotidine on renal transplant patients treated with ciclosporine A. Fundam Clin Pharmacol (1993) 7, 167–70.

Cyclosporin(e) + Cisapride

Abstract/Summary

Cisapride increases the serum levels of cyclosporin and also increases its bioavailability.

Clinical evidence, mechanism, importance and management

After taking 10 mg cisapride three times daily for 2 days, and then 10 mg just before and together with cyclosporin and a test meal, 10 renal transplant patients were found to have increased maximal serum cyclosporin levels (+ 24%) and increased 4 and 6 h AUCs (+ 50% and + 41% respectively). Peak serum levels also occurred earlier.[1] The reasons for these changes are not fully understood, but earlier gastric emptying may be involved. The clinical importance of these increases is uncertain, but it would be prudent to monitor concurrent use, reducing the dosages if necessary.

Reference

1 Finet L, Westeel PF, Hary G, Maurel M, Andrejak M, Dupas JL. Effects of cisapride on the intestinal absorption of cyclosporine in renal transplant recipients. Gastroenterology (1991) 100, A209

Cyclosporin(e) + Colchicine

Abstract/Summary

Two cases of cyclosporin toxicity have been reported when colchicine was given concurrently. Three cases of a serious muscle disorder (rhabdomyolysis) have also been seen.

Clinical evidence, mechanism, importance and management

A patient with a kidney transplant showed a transient (2–3 days) rise in creatinine and serum cyclosporin levels (from 100–200 to 1519 ng/ml) the day after receiving a total of 4 mg colchicine.[1] Another kidney transplant patient on cyclosporin, azathioprine and prednisone developed colchicine myoneuropathy (possibly rhabdomyolysis), cyclosporin nephrotoxicity and liver function abnormalities when treated with colchicine.[2] Another case suggestive of rhabdomyolysis has been published,[3] and Sandoz (the makers of cyclosporin) have another report on their records.[4] Rhabdomyolysis appears to be rare but Sandoz advise a change of treatment if any signs and symptoms develop.[4] Good monitoring is clearly necessary if both drugs are used.

References

1 Menta R, Rossi E, Guariglia A, David S, Cambi V. Reversible acute cyclosporine nephrotoxicity induced by colchicine administration. Neph Dial Transplant (1987) 2, 380–1.
2 Rieger EH, Halsaz NA, Wahlstrom HE. Colchicine neuromyopathy after renal transplantation. Transplantation (1990) 49, 1196–8.
3 Noppen M, Velkenirs B, Dierckx R, et al. Cyclosporin and myopathy. Ann Intern Med (1987) 107, 945–8.
4 Arello F, Krupp P. Muscular disorders associated with cyclosporin. Lancet (1991), 337, 915

Cyclosporin(e) + Corticosteroids

Abstract/Summary

Concurrent use is very common. Some evidence suggests that cyclosporin serum levels are raised but other evidence suggests the opposite (possibly an artefact of one assay method used ?) Cyclosporin can reduce the loss of the corticosteroids from the body and corticosteroid overdosage may occur. Convulsions have also been described during concurrent use, and the incidence of diabetes mellitus is said to be increased following the use of cyclosporin and methylprednisolone.

Clinical evidence

(a) Corticosteroid levels increased

A pharmacokinetic study in 40 patients showed that the clearance of prednisolone was reduced about 30% in those on cyclosporin when compared with those on azathioprine (1.9 compared with 2.6 ml/min/kg).[2]

Another study by the same group of workers reported a 25% reduction in clearance of prednisolone in the presence of cyclosporin in patients with kidney transplants.[6] Other studies[1,5,17] confirm that cyclosporin reduces the clearance of prednisolone from the body by about a third, as a result some patients develop signs of overdosage (cushingoid symptoms such as steroid diabetes, osteonecrosis of the hip joints).[1] These

studies have all been questioned in another study which found that the metabolism of prednisolone was not affected by cyclosporin.[8] A further study found that the pharmacokinetics of prednisolone in patients on cyclosporin and azathioprine varied widely between individual kidney transplant patients, but the mean values were similar to those found in normal subjects.[19]

(b) Cyclosporin levels increased or reduced

A comparative study over a year in two groups of kidney transplant patients taking cyclosporin and azathioprine, one group with and the other without prednisone, showed that the latter had higher trough cyclosporin levels (approximately 10–20%) despite using the same or lower doses of cyclosporin.[18] The serum cyclosporin levels of 22 out of 33 patients were reported to be more than doubled when given intravenous prednisolone. The cyclosporin dosage was reduced in six patients.[1,3] Another study found that high doses of methylprednisolone increased or more than doubled serum cyclosporin levels.[11,12,16] However a later study suggested quite the opposite: that the clearance of cyclosporin is increased by high dose steroids,[7] a possible explanation being that Radioimmunoassay (RIA) may give results which are different (higher) from those obtained with High Pressure Liquid Chromatography (HPLC) assay methods.[15] There is other evidence that low-dose steroids do not increase the immunosuppression of cyclosporin, but they can reduce the nephrotoxicity.[10]

(c) Convulsions

A report describes four young patients (aged 10, 12, 13 and 18) who had had bone marrow transplants for severe aplastic anaemia and who developed convulsions while treated with high dose methylprednisolone (5–20 mg/kg/day) and cyclosporin.[4] Convulsions also occurred in a woman of 25 when treated with cyclosporin and high dose methylprednisolone.[9]

(d) Hyperglycaemia and Diabetes mellitus

A study of 314 kidney transplant patients over the period 1979–87 found that the incidence of diabetes mellitus in those given cyclosporin and methylprednisolone was twice that of other patients treated with azathioprine and methylprednisolone. The diabetes developed within less than two months.[14]

Mechanisms

The evidence suggests that cyclosporin reduces the metabolism of the corticosteroids by the liver thereby reducing their loss from the body.[5,13]

Importance and management

None of these adverse interactions is well established, and the picture is confusing. Concurrent use is common and advantageous but be alert for any evidence of increased cyclosporin and corticosteroid effects. It is not clear whether high dose corticosteroids cause a rise in serum cyclosporin levels or not. Assay results should be interpreted with caution.[15] The authors of one report point out that this interaction could possibly lead to a misinterpretation of clinical data. In patients with kidney transplants a rise in serum creatinine levels is assumed to be due to rejection, unless proved otherwise. If a corticosteroid is then given, this could lead to increased cyclosporin levels which might be interpreted as cyclosporin nephrotoxicity.[3]

References

1 Ost L, Klintmalm G, Ringden O. Mutual interaction between prednisolone and cyclosporine in renal transplant patients. Transplant Proc (1985) 17, 1252–5.
2 Langhoff E, Madsen S, Olgaard K, Ladefoged J. Clinical results and cyclosporin effect on prednisolone metabolism. Kidney Int (1984) 26, 642.
3 Klintmalm G, Sawe J. High dose methylprednisolone increases plasma cyclosporin levels in renal transplant recipients. Lancet (1984) i, 731.
4 Durrant S, Chipping PM, Palmer S, Gordon-Smith EC. Cyclosporin A, methylprednisolone and convulsions. Lancet (1982) ii, 829–30.
5 Ost L. Effects of cyclosporin on prednisolone metabolism. Lancet (1984) i, 451.
6 Langhoff E, Madsen S, Flachs H, Olgaard K, Ladefoged J, Hvidberg EF. Inhibition of prednisolone metabolism by cyclosporine in kidney-transplanted patients. Transplantation (1985) 39, 107–9.
7 Ptachcinski RJ, Venkataramanan R, Burckart GJ, Hakal TR, Rosenthal JT, Carpenter BJ, Taylor RJ. Cyclosporine-high dose steroid interaction in renal transplant recipients: assessment by HPLC. Transplant Proc (1987) 19, 1728–9.
8 Frey FJ, Schnetzer A, Horber FF, Frey BM. Evidence that cyclosporine does not affect the metabolism of prednisolone after renal transplantation. Transplantation (1987) 43, 494–8.
9 Boogaerts MA, Zachee P, Verwilghen RL. Cyclosporin, methylprednisolone and convulsions. Lancet (1982) ii, 1216–17.
10 Nott D, Griffin PJA, Salaman JR. Low-dose steroids do not augment cyclosporine immunosuppression but do diminish cyclosporine nephrotoxicity. Transplant Proc (1985) 17, 1289–90.
11 Klintmalm G, Sawe J, Ringden O, Von Bah C, Magnusson A. Cyclosporine plasma levels in renal transplant patients. Association with renal toxicity and allograft rejection. Transplantation (1985) 39, 132–7.
12 Hall TG. Effect of methylprednisolone on cyclosporin blood levels. Pharmacotherapy (1990) 10, 248.
13 Henricsson S, Lindholm A, Aravoglou M. Cyclosporin metabolism in human liver microsomes and its inhibition by other drugs. Pharmacol Toxicol (1990) 66, 49–52.
14 Roth D, Milgrom M, Esquenazi V, Fuller L, BUrke G, Miller J. Posttransplant hyperglycaemia. Increased incidence in cyclosporine-treated allograft recipients. Transplantation (1989) 47, 278–81.
15 Ptachcinski RJ, Burckart GJ, Venkataramanan R, Rosenthal JT, Carpenter BJ, Hakala TR. Effect of high-dose steroids on cyclosporine blood concentrations using RIA and HPLC analysis. Drug Intell Clin Pharm (1987) 21, 20A.
16 Rogerson ME, Marsden JT, Reid KE, Bewick M, Holt DW. Cyclosporine blood concentrations in the management of renal transplant recipients. Transplantation (1986) 41, 276–8.
17 Ost L. Impairment of prednisolone metabolism by cyclosporine treatment in renal graft recipients. Transplantation (1987) 44, 533–35.
18 Hricik DE, Moritz C, Mayes JT, Schulak JA. Association of the absence of steroid therapy with increased cyclosporine blood levels in renal transplant recipients. Transplantation (1990) 49, 221–3.
19 Tornatore KM, Morse GD, Jusko WJ, Walshe JJ. Methylprednisolone disposition in renal transplant recipients receiving triple-drug immunosuppression. Transplantation (1989) 48, 962–5.

Cyclosporin(e) + Diuretics

Abstract/Summary

Nephrotoxicity has been described in three patients on cyclosporin when given either amiloride-chlorothiazide, metolazone or mannitol. Frusemide can possibly protect the kidney against cyclosporin damage.

Clinical evidence, mechanism, importance and management

A 39-year-old man on cyclosporin whose second kidney transplant functioned subnormally and who required treatment of hypertension with atenolol and minoxidil, developed ankle oedema which was resistant to increasing doses of frusemide (up to 750 mg daily). When metolazone (2.5 mg daily) was added for two weeks his serum creatinine levels more than doubled (from 193 to 449 µmol/l). When it was stopped the creatinine levels fell again. Cyclosporin serum levels were unchanged and neither graft rejection nor hypovolaemia occurred.[1] The kidney transplant of another patient on cyclosporin almost ceased to function when mannitol was used, and biopsy indicated severe cyclosporin nephrotoxicity. Transplant function recovered when the mannitol was stopped.[2] The same reaction was demonstrated in rats.[2] A woman showed a rise in serum creatinine levels from 121 to 171 mol/l three weeks after starting to take *Moduretic* (amiloride + chlorothiazide).[4] Trough serum cyclosporin levels were unchanged.[4] Although animal studies suggested that frusemide might increase the nephrotoxicity of cyclosporin,[3,] more recent human studies suggest that it may have a protective effect.[5]

The general importance of these adverse interactions is not clear, but good monitoring is obviously needed if these diuretics are given with cyclosporin.

References

1 Christensen P, Leski M. Nephrotoxic drug interaction between metolazone and cyclosporin. Br Med J (1987) 294, 578.
2 Brunner FP, Hermle M, Mihatsch MJ, Thiel G. Mannitol potentiates cyclosporine nephrotoxicity. Clin Nephrol (1986) 25 (Suppl 1) S130–6.
3 Whiting PH, Cunningham C, Thompson AW, Simpson JG. Enhancement of high dose cyclosporin A toxicity by frusemide. Biochem Pharmacol (1984) 7, 1075–9.
4 Deray G, Baumelou B, Le Hoang P, Aupetit B, Girard B, Baumelou A, Legrand JC, Jacobs C. Enhancement of cyclosporin nephrotoxicity by diuretic therapy. Clin Nephrol (1989) 32, 47.
5 Driscoll DF, Pinson CW, Jenkins RL, Bistrian BR. Potential protective effects of furosemide against early cyclosporine-induced renal injury in hepatic transplant recipients. Transplantation Proc (1989) 21, 3549–50.

Cyclosporin(e) + Fenofibrate

Abstract/Summary

Cyclosporin serum levels remained unchanged in heart transplant patients concurrently treated with fenofibrate for two weeks.

Clinical evidence, mechanism, importance and management

A study in 10 heart transplant patients on cyclosporin found that 200 mg fenofibrate effectively reduced blood cholesterol levels (from 7.7 to 6.5 mmol/l) without significantly altering serum cyclosporin levels over a 2 week period. The only possible adverse effect was an increase in creatinine levels from 145 to 157 mmol/l, suggesting some possible nephrotoxicity. No other clinically adverse effects were seen. The authors of this study suggest that longer follow-up studies are needed to confirm the safety of using these drugs together.[1]

Reference

1 de Lorgeril M, Boissonnat P, Bizollon CA, Guidollet J, Faucon G, Guichard JP, Levy-Prades-Sauron R, Renaud S, Dureau G. Pharmacokinetics of cyclosporine in hyperlipidaemic long-term survivors of heart transplantation. Lack of interaction with the lipid-lowering agent, fenofibrate. Eur J Clin Pharmacol (1992) 43, 161–5.

Cyclosporin(e) + Fluconazole, Itraconazole, Ketoconazole, Miconazole

Abstract/Summary

A very marked and rapid rise (up to 5–10-fold) in serum cyclosporin levels can occur if ketoconazole is given concurrently. Avoid combined use unless the cyclosporin dosage is markedly reduced because of the risk of nephrotoxicity. When controlled this interaction has been exploited to save costs. A less dramatic but still clinically important rise in cyclosporin serum levels (2–3-fold) has been seen in some patients when given fluconazole or itraconazole. A single report describes the same interaction with miconazole.

Clinical evidence

(a) Cyclosporin + Fluconazole

200 mg fluconazole daily for 14 days approximately doubled the trough serum cyclosporin levels (from 23 to 45 ng/ml) of eight kidney transplant patients. Their AUCs increased from 1900 to 3114 ng.h/ml but serum creatinine levels were unchanged.[19,24] Similar results were found by the same group of workers in a related studies.[20,21]

Other reports describe two to threefold rises in serum cyclosporin levels in kidney transplant patients within 6–11 days of starting treatment with 100–200 mg fluconazole daily.[6,13,39] One patient developed kidney toxicity which was solved by reducing the dosages of both drugs.[14]

In contrast, some patients showed little or no changes in serum cyclosporin or creatinine levels when fluconazole was given.[15,17,34,35,38,40] This may be because the interaction is dose-dependent.[40]

(b) Cyclosporin + Itraconazole

An average 56% reduction (range 33–84%) in the cyclosporin dosages in four heart-lung, two heart and one lung transplant patient were needed when itraconazole (dosage not stated) was given. Serum creatinine levels rose temporarily until the cyclosporin dosage had been readjusted.[22] Two three-fold rises were seen in two other patients given 200 mg itraconazole daily,[11,12] and in one case the raised levels persisted for more than 4 weeks after the itraconazole was stopped.[12] Unspecified reductions in the cyclosporin dosage are mentioned in another report.[32]

These reports contrast with another describing 14 bone marrow transplant patients taking cyclosporin. Those given 100 mg itraconazole twice daily showed no significant changes in cyclosporin or creatinine serum levels.[18]

(c) Cyclosporin + Ketoconazole

200 mg ketoconazole daily caused a marked and rapid rise in serum cyclosporin levels of 36 renal transplant patients. On the basis of experience with previous patients, the dosage was reduced by 70% when ketoconazole was started, and after a year the dosage reduction was 85% (from 420 mg to 66 mg daily). Minimal nephrotoxicity was seen.[16,23,41]

Other reports[1–3,5,7,8,25,27–31,41] describe essentially similar rises in serum cyclosporin levels during concurrent treatment with ketoconazole. See also 'Importance and management'. Topical ketoconazole (2% cream) has been found not interact with cyclosporin (1 mg/kg daily) in the treatment of contact allergic dermatitis. The cyclosporin dosage cannot be reduced.[33] Impaired glucose tolerance has been attributed to concurrent use in one patient.[26]

(d) Cyclosporin + miconazole

A single case report describes an approximately 65% rise in cyclosporin serum levels within three days of starting 1 g miconazole 8-hourly. Levels rose again during a subsequent treatment with miconazole.[36]

Mechanism

In vitro studies show that these azole antifungals inhibit the metabolism of cyclosporin by human liver microsomal enzymes, ketoconazole being the most potent.[4] As a result the loss of the cyclosporin from the body is reduced and its serum levels rise.

Importance and management

The cyclosporin/ketoconazole interaction is established and clinically important. Cyclosporin serum levels rise rapidly and sharply, but they can be controlled by markedly reducing the cyclosporin dosage by about 70–80%[3,9,10,16,32,42] thereby preventing kidney damage and also saving costs. A reduction of

68–89% (a 75% saving) over a 13-month period with no change in kidney, liver or immunosuppressive activity has been described, the total cost saving being about 65% because of the need to follow up more frequently and the cost of the ketoconazole.[16,23] Another study claimed an annual reduction in the 1991 costs from $6800 to $1862 (US) per heart transplant patient.[9] Reviews of the pros and cons of concurrent use have been published.[37,41] Ketoconazole may possibly have a kidney-protective effect.[16,23,42]

Information about cyclosporin with fluconazole, itraconazole or miconazole is less extensive but concurrent use should be closely monitored, anticipating the need to reduce the cyclosporin dosage by 50% or more, although some patients may demonstrate no significant changes at all. There is some evidence that with fluconazole the interaction may possibly depend on its dosage.[40]

References

1 Ferguson RM, Sutherland DE, Simmonds RL, Najarian JS. Ketoconazole-cyclosporin metabolism and renal transplantation. Lancet (1982) ii, 882–3

2 Morgenstern GR, Powles R, Robinson BL, McElwain TJ. Cyclosporin interaction with ketoconazole and melphalan. Lancet (1982) ii, 1342–3

3 Dieperink H, Moller J. Ketoconazole and cyclosporin A. Lancet (1982) ii, 1217

4 Back DJ, Tjia JF. Comparative effects of the antimycotic drugs ketoconazole, fluconazole, itraconazole and terbinafine on the metabolism of cyclosporin by human liver microsomes. Br J Clin Pharmac (1991) 32, 624–6.

5 Lokjec F. Pharmacokinetic monitoring during graft-versus-host disease treatment following bone marrow transplantation. International Symposium on Cyclosporin A (Trinity Hall, Cambridge. September 16–18, 1981). Quoted in reference 3.

6 Torregrosa V, De la Torre M, Campistol JM, Oppenheimer F, Ricart MJ, Vilardell J, Andreu J. Interaction of fluconazole with ciclosporin A. Nephron (1992) 60, 125–6.

7 Gluckman E, Devergie A, Lokiec F, Poirier O, Baumelon A. Nephrotoxicity of cyclosporin in bone marrow transplantation. Lancet (1981) ii, 144–5.

8 Shepard JH, Canafax DM, Simmons RL, Najarian JS. Cyclosporin-ketoconazole: a potentially dangerous drug-drug interaction. Clin Pharm (1986) 5, 468.

9 Butman SM, Wild JC, Nolan PE, Fagan TC, Finley PR, Hicks KJ, Mackie MJ, Copeland JG. Prospective study of the safety and financial benefit of ketoconazole as adjunctive therapy to cyclosporine after heart transplantation. J Heart Lung Transplant (1991) 10, 351–8.

10 Schroeder TJ, Melvin DB, Clardy CW, Myre SA, Reising JM, Wolf RK, Collins JA, Pesce AJ, First MR. The use of cyclosporine and ketoconazole without nephrotoxicity in two heart transplant recipients. J Heart Transplantation (1986) 5, 391.

11 Kwan JT C, Foxall PJD, Davidson DGC, Bending MR, Eisinger AJ. Interaction of cyclosporin and itraconazole. Lancet (1987) ii, 282.

12 Trenk D, Brett W, Jahnchen E, Birnbaum D. Time course of cyclosporin: itraconazole interaction. Lancet (1987) ii, 1335–6.

13 Sugar AM, Saunders C, Idelson BA, Bernard DB. Interaction of fluconazole and cyclosporine. Ann Intern Med (1989) 110, 844.

14 Collignon P, Hurley B, Mitchell D. Interaction of fluconazole with cyclosporin. Lancet (1989) ii, 1262.

15 Ehninger G, Jaschonek K, Schuler U, Kruger HU. Interaction of fluconazole with cyclosporin. Lancet (1989) ii, 104–5.

16 First MR, Schroeder TJ, Weiskittel P, Myre SA, Alexander JW, Pesce AJ. Concomitant administration of cyclosporin and ketoconazole in renal transplant patients. Lancet (1989) ii, 1198–1201.

17 Kruger HU, Schuler U, Zimmerman R, Ehninger G. Absence of significant interaction of fluconazole with cyclosporin. J Antimicrob Chemother (1989) 24, 781–6.

18 Novakova I, Donnelly P, de Witte T, de Pauw B, Boezeman J, Veltman G. Itraconazole and cyclosporin nephrotoxicity. Lancet (1987) ii, 920–1.

19 Carleton BC, Graves NM, Matas AJ, Hilligoss DM, Canafax DM. Managing the fluconazole and cyclosporine interaction: results of a double-blind randomized pharmacokinetic and safety study. Pharmacotherapy (1990) 10, 250.

20 Canafax DM, Graves NM, Hilligoss DM, Carleton BC, Gardner MJ, Matas AJ. Interaction between cyclosporine and fluconazole in renal allograft recipients. Transplantation (1991) 51, 1014–8.

21 Canafax DM, Graves NM, Hilligoss DM, Carleton BC, Gardner MJ, Matas AJ. Increased cyclosporine levels as a result of simultaneous fluconazole and cyclosporine therapy in renal transplant recipients: a double-blind, randomised pharmacokinetic and safety study. Transplant Proc (1991) 23, 1041–2.

22 Kramer MR, Marshall SE, Denning DW, Keogh AM, Tucker RM, Galgiani JN, Lewiston NJ, Stevens DA, Theodore J. Cyclosporine and itraconazole interaction in heart and lung transplant recipients. Ann Intern Med (1990) 113, 327–9.

23 First MR, Schroeder TJ, Alexander JW, Stephens GW, Weiskittel P, Myre SA, Pesce AJ. Cyclosporine dose reduction by ketoconazole administration in renal transplant recipients. Transplantation (1991) 51, 365–70.

24 Graves NM, Matas AJ, Hilligoss DM, Canafax DM. Fluconazole/cyclosporine interaction. Clin Pharmacol Ther (1990) 47, 208.

25 Schroeder TJ, Melvin DB, Clardy CW, Wadhwa NK, Myre SA, Reising JM, Wolf RK, Collins JA, Pesce AJ, First MR. Use of cyclosporine and ketoconazole without nephrotoxicity in two heart transplant recipients. J Heart Transplant (1987) 6, 84–9.

26 Kiss D, Thiel G. Glucose intolerance and prolonged renal-transplant insufficiency due to ketokonazole-cyclosporin A interaction. Clin Nephrol (1990) 33, 207–8.

27 Butman SM, Wild J, Nolan P, Fagan T, Mackie M, Finley P, Copeland JG. Cyclosporine and concomitant ketoconazole after cardiac transplantation: intermediate term findings and potential savings. J Am Coll Cardiol (1989) 13, 62A.

28 Girardet RE, Melo JC, Fox MS, Whalen C, Lusk R, Masri ZH, Lansing AM. Concomitant administration of cyclosporine and ketoconazole for three and a half years in one heart transplant recipient. Transplantation (1989) 48, 887–90.

29 Schroeder TJ, Weiskittle P, Pesce AJ, Myre SA, Alexadner JW. Cyclosporine pharmacokinetics with concomitant ketoconazole therapy. Clin Chem (1989) 35, 1176–7.

30 Charles BG, Ravenscroft PJ, Rigby RJ. The ketoconazole-cyclosporin interaction in an elderly renal transplant patient. Aust NZ J Med (1989) 19, 292–3.

31 Veraldi S, Menni S. Severe gingival hyperplasia following cyclosporin and ketoconazole therapy. (1988) 27, 730.

32 Faggian G, Livi U, Bortolotti U, Mazzucco A, Stellin G, Chiominto B, Viviani MA, Gallucci V. Itraconazole therapy for acute invasive pulmonary aspergillosis in heart transplantation. Transplant Proc (1989) 21, 2506–7.

33 McLelland J, Shuster S. Topical ketoconazole does not potentiate oral cyclosporin A in allergic contact dermatitis. Acta Derm Venereol (1992) 72, 285.

34 Conti DJ, Tolkoff-Rubin NE, Baker GP, Doran M, Cosinin AB, Delmonico F, Auchincloss H, Russell PS, Rubin RH. Successful treatment of invasive fungal infection with fluconazole in organ transplant recipients, Transplantation (1989) 48, 692–4.

35 Rubin RH, Debruin MF, Knirsch AK. Fluconazole therapy for patients with serious Candida infections who have failed standard therapies. Abs No.71. 29th ICAAC, Houston (1989).

36 Horton CM, Freeman CD, Nolan PE, Copeland JG. Cyclosporine interactions with miconazole and other azole-antimycotics: a case report and review of the literature. J Heart Lung Transplant (1992) 11, 1127–32.

37 Albengres E, Tillement JP. Cyclosporin and ketoconazole, drug interaction or therapeutic association ? Int J Clin Pharmacol Ther Tox (1992) 12, 555–70.

38 Rubin RH, Debruin MF, Knirsch AK. Fluconazole therapy for patients with serious candida infections who have failed standard therapy. 29th Intersci Conf Antimicrob Ag Chemother, Houston (1989), 112.

39 Barbar JAJ, Clarkson AR, LaBrooy J, MCNeil JD, Woodroffe AJ. *Candida albicans* arthritis in a renal allograft recipient with an interaction between cyclosporin and fluconazole. Nephrol Dial Transplant (1993) 8, 263–6.

40 López-Gil JA. Fluconazole-cyclosporine interaction: a dose-dependent effect ? Ann Pharmacotherapy (1993) 27, 427–30.

41 First MR, Schroder TJ, Michael A, Hariharan S, Weiskittle P, Alexander

JW. Cyclosporin-ketoconazole interaction. Long-term follow-up and preliminary results of a randomized trial. Transplantation (1993) 55, 1000–4.

42 First MR, Schroeder TJ, Michael A, Hariharan S, Weiskittel P, Alexander
JW. Randomized controlled study of coadministration of cyclosporine and
ketoconazole in renal transplant recipients. Clin Pharmacol Ther (1993)
53, 237.

Cyclosporin(e) + Macrolide and Related antibiotics

Abstract/Summary

Cyclosporin levels can be markedly raised by the concurrent
use of erythromycin. Toxicity will occur if the dosage of
cyclosporin is not reduced. Josamycin, ponsinomycin (miocamycin) and pristinamycin appear to interact similarly, but
no interaction is seen with spiramycin. Roxithromycin appears
to interact minimally. The behaviour of other macrolides is
uncertain but they possibly interact like erythromycin.

Clinical evidence

(a) Cyclosporin + Erythromycin

A study in nine patients with transplants on cyclosporin found
that when treated with erythromycin the mean trough serum
levels of the three patients with kidney transplants rose seven-
fold (from 147 to 1125 ng/ml) and in the six patients with heart
transplants 4–5-fold (from 185 to 815 ng/ml). Acute nephrotoxicity occurred in all nine patients and seven showed mild to
severe liver toxicity caused by the increased cyclosporin serum
levels.[1]

Markedly raised serum cyclosporin levels and/or toxicity
have been described in a number of other studies and case
reports with erythromycin given orally or intravenously in
about 40 other patients[2-13,27,30,31] and demonstrated in normal
subjects.[14]

(b) Cyclosporin + Josamycin

A man with a renal transplant on azathioprine, prednisone and
cyclosporin (330 mg daily) showed a marked rise in his serum
cyclosporin levels (from about 90 to 600 ng/ml) when treated
with 2 g josamycin daily for 5 days. He responded in the same
way when later rechallenged with josamycin. Another patient
reacted in the same way.[15] Two-four-fold rises have been seen
in four other patients given 3 g (50 mg/kg) josamycin daily.[23,32]

(c) Cyclosporin + Ponsinomycin (Miocamycin)

The steady-state serum cyclosporin levels of 10 kidney transplant patients were approximately doubled while taking
800 mg ponsinomycin twice daily.[24]

(d) Cyclosporin + Pristinamycin

A kidney transplant patient showed a ten-fold rise in serum
cyclosporin levels (from 30 to 290 ng/ml) after being given 2 g
pristinamycin daily for 8 days. Blood creatinine levels rose from
75 to 120 mmol/l. Another patient given 1.25 g pristinamycin
showed a rise in cyclosporin levels from 78 to 855 ng/ml after 6
days. Cyclosporin and creatinine levels fell to normal levels
within two days of stopping both drugs.[18]

50 mg/kg pristinamycin daily raised the serum cyclosporin
levels of 10 patients by 65% (from 560 to 925 ng/ml). Cyclosporin levels fell when the pristinamycin was stopped.[22,23]
Within five days of starting to take 4 g pristinamycin daily the
cyclosporin levels of another patient more than doubled. His
serum creatinine levels also rose. Both fell back to baseline
levels within three days of stopping the antibiotic.[19]

(e) Cyclosporin + Roxithromycin

Eight patients with heart transplants on cyclosporin (8 mg/kg
daily), prednisolone and azathioprine for at least a month, were
concurrently treated with 150 mg roxithromycin twice daily for
11 days. A rise in cyclosporin levels occurred, namely + 25% (a
rise from 176 to 242 ng/ml) at the time the cyclosporin was
given, and + 43% (from 294 to 469 ng/ml) 4 hours later.
Cyclosporin levels fell again when the roxithromycin was
stopped. A weak (10%) increase in serum creatinine levels
occurred. There was no evidence of a deterioration in renal
function.[25,26] The biological half-life of roxithromycin was
found on one study to be approximately doubled (from 17 to
34.4 h) in patients with kidney transplants on cyclosporin.[28]

(f) Cyclosporin + Spiramycin

The cyclosporin serum levels of six heart transplant patients on
steroids, azathioprine and cyclosporin remained unchanged
when given three MIU of spiramycin twice daily for 10 days.[16]
The same absence of an interaction was found in other studies
in patients with renal transplants.[17,20,21,29]

(g) Cyclosporin + Rokitamycin, Triacetyloleandomycin

In vitro studies (see Mechanism) suggest that these two macrolides may behave like erythromycin.[33] but as yet there seems
to be direct clinical evidence of an interaction.

Mechanism

Not fully understood. *In vitro* studies with human liver microsomes have shown that erythromycin, josamycin, rokitamycin, roxithromycin and troleandomycin (but not spiramycin)
inhibit cyclosporin metabolism which is catalyzed by cytochrome P4503A.[33] This would be expected to result in raised
cyclosporin levels. Erythromycin also possibly increases the
absorption of cyclosporin from the gut.[13]

Importance and management

The cyclosporin-erythromycin interaction is well documented, well established and potentially serious. If concurrent use is thought appropriate, monitor the cyclosporin serum levels closely and reduce the dosage appropriately. An approximately 60% reduction has been calculated for erythromycin.[30] The dosage should be increased again when the erythromycin is stopped to maintain adequate immunosuppression. A possible alternative is to give the cyclosporin intravenously which by-passes the effects of erythromycin on the absorption of cyclosporin from the gut.[13] Information about the interactions with josamycin, ponsinomycin and pristinamycin is more limited but they appear to behave like erythromycin.

Spiramycin does not interact, and roxithromycin appears only to interact very minimally, however bear in mind that the roxithromycin serum levels may be increased. There seems to be no direct clinical information about triacetyloleandomycin and rokitamycin but *in vitro* studies suggest that they may possibly interact like erythromycin.[33] Be on the alert if they are used.

References

1 Jensen CWB, Flechner SM, Van Buren CT, Frazier OH, Cooley DA, Lorber MI, Kahan BD. Exacerbation of cyclosporin toxicity by concomitant administration of erythromycin. Transplantation (1987) 43, 263–70.

2 Kohan DE. Possible interaction between cyclosporin and erythromycin. N Eng J Med (1986), 314, 448.

3 Hourmant M, Le Bigot JF, Vernillet L, Sagniez G, Remi JP, Souilou JP. Coadministration of erythromycin results in an increase of blood cyclosporine to toxic levels. Transplant Proc (1985) 17, 2723–7.

4 Wadhwa NK, Schroeder TJ, O'Flaherty E, Pesce AJ, Myre SA, Munda R, First MR. Interaction between erythromycin and cyclosporine in a kidney and pancreas allograft recipient. Ther Drug Monitor (1987) 9, 123–5.

5 Murray BM, Edwards L, Morse GD, Kohli RR, Venuto RC. Clinically important interaction of cyclosporin and erythromycin. Transplantation (1987) 43, 602–4.

6 Grino JM, Sabate I, Castelao AM, Guardia M, Seron D, Alsina J. Erythromycin and cyclosporine. Ann Intern Med (1986) 105, 467–8.

7 Gonwa TA, Nghiem DD, Schulak JA, Corry RJ. Erythromycin and cyclosporine. Transplantation (1986) 41, 797–9.

8 Harnett JD, Parfrey PS, Paul MD, Gault MH. Erythromycin-cyclosporine interaction in renal transplant patients. Transplantation (1987) 43, 316–18.

9 Kessler M, Louis J, Renoult E, Vigneron B, Netter P. Interaction between cyclosporin and erythromycin in a kidney transplant patients. Eur J Clin Pharmacol (1986) 30, 633–4.

10 Godin JRP, Sketris IS, Belitsky P. Erythromycin-cyclosporin interaction. Drug Intell Clin Pharm (1986) 20, 504–5.

11 Martell R, Heinrichs D, Stiller CR, Jenner M, Keown PA, Dupre J. The effects of erythromycin in patients treated with cyclosporin. Ann Intern Med (1986) 104, 660–1.

12 Ptachcinski PJ, Carpenter BJ, Burckart GJ, Venkataramana R, Rosenthal JT. Effect of erythromycin on cyclosporine levels. N Engl J Med (1985) 22, 1416–17.

13 Gupta SK, Bakran A, Johnson RWG, Rowland M. Erythromycin enhances the absorption of cyclosporin. Br J Clin Pharmac (1988) 25, 401–2.

14 Freeman DJ, Martell R, Carruthers SG, Heinrichs D, Keown PA, Stiller CR. Cyclosporin-erythromycin interaction in normal subjects. Br J Clin Pharmac (1987) 23, 776–8.

15 Kreft-Jais C, Billaud EM, Gaudry C, Bedrossan J. Effect of josamycin on plasma cyclosporine levels. Eur J Clin Pharmacol (1987) 32, 327–8.

16 Guillemain R, Billaud E, Dreyfus G, Amrein C, Kitzis M, Jebara VA, Kreft-Jais C. The effects of spiramycin on plasma cyclosporin A concentrations in heart transplant patients. Eur J Clin Pharmacol (1989) 36, 97–8.

17 Kessler M, Netter P, Zerrouki M, Renoult E, Trechot P, Dousset B, Jonon B, Mur JM. Spiramycin does not increase plasma cyclosporin concentrations in renal transplant. Eur J Clin Pharmacol (1988) 35, 331–2.

18 Gagnadoux MF, Loirat C, Pillion G, Bertheleme JP, Pouliquen M, Guest G, Broyer M. Nephrotoxicite due a l'interaction pristinamycine-cyclosporine chez le transplante renal. La Presse Med (1987) 16, 1761.

19 Garraffo R, Monnier B, Lapalus P, Duplay H. Pristinamycin increases cyclosporin blood levels. Med Sci Res (1987) 15, 461.

20 Vernillet L, Bertault-Peres P, Berland Y, Barradas J, Durand A, Olmer M. Lack of effect of spiramycin on cyclosporin pharmacokinetics. Br J Clin Pharmacol (1989) 27, 789–94.

21 Birmele B, Lebranchu Y, Beliveaau F, Rateau H, Furet Y, Nivet H, Bagros PH. Absence of interaction between cyclosporine and spiramycin. Transplantation (1989) 47, 927–8.

22 Herbrecht R, Garcia J-J, Bergerat J-P, Oberling F. Effect of pristinamycin on cyclosporin levels in bone marrow transplant recipients. Bone Marrow Transplant (1989) 4, 457–8.

23 Herbrecht R, Liu KL, Bergerat J-P. Interactions of cyclosporine with antimicrobial agents. Rev Infect Dis (1990) 12, 371.

23 Azanza J, Catalán M, Alvarez P, Honorato J, Herreros J, Llorens R. Possible interaction between cyclosporine and josamycin. J Heart Transplant (1990) 9, 265–6.

24 Couet W, Istin B, Seniuta P, Morel D, Potaux L, Fourtillan JB. Effect of ponsinomycin on cyclosporin pharmacokinetics. Eur J Clin Pharmacol (1990) 39, 165–67.

25 Billaud E M, Guillemain R, Fortineau N, Kitzis M-D, Dreyfus G, Amrein C, Kreft-Jaïs C, Husson J-M, Chrétien P. Interaction between roxithromycin and cyclosporin in heart transplant patients. Clin Pharmacokinet (1990) 19, 499–502.

26 Billaud E, Guillemain R, Kitzis M, Fortineau N, Dreyfus G, Amrein C, Kreft-Jaïs C, Chrétien P, Husson JM. Roxithromycin and cyclosporin; searching for an interaction. Thérapie (1990) 45, 41.

27 Morales JM, Andres A, Prieto C, Arenas J, Ortuño B, Praga M, Ruilope LM, Rodicio JL. Severe reversible cyclosporine-induced acute renal failure. A role for urinary PGE2 deficiency? Transplantation (1988) 46, 163–5.

28 Morávek J, Matousovic K, Prát V, Sedivy J. Pharmacokinetics of roxithromycin in kidney grafted patients under cyclosporin A or azathioprine immunosuppression and in healthy volunteers. Int J Clin Pharmacol Ther Tox (1990) 28, 262–7.

29 Kessler M, Netter P, Renoult E, Trechot P, Dousset B, Bannwarth B. Lack of effect of spiramycin on cyclosporin pharmacokinetics. Br J Clin Pharmac (1990) 29, 370–1.

30 Vereerstraeten P, Thiry P, Kinnaert P, Toussaint C. Influence of erythromycin on cyclosporine pharmacokinetics. Transplantation (1987) 44, 155–6.

31 Ben-Ari J, Eisenstein B, Davidovits M, Shmueli D, Shapira Z, Stark H. Effect of erythromycin on blood cyclsporine concentrations in kidney transplant patients. J Pediatr (1988) 112, 992–3.

32 Azanza JR, Catalán M, Alvarez MP, Sádaba B, Honorota J, Llorens R, Harreros J. Possible interaction between cyclosporine and josamycin: a description of three cases. Clin Pharmacol Ther (1992) 51, 572–5.

33 Marre R, de Sousa G, Orloff AM, Rahmani R. *In vitro* interaction between cyclosporin A and macrolide antibiotics. Br J Clin Pharmac (1993) 35, 447.

Cyclosporin(e) + Melphalan

Abstract/Summary

Melphalan appears to increase the nephrotoxic effects of cyclosporin.

Clinical evidence, mechanism, importance and management

A comparative study showed that 13 out of 17 patients receiving bone marrow transplants given cyclosporin (12.5 mg/

kg daily) and high-dose melphalan (single injection of 140–250 mg/m^2) developed kidney failure, compared with no cases of kidney failure in seven other patients given melphalan but no cyclosporin.[1] In another study one out of four patients given both drugs developed nephrotoxicity.[2] The reasons are not understood. The effects on kidney function of concurrent use should be very closely monitored.

References

1 Morgenstern GR, Powles R, Robinson B, McElwain TJ. Cyclosporin interaction with ketoconazole and melphalan. Lancet (1982) ii, 1342.
2 Dale BM, Sage RE, Norman JE, Barber S, Kotasek D. Bone marrow transplantation following treatment with high-dose melphalan. Transplantation Proc (1985) 17, 1711–12.

Cyclosporin(e) + Methotrexate

Abstract/Summary

Previous or concurrent treatment with methotrexate may possibly increase the risk of liver and other toxicity, but effective and valuable concurrent use has been reported.

Clinical evidence, mechanism, importance and management

A limited comparative study in patients with chronic plaque psoriasis suggested that prior treatment with methotrexate (which can cause liver damage) possibly increases the risk of cyclosporin toxicity (higher serum cyclosporin and creatinine levels, hypertension).[1] This was confirmed by another study in four patients with resistant psoriasis in whom concurrent use (5 mg cyclosporin daily, 2.5 mg methotrexate 12-hourly for three doses at weekly intervals) increased the serum levels of both drugs, and increased the side-effects (nausea, vomiting, mouth ulcers).[2] Rises in creatinine levels and liver enzymes (AST, ALT) also occurred. The reasons are not understood. The authors of the second study strongly recommend that combined use should be avoided, even in patients with severe unresponsive psoriasis.[2]

However another pilot study effectively used both drugs together for the control of acute graft-versus-host-disease in marrow transplant patients, with the cyclosporin dosage reduced by 50% (1.5 mg/kg/day) during the first 2 weeks. The methotrexate dosages were 10–15 mg/m^2 on days 1, 3, 6 and 11 after grafting. Hepatotoxicity appeared to be reduced.[3]

References

1 Powles AV, Baker BS, Fry L, Valdimarsson H. Cyclosporin toxicity. Lancet (1990) 335, 610.
2 Korstanje MJ, van Breda Vriesman CJP, van de Staak WJMB. Cyclosporine and methotrexate: a dangerous combination. J Am Acad Dermatol (1990) 23, 320–1.
3 Stockschlaeder M, Storb R, Pepe M, Longton G, McDonald G, Anasetti C, Appelbaum F, Doney K, Martin P, Sullivan K, Witherspoon R. A pilot

study of low dose cyclosporin for graft-versus-host prophylaxis in marrow transplantation. Br J Haematol (1991) 80, 49–54.

Cyclosporin(e) + Metoclopramide

Abstract/Summary

Metoclopramide increases the absorption of cyclosporin and raises the serum levels.

Clinical evidence, mechanism, importance and management

A study in 14 kidney transplant patients showed that when given metoclopramide and cyclosporin concurrently their peak serum cyclosporin levels were increased by 46% (from 388 to 567 ng/ml) and the AUC was increased by 29% (from 3370 to 4120 ng.h/ml).[1] The probable reason is that the metoclopramide hastens gastric emptying. Cyclosporin is largely absorbed by the small intestine. The clinical importance of this interaction is uncertain but it has been suggested that it could be used to save money because it might be possible to give smaller doses of the expensive cyclosporin. Concurrent use should be well monitored to ensure that cyclosporin levels do not rise to toxic levels.

Reference

1 Wadhwa NK, Schroeder TJ, O'Flaherty E, Pesce AJ, Myre SA, First MR. The effect of oral metoclopramide on the absorption of cyclosporin. Transplant Proc (1987) 18, 1730–3.

Cyclosporin(e) + Minoxidil

Abstract/Summary

The concurrent use of cyclosporin and minoxidil can cause excessive hairiness.

Clinical evidence, mechanism, importance and management

Six kidney transplant patients on cyclosporin (serum levels of 100–200 ng/ml) were additionally given methyldopa, a diuretic and 15–40 mg minoxidil daily for intractable hypertension. After 4 week's treatment all of them complained of severe and unpleasant hypertrichosis. Two months after stopping the minoxidil the hypertrichosis had significantly improved.[1] Both cyclosporin and minoxidil cause hypertrichosis and it would seem that their effects are additive. The authors of the report point out that this is not a life-threatening problem, but it limits concurrent use in both men and women.[1]

Reference

1 Sever MS, Sonmez YE, Kocak N. Limited use of minoxidil in renal transplant recipients because of additive side-effects of cyclosporine on hypertrichosis. Transplantation (1990) 50, 536.

Cyclosporin(e) + Miscellaneous drugs

Abstract/Summary

Isolated and unconfirmed interactions have been reported between cyclosporin and acetazolamide, acyclovir, allopurinol, cephalosporins, chloramphenicol, disopyramide, doxycycline, griseofulvin, imipenem/cilastatin, metronidazole, minocycline, moxalactam (latamoxef), propafenone, quinine, ticlopidine, simvastastin and sulphinpyrazone. Isotretinoin appears not to interact.

Clinical evidence, mechanism, importance and management

The Drug Monitoring Centre of Sandoz (the manufacturers of cyclosporin) in Basel has on record a number of previously unpublished spontaneous and isolated reports of interactions between cyclosporin and other drugs.[1] There are also other isolated case reports of interactions involving cyclosporin:

A man with a heart transplant demonstrated increased serum cyclosporin levels, marked renal impairment and neuro-toxicity when given oral acetazolamide for raised intra-ocular pressure secondary to panuveitis.[2] An increase in serum creatinine levels and in acyclovir levels accompanied by reversible acute tubular necrosis has been noted during the concurrent use of cyclosporin and acyclovir.[1] Nephrotoxicity has been described in three other patients given cyclosporin and acyclovir, and one died. Histological evidence suggested cyclosporin nephrotoxicity,[9] however no toxicity was observed in another study on 11 patients given both drugs.[10] The cyclosporin levels of a kidney transplant patient rose approximately three-fold after taking 100 mg allopurinol for 12 days, accompanied by signs of renal toxicity.[20] However another report describes a reduction in the frequency of acute kidney transplant rejections in patients on cyclosporin, prednisolone and azathioprine when low dose allupurinol (25 mg on alternate days) was added.[21] Two kidney transplant patients showed marked increases (almost doubled in one case) in serum cyclosporin levels when given chloramphenicol to treat urinary tract infections.[17] A woman treated with cyclosporin with a year old kidney transplant rapidly developed nephrotoxicity shortly after starting to take 100 mg disopyramide three times daily. She also experienced the anticholinergic side-effects of disopyramide (mouth dryness, dysuria).[3] A patient showed an increase in serum creatinine levels when treated with doxycycline,[1] whereas fish oil (Super EPA) seems to reduce the renal dysfunction due to cyclosporin in psoriasis.[14] An *in vitro* study using human liver microsomes indicated that no metabolic interaction occurs between cyclosporin and etretinate. They are probably metabolized by different P450 isoenzymes. No *in vivo* interaction

would be expected.[22] The cyclosporin levels of a man were roughly halved when given 500 mg griseofulvin daily despite an approximately 70% increase in the cyclosporin dosage. When 16 weeks later the griseofulvin was stopped, his serum cyclosporin levels rose again.[12] A woman with a kidney transplant and on cyclosporin developed a urinary tract infection for which 500 mg imipenem/cilastatin intravenously 12-hourly was given. 20 min after the second dose she became confused, disorientated, and agitated and developed motor aphasia and intense tremor. This was interpreted as being a combination of the adverse central nervous effects of both drugs. The imipenem/cilastatin was not given again and these adverse effects subsided over the next few days. However it was noted that the cyclosporin serum levels climbed over the next four days from about 400 to 1000 ng/ml.[5] In contrast imipenem/cilastin with ciprofloxacin was effectively and successfully used in another patient taking cyclosporin.[18] Reduced serum cyclosporin levels following the use of imipenem/cilastin have been seen in rats.[6] Two reports say that isotretinoin has been successfully and uneventfully used for severe acne in two patients on cyclosporin with heart transplants.[15,16] The serum cyclosporin levels of a kidney transplant patient more than doubled when metronidazole (2.25 g daily) and cimetidine (800 mg daily) were started. They fell about 50% when the metronidazole dosage was halved and the cimetidine stopped, and fell to their original levels when the metronidazole was withdrawn.[7] Increased cyclosporin levels associated with acute renal failure occurred in a patient given minocycline and amikacin.[18] Increased serum cyclosporin levels have been reported with moxalactam (latamoxef).[1] A kidney transplant patient on cyclosporin and prednisone experienced a marked fall in her serum cyclosporin levels on two occasions when treated with nafcillin (2 g 6-hourly). Trough serum levels fell from 229 to 119 and then to 68 ng/ml after three and seven days of nafcillin, before climbing again when the nafcillin was stopped. On the second occasion levels fell from 272 to 42 ng/ml after nine days treatment with nafcillin.[4] A patient showed a marked rise in serum cyclosporin levels (from 450 to 750 ng/ml) within a week of starting 600–750 mg propafenone daily. It was controlled by reducing the cyclosporin dosage to 200 mg daily.[8] A man with a kidney transplant and mild cerebral faciparum malaria showed a gradual decrease in his serum cyclosporin levels (from 328 to 107 ng/ml) over 7 days when treated with 600 mg quinine 8-hourly, and a gradual rise when the quinine was stopped.[11] Severe myopathy has been seen in one patient and rhabdomyolysis in another taking cyclosporin and simvastatin.[4,19] Increased serum cyclosporin levels have been reported with sulphinpyrazone, although there is the possibility that this may be an artefact due to interference with the assay method.[1] The serum cyclosporin levels of a patient with nephrotic syndrome were roughly halved on two occasions when given 500 mg ticlopidine daily.[13]

All of these reports need to be viewed in perspective because most of them are isolated and unconfirmed, and in some instances both drugs have been used uneventfully on a number of occasions. However it should also be appreciated that many now well-recognized interactions first came to light because someone took the trouble to make a report, even though it involved only one patient. The concurrent use of any of these drugs should be well monitored.

References

1 Cockburn I, (Sandoz, Basel). Cyclosporin A: a clinical evaluation of drug interactions. Transplantation Proc (1986) 18, (Suppl 5) 50–5.
2 Keogh A, Esmore D, Spratt P, Savdie E, McClusky P. Acetazolamide and cyclosporine. Transplantation (1988) 46, 478–9.
3 Nanni G, Magalini SC, Serino F, Castagneto M. Effect of disopyramide in a cyclosporine-treated patient. Transplantation (1988) 45, 257.
4 Blaison G, Weber JC, Sachs D, Korganow AS, Martin T, Kretz KG, Pasqauli JL. Rhabdomyolyse causee par la simvastatine chez un transplante cardiaque sous ciclosporine. Rev Med Interne (1992) 13, 61–3.
5 Zazgornik J, Schein W, Heimberger K, Shaheen FAM, Stockenhuber F. Potentiation of neurotoxic side-effects by coadministration of imipenem to cyclosporine therapy in a kidney transplant recipient-synergism or side-effects or drug interaction ? Clin Nephrol (1986) 26, 265–6.
6 Mraz W, Sido B, Knedel M, Hammer C. Concomitant immunosuppressive and antibiotic therapy-reduction of cyclosporin A blood levels due to treatment with imipenem/cilastin. Transplantation Proc (1987) 19, 4017–20.
7 Thaler F, Gotainer B, Teodori G, Dubois C, Loirat Ph. Mediastinitis due to *Nocardia asteroides* after cardiac transplantation. Intens Care Med (1992) 18, 127–8.
8 Spes CH, Angermann CE, Horn K, Strasser T, Mudra H, Landgraf R, Theisen K. Ciclosporin-propafenone interaction. Klin Wchschr (1990) 68, 872.
9 Shepp DH, Dandiker PS, Meyers JD. Treatment of varicella zoster virus infection in severely immunocompromised patients: a randomized comparison of acyclovir and vidarabine. N Engl J Med (1986) 314, 208–12.
10 Johnson PC, Kumor K, Welsh MS, Woo J, Kahan BD. Effects of coadministration of cyclosporine and acyclovir on renal function of renal allograft recipients. Transplantation. (1987) 44, 329–31.
11 Tan HW, Ch'ng SL. Drug interaction between cyclosporine A and quinine in a renal transplant patient with malaria. Singapore Med J (1991) 32, 189–90.
12 Abu-Romeh SH, Rashed A. Ciclosporin A and griseofulvin: another drug interaction. Nephron (1991) 58, 237.
13 Birmelé B, Lebranchu Y, Bagros Ph, Nivet H, Furet Y, Pengloan J. Interaction of cyclosporin and ticlopidine. Nephrol Dial Transplant (1991) 6, 150–1.
14 Stoof TJ, Korstanje MJ, Bilo HJG, Starink ThM, Hulsmans RFHJ, Donkder AJM. does fish oil protect renal function in cyclosporin-treated psoriasis patients ? J Intern Med (1989) 226, 437–41.
15 Bunker CB, Rustin MHA, Dowd PM. Isotretinoin treatment of severe acne in posttransplant patients taking cyclosporine. J Amer Acad Dermatol (1990) 22, 693–4.
16 Abel EA. Isotretinoin treatment of severe cystic acne in a heart transplant patient receiving cyclosporine: consideration of drug interactions. J Amer Acad Dermatol (1991) 24, 511.
17 Zawadzki J, Prokurat S, Smirska E, Jelonek A. Interaction between cyclosporine A and chloramphenicol after kidney transplantation. Pediat Nephrol (1991) 5, C49.
18 Zylber-Katz E, Rubinger D, Berlatsky Y. Cyclosporine interactions with metronidazole and cimetidine. Drug Intell Clin Pharm (1988) 22, 504.
19 Anon. In Focus, Simvastatin. Committee on Safety of Medicines, Current Problems Series (1992) 33, 3.
20 Stevens SL, Goldman MH. Cyclosporine toxicity associated with allopurinol. South Med J (1992) 85, 1265–6.
21 Chocair P, Duley J, Simmonds HA, Cameron JS, Ianhez L, Arap S, Sabbaga E. Low-dose allopurinol plus azathioprine cyclosporin prednisolone, a novel immunosuppressive regimen. Lancet (1993) 342, 83
22 Webber IR, Back DJ. Effect of etretinate on cyclosporine metabolism in vitro. Br J Dermatol (1993) 128, 42–4.

Cyclosporin(e) + Non-steroidal anti-inflammatory drugs (NSAIDs)

Abstract/Summary

There is limited evidence that some NSAIDs (diclofenac, ketoprofen, mefenamic acid, naproxen, piroxicam and possibly sulindac) can reduce kidney function and possibly increase the nephrotoxicity of cyclosporin, which is reflected in serum creatinine level rises and changes in cyclosporin levels.

Clinical evidence

(a) Cyclosporin + Diclofenac

A man with a kidney transplant and treated with cyclosporin, prednisolone, digoxin, frusemide and spironolactone showed a marked rise in serum creatinine levels immediately after starting to take 25 mg diclofenac three times daily. A fall in serum cyclosporin levels (from 409 to 285 ng/ml) also occurred. A study of 20 patients given both drugs found that seven of them had a high probability of an interaction (rises in serum creatinine levels and blood pressures), and nine possibly.[6] Increased nephrotoxicity was seen in another patient when given 150 mg diclofenac daily.[3]

(b) Cyclosporin + Ketoprofen, Mefenamic acid, Naproxen, Piroxicam, Sulindac

A patient with a kidney transplant showed a rise in serum creatinine levels when sulindac was used. Serum cyclosporin levels fell and rose again when the sulindac was stopped.[1] Another report states that the cyclosporin levels of a woman with a kidney transplant more than doubled within three days of starting to take 150 mg sulindac twice daily.[2] Both sulindac and naproxen increased serum creatinine levels of 11 patients on cyclosporin with rheumatoid arthritis by 24% with a reduction in renal function, but accompanied by clinical improvement,[7] while another report describes increased serum creatinine levels in a patient with rheumatoid arthritis when treated with ketoprofen, but not when given sulindac.[5] The serum cyclosporin levels of a patient approximately doubled, accompanied by rise in creatinine levels from 113 to 168 µmol/L within a day of starting to take mefenamic acid. Levels fell to normal within a week of stopping the mefenamic acid.[8] Piroxicam increased serum creatinine levels in another patient.[5]

Mechanism

Uncertain. One idea is that intact kidney prostacyclin synthesis is needed to maintain the glomerular filtration rate and renal blood flow in patients given cyclosporin which possibly may protect the kidney from the development of cyclosporin-induced nephrotoxicity. If NSAIDs are used which inhibit prostaglandin production in the kidney, the nephrotoxic effects of the cyclosporin manifest themselves, possibly independently of changes in serum cyclosporin levels.[1] A study in rats showed that indomethacin and cyclosporin together can cause rises in serum creatinine levels which are much greater than with either drug alone.[4]

Importance and management

Direct information is very limited (involving only diclofenac, ketoprofen, mefenamic acid, piroxicam, naproxen and sulindac) so that the general importance of these reactions is uncertain, but it has been suggested that all NSAIDs should be given to patients on cyclosporin with caution, and only if kidney function can be well monitored.[1]

References

1 Harris KP, Jenkins D, Walls J. Nonsteroidal antiinflammatory drugs and cyclosporine. A potentially serious adverse interaction. Transplantation (1988) 46, 598–9.
2 Sesin GP, O'Keefe E, Roberto P. Sulindac-induced elevation of serum cyclosporin concentration. Clin Pharm (1989) 8, 445–6.
3 Deray G, Le Hoang P, Aupetit B, Achour A, Rottembourg J, Baumelou A. Enhancement of cyclosporine A nephrotoxicity by diclofenac. Clin Nephrol (1987) 27, 213.
4 Whiting PH, Burke MD, Thomson AW. Drug interactions with cyclosporine. Implications from animal studies. Transplant Proc (1986) XVIII Suppl 5, 56–70.
5 Ludwin D, Bennett KJ, Grace EM, Buchanan WA, Bensen W, Bombardier C, Tugwell PX. Nephrotoxicity in patients with rheumatoid arthritis treated with cyclosporine. Transplant Proc (1988) XX Suppl 4, 367–70.
6 Branthwaite JP, Nicholls A. Cyclosporin and diclofenac interaction in rheumatoid arthritis. Lancet (1991) 337, 252.
7 Altman RD, Perez GO, Sfakianakis GN. Interaction of cyclosporin A and nonsteroidal antiinflammatory drugs on renal function in patients with rheumatoid arthritis. Am J Med (1992) 93, 396–402.
8 Agar JW MacD. Cyclosporin A and mefenamic acid in a renal transplant patient. Aust NZ Med J (1991) 21, 784–5.

Cyclosporin(e) + Octreotide

Abstract/Summary

Octreotide causes a marked fall in the serum levels of cyclosporin and inadequate immunosuppression may result.

Clinical evidence

A diabetic man with kidney and pancreatic segment transplants was successfully immunosuppressed with azathioprine, methylprednisolone and cyclosporin. When he was additionally treated twice daily with 100 g octreotide (a long-acting somatostatin analogue) subcutaneously to reduce fluid collection around the pancreatic graft, his trough serum cyclosporin levels fell below the assay detection limit of 50 ng/ml. Nine other diabetics similarly treated with octreotide for peripancreatic fluid collection and fistulas after pancreatic transplantation also showed significant falls in their serum cyclosporin levels within 24–48 hr, in three of them to undetectable levels.[1] A similar interaction was seen in another patient.[2]

Mechanism

Uncertain. A suggestion is that the octreotide reduces the intestinal absorption of the cyclosporin.[1,2]

Importance and management

An established and clinically important interaction, although the documentation is limited. The authors of the report cited recommend that before giving octreotide the oral dosage of cyclosporin should be increased on average by 50% and the serum levels monitored daily.[1]

References

1 Landgraf R, Landgraf-Leurs MMC, Nusser J, Hillebrand G, Illner WD, Abendroth D, Land W. Effect of somatostatin analogue (SMS 201–995) on cyclosporin levels. Transplantation (1987) 44, 724–5.
2 Rosenberg L, Dafoe DC, Schwartz R, Campbell DA. Administration of somatostatin analog (SMS 201–995) in the treatment of fistula occurring after pancreas transplantation. Transplantation (1987) 43, 764–6.

Cyclosporin + OKT3

Abstract/Summary

OKT3 increases serum cyclosporin levels.

Clinical evidence, mechanism, importance and management

When OKT3 (5 mg IV push daily for 10 days) was given to 10 kidney transplant patients to treat acute rejection, their mean trough cyclosporin levels on day 8 were still higher than before the OKT3 was started, despite a 50% reduction in the cyclosporin dosage. When the OKT3 was withdrawn, the cyclosporin dosage needed to be increased again.[1] The reasons are not understood. It is clearly necessary to titrate the dosage of cyclosporin downwards if OKT3 is given to prevent an excessive rise in cyclosporin levels with the attendant risks of kidney toxicity.

Reference

1 Vrahnos D, Sanchez J, Vasquez EM, Pollak R, Maddux MS. Cyclosporin levels during OKT3 treatment of acute renal allograft rejection. Pharmacotherapy (1991) 11, 278.

Cyclosporin + Omeprazole

Abstract/Summary

Omeprazole normally appears not to affect serum cyclosporin levels, but two isolated reports describe doubled serum cyclosporin levels in one patient, and more than halved serum cyclosporin levels in another.

Clinical evidence

Ten renal transplant patients showed no significant changes in cyclosporin levels when given 20 mg omeprazole daily for 2 weeks.[2,4]

In contrast, the serum cyclosporin levels of a liver transplant patient approximately doubled (from a range of 187–261, to 510 ng/ml) about two weeks after starting to take 40 mg omprezole daily. His cyclosporin levels were readjusted by reducing the dose from 130 to 80 mg twice daily. They then remained steady at about 171 ng/ml for the following four months.[1] Another patient with a bone marrow transplant showed just the opposite interaction. Her serum cyclosporin levels fell from 254 ng/ml to about 100 ng/ml over 14 days while taking 40 mg omeprazole daily, and climbed again rapidly when the omeprazole was stopped.[3]

Mechanism

Not understood.

Importance and management

The uncertainty of the outcome of giving omeprazole to patients on cyclosporin means that any patient given both drugs should be very well monitored to establish what will happen. Adjust the cyclosporin dosage if necessary. Note that in the study cited the dose of omeprazole was 20 mg daily whereas the two cases of interaction involved 40 mg daily.

References

1 Schouler L, Dumas F, Couzigou P, Janvier G, Winnock S, Saric J. Omeprazole-cyclosporin interaction. Am J Gastroenterol (1991) 86, 1097.
2 Blohmé I, Andersson T, Idström J-P. No interaction between omeprazole and cyclosporine. Gastroenterology (1991) 100, A721.
3 Arranz R, Yañez E, Franceschi JL, Fernandez-Rañada JM. More about omeprazole-cyclosporine interaction. Am J Gastroenterol (1993) 88, 154–5.
4 Blohmé I, Idström J-P, Andersson T. A study of the interaction between omeprazole and cyclosporine in renal transplant patients. Br J Clin Pharmac (1993) 35, 156–60.

Cyclosporin(e) + Penicillins

Abstract/Summary

Ampicillin does not interact adversely with cyclosporin. Increased nephrotoxicity has been seen in lung transplant patients given nafcillin prophylactically. Two isolated case reports describe a fall in serum cyclosporin levels in one patient treated with nafcillin, and a rise in another treated with ticarcillin.

Clinical evidence

(a) Ampicillin

Seventy-one renal transplant patients on cyclosporin showed no changes in serum urea, creatinine or serum cyclosporin levels when ampicillin was given and later withdrawn.[1]

(b) Nafcillin

A retrospective study of 19 lung transplant patients on cyclosporin found that those given prophylactic nafcillin for a week against staphylococci showed a greater degree of kidney dysfunction than the others without nafcillin. Serum creatinine levels climbed steadily over 6 days until the nafcillin was stopped, whereas the 'no nafcillin' patients showed no changes. Three of the nafcillin group temporarily needed haemodialysis. Cyclosporin doses in the nafcillin group were higher but the serum levels in both groups were not significantly different. The incidence of viral infections was also greater in the nafcillin group.[4]

A kidney transplant patient on cyclosporin and prednisone experienced a marked fall in her serum cyclosporin levels on two occasions when treated with nafcillin (2 g 6-hourly). Trough serum levels fell from 229 to 119 and then to 68 ng/ml after 3 and 7 days of nafcillin, before climbing again when the nafcillin was stopped. On the second occasion levels fell from 272 to 42 ng/ml after 9 days treatment with nafcillin.[2]

(c) Ticarcillin

Rises in serum cyclosporin levels from 90 to 230 ng/ml, and from 120 to 300 ng/ml occurred in a man within 5–10 days of starting to take 10 g ticarcillin daily.[3]

Mechanism

The authors of the study (b) postulate that the nafcillin may have interfered with the cyclosporin assay, resulting in an under-estimate of the actual levels, so that the nephrotoxicity was simply due to higher cyclosporin levels.[4] The fall in cyclosporin levels in the individual patient[2] is not understood, nor is the rise in levels seen in the patient on ticarcillin.[3]

Importance and management

Information seems to be limited to the studies cited. No special precautions would seem necessary with ampicillin, but an alternative to nafcillin should be used for antistaphylococcal prophylaxis. Close monitoring would seem necessary if either nafcillin or ticarcillin is given. More study is needed.

References

1 Xu F, Shi XH. Interaction between ampicillin, norfloxacin and cyclospo-

rine in renal transplant patients. Chinese Journal of Antibiotics (1992) 17, 290–2.

2 Veremis SA, Maddux MS, Pollak R, Mozes MF. Subtherapeutic cyclosporine concentrations during nafcillin therapy. Transplantation (1987) 43, 913–5.

3 Lambert C, Pointet P, Ducret F. Interaction ciclosporine-ticarcilline chez un transplanté rénal. La Presse Méd (1989) 18, 230.

4 Jahansouz F, Kriett JM, Smith CM, Jamieson SW. Potentiation of cyclosporin nephrotoxicity by nafcillin in lung transplant patients. Transplantation (1993) 55, 1045–8.

Cyclosporin(e) + Prazosin

Abstract/Summary

Preliminary studies show that prazosin causes a small reduction in the glomerular filtration rate of kidney transplant patients on cyclosporin.

Clinical evidence, mechanism, importance and management

A study in eight patients with kidney transplants showed that after taking 1 mg prazosin twice daily for a week, their serum cyclosporin levels remained unchanged, whereas arterial blood pressures and renal vascular resistance were reduced. However the glomerular filtration rate (GFR) was reduced by about 10% (from 47 to 42 ml/min).[1] Previous studies in kidney transplant patients treated with azathioprine, prednisone and prazosin found no reduction in GFR.[2] There would seem to be no strong reasons for totally avoiding prazosin in patients on cyclosporin, but the authors of the report point out that the fall in GFR makes prazosin a less attractive antihypertensive than a calcium channel blocker.

References

1 Kibord BA. Effects of prazosin therapy in renal allograft recipients receiving cyclosporine. Transplantation (1990) 49, 1200–1.

2 Curtis JR, Bateman FJA. Use of prazosin in management of hypertension in patients with chronic renal failure and in renal transplant recipients. Br Med J (1975) 4, 432.

Cyclosporin(e) + Probucol

Abstract/Summary

Probucol reduces blood cyclosporin levels.

Clinical evidence

A study in six heart transplant patients taking 2.44 mg/kg cyclosporin 12-hourly daily showed that the concurrent use of 500 mg probucol 12-hourly decreased whole blood cyclosporin levels and the AUC. The clearance was increased by 60% and volume of distribution also increased. Comparative whole blood cyclosporin levels in ng/ml before and while taking the probu-

col were as follows: 1034 v 786 (1 h), 1272 v 933 (3 h), 958 v 728 (5 h), 5995 v 413 (11 h).[1] This represents a 28% AUC decrease over 11 h.[1-3]

Mechanism

Not understood.

Importance and management

Information appears to be limited to these studies, but the conclusion to be drawn is that the cyclosporin dosage will need to be increased if probucol is added. Monitor the effects and adjust the dosage appropriately.

Reference

1 Corder CN, Sundarajan V, Liguori C, Cooper DKC, Muchmore J, Zuhdi N, Novitzky D, Barbi G, Larscheid P, Manion CV. Interference with steady state cyclosporine levels by probucol in heart transplant patients. Clin Pharmacol Ther (1990) 47, 204.

2 Sundararajan V, Cooper DKC, Muchmore J, Manion CV, Liguori C, Zuhdi N, Novitzky D, Chen P-N, Bourne DWA, Cordner CN. Interaction of cyclosporine and probucol in heart transplant patients. Transplant Proc (1991) 23, 2028–32.

3 Chen P, Bourne DWA, Corder CN, Larscheid P. Clinical pharmacokinetic interaction of cyclosporine and probucol studied using a HPLC assay procedure. Pharmaceutical Res (1990) 7, S-254.

Cyclosporin(e) + Quinolone antibiotics

Abstract/Summary

Cyclosporin serum levels are normally unchanged by the use of ciprofloxacin and kidney toxicity is not normally increased, but increased serum levels and nephrotoxicity may occur in a small number of patients. Two reports describe rises in cyclosporin levels in two patients given norfloxacin, but others state that no difficulties occurred. Enoxacin, ofloxacin and pefloxacin appear not to interact.

Clinical evidence

(a) Ciprofloxacin

A single dose study in 10 normal subjects found that after taking 500 mg ciprofloxacin twice daily for 7 days the pharmacokinetics of oral cyclosporin (5 mg/kg) were unchanged.[1] Four other studies in 10 renal transplant patients taking 750 mg ciprofloxacin twice daily for 13 days;[6] in 15 kidney transplant patients on 500 mg ciprofloxacin twice daily for 7 days;[10] in 10 bone marrow transplant patients given 500 mg ciprofloxacin twice daily for 4 days;[8] and in four heart transplant patients given 250–500 mg 7–140 days[12] also found no changes in serum cyclosporin levels nor evidence of kidney toxicity.

In contrast a handful of cases of nephrotoxicity have been

reported. A heart transplant patient developed acute renal failure within 4 days of being given ciprofloxacin (750 mg 8-hourly).[4] Another patient who had had a kidney transplant developed reversible nephrotoxicity.[2] Decreased renal function in a heart-lung transplant patient has been described in another report.[9] This patient and another also showed increased serum cyclosporin levels when given 500 mg ciprofloxacin three times daily.[9] A further report also describes a rise.[14]

(b) Enoxacin, Ofloxacin, Pefloxacin

A study in 10 subjects found that 400 mg enoxacin twice daily for five days had little effect on either blood or plasma levels of single doses of cyclosporin.[13] 39 patients with kidney transplants under treatment with cyclosporin and prednisolone showed no evidence of nephrotoxicity nor any other interaction when concurrently treated with 100–400 mg ofloxacin daily for periods of 3–500 days.[5] A study in kidney transplant patients treated with corticosteroids, azathioprine and cyclosporin found that the pharmacokinetics of the cyclosporin were not significantly changed by 400 mg pefloxacin twice daily for four days.[11]

(c) Norfloxacin

Six renal transplant patients given 400 mg norfloxacin twice daily for 3–23 days for urinary tract infections,[7] and four heart transplant patients given 400 mg for 7–140 days showed no changes in serum cyclosporin levels,[12] however two reports describe rises, one marked, in serum cyclosporin levels in a heart transplant patient and a kidney transplant patient when given norfloxacin.[3,14]

Mechanism

Not understood.

Importance and management

Information seems to be limited to these reports. They suggest that while concurrent use is usually uneventful and serum cyclosporin levels do not normally rise, kidney toxicity and increased cyclosporin levels occur occasionally and unpredictably with ciprofloxacin and norfloxacin. Concurrent use should therefore be very well monitored. There seem to be no reports of problems with enoxacin, ofloxacin or pefloxacin but the outcome should nevertheless be well monitored.

References

1 Tan KKC, Trull AK, Shawket S. Co-administration of ciprofloxacin and cyclosporin: lack of evidence for a pharmacokinetic interaction. Br J Clin Pharmacol (1989) 28, 185–7.
2 Elston RA, Taylor J. Possible interaction of ciprofloxacin with cyclosporin A. J Antimicrob Chemother (1988) 29, 679–80.
3 Thomson DJ, Menkis AH, McKenzie FN. Norfloxacin-cyclosporine interaction. Transplantation (1988) 46, 312–13.
4 Advent CK, Krinsky JK, Bourge RC, Figg WD. Synergistic nephrotoxicity due to ciprofloxacin and cyclosporine. Am J Med (1988) 85, 452.
5 Vogt P, Schorn T, Frei U. Ofloxacin in the treatment of urinary tract infection in renal transplant recipients. Infection (1988) 16, 175–8.
6 Lang J, Finaz de Villaine J, Garraffo R, Touraine J-L. Cyclosporine (cyclosporin A) pharmacokinetics in renal transplant patients receiving ciprofloxacin. Am J Med (1989) 87 (Suppl 5A) 82–85S.
7 Jadoul M, Pirson Y, van Ypersele de Strihou C. Norfloxacin and cyclosporine-a safe combination. Transplantation (1989) 47, 747–8.
8 Krüger HU, Schuler U, Proksch B, Göbel M, Ehninger G. Investigation of potential interaction of ciprofloxacin with cyclosporine in bone marrow transplant recipients. Antimicrob Ag Chemother (1990) 34, 1048–52.
9 Nasir M, Rotellar C, Hand M, Kulczycki L, Alijani MR, Winchester JF. Interaction between ciclosporin and ciprofloxacin. Nephron (1991) 57, 245–6.
10 van Buren DH, Koestner J, Adedoyin A, McCune T, MacDonell R, Johnson HK, Carroll J, Nylander W, Richie RE. Effect of ciprofloxacin on cyclosporine pharmacokinetics. Transplantation (1990) 50, 888–9.
11 Lang J, Finaz de Villaine J, Guemei A, Touraine JL, Faucon C. Absence of pharmacokinetic interaction between pefloxacin and cyclosporin A in patients with renal transplants. Rev Inf Dis (1989) II Suppl 5, S1094.
12 Robinson JA, Venezio FR, Costanzo-Nordin MR, Pifarre R, O'Keefe PJ. Patients receiving quinolones and cyclosporine after heart transplantation. J Heart Transplant (1990) 9, 30–1.
13 Ryerson BA, Toothaker RD, Posvar EL, Sedman AJ, Koup JR. Effect of enoxacin on cyclosporine pharmacokinetics in healthy subjects. 31st Intersci Conf Antimicrol Ag Chemother (1991) Abstracts, 198.
14 Castelao AM. Cyclosporine A — drug interactions. In Sunshine I (Ed.) Recent developments in therapeutic drug monitoring and clinical toxicology. 2nd Int Conf Therapeutic Drug Monitoring Toxicology, Barcelona, Spain, (1992) 203–9.

Cyclosporin(e) + Rifampicin (Rifampin) and Rifabutin (Ansamycin)

Abstract/Summary

Cyclosporin serum levels are markedly reduced by the concurrent use of rifampicin. Transplant rejection can rapidly develop if the cyclosporin dosage is not increased (3–5-fold). Rifabutin appears to interact minimally.

Clinical evidence

(a) Rifampicin

A heart transplant patient on cyclosporin was started on 600 mg rifampicin daily in addition to amphotericin B for the treatment of an *Aspergillus fumigatus* infection. Within 11 days her serum cyclosporin levels had fallen from 473 to less than 31 ng/ml and severe acute graft rejection occurred. The dosage of cyclosporin was increased stepwise and the levels climbed to a plateau before suddenly falling again. The dosage had to be increased to more than 30 mg/kg daily to achieve serum levels in the range 100–300 ng/ml.[1]

A considerable number of other reports about individual patients confirm that a very marked fall in serum cyclosporin levels occurs (often to undetectable levels), accompanied by transplantation rejection in many instances, if rifampicin is given without raising the cyclosporin dosage.[2–16,19,21] Even topical rifampicin used to irrigate a wound can have this effect.[16] Levels can rise to toxic proportions within 2 weeks of stopping the rifampicin unless the cyclosporin dosage is very much reduced.[2,4]

(b) Rifabutin (Ansamycin)

The clearance of cyclosporin in a patient with a kidney transplant approximately doubled (from 0.3 to 0.63 l/h/kg) when treated with isoniazid, ethambutol, pyridoxine and 600 mg daily rifampicin (rifampin). When replaced by 150 mg rifabutin and 100 mg clofazimine daily the clearance fell to approximately its former levels, but after about 3 weeks rose to 0.36 l/h/kg.[19]

Mechanism

Rifampicin stimulates the metabolism of the cyclosporin by the liver (increased amounts of cytochrome P450IIIA3)[17] resulting in a marked increase in its loss from the body, accompanied by a fall in its serum levels. In addition rifampicin decreases cyclosporin absorption from the gut by inducing its metabolism by the gut wall,[18] thus its immunosuppressant effects become markedly reduced. Rifabutin has some enzyme inducing properties but the extent is quite small compared with rifampicin, and is delayed.[20]

Importance and management

The cyclosporin-rifampicin interaction is well documented, well established and clinically important. Transplant rejection may occur unless the cyclosporin dosage is markedly increased. Monitor the effects of concurrent use and increase the cyclosporin dosage appropriately. 3–5-fold dosage increases (sometimes frequency-increases from two to three times daily) have proved to be effective. Remember to reduce the dosage if the rifampicin is stopped. Alternative tuberculostatics which are reported not to interact with cyclosporin include pyrazinamide (25 mg/kg)[4] and isoniazid,[10] however there is a case report describing a patient who showed a gradual rise in serum cyclosporin levels when isoniazid and ethambutol were stopped.[12] Rifabutin appears to interact minimally. Another alternative is to replace the cyclosporin with azathioprine and low-dose prednisolone for immunosuppression if using rifampicin.[11]

References

1 Modry DL, Stinson EB, Oyer PE, Jamieson SW, Baldwin JC, Shumway NE. Acute rejection and massive cyclosporine requirements in heart transplant recipients treated with rifampin. Transplantation (1985) 39, 313–14.

2 Langhoff E, Madsen S. Rapid metabolism of cyclosporin and prednisone in kidney transplant patients on tuberculostatic treatment. Lancet (1983) ii, 1303.

3 Cassidy MJD, Van Zyl-Smit R, Pascoe MD, Swanepoel CR, Jacobson JE. Effect of rifampicin on cyclosporin A blood levels in a renal transplant recipient. Nephron (1985) 41, 207–8.

4 Coward RA, Raferty AT, Brown CB. Cyclosporin and antituberculous therapy. Lancet (1985) i, 1342–3.

5 Howard P, Bixler TJ, Gill B. Cyclosporine-rifampin drug interaction. Drug Intell Clin Pharm (1985) 19, 763–4.

6 Van Buren D, Wideman CA, Reid M, Gibbons S, Van Buren CT, Jarowenko M, Flechner SM, Frazier OH, Cooley DA, Kahan BD. The antagonistic effect of rifampin upon cyclosporine bioavailability. Transplant Proc (1984) 16, 1642–5.

7 Allen RDM, Hunnisett AG, Morris PJ. Cyclosporin and rifampicin in renal transplantation. Lancet (1985) i, 980.

8 Langhoff E, Madsen S. Rapid metabolism of cyclosporin and prednisone in kidney transplant patient receiving tuberculostatic treatment. Lancet (1983) ii, 1031.

9 Offermann G, Keller F, Molzahn M. Low cyclosporin A blood levels and acute graft rejection in a renal transplant recipient during rifampin treatment. Am J Nephrol (1985) 5, 385–7.

10 Jurewicz WA, Gunson BK, Ismail T, Angrisani L, McMaster P. Cyclosporin and antituberculous therapy. Lancet (1985) i, 1343.

11 Daniels NJ, Dover JS, Schachter RK. Interaction between cyclosporin and rifampicin. Lancet (1984) ii, 639.

12 Leimenstoll G, Schlegelberger T, Fulde R, Niedermayer W. Interaktion von Ciclosporin und Ethambutol-Isoniazid. Dtsch med Wsch (1988) 113, 514–15.

13 Prado A, Ramirez M, Aguirre EC, Martin RS, Zucchini A. Interaccion entre ciclopsorina y rifampicina en un caso de transplante renal. Medicina (Buenos Aires) (1987) 47, 521–4.

14 Vandevelde C, Chang A, Andrews D, Riggs W, Jewesson P. Rifampin and ansamycin interactions with cyclosporine after renal transplantation. Pharmacotherapy (1991) 11, 88–9.

15 Al-Sulaiman MH, Dhar JM, Al-Khader A. Successful use of rifampicin in the treatment of tuberculosis in renal transplant patients immunosuppressed with cyclosporine. Transplantation (1990) 50, 597–8.

16 Renoult E, Hubert J, Trechot Ph, Hestin D, Kessler M, L'Hermite J. Effect of topical rifamycin SV treatment on cyclosporin A blood levels in a renal transplant patient. Eur J Clin Pharmacol (1991) 40, 433–4.

17 Pichard L, Fabre JM, Domergue J, Fabre G, Saint-Aubert B, Mourad G, Maurel P. Molecular mechanism of cyclosporine A drug interactions: inducers and inhibitors of cytochrome P450 screening in primary cultures of human hepatocytes. Transplant Proc (1991) 23, 978–9.

18 Hebert MF, Roberts JP, Prueksaritanont T, Benet LZ. Bioavailability of cyclosporine with concomitant rifampin administration is markedly less than predicted by hepatic enzyme induction. Clin Pharmacol Ther (1992) 52, 453–7.

19 Vandevelde C, Chang A, Andrews D, Riggs W, Jewesson P. Rifampin and ansamycin interactions with cyclosporine after renal transplantation. Pharmacotherapy (1991) 11, 88–9.

20 Perucca E, Grimaldi R, Frigo GM, Sardi A, Moning H, Ohnhaus EE. Comparative effects of rifabutin and rifampicin on hepatic microsomal enzyme activity in normal subjects. Eur J Clin Pharmacol (1988) 34, 595–9.

21 Sánchez DM, Rincón LC, Asensio JM, Serna AB. Interacción entre ciclosporina y rifampicina. Rev Clin Esp (1988) 183, 217.

Cyclosporin(e) + Sex hormones and Related drugs

Abstract/Summary

Hepatotoxicity has been described in two patients when concurrently treated with cyclosporin and oral contraceptives. Rises in serum cyclosporin levels may also occur. Hepatotoxicity occurred in two others given cyclosporin and norethandrolone. Marked increases in serum cyclosporin levels have been seen in three patients taking danazol and in two taking methyltestosterone. Some increase has been seen with norethisterone.

Clinical evidence

(a) Cyclosporin + Contraceptives (oral)

A woman treated for uveitis with cyclosporin (5 mg/kg daily) showed an increase in trough serum cyclosporin levels (very roughly doubled) on two occasions when given an oral contraceptive (levonorgestrel 150 µg + ethinyloestradiol 30 µg). She also experienced nausea, vomiting and heptalgia, and showed evidence of severe hepatotoxicity (very marked increases in aspartate and alanine aminotransferases, and rises in serum bilirubin and alkaline phosphatase).[4]

Another report describes hepatotoxicity in a patient when concurrently treated with cyclosporin and an oral contraceptive (desogestrel 150 ug + ethinyloestradiol 30 ug). Rises in serum cyclosporin levels were also seen.[5]

(b) Cyclosporin + Danazol

A 15-year-old girl who had had a kidney transplant for a year and taking cyclosporin and prednisone, showed a marked rise in serum cyclosporin levels over about 2 weeks (from a range of 250–325 to 700–850 mol/l) when given 200 mg danazol twice daily, even though the cyclosporin dosage was reduced from 350 to 250 mg daily.[1]

Similar rises in cyclosporin levels (from about 400 to 600 ng/ml, and from 150 to about 450 ng/ml) were seen in another patient on two occasions over about a 6-week period when given 400 mg and later 600 mg danazol daily.[2] A marked rise in serum cyclosporin levels has been described in another patient when given 200 mg danazol four times daily.[6]

(c) Cyclosporin + Methyltestosterone

A man with a kidney transplant was given methyltestosterone a few days before an attempt was made to change his immunosuppressive treatment from azathioprine and prednisone to cyclosporin. His serum cyclosporin levels rose to more than 2000 ng/ml and severe cyclosporin toxicity was seen (raised serum creatinine, bilirubin and alanine aminotransferase levels).[3] This interaction has been seen in another patient.[7]

(d) Cyclosporin + Norethandrolone

Three out of four patients with bone marrow aplasia treated with cyclosporin and prednisone developed liver toxicity. It developed in two of them when norethandrolone was added. No toxicity occurred when they were given either of the drugs singly.[9]

(e) Cyclosporin + Norethisterone

The 15-year-old girl on cyclosporin who had shown a marked increase in serum cyclosporin levels when given danazol (referred to above) continued to have elevated levels, but not as high, when the danazol was replaced by norethisterone, 5 mg

three times daily, and the levels fell once again when the norethisterone was stopped.[1] No changes in cyclosporin levels were seen in another patient when treated with norethisterone intermittently.[6] Two women showed a mild rise in cyclosporin with no changes in creatinine levels when given 10 mg norethisterone daily for 10 days.[8]

Mechanism

Uncertain. It seems possible that some of these compounds inhibit the metabolism of the cyclosporin by the liver, thereby reducing its loss from the body and leading to an increase in its serum levels. The mechanism of the hepatotoxicity is not understood.

Importance and management

Information is very limited indeed, but what is known indicates that the concurrent use of any of these drugs and cyclosporin should be well monitored for any evidence of increases in serum cyclosporin levels or hepatotoxicity.

References

1 Ross WB, Roberts D, Griffin PJA, Salaman JR. Cyclosporin interaction with danazol and norethisterone. Lancet (1986) i, 330.
2 Schroder O, Schmitz N, Kayser W, Euler HH, Loffler H. Erhohte Ciclosporin-A-Spiegel bei gleichzeitiger Therapie mit Danazol. Dtsch med Wsch (1986) 111, 602–3.
3 Moller BB, Ekelund B. Toxicity of cyclosporin during treatment with androgens. N Engl J Med (1985) 313, 1416.
4 Deray G, Le Hoang P, Cacoub P, Assogba U, Grippon P, Baumelou A. Oral contraceptive interaction with cyclosporin. Lancet (1987) i, 158–9.
5 Leimenstoll G, Jessen P, Zabel P, Niedermayer W. Arzneimittelschadigungder Leber bei Kombination von Cyclosporin A und einem Antikonzeptivum. Dtsch med Wsch (1984) 109, 1989.
6 Koneru B, Hartner C, Iwatsuki S, Starzl TE. Effect of danazol on cyclosporine pharmacokinetics. Transplantation (1988) 45, 1001.
7 Goffin E, Pirson Y, Geubel A, van Ypersele de Strihou C. Cyclosporine-methyltestosterone interaction. Nephron (1991) 59, 174–5.
8 Castelao AM. Cyclosporine A — drug interactions. In Sunshine I (Ed.) Recent developments in therapeutic drug monitoring and clinical toxicology. 2nd Int Conf Therapeutic Drug Monitoring Toxicology, Barcelona, Spain, (1992) 203–9.
9 Sahnoun Z, Frikha M, Zeghal KM, Souissi T. Toxicité hépatique de la ciclosporine et interaction médicamenteuse avec les androgènes. Sem Hôp Paris (1993) 69, 26–8.

Cyclosporin + Sulphonamides

Abstract/Summary

Sulphadiazine given orally or sulphadimidine/trimethoprim given intravenously can cause a marked fall in serum cyclosporin levels. Sulphamethoxydiazine can cause a minor fall. Although co-trimoxazole increases serum creatinine levels in kidney transplant patients on cyclosporin (normally interpreted as evidence of nephrotoxicity) it appears nevertheless normally to be safe and effective.

Clinical evidence

(a) Cyclosporin + Co-trimoxazole (Sulphamethoxazole/Trimethoprim)

A large-scale study in 132 kidney transplant patients on cyclosporin encompassing 33,876 patient-days found that co-trimoxazole was effective and well tolerated. Cyclosporin pharmacokinetics remained unchanged. A 15% rise in serum creatinine levels occurred which reversed when the co-trimoxazole was stopped. This rise was not interpreted as a sign of nephrotoxicity but appeared to be due to inhibition by the co-trimoxazole of the tubular excretion of creatinine.[7]

Other reports describe rises in creatinine levels (interpreted as evidence of nephrotoxicity)[1,5,6,8], interstitial nephritis,[9] granulocytopenia and thrombocytopenia[10,11] in a few patients during concurrent use of cyclosporin and co-trimoxazole. Apparent nephrotoxicity has also been seen with trimethoprim.[2]

(b) Cyclosporin + Sulphadiazine and Sulphamethoxydiazine

Three heart transplant patients under treatment for toxoplasmosis showed falls in their cyclosporin levels when given sulfadiazine (0.5–6.9 mg daily). Their dosage-to-level cyclosporin ratios rose by 58, 82 and 29% respectively. One out of two showed a minor fall when previously treated with sulphamethoxydiazine.[13]

Other reports mention the use of sulfadiazine without commenting about any interaction.[14,15]

(c) Cyclosporin + Sulphadimidine/Trimethoprim

A heart transplant patient on cyclosporin and prednisolone developed unmeasurably low serum cyclosporin levels seven days after starting sulphadimidine (2 g four times daily IV) and trimethoprim (300–500 mg twice daily). Doubling the cyclosporin dosage had little effect and evidence of transplant rejection was seen. Within 10 days of starting to take the anti-infective agents orally instead of intravenously the serum cyclosporin levels climbed to approximately their former levels and the rejection problems disappeared.[3]

Another report by some of the same authors similarly describes a marked fall in serum cyclosporin levels in five heart transplant patients (one of them the same as the report already cited[3]) when given sulphadimidine and trimethoprim intravenously.[4]

Mechanisms

Uncertain. (a) Co-trimoxazole and trimethoprim can raise serum creatinine levels, possibly due to inhibition of creatinine secretion by the kidney tubules.[12] (b & c) The reduction in serum cyclosporin levels is not understood.

Importance and management

Moderately documented, but established interactions of clinical importance. Be aware that intravenous sulphanilamide/trimethoprim and oral sulphadiazine can cause a marked reduction in serum cyclosporin levels with accompanying inadequate immunosuppression. The evidence suggests that oral sulphanilamide/trimethoprim, sulphamethoxydiazine and co-trimoxazole do not interact adversely and are normally safe and effective, although toxicity can apparently occur in a small number of patients. Until more information is available it would be prudent to keep a close check on cyclosporin levels if any sulphonamide is given.

References

1 Thompson JF, Chalmers DHJ, Hunnisett AGW, Wood RFM, Morris PJ. Nephrotoxicity of trimethoprim and cotrimoxazole in renal allograft recipients treated with cyclosporin. Transplantation (1983) 36, 204–6.

2 Nyberg G, Gabel H, Althoff P, Bjork S, Herlitz H, Brynger H. Adverse effect of trimethoprim on kidney function in renal transplant patients. Lancet (1984) i, 394–5.

3 Wallwork J, McGregor CGA, Wells FC, Cory-Pearce R, English TAH. Cyclosporin and intravenous sulphadimidine and trimethoprim therapy. Lancet (1983) i, 336–7.

4 Jones DK, Hakim M, Wallwork J, Higgenbottam TW, White DJG. Serious interaction between cyclosporin A and sulphadimidine. Br Med J (1986) 292, 728–9.

5 Ringden O, Myrenfors P, Klintmalm G, Tyden G, Ost L. Nephrotoxicity by co-trimoxazole and cyclosporin in transplanted patients. Lancet (1984) i, 1016–17.

6 Klintmalm G, Sawe J, Ringden O, von Bah C, Magnusson A. Cyclosporine plasma levels in renal transplant patients. Association with renal toxicity and allograft rejection. Transplantation (1985) 39, 132–7.

7 Maki DG, Fox BC, Kuntz J, Sollinger HW, Belzer FO. A prospective, randomized, double-blind study of trimethoprim-sulphamethoxazole for prophylais of infection in renal transplantation. Side effects of trimethoprim-sulphamethoxazole, interaction with cyclosporine. J Lab Clin Med (1992) 119, 11–24.

8 Klintmalm G, Ringdén O, Groth CG. Clinical and laboratory signs in nephrotoxicity and rejection in cyclosporine treated renal allograft recipients. Transplant Proc (1983) 15 Suppl 1) 2815–20.

9 Smith EJ, Light JA, Filo RS, Yum MN. Interstitial nephritis caused by trimethoprim-sulfamethoxazole in renal transplant recipients. J Amer Med Ass (1980) 244, 360–1.

10 Bradley PP, Warden GD, Maxwell JG, Rothstein G. Neuropenia and thrombocytopenia in renal allograft recipients treated with trimethoprim-sulfamethoxazole. Ann Intern med (1980) 93, 560–2.

11 Hulme B, Reeves DS. Leucopenia associated with trimethoprim-sulfa-methoxazole after renal transplantation. Br Med J (1971) 3, 610–2.

12 Berg KJ, Gjellestad A, Norby G, Rootwelt K, Djoseland O, Fauchald P, Mehl A, Narverud J, Talseth T. Renal effects of trimethoprim in ciclosporin- and azathioprine-treated kidney allografted patients. Nephron (1989) 53, 218–22.

13 Spes CH, Angermann CE, Stempfle HU, Wenke K, Theisen K. Sulfadiazine therapy for toxoplasmosis in heart transplant recipients decreases cyclosporine concentration. Clin Investi (1992) 70, 752–4.

14 Hakim M, Esmore D, Wallwork J, English TAH, Wreghitt T. Toxoplasmosis in cardiac transplantation. Br Med J (1986) 292, 1108.

15 Wreghitt TG, Hakim M, Gray JJ, Balfour AH, Gistovin P, Steward S, Scott J, English TAH, Wallwork J. Toxoplasmosis in heart and heart-lung transplant recipients. J Clin Pathol (1989) 42, 194–99.

Cyclosporin(e) + Vaccines

Abstract/Summary

Cyclosporin reduces the ability of the body to develop immunity when given influenza vaccine. Whether this is equally true for other vaccines is as yet uncertain.

Clinical evidence

(a) Cyclosporin + Influenza vaccine

A comparative study in 59 patients who had had kidney transplants showed that those who were on cyclosporin and prednisone (21 patients) had a significantly lower immune response to influenza vaccine (inactivated trivalent) than those on azathioprine and prednisone (38 patients) or normal subjects (29) taking no drugs. All of the immune response measurements made (mean antibody levels, four-fold titre rise, seroconversion to protective titres, the effects of booster immunization in those who responded poorly to the first vaccination) were reduced 20–30% in those on cyclosporin.[1]

Confirmation of the practical importance of this is described in a case report of a heart transplant patient on cyclosporin who twice failed to respond to influenza vaccination while receiving cyclosporin and prednisone.[2]

(b) Cyclosporin + Other vaccines

Since the effectiveness of influenza vaccination is reduced by cyclosporin it seems logical to expect that other vaccines will be similarly affected, however there seems to be no direct evidence confirming that this is so. It has been suggested that because cyclosporin can induce tolerance to antigens, this could lead to a situation where the patient becomes more (instead of less) susceptible to the infections against which one is trying to provide protection.[3]

Mechanism

Immunosuppression by cyclosporin diminishes the ability of the body to respond immunologically both to transplants and to influenza vaccination.

Importance and management

An established and clinically important interaction. The effectiveness of influenza vaccination may be reduced or abolished if cyclosporin is being used. One suggestion is that if patients remain unprotected after a single vaccination and a booster dose also fails to be effective, amantadine should be given during an influenza epidemic. It will protect against influenza A but not B infection. 200 mg daily is reported to be well tolerated.[2] It is not clear whether immunization with other vaccines is adversely affected by cyclosporin.

References

1 Versluis DJ, Beyer WEP, Masurel N, Wenting GJ, Weimar W. Impairment of the immune response to influenza vaccination in renal transplant recipients by cyclosporine, but not azathioprine. Transplantation (1986) 42, 376–9.
2 Beyer WEP, Diepersloot RJA, Masurel N, Simoons ML, Weimar W. Double failure of influenza vaccination in a heart transplant patient. Transplantation (1987) 43, 319.
3 Grabenstein JD, Baker JR. Comment: cyclosporine and vaccination. Drug Intell Clin Pharm (1985) 19, 679–80.

Tacrolimus (FK-506) + Clotrimazole

Abstract/Summary

An isolated report describes a marked increase in tacrolimus levels in a patient when given clotrimazole.

Clinical evidence, mechanism, importance and management

The serum tacrolimus levels of a liver transplant patient on 6 mg daily rose from 3.5 to 5.6 ng/ml within a day of starting 10 mg clotrimazole four times daily, and to more than 9 ng/ml within 8 days. Later studies and rechallenge confirmed that the clotrimazole was responsible. The tacrolimus AUC increased from 18 to 33 ng/ml/h. The reasons are not understood.[1] The general importance of this interaction is uncertain but monitor the effects of concurrent use in any patient, and reduce the tacrolimus dosage as necessary. The authors of the report suggest that this interaction might possibly be exploited to save tacrolimus costs.[1]

Reference

1 Mieles L, Venkataramanan R, Yokoyama I, Warty VJ, Starzl TE. Interaction between FK 506 and clotrimazole in a liver transplant recipient. Transplantation (1991) 52, 1086–7.

Tacrolimus (FK-506) + Danazol

Abstract/Summary

An isolated report describes an increase in tacrolimus levels in a patient when given danazol.

Clinical evidence, mechanism, importance and management

The serum tacrolimus levels of a kidney transplant patient on 10 mg daily rose from 0.7 to 2.7 ng/ml within 4 days of starting 400–1200 mg danazol daily. Despite a reduction in the dosage, her tacrolimus and creatinine serum levels remained high for a month until the danazol was withdrawn. The reason is not known but the authors suggest that danazol possibly inhibits the metabolism (demethylation and hydroxylation) of the tacrolimus by the liver so that it is cleared from the body more slowly. [1] The general importance of this interaction is uncertain but monitor the effects of concurrent use in any patient, and reduce the tacrolimus dosage as necessary.

Reference

1 Shapiro R, Venkataramanan R, Warty VS, Scantlebury VP, Rybka W, McCauley J, Fung JJ, Starzl TE. FK 506 interaction with danazol. Lancet (1993) 341, 1344–5.

Tacrolimus (FK-506) + Miscellaneous drugs

Abstract/Summary

It is not clear whether tacrolimus does or does not raise serum cyclosporin levels, but there is evidence that kidney damage is increased. There is evidence that tacrolimus possibly interacts with macrolides, calcium channel blockers and steroids, raising their serum levels. The effects of methylprednisolone on tacrolimus levels are variable.

Clinical evidence, mechanism, importance and management

One study found that the half life of cyclosporin was prolonged from a range of 6–15 h to 26–74 h by tacrolimus in patients with normal bilirubin levels, using a fluorescent polarization immunoassay, and it raised cyclosporin serum levels.[1] On the other hand another study found no changes in the pharmacokinetics of cyclosporin as measured by HPLC in patients given tacrolimus, but creatinine levels rose (suggesting kidney damage)[4] and confirming a previous report that severe renal dysfunction may develop.[5] The suggestion is that tacrolimus inhibits cyclosporin metabolism or its absorption.[1] Concurrent use should clearly be very closely monitored.

In vitro studies using human liver microsomes found that tacrolimus inhibits cytochrome P-450 dependent metabolism, in particular P-450IIIA and P-450IA.[2,3] This suggests that the metabolism of certain classes of drugs (eg macrolides such as erythromycin and triacetyloleandomycin, calcium channel blockers such as nifedipine and diltiazem, steroids such as ethinyloestradiol, cortisone, progesterone) might be reduced by tacrolimus, thereby increasing their effects. It would therefore be prudent to monitor concurrent use to find out if any of these potential interactions is clinically important.

Tacrolimus serum levels are said to have been increased on 10 occasions by methylprednisolone, decreased on 5 occasions, and unaltered on two out of a total of 17 occasions.[1]

Reference

1 Venkataramanan R, Jain A, Cadoff E, Warty V, Iwasaki K, Nagase K,

Krajack A, Imventaraza O, Todo S, Fung JJ, Starzl TE. Pharmacokinetics of FK 506: preclinical and clinical studies. Transplant Proc (1990) 22 (Suppl 1) 52–6.
2 Shah A, Whiting PH, Omar G, Thomson AW, Burke MD. Effects of FK 506 on human microsomal cytochrome P-450-dependent drug metabolism in vitro. Transplant Proc (1991) 23, 2783–5.
3 Pichard L, Fabre I, Domergue J, Joyeux H, Maurel P. Effect of FK 506 on human hepatic cytochromes P-450: interactions with CyA. Transplant Proc (1991) 23, 2791–3.
4 Jain AB, Venkataramanan R, Fung J, Burckart G, Emeight J, Diven W, Warty V, Abu-Almagd K, Todo S, Alessiani M, Starzl TE. Pharmacokinetics of cyclosporin and nephrotoxicity in orthoptic liver transplant patients rescued with FK 506. Transplant Proc (1991) 23, 2777–9.
5 McCauley J, Fung J, Jain A, Todo S, Starzl TE. The effects of FK506 on renal function after liver transplantation. Transplant Proc (1990) 22, 17–20.

OKT3 + Indomethacin

Abstract/Summary

Indomethacin may possibly increase the incidence of encephalopathy and psychosis in patients treated with OKT3.

Clinical evidence, mechanism, importance and management

A study of patient records found that four out of a total of 55 kidney transplant patients (7.3%) given OKT3 and indomethacin (50 mg orally or rectally 6–8 hourly) developed serious encephalopathy and psychosis compared with only two out of 173 patients (1.2%) who had had OKT3 without indomethacin.[1] The reasons are not understood. More study is needed to confirm the link between concurrent use and these serious adverse effects, but be particularly alert if both are used.

Reference

1 Chan GL, Weinstein SS, Wright CE, Bowers VD, Alveragna DY, Shires DL, Ackermann JR, LeFor WW, Kahana L. Encephalopathy associated with OKT3 administration. Possible interaction with indomethacin. Transplantation (1991) 52, 148–51.

Chapter 17
Lithium Drug Interactions

Lithium carbonate in dosages of about 400–600 mg daily is used to treat depressive illnesses, the dosage being adjusted to give plasma concentrations of 0.8–1.2 mmol/l for acute mania, and 0.4–0.8 for the prophylactic treatment of unipolar and bipolar affective illness. It is given under close supervision with regular monitoring of blood concentrations — initially at least once a week — because there is a narrow margin between therapeutic concentrations and those which are toxic.

Side-effects which are not usually considered serious include nausea, weakness, fine tremor, mild polydipsia and polyuria. If blood concentrations exceed about 1.5 mmol/l, more serious side-effects which amount to intoxication are seen: the gastrointestinal symptoms include abdominal pain, nausea, vomiting, diarrhoea, anorexia and thirst. Neurological symptoms include drowsiness, giddiness with ataxia, coarse tremor, slurred speech, blurred vision and muscular twitching. If concentrations rise as high as 3 mmol/l, life-threatening epileptic seizures, coma, hyperextension of the limbs, syncope and circulatory failure may occur.

In addition to these side-effects, lithium can induce diabetes insipidus and hypothyroidism in some patients, and is contraindicated in those with renal or cardiac insufficiency. Just how lithium exerts its beneficial effects is not known, but it may compete with sodium ions in various parts of the body and it alters the electrolyte composition of body fluids.

Table 17.1 Lithium salts: generic and proprietary names

Non-proprietary names	Proprietary names
Lithium acetate	*Quilonium, Quilonorm*
Lithium carbonate	*Camcolit, Carbolith, Ceglution, Eskalith, Hypnorex, Lentolith, Lithane, Lithicarb, Lithiobid, Litilent, Lithizine, Lithonate, Lithotabs, Lithuril, Manialith, Maniprex, Phasal, Plenur, Priadel, Quilonium Retard, Quilonorm-Retard, Teralithe*
Lithium chloride	
Lithium citrate	
Lithium gluconate	*Lithium Oligosol, Microplex Lithium, Neurolithium*
Lithium orotate	*Lithium Rotat*
Lithium sulphate	*Lithiofor, Lithionit, Lithium-Duriles*

Most of the interactions involving lithium are discussed in this chapter but a few are found elsewhere in this book. The index should be consulted for a full listing. Virtually all the reports are concerned with the carbonate, but sometimes lithium is given as the acetate, aspartate, chloride, citrate, gluconate, orotate or sulphate instead. There is no reason to believe that these lithium salts will not interact just like lithium carbonate.

Lithium carbonate + ACE inhibitors

Abstract/Summary

Concurrent use can be uneventful but at least 11 cases of lithium toxicity have been reported in patients when given captopril, enalapril or lisinopril, in some instances associated with decreased renal function. It has been suggested that concurrent use should be avoided in those with renal disease.

Clinical evidence

(a) Lithium + Captopril

A patient developed a serum lithium level of 2.35 mmol/L and intoxication (tremor, dysarthria, digestive problems) within 10 days of starting to take 50 mg captopril daily. He was restabilized on half his previous dose of lithium.[2]

(b) Lithium + Enalapril

5 mg enalapril for 9 days had no effect on the mean serum lithium levels of nine normal subjects taking 450 mg twice daily, but one subject showed a 31% increase.[12]

A woman developed signs of lithium intoxication (ataxia, dysarthria, tremor, confusion, etc.) within 2–3 weeks of starting to take 20 mg enalapril daily. After 5 weeks her serum lithium levels had risen from 0.88 to 3.3 mmol/l.[1] No toxicity occurred when the enalapril was later replaced by nifedipine.[1] Lithium toxicity following the use of enalapril, and associated in some cases with a decrease in renal function, has been seen in another five patients.[3,7–11]

(c) Lithium + Iisinopril

A woman on lithium developed intoxication and a trough serum level of 3.0 mmol/l within 3 weeks of stopping clonidine and starting 20 mg lisinopril daily.[4] Three other reports similarly describe acute lithium toxicity in three patients when given lisinopril.[5,6,11]

Mechanism

Not fully understood. One idea is that because the ACE-inhibitors reduce drinking behaviour, and both ACE-inhibitors and lithium cause sodium to be lost in the urine, fluid depletion can occur. The normal compensatory reaction to this would be the constriction of the efferent renal arterioles to maintain the glomerular filtration rate, but this mechanism is blocked by the ACE-inhibitor, as a result the excretion of lithium falls and toxicity develops.

Importance and management

An established but uncommon interaction. Some patients can certainly be stabilized on both drugs without any problems but because a serious reaction occurs unpredictably in a few individuals, concurrent use should be well monitored, particularly initially. There are risk factors: the authors of one of the reports say that '..use of this combination in patients with advanced age, congestive heart failure, renal insufficiency, or volume depletion is unjustified. If the combination is used, we would advise weekly serum lithium concentration monitoring for several weeks and reducing the dose of lithium by one half to one third before adding an ACE inhibitor.'[4]

References

1 Douste-Blazy Ph, Rostin M, Livarek B, Tordjman E, Montastruc JL, Galinier F. Angiotensin converting enzyme inhibitors and lithium treatment. Lancet (1986) i, 1448.
2 Pulik M, Lida H. Interaction lithium-inhibiteurs de l'enzyme de conversion. La Presse Med (1988) 17, 755.
3 Mahieu M, Houvenagel E, Leduc JJ, Choteau Ph. Lithium-inhibiteurs de conversion: une association a eviter? La Presse Med (1988) 17, 281.
4 Baldwin CM, Safferman AZ. A case of lisinopril-induced lithium toxicity. DICP Ann Pharmacotherapy (1990) 24, 946–7.
5 Griffin JH, Hahn SM. Lisinopril-induced lithium toxicity. DICP Ann Pharmacotherapy (1991) 25, 101.
6 Conrad AJ. Quoted as Written Communication, July 1st 1988, in Biol Therapies Psychiatry (1988) 11, 43.
7 Drouet A, Bouvet O. Lithium et inhibiteurs de l'enzyme de conversion. L'Encéphale (1990) XVI, 51–2.
8 Navis GJ, de Jong PE, de Zeeuw D. Volume homeostasis, angiotensin converting enzyme inhibition, and lithium therapy. Am J Med (1989) 86, 621.
9 Simon G. Combination angiotensin converting enzyme inhibitor/lithium therapy contraindicated in renal disease. Am J Med (1988) 85, 893–4.
10 Rimmer JM, Santella RN. A reply to reference 9. Am J Med (1988) 85, 894.
11 Correa FJ, Eiser A. Angiotensin-converting enzyme inhibitors and lithium toxicity. Am J Med (1992) 93, 108–9.
12 DasGupta K, Jefferson JW, Kobak KA, Greist JH. The effect of enalapril on serum lithium levels in healthy men. J Clin Psychiatry (1992) 53, 398–400.

Lithium carbonate + Baclofen

Abstract/Summary

Two patients with Huntington's chorea showed an aggravation of their hyperkinetic symptoms within a few days of starting concurrent treatment.

Clinical evidence, mechanism, importance and management

A patient with Huntington's chorea and under treatment with lithium and haloperidol, was additionally given baclofen. Another patient being treated with imipramine, clopenthixol, chlorpromazine and baclofen was additionally given lithium. Within a few days both patients showed a severe aggravation of their hyperkinetic symptoms which disappeared within three days of withdrawing the baclofen.[1] It is uncertain whether this is an interaction, but on the basis of this very limited evidence it would now seem prudent to monitor the effects of concurrent use carefully.

Reference

1 Anden N-E, Dalen P, Johansson B. Baclofen and lithium in Huntington's chorea. Lancet (1973) ii, 93.

Lithium carbonate + Benzodiazepines

Abstract/Summary

Preliminary evidence suggests that alprazolam is unlikely to cause a clinically important rise in serum lithium levels. Neurotoxicity may develop if clonazepam is added to treatment with lithium carbonate. An isolated case of serious hypothermia has been reported during concurrent treatment with lithium carbonate and diazepam.

Clinical evidence, mechanism, importance and management

(a) Lithium + Alprazolam

2 mg alprazolam daily for 4 days increased the steady-state AUC of lithium (from 10.3 to 11.1 mmol/h) in 10 normal subjects taking 900–1500 mg daily, and reduced its urinary clearance (from a 93.6 to 78.2% recovery). It is suggested that this is unlikely to be clinically significant, but confirmation of this is needed.[1]

(b) Lithium + Clonazepam

A retrospective study of patient records revealed five out of 30 with bipolar affective disorder under treatment with lithium carbonate (900–2400 mg) who had developed a neurotoxic syndrome with ataxia, dysarthria, drowsiness and confusion when their neuroleptic treatment (chlorpromazine, perphenazine, haloperidol) was replaced with clonazepam (2–16 mg). The syndrome was reversible. The reasons are not known but suggestions include lithium toxicity or synergistic toxicity. Whatever the explanation, the authors of the report suggest that the lithium levels should be more frequently measured if clonazepam is added, and the effects well monitored.[3]

(c) Lithium + Diazepam

A mentally retarded patient showed occasional hypothermic episodes (below 35°C) while taking lithium and diazepam, but not while on either drug alone. After taking both drugs for 17 days during a test (lithium 1 g and diazepam 30 mg daily) the patient experienced a temperature fall from 35.4 to 32°C over 2 h, and became comatose with reduced reflexes, dilated pupils, a systolic blood pressure of 40–60 mmHg, a pulse rate of 40 and no piloerector response.[2] The reasons are not known.

This is an isolated case so that concurrent use need not be avoided, but be alert for any evidence of hypothermia. There seems to be no evidence of this adverse interaction with any of the other benzodiazepines.

References

1 Naylor GJ, McHarg A. Profound hypothermia on combined lithium carbonate and diazepam treatment. Br Med J (1977) 3, 22.
2 Evans RL, Nelson MV, Melethil S, Townsend R, Hornstra RK, Smith RB. Evaluation of the interaction of lithium and alprazolam. J Clin Psychopharmacol (1990) 10, 355–9.
3 Koczerginski D, Kennedy SH, Swinson RP. Clonazepam and lithium — a toxic combination in the treatment of mania? Int Clin Psychopharmacol (1989) 4, 195–9.

Lithium carbonate + Calcium channel blockers

Abstract/Summary

Concurrent use can be uneventful but neurotoxicity and decreases in serum lithium levels have been seen in a few patients also given verapamil. Profound bradycardia occurred in two patients, and choreoathetosis in another on lithium when given verapamil. An acute parkinsonian syndrome developed in another patient on lithium and thiothixene when given diltiazem. Marked psychosis developed in yet another patient on lithium when given diltiazem.

Clinical evidence

(a) Increased Lithium effects, Neurotoxicity, Psychosis

A 42-year-old on 900 mg lithium carbonate daily developed toxicity (nausea, vomiting, muscular weakness, ataxia and tinnitus) within nine days of starting to take 80 mg verapamil three times daily although her bipolar depressive disorder improved. Her serum lithium levels remained unchanged at 1.1 mmol/l. The toxicity disappeared within 48 h of stopping the verapamil but her disorder worsened. The same pattern was repeated when the verapamil was re-started and then withdrawn.[1] A 74-year-old woman on lithium experienced similar toxicity two weeks after starting 240 mg verapamil daily. Her serum lithium level remained stable at 0.9 mmol/l. She was later well controlled on half the dose of lithium with a serum level of 0.3–0.5 mmol/l.[3] A woman on lithium developed progressive ataxia and dysarthria despite a steady serum lithium level (0.60 mmol/l) on two occasions when given 240 mg verapamil daily, but recovered when the verapamil was replaced by nifedipine.[9] A woman well controlled on lithium developed marked psychosis within a week of starting to take 90 mg diltiazem daily.[10]

(b) Reduced Lithium effects

A patient, well controlled on 900–1200 mg lithium daily for

over eight years, showed a marked fall in serum lithium levels when given 320 mg verapamil daily. He was restabilized on approximately double the dose of lithium. Another patient showed an increased lithium clearance when given verapamil for 3 days, and a fall in serum lithium levels from 0.61 to 0.53 mmol/l.[4]

(c) Other toxic effects

A man given lithium for 2 weeks was started on 120 mg verapamil. Within 4 days he developed marked choreoathetoid movements of his neck, trunk and all four limbs. The problem resolved when the verapamil was stopped.[8] An acute parkinsonism syndrome developed in a man of 58 within 4 days of adding 30 mg diltiazem three times daily to his treatment with lithium and thiothixene.[2] Two elderly patients on lithium developed profound bradycardia when given 320–480 mg verapamil daily. Fatal myocardial infarction followed in one case.[5]

Mechanisms

Not understood.

Importance and management

The adverse reactions cited above contrast with other reports describing uneventful concurrent use.[6,7] This unpredictability emphasises the need to monitor the effects closely where it is thought appropriate to give lithium and calcium channel blockers. It has been suggested that particular caution should be exercised in the elderly and those with cardiovascular disease.[5]

References

1 Price WA, Giannini AJ. Neurotoxicity caused by lithium-verapamil. J Clin Pharmacol (1986) 26, 717–19.
2 Valdiserri EV. A possible interaction between lithium and diltiazem: case report. J Clin Psychiatry (1985) 46, 540–1.
3 Price WA, Shalley JE. Lithium-verapamil toxicity in the elderly. J Amer Geriatr Soc (1987) 35, 177–9.
4 Weinrauch LA, Belok S, D'Elia JA. Decreased serum lithium during verapamil therapy. Amer Heart J (1984) 108, 1378–9.
5 Dubovsky SL, Franks RD, Allen S. Verapamil: a new antimanic drug with potential interactions with lithium. J Clin Psychiatry (1987) 48, 371–2.
6 Brotman AW, Farhadi AM, Gelenberg AJ. Verapamil treatment of acute mania. J Clin Psychiatry (1986) 47, 136–8.
7 Gitlin MJ, Weiss J. Verapamil as maintenance treatment in bipolar illness: a case report. J Clin Psychopharmacol (1984) 4, 341–3.
8 Helmuth D, Ljaljevic Z, Ramirez L, Metlzer HY. Choreoathetosis induced by verapamil and lithium treatment. J Clin Psychopharmacol (1989) 9, 454–5.
9 Wright BA, Jarrett DB. Lihium and calcium channel blockers: possible neurotoxicity. Biol Psychiatry (1991) 30, 635–6.
10 Binder EF, Cayabyab L, Ritchie DJ, Birge SJ. Diltiazem-induced psychosis and a possible diltiazem-lithium interaction. Arch Intern Med (1991) 151, 373–4.

Lithium carbonate + Carbamazepine

Abstract/Summary

Although combined use is beneficial in some patients, severe neurotoxicity is reported to have developed in a few others.

Clinical evidence

A patient on 1800 mg lithium daily developed severe neurotoxicity (ataxia, truncal tremors, nystagmus, limb hyperreflexia, muscle fasciculation) within three days of starting to take 600 mg carbamazepine daily. Blood levels of both drugs remained within the therapeutic range. The symptoms resolved when each drug was withdrawn in turn and re-occurred within three days of restarting concurrent treatment.[1]

Five rapid-cycling manic patients developed similar neurotoxic symptoms (confusion, drowsiness, generalized weakness, lethargy, coarse tremor, hyperreflexia, cerebellar signs) when concurrently treated with lithium carbonate and carbamazepine (doses not stated). Plasma levels of both drugs remained within the accepted range.[7] Other reports describe adverse neurological effects during concurrent use which were also not accompanied by changes in drug serum levels.[2,5,8]

In contrast, combined treatment in other patients is said to be well tolerated but beneficial,[3,4,6,10] but one report suggests that the dosages may need to be reduced to free the patient from side-effects.[10]

Mechanism

Not understood. A paper which plotted the serum levels of both drugs on a two-dimensional graph failed to find evidence of synergistic toxicity.[9] Another study found that concurrent use caused an approximately 10% rise in lithium levels and a 10% fall in carbamazepine levels.[11]

Importance and management

This interaction is established, but its incidence is not known. It may be quite small. If concurrent use is undertaken, the outcome should be closely monitored. This is particularly important because neurotoxicity can develop even though the drug serum levels remain within the accepted therapeutic range. The authors of one paper suggest that '...the risk factors appear to be a history of neurotoxicity with lithium therapies and the presence of concurrent compromised medical or neurological functioning.'[7]

References

1 Ghose K. Interaction between lithium and carbamazepine. Br Med J (1980) 250, 112.
2 Chaudhry RP, Waters BGH. Lithium and carbamazepine interaction: possible neurotoxicity. J Clin Psychiatry (1983) 44, 30–1.
3 MacCallum WAG. Interaction of lithium and phenytoin. Br Med J (1980) 280, 610–11.

4 Lipinski JF, Pope HG. Possible synergistic action between carbamazepine and lithium carbonate in the treatment of three acutely manic patients. Am J Psychiatry (1982) 139, 948–9.

5 Andrus PF. Lithium and carbamazepine. J Clin Psychiatry (1984) 45, 525.

6 Moss GR, James CR. Carbamazepine and lithium carbonate synergism in mania. Arch Gen Psychiatry (1983) 40, 588.

7 Shukla S, Godwin CD, Long EB, Miller MG. Lithium-carbamazepine neurotoxicity and risk factors. Am J Psychiatry (1984) 141, 1604–6.

8 Hassan MH, Thakar J, Weinberg AL, Grimes JD. Lithium-carbamazepine interaction: clinical and laboratory observations. Neurology (1987) 37 (Suppl 1) 172.

9 McGinness J, Kishimoto A, Hollister LE. Avoiding neurotoxicity with lithium-carbamazepine combinations. Psychopharmacol Bull (1990) 26, 181–4.

10 Lieber AI. Treatment of rapid cycling bipolar patients. Am J Psychiatry (1987) 144, 1619–20.

10 Kramlinger KG, Post RM. The addition of lithium to carbamazepine. Arch Gen Psychiatry (1989) 46, 794–800.

11 Rybakowski J, Lehmann W, Kanarkowski R, Matkowski K. Possible pharmacokinetic interaction of lithium and carbamazepine. Lithium (1991) 2, 183–6.

Lithium carbonate + Cisplatin

Abstract/Summary

A single case report describes a transient and clinically unimportant fall in serum lithium levels in a woman given cisplatin and a fluid load. No immediately important changes were seen in another patient.

Clinical evidence, mechanism, importance and management

A woman, well controlled for several years on 1200 mg lithium carbonate daily, showed a fall in serum lithium levels from 1.0 to 0.3, and from 0.8 to 0.5 mmol/l on two occasions over periods of two days when given $100 \, mg/m^2$ cisplatin IV over 2 h. Over the next 24 h she was also given one litre of normal saline over 4 h, 25 g sodium chloride and 20% mannitol over 4 h, and 5% dextrose in normal saline to prevent renal toxicity. Serum lithium levels returned to normal at the end of 2 days. No change in the control of the psychotic symptoms was seen.[1] It is not clear whether the fall in serum lithium levels was due to increased renal clearance caused by the cisplatin, the fluid-loading, or both. Another patient showed clinically insignificant changes in her serum lithium levels when treated with cisplatin, but 2 months later her deteriorating kidney function resulted in a rise in her serum lithium levels.[2]

Although neither of these interaction was clinically important, the authors of the first report pointed out that some regimens of cisplatin involve the use of higher doses ($40 \, mg/m^2$) with a normal saline fluid load over 5 days, and under these circumstances it would be prudent to monitor the serum lithium levels carefully. Concurrent use should be monitored in all patients.

Reference

1 Pietruszka LJ, Biermann WA, Vlasses PH. Evaluation of cisplatin-lithium interaction. Drug Intell Clin Pharm (1985) 19, 31–2.

2 Beijnen JH, Vlasveld, Wanders J, ten Bokkel Huinik WW, Rodenhuis S. Effect of cisplatin-containing chemotherapy on serum lithium concentrations. Ann Pharmacother (1992) 26, 488–90.

Lithium carbonate + Co-trimoxazole

Abstract/Summary

Two reports describe lithium intoxication in three patients given co-trimoxazole, paradoxically accompanied by a fall in serum lithium levels.

Clinical evidence, mechanism, importance and management

Two patients stabilized on lithium carbonate (serum levels 0.75 mmol/l) showed signs of lithium intoxication (tremor, muscular weakness and fasciculation, apathy) within a few days of being given co-trimoxazole (dose not stated), yet their serum lithium levels were found to have fallen to 0.3–0.4 mmol/l. Within 48 h of withdrawing the co-trimoxazole, the signs of intoxication had gone and their serum lithium concentrations had climbed to their former levels.[1] Another report[2] very briefly states that ataxia, tremor and diarrhoea developed in a patient on lithium and timolol when given co-trimoxazole. The reasons are not understood. The general importance of this interaction is uncertain but if concurrent use is undertaken it would clearly be prudent to monitor the clinical response closely because it would appear that serum level monitoring may not always be a reliable guide.

References

1 Desvilles M, Sevestre P. Effet paradoxal de l'association lithium et sulfamethoxazol-trimethoprime. Nouv Presse Med (1982) 11, 3267–8.

2 Edwards IR. Medicines Adverse Reactions Committee: Eighteenth annual report, 1983. NZ Med J (1984) 97, 729–32.

Lithium carbonate + Diuretics

Abstract/Summary

There is evidence that the excretion of lithium can be increased by triamterene and acetazolamide, but a case of lithium intoxication has also been seen. Chlormerodrin and amiloride are reported not to interact whereas serum lithium levels may rise if spironolactone is used. See also Lithium + Frusemide, and Lithium + Thiazides.

Clinical evidence, mechanism, importance and management

There is very little information about the possible interactions of any of these diuretics with lithium. A short-term study[1] on six subjects given lithium and acetazolamide demonstrated a 27–31% increase in the urinary excretion of lithium, and an increased clearance was found in another study.[5] A woman was successfully treated for a toxic overdose of lithium with acetazolamide, IV fluids, sodium bicarbonate, potassium chloride and mannitol,[4] but paradoxically lithium intoxication (a rise in serum levels from 0.8 to 5 mmol/l) occurred in another patient after treatment for a month with acetazolamide.[6] Amiloride has been found to have no significant effect on serum lithium levels when used in the treatment of lithium-induced polyuria.[7,8] Chlormerodrin was found not to interact.[1] The same study[1] found that spironolactone had no effect on the excretion of lithium, whereas in another report[2] the use of spironolactone was accompanied by a rise in serum lithium levels. Triamterene, administered to two patients taking lithium while on a salt-restricted diet, is said to have lead to a strong lithium diuresis.[3]

None of these reports gives a clear indication of the outcome of using these diuretics in patients on lithium, but they emphasize the need to monitor the response to concurrent use carefully.

References

1 Thomsen K, Schou M. Renal lithium excretion in man. Amer J Physiol (1968) 215, 823.
2 Baer L, Platman SR, Kassir S, Fieve RR. Mechanism of renal lithium handling and their relationship to mineralocorticoids: a dissociation between sodium and lithium ions. J Psychiat Res (1971) 8, 91–105.
3 Baer L, Platman S, Fieve RR. Lithium metabolism: its electrolyte actions and relationship to aldosterone. Recent Advances in the Psychobiology of the Depresssive Illnesses. Williams, Katz and Shield (eds) DHEW Publications, Washington DC (1972). p 49.
4 Horowitz LC, Fisher GU. Acute lithium toxicity. N Engl J Med (1969) 281, 1369.
5 Steele TH. Treatment of lithium intoxication with diuretics. In 'Clinical Chemistry and Chemical Toxicology of Metals.' (Ed SS Brown). Elsevier/North Holland (1977) p 289–93.
6 Gay C, Plas J, Granger B, Olie JP, Loo H. Intoxication au lithium. Deux interaction inedites: l'acetazolamide et l'acide niflumique. L'Encephale (1985) 11, 261–2.
7 Batlle DC, von Riotte AB, Gaviria M. Amelioration of polyuria by amiloride in patients receiving long-term lithium therapy. N Engl J Med (1985) 312, 408–14.
8 Kosten TR, Forrest JN. Treatment of severe lithium-induced polyuria with amiloride. Am J Psychiatry (1986) 143, 1563–8.

Lithium carbonate + Fluoxetine

Abstract/Summary

Elevated serum lithium levels have been seen in a handful of patients when additionally given fluoxetine. Toxicity, mania, somnolence and absence seizures may occur.

Clinical evidence, mechanism, importance and management

Although these drugs have been used together with apparent success,[3] problems have arisen in a handful of cases. A woman with a bipolar affective disorder, successfully maintained for 20 years on 1200 mg lithium carbonate daily, developed stiffness of her arms and legs, dizziness, unsteadiness in walking and speech difficulties within a few days of starting additional treatment with 20 mg fluoxetine daily. Her serum lithium levels had risen from a range of 0.75–1.15 mmol/l to 1.70 mmol/l. They fell and the toxic symptoms disappeared when the lithium dosage was reduced and the fluoxetine withdrawn.[1] Two other patients showed approximately 50% increases in serum lithium levels and developed mania (but no lithium toxicity) about a month after starting additional treatment with fluoxetine (20–40 mg daily). The problem resolved when the lithium dosage was reduced 25–33%.[2] Toxicity was seen in another patient when lithium was added to fluoxetine treatment, although the serum lithium levels remained in the therapeutic range,[4] and absence seizures occurred in another.[5]

The reasons for these adverse reactions are not understood, but it would clearly be prudent to monitor the effects if both drugs are given.

References

1 Salama AA, Shafey M. A case of severe lithium toxicity induced by combined fluoxetine and lithium carbonate. Am J Psychiatry (1989) 146, 278.
2 Hadley A, Cason MP. Mania resulting from lithium-fluoxetine combination. Am J Psychiatry (1989) 146, 1637–8.
3 Pope HG, McElroy SL, Nixon RA. Possible synergism between fluoxetine and lithium in refractory depression. Am J Psychiatry (1988) 145, 1292–4.
4 Noveske FG, Hahn KR, Flynn RJ. Possible toxicity of combined fluoxetine and lithium. Am J Psychiatry (1989) 146, 1515.
5 Sacristan JA, Iglesias C, Arellano F, Lequerica J. Absence seizures induced by lithium: possible interaction with fluoxetine. Am J Psychiatry (1991) 148, 146–7.

Lithium carbonate + Frusemide or Bumetanide

Abstract/Summmary

The concurrent use of lithium carbonate and frusemide can be safe and uneventful, but serious lithium intoxication has been described in a few individuals. Bumetanide can interact similarly.

Clinical evidence

Six normal subjects stabilized on 900 mg lithium carbonate daily (mean serum levels 4.3 mmol/l) were given 40 mg frusemide daily for 14 days. Five experienced some minor side-effects, probably attributable to the frusemide, but one subject experienced such a marked increase in the toxic effects of lithium that she withdrew from the study after taking both drugs for only 5 days. Her serum lithium levels were found to have risen by over 60% (from 0.44 to 0.71 mmol/l).[1]

There are four other case reports of individual patients who experienced serious lithium intoxication or other adverse reactions when given lithium and frusemide.[3–6] One of the patients was also on a salt-restricted diet.[3] In contrast, six patients who had been stabilized on lithium for over 6 years showed no significant changes in their serum lithium levels over a 12 week period while taking 20–80 mg frusemide daily.[2] Another study in normal subjects also found no significant changes in lithium levels when 40 mg frusemide daily was given.[9] Bumetanide has also been responsible for the development of lithium toxicity in two patients [8,10] one of whom was on a salt-restricted diet.[10]

Mechanism

Not fully understood. If and when a rise in serum lithium levels occurs, it may be related to the salt depletion which can accompany the use of frusemide. As with the thiazides, such an interaction would not be expected to be immediate but would take a few days to develop. This may explain why one study in subjects given a single dose of lithium failed to demonstrate any effect on the urinary excretion of lithium after the administration of frusemide.[7]

Importance and management

Information seems to be limited to the reports cited. The incidence of this interaction is uncertain and its development unpredictable. It would therefore be imprudent to give frusemide or bumetanide to patients stabilized on lithium unless the effects can be well monitored because the occasional patient may develop serious intoxication.

References

1 Jefferson JW, Kalin NH. Serum lithium levels and long term diuretic use. J Amer Med Ass (1979) 241, 1134–6

2 Safher D, Coppen A. Frusemide: a safe diuretic during lithium therapy? J Affective Disorders (1983) 5, 289–92.

3 Hurtig HI, Dyson WL. Lithium toxicity enhanced by diuresis. N Eng J Med (1974) 290, 748–9

4 Oh TE. Frusemide and lithium toxicity. Anaesth Intens Care (1977) 5, 60–2.

5 Segura EG, Ogne P, Peral MF. Intoxicacion por sales de litio. Presentacion de uno caso. Med Clin (Barc) (1984) 83, 294–6.

6 Thornton WE, Pray BJ. Lithium intoxication: a report of two cases. Can Psychiat Ass (1975) 20, 281–2.

7 Thomsen K, Schou M. Renal lithium excretion in man. Amer J Physiol (1968) 215, 823–7.

8 Kerry RJ, Ludlow JM, Owen G. Diuretics are dangerous with lithium. Br Med J (1980) 281, 371.

9 Crabtree BL, Mack JE, Johnson CD, Amyx BC. Comparison of the effects of hydrochlorothiazide and furosemide on lithium disposition. Am J Psychiatry (1991) 148, 1060–3.

10 Huang LG. Lithium intoxication with coadministration of a loop-diuretic. J Clin Psychopharmacol (1990) 10, 228.

Lithium carbonate + Haloperidol

Abstract/Summary

Although very serious adverse reactions have been described in some patients treated with lithium carbonate and haloperidol, there is ample evidence that concurrent use can be uneventful and therapeutically valuable.

Clinical evidence

(a) Adverse effects during concurrent use

Four patients with acute mania who were treated with 1500–1800 mg lithium carbonate daily and high doses of haloperidol (up to 45 mg per day), developed encephalopathic syndromes (lethargy, fever, tremulousness, confusion, extrapyramidal and cerebellar dysfunction) accompanied by leukocytosis and elevated levels of serum enzymes, blood urea nitrogen and fasting blood sugar.[1] Two of them suffered irreversible widespread brain damage and two others were left with persistent dyskinesias.

A woman patient was observed with neuromuscular symptoms, impaired consciousness and hyperthermia after 12 days treatment with 1500 mg lithium carbonate and 40 mg haloperidol daily. She recovered fully and uneventfully.[2] Three patients, two of them oligophrenic, who were given 1800 mg lithium carbonate with 10–20 mg haloperidol by injection for 10 days, 27 h and 24 h respectively, developed hypertonic-hypokinetic and extrapyramidal syndromes. All recovered.[3] There are other reports of adverse reactions including severe extrapyramidal symptoms and organic brain damage in individual patients when given both drugs.[5,6,8,9,11,15–17] Another report claims that measurable brain damage may have occurred in seven patients.[10] A small rise in serum lithium levels occurs in the presence of haloperidol, but it is almost certainly of little or no clinical significance.[12]

(b) Advantageous concurrent use

In contrast to the reports cited above, there are others describing successful and uneventful use.[7] Cohen and Cohen who first described the adverse interaction[1] have also written that '...at least 50 other patients have been similarly treated without reported adverse effects'.[1] They also say that '...a survey of the experiences of leading experts indicate that although hundreds of patients have been treated with various regimens of combined lithium carbonate/haloperidol, there have been no previous observations of substantial irreversible brain damage or persistent dyskinesia'. A retrospective search of Danish hospital records showed that 425 patients had been treated with both drugs and none of them had developed serious adverse reactions. There are other reports confirming that concurrent use can be useful and safe, involving 18 patients,[13] 59 patients[14] and 18 patients.[18]

Mechanism

Not understood. An unconfirmed suggestion is that the adverse effects are possibly due to the combined effects of lithium and haloperidol on basal striatal adenylate cyclase.[19] Another report claims that what is seen could be due to lithium toxicity alone.[21]

Importance and management

The advantageous effects of concurrent use are well documented, but the adverse effects are less clear. The Danish investigators offer the opinion that '..the combination of lithium and haloperidol is therapeutically useful when administered to diagnostically appropriate patients. To discourage or prohibit its use would, in our opinion, be injudicious, but treatment must be carried out under proper clinical control.'[4] This implies very close monitoring to detect any signs of adverse reactions. One review suggests that combined use seems to be safe if lithium levels are below 1.0 mmol/l.[20] At the moment there seems to be no way of identifying the apparently small number of patients who are particularly at risk, but possible likely factors include a previous history of extrapyramidal reactions with neuroleptics and the use of large doses of haloperidol.

References

1 Cohen WJ, Cohen NH. Lithium carbonate, haloperidol, and irreversible brain damage. J Amer Med Ass (1974) 230, 1283.
2 Thornton WE, Pray BJ. Lithium intoxication: a report of two cases. Canada Psychiat Ass J (1975) 20, 281.
3 Marhold J, Zimanova J, Lachman M, Kral J, Vojtechovsky M. To the incompatibility of haloperidol with lithium salts. Acta Nerv Super (Praha) (1974) 16, 199.
4 Baastrup PC, Hollnagel P, Sorensen R, Schou M. Adverse reactions in treatment with lithium carbonate and haloperidol. J Amer Med Ass (1976) 236, 2645.
5 Loudon JB, Waring H. Toxic reactions to lithium and haloperidol. Lancet (1976) ii, 1088.
6 Juhl RP, Tsuang MT, Perry PJ. Concomitant administration of haloperidol and lithium carbonate in acute mania. Dis Nerv Syst (1977) 38, 675.
7 Garfinkel PE, Stancer HC, Persad E. A comparison of haloperidol, lithium carbonate and their combination in the treatment of mania. J Affect Dis (1980) 2, 279.
8 Spring G, Frankel M. New data on lithium and haloperidol incompatibility. Amer J Psychiatry (1981) 138, 818–21.
9 Menes C, Burra P, Hoaken PCS. Untoward effects following combined neuroleptic-lithium therapy. Can J Psychiatry (1980) 25, 573.
10 Thomas C, Tatham A, Jakubowski S. Lithium/haloperidol combinations and brain damage. Lancet (1982) i, 626.
11 Keitner GI, Rahman S. Reversible neurotoxicity with combined lithium-haloperidol administration. J Clin Psychopharmacol (1984) 4, 104–5.
12 Schaffer CB, Batra K, Garvey MJ, Mungas DM, Schaffer LC. The effect of haloperidol on serum levels of lithium in adult manic patients. Biol Psychiatry (1984) 19, 1495–9.
13 Baptista T. Lithium-neuroleptic combination and irreversible brain damage. Acta Psychiatr Scand (1986) 73, 111.
14 Goldney RD, Spence ND. Safety of the combination of lithium and neuroleptic drugs. Am J Psychiatry (1986) 143, 882–4.
15 Kamlana SH, Kerry RJ, Khan IA. Lithium: some drug interactions. Practitioner (1980) 224, 1291–2.
16 Fetzer J, Kader G, Dahany S. Lithium encephalopathy: a clinical, psychiatric and EEG evaluation. Am J Psychiatry (1981) 138, 1622–3.
17 Thomas CJ. Brain damage with lithium/haloperidol. Br J Psychiatry (1979) 134, 552.
18 Biederman J, Lerner Y, Belmaker H. Combination of lithium and haloperidol in schizo-affective disorder. Arch Gen Psychiatry (1979) 36, 327.
19 Geisler A, Klysner R. Combined effect of lithium and flupenthixol on striatal adenylate cyclase. Lancet (1977) i, 430–1.
20 Batchelor DH, Lowe MR. Reported neurotoxicity with the lithium/haloperidol combination and other neuroleptics — a literature review. Human Psychopharmacology (1990) 5, 275–80.
21 von Knorring L. Possible mechanisms for the presumed interaction between lithium and neuroleptics. Human Psychopharmacology (1990) 5, 287–92.

Lithium carbonate + Iodides

Abstract/Summary

The hypothyroidic and goitrogenic effects of lithium carbonate, potassium iodide and possibly other iodides may be additive if given concurrently.

Clinical evidence

A man with normal thyroid function showed evidence of hypothyroidism after three weeks' treatment with lithium carbonate (750–1500 mg daily). After two further weeks' treatment with potassium iodide as well, the hypothyroidism became even more marked, but resolved completely within a fortnight of the withdrawal of both drugs.[1]

A number of other reports describe the antithyroid effect of lithium when given on its own[1–3,7–11] as well as with potassium iodide.[4,5,12] There is also a case on record involving lithium, isopropamide iodide and haloperidol.[6]

Mechanism

Lithium accumulates in the thyroid gland and blocks the release of the thyroid hormones by thyroid-stimulating hormone. The mechanism is not well understood. Potassium iodide temporarily prevents the production of the thyroid hormones but, as time goes on, synthesis recommences. Thus, both lithium ions and iodide ions can depress the production or release of the hormones and thereby have additive hypothyroidic effects.

Importance and management

The incidence and clinical importance of this interaction are difficult to assess. Hypothyroidism due to lithium treatment is not infrequent (variously reported as 12 out of 33 patients,[2] two out of 56 men[9] and 20 out of 93 women[9]) but there are very few reports of hypothyroidism due to the concurrent use of these drugs. Nevertheless the outcome of concurrent use should be monitored. Only potassium iodide and isopropamide iodide have been implicated but it would seem possible with other iodides. It should be remembered that some over-the-counter preparations contain iodine.

References

1 Shopsin B, Shenkman L, Blum M, Hollander CS. Iodine and lithium-induced hypothyroidism. Documentation of synergism. Amer J Med (1973) 55, 695.
2 Schou M, Amidsen A, Jensen SE, Olsen T. Occurrence of goitre during lithium treatment. Br Med J (1968) 3, 710.
3 Shopsin B, Blum M, Gershon S. Lithium-induced thyroid disturbance: case report and review. Compr Psychiatry (1969) 10, 215.
4 Jorgensen JD. Lithium-carbonate-induced myxedema. J Amer Med Ass (1971) 220, 587.
5 Weiner JD. Lithium carbonate-induced myxedema. J Amer Med Ass (1971) 220, 587.

6 Luby ED, Schwartz D, Rosenbaum H. Lithium carbonate-induced myxedema. J Amer Med Ass (1971) 218, 1298.

7 Emerson CH, Dyson WL, Utiger RD. Serum thyrotropin and thyroxine concentrations in patients receiving lithium carbonate. J Clin Endocrinol Metab (1973) 36, 338.

8 Candy J. Severe hypothyroidism — an early complication of lithium therapy. Br Med J (1972) 3, 277.

9 Villeneuve A, Grantier J, Jus A, Perron D. Effect of lithium on thyroid in man. Lancet (1973) ii, 502.

10 Lloyde GG, Rosser RM, Crowe MJ. Effect of lithium on thyroid in man. Lancet (1973) ii, 619.

11 Bocchetta A, Bernardi F, Pedditizi M, Loviselli A, Velluzzi F, Martino E, Del Zompo M. Thyroid abnormalities during lithium treatment. Acta Psychiat Scand (1991) 83, 193–8.

12 Spaulding SW, Burrow GN, Ramsey JN, Donabedian RK. Effect of increased iodide intake on thyroid function in subjects on chronic lithium therapy. Acta Endocrinol (1977) 84, 290–6.

Lithium carbonate + Ispaghula husk

Abstract/Summary

There is evidence that ispaghula (psyllium) can reduce serum lithium levels.

Clinical evidence

A woman, recently started on lithium, showed a fall in her serum lithium levels from 0.53 to 0.4 mmol/l when she started to take one teaspoonful of isphagula husk in water twice daily, despite an increase in her lithium dosage. Four days after the ispaghula was stopped, her serum lithium levels rose to 0.76 mmol/l with no change in her lithium dosage.[1]

A study in 6 normal subjects given isphagula similarly showed that the absorption of lithium (as measured by the urinary excretion) was reduced 14% by isphagula (*Metamucil*).[2]

Mechanism

Not understood. One idea is that the ispaghula may have reduced the absorption of the lithium from the gut.[1,2] An alternative is that the ispaghula preparation in question (not specifically named) might have had a high sodium content which would result in an increase in the excretion of the lithium by the kidneys.[2]

Importance and management

Information is limited and the general importance of this interaction is uncertain, but it would now seem prudent to monitor the serum lithium levels in patients given ispaghula preparations. Increase the lithium dosage if necessary.

References

1 Perlman BB. Interaction between lithium salts and ispaghula husk. Lancet (1990) 335, 416.

2 Toutoung M, Schulz P, Widmer J, Tissot R. Probable interaction entre le psyllium et le lithium. Therapie (1990) 45, 357–60.

Lithium carbonate + Mazindol

Abstract/Summary

An isolated case report describes lithium intoxication caused by the concurrent use of mazindol.

Clinical evidence

A manic depressive woman, well controlled on lithium carbonate, showed signs of lithium intoxication within three days of starting to take 2 mg mazindol daily. After 9 days concurrent treatment she developed twitching, limb rigidity and muscle fasciculation, and was both dehydrated and stuporose. Her serum lithium levels were found to have risen from 0.4–1.3 mmol/l to 3.2 mmol/l. She recovered when the mazindol was withdrawn.[1] The reason is not understood. This is an isolated case and its general importance is uncertain but the rapidity of onset and the potentially serious outcome are good reasons for not giving these drugs together unless the response can be well monitored.

Reference

1 Hendy MS, Dove AF, Arblaster PG. Mazindol-induced lithium toxicity. Br Med J (1980) 1, 684–5.

Lithium carbonate + Methyldopa

Abstract/Summary

Lithium intoxication has been described in four patients and three normal subjects when concurrently treated with methyldopa.

Clinical evidence

A manic-depressive woman, stabilized on lithium carbonate, rapidly developed signs of lithium intoxication (blurred vision, hand tremors, mild diarrhoea, confusion, and slurred speech) when additionally given 1 g methyldopa daily, although her serum lithium levels remained within the range 0.5–0.7 mmol/l.[1] Later the author of this report demonstrated this interaction on himself.[2] He found that within 2 days of starting to take 1 g methyldopa daily the signs of lithium intoxication had clearly developed, although his serum levels had risen only moderately, reaching a maximum of 0.9 mmol/l after only 4–5 days.

This interaction has been described in three other patients[3,4,6] and in three normal subjects.[5] In three cases the signs of intoxication developed although the serum lithium levels were within the normal therapeutic range.

Mechanism

Not understood.

Importance and management

Information appears to be limited to the reports cited, but the interaction would seem to be established. Avoid concurrent use whenever possible, but if not the effects should be closely monitored. Serum lithium measurements may be unreliable because intoxication can occur even though the levels remain within the accepted therapeutic range.

References

1 Byrd GJ. Methyldopa and lithium carbonate: suspected interaction. J Amer Med Ass (1975) 233, 320.
2 Byrd GJ. Lithium carbonate and methyldopa: apparent interaction in man. Clin Toxicol (1977) 11, 1–4.
3 Osanloo E, Deglin JH. Interaction of lithium and methyldopa. Ann Int Med (1980) 92, 433.
4 O'Regan JB. Adverse interaction of lithium carbonate and methyldopa. Can Med Ass J (1976) 115, 385
5 Walker N, White K, Tornatore F, Boyd JL, Cohen JL. Lithium-methyldopa interactions in normal subjects. Drug Intell Clin Pharm (1980) 14, 638.
6 Yassa R. Lithium-methyldopa interaction. Can Med Ass J (1986) 134, 141–2.

Lithium carbonate + Metronidazole

Abstract/Summary

Three patients have been described whose serum lithium levels rose (to toxic concentrations in two of them) when concurrently treated with metronidazole.

Clinical evidence, mechanism, importance and management

A woman of 40 taking 1800 mg lithium carbonate, 0.15 mg thyroxine and 60 mg propranolol daily whose serum lithium level two weeks previously was 1.3 mmol/l, developed signs of lithium intoxication (ataxia, rigidity, poor cognitive function, impaired co-ordination etc) while completing a one-week course of metronidazole (500 mg twice daily). Her serum lithium levels had climbed by 46% (to 1.9 mmol/l).[1] Two other patients are described in another report whose serum lithium levels rose by 20% and 125% respectively 12–19 days after starting a one-week course of metronidazole (500–750 mg daily).[3] Both of these two patients showed evidence of kidney abnormalities possibly caused by the concurrent use of these drugs. One other patient at least is said to have taken both drugs together uneventfully.[2]

There seem to be no strong reasons for totally avoiding concurrent use but the outcome should be well monitored. The authors of one of the reports also recommend frequent analysis of creatinine and electrolyte levels and urine osmolality in order to detect any renal problems.[3]

References

1 Brinkley JR. Quoted as personal communication by Ayd JF in Int Drug Ther Newsletter (1982) 17, 15–16.
2 Strathman I (GD Searle and Co). Quoted as personal communication by Ayd JF in Int Drug Ther Newsletter (1982) 17, 15.
3 Teicher MH, Altesman RI, Cole JO, Schatzberg AF. Possible nephrotoxic interaction of lithium and metronidazole. J Amer Med Ass (1987) 257, 3365–6.

Lithium carbonate + Non-steroidal anti-inflammatory drugs (NSAIDs)

Abstract/Summary

A marked and rapid rise in serum lithium levels (+ 60%) may occur and intoxication may develop in patients given clometacin or indomethacin. A more moderate rise (+ 15–34%) occurs with diclofenac and ibuprofen but much larger rises have been seen in a few patients. Increased serum lithium levels and/or intoxication has also been seen in a handful of patients when given ketoprofen, mefenamic acid, naproxen, niflumic acid, phenylbutazone and piroxicam. Sulindac is reported to reduce or have no effect on serum lithium levels. Aspirin, lysine acetylsalicylate and sodium salicylate do not interact.

Clinical evidence

(a) Aspirin and other Salicylates

10 normal women stabilized on lithium sulphate showed a slight fall in serum lithium levels (from 0.63 to 0.61 mmol/l), and a slight rise in their renal excretion of lithium (from 22.0 to 23.3 ml/min) when given 4 g aspirin daily for 7 days.[1] No interaction was seen in seven patients on lithium when given 3.9 g aspirin daily.[31] Another report states that 2.4 g aspirin daily had no effect on the absorption or renal excretion of single doses of lithium carbonate given to six normal subjects,[2] and a further report[3] very briefly describes the absence of an interaction between lithium carbonate and lysine acetylsalicylate or sodium salicylate.[4]

(b) Clometacin

The observation of lithium intoxication in three patients on lithium when given clometacin, prompted further study of this interaction. Six women stabilized on lithium showed an almost 60% rise (from 0.64 to 1.01 mmol/l) in their serum lithium levels after receiving 450 mg clometacin daily for five days.[5] The clearance of lithium by the kidney was found to be reduced.

(c) Diclofenac

Five normal subjects[6,7] stabilized on lithium showed a 26% rise in serum lithium levels after taking 150 mg diclofenac daily for 7–10 days. Lithium excretion by the kidney fell by 23%.

(d) Ibuprofen

The serum lithium levels of a patient rose by 25% (from 0.8 to 1.0 mEq/l) over a 7-day period while taking 2400 mg ibuprofen daily.[8,9] He experienced nausea and drowsiness. Two other patients in the study taking 1200–2400 mg ibuprofen daily did not show this interaction.

The serum lithium levels of 11 subjects rose by 15% when given 1600 mg ibuprofen daily.[10] 1800 mg ibuprofen daily for six days raised lithium levels in nine patients by 34% (range 12–66%)[21] Lithium toxicity developed in one patient within 24 h,[28] and in three others within 3–7 days of starting ibuprofen.[30] The serum lithium levels of the latter patients doubled or tripled. Lithium toxicity has been seen in other patients attributable to the use of ibuprofen.[33,34]

(e) Indomethacin

Indomethacin (50 mg three times a day) increased the serum lithium levels of five subjects taking 300–900 mg lithium carbonate daily by 43% after seven days. Renal clearance fell by 31%.[9]

Other studies have found rises of 59% and 61% in serum lithium levels in patients taking 150 mg indomethacin daily,[7,11] and lithium intoxication has been seen.[8,12] A similar rise in serum lithium levels was found in another study on 10 normal subjects taking lithium sulphate rather than carbonate.[1] Paradoxically indomethacin has also been successfully used to treat a lithium intoxicated patient who was polyuric, hypernatraemic and somnolent.[32]

(f) Ketoprofen

A manic-depressive patient stablized on lithium carbonate showed a rise in his serum lithium levels from 0.9 to 1.32 mmol/l over a 3-week period when treated with 400 mg ketoprofen daily.[3]

(g) Mefenamic acid

Acute lithium toxicity accompanied by a sharp deterioration in kidney function was seen in a patient when concurrently treated with lithium carbonate and 500 mg mefenamic acid three times daily.[25] Withdrawal of the drugs and subsequent re-challenge confirmed this interaction. Another case of toxicity was seen in a patient but his renal function was impaired before both drugs were given.[26] Another extremely brief report also describes this interaction in a patient.[23]

(h) Naproxen

Over a 6 day period while taking 760 mg naproxen daily the serum lithium levels of seven patients rose by 16% (from 0.81

to 0.94 mmol/l). The range was 0–42% and four showed a rise of over 20%. One patient whose levels rose from 0.95 to 1.13 mmol/l developed signs of toxicity (staggering gait and tremors).[22]

(i) Niflumic acid

An isolated report describes lithium intoxication in a woman after taking niflumic acid (three capsules) and 1.5 g aspirin daily for five days. Her serum lithium levels rose from 0.8 to 1.6 mmol/l.[24]

(j) Phenylbutazone and Oxyphenbutazone

The serum lithium levels of a manic depressive patient doubled (from 0.7 to 1.44 mmol/l), accompanied by signs of intoxication within three days of starting treatment with 750 mg phenyl-butazone daily in the form of suppositories.[14] Renal clearance of the lithium was found to have halved (from 10 to 5 ml/min./1.73 m). The patient was also taking viloxazine, clorazepate, spironolactone, isosorbide and dipyridamole. The same authors describe another patient who showed a sharp rise in serum lithium levels when given 500 mg oxyphenbutazone.[3]

In contrast, a study in 6 patients with bipolar affective illness found that 6 day's treatment with 300 mg phenylbutazone daily caused only a minor increase (0–15.35%) in serum lithium levels.[29] However some CNS-related side-effects (drowsiness, confusion etc) occurred.

(k) Piroxicam

A manic depressive woman, well controlled for over 9 years on lithium, experienced lithium toxicity (unsteadiness, trembling, confusion) and was admitted to hospital on three occasions after taking piroxicam. Her serum levels on two occasions had risen to 2.7 and 1.6 mmol/l, although in the latter instance the lithium had been withdrawn the previous day. In a subsequent study her serum lithium levels rose by one-third (from 1.0 to 1.5 mmol/l) when given 20 mg piroxicam daily while continuing to take the same dose of lithium (250 mg three time a day).[15]

This interaction has also been described in three other patients.[16–19,34] Another report describes lithium intoxication in a man given 20 mg piroxicam daily which apparently took four months to develop completely.[2]

(l) Sulindac

A patient stabilized on lithium showed a marked fall in serum lithium levels (from 0.65 to 0.39 mmol/l) after 2 weeks concurrent treatment with sulindac, 200 mg daily. His serum lithium levels gradually climbed over the next 6 weeks to 0.71 mmol/l and restabilized without any change in the dosage of either lithium or sulindac. The serum lithium levels of another patient were approximately halved a week after his dosage of sulindac was doubled to 400 mg daily.[20] Control of depression was not entirely lost in either patient.

In contrast three other studies found that serum lithium levels in one, four and six patients were unaffected by the use of sulindac.[13,22,27]

Mechanism

Not understood. One suggestion is that the interacting NSAIDs do so by inhibiting the synthesis of the renal prostaglandins (PGE$_2$) so that the renal blood flow is reduced, thereby reducing the renal excretion of the lithium. However this fails to explain why aspirin which blocks renal prostaglandin synthesis by 65–70% does not affect serum lithium levels.[1]

Importance and management

The documentation of these interactions is variable and limited, but what is known indicates that clometacin and indomethacin should be avoided unless serum lithium levels can be very well monitored and the dosage reduced appropriately. The other NSAIDs cited which have been reported to increase serum lithium levels and/or cause intoxication (diclofenac, ibuprofen, ketoprofen, mefenamic acid, naproxen, niflumic acid, phenylbutazone, oxyphenbutazone, piroxicam) seem to be a little less risky, but they should not be given with lithium unless the outcome can be well monitored and serum lithium dosages reduced as necessary. Sulindac appears not to increase lithium levels, but some loss of control of depression is a possibility in a few patients. Aspirin, lysine acetylsalicylate and sodium salicylate appear to be non-interacting alternatives. There seems to be nothing documented about other NSAIDs but be alert for evidence of an interaction with any of them because they have similar pharmacological characteristics.

References

1 Reimann IW, Diener U, Frohlich JC. Indomethacin but not aspirin increases plasma lithium ion levels. Arch Gen Psychiatry (1983) 40, 283–6.

2 Bikin D, Conrad KA, Mayersohn M. Lack of influence of caffeine and aspirin on lithium elimination. Clin Res (1982) 30, 249A.

3 Singer L, Imbs JL, Danion JM, Singer P, Krieger-Finance F, Schmidt M, Schwartz J. Risque d'intoxication par le lithium en cas de traitement associe par les anti-inflammatoires non steroidiens. Therapie (1981) 36, 323–6.

4 Reimann IW, Golbs E, Fischer C, Frohlich JC. Influence of intravenous acetylsalicylic acid and sodium salicylate on human renal function and lithium clearance. Eur J Clin Pharmacol (1985) 29, 435–41.

5 Edou D, Godin M, Colonna L, Petit M, Fillastre JP. Interaction medicamenteuse: clometacin-lithium. La Presse Med (1983) 12, 1551.

6 Reimann IW, Frohlich JC. Effects of diclofenac on lithium kinetics. Clin Pharmacol Ther (1980) 30, 348–52.

7 Reimann IW. Risks of non-steroidal anti-inflammatory drug therapy in lithium treated patients. Naunyn-Schmiedbergs Arch Pharmacol (1980) 3ll, R75.

8 Ragheb M, Ban TA, Buchanan D, Frohlich JC. Interaction of indomethacin and ibuprofen with lithium in manic patients under a steady-state lithium level. J Clin Psychiatry (1980) 41, 397–8.

9 Leftwich RB, Walker LA, Ragheb M, Oates JA, Frohlich JC. Inhibition of prostaglandin synthesis increases plasma lithium levels. Clin Res (1978) 26, 291A

10 Kristoff CA, Hayes PE, Barr WH, Small RE, Townsend RJ, Ettigi PG. Effect of ibuprofen on lithium plasma and red blood cell concentrations. Clin Pharm (1986) 5, 51–5.

11 Frohlich JC, Leftwich R, Ragheb M, Oates JA, Reimann I, Buchanan D. Indomethacin increases plasma lithium. Br Med J (1979) 2, 1115.

12 Herschberg SN, Sierles FS. Indomethacin-induced lithium toxicity. Am Fam Phys (1983) 28, 155–7.

13 Ragheb MA, Powell AL. Failure of sulindac to increase serum lithium levels. J Clin Psychiatry (1986) 47, 33–4.

14 Imbs JL, Schmidt M, Mack G, Sebban M, Danion JM. Baisse de la clearance renale du lithium sous l'effet de la phenylbutazone. L'Encephale (1978) IV, 33.

15 Kerry RJ, Owen G, Michaelson S. Possible interaction between lithium and piroxicam. Lancet (1983) i, 418–9.

16 Nadarajah J, Stein GS. Piroxicam induced lithium toxicity. Ann Rheum Dis (1985) 44, 502.

17 Walbridge DG, Bazire SR. An interaction between lithium carbonate and piroxicam presenting as lithium toxicity. Br J Psychiat (1985) 147, 206–7.

18 Harrison TM, Wynne Davies D, Norris CM. Lithium and Piroxicam. Brit J Psychiat (1986) 148, 124–5.

19 Shelley RK. Lithium and piroxicam. Brit J Psychiat (1986) 147, 343.

20 Furnell MM, Davies J. The effect of sulindac on lithium therapy. Drug Intell Clin Pharm (1986) 19, 374–6.

21 Ragheb M. Ibuprofen can increase serum lithium levels in lithium-treated patients. J Clin Psychiatry (1987) 48, 161–3.

22 Ragheb M, Powell AL. Lithium interaction with sulindac and naproxen. J Clin Psychopharmacol (1986) 6, 150–4.

23 Honey J. Lithium-mefenamic acid interaction. Pharmabulletin (1982) 59, 20. Quoted by Ayd FJ. in Int Drug Ther Newsletter (1982) 17, 16.

24 Gay C, Plas J, Granger B, Olie JP, Loo H. Intoxication au lithium. Deux interaction inedites: l'acetazolamide et l'acide niflumique. L'Encephale (1985) 11, 261–2.

25 MacDonald J, Neale TJ. Toxic interaction of lithium carbonate and mefenamic acid. Br Med J (1988) 297, 1339.

26 Shelley RK. Lithium toxicity and mefenamic acid: a possible interaction and the role of prostaglandin inhibition. Br J Psychiatry (1987) 151, 847–8.

27 Miller LG, Bowman RC, Bakht F. Sparing effect of sulindac on lithium levels. J Fam Prac (1989) 28, 592–3.

28 Bailey CE, Stewart JT, McElroy RA. Ibuprofen-induced lithium toxicity. S Med J (1989) 82, 1197.

29 Ragheb M. The interaction of lithium with phenylbutazone in bipolar affective patients. J Clin Psychopharmacol (1990) 10, 149–150.

30 Ayd FJ. Ibuprofen induced lithium intoxication. Int Drug Ther Newsletter (1985) 20, 16.

31 Ragheb MA. Aspirin does not significantly affect patients' serum lithium levels. J Clin Psychiatry (1987) 48, 425.

32 ter Wee PM, van Hoek B, Donker AJM. Indomethacin treatment in a patient with lithium-induced polyuria. Intensive Care Med (1985) 11, 103–4.

33 Khan IH. Lithium and non-steroidal anti-inflammatory drugs. Br Med J (1991) 302, 1537–8.

34 Kelly CB, Cooper SJ. Toxic elevation of serium lithium concentration by non-steroidal anti-inflammatory drugs. Ulster Med J (1991) 60, 240–2.

Lithium carbonate + Phenytoin

Abstract/Summary

Signs of lithium intoxication have been seen in three patients concurrently treated with phenytoin. The serum lithium levels may remain the same.

Clinical evidence, mechanism, importance and management.

A patient with a long history of depression and convulsions was treated with increasing doses of lithium carbonate and phenytoin over a period of about 12 years. Although the serum levels of both drugs remained within the therapeutic range, he eventually began to manifest signs of lithium intoxication (thirst, polyuria, polydipsia and tremor) which disappeared when the phenytoin was replaced by carbamazepine. The patient claimed that he felt normal for the first time in years.[1] Another report[2] describes a man on phenytoin who became ataxic within 3 days of starting to take lithium. He had no other toxic symptoms and his serum lithium level was 2.0 mEq/l. A further report states that intoxication can develop during concurrent use even though the serum levels remain within the normally accepted therapeutic range.[3]

Information seems to be limited to these reports and none of them presents a clear picture of the role of phenytoin in the reactions described.[1-3] The interaction is not well established. However it would be prudent to be alert for signs of intoxication during concurrent use, particularly because intoxication can apparently develop even though serum levels are within the therapeutic range.

References

1 MacCallum WAG. Interaction of lithium and phenytoin. Br Med J (1980) 280, 10.
2 Salem RB, Director K, Muniz CE. Ataxia as the primary symptom of lithium toxicity. Drug Intell Clin Pharm (1980) 14, 622
3 Spiers J, Hirsch SR. Severe lithium toxicity with normal serum concentrations. Br Med J (1978) 1, 185.

Lithium carbonate + Propranolol

Abstract/Summary

An isolated report describes marked bradycardia in a patient on lithium when additionally given propranolol.

Clinical evidence, mechanism, importance and management

A man of 70 who had taken lithium successfully for 16 years was additionally started on 30 mg propranolol daily for tremor. Six weeks later he was hospitalized because of vomiting, dizziness, headache and a fainting episode. His pulse rate was 35–40 bpm and his serum lithium was 0.3 mmol/l. When later discharged on lithium without propranolol his pulse rate had risen to 64–80 bpm. The authors point out that both drugs reduce the production of the second messenger, cyclic adenosine monophosphate, which inhibits the influx of calcium ions across cell membranes. Lithium also reduces the mobilization of calcium ions from intracellular pools by the inositol triphosphate dependent calcium channels. These combined effects could account for the decreased contraction rate of the heart muscle in this patient.

The general importance of this interaction is uncertain, but the authors of the report suggest careful monitoring in elderly patients with atherosclerotic cardiovascular problems.[1] This interaction seems possible with other beta-blockers because they also cause heart-slowing.

Reference

1 Becker D. Lithium and propranolol: possible synergism? J Clin Psychiatry (1989) 50, 473.

Lithium carbonate + Sodium chloride or Bicarbonate

Abstract/Summary

The ingestion of marked amounts of sodium as the chloride or bicarbonate can prevent the establishment or maintenance of adequate serum lithium levels. Conversely, dietary salt restriction can cause a serum lithium rise to toxic concentrations if the lithium dosage is not reduced appropriately.

Clinical evidence

(a) Lithium response reduced by the ingestion of sodium

A depressive man, initially given 250 mg lithium carbonate four times a day, achieved a serum lithium level of 0.5 mmol/l by the following morning. When the dosage frequency was progressively increased to five, and later six times a day, his serum lithium levels failed to exceed 0.6 mmol/l because, unknown to his doctor, he was also taking sodium bicarbonate. In the words of the patient's wife: '...he's been taking soda bic for years for an ulcer, doctor, but since he started on that lithium he's been shovelling it in...'. When the sodium bicarbonate was stopped, relatively stable serum lithium levels of 0.8 mmol/l were achieved on the initial dosage of lithium carbonate.[1]

An investigation to find out why a number of inpatients failed to reach, or maintain, adequate therapeutic serum lithium levels, revealed that a clinic nurse had been giving the patients a proprietary saline drink (*Efferdex*), used for 'upset stomachs' and containing about 50% sodium bicarbonate, because the patients complained of nausea. The depression in the expected serum lithium levels was as much as 40% in some cases.[6]

Other studies confirm that serum lithium levels fall and the effectiveness of treatment can lessen if the intake of sodium is increased.[4,9,11]

(b) Lithium response increased by sodium restriction

The serum lithium levels of four manic depressives rose more rapidly and to a higher peak when salt was restricted than when taking a dietary salt supplement.[2]

Other studies and observations confirm that salt restriction can, if the effects are not monitored, lead to lithium intoxication.[5,7,11]

Mechanism

Not fully established. One suggestion is as follows. Lithium is eliminated from the body almost exclusively in the urine. The proximal tubule does not readily distinguish between sodium and lithium ions and reabsorbs 60–70% of the filtered load. It seems possible that during sodium depletion, the extracellular volume of the body is contracted so that both ions are maximally reabsorbed, leading to an increased retention of the lithium. Conversely, when the sodium levels are high (e.g. when a salt supplement is used), the extracellular volume is expanded and both sodium and lithium are excreted rather than reabsorbed. Beyond the proximal tubule, lithium and sodium appear to be handled differently, but in any case lithium reabsorption is relatively small so that any interference by sodium is likely to be minimal.[3,8]

Importance and management

Well established and clinically important interactions. The establishment and maintenance of adequate serum lithium levels can be jeopardized if the intake of ionic sodium is increased. Warn patients not to take over-the-counter antacids or urinary alkalinizers without first seeking informed advice. Sodium bicarbonate comes in various guises and disguises (e.g. *Efferdex* (50%), *Eno's Fruit Salts* (56%), *Andrews Liver Salts* (22.6%), *Bismarex Antacid Powder* (65%), *BiSoDoL Powder* (58%)). Substantial amounts also occur in some urinary alkalinizing agents (e.g. *Citralka, Citravescent*).[12] There are many similar preparations available throughout the world. An antacid containing aluminium and magnesium hydroxides with simethicone has been found to have no effect on the bioavailability of lithium carbonate.[10]

Patients already stabilized on lithium should not begin to limit their intake of salt unless their serum lithium levels can be monitored and suitable dosage adjustments made because their lithium levels can rise quite rapidly.

References

1 Arthur RK. Lithium levels and 'Soda Bic'. Med J Aust (1975) 2, 918.
2 Platman SR, Fieve RR. Lithium retention and excretion. Arch Gen Psychiat (1969) 20, 285.
3 Thomsen K, Schou M. Renal lithium excretion in man. Am J Physiol (1968) 215, 823.
4 Bleiweiss H. Salt supplements with lithium. Lancet (1970) i, 416.
5 Hurtig HI, Dyson WL. Lithium toxicity enhanced by diuresis. N Eng J Med (1974) 290, 748.
6 McSwiggan C. Interaction of lithium and bicarbonate. Med J Aust (1978) 1, 38.
7 Corcoran AC, Taylor RD, Page IH. Lithium poisoning from the use of salt substitutes. J Am Med Ass (1949) 139, 685.
8 Singer I, Rotenburg D. Mechanisms of lithium action. N Eng J Med (1973) 289, 254.
9 Demers RG, Heninger GR. Sodium intake and lithium treatment in man. Am J Psychiatry (1971) 128, 100–4.
10 Goode DL, Newton DW, Ueda CT, Wilson JE, Wulf BG, Kafonek D. Effect of antacid on the bioavailability of lithium carbonate. Clin Pharm (1984) 3, 284–7.
11 Baer L, Platman SR, Kassir S, Fieve RR. Mechanisms of renal lithium handling and their relationship to mineralocorticoids: a dissociation between sodium and lithium ions. J Psychiat Res (1971) 8, 91–105.
12 Beard TC, Wilkinson SJ, Vial JH. Hazards of urinary alkalizing agents. Med J Aust (1988) 149, 723.

Lithium carbonate + Spectinomycin

Abstract/Summary

A single case report describes a patient who developed lithium intoxication when given spectinomycin.

Clinical evidence, mechanism, importance and management

A depressive woman[1] controlled on lithium developed intoxication (tremor, nausea, vomiting, ataxia and dysarthria) when given spectinomycin injections (dose not stated) for the treatment of gonorrhoea. Her serum lithium levels had climbed from a range of 0.8–1.1 mmol/l to 3.2 mmol/l. A likely explanation is that spectinomycin, particularly in multiple doses, decreases creatinine clearance, elevates BUN and reduces urine output which would be expected to reduce the excretion of lithium, resulting in a rise in serum levels. Information seems to be limited to this report, but it would now seem prudent to monitor the effects of concurrent use in any patient.

Reference

1 Conroy RW. Quoted as a personal communication by Ayd FJ. Possible adverse drug-drug interaction report. Int Drug Therapy Newsletter (1978) 13, 15.

Lithium carbonate + Tetracycline

Abstract/Summary

Concurrent use is normally uneventful, but an isolated report describes lithium intoxication in a woman attributed to the use of tetracycline.

Clinical evidence, mechanism, importance and management

An isolated report describes a manic depressive woman, well stabilized on lithium for 3 years, with serum concentrations within the range 0.5–0.84 mmol/l. Within 2 days of starting to take a sustained-release form of tetracycline (*Tetrabid*) her serum lithium levels had risen to 1.7 mmol/l, and two days later they had climbed to 2.74 mmol/l. By then she showed clear signs of lithium intoxication (slight drowsiness, slurring of the speech, fine tremor and thirst). The suggested reason is that the tetracycline (known to have nephrotoxic potentialities) may have adversely affected the renal clearance of lithium from the body.[1]

In contrast, 14 normal subjects taking 450 mg lithium carbonate twice daily showed a small reduction in serum lithium levels (from 0.51 to 0.47 mmol/l) when given 1 g tetracycline hydrochloride for seven days.[2] The incidence of adverse reactions remained largely unchanged except for a slight increase in

CNS and gastrointestinal side-effects. Another report describes the uneventful use of lithium and tetracyclines in patients.[3]

There seems to be no reason for avoiding concurrent use nevertheless it would be prudent to monitor the effects.

References

1 McGennis AJ. Lithium carbonate and tetracycline interaction. Br Med J (1978) 2, 1183.

2 Fankhauser MP, Lindon JL, Connolly B, Healey WJ. Evaluation of lithium-tetracycline interaction. Clin Pharm (1988) 7, 314–17.

3 Jefferson JW. Lithium and tetracycline. Br J Dermatol (1982) 107, 370.

Lithium carbonate + Theophylline

Abstract/Summary

Serum lithium levels are reduced by 20–30% by the concurrent use of theophylline and patients may relapse as a result. The interaction can be accommodated by raising the dosage of lithium.

Clinical evidence

The serum lithium levels of 10 normal subjects on 900 mg lithium carbonate daily fell by 20–30%, and the urinary clearance increased by 30%, when given 400–800 mg theophylline daily.[1,2]

A case report described a manic patient on lithium who very rapidly relapsed when given theophylline. It was found necessary to raise the dosage in a stepwise manner as the dosage of theophylline was increased in order to maintain the serum lithium levels and to control the mania.[3] Theophylline has also been used to treat lithium intoxication.[4,5]

Mechanism

Uncertain. Theophylline has an effect on the renal clearance of lithium.

Importance and management

Information is limited but the interaction appears to be established. Depressive and manic relapses may occur if the dosage of lithium is not raised appropriately when theophylline is given. Serum lithium levels should be monitored during concurrent use.

References

1 Perry PJ, Calloway RA, Cook BL, Smith RE. Theophylline precipitated alterations of lithium clearance. Acta Psychiatr Scand (1984) 69, 528–37.

2 Cook BL, Smith RE, Perry PJ, Calloway RA. Theophylline-lithium interaction. J Clin Psychiatry (1985) 46, 278–9.

3 Sierles FS, Ossowski MG. Concurrent use of theophylline and lithium in a patient with chronic obstructive lung disease and bipolar disorder. Am J Psychiat (1982) 139, 117.

4 Thomsen K, Schou M. Renal lithium excretion in man. Amer J Physiol (1968) 215, 823.

5 Jefferson JW, Greist JH. A Primer of Lithium Therapy. Williams and Wilkins Co., Baltimore (1977) p 204.

Lithium carbonate + Thiazides or Related diuretics

Abstract/Summary

Serum lithium levels can be increased by the concurrent use of the thiazides or related diuretics such as chlorthalidone and indapamide. Lithium intoxication will develop unless the lithium dosage is reduced appropriately. It seems probable that the same interaction will occur with a number of related diuretics.

Clinical evidence

A patient showed a rise in serum lithium concentrations from 1.3 to 2.0 mmol/l each time he was administered 500 mg chlorothiazide daily.[4]

A study carried out on 22 patients showed that long-term treatment with either hydroflumethiazide (25 mg daily) plus KCl (3.4 g daily) or bendrofluazide (2.5 mg daily) led to a 24% reduction in the urinary excretion of lithium.[2] A fall in the urinary excretion of lithium due to the use of chlorothiazide has been described elsewhere.[6] A study in normal subjects given low doses of lithium (300 mg twice daily) found that the addition of 25 mg hydrochlorothiazide twice daily for 5 days raised the serum lithium levels by 23% (from 0.30 to 0.37 mmol/l).[17]

Lithium toxicity arising from the use of thiazide diuretics either alone[10,11] (bendrofluazide[16]) or with other diuretics has been seen with *Moduretic* (hydrochlorothiazide + amiloride),[1,2,13,14] *Aldactazide* (hydrochlorothiazide + spironolactone),[3] and chlorothiazide with spironolactone and amiloride,[3] or triamterene.[12] It seems almost certain that in each case the thiazide component was principally responsible for the interaction. Chlorthalidone[9] and indapamide[15] have also been responsible for the development of lithium toxicity.

Mechanism

Not fully understood. The interaction occurs even though the thiazides and similar diuretics exert their major actions in the distal part of the kidney tubule whereas lithium is reabsorbed in the proximal part. A possible reason is that thiazide diuresis is accompanied by sodium loss which, within a few days, is compensated by a retention of sodium, this time in the proximal part of the tubule. Since both sodium and lithium ions are treated virtually indistinguishably, the increased reabsorption of sodium would include lithium as well, hence a significant and measurable reduction in its excretion. This would seem to be a long-term rather than an immediate effect which might explain why a short-term single-dose study in man with bendrofluazide failed to show any effect on lithium excretion.[5]

Importance and management

Established, well-documented and potentially serious interactions. None of the thiazides or the related diuretics cited (chlorthalidone, indapamide) should be given to patients on lithium unless the serum lithium levels can be closely monitored and appropriate dosage adjustments made. Concurrent use under controlled conditions has been advocated for certain psychiatric conditions and for the control of lithium-induced nephrogenic diabetes insipidus. Himmelhoch and his colleagues[13] calculate that 500 mg chlorothiazide daily would increase the serum lithium levels by 40% so that an approximately 40% reduction in lithium dosage would be necessary. Reductions of 60–70% would be necessary if 750–1000 mg were used.[8,13]

Quinethazone, metazolone, clorexolone, clopamide and several other diuretics are closely related to the thiazides and have similar actions. They may be expected to interact with lithium but so far there appear to be no reports confirming that they do so.

References

1 Macfie AC. Lithium poisoning precipitated by diuretics. Br Med J (1975) 1, 516.

2 Petersen V, Hvidt S, Thomsen K, Schou M. Effect of prolonged thiazide treatment on renal lithium excretion. Br Med J (1974) 2, 143.

3 Lutz EG. Lithium toxicity precipitated by diuretics. J Med Soc New Jersey (1975) 72, 439.

4 Levy ST, Forrest JN, Heninger GR. Lithium-induced diabetes insipidus: manic symptoms, brain and electrolyte correlates, and chlorothiazide treatment. Amer J Psychiat (1973) 130, 1014.

5 Thomsen K, Schou M. Renal lithium excretion in man. Amer J Physiol (1968) 215, 823.

6 Baer L, Platman S, Fieve RK. Lithium metabolism: its electrolyte actions and relationship to aldosterone. Recent Advances in the Psychobiology of the Depressive Illnesses. Williams, Katz and Shield (eds). DHEW Publications, Washington DC. (1972) p. 49.

7 Basdevant A, Beaufils M, Corvol P. Influence des diuretiques sur l'elimination renale du lithium. Nouv Presse Med (1976) 5, 2085.

8 Himmelhoch JM, Forrest J, Neil J, Detre TP. Thiazide-lithium synergy in refractory mood swings. Amer J Psychiat (1977) 134, 149.

9 Solomon JG. Lithium toxicity precipitated by a diuretic. Psychosomatics (1980) 21, 425.

10 Kerry RJ, Ludlow JM, Owen G. Diuretics are dangerous with lithium. Br Med J (1980) 281, 371.

11 Konig P, Kufferle B, Lenz G. Ein fall von Lithium-toxikation bei therapeutischen Lithium dosaen infolge zusatzlicher Gabe eines Diuretikums. Wien Klin Wochensch (1978) 90, 380.

12 Mehta BR, Robinson BHB. Lithium toxicity induced by triamterene-hydrochlorothiazide. Postgrad Med J. (1980) 56, 783.

13 Himmelhoch JM, Proust RI, Malinger AG. Adjustment of lithium dosage during lithium-chlorothiazide therapy. Clin Pharmacol Ther (1977) 22, 225.

14 Dorevitch A, Baruch E. Lithium toxicity induced by combined amiloride hydrochloride-hydrochlorothiazide administration. Am J Psychiatry (1986) 143, 257–8.

15 Hanna ME, Lobao CB, Steward JT. Severe lithium toxicity associated with indapamide therapy. J Clin Psychopharmacol (1990) 10. 379–80.

16 Aronson JK, Reynolds DJM. ABC of monitoring drug therapy. Lithium. Brit Med J (1992) 305, 1273–6.

17 Crabtree BL, Mack JE, Johnson CD, Amyx BC. Comparison of the effects of hydrochlorothiazide and furosemide on lithium disposition. Am J Psychiatry (1991) 148, 1060–3.

Lithium carbonate + Tricyclic antidepressants

Abstract/Summary

Tricyclic antidepressants added to lithium treatment can be successful in some patients, but a few may develop adverse side-effects.

Clinical evidence, mechanism, importance and management

Five out of nine depressed patients (all under 65) tolerated combined lithium/tricyclic antidepressants without significant side-effects, but severe neurotoxic side-effects developed in the other four elderly patients despite the use of therapeutic doses. One of them developed tremor, memory difficulties, disorganized thinking and auditory hallucinations when given 900 mg lithium carbonate daily and 50 mg nortriptyline daily. Another experienced severe tremor, ataxia and cogwheeling when given 400 mg lithium carbonate daily and 40 mg fluoxetine daily.[1] Another study in 14 elderly patients found that seven showed complete improvement and three showed partial improvement over a period from 3–21 days. Side effects occurred in six. In four of these the lithium was stopped as a result. One of them was successfully restarted at a lower dose. The other three accounted for three of the four non-responders. Tremor was the most frequent side-effect, and reversible neurotoxicity with a stroke-like syndrome was the most severe. The antidepressants used were amitriptyline, doxepin, maprotiline and trazodone.[2] These studies clearly show the potential advantages of concurrent use, but also illustrate the need to monitor the outcome for problematical side-effects.

References

1 Austin LS, Arana GW, Melvin JA. Toxicity resulting from lithium augmentation of antidepressant treatment in elderly patients. J Clin Psychiatry (1990) 51, 344–5.

2 Lafferman J, Solomon K, Ruskin P. Lithium augmentation for treatment-resistant depression in the elderly. J Geriat Psychiatry Neurol (1988) 1, 49–52.

Chapter 18
Monoamine Oxidase Inhibitor
Drug Interactions

Drugs with monoamine oxidase inhibitory activity were first developed as antidepressants because it was noticed that patients with tuberculosis given isoniazid, and more particularly iproniazid, showed some degree of mood elevation. A further development occurred when postural hypotension was seen to be one of the side-effects of treatment with iproniazid and, as a result, pheniprazine and later pargyline were introduced as antihypertensive agents.

Among the serious and unexpected problems with the first generation monoamine oxidase inhibitors (MAOIs) were the serious and potentially life-threatening interactions which occurred with the sympathomimetics found in some proprietary cough and cold remedies, and with tyramine-rich foods and drinks.

The intended target of the antidepressant MAOI is the MAO within the brain, but it is also found in other parts of the body, and in particularly high concentrations in the gut and liver where it acts as a protective detoxifying enzyme against tyramine and possibly other potentially hazardous amines which exist in foods which have undergone bacterial degradation. For this reason MAO was originally called tyramine oxidase. There are at least two forms of MAO: MAO-A metabolises (deaminates) noradrenaline and serotonin (5 HT), and MAO-B metabolises phenylethylamine. Substances like tyramine and dopamine are metabolized by both forms of MAO.

The older MAOIs are non-selective or non-specific. They inhibit both isoenzymes A and B, and are mostly irreversible and long-acting because the return of MAO-activity depends upon the regeneration of new enzymes. As a result they can continue to have activity (both beneficial and adverse) for 2–3 weeks after they have been withdrawn. Tranylcypromine differs in being a reversible inhibitor of MAO so that the onset and disappearance of its actions are much quicker than the other older MAOI.

Some of the newer and more recently developed MAOI are safer because they interact to a lesser extent than the first generation MAOI. This is because they are reversible and are largely selective, inhibiting either MAO-A or MAO-B. The reversible inhibitors of MAO-A such as moclobemide have been given the acronym RIMA (Reversible Inhibitors of Monoamine oxidase A). Table 18.1 is a list of the MAOI used for depression, hypertension and Parkinson's disease. Some of them are currently available,

Table 18.1 Monoamine oxydase inhibitors (MAOIs)

Non-proprietary (generic) names	Proprietary names
Older MAOI (Irreversible MAO-inhibitors)	
Iproclozide	*Sursum*
Iproniazid	*Marsilid*
Isocarboxazid	*Marplan*
Mebanazine	*Actomol*
Nialamide	*Niamid(e)*
Phenelzine	*Nardil, Nardelzine*
Phenelzine with pentaerythritol tetranitrate	*Perfenil*
Tranylcypromine	*Parnate*
Tranylcypromine with trifluoperazine	*Parstelin*
Newer MAOI RIMA (reversible inhibitors of MAO-A)	
Amiflamine	
Bromfaromine	
Cimoxatone	
Moclobemide	*Auroxix*
Toloxatone	*Humoryl, Perenum*
Selegiline (*Deprenyl*) (Reversible inhibitor of MAO-B)	*Eldepryl, Jumex, Jumexal, Movergan*

some are still undergoing trials and a few have been withdrawn.

If you look at the drug data sheets issued by manufacturers, you will frequently see warnings about interactions with MAOI. Blackwell, who has done so much work on the interactions of the MAOI, has rightly pointed out that the MAOI are among the drugs which '...have such a long history they accumulate much myth and misinformation. Lists of side-effects and interactions are lengthy but often unsupported by recent or creditable research to establish either a cause and effect relationship or to identify the underlying mechanism. Worse still, the MAOIs have developed such a sinister reputation that manufacturers often issue a reflexive admonition to avoid co-administration with new drugs.'[1] This means that many of the warnings about potential interactions with the MAOI may lack a sound scientific basis. Take note!

In addition to the interactions of the MAOI described in this chapter, there are others dealt with elsewhere. The index should be consulted for a full listing.

Reference

1 Blackwell B. Monoamine Oxidase Inhibitor interactions with other drugs. J Clin Psychopharmacology (1991) 11, 55–59.

Moclobemide + Miscellaneous drugs

Abstract/Summary

No serious adverse interactions were seen in patients and subjects given moclobemide with the drugs named below and no special precautions would seem necessary.

Clinical evidence, mechanism, importance and management

There was no evidence of any adverse interaction when mo-clobemide (150–675 mg daily) was given for 3–52 weeks to 50 patients on **lithium**.[1] A study in 24 normal subjects found that 150 mg moclobemide three times daily for 7 days had no effect on the absorption or disposition of **ibuprofen**, and the ibuprofen-induced blood loss was unaffected.[2] Studies in normal subjects found that 200 mg moclobemide three times daily increased the blood pressure lowering effects of **metoprolol** (systolic 10–15 mmHg, diastolic 5–10 mmHg), but no comparable effects were seen when given with **hydrochorothiazide** or **nifedipine**. No orthostatic hypotension occurred with any of the drug combinations.[1]

A study in 14 patients with decompensated heart failure found that 100 mg moclobemide three times daily for 8 days caused a non-significant 14% fall (from 0.99 to 0.85 ng/ml) in their serum **beta-acetyldigoxin** levels. No adverse effects attributable to an interaction were seen.[1] A study in seven women taking combined **oral contraceptives** found no evidence of any significant alterations in oestradiol, progesterone, FSH or LH levels while taking 200 mg moclobemide three times daily for one cycle. No serious adverse reactions occurred. The conclusion was reached that the efficacy of the oral contraceptives is likely to be maintained during concurrent use.[1] No serious adverse effects were seen in 110 patients given 150–400 mg moclobemide daily with **acepromazine, aceprometazine, bromperidol, chlorpromazine, chlorprothixene, clopenthixol, clothiapine, clozapine, cyamemazine, flupenthixol, fluphenazine, fluspirilene, haloperidol, methotrimeprazine, penfluridol, pipamperone, prothipendyl, sulpiride, thioridazine** or **trimeprazine**. However there was some evidence that hypotension, tachycardia, sleepiness, tremor and constipation were more common.[1] No serious adverse effects were reported in extensive clinical trials of moclobemide when used in patients taking antiparkinsonian drugs, antibiotics, anticonvulsants, hormones and others, but none was specifically named.[1]

References

1 Amrein R, Güntert TW, Dingemanse J, Lorscheid T, Stabl M, Schmid-Burgk W. Interactions of moclobemide with concomitantly administered medication: evidence from pharmacological and clinical studies. Psychopharmacology (1992) 106, S24–31.
2 Güntert TW, Schmitt M, Dingemanse J, Jonkman JHG. Influence of moclobemide on ibuprofen-induced faecal blood loss. Psychopharmacology (1992) 106, S40–2.

Moclobemide + Cimetidine

Abstract/Summary

Cimetidine increases the serum levels of moclobemide. Some dosage reduction may be necessary.

Clinical evidence, mechanism, importance and management

A study in normal subjects found that after taking 1 g cimetidine daily for 2 weeks the maximum serum levels of a single 100 mg dose of moclobemide was increased by 39% and the AUC (area under the curve) by 123%.[1] The probable reason is that the cimetidine (a well-recognized enyzme inhibitor) reduces the first-pass metabolism of the moclobemide. It has therefore been recommended that patients already taking cimetidine should be started on the lowest therapeutic dosage. If cimetidine is added to treatment with moclobemide, the dosage of the latter should initially be reduced by 50% and later adjusted as necessary.[2]

There seems to be nothing to suggest that an adverse interaction occurs with any other MAOI and cimetidine.

Reference

1 Schoerling M-P, Mayersohn M, Hoevels B, Eggers H, Dellenbach M, Pfefen J-P. Cimetidine alters the disposition kinetics of the monoamine oxidase-A inhibitor moclobemide. Clin Pharmacol Ther (1991) 49, 32–8.
2 Amrein R, Güntert TW, Dingemanse J, Lorscheid T, Stabl M, Schmid-Burgk W. Interactions of moclobemide with concomitantly administered medication: evidence from pharmacological and clinical studies. Psychopharmacology (1992) 106, S24–31.

Monoamine oxidase inhibitors + Amantadine

Abstract/Summary

An isolated report describes a rise in blood pressure in a patient on amantadine when given phenelzine.

Clinical evidence, mechanism, importance and management

A woman of 49 was treated for Parkinson's disease with amantadine (200 mg daily), haloperidol (5 mg daily) and flurazepam (30 mg at night). Within 72 h of starting to take 30 mg phenelzine daily for depression, her blood pressure rose from 140/90 to 160/110 mmHg and it remained high for a further 72 h after the amantadine and haloperidol had been withdrawn.[1] The reason for this hypertensive reaction is not understood. Another woman is reported to have been given amantadine (200 mg daily) and phenelzine (43 mg daily) successfully and uneventfully.[2] If concurrent use is undertaken the effects should be well monitored.

References

1 Jack RA, Daniel DG. Possible interaction between phenelzine and amantadine. Arch Gen Psychiatry (1984) 41, 726.

2 Greenberg R, Meyers BS. Treatment of major depression and Parkinson's disease with combined phenelzine and amantadine. Am J Psychiatry (1985) 142, 273.

Monoamine oxidase inhibitors + Barbiturates

Abstract/Summary

Although the MAOI can enhance and prolong the activity of the barbiturates in animals, only a few isolated cases attributed to an interaction have been described in man.

Clinical evidence

Kline has stated, without giving details, that on three or four occasions patients of his taking an MAOI continued, without his knowledge, to take their usual barbiturate hypnotic and thereby '...unknowingly raised their dose of barbiturate by five to ten times, and as a consequence barely managed to stagger through the day.'[3]

A patient on tranylcypromine was inadvertently given 250 mg sodium amylobarbitone (amobarbital) intravenously for sedation. Within an hour she became ataxic, fell to the floor repeatedly hitting her head. After complaining of nausea and dizziness the patient became semicomatose and remained in that state for a further 36 h. To what extent the head trauma played a part is uncertain.[5]

Two other cases of coma attributed to concurrent use have been described.[6,7] In contrast, mebanazine is reported not to have enhanced the hypnotic activities of quinalbarbitone (secobarbital) or butobarbitone (butobarbital) in a number of patients, nor was there any evidence of a hangover effect.[8]

Mechanism

Not known. Animal studies[1,2,4] suggest that the MAOI have a general inhibitory action on the liver microsomal enzymes, thereby prolonging the activity of the barbiturates, but whether this also occasionally occurs in man is uncertain.

Importance and management

The evidence for this interaction seems to be confined to a few unconfirmed anecdotal reports. There is no well-documented evidence showing that concurrent use should be avoided, although some caution is clearly appropriate. Mebanazine appears not to interact with quinalbarbitone or butobarbitone.

References

1 Wulfsohn NL, Politzer WM. 5-Hydroxytryptamine in anaesthesia. Anaesthesia (1962) 17, 64.

2 Lechat P, Lemergnan A. Monoamine oxidase inhibitors and potentiation of experimental sleep. Biochem Pharmacol (1961) 8, 8.

3 Kline NS. Psychopharmaceuticals: effects and side-effects. Bull WHO (1959) 21, 397.

4 Buchel L, Levy J. Mecanisme des phenomenes de synergie due sommeil experimental. II. Etude des associations iproniazide-hypnotique, chez le rat et la souris. Arch Sci Rech Sci Physiol (1965) 19, 161.

5 Domino EF, Sullivan TS, Luby E. Barbiturate intoxication in a patient treated with a MAO inhibitor. Amer J Psychiat (1962) 118, 941.

6 Etherington L. Personal communication (1973).

7 MacLeod I. Fatal reaction to phenelzine. Br Med J (1965) 1, 1554.

8 Gilmour SJG. Clinical trial of mebanazine — a new monoamine oxidase inhibitor. Br J Psychiat (1965) 111, 899.

Monoamine oxidase inhibitors + Benzodiazepines

Abstract/Summary

The concurrent use of the MAOI and the benzodiazepines is usually safe and effective, but a very small number of adverse reactions (chorea, severe headache, massive oedema, MAOI-toxicity) attributed to interactions have been described.

Clinical evidence, mechanism, importance and management

A patient with depression responded well when given 15 mg phenelzine and 10 mg chlordiazepoxide three times a day, but 4–5 months later developed choreiform movements of moderate severity and slight dysarthria. These symptoms subsided when the drugs were withdrawn.[1] Two patients on chlordiazepoxide and either isocarboxazid or phenelzine developed severe oedema which was attributed to the use of both drugs.[2,3] A patient on 60 mg phenelzine daily developed MAOI toxicity (excessive sweating, postural hypotension) within 10 days of increasing his daily dosage of nitrazepam to 15 mg. The patient was a slow acetylator.[7] A patient who had been taking 45 mg phenelzine daily for 9 years developed a severe occipital headache after taking 0.5 mg clonazepam. A similar but milder headache occurred the next night when she took the same dose. No blood pressure measurements were taken.[9] The reasons for the development of all of these reactions are unknown. A meta-analysis of 897 patients at 31 centres is reported to have found that the use of benzodiazepines appeared to double the incidence of adverse effects (insomnia, restlessness, agitation, anxiety) in patients on moclobemide, but it is suggested that the patient groups may possibly have been different.[10] Another report found no clinically relevant interaction between moclobemide and benzodiazepines.[8]

The general picture portrayed by the reports in the literature is that concurrent use is usually effective and uneventful.[4–6] The adverse interaction reports cited here appear to be the exception, and it is by no means certain that all the responses were due to drug interactions, however some caution is appropriate if these drugs are used together.

References

1 MacLeod DM. Chorea induced by tranquillizers. Lancet (1964) i, 388.
2 Goonewardene A, Toghill PJ. Gross oedema occurring during treatment for depression. Br Med J (1977) 1, 879.
3 Pathak SK. Gross oedema during treatment for depression. Br Med J (1977) 1, 1220.
4 Frommer EA. Treatment of childhood depression with antidepressant drugs. Br Med J (1967) 1, 729.
5 Mans J, Sennes M. L'isocarboxazide, le RO 5–0690 et chlordiazepoxide, le RO-4–0403 derive des thixanthenes. Etude sur leur effect propres et leurs possibilites d'association. J Med Bord (1964) 141, 1909.
6 Suerinck A, Suerinck E. Etats depressifs en milieu sanatorial et inhibiteurs de la mono-amine oxydase. (Resultats therepeutiques par l'association d'iproclozide et de chlodiazepoxide.) A propos de 146 observations. J Med Lyon (1966) 47, 573.
7 Harris AL, McIntyre N. Interaction of phenelzine and nitrazepam in a slow acetylator. Br J Clin Pharmac (1981) 12, 254–5.
8 Zimmer R, Gieschke R, Fischbach R, Gasic S. Interaction studies with moclobemide. Acta Psychiatr Scand (1990) Suppl 360, 84–6.
9 Eppel AB. Interaction between clonazepam and phenelzine. Can J Psychiatry (1990) 35, 647.
10 Amrein R, Güntert TW, Dingesmanse J, Lorsheid T, Stabl M, Schmid-Burgk W. Interactions of moclobemide with concomitantly administered medication: evidence from pharmacological and clinical studies. Psychopharmacology (1992) 106, S24–31.

Monamine oxidase inhibitors + Buspirone

Abstract/Summary

Elevated blood pressure has been reported in four patients taking buspirone and either phenelzine or tranylcypromine.

Clinical evidence, mechanism, importance and management

Four cases of significant blood pressure elevation during the concurrent use of buspirone and either phenelzine or tranylcypromine have been reported to the FDA's spontaneous Reporting System, and are described very briefly in Psychiatry Drug Alerts. One patient was a 75-year-old woman and the other three were men aged 30–42. The report does not say how much the pressures rose, or how quickly, and no other details are given.[1] On the basis of this rather sparse information the manufacturers say that "..the administration of *BuSpar* to a patient taking a MAOI may pose a hazard'[2]

Reference

1 Anon. *BuSpar* Update. Psychiatry Drug Alerts (1987) 1, 43.
2 *BuSpar* Product Information, Mead Johnson Pharmaceuticals. 1990

Monoamine oxidase inhibitors + Chloral hydrate

Abstract/Summary

A case of fatal hyperpyrexia and another of serious hypertension have been attributed to interactions between chloral and phenelzine.

Clinical evidence, mechanism, importance and management

A woman taking 45 mg phenelzine daily was found in bed deeply comatose with marked muscular rigidity, twitching down one side and a temperature of 41°C. She died without regaining consciousness. A postmortem failed to establish the cause of death, but it subsequently came to light that she had started drinking whisky again (she had been treated for alcoholism), and she had access to chloral hydrate. She may have taken a fatal dose.[1] Another patient, also taking 45 mg phenelzine daily and chloral hydrate for sleeping, developed an excruciating headache followed by nausea, photophobia and a substantial rise in blood pressure.[2] This latter reaction is similar to the 'cheese reaction', but at the time the authors of the report were unaware of this type of reaction so that they failed to find out if any tyramine-rich foods had been eaten on the day of the attack.[2]

There is no clear evidence that either of these adverse reactions was due to an interaction between phenelzine and chloral, and no other reports to suggest that an interaction between these drugs is normally likely.

References

1 Howarth E. Possible synergistic effects of the new thymoleptics in connection with poisoning. J Ment Sci (1961) 107, 100.
2 Dillon H, Leopold RL. Acute cerebro-vascular symptoms produced by an antidepressant. J Psychiatry (1965) 121, 1012.

Monoamine oxidase inhibitors + Cocaine

Abstract/Summary

An isolated report describes the delayed development of hyperpyrexia, coma, muscle tremors and rigidity in a patient on phenelzine after receiving a cocaine spray.

Clinical evidence, mechanism, importance and management

A man on 15 mg phenelzine twice daily underwent vocal chord surgery. He was anaesthetised with thiopentone and later nitrous oxide and 0.5% isoflurane in oxygen. Muscle paralysis was produced with suxamethonium and gallamine. During the operation his vocal chords were sprayed with 1 ml 10% cocaine spray. He regained consciousness 30 min after the surgery and was returned to the ward, but 30 min later he was found unconscious with generalized coarse tremors and marked muscle rigidity. Rectal temperature was 41.5°C. He was initially thought to have malignant hyperpyrexia and was treated accordingly with wet blankets, and largely recovered within 7 h. However later it seemed more likely that what occurred was probably due to an adverse interaction between the phenelzine and cocaine because he had been similarly and uneventfully treated with cocaine in the absence of phenelzine on two previous occasions. The reason is not understood, but a delayed excitatory reaction because of increased concentrations of 5-HT is suggested.[1] This is an isolated report and its general importance is not known.

Reference

1 Tordoff SG, Stubbing JF, Linter SPK. Delayed excitatory reaction following interaction of cocaine and monoamine oxidase inhibitor (phenelzine). Br J Anaesth (1991) 66, 516–8.

Monoamine oxidase inhibitors + Cyproheptadine

Abstract/Summary

An isolated report describes unexplained hallucinations which developed in a woman two months after cyproheptadine was added to her treatment with phenelzine.[1]

Reference

1 Kahn DA. Possible toxic interaction between cyproheptadine and phenelzine. Am J Psychiatry (1987) 144, 1242.

Monoamine oxidase inhibitors + Dextromethorphan

Abstract/Summary

Two fatal cases of hyperpyrexia and coma have occurred in patients on phenelzine who ingested dextromethorphan (in overdosage in one case). Three other serious but non-fatal reactions occurred in patients on isocarboxazid or phenelzine.

Clinical evidence

A woman on 60 mg phenelzine daily complained of nausea and dizziness before collapsing 30 min after drinking about 2 oz (55 ml) of a cough mixture containing 100 mg dextromethorphan. She remained hyperpyrexic (42°C), hypotensive (systolic pressure not above 70 mmHg) and unconscious for 4 h before dying of cardiac arrest.[1] A 15-year-old girl taking 45 mg

phenelzine daily (as well as thioridazine, procyclidine and metronidazole) took 13 capsules of *Romilar CF* (dextromethorphan 15 mg, phenylephrine 5 mg and acetaminophen 120 mg in each capsule). She became comatose, hyperpyrexic (103°F), had a blood pressure of 100/60 mmHg, a pulse of 160 and later developed cardiac fibrillation which appeared to be the cause of her death.[2] Neither of these cases is easily understood, the latter being complicated by the overdosage and multiplicity of drugs present, particularly the phenylephrine.

A woman taking 30 mg isocarboxazid daily ingested 1 mg diazepam and 10 ml *Robitussin DM* (15 mg dextromethophan + 100 mg guaiaphensin). Within 20 min she was nauseated and dizzy and within 45 min she began to have fine bilateral leg tremor and muscle spasms of the abdomen and lower back. These were followed by bilateral and persistent myoclonic jerks of legs, occasional choreoathetoid movements and marked urinary retention. These adverse effects persisted for about 19 h, gradually becoming less severe.[4] A further case has been described involving phenelzine and dextromethorphan (in *Robitussin-DM*).[6] Yet another patient on phenelzine also developed muscular rigidity, uncontrollable shaking, generalized hyperreflexia and sweating when given *Robitussin DM*. He responded within 2 h to 10 mg diazepam IV and oral activated charcoal.[5]

Mechanism

Uncertain. The authors of two of the reports[4–6] suggest that these effects may have been due to an increase in serotonin activity in the CNS (sometimes called the 'serotonin syndrome'). A reaction (hyperpyrexia, dilated pupils, hyperexcitability and motor restlessness) has been seen in rabbits treated with dextromethorphan and nialamide, phenelzine or pargyline,[3] and there is some similarity to the MAOI–pethidine interaction.

Importance and management

Despite the very limited information available and our lack of understanding of why it happens, the severity of the reactions indicates that patients on MAOI should avoid taking preparations containing dextromethorphan. Chlorpromazine opposes the development of this interaction in rabbits and has been used successfully in the clinical treatment of the MAOI-pethidine interaction. It might therefore also prove to be useful for this interaction. In one of the cases suxamethonium was used to cause paralysis, and lorazepam to reduced rigidity and myclonus.[6] Diazepam and activated charcoal was used in another.[5]

References

1 Rivers N, Horner B. Possible lethal reaction between Nardil and dextromethorphan. Can Med Ass J (1970) 103, 85.
2 Shamsie JC, Barriga C. The hazards of use of monoamine oxidase inhibitors in disturbed adolescents. Can Med Ass J (1971) 104, 715.
3 Sinclair JG. Dextromethorphan-monoamine oxidase inhibitor interaction in rabbits. J Pharm Pharmac (1973) 25, 803.
4 Sovner R, Wolfe J. Interaction between detromethorphan and monoamine

oxidase inhibitor therapy with isocarboxazid. N Eng J Med (1988) 319, 1671.

5 Sauter D, Macneil P, Weinstein E, Azar A. Phenelzine sulfate-dextromethorphan interaction: a case report. Vet Mum Toxicol (1991) 33, 365.

6 Nierenberg DW, Semprebon M. The central nervous system serotonin syndrome. Clin Pharmacol Ther (1993) 53, 84–9

Monoamine oxidase inhibitors + Dextropropoxyphene (Propoxyphene)

Abstract/Summary

An isolated report describes a marked increase in the sedative effects of dextropropoxyphene in a woman taking phenelzine. An adverse reaction may possibly occur with moclobemide.

Clinical evidence, mechanism, importance and management

A woman taking propranolol, an oestrogen and phenelzine became '...very sedated and groggy and had to lie down...' on two occasions within 2 h of taking dextropropoxyphene, 100 mg, and paracetamol (acetaminophen), 650 mg. She had had no problems with either paracetamol or dextropropoxphene-paracetamol before starting the phenelzine.[1] The mechanism of this interaction is not understood but the symptoms appear to be an increase in the effects of the dextropropoxyphene. There is also animal data suggesting that the effects of dextropropoxyphene are increased by moclobemide, and an ambiguous reference to a patient taking both drugs who may have developed moderate agitation.[2] In the light of these reports concurrent use should be undertaken with caution and good monitoring. More study is needed.

Reference

1 Garbutt JC. Potentiation of propoxyphene by phenelzine. Am J Psychiatry (1987) 144, 251–2.

2 Amrein R, Güntert TW, Dingemanse J, Lorscheid T, Stabl M, Schmid-Burgk W. Interactions of moclobemide with concomitantly administered medication: evidence from pharmacological and clinical studies. Psychopharmacology (1992) 106, S24–31.

Monoamine oxidase inhibitors + Erythromycin

Abstract/Summary

An isolated case report describes severe hypotension and fainting in a woman on phenelzine shortly after starting to take a course of erythromycin.

Clinical evidence, mechanism, importance and management

A woman taking 15 mg phenelzine daily experienced three syncopal episodes 4 days after starting to take 250 mg erythromycin four times daily for pneumonia. When admitted to hospital her systolic blood pressure while lying down was only 70 mmHg, and unrecordable when she sat up. Even though she was not dehydrated, she was given 4 litres normal saline, but without any effect on her blood pressure. Within 24 h of stopping the phenelzine her blood pressure had returned to normal.[1] The reasons for this severe hypotensive reaction are not known, but it is suggested that the erythromycin may have caused rapid gastric emptying which resulted in a very rapid absorption of the phenelzine (described by the author as rapid dumping into the blood stream), thereby allowing its hypotensive side-effects to develop.[1] This seems to be the first and only report of this interaction, so that its general importance is uncertain.

Reference

1 Bernstein A E. Drug interaction. Hosp Comm Psychiatry (1990) 41, 807–8.

Monoamine oxidase inhibitors + Fenfluramine

Abstract/Summary

A confusing situation: the manufacturers advise against combined use, but it has also been claimed that concurrent use is effective.

Clinical evidence, mechanism, importance and management

The recommendation of the manufacturers is that fenfluramine should not be used in patients with a history of depression and during treatment with antidepressants (especially the MAOIs) and there should be an interval of three weeks between stopping the MAOIs and starting fenfluramine.[1] Acute confusional states have been described when fenfluramine was used with phenelzine,[2] but it has also been claimed that in some instances fenfluramine has been used effectively with an MAOI.[3]

References

1 ABPI Data Sheet Compendium, 1985–6 p 1400. Datapharm publications, London.

2 Brandon S. Unusual effect of fenfluramine. Br Med J (1969) 4, 557.

3 Mason EC. Servier Laboratories Ltd. Personal communication (1976).

Monoamine oxidase inhibitors + Ginseng

Abstract/Summary

Two patients have been reported who developed adverse effects when concurrently treated with phenelzine and ginseng.

Clinical evidence, mechanism, importance and management

A woman of 64 treated with phenelzine developed headache and tremulousness when ginseng was added.[1] Another depressed woman of 42 taking ginseng and bee pollen experienced a relief of her depression and became active and extremely optimistic when she was started on phenelzine (45 mg daily), but this was accompanied by insomnia, irritability, headaches and vague visual hallucinations. When the phenelzine was stopped and then re-started in the absence of the ginseng and bee pollen, her depression was not relieved.[2] It is thought unlikely that the bee pollen had any part to play in these reactions and suspicion therefore falls on the ginseng. It would seem that the psychoactive effects of the ginsenosides from the ginseng and the MAOI were additive in some way as yet not understood. Ginseng has stimulant effects but its adverse effects include sleeplessness, nervousness, hypertension and euphoria. These two cases once again illustrate that over-the-counter herbal or 'green' medicines are not necessarily problem-free if combined with orthodox drugs.

References

1 Shader RI, Greenblatt DJ. Phenelzine and the dream machine, — ramblings and reflections. J Clin Psychopharmacol (1985) 5, 65.
2 Jones BD, Runikis AM. Interaction with ginseng. J Clin Psychopharmacol (1987) 7, 201–2.

Monoamine oxidase inhibitors + Lithium carbonate

Abstract/Summary

Four patients are reported to have been successfully and uneventfully treated with phenelzine and lithium carbonate.

Clinical evidence, mechanism, importance and management

Four severely depressed patients who had failed to respond to tricyclic antidepressants or to MAOI, did so when lithium was added to their MAOI treatment. Each of them was treated with relatively modest doses of phenelzine (30–60 mg daily) and lithium carbonate (600–900 mg daily). No adverse reactions were reported.[1]

Reference

1 Fein S, Paz V, Rao N, LaGrassa J. The combination of lithium carbonate and an MAOI in refractory depression. Am J Psychiatry (1988) 145, 249–50.

Monamine oxidase inhibitors + Mazindol

Abstract/Summary

An isolated report describes a marked rise in blood pressure in a patient on phenelzine when given a single dose of mazindol.

Clinical evidence, mechanism, importance and management

A woman on phenelzine (30 mg three times a day) showed a blood pressure rise from 110/60 to 200/100 mmHg within 2 h of receiving a 10 mg test dose of mazindol. The blood pressure remained elevated for another hour, but had fallen again after another 3 h. The patient experienced no subjective symptoms.[1] It is uncertain whether this hypertensive reaction was a direct response to the mazindol (the dose was large compared with the manufacturers recommended dosage of 2 mg daily) or to an interaction. The general importance is uncertain, but it would seem wise to avoid mazindol in patients on MAOI. This is in line with the manufacturers recommendations.

Reference

1 Oliver RM. Interaction between phenelzine and mazindol. Personal communication (1981).

Monoamine oxidase inhibitors + Methyldopa

Abstract/Summary

The concurrent use of pargyline and methyldopa appears to be safe, although an isolated report describes the delayed development of hallucinosis. The order of administration may be important. The concurrent use of antidepressant MAOI and methyldopa may not be desirable because methyldopa can sometimes cause depression.

Clinical evidence, mechanism, importance and management

A hypertensive woman on pargyline, 25 mg four times a day, developed hallucinosis about a month after starting to take 250 mg methyldopa daily, later increased to 500 mg.[5] However a number of other reports describe no unusual reactions or toxic effects during concurrent use.[1–4] The hypotensive response can be enhanced.[5]

The use of both drugs would therefore normally seem to be safe, but it has been suggested that the methyldopa should not be given after the pargyline so that the possibility of the sudden release by the methyldopa of the MAOI-accumulated stores of catecholamines can be avoided.[6] There seems to be nothing documented about the use of antidepressant MAOIs with methyldopa, but the potential depressant side-effects of methyldopa may make it an unsuitable drug for patients with depression.

References

1 Maronde RF, Haywood LJ, Feinstein D, Sobel C. The monoamine oxidase inhibitor, pargyline hydrochloride, and reserpine. J Amer Med Ass (1963) 184, 7.
2 Herting RL. Monoamine oxidase inhibitors. Lancet (1965) i, 1324.
3 Kinross-Wright J, Charolampous KD. Concurrent administration of dopa decarboxylase and monoamine oxidase inhibitors in man. Clin Res (1963) ii, 177.
4 Gillespsie L, Oates JA, Grout R, Sjoerdsma A. Clinical and chemical studies with alpha-methyldopa in patients with hypertension. Circulation (1962) 25, 281.
5 Paykel ES. Hallucinosis on combined methyldopa and pargyline. Br Med J (1966) 1, 803.
6 Natajaran S. Potential dangers of monoamine oxidase inhibitors and alpha-methyldopa. Lancet (1964) i, 1330.

Monoamine oxidase inhibitors + Miscellaneous drugs

Abstract/Summary

No adverse interactions between the MAOI and either anticholinergics, carbamazepine or doxapram have been reported, although the possibility has been suggested. Bradycardia has been reported in two patients on nadolol or metoprolol and phenelzine. An isolated report suggests that the CNS stimulant effects of caffeine may possibly be increased by the MAOI.

Clinical evidence, mechanism, importance and management

Drug manufacturers often include warnings in their data sheets and package inserts about alleged interactions with the MAOI, despite the absence of direct evidence in man that an interaction can actually take place (see the comment at the end of the introduction to this chapter). It is usually suggested that three weeks should elapse between stopping the MAOI and starting the other drug. This prudent precaution protects both the health of patients and the legal liability of manufacturers, but it also means that patients may sometimes be denied the use of a drug which may be perfectly safe. If you speak to the makers many will freely admit that this is the case.

(a) MAOI + Anticholinergics

Although some books and lists of drug interactions state that the effects of the anticholinergic drugs (by implication those which are adverse) used in the treatment of Parkinson's disease are increased by the MAOI, there appears to be no documentary evidence of this in man, although a hyperthermic reaction has been reported in animals.[6]

(b) MAOI + Beta-blockers

It has been claimed[1] that 'MAO inhibitors should be discontinued at least two weeks prior to the institution of propranolol therapy...', but studies in animals[2] using mebanazine as a representative MAOI failed to show '...any undesirable property of propranolol following MAO inhibition.' Bradycardia (46–53 bpm) has been described in two patients taking 40 mg nadolol or 150 mg metoprolol daily for hypertension within 8–11 days of starting 60 mg phenelzine daily. No noticeable ill effects were seen but the authors recommend careful monitoring particularly in the elderly who may tolerate bradycardia poorly.[9] Until the situation is quite clear it would prudent to monitor the concurrent use of any MAOI and beta-blocker.

(c) MAOI + Caffeine

It has been claimed that a patient who normally drank 10 or 12 cups of coffee daily, without adverse effects, experienced extreme jitteriness during treatment with an MAOI which subsided when the coffee consumption was reduced to two or three cups a day. The same reaction was also said to have occurred in other patients on MAOI who drank tea or some of the 'Cola' drinks which contain caffeine.[4] Another patient claimed that a single cup of coffee taken in the morning kept him jittery all day and up the entire night as well, a reaction which occurred on three separate occasions. Apart from this report and another[5] stating that the effects of caffeine in mice are enhanced by MAOI, the literature appears otherwise to be silent about this alleged interaction. Whether this reflects its mildness and unimportance, or its rarity, is not clear.

(d) MAOI + Doxapram

Based on animal studies which reportedly show that the actions of doxapram are potentiated by pretreatment with MAOI, the manufacturers[7] advise that concurrent use should be undertaken with great care. The adverse cardiovascular effects of doxapram (hypertension, tachycardia, arrhythmias) are said elsewhere[8] to be markedly increased in patients on MAOI, and it is also claimed that the pressor effects are enhanced[3] but no clinical data in support of these statements is cited.

References

1 Frieden J. Propranolol as an antiarrhythmic agent. Am Heart J (1967) 74, 283.
2 Barrett AM, Cullum VA. Lack of interaction between propranolol and mebanazine. J Pharm Pharmacol (1968) 20, 911.
3 Martindale's Extra Pharmacopoeia, 29th edn p 1442. Reynolds JEF (ed). Pharmaceutical Press, London (1989).
4 Kline NS. Psychopharmaceuticals: effects and side-effects. Bull WHO (1959) 21, 397.

5 Berkowitz BA, Spector S, Pool W. The interaction of caffeine, theophylline and theobromine with MAOI. Eur J Pharmacol (1971) 16, 315.

6 Pedersen V, Nielsen IM. Hyperthermia in rabbits caused by interaction between MAOI's, antiparkinson drugs and neuroleptics. Lancet (1975) i, 409.

7 ABPI Data Sheet Compendium 1985–6 p 1226. Datapharm Publications (1986).

8 Esplin DW, Zablocka-Esplin B. Central nervous stimulants. In 'The Pharmacological Basis of Therapeutics' 4th edn p 335. Goodman LS and Gillman A (eds). Macmillan NY (1970).

9 Reggev A, Vollhardt BR. Bradycardia induced by an interaction between phenelzine and beta-blockers. Psychosomatics (1989) 30, 106–8

Monoamine oxidase inhibitors + Monoamine oxidase inhibitors

Abstract/Summary

Two patients suffered strokes (one fatal) and another experienced a hypertensive reaction when phenelzine or isocarboxazid were replaced by tranylcypromine. Moclobemide and selegiline can safely be given together or sequentially but some dietary restrictions are necessary (no tyramine-rich foods and drinks). Marked orthostatic hypotension has been seen in two patients on iproniazid or *Parstelin* when given selegiline.

Clinical evidence, mechanism, importance and management

(a) Irreversible, Non-selective monoamine oxidase inhibitors

A patient on 30 mg isocarboxazid daily was switched to 10 mg tranylcypromine and on the following day to 30 mg daily. Later she complained of feeling 'funny', had difficulty in talking, developed a headache, was restless, flushed, sweating, had a blood pressure of 210/110 mmHg (normal for the patient) and a pulse rate of 130 bpm. She died the following day. The cause of death was either a subarachnoid haemorrhage or some other unidentified reaction.[1] Another patient, switched from 75 mg phenelzine daily to 10, 20, 30 and then 20 mg tranylcypromine daily, suffered a subcortical cerebral haemorrhage on the fourth day which resulted in total right-sided hemiplegia.[2,3] Another patient taking 45 mg phenelzine daily, followed by a 2-day drug free period and then 20 mg tranylcypromine daily, experienced a rise in blood pressure to 240/130 mmHg.[2]

The reasons for these reactions are not understood, but one idea is that the amphetamine-like properties of tranylcypromine may have had some part to play. Certainly there are cases of spontaneous rises in blood pressure and intracranial bleeding in patients given tranylcypromine, no other precipitating factor being known.[5] Not all patients experience adverse reactions when switched from one MAOI to another,[4] but until more is known it would seem prudent to have a drug-free wash-out interval when doing so, and to start dosing in a conservative and step-wise manner.

(b) Reversible, selective monoamine oxidase inhibitors

A study in 24 subjects to assess the safety and tolerability of giving 100–400 mg meclobemide and 10 mg selegiline daily, sequentially or combined, found that the adverse effects were no greater under steady-state conditions than with either drug alone, but the sensitivity to tyramine was considerably increased. The mean tyramine sensitivity factors for moclobemide alone, selegiline alone, and moclobemide + selegiline were 2–3, 1.4, and 8–9 respectively. One subject showed a value of 18 when given both drugs.[6] The reason would appear to be that in combination the two drugs inhibit both MAO-A and MAO-B.

In practical terms this means that patients taking both drugs should be given the same dietary restrictions about tyramine-rich foods and drinks (cheese, some wines and beers, etc) which relate to the non-selective MAOIs such as phenelzine and tranylcypromine, although the risks are less. The tyramine sensitivity of these latter MAOIs is about 25 or more.[7] On the basis of work done on the pig (said to be similar to man in relation to the MAO isoenzymes in the brain[8]) it is suggested that if selegiline is replaced by moclobemide, the dietary restrictions can be relaxed after a wash-out period of about 2 weeks. If switching from moclobemide to selegiline, a wash-out period of 1–2 days is sufficient.[6]

(c) Reversible + Irreversible monoamine oxidase inhibitors

A patient taking 150 mg iproniazid daily developed severe orthostatic hypotension on two occasions within an hour of taking 5 mg selegiline. Another patient similarly developed postural hypotension on two occasions within 2 h of taking 5 mg selegiline. He had stopped taking *Parstelin*, two tablets daily, 4 weeks previously.[9] The reasons are not understood. This evidence suggests that selegiline should be given with caution to patients taking irreversible MAOI, or who have recently stopped.

References

1 Bazire SR. Sudden death associated with switching monoamine oxidase inhibitors. Drug Intell Clin Pharm (1986) 20, 954–5.

2 Gelenberg AJ. Switching MAOI. Biol Ther Psychiatr (1984) 7, 36.

3 Gelenberg AJ. Switching MAOI. The sequel. Biol Ther Psychiatr (1985) 8, 41.

4 True BL, Alexander B, Carter BL. Comment: switching MAO inhibitors. Drug Intell Clin Pharm (1986) 20, 384.

5 Cooper AJ, Magnus RV, Rose MJ. A hypertensive syndrome with tranylcypromine medication. Lancet (1964) 1, 527–9.

6 Dingemanse J. An update of recent moclobemide interaction data. Int Clin Psychopharmacol (1993) 7, 167–180.

7 Bieck PR, Antonin KH. Tyramine potentiation during treatment with MAO inhibitors: brofaromine and moclobemide vs irreversible inhibitors. Psychopharmacology (1988) 96, S31.

8 Oreland L, Jossan SS, Hartvig P, Aquilonius SM, Lanström B. Turnover of monoamine oxidase B (MAO-B) in pig brain by positron emission tomography using ^{11}C-L-deprenyl. J Neural Transm (1990) 32, 55–9.

9 Pare CMB, Al Mousawi M, Sandler M, Glover V. Attempts to attenuate the 'cheese effect.' Combined drug therapy in depressive illness. J Affect Dis (1985) 9, 137–141.

Monoamine oxidase inhibitors + Monosodium glutamate

Abstract/Summary

Hypertension in patients on MAOI who have eaten certain foods (soy sauce, chicken nuggets) has been attributed in anecdotal reports to an interaction with monosodium glutamate, however a controlled study found no evidence to support this idea.

Clinical evidence

5 normal subjects were given 400–1600 mg monosodium glutamate or a placebo while taking no other drugs, and after taking tranylcypromine for at least 2 weeks. Episodes of hypertension were seen in 2 subjects on tranylcypromine alone, but no changes in blood pressure or heart rate occurred which could be attributed to an interaction while taking monosodium glutamate as well. The largest dose of monosodium glutamate used was about twice the amount usually found in meals containing large amounts of monosodium glutamate.[1]

There are anecdotal reports of hypertensive reactions attributed to interactions with the monosodium glutamate contained in soy sauce and chicken nuggets in patients on MAOI.[2,3]

Mechanism

None. Monosodium glutamate alone can cause a small rise in blood pressure, and MAOI alone very occasionally cause hypertensive episodes. The reactions reported with soy sauce and chicken nuggets may possibly have been due to a high tyramine content (see 'Monoamine oxidase inhibitors + Tyramine-rich foods').

Importance and management

The authors of the report cited suggest that any reaction is likely to be an idiosyncratic reaction and not due to an identifiable interaction between the MAOI and sodium glutamate.[1] No interaction is established. It should be pointed out that the number of subjects studied was very small.

References

1 Balon R, Pohl R, Yeragani K, Berchou R, Gershon S. Monosodium glutamate and tranylcypromine administration in healthy subjects. J Clin Psychiatry (1990) 51, 303–6.
2 Pohl R, Balon R, Berchou R. MAOI reaction to chicken nuggets. Am J Psychiatry (1988) 145, 651.
3 McCabe B, Tsuang M T. Dietary consideration in MAO inhibitor regimens. J Clin Psychiatry (1982) 43, 178–81.

Monoamine oxidase inhibitors + Morphine or Methadone

Abstract/Summary

No adverse interaction normally occurs in patients on MAOI given morphine, but there are two isolated and unexplained reports of patients on MAOI who showed hypotension, marked in one case and accompanied by unconsciousness. Some very limited evidence also suggests that no interaction occurs with methadone.

Clinical evidence

(a) MAOI + Morphine

A patient taking 40 mg tranylcypromine and 20 mg trifluoperazine daily and undergoing a preoperative test with morphine, became unconscious and unresponsive to stimuli with pinpoint pupils and showing a systolic blood pressure fall from 160 to 40 mmHg after receiving a total of 6 mg morphine. 2 min after being given 4 mg naloxone IV, the patient was awake and rational with a systolic blood pressure fully restored.[1] A moderate fall in blood pressure (from 140/90 to 90/60 mmHg) was seen in another patient on an MAOI given morphine.[6]

In contrast, a study in 15 patients who had been taking either phenelzine, isocarboxazid, iproniazid or *Parstelin* (tranylcypromine + trifluoperazine) for 3–8 weeks, showed no changes in blood pressure, pulse rate or state of awareness when given test doses of up to 4 mg morphine, or to test doses of up to 40 mg pethidine (meperidine).[7] Other patients on MAOI who reacted adversely to pethidine (meperidine), did not do so when given morphine.[3–5] For more information about the MAOI/pethidine interaction see the appropriate synopsis (see Index). Two other studies reported no adverse interaction in patients on MAOI given morphine.[8,9]

(b) MAOI + Methadone

A patient on methadone maintenance therapy (30 mg daily) was successfully and uneventfully treated for depression with tranylcypromine, initially 10 mg gradually increased to 30 mg daily.[2]

Mechanism

Not understood.

Importance and management

The serious MAOI-pethidine interaction also cast a shadow over morphine, and this probably accounts for its inclusion on a number of lists and charts of drugs said to interact with the MAOI, despite good evidence that patients on MAOI who had reacted adversely with pethidine did not do so when given morphine.[3–5] The hypotensive reactions cited here[1,6] are of a different character and appear to be rare. There seems to be no good reason for avoiding morphine in patients on MAOI, but be alert for the rare adverse response. Naloxone proved to be a rapid and effective treatment in one of the cases cited.[1] The extremely limited evidence available suggests that methadone can be given to patients on MAOI, but a stepwise dosing would seem to be a prudent precaution.

References

1 Barry BJ. Adverse effects of MAO inhibitors with narcotics reversed with naloxone. Anaesth Intens Care (1979) 7, 194.
2 Mendelson G. Narcotics and monoamine oxidase inhibitors. Med J Aust (1979) 1, 400.
3 Palmer H. Potentiation of pethidine. Br Med J (1960) 2, 944.
4 Denton PH, Borrelli VM, Edwards NV. Dangers of monoamine oxidase inhibitors. Br Med J (1962) 2, 1752.
5 Shee JC. Dangerous potentiation of pethidine by iproniazid and its treatment. Br Med J (1960) 2, 507.
6 Jenkins LC, Graves HB. Potential hazards of psychoactive drugs in association with anaesthesia. Can Anaesth Soc J (1965) 12, 121.
7 Evans-Prosser CDG. The use of pethidine and morphine in the presence of MAOI. Brit J Anaesth (1968) 40, 279–82.
8 El-Ganzouri A, Ivankovich AD, Braverman B, Land PC. Should MAOI be discontinued preoperatively? Anesthesiology (1983) 59, A384.
9 Ebrahim ZY, O'Hara J, Borden L, Tetzlaff J. Monoamine oxidase inhibitors and elective surgery. Cleveland J Med (1993) 60, 129–130.

Monoamine oxidase inhibitors + Oxtriphylline

Summary

An isolated report describes the development of tachycardia and apprehension in a patient on phenelzine after taking a cough syrup containing oxtriphylline (choline theophyllinate).

Interaction

A woman with agorophobia which was successfully treated with 45 mg phenelzine daily, developed tachycardia, palpitations and apprehension lasting about 4 h after taking a cough syrup (*Bronchodon*) containing oxtriphylline and guiaphenesin. The symptoms recurred when she was given the syrup, and again when given oxtriphylline (*Choledyl*) alone, but not when given guiaphenesin.[1] The reasons are not understood. An adverse reaction with an MAOI has also been reported with caffeine which is another xanthine (see Index), but MAOI-xanthine interactions seem to be rare. It would seem prudent to check that patients given these drugs together are not experiencing any adverse effects, but there would not appear to be a general need to avoid the xanthine bronchodilators.

Reference

1 Shader RI, Greenblatt DJ. MAOI's and drug interactions — A proposal for a clearing house. J Clin Psychopharmacol (1985) 5, A17.

Monoamine oxidase inhibitors (MAOI) + Pethidine (Meperidine)

Abstract/Summary

The concurrent use of pethidine (meperidine) and MAOI's has resulted in a serious and potentially life-threatening reaction in a few patients. Excitement, muscle rigidity, hyperpyrexia, flushing, sweating and unconsciousness occur very rapidly. Respiratory depression and hypotension are also seen. Pethidine should not be given to patients on MAOI unless a lack of sensitivity has been confirmed.

Clinical evidence

Severe, rapid and potentially fatal toxic reactions, both excitatory and depressant can occur:

A woman on 100 mg iproniazid daily became restless and incoherent almost immediately after being given 100 mg pethidine. She was comatose within 20 min. After an hour she was flushed, sweating and showed Cheyne-Stokes respiration. Her pupils were dilated and unreactive. Deep reflexes could not be initiated and plantar reflexes were extensor. Her pulse rate was 82 and blood pressure 156/110 mmHg. She was rousable within 10 min of receiving an intravenous injection of 25 mg prednisolone hemi-succinate.[1]

A woman who, unknown to her doctor, was taking tranylcypromine, was given 100 mg pethidine. Within minutes she became unconscious, noisy and restless, having to be held down by three people. Her breathing was stertorus and the pulse impalpable. Generalized tonic spasm developed with ankle clonus, extensor plantar reflexes, shallow respiration and cyanosis. On admission to hospital she had a pulse rate of 160, a blood pressure of 90/60 mmHg and was sweating profusely (temperature 38°C). Her condition gradually improved and 4 h after admission she was conscious but drowsy. Recovery was complete the next day.[10]

This interaction has been seen in other patients treated with iproniazid,[1,3–5] pargyline,[2] phenelzine,[6–9,18,20] tranylcypromine[10] and mebanazine.[11] Fatalities have occurred. It has also been seen with selegiline, a selective inhibitor of type B monoamine oxidase (MAO-B).[19] Animal data suggest that the effects of pethidine are increased by moclobemide but so far no human data seem to be available.[21]

Mechanism

Not understood, despite the extensive studies undertaken.[15–17] There is some evidence that the reactions may be due to an increase in levels of 5-HT (sertonin syndrome) within the brain, and that a critically high level must be reached before the toxicity manifests itself.

Importance and management

A well-documented, serious and potentially fatal interaction first observed in the mid-1950s. Its incidence is unknown, but it is probably quite low. One study found that 15 patients given various MAOI and pethidine failed to demonstrate the interaction.[12] No problems were also described in another study involving 45 patients on isocarboxazid given pethidine (25–75 mg) preoperatively.[22] Nevertheless it would seem imprudent to give pethidine to those on MAOI unless they are known not to be sensitive.

Churchill-Davidson has suggested[13] that sensitivity can be checked by giving a test dose of 5 mg pethidine, after which all the vital signs (pulse, respiration, blood pressure) are checked at 5 min intervals for 20 min, and then at 10 min intervals for the rest of the hour. If no obvious change has occurred, the whole check is repeated over the next hour with 10 mg pethidine, then with 20 mg, and after 3 h with 40 mg. It is not thought necessary to carry on further because by this stage any sensitivity should have revealed itself. A case is quoted of a patient who demonstrated sensitivity after 5 mg pethidine. The systolic blood pressure fell by 30 mmHg, the pulse rate rose by 20 beats/min and drowsiness developed.[13]

The interaction has been successfully treated with prednisolone hemisuccinate, 25 mg[1] or chlorpromazine.[4] Acidification of the urine would also effectively increase the rate of clearance.[14]

References

1 Shee JC. Dangerous potentiation of pethidine by iproniazid, and its treatment. Br Med J (1960) 2, 507.

2 Vigran IM. Dangerous potentiation of meperidine hydrochloride by pargyline hydrochloride. J Amer Med Ass (1964) 187, 953.

3 Clement AJ, Benazon D. Reactions to other drugs in patients taking monoamine oxidase inhibitors. Lancet (1962) ii, 197.

4 Papp C, Benaim S. Toxic effects of iproniazid in a patient with angina. Br Med J (1958) 2, 1070.

5 Mitchell RS. Fatal toxic encephalitis occurring during iproniazid therapy in pulmonary tuberculosis. An Inter Med (1955) 42, 417.

6 Palmer H. Potentiation of pethidine. Br Med J (1960) 2, 944.

7 Taylor DC. Alarming reaction to pethidine in patients on phenelzine. Lancet (1962) ii, 409.

8 Cocks DP, Passemore Rowe A. Dangers of monoamine oxidase inhibitors. Br Med J (1962) 2, 1545.

9 Reid NCRW, Jones D. Pethidine and phenelzine. Br Med J (1962) 1, 408.

10 Denton PH, Borrelli VM, Edwards NV. Dangers of monoamine oxidase inhibitors. Br Med J (1962) 2, 1752.

11 Anon. Death from drugs combination. Pharm J (1965) 195, 341.

12 Prosser Evans CDG. The use of pethidine and morphine in the presence of monoamine oxidase inhibitors. Br J Anest (1968) 40, 279.

13 Churchill-Davidson HC. Anaesthesia and monoamine oxidase inhibitors. Br Med J (1962) 1, 520.

14 London DR, Milne MD. Dangers of monoamine oxidase inhibitors. Br Med J (1962) 2, 1752.

15 Leander JD, Batten J, Hargis GW. Pethidine interaction with clorgyline, pargyline or 5-hydroxytryptophan: lack of enhanced pethidine lethality or hyperpyrexia in mice. J Pharm Pharmac (1978) 30, 396.

16 Rogers KJ, Thornton JA. The interaction between monoamine oxidase inhibitors and narcotic analgesics in mice. Br J Pharmacol (1969) 36, 470.

17 Gessher PK, Soble AG. A study of the tranylcypromine-meperidine interaction: effects of p-chlorophenylalanine and 1–5-hydroxytryptophan. J Pharmacol Exp Ther (1973) 186, 276.

18 Meyer D, Halfin V. Toxicity secondary to meperidine in patients on monoamine oxidase inhibitors: a case report and critical review. J Clin Psychopharmacol (1981) 1, 319–21.

19 Zornberg GL, Bodkin JA, Cohen BM. Severe adverse interaction between pethidine and selegiline. Lancet (1991) 337, 246.

20 Asch DA, Parker RM. Sounding board. The Libby Zion case. One step forward or two steps backward? N Engl J Med (1988) 318, 771–5.

21 Amrein R, Güntert TW, Dingemanse J, Lorscheid T, Stabl M, Schmid-Burgk W. Interactions of moclobemide with concomitantly administered medication: evidence from pharmacological and clinical studies. Psychopharmacology (1992) 106, S24–31.

22 Ebrahim ZY, O'Hara J, Borden L, Tetzlaff J. Monoamine oxidase inhibitors and elective surgery. Cleveland J Med (1993) 60, 129–130.

Monoamine oxidase inhibitors + Phenothiazines

Abstract/Summary

The concurrent use of the MAOI and phenothiazines is usually safe and effective. The exception appears to be methotrimeprazine which has been implicated in two fatal reactions with pargyline and tranylcypromine.

Clinical evidence, mechanism, importance and management

The concurrent use of MAOIs and phenothiazines has been recommended,[1–3] and a fixed combination (tranylcypromine with trifluoperazine, *Parstelin*) is marketed. Tranylcypromine with chlorpromazine has been found valuable in the treatment of schizophrenia and it may possibly prevent the occurrence of extra-pyramidal symptoms.[9] Promazine has been used safely and effectively in the treatment of overdosage with tranylcypromine.[4] A single report[5] describing the development of a severe occipital headache in a woman on an MAOI as a result of taking 30 ml of a child's cough linctus, attributed this reaction by inference to an interaction with promethazine, but it is now known that the linctus in question contained phenylpropanolamine which is much more likely to have been the cause,[6] (see 'MAOI + Sympathomimetic amines, indirectly-acting'). However unexplained fatalities while taking methotrimeprazine with pargyline,[7] another with methotrimeprazine and tranylcypromine[8] and the third with an unnamed MAOI-phenothiazine combination have been reported.[8]

No special precautions would normally seem to be necessary during the concurrent use of most MAOIs and phenothiazines, with the exception of methotrimeprazine which, because it has been implicated in two fatalities, should probably be regarded as contraindicated.

References

1 Winkelman NW. Three evaluations of an MAOI and phenothiazine (a methodological and clinical study). Dis Nerv Syst (1965) 26, 160.

2 Cheshrow EJ, Kaplitz SE. Anxiety and depression in the geriatric and chronically ill patient. Clin Med (1965) 72, 1281.

3 Janacek J, Schiele BC, Belville T, Anderson R. The effects of withdrawal of trifluoperazine on patients maintained on the combination of tranylcypromine and trifluoperazine. A double blind study. Curr Ther Res (1963) 5, 608.

4 Midwinter RE. Accidental overdose with 'Parstelin'. Br Med J (1962) 2, 1755.

5 Mitchell L. Psychotropic drugs. Br Med J (1968) 1, 381.

6 Mitchell L. (1977) Quoted as a personal communication in 'A Manual of

Adverse Drug Interactions' 2nd Edn p 174. Griffin JP, D'Arcy PF. Wright, Bristol (1979).

7 Barsa JA, Saunders JC. A comparative study of tranylcypromine and pargyline. Psychopharmacologia (1964) 6, 295.

8 McQueen EG. New Zealand Committee on Adverse Drug Reactions: 14th Annual Report (1979). NZ Med J (1980) 91, 226.

9 Bucci L. The negative symptoms of schizophrenia and the monoamine oxidase inhibitors. Psychopharmacology (1987) 91, 104–8.

Monoamine oxidase inhibitors (MAOI) + Phenylephrine

Abstract/Summary

The concurrent use of oral phenylephrine and the older MAOI can result in a potentially life-threatening hypertensive crisis. Phenylephrine is commonly found in proprietary cough, cold and influenza preparations. The effects of parenteral phenylephrine may be approximately doubled. No important interaction occurs between brofaromine and phenylephrine in nose drops, and none seems likely with moclobemide.

Clinical evidence

(a) Phenelzine and Tranylcypromine

A study in four normal subjects, given 45 mg phenelzine or 30 mg tranylcypromine daily for seven days, found that the blood pressure rise following oral phenylephrine was grossly enhanced. In three experiments with 45 mg given orally, the rise in blood pressure became potentially disastrous and had to be stopped with phentolamine. The enhancement was about 13 times in the only experiment which was not stopped, and 6–35 times in the two which were. The rise in blood pressure was accompanied by a severe headache. An approximately twofold increase was seen following parenteral administration.[1]

Another study describes a 2–2.5 times increase in the effects of parenteral phenylephrine,[2] and an exaggerated pressor response is described in a case report.[3] A hypertensive crisis occurred in a woman on phenelzine who took *Ribitussin-PE* which contains phenylephrine.[5]

(b) Brofaromine and Moclobemide

No clinically important interaction occurred in normal subjects taking 75 mg brofaromine twice daily when given 2.5 mg doses of phenylephrine (*Neo-Synephrine*) as nose drops.[6,8] Two studies in normal subjects found that 100–200 mg moclobemide three times daily for up to 3 weeks increased the blood pressure response to infusions of phenylephrine by a maximum of 1.8.[7]

Mechanism

Phenylephrine is given in large doses by mouth because a very large proportion is destroyed by the MAO in the gut and liver, and only a small amount gets into general circulation. If the MAO is inhibited, most of the oral dose escapes destruction and passes freely into circulation as an overdose. Hence the gross enhancement of the pressor effects. Phenylephrine has mainly direct sympathomimetic activity, but it may also have some minor indirect activity as well which would be expected to result in the release of some of the MAOI-accumulated noradrenaline (norepinephrine) at adrenergic nerve endings. This might account for the increased response to phenylephrine given parenterally.

Importance and management

The interaction between the older (irreversible) MAOI and oral phenylephrine is established, serious and potentially life-threatening. Phenylephrine commonly occurs in oral over-the-counter cough, cold and influenza preparations so that patients should be strongly warned about them. Whether the effects of nose drops and nasal sprays are also enhanced is uncertain, but it would be prudent to avoid them until they have been shown to be safe. The response to parenteral administration is also approximately doubled so that an appropriate dosage reduction is necessary.

If a hypertensive reaction occurs it can be controlled with an alpha-adrenoreceptor blocker such as phentolamine, 5 mg IV,[5] or failing that an intramuscular injection of 50 mg chlorpromazine. The simplest alternative is to chew a capsule of 10 mg nifedipine to release its contents, and wash it down with a drink of water.

No interaction occurs between brofaromine and phenylephrine as nose drops.[6] and no clinically important interaction would seem likely between phenylephrine and moclobemide.[4,7]

References

1 Boakes AJ, Laurence DR, Teoh PC, Barar FSK, Benedikter L, Prichard BNC. Interactions between sympathomimetic amines and antidepressant agents in man. Br Med J (1973) 1, 311.

2 Elis J, Laurence DR, Mattie H, Prichard BNC. Modification by monoamine oxidase inhibitors of the effect of some sympathomimetics on blood pressure. Br Med J (1967) 2, 75.

3 Jenkins LC, Graves HB. Potential hazards of psychoactive drugs in association with anaesthesia. Can Anaes Soc J (1965) 12, 121.

4 Korn A, Eichler HG, Gasic S. Moclobemide, a new specific MAO-inhibitor does not interact with direct adrenergic agonists. The Second Amine Oxidase Workshop, Uppsala. August 1986. Pharmacology and Toxicology (1987) 60, Suppl I, 31.

5 Harrison WM, McGrath PJ, Stewart JW, Quitkin F. MAOI's and hypertensive crises: the role of OTC drugs. J Clin Psychiatry (1989) 50, 64–5.

6 Mühlbauer B, Gradin-Frimmer G, Bieck P. Safety of reversible monoamine oxidase inhibitors (MAOI): interaction of brofaromine with sympathomimetic drugs in healthy volunteers. Naunyn-Schmiedebergs Arch Pharmacol (1990) 341 (Suppl) R113.

7 Amrein R, Güntert TW, Dingemanse J, Lorscheid T, Stabl M, Schmid-Burgk W. Interactions of moclobemide with concomitantly administered medication: evidence from pharmacological and clinical studies. Psychopharmacology (1992) 106, S24–31.

8 Gleiter CH, Mühlbauer B, Gradin-Frimmer G, Antonin KH, Bieck PR. Administration of sympathomimetic drugs with the selective MAO-A inhibitor brofaromine. Effect on blood pressure. Drug Invest (1992) 4, 149–54.

Monoamine oxidase inhibitors + Rauwolfia alkaloids or Tetrabenazine

Abstract/Summary

The use of potentially depressive drugs such as the rauwolfia alkaloids or tetrabenazine is generally contraindicated in patients needing treatment for depression. Central excitation and possibly hypertension can occur if the rauwolfia is given to patients already taking MAOI, but is unlikely if the rauwolfia is given first.

Clinical evidence

A chronically depressed woman treated firstly with nialamide (100 mg three times a day) and on the third day with reserpine as well (0.5 mg three times a day) became hypomanic on the following day and almost immediately went into frank mania.[1]

Seven days after stopping 25 mg nialamide daily, a patient was started on tetrabenazine. 6 h later he collapsed and demonstrated epileptiform convulsions, partial unconsciousness, rapid respiration and tachycardia.[2]

Other reports state that the administration of reserpine or tetrabenazine after pretreatment with iproniazid can lead to a temporary (up to 3 days) disturbance of affect and memory, associated with autonomic excitation, delerious agitation, disorientation and illusions of experience and recognition.[3,4]

A delayed 'reserpine-reversal' was seen in three schizophrenics treated firstly with phenelzine for 12 weeks, then a placebo for 16–33 weeks, and lastly reserpine. Their blood pressures rose slightly and persistently and their psychomotor activity was considerably increased, lasting in two cases throughout the 12-week period of treatment.[5]

Mechanism

Rauwolfia alkaloids such as reserpine cause adrenergic neurones to become depleted of their normal stores of noradrenaline (norepinephrine). In this way they prevent or reduce the normal transmission of impulses at the adrenergic nerve endings of the sympathetic nervous system and thereby act as antihypertensive agents. Since the brain also possesses adrenergic neurones, failure of transmission in the CNS could account for the sedation and depression observed. If these compounds are given to patients already taking MAOI, they can cause the sudden release of large amounts of accumulated noradrenaline (norepinephrine), and in the brain of 5-HT as well, resulting in excessive stimulation of the receptors which is seen as gross central excitation and hypertension. This would account for the case reports cited and the effects seen in animals.[7–9] These stimulant effects are sometimes called 'reserpine-reversal' because instead of the expected sedation or depression, excitation or delayed depression is seen. It depends upon the order in which the drugs are given.

Importance and management

The administration of potentially depressive drugs is generally contraindicated in patients needing treatment for depression. However if concurrent use is considered desirable, the MAOI should be given after, and not before, the other drug so that sedation rather than excitation will occur.[6] The documentation of this latter reaction in man is very limited.

References

1 Gradwell BG. Psychotic reactions and phenelzine. Br Med J (1960) 2, 1018.
2 Davies TS. Monoamine oxidase inhibitors and rauwolfia compounds. Br Med J (1960) 2, 739.
3 Voelkel A. Klinische Wirkung von Pharmaka mit Einfluss auf den Monoaminestoffwechsel de Gehirns. Confinia Neurol (1958) 18, 144.
4 Voelkel A. Experiences with MAO inhibitors in psychiatry. Ann NY Acad Sci (1959) 80, 680.
5 Esser AH. Clinical observations on reserpine reversal after prolonged MAO inhibition. Psychiat Neurol Neurochirugica (1967) 70, 59.
6 Natajaran S. Potential dangers of monoamine oxidase inhibitors and alpha-methyldopa. Lancet (1964) i, 1330.
7 Shore PA, Brodie BB. LSD-like effects elicited by reserpine in rabbits pretreated with isoniazid. Proc Soc Exp Biol NY (1957) 94, 433.
8 Chessin M, Kramer R, Scott CC. Modification of the pharmacology of reserpine and serotonin by iproniazid. J Pharmacol exp Ther (1957) 119, 453.
9 von Euler US, Bygoleman S, Persson N-A. Interaction of reserpine and monoamine oxidase inhibitors on adrenergic transmitter release. Biochem Biol Sper (1970) 9, 215.

Monoamine oxidase inhibitors + Sulphonamides

Abstract/Summary

An isolated report describes the development of weakness, ataxia and other adverse effects in a patient on phenelzine when additionally given sulphafurazole (sulfisoxazole).

Clinical evidence, mechanism, importance and management

A woman taking 45 mg phenelzine daily complained of weakness, ataxia, dizziness, tinnitus, muscle pains and parasthesias within seven days of starting to take 4 g of sulphafurazole (sulfisoxazole) daily. These adverse effects continued until the 10-day sulphonamide course was completed. All then disappeared.[1] The reasons are not understood, but as these adverse effects are a combination of the side-effects of both drugs, it seems possible that a mutual interaction (perhaps saturation of the acetylating mechanisms in the liver) was responsible. Concurrent use need not be avoided, but prescribers should be aware of this case.

Reference

1 Boyer WF, Lake CR. Interaction of phenelzine and sulfisoxazole. Am J Psychiatry (1983) 140, 264–5.

Monoamine oxidase inhibitors (MAOI) + Sympathomimetic amines (directly-acting)

Abstract/Summary

The pressor effects of adrenaline (epinephrine), isoprenaline (isoproterenol), noradrenaline (norepinephrine) and methoxamine may be unchanged or only moderately increased in patients taking MAOI. The increase may possibly be more marked in those who show a significant hypotensive response to the MAOI. An isolated case of tachycardia and apprehension has also been described in an asthmatic on phenelzine after taking salbutamol (albuterol). Hypomania was seen in another asthmatic after taking isoetharine. See also Phenylephrine + MAOI.

Clinical evidence

(a) Effects in normal subjects

Two subjects given 45 mg phenelzine daily, and another given 30 mg tranylcypromine daily, for 7 days showed no significant changes in their pressor responses to either adrenaline (epinephrine) or isoprenaline (isoproterenol). Another subject on tranylcypromine, similarly treated, showed a twofold increase in the pressor response in the mid-range of noradrenaline (norepinephrine) concentrations infused, but not in the upper or low ranges.[1]

These results confirm those from two other studies, one with noradrenaline (norepinephrine) and phenelzine[2] and the other with noradrenaline (norepinephrine) and methoxamine in patients taking nialamide.[3] However yet another study in three volunteers on tranylcypromine found that the effects of noradrenaline (norepinephrine) were slightly increased, while with adrenaline (epinephrine) a 2–4-fold increase in the effects on heart rate and diastolic pressure took place, but a less marked increase in systolic pressure. Isoprenaline behaved very much like adrenaline, but there was no enhancement of systolic pressure.[4] Moclobemide is reported not to interact with noradrenaline (norepinephrine)[8,9] or isoprenaline (isoproterenol).[8] Tachycardia and apprehension in a man on phenelzine after taking salbutamol (albuterol) has also been described,[5] and hypomania in a man on phenelzine while taking isoetharine.[6]

(b) Effects in patients with MAOI-induced hypotension

In a study in seven hypertensive patients who showed postural hypotension after being given either pheniprazine or tranylcypromine, it was demonstrated that the doses of noradrenaline (norepinephrine) required to produce a 25 mmHg rise in systolic pressure were reduced to 13–38% and of methoxamine to 30–39%.[3] However another study found no significant change when noradrenaline (norepinephrine) was given to two patients treated with pargyline.[7]

Mechanism

These sympathomimetic amines act directly on the receptors at the nerve endings which innervate arterial blood vessels, so that the presence of the MAOI-induced accumulation of noradrenaline (norepinephrine) within these nerve endings would not be expected to alter the extent of direct stimulation. The enhancement seen in those patients whose blood pressure was lowered by the MAOI might possibly be due to an increased sensitivity of the receptors which is seen if the nerves are cut, and is also seen during temporary 'pharmacological severance'. The reactions of the two patients given beta-adrenergic agonists (salbutamol, isoetherine) are not understood.

Importance and management

The evidence is limited, but the overall picture is that some slight to moderate enhancement of the effects of noradrenaline (norepinephrine) and adrenaline (epinephrine) may occur, but the authors of two of the reports cited[1,4] are in general agreement that the extent is normally not likely to be hazardous. Some caution is, however, appropriate. Direct evidence about methoxamine is even more limited but it seems to behave similarly. None of the studies demonstrated any marked changes in the effects of isoprenaline (isoproterenol).

The situation in patients who show a reduced blood pressure due to the use of an MAOI (this would seem to apply principally to pargyline) is less clear. One study found a very marked increase in the pressor efforts of noradrenaline (norepinephrine) and methoxamine[3] in hypertensive patients on pheniprazine or tranylcypromine, whereas another[7] found no changes in the pressor effects of noradrenaline (norepinephrine) in patients on pargyline. Some caution is clearly needed.

The cases involving salbutamol (albuterol) and isoetharine are isolated and possibly not of general importance. This needs confirmation. The interaction between phenylephrine and the MAOI is dealt with separately elsewhere (see Index).

References

1 Boakes AJ, Laurence DR, Teoh PC, Barar FSK, Benedikter L, Prichard BNC. Interactions between sympathomimetic amines and antidepressant agents in man. Br Med J (1973) 1, 311.
2 Elis J, Laurence DR, Mattie H, Prichard BNC. Modification by monoamine oxidase inhibitors of the effect of some sympathomimetics on blood pressure. Br Med J (1967) 2, 75.
3 Horwitz D, Goldberg LI, Sjoerdsma A. Increased blood pressure responses to dopamine and norepinephrine produced by monoamine oxidase inhibitors in man. J Lab Clin Med (1960) 56, 747.
4 Cuthbert MF, Vere DW. Potentiation of the cardiovascular effects of some catecholamines by a monoamine oxidase inhibitor. Brit J Pharmacol (1971) 43, 471P.
5 Shader RI, Greenblatt DJ. MAOI's and drug interactions-a proposal for a clearing house. J Clin Psychopharmacol (1985) 5, A17.
6 Goldman LS, Tiller JA. Hypomania related to phenelzine and isoetharine interaction in one patient. J Clin Psychiatry (1987) 48, 170.
7 Pettinger WA, Oates JA. Supersensitivity to tyramine during monoamine oxidase inhibition in man. Clin Pharmacol Ther (1968) 9, 341–4.
8 Zimmer R, Gieschke R, Fischbach R, Gasic S. Interaction studies with moclobemide. Acta Pschiatr Scand (1990) Suppl 360, 84–6.

9 Cusson JR, Goldenberg E, Larochelle P. Effect of a novel monoamine-oxidase inhibitor, moclobemide on the sensitivity to intravenous tyramine and norepinephrine in humans. J Clin Pharmacol (1991) 31, 462–7.

Monoamine oxidase inhibitors (MAOI) + Sympathomimetic amines (indirectly-acting)

Abstract/Summary

The concurrent use of sympathomimetic amines with indirect activity (amphetamines, ephedrine, phenylpropanolamine, pseudoephedrine, MDMA, metaraminol, etc.) and the older MAOI can result in a potentially fatal hypertensive crisis. These amines are found in many proprietary cough, cold and influenza preparations, or are used as appetite suppressants. No important interaction occurs with brofaromine and slow-release phenylpropanolamine but immediate-release preparations should be avoided. Indirectly-acting sympathomimetics should also be avoided in patients taking moclobemide.

Clinical evidence

Concurrent use can result in a rapid and serious rise in blood pressure accompanied by tachycardia, chest pains and severe occipital headache. Neck stiffness, flushing, sweating, nausea, vomiting, hypertonicity of the limbs and sometimes epileptiform convulsions can occur. Fatal intracranial haemorrhage, cardiac arrhythmias and cardiac arrest may result. Two examples from many:

A woman who, unknown to her doctors, was taking pargyline, was given phenylpropanolamine for nasal decongestion on the eve of surgery which promptly caused a hypertensive reaction. Her blood pressure rose rapidly from 130/80 to 220/160 mmHg and she complained of occipital headache, photophobia and nausea. She also exhibited sweating and vomited. Two intravenous injections of 5 mg phentolamine partially controlled her blood pressure.[1]

A 30-year-old depressed woman who was taking 45 mg phenelzine daily and 2 mg trifluoperazine at night, acquired some dexamphetamine tablets from a friend and took 20 mg. Within 15 min she complained of severe headache which she described as if 'her head was bursting'. An hour later her blood pressure was 150/100 mmHg. Later she became comatose and died. A postmortem examination revealed a haemorrhage in the left cerebral hemisphere, disrupting the internal capsule and adjacent areas of the corpus striatum.[2]

This interaction has been reported with amphetamine sulphate,[3] d-l amphetamine,[4] metaraminol,[11] methylamphetamine,[5–8] mephentermine,[19] ephedrine,[9,10] phenylpropanolamine,[12–15,24] pseudoephedrine,[18,22,24] and methylphenidate,[19] in patients on tranylcypromine,[3,5,6,9,10,13] phenelzine,[2,4–9,12,14,15,20,24] isocarboxazid,[6] iproniazid,[22] mebanazine,[12] and pargyline.[11] Nialamide is expected to behave similarly but reports seem to be lacking. There are other reports and studies of this interaction not listed here. Extreme hyper-

pyrexia, apparently without hypertension, has with described with tranylcypromine and amphetamines.[16,17]

No interaction was seen in subjects on brofaromine (75 mg twice daily for 10 days) when given slow-release 75 mg phenylpropanoloamine (*Acutrim Late Day*), but immediate-release phenylpropanolamine in gelatine capsules caused a 3.3-fold increase in pressor sensitivity.[28,31] The pressor effects of ephedrine in subjects taking moclobemide were increased by a factor of about three.[33]

Marked hypertension, diaphoresis, altered mental status and hypertonicity (slow forceful twisting and arching movements) occurred in one patient on phenelzine after taking MDMA (3,4-methylene-dioxy-methamphetamine).[27] Increased muscle tension, decorticate-like posturing and coma occurred in another.[32] Both recovered. MDMA is prescribed by some psychiatrists in dosages of 75–125 mg and is also 'street-available' as a recreational drug in doses of 50–100 mg. Its alternative names include AKA, ecstasy, XTC, MDM, Adam, doctor, M and Ms.

Mechanism

The reaction can be attributed to overstimulation of the adrenergic receptors of the cardiovascular system.[21] During treatment with MAOI, large amounts of noradrenaline (norepinephrine) accumulate at adrenergic nerve endings not only in the brain, but also within the sympathetic nerve endings which innervate arterial blood vessels. Stimulation of these nerve endings by sympathomimetic amines with indirect actions causes the release of the accumulated noradrenaline (norepinephrine) and in the massive stimulation of the receptors. An exaggerated blood vessel constriction occurs and the blood pressure rise is proportionately excessive. Intracranial haemorrhage can occur if the pressure is so high that a blood vessel ruptures.[2] The MAOI/MDMA reaction may also possibly be related to the 'serotonin syndrome'.

Importance and management

A very well-documented, serious, and potentially fatal interaction. Patients taking any of the older irreversible MAOI, whether for depression or hypertension, should not normally take any sympathomimetic amine with indirect activity. These include the amphetamines (dexamphetamine, hydroxyamphetamine, methylamphetamine), ephedrine, MDMA (ecstasy) mephentermine, metaraminol, methylphenidate, phenylpropanolamine and pseudoephedrine. Direct evidence implicating benzphetamine, chlorphentermine, cyclopentamine, diethylpropion, mazindol,[23] methylephedrine, phendimetrazine, phenmetrazine and pholedrine seems not to have been documented, but on the basis of their known pharmacology their concurrent administration with the MAOI should be avoided.

Many of these sympathomimetic amines occur in a over-the-counter cough, cold and influenza preparations, and as proprietary appetite suppressants. Patients should be strongly warned not to take any of these without first seeking informed advice. A possible exception to this prohibition is that under very well controlled conditions dexamphetamine and methyl-phenidate may sometimes be effectively (and apparently safely) used with MAOI for refractory depression.[29,30] No clinically important interaction appears to occur with brofaromine and slow-release phenylpropanolamine but immediate-release preparations should be avoided. Moclobemide can interact and the makers advise avoidance of sympathomimetics such as ephedrine, pseudoephedrine and phenylpropanolamine.

If a hypertensive reaction occurs it can be controlled with an alpha-blocker such as phentolamine (5 mg IV) or phenoxyben-zamine, or failing that an IM injection of 50 mg chlorpromazine. 20 mg labetolol given intravenously over 5 min. has also proved to be successful. An effective and simple alternative is to chew a 10 mg capsule of nifedipine to release its contents, and wash it down with a drink of water.[25,26]

References

1 Jenkins LC, Graves HB. Potential hazards of psychoative drugs in associ-ation with anaesthesia. Can Anaes Soc J (1965) 12, 121.
2 Lloyd JT, Walker DRH. Death after combined dexamphetamine and phenelzine. Br Med J (1965) 2, 168.
3 Zeck P. The dangers of some antidepressant drugs. Med J Aust (1961) 2, 607.
4 Tonks CM, Livingstone D. MAOI. Lancet (1963) i, 1323.
5 MacDonald R. Tranylcypromine. Lancet (1963) i, 269.
6 Mason A. Fatal reaction associated with tranylcypromine and methylam-phetamine. Lancet (1962) i, 1073.
7 Dally PJ. Fatal reaction associated with tranylcypromine and methylam-phetamine. Lancet (1962) i, 1235.
8 Nymark M, Nielsen IM. Reactions due to the combination of MAOI's with thymoleptics, pethidine or methylamphetamine. Lancet (1963) ii, 524.
9 Elis J, Laurence DR, Mattie H, Prichard BNC. Modification by monoamine oxidase inhibitors of the effects of some sympathomimetics on blood pressure. Br Med J (1967) 2, 75.
10 Low-Beer GA, Tidmarsh D. Collapse after *Parstelin*. Br Med J (1963) 2, 683.
11 Horler AR, Wynne NA. Hypertensive crisis due to pargyline and met-araminol. Br Med J (1965) 2, 460.
12 Tonks CM, Lloyd AT. Hazards with monoamine oxidase inhibitors. Br Med J (1965) 1, 589.
13 Cuthbert MF, Greenberg MP, Morley SW. Cough and cold remedies: potential danger to patients on monoamine oxidase inhibitors. Br Med J (1969) 1, 404.
14 Mason AMS, Buckle RM. 'Cold' cures and monoamine oxidase inhibitors. Br Med J (1969) 1, 845.
15 Humberstone PM. Hypertension from cold remedies. Br Med J (1969) 1, 846.
16 Lewis E. Hyperpyrexia with antidepressant drugs. Br Med J (1965) 1, 1671.
17 Krisko I, Lewis E, Johnson JE. Severe hyperpyrexia due to tranylcyprom-ine and amphetamine toxicity. Ann InternMed (1969) 70, 559.
18 Wright SP. Hazards with monoamine oxidase inhibitors: a persistent problem. Lancet (1978) i, 284.
19 Sherman M, Hauser GC, Glover BH. Toxic reactions to tranylcypromine. Ann J Psychiat (1964) 120, 1019.
20 Stark DCC. Effects of giving vasopressors to patients on monoamine oxidase inhibitors. Lancet (1962) i, 1405.
21 Simpson LL. Mechanism of the adverse interaction between monoamine oxidase inhibitors and amphetamine. J Pharm Exp Ther (1978) 205, 392.
22 Davies R. Patient medication records. Pharm J (1982) 287, 652.
23 Magrath SM (Sandoz Products Ltd). Personal communication (1987).
24 Harrison WM, McGrath PJ, Stewart JW, Quitkin F. MAOI's and hyperten-sive crises: the role of OTC drugs. J Clin Psychiatry (1989) 50, 64–5.
25 Clary C, Schweitzer E. Treatment of MAOI hypertensive crisis with sublingual nifedipine. J Clin Psychiatry (1987) 48, 249–50.
26 Fier M. Safer use of MAOI's. Am J Psychiatry (1991) 148, 391–2.
27 Smilkstein MJ, Smolinske SC, Rumack BH. A case of MAO inhibitor/

28 Mühlbauer B, Gradin-Frimmer G, Bieck P. Safety of reversible monoamine oxidase inhibitors (MAOI): interaction of brofaromine with sympathomi-metic drugs in healthy volunteers. Naunyn-Schmiedebergs Arch Pharma-col (1990) 341 (Suppl) R113.
29 Fawcett J, Kravitz HM, Zajecka JM, Schaff MR. CNS stimulant potentiation of monoamine oxidase inhibitors in treatment-refractory depression. J Clin Psychopharmacol (1991) 11, 127–32.
30 Feighner JP, Herbstein J, Damlouji N. Combined MAOI, TCA and direct stimulant therapy of treatment resistant depression. J Clin Psychiatry (1985) 46, 206–9.
31 Gleiter CH, Mühlbauer B, Gradin-Frimmer G, Antonin KH, Bieck PR. Administration of sympathomimetic drugs with the selective MAO-A inhibitor brofaromine. Effect on blood pressure. Drug Invest (1992) 4, 149–54.
32 Kaskey GB. Possible interaction between an MAOI and 'Ecstasy'. Am J Psychiatry (1992) 149, 411–2.
33 Dingemanse J. An update of recent moclobemide interaction data. Int Clin Psychopharmacol (1993) 7, 167–80.

MDMA interaction: agony after ecstasy. Clin Toxicol (1987) 25, 149–59.

Monoamine oxidase inhibitors + Tricyclic antidepressants

Abstract/Summary

Because of the very toxic and sometimes fatal reactions which have very occasionally taken place in patients taking both MAOI and tricyclic antidepressants, concurrent use came to be regarded as totally contraindicated, but informed opinion now considers that with extremely careful control it is permissible and advantageous for some refractory patients.

Clinical evidence

(a) Toxic reactions

The toxic reactions have included (with variations) sweating, flushing, hyperpyrexia, restlessness, excitement, tremor, mus-cle twitching and rigidity, convulsions and coma. An illustrative example:

A woman who had been taking 20 mg tranylcypromine daily for about three weeks, stopped taking it 3 days before taking a single tablet of imipramine. Within a few hours she complained of an excruciating headache, and soon afterwards lost con-sciousness and started to convulse. The toxic reactions mani-fested were a temperature of 40°C, pulse rate of 120, severe extensor rigidity, carpal spasm, opisthotonos and cyanosis. She was treated with amobarbital and phenytoin, and her temper-ature was reduced with alcohol-ice-soaked towels. The treat-ment was effective and she recovered.[11]

Similar reactions have been recorded on a number of other occasions with normal therapeutic doses of iproniazid,[1] isocarboxazid,[1,2] pargyline,[3] or phenelzine[4–9,22] with imi-pramine; phenelzine with desipramine[13] or clomipramine;[23,31] tranylcypromine[16,24,26] or moclobemide[29] with clomipramine. Some other reports are confused by overdosage with one or both drugs, or by the presence of other drugs and diseases. There have been fatalities.[13,16,21] In some instances the drugs were not taken together but were swapped without a washout period in between. There are far too many reports of these interactions to list them here, but they are extensively reviewed elsewhere.[10,12,20] Three patients with bipolar disorder developed mania when treated with isocarboxazid and amitriptyline.[25]

(b) Advantageous or uneventful concurrent use

Dr GA Gander of St Thomas's Hospital, London, has stated[14] that 98 out of 149 patients on combined therapy (phenelzine, isocarboxazid or iproniazid with imipramine or amitriptyline) over periods of 1–24 months improved significantly and that the side-effects were '...identical in nature and similar in frequency to those seen with a single antidepressant.... Side effects were easily controlled by adjusting the dosage. None of the serious side-effects previously reported, such as muscle twitching or loss of consciousness was seen.' He also states that more than 1400 patients having combined antidepressants over a period of 4 years '...tend to confirm these findings described.' Dr William Sargent from the same department has also written[15] that '...we have used combined antidepressant drugs for nearly 10 years now on some thousands of patients. We still wait to see any of the rare dangerous complications reported.'

Other reports and reviews describing the beneficial use of MAOI/tricyclic antidepressant combinations are listed elsewhere.[12,19,20,28] Moclobemide is reported not to interact with amitriptyline or desipramine[24,27] but a reaction similar to the serotonin syndrome occurred in one patient when given clomipramine.[29] Only a minor and clinically unimportant change in the pharmacokinetics of amitriptyline occurs in patients given toloxatone.[30]

Mechanism

Not understood. One idea is that both drugs cause grossly elevated monoamine levels (5-HT, noradrenaline, norepinephrine) in the brain which 'spill-over' into areas not concerned with mood elevation. Alternatively it may be related to the serotonin-syndrome seen with selective serotonin reuptake inhibitors.[31] Less likely suggestions are that the MAOI inhibit the metabolism of the tricyclic antidepressants, or that active and unusual metabolites of the tricyclic antidepressants are produced.[12]

Importance and management

An established, serious and life-threatening but apparently uncommon interaction. There is no precise information about its incidence but it is probably much lower than was originally thought. No detailed clinical work has been done to find out precisely what sets the scene for it to occur, but some general empirical guidelines have been suggested so that it can, as far as possible, be avoided when concurrent treatment is thought appropriate:[10,12,18,20,22]

1 Treatment with both types of drug should only be undertaken by those well aware of the problems and can undertake adequate supervision.

2 Only patients refractory to all other types of treatment should be considered.

3 Tranylcypromine, phenelzine, clomipramine and imipramine appear to be high on the list of drugs which have interacted adversely. Amitriptyline, trimipramine and isocarboxazid are possibly safer.

4 Drugs should be given orally, not parenterally.

5 It seems safer to give the tricyclic antidepressants first, or together with the MAOI, than to give the MAOI first. If the patient is already taking an MAOI, it may not be safe to start the tricyclic antidepressant until recovery from MAO-inhibition is complete.

6 Small doses should be given initially, increasing the levels of each drug, one at a time, over a period of 2–3 weeks to levels generally below those used for each one individually.

7 Do not exchange either the MAOI or the tricyclic antidepressant for other members of these drug groups without taking full precautions. A good washout period between the drugs is advisable.

50 mg chlorpromazine given intramuscularly has been used in the treatment of an adverse interaction[24] and one report suggests that patients should carry 300 mg chlorpromazine and take it if a sudden, throbbing, radiating occipital headache occurs, and seek medical help at once.[17]

References

1 Ayd FJ. Toxic somatic and psychopathological reactions to antidepressant drugs. J Neuropsychiat (1961) 2, (Suppl 1), 119.

2 Kane FJ, Freeman D. Non-fatal reaction to imipramine-MAO inhibitor combination. Amer J Psychiat (1963), 120, 79.

3 McCurdy A, Kane AB. Transient brain syndrome as a non-fatal reaction to combined pargyline-imipramine treatment. Amer J Psychiat (1964), 121, 397.

4 Loeb RH. Quoted in ref 10 below as written communication (1969).

5 Hills NF. Combining the antidepressant drugs. Br Med J (1965) 1, 859.

6 Davies G. Side effects of phenelzine. Br Med J (1960) 2, 1019.

7 Howarth E. Possible synergistic effects of the new thymoleptics in connection with poisoning. J Ment Sci (1961) 107, 1000.

8 Singh H. Atropine-like poisoning due to tranquillizing agents. Amer J Psychiat (1960) 117, 360.

9 Lockett MF, Milner G. Combining the antidepressant drugs. Br Med J (1965) 1, 921.

10 Schukit M, Robins E, Feighner J. Tricyclic antidepressants and monoamine oxidase inhibitors. Combination therapy in the treatment of depression. Arch Gen Psychiat (1971) 24, 509.

11 Brachfield J, Wirtschafter A, Wolfe S. Imipramine-tranylcypromine incompatibility. Near fatal toxic reaction. J Amer Med Ass (1963) 186, 1172.

12 Ponto LB, Perry PJ, Liskow BI, Seaba HH. Drug therapy reviews: tricyclic antidepressant and monoamine oxidase inhibitor combination therapy. Am J Hosp Pharm (1977) 34, 954.

13 Bowen LW. Fatal hyperpyrexia with antidepressant drugs. Br Med J (1964) 2, 1465.

14 Gander GA. In 'Antidepressant Drugs' Proc 1st Int Symp Milan (1966). Int Congr Ser No 122, p 336. Excerpta Medica.

15 Sargent W. Safety of combined antidepressant drugs. Br Med J (1971) 1, 555.

16 Beaumont G. Drug interactions with clomipramine (Anafranil). J Int Med Res (1973) 1, 480.

17 Schildkraut JJ, Klein DF. The classification and treatment of depressive disorders. In 'Manual of Psychiatric Therapeutics' p 61. Shader RI (ed). (1975). Little, Brown, Boston, Mass.

18 Beaumont G. Personal communication (1978).

19 Stockley IH. Tricyclic antidepressants. Part 1. Interaction with drugs

affecting adrenergic neurones. In 'Drug Interactions and Their Mechanisms' p 14. (1974) Pharmaceutical Press, London.

20 Anath J, Luchins D. A review of combined tricyclic and MAOI therapy. Compr Psychiatry (1977) 18, 221.

21 Wright SP. Hazards with monoamine oxidase inhibitors: a persistent problem. Lancet (1978) i, 284.

22 Graham PM, Potter JM, Patterson JW. Combination monoamine oxidase inhibitor/tricyclic antidepressant interaction. Lancet (1982) ii, 440.

23 Beeley L, Daly M (eds). Bulletin of the W. Midlands Centre for Adverse Drug Reaction Reporting. (1986) 23, 16.

24 Tackley RM, Tregaskis B. Fatal disseminated intravascular coagulation following a monoamine oxidase inhibitor/tricyclic interaction. Anaesthesia (1987) 42, 760–3.

25 De la Fuente JR, Berlanga C, Leon-Andrade C. Mania induced by tricyclic-MAOI combination therapy in bipolar treatment-resistant disorder. Case reports. J Clin Psychiatry (1986) 47, 40–1.

26 Richards GA, Fritz VU, Pincus P, Reyneke J. Unusual drug interactions between monoamine oxidase inhibitors and tricyclic antidepressants. J Neurol Neurosurg Psychiatry (1987) 50, 1240–1.

27 Zimmer R, Gieschke R, Fischbach R, Gasic S. Interaction studies with moclobemide. Acta Psychiatr Scand (1990) Suppl 360, 84–6.

28 White K, Pistole T, Boyd JL. Combined monoamine oxidase inhibitor-tricyclic antidepressant treatment: a pilot study. Am J Psychiatry (1980) 137, 1422–5.

29 Spigset O, Mjorndal T. Serotonin syndrome caused by a moclobemide-clomipramine interaction. Lancet (1993) 306, 248.

30 Vandel S, Bertschy G, Perault MC, Sandoz M, Bouguet S, Chakround R, Guibert S, Vandel B. Minor and clinically non-significant interaction between toloxatone and amitriptyline. Eur J Clin Pharmacol (1993) 44, 97–9.

31 Nierenberg DW, Semprebon M. The central nervous system serotonin syndrome. Clin Pharmacol Ther (1993) 53, 84–8.

Monoamine oxidase inhibitors + L-tryptophan

Abstract/Summary

Although the concurrent use of monoamine oxidase inhibitors and L-tryptophan can be both safe and effective, a number of patients have developed both severe behavioural and neurological signs of toxicity, and one patient died. L-tryptophan has been withdrawn in some countries because of possible toxicity.

Clinical evidence

A man on phenelzine (90 mg daily) developed behavioural and neurological toxicity within 2 h of being given 6 g tryptophan.[1] He showed shivering and diaphoresis, his psychomotor retardation disappeared and he became jocular, fearful and moderately labile. His neurological signs included bilateral Babinski signs, hyperreflexia, rapid horizontal ocular oscillations, shivering of the jaw, trunk and limbs, mild dysmetria and ataxia. The situation resolved on withdrawal of the drugs.[1]

Other reports describe patients who showed severe[8] or milder [3,7,11] symptoms of toxicity, hypomania[5] or delerium[9] when given beta-phenylisopropyl hydrazine, isocarboxazid, pargyline or phenelzine and tryptophan. Symptoms included alcohol-like intoxication, drowsiness, delerium, myoclonus, muscle twitching, hyper-reflexia, jaw quivering, teeth chattering, diaphoresis and ocular oscillations have been seen.[2,10,11,12,14] One patient showed toxicity with transient

hyperthermia when the dose of tryptophan was increased.[6] Fatal malignant hyperpyrexia occurred in another patient on phenelzine, tryptophan and lithium.[13]

In contrast, concurrent use is reported elsewhere to be both safe and effective,[4] however see the note below.

Mechanism

Not understood. The reactions appears to be related to the 'serotonin syndrome' which can occur with 5-HT uptake inhibitors.

Importance and management

Information seems to be confined to the reports listed. Concurrent use can be effective in the treatment of depression,[4] but occasionally and unpredictably severe and even life-threatening toxicity occurs. The authors of the report detailed above[1] recommend that patients on MAOI should be started on a low dose of L-tryptophan (0.5 g). This should be gradually increased while monitoring the mental status of the patient for mental changes suggesting hypomania, and neurological changes including ocular oscillations and upper motor neurone signs. However it should pointed out that most products containing L-tryptophan for the treatment of depression have been withdrawn in the USA and UK because of a possible association with the development of a serious eosinophilia-myalgia syndrome.

References

1 Thompson JN, Rubin EH. Case report of a toxic reaction from a combination of tryptophan and phenelzine. Am J Psychiatry (1984) 141, 281–3.

2 Hodge JV, Oates JA, Sjoerdsma A. Reduction of the central effects of tryptophan by a decarboxylase inhibitor. Clin Pharmacol Ther (1964) 5, 149–55.

3 Glassman AH, Platman SR, Potentiation of monoamine oxidase inhibitor by tryptophan. J Psychiatr Res (1969) 7, 83–8.

4 Klein DF, Gittelman R, Quitkin F. Diagnosis and drug treatment of psychiatric disorders: adults and children. Edition 2. Williams and Wilkins Co. (1980) 358.

5 Goff DC. Two cases of hypomania following the addition of L-tryptophan to a Monoamine oxidase inhibitor. Am J Psychiatry (1985) 142, 1487–8.

6 Price WA, Zimmer B, Kucas P. Serotonin syndrome: a case report. J Clin Pharmacol (1986) 26, 77–8.

7 Pare CMB. Potentiation of monoamine oxidase inhibitors by tryptophan. Lancet (1963) 2, 527–8.

8 Mueller PD. Life-threatening interaction between phenelzine and L-tryptophan. Vet Hum Toxicol (1989) 31, 370.

9 Alvine G, Black DW, Tsuang D. Case of delerium secondary to phenelzine/l-tryptophan combination. J Clin Psychiatry (1990) 51, 311.

10 Pope HG, Jonas JM, Hudson JI, Kafka MP. Toxic reactions to the combination of monoamine oxidase inhibitors and tryptophan. Am J Psychiatry (1985) 142, 491–2.

11 Baloh RW, Dietz J, Spooner JW. Myoclonus and ocular oscillations induced by L-tryptophan. Ann Neurol (1982) 11, 95–7.

12 Levy AB, Bucher P, Votolato N. Myoclonus, hyperreflexia and diaphoresis in patients on phenelzine-tryptophan combination treatment. Can J Psychiatry (1985) 30, 434–6.

13 Staufenberg EF, Tantam D. Malignant hyperpyrexia syndrome in combined treatment. Br J Psychiatry (1989) 154, 577–8.

14 Oates JA, Sjoerdsma A. Neurological effects of tryptophan in patients receiving a monoamine oxidase inhibitor. Neurology (1960) 10, 1076–8.

Monoamine oxidase inhibitors (MAOI) + Tyramine-rich drinks

Abstract/Summary

(a) Patients taking the older MAOI (tranylcypromine, phenelzine, nialamide, pargyline, etc.) may suffer a serious hypertensive reaction if they drink tyramine-rich drinks such as beer, lager or wine. (b) The hypotensive side-effects of the MAOI may be exaggerated in a few patients by alcohol and they may experience dizziness and faintness after drinking relatively modest amounts.

Interaction, mechanism, importance and management

(a) Hypertensive reactions

A severe and potentially life-threatening hypertensive reaction can occur in patients on MAOI if they have alcoholic drinks containing significant amounts of tyramine. The details of this reaction, its mechanism, the names of the older MAOI which interact and the newer ones which are unlikely to do so (see Table 18.1) are described in the synopsis ' Monoamine oxidase inhibitors + Tyramine-rich foods'. A dose of 10–25 mg tyramine is believed to be required before a serious rise in blood pressure takes place. Calculations made from the figures in Table 18.2 show that a litre (a little under two pints) of some samples of Canadian ale or beer, and about 400 ml of one early sample of Italian Chianti wine, contained enough tyramine to reach the 10–25 mg threshold dosage, and would represent a hazard to patients on MAOI. But some drinks contain too little tyramine to matter. The problem is that there is no way of knowing the probable tyramine-content without a detailed analysis.

The table can be used as broad general guide when advising patients, but it cannot be an absolute guide because all alcoholic drinks are the end-product of a biological fermentation process and no two batches are ever absolutely identical. There may be a 50-fold difference even between wines from the same grape stock.[7] It is claimed by the Chianti producers[4] and others[12] that the new methods which have replaced the ancient 'governo alla toscana' process result in negligible amounts of tyramine in today's Chianti. This seems to be borne out by the results of recent analyses[3,7,13,14] one of which found no tyramine in one sample.[14] Gin, whisky, vodka and other spirits do not contain significant amounts of tyramine because they are distilled and the volumes drunk are relatively small.[14] Alcohol-free beer and lager are not safe because their tyramine-content may be as much or even greater than ordinary beer and lager.[8,15] One patient on tranylcypromine suffered an acute cerebral haemorrhage after drinking a de-alcoholised Irish beer,[7] and hypertensive reactions occurred in four other patients after drinking not more than 375 ml (2/3rds pint) of alcohol-free beer or lager.[15,16]

The risk of a reaction with tyramine is very much less with

Table 18.2 The tyramine-content of some drinks.

Drink	Tyramine content (mg/L)	Ref
Ale (Canada)	8.8	1
Beer (Canada)	6.4, 11.1, 11.2	
Beer (UK)	1.34	7
Beer (USA)	1.8, 2.3, 4.4	1
Champagne (Canada)	0.2, 0.6	2
Chianti (Italy)		
Governo process	0.0, 1.76, 12.2, 10.36, 25.4	1–3,7
Newer process	0.0 – 4.7	3,7,13,14
Gin	0.0	14
Port	0.2	1
Reisling	0.6	1
Sauterne	0.4	1
Sherry (USA)	3.6	1
Sherry (Canada)	0.2	2
Sherry	2.65	14
Wine (from different regions in France)	5.17–3.70	6
Wine, red (Canada, France, Italy, Spain, USA)	3.51 – 8.64 (mean 5.18)	2,6
Wine, red (unstated origin)	1.36	7
Wine, white (Germany, Italy, Portugal, Spain)	1.26 – 5.87 (mean 4.41)	2,6
Wine, white (Germany, Former Yugoslavia)	1.22	7
Vodka	0.0	14
Whisky	0.0	14

the newer reversible and selective MAOI: see 'Importance and management' in the next synopsis. The next synopsis also explains what to do if a hypertensive crisis develops.

(b) Hypotensive reactions

Some degree of hypotension can occur in patients on MAOI (therapeutically exploited in the case of pargyline) and this may be exaggerated by the vasodilation and reduced cardiac output caused by alcohol. Patients should therefore be warned of the possibility of orthostatic hypotension and syncope if they drink.[5] They should be advised not to stand up too quickly, and to remain sitting or lying if they feel faint or begin to 'black out'.

(c) Other reactions

In addition to the hypertensive and hypotensive reactions described in (a) and (b), the possibility that the alcohol-induced deterioration in psychomotor skills (i.e. those associated with safe driving) might be increased by the MAOI has been studied. Moclobemide appears to have only a minor and clinically unimportant effect[9,10] and brofaromine does not interact.[11]

References

1 Horwitz D, Lovenberg W, Engelman K, Sjoerdsma A. Monoamine oxidase inhibitors, tyramine and cheese. J Amer Med Ass (1964) 188, 1108.

2 Sen NP. Analysis and significance of tyramine in foods. J Food Sci (1969) 34, 127.

3 Korn A, Eichler HG, Fischbach R, Gasic S. Moclobemide, a new reversible MAO inhibitor-interaction with tyramine and tricyclic antidepressants in healthy volunteers and depressive patients. Psychopharmacology (1986) 88, 153–7.

4 Anon. Statement from the Consorzio Vino Chianti Classico, London. Undated (circa 1984).

5 Anon. MAOI's — a patient's tale. Pulse (1981) December 5th, p 69.

6 Zee JA, Simard RE, L'Heureux L and Tremblay J. Biogenic amines in wines. Am J Enol Vitic (1983) 34, 6–9.

7 Hannah P, Glover V, Sandler M. Tyramine in wine and beer. Lancet (1988) i, 879.

8 Murray JA, Walker JF, Doyle JS. Tyramine in alcohol-free beer. Lancet (1988) i, 1167–8.

9 Berlin I, Cournot A, Zimmer R, Pedarriosse AM, Manfredi R, Molinier P, Puech AJ. Evaluation and comparison of the interaction between alcohol and moclobemide or clomipramine in healthy subjects. Psychopharmacology (1990) 100, 40–5.

10 Tiller JWG. Antidepressants, alcohol and psychomotor peformance. Acta Psychiatr Scand (1990) Suppl 360, 13–7.

11 Gilburt SJA, Sutton JA, Hindmarch I. The pharmacodynamics of brofaromine, alone and combination with alcohol in young healthy volunteers. Br J Clin Pharmacol (1991) 33, 245P.

12 Kalish G. Chianti myth. The Wine Spectator, July 31st (1981).

13 Da Prada M, Zürcher G, Wüthrich I, Haefely WE. On tyramine, food, beverages and the reversible MAO inhibitor moclobemide. J Neural Transm (1988) Suppl, 26, 31.

14 Shulman KI, Walker SE, MacKenzine S, Knowles S. Dietary restriction, tyramine, and use of monoamine oxidase inhibitors. J Clin Psychopharmacol (1989) 9, 397–402.

15 Thakore J, Dinan TG, Kelleher M. Alcohol-free beer and the irreversible monoamine oxidase inhibitors. Int Clin Psychopharmacol (1992) 7, 59–60.

16 Draper R, Sandler M, Walker PL. Clinical curio: monoamine oxidase inhibitors and nonalcoholic beer. Br Med J (1984) 289, 308

Monoamine oxidase inhibitors (MAOI) + Tyramine-rich foods

Abstract/Summary

A potentially life-threatening hypertensive crisis can develop in those on the older irreversible MAOI (nialamide, pargyline, phenelzine, tranylcypromine, etc.) who eat tyramine-rich foods. Deaths from intracranial haemorrhage have occurred. Significant amounts of tyramine occur in cheese, yeast extracts (e.g. *Marmite*) and some types of salami. Caviar, pickled herrings, chicken and beef livers, soy sauce and avacados have been implicated in this interaction. Some of the newer selective MAOI (amiflamine, brofaromine, cimoxatone, moclobemide, selegiline, toloxatone) interact only minimally or not at all.

Clinical evidence

A rapid, serious, and potentially fatal rise in blood pressure can occur in patients on MAOI who ingest tyramine-rich foods or drinks. A violent occipital headache, pounding heart, neck stiffness, flushing, sweating, nausea and vomiting may be experienced. Two illustrative examples: the first being one of the earliest recorded observations by Rowe, a pharmacist, in a letter after seeing the reaction in his wife who was taking *Parstelin* (tranylcypromine with trifluoperazine).

'After cheese on toast; within a few minutes face flushed, felt very ill; head and heart pounded most violently, and perspiration was running down her neck. She vomited several times, and her condition looked so severe that I dashed over the road to consult her GP. He diagnosed 'palpitations' and agreed to call if the symptoms had not subsided in an hour. In fact the severity diminished and after about 3 h she was normal, other than a severe headache — but 'not of the throbbing kind'. She described the early part of the attack 'as though her head must burst'.[1]

A man on pargyline who, despite eating Sweitzer cheese uneventfully on a number of previous occasions, experienced severe substernal chest pain and palpitations within 15 min. of eating the cheese. His blood pressure rose to 200/114 mmHg. Two other patients experienced headache after eating aged cheese. One of them had a severe nose-bleed and was found to have a blood pressure of 240/140 mmHg.[2]

There are too many reports of this interaction to list them here individually, but they are reviewed extensively elsewhere.[1,9] Blackwell and his colleagues list[5] a total of 110 instances caused by tyramine-rich foods which came to their attention during the 1963–66 period. There have been many since. Tranylcypromine, phenelzine, mebanazine or pargyline have been implicated in this interaction with cheese, yeast extracts, protein diet supplements, miso, pickled herrings, chicken livers, caviar, soy sauce, avocados, New Zealand prickly spinach, beef livers and chianti wine. Many patients recovered fully, but Blackwell lists 26 cases of intracranial haemorrhage and nine deaths.[1] Another review lists 38 cases of haemorrhage and 21 deaths.[8]

Mechanism

Tyramine is formed in foods such as cheese by the bacterial degradation of milk and other proteins, firstly to tyrosine and other amino acids, and the subsequent decarboxylation of the tyrosine to tyramine. This interaction is therefore not associated with fresh foods, but with those which have been allowed to 'mature' in some way (note that tyramine was first isolated from cheese in 1903 and is named after the Greek word for cheese: tyros).[21] Tyramine is an indirectly-acting sympathomimetic amine, one of its actions being to release noradrenaline (norepinephrine) from the adrenergic neurones associated with blood vessels which causes a rise in blood pressure by stimulating their constriction.

Normally any ingested tyramine is rapidly metabolized by the enzyme monoamine oxidase in the gut wall and liver before it escapes into general circulation. However, if the activity of the enzyme at these sites is inhibited (by the presence of an MAOI), any tyramine passes freely into circulation to cause not just a rise in blood pressure, but a highly exaggerated rise due to the release from the adrenergic neurones of the large amounts of noradrenaline which accumulate there during inhibition of the MAO. This final step in the interaction is identical with that which occurs with any other indirectly-acting sympathomimetic amine in the presence of an MAOI (see MAOI + Sympathomimetics'). The violent headache seems to occur when the blood pressure reaches about 200 mmHg. There is also some evidence that other amines such as tryptamine and phenylethylamine may play a part in this interaction.

Importance and management

An extremely well-documented, well-established, serious and potentially fatal interaction. The incidence is uncertain but estimates range from 1–20%.[6,7] Patients taking any of the older MAOI (isocarboxazid, nialamide, phenelzine, pargyline, tranycypromine, etc.) should not eat foods which contain substantial amounts of tyramine (see Tables 18.3, 18.4). As little as 6 mg can raise the blood pressure[3] and 10–25 mg would be expected to cause a serious hypertensive reaction.[3] Because tyramine levels vary so much it is impossible to guess the amount present in any food or drink. An old and mature cheese may contain trivial amounts of tyramine compared with one which is innocuous looking and even mild-tasting. The tyramine-content can even differ significantly within a single cheese between the centre and the rind.[4] There is no guarantee that patients who have risked eating these hazardous foodstuffs on many occasions uneventfully may not eventually experience a full-scale hypertensive crisis if all the many variables conspire together.[2]

A total prohibition should be imposed on the following: cheese and yeast extracts such as *Marmite* (tyramine content up to 3 mg/g), possibly *Bovril* (0.5 mg/g) and pickled herrings (3 mg/g) (see Table 18.3). Hypertensive reactions have been seen with chicken livers[17] and beef livers,[18] caviar,[13] pickled herrings,[16] avocados,[21] soy sauce,[28] miso,[35] a powdered protein diet supplement (*Ever-so-slim*)[31] and New Zealand prickly spinach (*tetragonia tetragonides*).[22] This is not a true spinach as found in the USA or Europe. A number of other foods should also be viewed with suspicion such as sauerkraut, fermented bolognas and salamis, pepperoni and summer sausage because some of them may contain significant amounts of tyramine (see Table 18.3). However the following are often viewed with unjustifiable suspicion: yoghourt, cream and possibly chocolate. It also seems very doubtful if either cream cheese or cottage cheese represent a hazard. Whole green bananas contain up to 65 g/g, but the pulp contains relatively small amounts. The need to plan a sensible and safe diet for those on MAOI is clear. Some, but not all, patients may be partially protected from the cheese reaction if they are also taking a tricyclic antidepressant.[48]

It is usual to recommend avoidance of the prohibited foods for 2–3 weeks after withdrawal of the MAOI to allow full recovery of the enzymes. If a hypertensive reaction occurs it can be controlled with an alpha-blocker such as phentolamine (5 mg IV) or phenoxybenzamine, or failing that an IM injection of 50 mg chlorpromazine. 20 mg labetolol given intravenously over 5 min has also proved to be successful.[28] The simplest alternative is to chew a 10 mg nifedipine capsule to release its contents, and wash it down with a drink of water.[35–7,39]

The newer MAOIs are safer than the earlier ones because they show some selectivity and reversibility. Low doses of selegiline (10 mg daily)[20] and toloxatone[26,47] have been shown not to interact at all, or only minimally with tyramine, however at higher doses selegiline (30 mg daily) has been shown to increase the sensitivity to tyramine 2–4-fold so that a tyramine-free diet has been advised.[41] Moclobemide, brofaromine, cimoxatone and toloxatone selectively inhibit MAO–A. The moclobemide-tyramine interaction is reduced with food present although a modest rise in blood pressure may occur,[27,29,31,38] however the risk of a serious hypertensive reaction with moclobemide,[42,43,45,46] cimoxatone or brofaromine[33,40] is considerably less than with the older non-selective MAOI. For example it has been calculated that patients taking 20 mg cimoxatone daily would need to ingest 57 g *Marmite*, 120 g average cheddar cheese or 3 litres of Chianti wine to reach the critical tyramine dosage level,[25,26] so that a clinically significant interaction is unlikely. The risk of an interaction is also very much reduced with amiflamine.[30]

Table 18.3 The tyramine-content of some foods

Food	Tyramine (µg/g)	Ref.
Avocado	23,0	15,32
Banana pulp	7,0	15,32
Banana (whole)	65	15
Caviar (Iranian)	680	13
Cheese-see Table 18.4		
Country cured ham	not detectable	
Farmer salami sausage	314	14
Genoa salami sausage	0-1237 (average 534)	14
Hard salami	0-392 (average 210)	14
Herring (pickled)	3030	16
Lebanon bologna	0-333 (average 224)	14
Liver-chicken	94–113	17
Liver-beef	0-274	18
Orange pulp	10	15
Pepperoni sausage	0-195 (average 39)	14
Plum, red	6	15
Sauerkraut	55	44
Soy sauce	0-663 ·	34,44
Smoked landjaeger sausage	396	14
Summer sausage	184	14
Tomato	4,0	15,32
Thuringer cervelat	0-162	14
Yeast extracts		
Barmene	157	5
Befit	419	5
Bovril	200–500	23
Bovril beef cubes	200–500	23
Bovril chicken cubes	50–200	23
Marmite	500–3000	23,32,44
Oxo chicken cubes	130	24
Red Oxo cubes	250	24
Yeastrel	101	5
Yex	506	5
Yoghurt	0.2, 3–4	19,32

Table 18.4 The tyramine-content of some cheeses. This table should not be used to predict the probable tyramine-content of a cheese. It is only intended to show the extent and the variation which can occur

Variety of cheese	Tyramine content (µg/g)	Ref.
American processed	50	3
Argenti	188	11
Blue	49, 203, 266, 997	10,11,44
Boursault	10	
Brick	194	11
Brie	21, 180	3, 44
Brie type (Danish)	0	10
Cambozola blue vein	18	44
Camembert	86,125	3, 11
Cheddar		
Australian	226	5
Canadian	120, 136, 192, 251, 535, 1000, 530	5,10
English	0,72, 182, 281, 332, 480, 953	5
Farmhouse	284	5
Kraft	214	5
New York State	1416	5
New Zealand	416, 580	5
Cream cheese	<0.2, 9	3,44
Cottage cheese	<0.2	3
Danish Blue (Gorgonzola type)	31, 93, 256, 369, 294	10, 44
d'Oka	100, 310	11
Edam	100, 214	11
Emmental	24, 225	11,44
Gorgonzola	56	44
Gouda	54, 95	11
Gouda type (Canadian)	20	10
Gourmandise	216	10
Gruyere	64 (mean of seven samples), 125, 514	12,44
Kashar	44 (mean of seven samples)	12
Liederkrantz	1226,1683	11
Limburger	204	11
Mozzarela	158, 410	10,44
Munster	101, 110	11,44
Mycelia	1340	11
Parmesan	15, 65	10,44
Parmesan type (USA)	4, 5, 290	10
Provolone	38	10
Romano	197, 238	10,11
Roquefort	27, 48, 520, 267	10,11
Stilton	466, 1156, 2170	10,44
Swiss	50, 434	11
Tulum	208 (mean of eight samples)	12
White (Turkish)	17.5	12

References

1 Blackwell B, Marley E, Price J, Taylor D. Hypertensive interactions between monoamine oxidase inhibitors and foodstuffs. Br J Psychiat (1967) 113, 349.

2 Hutchison JC. Toxic effects of monoamine oxidase inhibitors. Lancet (1964) ii, 150.

3 Horwitz D, Lovenberg W, Engelman K, Sjoerdsma A. Monoamine oxidase inhibitors, tyramine and cheese. J Amer Med Ass (1964) 188, 1108.

4 Price K, Smith SE. Cheese reaction and tyramine. Lancet (1971) i, 130.

5 Blackwell B, Marley E. Hypertensive interactions between MAOI and foodstuffs. In Neuropsychopharmacology. Proc 5th Int Congr Coll Int Neuro-psycho-pharmacologium. Brill H, Cole JO, Deniker P, Hippius H, Bradley PB (Eds). Int Congr Series no 129, Washington, March 1966. Excerpta Medica Foundation (1967).

6 Anon. Hypertensive reactions to monoamine oxidase inhibitors. Brit Med J (1964) i, 578.

7 Cooper AJ, Magnus RV, Rose MJ. A hypertensive syndrome with tranylcypromine medication. Lancet (1964) i, 527.

8 Sadusk JF. The physician and the Food and Drug Administration. J Amer Med Ass (1964) 190, 907.

9 Stockley IH. Drug Interactions and their Mechanisms. Pharmaceutical Press, London, (1974) p. 5.

10 Sen NP. Analysis and significance of tyramine in foods. J Food Sci (1969) 34, 127.

11 Kosikowsky FV, Dahlberg AC. The tyramine content of cheese. J Dairy Sci (1948) 31, 293.

12 Kayaalp SO, Renda N, Kaymarkcalan S, Ozer A. Tyramine content of some cheeses. Toxicol appl Pharmacol (1970) 16, 459.

13 Isaac P, Mitchell B, Grahame-Smith DG. Monoamine oxidase inhibitors and caviar. Lancet (1977) ii, 816.

14 Rice S, Eitenmiller RR, Koehler PE. Histamine and tyramine content of meat products. J Milk Food Technol (1975) 38, 256.

15 Udenfriend S, Lovenberg W, Sjoerdsma A. Physiologically active amines in common fruits and vegetables. Arch Biochem (1959) 85, 487.

16 Nuessle WF, Norman FC, Miller HE. Pickled herring and tranylcypromine reaction. J Amer Med Ass (1965) 192, 726.

17 Heberg DL, Gordon MW, Glueck BC. Six cases of hypertensive crisis in patients on tranylcypromine after eating chicken livers. Amer J Psychiatry (1966) 122, 933.

18 Boulton AA, Cookson B, Paulton R. Hypertensive crisis in a patient on MAOI antidepressants following a meal of beef liver. Can Med Ass J (1970) 102, 1394.

19 van Slyke L, Hart B. Conditions affecting the proportions of fat and proteins in cows milk. Amer Chem J (1903) 30, 8.

20 Elsworth JD, Glover V, Reynolds GP, Sandler M, Lees AJ, Phuapradit P, Shaw KM, Stern GM, Kumar P. *Deprenyl* administration in man: a selective monoamine oxidase B inhibitor without the cheese effect. Psychopharmacol (1978) 57, 33.

21 Generali JA, Hogan LC, McFarland M, Schwab S, Hartman CR. Hypertensive crisis resulting from avocados and a MAO inhibitor. Drug Intell Clin Pharm (1981) 15, 904–6.

22 Comfort A. Hypertensive reaction to New Zealand prickly spinach in a woman taking phenelzine. Lancet (1981) ii, 472.

23 Clarke A. (Bovril Ltd). Personal communication (1987).

24 Oxo Ltd. Personal communication (1987).

25 Dollery CT, Brown MJ, Davies DS, Lewis PJ, Strolin-Benedetti M. Oral absorption and concentration-effect relationship of tyramine with and without cimoxatone, a type-A specific inhibitor of monoamine oxidase. Clin Pharmacol Ther (1983) 34, 651–63.

26 Dollery CT, Brown MJ, Davies DS, Strolin Benedetti M. Pressor amines and monoamine oxidase inhibitors. In Monoamine Oxidase and Disease. Proc Conf Paris, Oct 1983. Tipton KF, Dostert P, Strolin Benedetti M. (Eds) Academic Press (1984) p 429–41.

27 Korn A, Eichler HG, Fischbach R, Gasic S. Moclobemide, a new reversible MAO inhibitor-interaction with tyramine and tricyclic antidepressants in healthy volunteers and depressive patients. Psychopharmacology (1986) 88, 153–7.

28 Abrams JH, Schulman P, White WB. Successful treatment of a monoamine oxidase inhibitor-tyramine hypertensive emergency with intravenous labetolol. N Engl J Med (1985) 313, 52.

29 Korn A, Da Prada M, Raffesberg W, Gasic S, Eichler HG. Tyramine

absorption and pressure response after MAO-inhibition with moclobemide. The Second Amine Oxidase Workshop, Uppsala, August 1986. Pharmacology and Toxicology (1987) 60, 30

30 Grind M, Alvan G, Graffner A, Gustavsson L, Helleday J, Lindgren JE, Selander H, Siwers B. Clinical investigation of the interaction between amiflamine and oral tyramine in man. In Monoamine Oxidase and Disease, p 497–503, Academic Press, London 1984.

31 Zetin M, Plon L, De Antonio M. MAOI reaction with powdered protein diet supplement. J Clin Psychiatry (1987) 48, 499.

32 Da Prada M, Zurcher G, Wuthrich I, Haefely WE. On tyramine, food, beverages and the reversible MAO inhibitor moclobemide. J Neural Transm (1988) (Suppl) 26, 31–56.

33 Bieck PR, Firkusny L, Schick C, Antonin K-H, Nilsson E, Schulz R, Schwenk M, Wollman H. Monoamine oxidase inhibition by phenelzine and brofaromine in healthy volunteers. Clin Pharmacol Ther (1989) 45, 260–9.

34 Lee S, Wing YK. MAOI and monosodium glutamate interaction. J Clin Psychiatry (1991) 52, 43.

35 Mesmer RE. Don't mix miso with MAOI's. J Amer Med Ass (!987) 258, 3515.

36 Clary C, Schweitzer E. Treatment of MAOI hypertensive crisis with sublingual nifedipine. J Clin Psychiatry (1987) 48, 249–50.

37 Fier M. Safer use of MAOI's. Am J Psychiatry (1991) 148, 391–2.

38 Burgess CD, Mellsop GW. Interaction between moclobemide and oral tyramine in depressed patients. Fundam Clin Pharmacol (1989) 3, 47–52.

39 Van Harten J, Burggraaf K, Danhof M, Van Brummelen P, Breimer DD. Negligible sublingual absorption of nifedipine. Lancet (1987) 2, 1363–4.

40 Bieck PR, Antonin KH. Tyramine potentiation during treatment with MAO inhibitors: brofaromine and moclobemide vs irreversible inhibitors. J Neural Transm (1989) [Suppl] 28, 21–31.

41 Prasad A, Glover V, Goodwin BL, Sandler M, Signy M, Smith SE. Enhanced pressor sensitivity to oral tyramine challenge following high dose selegiline treatment. Psychopharmacology (1988) 95, 540–3.

42 Berlin I, Zimmer R, Cournot A, Payan C, Pedarriosse AM, Puech AJ. Determination and comparison of tyramine during long-term moclobemide and tranylcypromine treatment in healthy volunteers. Clin Pharmacol Ther (1989) 46, 344–51.

43 Da Prada M, Zürcher G. Tyramine content of preserved and fermented foods or condiments of Far Eastern cuisine. Psychopharmacology (1992) 106, S32–4.

44 Shulman KI, Walker SE, MacKenzine S, Knowles S. Dietary restriction, tyramine, and the use of monoamine oxidase inhibitors. J Clin Psychopharmacology (1989) 9, 397–402.

45 Simpson GM, Gratz SS. Comparison of the pressor effect of tyramine after treatment with phenelzine and moclobemide in healthy male volunteers. Clin Pharmacol Ther (1992) 52, 286–91.

46 Warrington SJ, Turner P, Man TGK, Morrison P, Haywood H, Glover V, Goodwin BL, Sandler M, St John-Smith P, McClelland GR. Clinical Pharmacology of moclobemide, a new reversible monoamine oxidase inhibitor. J Psychopharmacology (1991) 5, 82–91.

47 Provost J-C, Funck-Brentano C, Rovei V, D'Estanque J, Ego D, Jaillon P. Pharmacokinetic and pharmacodynamic interaction between toloxatone, a new reversible monoamine oxidase-A inhibitor, and oral tyramine in healthy subjects. Clin Pharmacol Ther (1992) 52, 384–93.

48 Pare CMB, Al Mousawi M, Sandler M, Glover V. Attempts to attenuate the 'cheese effect.' Combined drug therapy in depressive illness. J Affect Dis (1985) 9, 137–141.

Chapter 19
Neuroleptic, Anxiolytic and
Tranquillizing Drug Interactions

The minor tranquillizers include the benzodiazepines, hydroxyzine and other agents used to treat psychoneuroses such as anxiety and tension, and are intended to induce calm without causing drowsiness and sleep. Some of the benzodiazepines and related drugs are also used as anticonvulsants and hypnotics. Table 19.1 contains a list of the benzodiazepines which are referred to in this book.

The major tranquillizers and neuroleptics are represented by chlorpromazine (and other phenothazines), butyrophenones and thioxanthenes. Their major use is in the treatment of psychoses such as schizophrenia and mania. These are listed in Table 19.2. Some of the phenothiazines are also used as antihistamines.

Most of the interactions involving tranquillizers and neuroleptics are listed in this chapter, but there are other synopses elsewhere in this book where the interacting agent is a tranquillizer or neuroleptic. A full listing is given in the Index.

Other benzodiazepines such as flunitrazepam (*Darkene, Flunipam, Rohnipnol*), flurazepam (*Dalmadorm, Dalmane, Dormodor, Felison, Somnol*), lormetazepam (*Loramet, Noctamid, Pronactan*), midazolam (*Dormicum, Hypnovel*), nitrazepam (*Alodorm, Mogadon*), temazepam (*Cerepax, Euhypnos, Lenal, Levanxene, Levanxol, Normison, Planum*) and triazolam (*Halcion, Novodorm*) may be used as sedatives and hypnotics, whereas clonazepam, (*Clonopin, Iktorivil, Klonopin, Rivotril*) and diazepam have application as anticonvulsants.

Table 19.1 Benzodiazepines and other minor tranquillizers

Non-proprietary names	Proprietary names
Benzodiazepines	
Alprazolam	*Tafil, Trankimazin, Valeans, Xanax*
Bromazepam	*Bartul, Brozam, Compendium, Durazanil, Gityl, Lectopam, Lexatin, Lexomil, Lexotan, Neo-Opt, Normoc*
Brotizolam	*Lendormin*
Chlordiazepoxide	*Ansiacal, A-poxide, Benzodiapin, Binomil, Calmoden, Cebrum, Chlotran, Corax, C-tran, Diazebrum, Diazepina, Elenium, Endequil, Equibral, Helogaphen, Huberplex, Karmoplex, Klopoxid, Labican, Liberans, Libritabs, Librium, Lixin, Medilium, Multum, Nack, Normide, Novopoxide, Omnalio, Paliatin, Philcorium, Psicofar, Psicoterina, Relaxil, Reliberan, Reposal, Risachief, Seren, Sintesdan, Smail, Solium, Trilium, Tropium, Viansin, Zeisin*
Clobazam	*Castilium, Clarmyl, Clopax, Frisin, Frisium, Karadium, Noiafren, Sederlona, Sentil, Urbadan, Urbanol, Urbanyl*
Clorazepate	*Azene, Belseren, Covengar, Enadine, Justum, Moderane, Nansius, Novoclopate, Tencilan, Transene, Tranxen(e), Tranxilen, Traxilium, Uni-tranxene*
Clotiazepam	*Clozan, Distensan, Rizen, Tienor, Trecalmo, Veratren*
Diazepam	*Aliseum, Alupram, Amiprol, Ansiolin, Antenex, Apozepam, Armonil, Atensine, Benzopin, Best, Cuadel, Cyclopam, Diaceplex, Dialar, Diapam, Diaquel, Diatran, Diazemuls, Diazepan, Dipam, Dipezona, Dizam, Domalium, Doval, Drenian, Ducene, E-pam, Eridan, Ethipam, Euphorin, Evacalm, Gubex, Lamra, Lorinon, Mandro-zep, Neo-calme, Neosorex, Neurolitryl, Noan, Notense, Novazam, Paceum, Pax(el), Pidan, Pro-pam, Quetinil, Quievita, Relanium, Relivan X, Rival, Saromet, Scriptopam, Sedapam, Sedaril, Serenack, Solis, Somasedan, Sonacon, Stesolid, Stress-pam, Tensium, Tranquase, Tranquirit, Valoxona, Valium, Valrelease, Vatran, Vivol*
Ketazolam	*Anxon, Contamex, Loftran, Marcen, Sedotime, Solatran, Unakalm*
Loprazolam	*Dormonct, Havlane, Sonin*
Lorazepam	*Almazine, Alzapam, Ativan, Control, Donix, Emotival, Idalprem, Kalmalin, Laubeel, Lorans, Lorax, Lorenin, Orfidal, Piralone, Placidia, Placinoral, Punktyl, Quait, Securit, Sedarkey, Sedatival, Sedicepan, Sidenar, Temesta, Tolid, Tranqil, Tranqipam, Trapaxm, Wypax*
Medazepam	*Anxitol, Azepamid, Benson, Elbrus, Lasazepam, Lerisum, Medacepan, Megasedan, Metonas, Narsis, Navizil, Nivelton, Nobrium, Resmit, Serenium, Siman, Templane*
Oxazepam	*Adumbran, Alepam, Anxiolit, Azutranquil, Aplakil, Benzotran, Durazepam, Enidrel, Isodin, Limbial, Murelax, Nesontil, Neurofren, Noctazepam, Novoxapam, Oxanid, Praxiten, Purata, Quen, Quilibrex, Sedokin, Serenid, Serepax, Seresta, Serpax, Sobile, Wakazepam*
Oxazolam	*Convertal, Hializan, Serenal, Tranquit*
Other drugs	
Alpidem	
Buspirone	*Bespar, Buspar*
Hydroxyzine	*Atarax, Atazina, Durrax, Multipax, Neocalma, Orgatrax, Paxistil, Sedaril, Vistaril*

Table 19.2 Phenothiazine, butyrophenone, thioxanthene and related neuroleptics

Non-proprietary names	Proprietary names
Phenothiazines	
Butaperazine	*Randolectil, Repoise*
Chlorpromazine	*Amazin, Ampliactil, Aspersinal, BayClor, Chloractil, Chlorazine, Chlorprom, Chlorpromanyl, Clopratets, Cloracin, Dozine, Hibanil, Klorazin, Klorpromex, Largactil, Megaphen, Novochlorpromazine, Procalm, Promacid, Promapar, Protran, Prozil, Prozin, Repazine*
Fluphenazine	*Anatenazine, Anatensol, Dapotum, Eutimox, Lyogen, Modecate, Moditen, Omca, Pacinol, Permitil, Prolixin, Sevinol*
Mesoridazine	*Imagotan, Serentil*
Methotrimeprazine	*Levonormal, Levoprome, Procrazine, Sinogan, Sofmin, Tisercin, Veractil*
Perphenazine	*Decentan, Fentazin, Trilafon*
Prochlorperazine	*Anti-naus, Buccastem, Compazine, Stemetil, Vertigon*
Promazine	*Calmotal, Neuroplegil, Prazine, Promabec, Promanyl, Protactyl, Sparine, Talofen*
Thioridazine	*Mallorol, Meleril, Mellaril, Melleretten, Melleril*
Trifluoperazine	*Calmazine, Clinazine, Eskazine, Flumatets, Jatroneural, Modalina, Nerolet, Novoflurazine, Pentazine, Solazine, Stelazine, Terfluzin, Triflurin, Tripazine*
Butyrophenones	
Benperidol	*Anquil, Frenactil, Glianimon, Psicoben*
Droperidol	*Dehyrobenperidol, Dridol, Droleptan, Inapsin(e), Sintodian*
Haloperidol	*Bioperidolo, Brotopon, Dozic, Duraperidol, Haldol, Halosten, Linton, Novoperidol, Pacedol, Peluces, Peridol, Serenace, Sigaperidol, Sylador, Tamide*
Thioxanthenes	
Chlorprothixene	*Taractan, Tarasan, Truxal, Truxaletten*
Flupenthixol	*Depixol, Emergil, Fluanxol*
Thiothixene	*Navane*
Other Drugs	
Clozapine	
Loxapine	*Daxolin, Desconex, Loxapac, Loxitane*
Molindone	*Lidone*
Sulpiride	*Abilit, Aiglonyl, Arminol, Biomaride, Championyl, Confidan, Coolspan, Digton, Dixibon, Dobren, Dogmatil, Dolmatil, Drominetas, Eglonyl, Euquilid, Eusulpid, Guastil, Kalpiride, Lebopride, Lusedan, Meresa, Miradol, Mirbanil, Misulvan, Neogama, Neoride, Omperan, Sato, Sernevin, Sicofrenol, Sulpitil, Tepavil, Vipral*

Ademetionine + Clomipramine

Abstract/Summary

A severe reaction, diagnosed as serotonin syndrome, developed in a woman on ademetionine (S-adenosylmethionine) shortly after her clomipramine dosage was raised.

Clinical evidence, mechanism, importance and management

An elderly woman with a major affective disorder was treated with 100 mg ademetionine (S-adenosylmethionine) daily, given intramuscularly, and 25 mg clomipramine daily for 10 days. About 2–3 days after the clomipramine dosage was raised to 75 mg daily, she became progressively agitated, anxious and confused. On admittance to hospital she was stuporous, with a pulse rate of 130, a breathing rate of 30 per min, and she had diarrhoea, myoclonus, generalized tremors, rigidity, hyperreflexia, shivering, profound diaphoresis and dehydration. Her temperature rose from 40.5 to 43° C. She had no infection, and the diagnosis was of serotonin syndrome. The drugs were withdrawn and she was given dantrolene 50 mg IV every 6 hours for 48 h. She made a complete recovery.[1] The reason for this severe adverse reaction is not understood.

Direct information is limited to this single case report, but clearly these two drugs should only be given together with great caution, if at all.

Reference

1 Iruela LM, Minguez L, Merino J, Monedero G. Toxic interaction of S-adenosylmethionine and clomipramine. Am J Psychiatry (1993) 150, 522.

Alpidem + Cimetidine

Abstract/Summary, clinical evidence, mechanism, importance and management

A study in normal subjects found no evidence that 1 g cimetidine for 22 days significantly affected the pharmacokinetics of single 50 mg doses of alpidem.[1] No special precautions seem necessary but more confirmatory study is needed.

Reference

1 Desager JP, Hulhoven R, Harvengt C, Bianchetti G. Effect of cimetidine on the pharmacodynamics, pharmacokinetics and biotransformation of a single oral dose of alpidem. Int J Clin Pharmacol Ther Tox (1990) 28, 498–503.

Benzodiazepines + Acetazolamide

Abstract/Summary

Although acetazolamide can be used to treat acute mountain sickness at very high altitudes, it may not protect climbers from the respiratory depressant effects of benzodiazepines such as triazolam.

Clinical evidence, mechanism, importance and management

Acetazolamide is sometimes used by climbers at very high altitudes as a prophylactic against acute mountain sickness, one of its effects being to improve sleep at high altitudes, probably because it improves oxygenation. Benzodiazepines, also used in this situation to treat insomnia, are believed to have the opposite effect because they reduce the normal respiratory response to hypoxia. This was demonstrated by a Japanese climber in the Himalayas who, while taking 500 mg acetazolamide daily and 0.5 mg triazolam, needed to be 'reminded' to hyperventilate in order to relieve his hypoxia while returning from a climb. The acetazolamide did not prevent and may possibly have increased the central ventilatory depression of the triazolam. The authors of the report advise against taking these two drugs together at high altitudes,[1] thus confirming a previous warning about the risks of taking acetazolamide and benzodiazepines in this situation.[2]

References

1 Masuyama S, Hirata K, Saito A. 'Ondine's curse': side-effect of acetazolamide? Amer J Med (1989) 86, 637.
2 Sutton JR, Powles ACR, Gray GW, Houston CS. Insomnia, sedation and high altitude cerebral oedema. Lancet (1979) 1, 165.

Benzodiazepines + Antacids

Abstract/Summary

The absorption of chlordiazepoxide and diazepam is slightly delayed by the concurrent use of aluminium and magnesium hydroxide or trisilicate antacids. The absorption of single doses of clorazepate may be reduced, but chronic dosing is unaffected. These interactions appear to be of little or no importance.

Clinical evidence

Ten healthy subjects taking 7.5 mg clorazepate nightly were given water, low dose *Maalox* (30 ml) or high dose *Maalox* (120 ml) for 10 days in random sequence. The mean steady-state serum levels of the active metabolite (desmethyldiazepam) were not affected by *Maalox*, although they varied widely between individuals.[1]

This is in line with another report[6] but contrasts with a

single-dose study in which the peak plasma concentration of desmethyldiazepam was delayed and reduced about one-third by the use of *Maalox*.[2] The 48-hour AUC was reduced about 10%. Chlordiazepoxide absorption (single dose) was delayed by *Maalox*, though the total amount of drug absorbed was not significantly affected.[3] Similar results have been found with diazepam.[4]

Mechanism

The delay in the absorption of chlordiazepoxide and diazepam is attributed to the effect of the antacid on gastric emptying. Clorazepate on the other hand is a 'pro-drug' which needs acid conditions in the stomach for conversion (hydrolysis and decarboxylation) to its active form. Antacids are presumed to inhibit this conversion by raising the pH of the stomach contents.[5]

Importance and management

Most of the reports describe single dose studies, but what is known suggests that no interaction of any clinical importance is likely during long-term treatment with chlordiazepoxide, diazepam or clorazepate. No special precautions seem to be necessary. Whether the delay in absorption (particularly with clorazepate) has an undesirable effect in those who only take benzodiazepines during acute episodes of anxiety and who need rapid relief is uncertain. Information about other benzodiazepines is lacking.

References

1 Shader RI, Ciraulo DA, Greenblatt DJ, Harmatz JS. Steady-state plasma desmethyldiazepam during long-term clorazepate use: effect of antacids. Clin Pharmacol Ther (1982) 31, 180–3.
2 Shader RI, Georgotas A, Greenblatt DJ, Harmatz JS, Allen MD. Impaired absorption of desmethyldiazepam from clorazepate by magnesium aluminium hydroxide. Clin Pharmacol Ther (1978) 24, 308–15.
3 Greenblatt DJ, Shader RI, Harmatz JS, Franke K, Koch-Weser J. Influence of magnesium and aluminium hydroxide mixture on chlordiazepoxide absorption. Clin Pharmacol Ther (1976) 19, 234–9.
4 Greenblatt DJ, Allen DA, MacLaughlin DS, Harmatz JS, Shader RI. Diazepam absorption: effect of antacids and food. Clin Pharmacol Ther (1978) 24, 600–9.
5 Abruzzo CW, Macasieb T, Weinfeld R, Rider JA, Kaplan SA. Changes in the oral absorption characteristics in man of dipotassium clorazepate at normal and elevated gastric pH. J Pharmacokinet Biopharm (1977) 5, 377.
6 Chun AHC, Carrigan PJ, Hoffman DJ, Kershner RP, Stuart JD. Effect of antacids on absorption of clorazepate. Clin Pharmacol Ther (1977) 22, 329.

Benzodiazepines + Anticonvulsants

Abstract/Summary

The concurrent use of benzodiazepines and non-benzodiazepine anticonvulsants is common and is possibly accompanied by changes in serum levels, but normally these changes are not of clinical importance. However barbiturate intoxication has been attributed in a single case report to the concurrent use of chlordiazepoxide, and another single case describes a marked fall in serum alprazolam levels due to the use of carbamazepine. Three patients developed phenytoin toxicity when given clobazam.

Clinical evidence

(a) Alprazolam + Carbamazepine

A patient with atypical bipolar disorder and panic attacks, being treated with 7.5 mg alprazolam daily, showed a more than 50% reduction in serum alprazolam levels (from 43 to 19.3 ng/ml) when concurrently treated with 300 mg carbamazepine daily, accompanied by a deterioration in his clinical condition.[5]

(b) Chlordiazepoxide + Phenobarbitone

A single case report describes a man given phenobarbitone and chlordiazepoxide who demonstrated drowsiness, unsteadiness, slurred speech, nystagmus, poor memory and hallucinations, all of which disappeared once the phenobarbitone was withdrawn. Substantial doses of chlordiazepoxide were well tolerated.[1]

(c) Clobazam + Anticonvulsants

A further study found that phenytoin and carbamazepine reduce the serum levels of clobazam and increase the levels of norclobazam, but phenobarbitone reduces the levels of both. Sodium valproate did not have a marked effect.[6] Since norclobazam retains some anticonvulsant activity the effect of carbamazepine may possibly have no clinical significance, but this needs further study. A report describes elevated phenytoin serum levels and toxicity in three patients when concurrently treated with clobazam.[7]

(d) Clonazepam + Anticonvulsants

Clonazepam in slowly increasing doses up to a maximum of 4–6 mg/day given over a 6-week period to patients on phenobarbitone or carbamazepine, alone or in combination, had no effect on either phenobarbitone or carbamazepine serum levels.[2] On the other hand a study in seven subjects given 1 mg clonazepam daily showed that carbamazepine (200 mg daily) over a 3-week period reduced clonazapam serum levels and its half-life.[3] A similar reduction in steady-state clonazepam levels but a rise in norclobazam levels in normal subjects is described in another study.[4]

Mechanisms

Uncertain. Changes in the drug metabolism (increases and decreases) due to enzyme induction and inhibition are probably responsible.

Importance and management

None of these interactions is well documented, nor do they appear to be of general importance. Nevertheless concurrent use should be well monitored for any evidence of changes in seizure frequency or increases in side-effects.

References

1 Kane FJ, McCurdy RL. An unusual reaction to combined Librium-barbiturate therapy. Am J Psychiatry (1964) 120, 816.
2 Johannessen SI, Strandjord RE, Muthe-Kaas AW. Lack of effect of clonazepam on serum levels of diphenylhydantoin, phenobarbital and carbamazepine. Acta Neurol Scand (1977) 55, 506.
3 Lai AA, Levy RH, Cutler RE. Time course of interaction between carbamazepine and clonazepam. Clin Pharmacol Ther (1978) 24, 316.
4 Levy RH, Lane EA, Guyot M, Brachet-Lierman A, Cenraud G, Loiseau P. Analysis of parent drug-metabolite relationship in the presence of an inducer. Application to the carbamazepine-clobazam interaction in normal man. Drug Metab Dispos (1983) 11, 286–92.
5 Arana GW, Epstein S, Molloy M, Greenblatt DJ. Carbamazepine-induced reduction of plasma alprazolam concentrations: a clinical case report. J Clin Psychiatry (1988) 49, 448–9.
6 Bun H, Monjanel-Mouterde S, Noel F, Durand A, Cano J-P. Effects of age and antiepileptic drugs on plasma levels and kinetics of clobazam and N-desmethylclobazam. Pharmacol Toxicol (1990) 67, 136–40.
7 Zifkin B, Sherwin A, Andermann F. Phenytoin toxicity due to interaction with clobazam. Neurology (1991) 41, 313–4.

Benzodiazepines + Atropine or Hyoscine

Abstract/Summary

Atropine and hyoscine do not affect the absorption of diazepam nor its sedative effects.

Clinical evidence, mechanism, importance and management

A study in eight normal subjects given single 10 mg oral doses of diazepam showed that serum diazepam levels were not significantly changed by the concurrent use of 1 mg atropine or 1 mg hyoscine, nor were the sedative effects of the diazepam altered.[1]

Reference

1 Gregoretti SM, Uges DRA. Influence of oral atropine or hyoscine on the absorption of oral diazepam. Br J Anaesth (1982) 54, 1231–4.

Benzodiazepines + Beta-blockers

Abstract/Summary

A small and probably clinically insignificant reduction in the metabolism of diazepam occurs if propranolol or metoprolol
are taken concurrently. Bromazepam and metoprolol also appear to interact but not to a clinically significant extent. More importantly there is some suggestion that patients on diazepam may possibly be more accident-prone while taking metoprolol.

Clinical evidence, mechanism, importance and management

The clearance from the body of diazepam in man is reduced 8% by propranolol[1] and 18% by metoprolol,[2] but propranolol has no effect on the clearance of alprazolam,[1] lorazepam[1] or oxazepam.[7] Labetalol also does not affect oxazepam.[7] Another study found that the AUC of diazepam was increased 2% by metoprolol, but no statistically significant changes were seen with atenolol or propranolol.[6] Studies with metoprolol, bromazepam and lorazepam found that the bromazepam AUC was increased 35% by metoprolol and bromazepam increased the effect of metoprolol on systolic blood pressures, but no important interactions occurred with lorazepam.[8]

All of these pharmacokinetic changes are either relatively small or appear not to be clinically unimportant, however studies of psychomotor performance in man have shown that simple reaction times with oxazepam combined with either propranolol or labetalol are increased,[7] and those taking diazepam and metoprolol have a reduced kinetic visual acuity (KVA).[3] The significance of this is that low KVA scores are associated with fatigue and accident-proneness in professional drivers.[4] Moreover, choice reaction times at 2 h were also found to be lengthened when taking diazepam and metoprolol, propranolol or atenolol, but at 8 h they only persisted with diazepam and metoprolol.[3,5] Information is very limited indeed, but what is known so far suggests that patients who drive and who are given diazepam and metoprolol in particular should be given some warning. There seems to be no information about other benzodiazepines and beta-blockers. More study is needed.

References

1 Ochs HR, Greenblatt DJ, Verburg-Ochs B. Propranolol interactions with diazepam, lorazepam and alprazolam. Clin Pharmacol Ther (1984) 36, 451–5.
2 Klotz U, Reimann IW. Pharmacokinetic and pharmacodynamic interaction study of diazepam and metoprolol. Eur J Clin Pharmacol (1984) 26, 223–6.
3 Betts TA, Crowe A, Knight R, Raffle A, Parson A, Blake A, Hawksworth G, Petrie JC. Is there a clinically relevant interaction between diazepam and lipophilic beta-blocking drugs? Drugs (1983) 25 (Suppl 2) 279–80.
4 Suzumura A. Visual aptitude tests with the use of the KVS tester. Annual Report of the Research Institute of Environmental Medicine, Nagoya Univeristy, Japan (1969) 17, 59–72.
5 Betts TA, Knight R, Crowe A, Blake A, Harvey P, Mortiboy D. Effect of beta-blockers on the psychomotor performance in normal volunteers. Eur J Clin Pharmacol (1985) 28 (Suppl) 39–49.
6 Hawksworth G, Betts T, Crowe A, Knight R, Nyemitei-Addo I, Parry K, Petrie JC, Raffle JC, Parsons A. Diazepam/beta-adrenoceptor antagonist interactions. Br J Clin Pharmac (1984) 17, 69–76S.
7 Sonne J, Dossing M, Loft S, Olesen KL, Vollmer-Larsen A, Victor MA, Hamberg O, Thyssen H. Single dose pharmacokinetics and pharmacodynamics of oral oxazepam during concomitant administration of propranolol and labetalol. Br J Clin Pharmac (1990) 29, 33–7.

8 Scott AK, Cameron GA, Hawksworth GM. Interaction of metoprolol with lorazepam and bromazepam. Eur J Clin Pharmacol (1991) 40, 405–9.

Benzodiazepines + Calcium channel blockers

Abstract/Summary

Diltiazem and felodipine appear not to interact significantly with diazepam, nor nitrendipine with midazolam.

Clinical evidence, mechanism, importance and management

Single 5 mg doses of diazepam and 60 mg diltiazem were given to six subjects. Plasma levels of each drug were not significantly altered by the presence of the other drug.[1] The pharmacokinetics of 10 mg diazepam IV were unchanged in 12 normal subjects after taking felodipine for 12 days but the AUC and peak serum levels of desmethyldiazepam were raised 14 and 18% respectively.[3] A study in nine subjects found that the pharmacokinetics and pharmacodynamics of midazolam were unaffected by a single 20 mg doses of nitrendipine.[2] No special precautions would seem necessary during concurrent use of any of these drugs. There seems to be no information about other benzodiazepines and calcium channel blockers.

Reference

1 Etoh A, Kohno K. Studies on the drug interaction of diltiazem. IV. Relationship between first pass metabolism of various drugs and the absorption enhancing effect of diltiazem. Yakugaku Zasshi (1983) 103, 581–8.
2 Handel J, Ziegler G, Gemeinhardt A, Stuber H, Fischer C, Klotz U. Lack of effect of nitrendipine on the pharmacokinetics and pharmacodynamics of midazolam during steady state. Br J Clin Pharmacol (1988) 25, 243–50.
3 Meyer BH, Muller FO, Hundt HK, Luus HG, de la Rey N, Rothig HJ. The effects of felodipine on the pharmacokinetics of diazepam. Int J Clin Pharmacol Ther Toxicol (1992) 30, 117–21.

Benzodiazepines + Cholestyramine/ Neomycin

Abstract/Summary

The loss of lorazepam from the body is increased by cholestyramine/neomycin.

Clinical evidence, mechanism, importance and management

A study in seven normal subjects found that neomycin (1 g 6 hourly) plus 4 g cholestyramine (4 g 4-hourly) reduced the half-life of oral lorazepam by 26% (from 15.8 to 11.7 hr) and increased the clearance of free lorazepam by 34% (from 8.5 to 11.39 ml/min/kg).[1] The reasons are not clear but parallel

studies using intravenous lorazepam[1] suggested that these two drugs may interfere with the possible enterohepatic circulation of lorazepam.

The clinical importance of this interaction is uncertain but probably small, however be alert for any evidence of a reduced lorazepam effect. Increase the dose if necessary. Separating the dosages may not prevent this interaction if it is true that the enterohepatic circulation is involved. There is no evidence as yet that other benzodiazepines interact similarly.

Reference

1 Herman RJ, Duc Van Pham J, Szakacs CBN. Disposition of lorazepam in human beings: enterohepatic recirculation and first-pass effect. Clin Pharmacol Ther (1989) 46, 18–25.

Benzodiazepines + Cimetidine, Ranitidine, Famotidine, Nizatidine

Abstract/Summary

The serum levels of adinazolam, alprazolam, chlordiazepoxide, clobazam, clorazepate, diazepam, flurazepam, midazolam (?), nitrazepam, triazolam (and probably halazepam and prazepam) are raised by cimetidine, but normally this appears to be of little or no clinical importance and only the occasional patient may experience an increase in the effects (sedation). Clotiazepam, lorazepam, lormetazepam, oxazepam and temazepam are not normally affected by cimetidine. Famotidine, nizatidine and ranitidine do not interact with most benzodiazepines, except possibly midazolam and triazolam.

Clinical evidence

Ten patients showed a combined serum level rise of 75% in diazepam and desmethyldiazepam (the active metabolite) after taking 1200 mg cimetidine daily for a fortnight, but reaction times and other motor and intellectual tests remained unaffected.[1]

Other reports also describe a rise in the serum levels of diazepam (associated with increased sedation in one report[19]) due to cimetidine.[2–4,30,36] Generalized incoordination has also been described in one individual.[22] Rises in serum levels occur with other benzodiazepines: adinazolam,[28] alprazolam,[9,10] chlordiazepoxide,[11] clobazam,[24] clorazepate,[12] flurazepam,[7] nitrazepam,[13] and triazolam.[9,10] Liver cirrhosis increases the effects of cimetidine on the loss of chlordiazepoxide.[39] Confusion has been reported in a man on clorazepate when given cimetidine,[27] and increased sedation in some patients on adinazolam.[28] Prolonged hypnosis in an elderly woman[21] and CNS toxicity[20] in a woman of 49 have been attributed to a triazolam-cimetidine interaction but this remains unconfirmed. In contrast cimetidine does not normally interact with lorazepam,[7] lormetazepam,[37] oxazepam[7] or temazepam,[8,32] although prolonged post-operative sedation was seen in one patient on oxazepam and cimetidine.[35]

Ranitidine,[5] and nizatidine[26,33,34] do not interact significantly with diazepam, nor ranitidine with adinazolam[29] or temazepam.[23,32] Famotidine does not interact with bromazepam,[38] clorazepate,[38] chlordiazepoxide,[38] diazepam[6] or triazolam,[38] but ranitidine can increase the bioavailability of oral triazolam.[31] There is some controversy about whether midazolam is or is not affected by cimetidine and ranitidine.[16,17,23,25,40,41]

Mechanism

Cimetidine inhibits the liver enzymes concerned with the metabolism (N-dealkylation plus oxidation or nitro-reduction) of diazepam, alprazolam, chlordiazepoxide, clorazepate, flurazepam, nitrazepam and triazolam.[18] As a result their clearance from the body is reduced and their serum levels rise. The metabolism of clobazam and clotiazepam seems to be unaffected.[14,15] Lorazepam,[7] oxazepam[7] and temazepam[8] are metabolized by a different metabolic pathway involving glucuronidation which is not affected by cimetidine. Ranitidine, famotidine and nizatidine appear not to inhibit liver microsomal enzymes.

Importance and management

The benzodiazepine/cimetidine interactions are well documented (not all the references are listed here) but normally they appear to be of little clinical importance, although a few patients may be adversely affected (increased effects, drowsiness, etc.). Reports of problems are very few indeed, particularly when viewed against the very common use of both drugs. Lorazepam, lormetazepam, oxazepam and temazepam are non-interacting alternative benzodiazepines. Ranitidine does not interact with diazepam or temazepam, and neither nizatidine, ranitidine nor famotidine would be expected to interact with other benzodiazepines which are metabolized similarly (see 'Mechanism' above), however the effects of oral triazolam are possibly increased. It is claimed that serum levels of midazolam and sedation are increased by ranitidine and/or cimetidine[17,25,41] whereas other reports claim that neither ranitidine nor cimetidine interact.[16,23,40]

References

1 Greenblatt DJ, Abernethy DR, Morse DS, Harmatz JS, Shader RI. Clinical importance of the interaction of diazepam and cimetidine. Anesth Analg (1986) 65, 176–80.
2 McGowan WAW, Dundee JW. The effect of intravenous cimetidine on the absorption of orally administered diazepam and lorazepam. Br J Clin Pharmacol(1982) 14, 207–11.
3 Klotz U, Reimann I. Elevation of steady-state diazepam levels by cimetidine. Clin Pharmacol Ther (1981) 30, 513–7.
4 Gough PA, Curry SH, Aranjo OE, Robinson JD, Dallman JJ. Influence of cimetidine on oral diazepam elimination with measurement of subsequent cognitive change. Br J Clin Pharmacol (1982) 14, 739–42.
5 Klotz U, Reimann IW, Ohnhaus EE. Effect of ranitidine on the steady state pharmacokinetics of diazepam. Eur J Clin Pharmacol(1983) 24, 357–60.
6 Locniskar A, Greenblatt DJ, Harmatz JS, Zinny MA. Influence of famotidine and cimetidine on the pharmacokinetic properties of intravenous diazepam. J Clin Pharmacol(1985) 25, 459–60.
7 Greenblatt DJ, Abernethy DR, Koepke HH, Shader RI. Interaction of cimetidine with oxazepam, lorazepam and flurazepam. J Clin Pharmacol (1984) 24, 187–93.
8 Greenblatt DJ, Abernethy DR, Divoll M, Locniskar A, Harmatz JS, Shader RI. Non-interaction of temazepam and cimetidine. J Pharm Sci (1984) 73, 399–401.
9 Pourbaix S, Desager JP, Hulhoven R, Smith RB, Harvengt C. Pharmacokinetic consequences of long-term co-administration of cimetidine and triazolobenzodiazepines, alprazolam and triazolam in healthy subjects. Int J Clin Pharmacol Ther Toxicol (1985) 23, 447–51.
10 Abernethy DR, Greenblatt DJ, Divoll M, Moschitto LJ, Harmatz JS, Shader RI. Interaction of cimetidine with the triazolobenzodiazepines alprazolam and triazolam. Psychopharmacol (1983) 80, 275–8.
11 Desmond PV, Patwardhan RV, Schneker S, Speeg KV. Cimetidine impairs elimination of chlordiazepoxide (Librium) in man. Ann Intern Med (1980) 93, 266–8.
12 Divoll M, Abernethy DR, Greenblatt DJ. Cimetidine impairs oxidising capacity in the elderly. Clin Pharmacol Ther (1982) 31, 218.
13 Ochs HR, Greenblatt DJ, Gugler R, Muntefering G, Locniskar A, Abernethy DR. Cimetidine impairs nitrazepam clearance. Clin Pharmacol Ther (1983) 34, 227–30.
14 Grigoleit H-G, Hajdu P, Hundt HK L, Koeppen D, Malerczyk BH, Muller FO, Witte PU. Pharmacokinetic aspects of the interaction between clobazam and cimetidine. Eur J Clin Pharmacol(1983) 25, 139–42.
15 Ochs HR, Greenblatt DJ, Verburg-Ochs B, Harmatz JS, Grehl H. Disposition of clotiazepam: influence of age, sex, oral contraceptives, cimetidine, isoniazid and ethanol. Eur J Clin Pharmacol(1984) 26, 55–9.
16 Greenblatt DJ, Locniskar A, Scavone JM, Blyden GT, Ochs HR, Harmatz JS, Shader RI. Absence of interaction of cimetidine and ranitidine with intravenous and oral midazolam. Anesth Analg (1986) 65, 176–80.
17 Ellwood RJ, Hildebrand PJ, Dundee JW, Collier PS. Ranitidine influences the uptake of oral midazolam. Br J Clin Pharmacol(1983) 15, 743–5.
18 Klotz U, Antilla V-J. Drug interactions with cimetidine: pharmacokinetic studies to evaluate its mechanism. Naunyn-Schmied Arch Pharmacol(1980) 311, R77.
19 Klotz U, Reimann I. Delayed clearance of diazepam due to cimetidine. N Engl J Med (1980) 302, 1012–13.
20 Britton ML, Waller ES. Central nervous system toxicity associated with concurrent use of triazolam and cimetidine. Drug Intell Clin Pharm (1985) 19, 666–8.
21 Parker WA, MacLachlan RA. Prolonged hypnotic response to triazolam-cimetidine combination in an elderly patient. Drug Intell Clin Pharm (1984) 18, 980–1.
22 Anon. Court warns on interaction of drugs. Doctor (1979) 9, 1.
23 Dundee JW, Wilson CM, Robinson FP, Thompson EM, Elliott P. The effect of ranitidine on the hypnotic action of single doses of midazolam, temazepam and zopiclone. Br J Clin Pharmac (1984) 20, 553P.
24 Pullar T, Edwards D, Haigh JRM, Peaker S, Feeley MP. The effect of cimetidine on the single dose pharmacokinetics of oral clobazam and N-desmethylclobazam. Br J Clin Pharmac (1987) 23, 317–21.
25 Fee JPH, Collier PS, Howard PJ, Dundee JW. Cimetidine and ranitidine increase midazolam bioavailability. Clin Pharmacol Ther (1987) 41, 80–4.
26 Klotz U, Gottlieb W, Keohance PP, Dammann HG. Nocturnal doses of ranitidine and nizatidine do not affect the disposition of diazepam. J Clin Pharmacol(1987) 27, 210–12.
27 Bouden A. El Hechmi Z, Douki S. Cimetidine-benzodiazepine association confusiogene: a propros d'une observation. La Tunisie médicale (1990) 68, 63–4.
28 Hulhoven R, Desager JP, Cox S, Harvengt C. Influence of repeated administration of cimetidine on the pharmacokinetics and pharmacodynamics of adinazolam in healthy subjects. Eur J Clin Pharmacol (1988) 35, 59–64.
29 Suttle AB, Songer SS, Dukes GE, Hak LJ, Koruda M, Fleishaker JC, Brouwer KLR. Ranitidine does not alter adinazolam pharmacokinetics or pharmacodynamics. Clin Pharmacol Ther (1991) 49, 178.
30 Bressler R, Carter D, Winters L. Enprostil, in contrast to cimetidine, does not affect diazepam pharmacokinetics. Adv Therapy (1988) 5, 306–12.
31 Vanderveen RP, Jirak JL, Peters GR, Cox SR, Bombardt PA. Effect of ranitidine on the disposition of orally and intravenously administered triazolam. Clin Pharm (1991) 10, 539–43.
32 Elliott P, Dundee JW, Collier PS, McClean E. The influence of two H2-receptor antagonists, cimetidine and ranitidine, on the systemic bioavailability of temazepam. Br J Anaesth (1984) 56, 880–1P.
33 Klotz U, Arvela P, Rosenkranz B. Famotidine, a new H2-receptor antago-

nist, does not affect hepatic elimination of diazepam or tubular secretion of procainamide. Eur J Clin Pharmacol (1985) 28, 671–5.

34 Klotz U, Damman HG, Gottlieb WR, Walter TA, Keohane P. Nizatidine (300 mg nocte) does not interfere with diazepam pharmacokinetics in man. Br J Clin Pharmac (1987) 23, 105–6.

35 Lam AM, Parkin JA. Cimetidine and prolonged post-operative somnolence. Canad Anaesth Soc J (1981) 28, 450–2.

36 Lima DR, Santos RM, Werneck E, Andrade GN. Effect of orally administered misoprostol and cimetidine on the steady state pharmacokinetics of diazepam and nordiazepam in human volunteers. Eur J Drug Metab Pharmacokinet (1991) 16, 161–70.

37 Doenicke A, Dorow R, Tauber U. Die Pharmakokinetik fon Lormetazepam nach Cimetidin. Anaesthetist (1991) 40, 675–9.

38 Chichmanian RM, Mignot G, Spreux A, Jean-Girard C, Hofliger P. Tolérance de la famotidine. Étude due réseau médecins sentinelles en pharmacovigilance. Therapie (1992) 47, 239–43.

39 Nelson DC, Schenker S, Hoyumpa AM, Speeg KV, Avant GR. The effects of cimetidine on chlordiazepoxide elimination in cirrhosis. Clin Res (1981) 29, 824A.

40 Ochs HR, Greenblatt DJ, Shader I. Absence of interaction of cimetidine and ranitidine with intravenous and oral midazolam. Dig Dis Sci (1986) 31, Suppl, 194S.

41 Sanders LD, Whitehead C, Gilcersleve CD, Rosen M, Robinson JO. Interaction of H$_2$-receptor antagonists and benzodiazepine sedation. Anaesthesia (1993) 48, 286–92.

Benzodiazepines + Ciprofloxacin

Abstract/Summary

One study suggested that no interaction occurs, but a later study found that ciprofloxacin markedly reduces the clearance of diazepam from the body.

Clinical evidence, mechanism, importance and management

A study in normal subjects found that 1 g ciprofloxacin daily had no effect on the loss of diazepam from the body.[1] However a later study found that 500 mg ciprofloxacin twice daily for a week increased the AUC of a single 5 mg intravenous dose of diazepam by 50% and reduced its clearance by 37%, possibly by inhibiting the metabolism of the diazepam.[2] This would be expected to result in increased diazepam effects (drowsiness, etc). More study is needed to find out whether this interaction is clinically important or not.

Reference

1 Wijnands WJA, Trooster JFG, Teunissen PC, Cats HA, Vree TB. Ciprofloxacin does not impair the elimination of diazepam in humans. Drug Metab Disp (1990) 18, 954–7.

2 Kamali F, Edwards C, Thomas HL, Rawlins MD. The effect of ciprofloxacin on diazepam pharmacokinetics. Br J Clin Pharmac (1993) 35, 78P.

Benzodiazepines + Contraceptives, oral

Abstract/Summary

Oral contraceptives can increase the effects of alprazolam, chlordiazepoxide, diazepam, nitrazepam and triazolam, and reduce the effects of oxazepam, lorazepam and temazepam, but whether in practice there is a need for dosage adjustments has not been determined. Chlordiazepoxide, diazepam, nitrazepam and meprobamate can possibly increase the incidence of break-through bleeding.

Clinical evidence

Effects of benzodiazepines increased

(a) Alprazolam, Chlordiazepoxide, Clotiazepam, Diazepam, Nitrazepam, Triazolam + Oral contraceptives

A controlled study in six women showed that the mean half-life of chlordiazepoxide (0.6 mg/kg IV) was virtually doubled while taking oral contraceptives (from 11.6 to 20.6 h) and the total clearance fell by almost two-thirds (from 33.2 to 13.4 ml/min).[1] Similar but less marked effects were found in other studies with chlordiazepoxide,[2] diazepam,[3,4] alprazolam[8] and to an even lesser extent with triazolam[8] and nitrazepam (a 30% reduction clearance)[5]. No changes were seen with clotiazepam[7] or midazolam given intramuscularly.[10] A behavioural study found that concurrent use impaired psychomotor performance.[12]

(b) Lorazepam, Oxazepam, Temazepam + Oral contraceptives

A controlled study in seven women showed that the mean half-life of lorazepam (2 mg IV) was more than halved while taking oral contraceptives (from 14 to 6 h) and the total clearance increased by a factor of three (from 77.4 to 288.9 ml/min.).[1]

A smaller change was seen in other controlled studies with lorazepam,[6,8] and temazepam,[8] and in two other studies both marked[1] and small[6] falls in the half-life of oxazepam were observed.

(c) Contraceptive effects decreased

A study in 72 patients taking combined oral contraceptives (*Rigevidon, Anteovin*) found that break-through bleeding occurred in 36.1% while taking daily doses of 10–20 mg chlordiazepoxide, 5–15 mg diazepam, 5–10 mg nitrazepam or 200–600 mg meprobamate, but no pregnancies occurred. Only three cases occurred with diazepam or nitrazepam.[11] The average values for break-through bleeding with these two oral contraceptives were 9.1% for Rigedon and 3.3% for *Anteovin* in the absence of other drugs. It was possible to establish a causal relationship between the bleeding and the use of the tranquilliser or hypnotic in 77% of the cases either by stopping the drug or exchanging it for another.[11]

Mechanisms

Oral contraceptives affect the metabolism of the benzodiazepines by the liver in different ways: oxidative metabolism is reduced (alprazolam, chlordiazepoxide, diazepam, etc.), whereas metabolism by glucuronide conjugation is increased (lorazepam, oxazepam, temazepam, etc.). Just why these tranquillizers should cause break-through bleeding is not understood.

Importance and management

Established interactions but of uncertain clinical importance. Long-term use of benzodiazepines which are highly oxidized (alprazolam, chlordiazepoxide, diazepam, nitrazepam, etc.) in women on the pill should be monitored to ensure that the dosage is not too high. Those taking glucuronidated benzodiazepines (lorazepam, oxazepam, temazepam, etc.) may need a dosage increase. Clotiazepam and midazolam appear not to interact. More study is needed to find out if any these interactions is of real practical importance. No firm conclusions could be drawn from the results of one study which set out to evaluate the importance of this interaction.[9]

The increased incidence of break-through bleeding (more than one-third) due to these tranquillizers, described in the report cited above, is an unpleasant reaction and it suggests that the contraceptive is possibly unreliable, but no outright contraceptive failures were actually reported.[11] Limited evidence from the study suggests that changing the tranquillizer or the contraceptive might be the answer.

References

1 Patwardhan RV, Mitchell MC, Johnson RF, Schenker S. Differential effects of oral contraceptive steroids on the metabolism of benzodiazepines. Hepatology (1983) 3, 248–53.
2 Roberts RK, Desmond PV, Wilkinson GR, Schenker S. Disposition of chlordiazepoxide: sex differences and effects of oral contraceptives. Clin Pharmacol Ther (1979) 25, 826–31.
3 Giles HG, Sellers EM, Naranjo CA, Frecker RC, Greenblatt DJ. Disposition of intravenous diazepam in young men and women. Europ J Clin Pharmacol(1981) 20, 207–13.
4 Abernethy DR, Greenblatt DJ, Divoll M, Arendt R, Ochs HR, Shader RI. Impairment of diazepam metabolism by low-dose estrogen-containing oral contraceptive steroids. N Engl J Med (1982) 306, 791–2.
5 Jochemsen R, Van der Graff M, Boejinga JK, Breimer DD. Influence of sex, menstrual cycles and oral contraception on the disposition of nitrazepam. Br J Clin Pharmacol(1982) 13, 319–24.
6 Abernethy DR, Greenblatt DJ, Ochs HR, Weyers D, Divoll M, Harmatz JS, Shader RI. Lorazepam and oxazepam kinetics in women on low-dose oral contraceptives. Clin Pharmacol Ther (1983) 33, 628–32.
7 Ochs HR, Greenblatt DJ, Verburg-Ochs B, Harmatz JS, Grehl H. Disposition of clotiazepam: influence of age, sex, oral contraceptives, cimetidine, isoniazid and ethanol. Eur J Clin Pharmacol(1984) 26, 55–9.
8 Stoeh GP, Kroboth PD, Juhl RP, Wender DB, Phillips P, Smith RB. Effect of oral contraceptives on triazolam, temazepam, alprazolam and lorazepam kinetics. Clin Pharmacol Ther (1984) 36, 683–90.
9 Kroboth PD, Smith RB, Stoeh GP, Juhl R. Pharmacodynamic evaluation of the benzodiazepine-oral contraceptive interaction. Clin Pharmacol Ther (1985) 38, 525–32.
10 Holazo AA, Winkler MB, Patel IH. Effects of age, gender and oral contraceptives on intramuscular midazolam pharmacokinetics. J Clin Pharmacol (1988) 28, 1040–5.
11 Somos P. Interaction between certain psychopharmaca and low-dose oral contraceptives. Ther Hung (1990) 38, 37–40.
12 Ellinwood EH, Easler ME, Linnoila M, Molter DW, Heatherly DG, Bjornsson TD. Effects of oral contraceptives on diazepam-induced psychomotor impairment. Clin Pharmacol Ther (1984) 35, 360–8.

Benzodiazepines + Dextropropoxyphene

Abstract/Summary

Some evidence suggests that the combined CNS depressant effects of alprazolam and dextropropoxyphene may be greater than with other benzodiazepines because the serum levels of alprazolam may be increased.

Clinical evidence, mechanism, importance and management

A study in 14 normal subjects showed that while taking 65 mg dextropropoxyphene 6-hourly the pharmacokinetics of single doses of diazepam and lorazepam were not significantly changed, but the half-life of alprazolam was prolonged from 11.6 to 18.3 h, and its clearance fell from 1.3 to 0.8 ml/min/kg.[1] It would seem that dextropropoxyphene inhibits the metabolism (hydroxylation) of the alprazolam by the liver, thereby reducing its loss from the body, but has little or no effect on the N-demethylation or glucuronidation of the other two benzodiazepines. The clinical importance of this is uncertain, but the inference to be drawn is that the CNS depressant effects of alprazolam will be increased, over and above the simple additive CNS depressant effects likely when other benzodiazepines and dextropropoxyphene are taken together. More study is needed.

Reference

1 Abernethy DR, Greenblatt DJ, Morse DS, Shader RI. Interaction of propoxyphene with diazepam, alprazolam and lorazepam. Br J Clin Pharmac (1985) 19, 51–7.

Benzodiazepines + Disulfiram

Abstract/Summary

The serum levels of chlordiazepoxide and diazepam are increased by the use of disulfiram and some patients may possibly experience increased drowsiness. Alprazolam, oxazepam and lorazepam are only minimally affected or not at all.

Clinical evidence

After taking 0.5 g disulfiram daily for 14–16 days, the plasma clearances of single doses of chlordiazepoxide and diazepam were reduced by 54 and 41% respectively in alcoholic and normal subjects. The half-lives were increased by 84 and 37% respectively. Serum levels of chlordiazepoxide were approximately doubled. Changes in the pharmacokinetic parameters of oxazepam were minimal.[1]

Another paper by the same workers shows that lorazepam behaves like oxazepam,[2] and the pharmacokinetics of alprazolam are unaffected by disulfiram.[3]

Mechanism

Disulfiram inhibits the initial metabolism (N-demethylation and oxidation) of both chlordiazepoxide and diazepam by the liver so that an alternative but slower metabolic pathway is used which results in the accumulation of these benzodiazepines in the body. In contrast, the metabolism (glucuronidation) of oxazepam and lorazepam is minimally affected by disulfiram so that their clearance from the body remains largely unaffected.[1,2] Just why alprazolam is affected is not understood.[3]

Importance and management

An established interaction, but the clinical effects are uncertain. Single dose studies are not necessarily reliable predictors of what happens in practice, however it seems probable that some patients will experience increased drowsiness (a) because of this interaction, and (b) because drowsiness is a very common side-effect of disulfiram. Reduce the dosage of the benzodiazepine if necessary. Other benzodiazepines which are metabolized similarly may possibly interact in the same way (bromazepam, clonazepam, clorazepate, prazepam, ketazolam, clobazam, flurazepam, nitrazepam, medazepam, triazolam) but this needs confirmation. Alprazolam, oxazepam and lorazepam appear to be non-interacting alternatives (and possibly temazepam which is also metabolized by glucuronidation)

References

1 MacLeod SM, Sellers EM, Giles HG, Billings BJ, Martin PR, Greenblatt DJ, Marshman JA. Interaction of disulfiram with benzodiazepines. Clin Pharmacol Ther (1978) 24, 583–9.
2 Sellers EM, Giles HG, Greenblatt DJ, Naranjo CA. Differential effects on benzodiazepine disposition by disulfiram and ethanol. Arzneim-Forsch/Drug Res (1980) 30, 882–6.
3 Diquet B, Gujadhur L, Lamiable D, Warot D, Hayound H, Choisy H. Lack of interaction between disulfiram and alprazolam in alcoholic patients. Eur J Clin Pharmacol (1990) 38, 157–60.

Benzodiazepines + Ethambutol

Abstract/Summary

Ethambutol appears not to interact with diazepam.

Clinical evidence, mechanism, importance and management

A study on six patients, newly diagnosed as having tuberculosis and treated with ethambutol (25 mg/kg), showed that although some of the pharmacokinetic parameters of diazepam were altered, the changes were not significant.[1] There seems to be nothing in the literature to suggest that ethambutol interacts with other benzodiazepines.

Reference

1 Ochs HR, Greenblatt DJ, Roberts GM, Dengler HJ. Diazepam interaction with antituberculous drugs. Clin Pharmacol Ther (1981) 29, 671.

Benzodiazepines + Food

Abstract/Summary

Food can delay and reduce the hypnotic effects of flunitrazepam and loprazolam.

Clinical evidence, mechanism, importance and management

A study in two groups of eight subjects found that when they took single 2.0 mg doses of flunitrazepam or loprazolam 2 h after an evening dinner (spaghetti, meat, salad, an apple and wine) and 1 h before going to bed, the peak plasma levels of the two hypnotics were reduced by 62% and 41% respectively. The time to reach these levels were delayed by 2.5 and 3.6 h respectively, and the absorption half-lives of the drugs were considerably prolonged.[1] It seems probable therefore in a 'real-life' situation the onset of sleep would be delayed and the effects reduced by food.

Reference

1 Bareggi SR, Pirola R, Truci G, Leva S, Smirna S. Effect of after-dinner administration on the pharmacokinetics of oral flunitrazepam and loprazolam. J Clin Pharmacol (1988) 28, 371–5.

Benzodiazepines + Granisetron

Abstract/Summary

Lorazepam impairs the performance of a number of psychometric tests, but the addition of granisetron appears not to make it worse.

Clinical evidence, mechanism, importance and management

2.5 mg lorazepam clearly affected the performance of a number of psychometric tests by 12 normal subjects. Statistically significant increases occurred in drowsiness, feebleness, muzziness, clumsiness, lethargy, mental slowness, relaxation, dreaminess, incompetence, sadness and withdrawal. But there was very little evidence that 160 µg/kg granisetron had any effect on the performance of these tests except that clumsiness and attentiveness were increased, nor was there evidence that granisetron added to these effects of lorazepam when taken concurrently.[1] No special precautions would seem to be necessary.

Reference

Leigh TJ, Link CGG, Fell GL. Effects of granisetron and lorazepam, alone and in combination, on psychometric performance. Br J Clin Pharmac (1991) 31, 333–6.

Benzodiazepines + Isoniazid

Abstract/Summary

Isoniazid reduces the loss of both diazepam and triazolam from the body. Some increase in their effects would be expected. No interaction occurs with oxazepam or clotiazepam.

Clinical evidence

(a) Diazepam and Triazolam

A study in nine normal subjects showed that after 3 day's treatment with 180 mg isoniazid daily, the half-life of a single dose of diazepam was increased from 34 to 45 h, and the total clearance reduced from 0.54 to 0.40 ml/min.[1] A study in six normal subjects showed that after taking 180 mg isoniazid daily for 3 days, the half-life of a single dose of triazolam was increased from 2.5 to 3.3 h, the AUC was increased from 26.5 to 38.6 ml^{-1}/h and the clearance was reduced from 6.8 to 3.9 ml/min/kg.[2]

(b) Oxazepam and Clotiazepam

A study in nine normal subjects showed that 180 mg isoniazid daily for three days had no effect on the pharmacokinetics of a single 30 mg oral dose of oxazepam.[2] Similarly the pharmacokinetics of clotiazepam were not altered in another study of the effects of isoniazid.[3]

Mechanism

What is known suggests that the isoniazid acts as an enzyme inhibitor, decreasing the metabolism and loss of diazepam and triazolam from the body, thereby increasing and prolonging their effects.

Importance and management

Information is limited but the interactions appear to be established. Their clinical importance is uncertain but be alert for the need to decrease the dosages of diazepam and triazolam if isoniazid is started. There seems to be no direct information about other benzodiazepines, but those undergoing high first-pass extraction and/or liver microsomal metabolism would be expected to interact similarly. Oxazepam and clotiazepam appear not to interact.

References

1 Ochs HR, Greenblatt DJ, Roberts GM, Dengler HJ. Diazepam interaction with antituberculous drugs. Clin Pharmacol Ther (1981) 29, 671.
2 Ochs HR, Greenblatt DJ, Knuchel M. Differential effect of isoniazid on triazolam and oxazepam conjugation. Br J Clin Pharmac (1983) 16, 743–46.
3 Ochs HR, Greenblatt DJ, Verburg-Ochs B, Harmatz JS, Grehl H. Disposition of clotiazepam: influence of age, sex, oral contraceptives, cimetidine, isoniazid and ethanol. Eur J Clin Pharmacol (1984) 26, 55–59.

Benzodiazepines + Ketoconazole

Abstract/Summary

Ketoconazole reduces the loss of chlordiazepoxide from the body, but the clinical effects of this seem unlikely to be of great importance.

Clinical evidence, mechanism, importance and management

After taking 400 mg ketoconazole daily for 5 days the clearance of chlordiazepoxide (0.6 mg/kg) in 12 normal subjects was decreased by 38%.[1] It seems unlikely that this will have a marked effect on the treatment of patients, but this needs confirmation. The effects of ketoconazole on other benzodiazepines seems not to have been studied.

Reference

1 Brown MW, Maldonado AL, Meredith CG, Speeg KV. Effect of ketoconazole on hepatic oxidative drug metabolism. Clin Pharmacol Ther (1985) 37, 290–7.

Benzodiazepines + Macrolide antibiotics

Abstract/Summary

The serum levels and effects of midazolam and triazolam are markedly increased and prolonged by the concurrent use of erythromycin. The same interaction has been seen between triazolam and both triacetyloleandomycin and josamycin.

Clinical evidence

(a) Midazolam + Erythromycin

A study in 12 subjects found that 500 mg erythromycin three times daily for 6 days almost tripled the peak serum levels of midazolam following a single 15 mg dose, more than doubled its half-life and increased the AUC more than four-fold. The subjects could hardly be wakened during the first hour after being given the midazolam, and most experienced amnesia lasting several hours.[10,12]

The serum midazolam levels (0.5 mg premedication) of a boy of 8 about to undergo surgery were approximately doubled when infused with erythromycin. He developed nausea and tachycardia, and after 40 min (200 mg erythromycin) he lost consciousness.[4] A patient in a coronary care unit given 300 mg midazolam IV over 14 h slept for about 6 days (apart from brief wakening when given flumazenil). The midazolam half-life was increased approximately 10-fold. This was attributed to the combined effects of 4 g erythromycin daily and 1.7 g amiodarone over 3 days.[5,7] An interaction between midazolam and erythromycin has been suspected in another report, but it was obscured by the state of the patient and the use of other drugs.[6] A study in normal subjects found that even a single 750 mg dose of erythromycin increased the sedative effects of midazolam.[11]

(b) Triazolam + Erythromycin

A study in 16 normal subjects found that 333 mg erythromycin daily for 3 days, reduced the clearance of a single 0.5 mg dose of triazolam by about 50%, increased the AUC by 106% (from 20.1 to 41.4 ng h/ml) and increased the maximum serum levels by about one-third (from 2.8 to 4.1 ng/ml).[1] Another study confirmed the marked decrease in clearance and an increase in peak serum levels.[8] Drowsiness, weakness and slowness were seen in a patient taking triazolam when treated with erythromycin for a dental abcess.[9]

(c) Triazolam + Triacetyloleandomycin and Josamycin

2 g triacetyloleandomycin daily given to seven normal subjects for 7 days increased the peak triazolam levels (0.25 mg) by 107%, increased the $AUC_{0-8\ h}$ by 275% and the half-life from 1.81 to 6.48 h, and reduced the apparent oral clearance by 74%. Marked psychomotor impairment and amnesia was seen.[3] Josamycin and triacetyloleandomycin have been reported to interact similarly in two patients on triazolam, causing an increase in its effects.[2]

Mechanism

The most probable explanation is that these macrolide antibiotics reduce the metabolism of midazolam and triazolam by the liver, thereby reducing their loss from the body, raising their serum levels and increasing and prolonging their effects. Possibly cytochrome P450IIIA is involved.

Importance and management

Information is limited but the midazolam/erythromycin, triazolam/erythromycin and triazolam/triacetyloleandomycin interactions appear to be established, and of clinical importance. The dosages of the midazolam and triazolam should be reduced 50–75% if these antibiotics are used to avoid excessive effects (marked drowsiness, memory loss). Remember too that the hypnotic effects are also prolonged so that patients should be warned about hangover effects next morning if they intend to drive.

Much less is known about triazolam/josamycin but the same precautions should be taken. Midazolam would also be expected to interact with both josmycin and triacetyloleandomycin but this needs confirmation.

References

1 Phillips JP, Antal EJ, Smith RB. A pharmacokinetic interaction between erythromycin and triazolam. J Clin Psychopharmacol (1986) 6, 297–9.

2 Carry PV, Ducluzeau R, Jourdan C, Bourrat C, Vigneou C, Descotes J. De nouvelles interactions avec les macrolides ? Lyon Med (1982) 248, 189–90.
3 Warot D, Bergougnan L, Lamiable D, Berlin I, Bensimon G, Danjou P, Puch AJ. Troleandomycin-triazolam interaction in healthy volunteers: pharmacokinetic and psychometric evaluation. Eur J Clin Pharmacol (1987) 32, 389–93.
4 Hiller A, Olkkola KT, Isohanni P, Saarnivaara L. Unconsciousness associated with midazolam and erythromycin. Br J Anaesthesia (1990) 65, 826–8.
5 Gascon P-M, Dayer P, Waldvogel F. Les interactions médicamenteuses du midazolam. Schweiz Med Wschr (1989) 119, 1834–6.
6 Byatt CM, Lewis LD, Dawling S, Cochrane GM. Accumulation of midazolam after repeated dosage in patients receiving mechanical ventiation in an intensive care unit. Br Med J (1984) 289, 799–800.
7 Gascon M-P, Dayer P. In vitro forecasting of drugs which may interfere with the biotransformation of midazolam. Eur J Clin Pharmacol (1991) 41, 573–8.
8 Hughes FC, LeJeunee CL, Munera Y. Therapeutic consequences of macrolide-induced inhibition of hepatic microsome. Sem Hop Paris (1987) 63, 2280–3.
9 Matera MG. Erythromycin inhibition of triazolam metabolism. Minerva Med (1987) 78, 1194.
10 Aranko K, Olkkola KT, Hiller A, Saarnivaara L. Clinically important interaction between erythromycin and midazolam. Br J Clin Pharmacol (1991) 33, 2178P.
11 Mattila MJ, Vanakoski J. Oral single doses of erythromycin enhance the effects of midazolam on human performance. Br J Clin Pharmac (1993) 35, 77P.
12 Oikkola KT, Aranko K, Luurila H, Hiller A, Saarnivaara L, Himberg J-J, Neuvonen PJ. A potentially hazardous interaction between erythromycin and midazolam. Clin Pharmacol Ther (1993) 53, 298–305.

Benzodiazepines + Metronidazole

Abstract/Summary

Metronidazole does not interact with alprazolam, diazepam or lorazepam.

Clinical evidence, mechanism, importance and management

One study in normal subjects found that 750 mg metronidazole (for an unstated time) had no effect on the pharmacokinetics of lorazepam or alprazolam.[1] Another study found that 800 mg metronidazole daily for 5 days also had no effect on the pharmacokinetics of a single 0.1 mg/kg intravenous dose of diazepam.[2] Interactions with other benzodiazepines seem unlikely. No special precautions seem necessary.

References

1 Blyden GT, Greenblatt DJ, Scavone JM. Metronidazole impairs clearance of phenytoin but not of alprazolam or lorazepam. Clin Pharmacol Ther (1986) 39, 181.
2 Jensen JC, Gugler R. Interaction between metronidazole and drugs eliminated by oxidative metabolism. Clin Pharmacol Ther (1985) 37, 407–10.

Benzodiazepines + Non-steroidal anti-inflammatory drugs

Abstract/Summary

Diazepam and indomethacin do not appear to interact adversely, but the feeling of dizziness may be increased. Diclofenac reduces both the sedative and hypnotic dosages of midazolam.

Clinical evidence, mechanism, importance and management

10–15 mg diazepam impaired the performance of a number of psychomotor tests (digit symbol substitution, letter cancellation, tracking and flicker fusion) in 119 healthy medical students. It also caused subjective drowsiness, mental slowness and clumsiness, but when 50 or 100 mg indomethacin was given as well, the effects were little different from diazepam alone except that the feeling of dizziness (common to both drugs) was increased.[1] A clinical study in patients found that 75 mg diclofenac given intravenously reduced both the sedative and hypnotic dosages of midazolam given by infusion by 35%.[2] The clinical importance of this is uncertain.

References

1 Nuotto E, Saarialho-Kere U. Actions and interactions of indomethacin and diazepam on performance in healthy volunteers. Pharmacol Toxicol (1988) 62, 293–7.
2 Carrero E, Castillo J, Bogdanovich A, Nalda MA. El diclofenac reduce las dosis dedante e hipnótica de midazolam. Rev Esp Anestesiol Reanim (1991) 38, 127.

Benzodiazepines + Omeprazole, Pantoprazole

Abstract/Summary

Gait disturbances (due to benzodiazepine intoxication?) occurred in two patients on triazolam, lorazepam or flurazepam when given omeprazole. The effects of diazepam are also possibly increased by omeprazole but not by pantoprazole.

Clinical evidence

Two elderly patients, both smokers, and taking triazolam and lorazepam or flurazepam, developed gait disturbances when concurrently treated with 20 mg omeprazole daily. They rapidly recoved when the benzodiazepines or the omeprazole were stopped.[4] After taking 40 mg omeprazole daily for a week, the clearance of a single dose of diazepam (0.1 mg/kg IV) in eight normal subjects was reduced by 54%. Another study found a 27% decrease in clearance while taking half this dose of omeprazole daily.[1,2] In contrast, pantoprazole was found to have no effect on the half-life, clearance or AUC of diazepam in 12 normal subjects.[5]

Mechanism

Not fully established, but it seems probable that the omeprazole inhibits the liver enzymes concerned with the metabolism and clearance of these benzodiazepines, as a result of which the benzodiazepines accumulate and their effects are increased. An *in vitro* study using human liver microsomes (from a healthy traffic accident victim) suggested that omeprazole may possibly interact similarly with midazolam.[3]

Importance and management

Information is very limited but what is currently known suggests that patients given omeprazole and the benzodiazepines cited should be monitored for any signs of increased benzodiazepine effects (sedation, unstable gait, etc). More study is needed. Pantoprazole appears not to interact with diazepam.

References

1 Gugler R, Jensen JC. Omeprazole inhibits elimination of diazepam. Lancet (1984) i, 1969.
2 Andersson T, Andrén K, Cederberg C, Edvardsson G, Heggelund A, Lundborg P. Effect of omeprazole and cimetidine on plasma diazepam levels. Eur J Clin Pharmacol (1990) 39, 51–4.
3 Li G, Klotz U. Inhibitory effect of omeprazole on the metabolism of midazolam *in vitro* Arzneim.-Forsch./Drug Res (1990) 40, 1105–7.
4 Martí-Massó JF, López de Munain A, López de Dicastillo G. Ataxia following gastric bleeding due to omeprazole-benzodiazepine interaction. Ann Pharmacother (1992) 26, 429–30.
5 Guler R, Hartmann M, Rudi J, Bliesath H, Brod I, Klotz U, Huber R, Steinijans VW, Wurst W. Lack of interaction of pantoprazole and diazepam in man. Gastroenterol (1992) 102, A77.

Benzodiazepines + Paracetamol (Acetaminophen)

Abstract/Summary

Paracetamol reduces the excretion of diazepam but plasma levels are little affected.

Clinical evidence, mechanism, importance and management

The 96 h urinary excretion of diazepam (a single 10 mg oral dose) and its metabolite (desmethyldiazepam) were reduced by 500 mg paracetamol in four normal subjects. The reductions were from 44 to 12% and 27 to 8% in the two female subjects, and from 11 to 4.5% in one of the males. The reasons are not understood. Plasma levels of diazepam and its metabolite were not significantly affected.[1] There would seem to be little reason for avoiding concurrent use. There seems to be no information about other benzodiazepines.

Reference

1 Mulley BA, Potter BI, Rye RM, Takeshita K. Interactions between diazepam and paracetamol. J Clin Pharmacy (1978) 3, 25–35.

Benzodiazepines + Probenecid

Abstract/Summary

Probenecid reduces the loss from the body of adinazolam, lorazepam and nitrazepam, but not temazepam. Increased therapeutic and toxic effects (sedation) may be expected.

Clinical evidence

(a) Adinazolam

2 g probenecid increased the psychomotor effects of 60 mg sustained-release adinazolam in 16 normal subjects. The tests used were symbol-digit substitution, digit span forwards and continuous performance.[3] An associated study using the same doses found that the peak serum levels of adinazolam and its active metabolite (N-desmethyl adinazolam) were increased (80% and 50% respectively) and the clearances were reduced (16% and 55% respectively).[4]

(b) Lorazepam

500 mg probenecid 6-hourly approximately halved the clearance of a single 2 mg IV dose of lorazepam in nine normal subjects (from 80.3 to 44 ml/min). The elimination half-life was more than doubled (from 14.3 to 33 h).[1]

(c) Nitrazepam and Temazepam

500 mg probenecid for 3 days reduced the clearance of nitrazepam by 25% in normal subjects but did not affect temazepam.[2]

Mechanism

Probenecid inhibits the clearance of many drugs and their metabolites (including some of the benzodiazepines) by the kidney tubules. It also inhibits the metabolism (glucuronidation) of nitrazepam and lorazepam by the liver.[1,2] The overall result is that the benzodiazepines accumulate and their effects are increased.

Importance and management

Established interactions but of uncertain clinical importance. Be alert for increases in both the therapeutic and toxic effects (sedation, antegrade amnesia). Reduce the dosage as necessary. There seems to be no direct information about other benzodiazepines but those which are metabolized like lorazepam (eg oxazepam) are possible candidates for this interaction. More study is needed.

References

1 Abernethy DR, Greenblatt DJ, Ameer B, Shader RI. Probenecid impairment of acetaminophen and lorazepam clearance: direct inhibition of ether glucuronide formation. J Pharmacol Exp Ther (1985) 234, 345–9.
2 Brockmeyer NH, Mertins L, Klimek K, Goos M, Ohnhaus EE. Comparative effects of rifampin and/or probenecid on the pharmacokinetics of temazepam and nitrazepam. Int J Clin Pharmacol Ther Tox (1990) 28, 387–93.
3 Golden PL, Brouwer KLR, Fleishaker JC, Warner PE, Milliken SP, Lyon JA, Jewell RC. Effect of probenecid on adinazolam II. Pharmacodynamics. Clin Pharmacol Ther (1993) 53, 165.
4 Warner PE, Jewell RC, Fleishaker JC, Golden PL, Milliken SP, Lyon JA, Brouwer KLR. Effect of probenecid on adinazolam I. Pharmacokinetics. Clin Pharmacol Ther (1993) 53, 165.

Benzodiazepines + Prostaglandins

Enprostil and misoprostol do not appear to interact significantly with diazepam.

Abstract/Summary, clinical evidence, mechanism, importance and management

Eight day's treatment with 35 µg enprostil twice daily had no statistically significant effect on pharmacokinetics of a single 10 mg oral dose of diazepam in 12 subjects although a 12.2% reduction in the diazepam AUC was seen. When the enprostil was given with 1200 mg cimetidine daily, the diazepam AUC was increased by 28.3% but this was attributed to the effects of the cimetidine.[1] Another study in 12 subjects found that 200 µg misoprostol four times daily for seven days had no effect on the steady-state serum levels of diazepam (10 mg daily) or nordiazepam.[2]

No special precautions would seem to be necessary if either enprostil or misoprostol is given with diazepam.

Reference

1 Bressler R, Carter D, Winters L. Enprostil, in contrast to cimetidine, does not affect diazepam pharmacokinetics. Adv Therapy (1988) 5, 306–12.
2 Lima DR, Santos RM, Werneck E, Andrade GN. Effect of orally administered misoprostol and cimetidine on the steady state pharmacokinetics of diazepam and nordiazepam in human volunteers. Eur J Drug Metab Pharmacokinet (1991) 16, 161–70.

Benzodiazepines + Rifampicin (Rifampin)

Abstract/Summary

Rifampicin causes a marked increase in the loss from the body of diazepam and nitrazepam, but not temazepam.

Clinical evidence

The mean half-life of diazepam was reduced to less than a third (from 58 to 14 h) in seven patients with TB when treated with daily doses of isoniazid (0.5–2.2 g), rifampicin (450–600 mg) and ethambutol (25 mg/kg). The clearance increased by more than 300%.[1] The total body clearance of nitrazepam in another study in normal subjects was increased 83% after taking 600 mg rifampicin daily for 3 days, but the pharmacokinetics of temazepam were unchanged.[2]

Mechanism

Rifampicin is a potent liver enzyme inducing agent which increases the metabolism of many drugs (including diazepam and nitrazepam) thereby hastening their loss from the body. Temazepam undergoes glucuronidation and is unaffected.

Importance and management

The documentation is limited but it is consistent with the way rifampicin interacts with many other drugs. The clinical importance has not been assessed but it seems likely that the diazepam and nitrazepam dosage will need to be raised. Monitor the outcome of concurrent use and raise the dosage accordingly. There seems to be no direct information about other benzodiazepines but if the mechanism suggested for diazepam and nitrazepam is correct, then those metabolized in a similar way (e.g. chlordiazepoxide, flurazepam) may possibly interact similarly, whereas those which undergo glucuronidation like temazepam (e.g. lorazepam, oxazepam) possibly do not. This needs confirmation. Ethambutol is a non-interacting alternative antitubercular.

References

1 Ochs HR, Greenblatt DJ, Roberts G-M, Dengler HJ. Diazepam interaction with antituberculous drugs. Clin Pharmacol Ther (1981) 29, 671–8.
2 Brockmeyer NH, Mertins L, Klimek K, Goos M, Ohnhaus EE. Comparative effects of rifampin and/or probenecid on the pharmacokinetics of temazepam and nitrazepam. Int J Clin Pharmacol Tox Ther (1990) 28, 387–93.

Benzodiazepines and related drugs + Theophylline and Caffeine

Abstract/Summary

Aminophylline can be used to antagonize the anaesthesia induced by benzodiazepines. Caffeine, and to a lesser extent theophylline, may reduce the sedative (and possibly also the anxiolytic) effects of diazepam, clonazepam. Caffeine also opposes the effects of triazolam and zoplicone.

Clinical evidence, mechanism, importance and management

A patient who was unarousable and unresponsive following anaesthesia with diazepam (60 mg over 10 min) and N_2O/O_2 (60%/40%), rapidly returned to consciousness when given 56 mg aminophylline intravenously.[1] Other reports confirm this antagonism by low doses of aminophylline (60 mg IV) of the anaesthesia induced by diazepam,[2] flunitrazepam,[11] lorazepam,[3] and midazolam.[12] There is some controversy about whether theophylline antagonizes midazolam anaesthesia/sedation or not.[4,5] No such interaction occurs if aminophylline is replaced by enprofylline.[2]

Caffeine, and to a lesser extent theophylline, counteract the drowsiness and mental slowness induced by diazepam in anxiolytic doses (10–20 mg).[6–9] This may be because they block adenosine receptors. There is also evidence that caffeine and clonazepam or triazolam have mutually opposing effects[10,13] and that caffeine similarly interacts with zoplicone.[13]

The aminophylline/benzodiazepine interaction can therefore be used with advantage if reversal of anaesthesia with some benzodiazepines is required, however bear in mind the likely effects of adding or withdrawing either theophylline or a benzodiazepine in patients in intensive care. The extent to which theophylline or caffeine (in strong coffee or tea) might reduce the anxiolytic effects of diazepam and other benzodiazepines is uncertain, but this too should be borne in mind. Enprofylline might be useful when an antiasthmatic is needed in combination with a benzodiazepine. Caffeine in tea or coffee also appears to reduce the sedative effects of triazolam and zoplicone. This would appear to be a disadvantage at night, but possibly useful the next morning.

References

1 Stirt JA. Aminophylline is a diazepam antagonist. Anesth Analg (1981) 60, 767–8.
2 Nieman D, Martinell S, Arvidsson S, Svedmyr N, Ekstrom-Jodal B. Aminophylline inhibition of diazepam sedation: is adenosine blockade of GABA-receptors the mechanism? Lancet (1984) i, 462–3.
3 Wangler MA, Kilpatrick DS. Aminophylline is an antagonist of lorazepam. Anesth Analg (1985) 64, 834–6.
4 Kanto J, Aaltonen L, Himberg J-J, Hovi-Viander M. Midazolam as an intravenous induction agent in the elderly: a clinical and pharmacokinetic study. Anesth Analg (1986) 65, 15–20.
5 Sleigh JW. Failure of aminophylline to antagonize midazolam sedation. Anesth Analg (1986) 65, 540.
6 Mattila MJ, Nuotto E. Caffeine and theophylline counteract diazepam effects in man. Med Biol (1983) 61, 337–43.
7 Mattila MJ, Palva E, Savolainen K. Caffeine antagonizes diazepam effects in man. Med Biol (1982) 60, 121–3.
8 Henauer SA, Hollister LE, Gillespie HK, Moore F. Theophylline antagonizes diazepam-induced psychomotor impairment. Eur J Clin Pharmacol(1983) 25, 743–7.
9 Meyer BH, Weis OF, Muller FO. Antagonism of diazepam by aminophylline in healthy volunteers. Anesth Analg (1984) 63, 900–2.
10 Gaillard J-M, Sovilla J-Y, Blois R. The effect of clonazepam, caffeine, and the combination of the two drugs on human sleep. In Sleep '84, Ed by Koella WP, Rüther E, Schulz H. Publ by Gustav Fischer Verlag, Stuttgart, NY (1985) pp 314–5
11 Gurel A, Elevli M, Hamulu A. Aminophylline reversal of flunitrazepam sedation. Anesth Analg (1987) 66, 333–6.

12 Gallen JS. Aminophylline reversal of midazolam sedation. Anesth Analg (1989) 69, 269.

13 Mattila ME, Mattila MJH, Nuotto E. Caffeine moderately antagonizes the effects of triazolam and zoplicone on the psychomotor performance of healthy subjects. Pharmacology & Toxicology (1992) 70, 286–9.

Benzodiazepines + Tobacco smoking

Abstract/Summary

Smokers may need larger doses of some benzodiazepines than non-smokers.

Clinical evidence, mechanism, importance and management

Some studies have suggested that smoking does not affect the pharmacokinetics of diazepam[1,11] chlordiazepoxide,[2] lorazepam,[11] midazolam,[11] or triazolam[10] but others have found that the clearance of diazepam[3] and lorazepam[8] from the body is increased in smokers.[3] A Boston Collaborative Drug Surveillance Program reported a decreased frequency of drowsiness in those on diazepam or chlordiazepoxide who smoked.[4] Smoking has also been found to increase the clearance of alprazolam,[5] lorazepam,[8] oxazepam[6,9] and clorazepate.[7] The probable reason is that some of the components of tobacco smoke are enzyme-inducing agents which increase the rate at which the liver metabolizes these benzodiazepines, thereby reducing their effects and side-effects. The inference to be drawn is that smokers may need larger doses than non-smokers to achieve the same therapeutic effects.

References

1 Klotz U, Avant GR, Hoyumpa A, Schenker S, Wilkinson GR. The effects of age and liver disease on the disposition and elimination of diazepam in adult man. J Clin Invest (1975) 55, 347–9.

2 Desmond PV, Roberts RK, Wilkinson GR, Schenker S. No effect of smoking on the metabolism of chlordazepoxide. N Engl J Med (1979) 300, 199–200.

3 Greenblatt DJ, Allen MD, Harmatz JS, Shader RI. Diazepam disposition determinants. Clin Pharmacol Ther (1980) 27, 301–12.

4 Boston Collaborative Drug Surveillance Program. Clinical depression of the central nervous system due to diazepam and chlordiazepoxide in relation to cigarette smoking and age. N Engl J Med (1973) 288, 277–80.

5 Smith RB, Gwilt PR, Wright CE. Single- and multiple dose pharmacokinetics of oral alprazolam in healthy smoking and non-smoking men. Clin Pharm (1983) 2, 139–43.

6 Greenblatt DJ, Divoll M, Harmatz JS, Shader RI. Oxazepam kinetics: effects of age and sex. J Pharmacol Exp Ther (1980) 215, 86–91.

7 Norman TR, Fulton A, Burrows GD, Maguire KP. Pharmacokinetics of N-desmethyldiazepam after a single oral dose of clorazepate: the effect of smoking. Eur J Clin Pharmacol(1981) 21, 229–33.

8 Greenblatt DJ, Allen MD, Locniskar A, Harmatz JS, Shader RI. Lorazepam kinetics in the elderly. Clin Pharmacol Ther (1979) 26, 103–13.

9 Ochs HR, Greenblatt DJ, Otten H. Disposition of oxazepam in relation to age, sex and cigarette smoking. Klin Wschr (1981) 59, 899–903.

10 Ochs HR, Greenblatt DJ, Burstein ES. Lack of influence of cigarette smoking on triazolam pharmacokinetics. Br J Clin Pharmac (1987) 23, 759–63.

11 Ochs HR, Greenblatt DJ, Knüchel M. Kinetics of diazepam, midazolam and lorazepam in cigarette smokers. Chest (1985) 87, 223–6.

Buspirone + Fluoxetine

Abstract/Summary

A single case report describes a reduction in the anxiolytic effects of buspirone when fluoxetine was given. Another describes a worsening of the control of obsessive-compulsive disorder when buspirone was added. Two other reports describe their effective concurrent use.

Clinical evidence, mechanism, importance · and management

A 35-year-old man with a long history of depression, anxiety and panic was started on 60 mg buspirone daily. His anxiety abated, but worsening depression prompted additional treatment for 3 weeks with 200 mg trazodone daily which had little effect. To this was added 20 mg fluoxetine daily for persistent dysphoria, but within 48 h his usual symptoms of anxiety had returned and persisted even when the dose was raised to 80 mg daily. Stopping the buspirone did not increase his anxiety.[1] Another patient with obsessive-compulsive disorder on fluoxetine experienced a marked worsening of the symptoms when 10 mg buspirone daily was added.[2] This contrasts with other patients with obsessive-compulsive disorder who were resistant to fluoxetine in whom buspirone had been effectively used as an adjunct.[3] Another report describes their effective concurrent use in three patients with treatment-resistant depression.[4] The reasons for these reactions are not understood.

There would seem to be little reason for avoiding concurrent use but the outcome should be monitored. More study is needed.

Reference

1 Bodkin JA, Teicher MH. Fluoxetine may antagonize the anxiolytic action of buspirone. J Clin Psychopharmacol (1989) 9, 150.

2 Tanquary J, Masand P. Paradoxical reaction to buspirone augmentation of fluoxetine. J Clin Psychopharmacol (1990) 10, 377.

3 Markovitz PJ, Stagno SJ, Calabrese JR. Buspirone augmentation of fluoxetine in obsessive-compulsive disorder. Presented at the annual meeting of the Society of Biological Psychiatry, San Francisco, CA May (1989).

4 Bakish D. Fluoxetine potentiation by buspirone: three case histories. Can J Psychiatry (1991) 36, 749–50.

Buspirone + miscellaneous drugs

Abstract/Summary

No adverse interaction occurs if buspirone and amitriptyline are given together, and with diazepam the side-effects are similar to those seen with diazepam alone. Buspirone and cimetidine appear not to interact. An isolated report describes mania in an alcoholic patient on buspirone when given disulfiram.

Clinical evidence, mechanism, importance and management

15 mg buspirone 8-hourly added to 25 mg amitriptyline 8-hourly for 10 days had no significant effect on the steady-state serum levels of amitriptyline or nortriptyline in normal subjects. No symptoms of a pharmacodynamic interaction were seen.[1] The same dosage of buspirone had no effect on serum diazepam levels (5 mg diazepam daily for 10 days) in 12 normal subjects but the nordiazepam levels were raised about 20%. All experienced some mild side-effects (headache, nausea, dizziness, and in two cases muscle twitching). These symptoms subsided after a few days.[1] Cimetidine (1 g daily for 7 days) had no effect on serum buspirone levels in 10 normal subjects nor on its excretion while taking 45 mg buspirone daily. Some small pharmacokinetic changes were seen, but the performance of three psychomotor function tests remained unaltered.[2] An isolated report describes mania in an alcoholic patient on 20 mg buspirone daily, possibly due to an interaction with 400 mg disulfiram daily[3], but buspirone on its own has also apparently caused mania.[4] The reasons are not understood.

There would seem to be no reason for avoiding the use of buspirone with either amitriptyline, cimetidine or diazepam but some caution is needed if disulfiram is used.

Reference

1 Gammans RE, Mayol RF, Labudde JA. Metabolism and disposition of buspirone. Amer J Med (1986) 80 (Suppl 3B) 41–51.
2 Gammans RE, Pfeffer M, Wetrick ML, Faulkner HC, Rehm KD, Goodson PJ. Lack of interaction between cimetidine and buspirone. Pharmacotherapy (1987) 7, 72–9.
3 McIvor RJ, Sinanan K. Buspirone induced mania. Br J Psychiatry (1991) 158, 136–7.
4 Price WA, Bielefeld M. Buspirone-induced mania. J Clin Psychopharmacol (1989) 9 150–1.

Clozapine + Anticonvulsants

Abstract/Summary

Preliminary evidence suggests that clozapine serum levels are markedly reduced by carbamazepine or phenytoin with a reduction in its antipsychotic effects. An isolated case of fatal pancytopenia and of neuroleptic malignant syndrome have been seen in two patients taking clozapine and carbamazepine

Clinical evidence

(a) Carbamazepine

The serum clozapine levels of two patients who had been on 600–800 mg clozapine daily and 600–800 mg carbamazepine daily for several months were approximately doubled (from 1.4 to 2.4 and from 1.5 to 3.0 µmol/l respectively) within 2 weeks of withdrawing the carbamazepine.[1]

A patient on carbamazepine, lithium, benztropine and clonazepam developed fatal pancytopenia about 10 weeks after starting clozapine (400 mg daily).[3] A man with mania on 1200 mg carbamazepine daily and lithium developed muscle rigidity, mild hyperpyrexia, tachycardia, sweating and somnolence (diagnosed as neuroleptic malignant syndrome) 3 days after the lithium was stopped and 25 mg clozapine daily started. The symptoms immediately improved when the clozapine was stopped.[4]

(b) Phenytoin

Two patients developed reduced clozapine levels (falls of 65–85%) and worsening psychoses when phenytoin was added to their treatment.[2]

Mechanism

Not established, but it seems likely that both anticonvulsants (recognized and potent enzyme inducers) increase the metabolism of the clozapine by the liver, thereby reducing its effects. The case of pantcytopenia may have been due to the additive bone marrow depressant effects of the clozapine and carbamazepine.

Importance and management

Information is limited and none of these interactions is firmly established. Anticipate the need to increase the clozapine dosage if carbamazepine or phenytoin is added, and to reduce the dosage if either anticonvulsant is withdrawn. The authors of one of the reports advise the use of oxcarbazepine or sodium valproate instead of carbamazepine, implying that these two anticonvulsants do not interact with clozapine, but they give no supporting evidence.[1] Be alert for any evidence of other adverse effects during concurrent use.

References

1 Raitasuo V, Lehtovaara R, Huttunen MO. Carbamazepine and plasma levels of clozapine. Am J Psychiatry (1993) 150, 169.
2 Miller DD. Effect of phenytoin on plasma clozapine concentrations in two patients. J Clin Psychiatry (1991) 52, 223–5.
3 Gerson SL, Lieberman JA, Friedenberg WR, Lee D, Marx JJ, Meltzer H. Polypharmacy in fatal clozapine-associated agranulocytosis. Lancet (1991) 338, 262–3.
4 Müller T, Becker T, Fritze J. Neuroleptic malignant syndrome after clozapine plus carbamazepine. Lancet (1988) 2, 1500.

Clozapine + Antiparkinson drugs

Abstract/Summary

Clozapine appears not to interact adversely with *Sinemet* and pergolide, and may be used advantageously in some patients.

Clinical evidence, mechanism, importance and management

Ten out of 13 patients with parkinson's disease with mild to moderate dementia which developed when treated with *Sinemet* (Levodopa + carbidopa), with or without pergolide, improved when they were additionally treated with clozapine.[1] There would therefore seem to advantages in some patients in giving these drugs in combination.

Reference

1 Greene P, Cote L, Fahn S. Treatment of drug-induced psychosis in Parkinson's disease with clozapine. In 'Advances In Neurology', Narabayashi H, Nagatsu T, Yanagisawa N, Mizuno Y (eds.), Raven Press, NY (1993) 703–6.

Clozapine + Benzodiazepines

Abstract/Summary

A handful of reports describe severe hypotension, respiratory depression and unconsciousness in patients on benzodiazepines when given clozapine.

Clinical evidence, mechanism, importance and management

A schizophrenic patient failed to respond to fluphenazine, diazepam, clobazam and lormetazepam. The fluphenazine was stopped and clozapine started, 25 mg at noon and 100 mg at night. 3 h later toxic delerium and severe hypersalivation developed. The patient collapsed (systolic pressure 50 mmHg, diastolic unrecordable), he stopped breathing and remained unconscious for 30 min. After a few drug-free days he was re-started on 12.5 mg clozapine and a low benzodiazepine dosage without problems.[1]

Three other cases of severe hypotension, respiratory depression and loss of consciousness have been seen in patients on clozapine and flurazepam, lorazepam or diazepam.[1] Two other patients on clozapine and lorazepam developed marked sedation, hypersalivation and ataxia.[2]

The authors of the first of these reports[1] say that the relative risk of the cardiovascular/respiratory reaction is 2.1%. Quite clearly concurrent use should be very well monitored.

References

1 Grohmann R, Ruuther E, Sassim N, Schmidt LG. Adverse effects of clozapine. Psychopharmacology (1989) 99, S101–4.
2 Cobb CD, Anderson CB, Seidel DR. Possible interaction between cloazepine and lorazepam. Am J Psychiatry (1991) 148, 1606–7.

Clozapine + Cimetidine

Abstract/Summary

A single case report describes increased serum clozapine levels and toxicity due to cimetidine, but not ranitidine.

Clinical evidence, mechanism, importance and management

A man with chronic paranoid schizophrenia was treated with atenolol and clozapine (900 mg daily). When 800 mg cimetidine daily was added for gastritis, his serum clozapine levels rose almost 60% (from a range of 1081–992 ng/ml to 1701–1559 ng/ml) but without any problems. Within 3 days of raising the cimetidine dosage to 1200 mg daily he developed evidence of clozapine toxicity (marked diaphoresis, dizziness, vomiting, weakness, orthorstatic hypotension), all of which resolved over five days when the clozapine dosage was lowered to 200 mg daily and the cimetidine stopped. The serum clozapine levels during this period are not available. When the cimetidine was replaced by 300 mg ranitidine daily his clozapine serum levels were not affected.[1] The suggested reason for this interaction is that the cimetidine (a potent enzyme inhibitor) reduces the liver metabolism of the clozapine so that it accumulates, causing toxicity. Ranitidine does not cause enzyme inhibition.

Information appears to be limited to this report but it is consistent with the way cimetidine interacts with many other drugs. Ranitidine, or possibly other H_2-blockers such as famotidine or nizatidine which do not inhibit liver enzymes, would seem to be preferable and safer alternatives. This needs confirmation. More study is needed.

Reference

1 Szymananski S, Lieberman JA, Picou D, Masiar S, Cooper T. A case report of cimetidine-induced clozapine toxicity. J Clin Psychiatry (1991) 52, 21–2.

Clozapine + Lithium

Abstract/Summary

An isolated report describes myoclonus in a man on clozapine when lithium was added. Two other reports describe neuroleptic malignant syndrome in two patients on lithium when given clozapine.

Clinical evidence, mechanism, importance and management

A schizophrenic man poorly controlled with 750 mg clozapine daily for 6 weeks was additionally given 900 and then 1200 mg lithium daily. His serum lithium level was 0.86 mEq/l. Within a week he began to experience paroxysmal jerky movements of his upper and lower extremities lasting about half an hour. This myoclonus resolved when both drugs were stopped, and did not recur when clozapine was restarted. The reasons are not known but the authors of the report suggest that what happened was possibly related to changes in 5-HT activity.[1] Another patient who had had neuroleptic malignant syndrome (stiffness, rigidity, tachycardia, diaphoresis, hypertension) while on fluphenazine developed it again 3–4 weeks after clozapine was added to his lithium treatment. The symptoms disappeared within 2–3 days of stopping the clozapine.[2] An elderly man also developed neuroleptic malignant syndrome three days after starting to take 25 mg clozapine daily. He was also taking carbamazepine and had stopped taking lithium three days before.[3] The reasons are not understood.

These are all isolated cases and there would seem to be little reason for avoiding concurrent use, but it should be well monitored for any sign of neuroleptic malignant syndrome (NMS).

Reference

1 Lemus CZ, Lieberman JA, Johns CA. Myoclonus during treatment with clozapine and lithium: the role of serotonin. Hillside J Clin Psychiatry (1989) 11, 127–30.
2 Pope HG, Cole JO, Choras PT, Fulwiler CE. Apparent neuroleptic malignant syndrome with clozapine and lithium. J Nerv Ment Dis (1986) 174, 493–5.
3 Müller T, Becker T, Fritze J. Neuroleptic malignant syndrome after clozapine plus carbamazepine. Lancet (1988) 2, 1500.

Clozapine + miscellaneous drugs

Abstract/Summary

Isolated cases of apparent interaction have been seen in patients taking clozapine. A severe urticarial rash developed in a patient given L-tryptophan, vitamin C and nicotinic acid. A fall in white cell counts occurred in a patient when given nitrofurantoin. Clozapine and chloroquine appear not to interact adversely.

Clinical evidence, mechanism, importance and management

A man with schizophrenia taking L-tryptophan, lorazepam, vitamin C, benztropine and niconitic acid, developed a severe urticarial rash covering his face, neck and trunk three days after starting 150 mg clozapine daily. All of the drugs except lorazepam were stopped and the rash subsided. It did not recur when clozapine was restarted and gradually increased to 600 mg daily, nor when small doses of benztriopine and fluphenazine were briefly added. The authors draw the inference that L-tryptophan, vitamin C and nicotinic acid may have been responsible for this 'interaction'.[1]

A patient who had been taking 500 mg clozapine daily for 8 months developed granulocytopenia within eight days of starting 200 mg nitrofurantoin daily. The problem resolved when the nitrofurantoin was stopped.[2]

A patient on clozapine, 25 mg daily, showed no significant changes in his white blood cell count while taking 23.5 g chloroquine for malarial prophylaxis over a month.[3]

These reports are isolated cases so that no general conclusions can be drawn from them except to confirm that close monitoring is necessary in any patient treated with clozapine.

References

1 Goumeniouk AD, Ancill RJ, MacEwan GW, Koczapski AB. A case of drug-drug interaction involving clozapine. Can J Psychiatry (1991) 36, 234.
2 Juul Povlsen U, Juul Poulsen U, Noring U, Fog R, Gerlach J. Tolerability and therapeutic effect of clozapine. Acta Psychiatr Scand (1985) 71, 176.
3 König P, Künz A. Compatibility of clozapine and chloroquine. Lancet (1991) 338, 948.

Droperidol/Hyoscine + Monoamine oxidase inhibitors (MAOI)

Abstract/Summary

An isolated and unexplained report describes hypotension in a patient given droperidol and hyoscine as premedication, shortly after the withdrawal of phenelzine and perphenazine.

Clinical evidence, mechanism, importance and management

Four days after the withdrawal of phenelzine and perphenazine, a patient was given operative premedication with 20 mg droperidol and 0.4 mg hyoscine. About 2 h later he was observed to be pale, sweating profusely, slightly cyanosed, with a blood pressure of 75/60 mmHg and a pulse rate of 60. No excitement or changes in respiration were seen. The blood pressure gradually rose to 115/80 mmHg over the next 45 min, but did not return to normal (160/100 mmHg) for 36 h. 11 days later, using the same premedication, the operation was successfully undertaken without any hypotensive episodes.[1] The response was attributed to the after-effects of phenelzine treatment, but there is no obvious explanation for this interaction (if indeed it is an interaction).

Reference

1 Penlington GN. Droperidol and monoamine oxidase inhibitors. Br Med J (1966) 1, 483.

Haloperidol + Anticonvulsants

Abstract/Summary

Haloperidol serum levels are approximately halved by carbamazepine, phenobarbitone and phenytoin. Neurotoxicity has been seen with haloperidol and carbamazepine. Sodium valproate appears not to interact.

Clinical evidence

(a) Haloperidol + Carbamazepine

Nine schizophrenics on haloperidol (averaging 30 mg daily) showed a 55% fall in serum haloperidol levels (a mean fall from 45.4 to 21.2 ng/ml) when given carbamazepine for five weeks (precise dose not stated, but said to be 5–6 tablets daily). They also had 10 mg benzhexol and 30 mg oxazepam at night as necessary. Carbamazepine serum levels and the control of the disease remained unchanged.[1]

Three other studies similarly found 50–60% falls in serum haloperidol levels while taking carbamazepine.[2,5,8] A few patients showed clinical worsening.[5,8,11] Three patients showed 2–5 fold increases in serum haloperidol levels and clinical improvement when carbamazepine (1200–1400 mg daily) was stopped but extrapyramidal side-effects developed within 1–30 days.[12] Three cases of of neurotoxicity (drowsiness, slurred speech) during concurrent use have also been described.[4,6,7]

(b) Haloperidol + Phenobarbitone and Phenytoin

A study in patients, two on phenobarbitone, three on phenytoin, and four on both, found that after 6 weeks their serum haloperidol levels (doses of 30 mg daily) were approximately half (19.4 ng/ml) of those in the control group who were not taking anticonvulsants (36.6 ng/ml). Their serum anticonvulsant levels remained unchanged.[9] Another patient showed a marked rise in serum haloperidol levels with clinical improvement when 300 mg phenytoin was stopped.[12]

(c) Haloperidol + Sodium valproate

A study in six patients given 6–10 mg haloperidol daily showed no significant interaction with sodium valproate.[10]

Mechanism

Carbamazepine, phenobarbitone and phenytoin are recognized enzyme inducing agents, therefore it seems almost certain that the reduced serum haloperidol levels occur because its metabolism by the liver is markedly increased by these anticonvulsants.

Importance and management

These interactions are moderately well documented and appear to be clinically important, although only a few patients have been reported to show clinical worsening. Although there are advantages in adding carbamazepine to haloperidol in treating manic patients or schizoaffective excited patients and others with excited psychoses and schizophrenia,[3] be alert for the need to increase the haloperidol dosage if carbamazepine, phenobarbitone or phenytoin are given concurrently. The authors of one study (with phenobarbitone and phenytoin) suggest a 200–300% increase in the haloperidol dosage.[9]

Remember too that if the anticonvulsants are withdrawn it may be necessary to reduce the haloperidol dosage. Also be alert for the development of dystonic reactions.

References

1 Jann MW, Ereshefsky L, Saklad SR, Seidel DR, Davis CM, Burch NR, Bowden CL. Effects of carbamazepine on plasma haloperidol levels. J Clin Psychopharmacol (1985) 5, 106–9.

2 Kidron R, Averbuch I, Klein E, Belmaker RH. Carbamazepine-induced reduction of blood levels of haloperidol in chronic schizophrenics. Biol Psychiatry (1985) 20, 219–22.

3 Klein E, Bental E, Lerer B, Belmaker RH. Combination of carbamazepine and haloperidol versus placebo and haloperidol in excited psychoses: a controlled study. Arch Gen Psychiatry (1984) 41, 165–70.

4 Kanter GL, Yerevanian BI, Ciccone JR. Case report of a possible interaction between neuroleptics and carbamazepine. Am J Psychiatry (1984) 141, 1101–2.

5 Arana GW, Goff DC, Friedman H, Ornstein M, Greenblatt DJ, Black B, Shader RI. Does carbamazepine-induced reduction of plasma haloperidol worsen psychotic symptoms. Am J Psychiatry (1986) 143, 650–1.

6 Brayley J, Yellowlees P. An interaction between haloperidol and carbamazepine in a patient with cerebral palsy. Aust NZ J Psychiatry (1987) 21, 605–7.

7 Yerevanian BI, Hodgeman CH. A haloperidol carbamazepine interaction in a patient with rapid-cycling disorder. Am J Psychiatry (1985) 142, 785–6.

8 Kahn EM, Schulz SC, Perel JM, Alexander JE. Change in haloperidol level due to carbamazepine — a complicating factor in combined medication for schizophrenia. J Clin Psychopharmacol (1990) 10, 54–7.

9 Linnoila M, Viukari M, Vaisanen K, Auvinen J. Effect of anticonvulsants on plasma haloperidol and thioridazine levels. Am J Psychiatry (1980) 137, 819–21.

10 Ishizaki T, Chiba K, Saito M, Kobayashi K, Iizuka R. The effects of neuroleptics (haloperidol and chlorpromazine) on the pharmacokinetics of valproic acid in schizophrenic patients. J Clin Psychopharmacol (1984) 4, 254–61.

11 Fast DK, Jones BD, Kusalic M, Erikson M. Effect of carbamazepine on neuroleptic plasma levels and efficacy. Am J Psychiatry (1986) 143, 117–8.

12 Jann MW, Fidone GS, Hernandez JM, Amrung S, Davis CM. Clinical implications of increased antipsychotic plasma concentrations upon anticonvulsant cessation. Psychiatry Res (1989) 28, 153–9.

Haloperidol + Antituberculars

Abstract/Summary

The serum levels of haloperidol can be reduced by the concurrent use of rifampicin (rifampin).

Clinical evidence, mechanism, importance and management

A study in 18 schizophrenic patients on haloperidol, some of whom were also being treated with a range of antitubercular drugs (ethambutol, isoniazid, rifampicin), showed that those on rifampicin had significantly reduced haloperidol serum levels. The half-life of haloperidol in two patients on rifampicin was 4.8 h compared with 9.4 h in three other patients not taking rifampicin. A likely explanation is that the rifampicin, a recognized enzyme inducing agent, increases the metabolism and loss of the haloperidol from the body. Three of the patients on isoniazid had increased serum haloperidol levels.[1] Information about this interaction is very limited but there is now enough evidence to suggest that the effects of concurrent use should be well monitored. Be alert for any evidence of reduced haloperidol effects if rifampicin is used. Increase the dosage if necessary. More study is needed.

Reference

1 Takeda M, Nishimura K, Yamasthita S, Matsubayashi T, Tamino S, Nishimura T. Serum haloperidol levels of schizophrenics receiving treatment for tuberculosis. Clin Neuropharmacol (1986) 9, 386.

Haloperidol + Buspirone

Abstract/Summary

Buspirone causes a modest rise in serum haloperidol levels.

Clinical evidence, mechanism, importance and management

Six chronic schizophrenic patients showed 15–122% rises in serum haloperidol levels after taking buspirone for 6 weeks. Another showed a 5% fall. The mean rise was 26%.[1] A single dose study in normal subjects found a 30% rise.[2] The reasons are not understood, nor is the clinical significance of this rise known, but it is probably small. No special precautions appear to be necessary.

References

1 Goff DC, Midha KK, Brotman AW, McCormick S, Waites M, Amico ET. An open trial of buspirone added to neuroleptics in schizophrenic patients. J Clin Psychopharmacol (1991) 11, 193–7.
2 Quoted in ref 1 as Mead Johnson Pharmaceuticals, personnal communication 1989.

Haloperidol + Granisetron

Abstract/Summary

Granisetron appears not to increase the adverse effects of haloperidol (drowsiness, mental slowness, etc).

Clinical evidence, mechanism, importance and management

A study in normal subjects found that while 3 mg haloperidol alone caused some impaired psychometric performance (increased drowsiness, muzziness, lethargy, mental slowness, etc), the addition of 160 μg/kg granisetron did not seem to make it significantly worse.[1] No special precautions would seem necessary, over and above those needed for haloperidol alone.

Reference

1 Leigh TJ, Link CGG, Fell GL. Effects of granisetron and haloperidol, alone and in combination, on psychometric performance and the EEG. Br J Clin Pharmac (1992) 34, 65–70.

Haloperidol + Indomethacin

Abstract/Summary

Profound drowsiness and confusion have been described in patients given haloperidol and indomethacin.

Clinical evidence

A double-blind crossover study on 20 patients to find out the possible advantages of combining haloperidol (5 mg daily) with indomethacin (75 mg daily) in the treatment of pain arising from osteoarthritis of the knee and/or hip was eventually abandoned because 13 patients (11 on haloperidol and two on placebo) failed to complete the trial, six of those on haloperidol being withdrawn because of profound drowsiness or tiredness. The authors of the paper said that the combined treatment '...produced drowsiness and confusion so severe that in some cases the patient's independent existence was in jeopardy; this side-effect was far more intense than anything which might have been expected with haloperidol alone'.[1]

I am personally aware of another anecdotal report of this marked drowsiness in a woman patient.

Mechanism

Not understood.

Importance and management

Evidence of this interaction appears to be very limited. The incidence (six out of 11) is high. If concurrent use is thought appropriate, keep a close watch to ensure that this severe side-effect does not develop. It might be wiser to avoid concurrent use because many patients requiring this type of treatment may not be hospitalized and under the day-to-day scrutiny of the prescriber.

Reference

1 Bird HA, Le Gallez P, Wright V. Drowsiness due to haloperidol/indomethacin combination. Lancet (1983) i, 830–1.

Haloperidol + Tobacco smoking

Abstract/Summary

Those who smoke may need more haloperidol than those who do not.

Clinical evidence

Steady-state haloperidol levels were found to be lower in a group of 23 cigarette smokers than in another group of 27 non-smokers (16.83 compared with 28.80 ng/ml) and the clearance was increased (1.58 compared with 1.10 l/min).[1] Another later study broadly confirmed these findings.[2] The probable reason is that some of the components of tobacco smoke act as liver enzyme inducers which increase the rate at which the liver metabolizes and clears the haloperidol from the body. It seems likely that smokers will need larger doses of haloperidol than non-smokers, and the dosage of haloperidol may need to be adjusted if patients start or stop smoking.

Reference

1 Jann MW, Sakald SR, Ereshefsky L, Richards AL, Harrington CA, Davis CM. Effects of smoking on haloperidol and reduced haloperidol plasma concentrations and haloperidol clearance. Psychopharmacol (1986) 90, 468–70.
2 Perry PJ, Miller DD, Arndt SV, Smith DA, Holman TL. Haloperidol dosing requirements: The contribution of smoking and nonlinear pharmacokinetics. J Clin Psychopharmacol (1993) 13, 46–51.

Hydroxyzine + miscellaneous drugs

Abstract/Summary

Hydroxyzine can cause ECG abnormalities in high doses. It has been suggested that concurrent use with other drugs which can cause cardiac abnormalities might increase the likelihood of dysrhythmias and sudden death.

Clinical evidence, mechanism, importance and management

A study in 25 elderly psychotic patients on 300 mg hydroxyzine over a nine-week period showed that ECG changes were mild except for alteration in T waves which were definite in nine patients and usually observed in leads 1,2 AVL and V_{3-6}. In each case the T-waves were lower in altitude, broadened and flattened and sometimes notched. The QT interval was usually prolonged. A repeat of the study in a few patients, one at least given 400 mg, gave similar results, the most pronounced change being a marked attentuation of the cardiac repolarization. On the basis of these observations the authors suggest that other drugs which cause ECG abnormalities (they mention antiparkinson drugs, atropine, lithium carbonate, phenothiazines, quinidine, procainamide, thioridazine, tricyclic antidepressants), might aggravate and exaggerate these hydroxyzine-induced changes and increase the risk of sudden death.[1] More study is needed to assess the practical importance of these potential interactions.

Reference

1 Hollister LE. Hydroxyzine hydrochloride: possible adverse cardiac interactions. Psychopharmacol Comm (1975) 1, 61.

Neuroleptics (Butyrophenones, Phenothiazines, Thioxanthenes) + Anticholinergics

Abstract/Summary

These drugs are very often given together advantageously and uneventfully, but occasionally serious and even life-threatening interactions occur. These include heat-stroke in hot and humid conditions, severe constipation and adynamic ileus, and atropine-like psychoses. Anticholinergics used to counteract the extrapyramidal side-effects of neuroleptics (e.g. chlorpromazine, haloperidol, etc.) may also reduce or abolish their therapeutic effects. See also 'Phenothiazines + Tricyclic antidepressants' and 'Anticholinergics + Anticholinergics'.

Clinical evidence

Concurrent use can result in a generalized, low grade, but not serious additive increase in the anticholinergic effects of these drugs (blurred vision, dry mouth, constipation, difficulty in urination), however sometimes serious intensification takes place. For the sake of clarity these have been subdivided here into (A) heat stroke, (B) constipation and adynamic ileus, (C) atropine-like psychoses and (D) antagonism of neuroleptic effects.

(A) Heat stroke in hot and humid conditions

Three patients were admitted to hospital in Philadelphia for drug-induced hyperpyrexia during a hot and humid period. In each case their skin and mucous membranes were dry and the pulse fast (120 bpm). The first was taking daily doses of 500 mg chlorpromazine, 200 mg chlorprothixene and 6 mg benztropine; the second was taking 600 mg chlorpromazine, 12 mg trifluoperazine and 2 mg benztropine daily; and the third was on 8 mg haloperidol and 2 mg benztropine daily. There was no evidence of infection.[1]

There are other reports of heat stroke, some of them fatal, in patients taking chlorpromazine, promazine, fluphenazine or other phenothiazines with benztropine or other atropine-like drugs and/or tricyclic antidepressants.[3-5] The danger of heat-stroke in patients on atropine or atropine-compounds was recognized more than half a century ago, and the warning has been repeated many times.[13,14]

Mechanism

Anticholinergic drugs inhibit the parasympathetic nervous system which innervates the sweat glands so that when the ambient temperature rises, the major body heat-losing mechanism can be partially or wholly put out of action.[2] Phenothiazines, thioxanthenes and butyrophenones may also have some anticholinergic effects, but additionally they impair to a varying extent the hypothalamic thermoregulatory mechanisms which control the body's ability to keep a constant temperature when exposed to heat or cold. Thus, when the ambient temperature rises, the body temperature also rises. The tricyclics can similarly disrupt the temperature control. So in very hot and humid conditions when the need to reduce the temperature is great, the additive effects of these drugs can make patients become '...little more able to control their internal responses to heat than are reptiles...'[5] but, unlike poikilothermic animals, they are unable to sustain life once the temperature reaches a certain point.

(B) Constipation and adynamic ileus

Eight cases of adynamic ileus with faecal impaction have been reported in patients treated with phenothiazines (chlorpromazine, levomepromazine, thioridazine, trifluoperazine, perphenazine), imipramine and benztropine or benzhexol, or a combination of two or more of these drugs. Five were treated successfully but three patients died because recognition of the condition was too late.[6]

A number of other cases have been described involving chlorpromazine with nortriptyline,[9] imipramine,[6] benzhexol,[6] trifluoperazine and benztropine,[7] or amitriptyline;[8] mesoridazine with benztropine;[25] trifluoperazine with bentropine or benzhexol;[6,26] imipramine with levomepromazine and benztropine,[6] or with thioridazine and benzhexol.[6] Seven of the cases had a fatal outcome. Severe constipation also occurred in a woman given thioridazine, biperiden and doxepin.[25]

Mechanism

Anticholinergic drugs reduce peristalsis which, in the extreme, can result in total gut stasis. Additive effects can occur if two or more anticholinergic drugs are taken.

(C) Atropine-like psychoses

Three patients taking part in a double-blind study of this interaction and given a phenothiazine and benztropine mesylate for the parkinsonian side-effects, developed an intermittent toxic confusional state (marked disturbance of short-term memory, impaired attention, disorientation, anxiety, visual and auditory hallucinations) with peripheral anticholinergic signs.[12]

Similar reactions occurred in three elderly patients given imipramine or desipramine with benzhexol.[11] A toxic psychosis was seen in a woman on meclozine three days after starting to use a transdermal preparation of hyoscine,[24] and in another man given chlorpromazine, benztropine and doxepin.[25]

Mechanism

These toxic psychoses resemble the CNS effects of atropine or belladonna poisoning and appear to result from the additive effects of the drugs used.

(D) Antagonism of the neuroleptic effects

Studies in psychiatric patients given 300–800 mg chlorpromazine daily showed that when 6–10 mg benzhexol daily was added, the plasma chlorpromazine levels fell from a range of 100–300 ng/ml to less than 30 ng/ml. When the benzhexol was withdrawn the plasma chlorpromazine levels rose again and clinical improvement was seen.[18,21]

Other studied confirm that benzhexol[17,22] and orphenadrine[10] reduce the plasma levels and effects of chlorpromazine. Some of the actions of haloperidol on social avoidance behaviour can be abolished by benztropine, but cognitive integrative function is unaffected.[15,16] In contrast to these reports, another found that benzhexol increased chlorpromazine levels by 41% in 20 young schizophrenics, but no clinical change was seen.[23]

Mechanism

Not understood. Animal studies suggest that the site of interaction is in the gut.[21]

Importance and management of (A)–(D)

Established and well-documented interactions. While these drugs have been widely used together with apparent advantage and without problems, prescribers should be aware that (i) an unspectacular low-grade anticholinergic toxicity can easily go undetected in the elderly because the symptoms can be so similar to the general complaints of old people; and (ii) also be aware of the serious problems which can develop, particularly if high doses are used. (A) Warn patients to minimize outdoor exposure and/or exercise in hot and humid climates, particularly if they are taking high doses of antipsychotic/anticholinergic drugs. (B) Be alert for severe constipation and for the development of complete gut stasis which can be fatal. (C) Be aware that the symptoms of central anticholinergic psychosis can be confused with the basic psychotic symptoms of the patient. Withdrawal of one or more of the drugs, or a dosage reduction and/or appropriate symptomatic treatment can be used to control these interactions. (D) Ensure that the concurrent use of anticholinergics to control the extrapyramidal side-effects of neuroleptics is necessary[19,20] and be aware that the therapeutic effects may possibly be reduced as a result. See also 'Phenothiazines + Tricyclic antidepressants'.

References

1 Westlake RJ, Rastegar A. Hyperpyrexia from drug combinations. J Amer Med Ass (1973) 225, 1250.

2 Kollias J, Bullard RW. The influence of chlorpromazine on the physical and chemical mechanism of temperature regulation in the rat. J Pharmacol Exp Ther (1964) 145, 373.

3 Zelman S, Guillan R. Heat stroke in phenothiazine-treated patients: a report of three fatalities. Am J Psychiat (1970) 126, 1787.

4 Sarnquist F, Larson CP. Drug induced heat stroke. Anesthesiology (1973) 39, 348.

5 Reimer DR, Mohan J, Nagaswami S. Heat dyscontrol syndrome in patients receiving antipsychotic, antidepressant and anti-parkinson drug therapy. J Florida Med Ass (1974) 61, 573.

6 Warnes H, Lehmann HE, Ban TA. Adynamic ileus during psychoactive medication. A report of three fatal and five severe cases. Canad Med Ass J (1976) 96, 1112.

7 Giorano J, Huang A, Canter JW. Fatal paralytic ileus complicating phenothiazine therapy. S Med J (1975) 68, 351.

8 Burkitt EA, Sutcliffe CK. Paralytic ileus after amitriptyline (Tryptizol). Br Med J (1961) 2, 1648.

9 Milner G, Hills NF. Adynamic ileus and nortriptyline. Br Med J (1966) 1, 841.

10 Loga S, Curry S, Lader M. Interactions of orphenadrine and phenobarbitone with chlorpromazine: plasma concentrations and effects in man. Br J Clin Pharmac (1975) 2, 197.

11 Roger SC. Imipramine and benzhexol. Br Med J (1967) 1, 500.

12 Davis JM. Psychopharmacology in the aged. Use of psychotropic drugs in geriatric patients. J Geriatric Psychiatry (1974) 7, 145.

13 Wilcox WH. The nature, prevention and treatment of heat hyper-pyrexia. Br Med J (1920) 1, 392.

14 Litman RE. Heat sensitivity due to autonomic drugs. J Amer Med Ass (1952) 149, 635.

15 Singh MM, Smith JM. Reversal of some therapeutic effects of an antipsychotic agent by an antiparkinsonian drug. J Nerv Ment Dis (1973) 157, 50.

16 Singh MM, Smith JM. Reversal of some therapeutic effects of haloperidol in schizophrenia by antiparkinson drugs. Pharmacologist (1971) 13, 207.

17 Chan T, Sakalis G, Gershon S. Some aspects of chlorpromazine metabolism in humans. Clin Pharmacol Ther (1973) 14, 133.

18 Rivera-Calimlim L, Castenada L, Lasagna L. Significance of plasma levels of chlorpromazine. Clin Pharmacol Ther (1973) 14, 144.

19 Priest RF. Unpublished surveys from the NIMH collaborative project on drug therapy in chronic schizophrenics and the VA collaborative project on interim drug therapy in chronic schizophrenics. Quoted in Int Drug Ther Newsletter (1974) 9, 29.

20 Klett CJ, Caffey EM. Evaluating the long-term need for antiparkinson drugs by chronic schizophrenics. Arch Gen Psychiatry (1972) 26, 374.

21 Rivera-Calimlim L, Castenada L, Lasagna L. Chlorpromazine and trihexiphenidyl interaction in psychiatric patients. Pharmacologist (1973) 15, 212.

22 Rivera-Calimlim L, Nasrallah H, Strauss J, Lasagna L. Clinical response and plasma levels: effect of dose, dosage schedules and drug interaction on plasma chlorpromazine levels. Am J Psychiat (1976) 133, 646.

23 Rockland L, Cooper T, Schwartz F, Weber D, Sullivan T. Effects of trihexyphenidyl on plasma chlorpromazine in young schizophrenics. Can J Psychiatry (1990) 35, 604–7.

24 Osterholm RK, Camoriano JK. Transdermal scopolamine psychosis. J Amer Med Ass (1982) 247, 3081.

25 Ayd FJ. Doxepin with other drugs. S Med J (1973) 66, 465–71.

26 Spiro RK, Kysilewsky RM. Iatrogenic ileus secondary to medication. J Med Soc NJ (1973) 70, 565.

Neuroleptics + Bromocriptine

Abstract/Summary

Concurrent use can be successful, but one report describes the re-emergence of schizophrenic symptoms in a patient when bromocriptine was added to molindone and imipramine.

Clinical evidence, mechanism, importance and management

Single low doses of bromocriptine have been found to improve the psychopathology of chronic schizophrenia in patients on neuroleptics[1] and a case report describes the successful concurrent use of bromocriptine and haloperidol.[2] Another report describes a schizoaffective schizophrenic on fluphenazine, benztropine, phenytoin and phenobarbitone whose psychiatric status was unaltered when bromocriptine was given to treat a pituitary adenoma, but the previously normal serum prolactin was reduced to less than detectable levels by the bromocriptine.[3] However a woman with schizoaffective schizophrenia stabilized on 100 mg molindone and 200 mg imipramine daily, relapsed (agitation, delusions, hallucinations) within five days of starting additional treatment with 7.5 mg bromocriptine daily for amenorrhoea-galactorrhoea.[4] Within three days of stopping the bromocriptine these symptoms vanished. The reason suggested by the authors of the report is that the bromocriptine (a dopamine agonist) opposed the actions of the antipsychotic medication (dopamine antagonists) thereby allowing the schizophrenia to re-emerge. If concurrent use is thought appropriate, the outcome should be well monitored.

References

1 Cutler NR, Jeste DV, Kaufmann CA, Karoum F, Schran HF, Wyatt RJ. Low dose bromocriptine: a study of acute effects in chronic medicated schizophrenics. Prog Neuro-Psycho-pharmacol Biol Psychiatry (1984) 8, 277–83.

2 Gattaz WF, Kollisch M. Bromocriptine in the treatment of neuroleptic-resistant schizophrenia. Biol Psychiatry (1986) 21, 519–21.

3 Kellner C, Harris P, Blumhardt C. Concurrent use of bromocriptine and fluphenazine. J Clin Psychiatry (1984) 46, 455.

4 Frye PE, Pariser SF, Kim MH, O'Shaughnessy RW. Bromocriptine associated with symptom exacerbation during neuroleptic treatment of schizoaffective schizophrenia. J Clin Psychiatry (1982) 43, 252–3.

Phenothiazines + Antacids

Abstract/Summary

Antacids containing aluminium hydroxide or magnesium trisilicate can reduce the serum levels of chlorpromazine which would be expected to reduce the therapeutic response. *In vitro* studies suggest that this may possibly also occur with other antacids and phenothiazines.

Clinical evidence

A study in 10 patients taking 600–1200 mg chlorpromazine daily showed that when concurrently treated with 30 ml *Aludrox* (aluminium hydroxide gel) their urinary excretion of chlorpromazine was reduced 10–45%.[3]

A study on six patients, prompted by the observation of one patient on chlorpromazine who relapsed within three days of starting to take an un-named antacid, showed that when 30 ml *Gelusil* (aluminium hydroxide + magnesium trisilicate) was given with a liquid suspension of chlorpromazine, the serum chlorpromazine levels measured 2 h later were reduced by 20% (from 168 to 132 ng/ml).[1,2] *In vitro* studies have also found that other phenothiazines (trifluperazine, fluphenazine, perphenazine, thioridazine) are adsorbed to a considerable extent onto a number of antacids (magnesium trisilicate, bismuth subnitrate, aluminium hydroxide-magnesium carbonate) but no clinical studies of the possible effects of these interactions appear to have been done.[5]

Mechanism

Chlorpromazine and other phenothiazines become adsorbed onto these antacids[1,4] which would seem to account for the reduced bioavailability.

Importance and management

Clinical information seems to be limited to the reports cited. Reductions in serum levels of up to 45% would be expected to be clinically important but so far only one case seems to have been reported.[1,2] Separating the dosages as much as possible (1–2 h) to avoid admixture in the gut should minimize any effects. An alternative would be to use one of the ionic antacids such as calcium carbonate-glycine or magnesium hydroxide gel which do not seem to affect the gastrointestinal absorption of chlorpromazine to any extent.[4] Other phenothiazines and antacids are known to interact *in vitro*,[5] but the clinical importance of these interactions awaits further study.

References

1 Fann WE, Davis JM, Janowsky DS, Sekerke HJ, Schmidt DM. Chlorpromazine: effects of antacids on its gastrointestinal absorption. J Clin Pharmacol (1973) 13, 388.
2 Fann WE, Davis JM, Janowsky DS, Schmidt DM. The effects of antacids on chlorpromazine levels. Ann Pharmacol Ther (1973) 14, 135.
3 Forrest FM, Forrest IS, Serra MT. Modification of chlorpromazine metabolism by some other drugs frequently administered to psychiatric patients. Biol Psychiat (1970) 2, 35.
4 Pinell OC, Fenimore DC, Davis CM, Fann WE. Drug-drug interaction of chlorpromazine and antacid. Clin Pharmacol Ther (1978) 23, 125.
5 Moustafa MA, Babhair SA, Kouta HI. Decreased bioavailability of some antipsychotic phenothiazines due to interactions with adsorbent antacid and antidiarrhoeal mixtures. Int J Pharmaceutics (1987) 36, 185–9.

Phenothiazines + Antimalarials

Abstract/Summary

Chloroquine, amodiaquine and *Fansidar* (sulphadoxine + pyrimethamine) can markedly increase serum chlorpromazine levels.

Clinical evidence

Fifteen schizophrenic patients (in three groups of five) given 400 or 500 chlorpromazine daily for at least 2 weeks were additionally given single doses of either chloroquine sulphate (400 mg), amodiaquine hydrochloride (600 mg) or three tablets of *Fansidar* (25 mg pyrimethamine + 500 mg sulphadoxine) an hour before the chlorpromazine. Serum chlorpromazine levels 3 h later were found to be raised approximately threefold by the chloroquine and amodiaquine, and almost fourfold by the *Fansidar*. The plasma levels of one of the major metabolites of chlorpromazine (7-OH-chlorpromazine) were also elevated, but not those of the other (chlorpromazine sulphoxide). Four days later the serum chlorpromazine levels of the patients given

chloroquine or *Fansidar* still remained elevated to some extent. There was subjective evidence that the patients were more heavily sedated when given the antimalarials.[1]

Mechanism

Not understood. Both chloroquine and *Fansidar* have relatively long half-lives compared with amodiaquine which may explain the persistence of their effects.

Importance and management

Direct information about this interaction seems to be limited to this study. Its clinical importance is uncertain but it seems possible that these antimalarials could cause chlorpromazine toxicity. Monitor the effects of concurrent use closely and anticipate the need to reduce the chlorpromazine dosage. More study is needed.

Reference

1 Makanjuola ROA, Dixon PAF, Oforah E. Effects of antimalarial agents on plasma levels of chlorpromazine and its metabolites in schizophrenic patients. Trop Geogr Med (1988) 40, 31–3.

Phenothiazines + Ascorbic acid

Abstract/Summary

A single case report describes a fall in serum fluphenazine levels and deterioration in a patient when given ascorbic acid (vitamin C).

Clinical evidence, mechanism, importance and management

A manic depressive man taking 15 mg fluphenazine daily showed a 25% fall (from 0.93 to 0.705 ng/ml) in his serum drug levels accompanied by a deterioration in behaviour over a 13-day period while taking 1 g ascorbic acid daily.[1] The reason is not understood. There seem to be no other reports of this interaction with fluphenazine or any other phenothiazine.

Reference

1 Dysken MW, Cumming RJ, Channon RA, Davis JM. Drug interaction between ascorbic acid and fluphenazine. J Amer Med Ass (1979) 241, 2008.

Phenothiazines + Attapulgite

Abstract/Summary

An attapulgite-pectin antidiarrhoeal preparation caused a fall in the absorption of promazine in one subject.

Clinical evidence, mechanism, importance and management

A study in a normal subject showed that attapulgite-pectin reduced the absorption of a single 50 mg dose of promazine by about 25%, possibly due to absorption of the phenothiazine onto the attapulgite.[1] The clinical importance of this and whether other phenothiazines behave similarly appears not to have been studied, but prescribers should be aware of this possible interaction if preparations containing attapulgite-pectin are given. Separating the administration as much as possible to avoid admixture in the gut has been shown with other drugs to minimize the effects of this type of interaction.

Reference

1 Sorby DL, Liu G. Effects of adsorbents on drug absorption. II. Effect of an antidiarrhoea mixture on promazine absorption. J Pharm Sci (1966) 55, 504–10.

Phenothiazines + Barbiturates

Abstract/Summary

The serum levels of each drug are reduced by the presence of the other, but the clinical importance of these reductions is uncertain. Pentobarbitone, promethazine and scopolamine in combination are said to increase the incidence of operative agitation.

Clinical evidence

(a) Serum phenothiazine levels reduced

A study in 12 schizophrenics on 300 mg chlorpromazine daily showed that when additionally treated with 150 mg phenobarbitone daily, there was a 25–30% fall in serum chlorpromazine levels accompanied by changes in certain physiological measurements which clearly reflected a reduced response. The conclusion was made that there was no advantage to be gained by concurrent use.[1]

In another study on seven patients the serum levels of thioridazine were observed to be reduced by phenobarbitone, the clinical effects of which were uncertain.[2] However another study found no changes in serum thioridazine levels, but the levels of its active metabolite (mesoridazine) were reduced.[6]

(b) Serum phenobarbitone levels reduced

A study in a large number of epileptic patients showed that their serum phenobarbitone levels fell by 29% when treated with phenothiazines including chlorpromazine, thioridazine or mesoridazine, and increased once more when the phenothiazine was withdrawn.[3]

This study confirms another in which 100–200 mg thioridazine daily was found to reduce serum phenobarbitone levels by about 25%.[4] There is also some limited evidence that the concurrent use of pentobarbitone, promethazine and scopolamine increases the incidence of pre-operative, operative and postoperative agitation, and it has been suggested that this triple combination should be avoided.[5]

Mechanisms

Uncertain. The barbiturates are potent liver enzyme inducing agents which, it is presumed, increase the metabolism of the phenothiazines by the liver.

Importance and management

These interactions appear to be established, but the documentation is limited. The importance of both interactions (a and b) is uncertain, but be alert for evidence of reductions in response during concurrent use, and to increased responses if one of the drugs is withdrawn. So far only chlorpromazine, thioridazine, mesoridazine and phenobarbitone are implicated, but it seems possible that other phenothiazines and barbiturates will behave similarly.

References

1 Loga S, Curry S, Lader M. Interactions of orphenadrine and phenobarbitone with chlorpromazine: plasma concentrations and effects in man. Br J Clin Pharmac (1975) 2, 197.
2 Ellenor GL, Musa MN, Beuthin FC. Phenobarbital-thioridazine interaction in man. Res Comm Chem Pathol Pharmacol (1978) 21, 185.
3 Haidukewych D, Rodin EA. Effect of phenothiazines on serum antiepileptic drug concentrations in psychiatric patients with seizure disorder. Ther Drug Monitor (1985) 7, 401–4.
4 Gay PE, Madsen JA. Interaction between phenobarbital and thioridazine. Neurology (1983) 33, 1631–2.
5 Macris SG, Levy L. Preanesthetic medication: untoward effects of certain drug combinations. Anesthesiology (1965) 26, 256.
6 Linnoila M, Viukari M, Vaisanen K, Auvinen J. Effect of anticonvulsants on plasma haloperidol and thioridazine levels. Am J Psychiatry (1980) 137, 819–21.

Phenothiazines + Cimetidine

Abstract/Summary

One study found that chlorpromazine serum levels are reduced by cimetidine. Another suggested that they can be increased.

Clinical evidence

A study in eight patients on 75-450 mg daily chlorpromazine found that 1 g cimetidine daily for a week decreased their steady-state serum chlorpromazine levels by a third (from 37 to 24 µg/ml). A two-thirds fall was noted in one patient.[1] The reasons are not understood but a decrease in absorption from the gut has been suggested.[1] In contrast another report describes two schizophrenic patients on 100 mg chlorpromazine four times daily who became excessively sedated when given

800 mg cimetidine. The sedation disappeared when the chlorpromazine dosage was halved. When the cimetidine was later withdrawn it was found necessary to give the original chlorpromazine dosage.[2] Chlorpromazine serum levels were not measured.[1] There is no simple explanation for these discordant reports, but they emphasise the need to monitor the concurrent use of chlorpromazine and cimetidine. More study is needed. There seems to be no information about other phenothiazines.

Reference

1 Howes CA, Pullar T, Sourindhrin I, Mistra PC, Capel H, Lawson DH, Tilstone WJ. Reduced steady-state plasma concentrations of indomethacin and chlorpromazine in patients receiving cimetidine. Eur J Clin Pharmacol (1983) 24, 99–102.
2 Byrne A, O'Shea B. Adverse interaction between cimetidine and chlorpromazine in two cases of chronic schizophrenia. Br J Psychiatry (1989) 155, 413–5.

Phenothiazines + Disulfiram

Abstract/Summary

A single case report describes a man on perphenazine whose psychotic symptoms re-emerged when he began to take disulfiram.

Clinical evidence, mechanism, importance and management

A psychotic man controlled on 16 mg perphenazine daily by mouth developed marked psychosis soon after starting to take 200 mg disulfiram daily.[1] His serum perphenazine levels had fallen from 2.3 to less than 1 nmol/l. Doubling the dosage of perphenazine had little effect and no substantial clinical improvement or rise in serum levels occurred until the perphenazine was given as the enanthate intramuscularly (50 mg weekly) when the levels rose to about 4 nmol/l. The results of clinical biochemical tests suggested that the disulfiram was acting as a liver enzyme-inducing agent, so that the perphenazine was being metabolized and cleared from the body more rapidly. Disulfiram normally acts as an enzyme inhibitor. Too little is known to assess the general importance of this interaction, but it would seem prudent to be on the alert during concurrent use. There seems to be no information about an interaction with other phenothiazines.

Reference

1 Hansen LB, Larsen N-E. Metabolic interaction between perphenazine and disulfiram. Lancet (1982) ii, 1472.

Phenothiazines + Lithium carbonate

Abstract/Summary

Serum levels of chlorpromazine can be reduced to non-therapeutic concentrations by the concurrent administration

of lithium. Dosage increases may be needed. The development of severe extrapyramidal side-effects or neurotoxicity has been seen in a few patients concurrently treated with lithium and chlorpromazine, thioridazine, thiothixene, flupenthixol, fluphenazine or loxapine. Sleep-walking has been described in some patients taking chlorpromazine-like drugs and lithium. See also Sulpiride + Lithium carbonate

Clinical evidence

Chlorpromazine + lithium carbonate

(i) Reduced serum chlorpromazine levels

In a double-blind study on psychiatric patients it was found that 400–800 mg daily doses of chlorpromazine (which normally produced serum levels of 100–300 ng/ml) only produced levels of 0–70 ng/ml during the concurrent use of lithium carbonate[1]

Other studies confirm the reduction in serum chlorpromazine levels by normal therapeutic serum levels of lithium carbonate.[2,3,6] Peak serum chlorpromazine levels in normal subjects were 40% lower and the areas under the time/concentration curves were 26% smaller.[2]

(ii) Toxic reactions

A paranoid schizophrenic maintained on 200–600 mg chlorpromazine daily for 5 years with no extrapyramidal symptoms developed stiffness of his face, arms and legs, and parkinsonian tremor of both hands within a day of starting to take 900 mg lithium daily. His serum lithium level after 3 days was 0.5 mEq/l. He was later maintained on daily doses of 1800 mg lithium (serum levels 1.17 mEq/l), 200 mg chlorpromazine and 2 mg benztropine, but he still complained of stiffness and had a persistent hand tremor.[16]

A number of other reports describe the emergence of severe extrapyramidal side-effects when chlorpromazine and lithium were used concurrently.[11,13,15] Ventricular fibrillation occurred in a patient taking both drugs when the lithium was suddenly withdrawn.[20]

Other phenothiazines + lithium carbonate

Four patients developed severe neurotoxic complications (seizures, encephalopathy, delerium, abnormal EEGs) while taking high doses of thioridazine (800 mg daily or more) and lithium. Serum lithium levels remained below 1.0 mmol/l. Three of them had used lithium and other phenothiazines uneventfully for extended periods without problems, and the fourth was subsequently successfully treated with lithium and fluphenazine.[4] The sudden emergence of extrapyramidal or other side-effects has been described in patients concurrently treated with lithium and flupenthixol,[5,18] fluphenazine,[12,18] thioridazine,[14] thiothixene[19] or loxapine.[17] Neurotoxicity developed in another patient on lithium when haloperidol was replaced by loxapine.[21] Irreversible brain damage has been reported in a patient taking fluphenazine decanoate and lithium.[6] The concurrent use of lithium and chlorpromazine, perphenazine, thioridazine or thiothixene has also been associated with sleepwalking episodes in 9% of a group of patients.[7]

Mechanisms

Not understood. One suggestion to account for the reduced serum levels of chlorpromazine, based on animal studies,[8,9] is that the lithium delays gastric emptying. This exposes the chlorpromazine to the metabolism by the gut wall for a longer time.

Importance and management

Information about the chlorpromazine/lithium interaction which results in reduced serum chlorpromazine levels is limited but it would seem to be established and of clinical importance. Serum chlorpromazine levels below 30 ng/ml have been shown to be ineffective, whereas clinical improvement is associated with levels within the 150–300 ng/ml range or more.[10] Thus a fall in levels to 0–70 ng/ml (study cited above) would be expected to result in a reduced therapeutic response. Monitor the effects and increase the dosage if necessary.

The development of severe neurotoxic and extrapyramidal side-effects with combinations of chlorpromazine or other phenothiazines (thioridazine, flupenthixol, fluphenazine, loxapine) and lithium appears to be very uncommon, but be alert for any evidence of toxicity if lithium is given with any of these drugs. One recommendation is that the onset of neurological manifestations such as excessive drowsiness or movement disorders warrants electroencephalography without delay. Much more study is needed to identify the patients at risk.

References

1 Kerzner B, Rivera-Calimlim L. Lithium and chlorpromazine (CPZ) interaction. Clin Pharmacol Ther (1976) 19, 109.
2 Rivera-Calimlim L, Kerzner B, Karach FE. Effect of lithium on plasma chlorpromazine levels. Clin Pharmacol Ther (1978) 23, 451.
3 Rivera-Calimlim L, Nasrallah H, Struss J, Lasagna L. Clinical response and plasma levels: effect of dose, dosage schedules and drug interactions on plasma chlorpromazine levels. Am J Psychiat (1976) 133, 646.
4 Spring GK. Neurotoxicity with combined use of lithium and thioridazine. J Clin Psychiat (1979) 40, 135.
5 West A. Adverse effects of lithium treatment. Br Med J (1977) 2, 642.
6 Singh SV. Lithium carbonate/fluphemazine decanoate producing irreversible brain damage. Lancet (1982) ii, 278.
7 Charney DS, Kales A, Soldatos CR, Nelson JC. Somnambulistic episodes secondary to combined lithium neuroleptic treatment. Br J Psychiat (1979) 135, 418–24.
8 Sundaresen PR, Rivera-Calimlim L. Distribution of chlorpromazine on the gastrointestinal tract of the rat and its effects on absorptive functions. J Pharmacol Exp Ther (1975) 194, 593.
9 Curry SH, O'Mello A, Mould GP. Destruction of chlorpromazine during absorption in the rat *in vivo* and *in vitro*. Br J Pharmacol (1971) 42, 403.
10 Rivera-Calimlim L, Castenada L, Lasagna L. Significance of plasma levels of chlorpromazine. Clin Pharmacol Ther (1973) 14, 978.
11 McGennis AJ. Hazards of lithium and neuroleptics in schizo-affective disorder. Br J Psychiatry (1983) 142, 99–100.
12 Sachdev PS. Lithium potentiation of neuroleptic-related extrapyramidal side-effects. Am J Psychiatry (1986) 143, 942.
13 Yassa R. A case of lithium-chlorpromazine interaction. J Clin Psychiatry (1986) 47, 90–1.
14 Bailine SH, Doft M. Neurotoxicity induced by combined lithium-thioridazine treatment. Biol Psychiatry (1986) 21, 834–7.
15 Habib M, Khalil R, Le Pensec-Bertrand, D, Ali-Cherif A, Bongrand MC, Crevat A. Syndrome neurologique persistant apres traitement par les sels de lithium. Rev Neurol(1986) 142, 1, 61–4.
16 Addonizio G. Rapid induction of extrapyramidal side-effects with combined use of lithium and neuroleptics. J Clin Psychopharmacol (1985) 5, 296–8.
17 de la Gandara J, Dominguez RA. Lithium and loxapine. A potential interaction. J Clin Psychiatry (1988) 49, 126.
18 Kamlana SH, Kerry RJ, Khan IA. Lithium: some drug interactions. Practitioner (1980) 224, 1291–2.
19 Fetzer J, Kader G, Dahany S. Lithium encephalopathy: a clinical, psychiatric and EEG evaluation. Am J Psychiatry (1981) 138, 1622–3.
20 Stevenson RN, Blanshard C, Patterson DLH. Ventricular fibrillation due to lithium withdrawal — an interaction with chlorpromazine? Postgrad Med J (1989) 65, 936–8.
21 Fuller MA, Sajatovic M. Neurotoxicity resulting from a combination of lithium and loxapine. J Clin Psychiatry (1989) 50, 187.

Phenothiazines + Naltrexone

Abstract/Summary

Extreme lethargy occurred in two patients on thioridazine when given naltrexone.

Clinical evidence, mechanism, importance and management

Two schizophrenic patients well stabilized on thioridazine (50–200 mg three times daily for 1–7 years) took part in a pilot project to assess the efficacy of naltrexone for the treatment of tardive dyskinesia. Both tolerated the first challenge dose of naloxone (0.8 mg IV) without problems but experienced extreme lethargy and slept almost continuously after the second dose (50–100 mg orally). The severe lethargy cleared up within 12 h of stopping the naltrexone.[1] The reasons for this reaction are not understood. Information seems to be limited to this report but this would seem to be a drug combination to be avoided. There seems to be nothing documented about other phenothiazines.

Reference

1 Maany I, O'Brien CP, Woody G. Interaction between thioridazine and naltrexone. Am J Psychiatry (1987) 144, 966.

Phenothiazines + Phenylpropanolamine

Abstract/Summary

A single case report describes fatal ventricular fibrillation attributed to the concurrent use of thioridazine and phenylpropanolamine.

Clinical evidence, mechanism, importance and management

A 27-year-old schizophrenic woman who was taking regular daily doses of 100 mg thioridazine and 5 mg procyclidine was found dead in bed 2 h after taking a single capsule of *Contac*C* (phenylpropanolamine 50 mg + chlorpheniramine maleate 4 mg). The principal cause of death was aspiration of the stomach contents attributed to ventricular fibrillation.[1] The mechanism is not understood but it is suggested that it may have been due to the combined effects of the thioridazine (known to be cardiotoxic and to cause T-wave abnormalities) and the phenylpropanolamine (possibly able to cause ventricular arrhythmias like adrenaline with anaesthetics).

The general importance of this alleged interaction is uncertain but the authors of the report suggest that ephedrine-like agents such as phenylpropanolamine should not be given to patients on thioridazine or mesoridazine.

Reference

1 Chouinard G, Ghadirian AM, Jones BD. Death attributed to ventricular arrhythmia induced by thioridazine in combination with a single *Contac*C* capsule. Can Med Ass J (1978) 119, 729.

Phenothiazines + Trazodone

Abstract/Summary

Undesirable hypotension occurred in two patients on chlorpromazine or trifluoperazine when given trazodone.

Clinical evidence, mechanism, importance and management

A depressed patient on chlorpromazine began to complain of dizziness and unstable gait within two weeks of starting to take 100 mg trazodone daily. His blood pressure had fallen to between 92/58 and 126/72 mmHg. Within two days of stopping the trazodone his blood pressure had restabilized.[1] Another patient on trifluoperazine was given 100 mg trazodone daily and within two days she complained of dizziness and was found to have a blood pressure of 86/52 mmHg. Within a day of withdrawing the trazodone her blood pressure was back to 100/65 mmHg.[1] It would seem that the hypotensive side-effects of the two drugs can be additive. Patients given both groups of drugs should be monitored for signs of excessive hypotension.

Reference

1 Asayesh K. Combination of trazodone and phenothiazines: a possible additive hypotensive effect. Can J Psychiatry (1986) 31, 857–8.

Phenothiazines, Butyrophenones or Tricyclic antidepressants + Tea or coffee

Abstract/Summary

Tea and coffee can cause some drugs to precipitate out of solution, but so far there is no clinical evidence to show that this normally affects the bioavailability of the drugs or that it has a detrimental effect on treatment.

Clinical evidence, mechanism, importance and management

Mikkelson[1] described two patients whose schizophrenia was said to have been exacerbated by an increased consumption of tea and coffee. Subsequent *in vitro* studies[2–5,8] showed that a number of drugs (chlorpromazine, diphenhydramine, promethazine, fluphenazine, orphenadrine, promazine, prochlorperazine, trifluoperazine, thioridazine, loxapine, haloperidol, droperidol, amitriptyline, imipramine) form a brown precipitate with tea or coffee due to the formation of a drug-tannin complex which it was thought might possibly lower the absorption of these drugs by the gut. Studies with rats also showed that tea abolished the cataleptic effects of chlorpromazine.[6]

However, the drug-tannin complex gives up the drug into solution if it becomes acidified, as in the stomach.[8] Moreover, a clinical study of this interaction showed that the serum levels of chlorpromazine, fluphenazine, trifluoperazine and haloperidol in a group of 16 mentally retarded patients were unaffected by the consumption of tea or coffee.[7] Their behaviour also remained unchanged.[7] So there appears to be little or no direct evidence that this physico-chemical interaction is normally of clinical importance.

References

1 Mikkelsen EJ. Caffeine and schizophrenia. J Clin Psychiat (1978) 39, 732–5.

2 Kulhanek F, Linde OK, Meisenberg G. Precipitation of antipsychotic drugs in interaction with coffee or tea. Lancet (1979) ii, 1130–1.

3 Hirsch SR. Precipitation of antipsychotic drugs in interaction with tea or coffee. Lancet (1979) ii, 1131.

4 Lasswell WL, Wilkins JM, Weber SS. *In vitro* interaction of selected drugs with coffee, tea and gallotannic acid. Drug-nutrient Interactions (1984) 2, 235–41.

5 Lasswell WL, Weber SS, Wilkins JM. *In vitro* interaction of neuroleptics and tricyclic antidepressants with coffee, tea and gallotannic acid. J Pharm Sci (1984) 73, 1056–8.

6 Cheesman HJ, Neal MJ. Interaction of chlorpromazine with tea and coffee. Br J Clin Pharm (1981) 12, 165–9.

7 Bowen S, Taylor KM, Gibb IAM. Effect of coffee and tea on blood levels and efficacy of antipsychotic drugs. Lancet (1981) i, 1217–18.

8 Curry ML, Curry SH, Marroum PJ. Interaction of phenothiazine and related drugs and caffeinate beverages. DICP Ann Pharmacother (1991) 25, 437–8.

Phenothiazines + Tobacco smoking

Abstract/Summary

Smokers may possibly need larger doses of chlorpromazine and fluphenazine than non-smokers.

Clinical evidence

A comparative study found that the frequency of drowsiness in 403 patients taking chlorpromazine was 16% in non-smokers, 11% in light smokers, and 3% in heavy smokers (more than 20 cigarettes daily).[1] Another report describes a patient on chlorpromazine who experienced increased sedation and dizziness, and higher serum chlorpromazine levels, when he gave up smoking.[2]

In a retrospective study in 61 psychiatric inpatients it was found that the serum fluphenazine levels of non-smokers were more than double those of smokers (1.83 compared with 0.89 ng/ml) when given fluphenazine hydrochloride by mouth, whereas when given fluphenazine decanoate intramuscularly the serum levels were little different (0.81 compared with 0.93 ng/ml). However in both cases the clearance of the fluphenazine was considerably greater in the smokers than in the non-smokers (clearance ratios of 1.67 (oral) and 2.33 (intramuscular)).[3] No behavioural differences were seen.[3]

Mechanism

Not established. The probable reason is that some of the components of tobacco smoke act as enzyme-inducing agents which increase the rate at which the liver metabolizes these phenothiazines, thereby reducing their serum levels and clinical effects.

Importance and management

Established interactions but of uncertain clinical importance. Be alert for the need to use increased dosages of these phenothiazines in patients who smoke, and reduced dosages if smoking is stopped.

References

1 Swett C. Drowsiness due to chlorpromazine in relation to cigarette smoking. A report from the Boston Collaborative Drug Surveillance Program. Arch Gen Psychiatry (1974) 31, 211–3.

2 Stimmel GL, Falloon IRH. Chlorpromazine plasma levels, adverse effects, and tobacco smoking: a case report. J Clin Psychiatry (1983) 44, 420.

3 Ereshefsky L, Jann MW, Saklad SR, Davis CM, Richards AL, Burch NR. Effects of smoking on fluphenazine clearance in psychiatric patients. Biol Psychiatry (1985) 20, 329–52.

Phenothiazines + Tricyclic antidepressants

Abstract/Summary

Concurrent treatment is common but a mutual interaction occurs which results in a rise in the serum levels of both drugs. Although fixed-dose combined preparations are available, it has been suggested that concurrent use might contribute to an increased incidence of tardive dyskinesia. A paradoxical reversal of the therapeutic effects of chlorpromazine after the addition of a tricyclic antidepressant has also been described.

Clinical evidence

(a) Effect of phenothiazines on tricyclic antidepressant serum levels

An extended study of four patients given 12.5 mg fluphenazine decanoate weekly, with 6 mg benztropine mesylate and 300 mg imipramine daily, showed that their mean combined plasma concentrations of imipramine and desipramine were 850 ng/ml compared with only 180 ng/ml in 60 other patients described elsewhere who were taking only 225 mg imipramine daily.[9]

A comparative study[11] of 99 patients taking only amitriptyline or nortriptyline and 60 other patients additionally taking an average of 10 mg perphenazine daily, showed that although the tricyclic antidepressant dosage levels were the same, the plasma tricyclic antidepressant levels of the latter group were up to 70% higher. Similar results were reported in another study on three patients,[3] but minimal or no changes were described in another.[14] Another found rises in nortriptyline levels but not in amitriptyline levels in 65 patients treated with perphenazine.[18] Other studies have demonstrated this interaction between imipramine and chlorpromazine,[2,4,13] between amitriptyline,[17] imipramine,[13] desipramine[15] and perphenazine, between desipramine and thioridazine,[16] and between nortriptyline and chlorpromazine.[12] In this last study on seven chronic schizophrenics it was also reported that the addition of full doses of nortriptyline (150 mg daily) to a course of chlorpromazine (300 mg daily) resulted in such a profound worsening of the clinical state, with marked increases in agitation and tension, that the nortriptyline was withdrawn.[12] A temporary reversion to a disruptive behaviour pattern has been seen in other patients on chlorpromazine when given amitriptyline.[10]

(b) Effect of tricyclic antidepressant on phenothiazine serum levels

In a controlled study on eight schizophrenic patients taking 20 mg butaperazine daily, six of them on 150 mg desipramine or more daily showed a rise in serum butaperazine levels of between 50 and 300%.[1]

Mechanism

The rise in the serum levels of both drugs is thought to be due to a mutual inhibition of the liver enzymes concerned with the metabolism of both drugs, resulting in the accumulation of both. The evidence available is consistent with this idea.[1-4,12]

Importance and management

Established interactions, but the advantages and disadvantages of concurrent use are still the subject of debate. These two groups of drugs are widely used together in the treatment of schizophrenic patients who show depression, and for mixed anxiety and depression. A number of fixed-dose combinations have been marketed, e.g. *Triptafen, Etrafon, Triaval* (amitriptyline and perphenazine), *Motival, Motipress* (nortriptyline, and fluphenazine), however the safety of using both drugs together has been questioned.

One of the problems of phenothiazine treatment is the development of tardive dyskinesia, and some evidence suggests that the higher the dosage, the greater the incidence.[6] The symptoms can be transiently masked by increasing the dosage,[7] thus the presence of a tricyclic antidepressant (which increases the levels of the phenothiazine) might not only be a factor causing the tardive dyskinesia to develop, but might also mask the condition and contribute towards its development (or so it has been suggested.[1,5]) Ayd has advised[5] that, until more is known, combined treatment should be the exception rather than the rule. It has also been recommended that the addition of full antidepressant doses of nortriptyline to average antipsychotic doses of chlorpromazine should be avoided because the therapeutic actions of the chlorpromazine may be reversed.[12] See also 'Neuroleptics + Anticholinergics'.

Attention has also been drawn to excessive weight gain associated with several months' use of amitriptyline with thioridazine for the treatment of chronic pain.[8]

References

1 El-Yousef MK, Manier DH. Tricyclic antidepressants and phenothiazines. J Amer Med Ass (1974) 229, 1419.
2 Gram LF, Overo KF. Drug interaction: inhibitory effect of neuroleptics on metabolism of tricyclic antidepressants in man. Br Med J (1972) 1, 463.
3 Gram LF, Overo KF, Kirk L. Influence of neuroleptics and benzodiazepines on metabolism of tricyclic antidepressants in man. Am J Psychiatry (1974) 131, 8.
4 Grammer JL, Rolfe B. Interaction of imipramine and chlorpromazine in man. Psychopharmacologia (1972) 26,(Suppl), 80.
5 Ayd FJ. Pharmacokinetic interaction between tricyclic antidepressants and phenothiazine neuroleptics. Int Drug Ther Newsletter (1974) 9, 31.
6 Crane GE. Persistent dyskinesia. Brit J Psychiatry (1973), 122, 395.
7 Crane GE. Tardive dyskinesia in patients treated with major neuroleptics: a review of the literature. Am J Psychiatry (1968) 124,(Suppl), 40.
8 Pfister AK. Weight gain from combined phenothiazine and tricyclic therapy. J Amer Med Ass (1978) 239, 1959.
9 Siris SG, Cooper TB, Rifkin AE, Brenner R, Lieberman JA. Plasma imipramine concentrations in patients receiving concomitant fluphenazine decanoate. Am J Psychiatry (1982) 193, 104.
10 O'Connor JW. Personal communication 1983.
11 Linnoila M, George L, Guthrie S. Interaction between antidepressants and perphenazine in psychiatric patients. Am J Psychiatry (1982) 139, 1329–31.
12 Loga S, Curry S, Lader M. Interaction of chlorpromazine and nortriptyline in patients with schizophrenia. Clin Pharmacokinetics. (1981) 6, 454–62.
13 Gram LF. Laegemiddelinteraktion: haemmende virkning af neurolepltica pa tricycliske antidepressivas metabolisering. Nord psykiat T. (1971) 25, 357–60.
14 Kragh-Sorensen P,Borga O, Hansen BV, Hansen CE, Hvidberg EF, Larsen N-E. Effect of simultaneous treatment with low doses of perphenazine on plasma and urine concentrations of nortriptyline and 10-hydroxynortriptyline. Europ J Clin Pharmacol (1977) 11, 479–483.
15 Nelson JC, Jatlow PI. Neuroleptic effect on desipramine steady-state plasma concentrations. Am J Psychiatry (1980) 137, 1232–34.
16 Hirschowitz J, Bennett JA, Zemlan FP, Garver DL. Thioridazine effect on desipramine plasma levels. J Clin Psychopharmacol (1983) 3, 376–9.
17 Perel JM, Stiller RL, Feldman BL. Therapeutic drug monitoring (TDM) of the amitriptyline (AT)/perphenazine interaction in depressed patients. Clin Chem (1985) 31, 939–40.
18 Cooper SF, Dugal R, Elie R, Albert J-M. Metabolic interaction between amitriptyline and perphenazine in psychiatric patients. Prog Neuro-Psychopharmacol (1979) 3, 369–76.

Prochlorperazine + Metoclopramide

Abstract/Summary

A case report describes tongue swelling and respiratory obstruction in a patient after being given prochlorperazine followed by metoclopramide.

Clinical evidence, mechanism, importance and management

A woman of 19 experienced progressive swelling of the tongue, partial upper airways obstruction and a sensation of choking over a period of 12 h following an intramuscular dose of 30 mg metoclopramide in divided doses. 24 h earlier she had had a 12.5 mg intramuscular dose of prochlorperazine for nausea and headaches. Her tongue on examination was strikingly blue, but within 15 min of receiving 2 mg benztropine it returned to its normal size and colour. The respiratory distress also disappeared.[1] The reason for the reaction, suggested by the authors of the report, is that the dystonic side-effects of both drugs were additive.[1] One of the authors had seen this reaction previously in a patient on large doses of haloperidol. Oedema of the tongue has also been described with metoclopramide alone.[2] Concurrent use of these drugs is not uncommon and need not be avoided, but prescribers should be aware of this adverse reaction, and know its simple antidote.

References

1 Alroe C, Bowen P. Metoclopramide and prochlorperazine: 'the blue-tongue sign'. Med J Aust (1989) 150, 724–5.
2 Robinson OPW. Metoclopramide — side effects and safety. Postgrad Med J (1973) 49 (suppl 4) 77–80.

Psychotropics + Fluoxetine

Abstract/Summary

Severe extrapyramidal symptoms developed in two patients on haloperidol or perphenazine when additionally given fluoxetine. Another patient on thiothixene and benztropine with fluoxetine developed marked urinary retention. Parkinson-like symptoms developed in a patient on sulpiride and maprotiline when given fluoxetine, and marked dystonia occurred in another when taking fluphenazine. Worsening extrapyramidal symptoms and bradycardia were seen in two patients given pimizode and fluoxetine.

Clinical evidence, mechanism, importance and management

A woman on 2–5 mg haloperidol daily for 2 years with only occasional mild extrapyramidal symptoms, started additionally to take 40 mg fluoxetine twice daily. After 5 days the haloperidol was stopped but restarted 9 days later. Two days later she began to experience severe extrapyramidal symptoms (tongue stiffness, parkinsonism, akathisia) and for three days was virtually incapacitated. Both drugs were stopped and she recovered over a period of a week while treated with benztropine, diphenhydramine and diazepam.[1] A severe dystonic reaction (painful jaw tightness and throat 'closing up') occurred in a man on 40 mg fluoxetine daily when he took 2.5 mg fluphenazine on two consecutive nights.[4] Another woman developed marked extrapyramidal symptoms within 2 weeks of starting 8 mg perphenazine daily and 20 mg fluoxetine.[2] A patient taking fluoxetine and pimozide showed a worsening of the extrapyramidal symptoms, and another developed marked sinus bradycardia (35–44 bpm) with somnolence. Parkinson-like symptoms developed in a patient taking sulpiride and maprotiline when fluoxetine was additionally given.[3] A woman developed severe urinary retention within two weeks of starting 20 mg thiothixene daily, 20 mg fluoxetine at bedtime and 2 mg benztropine daily. She was treated by replacing the benztropine with amantadine, urinary cathetarization and urecholine.[2]

The reasons for these reactions are not understood but most of them appear to be an exaggeration of the side-effects of the other drugs caused by the fluoxetine. All of these are individual and isolated reports and their general importance is uncertain, nevertheless if concurrent use is thought appropriate it should be very well monitored.

References

1 Tate JL. Extrapyramidal symptoms in a patient taking haloperidol and fluoxetine. Am J Psychiatry (1989) 146, 399–400.

2 Lock JD, Gwirtsman HE, Targ EF. Possible adverse drug interactions between fluoxetine and other psychotropics.

3 Touw DJ, Gernaat HBPE, van der Woude J. Parkinsonisme na toevoeging van fluoxetine aan behandeling met neuroleptica of carbamazepine. Ned Tijdschr Geneeskd (1992) 136, 332–3.

4 Ketai R. Interaction between fluoxetine and neuroleptics. Am J Psychiatry (1993) 150, 836–7.

Remoxipride + Miscellaneous drugs

Abstract/Summary

The performance of skilled tasks and the risks of car driving and handling other potentially dangerous machinery appear to be worsened if remoxipride is taken with alcohol, diazepam or possibly other benzodiazepines. Remoxipride appears not to interact with biperiden or warfarin. Remoxipride and imipramine do not affect the pharmacokinetics of each other.

Clinical evidence, mechanism, importance and management

(a) Remoxipride + Alcohol, Benzodiazepines

A double-blind cross-over study[1] in 12 normal subjects found that single 100 mg oral doses of remoxipride slightly impaired the performance of a number of psychomotor tests and caused drowsiness, clumsiness and mental slowness. 0.8 g/kg alcohol added to the remoxipride was found to worsen these effects. l5 mg diazepam had an even greater effect than alcohol. No changes in the serum levels of any of the drugs were seen during concurrent use in this study,[1] nor in another in which single doses were used.[2] In practical terms this means that the performance of skilled tasks will be made more difficult, and driving and handling other potentially dangerous machinery possibly made more hazardous if remoxipride is taken with alcohol, diazepam or possibly other benzodiazepines. Patients should be warned.

(b) Remoxipride + Biperiden, Imipramine, Warfarin

12 normal subjects were given single 100 mg doses of remoxipride with 4 mg biperiden. No interactions were seen.[2] After taking 100 mg remoxipride twice daily for 8 days in another study they were also given 25 mg warfarin. No interactions were seen.[2] These findings suggest that concurrent use need not be avoided, but confirmation of this is needed in patients given multiple doses of these drugs. A study in six fast-metabolizers and six slow-metabolizers of sparteine found that remoxipride and imipramine did not affect the pharmacokinetics of each other.[3]

References

1 Mattila M J, Mattila M E, Konno K, Saarialho-Kere U. Objective and subjective effects of remoxipride, alone and in combination with ethanol or diazepam, on performance in healthy subjects. J Psychopharmacol (1988) 2(3 & 4) 138–49.

2 Yisak W, von Bahr C, Farde L, Grind M, Mattila M, Ogenstad S. Drug interaction studies with remoxipride. Acta Psychiatr Scand (1990) 82, (Suppl 358) 58–62.

3 Yisak W, Lolk A, Hansen A, Nielsen S, Gram O-W, Gram L, v Bahr C, Ogenstad S, Harring M. Remoxipride imipramine interaction. Eur J Pharmacol (1990) 183, 2292.

Sulpiride + Antacids or Sucralfate

Abstract/Summary

Sucralfate and an aluminium-magnesium hydroxide antacid can reduce the absorption of sulpiride.

Clinical evidence, mechanism, importance and management

A study in six normal subjects showed that the bioavailability of a single 100 mg dose of sulpiride was reduced 40% by 1 g sucralfate and 32% by 30 ml of *Simeco* (an antacid containing 215 mg aluminium hydroxide, 80 mg magnesium hydroxide and 25 mg simethicone in each 5 ml) when taken together, and by 25% when either the sucralfate or the antacid were taken 2 h previously. No change in bioavailability was seen in one subject when the sucralfate was given 2 h after the sulpiride.[1] The mechanisms of these interactions are not understood. Their clinical importance is not established but it would seem reasonable to give the sulpiride 2 h after and not before these other drugs to avoid these interactions.

Reference

1 Gouda MW, Hikal AH, Babhair SA, ElHofy SA, Mahrous GM. Effect of sucralfate and antacids on the bioavailability of sulpiride in humans. Int J Pharmaceut (1984) 22, 257–63.

Sulpiride + Lithium

Abstract/Summary

Serious extrapyramidal reactions developed in two patients within a few hours of starting to take sulpiride and lithium carbonate concurrently.

Clinical evidence, mechanism, importance and management

A depressed woman who had been taking 2 g sulpiride daily for 4 weeks, then reduced to 1600 mg, developed a serious parkinsonian syndrome with choreiform movements of her arms after taking a single 800 mg of lithium carbonate at night. Next morning her serum lithium level was 0.5 mmol/l. The adverse effects disappeared within 2 days of stopping the lithium. A man with a manic episode who had started to take 1200 mg lithium at night, and with a stable serum lithium level of 0.6 mmol/l/l, developed marked orofacial dyskinesia and acute akathisia within 12 h of starting to take 800 mg sulpiride twice daily.[1] The reasons for these reactions are not understood. One theory is that the lithium may have increased the binding of the sulpiride to the dopamine D2 receptors in the brain, thereby causing extrapyramidal reactions to develop. Sulpiride is known to increase its binding in the presence of lithium.[2]

Information appears to be limited to these two cases. Its general importance is therefore uncertain, but the authors of the report advise caution when using this drug combination.

Reference

1 Dinan TG, O'Keane V. Acute extrapyramidal reactions following lithium and sulpiride co-administration: two case reports. Human Psychopharmacol (1991) 6, 67–9.
2 Jenner P, David A, Kilpatrick G, Kupniak NM, Chivers JK, Marsden CD. Selective interaction of sulpiride with brain dopamine receptors. In: Schizophrenia: New Pharmacology and Clinical Developments, Schiff AA, Roth M, Freeman HL (eds). RSM, London.

Tetrabenazine + Chlorpromazine

Abstract/Summary

An isolated report describes severe Parkinson-like symptoms in a woman with Huntington's Chorea when given tetrabenazine and chlorpromazine.

Clinical evidence, mechanism, importance and management

A woman with Huntington's Chorea, successfully treated with 100 mg tetrabenazine daily for nine years, became motionless, rigid, mute and only able to respond by blinking her eyes within a day of being given two intramuscular injections of 25 mg chlorpromazine. This was diagnosed as severe drug-induced parkinsonism which rapidly responded to withdrawal of both drugs and treatment with benztropine mesylate given intramuscularly and orally.[1] The reason for this reaction is not understood. The authors of this report advise caution if tetrabenazine and other neuroleptics are given.

Reference

1 Moss JH, Stewart DE. Iatrogenic Parkinsonism in Huntington's chorea. Can J Psychiatry (1986) 31, 865–6.

Thiothixene + miscellaneous drugs

Abstract/Summary

Carbamazepine, phenytoin, primidone and tobacco smoking increase the loss of thiothixene from the body, whereas cimetidine, doxepin, nortriptyline, propranolol and isoniazid reduce its loss.

Clinical evidence, mechanism, importance and management

A study in 42 patients found that the mean clearance of thiothixene in those taking enzyme-inducing drugs (carbamazepine, phenytoin, primidone) was three-fold greater than in the control group (92.5 compared with 32. 8 l/min). Five patients in the former group had non-detectable serum thiothixene levels and (not surprisingly) showed no clinical response. Another group taking enzyme inhibitors (cimetidine, doxepin, nortriptyline, propranolol, isoniazid) showed a clearance of only 9.51 l/min. Tobacco smoking (also an enzyme inducer) increased the clearance of thiothixene in those taking inhibitors and those taking no other drugs, but not in those taking inducers. Those who smoked were found to need on average 45% more thiothixene than the non-smokers.[1] The reasons for the different clearances are that enzyme inducers stimulate the liver enzymes to clear the thiothixene from the body more quickly, whereas enzyme inhibitors have the opposite effect.

The conclusion to be drawn from this study is that the dosage of thiothixene should be adjusted to accommodate these changes in clearance: bigger doses for those who take enzyme inducers and/or who smoke; smaller doses for those taking inhibitors. More study is needed to find out the individual effects of these drugs.

References

1 Ereshefsky L, Saklad SR, Watanabe MD, Davis CM, Jann MW. Thiothixene pharmacokinetic interactions: a study of hepatic enzyme inducers, clearance inhibitors, and demographic variable. J Clin Psychopharmacol (1991) 11, 296–301.

Trazodone + Tryptophan

Abstract/Summary

Concurrent use can effectively control aggression in patients with mental disorders, but a single case report describes the development of anorexia, psychosis and hypomania in one patient.

Clinical evidence, mechanism, importance and management

Trazodone with tryptophan can be used to treat aggressive behaviour in patients with dementia, mental retardation and other mental disorders.[1] A single report describes their effective use (100 mg and 500 mg respectively three times weekly) with clonazepam in a mildly mentally retarded patient with schizophrenia and congential defects, but the patient stopped eating and lost 4.5 kg in 3 weeks and developed signs of pychosis or hypomania. Soon afterwards she became drowsy and withdrawn. When the drugs were withdrawn the aggressive behaviour restarted, but she responded again to lower doses of trazodone and tryptophan although the signs of psychosis re-emerged.[2]

References

1 Wilcock GK, Stevens J, Perkins A. Trazodone/tryptophan for aggressive behaviour. Lancet (1987) 1, 929–30.
2 Patterson BD, Srisopark MM. Severe anorexia and possible psychosis or hypomania after trazodone-tryptophan treatment of aggression. Lancet (1989) 1, 1017.

Zolpidem + miscellaneous drugs

Abstract/Summary

Zolpidem does not interact with warfarin, cimetidine or ranitidine. The sedative effects of chlorpromazine and haloperidol (and probably other sedative drugs) are increased to some extent by zolpidem. Heavy smoking possibly reduces its effects.

Clinical evidence, mechanism, importance and management

A study on the possible interactions of zolpidem[1] (a non-benzodiazepine hypnotic) found that the prothrombin times of eight normal subjects on warfarin were unaffected by 4 days' treatment with 20 mg zolpidem. The pharmacokinetics of zolpidem in six normal subjects were unaffected by either 1 g cimetidine or 300 mg ranitidine daily for 17 days, although there was some increase in sleep duration with cimetidine.[3]

Single 20 mg doses of zolpidem had no effect on the pharmacokinetics of chlorpromazine, imipramine or haloperidol, and neither 50 mg chlorpromazine, 75 mg imipramine nor 2 mg haloperidol had any effect on the pharmacokinetics of zolpidem. However the elimination half-life of chlorpromazine was increased by 37% (from about 5 to 8 h). Both chlorpromazine and imipramine increased the sedative effects of zolpidem (as indicated by impaired performances of manual dexterity and Stroop's tests) and it seems likely that additive sedation will be seen with other sedative drugs. An anterograde amnesia was seen with zolpidem given with imipramine. There was no evidence that zolpidem could act as either an inducer or an inhibitor of liver microsomal enzymes.[1,2]

It was also noted in these studies that two heavy smokers had a very high zolpidem clearance and did not experience any sedative effect.[1] This suggests that smokers may need above average doses.

Reference

1 Harvengt C, Hulhoven R, Desager JP, Coupez JM, Guillet Ph, Fuseau E, Lambert D, Warrington SJ. Drug interactions investigated with zolpidem. In 'Imidazopyridines in Sleep Disorders', Sauvanet JP, Langer SZ, Morselli PL (eds.). Raven Press (1988) New York.
2 Desager JP, Hulhoven R, Harvengt C, Hermann P, Guillet P, Thiercelin JF. Possible interactions between zolpidem, a new sleep inducer, and chlorpromazine, a phenothiazine neuroleptic. Psychopharmacology (1988) 96, 63–6.
3 Hulhoven R, Desager JP, Harvengt C, Herman Ph, Guillet Ph, Thiercelin JF. Lack of interaction between zolpidem and H2 antagonists, cimetidine and ranitidine. Int J Clin Pharm Res (1988) VIII, 471–6.

Chapter 20
Neuromuscular Blocker and
Anaesthetic Drug Interactions

This chapter is concerned with the interactions where the effects of neuromuscular blocking drugs and anaesthetics, both general and local, are affected by the presence of other drugs. Where these drugs are responsible for an interaction they are dealt with under the heading of the drug affected. See the Index for a full listing.

Neuromuscular blockers are of two types. The non-depolarizing or competitive type of blocker (e.g. tubocurarine, gallamine, etc.) competes with acetyl-choline for the receptors on the endplate of the neuromuscular junction, thereby excluding the ace-

Table 20.1 Neuromuscular blockers

Non-proprietary names	Proprietary names
Non-depolarizing blockers	
Alcuronium chloride	*Alloferin(e), Aloferin*
Atracurium besylate	*Tacrium*
Fazadinium bromide	*Fazadon*
Gallium triethiodide	*Flaxedil, Miowas G*
Metocurine (dimethyltubocurarine)	*Metubine*
Pancuronium bromide	*Pavulon*
Pipecuronium bromide	
Tubocurarine chloride (curare, d-tubocurarine)	*Curarin(e), Intocostrin(e)-T, Jexin, Tubarine, Tubocuran*
Vecuronium bromide	*Norcuron*
Depolarizing blockers	
Carbolonium bromide (the blockade rapidly changes to non-depolarizing)	*Imbretil*
Decamethonium bromide	*Syncurine*
Decamethonium iodide (C10)	
Suxamethonium bromide/ chloride	*Anectine, Brevidil M, Celocurin(e), (succinylcholine), Celocurin-Chloride/ Klorid, Curalest, Clysthenon, Midarine, Mioflex, Muscuryl, Myoplegine, Pantolax, Paranoval, Scoline, Succinolin, Succinyl, Sucostrin*
Suxethonium bromide	*Brevidil-E*

Table 20.2 Anaesthetics

Non-proprietary names	Proprietary names
General anaesthetics	
Inhalation	
Cyclopropane	
Diethyl ether (ether)	
Enflurane	*Alyrane, Efrane, Ethrane, Inhelthran*
Fluroxene	
Halothane	*Fluopan, Fluothane, Halovis, Rhodialothan, Somnothane*
Isoflurane	*Aerrane, Forane*
Methoxyflurane	*Penthrane*
Nitrous oxide	*Etonox (N_2O/O_2)*
Trichloroethylene	*Trilene, Triklone*
Parenteral	
Alphaxalone/Alphadolone	*Alfatesin(e), Alfathesin, Alphadione, Althesin*
Ketamine hydrochloride	*Ketalar, Ketaject, Ketanest, Ketolar*
Propofol	*Diprivan*
Thiopentone sodium (thiopental)	*Farmotal, Hypnostan, Intraval Sodium, Leopental, Nesdonal, Pentothal (sodium), Thiobarbityral, Tiobarbital, Trapanal*
Local anaesthetics	
Bupivacaine	
Chloroprocaine	
Cocaine	
Lignocaine (lidocaine)	
Mepivacaine	
Procaine	
Propoxycaine	

tylcholine and preventing it from acting. A group of drugs called the anticholinesterases, such as neostigmine, can be used as an antidote to this type of blockade because they inhibit the enzymes which destroy acetylcholine so that the concentrations of acetylcholine build up. Thus the competition between the molecules of the blocker and the acetylcholine for occupancy of the receptors swings in favour of the acetylcholine and transmission is restored. The other type of blocker, the depolarizing type, also occupy the receptors on the endplate but they differ in that they act like acetylcholine to cause depolarization. However, they are not immediately removed by cholinesterase so that the depolarization is maintained and the muscle become paralyzed. Anticholinesterase drugs increase the levels of acetylcholine so that they would enhance and prolong this type of blockade. Under some circumstances depolarizing blockade (Type I) is converted to the competitive block (Type II). The different types of blocker are listed in Table 20.1.

The general and local anaesthetics mentioned in this chapter are listed in Table 20.2. Some of them are also used as antiarrhythmic agents and these are dealt with in the antiarrhythmics chapter.

Anaesthetics, general + Adrenaline, Noradrenaline and Terbutaline

Abstract/Summary

Patients anaesthetized with volatile anaesthetics (cyclopropane, enflurane, halothane, isoflurane, fluroxene, methoxyflurane, diethyl ether) can develop heart arrhythmias if given adrenaline (epinephrine) or noradrenaline (norepinephrine) unless the dosages are very low. Children appear to be less susceptible. Two patients developed arrhythmias when terbutaline was used with halothane. See also 'Anaesthetics + Phenylephrine'.

Clinical evidence, mechanism, importance and management

(a) Adrenaline and noradrenaline

Oliver and Schaefer were the first to observe in 1895 that an adrenal extract could cause ventricular fibrillation in a dog anaesthetized with chloroform,[1] and it is now very well recognized that similar cardiac dysrhythmias can be caused by adrenaline (epinephrine) and noradrenaline (norepinephrine) in man when anaesthetized with other volatile anaesthetics. A suggested listing of these anaesthetics in order of decreasing sensitivity is as follows: cyclopropane > halothane > enflurane = methoxyflurane > isoflurane = fluroxene > diethyl ether.[2]

The following recommendation has been made if adrenaline is used to reduce surgical bleeding in patients anaesthetized with halothane/nitrous oxide/oxygen: the dosage should not exceed 10 ml of 1:100,000 in any given 10 min period, nor 30 ml per h (i.e. about 100 μg or 1.5 μg/kg/10 min for a 70 kg person).[3] This dosage guide should also be safe for use with other volatile anaesthetics since halothane and adrenaline are more arrhythmogenic than the others.[2] Solutions containing 0.5% lignocaine (lidocaine) with 1:100,000 also appear to be safe because lignocaine may help to control the potential dysrhythmic effects. For example, a study in 15 adult patients showed that the dose of adrenaline needed to cause three premature ventricular contractions in half the group was 2.11 μg/kg in saline, but 3.69 μg/kg in 0.5% lignocaine (lidocaine).[4] However it should be borne in mind that the arrhythmogenic effects of adrenaline are increased if sympathetic activity is increased, and in hyperthyroidism and hypercapnia.[2]

Children appear to be much less susceptible than adults. A retrospective study of 28 children showed no evidence of dysrhythmia during halothane anaesthesia with adrenaline doses of up to 8.8 μg/kg, and a subsequent study on 83 children (three months to 17 years) found that 10 μg/kg doses were safe.[5]

(b) Terbutaline

Two patients have been described who developed ventricular arrhythmias while anaesthetized with halothane and nitrous oxide/oxygen when given 0.25–0.35 mg terbutaline subcutaneously for wheezing. Both developed unifocal premature ventricular contractions followed by bigeminy which responded to lignocaine.[6] Halothane was also replaced by enflurane in one case. See also 'Anaesthetics + Phenylephrine'.

References

1 Oliver G, Schaefer EA. The physiological effects of extracts of the suprarenal capsules. J Physiol (1895) 18, 230.
2 Wong KC. Sympathomimetic drugs. In 'Drug Interactions in Anesthesia' Smith NT, Miller RD, Corbascio AN (eds). Lea and Febiger, Philadelphia (1981) p 66.
3 Katz RL, Matteo RS, Papper EM. The injection of epinephrine during general anesthesia with halogenated hydrocarbons and cyclopropane in man. 2. Halothane. Anesthesiology (1962) 23, 597–600.
4 Johnston RR, Eger EI, Wilson C. A comparative interaction of epinephrine with enflurane, isoflurane and halothane in man. Anesth Analg (1976) 55, 709–12.
5 Karl HW, Swedlow DB, Leed KW, Downes JJ. Epinephrine-halothane interactions in children. Anesthesiology (1983) 58, 142–5.
6 Thiagarajah S, Grynsztejn M, Lear E, Azar I. Ventricular arrhythmias after terbutaline administration to patients anaesthetized with halothane. Anaesth Analg (1986) 65, 417–8.

Anaesthetics, general + Alcohol

Abstract/Summary

Those who regularly drink may need more thiopentone (thiopental) than those who do not drink.

Clinical evidence, mechanism, importance and management

A study in 532 healthy subjects aged 20–80 showed that those who normally drink alcohol need more thiopentone to achieve anaesthesia than non-drinkers. After adjusting for differences in age and weight distribution, men drinkers (40 g alcohol daily) needed 33% more thiopentone for induction than non-drinkers, and women drinkers needed 40% more.[1]

Reference

1 Dundee JW, Milligan KR. Induction dose of thiopentone: the effect of alcohol intake. Br J Clin Pharmac (1989) 27, 693–4P.

Anaesthetics, general + Alfentanil or Cocaine

Abstract/Summary

Opisthotonus and/or grand mal seizures have been associated with the use of propofol with alfentanil, or possibly cocaine.

Clinical evidence, mechanism, importance and management

A patient with no history of epilepsy, undergoing septorhinoplasty for cosmetic reasons, was premedicated with papaveretum and hyoscine, intubated after propofol and suxamethonium, and anaesthetised with nitrous oxide/oxygen with 2% isoflurane. 10% cocaine paste was applied to the nasal mucosa. After the surgery he experienced a dystonic reaction during recovery which developed into a generalized convulsion. The authors of the report suggest that a possible interaction between the propofol and cocaine might have been responsible.[1] Propofol has also been associated with opisthotonus and grand mal seizures in patients given alfentanil, in the absence of a history of epilepsy.[2,3]

References

1 Hendley BJ. Convulsions after cocaine and propofol. Anaesthesia (1990) 45, 788–9.
2 Laycock GJA. Opisthotonus and propofol: a possible association. Anaesthesia (1988) 43, 257.
3 Wittenstein U, Lyle DJR. Fits after alfentanil and propofol. Anaesthesia (1989) 44, 532–3.

Anaesthetics, general + Anaesthetics, general

Abstract/Summary

An isolated report describes myoclonic seizures in a man anaesthetized with Alfathesin (alphaxolone-alphadolone) when additionally given enflurane.

Clinical evidence

Anaesthesia was induced uneventfully in a normal man of 23 with 2.5 ml Alfathesin (alphaxolone and alphadolone) given intravenously over 2 min, and then maintained with 2% enflurane in oxygen through a circle absorber system. After 8 min the patient began to have intermittent myoclonic activity (violent flexion of the extremities and contraction of trunk and facial muscles). The enflurane was stopped and anaesthesia maintained with nitrous oxide and oxygen. The myclonic activity ceased within 3 min. After several minutes the enflurane was restarted and within 3 min the myclonus began again, but it resolved when the enflurane was stopped.[1]

Mechanism

Uncertain. Alfathesin can causes seizures even in normal subjects and enflurane can cause CNS excitation. It seems possible that these effects may be additive, and possibly exacerbated if hypocapnia also occurs.

Importance and management

Direct information seems to be confined to this single report. It has been suggested that concurrent use should be avoided, particularly in patients with known convulsive disorders.[1] Alfathesin has been withdrawn from general use.

Reference

1 Hudson R, Ethans CT. Alfathesin and enflurane: synergistic central nervous system excitation? Canad Anaesth Soc J (1981) 28, 55–60.

Anaesthetics (Methoxyflurane) + Antibiotics and Barbiturates

Abstract/Summary

The nephrotoxic effects of methoxyflurane appear to be increased by the use of barbiturates, tetracyclines and possibly some aminoglycoside antibiotics.

Clinical evidence, mechanism, importance and management

Methoxyflurane has been withdrawn in many countries because it causes kidney damage. This damage can be exacerbated by the concurrent use of some drugs. Five out of seven patients anaesthetized with methoxyflurane who had been given tetracycline before or after surgery showed rises in blood urea nitrogen and creatinine, and three died. Post-mortem examination showed pathological changes (oxalosis) in the kidneys.[1] Another study identified renal tubular necrosis associated with calcium oxalate crystals in six patients who had been anaesthetized with methoxyflurane and given tetracycline (four patients) and penicillin with streptomycin (two patients).[8] Other reports support the finding of increased nephrotoxicity with tetracycline.[2–4] Another study suggested that penicillin, streptomycin and chloramphenical appear not to increase the renal toxicity,[1] but gentamicin and kanamycin possibly do so.[5] There is also some evidence that barbiturates can exacerbate the renal toxicity because they alter the metabolism of the methoxyflurane and increase the production of nephrotoxic metabolites.[6,7]

The risk of kidney damage with methoxyflurane would therefore appear to be increased by some of these drugs and they should only be used with great caution, if at all.

References

1 Kuzucu EY. Methoxyflurane, tetracycline and renal failure. J Amer Med Ass (1970) 211, 1162.
2 Albers DD, Leverett CL, Sandin JH. Renal failure following prostatovesiculectomy related to methoxyflurane anesthesia and tetracycline-complicated by Candida infection. J Urol (1971) 106, 348.
3 Proctor EA, Barton FL. Polyuric acute renal failure after methoxyflurane and tetracycline. Br Med J (1971) 4, 661.
4 Stoelting RK, Gibbs PS. Effect of tetracycline therapy on renal function

after methoxyflurane anaesthesia. Anesth Analg (1973) 52, 431.

5 Cousins MJ, Mazze RI. Tetracycline, methoxyflurane anaesthetics and renal dysfunction. Lancet (1972) i, 751.

6 Churchill D, Yacoub JM, Siu KP, Symes A, Gault MH. Toxic nephropathy after low-dose methoxyflurane anesthesia: drug interaction with secobarbital? Canad Med Ass J (1976) 114, 326.

7 Cousins MJ, Mazze RI. Methoxyflurane nephrotoxicity: a study of dose response in man. J Amer Med Ass (1973) 225, 1611.

8 Dryden GE. Incidence of tubular degeneration with microlithiasis following methoxyflurane compared wih other anesthetic agents. Anesth Analg (1974) 53, 383–5.

Anaesthetics, general + Antihypertensives

Abstract/Summary

Concurrent use normally need not be avoided but it should be recognized that the normal homeostatic responses of the cardiovascular system will be impaired. Marked hypotension has been seen in patients on ACE inhibitors.

Clinical evidence, mechanism, importance and management

The antihypertensive drugs differ in the way they act, but they all interfere with the normal homeostatic mechanisms which control blood pressure and, as a result, the reaction of the cardiovascular system during anaesthesia to fluid and blood losses, body positioning, etc. is impaired to some extent. For example, enhanced hypotension was seen in a study of the calcium channel blocker nimodipine during general anaesthesia.[5] This instability of the cardiovascular system needs to be recognized and allowed for, but it is widely accepted that normally any antihypertensive treatment should be continued.[1,2] In some cases there is a real risk in stopping, for example a hypertensive rebound can occur if clonidine or the beta-blockers are suddenly withdrawn. See also 'Clonidine + Beta-blockers', and 'Anaesthetics + Beta-blockers'. However ACE inhibitors may possibly represent a risk.

Severe and unexpected hypotension has been seen during induction in patients on captopril.[3] Marked hypotension (75 mmHg systolic) occurred in a man of 42 on enalapril when anaesthetized with propofol which did not respond to surgical stimulation. He responded slowly to the infusion of 1 l of Hartmann's solution.[4] Although information is very limited, there would seem to be the need to take particular care with patients on ACE inhibitors. One recommendation is that intravenous infusion should be started in all patients on ACE inhibitors who are anaesthetised.[4]

References

1 Craig DB, Bose D. Drug interactions in anaesthesia: chronic antihypertensive therapy. Can Anaesth Soc J (1984) 31, 580–8.

2 Foex P, Cutfield GR, Francis CM. Interactions of cardiovascular drugs with inhalation anaesthetics. Anaesthesiol Intensivmed (Berlin) (1982) 150, 109–28.

3 McConachie I, Healy TEJ. ACE inhibitors and anaesthesia. Postgrad Med J (1989) 65, 273–4.

4 Littler C, McConachie I, Healey TEJ. Interaction between enalapril and propofol. Anaesth Intensive Care (1989) 17, 514–5.

5 Müller H, Kafurke H, Marck P, Zierski J, Hempelmann G. Interactions between nimodipine and general anaesthesia — clinical investigations in 124 patients during neurosurgical operations. Act Neurochirug (1988) Suppl, 45, 29–35.

Anaesthetics, general + Aspirin or Probenecid

Abstract/Summary

The induction of anaesthesia with midazolam is more rapid in patients who have been pretreated with aspirin or probenecid, while the anaesthetic dosage of thiopentone (thiopental) is reduced.

Clinical evidence

(b) Midazolam + Aspirin or Probenecid

A study in patients about to undergo surgery found that pretreatment with 1 g aspirin (given as IV lysine acetyl salicylate) 1 min before, or 1 g oral probenecid 1 h before induction, shortened the induction time with midazolam (0.3 mg/kg IV over 20 sec). Only 60% were 'asleep' within 3 min with midazolam alone, but 80–81% were 'asleep' within 3 min after the aspirin or probenecid pretreatment.[1]

(a) Thiopentone (thiopental) + Aspirin or Probenecid

The same study[1] cited above found that similar pretreatment with aspirin reduced the dosage of thiopentone by 34% (from 5.3 to 3.5 mg/kg). The thiopentone was given as a 2.5% solution intravenously, 2 mg/kg initially, followed by increments of 25 mg until the eyelash reflex was abolished.[1] The same study also found that 1 g oral probenecid 1 h before anaesthesia reduced the thiopentone dosage by 15% (from 5.3 to 4.1 mg/kg).[1]

A further double blind study in 86 women found that probenecid 3 h before surgery prolonged the duration of anaesthesia with thiopentone (7 mg/kg). Premedication with pethidine (1 mg/kg), atropine (0.0075 mg/kg) and either 0.5 mg or 1.0 g probenecid prolonged the duration of anaesthesia by 65% and 46% respectively. Without the pethidine, 0.5 mg probenecid caused a 26% prolongation. In patients without pethidine and given only 4 mg/kg thiopentone but no surgical stimulus during anaesthesia, probenecid increased the duration of anaesthesia by 109%.[3]

Mechanisms

Not understood. Among the suggestions are that it could be because the aspirin and the probenecid increase the amount of free (and active) midazolam and thiopentone in the plasma since they compete for the binding sites on the plasma albumins.[1,2]

Importance and management

Information is limited but what is known shows that the effects of both midazolam and thiopentone are increased by aspirin and probenecid. Be alert for the need to reduce the dosages.

References

1 Dundee JW, Halliday NJ, McMurray TJ. Aspirin and probenecid pretreatment influences the potency of thiopentone and the onset of action of midazolam. Eur J Anaesthesiol (1986) 3, 247–51.
2 Halliday NJ, Dundee JW, Collier PS, Howard PJ. Effects of aspirin pretreatment on the *in vitro* plasma binding of midazolam. Br J Clin Pharmacol (1985) 19, 581–2P.
3 Kaukinen S, Eerola M, Ylitalo P. Prolongation of thiopentone anaesthesia by probenecid. Br J Anaesth (1980) 52, 603–7.

Anaesthetics, general + Beta-blockers

Abstract/Summary

Anaesthesia in the presence of beta-blockers normally appears to be safer than withdrawal of the beta-blocker before anaesthesia, provided certain anaesthetics are avoided (methoxyflurane, cyclopropane, diethyl-ether, trichloroethylene) and atropine is used to prevent bradycardia. See also 'Anaesthetics + Timolol', and 'Beta-blockers + Anticholinesterases'.

Clinical evidence and mechanism

It used to be thought that beta-blockers should be withdrawn from patients before surgery because of the risk that their cardiac depressant effects would be additive with those of volatile anaesthetics, reducing cardiac output and lowering blood pressure, but it seems to depend on the anaesthetic used.[1] Lowenstein has drawn up a ranking order of compatibility (from the least to the most compatible) as follows: methoxyflurane, diethyl-ether, cyclopropane, trichloroethylene, enflurane, halothane, narcotics, isoflurane.[1]

(a) Cyclopropane, Diethyl-ether, Methoxyflurane, Trichloroethylene

A risk certainly seems to exist with cyclopropane and diethyl-ether because their depressant effects on the heart are normally counteracted by the release of catecholamines, which would be blocked by the presence of a beta-blocker. There is also evidence (both clinical and animal) that unacceptable cardiac depression may also occur with methoxyflurane and trichloroethylene when a beta-blocker is present.[2,3] For these four anaesthetics it has been stated that an absolute indication for their use should exist before giving them in combination with a beta-blocker.[1]

(b) Enflurane, Halothane, Isoflurane, Narcotics

The situation with enflurane is not clear because it has been widely used with propranolol without apparent difficulties,[1] but a marked reduction in cardiac performance has also been described.[2,3] Normally beta-blockers and halothane, isoflurane or narcotics appear to be safe, but a rare and severe life-threatening allergic reaction has been described in one patient on isoflurance, nitrous oxide and oxygen when given 0.25 mg propranolol.[4]

On the positive side there appear to be considerable benefits to be gained from the continued use of beta-blockers during anaesthesia. Their sudden withdrawal from patients treated for angina or hypertension can result in the development of acute and life-threatening cardiovascular complications (possibly due to the increased sensitivity of the receptors) whether the patient is undergoing surgery or not. In the peri-operative period patients benefit from beta-blockade because it can minimize the effects of sympathetic overactivity of the cardiovascular system during anaesthesia and surgery (for example during endotracheal intubation, laryngoscopy, bronchoscopy and various surgical manoeuvres) which can cause heart dysrrhythmias and hypertension.

Importance and management

The consensus of opinion is that beta-blockers should not be withdrawn before anaesthesia and surgery because the advantages of maintaining blockade and the risks accompanying withdrawal are considerable. But it is important to select the safest anaesthetics (isoflurane, halothane, narcotics), to avoid those which appear to be most risky (methoxyflurane, diethyl-ether, chloroform, cyclopropane, trichloroethylene) and to ensure that the patient is protected against bradycardia by atropine (1–2 mg IV). See also 'Anaesthetics + Timolol', and 'Beta-blockers + Anticholinesterases'.

References

1 Lowenstein E. Beta-adrenergic blockers. in 'Drug Interactions in Anesthesia.' Smith NT, Miller RD, Corbascio AN (eds). Lea and Febiger, Philadelphia (1981) p 83–101.
2 Foex P, Cutfield GR, Francis CM. Interactions of cardiovascular drugs with inhalation anaesthetics. Anaesthesiol Intensivemed (Berlin) (1982) 150, 109–28.
3 Foex P, Francis CM, Cutfield GR. The interactions between beta-blockers and anaesthetics. Experimental observations. Acta Anaesth scand (1982) Suppl 76, 38–46.
4 Parker SD, Curry CS, Hirshman CA. A life-threatening reaction after propranolol administration in the operating room. Anesth Analg (1990) 70, 220–1.

Anaesthetics, general + Calcium channel blockers

Abstract/Summary

Impaired myocardial conduction has been seen in two patients on diltiazem when anaesthetized with enflurane, but it has been suggested that the concurrent use of anaesthetics and calcium channel blockers is normally without problems.

Clinical evidence, mechanism, importance and management

The author of a review about calcium channel blockers and anaesthetics concluded that concurrent use is normally beneficial except where there are other complicating factors. Thus he warns about possible decreases in ventricular function in patients undergoing open chest surgery given intravenous verapamil or diltiazem.[1] A report describes a patient on diltiazem and atenolol who had impaired AV and sinus node function before anaesthesia which worsened when given enflurane.[2] Another patient also on diltiazem demonstrated severe sinus bradycardia which progressed to asystole when enflurane was used.[2] The authors of this latter report suggest that enflurane and diltiazem can have additive depressant effects on myocardial conduction. Some caution is clearly appropriate.

References

1 Merin RG. Calcium channel blocking drugs and anesthetics: is the drug interaction beneficial or detrimental? Anesthesiology (1987) 66, 111–13.
2 Hantler CB, Wilton N, Learned DM, Hill AEG, Knight PR. Impaired myocardial conduction in patients receiving diltiazem therapy during enflurane anesthesia. Anesthesiology (1987) 67, 94–6.

Anaesthetics, general + Fenfluramine

Abstract/Summary

An isolated case of fatal cardiac arrest has been attributed to halothane anaesthesia in a woman taking fenfluramine. Animal studies confirm that combined use can cause serious heart arrhythmias and myocardial depression.

Clinical evidence, mechanism, importance and management

A 23-year-old woman, premedicated with diazepam and hyoscine, anaesthetized initially with thiopentone followed by suxamethonium and later halothane with oxygen, became pulseless, cyanosed and showed acute pulmonary oedema within 5 min of induction. She failed to respond to resuscitative measures including cardiac massage. It was later discovered that she had been taking fenfluramine. Later studies in animals showed that during the concurrent use of halothane and fenfluramine, marked ECG changes, sinus bradycardia, heart block, ventricular asystoles, paroxysmal ventricular tachycardia and fibrillation occurred.[1] The reasons are not understood. The authors of this isolated report recommend that patients on fenfluramine should not be anaesthetized with halothane,[1] but to keep this serious reaction in perspective it should be said that the evidence for it has come under heavy fire from at least one author.[2]

References

1 Bennett JA, Eltingham RJ. Possible dangers of anaesthesia in patients receiving fenfluramine. Anesthesia (1977) 32, 8.
2 Winnie AP. Fenfluramine and halothane. Anesthesia (1979) 34, 79.

Anaesthetics, general + Monoamine oxidase inhibitors

Abstract/Summary

The usual advice is that MAOI should be withdrawn well before anaesthesia, but there is evidence that this is normally unnecessary in most patients, although individual cases of both hypo- and hypertension have been seen. The MAOI can however interact with other drugs sometimes used during surgery.

Clinical evidence and mechanism

The absence of problems during emergency general anaesthesia in two patients on MAOI prompted further study in six others taking un-named MAOI chronically. All six were premedicated with 10–15 mg diazepam 2 h before surgery. Anaesthesia was induced with thiopentone, intubation facilitated with suxamethonium (succinylcholine), and maintained with nitrous oxide/oxygen and either halothane or isoflurane. Pancuronium was used for muscle relaxation. Morphine was given postoperatively. One patient experienced hypotension which responded to repeated doses of 0.1 mg phenylephrine (IV) without hypertensive reactions. No untoward events occurred either during or after the anaesthesia.[1] A later anaesthetic study on 27 other patients on MAOI (tranylcypromine, phenelzine, isocarboxazid, pargyline) by the same group of workers also found no evidence of adverse reactions.[3] A single case report describes the safe use of propofol in a patient taking phenelzine.[5] Unexplained hypertension has been described in a patient taking tranylcypromine when etomidate and atracurium were used.[4]

Importance and management

There seems to be little or no documentary evidence that the withdrawal of MAOI before anaesthesia is normally necessary. Scrutiny of reports[2] alleging an adverse reaction usually shows that what happened could be attributed to an interaction between other drugs used during the surgery (e.g. pethidine, sympathomimetics) rather than with the anaesthetics. The authors of the reports cited[1,3] here offer the opinion that '...general and regional anesthesia may be provided safely without discontinuation of MAOI therapy, provided proper monitoring, adequate preparation, and prompt treatment of anticipated reactions are utilized.'[1] This implies that the possible interactions between the MAOI and other drugs are fully recognized but be alert for the rare unpredictable response.

References

1 El-Ganzouri A, Ivankovich AD, Braverman B, L, PC. Should MAOI be discontinued preoperatively? Anesthesiology (1983) 59, A384.

2 Jenkins LC, Graves HB. Potential hazards of psychoactive drugs in association with anesthesia. Can Anaesth Soc J (1965) 12, 121–8.

3 El-Ganzouri AR, Ivankovitch AD, Braverman B, McCarthy R. Monoamine Oxidase Inhibitors: should they be discontinued preoperatively? Anesth Analg (1985) 64, 592–6.

4 Sides CA. Hypertension during anaesthesia with monoamine oxidase inhibitors. Anaesthesia (1987) 42, 633–5.

5 Hodgson CA. Propofol and mono-amine oxidase inhibitors. Anaesthesia (1992) 47, 356.

Anaesthetics, general + Neuromuscular blockers

Abstract/Summary

The inhalation anaesthetics (diethyl ether, halothane, enflurane, isoflurane, etc.) increase neuromuscular blockade to differing extents, but nitrous oxide appears not to interact. Propofol can cause serious bradycardia if given with suxamethonium without adequate anticholinegic premedication, and asystole has been seen with fentanyl, propofol and suxamethonium given sequentially. Propofol in its new formulation does not interact with vecuronium.

Clinical evidence, mechanism, importance and management

(a) Increased blockade

Neuromuscular blockade is increased by inhalation anaesthetics, the greater the dosage of the anaesthetic the greater the increase in blockade. In broad terms diethyl ether, enflurane, isoflurane and methoxyflurane have a greater effect than halothane, which is more potent than fluroxene and cyclopropane, whereas nitrous oxide appears not to interact.[1-5] The reasons are not fully understood but the following mechanisms have been suggested: the anaesthetic may have an effect via the CNS, or it may affect the muscle membrane, or possibly that some change in blood flow to the muscle occurs. These anaesthetics do not seem to affect either the release of acetylcholine at neuromuscular junctions or the acetylcholine receptors. The dosage of the neuromuscular blocker may need to be adjusted according to the anaesthetic in use. For example, the dosage of atracurium can be reduced by 25–30% if, instead of balanced anaesthesia (with thiopentone, fentanyl and nitrous oxide/oxygen),[1] enflurane is used, and by up to 50% if isoflurane or desflurane are used.[2,8,9] Another study showed that the reversal of blockade by pancuronium with neostigmine was prolonged (roughly doubled) when using enflurane.[6] The effects of vecuronium are also increased by sevoflurane.[13]

(b) Bradycardia and asystole

Serious sinus bradycardia (heart rates of 30–40 bpm) developed rapidly in two young women when anaesthetised with a slow iv infusion of propofol (2.5 mg/kg), followed by suxamethonium (1.5 mg/kg). This was controlled with 0.6 mg IV atropine. Four other patients premedicated with 0.6 mg atropine IM 45 min before induction of anaesthesia showed no bradycardia.[7] It would appear that propofol lacks central vagolytic activity and can exaggerate the muscarinic effects of suxamethonium.[7] Another report describes asystole in a woman when given an anaesthetic induction sequence of fentanyl, propofol and suxamethonium.[10] Bradycardia and asystole have also been seen following the sequential administration of propofol-fentanyl in two patients.[11,12] All of these three drugs (fentanyl, propofol, suxamethonium) alone have been associated with bradycardia and their effects can apparently be additive. The authors of one report suggest that atropine or glycopyrrolate pretreatment should attenuate or prevent such reactions.[10]

(c) Propofol + Vecuronium: no interaction

The original formulation of propofol in Cremophor was found to increase the blockade due to vecuronium,[14] but the more recent formulation in soybean oil and egg phosphatide has been found in an extensive study in man not to interact with vecuronium.[15]

References

1 Ramsey FM, White PA, Stullken EH, Allen LL, Roy RC. Enflurane potentiation of neuromuscular blockade by atracurium. Anesthesiology (1982) 57, A255.

2 Sokoll MD, Gergis SD, Mehta M, Ali NM, Lineberry C. Safety and efficacy of atracurium (BW33A) in surgical patients receiving balanced or isoflurane anesthesia. Anesthesiology (1983) 58, 450–5.

3 Schuh FT. Differential increase in potency of neuromuscular blocking agents by enflurane and halothane. Int J Clin Pharmacol Ther Toxicol (1983) 21, 383–6.

4 Fogdall RP, Miller RD. Neuromuscular effects of enflurane alone and in combination with d-tubocurarine, pancuronium and succinylcholine in man. Anesthesiology (1975) 42, 173–8.

5 Miller RD, Way WL, Dolan WM, Stevens WC, Eger EI. Comparative neuromuscular effects of pancuronium, gallamine, and succinylcholine during Forane and halothane anaesthesia in man. Anesthesiology (1971) 35, 509–14.

6 Delisle S, Bevan DR. Impaired neostigmine antagonism of pancuronium during enflurane anaesthesia in man. Br J Anaesth (1982) 54, 441–5.

7 Baraka A. Severe bradycardia following propofol-suxamethonium sequence. Br J Anaesth (1988) 61, 482–3.

8 Lee C, Kwan WF, Chen B, Tsai SK, Gyermek L, Cheng M, Cantley E. Desflurane (I-653) potentiates atracurium in humans. Anesthesiology (1990) 73, A875.

9 Smiley RM, Omstein E, Matthews D, Matteo RS. A comparison of the effects of desflurane and isoflurane on the action of atracurium in man. Anesthesiology (1990) 73, A881.

10 Egan TD, Brock-Utne JG. Asystole after anesthesia induction with a fentanyl, profpol, and succinylcholine sequence. Anesth Analg (1991) 73, 818–20.

11 Guise PA. Asystole following propofol and fentanyl in an anxious patient. Anesth Intens Care (1991) 19, 116–7.

12 Dorrington KL. Asystole with convulsion following a subanaesthetic dose of propofol plus fentanyl. Anaesthesia (1989) 44, 658–9.

13 Izawa H, Takeda J, Fukushima K. The interaction between sevoflurane and vecuronium and its reversibility by neostigmine in man. Anesthesiology (1992) 77, A960.

14 Robertson EN, Fragen RJ, Booij LHDJ, Van Egmond J, Crul JF. Some effects of di-isopropyl phenol (ICI 35 868) on the pharmacodynamics of atracu-

rium and vecuronium in anaesthetised man. Br J Anaesth (1983) 55, 723–7.

15 McCarthy GJ, Mirakhur RK, Pandit SK. Lack of interaction between propofol and vecuronium. Anesth Analg (1992) 75, 356–8.

Anaesthetics, general + Nicotine

Abstract/Summary

A single report describes coronary vasospasm attributed to surgery, anaesthesia, and nicotine from a transdermal patch.

Clinical evidence, mechanism, importance and management

A 47-year-old woman recovering from surgery and general anaesthesia (etomidate, fentanyl, midazolam, vecuronium, lignocaine, nitrous oxide, isoflurane) complained of chest pain and demonstrated ECG changes which were interpreted as coronary vasospasm. The authors of the report linked this response to the possible use of a transdermal nicotine patch which was removed just before the induction of the anaesthesia. They postulated that the combination of the nicotine, the stress of surgery and the anaesthetic might have been responsible. They suggest that nicotine patches should be removed the night before surgery to ensure low levels of serum nicotine the next day.[1]

References

1 Williams EL, Tempelhoff R. Transdermal nicotine patch and general anaesthesia. Anesth Analg (1993) 76, 902–220.

Anaesthetics, general + Phenylephrine

Abstract/Summary

Phenylephrine eye drops caused marked cyanosis and bradycardia in a baby anaesthetized with halothane, and hypertension in a woman anaesthetized with isoflurane.

Clinical evidence, mechanism, importance and management

A three-week-old baby anaesthetized with halothane and nitrous oxide/oxygen became cyanosed shortly after the instillation of two drops of 10% phenylephrine solution in one eye. The heart rate decreased from 160 to 60 bpm, ST segment and T wave changes were seen, and blood pressure measurements were unobtainable. The baby recovered uneventfully when anaesthesia was stopped and oxygen administered. It was suggested that the phenylephrine caused severe peripheral vasodilatation and reflex bradycardia.[1] An adult patient aged 54 anaesthetized with isoflurane developed marked hypertension (a rise from 125/70 to 200/90 mmHg) shortly after having

two drops of 10% phenylephrine in one eye which responded to nasal nitroglycerin and increasing concentrations of isoflurane.[1] The authors of this report say that during anaesthesia the use of phenylephrine should be discouraged, but if necessary use the lowest concentrations of phenylephrine (2.5%). They also point out that the following are effective mydriatics: single drop combinations of 0.5% cyclopentolate and 2.5% phenylephrine or 0.5% tropicamide and 2.5% phenylephrine.

Reference

1 Van der Spek AFL, Hantler CB. Phenylephrine eyedrops and anaesthesia. Anaesthesiology (1986) 64, 812–4.

Anaesthetics, general + Phenytoin, Phenobarbitone, Rifampicin (Rifampin)

Abstract/Summary

Phenytoin intoxication occurred in a child following halothane anaesthesia, and fatal hepatic necrosis occurred in a woman on phenytoin, phenobarbitone and phenylbutazone after being anaesthetized with fluroxene. Near fatal hepatic shock occurred in a woman given rifampicin (rifampin) after halothane anaesthesia.

Clinical evidence

A 10-year-old girl on long-term treatment with phenytoin (300 mg daily) was found to have phenytoin serum levels of 25 µg/ml before surgery. Three days after anaesthesia with halothane her serum phenytoin levels had risen to 41 µg/ml and she had marked signs of phenytoin intoxication.[1] The probable reason is that the general toxic effects of halothane on the liver slowed the normal rate of phenytoin metabolism so that the serum levels rose. Another epileptic on 300 mg phenytoin, 120 mg phenobarbitone and phenylbutazone needed an increase in her phenytoin dosage to 2400 mg daily a week before surgery. She died of massive hepatic necrosis 36 h after anaesthesia with fluroxene.[2] A woman on promethazine and phenobarbitone (60 mg three times daily) died from halothane associated hepatitis within 6 days of having halothane for the first time.[4] A nearly fatal shock-producing hepatic reaction occurred in a woman 4 days after having halothane anaesthesia immediately followed by a course of 600 mg rifampicin and 300 mg isoniazid.[6]

Mechanism

A suggested explanation is that, just as in animals, pretreatment with phenobarbitone and phenytoin increases the rate of drug metabolism and the hepatotoxicity of halogenated hydrocarbons including chloroform and carbon tetrachloride.[3,5] The same may possibly apply to man. The reason for the halothane-rifampicin interaction is not clear but additive hepatotoxicity might be the explanation.

Importance and management

No firm conclusions can be drawn from these isolated cases, but they serve to emphasise the potential hepatotoxicity of these anaesthetics with other drugs. The authors of the second report[2] suggest that patients with similar drug histories may constitute a high-risk group for liver damage after halogen or vinyl-radical anaesthetics.

References

1 Karline JM, Kutt H. Acute diphenylhydantoin intoxication following halothane anesthesia. J Pediat (1970) 76, 941.
2 Reynolds ES, Brown BR, Vandam LD. Massive hepatic necrosis after fluroxene anesthesia-a case of drug interaction? N Engl J Med (1972) 286, 530.
3 Garner RC, McLean AEM. Increased susceptibility to carbon tetrachloride poisoning in the rat after pretreatment with oral phenobarbitone. Biochem Pharmacol (1969) 18, 645.
4 Patial RK, Sarin R, Patial SB. Halothane associated hepatitis and phenobarbitone. J Ass Phys India (1989) 37, 480.
5 Munson ES, Malagodi MH, Shields RP, Tham MK, Fiserova-Bergerova V, Holday DA, Perry JC, Embro WJ. Fluoxene toxicity induced by phenobarbital. Clin Pharmacol Ther (1976) 18, 687–99.
6 Most JA, Markle GB. A nearly fatal hepatotoxic reaction to rifampin after halothane anaesthesia. Am J Surg (1974) 127, 593–5.

Anaesthetics, general + Sparteine sulphate

Abstract/Summary

Patients induced with thiamyl sodium show a very marked increase in cardiac arrhythmias when given sparteine sulphate.

Clinical evidence, mechanism, importance and management

109 women undergoing dilatation and curretage were premedicated with atropine and fentanyl, induced with either 2% thiamyl sodium (5 mg/kg), 0.2% etomidate (0.3 mg/kg) or 2.5% thiopental (4 mg/kg), and given mask anaesthesia with nitrous oxide and oxygen. During the surgical procedure they were given a slow IV injection of 100 mg sparteine sulphate. 14 out of 45 patients given thiamyl sodium developed cardiac dysrhythmias, 10 had bigeminy and four had frequent VPCs, whereas only two patients given the other induction agents (etomidate or thiopental) showed any cardiac dysrhythmias. It is not understood why sparteine should interact with thiamyl sodium in this way. Although the dysrhythmias were effectively treated with xylocaine, the authors of this report suggest that the concurrent use of these drugs should be avoided.[1]

Reference

1 Cheng S-R, Chen S-Y, WU K-H, Wei T-T. Thiamyl sodium with sparteine sulfate inducing dysrhythmia in anesthetized patients. Anaesth Sinica (1989) 27, 297–8.

Anaesthetics, general and/or Neuromuscular blockers + Theophylline

Abstract/Summary

Cardiac arrhythmias can develop during the concurrent use of halothane and theophylline but this is possibly less likely with isoflurane. Seizures have been attributed to an interaction between ketamine and theophylline. Supraventricular tachycardia occurred in a patient on aminophylline when given pancuronium. The effects of pancuronium but not vecuronium can be opposed by aminophylline (theophylline).

Clinical evidence, mechanism, importance and management

(a) Development of arrhythmias

A number of reports describe arrhythmias apparently due to an interaction between halothane and theophylline. One describes intraoperative arrhythmias in four out of 67 adult asthmatics given theophylline and halothane (one had supraventricular tachycardia, two had bigeminy and one had multifocal premature ventricular contractions).[9] Nine out of another 45 patients developed heart rates exceeding 145 when given both drugs, whereas no tachycardia occurred in 22 other patients given only halothane.[9] There are other reports of individual adult and child patients who developed ventricular tachycardias[10] attributed to this interaction.[1,8,11,12] One child developed cardiac arrest.[12] The same interaction has been reported in animals.[2,3] Another report describes supraventricular tachycardia in a patient on aminophylline who was anaesthetized with thiopentone and fentanyl, followed by pancuronium. 3 min later his heart rate rose to 180 bpm and the ECG revealed that it was supraventricular in origin.[7] The authors of this report attributed this reaction to an interaction between the pancuronium and the aminophylline. The suggested reason for the interaction with halothane is that the theophylline causes the release of catecholamines (adrenaline-epinephrine, noradrenaline-norepinephrine) from the adrenal medulla which are known to sensitize the myocardium.

The authors of one of the reports advise the avoidance of concurrent use[1] but another says that: '...my own experience with the liberal use of these drugs has convinced me of the efficacy and wide margin of safety associated with their use in combination.'[4] A possibly safer anaesthetic may be isoflurane which in studies with dogs has been shown not to cause cardiac arrhythmias in the presence of aminophylline.[5]

(b) Development of seizures

Tachycardia and extensor-type seizures occurred in four patients initially anaesthetized with ketamine and later with halothane or enflurane.[6] The authors attributed the seizures to an interaction between ketamine and theophylline (aminophylline) and they suggest avoidance of the combination or the use of antiseizure premedication in patients at risk.

(c) Altered neuromuscular blockade

A study in rabbits showed that at therapeutic concentrations the effects of tubocurarine were increased by theophylline, but this does not seem to have been observed in man.[13] Marked resistance to the effects of pancuronium was seen in two patients infused with aminophylline,[14,17] but no resistance was seen in one of them when vecuronium was given instead.[14] Two other patients are reported to have shown a similar resistance but they had also had hydrocortisone which could have had a similar effect.[15,16]

References

1 Roizen MF, Stevens WC. Multiform ventricular tachycardia due to the interaction of aminophylline and halothane. Anesth Analg (1978) 57, 738.
2 Takori M, Loehning RW. Ventricular arrhythmias induced by aminophylline during halothane anaesthesia in dogs. Can Anesth Soc J (1967) 14, 79.
3 Stirt JA, Berger JM, Ricker SM, Sullivan SF. Halothane-induced cardiac arrhythmias following administration of aminophylline in experimental animals. Anesth Analg (1981) 60, 517–20.
4 Zimmerman BL. Arrhythmogenicity of theophylline and halothane used in combination. Anesth Analg (1979) 58, 259.
5 Stirt JA, Berger JM, Sullivan SF. Lack of arrhythmogenicity of isoflurane following administration of aminophylline in dogs. Anesth Analg (1983) 62, 568–71.
6 Hirshman CA, Krieger W, Littlejohn G, Lee R, Julien R. Ketamine-aminophylline-induced decrease in seizure threshold. Anesthesiology (1982) 56, 464–7.
7 Belani KG, Anderson WW, Buckley JJ. Adverse drug interaction involving pancuronium and aminophylline. Anesth Analg (1982) 61, 473–4.
8 Naito Y, Arai T, Miyake C. Severe arrhythmias due to the combined use of halothane and aminophylline in an asthmatic patient. Jpn J Anaesthesiol (1986) 35, 1126–9.
9 Barton MD. Anesthetic problems with aspirin-intolerant patients. Anesth Analg (1975) 54, 376.
10 Roizen MF, Stevens WC. Multiform ventricular tachycardia due to the interaction of aminophylline and halothane. Anesth Analg (1978) 57, 738.
11 Bedger RC, Chang JL, Larson CE. Increased myocardial irritability with halothane and aminophylline. Anesth Prog (1980) 27, 34.
12 Richards W, Thompson J, Lewis G, Levy DS, Church JA. Cardiac arrest associated with halothane anesthesia in a patient receiving theophylline. Ann Allergy (1988) 61, 83–4
13 Fuke N, Martyn J, Kim C, Basta S. Concentration-dependent interaction of theophylline with d-tubocurarine. J Appl Physiol (1987) 62, 1970–4.
14 Daller JA, Erstad B, Rosado L, Otto C, Putnam CW. Aminophylline antagonizes the neuromuscular blockade of pancuronium but not vecuronium. Crit Care Med (1991) 19, 983–5.
15 Doll DC, Rosenberg H. Antagonism of neuromuscular blockade by theophylline. Anesth Analg (1979) 58, 139.
16 Azar I, Kumar D, Betcher AM. Resistance to pancuronium in an asthmatic patient treated with aminophylline and steroids. Cab Anaesth Soc J (1982) 29, 280.
17 Doll DC, Rosenberg H. Antagonism of neuromuscular blockage by theophylline. Anesth Analg (1979) 58, 139–40.

Anaesthetics, general + Thyroid hormones

Abstract/Summary

Marked hypertension and tachycardia occurred in two patients taking levothyroxine when given ketamine.

Clinical evidence, mechanism, importance and management

Two patients on thyroid replacement treatment (levothyroxine) developed severe hypertension (240/140 and 210/130 mmHg respectively) and tachycardia (190 and 150 bpm) when given ketamine. Both were effectively treated with 1 mg IV propranolol.[1] It was not clear whether this was an interaction or simply a particularly exaggerated response to ketamine, but care is clearly needed if ketamine is given to patients in this category.

Reference

1 Kaplan JA, Cooperman LH. Alarming reactions to ketamine in patients taking thyroid medication — treatment with propranolol. Anesthesiol (1971) 35, 229–30.

Anaesthetics, general + Timolol

Abstract/Summary

Marked bradycardia and hypotension occurred in a man using timolol eye-drops when he was anaesthetized.

Clinical evidence, mechanism, importance and management

A 75-year-old man being treated with timolol eye drops for glaucoma developed bradycardia and severe hypotension when anaesthetized (agent not named) which responded poorly to atropine, dextrose-saline infusion and elevation of his feet.[1] It would seem that there was sufficient systemic absorption of the timolol for it to join with the anaesthetic to cause marked depression of cardiac activity. The authors of this report suggest that if patients are to be anaesthetized, low concentrations of timolol should be used (possibly withhold the drops preoperatively), and that '...induction agents should be used judiciously and beta-blocking antagonists kept readily available.' It is easy to overlook the fact that systemic absorption from eye-drops can be remarkably high. See also 'Anaesthetics + Beta-blockers'.

Reference

1 Mostafa SM. Ocular timolol and induction agents during anaesthesia. Br Med J (1985) 290, 1788.

Anaesthetics, general + Tricyclic antidepressants

Abstract/Summary

Some very limited evidence suggests that amitriptyline may increase the likelihood of enflurane-induced seizure activity. Tachyarrhythmias have been seen in patients on imipramine when given halothane and pancuronium.

Clinical evidence, mechanism, importance and management

(a) Enflurane + Amitriptyline

Two patients taking amitriptyline have been described who showed clonic movements of the leg, arm and hand during surgery while anaesthetized with enflurane and nitrous oxide. The movements stopped when the enflurane was replaced by halothane.[1] A possible reason is that amitriptyline can lower the seizure threshold at which enflurane-induced seizure activity occurs. It is suggested that it may be advisable to avoid enflurane in patients needing tricyclic antidepressants, particularly in those who have a history of seizure or when hyperventilation or high concentrations of enflurane are likely to be used.[1]

(b) Halothane + Imipramine and Pancuronium

Two patients taking imipramine developed marked tachyarrhthmias when anaesthetized with halothane and given pancuronium.[2] This adverse interaction was subsequently clearly demonstrated in dogs.[2] The authors concluded on the basis of their studies that (i) gallamine should be avoided but tubocurarine would be an acceptable alternative to pancuronium; (ii) caution is appropriate if patients are taking any tricyclic antidepressant and halothane is used; (iii) pancuronium is probably safe in the presence of a tricyclic if enflurane is used. More study is needed.

References

1 Sprague DH, Wolf S. Enflurane seizures in patients taking amitriptyline. Anesth Analg (1982) 61, 67–8.
2 Edwards RP, Miller RD, Roizen MF, Ham J, Way WL, Lake CR, Roderick L. Cardiac responses to imipramine and pancuronium during anesthesia with halothane and enflurane. Anesthesiology (1979) 50, 421–5.

Anaesthetics, local + Alcohol and Antirheumatics

Abstract/Summary

The failure rate of spinal anaesthesia with bupivacaine is markedly increased in patients who are receiving antirheumatic drugs and who drink.

Clinical evidence, mechanism, importance and management

The observation that regional anaesthetic failures seemed to be particularly high among patients undergoing orthopaedic surgery who were suffering from rheumatic joint diseases, prompted further study of a possible interaction involving antirheumatic drugs and alcohol. It was found that the failure rate of low-dose spinal anaesthesia with bupivacaine (2 ml of 0.5%) increased from 5% in the control group (no alcohol or treatment) to 32–45% in those who had been taking antirheumatic drugs for at least 6 months or who drank at least 80 g ethanol daily, or both. The percentage of those patients who had a reduced response (i.e. an extended latency period and a reduced duration of action). also increased from 3 to 39–42%. Indomethacin was the specific antirheumatic drug studied in one group.[1] The reasons are not understood.

Reference

1 Sprotte G, Weis KH. Drug interaction with local anaesthetics. Brit J Anaesth (1982) 54, 242P.

Anaesthetics, local + Anaesthetics, local

Abstract/Summary

Mixtures of local anaesthetics are sometimes used to exploit the most useful characteristics of each drug. This normally seems to be safe although it is sometimes claimed that it increases the risk of toxicity. There is a case report of a man who developed toxicity when bupivacaine and mepivacaine were mixed together. The effectiveness of bupivacaine in epidural anaesthesia is reduced if preceded by chloroprocaine

Clinical evidence and mechanism

(a) Evidence of no interaction

A study designed to assess the possibility of adverse interactions in man retrospectively studied the records of 10,538 patients over the 1952–72 period who had been given amethocaine (tetracaine) combined with chloroprocaine, lignocaine (lidocaine), mepivacaine, prilocaine, procaine or propoxycaine for caudal, epidural, brachial plexus, or peripheral nerve block. The incidence of systemic toxic reactions was found to be no greater than when used singly and the conclusion was reached that combined use was advantageous and safe.[1] An animal study using combinations of bupivacaine, lidocaine (lignocaine) and chloroprocaine also found no evidence that the toxicity was greater than if the anaesthetics were used singly.[3] Lignocaine does not affect the pharmacokinetics of bupivacaine in man.[4]

(b) Evidence of reduced analgesia

A study set up to examine the clinical impression that bupivacaine given epidurally did not relieve labour pain effectively if preceded by chloroprocaine confirmed that this was so. Using an initial 10 ml dose of 2% chloroprocaine followed by 8 ml 0.5% bupivacaine, the pain relief was less, the block was longer to set up, it had a shorter duration of action and had to be augmented more frequently than if only chloroprocaine was used.[5,6]

(c) Evidence of a toxic interaction

An animal study showed that if amethocaine (tetracaine) was combined with other local anaesthetics the incidence of systemic toxicity and deaths increased.[1] There is a single case report of a patient given 2% bupivacaine and 0.75% mepivacaine who demonstrated lethargy, dysarthria and mild muscle tremor which the authors of the report correlated with a marked increase in the percentage of unbound (active) bupivacaine. They attributed this to its displacement by the mepivacaine from protein binding sites.[2]

Importance and management

Well examined interactions. The overall picture is that combined use does not normally result in increased toxicity although the isolated case report cited above illustrates that the possibility cannot be entirely discounted. Reduced effectiveness is seen if bupivacaine is preceded by chloroprocaine.

References

1 Moore DC, Bridenbaugh LD, Bridenbaugh PO, Thompson GE, Tucker GT. Does compounding of local anaesthetic agents increase their toxicity in humans? Anesth Analg (1972) 51, 579–85.

2 Hartrick CT, Raj PP, Dirkes WE, Denson DD. Compounding of bupivacaine and mepivacaine for regional anaesthesia. A safe practice? Reg Anaesth (1984) 9, 94–7.

3 De Jong RH, Bonin JD. Mixtures of local anesthetics are no more toxic than the parent drugs. Anesthesiology (1981) 54, 177–81.

4 Freysz M, Beal JL, D'Athis P, Mounie J, Wilkening M, Escousse A. Pharmacokinetics of bupivacaine after axillary brachial plexus block. Int J Clin Pharmacol Ther Tox (1987) 25, 392–5.

5 Chen B-J, Kwan W-F. pH is not a determinant of 2-chloroprocaine-bupivacaine interaction: a clinical study. Reg Anaesthesia (1990) 15, (Suppl 1) 25.

6 Hodgkinson R, Husain FJ, Bluhm C. Reduced effectiveness of bupivacaine 0.5% to relieve labor pain after prior injection of chloroprocaine 2%. Anesthesiology (1982) 57, A201.

Anaesthetics, local + Acetazolamide

Abstract/Summary

Preliminary evidence suggests the possibility of procaine toxicity in patients given acetazolamide.

Clinical evidence, mechanism, importance and management

The mean plasma half-life of procaine in six normal subjects was increased by 66% (from 1.46 to 2.43 min) 2 h after being given 250 mg acetazolamide orally. The reason appears to be that the hydrolysis of the procaine is inhibited by the acetazolamide. The authors of the study suggest that higher than normal procaine levels (with toxicity) might possibly occur in patients given acetazolamide and (for example) large intramuscular doses of procaine penicillin G,[1] but thus far there appear to be no reports of adverse responses due to this interaction.

Reference

1 Calvo R, Carlos R, Erill S. Effects of disease and acetazolamide on procaine hydrolysis by red blood cell enzymes. Clin Pharmacol Ther (1980) 27, 179–83.

Anaesthetics, local + Benzodiazepines

Abstract/Summary

There is conflicting evidence about whether diazepam can increase or decrease serum bupivacaine levels. Midazolam causes a modest decrease in lignocaine (lidocaine) but not mepivacaine levels.

Clinical evidence, mechanism, importance and management

Twenty-one children aged 2–10 were given single caudal injections of 1 ml/kg of a mixture of 0.5% lignocaine (lidocaine) and 0.125% bupivacaine for regional anaesthesia. Pretreatment with 10 mg diazepam rectally 30 min before the surgery had no significant effect on the serum levels of lignocaine, but the AUC and maximal serum bupivacaine levels were increased by 70–75%.[1] A later study by the same workers similarly found that diazepam pretreatment in children raised serum bupivacaine levels.[5] These findings conflict with another in which IV diazepam in adult patients decreased the elimination half-life of epidural bupivacaine.[2] A later study in 20 children aged 2–7 receiving caudal block with 1 ml/kg of a 50:50 mixture of 1% lignocaine (lidocaine) and 0.25% bupivacaine, found that 0.4 mg/kg midazolam given rectally as premediction caused a slight but not significant reduction in the AUC and serum levels of bupivacaine, whereas the lignocaine AUC was reduced by 25%.[3] In contrast, 0.4 mg midazolam given rectally as a premedication was found to have no significant effect on plasma mepivacaine levels.[4]

The clinical importance of these interactions is uncertain, but anaesthetists should be aware that increased bupivacaine serum levels have been observed with diazepam, and reduced lignocaine levels with midazolam. More study is needed.

References

1 Giaufre E, Bruguerolle B, Morisson-Lacombe G, Rousset-Rouviere B. The influence of diazepam on the plasma concentrations of bupivacaine and lignocaine after caudal injection of a mixture of the local anaesthetics in children. Br J Clin Pharmac (1988) 26, 116–8.

2 Giasi RM, D'Agostino E, Covino BG. Interaction of diazepam in epidurally administered local anaesthetic agents. Reg Anesth (1980) 5, 8–11.

3 Giaufre E, Bruguerolle B, Morisson-Lacombe G, Rousset-Rouviere B. The influence of midazolam on the plasma concentrations of bupivacaine and lignocaine after caudal injection of a mixture of the local anaesthetics in children. Acta Anaesthesiol Scand (1990) 34, 44–6.

4 Giaufre E, Bruguerolle B, Morisson-Lacombe G, Rousset-Rouviere B. Influence of midazolam on the plasma concentrations of mepivacaine after lumber epidural injection in children. Eur J Clin Pharmacol (1990) 38, 91–2.

5 Bruguerolle B, Giaufre E, Morisson-Lacombe G, Rousset-Rouviere B, Arnaud C. Bupivacaine free plasma levels in children after caudal anaesthesia: influence of pretreatment with diazepam. Fundam Clin Pharmacol (1990) 4, 159–61.

Anaesthetics, local + Beta-blockers

Abstract/Summary

Propranolol reduces the clearance of bupivacaine and there is the theoretical possibility that the toxicity of bupivacaine may be increased. The coronary vasoconstriction caused by cocaine is increased by propranolol. See also Beta-blockers + Sympathomimetics, directly-acting.

Clinical evidence, mechanism, importance and management

(a) Bupivacaine + Propranolol

The clearance of bupivacaine (30–50 mg IV over 10–15 min) was reduced by 35% (from 0.33 to 0.21 l/min) in six normal subjects after taking 40 mg propranolol 6-hourly for a day. The reason is thought to be that the propranolol inhibits the activity of the liver microsomal enzymes, thereby reducing the metabolism of the bupivacaine. Changes in blood flow to the liver are unlikely to affect bupivacaine metabolism substantially because it is relatively poorly extracted from the blood. The clinical importance of this interaction is uncertain, but it is suggested that an increase in local anaesthetic toxicity might occur and caution should be exercised if multiple doses of bupivacaine are given.[1] Direct information about other beta-blockers is lacking, but some of them are known to reduce the metabolism of lignocaine (lidocaine). See 'Lignocaine (Lidocaine) + Beta-blockers'.

(b) Cocaine + Propranolol

A study in 30 patients being evaluated for chest pain found that cocaine (10% solution intra-nasally, 2 mg/kg) reduced coronary sinus flow by 14% and coronary artery diameter by 6–9%. The coronary vascular resistance increased by 21%. The addition of propranolol (0.4 mg/min by intracoronary infusion, total

2 mg) reduced coronary sinus flow by a further 15% and increased the coronary resistance by 17%. The probable reason is that the cocaine stimulates the alpha-receptors (vasoconstrictor) of the coronary blood vessels. When the beta-receptors (vasodilatory) are blocked by propranolol, the vasoconstriction is thereby increased. The clinical importance of these findings is uncertain but the authors of the report suggest that beta-blockers should be avoided in patients with myocardial ischaemia or infarction associated with the use of cocaine.[2] Remember that local anaesthetics preparations often contain adrenaline (epinephrine) as a vasoconstrictor which may interact with beta-blockers. See 'Beta-blockers + Sympathomimetics, directly-acting'.

References

1 Bowdle TA, Freund PR, Slattery JT. Propranolol reduces bupivacaine clearance. Anesthesiology (1987) 66, 36–8.

2 Lange RA. Cigarroa RG, Flores ED, McBride W, Kijm AS, Wells PJ, Bedotto JB, Danziger RS, Jillis LD. Potentiation of cocaine-induced coronary vasoconstriction by beta-adrenergic blockade. Ann Intern Med (1990) 112, 897–903.

Anaesthetics, local + Cimetidine or Ranitidine

Abstract/Summary

Some studies suggest that both cimetidine and ranitidine can raise bupivacaine levels whereas other evidence suggests that no significant interaction occurs. Neither H_2-blocker appears to affect lignocaine (lidocaine) when used an an anaesthetic, but see also Lignocaine + Cimetidine in Chapter 4 (Antiarrhythmic interactions).

Clinical evidence

(a) Cimetidine + Bupivacaine

Pretreatment with 300 mg cimetidine IM 1–4 h before undergoing caesarian section with 0.5% bupivacaine had no effect on the pharmacokinetics or bupivacaine of 36 women or their fetuses, although the unbound bupivacaine levels rose by 22%.[1] Another similar study[10] in 36 women pretreated with 400 mg cimetidine the night before or just before surgery, and yet another[7] in seven normal subjects given 400 mg cimetidine at 10.00 the previous evening and 6.00 the following morning confirmed these findings. However four normal male subjects who were given 400 mg cimetidine at 10.00 pm the previous evening and 8.00 am the following morning, followed by a 50 mg infusion of bupivacaine at 11.0 am, showed a 40% increase in the bupivacaine AUC.

(b) Cimetidine + Lignocaine (Lidocaine)

No changes in the pharmacokinetics of 400 mg lignocaine 2%

adrenaline 1:200,000 was seen in five women given epidural anaesthesia for caesarian section after a single 400 mg dose of cimetidine given about 2 h preoperatively.[6,8] Another very similar study in 11 women also found no statistically significant rises in whole blood lignocaine levels in the presence of cimetidine, 300 mg IM at least an hour preoperatively.[9]

(c) Ranitidine + Bupivacaine

Pretreatment with 150 mg ranitidine orally 2 h before bupivacaine for extradural anaesthesia for caesarian section increased the serum levels of bupivacaine in 16 patients at 40 min by about 20%.[3] Similar results by the same group of authors are reported elsewhere.[4] Another study found that 150 mg ranitidine caused a 25% increase but it was not statistically significant.[2] No increased bupivacaine toxicity was reported in any of these reports. However two other studies on 28[5] and 36[10] women undergoing caesarian section found no measurable effect on the bupivacaine disposition when given 50 mg ranitidine IM 2 h before or 150 mg the night before the morning of anaesthesia.[5]

(d) Ranitidine + Lignocaine (lidocaine)

No changes in the pharmacokinetics of 400 mg lignocaine (lidocaine) 2% adrenaline 1:200,000 was seen in a study on seven women given epidural anaesthesia for caesarian section after a single 150 mg dose of ranitidine given about 2 h preoperatively.[6,8] Another very similar study in 11 women also found no statistically significant rises in whole blood lignocaine levels in the presence of 150 mg ranitidine at least 2 h preoperatively.[9]

Mechanism

Not understood. A reduction in the metabolism of the bupivacaine by the liver caused by the cimetidine is one suggested explanation. Protein binding displacement is another.

Importance and management

A confusing situation. No clinically important interaction has been established but be alert for any evidence of increased bupivacaine toxicity resulting from raised total serum levels and rises in unbound levels during concurrent use. Cimetidine (but not ranitidine) can raise serum lignocaine (lidocaine) levels when used as an antiarrhythmic agent (see 'Lignocaine + Cimetidine' in Chapter 4) but this was not demonstrated in the studies cited above. More study is needed.

References

1 Kuhnert BR, Zuspan KJ, Kuhnert PM, Syracuse CD, Brashear WT, Brown DE. Lack of influence of cimetidine on bupivacaine levels during parturition. Anesth Analg (1988) 66, 986–90.
2 Noble DW, Smith KJ, Dundas CR. Effects of H$_2$-antagonists on the elimination of bupivacaine. Br J Anaesth (1987) 59, 735–7.
3 Wilson CM, Moore J, Ghaly RG, McLean E, Dundee JW. Plasma bupivacaine concentrations associated with extradural anaesthesia for Caesarian section: influence of pretreatment with ranitidine. Br J Anaesth (1986) 58, 1330P.
4 Flynn RJ, Moore J, Collier PS, McClean E. Does pretreatment with cimetidine and treatment with cimetidine and ranitidine affect the disposition of bupivacaine? Br J Anaesth (1989) 62, 87–91.
5 Brashear WT, Zuspan KJ, Lazebnik N, Kuhnert BR, Mann LI. Effect of ranitidine on bupivacaine disposition. Anesth Analg (1991) 72, 369–76.
6 Flynn RJ, Moore J, Collier PS, Howard PJ. Single dose oral H$_2$-antagonists do not affect plasma lignocaine levels in the parturient. Acta Anaesthsiol Scand (1989) 33, 593–6.
7 Pihlajamäki KK, Lindberg RLP, Jantunen ME. Lack of effect of cimetidine on the pharmacokinetics of bupivacaine in healthy subjects. Br J Clin Pharmac (1988) 26, 403–6.
8 Flynn RJ, Moore J. Lack of effect of cimetidine and ranitidine on lidocaine disposition in the parturient. Anesthesiology (1988) 69, A656.
9 Dailey PA, Hughes SC, Rosen MA, Healey K, Cheek DBC, Shnider SM. Effect of cimetidine and ranitidine on lidocaine concentrations during epidural anaesthesia for Cesarean section. Anaesthesiology (1988) 69, 1013–7.
10 O'Sullivan GM, Smith M, Morgan B, Brighouse D, Reynolds F. H2 antagonists and bupivacaine clearance. Anaesthesia (1988) 43, 93–5.

Anaesthetics, local + Carbamazepine, Lithium carbonate

Abstract/Summary

Lithium and carbamazepine appear to reduce the effects of cocaine when used as a drug of abuse.

Clinical evidence, mechanism, importance and management

Four patients were unable to get 'high' on cocaine while taking lithium.[1] A man who occasionally abused cocaine found that the acute cocaine experience (the euphoric 'rush') was very much less pleasurable while taking 1 g carbamazepine daily, and the 'high' was reduced.[2] Another report suggests that cocaine craving may be reduced by carbamazepine.[3] The reasons are not understood. The clinical importance of this is uncertain.

References

1 Cronson AJ, Flemenbaum A. Antagonism of cocaine highs by lithium. Am J Psychiatry (1978) 135, 856–7.
2 Sherer MA, Kumor KM, Mapou RL. A case in which carbamazepine attenuated cocaine 'rush'. Am J Psychiatry (1990) 147, 950.
3 Halakis J, Kemp K, Kuhn K. Carbamazepine for cocaine addiction ? Lancet (1989) 1, 623–4.

Neuromuscular blockers and/or Anaesthetics + Aminoglycoside antibiotics

Abstract/Summary

The aminoglycoside antibiotics (amikacin, gentamicin, kanamycin, neomycin, streptomycin, tobramycin, etc.) possess

neuromuscular blocking activity. Appropriate measures should be taken to accommodate the increased neuromuscular blockade and the prolonged and potentially fatal respiratory depression which can occur if these antibiotics are used with anaesthetics and conventional neuromuscular blocking drugs of any kind.

Clinical evidence

Two examples from many:

(a) Anaesthetic + Aminoglycoside Antibiotic

A 48-year-old patient anaesthetized with cyclopropane experienced severe respiratory depression after intraperitoneal irrigation with 500 mg 1% neomycin solution. This antibiotic-induced neuromuscular blockade was resistant to treatment with edrophonium but responded to neostigmine.[2]

(b) Anaesthetic + Neuromuscular Blocker + Aminoglycoside Antibiotic

A 56-year-old patient, initially anaesthetized with thiopentone followed by nitrous oxide, was given 160 mg gallamine as a muscle relaxant. His respiration was depressed for 18 h following the intraperitoneal administration of 2 g neomycin.[3]

Many other reports confirm that some degree of respiratory embarrassment or paralysis can occur if aminoglycosides are given to anaesthetized patients. When a conventional blocker is also used, the blockade is deepened and recovery prolonged. If the antibiotic is given towards the end of surgery the result can be that a patient who is recovering normally from neuromuscular blockade suddenly develops serious apnoea which can lead on to prolonged and in some cases fatal respiratory depression. Pittinger[1] lists more than a 100 cases in the literature over the 1955–70 period involving tubocurarine with neomycin or streptomycin; gallamine with neomycin, kanamycin or streptomycin; and suxamethonium with neomycin, kanamycin or streptomycin. The routes of antibiotic administration were oral, intraperitoneal, oesophageal, intraluminal, retroperineal, intramuscular, intrapleural, cystic, beneath skin flaps, intradural and intravenous. Later reports involve irrigation of the anterior chamber of the eye with framycetin;[4] gentamicin given alone[6] or with vecuronium,[23] tubocurarine[7] or pancuronium;[10] amikacin,[9] tobramycin[8] or ribostamycin[5,14] with tubocurarine or pancuronium,[16] but not ribostamycin with suxamethonium;[5] pancuronium with streptomcyin[11,15] or neomycin;[14,18] pipecuronium with netilmicin;[22] vecuronium with amikacin/polymyxin,[17] gentamicin alone[21] (and with clindamycin)[13] or tobramycin.[19,21] Dibekacin causes a small increase in the effects of tubocurarine and suxamethonium,[5,14] but tobramycin seems not to affect alcuronium[12] nor atracurium,[21] and gentamicin also seems not to affect atracurium.[21]

Mechanism

The aminoglycosides appear to reduce or prevent the release of acetylcholine at neuromuscular junctions (related to an impairment of calcium influx) and they may also lower the sensitivity of the postsynaptic membrane, thereby reducing transmission. These effects would be additive with those of conventional neuromuscular blockers which act at the post-synaptic membrane.

Importance and management

Extremely well documented, very long established, clinically important and potentially serious interactions. 10 out of the 111 cases cited by Pittinger[1] were fatal, related directly or indirectly to aminoglycoside-induced respiratory depression. Concurrent use need not be avoided but be alert for increased and prolonged neuromuscular blockade with every aminoglycoside and neuromuscular blocker although the potencies of the aminoglycosides differ. The neuromuscular blocking potencies of the aminoglycosides seem to be in descending order (based on animal studies): gentamicin > streptomycin > amikacin > sisomicin > kanamycin = tobramycin > kanendomycin = dibekacin.[20] The postoperative recovery period should also be closely monitored because of the risk of recurarization if the antibiotic is given during surgery. High risk patients appear to be those with renal disease and hypocalcaemia who may have elevated serum antibiotic levels, and those with pre-existing muscular weakness. Treatment of the increased blockade with anticholinesterases and calcium has met with variable success because the response seems to be inconsistent.

References

1 Pittinger CB, Eryasa Y, Adamson R. Antibiotic-induced paralysis. Anesth Analg (1970) 49, 487.
2 NY State Society of Anesthesiologists Clinical Anesthesia Conference: Postoperative neomycin respiratory depression. NY J Med (1960) 60, 1977.
3 LaPorte J, Mignault J, L'Allier R, Perron P. Un cas d'apnea a la neomycin. Un Med Canada (1959) 88, 149
4 Clark R. Prolonged curarization due to intraocular soframycin. Anesth Int Care (1975) 3, 79.
5 Arai T, Hashimoto Y, Shima Y, Matsukawa S, Iwatsuki K. Neuromuscular blocking properties of tobramycin, dibekacin and ribostamycin in man. Jap J Antibiot (1977) 30, 281.
6 Holtzman JL. Gentamicin and neuromuscular blockade. Ann Int Med (1976) 84, 55.
7 Warner WA, Sanders E. Neuromuscular blockade. J Amer Med Ass (1971) 215, 1157.
8 Waterman PM, Smith RB. Tobramycin-curare interaction. Anesth Analg (1977) 56, 587.
9 Singh YN, Marshall IG, Harvey AL. Some effects of the aminoglycoside antibiotic amikacin on neuromuscular and autonomic transmission. Br J Anaesth (1978) 50, 109.
10 Regan AG, Perumbetti PPV. Pancuronium and gentamicin interaction in patients with renal failure. Anesth Analg (1980) 59, 393.
11 Giala MM, Paradelis AG. Two cases of prolonged respiratory depression due to interaction of pancuronium with colistin and streptomycin. J Antimicrob Chemother (1979) 5, 234.
12 Boliston TA, Ashman R. Tobramycin and neuromuscular blockade. Anesthesia (1978) 33, 552.
13 Jedeikin R, Dolgunski E, Kaplan R, Hoffman S. Prolongation of neuromuscular blocking effect of vecuronium by antibiotics. Anaesthesia (1987) 42, 858–60.
14 Hashimoto T, Shima T, Matsukawa S, Iwatsuki K. Neuromuscular blocking properties of some antibiotics in man. Tohoku J Exp Med (1975) 117, 339.

15 Torresi E, Pasotti EM. Su un caso di curarizzazione prolungata da interazione tra pancuronio e streptomicina. Min Anest (1984) 50, 143–5.

16 Monsegur JC, Vidal MM, Beltran J, Felipe MAN. Paralsis neuromuscular prolongada tra administraction simultanea de amikacina y pancuronio. Rev Esp Anest Rean (1984) 31, 30–3.

17 Kronenfeld MA, Thomas SJ, Turndorf H. Recurrence of neuromuscular blockade after reversal of vecuronium in a patient receiving polymyxin/amikacin sternal irrigation. Anesthesiol (1986) 65, 93–4.

18 Giala M, Sareyiannis C, Cortsaris N, Paradelis A, Lappas DG. Possible interaction of pancuronium and tubocurarine with oral neomycin. Anaesthesia (1982) 37, 776.

19 Vanacker BF, Van de Walle J. The neuromuscular blocking action of vecuronium in normal patients and in patients with no renal function and interaction vercuronium-tobramycin in renal transplant patients. Acta Anaesth Belg (1986) 37, 95–9.

20 Paradelis AG, Triantaphyllidis C, Giala MM. Neuromuscular blocking activity of aminoglycoside antibiotics. Meth and Find Exptl Clin Pharmacol (1980) 2, 45–51.

21 Dupuis JY, Martin R, Tetrault JP. Atracurium and vecuronium interaction with gentamicin and tobramycin. Can J Anaesth (1989) 36, 407–11.

22 Stanley JC, Mirakhur RK, Clarke RSJ. Study of pipecuronium-antibiotic interaction. Anesthesiology (1990) 73, A898.

23 Harwood TN, Moorthy SS. Prolonged vecuronium-induced neuromuscular blockade in children. Anesth Analg (1989) 68, 534–6.

Neuromuscular blockers + Aprotinin

Abstract/Summary

Apnoea developed in a number of patients after being given aprotinin (Trasylol) while recovering from neuromuscular blockade with suxamethonium (succinylcholine) with or without tubocurarine.

Clinical evidence

Three patients underwent surgery in which either suxamethonium alone or with tubocurarine was used. At the end of, or shortly after, the operation when spontaneous breathing had recommenced, aprotinin (Trasylol) in doses of 2500–5000 kiu was given. In each case respiration rapidly became inadequate and apnoea lasting periods of 7, 30 and 90 min. occurred.[1] Seven other cases have been reported elsewhere.[2]

Mechanism

Not fully understood. Aprotinin is only a very weak inhibitor of serum pseudocholinesterase (100 000 kiu caused a maximal 16% inhibition in man)[3] and on its own would have little effect on the metabolism of suxamethonium. But it might tip the balance in those whose cholinesterase was already very depressed.

Importance and management

The incidence of this interaction is uncertain but probably low. Only a few cases have been reported. It seems probable that it only affects those whose plasma pseudocholinesterase levels are already very low for other reasons. No difficulties should arise in those whose plasma cholinesterase levels are normal.

References

1 Chasapakis G, Dimas C. Possible interaction between muscle relaxants and the kallikrein-trypsin inactivator 'Trasylol'. Br J Anaesth (1966) 38, 838.

2 Marcello B, Porati N. Trasylol e blocco neuromusculare. Minerva anest (Torino) 33, 814.

3 Doenicke A, Gesing H, Krumey I, Schmidinger St. Influence of aprotinin (Trasylol) on the action of suxamethonium. Br J Anaesth (1970) 42, 948–60.

Neuromuscular blockers + Bambuterol

Abstract/Summary

Bambuterol can prolong the recovery time from neuromuscular blockade with suxamethonium.

Clinical evidence

A double-blind study found that the recovery times of 25 patients from neuromuscular blockade with suxamethonium (succinylcholine) were prolonged about 30% in those who had had 10 mg bambuterol 10–16 h before surgery, and about 50% by 20 mg.[1] This confirms two previous studies,[2,3] one of which found that 30 mg bambuterol given about 10 h before surgery prolonged suxamethonium blockade by 100%.[2] In patients who are heterzygous for abnormal plasma cholinesterase, 20 mg bambuterol taken 2 h before surgery prolongs suxamethonium blockade 2–3 times, and in some patients a phase II block occurs.[4]

Mechanism

Bambuterol is an inactive prodrug which is slowly converted enzymatically in the body to its active form, terbutaline. The carbamate groups which are split off can selectively inhibit the plasma cholinesterase which is necessary for the metabolism of suxamethonium. As a result, the metabolism of the suxamethonium is reduced and its effects are thereby prolonged. The effect appears to be related to the dose of the bambuterol.

Importance and management

An established interaction but unlikely to be of great clinical importance in normal patients, although anaesthetists should certainly be aware of its existence. It may possibly be important where other factors reduce plasma cholinesterase activity or affect the extent of blockade in other ways (e.g. subjects heterozygous for abnormal plasma cholinesterase).

References

1 Staun P, Lennmarken C, Eriksson LI, Wirén J-E. The influence of 10 mg and 20 mg bambuterol on the duration of succinylcholine-induced neuromuscular blockade. Acta Anesthsiol Scand (1990) 34, 498–500.

2 Fisher DM, Caldwell JE, Sharma M, Wirén J-E. The influence of bambuterol (carbamylated terbutaline) on the duration of action of succinylcholine-induced paralysis in humans. Anesthesiology (1988) 69, 757–9.

3 Bang U, Viby-Mogensen J, Wirén JE, Theil-Slovgaard L. The effect of bambuterol (carbamylated terbutaline) on plasma cholinesterase activity and succinylcholine-induced neuromuscular blockade in genotypically normal patients. Acta Anaesthesiol Scand (1990) 34, 596–9.

4 Bang U, Viby-Mogensen J, Wirén JE. The effect of bambuterol on plasma cholinesterase activity and suxamethonium-induced neuromuscular blockade in subjects heterozygous for abnormal plasma cholinesterase. Acta Anaesth Scand (1990) 34, 600–4.

Neuromuscular blockers + Benzodiazepines

Abstract/Summary

Some studies report that diazepam and other benzodiazepines increase the effects of neuromuscular blockers, but others say that they do not. Patients given both drugs should be monitored for possible changes in the depth and duration of neuromuscular blockade.

Clinical evidence

(a) Increased blockade

A comparative study of 10 patients given gallamine and four others given gallamine and diazepam (0.15–0.2 mg/kg) showed that the duration of activity of the blocker was prolonged by a factor of three by the diazepam, and the depression of the twitch response was doubled. Persistent muscle weakness and respiratory depression was seen in two other patients on tubocurarine after premedication with diazepam.[1,2]

Increased neuromuscular blockade has been described with diazepam and tubocurarine,[3,4] suxamethonium[5] and gallamine.[3] Another study found that recovery from 25 to 75% of the twitch height after vecuronium was prolonged 25% by midazolam, and 45% by diazepam.[9] The same study found a 20% prolongation of recovery from the effects of atracurium by midazolam, and 20–35% by diazepam.[9]

(b) Reduced blockade or no effect

The duration of paralysis due to suxamethonium was reduced in one study by 20% when diazepam (0.15 mg/kg) was used and the recovery time was shortened.[2]

In other studies diazepam was found to have no significant effect on the blockade due to tubocurarine,[6] gallamine,[6] decamethonium,[6] pancuronium,[11] fazadinium,[11] alcuronium[11] or suxamethonium.[7,8,11] Lorazepam and lormetazepam have little or no effects on atracurium or vecuronium,[9] and midazolam has no effect on suxamethonium or pancuronium.[10]

Mechanism

Not understood. One suggestion is that where some alteration in response is seen it may be a reflection of a central depressant action rather than a direct effect on the myoneural junction.[6] Another study suggests instead a direct action on the muscle.[12]

Importance and management

There is no obvious explanation for these discordant observations. What is known shows that the benzodiazepines may sometimes unpredictably alter the depth and prolong the recovery period from neuromuscular blockade, but the extent may not be very great and may possibly be little different from the individual variations in the response of patients to neuromuscular blockers. Concurrent use need not be avoided but 'caution and monitoring' has been advised.

References

1 Feldman SA, Crawley BE. Diazepam and muscle relaxants. Br Med J (1970) 1, 691.

2 Feldman SA, Crawley BE. Interaction of diazepam with muscle-relaxant drugs. Br Med J (1970) 2, 336.

3 Vergano F, Zaccagna CA, Zuccaro G. Muscle relaxant properties of diazepam. Minerva Anest (1969) 35, 91.

4 Stovner J, Endresen R. Intravenous anesthesia with diazepam. Acta Anaesth Scand (1965), (Suppl) 24, 223.

5 Jorgensen H. Premedicinering med diazepam. Nord Med (1964) 72,1395.

6 Dretchen K, Ghoneim MM, Long JP. The interaction of diazepam with myoneural blocking agents. Anesthesiol (1971) 34, 463.

7 Stovner J, Endresen R. Diazepam in intravenous anaesthesia. Lancet (1965) ii, 1298.

8 Hunter AR. Diazepam as a muscle relaxant during general anaesthesia. Br J Anaesth (1967) 39, 633.

9 Driessen JJ, Cruhl JF, Vree TB van Egmond J, Booij LHDJ. Benzodiazepines and neuromuscular blocking drugs in patients. Acta Anaesthesiol Scand (1986) 30, 642–6.

10 Tassonyi E. Effects of midazolam (Ro 21–3981) on neuromuscular block. Pharmatherapeutica (1984) 3, 678–81.

11 Bradshaw EG, Maddison S. Effect of diazepam at the neuromuscular junction. A clinical study. Br J Anaesth (1979) 51, 955.

12 Ludin HP, Dubach K. Action of diazepam on muscular contraction in man. Z Neurol (1971) 199, 30–8.

Neuromuscular blockers + Beta-blockers

Abstract/Summary

Increases or decreases (often only modest) in the extent of neuromuscular blockade have been seen. The bradycardia and hypotension caused by anaesthetics and beta-blockers may possibly be increased by atracurium.

Clinical evidence

(a) Reduced neuromuscular blockade

A study in 31 patients given 1 mg/kg propranolol IV over a 4 min period during surgery showed that the effects of suxamethonium were slightly reduced. The mean period of apnoea fell from 4.4 min (without propranolol) to 3.6 min. Propranolol was also observed to shorten the recovery from tubocurarine.[1]

Other studies describe a shortened recovery period from tubo-curarine due to oxprenolol or propranolol, but pindolol affected only a few subjects.[2]

(b) Prolonged neuromuscular blockade

Two patients with thyrotoxicosis showed prolonged neuromuscular blockade with tubocurarine or suxamethonium when given 120 mg propranolol daily.[3]

(c) Bradycardia and hypotension

Eight out of 42 patients on un-named beta-blockers and given atracurium developed bradycardia (less than 50 bpm) and hypotension (systolic pressure less than 80 mmHg). Most of them had been premedicated with diazepam, induced with methohexitone, and anaesthetized with droperidol, fentanyl and nitrous oxide/oxygen. A further 24 showed bradycardia and eight showed hypotension. All responded promptly to atropine (0.3–0.6 mg IV).[6] Bradycardia and hypotension have been seen in other patients given alcuronium while using timolol eye drops for glaucoma or atenolol for hypertension.[7,8]

Mechanisms

The changes in the degree of blockade are not understood but it appears to occur at the neuromuscular junction. It has been seen in animal studies.[4,5] The bradycardia and hypotension (c) were probably due to the combined depressant effects on the heart of the anaesthetics, the beta-blocker and atracurium.

Importance and management

Information is limited. Be alert for changes in neuromuscular blockade (increases or decreases) if beta-blockers are used. They seem to be unpredictable and often only modest in extent. The combined cardiac depressant efects of beta-blockade and anaesthesia are well known (see 'Anaesthetics + Beta-blockers') and the possible additional effect of atracurium should also be recognized, but other neuromuscular blockers do not seem to have this effect. It is suggested in one report that it may be wise to avoid atracurium until more is known.[8] See also 'Beta-blockers + Anticholinesterases'.

References

1 Varma Y, Sharma PL, Singh HW. Effect of propranolol hydrochloride on the neuromuscular blocking action of d-tubocurarine and succinylcholine in man. Ind J Med Res (1972) 60, 266.
2 Varma Y, Sharma PL, Singh HW. Comparative effect of propranolol, oxprenolol and pindolol on neuromuscular blocking action of d-tubocurarine in man. Ind J Med Res (1973) 61, 1382.
3 Rozen MS, Whan FM. Prolonged curarization associated with propranolol. Med J Aust (1972) 1, 467.
4 Usubiaga JE. Neuromuscular blocking effects of beta-adrenergic blockers and their interaction with skeletal muscle relaxants. Anesthesiology (1968) 29,484.
5 Harrah MB, Walter LW, Katzune BC. The interaction of d-tubocurarine with anti-arrhythmic drugs. Anesthesiology (1970) 96, 99.

6 Rowlands DE. Drug interaction? Anaesthesia (1984) 39, 1252.
7 Glynne GL. Drug interaction? Anaesthesia (1984) 39, 293.
8 Yate B, Mostafa SM. Drug interaction? Anaesthesia (1984) 39, 728.

Neuromuscular blockers + Bretylium

Abstract/Summary

In theory there is the possibility of increased and prolonged neuromuscular blockade if bretylium is given with neuromuscular blockers.

Clinical evidence, mechanism, importance and management

Although case reports seem to be lacking, the muscular weakness seen in a few patients given bretylium[1] and the evidence from animal studies showing that the effects of tubocurarine can be increased and prolonged by bretylium, suggest that an interaction might occur in man.[2] One suggested possibility is that if the bretylium were to be given during surgery to control arrhythmias, its effects (which are delayed) might be additive with the residual effects of the neuromuscular blocker during the recovery period, resulting in apnoea. This needs confirmation.

References

1 Bowman WC. Effects of adrenergic activators and inhibitors on skeletal muscles. In 'Handbook of experimental pharmacology.' Szekeres L (ed). Springer-Verlag (1980) 47–128.
2 Welch GW, Waud BE. Effect of bretylium on neuromuscular transmission. Anesth Analg (1982) 61, 442–4.

Neuromuscular blockers + Calcium channel blockers

Abstract/Summary

Limited evidence indicates that diltiazem, nicardipine, nifedipine and verapamil can increase the neuromuscular blocking effects of vecuronium. Verapamil may similarly affect tubocurarine.

Clinical evidence

(a) Diltiazem

A study in 24 surgical patients anesthetised with nitrous oxide and isoflurane found that infusions of diltiazem (5 or 10 µg/kg/min) decreased the vecuronium requirements by up to 50%.[10]

(b) Nicardipine

A study in patients given 0.1 mg/kg^{-1} vecuronium for tracheal intubation found that 10μg nicardipine shortened the onset of blockade to the same extent as other patients given 0.15 mg/kg^{-1} vecuronium. Recovery times were unaffected.[9]

(c) Nifedipine

A study in 44 patients anaesthetised with isoflurane in nitrous oxide/oxygen showed that 1 mg nifedipine IV prolonged the neuromuscular blockade due to atracurium or vecuronium from 29 up to 40 min, and increased the neuromuscular blockade from 75 up to 90%.[6]

This contrasts with another study in which 30 predominantly elderly patients on chronic nifedipine treatment (mean daily dose 32 mg) showed no changes in the time of onset to maximum block nor the duration of clinical relaxation in response to atracurium or vecuronium.[7,8]

(d) Verapamil

A woman of 66, receiving 5 mg verapamil intravenously three times a day for superventricular tachycardia, underwent abdominal surgery during which she was initially anaesthetized with thiopentone and then maintained on nitrous oxide/oxygen with fentanyl. Vecuronium was used as the muscle relaxant. The effects of the vecuronium were increased and prolonged, and at the end of surgery reversal of the blockade using neostigmine was difficult and extended.[1]

Another report similarly describes increased blockade in a patient given tubocurarine which was difficult to reverse with neostigmine but which responded well to edrophonium.[2] However the authors of this report say that many patients on verapamil do not show a clinically significant increased sensitivity to muscle relaxants.[2] Verapamil alone caused respiratory failure in a patient with poor neuromuscular transmission (Duchenne's dystrophy).[3] An increase in the neuromuscular blocking effects of pancuronium, vecuronium, atracurium and suxamethonium by verapamil and nifedipine has been seen in animals.[3,5]

Mechanism

Not fully understood. One explanation for the increased blockade is as follows. Nerve impulses arriving at nerve endings release calcium ions which in turn causes the release of acetylcholine. Calcium channel blockers can reduce the concentration of calcium ions within the nerve so that less acetylcholine is released and this would be additive with the effects of a neuromuscular blocker.[4]

Importance and management

Direct information so far seems to be limited to the cases and reports cited here. The discord between the reports remains unexplained. Until the situation is resolved, be alert for increased blockade in any patient given nicardipine, nifedipine, verapamil or any other calcium channel blocker. More study is needed.

References

1 van Poorten JF, Dhasmana KM, Kuypers RSM, Erdmann W. Verapamil and reversal of vecuronium neuromuscular blockade. Anesth Analg (1984) 63, 155–7.
2 Jones RM, Cashman JN, Casson WR, Broadbent MP. Verapamil potentiation of neuromuscular blockade. Failure of reversal with neostigmine but prompt reversal with edrophonium. Anesth Analg (1985) 64, 1021–5.
3 Durant NN, Nguyen N, Katz RL. Potentiation of neuromuscular blockade by verapamil. Anesthesiology (1984) 60, 298–303.
4 Wali FA. Interactions of nifedipine and diltiazem with muscle relaxants and reversal of neuromuscular blockade with edrophonium and neostigmine. J Pharmacol (1986) 17, 244–53.
5 Bikhazi GB, Leung I, Foldes FF. Interaction of neuromuscular blocking agents with calcium blockers. Anesthesiology (1982) 57, A268.
6 Jelen-Esselborn S, Blobner M. Wirkungsverstärkung von nichtdepolarisierenden Muskelrelaxanzien durch Nifedipin i.v in Inhalationsanaesthesie. Anaesthetist (1990) 39, 173–8.
7 Bell PF, Mirakhur RK, Elliott P. Onset and duration of clinical relaxation of atrcurium and vecuronium in patients on chronic nifedipine therapy. Eur J Anaesthesiology (1989) 6, 343–6.
8 Mirakhur RK, Bell PF, Clarke RSJ. Chronic nifedipine therapy does not prolong the neuromuscular effects of vecuronium and atracurium. Anesthesiology (1988) 69, A506.
9 Yamada T; Takino Y. Can nicardipine potentiate vecuronium induced neuromuscular blockade ? Masui (1992) 41, 746–50.
10 Sumikawa K, Kawabata K, Aono Y, Kamibayashi T, Yoshiya I. Reduction in vecuronium infusion dose requirements by diltiazem in humans. Anesthesiology (1992) 77, A939.

Neuromuscular blockers + Carbamazepine

Abstract/Summary

Carbamazepine shortens the recovery time from neuromuscular blockade with atracurium, doxacurium, pancuronium and vecuronium.

Clinical evidence

The recovery from neuromuscular blockade with pancuronium in 18 patients undergoing craniotomy for tumours, seizure foci or cerebrovascular surgery was on average 65% shorter in those taking carbamazepine.[1] Another eight patients undergoing surgery and on carbamazepine for at least a week had a recovery time of 63 min compared with 161 min in the control group.[2,5] These findings are consistent with those of two other studies.[3,6] Yet another study in 18 patients found that the recovery time from atracurium (0.5 mg/kg IV) was 5.93 min in those on long-term carbamazepine compared with 8.02 min in the control group.[4] A further study found that carbamazepine almost halved the recovery time from vecuronium blockade, but had no effect on atracurium.[7]

Mechanism

Not understood. Competition for the same site(s) on the neuro-muscular junction has been suggested.

Importance and management

Information is limited but the interaction appears to be established. Anticipate a decreased response to atracurium, doxacurium, pancuronium and vecuronium in those taking carbamazepine, and an accelerated recovery.

References

1 Roth S, Ebrahim ZY. Resistance to pancuronium in patients receiving carbamazepine. Anesthesiol (1987) 66, 691–3.
2 Ornstein E, Matteo RS, Halevy JD, Young HL, Abou-Donia M. Accelerated recovery from doxacurium in carbamazepine treated patients. Anesthesiology (1989) 71, A785.
3 Desai P, Hewitt PB, Jones RM. Influence of anticonvulsant therapy on doxacurium and pancuronium-induced paralysis. Anesthesiology (1989) 71, A784.
4 Tempelhoff R, Modica PA, Jellish WS, Spitznagel EL. Resistance to atracurium-induced neuromuscular blockade in patients with intractable seizure disorders treated with anticonvulsants. Anesth Analg (1990) 71, 665–9.
5 Ornstein E, Matteo RS, Weinstein JA, Halevy JD, Young WL, Abou-Donia MM. Accelerated recovery from doxacurium-induced neuromuscular blockade in patients receiving chronic anticonvulsant therapy. J Clin Anesth (1991) 3, 108–11.
6 Modica P, Tempelhoff R. Effect of chronic anticonvulsant therapy on recovery from atracurium. Anesth Analg (1989) 68, S198.
7 Ebrahim Z, Bulkley R, Roth S. Carbamazepine therapy and neuromuscular blockade with atracurium and vecuronium. Anesth Analg (1988) 67, S55.

Neuromuscular blockers + Chloroquine

Abstract/Summary

A report describes respiratory insufficiency during the recovery period following surgery, attributed to the use of chloroquine diorotate.

Clinical evidence, mechanism, importance and management

Studies were carried on the possible neuromuscular blocking actions of chloroquine diorotate in animals because it was noticed that when it was used to prevent peritoneal adhesions following abdominal surgery in man, it caused respiratory insufficiency during the recovery period. These studies found that it has a non-depolarizing blocking action at the neuromuscular junction which can be opposed by neostigmine.[1] It would seem that during the recovery period the effects of the chloroquine were additive with the residual effects of the conventional neuromuscular blocker used during the surgery.

Although this appears to be the only report of this interac-

tion, it is consistent with the way chloroquine can unmask or aggravate myasthenia gravis, or oppose the effects of drugs used in its treatment. Be alert for this reaction if chloroquine is used.

Reference

1 Jui-Yen T. Clinical and experimental studies on mechanism of neuromuscular blockade by chloroquine diorotate. Japan J Anesth (1971) 20, 491–503.

Neuromuscular blockers + Cimetidine, Famotidine or Ranitidine

Abstract/Summary

One report says that recovery from the neuromuscular blocking effects of suxamethonium (succinylcholine) is prolonged by cimetidine but this may possibly have been due to the presence of metoclopramide. Four other reports say that no interaction occurs between suxamethonium and either cimetidine, ranitidine or famotidine. Cimetidine, but not ranitidine, is reported to increase the effects of vecuronium, and neither affects atracurium.

Clinical evidence

(a) Evidence of increased neuromuscular blockade

A controlled study in 10 patients given 300 mg cimetidine orally at bedtime and another 300 mg 2 h before anaesthesia, showed that while the onset of action of suxamethonium (1.5 mg/kg IV) was unchanged, the time to recover 50% of the twitch height was prolonged 2–2.5 times (from 8.6 to 20.3 min). One patient[1] took 57 min to recover. His serum pseudocholinesterase levels were found to be normal. It was later reported that some patients were also taking metoclopramide which is known to interact in this way.[6]

Another study in 24 patients found that 400 mg cimetidine significantly prolonged the recovery (T1–25 period) from vecuronium, but few patients showed any response to 200 mg cimetidine or 100 mg ranitidine.[8] This prolongation of recovery from vecuronium due to cimetidine was confirmed in another study (time to return of T1 30 v 22.5 min).[10] A study using a rat phrenic nerve diaphragm preparation found that cimetidine increased the neuromuscular blocking effects of tubocurarine and pancuronium, but there seem to be no reports confirming this in man.[2]

(b) Evidence of unchanged neuromuscular blockade

A controlled study in 10 patients given 400 mg cimetidine at bedtime and 400 mg 90 min before anaesthesia found no evidence of an effect on the neuromuscular blockade caused by suxamethonium, nor on its duration or recovery period.[5] Another controlled study in patients given 300 mg cimetidine or 150 mg ranitidine the night before and 1–2 h before surgery found no evidence that the duration of action of suxamethonium or the activity of plasma cholinesterase were altered.[6] A study in 15 patients undergoing Caesarian section also found no evidence that either cimetidine or ranitidine affected the neuromuscular blocking effects of suxamethonium.[7] A study in 70 patients found no changes in the neuromuscular blocking effects of suxamethonium in those given 400 mg cimetidine, 80 mg ranitidine or 20 mg famotidine.[9] Cimetidine and ranitidine appear not to affect atracurium, nor cimetidine affect atracurium.[10]

Mechanism

Not understood. Studies with human plasma failed to find any evidence that cimetidine in normal serum concentrations inhibits the metabolism of suxamethonium,[3,6] however metoclopramide does. *In vitro* studies with very high cimetidine concentrations found inhibition of pseudocholinesterase activity.[4] The cimetidine/vecuronium interaction is not understood.

Importance and management

Information seems to be limited to the reports cited. The most likely explanation for the discord between these results is that in the study reporting increased suxamethonium effects[1] some of the patients were also given metoclopramide which can inhibit plasma cholinesterase and prolong the effects of suxamethonium[6,9] (see also 'Neuromuscular blockers + Metoclopramide'). However until the situation is clarified the possibility of an interaction should be taken into account during concurrent use. The same precautions also apply in the case of cimetidine-vecuronium.

References

1 Kambam JR, Dymond R, Krestow M. Effect of cimetidine on duration of action of succinylcholine. Anesth Analg (1987) 66, 191–2.
2 Galatulas I, Bossa R, Benvenuti C. Cimetidine increases the neuromuscular blocking activity of aminoglycoside antibiotics: antagonism by calcium. Organ-directed toxic: Chem Indices Mech., Proc Symp (1981) 321–5. Pergamon Press, Oxford.
3 Cook DR, Stiller RL, Chakravorti S, Mannenhira T. Cimetidine does not inhibit plasma cholinesterase activity. Anesth Analg (1988) 67, 375–6.
4 Hansen WE, Bertl S. The inhibition of acetylcholinesterase and pseudocholinesterase by cimetidine. Arzneimittelforsch (1983) 33, 161–3.
5 Stirt JA, Sperry RJ, DiFazio CA. Cimetidine and succinylcholine: potential interaction and effect on neuromuscular blockade in man. Anesthesiology (1988) 69, 607–8.
6 Woodworth GE, Sears DH, Grove TM, Ruff RH, Kosek PS, Katz RL. The effect of cimetidine and ranitidine on the duration of action of succinylcholine. Anesth Analg (1989) 68, 295–7.
7 Bogod DG, Oh TE. The effect of H₂-antagonists on duration of action of suxamethonium in the parturient. Anaesthesia (1989) 44, 591–3.
8 Tryba M, Wruck G. Interaktionen von H₂-Antagonisten und nichtdepolarisierenden Muskelrelaxantien. Anaesthetist (1989) 38, 251–4.
9 Turner DR, Kao YJ, Bivona C. Neuromuscular block by suxamethonium following treatment with histamine type 2 antagonists or metoclopramide. Br J Anaesth (1989) 63, 348–50.
10 McCarthy G, Mirakhur RK, Elliott P, Wright J. Effect of H2-receptor antagonist pretreatment on vecuronium- and atracurium-induced neuromuscular blockade. Br J Anaesth (1991) 66, 713–5.

Neuromuscular blockers + Corticosteroids

Abstract/Summary

Three reports describe antagonism of the neuromuscular blocking effects of pancuronium by prednisone and hydrocortisone in patients with adrenocortical insufficiency. The dosage of vecuronium may need to be almost doubled in the presence of betamethasone.

Clinical evidence

A man undergoing surgery who was on 250 mg prednisolone daily had good muscular relaxation in response to 8 mg pancuronium early in the operation, but an hour later began to show signs of inadequate relaxation and continued to do so for the next 1.25 h despite being given four additional 2 mg doses of pancuronium.[1]

A hypophysectomized man on cortisone developed profound paralysis when given pancuronium which was rapidly reversed with 100 mg hydrocortisone sodium succinate.[2] Another patient on large doses of hydrocortisone, prenisolone and aminophylline proved to be resistant to the effects of pancuronium.[3]

Unexpected movements of head and arms occurred in a patient during surgery given vecuronium, and coughing in another. They had both been given betamethasone preoperatively (4 mg four times daily) to reduce raised intracranial pressure.[5] This prompted a retrospective search of the records of 50 other patients which revealed that those given betamethasone had needed almost double the dose of vecuronium (134 compared with 76 µg/kg/hr).[5]

These reports contrast with another in which 25 patients who had no adrenalcortical dysfunction or histories of corticosteroid therapy who were given pancuronium, metocurine, tubocurarine or vecuronium. They showed no changes in their neuromuscular blockade when given dexamethasone (0.4 mg/kg) or hydrocortisone (10 mg/kg) intravenously.[4]

Mechanism

Not understood. One idea, based on animal studies, is that adrenocortical insufficiency causes a defect in neuromuscular transmission (a decrease in the sensitivity of the end-plate) which is reversed by the corticosteroids. Another idea is that the effects seen are connected in some way with the steroid nucleus of the pancuronium and vecuronium, or that the effects are mediated presynaptically.

Importance and management

The evidence for an interaction seem to be limited to these reports, involving only pancuronium and vecuronium. Careful monitoring is clearly needed if either is used in patients who have been treated with corticosteroids, being alert for the need to increase the dosage of the neuromuscular blocker. Animal studies suggest that atracurium may possibly be affected by betamethasone.[6]

References

1 Laflin MJ. Interaction of pancuronium and corticosteroids. Anesthesiology (1977) 47, 471.
2 Meyers EF. Partial recovery from neuromuscular blockade following hydrocortisone administration. Anesthesiology (1977) 46, 148.
3 Azar I, Kumar D, Betcher AM. Resistance to pancuronium in an asthmatic patient treated with aminophylline and steroids. Canad Anesth Soc J (1982) 29, 280–2.
4 Schwartz AE, Matteo RS, Ornstein E, Silverberg PA. Acute steroid therapy does not alter non-depolarizing muscle relaxant effects in humans. Anesthesiology (1986) 65, 326–7.
5 Parr SM, Galletly DC, Robinson BJ. Betamethasone-induced resistance to vecuronium: a potential problem in neurosurgery ? Anaesth Intens Care (1991) 19, 103–5.
6 Robinson BJ, Lee E, Rees D, Purdie GL, Galletly DC. Betamethasone-induced resistance to neuromuscular blockade: a comparison of atracurium and vecuronium in vitro. Anesth Analg (1992) 74, 762–5.

Neuromuscular blockers + Cyclophosphamide

Abstract/Summary

The effects of suxamethonium (succinylcholine) can be increased and prolonged in patients under treatment with cyclophosphamide because their serum pseudocholinesterase levels are depressed. Respiratory insufficiency and prolonged apnoea have been reported.

Clinical evidence

Respiratory insufficiency and prolonged apnoea occurred in a patient on two occasions while receiving cyclophosphamide and undergoing anaesthesia during which suxamethonium and tubocurarine were used. Plasma pseudocholinesterase levels were found to be low. Anaesthesia without the suxamethonium was uneventful. Seven out of eight patients subsequently examined also showed depressed serum pseudocholinesterase levels while taking cyclophosphamide.[1] Respiratory depression and low serum pseudocholinesterase levels have been described in other reports.[2–4] One report described a 35–70% reduction.[2]

Mechanism

Cyclophosphamide irreversibly inhibits the activity of pseudocholinesterase in the serum, as a result the metabolism of the suxamethonium is reduced and its actions are enhanced and prolonged.[4]

Importance and management

A well-documented and established interaction of clinical importance. Whether all patients are affected to the same extent is uncertain. The depression of the serum pseudocholinesterase levels may last several days, possibly weeks, so that ideally serum pseudocholinesterase levels should be checked before using suxamethonium. It should certainly be used with caution, and the dosage should be reduced.[2] Some have suggested that concurrent use should be avoided.[1] Suxethonium probably interacts similarly, but not other neuromuscular blockers because they are not metabolized by serum pseudocholinesterase.

References

1 Walker IR, Zapf PW, Mackay IR. Cyclophosphamide, cholinesterase and anaesthesia. Aust NZ J Med (1972) 3, 247.
2 Zsigmond EK, Robins G. The effect of a series of anti-cancer drugs on plasma cholinesterase activity. Can Anaesth Soc J (1972) 19, 75.
3 Mone JG, Mathie WE. Qualitative and quantitative effects of pseudocholinesterase activity. Anaesthesia (1967) 22, 55.
4 Wolff H. Die Hemmung der Serumcholinesterase durch Cyclophosphamid (Endoxan). Klin Wsch (1965) 43, 819.

Neuromuscular blockers + Cyclosporin(e)

Abstract/Summary

There is evidence that the neuromuscular blocking effects of atracurium, vecuronium and pancuronium may be increased in some patients treated with cyclosporin.

Clinical evidence

(a) Atracurium

A retrospective study found 4 of 36 patients who experienced prolonged neuromuscular blockade when atracurium was used during anaesthesia for kidney transplantation. Some of them had had cyclosporin.[5] Extended recovery times are described in another report.[6]

(a) Pancuronium

A woman with a 2-year renal transplant controlled with 100 mg azathioprine, 300 mg cyclosporin and 10 mg prednisone and also taking nifedipine and furosemide for hypertension, underwent surgery during which she was initially anaesthetized with fentanyl and thiopentone, and later nitrous oxide/oxygen and isoflurane. Pancuronium was used as the neuromuscular blocker. She was also infused with cyclosporin before and after surgery. Residual paralysis was seen after surgery and she was re-intubated 20 min later because of increased respiratory distress.[1]

(b) Vecuronium

A girl of 15 on 20 mg cyclosporin IV twice daily and with serum levels of $138 \, \mu g.l^{-1}$ was anaesthetized for an endoscopy and bone marrow aspiration using fentanyl, thiopentone and 0.1 mg.kg^{-1} vecuronium. Anaesthesia was later maintained with nitrous oxide, oxygen and isoflurane. Attempts were later made to reverse the blockade with edrophonium, atropine and neostigmine but full neuromuscular function was not restored for 3 h and 20 min.[4]

A retrospective study of this interaction in other kidney transplant patients suggests that cyclosporin can increase the risk of prolonged neuromuscular blockade and ventilatory failure in those given vecuronium.[5] Extended recovery times are described in two other reports.[6,7]

Mechanism

Uncertain. One suggestion is that cremophor (polyoxyl 35 castor oil), a surface-active agent used as a vehicle for the cyclosporin[1] may increase the effective concentration of pancuronium at the neuromuscular junction. Both compounds have been observed in animal studies to increase vecuronium blockade[2] and cremophor has been seen to decrease the onset time of pancuronium blockade in patients given cremophor-containing anaesthetics.[3]

Importance and management

Direct information seems to be limited to the reports cited. The general importance is uncertain but be alert for an increase in the effects of atracurium, pancuronium or vecuronium in any patient receiving cyclosporin. Not all patients appear to develop this interaction.[5] More study is needed.

References

1 Crosby E, Robblee JA. Cyclosporine-pancuronium interaction in a patient with a renal allograft. Can J Anaesth (1988) 35, 300–2.
2 Gramstad L, Liileaasen P, Misaas B. Onset time for alcuronium and pancuronium after cremophor-containing anaesthetics. Acta Anaesth Scand (1981) 25, 484–6.
3 Viby-Mogensen J. Interaction of other drugs with muscle relaxants. Sem Anaesth (1985) 6, 52.
4 Wodd GG. Cyclosporine-vecuronium interaction. Can J Anaesth (1989) 36 (3 part 1), 358.
5 Sidi A, Kaplan RF, Davis RF. Prolonged neuromuscular blockade and ventilatory failure after renal transplantation and cyclosporine. Can J Anaesth (1990) 37, 543–8.
6 Lepage JY, Malinowsky JM, de Dieulevault C, Cozian A, Pinaud M, Souron R. Interaction cyclosporine atracurium et vecuronium. Ann Fr Anesth Reanim (1989) 8 (Suppl) R135.
7 Takita K, Goda Y, Kawahigashi H, Okuyama A, Kubota M, Kemmotsu O. Pharmacodynamics of vecuronium in the kidney transplant recipient and the patient with normal renal function. Jap J Anesthiol (1993) 42, 190–4.

Neuromuscular blockers + Dantrolene

Abstract/Summary

The muscle relaxant effects of dantrolene can be additive with those of conventional neuromuscular blockers.

Clinical evidence, mechanism, importance and management

A woman of 60, given a total of 350 mg dantrolene by mouth during the 28 h before surgery to control malignant hyperthermia, showed increased neuromuscular blockade and a slow recovery rate when vecuronium was used subsequently.[1] Dantrolene is a muscle relaxant which acts directly on the muscle by interfering with calcium uptake and release from the sarcoplasmic reticulum. It may also possibly interfere with the release of acetylcholine at the neuromuscular junction. These effects would appear to be additive with those of the neuromuscular blockers. This interaction should be taken into account during concurrent use.

Reference

1 Driessen JJ, Wuis EW, Gielen MJM. Prolonged vecuronium neuromuscular blockade in a patient receiving orally administered dantrolene. Anesthesiology (1985) 62, 523–4.

Neuromuscular blockers + Dexpanthenol

Abstract/Summary

An increase in the neuromuscular blocking effects of suxamethonium (succinylcholine) has been attributed to the concurrent use of dexpanthenol in one patient, but further studies failed to confirm this interaction.

Clinical evidence, mechanism, importance and management

A patient developed severe respiratory embarrassment following the intramuscular injection of 500 mg dexpanthenol during the recovery period from anaesthesia with nitrous oxide and cyclopropane, and neuromuscular blockade with suxamethonium.[1] However a later study on six patients under general anaesthesia showed that their response to suxamethonium was unaffected by the infusion of 500 mg pantothenic acid.[2]

Several manufacturers of products containing pantothenic acid have issued warnings about this interaction, but they seem to be solely based on the single unconfirmed report cited here,[1] and there seems to be little reason for avoiding concurrent use or for taking particular precautions. However users should be aware of this case.

References

1 Stewart P. Case reports. J Amer Ass Nurse Anesth (1960) 28, 56.
2 Smith RM, Gotthsall SC, Young JA. Succinylcholine-pantothenyl alcohol: a reappraisal. Anesth Analg (1969) 48, 205.

Neuromuscular blockers + Disopyramide

Abstract/Summary

An isolated case report suggests that disopyramide may oppose the effects of neostigmine when used to reverse neuromuscular blockade with vecuronium.

Clinical evidence, mechanism, importance and management

A case report suggests that therapeutic serum levels of disopyramide (5 µg/ml) may oppose the normal antagonism by neostigmine of vecuronium neuromuscular blockade.[1] Disopyramide has also been shown to decrease the antagonism by neostigmine of the neuromusuclar blockade of tubocurarine on the rat phrenic nerve-diaphragm preparation.[2] The general clinical importance of these observations are not known, but anaesthetists should be aware of these reports.

Reference

1 Baurain M, Barvais L, d'Hollander A, Hennart D. Impairment of the antagonism of vecuronium-induced paralysis and intra-operative disopyramide administration. Anaesthesia (1989) 44, 34–6.
2 Healy TEJ, O'Shea M, Massey J. Disopyramide and neuromuscular transmission. Br J Anaesth (1981) 53, 495–8.

Neuromuscular blockers + Ecothiopate iodide (Echothiophate)

Abstract/Summary

The neuromuscular blocking effects of suxamethonium (succinylcholine) are markedly increased and prolonged in patients under treatment with ecothiopate iodide. The dosage of suxamethonium should be reduced appropriately.

Clinical evidence

In 1965 Murray McGavi warned that the systemic absorption of ecothiopate iodide from eye drops could lower serum pseudocholinesterase levels to such an extent that '...within a few days of commencing therapy, levels are reached at which protracted apnoea could occur should these patients require general anaesthesia in which muscle relaxation is obtained with suxamethonium.'[1] Cases of apnoea due to this interaction were reported the following year[2,3] and the year after.[5] In one case a woman given 200 mg suxamethonium showed apnoea for 5½ hours. Other studies have confirmed that ecothiopate markedly reduces the levels of pseudocholinesterase and can prolong recovery.[4,6,8]

Mechanism

Suxamethonium is metabolized in the body by pseudocholinesterase. Ecothiopate iodide depresses the levels of this enzyme so that the metabolism of the suxamethonium is reduced and its effects are thereby enhanced and prolonged.[4] One study in 71 patients found that two drops of 0.06% ecothiopate iodide three times weekly in each eye caused a twofold reduction in pseudocholinesterase activity in about one-third of the patients, and a fourfold reduction in one out of every seven.[9]

Importance and management

An established, adequately documented and clinically important interaction. The dosage of suxamethonium should be reduced appropriately because of the reduced plasma pseudocholinesterase levels caused by ecothiopate. The study cited above[9] suggests that prolonged apnoea is only likely in about one in seven. One report describes the successful use of approximately one fifth of the normal dosage of suxamethonium in a patient receiving 0.125% ecothiopate iodide solution, one drop twice a day in both eyes, and with a plasma cholinesterase activity 62% below normal. Recovery from the neuromuscular blockade was rapid and uneventful.[7] Another report describes the successful and uneventful use of atracurium instead.[8]

References

1 McGavi DDM. Depressed levels of serum-pseudocholinesterase with ecothiopate-iodide eyedrops. Lancet (1965) ii, 272.
2 Gesztes T. Prolonged apnoea after suxamethonium injection associated with eye drops containing an anticholinesterase agent. Br J Anaesth (1966) 38, 408.
3 Pantuck EJ. Ecothiopate iodide eye drops and prolonged response to suxamethonium. Br J Anaesth (1966) 38, 406.
4 Cavallaro RJ, Krumperman LW, Kugler F. Effect of ecothiopate therapy on the metabolism of succinylcholine in man. Anesth Analg (1974) 47, 570.
5 Mone JG, Mathie WE. Qualitative and quantitative defects of pseudocholinesterase activity. Anaesthesia (1967) 22, 55.
6 de Roetth A, Dettbarn WD, Rosenberg P, Wilensky JG, Wong A. Effect of phopholine iodide on blood cholinesterase levels of normal and glaucoma subjects. Amer J Opthal (1965) 59, 586.
7 Donati F, Bevan DR. Controlled succinylcholine infusion in a patient receiving echothiophate eye drops. Can Anaesth Soc J (1981) 28, 488.
8 Messer GJ, Stoudemire A, Knos G, Johnson GC. Electroconvulsive therapy and the chronic use of pseudocholinesterase-inhibitor (echothiphate iodide) eye drops for glaucoma. A case report. Gen Hosp Psychiatry (1992) 14, 56–60.
9 Eilderton TE, Farmati O, Zsigmond EK. Reduction in plasma cholinesterase levels after prolonged administration of echothiophate iodide eyedrops. Can Anaesth Soc J (1968) 15, 291–6.

Neuromuscular blockers + Fentanyl citrate-droperidol (Innovar)

Abstract/Summary

Recovery from the neuromuscular blocking effects of suxamethonium is prolonged by fentanyl citrate-droperidol (*Innovar*).

Clinical evidence

The observation that patients who had had *Innovar* (fentanyl citrate-droperidol) before anaesthesia appeared to have a prolongation of the effects of suxamethonium, seen as apnoea, prompted further study of this interaction.[1] 19 patients were given suxamethonium and thiopentone during the induction of anaesthesia. The average time from end fasciculation to return of full tetanus was approximately doubled (from 5.83 to 10.45 min) in 10 patients given *Innovar* (2 ml intravenously 10 min before anaesthesia) when compared with nine patients not given Innovar.[1]

A much shorter delay in recovery was seen in a later study.[3] Another study[2] showed that the droperidol component of *Innovar* is responsible for this interaction.

Mechanism

Not understood. One suggestion[2] is that droperidol may act as a membrane stabilizer at neuromuscular junctions, and it may also reduce the levels of pseudocholinesterase which is responsible for the metabolism of suxamethonium.

Importance and management

An established interaction of moderate importance. Delayed recovery should be anticipated in patients on suxamethonium and other neuromuscular blockers if *Innovar* is used.

References

1 Wehner RJ. A case study: The prolongation of Anectine effect by Innovar. AANA Journal (1979) 47, 576–9.
2 Lewis RA. A consideration of prolonged succinylcholine paralysis with Innovar: Is the cause droperidol or fentanyl? AANA Journal (1982) 50, 55–9.
3 Moore GB, Ciresi S, Kallar S. The effect of Innovar versus droperidol or fentanyl on the duration of action of succinylcholine. AANA Journal (1986) 54, 130–6

Neuromuscular blockers + Frusemide (Furosemide)

Abstract/Summary

The effects of the neuromuscular blockers may be increased by low doses of frusemide but opposed by higher doses.

Clinical evidence

(a) Increased neuromuscular blockade

Three patients receiving kidney transplants showed increased neuromuscular blockade with tubocurarine (seen as a pronounced decrease in twitch tension) when given frusemide (40 or 80 mg) and mannitol (12.5 mg) intravenously. One of them showed the same reaction when later given only 40 mg frusemide but no mannitol. The residual blockade was easily antagonized with pyridostigmine (14 mg) or neostigmine (3 mg) with atropine (1.2 mg).[1]

(b) Decreased neuromuscular blockade

Ten patients given 1 mg/kg frusemide took 14.7 min to recover from 95 to 50% blockade with pancuronium (as measured by a twitch response) compared with 21.8 min in 10 other patients who had had no frusemide.[3]

Mechanism

Uncertain. Animal studies indicate that what happens probably depends on the dosage of frusemide: 0.1–10 g/kg increased the blocking effects of tubocurarine and suxamethonium whereas 1–4 mg/kg opposed the blockade.[2] One suggestion is that low doses of frusemide inhibit protein kinase, whereas higher doses cause inhibition of phosphodiesterase.

Importance and management

The documentation is very limited. Be on the alert for changes in the response to any blocker if frusemide is used. Animal studies suggest that increases occur with doses less than 10 g/kg, but decreases with doses of 1–4 mg/kg. Whether these same changes occur if frusemide is given orally seems not to have been studied.

Reference

1 Miller R, Sohn YJ, Matteo RS. Enhancement of d-tubocurarine neuromuscular blockade by diuretics in man. Anesthesiology (1976) 45, 422.
2 Scappaticci K, Ham JA, Sohn YJ, Miller RD, Dretchen KL. Effects of furosemide on the neuromuscular junction. Anesthesiology (1982) 57, 381–88.
3 Azar I, Cottbell J, Gupta B, Turndorf H. Furosemide facilitates recovery of evoked twitch response after pancuronium. Anesth Analg (1980) 59, 55–7.

Neuromuscular blockers + Immunosuppressants

Abstract/Summary

The neuromuscular blocking effects of tubocurarine are reduced by azathioprine and antilymphocytic globulin. The dosage may need to be increased 2–4-fold.

Clinical evidence, mechanism, importance and management

A retrospective study showed that patients on immunosuppressant drugs following organ transplantation needed an increased dosage of tubocurarine to achieve satisfactory muscle relaxation. A control group of 74 patients needed 0–10 mg tubo-curarine; 13 patients on azathioprine needed 12.5–25.0 mg; 11 patients on antilymphocytic globulin needed 10–20 mg and two patients on azathioprine and guanethidine needed 55–90 mg.[1] The reasons are not understood. Since azathioprine is converted within the body to mercaptopurine it is likely that it interacts similarly. Information is very sparse so it is not clear whether this interaction occurs with other neuromuscular blockers. More study is needed.

Reference

1 Vetten KB. Immunosuppressive therapy and anaesthesia. S Afr Med J (1973) 47, 767.

Neuromuscular blockers + Insecticides

Abstract/Summary

Exposure to organophosphate insecticides such as malathion and diazinon can markedly prolong the neuromuscular blocking effects of suxamethonium (succinylcholine).

Clinical evidence

A man admitted to hospital for an appendectomy became apnoeic during the early part of the operation when given 100 mg suxamethonium to facilitate tracheal intubation, and remained so throughout the 40 min surgery. Spontaneous restoration of neuromuscular activity did not return for 150 min. Later studies showed that he had an extremely low plasma cholinesterase activity (3–10%) although he had a normal phenotype. It subsequently turned out that he had been working with malathion for 11 weeks without any protection.[1]

Another report describes a man whose recovery from neuromuscular blockade with suxamethonium was very prolonged. He had attempted suicide 9 days earlier with diazinon (dimpylate), a household insecticide. His pseudocholinesterase was found to be 2.5 IU/l (normal values 7–19) and his dibucaine number was too low to be measured.[2]

Mechanism

Malathion and diazinon are organophosphate insecticides which inhibit the activity of plasma cholinesterase, thereby reducing the metabolism of the suxamethonium and prolonging its effects.

Importance and management

An established and well understood interaction. Particular care should be exercised if suxamethonium is used in individuals known to have been exposed to organophosphate insecticides such as malathion and diazinon. Insecticides of this type are found in sheep dips.

References

1 Guillermo FP, Pretel CMM, Royo FT, Macias MJP, Ossorio RA, Gomez JAA, Vidal CJ. Prolonged suxamethonium-induced neuromuscular blockade associated with organophosphate poisoning. Br J Anaesth (1988) 61, 233–6.
2 Ware MR, Frost ML, Berger JJ, Stewart RB, DeVane CL. Electroconvulsive therapy complicated by insecticide ingestion. J Clin Psychopharmacol (1990) 10, 72–3.

Neuromuscular blockers + Lignocaine, Procaine or Procainamide

Abstract/Summary

The neuromuscular blockade due to suxamethonium (succinylcholine) can be increased and prolonged by lignocaine (lidocaine), procaine and possibly procainamide.

Clinical evidence

A patient anaesthetized with fluroxene and nitrous oxide demonstrated 100% blockade with suxamethonium and tubocurarine. About 50 min later when twitch height had fully returned and tidal volume was 0.4 l, she was given 50 mg lignocaine intravenously for premature ventricular contractions. She immediately stopped breathing and the twitch disappeared. About 45 min later the tidal volume was 0.45 l. Later it was found that the patient had a dibucaine number of 23%.[3]

Other studies in man have confirmed that lignocaine and procaine prolong the apnoea following the use of suxamethonium (0.7 mg/kg). A dose-relationship was established. The duration of apnoea was approximately doubled by 7.5 mg/kg of lignocaine or procaine, and tripled by 16.6 mg/kg, although the effects of procaine at higher doses were more marked.[1]

Mechanism

Uncertain. Local anaesthetics appear to act on presynaptic, postsynaptic and muscle membranes. Procaine and lignocaine weakly inhibit pseudocholinesterase[2] which might prolong the activity of suxamethonium. There may additionally be competition between the suxamethonium and the procaine for hydrolysis by pseudocholinesterase which metabolizes them both.[1] Therapeutic serum levels of 4–12 g/ml procainamide have been found to inhibit cholinesterase activity by 15–30%.[6,7]

Importance and management

Information is limited but the suxamethonium-lignocaine and lignocaine-procaine interactions appear to be established and of clinical importance. Be alert for signs of increased blockade and/or recurarization with apnoea during the recovery period from suxamethonium blockade if either drug is used. Animal studies indicate that low and otherwise safe doses of lignocaine with other drugs having neuromuscular blocking activity (e.g. polymyxin B, aminoglycoside antibiotics) may possibly be additive with conventional neuromuscular blockers and cause problems.[4]

An increase in the effects of suxamethonium by procainamide has been reported in animals,[5] increased muscle weakness in a myasthenic patient[6] and reductions in serum cholinesterase activity in normal subjects but no marked interaction has yet been reported. Nevertheless be aware that some increase in the neuromuscular blocking effects is possible.

References

1 Usubiaga JE, Wikinski JA, Morales RL, Usubiaga LEJ. Interaction of intravenously administered procaine, lidocaine and succinylcholine in anesthetized subjects. Anesth Analg (1967) 46, 39–45.
2 Reina RA, Cannava N. Interazione di alcuni anestetici locali con la succinilcolina. Act Anaesth Ital (1972) 23, 1–10
3 Miller RD. Neuromuscular blocking agents. In 'Drug Interactions in Anesthesia', Smith NT, Miller RD, Corbascio AN (eds). Lea and Febiger, Philadelphia 1981, p 249.
4 Brueckner J, Thomas KC, Bikhazi GB, Foldes FF. Neuromuscular drug interactions of clinical importance. Anesth Anal (1980) 59, 533–4.
5 Cuthbert MF. The effect of quinidine and procainamide on the neuromuscular blocking action of suxamethonium. Br J Anaesth (1966) 38, 775.
6 Drachman DA, Skom JH. Procainimide-a hazard in myasthenia gravis. Arch Neurol (1965) 13, 316.
7 Kamban JR, Naukam RJ, Sastry BVR. The effect of procainimide on plasma cholinesterase acitivity. Can J Anaesth (1987) 34, 579–81.

Neuromuscular blockers + Lithium carbonate

Abstract/Summary

The concurrent use of neuromuscular blockers and lithium carbonate is normally safe and uneventful, but four patients have been described who experienced prolonged blockade and respiratory difficulties after receiving standard doses of pancuronium or suxamethonium (succinylcholine) or both.

Clinical evidence

A manic depressive woman on lithium carbonate and with a serum lithium concentration of 1.2 mmol/l, underwent surgery and was administered thiopentone, suxamethonium (a total of 310 mg over 2 h) and 0.5 mg pancuronium bromide. Prolonged neuromuscular blockade with apnoea occurred.[1,2]

Three other patients on lithium are described elsewhere who experienced enhanced neuromuscular blockade when given pancuronium alone[3] or with suxamethonium,[10] or with suxamethonium alone.[11] The authors of one of these reports say that '...We have seen potentiation of the neuromuscular blockade produced by succinylcholine in several patients...'[10] but give no further details. In contrast, a study in 17 patients failed to demonstrate any interaction in patients on lithium carbonate when given suxamethonium.[5] A lithium-pancuronium and lithium-suxamethonium interaction has been demonstrated in dogs[1,2,6] and a lithium-tubocurarine interaction in cats,[7] but no

clear interaction has been demonstrated with any other neuromuscular blocker.[8,9] A case of lithium toxicity has been described in a woman on lithium and suxamethonium, but it is doubtful if it arose because of an interaction.[4]

Mechanism

Uncertain. One suggestion is that, when the interaction occurs, it may be due to changes in the electrolyte balance caused by the lithium which results in a reduction in the release of acetylcholine at the neuromuscular junction.[7]

Importance and management

Information is limited. There are only four definite reports of this interaction in man and evidence that no adverse interaction normally occurs. Concurrent use need not be avoided but it would be prudent to be on the alert for evidence of this interaction in any patient on lithium carbonate who is given any neuromuscular blocker.

References

1 Hill G, Wong KC, Hodges M, Seutker C. Potentiation of succinylcholine neuromuscular blockade by lithium carbonate. Fed Proc (1976) 35, 729.
2 Hill G, Wong KC, Hodges MR. Potentiation of succinylcholine neuromuscular blockade by lithium carbonate. Anaesthesiol (1976) 44, 439.
3 Borden H, Clark M, Katz H. The use of pancuronium bromide in patients receiving lithium carbonate. Can Anaesth Soc J (1974) 21, 79.
4 Jephcott G, Kerry RJ. Lithium: an anaesthetic risk. Br J Anaesth (1974) 46, 389.
5 Martin BA, Kramer PM. Clinical significance of the interaction between lithium and a neuromuscular blocker. Am J Psychiatry (1982) 139, 1326–8.
6 Reimherr FW, Hodges MR, Hill GE, Wong KC. Prolongation of muscle relaxant effects by lithium carbonate. Am J Psychiatry (1977) 134, 205–6.
7 Basuray BN, Harris CA. Potentiation of d-tubocurarine (d-Tc) neuromuscular blockade in cats by lithium carbonate. Eur J Pharmacol (1977) 45, 79–82.
8 Waud BE, Farrell L, Waud DR. Lithium and neuromuscular transmission. Anesth Analg (1982) 61, 399–402.
9 Hill GE, Wong KC, Hodges MR. Lithium carbonate and neuromuscular blocking agents. Anesthesiol (1977) 46, 122–6.
10 Rosner TM, Rosenberg M. Anesthetic problems in patients taking lithium. J Oral Surgery (1981) 39, 282–5.
11 Rabolini V, Gatti G. Potenziamento del blocco neuro-muscolare di tipo depolarizzante da sali de litio (relazione su un case). Anest Rianim (1988) 29, 157–9.

Neuromuscular blockers + Magnesium salts

Abstract/Summary

The effects of tubocurarine, vecuronium, suxamethonium and possibly other neuromuscular blockers can be increased and prolonged by magnesium sulphate given parenterally.

Clinical evidence

A pregnant 40-year-old with severe pre-eclampsia and receiving magnesium sulphate by infusion, underwent emergency caesarian section during which she was initially anaesthetized with thiopentone, maintained with nitrous oxide/oxygen and enflurane, and given firstly suxamethonium and later vecuronium as muscle relaxants. At the end of surgery the patient rapidly recovered from the anaesthesia but the neuromuscular blockade was very prolonged (an eightfold increase in duration).[1]

Prolonged neuromuscular blockade has been described in two other women with pre-eclampsia given magnesium sulphate and either tubocurarine or suxamethonium.[2] Evidence of enhanced vecuronium neuromuscular blockade by magnesium sulphate is described in another report.[5] Another study in women undergoing caesarian section showed that those given magnesium sulphate for toxaemia needed less suxamethonium (4.73 compared with 7.39 mg/kg/h) than other normal patients.[3] Increased blockade has been demonstrated with decamethonium, tubocurarine and suxamethonium in animals.[2,4]

Mechanism

Not fully understood. Magnesium sulphate has direct neuromuscular blocking activity by inhibiting the normal release of acetylcholine from nerve endings, reducing the sensitivity of the postsynaptic membrane and depressing the excitability of the muscle membranes. These effects are possibly simply additive (or possibly more than additive) with the effects of conventional blockers.

Importance and management

An established interaction but the documentation is limited. Be alert for an increase in the effects of neuromuscular blockers if intravenous magnesium sulphate is used. Intravenous calcium gluconate was used to assist recovery in one case.[2] No interaction would be expected with magnesium sulphate given orally because its absorption is poor.

References

1 Sinatra RS, Philip BK, Naulty JS, Ostheimer GW. Prolonged neuromuscular blockade with vecuronium in a patient treated with magnesium sulphate. Anesth Analg (1985) 64, 1220–2.
2 Ghoneim MM, Long JP. The interaction between magnesium and other neuromuscular blocking agents. Anesthesiol (1970) 32, 23.
3 Morris R, Giesecke AH. Potentiation of muscle relaxants by magnesium sulphate in toxemia of pregnancy. South Med J (1968) 61, 25.
4 Giesecke AH, Morris RE, Dalton MD, Stephen CR. Of magnesium, muscle relaxants, toxemic parturients and cats. Anesth Analg (1968) 474, 689.
5 Baraka A, Yazigi A. Neuromuscular interaction of magnesium with succinylcholine-vecuronium sequence in the eclamptic parturient. anesthesiology (1987) 67, 806–8.

Neuromuscular blockers + Metoclopramide

Abstract/Summary

The neuromuscular blocking effects of suxamethonium (succinylcholine) can be increased and prolonged in patients taking metoclopramide.

Clinical evidence

A controlled study in 22 patients undergoing elective surgery showed that the recovery from neuromuscular blockade (time from 95% to 25% suppression of the activity of the adductor pollicis muscle) due to suxamethonium was prolonged in those patients who had also been given 10 mg metoclopramide IV.[1]

In another study of this interaction in patients undergoing postpartum tubal ligation it was found that mean block times after 1 mg/kg suxamethonium were 8.0 min (control), 9.83 min (10 mg metoclopramide), and 12.45 min (20 mg metoclopramide).[3] Prolongation of the actions of suxamethonium (+ 25%) by metoclopramide is described in another report and also briefly mentioned in another.[2]

Mechanism

Metoclopramide reduces the activity of plasma cholinesterase which is responsible for the metabolism of suxamethonium. As a result it is metabolized much more slowly and its effects are prolonged.[1,2] One study found that a metoclopramide serum concentration of 0.8 µg/ml inhibited plasma cholinesterase activity by 50%. A 10 mg dose of metoclopramide in a 70 kg adult produces serum concentrations of up to 0.14 µg/ml.[2]

Importance and management

An established but not extensively documented interaction of only moderate or minor clinical importance, however anaesthetists should be aware that some enhancement of blockade can occur (+ 25% has been reported). The authors of the first report cited[1] also point out that plasma cholinesterase activity is reduced in pregnancy and those taking ester-type local anaesthetics, which would be expected to be additive with the effects of metoclopramide.

References

1 Kao YJ, Turner DR. Prolongation of succinylcholine block by metoclopramide. Anesthesiology (1989) 70, 905–8.
2 Kambam JR, Parris WCV, Franks JJ, Sastry BVR, Naukam R, Smith BE. The inhibitory effect of metoclopramide on plasma cholinesterase activity. Can J Anaesth (1988) 35, 476–8.
3 Kao YJ, Tellez J, Turner DR. Dose-dependent effect of metoclopramide on cholinesterases and suxamethonium metabolism. Br J Anaesth (1990) 65, 220–4.

Neuromuscular blockers + Miscellaneous antibiotics

Abstract/Summary

Colistin, colistin sulphomethate sodium, polymyxins, lincomycin, some penicillins (apalcillin, azlocillin, mezocillin, piperacillin), clindamycin and vancomycin possess some neuromuscular blocking activity. Increased and prolonged neuromuscular blockade is possible if these antibiotics are used with anaesthetics and conventional neuromuscular blocking drugs. In theory amphotericin B might also interact, but the tetracyclines probably not. No interaction is seen with metronidazole, cefuroxime or chloramphenicol.

Clinical evidence

(a) Amphotericin B

Amphotericin B can induce hypokalaemia resulting in muscle weakness[2,3] which might be expected to enhance the effects of neuromuscular blockers, but there appear to be no reports in the literature confirming that this actually takes place. Check concurrent use carefully.

(b) Clindamycin or Lincomycin

Enhanced blockade has been demonstrated in patients given pancuronium and lincomycin which was reversed by neostigmine.[8] Respiratory paralysis was seen in a man recovering from blockade with tubocurarine[4] and this interaction was confirmed in another report.[5] Other reports describe the same interaction in patients on pancuronium or suxamethonium[12] while treated with clindamycin.

(c) Metronidazole

An increase in the neuromuscular blocking effects of vecuronium has been reported in cats,[13] but two later studies in patients failed to find any evidence of an interaction.[14,18]

(d) Penicillins

A study in patients showed that the neuromuscular blocking effects of vecuronium were prolonged by a number of acylaminopenicillins: alpacillin + 26%, azlocillin + 55%, mezlocillin + 38%, and piperacillin + 46%.[10] Recurarization occurred in a patient following vecuronium blockade when given piperacillin.[19]

(e) Polymyxins

Pittinger in his literature review of antibiotic-neuromuscular blocker interactions found 17 cases over the 1955–70 period in which colistin (polymyxin E) or colistin sulphomethate sodium,

with or without conventional neuromuscular blockers, were responsible for the development of increased blockade and respiratory muscle paralysis. Some of the patients had renal disease.[1] A later report describes prolonged respiratory depression in a patient on pancuronium and colistin.[9] Calcium gluconate was found to reverse the blockade.[9] Pittinger also lists five cases of enhanced neuromuscular blockade with polymyxin B. An increase in the blockade due to pancuronium by polymyxin B is described in another report,[11] and prolonged and fatal apnoea occurred in another patient on suxamethonium when his peritoneal cavity was instilled with a solution containing 100 mg polymyxin B and 100 000 U bacitracin.[15]

(f) Tetracyclines, Cefuroxime, Chloramphenicol

Pittinger lists four cases of enhanced neuromuscular blockade with rolitetracycline or oxytetracycline in myasthenic patients[1] but there seem to be no reports of interactions in normal patients given neuromuscular blocking drugs. No interaction was seen in the myasthenic patients when given chloramphenicol or penicillin,[6,7] nor in normal patients on cefuroxime when pipecuronium was being used.[18]

(f) Vancomycin

The neuromuscular blockade due to vecuronium was increased in a patient when given an infusion of vancomycin (1 g in 250 ml saline).[16] Transient apnoea and hypotension have also been described following rapid infusion of vancomycin during peritoneal dialysis of a patient.[17]

Mechanisms

Not fully understood but the following sites of action have been suggested.

Table 20.3 Neuromuscular blockers + Miscellaneous Antibiotics

Antibiotic	Prejunctional	Receptor block	Channel block	Muscle
Polymyxin B	+ +	+ + +		+
Colistin				+
Lincomycin	+ +	+ +	+	+
Tetracyclines				+

After Torda TA, Curr Clin Prac Ser (1983) 11, Clin Exper Norcuron, pp 72–8.

Importance and management

The interactions involving polymyxin B, colistin, colistin sulphomethate sodium, lincomycin, clindamycin and vancomycin are established and clinically important. The incidence is uncertain. Concurrent use need not be avoided, but be alert for increased and prolonged neuromuscular blockade with any neuromuscular blocker. The recovery period should be well monitored because of the risk of recurarization. Check the outcome of using amphotericin. No interaction would be expected with the tetracyclines, cefuroxime, chloramphenicol or metronidazole, but some caution would seem appropriate with apalcillin, azlocillin, mezocillin and piperacillin.

References

1 Pittinger CB, Eryasa Y, Adamson R. Antibiotic-induced paralysis. Anesth Analg (1970) 49, 487.
2 Holeman CW, Einstein H. The toxic effects of amphotericin B in man. Calif Med (1963) 99, 90.
3 Drutz DJ, Fan JH, Tai TY, Cheng JT, Hsien WC. Hypokalaemic rhabdomylosis and myoglobinuria following amphotericin therapy. J Amer Med Ass (1970) 211. 824.
4 Samuelson RJ, Giesecke AH, Kallus FT, Stanley VF. Lincomycin-curare interaction. Anesth Analg (1975) 54, 103.
5 Hashimoto Y, Iwatsuki N, Shima T. Neuromuscular blocking properties of lincomycin and kanamycin in man. Jap J Anesth (1971) 20, 407.
6 Gibbels E. Further observations on the side-effects of intravenous administration of rolitetracycline in myasthenia gravis pseudoparalytica. Deut Med Wsch (1967) 92, 1153.
7 Wullen F, Kast G, Bruck A. On the side-effects of tetracycline administration in myasthenic patients. Deut Med Wsch (1967) 92, 667.
8 Booij LHD, Miller RD, Crul JF. Neostigmine and 4-aminopyrimidine antagonism of lincomycin-pancuronium neuromuscular blockade in man. Anesth Analg (1978) 57, 316.
9 Giala MM, Paradelis AG. Two cases of prolonged respiratory depression due to interaction of pancuronium with colistin and streptomycin. J Antimicrob Chemother (1979) 5, 234.
10 Tryba M. Wirkungsverstärkung nicht-depolarisierender Muskelrelaxantien durch Acylaminopenicilline. Untersuchungen am Beispiel von Vecuronium. Anaesthetist (1985) 34, 651–55.
11 Fogdall RP, Miller RD. Prolongation of pancuronium-induced neuromuscular blockade by polymyxin B. Anesthesiol (1974) 41, 407.
12 Avery D, Finn R. Succinylcholine. Prolonged apnea associated with clindamycin and abonormal liver function tests. Dis Nerv Syst (1977) 38, 473.
13 McIndewar I, Marshall R. Interactions between the neuromuscular blocking drug ORGNC45 and some anaesthetic, analgesic and antimicrobial agents. Br J Anaesth (1981) 53, 785–92.
14 D'Hollander A, Agoston S, Capouet V, Barvais L, Bomblet JP, Esselen M. Failure of metronidazole to alter a vecuronium neuromuscular blockade in humans. Anesthesiology (1985) 63, 99–102.
15 Small GA. Respiratory paralysis after a large dose of intraperitoneal polymyxin B and bacitracin. Anesth Analg (1964) 43, 137–9.
16 Huang KC, Heise A, Shrader AK, Tsueda K. Vancomycin enhances the neuromuscular blockade of vecuronium. Anest Analg (1990) 71, 194–6.
17 Glicklich D, Figura I. Vancomycin and cardiac arrest. Ann Intern Med (1984) 101, 880.
18 Stanley JC, Mirakhur RK, Clarke RSJ. Study of pipecuronium-antibiotic interaction. Anesthesiology (1990) 73, A898.
19 Mackie K, Pavlin EG. Recurrent paralysis following piperacillin administration. Anesthesiology (1990) 72, 561–3.

Neuromuscular blockers + Monoamine oxidase inhibitors

Abstract/Summary

Three patients showed an enhancement of the effects of suxamethonium (succinylcholine) during concurrent treatment with phenelzine.

Clinical evidence, mechanism, importance and management

Two patients, one taking phenelzine and the other who had ceased to do so 6 days previously, developed apnoea following electroconvulsive therapy (ECT) during which suxamethonium was used. Both responded to injections of nikethamide and positive pressure ventilation with oxygen.[1] A later study observed the same response in another patient taking phenelzine.[2] This would appear to be explained by the finding that phenelzine caused a reduction in the levels of serum pseudocholinesterase in four out of 10 patients studied. Since the metabolism of suxamethonium depends on this enzyme, reduced levels of the enzyme would result in a reduced rate of suxamethonium metabolism and in a prolongation of its effects. None of 12 other patients taking tranylcypromine, isocarboxazid or mebanazine showed reduced pseudocholinesterase levels.

It would clearly be prudent to be on the alert for this interaction in patients on phenelzine, but on the basis of limited evidence it seems less likely to occur with the other MAOIs cited.

References

1 Bleaden FA, Czekanska G. New drugs for depression. Br Med J (1960) 1, 200.
2 Bodley PO, Halwax K, Potts L. Low serum pseudocholinesterase levels complicating treatment with phenelzine. Br Med J (1969) 3, 510.

Neuromuscular blockers and Anaesthetics + Morphine

Abstract/Summary

A patient experienced hypertension and tachycardia when given pancuronium bromide after induction of anaesthesia with morphine and nitrous oxide/oxygen. The respiratory depressant effects of ketamine and morphine may be additive.

Clinical evidence, mechanism, importance and management

A woman about to receive a coronary by-pass graft was premedicated with morphine and scopolamine. Morphine (1 mg/kg) was then slowly infused while the patient was ventilated with 50% N_2O/O_2. With the onset of neuromuscular relaxation with pancuronium, her blood pressure rose sharply from 120/60 to 200/110 mmHg and the pulse rate increased from 54 to 96, persisting for several minutes but restabilizing when 1% halothane was added.[1] The suggested reason is that pancuronium can antagonize the vagal tone (heart slowing) induced by the morphine, thus allowing the blood pressure and heart rate to rise. The authors of the report point out the undesirability of this in those with coronary heart disease. Ketamine is a respiratory depressant like morphine but less potent, and its effects can be additive with morphine.[2]

References

1 Grossman E, Jacobi AM. Hemodynamic interaction between pancuronium and morphine. Anesthesiology (1974) 40, 299.
2 Bourke DL, Malit LA, Smith TC. Respiratory interactions of ketamine and morphine. Anesthesiology (1987) 66, 153–6.

Neuromuscular blockers + Phenytoin

Abstract/Summary

The neuromuscular blocking effects of doxacurium, metocurine, pancuronium and vecuronium are reduced by the concurrent use of phenytoin given chronically. The effects on atracurium seem to be small and tubocurarine is only minimally affected. In contrast, if the phenytoin is given acutely, the effects of vecuronium are increased.

Clinical evidence

(a) Phenytoin given chronically: Neuromuscular blocking effects reduced

A comparative study in patients showed that those on phenytoin were resistant to the effects of certain neuromuscular blockers, as measured by the time to recover from 25 to 75% of the response to ulnar nerve stimulation. Compared with the controls, the recovery time for metocurine was reduced by 58%, for pancuronium by 40%, for tubocurarine by 24% and for atracurium by 8% (the last two were deemed not to be statistically significant).[1] Similar results for metocurine are described elsewhere by the same authors.[4] Another study in nine patients on phenytoin showed that on average they needed 80% more pancuronium (0.058 mg/kg/h) than 18 other patients not taking phenytoin (0.032 mg/kg/h),[2] while yet another found that in the presence of phenytoin 50% more vecuronium was needed but atracurium was not affected.[6] Only a small reduction in the effects of atracurium by phenytoin was seen in two other studies,[7,16] however 18 patients on carbamazepine and either phenytoin or sodium valproate had a recovery time of 1.96 min compared with 8.02 min in the control group.[10] Resistance to pancuronium due to phenytoin has also been described in three other reports,[3,8,9] and a shortening of the recovery period in yet another.[5] Doxacurium seems to be affected even more than pancuronium.[9] One study found that the time to recover from 75 to 25% blockade with doxacurium was decreased by 53%.[15]

(b) Phenytoin given acutely: neuromuscular blocking effects increased

A comparative retrospective review of 8 patients on chronic phenytoin treatment and 3 others given phenytoin acutely (within 8 h of surgery) showed that the average doses of vecuronium used from induction to extubation were 0.155 and 0.0615 mg/kg/hr respectively.[11] Another study with vecuronium also found that phenytoin given acutely increased the patients' sensitivity to the neuromuscular blocker.[12] A further study in 10 patients similarly found an increase in vecuronium blockade when given 10 mg/kg phenytoin intravenously.[14] Animal studies have also shown that phenytoin given acutely increases tubocurarine blockade.[13]

Mechanisms

Not understood. Suggestions include induction of liver enzyme activity which would increase the metabolism of the neuromuscular blocker, increases in the number of acetylcholine receptors on the muscle membrane, and changes in plasma protein binding.[17]

Importance and management

Established and clinically important interactions. (a) Anticipate the need to use more doxacurium, pancuronium, metocurine and vecuronium in patients on long-term treatment with phenytoin, and expect an accelerated recovery. The effects on tubocurarine and atracurium appear only to be moderate. (b) Anticipate the need to use less vecuronium (and possibly other neuromuscular blockers) if phenytoin is given acutely.

References

1 Ornstein E, Matteo RS, Silverberg PA, Shwartz AE, Young WL, Diaz J. Chronic phenytoin therapy and non-depolarizing muscular blockade. Anesthesiology (1985) 63, A331.
2 Chen J, Kim YD, Dubois M, Kammerer W, Macnamara TE. The increased requirement of pancuronium in neurosurgical patients receiving Dilantin chronically. Anesthesiology (1983) 59, A288.
3 Callan DL. Development of resistance to pancuronium in adult respiratory distress syndrome. Anesth Analg (1985) 64, 1126–8.
4 Ornstein E, Matteo RS, Young WL, Diaz J. Resistance to metocurine-induced neuromuscular blockade in patients receiving phenytoin. Anesthesiology (1985) 63, 294–8.
5 Messick J, Maass L, Faust R, Cucchiara R. Duration of pancuronium neuromuscular blockade in patients taking anticonvulsant medication. Anesth Analg (1982) 61, 203–4.
6 Ornstein E, Matteo RS, Schwartz AE, Silverberg PA, Young WL, Diaz J. The effect of phenytoin on the magnitude and duration of neuromuscular block following atracurium or vecuronium. Anesthesiology (1987) 67, 191–6.
7 deBros F, Okutani R, Lai A, Lawrence KW, Basts S. Phenytoin does not interfere with atracurium phamacokinetics and pharmacodynamics. Anesthesiology (1987) 67, A607.
8 Liberan BA, Norman P, Hardy BG. Pancuronium-phenytoin interaction: a case of depressed duration of neuromuscular blockade. Int J Clin Pharmacol Ther Toxicol (1988) 26, 371–4.
9 Desai P, Hewitt PB, Jones RM. Influence of anticonvulsant therapy on doxacurium and pancuronium-induced paralysis. Anesthesiology (1989) 71, A784.
10 Tempelhoff R, Modica PA, Jellish WS, Spitznagel EL. Resistance to atracurium-induced neuromuscular blockade in patients with intractable seizure disorders treated with anticonvulsants. Anesth Analg (1990) 71, 665–9.
11 Baumgardner JE, Bagshaw R. Acute versus chronic phenytoin therapy and neuromuscular blockade. Anesthesia (1990) 45, 493–4.
12 Gray HSJ, Slater RM, Pollard BJ. The effect of acutely administered phenytoin on vecuronium-induced neuromuscular blockade. Anaesthesia (1989) 44, 491–81.
13 Gandhi IC, Jindal MN, Patel VK. Mechanism of neuromuscular blockade with some antiepileptic drugs Arneim Forsch (1976) 26, 258–61.
14 Gray H StJ, Slater RM, Pollard BJ. The effect of acutely administered

phenytoin on vecuronium-induced neuromuscular blockade. Anaesthesia (1989) 44, 379–81.

15 Ornstein E, Matteo RS, Weinstein JA, Halevy JD, Young WL, Abou-Donia MM. Accelerated recovery from doxacurium-induced neuromuscular blockade in patients receiving chronic anticonvulsant therapy. J Clin Anesth (1991) 3, 108–11.

16 Modica P, Tempelhoff R. Effect of chronic anticonvulsant therapy on recovery from atracurium. Anesth Analg (1989) 68, S198.

17 Kim CS, Arnold FJ, Itani MS, Martyn JAJ. Decreased sensitivity to metocurine during long-term phenytoin therapy may be attributable to protein binding and acetylcholine receptor changes. Anesthesiology (1992) 77, 500–6.

Neuromuscular blockers + Promazine

Abstract/Summary

An isolated report describes prolonged apnoea in a patient given promazine while recovering from neuromuscular blockade with suxamethonium (succinylcholine).

Clinical evidence, mechanism, importance and management

A woman, recovering from surgery during which she had received suxamethonium, was given 25 mg promazine IV for sedation. Within 3 min she had become cyanotic and dyspnoeic, and required assisted respiration for 4 h.[1] The reason is not understood but one suggestion is that promazine possibly depresses pseudocholinesterase levels which would reduce the metabolism of the suxamethonium and thereby prolong recovery. Some caution would seem appropriate if promazine is given to any patient who has had suxamethonium. There seems to be no information about other phenothiazines and other neuromuscular blockers.

Reference

1 Regan AG, Aldrete JA. Prolonged apnea after administration of promazine hydrochloride following succinylcholine infusion. A case report. Anesth Analg (1967) 46, 315.

Neuromuscular blockers + Quinidine

Abstract/Summary

The effects of both depolarizing (e.g. suxamethonium) and non-depolarizing (e.g. tubocurarine) neuromuscular blockers can be increased by quinidine. Recurarization and apnoea have been seen in patients when quinidine was given during the recovery period from neuromuscular blockade.

Clinical evidence

A patient given metocurine (dimethyltubocurarine) during surgery regained her motor functions and was able to talk coherently during the recovery period. Within 15 min of additionally being given 200 mg quinidine sulphate by injection she developed muscular weakness and respiratory embarrassment. She needed intubation and assisted respiration for a period of 2½ h. Edrophonium and neostigmine were used to aid recovery.[1] This interaction has been described in man in reports involving tubocurarine[2] and suxamethonium.[3,4] It has also been seen in animals.[5–8]

Mechanism

Not fully understood, but it has been shown that quinidine can inhibit the enzyme (choline acetyltransferase) which is concerned with the synthesis of acetylcholine at nerve endings.[9] Neuromuscular transmission would be expected to be reduced if the synthesis of acetylcholine is reduced.

Importance and management

An established interaction but the documentation in man is limited. The incidence is uncertain but it was seen to a greater or lesser extent in five of six patients studied.[3] It has only been reported in man with metocurine, tubocurarine and suxamethonium, but it occurs in animals with gallamine and decamethonium and it seems possible that it will occur in man with any depolarizing or non-depolarizing neuromuscular blocker. This needs confirmation. Care should clearly be exercised if quinidine is used with any neuromuscular blocking drug.

References

1 Schmidt JL, Vick NA, Sadove MS. The effect of quinidine on the action of muscle relaxants. J Amer Med Ass (1963) 183, 669.

2 Way WL, Katzung BG, Larson CP. Recurarization with quinidine. J Amer Med Ass (1967) 200, 163.

3 Grogono AW. Anesthesia for atrial defibrillation. Effect of quinidine on muscular relaxation. Lancet (1963) ii, 1039.

4 Boere LA. Fehler und Gefahren. Recurarisation nach Chinidinsulfat. Anaesthetist (1964) 13, 368.

5 Miller RD, Way WL, Katzung BG. The neuromuscular effects of quinidine. Proc Soc Exp Biol Med (1968) 129, 215.

6 Miller RD, Way WL, Katzung BG. The potentiation of neuromuscular blocking agents by quinidine. Anesthesiol (1967) 28, 1036.

7 Cuthbert MF. The effect of quinidine and procainamide on the neuromuscular blocking action of suxamethonium. Br J Anaesth (1966) 38, 775.

8 Usubiaga JE. Potentiation of muscle relaxants by quinidine. Anaesthesiol (1968) 29, 1068.

9 Kambam JR, Day P, Jansen VE, Sastry BVR. Quinidine inhibits choline acetyltransferase activity. Anaesthesiology (1989) 71, A818.

Neuromuscular blockers + Quinine

Abstract/Summary

An isolated report describes recurarization and apnoea in a patient given intravenous quinine after recovering from neuromuscular blockade with suxamethonium and pancuronium.

Clinical evidence, mechanisms, importance and management

A patient with acute pancreatitis, taking 1800 mg quinine daily, was given penicillin and gentamicin before undergoing surgery during which pancuronium and suxamethonium were used uneventfully. After the surgery the neuromuscular blockade was reversed with neostigmine and atropine, and the patient awoke and was breathing well. After an 1½ h an IV infusion of 500 mg quinine in 500 ml isotonic saline (to run over 6 h) was started. Within 10 min (about 15 mg quinine) he became dyspnoeic, his breathing became totally ineffective and he needed re-intubation. Muscle flaccidity persisted for 3 h.[1] The reason for this reaction is not understood. A possible explanation is that it may have been the additive neuromuscular blocking effects of the gentamicin (well recognized as having neuromuscular blocking activity), the quinine (an optical isomer of quinidine which has blocking actions) and the residual effects of the pancuronium and suxamethonium.

There seem to be no other reports of problems in patients on neuromuscular blockers when given quinine, but this isolated case serves to emphasize the importance of being alert for any signs of recurarization in patients concurrently treated with one or more drugs possessing some neuromuscular blocking activity.

Reference

1 Sher MH, Mathews PA. Recurarization with quinine administration after reversal from anaesthesia. Anaesth Intens Care (1983) 11, 241–3.

Neuromuscular blockers + Testosterone

Abstract/Summary

An isolated report describes marked resistance to the effects of suxamethonium and vecuronium, apparently due to the long-term use of testosterone.

Clinical evidence, mechanism, importance and management

A woman trans-sexual who had been receiving 200 mg testosterone enanthate intramuscularly twice monthly for 10 years was resistant to 100 mg suxamethonium and needed 0.1 mg/kg vecuronium for effective tracheal intubation before surgery. During the surgery it was found necessary to use a total of 22 mg vecuronium over a 50 min period to achieve acceptable relaxation of the abdominal muscles for hysterectomy and salpingo-oophorectomy to be carried out. The reasons are not understood.[1]

Reference

1 Reddy P, Guzman A, Robalino J, Shevde K. Resistance to muscle relaxants in a patient receiving prolonged testosterone therapy. Anesthesiology (1989) 70, 871–3.

Neuromuscular blockers + Thiotepa

Abstract/Summary

An isolated report describes a marked increase in the neuromuscular blocking effects of pancuronium in a myasthenic patient when given thiotepa, but it normally appears not to interact with neuromuscular blocking agents.

Clinical evidence, mechanism, importance and management

A myasthenic patient rapidly developed very prolonged respiratory depression when given thiotepa intraperitoneally after receiving pancuronium.[1] Thiotepa has also been shown to increase the duration of succinylcholine neuromuscular blockade in dogs.[2] However *in vitro* studies show that thiotepa is a poor inhibitor of pseudocholinesterase[3] and in a normal patient it was found not to decrease serum levels significantly.[4] The general silence in the literature would seem to confirm that no special precautions are normally necessary.

References

1 Bennett EJ, Schmidt GB, Patel KP, Grundy EM. Muscle relaxants, myasthenia and mustards? Anesthesiology (1977) 46, 220–1
2 Cremonesi E, Rodrigues I de J. Interacao de agentes curarizantes com antineoplasico. Rev Bra Anest (1982) 32, 313–15.
3 Zsigmond EK, Robins G. The effects of a series of anti-cancer drugs on plasma cholinesterase activity. Can Anesth Soc J (1972) 19, 75–8.
4 Mone JG, Mathie WE. Qualitative and quantitative defects of pseudocholinesterase activity. Anaesthesia (1967) 22, 55–7.

Neuromuscular blockers + Trimetaphan

Abstract/Summary

Trimet(h)aphan can increase the effects of suxamethonium (succinylcholine) which may result in prolonged apnoea. This may possibly occur with other neuromuscular blocking drugs (seen also with alcuronium).

Clinical evidence

A man undergoing neurosurgery was given tubocurarine and suxamethonium. During the recovery period he developed apnoea lasting about 2.5 h attributed to the concurrent use of trimetaphan (4500 mg over a 90 min period). Later when he underwent further surgery using essentially the same anaesthetic techniques and drugs but with a very much smaller dose of trimetaphan (35 mg over a 10 min period) the recovery was normal.[1]

Nine out of 10 patients receiving ECT treatment and given suxamethonium showed an almost 90% prolongation in apnoea (from 142 to 265 s) when 10–20 mg trimetaphan was used instead of 1.2 mg atropine.[2] Prolonged apnoea has been seen in another patient given suxamethonium and trimetaphan.[6] On the basis of an *in vitro* study it was calculated that a typical dose of trimetaphan would double the duration of paralysis due to suxamethonium.[9] Prolonged neuromuscular blockade was also seen in a man given alcuronium and trimetaphan.[10]

Mechanism

Not fully understood. Trimetaphan can inhibit serum pseudocholinesterase to some extent[2] which would reduce the metabolism of the suxamethonium and thereby prolong its activity. Studies in dogs[5] and rats[3,4,8] and case reports in man[7] also indicate that trimetaphan has direct neuromuscular blocking activity. Its effects are additive with the neuromuscular blocking effects of the aminoglycosides.[8]

Importance and management

Information is limited but the interaction appears to be established. If trimetaphan and suxamethonium are used concurrently, be alert for enhanced and prolonged neuromuscular blockade. This has also been seen with alcuronium in man, and with other non-depolarizing blockers such as tubocurarine in animals.[3–5] Respiratory arrest has been seen in man when large doses of trimetaphan were given in the absence of a neuromuscular blocker so that caution is certainly needed.[7] Animal studies suggested that the blockade might not be reversed by neostigmine or calcium chloride,[8] but one study in man successfully used neostigmine and calcium gluconate to reverse the effects of alcuronium and trimetaphan.[10]

References

1 Wilson SL, Miller RN, Wright C, Hasse D. Prolonged neuromuscular blockade with trimethaphan: a case report. Anesth Analg (1976) 55, 353.
2 Tewfik GI. Trimethaphan. Its effect on the pseudocholinesterase level of man. Anaesthesia (1957) 12, 326.
3 Pearcy WC, Wittenstein ES. The interactions of trimethaphan (Arfonad), suxamethonium and cholinesterase inhibition in the rat. Br J Anaesth (1960) 32, 156.
4 Deacock AR, Davies TDW. The influence of certain ganglionic blocking agents on the neuromuscular transmission. Br J Anaesth (1958) 30, 217.
5 Randall LD, Peterson WG, Lebmann G. The ganglionic blocking action of thiophan dervatives. J Pharmacol Exp Ther (1949) 97, 48.
6 Poulton TJ, James FM, Lockridge O. Prolonged apnoea following trimethaphan and succinylcholine. Anesthesiology (1979) 50, 54.
7 Dale RC, Schroeder ET. Respiratory paralysis during treatment of hyper-

tension with trimethaphan camsylate. Arch Intern Med (1976) 136, 816.
8 Paradelis AG, Crassaris LG, Karachalios DN, Triantaphyllidis CJ. Aminoglycoside antibiotics: interaction with trimethaphan at the neuromuscular junctions. Drugs Exptl Clin Res (1987) 8, 233–6.
9 Sklar GS, Lanks KW. Effects of trimethaphan and sodium nitroprusside on hydrolysis of succinylcholine in vitro. Anesthesiology (1977) 47, 31–3.
10 Nakamura K, Koide M, Imanaga T, Ogasawara H, Takahashi M, Yoshikawa M. Prolonged neuromuscular blockade following trimethaphan infusion. Anaesthesia (1980) 35, 1202–7.

Vecuronium + Miscellaneous drugs

Abstract/Summary

Bradycardia has been seen in patients given vecuronium with alfentanil, fentanyl, sufentanil, thiopentone and etomidate.

Clinical evidence, mechanism, importance and management

Two patients, one aged 72 and the other aged 84 undergoing elective carotid endarterectomy developed extreme bradycardia following induction with alfentanil and vecuronium. The first was taking 20 mg propranolol 8-hourly and as the drugs were injected his heart rate fell from 50 to 35 bpm, and his blood pressure fell from 170/70 to 75/35 mmHg. He responded to ephedrine and phenylephrine. The other was taking nifedipine and quinidine. His heart rate fell from 89 to 43 bpm, and his blood pressure dropped from 210/80 to 140/45 mmHg. Both heart rate and blood pressures responded following skin incision.[1]

Bradycardia in the presence of vecuronium has been seen during induction with other drugs including fentanyl,[2,4] sufentanil,[3] thiopentone[4] and etomidate,[4] and may possibly be due to some effect on the CNS. Be alert for this effect if vecuronium is given with any of these agents.

References

1 Lema G, Sacco C, Urzúa J. Bradycardia following induction with alfentanil and vecuronium. J Cardiothorac Vasc Anesth (1992) 6, 774–5.
2 Mirakhur RK, Ferres CJ, Clarke RSJ et al. Clinical evaluation of Org NC 45. Br J Anaesthesia (1983) 55, 119.
3 Starr NJ, Sethna DH, Estafanous FG. Bradycardia and asystole following the rapid elimination of sufentanil with vecuronium. Anesthiology (1986) 64, 521–3.
4 Inoue K, El-Banayosy A, Stolarksi L, Teichelt W. Vecuronium-induced braycardia following induction of anesthesia with etomidate or thiopentone, with or without fentanyl. Br J Anesth (1988) 60, 10–17.

Chapter 21
Sympathomimetic Drug Interactions

Noradrenaline (norepinephrine, levarterenol) is the principal neurotransmitter involved in the final link between nerve endings of the sympathetic nervous system and the adrenergic receptors of the organs or tissues innervated. The effects of stimulation of this system can be reproduced or mimicked by noradrenaline itself and by a number of other drugs which can also cause stimulation of these receptors. The drugs which can behave in this way are described as 'sympathomimetics' and act either directly on the adrenergic receptors like noradrenaline itself or indirectly by releasing stored noradrenaline from the nerve endings. Some of them do both. This is very simply illustrated in Fig. 21.1.

We now know that the adrenergic receptors of the sympathetic system are not identical but can be subdivided into at least four main types, alpha-1, alpha-2, beta-1 and beta-2, and it is now possible broadly to categorize the sympathomimetics into groups according to their activity. The value of this categorization is that individual sympathomimetic drugs can be selected for their stimulant actions on articular organs or tissues. For example, salbutamol and terbutaline are so-called beta-agonists which selectively stimulate the beta-2 receptors in bronchi causing bronchodilation. This represents a significant improvement on both isoprenaline (isoproterenol) which also stimulates beta-1 receptors in the heart, and on ephedrine, which stimulates alpha receptors as well. Although the sympathomimetics are categorized together in this chapter, it is important to appreciate that they have a very wide range

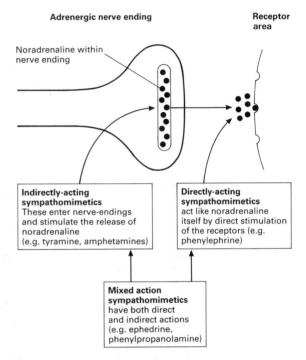

Fig. 21.1 A very simple illustration of the modes of action of indirectly-acting, directly-acting and mixed action sympathomimetics at adrenergic neurones.

of actions and uses. One should not, therefore, extrapolate the interactions seen with one drug to any other without fully taking into account their differences and similarities. The Index should be consulted for a full listing of all interactions involving drugs with sympathomimetic activity.

Table 21.1 A categorization of some sympathomimetic drugs

Drug	Receptors stimulated
Direct stimulators of alpha and beta receptors	
Adrenaline (epinephrine)	Beta more marked than alpha
Mainly direct stimulators of alpha receptors	
Phenylephrine	Predominantly alpha
Methoxamine	Premoninantly alpha
Metaraminol	Predominantly alpha
Noradrenaline (norepinephrine)	Predominantly alpha
Mainly direct stimulators of beta-1 receptors	
Dopamine	Predominantly beta-1, some alpha
Dobutamine	Predominantly beta-1, some beta-2 and alpha
Direct stimulators of beta-1 and beta-2 receptors (beta-agonist bronchodilators)	
Fenoterol	Predominantly beta-2
Formoterol	Predominantly beta-2
Isoetharine	Predominantly beta-2
Isoprenaline (Isoproterenol)	Beta-1 and beta-2
Orciprenaline	Predominantly beta-2
Pirbuterol	Predominantly beta-2
Reproterol	Predominantly beta-2
Rimiterol	Predominantly beta-2
Ritodrine	Predominantly beta-2
Salbutamol	Predominantly beta-2
Salmeterol	Predominantly beta-2
Terbutaline	Predominantly beta-2
Tolbuterol	Predominantly beta-2
Direct and indirect stimulators of alpha and beta receptors	
Ephedrine	Alpha and beta
Etefedrine	Alpha and beta
Phenylpropanolamine	Alpha and beta
Pseudoephedrine	Alpha and beta
Mainly indirect stimulators of alpha and beta receptors	
Amphetamine	Alpha and beta ⎫
Mephentermine	Alpha and beta ⎪ also central stimulants
Methylphenidate	Alpha and beta ⎬
Tyramine	Alpha and beta ⎭

Amphetamines and Related drugs + Chlorpromazine

Abstract/Summary

The appetite suppressant and other effects of amphetamines, chlorphentermine and phenmetrazine are opposed by chlorpromazine. The antipsychotic effects of chlorpromazine can be opposed by amphetamine.

Clinical evidence

(a) Dextroamphetamine + Phenothiazines

20 obese schizophrenic patients being treated with phenothiazines and other drugs (including chlorpromazine, thioridazine, imipramine and chlordiazepoxide) failed to respond to concurrent treatment with dextroamphetamine for obesity, and the expected sleep disturbance was not seen.[3] Antagonism of the effects of amphetamines by chlorpromazine has been described in other reports.[2,4]

A study in a very large number of patients taking 200–600 mg chlorpromazine daily indicated that the addition of 10–40 mg amphetamine had a detrimental effect on the control of their schizophrenic symptoms.[1]

(b) Chlorphentermine or Phenmetrazine + Chlorpromazine

Chlorpromazine was found in a double-blind controlled study in patients to diminish the weight reducing effect of phenmetrazine.[5] The effects of both phenmetrazine and chlorphentermine on the control of obesity were found in another study to be reduced by chlorpromazine.[6]

Mechanism

Not understood. It is known that phenothiazines can inhibit the uptake mechanism by which the amphetamines enter neurones. If this occurs at peripheral adrenergic neurones and centrally at both adrenergic and dopaminergic neurones, some part of the antagonism of the amphetamines can be explained.

Importance and management

Established interactions. These reports amply demonstrate that it is not desirable to attempt to treat patients with chlorpromazine and amphetamines, phenmetrazine or chlorphentermine concurrently. It is not clear whether this interaction takes place with phenothiazines other than chlorpromazine, but it seems possible.

This interaction has been deliberately exploited, and with success, in the treatment of 22 children poisoned with various amphetamines (dexamphetamine, methamphetamine, phenmetrazine).[2] They were given 1 mg/kg chlorpromazine intramuscularly initially, followed by further doses as necessary.

References

1 Casey JF, Hollister LE, Klett CJ, Lasky JJ, Caffrey EM. Combined drug therapy of chronic schizophrenics. Controlled evaluation of placebo, dextroamphetamine, imipramine, isocarboxazid and trifluoperazine added to maintenance doses of chlorpromazine. Am J Psychiat (1961) 117, 997.

2 Espelin DE, Done AK. Amphetamine poisoning: effectiveness of chlorpromazine. N Engl J Med (1968) 278, 1361.

3 Modell W, Hussar AE. Failure of dextroamphetamine sulphate to influence eating and sleeping patterns in obese schizophrenic patients: clinical and pharmacological significance. J Amer Med Ass (1965) 193, 275.

4 Jonsson LE. Pharmacological blockade of amphetamine effects in amphetamine-dependent subjects. Eur J Clin Pharmacol (1972) 4, 206.

5 Reid AA. Pharmacological antagonism between chlorpromazine and phenmetrazine in mental hospital patients. Med J Aust (1964) 1, 187.

6 Sletten IW, Orgnjanov V, Menendez S, Sunderland D, El-Toumi A. Weight reduction with chlorphentermine and phenmetrazine in obese psychiatric patients during chlorpromazine therapy. Curr Ther Res (1967) 9, 570.

Amphetamines + Lithium carbonate

Abstract/Summary

The effects of the amphetamines can be opposed by lithium carbonate.

Clinical evidence, mechanism, importance and management

Two depressed patients spontaneously abandoned abusing amphetamines (methamphetamine with cannabis and phenmetrazine) because, while taking lithium carbonate, they were unable to get 'high'. Another patient complained of not feeling any effects from amphetamines taken for weight reduction until lithium carbonate was withdrawn.[1] A controlled study in nine depressed patients confirmed these findings.[2] The reasons for these reactions is not known, but one suggestion is that amphetamines and lithium have mutually opposing pharmacological actions on noradrenaline uptake at adrenergic neurones.[1] Information is very limited, but reduced amphetamine effects seem probable in the presence of lithium.

References

1 Flemenbaum A. Does lithium block the effects of amphetamine? A report of three cases. Am J Psychiatry (1974) 131, 820.

2 Van Kammen DP, Murphy D. Attenuation of the euphoriant and activating effects of d- and l-amphetamine by lithium carbonate treatment. Psychopharmacologia (1975) 44, 215.

Amphetamines + Nasal decongestants

Abstract/Summary

An isolated report describes the antagonism of l-amphetamine in a hyperactive child by nasal decongestants containing phenylpropanolamine and chlorpheniramine.

Clinical evidence

Maintenance therapy with 42 mg levoamphetamine succinate daily in a 12-year-old hyperactive boy was found to be ineffective on two occasions when he was concurrently treated with *Contac* and *Allerest* for colds. Both of these proprietary nasal decongestants contain phenylpropanolamine and chlorpheniramine.[1] The reason is not understood. There is too little information to make any statement about the general importance of this reaction.

Reference

1 Heustis RD, Arnold LE. Possible antagonism of amphetamine by decongestant-antihistamine compounds. J Pediatrics (1974) 85, 579.

Amphetamines + Urinary acidifiers or Alkalinizers

Abstract/Summary

The loss of amphetamine in the urine is increased by urinary acidifiers, and reduced by urinary alkalinizers.

Clinical evidence

A study in six normal subjects given 10–15 mg amphetamine by mouth showed that when the urine was made alkaline (approximately pH 8) by giving sodium bicarbonate, only 3% of the original dose of amphetamine was excreted over a 16 h period compared with 54% when the urine was made acid (approximately pH 5) by taking ammonium chloride.[1]

Similar results have been reported elsewhere.[3] Psychoses resulting from amphetamine retention in patients with alkaline urine have been described.[2]

Mechanism

Amphetamine is a base which is excreted by the kidneys. In alkaline solution most of it exists in the un-ionized form which is readily reabsorbed by the kidney tubules so that little is lost in the urine. In acid solution, little of the drug is in the un-ionized form so that little can be reabsorbed and much is lost in the urine. A more detailed and illustrated account of this interaction mechanism is given in the introductory chapter.

Importance and management

A well-established interaction. It can be usefully exploited to clear amphetamine from the body more rapidly in cases of overdosage by acidifying the urine with ammonium chloride. Conversely it can represent an undesirable interaction if therapeutic doses of amphetamine are excreted too rapidly. Care is also needed to ensure that amphetamine intoxication does not develop if the urine is made alkaline with, for example, sodium bicarbonate or acetazolamide.

References

1 Beckett AH, Rowland M, Turner P. Influence of urinary pH on excretion of amphetamine. Lancet (1965) i, 303.
2 Änggård E, Jönsson L-E, Hogmark A-L, Gunne L-M. Amphetamine metabolism in amphetamine psychosis. Clin Pharmacol Ther (1973) 14, 870.
3 Rowland M, Beckett AH. The amphetamines: clinical and pharmacokinetic implications of recent studies of an assay procedure and urinary excretion in man. Arzneim-Forsch (1966) 16, 1369.

Beta-agonist brochodilators + Potassium-depleting drugs

Abstract/Summary

Beta-agonists (e.g. fenoterol, terbutaline, salbutamol (albuterol)) can cause hypokalaemia. This can be increased by other potassium-depleting drugs such as the corticosteroids, diuretics (bumetanide, ethacrynic acid, frusemide, thiazides, etc) and theophylline. The risk of serious heart arrhythmias in asthmatic patients may be increased.

Clinical evidence

(a) Beta-agonist bronchodilators + Corticosteroids

24 normal healthy subjects showed a fall in serum potassium levels when given either 5 mg salbutamol (albuterol) or 5 mg fenoterol by nebulizer over 30 min. These falls were increased after taking 30 mg prednisone daily for a week. The greatest fall (from 3.75 to 2.78 mmol/l) was found 90 min after fenoterol and prednisone. The ECG effects observed included ectopic beats and transient T wave inversion, but no significant interaction was noted for ECG disturbances in these healthy subjects.[4] However there is evidence that the risk of mortality may be increased in corticosteroid-dependent asthmatics who take beta-agonists.[5]

(b) Beta-agonist bronchodilators + Diuretics

The serum potassium levels of 15 normal subjects were measured after inhaling 5000 µg terbutaline while taking either a placebo, or 40 mg frusemide daily, or 40 mg frusemide + 50 mg triamterene daily for 4 days. With terbutaline alone the levels fell from 3.88 to 3.35 mmol^{-1}; after taking frusemide as well they fell to 3.13 mmol^{-1}; and after frusemide and triamterene they fell to only 3.29 mmol.$^{-1}$ These falls were reflected in some ECG (T wave) changes.[1]

After 7 days treatment with 5 mg bendrofluazide daily for a week the serum potassium levels of 10 normal subjects had fallen from 3.78 to 3.07 mmol/l. After taking 100–2000 mg inhaled salbutamol (albuterol) as well, the levels fell to 2.72 mmol/l. ECG changes consistent with hypokalaemia and hypomagnasaemia were also seen.[3]

Other diuretics which can cause potassium loss include bumetanide, frusemide, ethacrynic acid, the thiazides, and many other related diuretics. See Table 14.2.

(c) Beta-agonist bronchodilators + Theophylline

The concurrent use of salbutamol (albuterol) or terbutaline and theophylline can cause a fall in serum potassium levels. See details under 'Theophylline + Beta-agonist bronchodilators' (refer to Index).

Mechanism

Additive potassium-losing effects.

Importance and management

Established interactions. The CSM in the UK issue the following advice: 'Potentially serious hypokalaemia may result from beta$_2$-adrenoceptor stimulant therapy. Particular caution is required in severe asthma, as this effect may be potentiated by concomitant treatment with theophylline and its derivatives, corticosteroids, and diuretics, and hypoxia. Plasma potassium concentrations should therefore by monitored in severe asthma.'[2] Hypokalaemia may result in heart arrhythmias in patients with ischaemic heart disease and may also affect the response of patients to drugs such as the digitalis glycosides and antiarrhythmics.

Reference

1 Newnham DM, McDevitt DG, Lipworth BJ. The effects of frusemide and triamterene on the hypokalaemic and electrocardiographic responses to inhaled terbutaline. Br J Clin Pharmac (1991) 32, 630–2.
2 British National Formulary (March 1992) 23, 108. Published by The British Medical Association and The Pharmaceutical Press, London.
3 Lipworth BJ, Mc Devitt DG, Struthers AD. Prior treatment with diuretic augments the hypokalemic and electrocardiographic effects of inhaled albuterol. Am J Med (1989) 86, 653–7.
4 Taylor DR, Wilkins GT, Herbison GP, Flannery EM. Interaction between corticosteroid and beta-agonist drugs. Biochemical and cardioavascular effects in normal subjects. Chest (1992) 102, 519–24.
5 Crane J, Pearce N, Flatt A, Burgess C, Jackson R, Kwong T. Prescribed fenoterol and death from asthma in New Zealand, 1981–1983; case control study. Lancet (1989) 1, 917–22.

Dobutamine + Calcium chloride

Abstract/Summary

Calcium chloride infusion reduces the cardiotonic effects of dobutamine but not those of amrinone.

Clinical evidence, mechanism, importance and management

An experimental study of the mode of action of dobutamine in 22 patients recovering from aortocoronary bypass surgery found that an infusion of calcium chloride (1 mg/kg/min initially, later 0.25 mg/kg/min) reduced by 30% the increase in cardiac output produced by dobutamine (an infusion of 2.5 – 5.0 µg/kg/min). The cardiotonic actions of amrinone (a phos-phodiesterase inhibitor) in a group of 24 similar patients were unaffected by the calcium infusion.[1] Just how the calcium alters the dobutamine effects is not known but since dobutamine is a beta-receptor agonist it is reasonable to postulate that it interferes with the signal transduction through the beta-adrenergic receptor complex. The clinical importance of these findings is uncertain.

Reference

1 Butterworth JF, Zaloga GP, Prielipp RC, Tucker WY, Royster RL. Calcium inhibits the cardiac stimulating properties of dobutamine but not of amrinone. Chest (1992) 101, 174–80.

Dobutamine + Cimetidine

Abstract/Summary

An isolated report describes an exaggerated hypertensive response to dobutamine in a patient on cimetidine while undergoing anaesthetic induction before surgery

Clinical evidence, mechanism, importance and management

A patient developed unexpectedly marked hypertension (210/100 mmHg) in response to the infusion of dobutamine (5 µg/kg/min) during induction of anaesthesia (with midazolam, fentanyl, vecuronium and oxygen) for coronary artery bypass grafting. The infusion was stopped and over the next 15 min the blood pressure fell to 90/59 mmHg. A new infusion had just the same effect, and his blood pressure was subsequently controlled at 120/80 mmHg with only 1 µg/kg/min of dobutamine.[1]

The authors of the report suggest that this exaggerated response to dobutamine may have been due to the 1 g cimetidine which the patient was taking. The cimetidine may possibly have inhibited the metabolism and clearance of the dobutamine by the liver, thereby increasing its effects.[1] This is an isolated case but it would now seem prudent to reduce the dosage of dobutamine initially in patients taking cimetidine.

References

1 Baraka A, Nauphal M, Arab W. Cimetidine-dobutamine interaction ? Anaesthesia (1992) 47, 965–66.

Dopamine + Ergometrine (Ergonovine)

Abstract/Summary

A single report attributes the development of gangrene in a patient to the infusion of dopamine after ergometrine.

Clinical evidence, mechanism, importance and management

Gangrene of the extremities (hands and feet) has been described in one patient who was given an infusion of dopamine following the administration of ergometrine.[1] This would seem to have resulted from the additive peripheral vasoconstrictor effects of both drugs which reduced the circulation to such an extent that infection became unchecked. It would seem prudent to avoid concurrent use.

Reference

1 Buchanan N, Cane RD, Miller M. Symmetrical gangrene of the extremities associated with the use of dopamine subsequent to ergometrine administration. Intens Care Med (1977) 3, 55.

Dopamine + Phenytoin

Abstract/Summary

There is evidence that patients needing dopamine to support their blood pressure can become severely hypotensive if phenytoin is added to their treatment.

Clinical evidence, mechanism, importance and management

Five critically ill patients with a variety of conditions and under treatment with a number of different drugs, were given dopamine hydrochloride to maintain an adequate blood pressure. When seizures developed they were additionally given phenytoin. Coincidentally their hitherto stable blood pressures fell rapidly and one patient died from cardiorespiratory arrest. A similar reaction was demonstrated in dogs made hypovolemic and hypotensive by bleeding.[1] The reason for this reaction is not understood, but one suggestion is that the phenytoin may have a greater myocardial depressant effect during dopamine-induced catecholamine depletion.

The documentation is limited to this single report. This suspected interaction is not fully established, but there is enough evidence to indicate that phenytoin should only be used with great caution, if at all, in those requiring dopamine to maintain their blood pressure.

Reference

1 Bivins BA, Rapp RP, Griffin WO, Bloudin R, Bustrack J. Dopamine-phenytoin interaction. A cause of hypotension in the critically ill. Arch Surg (1978) 113, 245.

Dopamine + Tolazoline

Abstract/Summary

Acute and eventually fatal hypotension occured in a patient given dopamine and tolazoline concurrently

Clinical evidence

A patient who had undergone surgery three days before was given dopamine to maintain his cardiac index at about 3.5 l/min/m^2. Pulmonary arterial pressure had been steadily rising since the surgery so that on day 4 he was given a slow bolus of tolazoline (2 mg/kg) to reduce the afterload of the right ventricle. Systemic arterial pressure immediately fell to 50/30 mmHg whereupon the dopamine infusion was increased, but the arterial pressure then fell even further to 38/15 mmHg. The dopamine was stopped and ephedrine, methoxamine and fresh frozen plasma were given. Two hours later his blood pressure was 70/40 mmHg. Two further attempts were made to infuse dopamine, but the arterial pressure fell to 40/15 mmHg on the first occasion, and to 38/20 mmHg on the second. The patient died of cardiac arrest.[1]

Mechanism

Not fully understood. Dopamine has both alpha (vasconstrictor) and beta (vasodilator) activity. With the alpha effects on the systemic circulation competitively blocked by the tolazoline, its vasodilatory actions would predominate, resulting in paradoxical hypotension.

Importance and management

Information is limited but this interaction would appear to be established. The authors of this report warn that infusion of dopamine should not be considered for several hours after giving even a single small dose of tolazoline. They point out that impaired renal function often accompanies severe respiratory failure which may significantly prolong the half-life of tolazoline.

Reference

1 Carlon GC. Fatal association of tolazoline and dopamine. Chest (1975) 76, 336.

Ephedrines + Adsorbents, Antacids, Urinary acidifiers and Alkalinizers

Abstract/Summary

Alkalinization of the urine by sodium bicarbonate or other urinary alkalinizers causes retention of ephedrine and pseudoephedrine in the body, leading to the possible development of toxicity (tremors, anxiety, insomnia, tachycardia). Acidification of the urine with ammonium chloride has the opposite effect because the loss is increased. Kaolin does not appear to interact significantly with pseudoephedrine but aluminium hydroxide may possibly cause a more rapid onset of activity.

Clinical evidence

(a) Ephedrine + Urinary acidifiers and Alkalinizers

The excretion of ephedrine in the urine of three normal subjects, made acidic (about pH 5) with ammonium chloride, was two-fourfold higher than when the urine was made alkaline (about pH 8) with 3 g oral sodium bicarbonate.[4]

(b) Pseudoephedrine + Antacids or Urinary acidifiers and Alkalinizers

Prompted by the observation of a patient with renal tubular acidosis and persistently alkaline urine who developed unexpected toxicity when given ordinary doses of pseudoephedrine, a study was made on eight adult and child subjects of the possible effects of changing the urinary pH on the loss or retention of pseudoephedrine by the body. When the urinary pH was made alkaline with sodium bicarbonate, the half-life of a single 0.5 mg/kg dose of pseudoephedrine increased from 1.9 to 21 h.[1]

This confirms an earlier study in which it was found that when the urinary pH of three subjects was made about 8 (using sodium bicarbonate), the half-lives of pseudoephedrine were 16, 9.2 and 15 h respectively. When the pH was made about 5 (using ammonium chloride), the half-lives were 4.8, 3.0 and 6.4 respectively.[2]

Another study found that 5 g sodium bicarbonate increased the absorption rate at 2–4 h of a single 60 mg dose of pseudoephedrine.[3] The same study also found that 30 ml aluminium hydroxide gel did not affect the total amount of pseudoephedrine absorbed over 24 h but the rate of absorption was briefly increased.[3]

(c) Pseudoephedrine + kaolin

30 ml of a 30% suspension of kaolin was found in a study in 6 normal subjects to cause a small decrease (about 10%) in the absorption of a single 60 mg dose of pseudoephedrine. The rate of absorption was also decreased.[3]

Mechanism

The ephedrines are basic drugs mainly excreted unchanged in the urine. In acid urine, most of the drug is ionized in the tubular filtrate and unable to diffuse passively back into the circulation, and is therefore lost in the urine. In alkaline urine, it mostly exists in the lipid-soluble form which is retained. As a result they are lost much more slowly and accumulate. The increased rate of absorption of pseudoephedrine in the gut seen with sodium bicarbonate and aluminium hydoxide is probably also due to pH rises which favour the formation of the lipid-soluble absorbable form of pseudoephedrine. The reduced absorption with kaolin is probably due to adsorption of the pseudoephedrine onto the surface of the kaolin.

Importance and management

The ephedrines/urinary alkalinizer interaction is established but reports of adverse reactions in patients appear to be rare. Monitor the outcome of alkalinizing the urine for any evidence of toxicity due to drug retention (tremor, anxiety, insomnia, tachycardia, etc), reducing the dosage if necessary. Acidification of the urine with ammonium chloride increases the loss of the ephedrines in the urine and could be exploited in cases of drug overdosage. Aluminium hydroxide may possibly cause a more rapid onset of pseudoephedrine activity (but this needs confirmation) whereas the effects of kaolin on absorption are small and unlikely to be clinically important.

References

1 Brater D C, Kaojararern S, Benet L Z, Lin E T, Lockwood T, Morris R C, McSherry E J, Melmon K L. Renal excretion of pseudoephedrine. Clin Pharmacol Ther (1980) 28, 690–4.

2 Kuntzman R G, Tsai I, Brand L, Mark L C. The influence of urinary pH on the plasma half-life of pseudoephedrine in man and dog and a sensitive assay for its determination in human plasma. Clin Pharmacol Ther (1971) 12, 62–7.

3 Lucarotti R L, Claizzi J L, Barry H, Poust R I. Enhanced pseudoephedrine absorption by concurrent administration of aluminium hydroxide gel in humans. J Pharm Sci (1972) 61, 903–5.

4 Wilkinson GR, Beckett AH. Absorption, metabolism and excretion of the ephedrines in man. I. The influence of urinary pH and urine volume output. J Pharmacol Exp Ther (1968) 162, 139–47.

Phenmetrazine + Amylobarbitone (Amobarbital)

Abstract/Summary

The CNS side-effects and the weight-reducing effects of phenmetrazine are reduced by amylobarbitone

Clinical evidence, mechanism, importance and management

A comparative study in 50 overweight adults of the effects of either 75 mg phenmetrazine daily or 50 mg phenmetrazine plus 30 mg amylobarbitone (amobarbital) daily found that although the adverse CNS side-effects, particularly insomnia, headache and nervousness, were decreased by the presence of the barbiturate, the weight reducing effects were also decreased (by 65%)[1]

Reference

1 Hadler AJ. Phenmetrazine vs. phenmetrazine with amobarbital for weight reduction: a double blind study. Curr Ther Res (1969) 11, 750–4.

Phenylpropanolamine + Caffeine

Abstract/Summary

Phenylpropanolamine can raise blood pressure and this may be further increased by caffeine. Phenylpropanolamine can also markedly raise serum caffeine levels. Combined use may result in a hypertensive crisis in a few particularly susceptible individuals and increase the risk of intracranial haemorrhage. Manic psychosis has also been seen.

Clinical evidence, mechanism, importance and management

After taking 75 mg phenylpropanolamine or 400 mg caffeine alone, or both together, the blood pressures of 16 normal subjects rose from 137/85 mmHg to 148/97 mmHg, and after 150 mg phenylpropanolamine alone they rose to 173/103 mmHg. One of the subjects had a hypertensive crisis after 150 mg phenylpropanolamine and again 2 h after 400 mg caffeine. This needed antihypertensive treatment.[1] The same group of workers describe a similar study in which the AUC of caffeine increased more than 20-fold (from 0.8 to 18.5 μg h/ml) when taken with 75 mg phenylpropanolamine, and the peak serum caffeine level increased almost fourfold (from 2.1 to 8.0 μg/ml).[2] Additive effects on blood pressure are described in another report.[4]

Mania with psychotic delusions occurred in a healthy woman (who normally drank 8–10 cups of coffee daily) within 4 days of starting to take a phenylpropanolamine-containing decongestant. She recovered within a week of stopping both the coffee and the phenylpropanolamine.[3,4]

Mechanism

Uncertain. Simple additive hypertensive effects would seem to be part of the explanation.

Importance and management

Established interactions. These studies illustrate the potential hazards of these drugs, even in normal healthy individuals. The authors of one report[1] advise that likely users of phenylpropanolamine (those with allergies, or overweight, or postpartum women) and those particularly vulnerable (elderly or hypertensive) should be warned about taking more than the recommended doses, and of taking caffeine at the same time, because of the possible risk of intracranial haemorrhage. The effects of high levels of caffeine (insomnia, jitteriness, nervousness, agitation) are undesirable and unpleasant.

References

1 Lake CR, Zaloga G, Bray J, Rosenberg D, Chernow B. Transient hypertension after two phenylpropanolamine diet aids and the effects of caffeine: a placebo-controlled follow-up study. Am J Med (1989) 86, 427–32.
2 Lake CR, Rosenberg DB, Gallant S, Zaloga G, Chernow B. Phenylpropano-
lamine increases plasma caffeine levels. Clin Pharmacol Ther (1990) 47, 675–85.
3 Lake CR. Organic manic psychosis after ENTEX and coffee. J Clin Psychiatry. Quoted as In press in reference 2].
3 Lake CR. Manic psychosis after coffee and phenylpropanolamine. Biol Psychiatry (1991) 30, 401–4.
4 Brown NJ, Ryder D, Branch RA. A pharmacodynamic interaction between caffeine and phenylpropanolamine. Clin Pharmacol Ther (1991) 50, 363–71.

Phenylpropanolamine + Indomethacin

Abstract/Summary

An isolated case report describes a patient on phenylpropanolamine who developed serious hypertension after taking a single dose of indomethacin, but a controlled study in other subjects failed to find any evidence of an adverse interaction.

Clinical evidence

A woman who had been taking one *Trimolet* (85 mg D-phenylpropanolamine) daily for several months as an appetite suppressant, developed a severe bifrontal headache within 15 min of taking 25 mg indomethacin. 30 min later her systolic blood pressure was 210 mmHg and the diastolic was unrecordable. A later study on her confirmed that neither drug on its own caused this response, but when taken together the blood pressure rose to a maximum of 200/150 mmHg within 30 min of taking the indomethacin, and was associated with bradycardia. The blood pressure was rapidly reduced by phentolamine.[1]

In contrast, a controlled study, carried out to study this possible interaction, failed to find any evidence that the concurrent use of 75 mg indomethacin twice daily and 75 mg slow release phenylpropanolamine daily in 14 healthy young women caused a rise in blood pressure.[5]

Mechanism

Not understood.

Importance and management

Direct information seems to be limited to these reports. They suggest that an adverse hypertensive response is unlikely in most normal individuals given these doses, but it should be borne in mind that phenylpropanolamine, even on its own, can sometimes cause severe hypertension.[2–4]

References

1 Lee KY, Bellin LJ, Vandongen R. Severe hypertension after ingestion of an appetite suppressant (phenylpropanolamine) with indomethacin. Lancet (1979) i, 1110.
2 Livingstone PH. Transient hypertension and phenylpropanolamine. J Am Med Ass (1966) 196, 1159.
3 Duvernoy WFC. Positive phentolamine test in hypertension induced by a nasal decongestant. N Engl J Med (1969) 280, 877.

4 Shapiro SR. Hypertension due to anorectic agent. N Engl J Med (1969) 280, 1363.

5 McKenney JM, Wright JT, Katz GM, Goodman RP. The effect of phenylpropanolamine on 24-hours blood pressure in normotensive subjects administered indomethacin. DICP Ann Pharmacotherapy (1991) 25, 234–9.

Sympathomimetics (directly and indirectly-acting) + Rauwolfia alkaloids

Abstract/Summary

The pressor and other effects of directly acting sympathomimetics (adrenaline, epinephrine, noradrenaline, norepinephrine, phenylephrine, etc.) are slightly increased in the presence of the rauwolfia alkaloids. The effects of indirectly acting sympathomimetics or those with mixed activity (amphetamines, mephentermine, ephedrine, phenylpropanolamine, etc.) may be reduced or abolished.

Clinical evidence

After taking 0.25–1.0 mg reserpine daily for two weeks the pressor responses of seven normal subjects to noradrenaline (norepinephrine levarterenol) were slightly increased (20–40%) but their responses to tyramine (an indirectly acting amine) were reduced about 75%.[9] A man on reserpine who became hypotensive while undergoing surgery failed to respond to an intravenous injection of ephedrine, but did so after 30 min treatment with noradrenaline (norepinephrine), presumably because the stores of noradrenaline at adrenergic neurones had become replenished.[1] A child who had accidentally taken reserpine (thought to be about 6.5 mg) also failed to respond to an intramuscular injection of ephedrine (16 mg).[3] The mydriatic effects of ephedrine in man were shown to be antagonized by pretreatment with reserpine,[2] but a number of patients on reserpine were found to have increased blood pressures (+30/+13 mmHg) during surgery if pretreated with phenylephrine eyedrops.[10]

Experiments with dogs have demonstrated that adrenaline (epinephrine), noradrenaline (norepinephrine) and phenylephrine — all with direct actions — remain effective vasopressors after treatment with reserpine and their actions are enhanced to some extent, whereas the vasopressor actions of ephedrine, amphetamine, methamphetamine, tyramine and mephentermine — all with indirect actions — are reduced or abolished by reserpine.[5–7]

Mechanism

The rauwolfia alkaloids cause adrenergic neurones to lose their stores of noradrenaline (norepinephrine), so that they can no longer stimulate adrenergic receptors and transmission ceases. Indirectly acting sympathomimetics (which depend on their ability to stimulate the release of stored noradrenaline) may therefore be expected to become ineffective, whereas the effects of directly acting sympathomimetics should remain unchanged or possibly even enhanced because of the supersensitivity of the receptors which occurs when they are deprived of stimulation by noradrenaline for any length of time. Drugs with mixed direct and indirect actions, such as ephedrine, should fall somewhere between the two, although the reports cited seem to indicate that ephedrine has predominantly indirect activity in man.[1–3]

Importance and management

These are established interactions, but the paucity of clinical information suggests that in practice these interactions have not presented many problems. If a pressor drug is required, a directly acting drug such as noradrenaline (noradrenaline) or phenylephrine may be expected to be effective. Metaraminol has also been successfully used as a pressor drug in reserpine-treated patients.[8] The receptors may show some supersensitivity so that a dosage reduction may be required. Somewhat surprisingly in the light of the other evidence, one report claims that 25 mg ephedrine given orally or intramuscularly, once or twice a day, proved to be an effective treatment for reserpine-induced hypotension and bradycardia in schizophrenic patients.[4]

References

1 Ziegler CH, Lovette JB. Operative complications after therapy with reserpine and reserpine compounds. J Amer Med Ass (1961) 176, 916.

2 Sneddon JM, Turner P. Ephedrine mydriasis in hypotension and the response to treatment. Clin Pharmacol Ther (1969) 10, 64.

3 Phillips T. Overdose of reserpine. Br Med J (1955) 2, 969.

4 Noce RH, Williams DB, Rapaport W. Reserpine (Serpasil) in the management of the mentally ill. J Amer Med Ass (1955) 158, 11–15.

5 Stone CA, Ross AC, Wenger HC, Ludden CT, Blessing JA, Totaro JA, Porter CC. Effect of alpha-methyl-3,4-dihydroxyphenylalanine (methyldopa), reserpine, and related agents on some vascular responses in the dog. J PharmacolExp Ther (1962) 136, 80.

6 Eger EI, Hamilton WK. The effect of reserpine on the action of various vasopressors. Anaesthesiology (1959) 20, 641.

7 Moore JI, Moran NC. Cardiac contractile force responses to ephedrine and other sympathomimetic amines in dogs after pretreatment with reserpine. J Pharmacol Exp Ther (1962) 136, 89.

8 Smessaert AA, Hicks RG. Problems caused by rauwolfia drugs during anaesthesia and surgery. NY State J Med (1961) 61, 2399.

9 Abboud FM, Ekstein JW. Effects of small oral doses of reserpine on vascular responses to tyramine and norepinephrine in man. Circulation (1964) 29, 219–23.

10 Kim JM, Stevenson CE, Matthewson HS. Hypertensive reactions to phenylephrine eyedrops in patients with sympathetic denervation. Am J Ophthalmol (1978) 85, 862–8.

Ritodrine + Miscellaneous drugs

Abstract/Summary

Supraventricular tachycardia developed in a woman on ritodrine when given glycopyrronium. The abuse of cocaine does not appear to increase the incidence of side-effects in patients given ritodrine.

Clinical evidence, mechanism, importance and management

Premature labour in a 39-year-old who was 28 weeks pregnant was arrested with an IV infusion of ritodrine hydrochloride. Two weeks later while on the maximum dose of ritodrine (0.3 mg/min) her uterine contractions began again and she was scheduled for emergency caesarian section. It was noted in the operating room that she had copious oral secretions so she was given 100% oxygen by mask and 0.2 mg glycopyrronium intravenously. Shortly afterwards she developed superventricular tachycardia (a rise from 80 to 170–180 bpm) which was converted to sinus tachycardia (130 bpm) with 0.5 mg propranolol IV in divided doses.[1] The reason for this reaction is not understood. Ritodrine alone has been responsible for tachyarrhythmias and a possible explanation is that the effects of these two drugs were additive. Two other cases of tachyarrhythmia have been described in patients premedicated with atropine who were given ritodrine as a single IV bolus.[2]

Information is very limited and the interaction is not well established but some caution is clearly appropriate if both drugs are used. The authors of the first report advise avoidance.

A study in patients found no evidence of an increase in adverse side-effects in pregnant patients given ritodrine for premature labour who had been abusing cocaine.[3]

References

1 Simpson JI, Giffin JP. A glycopyrrolate-ritodrine drug-drug interaction. Can J Anaesth (1988) 35, 187–9.
2 Sheybany S, Murphy JF, Evans D, Newcombe RG, Pearson JF. Ritodrine in the management of fetal distress. Br J Obstet Gynaecol (1982) 89, 723–6.
3 Darby MJ, Mazdisnian F. Does recent cocaine use increase the risk of side-effects with beta-adrenergic tocolysis ? Am J Obst Gyn (1991) 164, 377.

Tyramine-rich foods + Cimetidine

Abstract/Summary

A woman on cimetidine experienced a severe headache with hypertension when she drank *Bovril* and ate some cheese.

Clinical importance, mechanism, importance and management

A woman of 77 with hiatus hernia, on 400 mg cimetidine four times daily for 3 years, experienced a severe frontal headache and hypertension which appeared to be related to the ingestion of a cup of *Bovril* and some English cheddar cheese, both of which can contain substantial amounts of tyramine.[1] Although the authors point out the similarity between this reaction and that which is seen in patients on MAOI who eat tyramine-rich foods (see' MAOI + Tyramine-rich foods'), there is no satisfactory explanation for what occurred. This is an isolated report and there is no reason why patients in general on cimetidine should avoid tyramine-rich foods.

Reference

1 Griffin MJJ, Morris JS. MAOI-like reaction associated with cimetidine. Drug Intell Clin Pharm (1987) 21, 219.

Xamoterol + Flosequinan

Abstract/Summary, clinical evidence, mechanism, importance and management

No significant haemodynamic interactions occurred in nine normal subjects when given 100 mg flosequinan and 200 mg xamoterol.[1] No special precautions seem necessary.

Reference

1 Lack of interaction of flosequinan and xamoterol in central and peripheral haemodynamics at supine rest in normal subjects. Br J Clin Pharmac (1992), 557P.

Chapter 22
Theophylline and Related Xanthine Drug Interactions

The main xanthines used in medicine are theophylline and aminophylline, the latter being used when greater water solubility is needed. They are of particular value in the treatment of asthma because they relax the bronchial smooth muscle. In an attempt to overcome the gastrointestinal irritation caused by theophylline, various formulations have been devised and different derivatives have been made such as diprophylline and enprofylline which do not liberate theophylline in the body. Within the context of interactions, aminophylline would be expected to behave like theophylline because it is a complex of theophylline with ethylenediamine, but other derivatives of theophylline seem to act differently and it should not be assumed that they all share common interactions.

Caffeine is also a xanthine and it is principally used because it stimulates the central nervous system, increasing wakefulness, mental and physical activity. There are hundreds of over-the-counter preparations containing caffeine with other ingredients such as aspirin, codeine and paracetamol, but caffeine is most commonly taken in the form of tea, coffee, cola drinks and cocoa.

Table 22.1 Caffeine-containing herbs and caffeine-containing drinks[1]

Source	Caffeine-content (%)	Caffeine-content of drink[1]
Cocoa		Up to 30 mg/100 ml
Coffee beans	1–2	Up to 100 mg/100 ml decaffeinated about 3 mg/100 ml
Guarana		
Kola	1.5–2.5	Up to 20 mg/100 ml in 'Coke' drinks
Maté	0.2–2.0	
Tea	1–4	Up to 60 mg/100 ml

[1] After Martindale. The Extra Pharmacopoeia. Edn 29 (1989) p 1535.

Table 22.2 Theophylline and related xanthines

Non-proprietary names	Proprietary names
Aminophylline	Afonilum, Aminocont, Aminodur, Aminomal, Aminophyl(lin), Androphyllin, Cardophyl(l)in, Carine, Corophyllin, Corophyllamin, Duraphyllin, Escophyllin, Eufilina, Euphyllin(a), Fergupina, Lixaminoil, Mini-lix, Paralon, Peterphyllin, Phyldrox, Phyllocontin, Phyllotemp, Planophylline, Tefamin, Teofylamin, Variaphylline, Vernaphyllin
Diprophylline (diphylline)	Aerophylline, Airet, Asthmolysin, Astmamasitt, Brosema, (dyphylline), Dicoryllin, Difilina, Difillin, Dilin, Dilor, Droxine, Dyflex, Emfabid, Glyfillin, Katasma, Lancephylline, Lufylin, Neophyllin, Neothylline, Neo-vasophylline, Neothylline, Neutralfillina, Neutraphylline, Prophyllen, Protophylline, Silbephylline, Synthophylline, Thylline
Doxofylline	Ansimar
Enprofylline	
Theophylline	Accurbron, Aerobin, Aerolate, Afonilum, Aminomal, Aminomed, Aquaphyllin, Armophylline, Asmafil, Aspertal-t, Asthmophylline, Bilordyl, Biophylline, Bronchoparat, Bronchoretard, Brokodyl, Cetraphylline, Cronasma, Diffumal, Dilatrane, Duraphyl(llin), Elexicon, Elexomin, Elixophyllin, Englate, Euphyllin, Godafilin, Inophyline, Labid, Labophylline, Lasma, Lodrane, Neulin, Oxyphyllin, Physpan, Pro-vent, Pulmidur, Pulmophylline, Respid, Rona-phyllin, Slo-phyllin, Sodiphylline, Solosin, Somophyllin, Sustaire, Synophylate, Tagilen, Techniphylline, Tefamin, Teoclasma, Teolix, Teonova, Theobid, Theocap, Theoclear, Theocontin, Theocot, Theo-dur, Theofrenon, Theograd, Theolair, Teolixir, Theospan, Theovent, Unifyl, Uniphyl(llin), Unixan, Xantivent

Caffeine + Antiarrhythmics

Abstract/Summary

The clearance of caffeine from the body is reduced 30–60% by the concurrent use of mexiletine, resulting in raised serum caffeine levels. Whether this might result in caffeine toxicity is uncertain. Lignocaine, flecainide and tocainide appear not to interact with caffeine.

Clinical evidence

(a) Mexiletine

Seven patients with cardiac arrhythmias showed a 48% reduction in caffeine clearance when given long-term treatment with 600 mg mexiletine daily.[1] The clearance of a single 366 mg dose of caffeine was reduced by 57% (from 126 to 54 ml/min) in five normal subjects by a single 200 mg dose of mexiletine. The elimination half-life rose from 246 to 419 min.[1] In a similar study by the same authors the caffeine clearance was reduced 30% (from 77 to 54 ml/min) in seven normal subjects by 200 mg mexiletine, and by 48% (from 71 to 37 ml/min) in five patients taking 600 mg mexiletine daily. Fasting caffeine levels were almost six-fold higher during than after mexiletine treatment (1.99 compared with 0.35 g/ml).[2]

(b) Flecainide, lignocaine (lidocaine), tocainide

200 mg lignocaine (lidocaine), 100 mg flecainide and 500 mg tocainide have no effect on the caffeine clearance.[2]

Mechanism

Not understood. The pharmacokinetics of the mexiletine are unaffected by the caffeine.

Importance and management

The caffeine/mexiletine interaction appears to be established but its clinical importance is uncertain. Some of the side-effects of mexiletine treatment might be partially due to caffeine-retention (from drinking tea, coffee, *Coca-Cola*, etc).[1] In excess caffeine can cause jitteriness, tremor and insomnia. It has also been suggested that the caffeine test for liver function might be impaired by mexiletine.[1] Be alert for these possible changes.

References

1 Joeres R, Klinker H, Heusler H, Epping J, Richter E. Influence of mexiletine on caffeine elimination. Pharmac Ther (1987) 33, 163–9.
2 Joeres R, Richter E. Mexiletine and caffeine elimination. N Engl J Med (1987) 317, 117.

Caffeine + Anticonvulsants

Abstract/Summary

Phenytoin can increase the loss of caffeine from the body, and possibly invalidate the caffeine liver function test.

Clinical evidence, mechanism, importance and management

A comparative study in non-epileptic patients and epileptics taking anticonvulsants found that phenytoin increased the clearance of caffeine about two-fold and reduced its half-life by 49% because it acts as an enzyme inducer, thereby increasing the metabolism and loss of caffeine from the body. Carbamazepine and sodium valproate had no effect.[1] The practical consequence of this interaction is that phenytoin may possibly invalidate the caffeine liver function test but normally no special precautions are needed if both drugs are taken.

References

1 Wietholtz H, Zysset Th, Kreiten K, Kohl D, Büchsel R, Matern S. Effect of phenytoin, carbamazepine and valproic acid on caffeine metabolism. Eur J Clin Pharmacol (1989) 36, 401–6.

Caffeine + Calcium channel blockers

Abstract/Summary

A small and relatively unimportant increase in the effects of caffeine may occur in patients given verapamil,

Clinical evidence, mechanism, importance and management

80 mg verapamil three times daily for 2 days decreased the total clearance of single 200 mg doses of caffeine in six normal subjects by 25% (from 4.6 to 5.8 h).[1] These changes are not large and unlikely to be of much importance in most patients. In excess the caffeine from tea, coffee and 'Coke' can cause jitteriness and insomnia.

Reference

1 Nawoot S, Wong D, Mays DC, Gerber N. Inhibition of caffeine elimination by verapamil. Clin Pharmacol Ther (1988) 43, 148.

Caffeine + Cimetidine

Abstract/Summary

The stimulant effects of caffeine may be increased to some extent by cimetidine.

Clinical evidence, mechanism, importance and management

1 g cimetidine daily for 6 days increased the half-life of caffeine in five subjects by about 70% and the average plasma levels were estimated as being about 1.7 times higher.[1] Another study confirmed that the caffeine half-life is increased by cimetidine.[2] The probable reason is that the cimetidine inhibits the metabolism of the caffeine by the liver, resulting in its accumulation in the body. Such an increase is unlikely to be of much importance in most patients, but it might have a part to play in exaggerating the undesirable effects of caffeine-containing drinks (tea, coffee, *Coca-Cola*) in a few patients who have insomnia or anxiety.

References

1 Broughton LJ, Rogers HJ. Decreased systemic clearance of caffeine due to cimetidine. Br J Clin Pharmacol (1981) 12, 155–9.
2 Beach CA, Gerber N, Ross J, Bianchine JR. Inhibition of elimination of caffeine by cimetidine. Clin Res (1982) 30, 438A.

Caffeine + Contraceptives (oral)

Abstract/Summary

The stimulant effects of caffeine may be increased to some extent in women taking combined oral contraceptives.

Clinical evidence, mechanism, importance and management

A study over 3 months in nine women showed that, while using low dose combined oral contraceptives, the clearance of single 162 mg doses of caffeine was reduced, the half-life prolonged (from 5.4 to 7.9 h) and the serum levels raised.[1] This finding is confirmed by three other studies,[2–4] two of which found that the caffeine elimination was prolonged from 4–6 to about 9 h by the end of the first cycle, and to about 11 h by the end of the third cycle.[3,4] The probable mechanism of this interaction is that these contraceptives inhibit the metabolism of caffeine by the liver resulting in its accumulation in the body. Women on the pill who drink caffeine-containing drinks (tea, coffee, *Coca-Cola*, etc.) may find the stimulant effects of caffeine increased. In excess caffeine can cause jitteriness and insomnia.

References

1 Abernethy DR, Todd EL. Impairment of caffeine clearance by chronic use of low-dose oestrogen-containing oral contraceptives. Eur J Clin Pharmacol (1985) 28, 425–8.
2 Patwardhan RV, Desmond PV, Johnson RF, Schenker S. Impaired elimination of caffeine by oral contraceptive steroids. J Lab Clin Med (1980) 95, 603–8.
3 Meyer FP, Canzler E, Giers H, Walther H. Langzeituntersuchung zum Einfluss von Non-Ovlon auf die Pharmakokinetik von Coffein im intraindividuellen Vergleich. Zent bl Gynäkol (1988) 110, 1449–54.
4 Rietveld EC, Broekman MMM, Houben JJG, Eskes TKAB, van Rossum JM.

Rapid onset of an increase in caffeine residence time in young women due to oral contraceptive steroids. Eur J Clin Pharmacol (1984) 26, 371–3.

Caffeine + Disulfiram

Abstract/Summary

Disulfiram reduces the loss of caffeine from the body which might complicate the withdrawal from alcohol, particularly in a few individuals.

Clinical evidence, mechanism, importance and management

A study in normal subjects and recovering alcoholics found that disulfiram treatment (250 mg maintenance dose) reduced the clearance of caffeine by about 30%, but a few of the alcoholics had a more than 50% reduction.[1] As a result the levels of caffeine in the body increase. Raised levels of caffeine can cause irritability, insomnia and anxiety, and as coffee consumption is often particularly high among recovering alcoholics, there is the risk that they may turn to alcohol to calm them down. To avoid this possible complication it might be wise for recovering alcoholics not to drink too much tea or coffee. De-caffeinated coffee and tea are widely available.

Reference

1 Beach CA, Mays DC, Guiler RC, Jacober CH, Gerber N. Inhibition of elimination of caffeine by disulfiram in normal subjects and recovering alcoholics. Clin Pharmacol Ther (1986) 39, 265–70.

Caffeine + Fluconazole

Abstract/Summary

Fluconazole causes a modest rise in serum caffeine levels.

Clinical evidence, mechanism, importance and management

A study in six young subjects (average age 24) and five elderly subjects (average age 69) found that 400 or 200 mg fluconazole respectively daily for 10 days, reduced the clearance of the caffeine from the plasma by 25% (32% in the young and 17% in the old).[1] It seems unlikely that the moderately increased serum caffeine levels will have a clinically important effect, but this needs confirmation.

Reference

1 Nix DE, Zelenitsky SA, Symonds WT, Spivey JM, Norman A. The effect of fluconazole on the pharmacokinetics of caffeine in young and elderly subjects. Clin Pharmacol Ther (1992) 51,183.

Caffeine + Idrocilamide

Abstract/Summary

Idrocilamide causes the marked retention in the body of caffeine from tea, coffee and other drinks. This can lead to caffeine intoxication (insomnia, extreme nervousness, jitteriness, anxious agitation).

Clinical evidence

The possibility that caffeine ingestion might have had some part to play in the development of psychiatric disorders seen in patients on idrocilamide, prompted a pharmacokinetic study in four normal subjects. While taking 400 mg idrocilamide three times a day, the half-life of caffeine from a cup of coffee (150–200 mg caffeine) was prolonged by a factor of nine (from about 7 to 59 h). The overall clearance of caffeine was decreased about 90%.[1,2]

Mechanism

Idrocilamide causes very marked inhibition of the metabolism and clearance of caffeine from the body, leading to its accumulation.

Importance and management

Evidence is limited but the interaction appears to be established. Patients on idrocilamide should avoid caffeine-containing drinks (tea, coffee, *Coca-Cola*, etc.) or only take very small amounts, otherwise caffeine intoxication may develop. Decaffeinated teas and coffee are widely available.

References

1 Brazier JL, Descotes J, Lery N, Ollagnier M, Evreux J-Cl. Inhibition by idrocilamide of the disposition of caffeine. Eur J Clin Pharmacol (1980) 17, 37.
2 Evreux JC, Bayere JJ, Descotes J, Lery N, Ollagnier M, Brazier JL. Les accidents neuropsychiques de l'idrocilamide: consequences d'une inhibition due metabolisme de la cafeine? Lyon Medical (1979) 241, 89.

Caffeine + Methoxsalen

Abstract/Summary

Methoxsalen markedly reduces the loss of caffeine from the body. Increased caffeine effects and possibly intoxication may occur.

Clinical evidence, mechanism, importance and management

A single 1.2 mg/kg oral dose of methoxsalen given to five subjects with psoriasis 1 h before a single 200 mg oral dose of caffeine reduced the caffeine clearance by 69% (from 110 to 34 ml/min). The elimination half-life of caffeine over the period 2–16 h after taking the methoxsalen increased tenfold (from 5.6 to 57 h).[1] The reason is believed to be that the methoxsalen acts as a potent inhibitor of the metabolism of the caffeine by the liver, thereby markedly reducing its loss from the body. The practical consequences of this interaction are as yet uncertain, but it seems possible that the toxic effects of caffeine will be increased. In excess the caffeine from tea, coffee and *Coca-Cola* can cause jitteriness, headache and insomnia. More study is needed.

Reference

1 Mays DC, Camisa C, Cheney P, Pacula CM, Nawoot S, Gerber N. Methoxsalen is a potent inhibitor of the metabolism of caffeine in humans. Clin Pharmacol Ther (1987) 42, 621–6.

Caffeine + Quinolone antibiotics

Abstract/Summary

Enoxacin and, to a much lesser extent, pipemidic acid can increase the blood levels of caffeine. The side-effects of caffeine (restlessness, insomnia, jitteriness, etc.) derived from drinks such as tea, coffee or '*Coke*' would be expected to be increased. Ciprofloxacin and norfloxacin interact very much less, and lomefloxacin and ofloxacin not at all.

Clinical evidence

(a) Ciprofloxacin

500 mg ciprofloxacin for 5 days increased the AUC (area under the curve) of caffeine in 12 normal subjects about 60%.[1] Another study found that the AUC of caffeine increased by 16.8, 57.1 and 57.8% respectively when given 100 mg, 250 mg and 500 mg ciprofloxacin twice daily for four days.[3] Yet another study found a 59% increase in the AUC after taking three 750 mg doses of ciprofloxacin.[9] A further study found a 51% increase in the caffeine AUC after 5 days use of 750 mg ciprofloxacin twice daily.

(b) Enoxacin

The AUCs of a single 230 mg dose of caffeine in 12 normal subjects increased by 138%, 176% and 346% respectively after taking 100 mg, 200 mg or 400 mg enoxacin twice daily for three days.[3] 400 mg enoxacin twice daily for 5 days doubled the peak serum levels of caffeine (200 mg dose) in 14 normal subjects and increased the AUC almost 5-fold (from 51 to 240 mg/h/l).[7]

(c) Lomefloxacin

Five days treatment with 400 mg lomefloxacin daily had no

significant effect on the pharmacokinetics of caffeine in 16 normal subjects.[5]

(d) Norfloxacin

800 mg norfloxacin twice daily for a day reduced the clearance of 350 mg caffeine in six normal subjects by about one third (from 9.7 to 3.56 l/h).[2] Another study found no statistically significant change in the AUC of caffeine in subjects given 400 mg nofloxacin daily for 3 days.[3]

(e) Ofloxacin

400 mg ofloxacin daily for five days had no significant effect on the pharmacokinetics of a single dose of caffeine in 12 subjects.[1] This was confirmed in another study.[3]

(f) Pipemidic acid

800 mg pipemidic acid twice daily for a day reduced the clearance of 350 mg caffeine in six normal subjects by two-thirds (from 9.7 to 3.56 l/h). The steady-state caffeine levels after repeated doses in two of the subjects rose about three-fold.[2] Another study found that 400 mg pipemidic acid twice daily for three days increased the AUC of a single 230 mg dose by 179%.[3]

Mechanism

It would seem that the metabolism (N-demethylation) of caffeine is markedly reduced by some quinolones (pipemidic acid, enoxacin) so that it accumulates in the body, thereby enhancing its effects. Other quinolones have a much smaller effect or none at all.[4] There appears to be a competitive interaction between the quinolones and the cytochrome p-450 iso-enzymes.[6]

Importance and management

Established interactions. On a scale of 100 to 0, the relative potencies of these quinolones for an interaction with caffeine have been determined as follows: enoxacin (100), pipemidic acid (29), ciprofloxacin (11), norfloxacin (9), ofloxacin (0). Lomefloxacin appears to behave like ofloxacin. Patients taking enoxacin may therefore possibly experience an increase in the side-effects of caffeine (headache, jitteriness, restlessness, insomnia) if they continue to drink normal amounts of caffeine-containing drinks (tea, coffee, 'Coke', etc.). They should be warned to cut out or reduce their intake of caffeine. The authors of one report[1] suggest that patients with hepatic disorders, cardiac arrhythmias or latent epilepsy should avoid caffeine if they take enoxacin for a week or more. The effects of pipemidic acid are considerably less, and those of ciprofloxacin and norfloxacin probably of little importance. Lomefloxacin and ofloxacin are non-interacting alternatives.

References

1 Staib AH, Stille W, Dietlin G, Shah PM, Harder S, Mieke S, Beer C. Interaction between quinolones and caffeine. Drugs (1987) 34 (Suppl 1) 170–4.
2 li Carbo M, Segura J, De la Torre R, Badenas JM, Cami J. Effect of quinolones on caffeine disposition. Clin Pharmacol Ther (1989) 45, 234–40.
3 Harder S, Staib AH, Beer C, Papenburg A, Stille W, Shah PM. 4-quinolones inhibit biotransformation of caffeine. Eur J Clin Pharmacol (1988) 35, 651–6.
4 Still W, Harder S, Mieke S, Beer C, Shah PM, Frech K, Staib AH. Decrease of caffeine elimination in many patients during co-administration of 4-quinolones. J Antimicrob Chemother (1987) 20, 729–34.
5 Healey DP, Schoenle JR, Stotka J, Polk RE. Lack of interaction between lomefloxacin and caffeine in normal volunteers. Antimicrob Ag Chemother (1991) 35, 660–4.
6 Fuhr U, Wolff T, Harder S, Schymanski P, Staib AH. Quinolone inhibition of cytochrome P-450 dependent caffeine metabolism in human liver microsomes. Drug Metab Disp (1990) 18, 1005–10.
7 Peloquin CA, Nix DE, Sedman AJ, Wilton JH, Toothaker RD, Harrison NJ, Schentag JJ. Pharmacokinetics and clinical effects of caffeine alone and in combination with oral enoxacin. Rev Infect Dis (1989) II, Suppl 5, S1095.
8 Barnett G, Segura J, de la Torre R, Carbó M. Pharmacokinetic determination of relative potency of quinolone inhibition of caffeine disposition. Eur J Clin Pharmacol (1990) 39, 63–9.
9 Healey DP, Polk RE, Kanawati L, Rock DT, Mooney ML. Interaction between oral ciprofloxacin and caffeine in normal volunteers. Antimicrob Ag Chemother (1989) 33, 474–8.

Doxofylline + Digitalis glycosides

Abstract/Summary

Digoxin lowers serum doxofylline levels at steady-state after an initial rise, but the bronchodilator effects do not appear to be significantly affected.

Clinical evidence, mechanism, importance and management

A comparative study in 10 patients, five given digoxin (0.5 mg daily) and five without, found that the digoxin increased the serum levels of doxofylline (800 mg daily) on the first day of treatment by about 50%, but at steady-state (30 days) the serum levels were reduced about 60%. Nevertheless the bronchodilating effects of the doxofylline were little different between the two groups. It was concluded that concurrent use is normally safe and effective, but the initial doxofylline dose should be chosen to avoid too high a serum level on the first day, and pulmonary function should be well monitored.[1]

Reference

1 Provvedi D, Rubegni M, Biffignandi P. Pharmacokinetic interaction between doxofylline and digitalis in elderly patients with chronic obsructive bronchitis. Acta Ther (1990) 16, 239–46

Theophylline + Allopurinol

Abstract/Summary

Limited evidence from clinical studies and a single case report indicate that the effects of theophylline may be increased by the concurrent use of allopurinol.

Clinical evidence

A patient on 450 mg theophylline daily showed a 38% increase in peak serum levels after taking 100 mg allopurinol for 2 days.[4] 600 mg allopurinol daily for 14 days increased the half-life of theophylline in 12 normal subjects (5 mg/kg) by 25% and increased the AUC by 27%.[1] Two other studies with 300 mg allopurinol daily failed to show any effect on the pharmacokinetics of theophylline,[2,3] possibly because the dosage was smaller and the trials lasted only a week.

Mechanism

Uncertain. One suggestion is that the allopurinol inhibits the metabolism of the theophylline by the liver.[4]

Importance and management

Evidence appears to be limited to a single case report and the studies on normal healthy subjects. The clinical importance of this interaction is uncertain, but it would now seem prudent to check for any signs of theophylline overdosage during concurrent use, particularly in patients whose disease condition may result in a reduction in the metabolism of the theophylline or where high doses of allopurinol are used.

References

1 Manfredi RL, Vessell ES. Inhibition of theophylline metabolism by long-term allopurinol administration. Clin Pharmacol Ther (1981) 29, 224.
2 Vozeh S, Powell RJ, Cupit GC, Riegelman S, Sheiner LB. Influence of allopurinol on theophylline disposition in adults. Clin Pharmacol Ther (1980) 27, 194.
3 Grygiel JJ, Wing LMH, Farkas J, Birkett DJ. Effects of allopurinol on theophylline metabolism and clearance. Clin Pharmacol Ther (1979) 26, 660.
4 Barry M, Feeley J. Allopurinol influences amiphenazone elimination. Clin Pharmacokinet (1990) 19, 167–9.

Theophylline + Aminoglutethimide

Abstract/Summary

The loss of theophylline from the body is increased by the concurrent use of aminoglutethimide and some reduction in its serum levels and therapeutic effects seems probable.

Clinical evidence

Aminoglutethimide (250 mg four times a day) for 2–12 weeks increased the theophylline clearance in three patients taking a sustained release preparation (200 mg twice daily) by 32%.[1]

Mechanism

Uncertain. It seems probable that the aminoglutethimide, a known enzyme inducing agent, increases the metabolism of theophylline by the liver, thereby increasing its loss from the body.

Importance and management

Direct information is limited to this study. Its clinical importance is uncertain, but the effects of theophylline would be expected to be reduced to some extent by the addition of aminoglutethimide. Monitor the effects and increase the theophylline dosage if necessary.

Reference

1 Lonning PE, Kvinnsland S, Bakke OM. Effect of aminoglutethimide on antipyrine, theophylline and digitoxin disposition in breast cancer. Clin Pharmacol Ther (1984) 36, 796–802.

Theophylline + Amiodarone

Abstract/Summary

An isolated report describes raised theophylline levels and toxicity in an old man when amiodarone was added.

Clinical evidence, mechanism, importance and management

An 86-year old man on frusemide (furosemide), digoxin, domperidone and theophylline developed signs of theophylline toxicity when amiodarone (600 mg daily) was added. After 9 days' concurrent use his serum theophylline levels had doubled (from 93 to 194 μmol/l). The toxicity disappeared when the theophylline was stopped.[1] The reason for this adverse reaction is not understood but a reduction in the metabolism of the theophylline by the liver is suggested.[1] There was no evidence of liver dysfunction. This is an isolated case and its general importance is uncertain, but it would now seem prudent to monitor serum theophylline levels if amiodarone is given to any patient. More study is needed.

Reference

1 Soto J, Sacristán JA, Arellano F, Hazas J. Possible theophylline-amiodarone interaction. DICP Ann Pharmacotherapy (1990) 24, 1115.

Theophylline + Albendazole and Mebendazole

Abstract/Summary

Neither albendazole nor mebendazole appear to interact with theophylline.

Clinical evidence, mechanism, importance and management

Studies in 12 and six normal subjects found that the pharmacokinetics of theophylline were unaffected by 100 mg mebendazole twice daily for 3 days or a single 400 mg dose of albendazole.[1] No special precautions would seem to be needed if either of these anthelmintics is given to patients taking theophylline but more study is needed to confirm the absence of an interaction.

Reference

1 Adebayo GI, Mabadeje AFB. Theophylline disposition — effects of cimetidine, mebendazole and albendazole. Aliment Pharmacol Ther (1988) 2, 341–6.

Theophylline + Ampicillin or Amoxycillin

Abstract/Summary

Neither ampicillin, amoxycillin nor sulbactam interacts adversely with theophylline, nor amoxycillin with enprofylline.

Clinical evidence, mechanism, importance and management

A study on 11 asthmatic children aged 3 months to 6 years found that the mean half-life of theophylline was unchanged by the concurrent use of ampicillin.[1] 12 adult patients with chronic obstructive pulmonary disease showed no changes in the pharmacokinetics of theophylline when given ampicillin 1 g plus sulbactam 500 mg 12-hourly for seven days.[5] Another study[2,3] on nine normal adults similarly showed that the concurrent use of amoxycillin (750 mg daily for 9 days) did not affect the pharmacokinetics of theophylline. Amoxycillin causes a small but not statistically significant reduction in the renal clearance of enprofylline.[4] No special precautions would seem to be necessary during concurrent use.

References

1 Kadlec GJ, Ha Le Thanh, Jarboe CH, Richard D, Karibo JM. Effect of ampicillin on theophylline half-life in infants and young children. South Med J (1978) 71, 1584.

2 Jonkman JHG, van der Boon WJV, Schoenmaker R, Holtkamp A, Hempenius J. Lack of effect of amoxicillin on theophylline pharmacokinetics. Br J Clin Pharmac (1985) 19, 99–101.

3 Jonkman JHG, van der Boon WJV, Schoenmaker R, Holtkamp AH, Hempenius J. Clinical pharmacokinetics of amoxicillin and theophylline during cotreatment with both medicaments. Chemotherapy (1985) 31, 329–35.

4 Sitar DS, Aoki FY, Hoban DJ, Hidinger K-G, Montgomery PR, Mitenko PA. Enprofylline disposition in the presence and absence of amoxicillin and erythromycin. Br J Clin Pharmac (1987) 24, 57–61.

5 Cazzola M, Santangelo G, Guidetti E, Mattina R, Caputi M, Girbino G. Influence of sulbactam plus ampicillin on theophylline clearance. Int J Clin Pharm Res (1991) XI, 11–15.

Theophylline + Antacids

Abstract/Summary

The absorption of theophylline from the gut does not normally appear to be significantly affected by the concurrent use of aluminium or magnesium hydroxide antacids such as *Maalox*, *Mylanta* or *Amphojel*, but a significant rise in theophylline levels has been described with one sustained-release theophylline preparation (*Nuelin Depot*).

Clinical evidence, mechanism, importance and management

A study[1] in 12 normal subjects showed that the absorption of aminophylline (200 mg) was slightly reduced by the concurrent use of 30 ml *Maalox* (magnesium-aluminium hydroxide gel) but the extent was considered to be clinically unimportant. Another three-day study[2] on nine asthmatic patients showed that neither 30 ml *Mylanta* nor 60 ml *Amphojel* had a predictable or significant effect on the steady-state serum levels of theophylline when administered as aminophylline or as a sustained-release preparation of theophylline. The absence of a significant interaction was confirmed in another study using an aluminium-magnesium hydroxide antacid and a sustained release theophylline preparation (un-named).[3] No changes were seen in the pharmacokinetics of *K1-b Riker*, a sustained-release preparation, in another study using an un-named antacid,[5] nor any significant changes when *Maalox* was given with another slow release preparation, *Armophylline*.[6,7] In contrast, in another study[4] it was found that serum theophylline levels from a sustained-release formulation (*Nuelin Depot*) but not from *Theodur*, were raised when an antacid (*Novalucid*-magnesium and aluminium hydroxides, and magnesium carbonate) was given concurrently.

In this last instance the side-effects of theophylline might be increased in those with serum levels at the top end of the range, but generally speaking no special precautions seem to be necessary during the concurrent use of theophylline and antacids.

References

1 Arnold LA, Spurbeck GH, Shelver WH, Henderson WM. Effect of an antacid on gastrointestinal absorption of theophylline. Am J Hosp Pharm (1979) 36, 1059–62.

2 Reed RC, Schwartz HJ. Lack of influence of an intensive antacid regimen on theophylline bioavailability. J Pharmacokinetic Biopharm (1984) 12, 315–331.

3 Darzentas LJ, Stewart RB, Curry SH, Yost RL. Effect of antacid on bioavailability of a sustained-release theophylline tablet preparation. Drug Intell Clin Pharm (1982) 16, 4714

4 Myhre KI, Walstad RA. The influence of antacid on the absorption of two different sustained-release formulations of theophylline. Br J Clin Pharmac (1983) 15, 683–7.

5 Moreland TA, McMurdo MET, McEwen J. The effect of food and antacid on the pharmacokinetics of a sustained release theophylline preparation. Br J Clin Pharmac (1987) 24, 275–6.

6 Muir JF, Moore N, Pfeiffer G, Andrejak M, Richard MO, Ulmann A, Abella ML. Is there an interaction between slow-release theophyllin (*Armophylline®*) and an antacid treatment (*Maalox®*)? Thérapie (1990) 45, 42.

7 Muir JF, Peiffer G, Richard MO, Benhamou D, Adrejak M, Hary L, Moore N. lack of effect of magnesium-aluminium hydroxide on the absorption of theophylline given as a pH-dependent sustained release preparation. Eur J Clin Pharmacol (1993) 44, 85–8.

Theophylline + Antihistamines and Related drugs

Abstract/Summary

Ketotifen, mequitazine, picumast dihydrochloride, terfenadine and temelastine appear not to interact adversely with theophylline.

Clinical evidence, mechanism, importance and management

Two studies showed that ketotifen does not affect the pharmacokinetics of theophylline.[3,4] No adverse effects were seen and the symptom score was improved.[4] The steady-state serum levels of theophylline were found to be unchanged in seven asthmatic patients when given 6 mg mequitazine daily for three weeks.[6] Four studies in normal subjects showed that the pharmacokinetics of theophylline were unchanged by the concurrent use of 200 mg temelastine daily[1] or 60 mg terfenadine.[2,5,7] 10 mg picumast dihydrochloride was found not to affect the pharmacokinetics of theophylline, although the bioavailability of the picumast was slightly, but not clinically significantly, reduced.[8]

References

1 Charles BG, Schneider JJ, Norris RLG, Ravenscroft PJ. Temelastine does not affect theophylline pharmacokinetics in normal subjects. Br J Clin Pharmac (1987) 24, 673–5.

2 Luskin AT, Fitzsimmons WE, Luskin S, MacLeod CM. Single dose study of the effect of terfenadine on theophylline absorption and disposition. Ann Allergy (1987) 60, 184.

3 Garty M, Scolnik D, Danziger Y, Volovitz B, Ilfeld DN, Varsano I. Non-interaction of ketotifen and theophylline in children with asthma-an acute study. Eur J Clin Pharmacol (1987) 32, 187–9.

4 Hendy MS, Burge PS, Stableforth DE. Effects of ketotifen on the bronchodilating action of aminophylline. Respiration (1986) 49, 296–9.

5 Brion N, Naline E, Beaumont D, Pays M, Advenier C. Lack of effect of terfenadine on theophylline pharmacokinetics and metabolism in normal subjects. Br J Clin Pharmac (1989) 27, 391–5.

6 Hasegawa T, Takagi K, Kuzuya T, Nadai M, Apichartpichean R, Muraoka I. Effect of mequitazine on the pharmacokinetics of theophylline in

asthmatic patients. Eur J Clin Pharmacol (1990) 38, 255–8.

7 Luskin SS, Fitzsimmons WE, MacLeeod CM, Luskin AT. Pharmacokinetic evaluation of the terfenadine-theophylline interaction. J Allergy Clin Immunol (1989) 83, 406–11.

8 Wittenbrink-Dix AM, Neugebauer G, Fuhr U, Neubert P, Besenfelder E, Woelke-Seidl E. Harder S, Staib AH. Study of potential kinetic interactions of picumast dihydrochloride and theophylline *in vitro* and after oral administration in man. Arzneim.-Forsch/Drug Res (1989) 39, 1339–43.

Theophylline + Barbiturates

Abstract/Summary

Theophylline serum levels can be reduced by the concurrent use of phenobarbitone (phenobarbital) or pentobarbitone (pentobarbital). A single report describes a similar interaction with quinalbarbitone (secobarbital) and would be expected with other barbiturates.

Clinical evidence

(a) Pentobarbitone (Pentobarbital)

A single case report describes a man who showed a 95% rise in the clearance of theophylline when treated with high dose pentobarbitone.[6] 100 mg pentobarbitone given to normal subjects for 10 days increased the clearance of theophylline by 40% (range 4–79%) and reduced the AUC by 26% (range + 3.6 to – 44%).[9]

(b) Phenobarbitone (Phenobarbital)

After taking phenobarbitone (2 mg/kg daily) for 19 days the mean steady-state serum theophylline levels in seven asthmatic children (6–12 years old) were reduced by 30%, and the clearance was increased 35% (range 12–71%).[1]

Increases in theophylline clearance of up to 34% and decreases in half-life have been seen in other studies in normal subjects given phenobarbitone for periods of 2–4 weeks.[2–4] The effects of phenobarbitone can be additive with the effects of phenytoin and smoking.[12] One study found that premature babies needed more theophylline if treated with phenobarbitone,[8] but a later study failed to confirm this.[10] In contrast, an early study found no significant change in the half-life of theophylline in asthmatic children given 16 or 32 mg phenobarbitone three times daily.[11]

(c) Quinalbarbitone (Secobarbital)

A 337% increase in the clearance of theophylline occurred over a 4-week period in a child treated with quinalbarbitone (secobarbital).[7]

Mechanism

Barbiturates are potent liver enzyme inducing agents which increase the metabolism of theophylline by the liver, thereby hastening its removal from the body. This has been shown in animal studies[5] and is almost certainlyt true for man.

Importance and management

A moderately well documented, established and clinically important interaction. Patients treated with phenobarbitone or pentobaribitone may need above-average doses of theophylline to achieve and maintain adequate serum levels. Concurrent use should be monitored and appropriate dosage increases made. All of the barbiturates can cause enzyme induction and may, to a greater or lesser extent, be expected to behave similarly. This is illustrated by the single report involving quinalbarbitone.

References

1 Saccar CL, Danish M, Ragni MC, Rocci ML, Greene J, Yaffe SJ, Mansmann HC. The effects of phenobarbital on theophylline disposition in children with asthma. J Allergy Clin Immunol (1985) 75, 716–9.
2 Landay RA, Gonzalez MA, Taylor JC. Effect of phenobarbital on theophylline disposition. J Allergy Clin Immunol (1978) 62, 27.
3 Piafsky KM, Sitar DS, Ogilvie RI. Effect of phenobarbital on the disposition of intravenous theophylline. Clin Pharmacol Ther (1977) 22, 336.
4 Jacobs MH, Senior R. Personal communication (1978) cited by Ogilvie RI in Clin Pharmacokinetics (1978) 3, 267–93.
5 Williams JF, Szentivanyi A. Implications of hepatic metabolising activity in the therapy of bronchial asthma. J Allergy Clin Immunol (1975) 55, 125.
6 Gibson GA, Blouin RA, Bauer LA, Rapp RP, Tibbs PA. Influence of high dose pentobarbital on theophylline pharmacokinetics: a case report. Ther Drug Monit (1985) 7, 181–4.
7 Paladino JA, Blumer NA, Maddox RR. Effect of secobarbital on theophylline clearance. Ther Drug Monit (1983) 5, 133–9.
8 Yazdani M, Kissling GE, Tran TH, Gottschalk SK, Schuth CR. Phenobarbital increases the theophylline requirements of premature infants being treated for apnea. Am J Dis Child (1987) 141, 97–9.
9 Dahlqvist R, Steiner E, Koike Y, von Bahr C, Lind M, Billing B. Induction of theophylline metabolism by pentobarbital. Ther Drug Monitor (1989) 11, 408–10.
10 Kandrotas RJ, Cranfield TL, Gal P, Ransom L, Weaver RL. Effect of phenobarbital administration on theophylline clearance in premature neonates. Ther Drug Monit (1990) 12, 139–43.
11 Goldstein EO, Eney RD, Mellits ED, Solomon H, Johnson G. Effect of phenobarbital on theophylline metabolism in asthmatic children. Ann Allergy (1977) 39, 69.
12 Nicholson JP, Basile SA, Cury JD. Massive theophylline dosing in a heavy smoker receiving both phenytoin and phenobarbital. Ann Pharmacother (1992) 26, 334–6.

Theophylline + BCG vaccine

Abstract/Summary

There is evidence that BCG vaccine can cause a small increase in the serum levels of theophylline but the clinical importance of this is uncertain.

Clinical evidence, mechanism, importance and management

Two weeks after receiving BCG vaccination (0.1 ml *Tubersol*, equivalent to five TU of tuberculin PPD), the clearance of single doses of theophylline in 12 normal subjects was reduced by 21% and the theophylline half-life was prolonged by 14% (range 4 to 47%).[1] It seems possible therefore that the occasional patient may develop some signs of theophylline toxicity, particularly if their serum levels are already towards the top end of the therapeutic range. More study is needed to determine the clinical importance of this interaction.

Reference

1 Gray JD, Renton KW, Hung OR. Depression of theophylline elimination following BCG vaccination. Br J Clin Pharmac (1983) 16, 735–7.

Theophylline + Beta-agonist bronchodilators

Abstract/Summary

The concurrent use of theophylline and beta-agonist bronchodilators is common and considered advantageous but some adverse reactions can occur, the most serious being hypokalaemia (with salbutamol (albuterol) and terbutaline) and increased heart rate. Some patients may show a significant fall in serum theophylline levels if given oral salbutamol (albuterol) or isoprenaline (isoproterenol). See also Theophylline + Phenylpropanolamine.

Clinical evidence, mechanism, importance and management

Concurrent use is very common and is regarded as advantageous, but the reports outlined below illustrate some of the disadvantages and adverse effects which have been identified:

(a) Theophylline + Ephedrine

A double-blind randomized study of theophylline, ephedrine and hydroxyzine given separately and together (conventional ephedrine/theophylline ratios of 25:130) to 23 children showed that given singly none of the drugs caused a significant number of adverse reactions, but ephedrine/theophylline in combination was associated with insomnia (14 patients), nervousness (13 patients) and gastrointestinal complaints (18 patients) including vomiting (12 patients). This combination was also no more effective than theophylline alone.[1,2] A previous study in 12 asthmatic children produced essentially similar results,[3] however a later study suggested that no adverse effects occurred if lower doses of ephedrine were used.[14]

(b) Theophylline + Isoprenaline (Isoproterenol)

The infusion of isoprenaline increased the clearance of theophylline (given as IV aminophylline) by 19% in six asthmatic children with status asthmaticus and respiratory failure.[13] Another study in 12 patients with severe status asthmaticus found that an isoprenaline infusion (0.77 µg/kg/min) caused a mean fall in serum theophylline levels of almost 6 μg/ml.[16] The levels rose again when the isoprenaline was stopped.[16] A very marked increase in clearance (+354%) was seen in another patient also taking phenytoin, methylprednisolone and terbutaline.[15]

(c) Theophylline + Orciprenaline (Metaproterenol)

Orciprenaline given orally (20 mg 8-hourly) or by inhalation (1.95 mg 6-hourly) had no effect on the clearance of theophylline in six normal subjects.[11] This confirms a previous finding in asthmatic children in whom it was shown that orciprenaline does not alter serum theophylline levels.[12]

(d) Theophylline + Salbutamol (Albuterol)

Theophylline significantly increased the hypokalaemia and tachycardia caused by infusions of salbutamol in normal subjects, suggesting an increased risk of profound hypokalaemia and cardiac arrhythmias in acutely ill hypoxic patients.[5] A potentially dangerous additive effect on heart rate was seen in one study in nine patients given aminophylline and salbutamol[20] and increased tachycardia in two others,[8,9] whereas another study found that neither the occurrence nor the severity of arrhythmias seem to be changed.[18] Respiratory arrest possibly related to hypokalaemia occurred in a girl of 10 given theophylline and salbutamol.[19]

Reduced theophylline levels (clearance increased 14%[21]), worsened peak flow rates[8,9] but no changes in clearance when given by inhalation[21] have also been described. A 25% reduction in serum theophylline levels while taking 16 mg oral salbutamol were described in one study in patients.[17] A child of 19 months needed a threefold increase in theophylline dosage given intravenous salbutamol and theophylline because of an increase in the theophylline clearance.[6] These reports contrast with another in normal subjects which found no change in the pharmacokinetics of theophylline.[10]

(e) Theophylline + Terbutaline

Intravenous terbutaline caused a fall in serum potassium levels and rises in blood glucose, pulse rates and systolic blood pressures of normal subjects given theophylline.[4] Terbutaline was found in another study to decrease serum theophylline levels by about 10% in asthmatics, but the control of asthma was improved.[7] Another study in children given slow-release theophylline and terbutaline found no increases in side-effects and simple additive effects on the control of their asthma.[22] Yet another study found no changes in the pharmacokinetics of aminophylline in asthmatic children when given terbutaline.[23]

References

1 Weinberger M, Bronsky E. Interaction of ephedrine and theophylline. Clin Pharmacol Ther (1974) 15, 223.
2 Weinberger M, Bronsky E, Bensch GW, Brock GN, Yeckles JJ. Interaction of ephedrine and theophylline. Clin Pharmacol Ther (1975) 17, 585.
3 Weinberger M, Bronsky EA. Evaluation of oral bronchodilator therapy in asthmatic children. J Pediat (1974) 84, 421.
4 Smith SR, Kendall MJ. Potentiation of the adverse effects of intravenous terbutaline by oral theophylline. Br J Clin Pharmac (1986) 21, 451–3.
5 Whyte KF, Reid C, Addis GJ, Whitesmith R, Reid JL. Salbutamol induced hypokalaemia: the effect of theophylline alone and in combination with adrenaline. Br J Clin Pharmac (1988) 25, 571–8.
6 Amirav I, Amitai Y, Avital A, Godfrey S. Enhancement of theophylline clearance by intravenous albuterol. Chest (1988) 94, 444–5.
7 Garty MS, Keslin LS, Ilfeld DN, Mazar A, Spitzer S, Rosenfeld JB. Increased theophylline clearance by terbutaline in asthmatic adults. Clin Pharmacol Ther (1988) 43, 150.
8 Danziger Y, Garty M, Volwitz B, Ilfeld D, Versano I, Rosenfeld JB. Reduction of serum theophylline levels by terbutaline in children with asthma. Clin Pharmacol Ther (1985) 37, 469–71.
9 Dawson KP, Fergusson DM. Effects of oral theophylline and oral salbutamol in the treatment of asthma. Arch Dis Child (1982) 57, 674–6.
10 McCann JP, McElnay JC, Nicholls DP, Scott MG, Stanford CF. Oral salbutamol does not affect theophylline kinetics. Br J Pharmac (1986) 89 (Proc Suppl) 715P.
11 Conrad KA, Woodworth JR. Orciprenaline does not alter theophylline elimination. Br J Clin Pharmac (1981) 12, 756–7.
12 Rachelefsky GS, Katz RM, Mickey MR, Siegel SC. Metaproterenol and theophylline in asthmatic children. Ann Allergy (1980) 45, 207–12.
13 Hemstreet MP, Miles MV, Rutland RO. Effect of intravenous isoproterenol on theophylline kinetics. J Allerg Clin Immunol (1982) 69, 360–4.
14 Tinkelman DG, Avener SE. Ephedrine therapy in asthmatic children. J Amer Med Ass (1977) 237, 553.
15 Griffith JA, Kozloski GD. Isoproterenol-theophylline interaction: possible potentiation by other drugs. Clin Pharm (1990) 9, 54–7.
16 O'Rourke PP, Crone RK. Effect of isoproterenol on measured theophylline levels. Crit Care Med (1984) 12, 373–5.
17 Terra Filho M, Santos SR, Cukier A, Verrastro C, Carvalho-Pinto RM, Fiss E, Vargas FS. Effects of adrenergic beta-2 agonists by oral route on theophylline blood levels. Revista Do Hospital Das Clinicas; Faculdade De Medicina Da Universidade De Sao Paulo (1991) 46, 170–2.
18 Poukkula A, Korhonen UR, Huikuri H, Linnaluoto M. Theophylline and salbutamol in combination in patients with obstructive pulmonary disease and concurrent heart disease: effect on cardiac arrhythmias. J Int Med (1989) 226, 229–34.
19 Epelbaum S, Benhamou PH, Pautard JC, Devoldere C, Kremp O, Piussan Ch. Arrêt respiratoire chez une enfant asthmatique traitée par bêta-2-mimétiques et théophylline. Rôle possible de l'hypokaliémie dans les décès subits des asthmatiques. Ann Pédiatr (Paris) (1989) 36, 473–5.
20 Georgopoulos D, Wong D, Anthonisen NR. Interactive effects of systemically adminstered salbutamol and aminophylline in patients with chronic obstructive pulmonary disease. Am Rev Respir Dis (1988) 138, 1499–1503.
21 Amitai Y, Glustein J, Godfrey S. Enhancement of theophylline clearance by oral albuterol. Chest (1992) 102, 786–9.
22 Chow OKW, Fung KP. Slow-release terbutaline and theophylline for the long-term therapy of children with asthma: a latin square and factorial study of drug effects and interactions. Pediatrics (1989) 84, 119–25.
23 Wang Y, Yin A, Yu Z. Effects of bricanyl on the pharmacokinetics of aminophylline in asthmatic patients. Zhongguo Yiyuan Yaoxue Zazhi (1992) 12, 389–90.

Theophylline + Beta-blockers

Abstract/Summary

Propranolol reduces the clearance of theophylline. More importantly, non-selective beta-blockers such as nadolol and propranolol should not be given to asthmatic patients because they can cause bronchospasm. The concurrent use of theophylline and selective beta-blockers such as atenolol, bisoprolol or metoprolol is not totally contraindicated, but some

caution is still appropriate. See also 'Antiasthmatics + Beta-blockers' in Chapter 10.

Clinical evidence

Pharmacokinetics

A study in nine normal subjects (six of whom smoked 10–30 cigarettes daily) found that the clearance of theophylline was reduced 37% by propranolol (40 mg 6-hourly) but not in the group as a whole by metoprolol (50 mg 6-hourly), although the smokers did show some reduction in clearance.[1]

Three other studies found that atenolol[4,5] and bisoprolol,[3] both selective beta-blockers, and nadolol,[4] a non-selective blocker, do not affect the pharmacokinetics of theophylline.

Mechanism

Those beta-blockers which interact with theophylline do so by inhibiting its metabolism (demethylation).[6] The non-selective beta-blockers can cause serious bronchoconstriction which opposes the bronchodilatory effects of theophylline.

Importance and management

The risk of severe, possibly even fatal, bronchospasm in asthmatics would seem to be far more important than any pharmacokinetic interaction (see the warning in 'Antiasthmatics + Beta-blockers' in Chapter 24). The non-selective beta-blockers such as propranolol (see the list at the beginning of Chapter 10) are normally contraindicated in asthmatic patients. Bronchospasm can occur whether given orally or even as eye drops. The clinical importance of a possible interaction between theophylline and selective beta-blockers such as metoprolol in smokers awaits assessment. Some caution would seem appropriate because metoprolol can block the inotropic effects of theophylline,[2] and also because the safety of the selective (beta-1 selective) beta-blockers in asthmatic patients is by no means certain.

References

1 Conrad KA, Nyman DW. Effects of metoprolol and propranolol on theophylline elimination. Clin Pharmacol Ther (1980) 28, 463.
2 Conrad KA, Prosnitz EH. Cardiovascular effects of theophylline. Partial attenuation by beta-blockade. Eur J Clin Pharmacol (1981) 21, 109.
3 Warrington SJ, Johnston A, Lewis Y, Murphy M. Bisoprolol: studies of potential interactions with theophylline and warfarin in healthy volunteers. J Cardiovasc Pharmacol (1990) 16 (Suppl 5) S164–8.
4 Corsi CM, Nafziger AN, Pieper JA, Bertino JS. Lack of effect of atenolol and nadolol on the metabolism of theophylline. Br J Clin Pharmac (1990) 29, 265–8.
5 Ceresa LA, Bertino JS, Ludwig EA, Savliwala M, Middleton E, Slaughter RL. Lack of effect of atenolol on the pharmacokinetics of theophylline. Br J Clin Pharmac (1988) 26, 800–2.
6 Greenblatt DJ. Impairment of antipyrine clearance in humans by propranolol. Circulation (1978) 57, 1161.

Theophylline and Related drugs + Caffeine

Abstract/Summary

Caffeine can raise serum theophylline levels and a few individuals may experience some adverse effects. Furafylline, a new xanthine, causes a very marked rise in caffeine levels accompanied by toxicity.

Clinical evidence, mechanism, importance and management

(a) Theophylline + Caffeine

Coffee can decrease the clearance of theophylline by 18–27%, prolong its half-life by up to 44% and increase its steady-state serum levels by as much as 23%.[1,3,4] The subjects under study drank 2–10 cups of coffee daily. Two of the subjects who did not normally drink coffee experienced headaches and nausea.[3]

The probable mechanism of the interaction is that the two drugs compete for the same metabolic pathway so that they accumulate, and when caffeine levels are high some of it is converted to theophylline. There would however seem to be no good reason for those on theophylline to avoid caffeine (in coffee, tea, 'Coke', etc), but if otherwise unexplained adverse effects occur it might be worth checking if caffeine is responsible.

(b) Theophylline + Furafylline

A study on furafylline, a new theophylline-like xanthine compound, found that it causes caffeine (ingested in coffee) to accumulate in the body to a very marked extent (a 5–10-fold rise) accompanied by a number of unacceptable side-effects.[2] The probable reason is that the furafylline inhibits the metabolism and clearance of caffeine from the body. It seems likely therefore that patients on furafylline may need to limit their caffeine consumption very considerably. The authors of this report also point out that the toxic side-effects of some other new drugs may be related to caffeine-intoxication.

References

1 Loi CM, Jue SG, Bush ED, Crowley JJ, Vestal RE. Effect of caffeine dose on theophylline metabolism. Clin Res (1987) 35, 377A.
2 Tarrus E, Cami J, Roberts DJ, Spickett RGW, Celdran E, Segura J. Accumulation of caffeine in healthy volunteers treated with furafylline. Br J Clin Pharmac (1987) 23, 9–18.
3 Jonkman JHG, Sollie FAE, Sauter R, Steinijans VW. The influence of caffeine on the steady-state pharmacokinetics of theophylline. Clin Pharmacol Ther (1991) 49, 248–55.
4 Sato J, Nakata H, Owada E, Kikuta T, Umetsu M, Ito K. Influence of usual intake of dietary caffeine on single-dose kinetics of theophylline in healthy human subjects. Eur J Clin Pharmacol (1993) 44, 295–8.

Theophylline + Calcium channel blockers

Abstract/Summary

Concurrent use normally seems to have no adverse effect on the control of asthma, despite the small or modest changes (increases or decreases) in serum theophylline levels reported with diltiazem, felodipine, nifedipine and verapamil. However there are isolated case reports of unexplained intoxication in two patients given nifedipine and one patient given verapamil.

Clinical evidence

(a) Theophylline + Diltiazem

90 mg diltiazem twice daily for 10 days reduced the clearance of theophylline (given as aminophylline) by 21% in nine normal subjects, and increased its half-life from 6.1 to 7.5 hr.[8] A 12% fall in clearance was found in another study,[9] whereas other studies found no clinically significant changes in theophylline levels in 18 patients given 480 mg daily for 7 days[17] or in the theophylline half-life.[5] A very small rise in serum theophylline was seen in another study.[19]

(b) Theophylline + Felodipine

5 mg felodipine 8-hourly for 4 days reduced the plasma AUC of theophylline in 10 normal subjects by 18.3% (from 270 to 220 μmol.h.l^{-1}).[13]

(c) Theophylline + Nifedipine

20 mg slow-release nifedipine twice daily reduced the serum theophylline levels of eight asthmatics by 30% (from 9.7 to 6.8 μg/ml). Levels fell below the therapeutic range (Ld4 μg/ml) in three of the patients, but no changes in the control of the asthma were seen as measured by peak flow determinations and symptom scores.[4] No changes or only small or modest changes in the pharmacokinetics of theophylline were seen in other studies in normal subjects[2,7,18,19] or asthmatic patients also given nifedipine.[6,10,17,21] The control of the asthma remained unchanged.[6,21]

In contrast there are two case reports of patients who developed theophylline intoxication apparently due to the addition of nifedipine.[11,12] During a Swan Ganz catheter study of patient response to nifedipine for pulmonary hypertension, two patients developed serious nifedipine side-effects which responded dramatically to intravenous aminophylline.[14]

(d) Theophylline + Verapamil

80 mg verapamil 6-hourly for 2 days had no effect on the pharmacokinetics of theophylline (200 mg aminophylline 6-hourly) given to five asthmatics, and no effect on their spiro-metric measurements(FVC, FEV1, FEF25-7).[1] Other studies found reductions in theophylline clearance ranging between 11.5% and 23%,[2,5,9,15,16,20,23] one of which showed that the extent depended on the verapamil dosage.[23] An isolated report describes a woman on digoxin and theophylline who developed signs of toxicity (tachycardia, nausea, vomiting) which was attributed to the concurrent use of verapamil.[3] Her theophylline serum levels doubled over a 6-day period.

Mechanism

It is believed that diltiazem, nifedipine and verapamil can alter (increase or decrease) the metabolism of theophylline by the liver to a small extent, as a result its loss from the body may be changed. The P450 isoform CYP1A2 possibly has a small part to play in the verapamil interaction.[22] Felodipine possibly reduces theophylline absorption.

Importance and management

Well documented. The results are not entirely consistent but the overall picture is that concurrent use is normally safe. Despite the small or modest decreases in the clearance or absorption of theophylline seen with diltiazem, felodipine and verapamil, and the quite large reductions in serum levels seen in one study with nifedipine, no adverse changes in the control of the asthma were seen in any of the studies. However, very occasionally and unpredictably theophylline levels have risen enough to cause intoxication in patients given nifedipine (two patients) or verapamil (one patient), so that it would be prudent to monitor the effects. There seems to be no information about other calcium channel blockers.

References

1 Gotz VP, Russell WL. Effect of verapamil on theophylline disposition. Chest (1987) 92, 75S.

2 Robson RA, Miners JO, Birkett DJ. Selective inhibitory effects of nifedipine and verapamil on oxidative metabolism: effects on theophylline. Br J Clin Pharmac (1988) 25, 397–400.

3 Burnakis TG, Seldon M, Czaplicki AD. Increased serum theophylline concentrations secondary to oral verapamil. Clin Pharm (1983) 2, 458–61.

4 Smith SR, Wiggins J, Stableforth DE, Skinner C, Kendall MJ. Effect of nifedipine on serum theophylline concentrations and asthma control. Thorax (1987) 42, 794–6.

5 Abernethy DR, Egan JM, Dickinson TH, Carrum G. Substrate-selective inhibition by verapamil and diltiazem: differential disposition of antipyrine and theophylline in humans. J Pharmacol Exp Ther (1988) 244, 994–9.

6 Garty M, Cohen E, Mazar A, Ilfeld DN, Spitzer S, Rosenfeld JB. Effect of nifedipine and theophylline in asthma. Clin Pharmacol Ther (1986) 40, 195–8.

7 Jackson SHD, Shah K, Debbas NMG, Johnston A, Peverel-Cooper CA, Turner P. The interaction between IV theophylline and chronic oral dosing with slow release nifedipine in volunteers. Br J Clin Pharmac (1986) 21, 389–92.

8 Nafziger AN, May JJ, Bertino JS. Inhibition of theophylline elimination by diltiazem therapy. J Clin Pharmacol (1987) 27, 862–5.

9 Sirmans A, Pieper JA, Lalonde RL, Self TH, Smith D. Effect of calcium channel antagonists on theophylline disposition. Drug Intell Clin Pharm (1987) 21, 16A.

10 Christopher MA, Harman E, Bell JA, Hendeles L. Measurement of

steady-state theophylline concentrations before and during concurrent therapy with diltiazem or nifedipine. Drug Intell Clin Pharm (1987) 21, 4A.

11 Parrillo SJ, Venditto SJ. Elevated theophylline blood levels from institution of nifedipine therapy. Ann Emerg Med (1984) 43, 216–17.

12 Harrod CS. Theophylline toxicity and nifedipine. Ann Intern Med (1987) 106, 480.

13 Bratel T, Billing B, Dahlqvist R. Felodipine reduces the absorption of theophylline in man. Eur J Clin Pharmacol (1989) 36, 481–5.

14 Kalar L, Bone MF, Ariaraj SJP. Nifedipine-aminophylline interaction. J Clin Pharmacol (1988) 28, 1056–7.

15 Nielsen-Kudsk J, Buhl JS, Johannessen AC. Verapamil-induced inhibition of theophylline elimination in healthy humans. Pharmacol Toxicol (1990) 66, 101–3.

16 Rindone JP, Zuniga R, Sock JA. The influence of verapamil on theophylline serum concentrations. Drug Metab Drug Interact (1989) 7, 143–7.

17 Christopher MA, Harman E, Hendeles L. Clinical relevance of the interaction of theophylline with diltiazem or nifedipine. Chest (1989) 95, 309–13.

18 Adebayo GI, Mabadeje FB. Effect of nifedipine on antipyrine and theophylline disposition. Biopharm Drug Disp (1990) 11, 157–64.

19 Smith SR, Haffner CA, Kendall MJ. The influence of nifedipine and diltiazem on serum theophylline concentration-time profiles. J Clin Pharmacol Ther (1989) 14, 403–8.

20 Gin AS, Stringer KA, Welage LS, Wilton JH, Matthews GE. The effect of verapamil on the pharmacokinetic disposition of theophylline in cigarette smokers. J Clin Pharmacol (1989) 29, 728–32.

21 Yilmaz E, Canberk A, Eroglu L. Nifedipine alters serum theophylline levels in asthmatic patients with hypertension. Fundam Clin Pharmacol (1991) 5, 341–5.

22 Fuhr U, Woodcock BG, Siewert M. Verapamil and drug metabolism by the cytochrome P450 isoform CYP1A2. Eur J Clin Pharmacol (1992) 42, 463–4.

23 Stringer KA, Mallet J, Clarke M, Lindenfeld JA. The effect of three different oral doses of verapamil on the disposition of theophylline. Eur J Clin Pharmacol (1992) 43, 35–8.

Theophylline + Carbamazepine

Abstract/Summary

Two case reports describe a marked fall in serum theophylline levels during the concurrent use of carbamazepine. Another single case report describes a fall in serum carbamazepine levels when theophylline was given.

Clinical evidence

(a) Theophylline serum levels reduced

An asthmatic girl of 11 was well controlled for 2 months with theophylline until the phenobarbitone she was taking was replaced by carbamazepine. The asthma worsened, her theophylline serum levels became subtherapeutic and the half-life of the theophylline halved (from 5.25 to 2.75 h). Asthmatic control was restored when the carbamazepine was replaced by ethotoin.[1] The clearance of theophylline in another patient was doubled when carbamazepine (600 mg daily) was withdrawn.[3]

(b) Carbamazepine serum levels reduced

A girl of 10 showed a fall in serum carbamazepine levels (trough concentrations roughly halved) when given theophylline, and

she experienced grand mal convulsions. Her serum theophylline levels were also unusually high (142 mol/l) for the dosage taken (5 mg/kg 6-hourly), so it may be that the convulsions were as much due to this as to the fall in carbamazepine levels.[2]

Mechanism

Not understood, but it has been suggested that each drug possibly increases the liver metabolism and clearance of the other drug, resulting in a reduction in their effects.[1,2]

Importance and management

Information seems to be limited to the reports cited so that their general importance is uncertain. Concurrent use need not be avoided, but it would be prudent to check that the serum concentrations of each drug (and their effects) are not reduced to subtherapeutic levels.

References

1 Rosenberry KR, Defusco CJ, Mansmann HC, McGeady SJ. Reduced theophylline half-life induced by carbamazepine therapy. J Ped (1983) 102, 472–4.

2 Mitchell EA, Dower JC, Green RJ. Interaction between carbamazepine and theophylline. NZ Med J (1986) 99, 69–70.

3 Reed RC, Schwartz HJ. Phenytoin-theophylline-quinidine interaction. N Engl J Med (1983) 308, 724–5.

Theophylline + Cephalosporins, Lincomycin

Abstract/Summary

Ceftibuten, cephalexin and lincomycin appear not to interact with theophylline. Cefaclor has been implicated in the development of theophylline toxicity in a child but other studies failed to confirm that this normally occurs.

Clinical evidence, mechanism, importance and management

A trial on nine healthy adults given single doses of aminophylline (5 mg/kg IV) found that the concurrent use of cephalexin, 250 mg 6-hourly for 48 h, had no significant effect on the kinetics of theophylline.[1] 200 mg ceftibuten twice daily for 7 days was also found to have no significant effect on the pharmacokinetics of single IV doses of theophylline given to 12 normal subjects.[5] A single case report suggested that cefaclor might have been responsible for the development of theophylline toxicity in a child,[6] but a single dose and a steady-state study found that 750 mg cefaclor daily for 8 and 9 days respectively had no effect on the pharmacokinetics of theophylline.[2,3] This was confirmed in another study.[4] Another study found that lincomycin did not have an important effect on theophylline.[7]

No special precautions, apart from those normally taken with theophylline, seem to be necessary with any of these antibiotics.

References

1 Pfeifer HJ, Greenblatt DJ, Friedman P. Effects of three antibiotics on theophylline kinetics. Clin Pharmacol Ther (1979) 26, 36.

2 Bachmann K, Schwartz J, Forney RB, Jauregui L. Impact of cefaclor on the pharmacokinetics of theophylline. Ther Drug Monit (1986) 8, 151–4.

3 Jonkman JHG, van der Boon WJV, Schoenmaker R, Holtkamp A, Hempenius J. Clinical pharmacokinetics of theophylline during co-treatment with cefaclor. Int J Clin Pharmacol Ther Toxicol (1986) 24, 88–92.

4 Jauregui L, Bachmann K, Forney R, Bischoff M, Schwartz J. The impact of cefaclor on the pharmacokinetics of theophylline. Recent Adv Chemother. Proc Int Congr Chemother 14th Antimicrob Section 1 (1985) 694–5.

5 Bachmann K, Schwartz J, Jauregui L, Martin M, Nunlee M. Failure of ceftibuten to alter single dose theophylline clearance. J Clin Pharmacol (1990) 30, 444–8.

6 Hammond D, Abate MA. Theophylline toxicity, acute illness, and cefaclor administration. DICP Ann Pharmacotherapy (1989) 23, 339–40.

7 Halawa B. Interakcje teofiliny z erytromycna, ryfampicyna i linkomycyna. Polski Tygodnik Lekarski (1988) XLIII, 854–7.

Theophylline + Cimetidine, Etintidine, Famotidine or Ranitidine

Abstract/Summary

Theophylline serum levels are raised by cimetidine and toxicity may develop if appropriate reductions (one third to a half) are not made in the theophylline dosage, however aminophylline and low-dose intravenous cimetidine appear not to interact significantly. Etintidine behaves like cimetidine. Ranitidine and famotidine would not be expected to interact like cimetidine but there is evidence that sometimes they do so.

Clinical evidence

(a) Cimetidine

A number of case reports describe the development of toxic theophylline levels in patients treated with cimetidine.[1,7,8,11] Well-controlled pharmacokinetic studies in groups of healthy subjects[2,4–6,9,21,31,42] and patients[3,4,10,13,18,30,38] also all clearly demonstrate that cimetidine (800–1200 mg daily) prolongs the theophylline half-life by about 60% and reduces the clearance by 30–40%. Trough serum levels are raised about one-third.[13] The extent of the interaction does not depend on the dosage of cimetidine within the 1200–2400 mg daily range[9] but appears to be dose-dependent below 800 mg daily.[45] One study found that the inhibitory effects of cimetidine and ciprofloxacin were additive.[41] No clinically important interaction seems to occur with intravenous aminophylline and low-dose iv cimetidine or intermittent infusion.[39]

(b) Etintidine

800 mg etintidine daily for 4 days in 10 normal subjects almost

tripled the half-life of theophylline (from 6 to 16.8 h) and reduced the clearance by about 65% (from 0.0564 to 0.02 l/h/kg).[28]

(c) Famotidine

40 mg famotidine twice daily for 5 days had no effect on the pharmacokinetics of theophylline in 10 healthy subjects.[23] Four asthmatics on theophylline were treated with famotidine without problems for 4–8 weeks.[44] In contrast, another study in a patient with chronic obstructive lung disease and liver impairment found that after taking 40 mg famotidine daily for eight days, his serum theophylline levels and the AUC after an intravenous dose were raised (+78%) and the clearance lowered (halved).[32] A later study by the same authors in seven patients with COPD similarly treated but with normal liver function found that the theophylline AUC was increased 57% and the clearance reduced by 35%.[46] This interaction has also been described in one other patient.[36]

(d) Ranitidine

Pharmacokinetic studies on considerable numbers of subjects and patients failed to find that ranitidine affects the pharmacokinetics of theophylline,[8,12,14,16,24,30,31,34,35,42] even in daily doses up to 4200 mg daily.[22] However seven reports describe a total of eight patients who developed theophylline toxicity when given ranitidine.[19,20,26,27,29,33,37] The validity of these reports has been challenged.[40,43]

Mechanism

Cimetidine is a well-recognised enzyme inhibitor which depresses the metabolism of theophylline by the liver, thereby prolonging its stay in the body and raising its serum levels. It has also been suggested that a theophylline-cimetidine complex may be formed in the body which is less easily metabolized than theophylline.[17] Etintidine behaves similarly. Famotidine and ranitidine do not have enzyme inhibiting effects so that it is no clear why they sometimes appear to behave like cimetidine.

Importance and management

The theophylline-cimetidine interaction is very well documented (not all the references being listed here), very well established and clinically important. Theophylline serum levels normally rise by about one-third, but much greater increases have been seen in individual patients. Reduce the dosage to avoid toxicity (initial reductions of 30–50% have been suggested[8]) and monitor the effects. There is some disagreement about whether smokers do or do not need a greater reduction.[15,25] The extent of the interaction appears to be greatest in the elderly.[45] Aminophylline and low dose cimetidine appear not to interact significantly.[39] Etintidine appears to behave like cimetidine.

The situation with ranitidine is not totally clear. It would not be expected to interact but it is claimed to do so very occasionally and unpredictably. Current opinion is that normally no special precautions are needed.[43] Famotidine would also not be expected to interact but, as with ranitidine, the effects should be monitored because there is evidence that serum theophylline levels can increase.

References

1 Weinberger MM, Smith G, Milavetz G, Hendeles L. Decreased theophylline clearance due to cimetidine. N Engl J Med (1981) 304, 672.
2 Jackson JE, Powell JR, Wandell M, Bentley J, Dorr R. Cimetidine-theophylline interaction. Pharmacologist (1980) 22, 231.
3 Campbell MA, Platetka JR, Jackson JE, Moon JF, Finley PR. Cimetidine decreases theophylline clearance. Ann Intern Med (1981) 95, 68.
4 Wood L, Grice J, Petroff V, McGuffie C, Roberts RK. Effect of cimetidine on the disposition of theophylline. Aust NZ J Med (1980) 10, 586.
5 Roberts RK, Grice J, Wood L, Petroff V, McGuffie C. Cimetidine impairs the elimination of theophylline and antipyrine. Gastroenterol (1981) 81, 19.
6 Reitberg DP, Bernhard H, Schentag JJ. Alteration of theophylline clearance and half-life by cimetidine. Ann Intern Med (1981) 95, 582.
7 Lofgren RP, Gilbertson A. Cimetidine and theophylline. Ann Intern Med (1982) 96, 378.
8 Bauman JH, Kimelblatt BJ, Carracio DR, Silverman HM, Simon GI, Beck GJ. Cimetidine-theophylline interaction. Report of four patients. Ann Allergy (1982) 48, 100–2.
9 Powell JR, Rogers JF, Wargin WA, Cross RE, Eshelman FN. The influence of cimetidine vs ranitidine on theophylline pharmacokinetics. J Pharmacol Ther (1982) 31, 261.
10 Fenje PC, Isles AF, Baltodan A, Macleod SM, Soldin S. Interaction of cimetidine and theophylline in two infants. Can Med Ass J (1982) 126, 1178.
11 Uzzan D, Uzzan B, Bernard N, Caubarrere I. Interaction medicamenteuse de la cimetidine et de la theophylline. Nouv Presse Med (1982) 11, 1950.
12 Ruff F. Interferences medicamenteuses de la theophylline. Absence d'interaction theophylline-ranitidine. Nouv Presse Med (1982) 11, 3512.
13 Vestal RE, Thummel KE, Musser B, Mercer GD. Cimetidine inhibits theophylline clearance in patients with chronic obstructive pulmonary disease. A study using stable isotope methodology during multiple oral dose administration. Br J Clin Pharmacol (1983) 15, 411–18.
14 Powell JR, Rogers JF, Wargin WA, Cross RE, Eshelman FN. Inhibition of theophylline clearance by cimetidine but not ranitidine. Arch Intern Med (1984) 144, 484–6.
15 Grygiel JJ, Miners JO, Drew R, Birkett DJ. Differential effects of cimetidine on theophylline metabolic pathways. Eur J Clin Pharmacol (1984) 26, 335–40.
16 Ferrari M, Angelili GP, Barozzi E, Olivieri M, Penna S, Accardi R. A comparative study of ranitidile and cimetidine effects on theophylline metabolism. Giornale Italialo Malattie del Torace (1184) 38, 31–4.
17 Ritschel WA, Alcorn GJ, Streng WH, Zoglio MA. Cimetidine-theophylline complex formation. Meth Find Exptl Clin Pharmacol (1983) 5, 55–8.
18 Cohen IA, Johnson CE, Berardi RR, Hyneck ML, Achem SR. Cimetidine-theophylline interaction: effects of age and cimetidine dose. Ther Drug Monit (1985) 7, 426–34.
19 Fernandes E, Melewicz FM. Ranitidine and theophylline. Ann Intern Med (1984) 100, 459.
20 Gardner ME, Sikorski GW. Ranitidine and theophylline. Ann Intern Med (1985) 102, 559.
21 Mulkey PM, Murphy JE, Shleifer NH. Steady-stade theophylline pharmacokinetics during and after short-term cimetidine administration. Clin Pharm (1983) 2, 439–41.
22 Kelly HW, Powell JR, Donohue JF. Ranitidine at very large doses does not inhibit theophylline elimination. Clin Pharmacol Ther (1986) 39, 577–81.
23 Chremos AN, Lin JH, Yeh KC, Chiou WF, Bayne WF, Lipschutz K, Williams RL. Famotidine does not interfere with the disposition of theophylline in man. Comparison with cimetidine. Clin Pharmacol Ther (1986) 39, 187.
24 Seggev JS, Barzilay M, Schey G. No evidence for interaction between ranitidine and theophylline. Arch Intern Med (1987) 147, 179–80.
25 Cusack BJ, Dawson GW, Mercer GD, Vestal RE. Cigarette smoking and theophylline metabolism: effects of cimetidine. Clin Pharmacol Ther (1985) 37, 330–6.
26 Roy AK, Cuda MP, Levine RA. Induction of theophylline toxicity and inhibition of clearance rates by ranitidine. Am J Med (1988) 85, 525–7.
27 Dietemann-Molard A, Popin E, Oswald-Mammosser M, Colas des Francs V, Pauli G. Intoxication a la theophylline par interaction avec la ranitidine a dose elevee. La Presse Med (1988) 17, 280.
28 Huang S-M, Weintraub HS, Marriott TB, Marinan B, Abels R, Leese PT. Etintidine-theophylline interaction study in humans. Biopharm and Drug Disp (1987) 8, 561–9.
29 Skinner MH, Lenert L, Blaschke TT. Theophylline toxicity subsequent to ranitidine administration: a possible drug-drug interaction. Am J Med (1989) 86, 129–32.
30 Boehning W. Effect of cimetidine and ranitidine on plasma theophylline in patients with chronic obstructive airways disease treated with theophylline and corticosteroids. Eur J Clin Pharmacol (1990) 38, 43–5.
31 McEwen J, McMurdo MET, Moreland TA. The effects of once-daily dosing with ranitidine and cimetidine on theophylline pharmacokinetics. Eur J Drug Metab Pharmacokinet (1988) 13, 201–5.
32 Dal Nego R, Turco P, Pomari C, Trevisan F. Famotidina e teofilina: interferenza farmacocinetica cimetidino-simile ? G Ital Malattie del Torace (1988) 42, 185–6.
33 Hegman GW, Gilbert RP. Ranitidine-theophylline interaction — fact or fiction ? DICP Ann Pharmacotherapy (19910 25, 21–5.
34 Vargas FS, Costa A, Costa JN, Santos SRCJ, Varvalho CRR. Theophylline-ranitidine interaction in elderly COPD patients. Am Rev Resp Dis (1991) 143, A446.
35 Zarogoulidis K, Economidis D, Paparoglou A, Pneumaticos I, Sevastou P, Tsopouridis A, Papaioanou A. Effect of ranitidine on theophylline plasma levels in patients with COPD. Eur Resp J (1988) Suppl 2, 195s.
36 Verdiani P, DiCarlo S, Baronti A. Famotidine effects on theophylline pharmacokinetics in subjects affected by COPD: comparison with cimetidine and placebo. Chest (1988) 94, 807–10.
37 Murialdo G, Piovano PL, Costelli P, Fonzi S, Barberis A, Ghia M. Seizures during concomitant treatment with theophylline and ranitidine: a case report. Ann Ital Med Int (1990) 5, 413–7.
38 Roberts RK, Grice J, McGuffie C. Cimetidine-theophylline interaction in patients with chronic obstructive airways disease. Med J Aust (1984) 140, 279–80.
39 Gastka JA, Tietze KJ, Rocci ML, Vlasses PH. Theophylline pharmacokinetics: effect of continuous versus intermittent cimetidine IV infusion. J Clin Pharmacol (1991) 31, 668–72.
40 Muir JG, Powell JR, Baumann JH. Induction of theophylline toxicity and inhibition of clearance rates by ranitidine. Am J Med (1989) 86, 513–4.
41 Davis RL, Quenzer RW, Kelly W, Powell JR. Effect of the addition of ciprofloxacin on theophylline pharmacokinetics in subjects inhibited by cimetidine. Ann Pharmacother (1992) 26, 11–3.
42 Adebayo GI. Effects of equimolar doses of cimetidine and ranitidine on theophylline elimination. Biopharm Drug Dis (1991) 10, 77–85.
43 Kelly HW; Williams DM, Figg WD, Pleasants RA; Hegman GW. Comment: ranitidine does not inhibit theophylline metabolism. Ann Pharmacother (1991) 25, 1139–41.
44 Chichmanian RM, Mignot G, Spreux A, Jean-Girard C, Hofliger P. Tolérance de la famotidine. Étude due réseau médecins sentinelles en pharmacovigilance. Therapie (1992) 47, 239–43.
45 Seaman JJ, Randolph WC, Peace KE, Rank WO, Dickson B, Putterman K, Young MD. Effects of two cimetidine dosage regimens on serum theophylline levels. Postgrad Med Custom Comm (1985) 78, 47–53.
46 Dal Negro R, Pomari C, Turco P. Famotidine and theophylline pharmacokinetics. An unexpected cimetidine-like interaction in patients with chronic obstructive pulmonary disease. Clin Pharmacokinet (1993) 24, 255–8.

Theophylline + Contraceptives (oral)

Abstract/Summary

Serum theophylline levels are raised to some extent in women taking oral contraceptives, but no toxicity has been reported.

Clinical evidence

The total plasma clearance of a single oral dose of aminophylline (4 ml/kg) in eight women on oral contraceptives was about 30% lower than in eight other women not on oral contraceptives (35.1 compared with 53.1 ml/h/kg).[1] The theophylline half-life was also prolonged by about 30% (from 7.34 to 9.79 h).

These findings are confirmed by other studies[2–4,7] which also showed a 30% decrease in the plasma clearance of theophylline due to oral contraceptives. In contrast, no significant changes were seen in 10 adolescent women (16–18 years).[6]

Mechanism

Uncertain, but it seems possible that the oestrogenic component (rather than the progestogen[5]) may inhibit the metabolism of the theophylline by the liver microsomal enzymes, thereby reducing its clearance.

Importance and management

An established interaction but there seem to be no reports of theophylline toxicity resulting from concurrent use. Women on oral contraceptives may need less theophylline than those not taking oral contraceptives. There is a small risk that patients with serum theophylline at the top end of the range may show some toxicity.

References

1 Tornatore KM, Kanarkowski R, McCarthy TL, Gardner MJ, Yurchak AM, Jusko WJ. Effect of chronic oral contraceptive steroids on theophylline disposition. Eur J Clin Pharmacol (1982) 23, 129–34.
2 Jusko WJ, Gardner MJ, Mangione A, Schentag JJ, Koup JR, Vance JW. Factors affecting theophylline clearances: age, tobacco, marijuana, cirrhosis, congestive heart failure, obesity, oral contraceptives, benzodiazepines, barbiturates and ethanol. J Pharm Sci (1979) 68, 1358–66.
3 Roberts RK, Grice J, McGuffie C, Heilbron L. Oral contraceptive steroids impair the elimination of theophylline. J Lab Clin Med (1983) 101, 821–5.
4 Gardner MJ, Tornatore KM, Jusko WJ, Karnankowski R. Effects of tobacco smoking and oral contraceptive use on theophylline disposition. Br J Clin Pharmacol (1983) 16, 271–80.
5 Gotz VP, Dolly FR, Block AJ. Influence of medroxyprogesterone on theophylline disposition. J Clin Pharmacol (1983) 23, 281–4.
6 MacLeod S, Koren G, Chin T, Correia J, Tesoro A. Theophylline pharmacokinetics in adolescent females following coadministration of oral contraceptives. Clin Pharmacol Ther (1985) 37, 209.
7 Long DR, Roberts EA, Brill-Edwards M, Quaggin S, Correia J, Koren G, MacLeod SM. The effect of the oral contraceptive Ortho 7/7/7 on theophylline clearance in non-smoking women aged 18–22. Clin Invest Med (1987) 10 (4 Suppl B) B59.

Theophylline + Corticosteroids

Abstract/Summary

Concurrent use is not uncommon but increases in serum theophylline levels (sometimes associated with toxicity), decreases and no changes have been described during concurrent use. The general clinical importance of these interactions is uncertain.

Clinical evidence

(a) Increased serum theophylline levels

Six patients in status asthmaticus with stable serum concentrations of theophylline (by infusion) were given an intravenous 500 mg bolus of hydrocortisone followed 6 h later by three two-hourly doses of 200 mg. In each case the serum theophylline levels rapidly climbed from about 20 to between 30 and 50 μg/ml. At least two of the patients complained of nausea and headache.[1] Another study on 10 children (aged 2–6) with status asthmaticus showed that methylprednisolone increased the half-life of theophylline.[4] Another study using an unnamed corticosteroid also reported a prolonged theophylline half-life (from 4.98 to 6.18 h) and a clearance reduced by about one-third.[6]

(b) Reduced serum theophylline levels

Seven normal subjects stabilized on theophylline given intravenous methylprednisolone (1.6 mg/kg) and hydrocortisone (33 mg/kg) separately showed a 21% increase in clearance when the results of the two were combined.[2] An increase in the clearance of theophylline was seen in a normal subject given methylprednisolone but no changes in the kinetics of theophylline were seen in two subjects given methylprednisolone.[5] Another study[3] on six normal subjects showed that prednisone (20 mg) caused a small but clinically trivial reduction in the serum levels of theophylline.

(c) Theophylline levels unchanged

Nine patients with chronic airflow obstruction showed no changes in the pharmacokinetics of a single IV dose of aminophylline (5.6 mg/kg) when treated with 20 mg prednisolone daily for 3 weeks.[7] Intravenous bolus doses of 500 or 1000 mg hydrocortisone were found not to affect theophylline levels in patients taking 400 mg choline theophyllinate 12-hourly.[8]

Mechanism

Not understood.

Importance and management

The interactions of theophylline with the various corticosteroids are poorly documented and their clinical importance is difficult to assess because both increases, small decreases and no changes in the serum levels of theophylline have been reported. It is also questionable whether the results of studies in normal healthy subjects can validly be extrapolated to patients with status asthmaticus. There is no good reason for avoiding concurrent use, but the effects and/or serum theophylline levels should be checked.

References

1 Buchanan N, Hurwitz S, Butler P. Asthma — a possible interaction between hydrocortisone and theophylline. S Afr Med J (1979) 56, 1147.
2 Leavengood DC, Bunker-Soler AL, Nelson HS. The effect of corticosteroids on theophylline metabolism. Ann Allergy (1983) 50, 249.
3 Anderson JL, Ayres JW, Hall CA. Potential pharmacokinetic interaction between theophylline and prednisone. Clin Pharm (1984) 3, 187–8.
4 De La Morena E, Borges MT, Rebollar CG, Escorihuela R. Efecto de la metil-prednisolona sobre los niveles sericos de teofilina. Rev Clin Esp (1982) 167, 297–300.
5 Squire EN, Nelson HS. Corticosteroids and theophylline clearance. NER Allergy Proc (1987) 8, 113–15.
6 Elvey SM, Saccar CL, Rocci ML, Mansmann HC, Martynec DM, Kester MB. The effect of corticosteroids on theophylline metabolism in asthmatic children. Ann Allergy (1986) 56, 520.
7 Fergusson RJ, Scott CM, Rafferty P, Gaddie J. Effect of prednisolone on theophylline pharmacokinetics in patients with chronic airflow obstruction. Thorax (1987) 42, 195–8.
8 Tatsis G, Orphanidou D, Douratsos D, Mellissinos C, Pantelakis D, Pipini E, Jordanoglou J. The effect of steroids on theophylline absorption. J Int Med Res (1991) 19, 326–9.

Theophylline + Co-trimoxazole

Abstract/Summary

Co-trimoxazole does not interact with theophylline.

Clinical evidence, mechanism, importance and management

Eight days treatment with co-trimoxazole (960 mg twice daily) had no effect on the pharmacokinetics of theophylline given intravenously to six normal subjects.[1] Another study found that co-trimoxazole (960 mg twice daily) for 5 days had no effect on the pharmacokinetics of theophylline given orally.[2] No special precautions would seem necessary if these two drugs are given concurrently.

Reference

1 Jonkman JHG, van der Boon WJV, Schoenmaker R, Holtkamp AH, Hempenius J. Lack of influence of co-trimoxazole on theophylline pharmacokinetics. J Pharm Sci (1985) 74, 1103–4.
2 Lo KF, Nation RL, Sansom LN. Lack of effect of co-trimoxazole on the pharmacokinetics of orally administered theophylline. Biopharm Drug Disp (1989) 10, 573–80.

Theophylline + Dextropropoxyphene

Abstract/Summary

Dextropropoxyphene does not interact significantly with theophylline.

Clinical evidence, mechanism, importance and management

65 mg dextropropoxyphene 8-hourly for 5 days did not significantly change the plasma clearance of theophylline (125 mg 8-hourly) of six normal subjects.[1] There would seem to be no need to avoid concurrent use or to take particular precautions.

Reference

1 Robson RA, Miners JO, Whitehead AG, Birkett DJ. Specificity of the inhibitory effect of dextropropoxyphene on oxidative drug metabolism in man: effects on theophylline and tolbutamide disposition. Br J Clin Pharmac (1987) 23, 772–5.

Theophylline + Disulfiram

Abstract/Summary

Blood theophylline levels are increased by disulfiram. The theophylline dosage may need to be reduced to avoid toxicity.

Clinical evidence

After taking 250 mg disulfiram daily for a week, the clearance of theophylline (5 mg/kg infused IV) in 20 recovering alcoholics was decreased by 21% (from 105.7 to 83.1 ml/kg/h). Those taking 500 mg disulfiram daily showed a decrease of 32.5% (from 94.3 to 65.4 ml/kg/h).[1,2] Smoking appeared to have no important effects on the extent of this interaction.

Mechanism

Disulfiram inhibits the liver enzymes concerned with the metabolism of the theophylline, thereby reducing its clearance from the body.

Importance and management

Information appears to be limited to this study but it would seem to be an established and clinically important interaction. Monitor the serum levels of theophylline and its effects if disulfiram is added, anticipating the need to reduce the theophylline dosage, bearing in mind that the extent of this interaction depends upon the dosage of disulfiram used. Some individuals on 500 mg disulfiram showed a 50% reduction in clearance.

References

1 Loi C-M, Day JD, Jue SG, Costello P, Vestal RE. The effect of disulfiram on theophylline disposition. Clin Pharmacol Ther (1987) 41, 165.
2 Loi C-M, Day JD, Jue SG, Bush ED, Costello P, Dewey LV, Vestal RE. Dose-dependent inhibition of theophylline metabolism by disulfiram in recovering alcoholics. Clin Pharmacol Ther (1989) 45, 476–86.

Theophylline + Enprostil and Rioprostil

Abstract/Summary

Enprostil and rioprostil do not interact with theophylline.

Clinical evidence, mechanism, importance and management

70 µg enprostil daily for 5 days had no effect on serum theophylline levels, vital capacity or FEV_1 of 10 asthmatics.[1] 300 µg rioprostil twice daily for 6 days did not significantly alter the pharmacokinetics or the steady-state serum levels of theophylline in 8 normal subjects when given a micronized slow-release formulation (*Techniphylline*).[2] No special precautions would seem necessary during concurrent use.

References

1 Gross G, Bynum L. Use of enprostil in asthmatics taking theophylline. Gastroenterol (1985) 88, 1407.
2 de Lauture D, Rey E, d'Athis P, Richard MO, Paccaly D, Prunieras F, Strauch G, Olive G. Pharmacokinetic interactions between theophylline and rioprostil. Scand J Gastroenterol (1989) 24 (Suppl 164) 63–7.

Theophylline + Erythromycin

Abstract/Summary

Theophylline serum levels can be increased by the concurrent use of erythromycin. Intoxication may develop in those patients whose serum levels are already high unless the dosage is reduced. Not all patients demonstrate this interaction. Erythromycin levels may possibly fall to subtherapeutic concentrations.

Clinical evidence

(a) Theophylline serum levels increased

The peak serum theophylline levels of 12 patients with chronic bronchitis given aminophylline (4 mg/kg/day) were raised 28% when concurrently treated with erythromycin stearate (500 mg 6-hourly). The clearance was reduced 22%.[1]

Rises in serum theophylline levels of up to 40% as a result of this interaction have been described in numerous studies[2–10,16,21,22] some of which report the development of theophylline toxicity. Not all patients show this interaction. Two reports state that it occurred in only three of the nine subjects and five out of 15 patients studied[11,21] Two other studies[12,13,15] involving eight and 13 subjects failed to demonstrate this interaction.

(b) Erythromycin serum levels reduced

The peak serum erythromycin levels of six normal subjects taking 500 mg 8-hourly were almost halved when given a single 250 mg dose of theophylline intravenously. Over an 8 h period the AUC was reduced 38%.[14]

Another pharmacokinetic study found that serum erythromycin levels fell by more than 30% when theophylline was given concurrently,[18] whereas an earlier studies found no changes apart from an increase in renal clearance.[16,20]

Mechanisms

Not fully understood. It seems most likely that erythromycin inhibits the metabolism of theophylline by the liver resulting in a reduction in its clearance from the body and in a rise in its serum levels. It also seems possible that theophylline can affect both the absorption and the elimination of erythromycin.[17,18]

Importance and management

(a) The effects of erythromycin on theophylline are established (but still debated) and well documented. Not all the reports are referenced here. It does not seem to matter which erythromycin salt is used. Monitor concurrent use and anticipate the need to reduce the theophylline dosage to avoid toxicity. Not all will show this interaction but remember it may take several days to manifest itself. Those particularly at risk are patients with high serum theophylline levels and/or taking high dosages (20 mg/kg body weight or more). A 25% reduction has been recommended for those in the 15–20 µg/ml range,[1,5,22] but little dosage adjustment is probably needed for those at the lower end of the range (8–15 µg/ml) unless toxic symptoms appear.[1,9] Enprofylline appears not to interact with erythromycin and is a possible alternative.[19] (b) The fall in erythromycin levels caused by theophylline is not well documented but what is known suggests that it may be clinically important. Be alert for any evidence of an inadequate response to the erythromycin and increase the dosage if necessary. More study is needed.

References

1 Reisz G, Pingleton SK, Melethil S, Ryan P. The effect of erythromycin on theophylline pharmacokinetics in chronic bronchitis. Am Rev Resp Dis (1983) 127, 581–4.
2 Cummins LH, Kozak PP, Gillman SA. Erythromycin's effects on theophylline blood levels. Pediatric (1977) 59, 144.
3 Cummins LH, Kozak PP, Gillman SA. Theophylline determinations. Ann Allergy (1976) 37, 450.
4 Anderson RJ. Review of antimicrobial drug interactions. Clin Med (1978) 85, 13.
5 Prince RA, Wing DS, Weinberger MM, Hendeles LS and Riegleman S. Effect of erythromycin on theophylline kinetics. J Allergy Clin Immunol (1981) 68, 427–31.
6 May DC, Jarboe CH, Ellenberg DT, Roe EJ, Karibo J. The effects of erythromycin on theophylline elimination in normal males. J Clin Pharmacol (1982) 22, 125–30.
7 Branigan TA, Robbins RA, Cady WJ, Nickols JG, Ueda CT. The effects of erythromycin on the absorption and disposition kinetics of theophylline. Eur J Clin Pharmac (1981) 21, 115–20.
8 Green JA, Clementi WA. Decrease in theophylline clearance after the

administration of erythromycin to a patient with obstructive lung disease. Drug Intell Clin Pharm (1983) 17, 370–2.

9 Zarowitz BJM, Szefler SJ, Lasezkay GM. Effect of erythromycin base on theophylline kinetics. Clin Pharmacol Ther (1981) 29, 601–5.

10 Richer C, Matthieu M, Bah H, Thuillez C, Duroux P, Guidicelli J-F. Theophylline kinetics and ventilatory flow in bronchial asthma and chronic airflow obstruction: influence of erythromycin. Clin Pharmacol Ther (1982) 31, 579–86.

11 Pfeifer HJ, Greenblatt DJ, Friedman P. Effects of three antibiotics on theophylline kinetics. Clin Pharmacol Ther (1979) 26, 36.

12 Kelly SJ, Pingleton SK, Ryan PB, Sri M. The lack of influence of erythromycin on plasma theophylline serum levels. Chest (1980) 78, 523.

13 Maddux M, Organek H, Hasegawa G, Leeds N, Bauman J. Erythromycin alteration of theophylline pharmacokinetics. Lack of effect at steady-state. Am Rev Resp Dis (1981) 123, 60.

14 Iliopoulou A, Aldhous ME, Johnston A, Turner P. Pharmacokinetic interaction between theophylline and erythromycin. Br J Clin Pharmac (1982) 14, 495–9.

15 Maddux MS, Leeds NH, Organek HW, Hasegawa GR, Bauman JL. The effect of erythromycin on theophylline pharmacokinetics at steady-state. Chest (1982) 81, 563–5.

16 LaForce CF, Miller MF, Chai H. Effect of erythromycin on theophylline clearance in asthmatic children. J Ped (1981) 99, 153–6.

17 Hildebrandt R, Moller H, Gundert-Remy U. Influence of theophylline on the renal clearance of erythromycin. Int J Clin Pharmacol Ther Tox (1987) 25, 601–4.

18 Paulsen O, Hoglund P, Nilsson L-G, Bengtsson H-I. The interaction of erythromycin with theophylline. Eur J Clin Pharmacol (1987) 32, 493–8.

19 Sitar DS, Aoki FY, Hoban DJ, Hidinger K-G, Montgomery PR, Mitenko PA. Enprofylline disposition in the presence and absence of amoxycylline and erythromycin. Br J Clin Pharmac (1987) 24, 57–61.

20 Pasic J, Jackson HD, Johnston A, Peverel-Cooper CA, Turner P, Downey K, Chaput de Saintonge DM. The interaction between chronic oral slow-release theophylline and single-dose intravenous erythromycin. Xenobiotica (1987) 17, 493–7.

21 Stults BM, Felice-Johnson J, Higbee MD, Hardigan K. Effect of erythromycin stearate on serum theophylline concentration in patients with chronic obstructive lung disease. S Med J (1983) 76, 714–8.

22 Aronson JK, Hardman M, Reynolds DJM. ABC of monitoring drug therapy. Theophylline. Br Med J (1992) 305, 1355–8.

Theophylline + Fluvoxamine

Abstract/Summary

Three reports describe markedly elevated theophylline levels associated with toxicity (in a boy and two old men) when additionally given fluvoxamine.

Clinical evidence

Theophylline toxicity (agitation, tachycardia) developed in a man of 83 about a week after starting to take 100 mg fluvoxamine daily. His serum theophylline levels were found to have risen from a range of about 10–14 mg/l to 39.8 mg/l.[1] A man of 70 similarly developed theophylline toxicity (177 μmol/l) when fluvoxamine was added. Subsequently the theophylline concentrations were found closely to parallel a number of changes in fluvoxamine dosages.[3] A boy of 11 complained of headaches, tiredness and vomiting within a week of starting to take fluvoxamine. His serum theophylline levels were found to have doubled (from 14.2 to 27.4 mg/l).[2]

Mechanism

In vitro studies with human liver microsomes have found that fluvoxamine inhibits cytochrome P4501A2 (CYP1A2) which is concerned with the metabolism of theophylline.[4] *In vivo* this would have the effect of raising serum theophylline levels, resulting in the development of toxicity.

Importance and management

Information is very limited and the general importance of this interaction is still uncertain, but close monitoring during their concurrent use in any patient would now seem advisable, anticipating the need to reduce the theophylline dosage.

References

1 Diot P, Jonville AP, Gerard F, Bonnelle M, Autret E, Bretau M, Lemarie E, Lavnadier M. Possible interaction entre théophylline et fluvoxamine. Therapie (1991) 46, 170–71.

2 Sperber AD. Toxic interaction between fluvoxamine and sustained release theophylline in an 11-year-old boy. Drug Saf (1991) 6, P460–2.

3 Thomson AH, McGovern EM, Bennie P, Caldwell G, Smith M. Interaction between fluvoxamine and theophylline. Pharm J (1992) 248,137.

4 Brdosen K, Skjelbo E, Rasmussen BB, Poulsen HE, Loft S. Fluvoxamine is a potent inhibitor of cytochrome P4501A2. Biochem Pharmacol (1993) 45, 1211–14.

Theophylline + Food

Abstract/Summary

The bioavailability of theophylline from a number of sustained-release formulations can be increased or decreased by food and by the type of food eaten. High protein diets increase the loss of theophylline from the body, whereas high carbohydrate diets reduce the loss. No interaction appears to occur with dietary fibre. Changes in the bioavailability of theophylline can occur in patients fed by nasogastric tube or intravenously.

Clinical evidence

(a) Theophylline and food given orally

The absorption of theophylline from a controlled release tablet (*Theograd*) in seven normal subjects increased from 65 to 87% when taken after a meal.[1] Food was shown not to affect the bioavailability of theophylline in *Theolin Retard*[4] but increased it from 53 to 96% with *Uniphyl*.[6] The AUC of theophylline given as *Nuelin SA* increased by 33% in eight patients with airways obstruction after eating a high carbohydrate/low protein diet for a week when compared with a high protein/low carbohydrate diet.[2] Carbohydrate delayed the absorption of theophylline from *Teovent* of 18 normal subjects.[3] Food but not *Ensure* is reported to increase the absorption of theophylline from *Theo-24* [5,16] but it reduced (by 53%) the bioavailability of

Theo-Dur Sprinkle.[6] *Osmolite* is reported not to affect the absorption of a slow-release preparation (*Slo-bid Gyrocaps*).[14] A patient with chronic obstructive pulmonary disease showed a two-thirds fall in his serum theophylline levels accompanied by bronchospasm when he was fed through a nasogastric tube with *Osmolite*. The interaction occurred with both theophylline tablets (Theo-Dur) and liquid theophylline, but not when the theophylline was given intravenously as aminophylline.[7] Food was found to alter the absorption pattern of *Uniphyll*ine in children but not adults. 'Dose dumping' and toxic serum theophylline levels occurred in some children and it was concluded that children should not take this sustained release preparation in large doses with food.[11] Only slight and clinically unimportant changes in absorption were seen in studies of *Theostat 300, Uniphyl* and *Teonova* in normal adults when given with food,[12,15] but *Theolair* serum levels were markedly reduced.[20] One study suggested that food could have as large an effect on the metabolism of theophylline as cimetidine.[17] Fibre (non-soluble cellulose) apparently does not affect absorption of theophylline.[13]

(b) Theophylline and food given parenterally

An isolated report describes an elderly woman treated with aminophylline by intravenous infusion who showed a marked fall in her serum theophylline levels (from 16.3 to 6.3 mg/l) when the amino acid concentration of her parenteral nutrition regimen was increased from 4.25 to 7%.[8]

Mechanism

Not fully understood. One suggestion is that high protein diets stimulate liver enzymes (the cytochrome P-450 mono-oxygenase system) thereby increasing the metabolism of the theophylline and hastening its loss from the body. High carbohydrate diets have the opposite effect.[9,10]

Importance and management

The theophylline-food interactions have been thoroughly studied but there seems to be no consistent pattern in the way the absorption of different theophylline preparations is affected. Be alert for any evidence of an inadequate response which can be related to food intake, and monitor the effects if one preparation is exchanged for another. Encourage patients to take their theophylline consistently in relation to meals, and not to make major changes in their diet without consultation.

References

1 Lagas M, Jonkman JHG. Influence of food on the rate and extent of absorption of theophylline after a single dose oral administration of a controlled release tablet. Int J Clin Pharmacol Ther Tox (1985) 23, 424–6.
2 Thompson PJ, Skypala I, Dawson S, McAllister WAC, Warwick MT. The effect of diet upon serum concentrations of theophylline. Br J Clin Pharmac (1983) 16, 267–70.
3 Johansson O, Lindberg T, Melander A, Whalin-Boll E. Different effects of different nutrients on theophylline absorption in man. Drug-Nutr Interactions (1985) 3, 205–11.
4 Sips AP, Edelbroek PM, Kulstad S, de Wolff FA, Dijkman JH. Food does not effect bioavailability of theophylline from *Theolin Retard*. Eur J Clin Pharmacol (1984) 26, 405–7.
5 Vaughan L, Milavetz G, Hill M, Weinberger M, Hendeles L. Food-induced dose-dumping of *Theo-24*, a 'once-daily' slow release theophylline product. Drug Intell Clin Pharm (1984) 18, 510.
6 Karim A, Burns T, Wearley L, Streicher J, Palmer M. Food-induced changes in theophylline absorption from controlled release formulations. Part I. Substantial increased and decreased absorption with *Uniphyl* tablets and *Theo-Dur Sprinkle*. Clin Pharmacol Ther (1985) 38, 77–83.
7 Gal P, Layson R. Interference with oral theophylline absorption by continuous nasogastric feedings. Ther Drug Monitor (1986) 8, 421–3.
8 Ziegenbein RC. Theophylline clearance increase from increased amino acid in a CPN regimen. Drug Intell Clin Pharm (1987) 21, 220–1.
9 Kappas A, Anderson KE, Conney AH, Alvares AP. Influences of dietary protein and carbohydrate on antipyrine and theophylline metabolism in man. Clin Pharmacol Ther (1976) 20, 643–53.
10 Feldman CH, Hutchinson VE, Pippenger CE, Blumenfeld TA, Feldman BR, Davis WJ. Effect of dietary protein and carbohydrate on theophylline metabolism in children. Pediatrics (1980) 66, 956–62.
11 Steffensen G, Pedersen S. Food induced changes in theophylline absorption from a once-a-day theophylline product. Br J Clin Pharmac (1986) 22, 571–7.
12 Thebault JJ, Aiache JM, Mazoyer F, Cardot JM. The influence of food on the bioavailability of a slow release theophylline preparation. Clin Pharmacokinet (1987) 13, 267–72.
13 Fassihi AR, Dowse R, Robertson SSD. Effect of dietary cellulose on the absorption and bioavailability of theophylline. Int J Pharmaceutics (1989) 50, 79–82.
14 Bhargava VO, Schaaf LJ, Berlinger WG, Jungnickel PW. Effect of an enteral nutrient formula on sustained release theophylline absorption. Ther Drug Monit (1989) 11, 515–9.
15 Lefebrve RA, Belpaire FM, Bogaert MG. Influence of food on steady state serum concentrations of theophylline from two controlled-release preparations. Int J Clin Pharmacol Ther Toxicol (1988) 26, 375–9.
16 Plezia PM, Thornley SM, KRamer TH, Armstrong EP. The influence of enteral feedings on sustained-release theophylline absorption. Pharmacotherapy (1990) 10, 356–61.
17 Anderson KE, McCleery RB, Vesell ES, Vickers FF, Kappas A. Diet and cimetidine induce comparable changes in theophylline metabolism in normal subjects. Hepatology (1991) 13, 941–6.

Theophylline + Frusemide

Abstract/Summary

The outcome of concurrent use is uncertain. Frusemide is reported to increase, decrease or to have no effect on serum theophylline levels.

Clinical evidence

The mean serum theophylline levels of eight asthmatics, given 300 mg of sustained release formulation, and measured at 1 and 6 h, were reduced by 41% (from 12.14 to 7.16 g/ml) by 25 mg frusemide.[1] Four premature neonates, two given theophylline and frusemide orally and the other two intravenously, showed a fall in steady-state serum theophylline levels from 8 to 2–3 g/ml when the frusemide was given within 30 min of the theophylline.[2] 10 patients with asthma, chronic bronchitis or emphysema on continuous maintenance infusion with aminophylline showed a 21% rise in their serum theophylline levels (from 13.7 to 16.6 g/ml) 4 h after being given a 40 mg dose of frusemide (intravenously over 2 min).[3]

A study in 12 normal subjects given theophylline failed to

find any change in serum theophylline levels when given 40 mg frusemide orally.[4]

Mechanism

Not understood.

Importance and management

Information is limited and the outcome of concurrent use is inconsistent and uncertain. If both drugs are used the serum theophylline levels should be monitored and appropriate dosage adjustments made as necessary.

References

1 Carpentiere G, Marino S, Castello F. Furosemide and theophylline. Ann Intern Med (1985) 103, 957.
2 Toback JW, Gilman ME. Theophylline-furosemide inactivation? Pediatrics (1983) 71, 140–1.
3 Conlon PF, Grambau GR, Johnson CE, Weg JR. Effect of intravenous furosemide on serum theophylline concentration. Am J Hosp Pharm (1981) 38, 1345–7.
4 Janicke U-A, Gundert-Remy U. Failure to detect a clinically significant interaction between theophylline and furosemide. Naunyn-Schmied Arch Pharmacol (1986) 332, R100.

Theophylline + Idrocilamide

Abstract/Summary

Idrocilamide can increase serum theophylline levels. A reduction in the theophylline dosage may be needed to avoid intoxication.

Clinical evidence, mechanism, importance and management

Idrocilamide (600 mg daily for 7 days) increased the half-life of a single dose of theophylline by 2.5 (from 8.5 to 21.6 h) in six normal subjects due, so it is suggested, to a reduction in the liver metabolism caused by the idrocilamide.[1] Information is very limited but it indicates that concurrent use should be closely monitored. The need to reduce the theophylline dosage should be anticipated.

Reference

1 Lacroix C, Nouveau J, Hubscher Ph, Tardif D, Ray M, Goulle JP. Influence de l'idrocilamide sur le metabolisme de la theophylline. Rev Pneumol Clin (1986) 42, 164–6.

Theophylline + Imipenem

Abstract/Summary

Seizures developed in three patients on theophylline when given imipenem.

Clinical evidence, mechanism, importance and management

Three patients on theophylline developed seizures within 2–3 days of starting treatment with imipenem (500 mg 6–8-hourly IV).[1] The reasons are not know. Imipenem was associated with seizures in about 1% of patients in one clinical study.[2] The general importance of these observations is uncertain but you should be aware of these cases.

References

1 Semel JD, Allen N. Seizures in patients simultaneously receiving theophylline and imipenem or ciprofloxacin or metronidazole. S Med J (1991) 84, 465–8.
2 Calandra G, Lydick E, Carrigan J. Factors predisposing to seizures in seriously ill infected patients receiving antibiotics: experience with imipenem/cilastin. Am J Med (1988) 84, 911–8.

Theophylline + Influenza vaccines

Abstract/Summary

Normally none of the influenza vaccines (whole virus, split virus and purified subunit) interact with theophylline, but there are three reports describing rises in serum theophylline levels in a few patients attributed to the use of an influenza vaccine, accompanied by toxicity in some instances.

Clinical evidence

(a) Evidence of no interaction

No evidence of a rise in serum theophylline levels was seen in 12 patients given influenza vaccine, trivalent, Types A and B[9] or in 119 elderly people given an un-named influenza vaccine.[4] No evidence of an interaction was found in a number of other studies involving 23 normal subjects (split virus vaccine),[5] nine patients (tween-ether split virion vaccine)[14] seven subjects and five patients (purified subunit vaccine),[6] 12 patients (trivalent vaccine-*Fluzone*),[7] 11 patients, eight child patients and 12 normal subjects (trivalent vaccine-*Fluogen*),[8,15] 16 normal subjects (whole virus vaccine),[10] 16 patients (trivalent vaccine-*Fluzone*),[11] seven patients (inactivated subvirion trivalent vaccine)[16] or 49 asthmatic children (trivalent subvirion influenza V).[12]

(b) Evidence of an interaction

Three patients taking 200 mg oxytriphylline (equivalent to 128 mg theophylline) orally 6-hourly for at least 7 days showed a rise in their serum theophylline levels of 219, 89 and 85% respectively within 12–24 h of receiving 0.5 ml trivalent influenza vaccine (*Fluogen*-Parke Davis). Two of them showed signs of theophylline toxicity. A subsequent study on four normal subjects showed that the same dose of vaccine more than doubled the half-life of theophylline (from 3.3 to 7.3 h) and /halved its clearance (from 52 to 25 mg/kg/h).[1] A girl of 15 showed a transient rise in theophylline levels (no sign of toxicity) when given a split-virus vaccine,[3] and a woman showed a rise accompanied by headaches and palpitations.[7] Theophylline intoxication has been seen in children during an influenza epidemic accompanied by changes in serum theophylline levels.[2]

Mechanism

Uncertain. If an interaction occurs it is probably due to inhibition by the vaccine of the activity of the liver enzymes concerned with the metabolism of theophylline, resulting in its accumulation in the body.[1] One suggestion is that the vaccine contaminants (rather than the vaccine itself) may be responsible so that an interaction would seem to be less likely with highly purified subunit vaccines.[13]

Importance and management

A very thoroughly investigated interaction, the weight of evidence being that no adverse interaction normally occurs with any type of influenza vaccine in children, adults or the elderly. Even so, bearing in mind the occasional and unexplained reports of interaction,[1,3,7] it would seem prudent to monitor the effects of concurrent use although problems are very unlikely to arise now that purer vaccines are available (see 'Mechanism').

References

1 Renton KW, Gray JD, Hall RI. Decreased elimination of theophylline after influenza vaccination. Can Med Ass J (1980) 123, 288.
2 Kraemer MJ, Furukawa CT, Koup JR, Shapiro GG, Pierson WE, Bierman CW. Altered theophylline clearance during an influenza B outbreak. Paediatrics (1982) 69, 476–80.
3 Walker S, Schreiber L, Middelkamp JN. Serum theophylline levels after influenza vaccination. Can Med Ass J (1981) 125, 243–4.
4 Patriarca PA, Kendal AP, Stricof RL, Weber JA, Meissner MK, Dateno B. Influenza vaccination and warfarin or theophylline toxicity in nursing home residents. N Engl J Med (1983) 308, 1601–2.
5 Grabowski N, May JJ, Pratt DS, Richtmeier WJ, Bertino JS, Sorge KF. The effect of split virus influenza vaccination on theophylline pharmacokinetics. Am Rev Resp Dis (1985) 131, 934–8.
6 Winstanley PA, Tjia J, Back DJ, Hobson D, Breckenridge AM. Lack of effect of highly purified subunit influenza vaccination on theophylline metabolism. Br J Clin Pharmac (1985) 20, 47–53.
7 Fischer R, Booth B, Mitchell D, Kibbe A. Influence of trivalent influenza vaccine on serum theophylline levels. Can Med Ass J (1982) 126, 1312–13.
8 Bukowskyj M, Munt P, Wigle R, Nakatou K. Theophylline clearance: lack of effect of influenza vaccination and ascorbic acid. Am Rev Resp Dis (1984) 129, 672–5.
9 Gomolin IH, Chapron DJ, Luhan PA. Effects of influenza virus vaccine on theophylline and warfarin clearance in institutionalised elderly. J Amer Ger Soc (1984) 32, Suppl S21.
10 Hannan SE, May JJ, Pratt DS, Richtsmeier WJ, Bertino JS. Lack of effect of whole virus influenza vaccine on theophylline pharmacokinetics. Am Rev Resp Dis (1986) 133, A61
11 Goldstein RS, Cheung OT, Seguin R, Lobley G, Johnson AC. Decreased elimination of theophylline after influenza vaccination. Can Med Ass J (1981) 126, 470.
12 Feldman CH, Rabinowitz A, Levison M, Klein R, Feldman BR, Davis WJ. Effects of influenza vaccine on theophylline metabolism in children with

asthma. Am Rev Respir Dis (1985) 131 (4 Suppl) A9.
13 Winstanley PA, Back DJ, Breckenridge AM. Inhibition of theophylline metabolism by interferon. Lancet (1987) ii, 1340.
14 Bryett KA, Levy J, Pariente R, Gobert P, Falquet JCV. Influenza vaccine and theophylline metabolism. Is there an interaction ? Acta Therapeutica (1989) 15, 49–58.
15 San Joaquin VH, Reyes S, Marks MI. Influenza vaccination in asthmatic children on maintenance theophylline therapy. Clin Paed (1982) 724–6.
16 Stults BM, Hashisaki PA. Influenza vaccination and theophylline pharmacokinetics in patients with obstructive lung disease. Western J Med (1983) 139, 651–4.

Theophylline + Interferon

Abstract/Summary

The clearance of theophylline from the body is reduced by interferon. One study found that it was halved. This suggests that theophylline intoxication might occur if the dosage is not reduced appropriately.

Clinical evidence

A study in five patients with stable chronic active hepatitis B and four healthy subjects showed that 20 h after being given a single 9 or 18 mega unit IM injection of interferon (recombinant alpha A, Hoffman La Roche), the theophylline clearance in eight of them was approximately halved (from 0.7 to 0.36 ml/kg/min) with a range of 33–81%. The mean theophylline elimination half-life was increased from 6.3 to 10.7 h (1.5 to 6-fold increases). One healthy subject showed no change. Four weeks after the study the theophylline clearances were noted to have returned to their former values.[1] Another study using alpha-interferon (*Roferon-A®*) found that the terminal half-life, AUC and mean residence time of the theophylline was only increased by 15%.[3]

Mechanism

Interferon inhibits the liver enzymes[2] concerned with the metabolism of some drugs, including theophylline, so that it is cleared from the body more slowly and accumulates.[1]

Importance and management

Direct information appears to be limited to these reports, only one of which found evidence of a clinically important interaction. So far there appear to be no reports of toxicity but it would seem prudent to monitor concurrent use closely, reducing the theophylline dosage if necessary.

References

1 Williams SJ, Baird-Lambert JA, Farrell GC. Inhibition of theophylline metabolism by interferon. Lancet (1987) ii, 939–41.
2 Williams SJ, Farrell GC. Inhibition of antipyrine metabolism by interferon. Br J Clin Pharmacol (1986) 22, 610–12.
3 Jonkman JHG, Nicholson KG, Farrow PR, Eckert M, Grasmeijer G, Oosterhuis B, De Noorde OE, Guentert TW. Effects of alpha-interferon on

theophylline pharmacokinetics and metabolism. Br J Clin Pharmac (1989) 27, 795–802.

Theophylline + Ipriflavone

Abstract/Summary

An isolated report describes increased theophylline levels in a patient when given ipriflavone.

Clinical evidence, mechanism, importance and management

The theophylline serum levels of a patient with chronic airways disease, taking 600 mg daily, rose from 9.5 to 17.3 µg/ml after additionally taking 600 mg ipriflavone daily for about 4 weeks. No toxicity occurred. The serum theophylline levels fell when the ipriflavone was stopped and rose again when it was restarted. The suggested reason is that ipriflavone can inhibit the metabolism of the theophylline by the liver, thereby reducing its loss from the body.[1] Monitor the theophylline levels of any patient given ipriflavone and make dosage reductions as necessary. More study is needed.

Reference

1 Takahashi J, Kawakatsu K, Wakayama T, Savaoka H. Elevation of serum theophylline levels by ipriflavone in a patient with chronic obstructive pulmonary disease. Eur J Clin Pharmacol (1992) 43, 207–8.

Theophylline + Isoniazid

Abstract/Summary

Two short term studies found that theophylline serum levels were increased by the concurrent use of isoniazid. Theophylline intoxication occurred in one patient a month after starting to take isoniazid. However another study found that isoniazid increased rather than decreased theophylline clearance.

Clinical evidence

Theophylline toxicity a month after starting to take isoniazid has been described in one patient, subsequently demonstrated again in a re-challenge study.[3]

10 mg/kg isoniazid daily for the 10 days in seven normal subjects increased the half-life and AUC of theophylline by 15% (from 152 to 175 min) and 31% (from 439–620 mol/h/l) respectively. The theophylline was given as an IV infusion and the serum levels after 6 h were 22% higher (58 mol/l compared with 48.5 mol/l). Five subjects also showed an increase in isoniazid half-life and AUC but they were not statistically significant.[1] Another study found that 400 mg isoniazid daily for two weeks reduced the mean clearance of theophylline in 13 subjects by 21%.[4] However another study on four normal subjects, given 300 mg isoniazid daily for 6 days, found that the clearance of theophylline given orally was increased by 16%, but no consistent changes were seen in any of the other pharmacokinetic parameters measured.[2]

Mechanism

Isoniazid is believed to inhibit the metabolism of theophylline by the liver, thereby reducing its loss from the body and increasing its serum levels.

Importance and management

The reason for these inconsistent results is not understood nor is this interaction well established, however it has been suggested that it may take 3–4 weeks for any significant increase in theophylline levels to occur.[3] Both of the studies cited covered a period of only 6–14 days whereas the case report describes the effects over a period up to 55 days.[3] The outcome of concurrent use is uncertain but it would clearly be prudent to be alert for any evidence of increased theophylline levels and toxicity if isoniazid is given.

References

1 Hoglund P, Nilsson L-G, Paulsen O. Interaction between isoniazid and theophylline. Eur J Resp Dis (1987) 70, 110–6.
2 Thompson JR, Burckart GJ, Self TH, Brown RE, Straughn AB. Isoniazid-induced alterations in theophylline pharmacokinetics. Curr Ther Res (1982) 32, 921–5.
3 Torrent J, Izquierdo I, Cabezas R, Jané F. Theophylline-isoniazid interaction. DICP Ann Pharmacotherapy (1989) 23, 143–5.
4 Samigun, Mulyono, Santos B. Lowering of theophylline clearance by isoniazid in slow and rapid acetylators. Br J Clin Pharmac (1990) 29, 570–3.

Theophylline + Ketoconazole, Fluconazole

Abstract/Summary

Although ketoconazole normally appears not to interact with theophylline in normal subjects, one report says that it can reduce theophylline levels in asthmatics. An isolated report describes increased theophylline levels in a patient given fluconazole.

Clinical evidence, mechanism, importance and management

No changes in the pharmacokinetics of theophylline (3 mg/kg IV) were seen in 12 normal subjects after taking 400 mg ketoconazole daily for five days.[1] Similar results were found in another study in 10 normal subjects.[2] However a case report describes a man whose serum theophylline levels fell sharply from about 16.5 to 9 mg/l (a subtherapeutic level) over the 2 h immediately after taking 200 mg ketoconazole. A less striking fall was seen in two other patients.[3] An isolated and undetailed report says that one of two patients given theophylline and fluconazole showed a rise in serum theophylline levels.[4] It would now seem prudent therefore to monitor the effects of concurrent use in any patient. More study is needed.

References

1 Brown MW, Maldonado AL, Meredith CG, Speeg KV. Effect of ketoconazole on hepatic oxidative drug metabolism. Clin Pharmacol Ther (1985) 37, 290–7.
2 Heusner JJ, Dukes GE, Rollins DE, Tolman KG, Galinsky RE. Effect of chronically administered ketoconazole on the elimination of theophylline in man. Drug Intell Clin Pharm (1987) 21, 514–7.
3 Murphy E, Hannon D, Callaghan B. Ketoconazole-theophylline interaction. Irish Med J (1987) 80, 123–4.
4 Tett S, Carey D, Lee H-S. Drug interactions with fluconazole. Med J Aust (1992) 156, 365.

Theophylline + Macrolide antibiotics

Abstract/Summary

Triacetyloleandomycin (troleandomycin, TAO) can increase serum theophylline levels, causing toxicity if the dosage is not reduced. Clarithromycin, josmycin, midecamycin, miocamycin (ponsinomycin), rokitamycin, roxithromycin and spiramycin normally only cause modest changes in theophylline levels or do not interact at all. There is an unexplained and isolated case report of theophylline toxicity with josamycin. See also 'Theophylline + Erythromycin'.

Clinical evidence

(a) Clarithromycin, Dirithromycin, Midecamycin, Miocamycin (Ponsinomycin), Rokitamycin, Roxithromycin and Spiramycin

250 mg clarithromycin twice daily for seven days had no effect on the serum theophylline levels of 30 patients.[24] Another study found a 17% rise in the AUC, but this was considered clinically unimportant.[25] However two studies suggest that a modest reduction in theophylline dosage may be necessary in a few patients.[26,27] 14 normal subjects showed a steady-state theophylline trough serum level fall of 18%, and a peak serum level fall of 26% while taking 500 mg dirithromycin daily for 10 days.[17] 18 asthmatic children showed a slight decrease in serum theophylline levels when given midecamycin (40 mg/kg/day) for 10 days for a bronchopulmonary infection, but no changes were seen in a pharmacokinetic study in five normal adults.[9] No significant changes in serum theophylline levels were seen in 20 patients on slow-release theophylline (*Theodur*), 600 mg daily, or 4 mg/kg intravenous theophylline, three times daily, when concurrently treated with 1200 mg miocamycin daily for 10 days.[10] A number of other studies confirm the absence of a clinically important interaction between theo-

phylline and miocamycin in children and adults.[12,15,16,21] Two studies in 12 adults and 11 elderly patients on theophylline showed no significant changes in serum theophylline levels when given 600 mg rokitamycin daily for a week.[13,22] A study in 12 normal subjects and another in 16 patients showed only minor changes in the pharmacokinetics of theophylline when given 300 mg roxithromycin daily.[14,19] A study in 15 asthmatic patients on theophylline showed that the concurrent use of 1 g spiramycin for at least 5 days had no significant effect on their steady-state serum theophylline levels.[11]

(b) Josamycin

No significant changes in the serum theophylline levels were seen in four studies in adult and child patients given josamycin concurrently.[4–6,7] but a modest rise was described in another study in children.[29] Another study reported a fall of 23% in five patients with particularly severe respiratory impairment, but no significant effect in five other patients with less severe disease.[8] However an isolated report describes unexplained theophylline toxicity in a man of 80 when given josamycin.[18]

(c) Triacetyloleandomycin

Eight patients with severe chronic asthma showed a 50% reduction in their theophylline clearance when treated with 250 mg triacetyloleandomycin four times daily. One of them had a theophylline-induced seizure after 10 days with a serum theophylline level of 40 µg/ml (normal range 10–20 µg/ml). The theophylline half-life in this patient had increased from 4.6 to 11.3 h.[1–3] Other studies in adult and child patients have found reductions in theophylline clearance of 24–26% and marked rises in serum theophylline levels due to triacetyloleandomycin.[20,23,28]

Mechanism

It is believed that triacetyloleandomycin forms inactive cytochrome P-450-metabolite complexes within the liver cells, the effect of which is to reduce the metabolism of theophylline, thereby reducing its loss from the body. Josamycin, midecamycin, ponsinomycin, rokitamycin and spiramycin have different molecular structures which apparently do not behave like triacetyloleandomycin.[11]

Importance and management

The theophylline/triacetyloleandomycin interaction is established and well documented. If triacetyloleandomycin is added, reduce the theophylline dosage by 25% initially, monitor the effects closely and 'titrate' the dosage as necessary.[28] Alternative macrolides which interact only modestly, or not at all, are dirithromycin, josamycin, midecamycin, miocamycin, rokitamycin, roxithromycin and spiramycin. Even with these it would be prudent to monitor the outcome because a few patients may need some theophylline dosage adjustment.

References

1 Weinburger M, Hudgel D, Spector S, Chidsey C. Troleandomycin (TAO): an inhibitor of theophylline metabolism. J Allergy Clin Immunol (1976) 57, 262.

2 Weinburger M, Hudgel D, Spector S, Chidsey C. Effect of triacetyloleandomycin (TAO) on the metabolism of theophylline. Clin Pharmacol Ther (1976) 19, 118.

3 Weinburger M, Hudgel D, Spector S, Chidsey C. Inhibition of theophylline clearance by troleandomycin. J Allergy Clin Immunol (1977) 59, 228.

4 Ruff F, Prosper M, Pujet JC. Theophylline et antibiotiques. Absence d'interaction avec la josamycine. Therapie (1984) 39, 1–6.

5 Baos RJ, de Frias EC, Cadorniga R, Moreno M. Estudio de posibles interaccinones entre josamicina y teofilina en ninos. Rev Farmacol Clin Exp (1985) 2, 345–8.

6 Ruff F, Santais MC, Chastagnol D, Huchon G, Durieux P. Macrolide et theophylline: absence d'interaction josamycine-theophylline. Nouv Presse Med (1981) 10, 175.

7 Brazier JL, Kofman J, Faucon G, Perrin-Fayolle M, Lepape A, Lanove R. Retard d'elimination de la theophylline du a la troleandomycine. Absence d'effet de la josamycine. Therapie (1980) 35, 545.

8 Bartolucci L, Gradoli C, Vincenzi V, Iapadre M, Valori C. Macrolide antibiotics and serum theophylline levels in relation to the severity of the respiratory impairment: a comparison between the effects of erythromycin and josamycin. Chemioterapia (1984) 3, 286–90.

9 Lavarenne J, Paire M, Talon O. Influence d'un nouveau macrolide, la mydecamycine, sur les taux sanguins de theophylline. Therapie (1981) 36, 451–6.

10 Rimoldi R, Babdera M, Fioretti M, Giorcelli R. Miocamycin and theophylline blood levels. Chemioterapia (1986) 5, 213–6.

11 Debruyne D, Jehan A, Bigot M-C, Lechevalier B, Prevost J-N and Moulin M. Spiramycin has no effect on serum theophylline in asthmatic patients. Eur J Clin Pharmacol (1986) 30, 505–7.

12 Principi N, Onorato J, Giuliani MG, Vigano A. Effect of miocamycin on theophylline kinetics in children. Eur J Clin Pharmacol (1987) 31, 701–4.

13 Ishioka T. Effect of a new macrolide antibiotic, 3'-O-propionyl-leucomycin A5 (Rokitamycin), on serum concentrations of theophylline and digoxin in the elderly. Acta Therapeutica (1987) 13, 17–23.

14 Saint-Salvi B, Tremblay D, Surjust A, Lefebvre MA. A study of the interaction of roxithromycin with theophylline and carbmazepine. J Antimicrob Chemother (1987) 20, Suppl B, 121–9.

15 Couet W, Ingrand I, Reigner B, Girault J, Bizouard J, Fourtillan JB. Lack of effect of ponsinomycin on the plasma pharmacokinetics of theophylline. Eur J Clin Pharmacol (1989) 37, 101–4.

16 Dal Negro R, Turco P, Pomari C, de Conti F. Miocamycin doesn't affect theophylline serum levels in COPD patients. Int J Clin Pharmacol Ther Tox (1988) 26, 27–9.

17 Bachmann K, Nunless M, Martin M, Sullivan T, Jauregui L, DeSante K, Sides GD. Changes in steady-state pharmacokinetics of theophylline during treatment with dirithromycin. J Clin Pharmacol (1990) 30, 1001–5.

18 Barbare JC, Martin F, Biour M. Surdosage en théophylline at anomalies des tests hépatiques associés à la prise de josamycine. Therapie (1990) 45, 357.

19 Bandera M, Fioretti M, Rimoldi R, Lazzarini A, Anelli M. Roxithromycin and controlled release theophylline, an interaction study. Chemioterapia (1988) 7, 313–6.

20 Eitches RW, Rachelefsky GS, Katz RM, Mendoza GR, Siegel SC. Methylprednisolone and troleandomycin in treatment of steroid-dependent asthmatic children. Am J Dis Child (1985) 139, 264–8.

21 Principi N, Onorato J, Giuliani M, Vigano A. Effect of miocamycin on theophylline kinetics in asthmatic children. Chemioterapia (1987) 6 (Suppl 2) 339–40.

22 Cazzola M, Matera MG, Paternò E, Scaglione F, Santangelo G, Rossi F. Impact of rokitamycin, a new 16-membered macrolide, on serum theophylline. J Chemother (1991) 3, 240–4.

23 Kamada AK, Hill MR, Brenner AM, Szefler SJ. Inhibition of theophylline clearance by trolandomycin: clinical impact in severe asthmatics. Pharmacotherapy (1990) 10, 255.

24 Valentino G-R, Fabio C, Guffanti EE. Theophylline interaction with new quinolones and macrolides in COPD patients. Am Rev Resp Dis (1991) 143, A498.

25 Ruff SY, Chu SY, Sonders RC et al. Effect of multiple doses of clarithromycin on the pharmacokinetics of theophylline. 30th Ann Intersc Conf Antimicrob Ag Chemother, Atlanta, GA, October 23rd, 1990, 213

26 Bachand RT. Comparative study of clarithromycin and ampicillin in the treatment of patients with acute bacterial exacerbations of chronic bronchitis. J Antimicrol Chemother (1991) 27, Suppl A, 91–100.

27 Aldons PM. A comparison of clarithromycin with ampicillin in the treatment of outpatients with acute bacterial exacerbations of chronic bronchitis. J Antimicrob Chemother (1991) 27, Suppl A, 101–8.

28 Kamada AK, Hill MR, Brenner AM, Szefler SJ. Effect of low dose troleandomycin on theophylline clearance: implications for therapeutic monitoring. Pharmacotherapy (1992) 12, 98–102.

29 Vallarino G, Merlini M, Vallarino R. Josamicina e teofillinici nella patologia respiratoria pediatrica. Giornale Italiano Chemioterapia (1982) 29, Suppl 1, 129–33.

Theophylline + Methotrexate

Abstract/Summary

Methotrexate causes a modest reduction (19%) in the loss of theophylline from the body.

Clinical evidence

The apparent clearance of theophylline was reduced by 19% (from 48 to 38.9 ml/hr/kg) in 15 severe steroid dependent asthmatics on prednisolone sodium phosphate (40 mg/1.73 m^2) after 6 weeks treatment with 15 mg IM methotrexate weekly. Three patients complained of nausea and the theophylline dosage was reduced in one of them.[1]

Mechanism

Not known.

Importance and management

Information seems to be limited to this study and its clinical importance is uncertain, but it would be prudent to monitor concurrent use for any increase in theophylline side-effects.

Reference

1 Glynn-Barnhart AM, Erzurum SC, Leff JA, Martin RJ, Cochran JE, Cott GR, Szefler SJ. Effect of low-dose methotrexate on the disposition of glucocorticiods and theophylline. J Allergy Clin Immunol (1991) 88, 180–6.

Theophylline + Metoclopramide

Abstract/Summary

Metoclopramide causes a slight but unimportant fall in the bioavailability of *TheoDur* but the incidence of theophylline side-effects may possibly be increased.

Clinical evidence, mechanism, importance and management

10 mg metoclopramide taken 20 min before two 300 mg tablets of slow-release theophylline (*TheoDur*) caused a small (14.5%) but not statistically significant fall in the bioavailability of the theophylline in eight normal subjects. Adverse side-effects (nausea, headache, tremors, CNS stimulation) were seen more often in those taking metoclopramide than in those taking a placebo, possibly because of an earlier rise in the theophylline levels, and because the effects of the two drugs may be additive.[1] There would seem to be no reason for avoiding the concurrent use but the outcome should be monitored. The authors of this report point out that these results should not extrapolated to patients with gastric stasis or receiving other slow-release theophylline preparations.

Reference

1 Steeves RA, Robinson JD, McKenzie MW, Justus PG. Effects of metoclpramide on the pharmacokinetics of a slow-release theophylline product. Clin Pharm (1982) 1, 356–60.

Theophylline + Metronidazole

Abstract/Summary

No interaction of clinical importance normally takes place if metronidazole is given to patients taking theophylline, but an isolated report describes seizures in one patient also taking ciprofloxacin.

Clinical evidence, mechanism, importance and management

While taking metronidazole (250 mg three times a day) for trichmoniasis, the pharmacokinetics of theophylline in five women were slightly but not significantly changed.[1] Another study in five normal subjects confirmed this finding.[2] Seizures developed in one patient when given metronidazole and ciprofloxacin,[3] but seizures have also been seen (though very rarely) in patients on theophylline and ciprofloxacin in the absence of metronidazole. Although the evidence is limited, no special precautions would seem to be necessary during concurrent use.

References

1 Reitberg DP, Klarnet JP, Carlson JK, Schentag JJ. Effect of metronidazole on theophylline pharmacokinetics. Clin Pharm (1983) 2, 441–4.
2 Adebayo GI. Lack of inhibitory effect of metronidazole on theophylline disposition in healthy subjects. Br J Clin Pharmacol (1987) 24, 110–13.
3 Semel JD, Allen N. Seizures in patients simultaneously receiving theophylline and imipenem or ciprofloxacin or metronidazole. S Med J (1991) 84, 465–8.

Theophylline + Mexiletine, Tocainide

Abstract/Summary

Serum theophylline levels are increased by mexiletine. The theophylline dosage will need to be reduced (approximately halved) to avoid toxicity. Tocainide has only a small and probably clinically unimportant effect on theophylline.

Clinical evidence

(a) Mexiletine

A man developed theophylline toxicity within a few days of starting 200 mg mexiletine three times daily. His serum theophylline levels had risen from 15.3 to 25 µg/ml, but they fell to 14.2 µg/ml with the disappearance of the toxicity when the theophlline dosage was reduced from 600 to 200 mg daily.[1]

Other reports describe approximately doubled theophylline serum levels (accompanied by clear signs of toxicity in some instances) in a total of six patients when additionally given mexiletine.[2,4,6,13] One patient also showed arrhythmia aggravation even at therapeutic theophylline serum levels.[6]

600 mg mexiletine daily for 5 days in 15 normal subjects reduced the clearance of an IV infusion of theophylline (5 mg/kg) by 46% in the women and 40% in the men. The theophylline half-life was prolonged by 96% in the women and 71% in the men.[3,7] Two other studies found falls of 37 and 44% in the clearance of theophylline,[8] while two further studies found increases in theophylline AUCs of 58 and 65% when mexiletine was given, associated with a marked increase in theophylline side-effects.[9,10,11]

(b) Tocainide

After taking 400 mg tocainide 8-hourly for 5 days, the pharmacokinetics of a single 5 mg/kg IV dose of theophylline was measured in eight subjects. The clearance was decreased about 10% (from 37.5 to 33.7 ml/hr/kg) and the half-life slightly prolonged (from 9.7 to 10.4 hr).[12]

Mechanism

Mexiletine inhibits the metabolism (demethylation) of theophylline by the liver, thereby reducing its loss from the body and increasing its effects.[3,5,7,11] Studies in rats have shown that tocainide has a substantially smaller effect on the P450IA (CYP1A) family of isoenzymes than mexiletine.[14]

Importance and management

The theophylline-mexiletine interaction is established and of clinical importance. Monitor concurrent use and reduce the theophylline dosage as necessary (to approximately half[1,7]) to prevent the development of theophylline toxicity. It seems doubtful if the theophylline/tocainide interaction is of clinically important but this needs confirmation.

References

1 Katz A, Buskila D, Sukenik S. Oral mexiletine-theophylline interaction. Int J Cardiol (1987) 17, 227–8.
2 Stanley R, Comer T, Taylor JL, Saliba D. Mexiletine-theophylline interaction. Amer J Med (1989) 86, 733–4.
3 Loi CM, Vestal RE. Effect of mexiletine on theophylline metabolism. Clin Pharmacol Ther (1990) 45, 130.
4 Ueno K, Miyai K, Seki T, Kawaguchi Y. Interaction between theophylline and mexiletine. DICP Ann Pharmacother (1990) 24, 471–2.
5 Ueno K, Miyai K, Kato M, Kawaguchi Y, Suzuki T. Mechanism of interaction between theophylline and mexiletine. DICP Ann Pharmacother (1991) 25, 727–30.
6 Kessler KM, Interian A, Cox M, Topaz O, De Marchena EJ, Myerburg RJ. Proarrhythmia related to a kinetic and dynamic interaction of mexiletine and theophylline. Am Heart J (1989) 117, 964–6.
7 Loi CM, Wei X, Vestal RE. Inhibition of theophylline metabolism by mexiletine in young male and female non-smokers. Clin Pharmcol Ther (1991) 49, 571–80.
8 Gannon JM, Mohiuddin SM, Destache CJ, Stoysich AM, Hilleman DE. Interaction between theophylline and mexiletine. Clin Pharmacol Ther (1991) 49, 142.
9 Stoysich AM, Mohiuddin SM, Destache CJ, Nipper HC, Hilleman DE. Influence of mexiletine on the pharmacokinetics of theophylline in healthy volunteers. J Clin Pharmacol (1991) 31, 354–7.
10 Vacek JL, Sztern MI, Botteron GW, Hurwitz A, Hughes EM, Jayaraj A. Mexiletine-theophylline interaction. J Am Coll Cardiol (1990) 15, 39A.
11 Hurwitz A, Vacek JL, Botteron GW, Sztern MI, Hughes EM, Jayaraj A. Mexiletine effects on theophylline disposition. Clin Pharmacol Ther (1991) 50, 299–307.
12 Loi CM, Wei X, Parker BM, Korrapati MR, Vestal RE. Effect of tocainide on theophylline elimination. Br J Clin Pharmac (1993) 35, 437–40.
13 Kendall JD, Chrymko MM, Cooper BE. Theophylline-mexiletine interaction: a case report. Pharmacotherapy (1992) 12, 416–8.
14 Wei X, Loi CM, Jarvi E, Vestal RE. Relative potency of mexiletine, lidocaine and tocainide as inhibitors of rat liver cytochrome P4501A activity. FASEBJ (quoted in Ref 12 as in press).

Theophylline + Moricizine

Abstract/Summary

Moricizine increases the loss of theophylline from the body. An increase in the theophylline dosage may possibly be necessary during concurrent use.

Clinical evidence

Prompted by the observation that theophylline levels decreased in four patients when treated with moricizine, a further study was undertaken on 15 normal subjects using single doses of aminophylline and a sustained-release preparation (*TheoDur*). After taking moricizine for 2 weeks (dosage not stated) the AUC fell by about 40%, theophylline clearance increased by 46–68% and the elimination half-life decreased by 20–34%.[1]

Another study found decreases in theophylline AUCs of 32% (immediate-release preparation) and 36% (controlled release preparation) when given 250 mg moricizine 8-hourly for 2 weeks.[2]

Mechanism

Uncertain. A likely reason is that moricizine increases the metabolism of theophylline.

Importance and management

Information seems to be limited to these studies. The clinical importance of this interaction has not been assessed, but monitor the effects of concurrent use and be alert for the need to increase the theophylline dosage. More study is needed.

References

1 Quoted as data on file, Du Pont Pharmaceuticals, by Siddoway LA, Schwartz SL, Barbey JT, Woosley RL. Clinical pharmacokinetics of moricizine. Am J Cardiol (1990) 65, 21–25D.
2 Benedek IH, Pieniaszek HJ, Davidson AF. Effect of moricizine on the pharmacokinetics of theophylline in healthy volunteers. Pharm Res (1989) 6, S-234.

Theophylline + Nizatidine

Abstract/Summary

Increased serum theophylline levels in a handful of cases have been attributed to the concurrent use of nizatidine.

Clinical evidence, mechanism, importance and management

Five reports of apparent interactions occur in the FDA Spontaneous Adverse Drug Reaction Database. Three patients aged 61–79 on theophylline developed elevated serum theophylline levels, with toxicity in at least one case, when given nizatidine. The problems resolved when both drugs or nizatidine were stopped. Two other possible cases are briefly mentioned.[1] Nizatidine would not be expected to interact this way because, unlike cimetidine, it is not an enzyme inhibitor, however these cases underline the importance of monitoring concurrent use so that the occasional interaction can be identified and dealt with accordingly.

Reference

1 Shinn AF. Unrecognized drug interactions with famotidine and nizatidine. Arch intern Med (1991) 151, 810–1.

Theophylline + Non-steroidal anti-inflammatory drugs (NSAIDs)

Abstract/Summary

Neither nimesulide nor piroxicam appear to interact with theophylline.

Clinical evidence, mechanism, importance and management

20 mg piroxicam daily for 7 days had no effect on the pharmacokinetics of theophylline, given as aminophylline 6 mg/kg intravenously, in six normal subjects.[1] Nimesulide did not affect lung function in patients taking slow-release theophylline with chronic obstructive airways disease, although there was a slight, clinically insignificant fall in theophylline levels, possibly due to enzyme induction. The pharmacokinetics of the nimesulide were unchanged.[2] No special precautions seem to be necessary with either of these NSAIDs.

References

1 Maponga C, Barlow JC, Schentag JJ. Lack of effect of piroxicam on theophylline clearance in healthy volunteers. DICP Ann Pharmacotherapy (1990) 24, 123–6.
2 Auteri A, Blardi P, Bruni F, Domini L, Pasqui AL, Saletti M, Verzuri MS, Scaricabarozzi I, VArgui G, Di Perri T. Pharmacokinetics and pharmacodynamics of slow-release theophylline during treatment with mimesulide. Int J Clin Pharmacol Res (1991) 11, 211–7.

Theophylline + Ozagrel

Abstract/Summary

Ozagrel appears not to interact with theophylline.

Clinical evidence, mechanism, importance and management

Twice daily dosing for 24 weeks of 200 mg ozagrel to four asthmatic patients on theophylline was found not to alter their serum theophylline levels. Seven days treatment with the same dose of ozagrel in another eight asthmatic patients was also found not to affect the pharmacokinetics of a single infusion of aminophylline.[1] No special precautions would seem to be needed during concurrent use.

Reference

1 Kawakatsu K, Kino T, Yasuba H, Kawaguchi H, Tsubata R, Satake N. Effect of ozagrel (OKY-046), a thromboxane synthetase inhibitor, on theophylline pharmacokinetics in asthmatic subjects. Int J Clin Pharmacol Ther Toxicol (1990) 28, 158–63.

Theophylline + Pantoprazole

Abstract/Summary

Pantoprazole appears not to interact with theophylline.

Clinical evidence, mechanism, importance and management

Repeated once daily IV injections of 30 mg pantoprazole had no clinically important effect on the steady-state serum theophylline concentrations in eight normal subjects.[1] No special precautions would seem necessary during concurrent use.

Reference

1 Schulz H-U, Hartmann M, Steinijans VW, Huber R, Lührmann B, Bliessath H, Wurst W. Lack of influence of pantoprazole on the disposition kinetics of theophylline in man. Int J Clin Pharmacol Ther Toxicol (1991) 29, 369–75.

Theophylline + Oxpentifylline or Theophylline

Abstract/Summary

Oxpentifylline (pentoxifylline) can raise serum theophylline serum levels. Patients on theophylline should not take other medications containing theophylline unless the total dosage of theophylline can be adjusted appropriately.

Clinical evidence, mechanism, importance and management

(a) Oxpentifylline

The mean trough steady-state theophylline serum levels of nine normal subjects on 300 mg *TheoDur* daily were 30% higher (range 0–95%) while taking 400 mg oxpentifylline three times daily. The subjects complained of insomnia, nausea, diarrhoea and tachycardia more frequently while taking both drugs, but this did not reach statistical significance.[1] The mechanism of this interaction is not understood. Patients should be well monitored while taking both drugs. More study is needed.

(b) Theophylline

A report of a patient on theophylline for bronchospasm who developed elevated serum theophylline levels when additionally given *Quinamm* for leg cramps (old formulation containing quinine and aminophylline), highlights the need to avoid the inadvertent intake of additional doses of theophylline if toxicity is to be avoided. The newer formulation of *Quinamm* does not contain theophylline.[2] Theophylline preparations are available over the counter in some countries. Patients should be warned.

References

1 Ellison MJ, Horner RD, Willis SE, Cummings DM. Influence of pentoxifylline on steady-state theophylline serum concentrations from sustained-release formulations. Pharmacotherapy (1990) 10, 383–6.
2 Shane R. Potential toxicity of theophylline in combination with *Quinamm*. Amer J Hosp Pharm (1982) 39, 40.

Theophylline + Phenylpropanolamine

Abstract/Summary

There is evidence that phenylpropanolamine can markedly reduce the clearance of theophylline from the body. Increases in serum theophylline levels and toxicity may occur.

Clinical evidence, mechanism, importance and management

150 mg phenylpropanolamine given orally decreased the clearance of theophylline in 8 subjects by 50% (a reduction from 0.88 to 0.44 µg/ml/h) when given as a 4 mg/kg IV aminophylline bolus 1 h after taking the phenylpropanolamine.[1] Such a large reduction would be expected to cause a marked rise in serum theophylline levels, but so far no studies of this potentially clinically important interaction seem to have been carried out in patients. Be alert for evidence of toxicity if both drugs are used. More study is needed.

Reference

1 Wilson HA, Chin R, Adair NE, Zaloga GP. Phenylpropanolamine significantly reduces the clearance of theophylline. Am Rev Resp Dis (1991) 143, A629.

Theophylline + Pinacidil

Abstract/Summary

Pinacidil appears not to interact with theophylline.

Clinical evidence, mechanism, importance and management

After taking 25 mg pinacidil daily for a week, and then 50 mg daily for a further week, the pharmacokinetics and metabolism of single iv 5 mg/kg doses of theophylline were not significantly changed in six normal subjects.[1] This suggests that concurrent use in patients is likely to be safe, but further confirmation is needed.

Reference

1 Nielsen-Kudsk JE, Nielsen CB, Mellemkj'ber S, Siggard C. Lack of effect of pinacidil on theophylline pharmacokinetics and metabolism in man. Pharmacol & Toxicol (1990) 67, 156–8.

Theophylline + Pirenzepine

Abstract/Summary

Pirenzepine does not interact with theophylline.

Clinical evidence, mechanism, importance and management

50 mg pirenzepine daily for 5 days had no effect on the pharmacokinetics of theophylline (given as aminophylline, 6.5 mg/kg body weight, intravenously) in five normal subjects.[1] This would suggest that concurrent use need not be avoided.

Reference

1 Sertl K, Rameis H, Meryn S. Pirenzepin does not alter the pharmacokinetics of theophylline. Int J Clin Pharmacol Ther Toxicol (1987) 25, 15–17.

Theophylline + Pneumococcal vaccine

Abstract/Summary

Pneumococcal vaccination appears not to affect theophylline.

Clinical evidence, mechanism, importance and management

The pharmacokinetics of theophylline (250 mg given orally three times daily for 10 days) were unaltered in six normal subjects the day after receiving 0.5 ml of a pneumococcal vaccine, and week later.[1,2] These findings need confirmation in patients, but what is known suggests that no special precautions are needed during concurrent use.

References

1 Cupit GC, Self TH, Pieper JA, Pieper JA, Bekemayer WB. Effect of pneumococcal vaccine (PV) on theophylline (T) disposition. Clin Pharmacol Ther (1987) 41, 199.
2 Cupit GC, Self TH, Bekemayer WB. The effect of pneumococcal vaccine on the disposition of theophylline. Eur J Clin Pharmacol (1988) 34, 505–7.

Theophylline and Related drugs + Probenecid

Abstract/Summary

Serum levels of theophylline are unaffected by the concurrent use of probenecid, but serum diprophylline (dyphylline) and enprofylline levels can be raised.

Clinical evidence, mechanism, importance and management

A study in 12 subjects showed that the half-life of dyphylline (dihydroxypropyl theophylline) (20 mg/kg) was doubled (from 2.6 to 4.9 h) and the clearance halved (from 173 to 95 ml/h/kg) by the concurrent use of 1 g probenecid, resulting in raised serum dyphylline levels.[1] In another study in six normal subjects the total body clearance of enprofylline was halved (from 21 to 9.8 l/h) by the concurrent use of 1 g probenecid.[3] In contrast, a study in seven normal subjects showed that 1 g probenecid given 30 min before an oral dose of aminophylline (5.6 mg/kg) had no significant effect on the pharmacokinetics of theophylline.[2] The probable reason for the difference is that theophylline is largely cleared from the body by liver metabolism, whereas dyphylline and enprofylline are mostly lost in the urine which is where probenecid is most likely to interfere.

These are single doses studies and the outcome of chronic concurrent use is therefore uncertain, but it would seem to be prudent to monitor serum dyphylline and enprofylline levels if probenecid is started or stopped.

References

1 May DC, Jarboe CH. Inhibition of clearance of dyphylline by probenecid. N Engl J Med (1981) 304, 791.
2 Chen TWD, Patton TF. Effect of probenecid on the pharmacokinetics of aminophylline. Drug Intell Clin Pharm (1983) 17, 465–6.
3 Borga O, Parsson R, Lunell E. Effects of probenecid on enprofylline kinetics in man. Eur J Clin Pharmacol (1986) 30, 221–3.

Theophylline + Propafenone

Abstract/Summary

Two isolated reports describe theophylline toxicity and raised serum levels in two patients when given propafenone.

Clinical evidence

The theophylline serum levels of a 71-year old man taking 300 mg twice daily rose from 10.2–12.8 µg/ml to 19 µg/ml with signs of theophylline toxicity when given 150 mg propafenone three times daily, and fell again when it was withdrawn. When the propafenone was later restarted, the theophylline levels rose again within a week to 17.7 µg/ml, but fell again when the theophylline dosage was reduced to 200 mg twice daily.[1] Another report describes a marked reduction in the clearance of theophylline and rises in serum theophylline levels in a patient when propafenone in doses up to 300 mg 8-hourly was started.[2]

Mechanism

Uncertain. The probably reason is that the propafenone reduces the metabolism of the theophylline by the liver, thereby reducing its loss from the body.

Importance and management

Information is limited to these two reports. The unpredictability of this interaction means that the effect of adding propafenone to established treatment with theophylline in any patient should be monitored. Be alert for increased serum levels and signs of toxicity. Lower the theophylline dosage if necessary.

References

1 Lee BL, Dohrmann ML. Theophylline toxicity after propafenone treatment: evidence for drug interaction. Clin Pharmacol Ther (1992) 51, 353–5.
2 Spinler SA, Gammaiton A, Charland SL, Hurwitz J. Propafenone-theophylline interaction. Pharmacotherapy (1993) 13, 68–71.

Theophylline + Pyrantel

Abstract/Summary

A single case report describes increased serum theophylline levels in a child when given pyrantel embonate (pyrantel pamoate).

Clinical evidence

A boy of eight with status asthmaticus was treated firstly with aminophylline and then switched to oral theophylline on day three. On day four he was additionally given a single 160 mg dose of pyrantel embonate for an *Ascaris Lumbricoides* infection at the same time as his second theophylline dose. About 2.5 h later his serum theophylline level had risen from 15 to 24 µg/ml. The theophylline was stopped. 1.5 h later it had risen to 30 µg/ml. No theophylline toxicity occurred and the patient was discharged later in the day without theophylline.[1]

Mechanism

Not understood. One suggestion is that the pyrantel inhibited the liver enzymes concerned with the metabolism of the theophylline, thereby reducing its loss from the body. Another is that it increased drug release from the sustained-release theophylline preparation.

Importance and management

Information is limited to this single case report. No general conclusions can be based on such slim evidence but concurrent use should be well monitored because in this case the serum theophylline concentration increase was very rapid. More study is needed.

Reference

1 Hecht L, Murray WE. Theophylline-pyrantel pamoate interaction. DICP Ann Pharmacotherapy (1989) 23, 258.

Theophylline + Quinolone antimicrobials and other quinolones

Abstract/Summary

Theophylline serum levels can be markedly increased (two-three-fold) in some patients by the concurrent use of enoxacin or ciprofloxacin. The theophylline dosage may need to be approximately halved if toxicity is to be avoided. OPC-17116, pipemidic acid and tosufloxacin also interact but to a lesser extent. No theophylline dosage adjustment will probably be needed in most patients given fleroxacin, flosequinan, levofloxacin (DR3355), lomefloxacin, nalidixic acid, norfloxacin, ofloxacin, pefloxacin, or sparfloxacin because they normally cause a much smaller rise in theophylline levels, or even no rise at all. However serious toxicity has been seen in few patients given norfloxacin. The situation with rufloxacin is as yet uncertain.

Clinical evidence

(a) Theophylline + Ciprofloxacin

A study in 33 patients on theophylline found that ciprofloxacin, 750 mg twice daily, doubled their serum theophylline levels (from 7.8 to 14.6 μg/ml). Seven of the older patients showed symptoms of theophylline toxicity.[1]

Numerous case reports and studies in normal subjects and patients confirm this interaction.[2,3,8,22–5,29,30,34,44,51,59] with up to threefold increases in serum theophylline levels and/or toxicity. Three of the subjects showed 42–113% decreases.[2] The CSM in the UK had eight reports of clinically important toxic interactions in 1988 between these two drugs.[3] Two elderly women on theophylline daily died with toxic serum levels shortly after starting to take ciprofloxacin.[3,34] By1992 the FDA had 39 reports, 36% of which involved seizures. Three patients died.[61] In contrast an unexplained report found no increases in theophylline levels and no toxicity in 20 patients given 500–750 mg ciprofloxacin twice daily.[4] Seizures occurred in five patients given both drugs,[44,56,60] two of whom were epileptics, and in another also taking metronidazole.[57]

(b) Theophylline + Enoxacin

Two to 3-fold rises in serum theophylline levels and/or theophylline toxicity (nausea, vomiting) have been seen in patients and subjects within 3–5 days of starting 600–1200 mg enoxacin daily.[5,6,7,8,11,18,38,48,54] Constant theophylline serum levels in the presence of 800 mg enoxacin daily were achieved in one study by reducing the theophylline dosage from 400 to 200 mg daily.[35]

(c) Theophylline + Fleroxacin

The theophylline pharmacokinetics of 5 subjects were unchanged by 200 mg fleroxacin given twice daily for 3 days.[28] Another study in 12 subjects given 400 mg fleroxacin daily found that most of the pharmacokinetic parameters of theophylline were unchanged, but the clearance was reduced and half-life increased but only minimally (< 10%).[32] Four other studies found that 400 mg fleroxacin daily had little or no effect on steady-state serum theophylline levels or its clearance in normal subjects.[33,42,45,46,50]

(d) Theophylline + Flosequinan

14 days treatment with 50–100 mg flosequinan in 21 subjects had no significant effect on the pharmacokinetics of theophylline.[39]

(e) Theophylline + Levofloxacin (DR3355)

300 mg levofloxacin daily for 5 days was found to cause rises of only 2–3% in the theophylline AUC and serum levels after 5 days use.[59] Another study also found only trivial rises in theophylline serum levels after taking 300 mg levofloxacin daily for five days.[64]

(f) Theophylline + Lomefloxacin (NY-198)

400 mg lomefloxacin daily for 7 days had little or no effect on the pharmacokinetics of theophylline in 25 normal subjects, although the half-life was slightly increased (from 6.72 to 7.02 h).[17] Other studies in normal subjects similarly found that 200–400 mg lomefloxacin twice daily for up to 7 days did not significantly affect the pharmacokinetics of theophylline.[21,26,31,47,55,58]

(g) Theophylline + Nalidixic acid

500 mg nalidixic acid four times daily for 7 days did not significantly affect the pharmacokinetics of theophylline.[49]

(h) Theophylline + Norfloxacin

Four studies found that 800 mg norfloxacin daily did not affect theophylline levels[12,13,14,29] but some modest changes were found in others. For example 800 mg norfloxacin daily for 6 days increased the half-life of aminophylline and AUC by 16% and 14% respectively, and decreased the clearance 15%.[15] The greatest individual change in clearance was 29%.[15] Other studies found clearance decreases of 8–16%.[43,49] No clinically significant changes in theophylline levels occurred in a patient given norfloxacin who subsequently showed marked changes when given ciprofloxacin.[22] These studies contrast with the FDA records of nine patients who experienced theophylline level increases ranging from 32 to 308% (mean 114%). Three developed seizures and one died.[52,61]

(i) Theophylline + Ofloxacin

400 mg ofloxacin twice daily for 8 days increased the steady-state theophylline levels of 15 subjects by 10.3% and the AUC by 9.9%.[10] In another study an 11% decrease in clearance was seen,[2] and no changes were seen in eight other studies.[11,13,19,29,36,44,53,62]

(j) Theophylline + OPC-17116 (Otsuka Pharmaceutical)

200 mg OPC-17116 caused rises in the theophylline serum levels and AUC of 28–33%.[57]

(k) Theophylline + Pefloxacin

800 mg pefloxacin daily for 5½ days in eight patients raised their serum theophylline levels by 19.6% while the clearance fell by 29.4%.[9,11] No changes were seen in another study.[13] An isolated report describes convulsions in a patient attributed to the concurrent use of theophylline and pefloxacin.[27]

(l) Theophylline + Pipemidic acid

800 mg pipemidic acid for 5 days in 12 subjects prolonged the elimination half-life of theophylline by 75% (from 6.2 to 10.8 h).[37] Another study found 800 mg daily for 5 days approximately doubled the theophylline half-life.[55] 1500 mg daily increased the theophylline AUC by 79% and the maximal serum level by 71% by 5 days in yet another study.[59]

(m) Theophylline + Rufloxacin

Studies with single doses of theophylline (300 mg) and rufloxacin (400 mg) found no evidence of a significant pharmacokinetic interaction.[40]

(n) Theophylline + Sparfloxacin

A study in six asthmatic patients taking theophylline showed that concurrent treatment for one week with 200 mg sparfloxacin daily did not significantly affect the clearance or the plasma levels of the theophylline.[41]

(o) Theophylline + Tosufloxacin (T-3262, Toyama)

A study in seven normal subjects on theophylline showed that concurrent treatment with 150 mg tosufloxacin three times daily for 10 days increased steady-state theophylline levels by about 50%.[48] Another study found that 450 mg daily caused a 23% rise in serum levels and an AUC rise of 24% after 5 days use,[59] and a further study found an AUC increase of 60% after four days of 900 mg daily.[61]

Mechanism

These quinolone antibiotics appear to inhibit the metabolism of theophylline by the liver to different extents (some hardly at all), so that it is cleared from the body more slowly and its serum levels rise. The renal clearance may also be reduced.[16] There is also some evidence that combined use may also amplify the epileptogenic activity of the quinolones.[63]

Importance and management

The theophylline/enoxacin and /ciprofloxacin interactions are well documented, well established and of clinical importance. The incidence is uncertain but it does not cause problems in all patients.[7] The risk seems greatest in the elderly[1] and those with theophylline levels already towards the top end of the therapeutic range. Toxicity may develop rapidly (within 2–3 days) unless the dosage of theophylline is reduced. Reductions of 25–50% have been suggested,[6,11,29,35] although reductions of 75% may possibly be necessary for those with high theophylline clearances.[35] One study found that new steady-state serum theophylline levels were achieved within about three days of starting and stopping enoxacin.[20] Direct information about pipemidic acid and tosufloxacin is more limited, but they also appear to cause a considerable rise in serum theophylline levels.[37,48,61] A smaller rise has been seen with OPC-17116.[59]

Keep a check on the effects if norfloxacin, ofloxacin or pefloxacin are used because theophylline serum levels may possibly rise to a small extent (10–20%[10,11]) but these antibiotics normally appear to be much safer. However be aware that norfloxacin on occasions has caused a much larger rise.[52,61] Fleroxacin, flosequinan (a vasodilator), levofloxacin, lomefloxacin, nalidixic acid and sparfloxacin appear not to interact significantly and no special precautions seem necessary. The situation with rufloxacin is as yet uncertain.

References

1 Raoof S, Wollschlager C, Khan FA. Ciprofloxacin increases serum levels of theophylline. Am J Med (1987) 82 (Suppl 4A) 115–18.
2 Nix DE, DeVito JM, Whitbread MA, Schentag JJ. Effect of multiple dose oral ciprofloxacin on the pharmacokinetics of theophylline and indocyanine green. J Antimicrob Chemother (1987) 19, 263–9.
3 Bem JL, Mann RD. Danger of interaction between ciprofloxacin and theophylline. Br Med J (1988) 296, 1131.
4 Maesen FPV, Teengs JP, Bauer C, Davies BI. Quinolones and raised concentrations of theophylline. Lancet (1984) ii, 530.
5 Wijnands WJA, van Herwaarden CLA, Vree TB. Enoxacin raises plasma theophylline concentrations. Lancet (1984) ii, 108.
6 Wijnands WJA, Vree TB, van Herwaarden CLA. Enoxacin decreases the clearance of theophylline in man. Br J Clin Pharmac (1985) 20, 583–8.
7 Davies BI, Maessen FP, Teengs JP. Serum and sputum concentrations of enoxacin after oral single dosing in a clinical and bacteriological study. J Antimicrob Chemother (1984) 14 (Suppl C), 83–9.
8 Thomsen AH, Thompson GD, Hepburn M, Whiting BA. Clinically significant interaction between ciprofloxacin and theophylline. Eur J Pharmacol (1987) 33, 435–6.
9 Wijnands WJA, Vree TB, van Herwaarden CLA. Comment: potential theophylline toxicity with enoxacin. Drug Intell Clin Pharm (1987) 21, 383.
10 Gregoire SL, Grasela TH, Freer JP, Tack KJ, Schentag JJ. Inhibition of theophylline clearance by coadministered ofloxacin without alteration of theophylline effects. Antimicrob Ag Chemother (1987) 31, 375–8.
11 Wijnands WJA, Vree TB, van Herwaarden CLA. The influence of quinolone derivatives on theophylline clearance. Br J Clin Pharmac (1986) 22, 677–83.
12 Bowles SK, Popovski Z, Rybak MJ, Beckman H, Edwards DJ. Effect of norfloxacin on theophylline pharmacokinetics. Clin Pharmacol Ther (1988) 43, 156.
13 Niki Y, Soejima R, Kawane H, Sumi M, Umeki S. New synthetic quinolone antibacterial agents and serum concentration of theophylline. Chest (1987) 92, 663–9.
14 Sano M, Yamamoto I, Ueda J, Yoshikawa E, Yamashinia H, Goto M. Comparative pharmacokinetics of theophylline following two fluoroquinolones co-administration. Eur J Clin Pharmacol (1987) 32, 431–2.
15 Tierney MG, Ho G, Dales RE. Effect of norfloxacin on theophylline pharmacokinetics. Clin Pharmacol Ther (1988) 43, 156.
16 Beckmann J, Elsasser W, Gundert-Remy U, Hertrampf R. Enoxacin-a potent inhibitor of theophylline metabolism. Eur J Clin Pharmacol (1987) 33, 227–30.
17 Nix DE, Norman A, Schentag JJ. Effect of lomefloxacin on theophylline pharmacokinetics. Antimicrob Ag Chemother (1989) 33, 1006–8.

18 Takagi K, Hasegawa T, Yamaki K, Suzuki R, Watanabe T, Satake T. Interaction between theophylline and enoxacin. Int J Clin Pharmacol Ther Tox (1988) 26, 288–92.

19 Al-Turk WA, Shaheen OM, Othman S, Khalaf RM, Awidi AS. Effect of ofloxacin on the pharmacokinetics of a single intravenous theophylline dose. Ther Drug Monit (1988) 10, 160–3.

20 Rogge MC, Solomon WR, Sedman AJ, Welling PG, Koup JR, Wagner JG. The theophylline-enoxacin interaction: II. Changes in the disposition of theophylline and its metabolites during intermittent administration of enoxacin. Clin Pharmacol Ther (1989) 46, 420–8.

21 Nix DE, Norman A, Schentag JJ. Effect of lomefloxacin on theophylline pharmacokinetics. Antimicrob Ag Chemother (1989) 33, 1006–8.

22 Richardson JP. Theophylline toxicity associated with the administration of ciprofloxacin in a nursing home patient. J Amer Geriatr Soc (1990) 38, 236–8.

23 Duraski RM. Ciprofloxacin-induced theophylline toxicity. S Med J (1988) 81,1206.

24 Holden R. Probable fatal interaction between ciprofloxacin and theophylline. Br Med J (1988) 297, 1339.

25 Rybak MJ, Bowles SK, Chandraseker PH. Increased theophylline concentrations secondary to ciprofloxacin. Drug Intell Clin Pharm (1987) 21, 879.

26 Wijnands GJA, Cornel JH, Martea M, Vree TB. The effect of multiple dose oral lomefloxacin on theophylline metabolism. Chest (1990) 98, 1440–4.

27 Conri Cl, Lartigue MC, Abs L, Mestre MC, Vincent MP, Haramburu F, Constans J. Convulsions chez une malade traitée par péfloxacine et théophylline. Therapie (1990) 45, 358.

28 Niki Y, Tasaka Y, Kishimoto T, Nakajima M, Tsukiyama K, Nakagawa Y, Umeki S, Hino J, Okimoto N, Yagi S, Kawane H, Soejma R. Effect pf fleroxacin on serum concentrations of theophylline. Chemotherapy (1990) 38, 364–71.

29 Sano M, Kawakatsu K, Ohkita C, Yamamoto I, Takeyama M, Yamashina H, Goto M. Effects of enoxacin, ofloxacin and norfloxacin on theophylline disposition in humans. Eur J Clin Pharmacol (1988) 35, 161–5.

30 Schwartz J, Jauregui L, Lettieri J, Bachmann K. Impact of ciprofloxacin on theophylline clearance and steady-state concentrations in serum. Antimicrob Ag Chemother (1988) 32, 75–7.

31 LeBel M, Vallée F, St-Laurent M. Influence of lomefloxacin on the pharmacokinetics of theophylline. Antimicrob Ag Chemother (1990) 34, 1254–6.

32 Seelman R, Mahr G. Gottschalk B, Stephan U, Sörgel F. Influence of fleroxacin on the pharmacokinetics of theophylline. Rev Inf Dis (1989) II, Suppl 5, S1100.

33 Soejima R, Niki Y, Sumi M. Effect of fleroxacin on serum concentrations of theophylline. Rev Inf Dis (1989) II Suppl 5, S1099.

34 Paidipaty B, Erickson S. Ciprofloxacin-theophylline drug interaction. Crit Care Med (1990) 18, 685–6.

35 Koup JR, Toothaker RG, Posvar E, Sedman AJ, Colburn WA. Theophylline dosage adjustment during enoxacin administration. Antimicrob Ag Chemother (1990) 34, 803–7.

36 Wijnands WJA, Janssen TJ, Guelen PMJ, Vree TB, De Witte TMC. The influence of ofloxacin and enoxacin on the metabolic pathways of theophylline in healthy subjects. Pharm Weekbl [Sci] (1988) 10, 272–6.

37 Staib AH, Harder S, Fuhr U, Wack C. Interaction of quinolones with the theophylline metabolism in man: investigations with lomefloxacin and pipemidic acid. Int J Clin Pharmacol Ther Toxicol (1989) 27, 289–93.

38 Takagi K, Hasegawa T, Yamaki K, Suzuki R, Watanbe T, Satake T. Interaction between theophylline and enoxacin. Int J Clin Pharmacol Ther Tox (1988) 26, 288–92.

39 Kamali F, Edwards C, Rawlins MD. Lack of effect of flosequinan on the pharmacokinetics of theophylline. Br J Clin Pharmac (1991) 32, 124–6.

40 Cesana M, Broccali G, Imbimbo BP, Crema A. Effect of single doses of rufloxacin on the disposition of theophylline and caffeine after single administration. Int J Clin Pharmacol Ther Tox (1991) 29, 133–8.

41 Takagi K, Yamaki K, Nadai M, Kuzuya T, Hasegawa T. Effect of new quinolone, sparfloxacin, on the pharmacokinetics of theophylline in asthmatic subjects. Antimicrob Ag Chemother (1991) 35, 1137–41.

42 Parent M, St-Laurent M, Bergeron MG, LeBel M. Safety of fleroxacin co-administered with theophylline in young and elderly volunteers. Clin Pharmacol Ther (1989) 45, 164.

43 Davis RL, Kelly HW, Quenzer RW, Standefer J, Steinberg B, Gallegos J. Effect of norfloxacin on theophylline metabolism. Antimicrob Ag Chemother (1989) 33, 212–4.

44 Semel JD, Allen N. Seizures in patients simultaneously receiving theophyl-

line and imipenem or ciprofloxacin or metronidazole. S Med J (1991) 84, 465–8.

45 Seelmann R, Mahr G, Gottschal B, Stephan U, Sörgel F. Influence on the pharmacokinetics of fleroxacin on the pharmacokinetics of theophylline. Rev Infect Dis (1989) II Suppl 5, S1100.

46 Soejima R, Nike Y, Sumi M. Effect of fleroxacin on serum concentrations of theophylline. Rev Infect Dis (1989) II Suppl 5, S1099.

47 Robson RA, Begg EJ, Atkinson HC, Saunders DA, Frampton CM. Comparative effects of ciprofloxacin and lomefloxacin on the oxidative metabolism of theophylline. Br J Clin Pharmac (1990) 29, 491–3.

48 Takagi K, Hasegawa T, Ogura Y, Suzuki R, Yamaki K, Watanabe T, Kitazawa S, Satake T. Comparative studies on interaction between theophylline and quinolones. J Asthma (1988) 25, 63–71.

49 Prince RA, Casabar E, Adair CG, Wexler DB, Lettieri J, Kasik JE. Effect of quinolone antimicrobials on theophylline pharmacokinetics. J Clin Pharmacol (1989) 29, 650–4.

50 Parent M, St-Laurent M, LeBel M. Safety of fleroxacin coadministered with theophylline to young and elderly volunteers. Antmicrob Ag Chemother (1990) 34, 1249–53.

51 Spivey JM, Laughlin PH, Goss TF, Nix DE. Theophylline toxicity secondary to ciprofloxacin administration. Ann Emerg Med (1991) 20, 1131–4.

52 Green L, Clark J. Fluoroquinolones and theophylline toxicity: norfloxacin. J Amer Med Ass (1988) 262, 2383.

53 Fourtillan JB, Granier J, Saint-Salvi J, Slamon J, Surjus A, Tremblay D, Du Laurier MV, Beck S. Pharmacokinetics of ofloxacin and theophylline alone and in combination, Infection (1986) Suppl 1, S67–9.

54 Mahr G, Seelmann R, Granneman R, Sylvester J, Gottschalf B, Jürgens C, Muth P, Stephan U, Sörgel F. The effect of temafloxacin and enoxacin on the pharmacokinetics of theophylline. Proc 29th Intersci Conf Antimicrob Ag Chemother (1989) Houston, Texas, p 137.

55 Staib AH, Harder S, Fuhr U, Wack C. Interaction of 4-quinolones with theophylline metabolism in man: investigations with lomefloxacin and pipemidic acid. Proc 29th Intersci Conf Antimicrob Ag Chemother (1989) Houston, Texas, p 137.

56 Slavich IL, Gleffe RF, Haas EJ. Grand mal seizures during ciprofloxacin therapy. J Amer Med Ass (1989) 261, 558–9.

57 Niki Y, Hashiguchi K, Okimoto N, Soejima R. Quinolone antimicrobial agents and theophylline. Chest (1992) 101, 891.

58 Kuzuya T, Takagi K, Aiochartoichean R, Muraoka I, Nadai M, Hasegawa T. Kinetic interaction between theophylline and a new developed quinolone NY-198. J Pharmacobiodyn (1989) 12, 405–9.

59 Grasela TH, Dreis MW. An evaluation of the quinolone-theophylline interaction using the Food and Drug Administration spontaneous reporting system. Arch Intern Med (1992) 152, 617–621.

60 Bader MB. Role of ciprofloxacin in fatal seizures. Chest (1992) 101, 883–4.

61 Muralidharan G, Kinzig M, Kazempour, Faulkner R, Kinchelow T, Lockhart S, Sörgel F. Effects of tosufloxacin on the metabolism of theophylline and the relationship to TOS drug levels. Int Sci Conf Antimicrob Ag Chemother (1992) Abstracts, p 355

62 Petermann W. Ofloxacin in lower respiratory tract infections. Infection (1991) 19, Suppl 7, S372–7.

63 Segev S, Rehavi M, Rubinstein E. Quinolones, theophylline and diclofenac interactions with gamma-aminobutyric acid receptor. Antimicrob Ag Chemother (1988) 32, 1624–6.

64 Okimoto N, Niki Y, Soejima R. Effect of levofloxacin on serum concentrations of theophylline. Chemotherapy (1992) 40, 68–74.

Theophylline + Repirinast

Abstract/Summary

Repirinast appears not to interact adversely with theophylline.

Clinical evidence, mechanism, importance and management

A study in seven adult asthmatics given 400–800 mg theophylline twice daily found that repirinast (dosage not clearly stated but by implication 150 mg twice daily) for 3 weeks had no effects on the pharmacokinetics of the theophylline.[1] 300 mg repirinast daily had no effect on the pharmacokinetics of theophylline in 10 asthmatics.[2] No special precautions would seem necessary if both drugs are given.

Reference

1 Tagaki K, Kuzuya T, Horiuchi T, Nadai M, Apichartpichean R, Ogura Y, Hasegawa T. Lack of effect of repirinast on the pharmacokinetics of theophylline in asthmatic patients. Eur J Clin Pharmacol (1989) 37, 301–3.
2 Nagata M, Tabe K, Houya I, Kiuchi H, Sakomoto Y, Yamamoto K, Dohi Y. The influence of repirinast, an anti-allergic drug, on theophylline pharmacokinetics in patients with bronchial asthma. Jap J Thoracic Dis (1991) 29, 413–9.

Theophylline + Ribavirin

Abstract/Summary

Ribavirin does not interact with theophylline.

Clinical evidence, mechanism, importance and management

200 mg ribavirin 6-hourly had no effect on the serum theophylline levels of 13 normal subjects given aminophylline, nor of six children with either influenza superimposed on bronchial asthma or an asthmatic syndrome treated with theophylline.[1] No special precautions seem necessary.

Reference

1 Fraschini F, Scaglione F, Maierna G, Cogo R, Furcolo F, Gattei R, Borghu C, Palazzini E. Ribavirin influence on theophylline plasma levels in adults and children. Int J Clin Pharmacol Ther Toxicol (1988) 26, 30–2.

Theophylline + Rifampicin (Rifampin)

Abstract/Summary

Serum theophylline levels can be reduced by the concurrent use of rifampicin. An increase in the theophylline dosage may be necessary.

Clinical evidence

After taking 600 mg rifampicin daily for a week, the AUC following 450 mg of a sustained-release aminophylline preparation of seven normal subjects was reduced by 18%. A parallel study with eight normal subjects showed that the metabolic clearance of intravenous aminophylline was increased by 45%.[1]

Other studies in normal subjects given 600 mg rifampicin daily for 1–2 weeks showed that rises in theophylline clearance of 25–82% occurred.[2-7] A 61% fall in serum theophylline levels occurred in a 15-month-old boy when given rifampicin.[8] An unusual report paradoxically describes markedly increased serum theophylline levels in a patient treated with rifampicin and isoniazid.[9]

Mechanism

Rifampicin is a potent liver enzyme inducing agent which increases the metabolism of the theophylline, thereby speeding up its clearance from the body resulting in reduced serum levels.[4] Raised theophylline levels in the isolated case may have been due to liver impairment brought about by the combined use of rifampicin and isoniazid.[9]

Importance and management

An established interaction. Serum theophylline levels and its therapeutic effects may be expected to be reduced during concurrent treatment with rifampicin. It can occur within 36 h.[8] The wide range of increases in clearance which have been reported (25–82%) makes it difficult to predict the increase in theophylline dosage required, but in some instances it may possibly need to be doubled.[4]

References

1 Powell-Jackson PR, Jamieson AP, Gray BJ, Moxham J, Williams R. Effect of rifampicin administration on theophylline pharmacokinetics in humans. Am Rev Resp Dis (1985) 131, 939–40.
2 Boyce EG, Dukes GE, Rollins DE, Sudds TW. The effect of rifampin on theophylline kinetics. Clin Pharmacol Ther (1985) 37, 183.
3 Straughn AB, Henderson RP, Lieverman PL, Self TH. Effect of rifampin on theophylline disposition. Ther Drug Monit (1984) 6, 153–6.
4 Robson RA, Miners JO, Wing LMH, Birkett DJ. Theophylline-rifampicin interaction: non-selective induction of theophylline metabolic pathways. Br J Clin Pharmac (1984) 18, 445–8.
5 Lofdahl CG, Mellstrad T, Svedmyr N. Increased metabolism of theophylline by rifampicin. Respiration (1984) 46 (Suppl 1), 104.
6 Hauser AR, Lee C, Teague RB, Mullins C. The effect of rifampin on theophylline disposition. Clin Pharmacol Ther (1983) 33, 254.
7 Boyce EG, Dukes GE, Rollins DE, Sudds TW. The effect of rifampin on theophylline kinetics. J Clin Pharmacol (1986) 26, 696–9.
8 Brocks DR, Lee KC, Weppler CP, Tam YK. Theophylline-rifampin in a pediatric patient. Clin Pharm (1986) 5, 602–4.
9 Dal Negro R, Turco P, Trevisan F, De Conti F. Rifampicin-isoniazid and delayed elimination of theophylline: a case report. Int J Clin Pharm Res (1988) VIII, 275–7.

Theophylline + Sucralfate

Abstract/Summary

One study indicates that no interaction occurs. Two others suggest that the absorption of sustained-release theophylline is reduced by sucralfate.

Clinical evidence, mechanism, importance and management

While taking 1 g sucralfate four times daily, no clinically important changes occurred in the absorption of a single 5 mg/kg dose of an oral non-sustained release theophylline preparation (*Slo-Phyllin*) in normal subjects.[1] In contrast, another group of workers found that when 1 g sucralfate was given 30 min before a 350 mg sustained-release theophylline preparation, the theophylline absorption was reduced by 40%.[2] Yet another found that 1 g sucralfate four times daily reduced the absorption of another sustained release preparation (*TheoDur*) by 9%.[3] The reasons are not understood.

Many patients are given sustained-release preparations but none of these studies clearly shows what is likely to happen in clinical practice, so be alert for any evidence of a reduced response to theophylline. Increase the dosage if necessary.

Reference

1 Cantral KA, Schaaf LJ, Jungnickel PW, Monsour HP. Effect of sucralfate on theophylline absorption in healthy volunteers. Clin Pharm (1988) 7, 58–61.
2 Fleischmann R, Bozler G, Boekstegers P. Bioverfugbarkeit von Theophyllirie unter Ulkustherapeutika. Verh Dtsch Ges Inn Med (1984) 90 (II), 1876–9.
3 Kisor DF, Livengood B, Vieira-Fattahi S, Sterchele JA. Effect of sucralfate administration on the absorption of sustained released theophylline. Pharmacotherapy (1990) 10, 253.

Theophylline + Sulphinpyrazone

Abstract/Summary

Sulphinpyrazone can cause a small reduction in serum theophylline levels.

Clinical evidence, mechanism, importance and management

800 mg sulphinpyrazone daily increased the total clearance of theophylline in six normal subjects (125 mg 8-hourly for 4 days) by 22% (range 8.5 to 42%).[1] This appears to be the sum of an increase in the metabolism of the theophylline by the liver, and a decrease in its renal clearance.

Information seems to be limited to this study. The fall in serum theophylline levels in most patients is unlikely to be very important, but it may possibly affect a few. Concurrent use should be monitored.

Reference

1 Birkett DJ, Miners JO, Attwood J. Evidence for a dual action of sulphinpyrazone on drug metabolism in man: theophylline-sulphinpyrazone interaction. Br J Clin Pharmac (1983) 15, 567–9.

Theophylline + Teicoplanin

Abstract/Summary, clinical evidence, mechanism, importance and management

Experimental and clinical studies in patients with chronic obstructive pulmonary disease found that teicoplanin and theophylline (given together as intravenous infusions) had no effect on the steady-state serum levels of either drug.[1] No special precautions would seem necessary during concurrent use.

Reference

1 Angrisani M, Cazzola M, Loffreda A. Losasso C. Lucarelli C, Rossi F. clinical pharmacokinetics of teicloplanin and aminophylline during cotreatment with both medicaments. Int J Clin Pharmacol Res (1992) 12, 165–71.

Theophylline + Tetracyclines

Abstract/Summary

Serum theophylline levels can be increased in a few patients given doxycycline, minocycline or tetracycline although toxicity seems to be uncommon.

Clinical evidence

(a) Doxycycline

A study on 10 asthmatic subjects given doxycycline (100 mg twice daily on day 1 and then 100 mg four times daily for three days) showed that on average their serum theophylline levels were not significantly altered, although four of them showed rises of more than 20%.[2] Another study in nine normal subjects failed to find evidence of a significant interaction with theophylline.[3]

(b) Minocycline

The serum theophylline levels of a woman of 70 with normal liver function increased from 9.8 to 15.5 µg/ml after being given 100 mg minocycline twice daily by infusion for 6 days. No signs of intoxication occurred. The serum concentrations fell to 10.9 µg/ml 14 days after the minocycline was stopped.[7] Another report suggests that minocycline inhibits the formation of theophylline metabolites.[8]

(c) Tetracycline

After taking tetracycline hydrochloride (250 mg four times daily) for eight days an asthmatic patient showed evidence of theophylline toxicity, and after 10 days her serum theophylline levels had risen from about 12–13 mg/l to 30.8 mg/l. A later study in this patient confirmed that the tetracycline was responsible.[5] In an earlier study in eight normal subjects the same dose of tetracyline for 7 days was found to have decreased the clearance of single doses of aminophylline in 4 subjects by 15% and in one subject by 32%. Such a large reduction in clearance in this last subject would be expected to increase steady-state serum theophylline levels by almost 50%.[6]

Other studies in subjects and patients given tetracycline for less than 7–8 days failed to demonstrate important interactions. A trial on nine healthy adults given single doses of aminophylline (5 mg/kg IV) showed that the concurrent use of tetracycline 250 mg 6-hourly for 48 h, had no significant effect on the kinetics of theophylline.[1] Five non-smoking patients with chronic obstructive airway disease showed an average 14% rise in serum theophylline levels after 5 days' treatment with 1000 mg tetracycline daily, but when a sixth patient was included (a smoker) the results were deemed not to be statistically significant.[4]

Mechanism

Not understood. Inhibition of theophylline metabolism and clearance by the tetracyclines has been suggested.[5,8]

Importance and management

Information seems to be limited to these reports. These suggest that a clinically important interaction possibly only occurs in a few patients. Since the reaction is unpredictable, the effects of concurrent use in all patients should be monitored. There seems to be no evidence of adverse interactions with any of the other tetracyclines not already cited here.

References

1 Pfeifer HJ, Greenblatt DJ, Friedman P. Effects of three antibiotics on theophylline kinetics. Clin Pharmacol Ther (1979) 26, 36.
2 Seggev JS, Shefi M, Schey G, Farfel Z. Serum theophylline concentrations are not affected by coadministration of doxycycline. Ann Allergy (1986) 56, 156–7.
3 Jonkman JHG, van der Boom WJV, Schoenmaker R, Holtkamp A, Hempenius J. No influence of doxycycline on theophylline pharmacokinetics. Ther Drug Monit (1985) 7, 92–4.
4 Gotz VP, Ryerson GG. Evaluation of tetracycline on theophylline disposition in patients with chronic obstructive airways disease. Drug Intell Clin Pharm (1986) 20, 694–7.
5 McCormack JP, Reid SE, Lawson LM. Theophylline toxicity induced by tetracycline. Clin Pharm (1990) 9, 546–9.
6 Mathis JW, Prince RA, Wienberger MM. Effect of tetracycline on hydrochloride on theophylline kinetics. Clin Pharm (1982) 1, 446–8.
7 Kawai M, Honda A, Yoshida H, Goto M, Shimokata T. Possible theophylline-minocycline interaction. Ann Pharmacother (1992) 26, 1300–1.
8 Ueno K, Miyai K, Bito K. Interaction between theophylline and minocycline. Jpn J Ther Drug Monit (1991) 7, 140–3.

Theophylline + Thiabendazole

Abstract/Summary

Theophylline serum levels can be markedly increased by the concurrent use of thiabendazole. Toxicity may develop if the theophylline dosage is not reduced appropriately. A 50% reduction has been suggested.

Clinical evidence

An elderly man on prednisone, frusemide, terbutaline and orciprenaline was additionally given theophylline by infusion (40–50 mg/h). When he was also given 4 g thiabendazole daily for five days for a *Strongloides stercoralis* infestation he developed theophylline toxicity and his serum levels were found to have more than doubled (from 19.2 to 46 µg/ml), although he had previously been treated with 3 g thiabendazole daily for three days uneventfully (and unsuccessfully).[1]

Another patient developed elevated serum theophylline levels when started on 1.8 g thiabendazole twice daily, despite a dosage reduction. Theophylline levels fell when the thiabendazole was stopped.[2]

A retrospective study of patients given both drugs found that nine out of forty (23%) had developed elevated serum theophylline levels and five of the nine experienced toxicity.[4] A study in six normal subjects found that 1.5 mg thiabendazole twice daily for 3 days markedly affected the pharmacokinetics of aminophylline; the half-life increased (from 6.72 to 18.60 h), the clearance fell (from 0.067 to 0.023 l/h/kg) and the elimination rate constant also decreased (from 0.11 to 0.039 h^{-1}). Two of the subjects experienced severe nausea, vomiting and dizziness.[3]

Mechanism

Uncertain. It is suggested that the thiabendazole inhibits the metabolism of the theophylline by the liver thereby prolonging its stay in the body and raising its serum levels. The nausea and vomiting may have been due to both the theophylline and the thiabendazole.[2]

Importance and management

An established interaction of clinical importance. Monitor the effects of concurrent use and reduce the theophylline dosage accordingly. The authors of the second report suggest a 50% theophylline dosage reduction.[2]

References

1 Sugar AM, Kearns PJ, Haulk AA, Rushing JL. Possible thiabendazole-induced theophylline toxicity? Amer Rev Resp Dis (1980) 122, 501.
2 Lew G, Murray WE, Lane JR, Haeger E. Theophylline-thiabendazole drug interaction. Clin Pharm (1989) 8, 225–7.
3 Schneider D, Gannon R, Sweeney K, Shore E. Theophylline and antiparasitic drug interactions. A case report and a study of the influence of

thiabendazole and mebendazole on theophylline kinetics in adults. Chest (1990) 97, 84–7.

4 German T, Berger R. Interaction of theophylline and thiabendazole in patients with chronic obstructive lung disease. Am Rev Resp Dis (1992) 145, A807.

Theophylline + Thyroid and Antithyroid compounds

Abstract/Summary

The serum levels of theophylline can increase and toxicity may develop if hyperthyroidic patients are treated with antithyroid compounds without reducing the theophylline dosage. An increase in the theophylline requirements may occur if thyroid hormones are given to hypothyroidic patients.

Clinical evidence

The clearance of theophylline is much greater in hyperthyroidic patients (0.155 h^{-1}) than in euthyroidic (0.107 h^{-1}) or hypothyroidic patients (0.60 h^{-1}).[1] Drug-induced changes in the thyroid status will therefore alter the amount of theophylline which is needed to maintain therapeutic levels.

(a) Theophylline + Antithyroid compounds

The serum theophylline levels of an asthmatic patient doubled (from 16.8 to 30.9 µg/ml) accompanied by toxicity, following treatment for hyperthyroidism with radioactive iodine (I^{131}).[2] Five hyperthyroidic patients showed a reduction in their clearance of theophylline from 3.98 to 3.17 l/h, and a rise in the theophylline half-life from 4.6 to 5.9 h when treated with carbimazole.[3]

(b) Theophylline + Thyroid hormones

A patient taking 1 g theophylline daily and who was hypothyroidic (serum thyroxine 1.4 g/100 ml) developed severe theophylline intoxication (serum levels 34.7 g/ml) accompanied by life-threatening cardiac arrhythmia. Two months later after treatment with thyroid hormones which increased his serum levels to 4.3 g/100 ml, his serum theophylline levels had fallen to 13.5 g/ml while continuing to take the same theophylline dosage (1 g daily).[4]

Mechanism

The thyroid status affects the rate at which theophylline is metabolized. In hyperthyroidism it is increased, whereas in hypothyroidism it is decreased.

Importance and management

It is well established that changes in thyroid status affect how the body handles theophylline. Monitor the effects and anticipate the need to reduce the theophylline dosage if treatment for hyperthyroidism is started (e.g. with radioactive iodine, carbimazole, etc.). Similarly anticipate the need to increase the theophylline dosage if treatment is started for hypothyroidism (e.g. with levothyroxine).

References

1 Pokrajac M, Simic D, Varagic VM. Pharmacokinetics of theophylline in hyperthyroid and hypothyroid patients with chronic obstructive pulmonary disease. Eur J Clin Pharmacol (1987) 33, 483–6.

2 Johnson CE, Cohen IA. Theophylline toxicity after iodine 131 treatment for hyperthyroidism. Clin Pharm (1988) 7, 620–2.

3 Vozeh S, Otten M, Staub J-J, Follath F. Influence of thyroid function on theophylline kinetics. Clin Pharmacol Ther (1984) 36, 634–40.

4 Aderka D, Shavit G, Garfinkel D, Santo M, Gitter S, Pinkhas J. Life-threatening theophylline intoxication in a hypothyroidic patient. Respiration (1983) 44, 77–80.

Theophylline + Ticlopidine

Abstract/Summary

Ticlopidine reduces the loss of theophylline from the body.

Clinical evidence, mechanism, importance and management

250 mg ticlopidine twice daily for 10 days in 10 subjects reduced the clearance of a single 5 mg/kg oral dose of theophylline by 37% (from 0.682 to 0.431 ml/kg/min) and increased the half-life by 42% (from 514 to 731 min).[1] The reason is not known but it seems possible that the ticlopidine inhibits the metabolism of the theophylline by the liver. Information is very limited, but it would now seem prudent to monitor the effects of concurrent use. It may be necessary to reduce the dosage of the theophylline.

Reference

1 Colli A, Buccino G, Cocciolo M, Parravicini R, Elli GM, Scaltrini G. Ticlopidine-theophylline interaction. Clin Pharmacol Ther (1987) 41, 358–62.

Theophylline + Tobacco or Cannabis smoking

Abstract/Summary

Tobacco or cannabis smokers and non-smokers heavily exposed to smoke may need more theophylline than other non-smokers to achieve the same therapeutic benefits because the theophylline is cleared from the body more quickly. This may also occur in those who chew tobacco or take snuff but not if they chew nicotine gum.

Clinical evidence

A study found that the mean half-life of theophylline in a group of smokers was 4.3 h compared with 7 h in a group of non-smokers.[1] Almost identical results were found in another study,[2] and a number of other studies confirm these findings.[3–5] The same increased clearance has been seen in a patient who chewed tobacco (1.11 compared with the more usual 0.59 ml/kg/min).[8] The theophylline half-life in passive smokers (non-smokers regularly exposed to tobacco smoke in the air they breathe) is reported to be shorter than in non-smokers (6.93 compared with 8.69 h).[10] One study found that tobacco or cannabis smoking increased the total clearance of theophylline from 52 to 74 ml/kg/hr. It rose to 93 ml/kg/hr in those who smoked both.[5]

Mechanism

Tobacco and cannabis smoke contain polycyclic hydrocarbons which act as liver enzyme inducing agents, and this results in a more rapid clearance of theophylline from the body.[6]

Importance and management

An established interaction of moderate clinical importance. Smokers may have (explicably) fewer theophylline side-effects than non-smokers,[7] even so they should clearly be encouraged not to smoke. Heavy smokers (20–40 cigarettes daily) may need double the theophylline dosage of non-smokers, and increased doses are likely for those who chew tobacco or take snuff, but not those who chew nicotine gum.[8,11] One report says that a week after stopping smoking the clearance of theophylline falls by almost 40% so that a dosage reduction may be needed,[9] whereas another says that recovery takes many months.[1]

Investigators of the possible interactions of theophylline with other drugs should take into account the theophylline/tobacco[10] and cannabis's interaction in both smokers and passive smokers when selecting their subjects.

References

1 Hunt SN, Jusko WJ, Yurchak AM. Effect of smoking on theophylline disposition. Clin Pharmacol Ther (1976) 19, 546.
2 Jenne J, Nagasawa H, McHugh R, Macdonald F, Wyse E. Decreased theophylline half-life in cigarette smokers. Life Sci (1975) 17, 195.
3 Powell JR, Thiercelin J-F, Vozeh S, Sansom L and Riegelman S. The influence of cigarette smoking and sex on theophylline disposition. Am Rev Resp Dis (1977) 116, 17–23.
4 Cusack B, Kelly JG, Lavan J, Noel J, O'Malley K. Theophylline kinetics in relation to age; the importance of smoking. Br J Clin Pharmac (1980) 10, 109–14.
5 Jusko WJ, Schentag JJ, Clark JH, Garndern M, Yurchak AM. Enhanced biotransformation of theophylline in marihuana and tobacco smokers. Clin Pharmacol Ther (1978) 24, 406–10.
6 Grygiel J, Birkett DJ. Cigarette smoking and theophylline clearance and metabolism. Clin Pharmacol Ther (1981) 30, 491–6.
7 Pfeifer HJ, Greenblatt DJ. Clinical toxicity of theophylline in relation to cigarette smoking. Chest (1978) 73, 455–9.
8 Rockwood R, Henann N. Smokeless tobacco and theophylline clearance. Drug Intell Clin Pharm (1986) 20, 624–5.
9 Lee BL, Benowitz NL, Jacob P. Cigarette abstinence, nicotine gum and

theophylline metabolism. Clin Pharmacol Ther (1987) 41, 245.
10 Matsunga SK, Plezia PM, Karol MD, Katz MD, Camilli AE, Benowitz NL. Effects of passive smoking on theophylline clearance. Clin Pharmacol Ther (1989) 46, 399–407.
11 Benowitz NL, Lee BL, Jacob P. Nicotine gum and theophylline metabolism. Biomed & Pharmacother (1989) 43, 1–3.

Theophylline + Vidarabine

Abstract/Summary

A single case report describes a woman who showed a rise in serum theophylline levels when concurrently treated with vidarabine.

Clinical evidence, mechanism, importance and management

A woman under treatment with several drugs (ampicillin, gentamicin, clindamycin, digoxin and aminophylline for congestive heart failure, chronic pulmonary disease and suspected abdominal sepsis) developed elevated serum theophylline levels 4 days after starting to take vidarabine (400 mg daily) for herpes.[1] The suggestion is that the vidarabine inhibited the metabolism of the theophylline. Whether this is an interaction is uncertain, but it would now seem prudent to be on the alert for a rise in serum theophylline levels if vidarabine is given concurrently.

Reference

1 Gannon R, Sullman S, Levy RM, Grober J. Possible interaction between vidarabine and theophylline. Ann Intern Med (1984) 101, 148.

Theophylline + Viloxazine

Abstract/Summary

Viloxazine increases serum theophylline levels and intoxication may occur unless the theophylline dosage is reduced.

Clinical evidence

A study in eight normal subjects given a single 200 mg dose of theophylline showed that the concurrent use of 300 mg viloxazine daily increased the 24-h AUC of the theophylline by 47%, increased the maximal serum concentration and reduced its clearance.[3]

An elderly woman on theophylline developed acute intoxication (a grand mal seizure) 2 days after starting to take 200 mg viloxazine daily. Her serum theophylline levels had increased threefold (from about 10 to 28 mg/l) and fell again when the viloxazine was withdrawn.[1] Nausea and vomiting, associated with raised serum theophylline levels, occurred in another patient when treated with viloxazine.[2] The theophylline fell to subtherapeutic levels when the viloxazine was eventually stopped.

Mechanism

The suggestion is that the viloxazine competitively antagonizes the metabolism of the theophylline by the liver, thereby reducing its loss from the body and resulting in an increase in its serum levels.

Importance and management

Information seems to be limited to these reports but it would seem to be a clinically important interaction. Theophylline serum levels should be monitored if viloxazine is added, anticipating the need to reduce the dosage.

References

1 Laaban JP, Dupeyron JP, Lafay M, Sofeir M, Rochemaure J, Fabiani P. Theophylline intoxication following viloxazine induced decrease in clearance. Eur J Clin Pharmacol (1986) 30, 351–3.
2 Thompson AH, Addis GJ, McGovern EM, McDonald NJ. Theophylline toxicity following coadministration of viloxazine. Ther Drug Monitor (1988) 10, 359–60.
3 Perault MC, Griesemann E, Bouquet S, Lavoisy J, Vandel B. A study of the interaction of viloxazine with theophylline. Ther Drug Monit (1989) 11, 520–2.

Chapter 23
Tricyclic, Selective Serotonin Uptake Inhibitor and Related Antidepressant Drug Interactions

The development of the tricyclic antidepressants arose out of work carried out on phenothiazine compounds related to chlorpromazine. The earlier ones possessed two benzene rings joined by a third ring of carbon atoms, with sometimes a nitrogen, and of having antidepressant activity (hence their name), however some of the later ones have one, two or even four rings. Table 23.1 lists the common tricyclic antidepressants, the related selective serotonin uptake inhibitors (SSUI) and a number of other compounds which are also used for depression.

Antidepressant activity

The tricyclic antidepressants inhibit the activity of the 'uptake' mechanism by which some chemical transmitters (5-HT or sertonin, noradrenaline or norepinephrine) re-enter nerve endings in the CNS. In this way they raise the concentrations of the chemical transmitter in the receptor area. If depression represents some inadequacy in transmission between the nerves in the brain, increasing amounts of transmitter may go some way towards reversing this inadequacy by improving transmission.

Other properties of the tricyclic antidepressants

The tricyclics also have anticholinergic (atropine-like) activity and can cause dry mouth, blurred vision, constipation, urine retention and an increase in ocular tension. Postural hypotension occurs sometimes and there are also cardiotoxic effects. Among the central side-effects are sedation, the precipitation of seizures in certain individuals, and extrapyramidal reactions.

Selective serotonin uptake inhibitor antidepressants (SSUI)

These antidepressants (citalopram, fluvoxamine, fluoxetine, paroxetine, sertraline etc) act on neurones in a similar way to the tricyclics but they selectively inhibit the re-uptake of serotonin (5-hydroxy-tryptamine or 5HT) and have fewer anticholinergic effects and are also less sedative and cardiotoxic.

Table 23.1 Cyclic and other antidepressants

Non-proprietary names	Proprietary names
Tricyclic compounds	
Amoxapine	*Asendin, Demolox, Omnipress*
Amitriptyline	*Adepril, Amival, Amilent, Amiline, Amilit, Amitid, Amitril, Amitrip(tol), Annolytin, Deprestat,Deprex, Domical, Elavil, Endep, Equilibrin, Laroxyl, Lentizol, Levate, Miketorin, Novotryptin, Redomox, Saroten, Sarotex, Teperin, Trepiline, Triptizol, Tryptanol, Tryptizol*
Butriptyline	*Centrolyse, Evadene, Evadyne*
Clomipramine	*Anafranil*
Desipramine	*Nebril, Norpramin, Nortimil, Pertofran(a), Pertofrin, Sertofren*
Dibenzepin	*Deprex, Ecatril, Noveril*
Dimetacrine	*Istonil, Linostil*
Dothiepin	*Idom, Prothiaden, Protiaden*
Doxepin	*Adapin, Aponal, Co-Dox, Novoxapin, Quitaxon, Sin(e)quan, Sinquane, Spectra, Toruan, Triadapin*
Imipramine	*Antipress, Berkomine, Chimoreptin, Dimipressin, Dynaprin, Efuranol, Ethipramine, Imavate, Imidol, Imiprin, Iramil, Janimine, Medipramine, Melipramine, Norpramine, Novopramine, Oppanyl, Panpramine, Praminil, Presamine, Prodepress,*
Lofepramine	*Amplit, Deftan, Deprimil, Didalen-70, Gamanil, Gamonil, Tymelyt*
Melitracen	*Dixeran, Melixeran, Trausabun*
Nortriptyline	*Allegron, Altilev, Ateben, Aventyl, Kareon, Martimil, Noritren, Nortab, Nortrilen, Pamelor, Paxtibi, Psychostyl, Sensaval, Sensival, Vividyl*
Protriptyline	*Concordin, Maximed, Triptil*
Trimipramine	*Stangyl, Surmontil, Tydamine*
Tetracyclic compound	
Maprotiline	*Ludiomil*
Mianserin	*Athimil, Athymil, Bolvidon, Lantanon, Lerivon, Norval, Tetramide, Tolvin, Tolvon*
Bicyclic compounds	
Viloxazine	*Vicilan, Vivalan*
Selective Serotonin uptake inhibitors	
Citalopram	
Femoxetine	*Malexil*
Fluoxetine	*Prozac*
Fluvoxamine	*Faverin, Fevarin, Floxyfal*
Paroxetine	*Seroxat*
Sertraline	*Lustral*
Other compounds	
Iprindole	*Prondol*
Trazodone	*Deprax, Desyrel, Manegan, Molipaxin, Pragmarel, Thomban, Tramensan, Trittico*
Nomifensine	(withdrawn 1986)
Zimeldine	(withdrawn 1983)

Citalopram + Miscellaneous drugs

Abstract/Summary

Levopromazine decreases the metabolism of citalopram whereas lithium has no effect. There is preliminary evidence that citalopram may possibly increase the effects of imipramine.

Clinical evidence, mechanism, importance and management

A study in three groups of eight normal subjects taking 40 mg citalopram daily for 10 days found that a single 50 mg oral dose of levopromazine increased the initial steady-state levels of the primary metabolite of citalopram (desmethylcitalopram) by 10–20%. The citalopram caused an approximately 50% increase in the AUC (area under the curve) of desipramine (the primary metabolite of imipramine) after a single 100 mg oral dose of imipramine, and a reduction in the levels of the subsequently formed metabolite of desipramine. No changes were seen when 30 mmol/day of lithium was given.[1]

The practical consequences of these changes are still uncertain, but if (as seems likely) the citalopram inhibits the activity of CYP2D6 in the liver, then an increase in the serum levels, the activity and the toxicity of imipramine and other tricyclic antidepressants seems a possibility (as with fluoxetine and the tricyclic antidepressants). Be alert for this potential interaction if citalopram and any of the tricyclic antidepressants are given concurrently. More study is needed to confirm the extent and importance of this possible interaction.

Reference

1 Gram LF, Hansen MG, Sindrup SH, Brosen K, Poulsen JH, Aaes-Jorgensen T, Overo KF. Citalopram: interaction studies with levopromazine, imipramine and lithium. Ther Drug Monit (1993) 15, 18–24.

Femoxetine + Cimetidine

Abstract/Summary

Femoxetine serum levels are increased by cimetidine.

Clinical evidence, mechanism, importance and management

1 g cimetidine daily for 7 days raised the steady-state serum trough levels of femoxetine in six normal subjects taking 600 mg daily by 140% (from 10 to 24 ng/ml). The AUC was increased but not significantly.[1] The probable reason for this interaction is that the cimetidine inhibits the oxidative metabolism of the femoxetine by the liver, reducing its loss from the body and thereby raising the serum levels. The authors of the paper recommend that the initial femoxetine dosage should be reduced from 600 to 400 mg daily. More study is needed to confirm this interaction.

Reference

1 Schmidt J, Sorensen AS, Gjerris A, Rafaelsen OJ, Mengel H. Femoxetine and cimetidine: interaction in healthy volunteers. Eur J Clin Pharmacol (1986) 31, 299–302.

Fluoxetine + Benzodiazepines

Abstract/Summary

Some preliminary evidence suggests that diazepam and alprazolam serum levels (but not clonazepam or triazolam) may be raised by fluoxetine, and that combined use may impair the performance of some psychomotor tests.

Clinical evidence, mechanism, importance and management

One study found that fluoxetine given as single doses or in multiple doses over 8 days had no effect on the pharmacokinetics of 10 mg diazepam,[1] but a later study by the same group suggested that the diazepam half-life and the AUC were increased, possibly because the fluoxetine reduces the metabolism of the diazepam.[2] Another study found that fluoxetine alone did not affect psychomotor performance but fluoxetine plus diazepam impaired the Divided Attention tracking test and Vigilance test more than with diazepam alone.[3] The concurrent use of fluoxetine (60 mg) has been found to reduce alprazolam clearance by almost 30% and increase its plasma levels (1 mg four times daily) also by about 30%[4] while psychomotor impairment is also increased.[4] The pharmacokinetics of clonazepam[6] and triazolam[5] are unaffected by fluoxetine.

The practical importance of all of these findings is uncertain, but the possibility should be borne in mind that combined use of the interacting drugs (diazepam, alprazolam) might adversely affect driving and other skills. Patients should be warned. More study is needed.

References

1 Lemberger L, Bergstrom RF, Wolen RL, Farid NA, Enas GG, Aronoff GR. Fluoxetine: clinical pharmacology and physiologic disposition. J Clin Psychiatry (1985) 46, 3 (Sec 2), 14–19.
2 Lemberger L, Rowe H, Bosomworth JC, Tenbarge JB, Bergstrom RF. The effect of fluoxetine on the pharmacokinetics and psychomotor resposnes of diazepam. Clin Pharmacol Ther (1988) 43, 412–19.
3 Moskowitz H, Burns M. The effects on performance of two antidepressants, alone and in combination with diazepam. Prog Neuropsychopharmacol Biol Psychiatry (1988) 12, 783–92.
4 Lasher TA, Fleishaker JC, Steenwijk RC, Antal EJ. Pharmacokinetic pharmadcodynamic evaluation of the combined administration of alprazolam and fluoxetine. Psychopharmacology (1991) 104, 323–7.
5 Wright CE, Lasher-Sisson TA, Steenwyk RC, Swanson CN. A pharmacokinetic evaluation of the combined administration of triazolam and fluoxetine. Pharmacotherapy (1992) 12, 103–6.

6 Greenblatt DJ, Preskorn SH, Cortreau MM, Horst WD, Harmatz JS. Fluoxetine impairs clearance of alprazolam but not of clonazepam. Clin Pharmacol Ther (1992) 52, 479–86.

Fluoxetine + Bupropion

Abstract/Summary

An isolated report describes severe psychosis in a patient when fluoxetine was replaced by bupropion. Another developed mania on bupropion after fluoxetine was stopped. Yet another patient had grand mal seizures.

Clinical evidence, mechanism, importance and management

The day after stopping 60 mg fluoxetine daily, a man of 41 was started on 75 and later 100 mg bupropion three times daily. After 10 days he became 'edgy and anxious'and after 12 days he developed myoclonus. After 14 days he became severely agitated and psychotic with delerium and hallucinations. His behaviour returned to normal 6 days after the bupropion was stopped.[1] It was suggested that the fluoxetine may have inhibited the metabolism of the bupropion, leading to toxic levels. A little over a week after stopping fluoxetine and starting bupropion, another patient developed anxiety, panic and eventually mania.[3] Yet another patient developed a grand mal seizure after being given fluoxetine and 300 mg bupropion daily.[2] If concurrent or sequential use is thought appropriate, monitor the effects closely. More study is needed.

References

1 Van Putten T, Shaffer I. Delerium associated with bupropion. J Clin Psychopharmacol (1990) 10, 234.
2 Ciraulo DA, Shader RI. Fluoxetine drug-drug interactions.II. J Clin Psychopharmacol (1990) 10, 213–5.
3 Zubiata JK, Demitrack MA. Possible bupropion precipitation of mania and a mixed affective state. J Clin Psychopharmacol (1991) 11, 327.

Fluoxetine + Cannabis

Abstract/Summary

An isolated report describes mania in a patient on fluoxetine after smoking cannabis.

Clinical evidence, mechanism, importance and management

A woman of 21 with a 9-year history of bulimia and depression was treated with 20 mg fluoxetine. A month later, about 2 days after smoking two 'joints' of cannabis (marijuana), she experienced a persistent sense of well-being, increased energy, hypersexuality and pressured speech. These symptoms progressed into grandiose delusions for which she was hospitalized. Her mania and excitement were controlled with lorazepam and perphenazine, and she largely recovered after about 8 days. The reasons for this reaction are not understood but the authors of the report point out that one of the active components of cannabis, Δ–9-tetrahydrocannabinol, is, like fluoxetine, a potent inhibitor of serotonin uptake. Thus a synergistic effect on central serotonergic neurones might have occurred.[1] This seems to be the first and only report of an apparent adverse interaction between cannabis and fluoxetine, but it emphasises the risks of concurrent use.

Reference

1 Stoll AL, Cole JO, Lukas SE. A case of mania as a result of fluoxetine-marijuana interaction. J Clin Psychiatry (1991) 52, 280–1.

Fluoxetine + Cyproheptadine

Abstract/Summary

Two reports say that cyproheptadine can oppose the antidepressant effects of fluoxetine. Another failed to observe this response.

Clinical evidence

Three depressed men complained of anorgasmia when treated with fluoxetine. When this was treated with cyproheptadine their depressive symptoms returned.[1] Two women also complained of anorgasmia within 1–3 months of starting treatment with 40–60 mg fluoxetine daily for bulimia nervosa. When cyproheptadine was added to treat this sexual dysfunction, the urge to binge on food returned in both of them and one experienced increased depression.[3] In contrast, no exacerbation of depression was seen in a previous study in which both cyproheptadine and fluoxetine were used in two patients.[2]

Mechanism

Not fully understood. Cyproheptadine is a serotonin antagonist which appears to block or oppose the serotoninergic effects of fluoxetine.

Importance and management

Information about this interaction appears to be limited to these studies. If concurrent use is thought appropriate, the outcome should be well monitored for evidence of a reduced antidepressant response.

References

1 Feder R. Reversal of antidepressant activity of fluoxetine by cyproheptadine in three patients. J Clin Psychiatry (1991) 52, 163–4.
2 McCormick S, Olin J, Brotman AW. Reversal of fluoxetine-induced anorgasmia by cyproheptadine in two patients. J Clin Psychiatry (1990) 51, 383–4.
3 Goldbloom DS, Kennedy SH. Adverse interaction of fluoxetine and cypro-

heptadine in two patients with bulimia nervosa. J Clin Psychiatry (1991) 52, 261–2.

Fluoxetine + Miscellaneous drugs

Abstract/Summary

Fluoxetine normally appears not to interact with warfarin, dextromethophan or hypoglycaemic agents, but isolated interactions have been seen with warfarin (bleeding, bruising), chloral (prolonged drowsiness), dextromethorphan (hallucinations), insulin (hypoglycaemia), LSD (convulsions) and phenylpropanolamine (dizziness, weight loss, hyperactivity). There is *in vitro* evidence that the effects of flecainide, propafenone and thioridazine may possibly be increased by fluoxetine. Chlorothiazide appears not to interact. See also 'Psychotropics + Fluoxetine'.

Clinical evidence, mechanism, importance and management

(a) Fluoxetine + Anticoagulants

Fluoxetine given as a single dose or in multiple doses over 8 days had no effect on the pharmacokinetics or the anticoagulant effects of 20 mg warfarin.[1] In another study in 3 normal subjects, the half-life of warfarin was not significantly changed by either a single 30 mg dose of fluoxetine given 3 h before the warfarin, or by 30 mg fluoxetine daily for a week.[2] In contrast, a very brief report describes an increase in the effects of warfarin and small bowel haemorrhage in one patient on fluoxetine. The concurrent use of mefenamic acid may have been a contributory factor.[3] Another patient on fluoxetine developed severe bruising when given warfarin.[4] Concurrent use need not be avoided but the effects should be monitored because apparently a few individuals may react adversely.

(b) Fluoxetine + Chlorothiazide

Fluoxetine is reported not to affect the pharmacokinetics of chlorothiazide.[1] No special precautions would seem necessary.

(c) Fluoxetine + Chloral hydrate

Marked drowsiness occurred for a whole day in a patient taking 20 mg fluoxetine daily after being given 500 mg chloral hydrate the night before. She later tolerated 1 g chloral hydrate in the absence of fluoxetine without adverse effects. The reason for this adverse response is not known, but the author suggests the possibility of protein binding displacement, reduced chloral metabolism, or the additive sedative effects of both drugs.[10] The general importance of this interaction is unknown but concurrent use should now be well monitored.

(d) Fluoxetine + Dextromethorphan

A woman who had been on 20 mg fluoxetine daily for 17 days took two teaspoonfuls of a cough syrup containing dextromethorphan, and two more the next morning with the next capsule of fluoxetine. Within 2 h vivid hallucinations developed (bright colours, distortions of shapes and sizes) which lasted 6–8 h. The patient said they were similar to her past experience with LSD 12 years earlier.[9] The reasons for this reaction are not known. This seems to be the first and only report of this interaction. No adverse effects were reported in a metabolic study[11] of fluoxetine with dextromethorphan in large numbers of normal subjects and patients which suggests that the case cited here[9] is unusual. Nevertheless concurrent use should be well monitored.

(e) Fluoxetine + Flecainide, Propafenone, Thioridazine

Studies using human liver microsomes have shown that fluoxetine and its metabolite, norfluoxetine have a strong inhibitory effect on the activity of cytochrome P450IID6 in the liver.[12] The practical consequences of this are that the effects of other drugs whose liver metabolism depends on this particular P450 isoenzyme are likely to be increased and prolonged. A clear example of this is the increase in the effects of the tricyclic antidepressants when fluoxetine is given concurrently (see 'Tricyclic Antidepressants + Fluoxetine'). There is also a single case of markedly increased extrapyamidal side-effects in a patient given perphenazine and fluoxetine (see 'Psychotropics + Fluoxetine'). Other drugs, the effects of which are largely or partly metabolized by P450IID6, include thioridazine, propafenone and flecainide.[13] So far there appear to be no clinical cases of interactions between these drugs and fluoxetine, but it would now be prudent to be alert for increased and prolonged effects if fluoxetine is added.

(f) Fluoxetine + Hypoglycaemic agents

Although one study found that single or multiple doses of fluoxetine over eight days did not affect the pharmacokinetics or the hypoglycaemic effects of 1 g tolbutamide,[1] the makers of fluoxetine say that hypoglycaemia has been seen in patients when fluoxetine was started, and hyperglycaemia when it was stopped.[6] An insulin-dependent diabetic experienced signs of hypoglycaemia (nausea, tremor, sweating, anxiety, lightheadedness) after starting to take 20 mg fluoxetine nightly. These disappeared when the fluoxetine was stopped and reappeared when it was restarted, however blood sugar levels were found to be normal (9–11 mmol/l).[5] The reasons are not understood. Concurrent use need not be avoided but the diabetic control should be monitored if fluoxetine is added.

(g) Fluoxetine + LSD

An isolated report describes grand mal convulsions in a patient while taking fluoxetine, tentatively attributed to the concurrent abuse of LSD.[7]

(h) Fluoxetine + Phenypropanolamine

A 16 year-old-girl with an eating disorder and taking 20 mg fluoxetine four time daily developed vague medical complaints of dizziness, 'hyper' feelings, diarrhoea, palpitations and a reported weight loss of 14 lbs within two weeks. The author of the report suggested that these might have been the result of an interaction with phenylpropranolamine (1–2 capsules of *Dexatrim®* four time daily) which the patient was surreptitiously taking, associated with a restricted food and fluid intake.[8] The general importance of this alleged interaction is uncertain.

References

1 Lemberger L, Bergstrom RF, Wolen RL, Farid NA, Enas GG, Aronoff GR. Fluoxetine: clinical pharmacology and physiologic disposition. J Clin Psychiatry (1985) 46, 3 (Sec 2), 14–19.

2 Rowe H, Carmichael R, Lemberger L. The effect of fluoxetine on warfarin metabolism in the rat and man. Life Sci (1978) 23, 807–12.

3 Beeley L, Magee P, Hickey FN. Bulletin of the West Midlands Centre for Adverse Drug Reaction Reporting (1990) 30, 32.

4 Claire RJ, Servis ME, Cram DL. Potential interaction between warfarin sodium and fluoxetine. Am J Psychiatry (1991) 148, 1604.

5 Lear J, Burden AC. Fluoxetine side-effects mimicking hypoglycaemia. Lancet (1992) 339, 1296.

6 Prozac (Dista Products). ABPI Datasheet Compendium 1991–2, p 397.

7 Picker W, Lerman A, Hajal F. Potential interaction of LSD and fluoxetine. Am J Psychiatry (1992) 129, 843–4.

8 Walters AM. Sympathomimetic-fluoxetine interaction. J Am Acad Child Adolesc Psychiatry (1992) 31, 565–6.

9 Achamallah NS. Visual hallucinations after combining fluoxetine and dextromethorphan. Am J Psychiatry (1992) 149, 1406.

10 Devarajan S. Interaction of fluoxetine and chloral hydrate. Can J Psychiatr (1992) 37, 590–1.

11 Otton SV, Wu D, Joffe RT, Cheung SW, Sellers EM. Inhibition of fluoxetine of cytochrome P450 2d6 activity. Clin Pharmacol Ther (1993) 53, 401–9.

12 Brøsen K, Skjelbo E. Fluoxetine and norfloxetine are potent inhibitors of P450IID6 — the source of the sparteine/debrisoquine oxidation polymorphism. Br J Clin Pharmac (1991) 32, 136.

13 Brdosen K, Gram LF. Clinical significance of the sparteine/debrisoquine oxidation polymophism. Eur J Clin Pharmac (1989) 36, 537–47.

Fluoxetine + Monoamine oxidase inhibitors (MAOIs)

Abstract/Summary

Serious and potentially life-threatening reactions (the serotonin syndrome) can develop if fluoxetine and the non-selective, irreversible MAOI are given concurrently, or even sequentially if insufficient time is left in between. Phenelzine, tranylcypromine and selegiline have all been implicated, but moclobemide appears not to interact.

Clinical evidence

(a) Fluoxetine + Phenelzine or Tranylcypromine

A very high incidence (25–50%) of adverse effects occurred in 12 patients taking fluoxetine (10–100 mg daily) with either phenelzine (30–60 mg daily) or tranylcypromine (10–140 mg daily), and in six other patients started on either of these MAOI 10 days or more after stopping the fluoxetine. There were mental changes such as hypomania, racing thoughts, agitation, restlessness and confusion. The physical symptoms included myoclonus, hypertension, tremor, teeth chattering and diarrhoea.[4]

Uncontrollable shivering, teeth chattering, double vision, nausea, confusion, and anxiety developed in a woman given tranylcypromine after stopping fluoxetine. The problem resolved within a day of stopping the tranylcypromine, and did not recur when fluoxetine was tried again 6 weeks later.[1] Another patient developed feverishness, shivering, tremor and rigidity on the second day of replacing fluoxetine, 60 mg daily, by *Parstelin* (tranylcypromine + trifluoperazine).[5] Confusion, agitation and diaphoresis occurred in yet another patient when fluoxetine was stopped and tranylcypromine started.[6] Fever, chills, flushes, confusion, abdominal cramping, diarrhoea and other signs of the serotonin syndrome developed in a woman taking 20 mg tranylcypromine daily 6 weeks after stopping fluoxetine. Her blood levels of norfluoxetine were still very high (84 ng/ml).[11] The makers of fluoxetine have on record three unpublished reports of fatal toxic reactions attributed to the use of an MAOI after fluoxetine was stopped.[1] Another fatality occurred in a woman on tranylcypromine, fluoxetine, tryptophan and thioridazine.[7]

(b) Fluoxetine + Moclobemide

A placebo-controlled trial in 18 subjects found that the concurrent use of 20 mg fluoxetine and 100–600 mg moclobemide daily for 9 days gave no evidence of an adverse interaction.[9,11] A post-marketing analysis found that at least 30 patients switched from fluoxetine to moclobemide within a week had experienced no ill-effects.[9,12]

(c) Fluoxetine + Selegiline

A woman with parkinson's disease on selegiline, bromocriptine and levodopa-carbidopa was additionally started on 20 mg fluoxetine. Several days later she developed episodes of shivering and sweating in the mid-afternoon which lasted several hours. Her hands became blue, cold and mottled and her blood pressure was elevated (200/120 mmHg). These episodes disappeared when both fluoxetine and selegiline were stopped, and did not reappear when the fluoxetine was restarted.[3]

Another patient became hyperactive and apparently manic about a month after starting to take selegiline and fluoxetine.[3] The makers of fluoxetine are said to know of other cases of interaction.[3] Ataxia developed in a woman with parkinson's disease on multiple therapy which appeared to be related to the concurrent use of fluoxetine and selegiline. No other toxic symptoms developed.[8] Another patient on levodopa, carbidopa, bromocriptine, selegiline and domperidone developed a probable tonic-clonic seizure and a pseudophaeochromocytoma syndrome (headache, flushes, palpitations, blood pressure 250/130 mmHg) when additionally given 20 mg fluoxetine daily.[10]

Mechanisms

Not understood. The symptoms seen in some (but not all) of the patients was not typical of the MAOI-sympathomimetic reaction (no headache, chest pain or raised blood pressure) and appear to be the 'serotonin-syndrome' which is typified by CNS irritability, increased muscle tone, shivering, altered consciousness and mycolonus. Toxicity of this kind has been seen in patients on fluoxetine within a few days of starting additional treatment with L-tryptophan which is a precursor of serotonin (see 'Fluoxetine + L-tryptophan'). A not dissimilar reaction has been seen with phenelzine and tryptophan (see 'MAOI + Tryptophan').

Importance and management

Established interactions of uncertain incidence. Because of the serious nature of the reactions, the concurrent use of the older, non-selective irreversible MAOI or selegiline and fluoxetine should be avoided, and sequential use only undertaken with great care. Dista, the makers of fluoxetine, recommend that (a) 5 weeks should elapse between stopping the fluoxetine and starting the MAOI because the effects of fluoxetine are very persistent, and (b) 2 weeks between stopping an MAOI and starting fluoxetine.[2] Clonazepam has been successfully used to alleviate myoclonus, and 10 mg nifedipine to correct hypertension.[4] Other treatment has included the use of diazepam, pancuronium and cooling.[5] Moclobemide, which is a selective, reversible inhibitor of MAO A, appears not to interact adversely with fluoxetine and would therefore seem to be a safer alternative.[9] A report originating from the makers says that 'after discontinuation of fluoxetine therapy, moclobemide treatment can be started immediately.'

References

1 Sternbach H. Danger of MAOI therapy after fluoxetine withdrawal. Lancet (1988) ii, 850–1.

2 Doyle MJ (Dista Products). Personal communication (1988).

3 Suchowersky O, de Vries JD. Interaction of fluoxetine and selegiline. Can J Psychiatry (1990) 35, 571–2.

4 Feighner JP, Boyer WF, Tyler DL, Neborsky RJ. Adverse consequences of fluoxetine-MAOI combination therapy. J Clin Psychiatry (1990) 51, 222–5.

5 Ooi, TK. The serotonin syndrome. Anaesthesia (1991) 46, 507–8.

6 Spiller HA, Morse S. Fluoxetine ingestion: A one year retrospective study. Vet Hum Toxicol (1990) 32, 153–5.

7 Kline SS, Mauro LS, Scala-Barnett DM, Zick D. Serotonin syndrome versus neuroleptic malignant syndrome as a cause of death. Clin Pharm ((1989) 8, 510–4.

8 Jermain DM, Hughes PL, Follender AB. Potential fluoxetine-selegiline interaction. Ann Pharmacother (1992) 26, 1300.

9 Dingemanse J. An update of recent moclobemide interaction data. Int Clin Psychopharmacol (1993) 7, 167–80.

10 Montastruc JL, Chamontin B, Senard JM, Tran MA, Rascol O, Llau ME, Rascol A. Pseudophaeochromocytoma in parkinsonian patient treated with fluoxetine plus selegiline. Lancet (1993) 341, 555.

11 Coplan JD, Gorman JM. Detectable levels of fluoxetine metabolites after discontinuation: an unexpected serotonin syndrome. Am J Psychiatry (1993) 150, 837.

12 Dingemanse J, Guentert TW, Moritz E, Eckernas S-A. Pharmacodyamic and pharmacokinetic interactions between fluoxetine and moclobemide. Clin Pharmacol Ther (1993) 53, 178

Fluoxetine + Pentazocine

Abstract/Summary

A man on fluoxetine experienced an adverse excitatory reaction when given a single dose of pentazocine.

Clinical evidence, mechanism, importance and management

A man who had been taking 10 mg fluoxetine daily for 10 days, later increased to 40 mg daily, was given a single 100 mg oral dose of pentazocine (*Talwin Nx* containing 50 mg pentazocine and 0.5 mg naloxone) for a severe headache. Within 30 min he complained of lightheadedness, anxiety, nausea and parasthesias of the hands. He was diaphoretic, flushed, ataxic and showed a mild tremor of his arms. His blood pressure was 178/114 mmHg, pulse 62 bpm and respiration 16. He was given 50 mg diphenhdyramine intramuscularly and recovered over the following 4 h. The reasons for this reaction are not understood, but the authors of the report suggest that it may have been due to increased serotoninergic activity in the CNS.[1] The general importance of this possible interaction is uncertain, but the authors of the report advise caution if the use of both drugs is being considered.

Reference

1 Hansen T E, Dieter K, Keepers G A. Interaction of fluoxetine and pentazocine. Am J Psychiatry (1990) 147, 949–50

Fluoxetine + L-tryptophan

Abstract/Summary

Central and peripheral toxicity developed in five patients on fluoxetine when given L-tryptophan.

Clinical evidence, mechanism, importance and management

Concurrent use with low doses of fluoxetine (20 mg daily) is said to be tolerated,[2] but problems have been seen with higher doses. Five patients on fluoxetine (50–100 mg daily) for at least three months developed a number of reactions including central toxicity (agitation, restlessness, aggressivity, worsening of obsessive-compulsive disorders) and peripheral toxicity (abdominal cramps, nausea, diarrhoea) within a few days of starting 1–4 g L-tryptophan daily. These symptoms disappeared when the tryptophan was stopped. Some of the patients had had tryptophan before without problems.

The reason for this reaction is not understood but the authors point out that the symptoms resemble the 'serotonin syndrome' seen in animals when serotonin levels are increased, and warn against the concurrent use of tryptophan with fluoxetine or other serotonin re-uptake inhibitors.[1] Most products containing L-tryptophan for the treatment of depression have been withdrawn in the USA and UK because of a possible association with the development of an eosinophilia-myalgia syndrome.

References

1 Steiner W, Fontaine R. Toxic reaction following the combined administration of fluoxetine and L-tryptophan: five case reports. Biol Psychiatry (1986) 21, 1067–71.
2 Ciraulo DA, Shader RI. Fluoxetine drug-drug interactions II. J Clin Psychopharmacol (1990) 10, 213–7.

Fluvoxamine + Antidepressants

Abstract/Summary

On theoretical grounds an adverse reaction seems possible between fluvoxamine and the irreversible non-selective MAOI's or tryptophan, but moclobemide appears not to interact. Adverse reactions have been reported between fluvoxamine and lithium.

Clinical evidence, mechanism, importance and management

(a) Fluvoxamine + Monoamine oxidase inhibitors

The Committee on the Safety of Medicines in the UK has warned of possible adverse reactions if fluvoxamine is given with antidepressants such as the MAOI,[2] but this is probably an extrapolation from the serious serotonin syndrome reaction seen with fluoxetine, another serotonin re-uptake inhibitor. As yet there seems to be no direct evidence of a similar interaction involving fluvoxamine and an MAOI.

2 normal subjects given 100 mg fluvoxamine and increasing doses of moclobemide from 50 to 400 mg developed no serious adverse reactions. Any adverse events were mild to moderate and were those normally seen with both drugs.[1] Moclobemide is a reversible and selective inhibitor of MAO A (RIMA) so that it would be unwise to assume from its apparent safety with fluvoxamine that the same is true for irreversible non-selective MAOI's.

(b) Fluvoxamine + Lithium

Nineteen reports have been received of adverse reactions when fluvoxamine was given with lithium (five reports of convulsions and one of hyperpyrexia).[2] A patient on fluvoxamine became somnolent within a day of starting additional treatment with lithium and could not stay awake. The serum lithium level 20 h after the last dose was 0.2 mmol/l. She recovered when both drugs were stopped and was discharged on lithium alone.[3] If concurrent use is thought to appropriate, it should be very well monitored.

(c) Fluvoxamine + Tryptophan

The warning about the MAOI and tryptophan by the CSM also appears to be an extrapolation from the reaction (a serotonin-syndrome) which has been seen with fluoxetine, another serotonin re-uptake inhibitor (see 'Fluoxetine + Tryptophan').[2] Most products containing L-tryptophan for the treatment of depression have been withdrawn in the USA and UK because of a possible association with the development of an eosinophilia-myalgia syndrome.

References

1 Dingemanse J. An update of recent moclobemide interaction data. Int Clin Psychopharmacol (1993) 7, 167–80.
2 Committee on the Safety of Medicines. Current Problems, May 1989, 26, 3.
3 Evans M, Marwick P. Fluvoxamine and lithium: an unusual interaction. Br J Psychiatry (1990) 156, 286.

Fluvoxamine + Miscellaneous drugs

Abstract/Summary

Warfarin serum levels are increased by fluvoxamine and bleeding may occur if the anticoagulant dosage is not reduced. No clinically important interaction appears to occur if fluvoxamine is used with propranolol, atenolol, chloral hydrate or the benzodiazepines.

Clinical evidence, mechanism, importance and management

(a) Fluvoxamine + Anticoagulants

The concurrent use of fluvoxamine can increase serum warfarin levels by 65% and a few cases of bleeding have been described.[1,3] The reasons are not understood. Concurrent use need not be avoided but monitor the effects, anticipating the need to decrease the warfarin dosage. Until more information becomes available, apply the same precautions if any other anticoagulant is used.

(c) Fluvoxamine + Beta-blockers, Benzodiazepines, Chloral hydrate

100 mg fluvoxamine daily raised the serum levels of propranolol (160 mg) 5-fold in normal subjects, but the heart-slowing effects were only slightly increased (3 bpm). The diastolic pressure following exercise was slightly reduced but the general hypotensive effects remained unaltered.[1] The probable reason is that the fluvoxamine inhibits the activity of the cytochrome P450 concerned with the metablism of propranolol.[5] No changes in plasma levels of atenolol were seen but the heart-slowing effects were slightly increased and the hypotensive effects slightly decreased.[1] There would seem to be little reason to avoid the concurrent use of fluvoxamine and beta blockers.

Fluvoxamine has also been found not to interact adversely with either chloral hydrate or benzodiazepines.[2,4]

References

1 Duphar files, quoted by Benfield P, Ward A. Fluvoxamine, a review of its pharmacodynamic and pharmocokinetic properties and therapeutic efficacy in depressive illness. Drugs (1986) 32, 313–34.
2 Wagner W, Cimander K, Schnitker J, Koch HF. Influence of concomitant psychotropic medication on the efficacy and tolerance of fluvoxamine. Adv Pharmacotherapy (1986) 2, 34–56.
3 Ashford G (Duphar). Personal communication(s) 1989.
4 Amin MM, Ananth JV, Coleman BS, Darcourt G, Farkas T et al. Fluvoxamine: antidepressant effects confirmed in a placebo-controlled international study. Clin Neuropharmacol (1984) 7 (Suppl 1) S312–9.
5 Brdosen K, Skjelbo E, Rasmussen BB, Poulsen HE, Loft S. Fluvoxamine is a potent inhibitor of cytochrome P4501A2. Biochem Pharmacol (1993) 45, 1211–14.

Mianserin or Nomifensine + Anticonvulsants

Abstract/Summary

The serum levels of both mianserin and nomifensine can be markedly reduced by the concurrent use of phenytoin, phenobarbitone or carbamazepine. Nomifensine has been withdrawn.

Clinical evidence

A comparative study in six epileptics and six normal subjects showed that phenytoin with either phenobarbitone or carbamazepine markedly reduced the serum levels of single doses of mianserin and nomifensine. The mean half-life of mianserin was reduced by 75% (from 16.9 to 4.8 h) and the AUC by 86%. The half-life of nomifensine was not significantly altered, despite the fact that the AUC was reduced by almost 50%.[1,2] Another study in four patients found that carbamazepine reduced serum mianserin concentrations by 70%.[3]

Mechanism

It seems probable that these anticonvulsants increase the metabolism of mianserin and nomifensine by the liver, thereby increasing their loss from the body.

Importance and management

Information appears to be limited to these studies, but the interaction appears to be established and of clinical importance. Monitor concurrent use and increase the dosage of mianserin as necessary. Nomifensine was withdrawn world-wide in January 1986 by the manufacturers because it has been associated with acute immune haemolytic anaemia and intravascular haemolysis

References

1 Nawishy S, Hathaway N, Turner P. Interactions of anticonvulsant drugs with mianserin and nomifensine. Lancet (1981) ii, 871.
2 Richens A, Nawishy S, Trimble M. Antidepressant drugs, convulsions and epilepsy. Br J Clin Pharmac (1983) 15, 295–8S.
3 Leinonen E, Lillsunde P, Laukkanen V, Ylitalo P. Effects of carbamazepine on serum antidepressant concentrations in psychiatric patients. J Clin Psychopharmacol (1991) 11, 313–8.

Maprotiline, Mianserin or Trazodone + Sympathomimetics (directly and indirectly-acting)

Abstract/Summary

No adverse interaction would be expected in patients on maprotiline, mianserin or trazodone who are treated with sympathomimetic amines, however a single report describes toxicity in a woman on trazodone when she took pseudoephedrine.

Clinical evidence, mechanism, importance and management

The pressor (increased blood pressure) responses to tyramine and noradrenaline (norepinephrine) in depressed patients remained virtually unchanged after 14 days treatment with 60 mg mianserin daily.[1–4] In five normal subjects on maprotiline the pressor response to tyramine was reduced three-fold while the noradrenaline response remained unchanged.[7] Other studies on normal subjects given 50 mg trazodone three times a day found that the pressor response to tyramine remained unchanged whereas the response to noradrenaline was reduced.[5] However an isolated report describes a woman who had been taking 250 mg trazodone daily for 2 years who took two doses of an over-the-counter medicine containing pseudoephedrine. Within 6 h she experienced dread, anxiety, panic, confusion, depersonalization and the sensation that parts of her body were separating. None of these symptoms had been experienced in the past on either preparation alone.[6] The reasons for this reaction are not understood.

The practical importance of these observations is that, unlike the tricyclic antidepressants, no special precautions normally seem necessary if patients on maprotiline, mianserin or trazodone are given noradrenaline (norepinephrine) or other directly-acting sympathomimetics. Similarly, none of the dietary precautions against eating tyramine-rich foods or drinks, or the administration of indirectly-acting sympathomimetics such as phenypropranolamine in cough and cold remedies, need to be imposed. However the isolated report cited indicates that the occasional patient may possibly experience unpleasant adverse effects.

References

1 Ghose K, Coppen A, Turner P. Autonomic actions and interactions of

mianserin hydrochloride (Org GB94) and amitriptyline in patients with depressive illness. Psychopharmacology (1976) 49, 201.

2 Coppen A, Ghose K, Swade C, Wood K. Effect of mianserin hydrochloride on peripheral uptake mechanisms for noradrenaline and 5-hydroxytryptamine in man. Br J Clin Pharmac (1978) 5, 13s.

3 Ghose K. Studies on the interaction between mianserin and noradrenaline in patients suffering with depressive illness. J Clin Pharmacol (1977) 4, 712.

4 Coppen AJ, Ghose K. Clinical and pharmacological effects of treatment with a new antidepressant. Arzneim-Forsch/Drug Res (1976) 26, 1166.

5 Larochelle P, Hamet P, Enjalbert M. Responses to tyramine and norepinephrine after imipramine and trazodone. Clin Pharmacol Ther (1979) 26, 24.

6 Weddige RL. Possible trazodone-pseudoephedrine toxicity: a case report. Neurobehav toxicol teratol (1985) 7, 201.

7 Briant RH, George CF. The assessment of potential drug interactions with a new tricyclic antidepressant drug. Br J Clin Pharmac (1974) 1, 113–8.

Paroxetine + miscellaneous drugs

Abstract/Summary

Some, but not all, individuals may show increased paroxetine serum levels if given cimetidine, and possibly reduced serum levels if given carbamazepine, phenobarbitone or phenytoin. The serum levels and effects of these anticonvulsants and sodium valproate appear to be unaffected by paroxetine. An increased bleeding tendency has been seen with warfarin, but paroxetine appears not to interact to a clinically important extent with aluminium hydroxide, amylobarbitone, diazepam, digoxin, haloperidol, sodium valproate or food. There may possibly be a modest loss of attentiveness with oxazepam and alcohol.

Clinical evidence, mechanism, importance and management

(a) Paroxetine + Alcohol, Amylobarbitone, Haloperidol.

Studies in human subjects[4,5] found that paroxetine alone caused little impairment of a series of psychomotor tests related to car driving, and with alcohol the effects were unchanged except for a small decrease in attentiveness.[4] The sedative effects and impairment of psychomotor performance caused by 100 mg amylobarbitone and 3 mg haloperidol were not increased by 30 mg paroxetine.[4] No special precautions seem necessary.

(b) Paroxetine + Aluminium hydroxide

15 ml *Aludrox* (aluminium hydroxide) twice daily increased the absorption of a single 30 mg dose of paroxetine in normal subjects by about 12% and the maximal serum concentration by 14%.[3] This is unlikely to be clinically important. No particular precautions would seem to be necessary.

(c) Paroxetine + Anticonvulsants

100 mg phenobarbitone twice daily for 14 days given to 10 normal subjects caused paroxetine AUC reductions of 10–86% in 6 subjects, but the mean values were unaltered. One subject showed a 56% increase.[1] 16 day's treatment with 30 mg paroxetine daily in 20 epileptics caused no changes in the serum levels or therapeutic effects of carbamazepine, phenytoin or sodium valproate. Steady-state paroxetine serum levels were lower in those taking phenytoin (16 μg/ml) than in those on carbamazepine (27 μg/ml) or sodium valproate (73 μg/ml).[6] A possible explanation is that phenobarbitone, phenytoin and carbamazepine (well recognized enzyme inducing agents) increase the metabolism and loss of paroxetine from the body. Although there seems to be little correlation between plasma paroxetine levels and its efficacy, but be alert for the need to increase its dosage if any of these anticonvulsants is given.

(d) Paroxetine + Cimetidine

200 mg cimetidine four times daily for 8 days did not affect the mean pharmacokinetic values or bioavailability of single 30 mg doses of paroxetine in 10 normal subjects. However two subjects showed AUC increases of 55% and 81% respectively while on cimetidine and four others also showed some increases.[1] Another study in 11 subjects found that 300 mg cimetidine three times a day increased the AUC of a single 30 mg dose of paroxetine by 50%.[2] A likely reason is that cimetidine (a known enzyme inhibitor) reduces the metabolism of the paroxetine and its loss from the body, thereby increasing its serum levels. Monitor concurrent use and reduce the paroxetine dosage if necessary.

(e) Paroxetine + Diazepam or oxazepam

No important changes in the pharmacokinetics of either paroxetine or diazepam were seen when two groups of 12 subjects were given 30 mg paroxetine daily and 5 mg diazepam three times a day.[2] Paroxetine did not increase the impairment by oxazepam of a number of psychomotor tests, but the subjects said that they felt less alert and capable while taking both drugs.[4] There is no reason for avoiding concurrent use, but until more is known about the effects in a real clinical context, it would seem prudent to monitor the outcome.

(f) Paroxetine + Digoxin

No important changes in the pharmacokinetics of either paroxetine or digoxin were seen when two groups of 10 and 13 subjects were given 30 mg paroxetine and 0.25 mg digoxin daily.[2] No special precautions would seem to be needed.

(g) Paroxetine + Food

A study in normal subjects found that paroxetine was not markedly changed by the concurrent ingestion of food. A 40% reduction in absorption was seen when taken with 1 litre of milk, but few people are likely to drink such a large amount.[3]

(h) Paroxetine + Warfarin

30 mg paroxetine daily given to subjects on 5 mg warfarin daily

did not significantly increase their mean prothrombin times, but mild, clinically significant bleeding was seen in 5 out of 27 subjects. Two withdrew from the study because of increased prothrombin times, and another because of haematuria. The disposition of the warfarin and the paroxetine remained unchanged.[2] The reasons for these reactions are not understood. This preliminary information suggests that prothrombin times should be well monitored during concurrent use.

References

1 Greb W H, Buscher G, Dierdorf H-D, Köster F E, Wolf D, Mellows G. The effect of liver enzyme inhibition by cimetidine and enzyme induction by phenobarbitone on the pharmacokinetics of paroxetine. Acta psychiatr scand (1989) 80, (supp 350) 95–8.

2 Bannister S J, Houser V P, Hulse J D, Kisicki J C, Rasmussen J G C. Evaluation of the potential interactions of paroxetine with diazepam, cimetidine, warfarin and digoxin. Acta psychiatr scand (1989) 80, (supp 350) 102–6.

3 Greb W H, Brett M A, Buscher G, Dierdorf H-D, von Schrader H W, Wolf D, Mellows G, Zussman B D. Absorption of paroxetine under various dietary conditions and following antacid intake. Acta psychiatry scand (1989) 80, (supp 350) 99–101.

4 Cooper S M, Jackson D, Loudon J M, McClelland G R, Raptopoulos P. The psychomotor effects of paroxetine alone and in combination with haloperidol, amylobarbitone, oxazepam, or alcohol. Acta psychiatry scand (1989) 80, (supp 350) 53–55.

5 Hindmarch I, Harrison C. The effects of paroxetine and other antidepressants in combination with alcohol on psychomotor activity related to car driving. Acta psychiatry scand (1989) 80, (supp 350) 45.

6 Andersen BB, Mikkelsen M, Versterager A, Dam M, Kristensen HB, Pedersen B, Lund J, Mengel H. No influence of the antidepressant paroxetine on carbamazepine, valproate and phenytoin. Epilepsy Rev (1991) 10, 201–4.

Sertraline + miscellaneous drugs

Abstract/Summary

Sertraline appears not to interact with alcohol, atenolol, diazepam, digoxin, glibenclamide, tolbutamide or warfarin, but concurrent use should be monitored until more experience has been gained in normal clinical situations. The side-effects of lithium (tremor) are possibly increased.

Clinical evidence, mechanism, importance and management

(a) Sertraline + Alcohol

Sertaline has been found not to impair psychomotor performance, including simulated car driving. It also appears not to increase the effects of alcohol.[6] No special precautions would seem necessary.

(b) Sertraline + Atenolol, Diazepam

No clinically relevant effects were found in interaction studies in which sertraline was given with atenolol or diazepam.[6] No special precautions would seem necessary.

(c) Sertraline + Digoxin

A 17-day course of sertraline in doses of up to 200 mg daily had no significant effect on the pharmacokinetics of digoxin (0.25 mg daily) in 10 normal subjects, with the exception of a small decrease in the time taken to achieve maximum serum levels.[5] Sertraline does not significantly alter steady-state serum digoxin levels nor its renal clearance.[5] There would therefore seem to be no good reason for avoiding concurrent use but the outcome should be monitored.

(d) Sertraline + Hypoglycaemic agents

After taking 200 mg sertraline daily for 22 days the clearance of a single IV dose of tolbutamide in 25 subjects was decreased by 16%.[3] In another study in 11 normal subjects the pharmacokinetics of a single 5 mg dose of glibenclamide were found to be unaffected by sertraline taken in increasing doses up to 200 mg daily over 15 days. Blood glucose levels levels were also unchanged.[4] There would seem to be little reason for avoiding concurrent use, but until more is known it would seem prudent to monitor the outcome.

(e) Sertraline + Lithium

After taking 600 mg lithium twice daily for 8 days, a single 100 mg dose of sertraline caused a small but statistically insignificant fall in steady-state serum levels in 8 normal subjects, and a statistically insignificant rise in renal lithium excretion. 7 out of the 8 subjects also experienced side-effects (mainly tremor and nausea) whereas no side-effects were reported in the placebo group.[2] The makers of sertraline advise caution if both drugs are used. Study in patients is needed.

(f) Sertraline + Warfarin

After taking sertraline in stepwise increasing doses up to 200 mg daily for 22 days, the prothrombin time AUC in response to a single 0.75 mg/kg dose of warfarin in 12 normal subjects was increased by 7.9%. This was statistically significant, but regarded as too small to be clinically important, nevertheless concurrent use should be monitored to confirm that this is so when repeated doses of warfarin are given to patients.[1]

References

1 Invicta Pharmaceuticals. Phase I study to assess the potential of sertraline to alter the pharmacokinetics and plasma protein binding of warfarin in healthy male volunteers. Data on file (Study 018), 1991.

2 Invicta Pharmaceuticals. Determination of the effects of sertraline on steady state lithium levels and renal clearance of lithium in healthy volunteers. Data on file (Study 017), 1990.

3 Invicta Pharmaceuticals. Phase I study to assess the potential of sertraline to alter the clearance of plasma protein binding of tolbutamide in healthy volunteers. Data on file (Study 011), 1990.

4 Invicta Pharmaceuticals. A double blind placebo controlled, multiple dose study to assess potential interaction between oral sertraline (200 mg) and

glibenclamide (5 mg) in healthy male volunteers. Data on file (Study 223), 1991.

5 Invicta Pharmaceuticals. A double blind, placebo controlled, parallel group study to investigate the effects of orally administered sertraline on the plasma concentration profile and renal clearance of digoxin. Data on file. (Study 224), 1991.

6 Warrington SJ. Clinical implications of the pharmacology of sertraline. Int Clin Psychopharmacol (1991) 6, Suppl 2, 11–21.

Sertraline + Monoamine oxidase inhibitors (MAOI)

Abstract/Summary

An isolated report describes the development of adverse reactions attributed to the serotonin syndrome in a patient on tranylcypromine and clonazepam when given sertraline.

Clinical evidence, mechanism, importance and management

A depressed man on tranylcypromine and clonazepam was additionally given 25–50 mg sertraline daily. Within 4 days had began to experience chills, increasing confusion, sedation, exhaustion, unsteadiness and incordination. Other symptoms included impotence, urinary hesitancy and constipation. These problems resolved when the sertraline was stopped and the tranycypromine dosage reduced from 30 mg to 20 mg daily. The authors of the study attributed these reactions to the serotonin syndrome which in a more severe form has been seen with other sertoninin reuptake inhibitors (e.g. fluoxetine) and MAOI.[1]

The general importance of this adverse interaction is uncertain, but when set against the background of the severe reactions seen with other sertoninin reuptake inhibitors and MAOI, it would seem prudent not to give sertraline without waiting two weeks after stopping an MAOI. A wait of 5 weeks (recommended for fluoxetine) may not be necessary between stopping sertraline and starting an MAOI because the half-life of sertraline is much shorter than fluoxetine. More study is needed.

Reference

1 Bhatara VS, Bandettini FC. Possible interaction between sertraline and tranylcypromine. Clin Pharm (1993) 12, 222–5.

Tetracyclic antidepressants + Beta-blockers

Abstract/Summary

Maprotiline toxicity attributed to the concurrent use of propranolol has been described in three patients.

Clinical evidence

A patient experienced maprotiline toxicity (dizziness, hypotension, dry mouth, blurred vision, etc.) after taking 120 mg propranolol daily for two weeks. His trough serum maprotiline levels had risen by 40%. The serum levels fell and the side-effects disappeared when the propranolol was withdrawn.[2] A man on 120 mg propranolol daily began to experience visual hallucinations and psychomotor agitation with a few days of starting to take 200 mg maprotiline daily.[3] Another man on haloperidol, benztropine, triamterene, hydrochlorothiazide and propranolol became disorientated, agitated and uncooperative with visual hallucinations and incoherent speech within a week of starting to take 150 mg maprotiline daily. These symptoms disappeared when all the drugs were withdrawn. Reintroduction of the antihypertensive drugs with haloperidol and desipramine proved effective and uneventful.[1]

Mechanism

Not understood. A suggested reason is that the propranolol reduces the blood flow to the liver so that the metabolism of the maprotiline is reduced, leading to its accumulation in the body.

Importance and management

Information seems to be limited to the cases cited. The general importance of this interaction is uncertain, but if concurrent use it thought appropriate the outcome should be well monitored. The authors of one of the reports[3] say that simultaneous use is inadvisable. Another tetracyclic antidepressant, mianserin, appears not to interact with propranolol. See Index.

References

1 Malkek-Ahmadi P, Tran T. Propranolol and maprotiline toxic interaction. Neurobehav Toxicol Teratol (1985) 7, 203–9.

2 Tollefson G, Lesar T. Effect of propranolol on maprotiline clearance. Am J Psychiatry (1984) 141, 148–9.

3 Saiz-Ruiz J, Moral L. Delerium induced by association of propranolol and maprotiline. J Clin Psychopharmacol (1988) 8, 77–8.

Tetracyclic Antidepressants + Contraceptives (oral) or Tobacco smoking

Abstract/Summary

Neither tobacco smoking nor the oral contraceptives affect maprotiline.

Clinical evidence, mechanism, importance and management

A study in women showed that, over a 28-day period, the use of oral contraceptives did not significantly affect the steady-state serum levels of maprotiline (75 mg nightly), nor was its therapeutic effectiveness changed.[1] Smoking also has no effect on maprotiline serum levels nor on its effectiveness.[1,2]

References

1 Luscombe DK. Interaction studies: the influence of age, cigarette smoking and the oral contraceptive on blood concentrations of maprotiline. In 'Depressive Illness — Far Horizons?' McIntyre JNM (ed), Cambridge Med Publ, Northampton 1982, p 62–3.
2 Holman RM. Maprotiline and cigarette smoking: an interaction study: clinical findings. In 'Depressive Illness — Far Horizons?' McIntyre JNM (ed), Cambridge Med Publ, Northampton 1982, p 66–7.

Tianeptine + Alcohol

Abstract/Summary

Alcohol reduces the absorption of tianeptine by about 30%.

Clinical evidence, mechanism, importance and management

The absorption and peak serum levels of tianeptine after a single 12.5 mg dose were reduced about 30% in 12 normal subjects by the concurrent of alcohol. The subjects were given vodka diluted in orange juice to give blood levels between 0.77 and 0.64 mg%. The serum levels of its major metabolite were unchanged.[1] No behavioral studies were done so that the clinical significance of these studies is as yet uncertain.

Reference

1 Salvadori C, Ward C, Defrance R, Hopkins R. The pharmacokinetics of the antidepressant tianeptine and its main metabolite in healthy humans — influence of alcohol co-administration. Fund Clin Pharmacol (1990) 4, 115–25.

Trazodone + Phenothiazines

Abstract/Summary

Undesirable hypotension occurred in two patients on chlorpramazine or trifluoperazine when given trazodone.

Clinical evidence, mechanism, importance and management

A depressed patient on chlorpramazine began to complain of dizziness and unstable gait within 2 weeks of starting 100 mg trazodone daily. His blood pressure had fallen to between 92/58 and 126/72 mmHg. Within 2 days of stopping the trazodone his blood pressure had restabilized.[1] Another patient on trifluoperazine was given 100 mg trazodone daily and within 2 days she complained of dizziness. Her blood pressure had fallen to 86/52 mmHg. Within a day of withdrawing the trazodone her blood pressure was back to 100/65 mmHg.[1] It would seem from this that the hypotensive side-effects of the two drugs can be additive. Patients given both groups of drugs should be monitored for signs of excessive hypotension.

Reference

1 Asayesh K. Combination of trazodone and phenothiazines: a possible additive hypotensive effect. Can J Psychiatry (1986) 31, 857–8.

Tricyclic antidepressants + ACE inhibitors

Abstract/Summary

Preliminary evidence from two patients suggests that enalapril may increase the effects of clomipramine with the development of toxicity.

Clinical evidence

Two patients taking enalapril (one on 20 mg daily and the other taking 20 mg five times weekly) were additionally given clomipramine for depression. The clomipramine dosage of one of them was increased from 25 to 50 mg, and 10 days later he became euphoric and exalted. The problem resolved when the clomipramine dosage was reduced again. The other patient was given clomipramine and disulfiram 400 mg daily, and within two weeks he developed confusion, irritability and insomnia. These adverse effects diminished when the clomipramine dosage was reduced.[1]

Mechanism

The ratio of clomipramine to its metabolite (desmethylclomipramine), is normally less than 1, but both of these patients demonstrated a ratio of more than 1. This suggests that the normal metabolism (demethylation) of the clomipramine was inhibited, thus allowing the clomipramine to accumulate and its toxic effects to manifest themselves. In the second patient the disulfiram may also have had an additional enzyme inhibitory effect.[1]

Importance and management

Information is limited to these two cases and the interaction is not firmly established, however it would now be prudent to monitor the outcome of giving clomipramine to any patient taking enalapril. More study is needed. There seems to be nothing documented about adverse effects from the concurrent use of the other ACE inhibitors and tricyclic antidepressants.

Reference

1 Toutoungi M. Potential effect of enalapril on clomipramine metabolism. Human Pscyphopharmacology (1992) 7, 347–9.

Tricyclic antidepressants + Baclofen

Abstract/Summary

An isolated report describes a patient with multiple sclerosis on baclofen who was unable to stand within a few days of starting to take nortriptyline, and later imipramine.

Clinical evidence, mechanism, importance and management

A man with multiple sclerosis who was taking 10 mg baclofen four times a day to relieve spasticity, complained of leg weakness and was unable to stand within six days of starting to take 50 mg nortriptyline at bedtime. 48 h after stopping the nortriptyline his muscle tone returned. Two weeks later he was given 75 mg imipramine daily and once again his muscle tone was lost.[1] The reason is not understood. Prescribers should be aware of this report if the concurrent use of baclofen and any tricyclic antidepressant is being considered.

Reference

1 Silverglat MJ. Baclofen and tricyclic antidepressants: possible interaction. J Am Med Ass (1981) 246, 1659.

Tricyclic antidepressants + Barbiturates

Abstract/Summary

The serum levels of amitriptyline, desipramine and nortriptyline are reduced by the concurrent use of barbiturates. A reduced therapeutic response would be expected. The tricyclics also lower the convulsive threshold and may be inappropriate for patients with convulsive disorders.

Clinical evidence

A comparative study in five pairs of twins given nortriptyline found that the twins concurrently treated with un-named barbiturates developed steady-state serum nortriptyline levels which were reduced by 14–60%.[2] Similar observations have been made in patients and normal subjects taking nortriptyline with amylobarbitone[3,5] pentobarbitone,[10] and protriptyline with sodium amylobarbitone.[4] A patient showed a 50% reduction in serum desipramine levels when given 100 mg phenobarbitone each night as a hypnotic.[1]

Mechanism

The barbiturates are potent liver enzyme inducing agents which increase the metabolism and clearance of the tricyclic antidepressants from the body, thereby reducing their serum levels.

Importance and management

An established interaction but of uncertain clinical importance. Be alert for a reduced antidepressant response if both drugs are given. The barbiturates are potent liver enzyme inducers so that this interaction would be expected with any of them. This needs confirmation. Toxic overdosage with the tricyclics can cause convulsions and other effects, including respiratory depression, which may be increased by the use of a barbiturate. It is thought that diazepam[6] may be a better choice of anticonvulsant in this situation, although sodium amylobarbitone[7,8] and paraldehyde[9] have been used successfully. Remember too that the tricyclics lower the convulsive threshold.

References

1 Hammer W, Idestrom CM, Sjoqvist F. In 'Antidepressant Drugs' p 301, Garattini S, Dukes MNG (eds) Proc 1st Int Symp, Milan (1966). Int Congr Series no 122, Excerpta Medica.
2 Alexanderson A, Evans DAP, Sjoqvist F. Steady state plasma levels of nortriptyline in twins: influence of genetic factors and drug therapy. Br Med J (1969) 4, 764.
3 Burrows GD, Davies B. Antidepressants and barbiturates. Br Med J (1971) 4, 113.
4 Moody JP, Whyte SF, MacDonald AJ, Naylor GJ. Pharmacokinetic aspects of protriptyline plasma levels. Eur J Clin Pharmacol (1977) 11, 51.
5 Silverman G, Braithwaite R. Interaction of benzodiazepines and tricyclic antidepressants. Br Med J (1972) 4, 111.
6 Crocker J, Morton B. Tricyclic (antidepressant) drug toxicity. Clin Toxicol (1969) 2, 397.
7 Arneson GAA. A near fatal case of imipramine overdosage. Am J Psychiat (1961) 177, 934.
8 Luby ED, Domino EF. Toxicity from large doses of imipramine and MAO inhibitor in suicidal intent. J Am Med Ass (1961) 117, 68.
9 Connelly JF, Venables AA. A case of poisoning with 'Tofranil'. Med J Aust (1961) 1, 108.
10 Steiner E, Koike Y, Lind M, von Bahr C. Increased nortriptyline metabolism after treatment with pentobarbital in man. Acta Pharmacol Toxicol (1986) 59, Suppl 4, 91.

Tricyclic antidepressants + Benzodiazepines

Abstract/Summary

Concurrent use is not uncommon and normally appears to be uneventful. Roche markets a combined amitriptyline-chlordiazepoxide preparation (*Limibitrol*) but its advantages have been questioned. However three patients have been described who became drowsy, forgetful and appeared uncoordinated and drunk while taking amitriptyline and chlordiazepoxide, and four others have been described who showed toxic effects while taking *Limibitrol*. Diazepam may increase the risks of carrying out complex tasks (e.g. driving) if added to amitriptyline.

Clinical evidence

(a) Amitriptyline + Chloridazepoxide

Clinical trials on large numbers of patients have shown that the incidence of adverse reactions while taking amitriptyline and chlordiazepoxide was no greater than might have been expected with either of the drugs used singly,[3,4] but a few adverse reports have been documented. A depressed patient on 150 mg amitriptyline and 40 mg chlordiazepoxide daily became confused, forgetful and uncoordinated. He acted as though he was drunk.[1] Two other patients taking amitriptyline and chlordiazepoxide experienced drowsiness, memory impairment, slurring of the speech and an inability to concentrate. Both were unable to work and one described himself as feeling drunk.[2] Four patients on *Limibitrol* are reported to have experienced some manifestations of toxicity (delusions, confusion, agitation, disorientation, dry mouth, blurred vision).[8] Some of these effects seem to arise from increased CNS depression (possibly additive) and/or an increase in the anticholinergic side-effects of the tricyclic.

(b) Other Tricyclics and Benzodiazepines

Studies on the effects of nitrazepam, diazepam, oxazepam and chlordiazepoxide on steady-state plasma levels of nortriptyline and amitriptyline,[5] of diazepam and chlordiazepoxide on nortriptyline,[6] and alprazolam on clomipramine[14] failed to find any interaction, but alprazolam possibly raises imipramine levels (+ 30%).[14] Another study demonstrated an increase in amitriptyline levels when diazepam was given,[7] and two others found that 50–75 mg amitriptyline alone reduced attention and performance of a number of psychomotor tests; a worsening of performance and a deterioration in vigilance occurred if diazepam was added.[10,11] An isolated report describes a patient whose serum desipramine levels (300 mg daily) were halved when he was given 3 mg clonazepam daily and rose again when it was withdrawn.[9] Triazolam is effective in treating insomnia in depressed patients on imipramine, and does not reduce the effects of the antidepressant.[12,13]

Mechanisms

Uncertain. Additive CNS depression is a possibility with some combinations, and increased anticholinergic effects.

Importance and managment

There seems to be no strong reason for avoiding the concurrent use of some of these drugs although the advantages and disadvantages remain the subject of debate. Other tricyclic antidepressant/benzodiazepine combinations would not be expected to behave differently from those described here. Some patients will possibly experience increased drowsiness and inattention with the more sedative antidepressants such as amitriptyline, particularly during the first few days, and this may be exaggerated by benzodiazepines such as diazepam. This may increase the risk of driving.

References

1 Kane FJ, Taylor TW. A toxic reaction to combined Elavil-Librium therapy. Am J Psychiat (1963) 119, 1179.
2 Abdon FA. Elavil-Librium combination. Am J Psychiat (1964) 120, 1204.
3 Haider IA. A comparative trial of RO-4–6270 and amitriptyline in depressive illness. Br J Psychiat (1967) 113, 993.
4 General Practitioner Clinical Trials. Chlordiazepoxide with amitriptyline in neurotic depression. Practitioner (1969) 202, 437.
5 Silverman G, Braithwaite R. Benzodiazepines and tricyclic antidepressant plasma levels. Br Med J (1973) 2, 18.
6 Gram LF, Overo KF, Kirk L. Influence of neuroleptics and benzodiazepines on metabolism of tricyclic antidepressants in man. Am J Psychiat (1974) 131, 863.
7 Dugal R, Caille G, Albert J-M, Cooper SF. Apparent pharmacokinetic interaction of diazepam and amitriptyline in psychiatric patients: a pilot study. Curr Ther Res (1975) 18, 679.
8 Beresford TP, Feinsilver DL, Hall RCW. Adverse reactions to a benzodiazepine-tricyclic antidepressant compound. J Clin Psychopharmacol (1981) 1, 392.
9 Deicken RF. Clonazepam-induced reduction in serum desipramine concentrations. J Clin Psychopharmacol (1988) 8, 71–2.
10 Patat A, Klein MJ, Hucher M, Granier J. Acute effects of amitriptyline on human performance and interactions with diazepam. Eur J Clin Pharmacol (1988) 35, 585–92.
11 Moskowitz H, Burns M. The effects on performance of two antidepressants, alone and in combination with diazepam. Prog Neuro-Psychopharmacol & Biol Pschiat (1988) 12, 783–92.
12 Cohn JB. Triazolam treatment of insomnia in depressed patients taking tricyclics. J Clin Psychiatry (1983) 44, 401–6.
13 Dominguez RA, Jacobson AF, Goldstein BJ. Comparison of triazolam and placebo in the treatment of insomnia in depressed patients. Curr Ther Res (1984) 36, 1–10.
14 Carlson SW, Wright CE, Millikin SP, Lyon J, Chambers JH. Pharmacokinetic evaluation of the combined administration of alprazolam and clomipramine. Clin Pharmacol Ther (1992) 51, 154.

Tricyclic antidepressants + Calcium channel blockers or Labetalol

Abstract/Summary

Diltiazem, verapamil and labetalol increase serum imipramine levels, possibly accompanied by undesirable ECG changes.

Clinical evidence, mechanism, importance and management

13 normal subjects were given a 7-day course of verapamil (120 mg 8-hourly), diltiazem (90 mg 8-hourly) or labetalol (200 mg 12-hourly). The AUCs of single 100 mg doses of imipramine given on day 4 were increased follows: verapamil (+ 15%), diltiazem (+ 30%) and labetalol (+ 53%). 1 h after taking imipramine (2 h after taking the calcium channel blockers), the average PR interval on the ECG was > 200 msec, i.e. first-degree heart block, and two subjects given verapamil and imipramine developed second-degree heart block.[1] Labetalol and imipramine had no effect on atrioventricular conduction.[1]

Mechanism

Each drug apparently decreases the metabolism of the imipramine by the liver (in the case of labetalol the activity of cytochrome P4550IID6 is reduced). As a result the imipramine is lost from the body more slowly. The ECG changes appear to result from the increased imipramine levels and the additive effects of both drugs on the atrioventricular conduction time.

Importance and management

Information appears to be limited to this study. Single dose studies may not necessarily reliably predict what will happen if drugs are taken chronically, but the authors suggest that the use of verapamil and diltiazem could lead to 33% and 54% increases respectively in the average steady-state levels of imipramine. Moreover the ECG changes are by no means unimportant. The authors of the study suggest that these changes could lead to an increased risk of arrhythmias in some patients and they advise rigorous monitoring if any of these drugs is given with imipramine. More study is needed. Information about other tricyclics is lacking.

Reference

1 Hermann DJ, Krol TF, Dukes GE, Hussey EK, Danis M, Han Y-H, Powell JR, Hak LJ. Comparison of verapamil, dilitazem, and labetalol on the bioavailability and metabolism of imipramine. J Clin Pharmacol (1992) 32, 176–83.

Tricyclic antidepressants + Cannabis

Abstract/Summary

Marked tachycardia has been described in two patients, one taking imipramine and the other nortriptyline, when they smoked cannabis.

Clinical evidence, mechanism, importance and management

A 21-year-old student who had had no problems with either nortriptyline or cannabis separately, experienced marked tachycardia (160 bpm) when used together.[1] It was controlled with propranolol.[1] A man of 25 complained of restlessness, dizziness and tachycardia (120 bpm) after smoking cannabis while taking 50 mg imipramine daily.[2] Increased heart rates are well-documented side-effects of both the tricyclic antidepressants and cannabis, and what occurred was probably due to the additive beta-adrenergic and anticholinergic effects of the tricyclic antidepressants, with the beta-adrenergic effect of the cannabis. Direct information is limited but it has been suggested that concurrent use should be avoided.[1]

References

1 Hillard JR, Vieweg WVR. Marked sinus tachycardia resulting from the synergistic effects of marijuana and nortriptyline. Am J Psychiatry (1983) 140, 626–7.
2 Kizer KW. Possible interaction of TCA and marijuana. Ann Emerg Med (1980) 19, 444.

Tricyclic antidepressants + Carbamazepine

Abstract/Summary

The serum levels of amitriptyline, doxepin, imipramine and possibly desipramine can be more than halved by the concurrent use of carbamazepine. Clomipramine appears to be the exception. An isolated report describes carbamazepine toxicity in a patient shortly after starting to take desipramine.

Clinical evidence

(a) Serum tricyclic antidepressant levels reduced

The addition of carbamazepine reduced the serum levels of nortriptyline to 42% and of amitriptyline + nortriptyline to 40% in 8 psychiatric patients. In 17 other patients on doxepin the addition of carbamazepine reduced serum doxepin levels to 46% and of doxepin + nordoxepin to 45%.[4]

Thirty-six children (aged 5–16) with attention-deficit disorder on imipramine and carbamazepine for 1–6 months had total serum antidepressant levels which were approximately half those found in other children not taking carbamazepine, necessitating a doubling of the imipramine dosage.[1,2] A patient given desipramine and carbamazepine is reported to have had exceptionally low serum desipramine levels and cardiac complaints which may have been due to the presence of increased levels of the hydroxy metabolite of despramine.[5]

(b) Serum clomipramine levels increased

In contrast to (a), a study confirming the value of carbamazepine and clomipramine in the treatment of post-herpetic neuralgia found that the carbamazepine appeared to raise the clomipramine serum levels and those of its major metabolite (desmethylclomipramine).[6]

(c) Serum carbamazepine levels increased

A woman on long-term treatment with carbamazepine developed intoxication (nausea, vomiting, blurred vision, slurred speech, ataxia) within 6 days of starting to take 150 mg desipramine daily. Her serum carbamazepine levels were found to have doubled (from 7.7 to 15 μg/ml).[3]

Mechanism

It seems likely that the carbamazepine (a recognized enzyme-inducing agent) increases the metabolism and loss of these tricyclics from the body, thereby reducing their serum levels. The reason for the increased serum carbamazepine and clomipramine levels is not understood.

Importance and management

Information seems to be limited to these reports. Monitor the effects if carbamazepine is combined with these or any other tricyclic antidepressant (except clomipramine) and be alert for a reduction in the effects of the tricyclic. An increased dosage may be needed. Also be alert for any evidence of carbamazepine toxicity if desipramine or any other tricyclic is added to established treatment with carbamazepine. Remember too that the tricyclics lower the convulsive threshold.

References

1 Brown CS, Wells BG, Self TH, Jabbour JT. Influence of carbamazepine on plasma imipramine concentration in children with attention-deficit hyperactivity disorder. Pharmacotherapy (1988) 8, 135.
2 Brown CS, Wells BG, Cold JA, Froemming JH, Self TH, Jabbour JT. Possible influence of carbamazepine on plasma imipramine concentrations in children with attention deficit hyperactivity disorder. J Clin Psychopharmacol (1990) 10, 359–62.
3 Lesser I. Carbamazepine and desipramine: a toxic reaction. J Clin Psychiatry (1984) 45, 360.
4 Leinonen E, Lillsunde P, Laukkanen V, Ylitalo P. Effects of carbamazepine on serum antidepressant concentrations in psychiatric patients. J Clin Psychopharmacol (1991) 11, 313–8.
5 Baldessarini RJ, Teicher MH, Cassidy JW, Stein MH. Anticonvulsant cotreatment may increase toxic metabolites of antidepressants and other psychotropic drugs. J Clin Psychopharmacol (1988) 8, 381–2.
6 Gerson GR, Jones RB, Luscombe DK. Studies on the concomitant use of carbamazepine and clomipramine for the relief of post-herpetic neuralgia. Postgrad Med J (1977) 53 Suppl 4, 104–9.

Tricyclic antidepressants + Cholestyramine

Abstract/Summary

A single case report describes a marked reduction in the serum levels and antidepressant effectiveness of doxepin caused by the concurrent use of cholestyramine.

Clinical evidence

A man whose depression was controlled with doxepin relapsed within a week of starting to take 6 g cholestyramine twice daily. Within three weeks of increasing the dosage separation of the doxepin and cholestyramine from 4 to 6 h his combined serum antidepressant (i.e. doxepin plus n-desmethyldoxepin) levels had risen from 39 to 81 ng/ml and his depression had improved. Reducing the cholestyramine dosage to a single 6 g dose daily, separated from the doxepin by 15 h, resulted in a further rise in his serum antidepressant levels to 117 ng/ml accompanied by relief of his depression.[1]

Mechanism

The most likely explanation is that the doxepin became bound to the cholestyramine within the gut, thereby reducing its absorption. An in vitro study with simulated gastric fluid (1.2 mol/L HCl) found an approximately 75–90% binding at pH 1 with amitriptyline, desipramine, doxepin, imipramine and nortriptyline, 35–50% at pH 4, and 65–70% at pH 6.5.[2,3]

Importance and management

Direct information seems to be limited to this single report.[1] As the authors point out, it is difficult to generalize from this case because the patient had an abnormal gastrointestinal tract (hemigastrectomy with pyloroplasty and chronic diarrhoea), nevertheless be alert for reduced antidepressant levels and reduced effects in patients treated with any tricyclic antidepressant and cholestyramine because in vitro studies suggest that it may possibly occur with other tricyclics. A 6-hour dosage separation may only be partially effective.

References

1 Geeze DS, Wise MG, Stigelman WH. Doxepin-cholestyramine interaction. Psychosomatics (1988) 29,233–5.
2 Bailey DN, Coffee JJ, Anderson B, Manoguerra As. Interactions of tricyclic antidepressants with cholestyramine in vitro. Ther Drug Monit (1992) 14, 339–42.
3 Bailey DN. Effect of pH changes and ethanol on the binding of tricyclic antidepressants to cholestyramine in simulated gastric fluid. Ther Drug Monit (1992) 14, 343–6

Tricyclic antidepressants + Cimetidine or Ranitidine

Abstract/Summary

The concurrent use of cimetidine can raise the serum levels of amitriptyline, desipramine, doxepin, imipramine and nortriptyline. Toxicity may develop if the dosage of the tricyclic antidepressant is not reduced appropriately. Other tricyclic antidepressants are expected to interact similarly. Ranitidine does not interact.

Clinical evidence

(a) Amitriptyline + Cimetidine or Ranitidine

After taking 1200 mg cimetidine daily for two days, peak serum levels and the AUC of amitriptyline in a group of normal subjects following a single 25 mg dose were raised by 37% and 80% respectively.[1] Another study by the same authors found that ranitidine does not interact with amitriptyline.[12]

(b) Desipramine + Cimetidine

After taking 1200 mg cimetidine daily for 4 days, the serum desipramine levels of eight patients taking 100–250 mg daily were raised by 51%, and its hydroxylated metabolite (2-hydroxydesipramine) by 46%.[2] Another study showed that this interaction only occurs in those individuals who are 'rapid' hydroxylators.[3]

(c) Doxepin + cimetidine or ranitidine

A study in 10 normal subjects showed that 12 h after starting to take 300 mg cimetidine daily, peak serum levels and the AUC of doxepin after a single 100 mg oral dose were raised by 28% and 31% respectively.[4]

In another study 1200 mg cimetidine daily was found to double the steady-state serum levels of doxepin (50 mg daily) whereas 300 mg ranitidine daily had no effect.[13] A patient being treated with doxepin complained that the normally mild side-effects (urinary hesitancy, dry mouth and decreased visual acuity) became incapacitating when additionally treated with cimetidine. His serum doxepin levels were found to be elevated.[5]

(d) Imipramine + Cimetidine or Ranitidine

After taking 1200 mg cimetidine daily for 3 days, the peak serum levels and the AUC of imipramine in 12 normal subjects following a single 100 mg dose were raised by 65% and 172% respectively. After taking 300 mg ranitidine daily for 3 days the pharmacokinetics of imipramine were unaltered.[6] These findings with cimetidine confirm those of previous studies.[9,14] There are case reports of patients taking imipramine who developed severe anticholinergic side-effects (dry mouth, urine retention, blurred vision) associated with very marked rises in serum imipramine levels when concurrently treated with cimetidine.[7,8]

(e) Nortriptyline + cimetidine

After taking 1200 mg cimetidine daily for 2 days, the peak serum nortriptyline levels of six normal subjects were not significantly raised, but the AUC was increased by 20%.[9] A case report describes a patient whose serum nortriptyline levels were raised about one-third while taking cimetidine.[10] Another patient complained of abdominal pain and distention (but no other anticholinergic side-effects) when treated with nortriptyline and cimetidine.[11]

Mechanism

Cimetidine is a potent liver enzyme inhibitor which reduces the metabolic clearance of the tricyclic antidepressants from the body. This results in a rise in their serum levels. Ranitidine does not interact because it is not an enzyme inhibitor.

Importance and management

The interactions with cimetidine are well established, well documented and of clinical importance. The incidence is uncertain but a study with desipramine[3] showed that only 'rapid' hydroxylators demonstrate this interaction so that not all patients will be affected. Those taking amitriptyline, desipramine, doxepin, imipramine or nortriptyline who are given cimetidine should be monitored for evidence of increased toxicity (an excessive increase in mouth dryness, urine retention, blurred vision, constipation, tachycardia, postural hypotension). Other tricyclic antidepressants would be expected to be similarly affected. Ideally the antidepressant serum levels should be monitored. Reduce the dosage of the antidepressant

by 33–50% where necessary or replace the cimetidine with ranitidine which, because it is not an enzyme inhibitor, does not interact with amitriptyline, doxepin or imipramine and would not be expected to interact with other tricyclic antidepressants. Other H_2-blockers which do not cause enzyme inhibition include famotidine and nizatidine.

References

1 Curry SH, CL De Vane, Wolfe MM. Cimetidine interaction with amitriptyline. Eur J Clin Pharmacol (1985) 29, 429–33.
2 Amsterdam JD, Brunswick DJ, Potter L, Kaplan MJ. Cimetidine-induced alterations in desipramine plasma concentrations. Psychopharmacology (1984) 83, 373–5.
3 Steiner E, Spina E. Differences in the inhibitory effect of cimetidine on desipramine metabolism between rapid and slow debrisoquin hydroxylators. Clin Pharmacol Ther (1987) 42, 278–82.
4 Abernethy DR, Todd EL. Doxepin-cimetidine interaction: increased bioavailability during cimetidine treatment. J Clin Psychopharmacol (1986) 6, 8–12.
5 Brown MA, Haight KR, McKay G. Cimetidine-doxepin interaction. J Clin Psychopharmacol (1985) 5, 245–7.
6 Wells BG, Pieper JA, Self TH, Stewart CF, Waldon SL, Bobo L and Warner C. The effect of ranitidine and cimetidine on imipramine disposition. Eur J Clin Pharmacol (1986) 31, 285–90.
7 Shapiro PA. Cimetidine-imipramine interaction: case report and comments. Am J Psychiatry (1984) 141, 152.
8 Miller DD, Macklin M. Cimetidine-imipramine interaction: a case report. Am J Psychiatry (1983) 140, 351.
9 Henauer SA, Hollister LE. Cimetidine interaction with imipramine and nortriptyline. Clin Pharmacol Ther (1984) 35, 183–7.
10 Miller DD, Macklin M. Cimetidine-imipramine interaction: case report and comments. Am J Psychiatry (1984) 141, 153.
11 Lerro FA. Abdominal distention syndrome in a patient receiving cimetidine-nortriptyline therapy. J Med Soc New Jersey (1983) 80, 631–2.
12 Curry SH, DeVane CL, Wolfe MM. Lack of interaction of ranitidine with amitriptyline. Eur J Clin Pharmacol (1987) 32, 317–20.
13 Sutherland DL, Remillard AJ, Haight KR, Brown MA, Old L. The influence of cimetidine versus ranitidine on doxepin pharmacokinetics. Eur J Clin Pharmacol (1987) 32, 159–64.
14 Abernethy DR, Greenblatt DJ, Shader RI. Imipramine-cimetidine interaction: impairment of clearance and enhanced absolute bioavailability. J Pharmacol Exptl Ther (1984) 229, 702–5.

Tricyclic and Related antidepressants + Co-trimoxazole

Abstract/Summary

Four patients on tricyclics and one on viloxazine relapsed when given co-trimoxazole.

Clinical evidence, mechanism, importance and management

Four patients taking tricyclic antidepressants (imipramine, clomipramine, dibenzepine) and one taking viloxazine relapsed into depression when they were concurrently treated with co-trimoxazole (trimethoprim + sulphamethoxazole) for 2–9 days.[1] The reasons are not known. This seems to be the first and only report of a possible interaction between these very commonly prescribed drugs so that its general importance is very uncertain, but it would now seem prudent to monitor the outcome of concurrent use.

Reference

1 Brion S, Orssaud E, Chevalier JF, Plas J, Waroquaux O. Interaction entre le cotrimoxazole et les antidepresseurs. L'Encephale (1987) 8, 123–6.

Tricyclic antidepressants + Dextropropoxyphene

Abstract/Summary

An elderly patient on doxepin experienced increased lethargy and daytime sedation when additionally given dextropropoxyphene. No marked effects were seen in other patients given amitriptyline and dextropropoxyphene.

Clinical evidence, mechanism, importance and management

An elderly man on 150 mg doxepin daily developed lethargy and daytime sedation when he started to take 65 mg dextropropoxyphene every 6 h. His plasma doxepin levels rose by almost 150% (from 20 to 48.5 ng/ml) and desmethyldoxepin levels were similarly increased (from 8.8 to 20.7 ng/ml). A later study on 10 young normal subjects found that the same dose of dextropropoxyphene reduced the metabolism of antipyrine (a marker of drug inhibition) by 16%.[1]

Fifteen patients with rheumatoid arthritis given small doses of amitriptyline (25 mg) and dextropropoxyphene (up to 65 mg three times daily) experienced some drowsiness and mental slowness. They complained of being clumsier and had more pain, but these effects were said to be mild.[2]

The general clinical significance of these interactions is uncertain but patients should be warned that some increase in CNS depression may occur.

Reference

1 Abernethy DR, Greenblatt DJ, Steel K. Propoxyphene inhibition of doxepin and antipyrine metabolism. Clin Pharmacol Ther (1982) 31, 199.
2 Saarialho-Kere U, Julkuenen H, Mattila MJ, Seppälä T. Psychomotor performance of patients with rheumatoid arthritis: cross over comparison of dextropropoxyphene, dextropropoxyphene plus an itriptyline, indomethacin and placebo. Pharmacol Toxicol (1988) 63, 286–92.

Tricyclic antidepressants + Disulfiram

Abstract/Summary

Disulfiram reduces the clearance of imipramine and desipramine from the body. The concurrent use of amitriptyline and disulfiram is reported to cause a therapeutically useful increase in the effects of disulfiram but organic brain syndrome has been seen in two patients.

Clinical evidence, mechanism, importance and management

Amitriptyline is reported to have been successfully used to increase the effects of both disulfiram and citrated calcium carbimide without any increase in side-effects,[1,2] however there is also some evidence that an adverse interaction can occur. A study in two men showed that while taking 500 mg disulfiram daily, the AUC of imipramine given intravenously increased by 32.5 and 26.7%, and of despramine in one subject by 32.3%.[3] Peak serum levels were also increased. The suggested reason is that the disulfiram inhibits the metabolism of the antidepressants by the liver. There is also a report of a man taking disulfiram who, when given amitriptyline, complained of dizziness, visual and auditory hallucinations, and who became disorientated to person, place and time. A not dissimilar reaction was seen in another patient.[4] Concurrent use should therefore be well monitored for any evidence of toxicity. More study is needed to establish the importance and extent of this interaction.

References

1 MacCallum WAG. Drug interactions in alcoholism treatment. Lancet (1969) i, 313.
2 Pullar-Strecker H. Drug interactions in alcoholism treatment. Lancet (1969) i, 735.
3 Ciraulo DA, Barnhill J, Boxenbaum H. Pharmacokinetic interaction of disulfiram and antidepressants. Am J Psychiatry (1985) 142, 1373–4.
4 Maany I, Hayashida M, Pfeffer SL. Possible toxic interaction between disulfiram and amitriptyline. Arch Gen Psychiatry (1982) 39, 743–4.

Tricyclic antidepressants + Erythromycin, Josamycin

Abstract/Summary

Erythromycin is reported not to interact with tricyclic antidepressants, but an isolated report suggests that josamycin may possibly increase amitriptyline serum levels.

Clinical evidence, mechanism, importance and management

Six day's treatment with 250 mg erythromycin four times daily was found not to affect the serum levels of eight patients taking tricyclic antidepressants (desipramine, imipramine, doxepin, nortriptyline).[1] No special precautions seem to be necessary. A patient taking amitriptyline showed a marked increase in total amitriptyline/nortriptyline serum levels after being treated with josamycin, enzyme inhibition being the suggested reason, but no toxicity was reported.[2] Nevertheless be alert for any evidence of increased tricyclic side-effects and toxicity if josamycin is given. More study is needed.

Reference

1 Amsterdam JD, Maislin G. Effect of erythromycin on tricyclic antidepressant metabolism. J Clin Psychopharmacol (1991) 11, 204–6.

2 Romero AS, Solaz CC. Posible interacción entre josamicina y amitriptilina. Med Clin (1992) 98, 279

Tricyclic antidepressants + Ethchlorvynol

Abstract/Summary, clinical evidence, mechanism, importance and management

Transient delerium has been attributed to the concurrent use of amitriptyline and ethchlorvynol,[1] but no details are given and there appear to be no other reports confirming this alleged interaction.

Reference

1 Hussar DA. Tabular compilation of drug interactions. Am J Pharm (1969) 141, 109.

Tricyclic antidepressants + Fenfluramine

Abstract/Summary

A confusing situation: some say that concurrent use is safe and effective while others say that fenfluramine can cause depression and should not be used in patients with depression.

Clinical evidence, mechanism, importance and management

Depression has been seen in some patients given fenfluramine[2] and several cases of withdrawal depression have been observed in patients on amitriptyline and fenfluramine, following episodes of severe depression.[3] The manufacturers say that fenfluramine should not be used in patients with a history of depression or while being treated with antidepressants.[1] On the other hand it has also been claimed that depression is not a serious problem in most patients taking fenfluramine[6] and that it can be used safely and effectively with tricyclic antidepressants.[5–7] One report describes a rise in the serum levels of amitriptyline when 60 mg fenfluramine was given to patients on 150 mg amitriptyline daily for depression.[4]

References

1 ABPI Data Sheet Compendium, 1985–6 p 1400. Datapharm publications, London.

2 Gaind R. Fenfluramine (Ponderax) in the treatment of obese psychiatric outpatients. Br J Psychiatry (1969) 115, 963.

3 Harding T. Fenfluramine dependence. Br Med J (1971) 3, 305.

4 Gunne LM, Antonijevic S, Jonsson J. Effect of fenfluramine on steady state

plasma levels of amitriptyline. Postgrad Med J (1975) 51 (Suppl 1) 113.

5 Pinder RM, Brogden RN, Sawyer PR, Speight TM, Avery GS. Fenfluramine: a review of its pharmacological properties and therapeutic efficacy in obesity. Drugs (1975) 10, 241.

6 Poire R, Rombach F, Crance JP. Obesite et fenfluramine (768 S). Experiences de trois ans d'utilisation prolongee et controlee du medicament en milieu psychiatrique hospitalies. Ann Medicopsychologiques (1966) 1, 26.

7 Mason EC. Servier Laboratories Ltd. Personal Communication (1976).

Tricyclic antidepressants + Fluconazole

Abstract/Summary

An isolated report describes increased serum nortriptyline levels due to the concurrent use of fluconazole.

Clinical evidence, mechanism, importance and management

An elderly woman on nortriptyline and other drugs (cyclosporin, morphine, metoclopramide, bumetanide as well an un-named antibiotic and antifungal) was additionally started on 100 mg fluconazole daily. After 13 days concurrent use her trough serum nortriptyline levels had risen by 70% (from 149 to 252 ng/ml). The reason is not understood but inhibition by the fluconazole of the liver enzymes concerned with the metabolism of the nortriptyline is suggested.[1] The general clinical importance of this reaction is unknown, but concurrent use in any patient should now be monitored for any sign of increased nortriptyline effects.

Reference

1 Gannon RH, Anderson ML. Fluconazole-nortriptyline drug interaction. Ann Pharmacother (1992) 26, 1456–7.

Tricyclic and related antidepressants + Fluoxetine

Abstract/Summary

The serum levels of amitriptyline, clomipramine, desipramine, imipramine and nortriptyline can be markedly increased (two-fourfold or even more) by the concurrent use to fluoxetine. Toxicity may occur unless the tricyclic antidepressant dosage is considerably reduced. This interaction can continue for many days after fluoxetine has been withdrawn. Trazodone and fluoxetine have been used concurrently with advantage, but two reports describe increased side-effects in some patients.

Clinical evidence

(a) Amitriptyline, Clomipramine, Desipramine, Imipramine and Nortriptyline

Four patients on 250 mg desipramine daily, 150 mg imipramine daily or 100 mg nortriptyline daily showed 2–4-fold increases in serum tricyclic antidepressant levels within 1–2 weeks of additionally taking 50–400 mg fluoxetine daily. Two of them developed typical tricyclic antidepressant anticholinergic side-effects (constipation, urinary hesitancy).[1]

A number of other reports and studies clearly confirm that marked increases (two-threefold) occur in the serum levels of amitriptyline,[8,27] clomipramine,[27] desipramine,[2,4,10,13,14,16,21,24,25,26] imipramine[3,14,16,18,21,24,27] and nortriptyline,[5–7,10,12,13] accompanied by toxicity if fluoxetine is added without reducing the dosage of the tricyclic antidepressant. Delerium and seizures have also been described.[16] Parkinson-like symptoms developed in a patient on amitriptyline and flupenthixol when given fluoxetime.[23]

(b) Trazodone

A patient on trazodone showed a 31% increase in the antidepressant/dose ratio when given 40 mg fluoxetine daily. She experienced sedation and an unstable gait.[1] Five patients out of 16 stopped their medication (25–75 mg trazodone used for insomnia) because of excessive sedation next day.[17] Three out of eight patients had improvement in sleep and depression when given both drugs but the other five were either unaffected or had intolerable side-effects (headahces, dizziness, daytime sedation, fatigue).[22] However another report described advantageous concurrent use in six patients without an increase in side-effects.[11]

Mechanism

Fluoxetine appears to inhibit the metabolism (oxidation and N-demethylation) of these antidepressants by the liver, possibly involving inhibition of P450IID6 isoenzyme, resulting in a reduction in their loss from the body.[28] A ten-fold reduction in clearance was found in one study.[24]

Importance and management

The tricyclic antidepressant/fluoxetine interaction is established and clinically important. Monitor concurrent use (measure plasma levels), be alert for any evidence of antidepressant toxicity and reduce the dosage appropriately. Initial dosage reductions to a quarter[14] have been advised if 20 mg fluoxetine daily is added, and regular monitoring for several weeks or even months.[14] Fluoxetine's active metabolite (norfluoxetine) has a long half-life (7–15 days) and persists in the body so that this interaction can occur or continue for days or even weeks after the fluoxetine has been withdrawn.[9,15,16,19] Both concurrent and sequential use can therefore carry a risk. Also be aware that after fluoxetine withdrawal the tricyclic dosage may eventually need to be increased when the fluoxetine effects finally disappear.[20] Information about other tricyclics seems to be lacking but be alert for this interaction with any of them. Monitor the outcome of using trazodone and fluoxetine together for any evidence of increased side-effects (excessive sedation).

References

1 Aranow RB, Hudson JI, Pope HG, Grady TA, Laage TA, Bell IR, Cole JD. Elevated antidepressant plasma levels after addition of fluoxetine. Am J Psychiatry (1989) 146, 911–13.

2 Bell IR, Cole JD. Fuoretine induces elevation of desipramine and exacerbation of geriatric non-psychotic symptoms. J Clin Psychopharmacol (1988) B, 447–8.

3 Faynor SM, Espina V. Fluoxetine inhibition of imipramine metabolism. Clin Chem (1989) 35, 1180.

4 Goodrick PJ. Influence of fluoxetine on plasma levels of desipramine. Am J Psychiatry (1989) 146, 552.

5 Kahn DG. Increased plasma nortriptyline concentration in a patient cotreated with fluoxetine. J Clin Psychiatry (1990) 51, 36.

6 Vaughan DA. Interaction of fluoxetine with tricyclic antidepressants. Am J Psychiatry (1989) 145, 1478.

7 Schraml F, Benedetti G, Hoyle K, Clayton A. Fluoxetine and nortriptyline combination. Am J Psychiatry (1989) 146,

8 March JS, Moon RL, Johnston H. Fluoxetine-TCA interaction. J Am Acad Child Adolesc Pscyhiatry (1990) 29, 985–6.

9 Downs JM, Dahmer SK. Fluoxetine and elevated plasma levels of tricyclic antidepressants. Am J Psychiatry (1990) 147, 1251.

10 Cavanaugh S von A. Drug-drug interactions of fluoxetine with tricyclics. Psychosomatics (1990) 31, 273–6.

11 Swerdlow NR, Andia AM. Trazodone-fluoxetine combination for treatment of obsessive-compulsive disorder. Am J Psychiatry (1989) 146, 1637.

12 Downs JM, Downs AD, Rosenthal TL, Deal N, Akiskal HS. Increased plasma tricyclic antidepressant concentrations in two patients concurrently treated with fluoxetine. J Clin Psychiatry (1989) 50, 226–7.

13 Vaughan DA. Interaction of fluoxetine with tricyclic antidepressants. Am J Psychiatry (1988) 145, 1478.

14 Westermeyer J. Fluoxetine-induced tricyclic toxicity: extent and duration. J Clin Pharmacol (1991) 31, 388–92.

15 Skowron DM, Gutierrez MA, Epstein S. Precaution with titrating nortriptyline after the use of fluoxetine. DICP Ann Pharmacotherapy (1990) 24, 1008.

16 Preskorn SH, Beber JH, Faul JC, Hirschfeld RMA. Serious adverse effects of combining fluoxetine and tricyclic antidepressants. Am J Psychiatry (1990) 147, 532–3.

17 Metz A, Shader RI. Adverse interactions encountered when using trazodone to treat insomnia associated with fluoxetine. Int Clin Psychopharmacol (1990) 5, 191–4.

18 Hahn SM, Griffin JH. Comment: fluoxetine adverse effects and drug interactions. DICP Ann Pharmacotherapy (1991) 25, 1273–4.

19 Müller N, Brockmöller J, Roots I. Extremely long plasma half-life of amitriptyline in a woman with the cytochrome P450IID6 29/29-kilobase wild-type allele — a slowly reversible interaction with fluoxetine. Ther Drug Monit (1991) 13, 535–6.

20 Extein IL. Recent fluoxetine treatment and complications of tricyclic therapy. Am J Psychiatry (1991) 148, 1602.

21 Bergstrom RF, Lemberger L, Peyton AL. Drug interaction between fluoxetine and the tricyclic antidepressants imipramine and desipramine. Pharmaceutical Res (1990) 7, S-254.

22 Nierenberg AA, Cole JO, Glass L. Possible trazodone potentiation of fluoxetine: a case series. J Clin Psychiatry (1992) 53, 83–5.

23 Touw DJ, Gernaat HBPE, van der Woude J. Parkinsonisme na toevoeging van fluoxetine aan behandeling met neuroleptica of carbamazepine. Ned Tijdschr Geneeskd (1992) 136, 332–3.

24 Bergstrom RF, Peyton AL, Lemberger L. Quantification and mechanism of the fluoxetine and tricyclic antidepressant interaction. Clin Pharmacol Ther (1992) 51, 239–48.

25 Nelson JC, Mazure CM, Bowers MB, Jatlow OI. A preliminary open study of the combination of fluoxetine and desipramine for rapid treatment of major depression. Arch Gen Psychiatry (1991) 48, 303–7.

26 Wilens T, Biederman J, Baldessarini RJ, McDermott SP, Puopolo PR, Flood JG. Fluoxetine inhibits desipramine metabolism. Arch Gen Psychiatry (1992) 49, 752.

27 Vandel S, Bertschy G, Bonin B, Nezelof S, Francois TH, Vandel B, Sechter D, Bizouard P. Tricyclic antidepressant levels after fluoxetine addition. Neuropsychobiol (1992) 25, 202–7

28 Brøsen K, Skjelbo E. Fluoxetine and norfloxetine are potent inhibitors of P450IID6 — the source of the sparteine/debrisoquine oxidation polymorphism. Br J Clin Pharmac (1991) 32, 136.

Tricyclic antidepressants + Fluvoxamine

Abstract/Summary

Fluvoxamine can markedly raise the serum levels of amitriptyline, clomipramine, desipramine, imipramine and maprotiline. Toxicity may occur if their dosages are not reduced.

Clinical evidence

Five patients on amitriptyline and four on clomipramine more than doubled their serum tricyclic antidepressant levels when given fluvoxamine while taking tricyclic dosages which were the same or slightly lower. No toxicity was seen.[1,2]

Very marked increases in tricyclic antidepressant levels (50–100% or more) were seen in another four other patients on imipramine or desipramine, associated with marked side-effects in two of them (one case of seizure, tremor, confusion, anticholinergic effects).[3] Eight other patients taking amitriptyline, clomipramine, imipramine or maprotiline also demonstrated this interaction with fluvoxamine. Fluvoxamine levels were seen to rise.[6]

Mechanism

In vivo and *in vitro* studies with human liver microsomes show that fluvoxamine inhibits cytochrome P4501A2 (CYP1A2) which is concerned with the metabolism (N-demethylation) of tricyclic antidepressants.[4–6] This has the effect of raising their levels, resulting in the possible development of toxicity.

Importance and management

An established interaction but still with limited documentation. The authors of one of the reports advise a reduction in the tricyclic antidepressant dosage based on plasma level monitoring, with an initial reduction of at least one third to avoid toxicity.[3] The effects of the interaction disappear within 1–2 weeks of withdrawing the fluvoxamine.[6]

References

1 Vandel S, Bertschy G, Allers G. Fluvoxamine tricyclic antidepressant interaction. Therapie (1990) 45, 21.
2 Bertchy G, Vandel S, Vandel B, Allers G, Vomat R. Fluvoxamine-tricyclic antidepressant interaction. An accidental finding. Eur J Clin Pharmacol (1991) 40, 119–120.
3 Spina E, Campo GM, Avenoso A, Pollicin MA, Caputi AP. Interaction between fluvoxamine and imipramine/desipramine in four patients. Ther Drug Monit (1992) 14, 194–6.
4 Brøsen K, Skjelbo E, Rasmussen BB, Poulsen HE, Loft S. Fluvoxamine is a potent inhibitor of cytochrome P4501A2. Biochem Pharmacol (1993) 45, 1211–14.
5 Skelbo E, Brøsen K. Inhibitors of imipramine metabolism by human liver microsomes. Br J Clin Pharmac (1992) 34, 256–61.
6 Härtter S, Wetzel H, Hammes E, Hiemke C. Inhibition of antidepressant demethylation and hydroxylation by fluvoxamine in depressed patients. Psychopharmacology (1993) 110, 302–8.

Tricyclic antidepressants + Food

Abstract/Summary

Some preliminary evidence suggests that very high fibre diets can reduce the serum levels of doxepin and desipramine, and thereby prevent the relief of depression.

Clinical evidence, mechanism, importance and management

Three patients showed no response to doxepin or desipramine and had depressed serum tricyclic antidepressant levels while taking very high fibre diets (wheat bran, wheat germ, oat bran, rolled oats, sunflower seeds, coconut shreds, raisins, bran muffins). When the diet was changed or stopped, the serum tricyclic antidepressant levels rose and the depression was relieved.[1] The reason is not known. This interaction may possibly provide an explanation for otherwise unaccountable relapses or inadequate responses to tricyclic antidepressant treatment. Another study found that the ingestion of food (breakfast) had no effect on the bioavailability of imipramine, its peak serum concentrations or the time to peak concentrations in 12 normal subjects following a 50 mg oral dose.[2]

References

1 Stewart DE. High-fiber diet and serum tricyclic antidepressant levels. J Clin Pyschopharmacol (1992) 12, 438–40.
2 Abernethy DR, Divoll M, Greenblatt DJ, Shader RI. Imipramine pharmacokinetics and absolute bioavailability. Clin Res (1983) 31, 626A.

Tricyclic antidepressants + Furazolidone

Abstract/Summary

A report describes the development of toxic psychosis, hyperactivity, sweating and hot and cold flushes in a woman on amitriptyline when given furazolidone with diphenoxylate and atropine.

Clinical evidence, mechanism, importance and management

A depressed woman taking daily doses of 1.25 mg conjugated oestrogen substances and 75 mg amitriptyline, was additionally given 300 mg furazolidone and diphenoxylate with atropine sulphate. Three days later she began to experience blurred vision, profuse perspiration followed by alternate chills and hot flushes, restlessness, motor activity, persecutory delusions, auditory hallucinations and visual illusions. The symptoms cleared within a day of stopping the furazolidone.[1] The reasons are not understood but the authors point out that furazolidone has MAO-inhibitory properties and that the symptoms were similar to those seen when the tricyclic antidepressants and MAOI interact. However the MAO-inhibitory activity of furazolidone normally takes about five days to develop. Whether the concurrent use of atropine and amitriptyline (both of which have anticholinergic activity) had some part to play in the reaction is uncertain. No firm conclusions can be drawn from this slim evidence, but prescribers should be aware of this case when considering the concurrent use of tricyclic antidepressants and furazolidone.

Reference

1 Aderhold RM, Munitz CE. Acute psychosis with amitriptyline and furazolidone. J Am Med Ass (1970) 213, 2080.

Tricyclic antidepressants + Haloperidol

Abstract/Summary

Serum tricyclic antidepressant levels can be considerably increased in a few patients by the concurrent use of haloperidol. This may have caused a grand mal seizure in one case but toxic reactions appear to be uncommon.

Clinical evidence

A comparative study of 30 patients on similar doses of desipramine (2.5–2.55 mg/kg) showed that two of them concurrently treated with haloperidol had steady-state serum desipramine levels which were more than double those of 15 others not taking haloperidol (255 compared with 110 ng/ml).[3] A case report describes a patient who had a grand mal seizure when concurrently treated with desipramine and haloperidol. Her serum desipramine levels were unusually high (610 ng/ml).[4]

Mechanism

Haloperidol reduces the metabolism of the tricyclic antidepressants, thereby reducing their loss from the body and resulting in a rise in their serum levels. For example, the urinary excretion of a test dose of C^{14}-imipramine given to two schizophrenic patients was reduced 35–40% while taking 12–20 mg haloperidol daily.[1] In a similar study on another schizophrenic patient given C^{14}-nortriptyline it was found that the urinary excretion and plasma metabolite levels of nortriptyline fell while taking 16 mg haloperidol daily, while plasma levels of unchanged nortriptyline rose.[2]

Importance and management

An established interaction though its documentation is small. Concurrent use is common whereas adverse reactions are uncommon but be aware that the serum tricyclic levels will be elevated. This may have been the cause of the grand mal seizure in the case cited.[4]

References

1 Gram LF and Overo KF. Drug interaction: inhibitory effect of neuroleptics on metabolism of tricyclic antidepressants in man. Br Med J (1972) 1, 463.
2 Gram LF, Overo KF, Kirk L. Influence of neuroleptics and benzodiazepines on metabolism of tricyclic antidepressants in man. Am J Psychiatry (1974) 131, 8.
3 Nelson JC, Jatlow I. Neuroleptic effect on desipramine on steady-state plasma concentrations. Am J Psychiatry (1980) 137, 1232–4.
4 Mahr GC, Berchon R, Balon R. A grand mal seizure associated with desipramine and haloperidol. Can J Psychiatry (1987) 32, 463–4.

Tricyclic antidepressants + Isoprenaline

Abstract/Summary

Although isoprenaline (isoproterenol) and amitriptyline have been used together safely and with advantage in the treatment of asthma, an isolated case has been reported of death arising from their current use (or abuse?).

Clinical evidence, mechanism, importance and management

Amitriptyline alone[2,3] and with isoprenaline[4] is beneficial in the treatment of asthma, and in a study of possible adverse interactions between the two, no abnormalities of heart rhythm were seen, although one out of the four patients studied showed tachycardia.[5] However a woman taking *Tedral* (theophylhine, ephedrine and phenobarbitone), twice daily, died as a result of aspiration of vomit in response to cardiac arrhythmias induced by the use of amitriptyline and isoprenaline.[1] It was estimated that she had taken forty 125 μg doses of isoprenaline daily for several days prior to her death. Amitriptyline, isoprenaline, ephedrine and the fluorocarbon inhaler propellant appear to have had additive cardiotoxic effects, but just why cardiac arrhythmias should cause vomiting is not understood. This fatal interaction would seem to be due to the abuse rather than the responsible use of these drugs. However the case serves to emphasize the risk attached to the over-use of isoprenaline inhalers if cardiotoxic drugs such as the tricyclic antidepressants are being used concurrently.

References

1 Kadar D. Amitriptyline and isoproterenol: a fatal combination. Can Med Ass J (1975) 112, 556.
2 Ananth J. Antiasthmatic effect of amitriptyline. Can Med Ass J (1974) 110, 1131.
3 Meares RA, Mills JE, Horvath TB. Amitriptyline and asthma. Med J Aust (1971) 2, 25.
4 Matilla MJ, Muittari A. Modification by imipramine of the bronchodilator response to isoprenaline in asthmatic patients. Ann Med Int Fenn (1968) 57, 185.
5 Boakes AJ, Laurence DR, Teoh PC, Barar FSK, Benedikter LT and Prichard BNC. Interactions between sympathomimetic amine and antidepressant agents in man. Br Med J (1973) 1, 311.

Tricyclic antidepressants + Methadone

Abstract/Summary

Methadone can double the serum desipramine levels.

Clinical evidence

After taking 0.5 mg/kg methadone daily for two weeks, the mean serum desipramine levels of five men on 2.5 mg/kg daily had risen by 108%. Previous observations on patients given both drugs had shown that desipramine levels were higher than expected and desipramine side-effects developed at relatively low doses.[1] Further evidence of an increase in serum despramine levels due to methadone is described in another study.[2]

Mechanism

Not understood. It is suggested that the methadone may possibly inhibit the hydroxylation of the despramine, thereby reducing its loss from the body.[2]

Importance and management

Information seems to be limited to these two studies but the interaction would seem to be established. Monitor the effects of concurrent use and anticipate the need to reduce the desipramine dosage. There seems to be nothing reported about the effects of methadone on other tricyclic antidepressants.

References

1 Maany I, Dhopesh V, Arndt IO, Burke W, Woody G, O'Brien CP. Increase in desipramine serum levels associated with methadone treatment. Am J Psychiatry (1989) 146, 1611–13.

2 Kosten TR, Gawin FH, Morgan C, Nelson JC, Jatlow P. Desipramine and its 2-hydroxy metabolite in patients taking or not taking methadone. Am J Psychiatry (1990) 147, 1379–80.

Tricyclic antidepressants + Methylphenidate

Abstract/Summary

Methylphenidate can cause a marked increase in the blood levels of imipramine resulting in clinical improvement. Whether levels can rise to toxic concentrations appears not to be documented but two adolescents have been described who experienced severe mood deterioration while taking both drugs.

Clinical evidence

A study in '... several patients...' demonstrated a dramatic increase in the blood levels of desipramine and imipramine during concurrent treatment with imipramine and methylphenidate. In one patient taking 150 mg imipramine daily it was observed that 20 mg methylphenidate a day increased the blood levels of the imipramine from 100 to 700 g/l and of desipramine from 200 to 850 g/l over a period of 16 days.[1]

Similar effects have been described in other reports.[2,3] A 9-year-old and a 15-year-old exhibited severe behavioural problems until the imipramine and methylphenidate they were taking were stopped.[4]

Mechanism

In vitro experiments with human liver slices indicate that methylphenidate inhibits the metabolism of imipramine, resulting in its accumulation, and this is reflected in raised blood levels.[3]

Importance and management

Information is limited. Some therapeutic improvement is seen because of the very marked rise in the blood levels of the antidepressant, but whether this also can lead to tricyclic antidepressant toxicity is uncertain. It does not seem to have been reported, but the possibility should be considered. Information about other tricyclic antidepressants is lacking. It has been suggested that concurrent use in children and adolescents may be undesirable.[3]

References

1 Dayton PG, Perel JM, Israili ZH, Faraj BA, Rodewig K, Black N, Goldberg LI. Studies with methylphenidate: drug interactions and metabolism. In 'Clinical Pharmacology of Psychoactive Drugs', Sellers EM (ed). Alcoholism and Drug Addiction Reseach Foundation. Toronto (1975) p 183.

2 Cooper TB, Simpson GM. Concomitant imipramine and methylphenidate administration: a case report. Am J Psychiat (1973) 130, 721.

3 Wharton RN, Perel JM, Dayton PG, Malitz S. A potential use for the interaction of methylphenidate with tricyclic antidepressants. Am J Psychiat (1971) 127, 1619.

4 Grob CS, Coyle JT. Suspected adverse methylphenidate-imipramine interactions in children. J Dev Behav Pediatrics (1986) 7, 265–7.

Tricyclic antidepressants + Oestrogens (estrogens)/Contraceptives (oral)

Abstract/Summary

There is evidence that oestrogens can sometimes paradoxically reduce the effects of imipramine yet at the same time cause imipramine toxicity. The general clinical importance of this interaction has yet to be evaluated.

Clinical evidence

A study in 10 women taking 150 mg imipramine daily for primary depression found that those given 50 g ethinyloestradiol daily for a week showed less improvement than other women given only 25 g or a placebo. Four out of the 10 developed signs of imipramine toxicity which was dealt with by halving the imipramine dose.[1] Another study found that oral contraceptives increased the absolute bioavailability by 60%.[3] Long-standing imipramine toxicity was also relieved in a woman taking 100 mg daily when her dosage of conjugated oestrogen was reduced to a quarter.[2] In contrast, several studies which showed that serum clomipramine levels were raised or remained unaffected by the concurrent use of oestrogen-containing contraceptives, failed to confirm that tricyclic antidepressant toxicity occurs more often in those on the pill than those who are not.[5-8] Akathisia in three patients has been attributed to an interaction betwen conjugated oestrogens and amitriptyline or chlorimipramine.[9]

Mechanism

Among the possible reasons for these effects are that the oestrogens increase the bioavailability of imipramine,[3] or inhibit its metabolism.[4]

Importance and management

These interactions are inadequately established. There is no obvious reason for avoiding concurrent use, but it would seem reasonable to be alert for any evidence of toxicity and/or lack of response to tricyclic antidepressant treatment. One study suggested that the imipramine dosage should be reduced by about a third.[3] More study is needed.

References

1 Prange AJ, Wilson JC, Alltop A. Estrogen may well affect response to antidepressant. J Amer Med Ass (1972) 219, 143.
2 Khurana RC. Estrogen-imipramine interaction. J Amer Med Ass (1972) 222, 702.
3 Abernethy DR, Greenblatt DJ, Shader RI. Imipramine disposition in users of oral contraceptives. Clin Pharmacol Ther (1984) 35, 792.
4 Somani SM, Khurana RC. Mechanism of estrogen-imipramine interaction. J Amer Med Ass (1973) 223, 560.
5 Beaumont G. Drug interactions with clomipramine (Anafranil). J Int Med Res (1973) 1, 480.
6 Gringras M, Beaumont G, Grieve A. Clomipramine and oral contraceptives: an interaction study--clinical findings. J Int Med Res (1980) 8, (Suppl 3), 76.
7 Luscombe DK, Jones RB. Effects of concomitantly administered drugs on plasma levels of clomipramine and desmethyl-clomipramine in depressive patients receiving clomipramine therapy. Postgrad Med J (1977) 53 (Suppl 4), 77.
8 John VA, Luscombe DK, Kemp H. Effects of age, cigarette smoking and oral contraceptives on the pharmacokinetics of clomipramine and its desmethyl metabolite during chronic dosing. J Int Med Res (1980) 8,(Suppl 3), 88.
9 Krishnan KRR, France RD, Ellmwood EH. Tricyclic-induced akathisia in patients taking conjugated estrogens. Am J Psychiatry (1984) 141, 696-7.

Tricyclic antidepressants + Propafenone

Abstract/Summary

An isolated report describes markedly raised serum desipramine levels in a patient when concurrently treated with propafenone.

Clinical evidence, mechanism, importance and management

A man with major depression responded well to 175 mg desipramine daily with serum desipramine levels in the range 500–1000 nmol/l. When later he was treated for paroxysmal atrial fibrillation with digoxin (0.25 mg daily) and propafenone (150 mg twice daily and 300 mg qhs) he developed markedly elevated serum desipramine levels (2092 nmol/l) and toxicity (dry mouth, sedation, shakiness) while taking 150 mg desipramine daily. The side-effects resolved when the desipramine was stopped for 5 days, but when restarted at 75 mg daily his serum desipramine levels were still raised (1130 nmol/l). The reason is thought to be that the propafenone reduced the metabolism and clearance of the desipramine from the body.[1] The general importance of this case is uncertain, but be alert for signs of desipramine toxicity in any patient given propafenone concurrently. Reduce the desipramine dosage appropriately.

Reference

1 Katz MR. Raised serum levels of desipramine with the antiarrhythmic propafenone. J Clin Psychiatry (1991) 52, 432–3.

Tricyclic antidepressants + Quinidine

Abstract/Summary

Quinidine can reduce the loss of desipramine, imipramine and nortriptyline from the body, thereby increasing their serum levels.

Clinical evidence

50 mg quinidine given 1 h before a single 50 mg dose of nortriptyline increased the AUC of the nortriptyline in five normal subjects[1] fourfold (from 0.6 to 2.8 mg l^{-1} h), and the half-life three-fold (from 14.2 to 44.7 h). The clearance fell from 5.4 to 1.9 ml min.$^{-1}$

Another study in normal subjects found that 200 mg quinidine daily reduced the clearance of single doses of 100 mg imipramine by 30% and of 25 mg desipramine by 85%.[2]

Mechanism

Quinidine reduces the metabolism (hydroxylation) of these tricyclic antidepressants, involving inhibition of cytochrome P450dbl, thereby reducing their loss from the body.[3]

Importance and management

The clinical importance of these interactions awaits assessment, but be alert for evidence of increased tricyclic antidepressant effects, and possibly the toxicity, if quinidine is added. One report suggested steady-state increases of 30% with imipramine and more than 500% with desipramine in extensive metabolizers.[2] More study is needed.

Reference

1 Ayesh R, Dawling S, Widdop B, Idle JR, Smith RL. Influence of quinidine on the pharmacokinetics of nortriptyline and desipramine. Br J Clin Pharmac (1988) 25, 140–1P.

2 Brøsen K, Gram LF. Quinidine inhibits the 2-hydroxylation of imipramine and desipramine, but not the demethylation of imipramine. Eur J Clin Pharmacol (1989) 37, 155–60.

3 Pfandl B, Mörike K, Winne D, Schareck W, Breyer-Pfaff U. Stereoselective inhibition of nortriptyline hydroxylation in man by quinidine. Xenobiotica (1992) 22, 721–30.

Tricyclic antidepressants + Rifampicin (Rifampin)

Abstract/Summary

A single case report describes a marked reduction in serum nortriptyline levels in a patient given rifampicin.

Clinical evidence, mechanism, importance and management

A man with tuberculosis needed large doses of nortriptyline (175 mg daily) to achieve therapeutic concentrations while taking 300 mg isoniazid, 600 mg rifampicin, 1500 mg pyrazinamide and 25 mg pyridoxine daily. Three weeks after stopping the antitubercular drugs, the patient suddenly became drowsy and his nortriptyline serum levels were found to have risen from 193 to 562 nmol/l and later to 671 nmol/l. It was then found possible to maintain his nortriptyline serum levels in the range 200–300 nmol/l with only 75 mg nortriptyline daily.[1]

The probable reason is that the rifampicin (a potent liver enzyme inducing agent) increases the liver metabolism of the nortriptyline by the liver and hastens its loss from the body. When the rifampicin was stopped the previous nortriptyline dosage became an overdosage. This seems to be the first and only report of an interaction between a tricyclic antidepressant and rifampicin, but it would now seem prudent to monitor the concurrent use of any of them, being alert for reduced antidepressant effects.

Reference

1 Bebshuk JM, Stewart DE. Drug interaction between rifampin and nortriptyline: a case report. Int J Psychiatry in Medicine (1991) 21, 183–7.

Tricyclic antidepressants + Sertraline

Abstract/Summary

A case report describes increased desipramine serum levels in a man when additionally given sertraline.

Clinical evidence, mechanism, importance and management

A depressed man taking desipramine was additionally given 50 mg sertraline daily. Within a week his serum desipramine levels had risen from 152 to 204 ng/ml, and after a month to 240 ng/ml. No adverse effects were seen and the patient said he felt more energetic and motivated.[1] The reasons are not understood. On the basis of this report there would seem to be no reason to avoid concurrent use, but the outcome should be well monitored. More study is needed.

Reference

1 Lydiard RB, Anton RF, Cunningham T. Interactions between sertraline and tricyclic antidepressants. Am J Psychiatry (1993) 150, 1125–6.

Tricyclic antidepressants + Sucralfate

Abstract/Summary

Sucralfate causes a marked reduction in the absorption of amitriptyline.

Clinical evidence, mechanism, importance and management

When a single 75 mg dose of amitriptyline was taken by six normal subjects with a single 1 g dose of sucralfate, the AUC of the amitriptyline was reduced by 50% (from 680 to 320 ng h/ml).[1] Concurrent use should be monitored to confirm that the therapeutic effects of the antidepressant are not lost. An increase in the dosage may be needed. There seems to be nothing documented about other tricyclic

Reference

1 Ryan R, Carlson J, Farris F. Effect of sucralfate on the absorption and disposition of amitriptyline in humans. Fed Proc (1986) 45, 205.

Tricyclic antidepressants + Sympathomimetics (directly-acting)

Abstract/Summary

Patients being treated with tricyclic antidepressants show a grossly exaggerated response (hypertension, cardiac arrhythmias, etc.) to injections of noradrenaline (norepinephrine, levarterenol), adrenaline (epinephrine) or, to a lesser extent, to phenylephrine. Local anaesthetics containing these vasoconstrictors and levonordefrin should not be used, but felypressin is a safe alternative. Doxepin and maprotiline appear not to interact to the same extent as most tricyclic antidepressants.

Clinical evidence

The effects of intravenous infusions of noradrenaline were increased approximately nine-fold, and of adrenaline approximately sixfold, in six healthy subjects who had been taking 60 mg protriptyline daily for 4 days.[1,2]

The effects of intravenous infusions of noradrenaline were increased 4–8-fold, of adrenaline 2–4-fold, and of phenylephrine 2–3-fold in four healthy subjects who had been taking 75 mg imipramine daily for 5 days. There were no noticeable or consistent changes in their response to isoprenaline (isoproterenol).[5]

Five patients taking nortriptyline, desipramine or other un-named tricyclic antidepressants experienced adverse reactions, some of them severe (throbbing headache, chest pain) following the injection of *Xylestin* (lignocaine with 1:25,000 noradrenaline) during dental treatment.[4] Several episodes of marked increases in blood pressure, dilated pupils, intense malaise, violent but transitory tremor and palpitations have been reported in patients taking un-named tricyclic antidepressants when they were given local anaesthetics containing adrenaline or noradrenaline for dental treatment.[3]

There are other reports describing this interaction of noradrenaline with imipramine,[6,9] desipramine,[9,10] nortriptyline,[8] protriptyline[10] and amitriptyline;[9,10] of adrenaline with amitriptyline,[7] and of levonordefrin with desipramine (in dogs).[19]

Mechanism

The tricyclics and some related antidepressants block or inhibit the uptake of noradrenaline into adrenergic neurones. Thus the most important means by which noradrenaline is removed from the adreno-receptor area is inactivated and the concentration of noradrenaline outside the neurone can rise. If therefore more noradrenaline (or one of the other directly acting alpha or alpha/beta agonists) is infused into the body, the adreno-receptors of the cardiovascular system concerned with raising blood pressure become grossly stimulated by this superabundance of amines, and the normal response is accordingly exaggerated.

Importance and management

A well-documented, well-established and potentially serious interaction. The parenteral administration of noradrenaline (norepinephrine, levarterenol), adrenaline (epinephrine), phenylephrine or any other sympathomimetic amine with predominantly direct activity should be avoided in patients under treatment with tricyclic antidepressants. If these sympathomimetics must be used, the rate and amount injected must be very much reduced to accommodate the exaggerated responses which will occur. Local anaesthetics containing conventional vasoconstrictors (noradrenaline, adrenaline, levonordefrin) should not be given to patients taking tricyclic antidepressants, but felypressin has been shown to be a safe alternative.[11,12,16] If an adverse interaction occurs it can be controlled by the use of an alpha-receptor blocking agent such as phentolamine.

Doxepine in doses of less than 200 mg daily blocks neuronal uptake much less than other tricyclic antidepressants and so is unlikely to show this interaction to the same degree, but in larger doses it will interact like other tricyclics.[13,15] Maprotiline (a tetracyclic antidepressant) also blocks uptake much less than most of the tricyclics and in normal therapeutic doses in one study on three subjects was shown not to increase the pressor response to noradrenaline.[14] The pressor response to noradrenaline is also not significantly increased in the presence of mianserin (see 'Noradrenaline + Mianserin') or iprindole,[18] and is reported to be reduced in the presence of trazodone.[17] It does not seem to have been established whether the response to oral doses of phenylephrine is enhanced.

References

1 Svedmyr N. The influence of a tricyclic antidepressive agent (protriptyline) on some circulatory effects of noradrenaline and adrenaline in man. Life Sci (1968) 7, 77.

2 Svedmyr N. Potentieringsvisker vid tillforsel au katekolaminer till patienter som behandlas med tricykliska antidepressiva medel. Svenska Lak Tidn (1968) 65, 72.

3 Dam WH. Personal communication cited by Kristoffersen MB. Antidepressivas potensering af Katekolaminvirkning. Ugeskr Laeg (1969) 131, 1013.

4 Boakes AJ, Laurence DR, Lovel KW, O'Neil R, Verrill PJ. Adverse reactions to local anaesthetic/vasoconstrictor preparations. A study of the cardiovascular responses to Xylestin and hostacain-with-adrenaline. Brit Dent J (1972) 133, 137.

5 Boakes AJ, Laurence DR, Teoh PC, Barar FSK, Benedikter LT and Prichard BNC. Interactions between sympathomimetic amines and antidepressant agents in man. Br Med J (1973) 1, 311.

6 Gershon S, Holmberg G, Mattsson E. Mattsson N, Marshall A. Imipramine hydrochloride. Its effects on clinical, autonomic and psychological functions. Arch Gen Psychiat (1962) 6, 96.

7 Siemkowicz E. Hjertestop efter amitriptylin og adrenalin. Ugeskrift Laeg (1975) 137, 1403.

8 Persson G, Siwers B. The risk of potentiating effect of local anaesthesia with adrenalin in patients treated with tricyclic antidepressants. Sven Tanlak Tiskr (1975) 68, 9.

9 Fischbach R, Harrer G, Harrer H. Verstarkung der Noradrenalin-wirkung durch Psychopharmaka beim Menschen. Arzneim-Forsch (1966) 16, 263.

10 Mitchell JR, Cavanaugh JH, Arias L and Oates JA. Guanethidine and related agents. III. Antagonism by drugs which inhibit the norepinephrine pump in man. J Clin Invest (1970) 49, 1596.

11 Aelig WH, Laurence DR, O'Neil R, Verrill PJ. Cardiac effects of adrenaline and felypressin as vasoconstrictors in local anaesthesia for oral surgery under diazepam sedation. Br J Anaesth (1970) 42, 174.

12 Goldman V, Astrom A, Evers H. The effects of a tricyclic antidepressant on the cardiovascular effects of local anaesthetic solutions containing different vasoconstrictors. Anesthesia (1971) 26, 91.

13 Fann WE, Cavanaugh JH, Kaufmann JS, Griffith JD, Davis JM, Janowsky DS, Oates JA. Doxepin: effects on transport of biogenic amines in man. Psychopharmacologia (1971) 22, 111.

14 Briant RH, George CF. The assessment of potential drug interactions with a new tricyclic antidepressant drug. Br J Clin Pharmacol (1974) 1, 113.

15 Oates JA, Fann WE, Cavanaugh JH. Effect of doxepin on the norepinephrine pump. Psychosomatics (1969) 10 (Suppl) 12.

16 Perovic J, Terzic M, Todorovic L. Safety of local anaesthesia induced by prilocaine with felypressin in patients on tricyclic antidepressants. Bull Group Int Rech Sci Stomatol Odontol (1979) 22, 57.

17 Larochelle P, Hamet P, Enjalbert M. Responses to tyramine and norepinephrine after imipramine and trazodone. Clin Pharmacol Ther (1979) 26, 24.

18 Fann WE, Davis JM, Janowsky DS, Kaufmann JS, Griffith JD, Oates JA. Effect of iprindole on amine uptake in man. Arch Gen Psychiatry (1972) 26, 158–62.

19 Dreyer AC, Offermeier J. The influence of desipramine on the blood pressure elevation and heart rate stimulation of levonordefrin and felypressin alone and in the presence of local anaesthetics. J Dent Ass SA (1986) 41, 615–18.

Tricyclic antidepressants + Sympathomimetics (indirectly-acting)

Abstract/Summary

The effects of indirectly acting sympathomimetics (amphetamines, phenylpropanolamine, etc.) would be expected to be reduced by the tricyclic antidepressants, but so far only one case involving ephedrine and amitriptyline seems to have been reported.

Clinical evidence, mechanism, importance and management

Indirectly-acting sympathomimetic amines like tyramine exert their effects by causing the release of noradrenaline (norepinephrine) from adrenergic neurones rather than by a direct stimulant action on the receptors. In the presence of a tricyclic antidepressant, the uptake of these amines into adrenergic neurones is partially or totally prevented and the noradrenaline-releasing effects are therefore blocked. The reduction in the pressor response to tyramine has been used to monitor the efficacy of treatment with the tricyclic antidepressants.[1] However tyramine itself is only used as a research tool, or as a model of the behaviour of the indirectly acting sympathomimetics. The activity of other similar sympathomimetics might be expected to be blocked by the tricyclics in the same way, but only one case seems to have been reported. An elderly woman on 75 mg amitriptyline daily developed hypotension (70 mmHg systolic) during subarachnoid anaesthesia. Her blood pressure rose only minimally when given IV boluses of ephedrine (a mixed action sympathomimetic) totalling 90 mg but she responded normally when given adrenaline (a directly-acting sympathomimetic).[2]

References

1 Mulgirigama LD, Pare CMB, Turner P, Wadsworth J, Witts DJ. Tyramine pressor responses and plasma levels during tricyclic antidepressant therapy. Postgrad Med J (1977) 53 (Suppl 4) 30.

2 Serle DG. Amitriptyline and ephedrine in subarachnoid anesthesia. Anaesth Int Care (1985) 13, 214

Tricyclic antidepressants + Thioxanthenes

Abstract/Summary, clinical evidence, mechanism, importance and management

A study using C^{14}-imipramine showed that, unlike the situation between the tricyclic antidepressants and phenothiazines, no interaction occurred with flupenthixol.[1]

Reference

1 Gram LF and Overo KF. Drug interaction: inhibitory effect of neuroleptics on metabolism of tricyclic antidepressants in man. Br Med J (1972) 1, 463.

Tricyclic antidepressants + Thyroid preparations

Abstract/Summary

The antidepressant response to imipramine, amitriptyline and possibly other tricyclics can be accelerated by the use of thyroid preparations. An isolated case of paroxysmal atrial tachycardia, another of thyrotoxicosis and yet another of hypothyroidism due to concurrent therapy have been described.

Clinical evidence, mechanism, importance and management

Normally an advantageous interaction. The addition of 25 g tri-iodothyronine daily was found to increase the speed and efficacy of imipramine in relieving depression.[1] Similar results have been described in other studies with imipramine, desipramine[2] and amitriptyline[3] but the reasons are not understood. However adverse reactions have also been seen. A patient being treated for both hypothyroidism and depression with 60 mg thyroid and 150 mg imipramine daily complained of dizziness and nausea. She was found to have developed paroxysmal atrial tachycardia.[4] A 10-year-old girl with congenital hypothyroidism, well controlled on 150 mg desiccated thyroid daily, developed severe thyrotoxicosis after taking 25 mg imipramine daily for 5 months for enuresis. The problem disappeared when the imipramine was withdrawn.[5] In another patient the effect of thyroxine was lost and hypothyroidism developed when given dothiepin.[6] These apparent interactions remain unexplained.

References

1 Wilson IC, Prange AJ, McLane TK, Rabon AM, Lipton MA. Thyroid-hormone enhancement of imipramine in non-retarded depressions. N Engl J Med (1960) 282, 1063.

2 Extein I. Case reports of L-triiodothyronine potentiation. Am J Psychiatry (1982) 139, 966–7.

3 Wheatley D. Potentiation of amitriptyline by thyroid hormone. Arch Gen Psychiatb (1972) 26, 229.

4 Prange AJ. Paroxycmal auricular tachycardia apparently resulting from combined thryoid-imipramine treatment. Am J Psychiatry (1963) 119, 994.

5 Colantonio LA and Orson JM. Triiodothyronine thyrotoxicosis. Induction by desiccated thyroid and imipraminE, Am J Dis Child (1974) 128, 396.

6 Beeley L, Beadle F, Lawrence R. Bull West Midl Centre for Adverse Drug Reaction Reporting (1984) 19, 11.

Tricyclic antidepressants + Tobacco smoking

Abstract/Summary

Smoking reduces the serum levels of amitriptyline, clomipramine, desipramine, imipramine and nortriptyline, but the concentration of the free and unbound antidepressant rises which appears to offset the effects of this interaction.

Clinical evidence

Two studies failed to find any difference between the steady-state nortriptyline serum levels of smokers and non-smokers,[1,2] but others have found that smoking lowers the serum levels of amitriptyline, clomipramine,[5] desipramine, imipramine[4] and nortriptyline.[3] For example a 25% reduction in serum nortriptyline levels was found in one study,[3] and a 45% reduction in imipramine/desipramine levels.[4]

Mechanism

The probable reason is that some of the components of tobacco smoke are enzyme inducing agents which increase the metabolism of these antidepressants by the liver.

Importance and management

An established interaction, however it might wrongly be concluded from the figures quoted that smokers need larger doses to control their depression. Preliminary data show that the serum concentrations of free (and pharmacologically active) nortriptyline are greater in smokers than non-smokers (10.2 compared with 7.4%) which probably offsets the fall in total serum levels.[3] Thus the lower serum levels in smokers may be as therapeutically effective as the higher levels in non-smokers, so that there is probably no need to raise the dosage to accommodate this interaction.

References

1 Norman TR, Burrows GD, Maguire KP, Rubinstein G, Scoggins BA, Davies

B. Cigarette smoking and plasma nortriptyline levels. Clin Pharmacol Ther (1977) 21, 453–6.

2 Alexander B, Price-Evans and Sjoqvist F. Steady-state plasma levels of nortriptyline in twins: influence of genetic factors and drug therapy. Br Med J (1969) 4, 764–8.

3 Perry PJ, Browne JL, Prince RA, Alexander B, Tsuang MT. Effects of smoking on nortriptyline plasma concentrations in depressed patients. Ther Drug Monit (1986) 8, 279–84.

4 Perel JM, Hurwie MJ, Kanzler MB. Pharmacodynamics of imipramine in depressed patients. Psychopharmacol Bull (1975) 11, 16–18.

5 John VA, Luscombe DK, Kemp H. Effects of age, cigarette smoking and the oral contraceptive on the pharmacokinetics of clomipramine and its desmethyl metabolite during chronic dosing. J Int Med Res (1980) 8, (Suppl 3) 88–95.

Tricyclic antidepressants + Urinary alkalinizers or Acidifiers

Abstract/Summary

Blood levels of desipramine, nortriptyline and other tricyclic antidepressants are not significantly affected by agents which alter urinary pH.

Clinical evidence, mechanism, importance and management

Because the tricyclics are bases it might be expected that changes in the urinary pH would have an effect on their excretion, but in fact the excretion of unchanged drug is small (less than 5% with nortriptyline and desipramine) compared with the amounts metabolized by the liver.[1] No significant changes in blood levels occur with agents such as acetazolamide or ammonium chloride which can have a marked effects on the pH of the urine.[1] Even in cases of poisoning '...vigorous procedures such as forced diuresis, peritoneal dialysis, or haemodialysis can therefore not be expected to markedly accelerate the elimination of these drugs.'[1] Only in the case of hepatic dysfunction is simple urinary clearance likely to take on a more important role.

Reference

1 Sjoqvist F, Berglund F, Borga O, Hammer W, Andersson S, Thorstrad C. The pH-dependent excretion of monomethylated tricyclic antidepressants. Clin Pharmacol Ther (1969) 10, 826.

Tricyclic antidepressants + Valpromide

Abstract/Summary

Valpromide can increase the serum levels of amitriptyline and nortriptyline.

Clinical evidence, mechanism, importance and management

The addition of 600 mg valpromide daily for 10 days caused a 65% rise in the serum levels of nortriptyline (from 61 to 100.5 ng/ml) and a 50% rise in the levels of amitriptyline (from 70.5 to 105.5 ng/ml) in two groups of ten patients.[1,2] The clinical importance of this interaction awaits assessment, but one patient developed delerium within three days which suggests that it would be prudent to monitor the outcome of concurrent use.

Reference

1 Bertschy G, Vandel S, Jounet JM, Allers G. Interaction valpromide-amitriptyline. Augmentation de la biodisponibilité de l'amitriptyline et del a nortriptyline par le valpromide. L'Encéphale (1990) XVI, 43–5.
2 Vandel S, Bertschy G, Jounet JM, Allers G. Valpromide increases the plasma concentrations of amitriptyline and its metabolite nortriptyline in depressive patients. Ther Drug Monit (1988) 10, 386–9.

Tricyclic antidepressants + Vinpocetine

Abstract/Summary

Vinpocetine does not affect serum imipramine levels.

Clinical evidence, mechanism, importance and management

The steady-state plasma imipramine levels (25 mg three times daily) of 18 normal subjects were unaffected by 10 mg vinpocetine three times daily, taken concurrently for 10 days.[1] No special precautions would seem to be necessary. There seems to be nothing documented about any of the other tricyclic antidepressants.

References

1 Hitzenberger G, Schmid R, Braun W, Grandt R. Vinpocetine therapy does not change imipramine pharmacokinetics in man. Int J Clin Pharmacol Ther Toxicol (1990) 28, 99–104.

Chapter 24
Miscellaneous Drug Interactions

Acipimox + Cholestyramine

Abstract/Summary

Acipimox does not interact significantly with cholestyramine

Clinical evidence, mechanism, importance and management

A randomized cross-over study in seven normal subjects given 150 mg of acipimox with 4 g cholestyramine, followed by two additional 4 g doses of cholestyramine 8 and 16 h later showed that the pharmacokinetics of acipimox were slightly but not significantly altered by the cholestyramine.[1] There would seem to be no good reason for avoiding concurrent use.

Reference

1 De Paolis C, Farina R, Pianezzola E, Valzelli G, Celotti F, Pontiroli AE. Lack of pharmacokinetic interaction between cholestyramine and acipimox, a new lipid lowering agent. Br J Clin Pharmac (1986) 22, 496–7.

Acitretin + Food

Abstract/Summary

Fatty foods increase the absorption of acitretin.

Clinical evidence, mechanism, importance and management

The absorption of 50 mg acitretin was increased by 90% (from 1175 to 2249 ng/ml.h) and peak serum concentrations by 70% when taken by 18 normal subjects with a standard breakfast. The breakfast consisted of two poached eggs, two slices of toast, two pats of margarine and 8 oz skimmed milk.[1] Other studies have found that high fat meals and milk increase the absorption when compared with high carbohydrate meals or when fasting.[2,3] The reason is thought to be that, like other retinoids, acitretin (which is lipid soluble) is absorbed into the lymphatic system by becoming incorporated into the bile-acid micelles of the fats in the food. In this way losses due to first-pass liver metabolism and gut wall metabolism are minimized. The makers of acitretin recommend taking it with food. No special precautions appear to be necessary.

References

1 McNamara PJ, Jewell RC, Jensen BK, Brindley CJ. Food increases the bioavailability of acitretin. J Clin Pharmaacol (1988) 28, 1051–5.
2 DiGiovanna JJ, Cross EG, McClean SW, Ruddel ME, Gantt G, Peck GL. Etretinate: effect of milk intake on absorption. J Invest Dermatol (1984) 82, 636–40.
3 Colburn WA, Gibson DM, Weins RE, Hanigan JJ. Effect of meals on the kinetics of etretinate. J Clin Pharmacol (1983) 23, 534–9.

Alfacalcidol + Danazol

Abstract/Summary

An isolated report describes hypercalcaemia in a woman on alfacalcidol when additionally treated with danazol.

Clinical evidence, mechanism, importance and management

A woman with idiopathic hypoparathyroidism treated with alfacalcidol (1 alpha hydroxycholecalciferol) developed hypercalcaemia when additionally given 400 mg danazol daily for endometriosis. This required a reduction in the dosage of alfacalcidol from 4 to 0.75 µg daily. When the danazol was stopped six months later, she remained normocalcaemic with the alfacalcidol dosage again raised to 4 µg daily.[1] The reasons are not understood. The general importance of this apparent interaction is unknown but concurrent use in any patient should be well monitored.

Reference

1 Hepburn NC, Abdul-Aziz LAS, Whiteoak R. Danazol-induced hypercalcaemia in alphacalcidol-treated hypoparathyroidism. Postgrad Med J (1989) 65, 849–50.

Allopurinol + Antacids

Abstract/Summary

Three haemodialysis patients showed a marked reduction in the effects of allopurinol while concurrently taking an aluminium hydroxide antacid. Separating the dosages by 3 h reduced the effects of this interaction.

Clinical evidence, mechanism, importance and management

Three patients on chronic haemodialysis, taking 5.7 g aluminium hydroxide daily and 300 mg allopurinol daily for high uric acid and phosphate levels, failed to show any fall in their hyperuricaemia until the antacid was given 3 h before the allopurinol, whereupon their uric acid levels fell by 40–65%. When one of them started once again to take both preparations together, his uric acid levels began to climb.[1] It would appear that the aluminium hydroxide considerably reduces the absorption of allopurinol from the gut by some as yet unknown mechanism.

Information seems to be limited to this report. Advise patients on haemodialysis to separate the administration of these two drugs by 3 h or more to avoid admixture in the gut. Monitor the outcome. Follow the same precautions with any other antacid until more information becomes available. There seems to be no information about other patients.

Reference

1 Weissman I, Krivoy N. Interaction of aluminium hydroxide and allopurinol in patients on chronic haemodialysis. Ann Intern Med (1987) 107, 787.

Allopurinol + Iron

Abstract/Summary

No adverse interaction occurs if iron and allopurinol are given concurrently.

Clinical evidence, mechanism, importance and management

Some early animal studies suggested that allopurinol might have an inhibitory effect on the metabolism of iron. This led the makers of allopurinol in some countries to issue a warning about their concurrent use,[1,2] however it would now seem that no special precautions are necessary.[3]

References

1 Emmerson BT. Effects of allopurinol on iron metabolism in man. Ann Rheum Dis (1966) 25, 700.

2 Davis PS, Deller DJ. Effect of a xanthine oxidase inhibitor (allopurinol) on radio-iron absorption in man. Lancet (1966) ii, 470.

3 Ascione FJ. Allopurinol and iron. J Amer Med Ass (1975) 232, 1010.

Allopurinol + Probenecid

Abstract/Summary

The theoretical possibility of an adverse interaction between allopurinol and probenecid which could lead to uric acid precipitation in the kidneys appears not to be realized in practice.

Clinical evidence, mechanism, importance and management

Probenecid appears to increase the renal excretion of allopurinol or its active metabolite (oxipurinol, or alloxanthine),[1] while allopurinol is thought to inhibit the metabolism of probenecid. It increases the half-life of probenecid by 50% and raises serum plateau levels of allopurinol by about 20%.[2–4] It has been suggested that the outcome might be an increase in the excretion of uric acid which could result in the precipitation of uric acid in the kidneys. However the clinical importance of these mutual interactions seems to be minimal. No problems were reported in two studies in patients given 200–600 mg allopurinol and 500–1000 mg probenecid daily.[3,4]

References

1 Elion GB, Yu T-F, Gutman AB, Hitchings GH. Renal clearance of oxipurinol, the chief metabolite of allopurinol. Amer J Med (1968) 45, 69.

2 Horwitz D, Thorgeirsson SS, Mitchell JR. The influence of allopurinol and size of dose on the metabolism of phenylbutazone in patients with gout. Eur J Clin Pharmacol (1977) 12, 133.

3 Yu T-F and Gutman AB. Effect of allopurinol (4-hydroxypyrazolo(3,4-dl) pyrimidine) on serum and urinary uric acid in primary and secondary gout. Amer J Med (1964) 37, 885.

4 Tjandramaga TB, Cucinell SA. Interaction of probenecid and allopurinol in gouty subjects. Fed Proc (1971) 30, 392 Abs.

Allopurinol + Tamoxifen

Abstract/Summary

A single case report describes a marked exacerbation of allopurinol hepatotoxicity in a man when given tamoxifen

Clinical evidence, mechanism, importance and management

An elderly man who had been taking 300 mg allopurinol daily for 12 years and who had mild chronic allopurinol hepatotoxicity, developed fever and marked increases in his serum levels of lactic dehydrogenase and alkaline phosphatase within a day of starting to take 10 mg tamoxifen twice daily.[1] This was interpreted as an exacerbation of the heptatotoxicity. He rapidly recovered when the allopurinol was stopped. The reasons for the reaction are not understood. It would now seem prudent to monitor the effects of concurrent use, but the general importance of this interaction is not known.

Reference

1 Shad KA, Levin J, Rosen N, Greenwald E, Zumoff B. Allopurinol hepatotoxicity potentiated by tamoxifen. NY State J Med (1982) 82, 1745–6.

Allopurinol + Thiazides

Abstract/Summary

Severe allergic reactions to allopurinol have been seen in a few patients, tentatively attributed to renal failure and the use of thiazide diuretics.

Clinical evidence, mechanism, importance and management

Most patients tolerate allopurinol very well, but life-threatening hypersensitivity reactions (rash, vasculitis, hepatitis, eosinophilia, progressive renal insufficiency, etc.) develop very occasionally even with standard doses of 200–400 mg. Most of the reported cases are associated with renal insufficiency and about half were taking thiazide diuretics.[4] For example, four patients developed a hypersensitivity vasculitis while taking allopurinol and hydrochlorothiazide.[1] Renal failure impairs the loss of oxipurinol (the major metabolite of allopurinol) but a study in normal subjects failed to find any alteration in its clearance by thiazides which might provide a pharmacokinetic link between thiazide use and allopurinol toxicity.[3] Other studies have shown that the effects of allopurinol on pyrimidine metabolism are enhanced by the use of thiazides.[2] Some caution is therefore appropriate if both drugs are used, particularly if renal function is abnormal, but more study is needed to confirm this possible interaction.

References

1 Young JL, Boswell RB, Nies AS. Severe allopurinol sensitivity. Association with thiazides and prior renal compromise. Arch Intern Med (1974) 134, 553.
2 Wood MH, O'Sullivan WJ, Wilson M, Tiller DJ. Potentiation of an effect of allopurinol on pyrimidine metabolism by chlorothiazide in man. Clin Exp PharmacolPhysiol (1974) 1, 53.
3 Hande KR. Evaluation of a thiazide-allopurinol drug interaction. Am J Med Sci (1986) 292, 213–16.
4 Hande KR, Noon RM, Stone WJ. Severe allopurinol toxicity: description and guidelines for prevention in patients with renal insufficiency. Am J Med (1984) 76, 47–56.

Aluminium hydroxide + Citrates and Vitamin C (ascorbic acid)

Abstract/Summary

Patients with kidney failure given aluminium antacids and oral citrate can develop a potentially fatal encephalopathy due to a very marked rise in blood aluminium levels. Some drug formulations (including many over-the-counter remedies) contain citrates as the effervescing or dispersing agent. There is evidence that vitamin C may interact similarly.

Clinical evidence

(a) Citrates

A retrospective study of haemodialysis patient's records identified eight who developed a rapidly progressive encephalopathy, characterized by confusion, myoclonus, seizures, coma and death. All of them had renal failure and had received an oral solution of citrate and aluminium hydroxide concurrently. Two of them had very markedly elevated blood aluminium levels.[2] Other patients with renal failure who had developed seizures or puzzling changes in mental status were also noted to have had aluminium-containing antacids and oral citrate.[2]

Seven other cases of encephalopathy (three of them fatal) due to an aluminium/citrate interaction in patients with renal failure have been described elsewhere.[3,11] A 10-fold rise in serum aluminium levels occurred in a haemodialysis patient given effervescent co-codamol, due to the presence of sodium citrate in the formulation used to cause the effervescence.[10]

(b) Vitamin C (ascorbic acid)

A study in normal subjects given 900 mg aluminium hydroxide three times daily found that 2 g vitamin C daily increased the urinary excretion of aluminium threefold.[8] Ascorbic acid has been shown significantly to increase the concentration of aluminium in the liver, brain and bones of rats given aluminium hydroxide.[9]

Mechanism

Studies in normal subjects clearly demonstrate that citrate markedly increases the absorption of aluminium from the gut.[1,4,11] The absorption is increased 8–50 fold if taken with orange juice or citrate,[1,4–6,11] but the reason is not understood. It is possible that a highly soluble aluminium citrate complex is formed.[1]

Importance and management

The aluminium antacid/citrate interaction in patients with renal failure is established and clinically important. It is potentially fatal. Concurrent use should be strictly avoided. The authors of one report emphasise the risks associated with any of the commonly used citrates (sodium, calcium or potassium citrates, citric acid, Shohl's solution (citric acid/sodium citrate), etc).[1] Remember too that some effervescent and dispersible tablets (including many proprietary over-the-counter analgesics, indigestion and hangover remedies such as *Alka-Seltzer*) contain citric acid or citrates,[9] and they may also occur in soft drinks.[7] Haemodialysis patients should be strongly warned about these.

The aluminium antacid/vitamin C interaction is not yet well established but the information available so far suggests that this combination should also be avoided.

References

1 Coburn JW, Mischel MG, Goodman WG, Salusky IB. Calcium citrate markedly enhances aluminium absorption form aluminium hydroxide. Am J Kid Dis (1991) XVII, 708–11.
2 Kirschbaum HB, Schoolwerth AC. Acute aluminum toxicity associated with oral citrate and aluminum-containing antacids. Am J Med Sci (1989) 297, 9–11.
3 Bakir AA, Hryhorczuk DO, Berman E. Acute fatal hyperaluminemic encephalopathy in undialyzed and recently dialyzed uremic patients. Trans Am Soc Artif Intern Organs (1986) 32, 171–6.
4 Walker JA, Sherman RA, Cody RP. The effect of oral bases on enteral aluminium absorption. Arch intern Med (1990) 150, 2037–9.
5 Slanina P, Frech W, Ekstrom L. Dietary citric acid enhances absorption of aluminium in antacids. Clin Chem (1986) 32, 539–41.
6 Weberg R, Berstad A. Gastrointestinal absorption of aluminium from single doses of aluminium containing antacids in man. Eur J Clin Invest (1986) 16, 428–32.
7 Dorhout Mees EJ, Basci A. Citric acid in calcium effervescent tablets may favour aluminium intoxication. Nephron (1991) 59, 322.
8 Domingo JL, Gomez M, Llobet JM, Richart C. Effect of ascorbic acid on gastrointestinal aluminium absorption. Lancet 91991) 338, 1467.
9 Domingo JL, Gomez M, Llobet JM, Corbella J. Influence of some dietary constituents on aluminium absorption and retention in rats. Kidney Int (1991) 39, 598–601.
10 Main J, Ward MK. Potentiation of aluminium absorption by effervescent analgesic tablets in haemodialysis patient. Br Med J (1992) 304, 1686.
11 Bakir AA, Hryhorczuk DO, Ahmed S, Hessl SM, Levy PS, Spengler R, Dunea G. Hyperaluminemia in renal failure: the influence of age and citrate intake. Clin Nephrol (1989) 31, 40–4.

Anistreplase (APSAC) + Streptokinase

Abstract/Summary

The effects of streptokinase are likely to be reduced or abolished if given within 6 months of streptokinase or anistreplase because the persistently high levels of streptokinase antibodies reduce or prevent its activation.

Clinical evidence

A study in 25 patients who had been given streptokinase for the treatment of acute myocardial infarction found that 12 weeks later they still had enough anti-streptokinase antibodies in circulation to neutralize an entire 1.5 million unit dose. At 4–8 months 18 out of 20 still had enough to neutralize half of a 1.5 million unit dose, and after 8 months the neutralization ranged from 0.4 to two million units.[1]

Mechanism

The administration of streptokinase causes the production of anti-streptokinase antibodies. These persist in the circulation so that the clot-dissolving effects of another dose of streptokinase given many months later may be ineffective or less effective because it becomes bound and neutralised by these antibodies before it can activate the plasmin which dissolves the fibrin of the clot. Many people already have a very low titre of antibodies against streptokinase even before they are given a first dose because they have become sensitized by a previous streptococcal infection, yet the incidence of allergic and anaphylactic reactions to anistreplase and streptokinase seems to be low (3% or less). At-risk patients can be identified by means of a skin test.[3]

Importance and management

An established and clinically important interaction. One author says that 'the real practical reason why therapy is not repeated within a year is that it simply would not work',[2] whereas the authors of the report cited[1] suggest that the streptokinase neutralization titres should be measured before giving a second dose within a year so that an effective dosage can be calculated.

References

1 Jalihal S, Morris GK. Antistreptokinase titres after intravenous streptokinase. Lancet (1990) i, 184–5.
2 Moriarty AJ. Anaphylaxis and streptokinase. Hosp Update (1987) 13, 342.
3 Dykewicz MS, McGrath KG, Davison R, Kaplan KJ, Patterson R. Identification of patients at risk for anaphylaxis due to streptokinase. Arch Intern Med (1986) 146, 305–7.

Antiasthmatic drugs + Beta-blockers

Abstract/Summary

Asthmatic patients and others with a history of obstructive airways disease may experience marked, possibly life-threatening, bronchospasm if given beta-blocking drugs, on rare occasions even with those which are classed as cardioselective, whether given orally or as eye drops.

Clinical evidence, mechanism, importance and management

The CSM in the UK has issued the following advice: 'Beta-blockers, even those with apparent cardioselectivity, should not be used in patients with asthma or a history of obstructive airways disease, unless no alternative treatment is available. In such cases the risk of inducing bronchospasm should be appreciated and appropriate precautions taken.'[1] An example of the danger is illustrated by an asthmatic patient who developed fatal status asthmaticus after taking just one dose of propranolol.[2]

The warning applies particularly to the non-selective beta-blockers because asthmatics and others with chronic obstructive airways disease are particularly sensitive to the effects of beta-blockade on the bronchi. However it also extends to the so-called selective (cardioselective) beta-blockers because while they are unquestionably much safer, occasionally they also cause severe bronchospasm (particularly with high doses). The warning also applies to eye drops because, perhaps unexpectedly, the systemic absorption can be very considerable. Strictly speaking this is not a drug-drug interaction, but a drug-disease interaction. The beta-blockers are classified in the introduction to Chapter 10. Celiprolol is an unusual selective beta-blocker which has been shown to cause bronchodilation rather than bronchoconstriction[3] with apparently some reduced risks for asthmatics. This needs confirmation.

Reference

1 Committee on the Safety of Medicines advice. British National Formulary, No 23 (March) 1992, p70.
2 Anon. Beta-blocker caused death of asthmatic. Pharm J (1991) 284, 185.
3 Pujet JC, Dubreuill C, Fluery B, Provendier O, Abella ML. Effects of celiprolol, a cardioselective beta-blocker, on respiratory function in asthmatic patients. Eur Resp J (1992) 5, 196–200.

Antiasthmatics + Betel nuts

Abstract/Summary

The chewing of betel nuts may worsen the symptoms of asthma.

Clinical evidence

A study of this possible interaction was prompted by the observation of two Bangladeshi patients with severe asthma which appeared to have been considerably worsened by chewing betel nuts. One out of four other asthmatic patients who regularly chewed betel nuts developed severe bronchoconstriction (a 30% fall in the FEV1) on two occasions when given betel nut to chew, and all four said that prolonged betel nut chewing induced coughing and wheezing. A double-blind study found that inhalation of arecoline (the major constituent of the nut) caused bronchoconstriction in six of seven asthmatics, and one of six controls.[1]

Mechanism

Betel nut 'quids' consist of areca nut (*Areca catechu*) wrapped in betel vine leaf (*Piper betle*) and smeared with a paste of burnt (slaked) lime. It is chewed for the euphoric effects of the major constituent, arecoline, a cholinergic alkaloid which appears to be absorbed through the mucous membrane of the mouth. Arecoline has identical properties to pilocarpine and normally has only mild systemic cholinergic properties, however asthmatic subjects seem to be particularly sensitive to the bronchoconstrictor effects of this alkaloid and possibly other substances contained in the nut.

Importance and management

Direct evidence appears to be limited to the reports cited, but the interaction seems to be established. It would appear normally not to be a serious interaction, but asthmatics should be encouraged to avoid betel nuts if it worsens their asthma. Strictly speaking this is a drug-disease interaction rather than a drug-drug interaction.

References

1 Taylor RFH, Al-Jarad N, John LME, Conroy DM, Barnes NC. Betel-nut chewing and asthma. Lancet (1992) 339, 1134–6.

Anticholinesterases + Antimalarials

Abstract/Summary

On theoretical grounds, the neuromuscular blocking effects occasionally seen with chloroquine and quinine may be expected to worsen the symptoms of myasthenia gravis, and oppose the effects of drugs (anticholinesterases) used in its treatment.

Clinical evidence, mechanism, importance and management

Quinine and chloroquine[1-4] very occasionally cause muscular weakness similar to that seen in myasthenia gravis, and rarely this neuromuscular blocking effect has been seen to be additive with the effects of conventional neuromuscular blockers (see 'Neuromuscular blockers + Quinine' and 'Neuromuscular blockers + Chloroquine'). One patient developed a myasthenic syndrome within a week of starting 300 mg chloroquine daily which was controllable with edrophonium, and which disappeared within a few days of stopping the chloroquine.[2]

There seem to be no cases on record of myasthenic patients who have shown increased muscular weakness when given either of these antimalarial drugs so that the risk is still uncertain, but be alert for evidence of worsening myasthenia if either drug is used. Martindale suggests that quinine should be avoided by myasthenics.[5] Strictly speaking this is a drug-disease rather than a drug-drug interaction.

References

1 De Bleeker J, De Reuck J, Quatacker J, Meire F. Persisting chloroquine-induced myasthenia ? Acta Clin Belg (1991) 46, 401–6.
2 Robberecht W, Bednarik J, Bourgeois P, van Hees J, Carton H. Myasthenic syndrome caused by direct effect of chloroquine on neuromuscular junction. Arch Neurol (1989) 46, 464–8.
3 Sghirlanzoni A, Mantegazza R, Mora M, Pareyson D, Cornelio F. Chloroquine myopathy and myasthenia-like syndrome. Muscle Nerve (1988) 11, 114–9.
4 Pichon P, Soichot P, Loche D, Chapelon M. Syndrome myasthenique induit par une intoxication á la choroquine: une forme clinique inhabituelle confirmée par une atteinte oculaire. Bull Soc Ophtalmol Fr.(1984) 84, 219–22.

5 Reynolds JE (Ed). Martindale. The Extra Pharmacopoeia. Edn 30, 1993, p 409.

Anticholinesterases + Methocarbamol

Abstract/Summary

An isolated report describes a reduction in the effects of pyridostigmine in a myasthenic patient when treated with methocarbamol.

Clinical evidence, mechanism, importance and management

A woman with myasthenia gravis controlled with pyridostigmine developed weakness when started on 1 g methocarbamol and 130 mg dextropropoxyphene 6-hourly for constant back pains, but recovered over 4 days when the methocarbamol was stopped and the dextropropoxyphene reduced to 65 mg 4-hourly. Rechallenge with 1 g methocarbamol five times daily resulted in 'overwhelming weakness' 2 days later, and recovery when it was withdrawn.[1] The reasons are not understood. This seems to be the only report of this interaction but it would be prudent to monitor the effects of methocarbamol in any myasthenic patient or avoid its use.

Reference

1 Podrizki A. Methocarbamol and myasthenia gravis. J Amer Med Ass (1968) 205, 938.

Anticholinesterases + miscellaneous drugs

Abstract/Summary

Diuretic doses of acetazolamide can oppose the actions of anticholinesterases used in the treatment of myasthenia gravis. Dipyridamole, procainamide, quinidine and possibly chlorpromazine can also oppose the activity of drugs used to treat myasthenia gravis, or unmask the disease. See Index for other drugs which may cause myasthenia.

Clinical evidence, mechanism, importance and management

Acetazolamide (500 mg intravenously) given as a diuretic has been observed to worsen the muscular weakness of patients with myasthenic gravis who are taking anticholinesterase drugs.[1] This was confirmed in an electromyographic study in patients taking edrophonium, and in an isolated animal nerve-muscle preparation.[1] A patient well maintained on distigmine bromide experienced an aggravation of his myasthenic symptoms on two occasions when additionally given 75 mg dipyridamole three times daily.[4] The mechanisms of these interactions are not understood. Chlorpromazine,[6] lithium carbonate,[9] procainamide[2,7] and quinidine[3,5,7,8] have also been observed to increase the muscular weakness of a few patients with myasthenia gravis, or to unmask the disease, and should therefore only be used with caution. Care is therefore needed if concurrent use it undertaken. Penicillamine,[8,11] phenytoin[12] and trimethadione[10] have been associated with the development of myasthenia in a few patients, the subsequent treatment included the use of anticholinesterase drugs.

References

1 Carmignani M, Scoppetta C, Ranelletti FO, Tonali P. Adverse interaction between acetazolamide and anticholinesterase drugs at the normal and myasthenic neuromuscular junction. Int J Clin Pharmacol Ther Toxicol (1984) 22, 140–4.
2 Drachman DA, Skom JH. Procainamide — a hazard in myasthenia gravis. Arch Neurol (1965) 13, 316.
3 Aviado DM, Salem H. Drug action, reaction and interaction. I. Quinidine for cardiac arrhythmias. J Clin Pharmacol (1975) 15, 477.
4 Haddad M, Zelikovski A, Reiss R. Dipyridamole counteracting distigmine in a myasthenic patient. IRCS Med Sci (1986) 14, 297.
5 Stoffer SS, Chandler JH. Quinidine-induced exacerbation of myasthenia gravis in patient with Grave's disease. Arch Intern Med (1980) 140, 283–4.
6 McQuillen MP, Gross M, Johns RJ. Chlorpromazine-induced weakness in myasthenia gravis. Arch Neurol (1963) 8, 70–4.
7 Kornfeld P, Horowitz SH, Genkins G, Paptestas AE. Myasthenia gravis unmasked by antiarrhythmic agents. Mt Sinai J Med (1976) 43, 10–4.
8 Weisman SJ. Masked myasthenia gravis. J Amer Med Ass (1949(141, 917–8.Masters CL, Dawkins RL, Zilko PJ, Simpson JA, Leedman RJ, Lindstrom J. Penicillamine-associated myasthenia gravis, antiacetylcholine receptor and antistriational antibodies. Amer J Med (1977) 63, 689–94.
9 Neil JF, Himmelhoch JM, Licata SM. Emergence of myasthenia gravis during treatment with lithium carbonate. Arch Gen Psychiatry (1976) 33, 1090–1.
10 Booker HE, Chun RWM, Sanguino M. Myasthenia gravis syndrome associated with trimethadione. J Amer Med Ass (1970) 212, 2262–3.
11 Vincent A, Newsome-Davis J, Martin V. Anti-acetylcholine receptor antibodies in D-penicillamine-associated myasthenia gravis. Lancet (1978) 1, 1254.
12 Brumlik J, Jacobs RS. Myasthenia gravis associated with diphenylhydantoin therapy for epilepsy. Can J Neurol Sci (1974) 1, 127–9.

Anticholinesterases + Quinolone antibiotics

Abstract/Summary

Three reports describe a worsening of the symptoms of myasthenia gravis in one patient given norfloxacin, and two given ciprofloxacin.

Clinical evidence

A woman with myasthenia gravis on 360 mg pyridostigmine and 20 mg prednisone daily, was started on 400 mg norfloxacin twice daily for a urinary tract infection. Over the next 4 h she progressively developed double vision, weakness of the neck and proximal muscles of the arms and legs, dysphagia, weakness of the chest wall muscles and shortness of breath. She complained of increasing fatigue and shortness of breath with each subsequent dose. It was necessary to double the pyridostigmine dosage to control the symptoms. The symptoms vanished within 2 days of stopping the norfloxacin. Rechallenge with 400 mg norfloxacin 6 months later in the absence of the prednisone produced essentially the same response.[1]

Another woman with myasthenia controlled with 180 mg pyridostigmine 4–6 hourly, IV cyclophosphamide and prednisone, developed shortness of breath and weakness of limb and neck muscles within 8 h of starting to take 750 mg ciprofloxacin twice daily for a respiratory tract infection. The symptoms were initially tolerable when the dosage was reduced to 500 mg but over the next few days it was found necessary to continue to reduce the dosage and eventually to stop the ciprofloxacin because of worsening myasthenia. Improvement occurred once the ciprofloxacin was stopped.[2] Another report describes a man who developed myasthenic symptoms (severe dysphagia, dysarthria and ptosis) within 48 h of starting to take 250 mg ciprofloxacin twice daily, which was later relieved by edrophonium and pyridostigmine. He appeared to have had mild undiagnosed myasthenia for several months.[3]

Mechanism

Not understood. The inference to be drawn is that these quinolones have sufficient neuromuscular blocking activity in some myasthenic patients to oppose the actions of anticholinesterases.

Importance and management

Information seems to be limited to these three reports. Until more is known it would be prudent to monitor the effects of ciprofloxacin and norfloxacin in any patient with myasthenia gravis. There seems to be no information about any of the other quinolones.

References

1 Rauser E H, Ariano R E, Anderson B A. Exacerbation of myasthenia gravis by norfloxacin. DICP Annals of Pharmacotherapy (1990) 24, 208–9.
2 Moore B, Safani M, Keesey J. Possible exacerbation of myasthenia gravis by ciprofloxacin. Lancet (1988) 1, 882.
3 Mumford C J, Ginsberg L. Ciprofloxacin and myasthenia gravis. Br Med J (1990) 301, 818.

Antihistamines + Contraceptives (oral)

Abstract/Summary

The effects of doxylamine and diphenhydramine appear not to be affected by the concurrent use of oral contraceptives.

Clinical evidence, mechanism, importance and management

The pharmacokinetics of 25 mg doxylamine and 50 mg diphenhydramine were unaltered by the use of low dose oestrogen-containing contraceptives in two groups of women (13 and 10).[1] One case of oral contraceptive failure has been attributed to the use of un-named antihistamines[2] but this remains unconfirmed. No particular precautions would seem to be necessary during concurrent use.

Reference

1 Luna BG, Scavone JM, Greenblatt DJ. Doxylamine and diphenhydramine pharmacokinetics in women on low-dose estrogen oral contraceptives. J Clin Pharmacol (1989) 29, 257–60.
2 DeSano EA, Hurley SC. Possible interactions of antihistamines and antibiotics with oral contraceptive effectiveness. Fertil Steril (1982) 37, 853–4.

Antihistamines + miscellaneous drugs

Abstract/Summary

The risk of ventricular arrhythmias in those taking astemizole or terfenadine is believed to be increased by macrolide antibiotics, some imidazole antifungals, antiarrhythmics, tricyclics, neuroleptics and possibly diuretics.

Clinical evidence, mechanism, importance and management

The development of torsades de pointes arrhythmias and QT interval prolongation in a few patients on terfenadine when given erythromycin or ketoconazole (see Index for the detailed synopses) centred attention on the other risk factors which might be associated with this serious and potentially life-threatening adverse effect. Astemizole seems not to have been directly implicated, but in overdosage it has been associated with QT interval prolongation and torsades de pointes arrhythmias. For these reasons, the CSM now strongly advises[1] the avoidance of both of these antihistamines in those with significant liver diseases, pre-existing QT interval prolongation, and while taking erythromycin, ketoconazole or drugs with arrhythmogenic potential, e.g. antiarrhythmics (amiodarone, disopyramide, procainamide, quinidine, etc), neuroleptics, tricyclic antidepressants and drugs such as diuretics which can produce an electrolyte imbalance, although direct evidence about these latter drugs is lacking.[2] They also advise the avoidance of other macrolide antibiotics and imidazole antifungals.[1] More study is needed to establish the extent of the risk with all of these drugs. See also 'Terfenadine + Imidazole antifungals'.

References

1 Anon. Ventricular arrhythmias due to terfenadine and astemizole. CSM Current Problem Series (1992) 35, 1–2.
2 Marion Merrell Dow. Triludan Datasheet, November (1992).

Anti-ulcer preparation + Milk

Abstract/Summary

Hypercalcaemia, alkalosis and renal insufficiency (milk-alkali syndrome) developed in a man while taking *Caved-S* and large amounts of milk.

Clinical evidence

A man presented with nausea, vomiting, constipation, polyuria and polydipsia, which was diagnosed as milk-alkali syndrome (hypercalcaemia, alkalosis, renal insufficiency) due to daily treatment with six tablets of *Caved-S* and 3.5 pints of milk for dyspepsia caused by a peptic ulcer.[1] Each tablet of *Caved-S* contains 100 mg aluminium hydroxide, 100 mg sodium bicarbonate, 100 mg bismuth subnitrate, 200 mg magnesium carbonate and 380 mg deglycyrrhinated liquorice.

Mechanism

The hypercalcaemia occurred because the absorbed alkali decreased the excretion of calcium by the kidneys, while the intake of calcium (in the milk) remained high. The excessive amount of calcium increased the reabsorption of bicarbonate by the kidneys (through salt and water depletion) so that the alkalosis was maintained. Hypermagnasaemia may also have had a part to play.

Importance and management

The milk-alkali syndrome is well documented but very uncommon these days because there are now other and better ways of treating peptic ulcers. This case amply illustrates that while taking an anti-ulcer preparation, well within the recommended dosage range (up to 12 tablets daily), it is still possible to develop a serious and potentially life-threatening reaction if the intake of calcium (in milk for example) is high.

Reference

1 Gibbs CJ, Lee HA. Milk-alkali syndrome due to *Caved-S*. J Roy Soc Med (1992) 85, 498–9.

Baclofen + Ibuprofen

Abstract/Summary

A man developed baclofen toxicity when given ibuprofen.

Clinical evidence, mechanism, importance and management

An isolated report describes a man taking 20 mg baclofen three times a day who developed baclofen toxicity (confusion, disorientation, bradycardia, blurred vision, hypotension and hypothermia) after taking eight 600 mg doses of ibuprofen (600 mg three times daily). It appeared that the toxicity was caused by baclofen accumulation arising from acute renal insufficiency caused by the ibuprofen.[1] The general importance of this interaction is likely to be small, but concurrent use should be monitored.

Reference

1 Dahlin PA, George J. Baclofen toxicity associated with declining renal clearance after ibuprofen. Drug Intell Clin Pharm (1984) 18, 805–8.

Betahistidine + Terfenadine

Abstract/Summary

A single report describes the re-mergence of the labyrinthine symptoms in a patient taking betahistidine when given terfenadine.

Clinical evidence, mechanism, importance and management

An isolated and very brief report says that the effects of betahistidine were opposed in a patient by the concurrent use of terfenadine and a multi-drug regimen (not detailed), with the return of the labyrinthine symptoms.[1] This interaction had been predicted on theoretical grounds because betahistidine is an analogue of histamine which would be expected to interact with any antihistamine.[2] Antihistamines should be avoided by patients taking betahistidine.

Reference

1 Beeley L, Cunningham H, Brennan A. Bull W Midlands Centre of Adverse Drug Reporting. (1993) 36, 28.
2 SERC (Duphar Labs). ABPI Datasheet Compendium 1991–2, Datapharm Publications, London (1991), 423.

Bezafibrate + Frusemide

Abstract/Summary, clinical evidence, mechanism, importance and management

An isolated report describes acute renal failure and rhabdomyolysis in a patient attributed to treatment with 400 mg bezafibrate daily and 25 mg frusemide on alternate days.[1]

Reference

1 Venzano C, Cordi GC, Corsi L, Dapelo M, De Micheli A, Grimaldi GP. Un caso di rabdomiolisi acuta con insufficienza renale acuta da assunzione contemporanea di furosemide e bezafibrato. Minerva Med (1990) 81, 909–11.

Benzbromarone + miscellaneous drugs

Abstract/Summary

Benzbromarone appears not to interact with the oral anticoagulants but aspirin antagonizes its uricosuric effects. It is also not clear whether benzbromarone remains effective in the presence of pyrazinamide, but it is not affected by chlorothiazide.

Clinical evidence, mechanism, importance and management

Although there seems to be no direct evidence that benzbromarone interacts with the oral anticoagulants, concurrent use should be monitored because increased anticoagulant effects occur with other benzofuran derivatives (e.g. benziodarone, amiodarone). However it is claimed that no increases in the anticoagulant effects of nicoumalone, ethylbiscoumacetate or phenindione were seen in a few patients given benzbromarone.[1]

A single 600 mg dose of aspirin reduced the peak ratio of urate to creatinine clearance with 160 mg benzbromarone in six gouty subjects by a half (23 compared with 12%).[2] 2600 mg aspirin daily given to 29 normal subjects on 40–80 mg benzbromarone daily reduced the urate lowering effects by 20–40%.[3] Aspirin should be avoided by patients taking benzbromarone.

It is not clear whether benzbromarone remains effective in patients taking pyrazinamide. One report claims that when 50 mg benzbromarone was given to 10 patients taking 35 mg/kg pyrazinamide daily, uric acid levels were reduced in all of them (averaging 24.3%) and were normal in four of the 10.[6] However another report says that 160 mg benzbromarone daily had no uricosuric effect on 5 patients taking 3 g pyrazinamide daily,[2] and other authors also refer to this failure to reduce uric acid levels.[3]

The uricosuric effects of benzbromarone appear to be unaffected by the concurrent use of chlorothiazide.[4,5]

References

1 Masbernard A. Quoted as personal communication (1977) by Heel RC, Brogden RN, Speight TM, Avery GS. Benzbromarone: a review of its pharmacological properties and their use in gout and hyperuricaemia. Drugs (1977) 14, 349–66.
2 Sinclair DS, Fox IH. The pharmacology of hypouricaemic effect of benzbromarone. J Rheumatol (1975) 2, 437.
3 Sorensen LB and Levinson DJ. Clinical evaluation of benzbromarone. Arth Rheum (1976) 19, 183.
4 Lee IK. Mead Johnson Research Centre. A clinical study of benzbromarone, unpublished data 1977. Quoted by Heel et al (reference 1).
5 Gross A, Giraud V. Uber die Wirkung von Benzbromaron auf Urikamie und Urikosurie. Med Welt (1972) 23, 133–6.
6 Kropp A. Uricosuric action of benzbromarone upon pyrazinamide-induced hyperuricaemia. Med Welt (1970) 65, 1448.

Bismuth subcitrate + miscellaneous drugs

Abstract/Summary

Antacids, food and large amounts of milk can reduce the effects of bismuth subcitrate. It is as yet uncertain whether other drugs which raise gastric pH can reduce its ulcer-healing effects.

Clinical evidence, mechanism, importance and management

Bismuth subcitrate (bismuth chelate, tripotassium dicitratobismuthate, TDB) is believed to act by precipitating within the stomach where it coats and binds to the ulcerated site, thereby blocking the irritant actions of stomach acid. If the pH of the stomach rises above 3.5, precipitation does not occur to any great extent[1] so that the ulcer-healing properties are reduced or lost. Bismuth subcitrate can also bind to antacids and for these reasons the makers suggest that antacids should not be taken 30 min before or after bismuth subcitrate. On theoretical grounds H_2-blockers (e.g. cimetidine, ranitidine) or proton pump inhibitors (e.g. omeprazole) which can raise gastric pH should also be avoided but there seems as yet to be no direct evidence confirming this.[4] The makers also suggest that large amounts of milk should not be taken with bismuth subcitrate but say that small amounts on breakfast cereals, or in tea or coffee do not matter.[3] One recommendation is that the bismuth subcitrate should be taken 30 min before food, and any antacid 30 min after food to minimize any interactions.[2] Bismuth subcitrate would also be expected to interact with tetracyclines given orally (see 'Tetracyclines + Antacids').

References

1 Lee SP. A potential mechanism of action of colloidal bismuth subcitrate: diffusion barrier to hydrochloric acid. Scand J Gastroenterol (1982) 17 (Suppl 80) 17–21.
2 Baguley J. Ranitidine interactions. Pharm J (1990) 244, 5.
3 Data Sheet Compendium 1989–90. Datapharm Publications (1989)
4 Baxter GF. Ranitidine interactions. Pharm J (1990) 244,117.

Calcium/Vitamin D + Thiazide diuretics

Abstract/Summary

Hypercalcaemia and possibly metabolic alkalosis (milk-alkali syndrome) can develop in patients given vitamin D and/or large amounts of calcium if they are additionally treated with diuretics such as the thiazides which can reduce the urinary excretion of calcium.

Clinical evidence

(a) Calcium/vitamin D + Thiazides

An elderly woman on hydrochlorothiazide 25 mg and triamterene 50 mg daily for hypertension, and 5000 U vitamin D_2 with 1.5 g calcium daily for osteoporosis, became confused, disorientated and dehydrated. Her serum calcium level had risen to 13.9 mg/dl (normal 8.2–10.5 mg/dl).[1]

Another elderly woman with normal kidney function on hydrochlorothiazide, 50 mg daily, and 2.5–7.5 mg calcium daily also developed hypercalcaemia.[2] A young woman with osteoporosis taking 120,000 IU vitamin D_2 and 2 g calcium daily became hypercalcaemic when given chlorothiazide.[3] 5 out of 12 patients under treatment for hypoparathyroidism with vitamin D became hypercalcaemic when treated with thiazides.[4]

(b) Calcium carbonate + Thiazides

A 47-year-old man was admitted to hospital complaining chiefly of dizziness and general weakness which had begun two months previously. He was taking 500 mg chlorothiazide daily for hypertension, 120 mg thyroid daily for hypothyroidism and 7.5–10.0 g calcium carbonate daily for 'heartburn'. On examination he was found to have metabolic alkalosis with respiratory compensation, a total serum calcium concentration of 6.8 meq/l (normal 4.3–5.2 meq/l) and an abnormal ECG. He was diagnosed as having the milk-alkali syndrome. Recovery was rapid when the thiazide and calcium carbonate were withdrawn and sodium chloride was given by infusion, and frusemide with oral phosphates.[5]

Another patient developed similar symptoms while taking large amounts of calcium carbonate and hydrochlorothiazide.[6]

Mechanism

The thiazide diuretics (and triamterene) can cause calcium-retention by reducing the urinary excretion. This, added to the increased intake of calcium, resulted in excessive calcium levels. Alkalosis (the Milk-alkali syndrome associated with hypercalcaemia, alkalosis, renal insufficiency) may also occur in some individuals because the thiazide limits the excretion of bicarbonate.

Importance and management

An established interaction. The incidence is unknown. Concurrent use need not be avoided but the serum calcium levels should be regularly monitored to ensure that they do not become excessive. Patients should be warned about the ingestion of very large amounts of calcium carbonate (readily available over the counter) if they are taking thiazide diuretics.

References

1 Drinka PJ, Nolten WE. Hazards of treating osteoporosis and hypertension concurrently with calcium, vitamin D and distal diuretics. J Am Geriat Soc (1984) 32, 405–7.
2 Hakim R, Tolis G, Golzman D et al. Severe hypercalcemia associated with hydrochlorothiazide and calcium carbonate therapy. Can Med Ass J (1979) 121, 591.
3 Parfitt AM. Chlorothiazide-induced hypercalcaemia in juvenile osteoporosis and hyperparathyroidism. N Engl J Med (1969) 281, 55.
4 Parfitt AM. Thiazide-induced hypercalcaemia in vitamin D-treated hypoparathyroidism. Ann Intern Med (1972) 77, 557.
5 Gora ML, Seth SK, Bay WH, Visconti JA. Milk-alkali syndrome associated with use of chlorothiazide and calcium carbonate. Clin Pharm (1989) 8, 227–9.
6 Hakim R, Tolis G, Goltzman A, Meltzer S, Friedman R. Severe hypercalcaemia associated with hydrochlorothiazide and calcium carbonate therapy. Can Med Ass J (1979) 8, 591–4.

Cannabis + Disulfiram

Abstract/Summary

An isolated case report describes a hypomanic-like reaction in a man on disulfiram when he used cannabis.

Clinical evidence, mechanism, importance and management

A man with a 10-year history of drug abuse (alcohol, amphetamines, cocaine, cannabis) experienced a hypomanic-like reaction (euphoria, hyperactivity, insomnia, irritability) on two occasions while being treated with 250 mg disulfiram daily which was attributed to the concurrent use of cannabis. The patient said that he felt as though he had been taking amphetamine.[1] The reason for this reaction is not understood.

Reference

1 Lacoursiere RB, Swatek R. Adverse interaction between disulfiram and marijuana: a case report. Am J Psychiatry (1983) 140, 242–4.

Carbenoxolone + Antacids

Abstract/Summary

There is some evidence that antacids may possibly reduce the effects of carbenoxolone.

Clinical evidence, mechanism, importance and management

The bioavailability of carbenoxolone combined with magnesium and aluminium hydroxide antacids in a liquid formulation was found to be approximately half that of carbenoxolone in granular and capsule formulations.[1] The extent to which antacids might reduce the ulcer-healing effects of carbenoxolone given in other formulations seems not to have been assessed but the possibility should be borne in mind.

Reference

1 Crema F, Parini J, Visconti M, Perucca E. Effetto degli antiacidi sulla biodisponibilita del carbenoxolone. Il Farmaco (1987) 42, 357–64.

Carbenoxolone + Antihypertensives and Diuretics

Abstract/Summary

Carbenoxolone causes fluid retention and raises the blood pressure in some patients. This may be expected to oppose the effects of antihypertensive drugs. Thiazides can be used to treat the adverse side-effects of carbenoxolone, but not spironolactone or amiloride which oppose its ulcer-healing effects. The potassium-losing effects of the thiazides, related diuretics and carbenoxolone can be additive so that a potassium supplement may be needed to prevent hypokalaemia.

Clinical evidence, mechanism, importance and management

(a) Antihypertensives + Carbenoxolone

Carbenoxolone can raise the blood pressure. Five out of 10 patients on 300 mg carbenoxolone daily, and two out of 10 taking 150 mg daily, showed a rise in diastolic blood pressure of 20 mmHg or more.[1] Other reports[2–8] confirm that fluid retention and hypertension commonly occur, the incidence of the latter being variously reported as being as low as 4%[10] or as high as 50%,[8] and fluid retention as absent[2] or affecting 46%.[8] The reason for the blood pressure rise is that carbenoxolone has mineralocorticoid-like activity. There appear to be few direct reports of adverse interactions between antihypertensive drugs and carbenoxolone, but patients on carbenoxolone should have regular checks on their weight and blood pressure, whether taking an antihypertensive agent or not. An increase in the dosage of the antihypertensive agent may be necessary.

(b) Carbenoxolone + Diuretics

Thiazide diuretics can be used to control the oedema and hypertension caused by carbenoxolone, but not spironolactone (an aldosterone-antagonist) or amiloride[11] because they oppose its ulcer-healing effects.[4] Deglycyrrhizinated liquorice which is an analogue of carbenoxolone has reduced mineralocorticoid activity and fewer side-effects.[8,9] If thiazides or related drugs are used it should be remembered the potassium-losing effects of the carbenoxolone and the diuretic will be additive so that a potassium supplement may be needed to prevent hypokalaemia. For example, severe hypokalaemia associated with rhabdomyolysis and acute tubular necrosis occurred in a patient given carbenoxolone and chlorthalidone without a potassium supplement.[12] Other potassium-depleting diuretics which would be expected to interact similarly are listed in table 14.2. Alternative drugs for the treatment of ulcers are the

H_2-blockers, ranitidine being one which interacts with very few other drugs.

References

1 Turpie AGG and Thomson TJ. Carbenoxolone sodium in the treatment of gastric ulcer with special reference to side-effects. Gut (1965) 6, 591.

2 Bank S, Marks IN. Maintenance carbenoxolone sodium in the treatment of gastric ulcer recurrence. In 'Carbenoxolone Sodium', Baron A, Sullivan (eds), Butterworths, London (1970) p.103.

3 Doll R, Langman MJS and Shawdon HH. Effect of different doses of carbenoxolone and different diuretics. In 'A Symposium on Carbenoxolone Sodium', Robson A, Sullivan S (eds), Butterworths, London (1968) p 51.

4 Doll R, Langman MJS and Shawdon HH. Treatment of gastric ulcer with carbenoloxone: antagonistic effect of spironolactone. Gut (1968) 9, 42.

5 Montgomery RD, Cookson JB. Comparative trial of carbenoxolone and a deglycyrrhizinated liquorice preparation (Cavid-S). Clin Trials J (1972) 9, 33.

6 Langman MJS, Knapp DR, Wakley EJ. Treatment of chronic gastric ulcer with carbenoxolone and gefarnate; a comparative trial. Br Med J (1973) 3, 84.

7 Horwich L and Galloway R. Treatment of gastric ulcer with carbenoxolone sodium. Clinical and radiological evaluation. Br Med J (1965) 2, 1272.

8 Fraser PM, Doll R, Langman MJS, Misiewicz JJ, Shawdon HH. Clinical trial of a new carbenoxolone analogue BX-24, zinc sulphate and vitamin A in the treatment of gastric ulcer. Gut (1972) 13, 459.

9 Brogden RN, Speight TM, Avery GS. Deglycyrrhinized liquorice: a report of its pharmacological properties and therapeutic efficacy in peptic ulcer. Drugs (1974) 8, 330.

10 Montgomery RD. Side-effects of carbenoxolone sodium: a study of ambulant therapy of gastric ulcer. Gut (1967) 8, 148.

11 Reed PI, Lewis SI, Vincent-Brown A, Holdstock DJ, Gribble RJN, Murgatroyd RE, Baron JH. The influence of amiloride on the therapeutic and metabolic effects of carbenoxolone in patients with gastric ulcer. Scand J Gastroenterol (1980) 15, Suppl 65, 51.

12 Descamps C. Rhabdomyolysis and acute tubular necrosis associated with carbenoxolone and diuretic treatment. Br Med J (1977) 1, 272.

Carbenoxolone + Chlorpropamide, Tolbutamide, Phenytoin, Warfarin

Abstract/Summary

Of these drugs, only chlorpropamide appears to have an effect on the pharmacokinetics of carbenoxolone, causing a small reduction in serum levels.

Clinical evidence, mechanism, importance and management

Single doses of 500 mg tolbutamide, 100 mg phenytoin or 10 mg warfarin had no significant effect on the half-life of single 100 mg doses of carbenoxolone in four normal subjects. A single 250 mg dose of chlorpropamide delayed the absorption of carbenoxolone and this was confirmed in six patients with benign gastric ulcers taking 300 mg carbenoxolone daily who showed a depression in their serum levels (about 20%). Some delay in absorption also occurred.[1] The clinical importance of this is uncertain. More study is needed.

Reference

1 Thornton PC, Papouchado M, Reed PI. Carbenoxolone interactions in man-preliminary report. Scand J Gastroenterol (1980) 15, Suppl 65, 35.

Charcoal + miscellaneous drugs

Abstract/Summary

Charcoal adsorbs drugs onto its surface and in large doses (8–50 g) can markedly reduce their absorption by the gut, but smaller doses (1–2 g) possibly interact minimally or not at all.

Clinical evidence

In a series of human studies it was found that 118 g charcoal in five divided doses given over 10–48 h reduced the half-life of phenobarbitone by 82%, of carbamazepine by 45%, of phenylbutazone by 29% and of dapsone by 47%.[12] 140 g activated charcoal in divided doses halved the AUC (area under the curve) of theophylline.[13] 50 g activated charcoal adsorbed 98% of 0.5 mg digoxin, 98% of 500 mg phenytoin, 70% of 1 g aspirin,[1] 90% of 250 mg chlorpropamide,[3] 90% of 500 mg tolbutamide and 65% of 300 mg sodium valproate.[5] 40 g charcoal almost totally reduced the absorption of 60 mg paroxetine. 10 g charcoal reduced the absorption of 2 g paracetamol (acetaminophen) by 63% over a 2 h period, but by only 23% over an 80 min period when the paracetamol was given 1 h before the charcoal.[9] 10 g charcoal in another study absorbed 70% of a single 975 mg dose of aspirin.[11] In other human studies 8 g activated charcoal adsorbed 81% of 10 mg glipizide,[2] 98% of 0.25 g digoxin, 92% of 400 mg carbamazepine and 99.1% of 40 mg frusemide.[4] 2 g charcoal reduced the absorption of 150 mg nizatidine by about 30%.[10] *In vitro* studies have found that carbutamide, chlorpropamide, tolazamide, tolbutamide, glibenclamide and glipizide are all extensively adsorbed onto charcoal.[6] However 1 g charcoal has been reported not to affect the pharmacokinetics of 500 mg ciprofloxacin.[8,14]

Mechanism

Activated charcoal can adsorb gases, toxins and drugs onto its surface so that less is available for absorption through the gut wall. Separating the dosages reduces admixture in the gut.

Importance and management

Very well established interactions. Most of the reports are about the treatment of drug poisoning and overdosage where relatively large amounts of charcoal (50 g or more) are given to adsorb as much of the drug as possible, only a few being concerned with smaller therapeutic doses. Activated charcoal in doses of 8 g three times a day has been used for primary hypercholesterolaemia[7] and would be expected to interact with any of the drugs cited above (aspirin, carbamazepine, digoxin, glipizde, frusemide, paracetamol) so that concurrent use should be avoided or the dosages separated as much as possible. There seems to be little reported about the effects of small doses of charcoal (1–2 g daily) given to absorb intestinal gas or for the treatment of diarrhoea and dysentery, except that ciprofloxacin[8] is apparently not affected by 1 g charcoal, while nizatidine absorption is reduced about 30%.[10] More study is needed to define the situation more clearly and to find out the extent to which separating the dosages to prevent admixture in the gut reduces the effects of this interaction. A one hour separation was partially effective with paracetamol.[9]

References

1 Neuvonen P J, Elfving S M, Elonen E. Reduction of adsorption of digoxin, phenytoin and aspirin by activated charcoal. Eur J Clin Pharmacol (1978) 13, 213.

2 Kivisto K T, Neuvonen P J. The effect of cholestyramine and activated charcoal on glipizide absorption. Br J Clin Pharmac (1990) 30, 733–6.

3 Neuvonen P J, Kärkkäinen S. Effects of charcoal, sodium bicarbonate and ammonium chloride on chlorpropamide kinetics. Clin Pharmac Ther (1983) 33, 386–93.

4 Neuvonen P J, Kivistö K, Hirvisalo E L. Effects of resins and activated charcoal on the adsorption of digoxin, carbamazepine and frusemide. Br J Clin Pharmac (1988) 25, 229–33.

5 Neuvonen P J, Kannisto H, Hirvisalo E L. Effect of activated charcoal on the absorption of tolbutamide and valproate in man. Eur J Clin Pharmacol (1983) 24, 243–6.

6 Kannisto H, Neuvonen P J. Adsorption of sulphonylureas onto activated charcoal. J Pharm Sci (1984) 73, 253–6.

7 Kuusisto P, Vapaatalo H, Manninen V, Huttunen J K, Neuvonen P J. Effect of activated charcoal on hypercholesterolaemia. Lancet (1986) 2, 366–7.

8 Torre D. Influence of charcoal on ciprofloxacin activity. Rev Infect Dis (1988) 10, 1231.

9 Dordoni B, Willson R A, Thompson R P H, Williams R. Reduction of absorption of paracetamol by activated charcoal and cholestyramine: a possible therapeutic measure. Br Med J (1973) 3, 86–7.

10 Knadler M P, Bergstrom R F, Callaghan J T, Obermeyer B D, Rubin A. Absorption studies of the H2-blocker nizatidine. Clin Pharmacol Ther (1987) 42, 514–20.

11 Juhl RP. Comparison of kaolin-pectin and activated charcoal for inhibition of aspirin absorption. Am J Hosp Pharm (1979) 36, 1097–8.

12 Neuvonen PJ, Elonen E, Mattila MJ. Orally given charcoal increases the rate of elimination of phenobarbital, carbamazepine, phenylbutazone and dapsone in man. Clin Pharmacol Ther (1980) 27, 275–6.

13 Berlinger WG, Spector R, Goldberg MJ, Johnson GF, Quee CK, Berg MJ. Enhancement of theophylline clearance by oral activated charcoal. Clin Pharmacol Ther (1981) 33, 351–4.

14 Torre D, Sampietro C, Rossi S, Bianchi W, Maggiolo F. Ciprofloxacin and activated charcoal; pharmacokinetic data. Rev Infect Dis (1989) 11 Suppl 5, S1015–6.

15 Greb WH. Ability of charcoal to prevent absorption of paroxetine. Acta psychiatr scand (1993) 80 (Suppl 350) 156–7.

Chlormethiazole (Clomethiazole) + Cimetidine or Ranitidine

Abstract/Summary

The sedative and hypnotic effects of chlormethiazole are markedly increased by cimetidine, but not by ranitidine.

Clinical evidence

After one week's treatment with 1 g cimetidine daily the clearance of a single 1 g oral dose of chlormethiazole (the normal hypnotic dose) in eight normal subjects was reduced by 69%, and the elimination half-life and AUC were increased by 60 and 55% respectively. Without the cimetidine the subjects slept for 30–60 min after taking the chlormethiazole, whereas after the cimetidine treatment most of them slept for at least 2 h.[1,2] Subsequent studies showed that 300 mg ranitidine daily does not interact significantly with chlormethiazole.[3,4]

Mechanism

Cimetidine not only inhibits the liver enzymes concerned with the metabolism of the chlormethiazole but it also reduces the flow of blood through the liver, both of which results in a reduction in the rate at which the chlormethiazole is removed from the body. Ranitidine does not inhibit liver enzymes.

Importance and management

The chlormethiazole/cimetidine interaction is established, but the documentation is limited. What occurred is consistent with the way cimetidine increases and prolongs the activity of other drugs. The authors emphasize that the risks of over-sedation and respiratory depression are likely to be greatest in the elderly and those with liver disease. Reduce the chlormethiazole dosage (to approximately half) or replace the cimetidine with ranitidine or another H_2-blocker which lacks enzyme inhibitory activity.

References

1 Shaw G, Bury RW, Mashford ML, Breen KJ, Desmond PV. Cimetidine impairs the elimination of chlormethiazole. Eur J Clin Pharmacol (1981) 21, 83.
2 Desmond PV, Shaw RG, Bury RW, Mashford ML and Breen KJ. Cimetidine impairs the clearance of an orally administered high clearance drug, chlormethiazole. Gastroenterol (1981) 80, 21.
3 Desmond PV, Breen KJ, Harman P, Mashford ML and Morphett B. No effect of ranitidine on the disposition or elimination of chlormethiazole or indocyanin green (ICG). Scand J Gastroenterol (1982) 17, Suppl 78, A50.
4 Mashford ML, Harman PJ, Morphett BJ, Breen KJ, Desmond PV. Ranitidine does not affect chlormethiazole or indocyanine green disposition. Clin Pharmacol Ther (1983) 34, 231–3.

Chlormethiazole (Clomethiazole) + miscellaneous drugs

Abstract/Summary

Chlormethiazole and frusemide do not appear to interact adversely, nor does chlormethiazole appear to interact with any of the other drugs listed below.

Clinical evidence, mechanism, importance and management

Ten women patients aged 66–99 were given 10 ml chlormethiazole syrup (500 mg) each evening at 10.0 pm as a sedative, and 5 ml each morning with frusemide (20–80 mg). Other drugs being taken included slow-release potassium chloride, ferrous sulphate, thyroxine, lactulose, hydroxycobalamin, benzhexol, levodopa, digoxin, amitriptyline, folic acid, ferrous sulphate, calcium with vitamin D, and carbidopa. No significant changes in the serum levels or effects of chlormethiazole or frusemide were detected, and no other significant adverse reactions were seen.[1]

Reference

1 Reid J, Judge TG. Chlormethiazole night sedation in elderly subjects receiving other medications. Practitioner (1980) 224, 751–3.

Cholestyramine + Spironolactone

Abstract/Summary

Hyperchloraemic metabolic acidosis has been seen in two patients associated with the use of cholestyramine and spironolactone.

Clinical evidence, mechanism, importance and management

Two case reports describe the development of hyperchloraemic metabolic acidosis in two elderly patients with hepatic cirrhosis treated with cholestyramine (up to four sachets daily) who were concurrently receiving spironolactone. Other predisposing factors included mild renal impairment and upper respiratory tract infection.[1,2] This adverse reaction appears to be rare, but electrolyte monitoring during concurrent use has been advised.[1]

References

1 Eaves ER, Korman MG. Cholestyramine induced hyperchloremic metabolic acidosis. Aust NZ J Med (1984) 14, 670–1.
2 Clouston WM, LLoyd HM. Cholestyramine induced hyperchloremic metabolic acidosis. Aust NZ J Med (1985) 15, 271.

Cimetidine + Rifampicin

Abstract/Summary, clinical evidence, mechanism, importance and management

The rifampicin component of triple anti-tubercular treatment (rifampicin, isoniazid, ethambutol) has been shown to increase the non-renal clearance of cimetidine by about 50% (probably due to enzyme induction) but the total clearance is unchanged.[1] This interaction appears to be of little clinical importance.

Reference

1 Kellter E, Schollmeyer P, Brandenstein U, Hoppe-Seyler G. Increased non-renal clearance of cimetidine during antituberculous therapy. Int J Clin Pharmacol Ther Toxicol (1984) 22, 307–11.

Cinnarizine + Phenylpropanolamine

Abstract/Summary, clinical evidence, mechanism, importance and management

Phenylpropanolamine counteracts the mild sedation caused by cinnarizine and improves the performance of some skills related to driving.[1] There would seem to be some possible advantage in giving these two drugs together.

Reference

1 Savolainen K, Mattila MJ, Mattila ME. Actions and interactions of cinnarizine and phenylpropanolamine on human psychomotor performance. Curr Ther Res (1992) 52, 160–8.

Cisapride + miscellaneous drugs

Abstract/Summary

Cisapride increases the rate of absorption of diazepam and disopyramide. No clinically important interactions are apparent with acetaminophen, antacids, cimetidine, morphine, paracetamol, phenytoin, propranolol or ranitidine.

Clinical evidence, mechanism, importance and management

Cisapride speeds up gastrointestinal motility. This would be expected to accelerate drug transit through the gut, to increase the absorption rate of some drugs and reduce the extent of absorption. For this reason the manufacturers of cisapride suggest[10] that for drugs which need careful individual titration (e.g. anticonvulsants) it may be useful to measure their plasma concentrations, however there seems to be no direct evidence that a clinically important interaction actually occurs. In fact a study in a child of 3 found that four days after withdrawing cisapride, the total serum **phenytoin** levels and free phenytoin fraction were unchanged.[11]

Cisapride does not cause sedation but it accelerates the absorption of **diazepam**[3] so that its sedative effects occur more quickly and may possibly be transiently increased.[4] Cisapride was found not to affect serum **propranolol** levels nor the blood pressure control of 10 mildly hypertensive patients given a sustained-release propranolol preparation.[9] 20 mg cisapride was found to increase the serum levels of **morphine** (20 mg

MST Continus, a sustained release preparation) but the effects (as measured by pupil-constriction and sedation) were unchanged.[4] Cisapride also causes no significant changes in the pharmacokinetics of **paracetamol (acetaminophen)**.[12]

Cisapride and anticholinergics have opposite effects on gastrointestinal motility (increased and decreased effects respectively). Thus one study found that cisapride (2.5 mg three times daily) increased the gastric emptying reduced by the anticholinergic **disopyramide** (100 mg three times daily), thereby markedly increasing the absorption and the serum levels of disopyramide. Its absorption rate constant was doubled and the lag time was halved.[13] The clinical significance of this is uncertain but be alert for increased disopyramide effects.

Peak serum cisapride levels are increased 22% by **cimetidine** (possibly by enzyme inhibition) whereas the bioavailabity of cimetidine is reduced (17%).[1,5] Cisapride enhances the absorption rate of **ranitidine** but reduces its absorption (AUC reduced 26%).[6,8] The increase in the bioavailability of cisapride by ranitidine[6] was not confirmed in one study.[8] The concurrent use of **aluminium oxide** and **magnesium hydroxide** was found in another study not to affect the absorption of cisapride.[7] It seems doubtful if the concurrent use of these drugs and cisapride is likely to result in a clinically relevant adverse interaction but this needs confirmation.

15 normal subjects were given 30 mg cisapride daily for 28 days to find out if it induces or inhibits liver microsomal enzymes, using antipyrine as a marker or index drug. No changes in metabolism were found.[2]

References

1 Kirsch W, Rose I, Ohnhaus EE. Cispride and cimetidine. Both drugs alter the pharmacokinetics of each other. Clin Pharmacol Ther (1986) 39, 202.
2 Davies DS, Mills FJ, Welburn PJ. Cisapride has no effect on antipyrine clearance. Br J Clin Pharmac (1988) 26, 808–9.
3 Bateman DN. The action of cisapride on gastric emptying and the pharmacodynamics and pharmacokinetics of oral diazepam. Eur J Clin Pharmacol (1986) 30, 205–8.
4 Rowbotham DJ, Milligan K, McHugh P. Effect of cisapride on morphine absorption after oral administration of sustained-release morphine. Br J Anaesth (1991) 67, 421–5.
5 Kirch W, Janisch HD, Ohnhaus EE, Van Peer A. Cisapride-cimetidine interaction: enhanced cisapride bioavailability and accelerated cimetidine absorption. Ther Drug Monit (1989) 11, 411–14.
6 Castelli G, van Peer A, Gasparini R, Woestenborghs R, Heykants J, Verlinden M, Capozzi C. Cisapride-ranitidine interaction. Unpublished report N49638 on file, Janssen Pharmaceuticals (1986).
7 Verlinden M, Van Peer A, Gasparini R, Woestenborghs R, Heykants J, Reyntjens A. Unaltered oral absorption of cisapride on coadministration of antacids. Unpublished report N49374 on file, Janssen Pharmaceuticals (1986).
8 Milligan KA, McHugh P, Rowbotham DJ. Effects of concomitant administration of cisapride and ranitidine on plasma concentrations in volunteers. Br J Anaesth (1989) 63, 628P.
9 Van der Kleijn E, Van Mameren C. Effect of cisapride on the plasma concentrations of a delayed formulation of propranolol and on its clinical effects on blood pressure in mildly hypertensive patients. Unpublished report N46957 on file, Janssen Pharmaceuticals (1986).
10 Prepulsid (cisapride). Data sheet, Janssen Pharmaceuticals (1989).
11 Roberts GW, Kowlaski SR, Calabretto JP. Lack of effect of cisapride on phenytoin free fraction. Ann Pharmacother (1992) 26, 1016–7.
12 Rowbotham DJ, Parnacott S, Nimmo WS. No effect of cisapride on paracetamol absorption after oral simultaneous administration. Eur J Clin Pharmacol (1992) 42, 235–6.
13 Kuroda T, Yoshihara Y, Nakamura H, Asumi T, Inatome T, Fukuzaki H,

Takanashi H, Yogo K, Akima M. Effects of cispapride on gastrointestianl motor activity and gastric emptying of disopyramide. J Pharmacobio Dyn (1992) 15, 395–402.

Clofibrate + Cholestyramine

Abstract/Summary

No significant interaction occurs between clofibrate and cholestyramine.

Clinical evidence, mechanism, importance and management

16 g cholestyramine daily had no effect on the fasting plasma levels, urinary and faecal excretion, or the half-life of clofibrate in 15 patients taking 1 g clofibrate twice daily.[1] No special precautions are needed.

Reference

1 Sedaghat A, Ahrens EH. Lack of effect of cholestyramine on the pharmacokinetics of clofibrate in man. Eur J Clin Invest (1975) 5, 177.

Clofibrate + Contraceptives (oral)

Abstract/Summary

Serum cholesterol and triglyceride levels can be increased by the oral contraceptives, and in two cases this is reported to have opposed the cholesterol-lowering effects of clofibrate. Oral contraceptives increase the loss of clofibrate from the body.

Clinical evidence, mechanism, importance and management

A woman with hypercholesterolaemia, taking clofibrate, showed a rise in her serum cholesterol levels on two occasions when concurrently using an oral contraceptive.[1] Another patient with type IV hyperlipoproteinaemia reacted similarly.[2] Rises in serum levels of cholesterol and triglycerides in women taking oral contraceptives are well recognized.[3,4] A comparative study in men, women, and women taking oral contraceptives found that the clearance of clofibrate was increased by 48% in those taking oral contraceptives, apparently due to an increase in its metabolism (glucuronidation).[5] Another study found that oral contraceptives increased the excretion of clofibrate glucuronide by 25%.[6] None of these studies addressed the question of whether oral contraceptives are appropriate for women needing to take clofibrate, or whether concurrent use significantly reduces the effectiveness of the clofibrate, but it would seem prudent to monitor for increases in blood lipid levels. More study is needed.

References

1 Smith RBW and Prior IAM. Oral contraceptive opposition to hypercholesterolaemic action of clofibrate. Lancet (1968) i, 750.
2 Robertson-Rintoul J. Raised serum-lipids and oral contraceptives. Lancet (1972) ii, 1320.
3 Wynn V, Doar JWH, Mills GL and Stokes T. Fasting serum triglyceride, cholesterol and lipoprotein levels during oral contraceptive therapy. Lancet (1969) ii, 756.
4 Stokes T, Wynn V. Serum lipids in women on oral contraceptives. Lancet (1971) ii, 677.
5 Miners JO, Robson RA, Birkett DJ. Gender and oral contraceptive steroids as determinants of drug glucuronidation: effects on clofibric acid elimination. Br J Clin Pharmac (1984) 18, 240–3.
6 Liu H-F, Magdalou J, Nicholas A, Lafuarie C, Siest G. Oral contraceptives stimulate the excretion fo clofibric acid glucuronide in women and female rats. Gen Pharmac (1991) 22, 393–7.

Clofibrate + Probenecid

Abstract/Summary

Serum clofibrate levels can be approximately doubled by probenecid.

Clinical evidence, mechanism, importance and management

A pharmacokinetic study in four normal subjects taking 500 mg clofibrate 12-hourly showed that 500 mg probenecid six-hourly almost doubled steady-state clofibric acid levels (from 72 to 129 mg/l) and raised free clofibric acid levels from 2.5 to 9.1 mg/l. The suggested reason is that the probenecid reduces the renal and metabolic clearance of the clofibrate by inhibiting its conjugation with glucuronic acid.[1] The clinical importance of this interaction is uncertain. It appears not to have been assessed.

Reference

1 Veenendaal JR, Brooks PM, Meffin PJ. Probenecid-clofibrate interaction. Clin Pharmacol Ther (1981) 29, 351.

Clofibrate + Rifampicin (Rifampin)

Abstract/Summary

Preliminary evidence shows that rifampicin can reduce the serum levels of the active metabolite of clofibrate.

Clinical evidence, mechanism, importance and management

Five subjects showed a 35% reduction in the steady-state serum levels of the active metabolite of clofibrate (chlorophenoxyisobutyric acid, CIPB) after taking 600 mg rifampicin daily for seven days.[1] The reason appears to be that CIPB metabolism by the liver and/or the kidneys is increased.[1] This is consistent with the well recognized and potent enzyme inducing activity of rifampicin. Whether long-term use of rifampicin would have the same effect is uncertain, but it would now be prudent to monitor serum lipid levels of patients if rifampicin is added, increasing the clofibrate dosage if necessary.

Reference

1 Houin G, Tllement J-P. Clofibrate and enzyme induction. Int J Clin Pharmacol (1978) 16, 150–4.

CNS depressants + CNS depressants

Abstract/Summary

The concurrent use of two or more drugs which depress the central nervous system may be expected to result in increased depression. This may have undesirable and even life-threatening consequences.

Clinical evidence, mechanism, importance and management

The primary effect of some drugs and the unwanted, secondary or side-effect of many other drugs is depression of the activity of the central nervous system. If taken together their effects may be additive. It is not uncommon for patients, particularly the elderly, to be taking half-a-dozen drugs or more (possibly alcohol as well) causing a culmulative CNS depression ranging from mild drowsiness through to a befuddled stupor which can make the performance of the simplest everyday task more difficult or even impossible. The importance of this will depend on the context: at home and at bedtime it may even be advantageous, whereas it may considerably increase the risk of accident in the kitchen, at work, in a busy street, driving a car or handling other potentially dangerous machinerywhere alertness is at a premium. An example of the lethal effects of combining an antihistamine, a benzodiazepine tranquillizer and alcohol is briefly mentioned in the synopsis 'Alcohol + Antihistamines'. A less spectacular but socially distressing example is that of a woman accused of shop-lifting while in a confused state arising from the combined sedative effects of *Actifed*, a *Beechams Powder* and *Dolobid* (containing triprolidine, salicylamide and diflunisal respectively).[1]

Few if any well-controlled studies have been made on the cumulative or additive detrimental effects of CNS depressants (except with alcohol), but the following is a list of some of the groups of drugs which to a greater or lesser extent possess CNS depressant activity and which may be expected to interact in this way: alcohol, analgesics, antibiotics, anticonvulsants, antidepressants, antihistamines, antinauseants, antipsychotics, anxiolytics, cough and cold preparations, hypnotics, narcotics, sedatives and tranquillizers. Some of the interactions of alcohol with these drugs are dealt with in individual synopses. The Index should be consulted.

Reference

1 Herxheimer A, Haffner BD. Prosecution for alleged shoplifting: successful pharmacological defence. Lancet (1982) i, 634.

Colestipol + Clofibrate or Fenofibrate

Abstract/summary, clinical evidence, mechanism, importance and management

Over a 6-day period no adverse interaction occurred in six normal subjects when given daily doses of 10–15 g colestipol with either 500 mg clofibrate or 300 mg fenofibrate.[1,2]

References

1 Harvengt C, Desager JP. Lack of pharmacokinetic interaction of colestipol and fenofibrate in volunteers. Eur J Clin Pharmacol (1980) 17, 459.
2 DeSante KA, Disanto AR, Albert KS, Weber DJ, Welch RD, Vecchio TJ. The effect of colestipol hydrochloride on the bioavailability and pharmacokinetics of clofibrate. J Clin Pharmacol (1979) 11–12, 721.

Colestipol + miscellaneous drugs

Abstract/Summary

Colestipol is reported not to interact significantly with aspirin or methyldopa. A report suggests that colestipol is active in insulin-treated diabetics but may be ineffective in those treated with phenformin and sulphonylureas.

Clinical evidence, mechanism, importance and management

Although colestipol can undoubtedly bind to a number of drugs in the gut, the effects on the bioavailability of most of them is usually small and clinically unimportant. The rate of absorption of aspirin is increased by 10 g colestipol but the extent is unaltered and no particular precautions seem to be necessary.[3] Colestipol is also reported to have no important effect on the absorption of methyldopa.[1]

The concurrent use of phenformin and a sulphonylurea (chlorpropamide, tolbutamide or tolazamide) inhibited the normal hypocholesterolaemic effects of the colestipol in 12 diabetics with elevated serum cholesterol levels. No such antagonism was seen in two maturity-onset diabetics treated with insulin. The control of diabetes was not affected by the colestipol.[2] This suggests that colestipol may not be suitable for lowering the blood cholesterol levels of diabetics treated with these oral hypoglycaemic agents. More study is needed to confirm these findings.

References

1 Hunninghake DB, King S. Effect of cholestyramine and colestipol on the absorption of methyldopa and hydrochlorothiazide. Pharmacologist (1978) 20, 220.

2 Bandisole MS, Boshell BR. Hypocholesterolemic activity of colestipol in diabetics. Curr Ther Res (1975) 18, 276.

3 Hunningshake DB, Pollack E. Effect of bile acid sequestering agents on the absorption of aspirin, tolbutamide and warfarin. Fed Proc (1977) 36, 996.

ocular toxicity induced by desferrioxamine. Quart J Med (1985) 56, 345–55.

5 Pall H, Blake DR, Good PA, Wynyard AC. Copper chelation and the neuro-ophthalmic toxicity of desferrioxamine. Lancet (1986) ii, 1279.

Desferrioxamine (Deferoxamine) + miscellaneous drugs

Abstract/Summary

Vitamin C may cause cardiac disorders in some patients treated with desferrioxamine. Prochlorperazine caused unconsciousness in two patients being treated with desferrioxamine.

Clinical evidence, mechanism, importance and management

(a) Desferrioxamine + Vitamin C (ascorbic acid)

Sometimes vitamin C is given to increase the excretion of iron when desferrioxamine is being used, however some patients given 500 mg vitamin C daily have shown a striking, but often transitory, deterioration in left ventricular function. For this reason it has been suggested that extreme caution should be used in patients with excess tissue iron.[1,2] The need for the use of the vitamin needs to be clearly established. Patients with advanced primary or secondary hemochromatosis, particularly those with overt cardiac disease, should reduce their vitamin C intake to a minimum. It has also been stated that the use of orange juice as a source of potassium in those receiving diuretic therapy is most injudicious.[2] The need for the use of vitamin C needs to be clearly established, but under very well controlled conditions concurrent use can be undertaken.[3]

(b) Desferrioxamine + Prochlorperazine

Two out of seven patients treated for rheumatoid arthritis with desferrioxamine lost consciousness for 48–72 h when given prochlorperazine, the presumed reason being that this drug combination removes essential iron from the nervous system.[4] It has also been suggested that desferrioxamine-induced damage of the retina may be more likely in the presence of phenothiazines.[5] The concurrent use of desferrioxamine and prochlorperazine should be avoided, but there seems to be no direct evidence of adverse interactions with any of the other phenothiazines.

References

1 Henry W. Echocardiographic evaluation of the heart in thalassaemia major. In Nienhaus AW, moderator. Thalassaemia major: molecular and clinical aspects. Ann Intern Med (1979) 91, 892–4.

2 Nienhaus A W. Vitamin C and iron. N Engl J Med (1981) 304. 170–1.

3 Cohen A, Cohen IJ, Schwartz E. Scurvy and altered iron stores in Thalassaemia major. N Engl J Med (1981) 304, 150–60.

4 Blake DR, Winyard P, Lunec A, Williams A, Good PA, Crewers S J, Gutteridge J, Rowley D, Halliwell B, Cornish A, Hidor RC. Cerebral and

Dextromethorphan + Amiodarone

Abstract/Summary

Amiodarone can increase the serum levels of dextromethorphan.

Clinical evidence

A study in eight patients with heart arrhythmias (all extensive metabolizers) found that amiodarone (1 g daily for 10 days followed by 200–400 mg daily for a mean time of 76 days) changed their excretion of dextromethophan and its metabolite following a 40 mg dose. The amount of unchanged dextromethorphan in the urine rose from 0.084 to 205 μmol/8 h whereas the amount of its metabolite (dextrophan) fell from 26 to 20 μmol/8 h. The same study found that amiodarone did not affect the metabolism of methoin (mephenytoin) or isoniazid.[1]

Mechanism

In vitro studies using liver microsomes showed that amiodarone inhibits the metabolism (O-demethylase) of the dextromethorphan by decreasing the activity of cytochrome P450 (CYP2D6) within the liver.[1] Thus the dextromethorphan is cleared from the body more slowly.

Importance and management

Information seems to be limited to this study. The clinical implications are (a) that amiodarone may interfere with the results of phenotyping if dextromethorphan is used to determine CYP2D6 activity, and (b) that dextromethorphan toxicity (excitation, confusion) may possibly develop in patients taking amiodarone. Be alert for any signs of toxicity if both are used. As yet too little is known about this interaction to say by how much the dextromethorphan dosage should be reduced. Remember that dextromethorphan occurs in a considerable number of proprietary cough preparations.

Reference

1 Funck-Bretano C, Jacqz-Aigrain E, Leenhardt A, Roux A, Poirier J-M, Jaillon P. Influence of amiodarone on genetically determined drug metabolism in humans. Clin Pharmacol Ther (1991) 50, 259–66.

Dextromethorphan + Quinidine

Abstract/Summary

Quinidine markedly increases the serum levels of dextromethorphan.

Clinical evidence

Preliminary studies found that three out of five patients given 120 mg dextromethorphan daily developed steady-state serum levels of less than 5 ng/ml, whereas seven other patients additionally stabilized on 150 mg quinidine daily and given the same dose of dextromethorphan had serum levels of 252 ng/ml.[1] A subsequent (extended ?) study by the same workers in six patients with amyotrophic lateral sclerosis found that the serum levels of dextromethorphan while taking 120 mg daily averaged only 12 ng/ml (it was actually undetectable in three of them), but when additionally given 150 mg quinidine daily for a week with only half the dose of dextromethorphan, their serum levels averaged 38 ng/ml.[2] Some of the patients experienced dextromethorphan toxicity (nervousness, tremors, restlessness, dizziness, shortness of breath, confusion, etc).[2]

Mechanism

Quinidine inhibits cytochrome P4502D6 which is involved with the metabolism of the dextromethorphan by the liver.[1,2] As a result, the dextromethorphan accumulates, its serum levels rise and its toxic effects manifest themselves.

Importance and management

An established and clinically important interaction but with limited documentation. Quinidine can be exploited to increase the serum levels of dextromethorphan, but concurrent use should be well monitored for evidence of toxicity (see above). Other patients on quinidine should be told to avoid dextromethorphan.

References

1 Zhang Y, Britto MR, Wedlund PJ, Vanderhaug KL, Smith RA. Dextromethorphan and quinidine: a drug interaction of potential therapeutic utility. Pharm Res (1991) 8, (10 Suppl), S-314.
2 Zhang Y, Britto M, Valderhaug KL, Wedlund PJ, Smith RA. Dextromethorphan: enhancing its systemic bioavailability by way of low-dose quinidine-mediated inhibition of cytochrome P4502D6. Clin Pharmacol Ther (1992) 51, 647–55.

Dimethicone + Cimetidine or Doxycycline

Abstract/Summary

The bioavailabilities of cimetidine and doxycycline are not affected by dimethicone.

Clinical evidence, mechanism, importance and management

The pharmacokinetics of a 200 mg dose of cimetidine were not significantly changed by 2.25 g dimethicone in 11 normal subjects.[1] Another study in eight subjects found that 2.25 g dimethicone did not alter the bioavailability of doxycycline.[2]

References

1 Boismare F, Flipo JL, Moore N, Chanteclair G. Etude de l'effet du dimeticone sur la disponibilite de la cimetidine. Therapie (1987) 42, 9–11.
2 Bistue C, Perez P, Becquart D, Vincon G, Albin H. Effet du dimeticone sur la biodisponibilite de la doxycycline. Therapie (1987) 42, 13–16.

Dinoprostone (Prostaglandin E2) + Oxytocin

Abstract/Summary

Concurrent use may result in uterine hypertonus.

Clinical evidence, mechanism, importance and management

The makers of *Propess*, a slow-release pessary containing dinoprostone for the initiation or continuation of cervical ripening in patients at term (38–40 weeks gestation), say that concurrent or close sequential use of these drugs should only be undertaken under exceptional circumstances because it is known that the prostaglandins potentiate the uterotonic effects of oxytocics. Uterine activity should be monitored for evidence of hypertonus. Normally the pessary is removed when labour is established.[1] *Propess* was withdrawn in the UK in July 1990 because of an unacceptable incidence of hypertonus and foetal distress.[2]

Reference

1 Propess data sheet (1989), Rousell Labs.
2 CSM current problems series, no 29, Aug 1990.

Dipyridamole + Caffeine

Abstract/Summary

Caffeine (in tea, coffee, Cola, etc) may interfere with dipyridamole-thallium 201 scintigraphy tests.

Clinical evidence, mechanism, importance and management

250 mg caffeine (roughly equivalent to 2–3 cups of coffee) before dipyridamole-thallium 201 scintigraphy caused a false-

negative test result in a patient.[1] Futher studies in normal subjects confirmed that caffeine inhibits the haemodynamic response to the infusion of dipyridamole.[2] The authors of the report therefore say that patients should abstain from caffeine (tea, coffee, chocolate, cocoa, cola, etc) for at least 24 h before a test, and if during the test the haemodynamic response is low (ie no increase in heart rate) the presence of caffeine should be suspected.[2] It is not known whether caffeine has a deleterious effect on the antiplatelet effects of dipyridamole.

References

1 Smits P, Aengevaeren WRM, Corstens FHM, Thien T. Caffeine reduces dipyridamople-induced myocardial ischemia. J Nucl Med (1989) 30, 1723–6.
2 Smits P, Straatman C, Pijpers E, Thien T. Dose-dependent inhibition of the hemodynamic response to dipyridamole by caffeine. Clin Pharmacol Ther (1991) 50, 529–37.

Doxapram + Theophylline

Abstract/Summary

Doxapram pharmacokinetics are unchanged in babies by theophylline, but agitation and increased muscle activity may occur in adults.

Clinical evidence, mechanism, importance and management

Theophylline does not affect the pharmacokinetics of doxapram when used to treat apnoea in premature babies. No adjustment of the dosage of doxapram is needed in the presence of theophylline.[1] However the makers of doxapram say that clinical data suggests there may be an interaction between doxapram and aminophylline which is manifested by agitation and increased skeletal muscle activity. Care should be taken if used together.[2]

Reference

1 Jamali F, Coutts RT, Malek F, Finer NN, Peliowski A. Lack of a pharma-cokinetic interaction between doxapram and theophylline in apnea of prematurity. Dev Pharmacol Ther (1991) 16, 78–82.
2 ABPI Datasheet Compendium 1991–2, p 1226.

Ebastine + Diazepam

Abstract/Summary, clinical evidence, mechanism, importance and management

20 mg doses of ebastine daily were found not to impair the performance of a number of tests (simulated driving, body balance, digital symbol substitution) by 12 normal subjects, nor did it importantly increase the effects of diazepam.[1,2] No

special precautions during concurrent use would seem to be necessary.

Reference

1 Mattila MJ, Ebastine administered subacutely does not impair human performance or enhance diazepam effects. Br J Clin Pharmacol (1992) 33, 244P.
2 Mattila MJ, Aranko K, Kuitunen T. Diazepam effects on the performance of healthy subjects are not enhanced by treatment with the antihistamine ebastine. Br J Clin Pharmac (1993) 35, 272–77.

Enisoprost + Cyclosporin(e)

Abstract/Summary, clinical evidence, mechanism, importance and management

350 mg cyclosporin increased the AUC of a single 400 µg dose of enisoprost in 24 subjects by 93%.[1] The clinical importance of this awaits assement.

Reference

1 Garnett WR, Venitz J, Karim A, Neuhaus J, Moran MS, Hyndman V. Effect of cyclosporine on the pharmacokinetics of enisoprost in healthy male subjects. Pharm Res (1991) 8 (Suppl 10), S-65.

Enoximone + Theophylline

Abstract/Summary

Aminophylline reduces the beneficial cardiovascular effects of enoximone.

Clinical evidence, mechanism, importance and management

An experimental study of the mechanism of action of enoxi-mone in 14 patients with ischemic or idiopathic dilative cardi-omyopathy found that pretreatment with aminophylline (7 mg/kg IV over 15 min) reduced the beneficial haemodynamic effects of enoximone (1 mg/kg IV over 15 min).[1] The reason appears to be that each drug competes for inhibition of cAMP specific phosphodiesterases in cardiac and vascular smooth muscle. The clinical importance of this awaits evaluation.

Reference

1 MorgagniGL, Bugiardini R, Borghi A, Pozzati A, Ottani F, Puddu P. Aminophylline counteracts the hemodynamic effects of enoximone. Clin Pharmacol Ther (1990) 47, 140.

Enteral tube feeding + Antacids

Abstract/Summary

Aluminium-containing antacids can interact with high protein liquid enteral feeds within the oesophagus to produce an obstructive plug.

Clinical evidence, mechanism, importance and management

Three patients who were being fed with a liquid high protein nutrient (*Fresubin liquid*) through an enteral tube developed an obstructing protein-aluminium complex oesophageal plug when intermittently given an aluminium/magnesium hydroxide antacid (*Alucol-Gel*). The authors of the report advise that high molecular protein solutions should not be mixed with antacids or followed by antacids, and if an antacid is needed it should be given some time after the nutrients and the tube should be vigorously flushed beforehand.[1]

Reference

1 Valli C, Schulthess H-K, Asper R, Escher F, Hacki WH. Interaction of nutrients with antacids: a complication during enteral tube feeding. Lancet (1986) i, 747.

Ergot + Glyceryl trinitrate (GTN)

Abstract/Summary

The ergot alkaloids such as dihydroergotamine would be expected to oppose the anti-anginal effects of glyceryl trinitrate (nitroglycerin).

Clinical evidence, mechanism, importance and management

There seem to be no clinical reports of adverse interactions between these drugs but since ergot causes vasoconstriction and can provoke angina, it would be expected to oppose the effects of glyceryl trinitrate used as a vasodilator in the treatment of angina. Glyceryl trinitrate has also been shown to increase the bioavailability of dihydroergotamine in hypotensive subjects[1] which would increase its vasoconstrictor effects.

Reference

1 Bobik A, Jennings G, Skews H, Esler M, McLean A. Low oral bioavailability of dihydroergotamine and first-pass extraction in patients with orthostatic hypotension. Clin Pharmacol Ther (1981) 30, 673–9.

Ergot + Macrolide antibiotics

Abstract/Summary

Ergot toxicity can develop rapidly in patients on ergotamine or dihydroergotamine if they are given erythromycin or triacetyloleandomycin. A similar response is expected with ponsinomycin. A single case has occurred with josamycin but none appear to have been described with midecamycin or spiramycin and none would be expected.

Clinical evidence

(a) Ergot + Erythromycin

A woman who had regularly and uneventfully taken *Migral* (ergotamine tartrate 2 mg, cyclizine hydrochloride 50 mg, caffeine 100 mg) on a number of previous occasions, took one tablet during a course of treatment with erythromycin (250 mg every 6 hours). Within 2 days she developed severe ischaemic pain in her arms and legs during exercise, with a burning sensation in her feet and hands. When admitted to hospital 10 days later her extremities were cool and cyanosed. Her pulse could not be detected in the lower limbs.[3]

Five other cases of acute ergotism are reported elsewhere[1,2,4–6] involving ergotamine tartrate or dihydroergotamine with erythromycin. The reaction developed within a few hours[5] or days.[2] The spasm of the blood vessels was moderate or severe, and prolonged.

(b) Ergot + Josamycin

An isolated report describes a woman of 33 who developed severe ischaemia of the legs within 3 days of starting to take 2 g josamycin daily and capsules containing 0.3 mg ergotamine tartrate. Her legs and feet were cold, white and painful, and most of her peripheral pulses were impalpable.[16]

(c) Ergot + Ponsinomycin

After taking 800 mg ponsinomycin twice daily for 8 days, peak concentrations of dihydroergotamine following single 9 mg doses were raised 3–40 fold in 12 normal subjects.[18]

(d) Ergot + Triacetyloleandomycin

A woman of 40 who had been taking dihydroergotamine, 90 drops daily, for 3 years without problems, developed cramp in her legs within a few hours of starting to take triacetyloleandomycin (250 mg four times a day). Five days later she was admitted to hospital as an emergency with severe ischaemia of her arms and legs. Her limbs were cold and all her peripheral pulses were impalpable[1]

There are reports[2–12,14,17] of at least 11 other patients taking normal doses of ergotamine tartrate or dihydroergotamine for months or years without problems who developed severe ergotism within hours or days of starting to take normal doses of triacetyloleandomycin. Myocardial infarction developed in one patient.[19]

Mechanism

Erythromycin and triacetyloleandomycin form metabolites in the liver which make stable complexes with the iron of cytochrome P-450 so that the normal metabolizing activity of the liver enzymes is reduced.[15] As a result the ergot is poorly metabolized so that it accumulates in the body, thus increasing its vasoconstrictive effects. Spiramycin, midecamycin and josamycin normally do not form these complexes.[15]

Importance and management

The interactions of ergot alkaloids with erythromycin and triacetyloleandomycin are well documented, well established and clinically important. Ponsinomycin is expected to interact similarly. Concurrent use should be avoided because the outcome can be serious. Some of the cases cited were effectively treated with sodium nitroprusside or naftidrofuryl oxalate.[2,5,13] Spiramycin, midecamycin and josamycin would not be expected to interact because they do not form cytochrome P-450 complexes (see 'Mechanism'), however there is one unexplained and unconfirmed report of an interaction with josamycin (cited above[17]).

References

1 Lagier G, Castot A, Riboulet G, Bosesh C. Un cas d'ergotisme mineur semblant en rapport avec une potentialisation de l'ergotisme par l'ethylsuccinate d'erythromcyine. Therapie (1979) 34, 515.
2 Neveux E, Lesgourgues B, Luton J-P, Guilhaume B, Bertagna A, Picard J. Ergotisme aigu par association propionate d'erythromycine-dihydroergotamine. Nouv Presse méd (1981) 10, 2830.
3 Francis H, Tyndall A, Webb J. Severe vascular spasm due to erythromycin-ergotamine interaction. Clin Rheumatol (1984) 3, 243–6.
4 Collet AM, Moncharmont D, San Marco JL, Eissinger F. Pinot JJ, Laselve L. Ergotisme iatrogene: role de l'association tartrate d'ergotamine-propionate d'erythromycine. Semm Hop Paris (1982) 58, 1624–6.
5 Boucharlat J, Franco A, Carpentier P, Charignon Y, Denis B, Hommel M. Ergotisme en milieu psychiatrique par association DHE propionate d'erythromycine. Ann Med Psychol (1980) 138, 292–6.
6 Leroy F, Asseman P, Pruvost P, Adnet P, Lacroix D , Thery C. Dihydroergotamine-erythromycin-induced ergotism. Ann Intern Med (1988) 109, 249.
7 Franco A, Bourland P, Massot C, Lecoeur J, Guidicelli H, Bessard G. Ergotisme aigu par association dihyroergotamine-triacetyloleandomycine. Nouv Presse méd (1978) 7, 205.
8 Lesca H, Ossard D, Reynier Ph. Les risques de l'association tri-acetyl oleandomycine et tartrate d'ergotamine. Nouv Presse med (1976) 5, 1832.
9 Hayton AC. Precipitation of acute ergotism by triacetyloleandomycin. NZ Med J (1969) 69, 42.
10 Dupuy JC, Lardy Ph, Seaulau P, Kervoelen O, Paulet J. Spasmes arteriels systemiques. Tartrate d'ergotamine. Arch Mal Coeur (1979) 72, 86.
11 Bigorie B, Aimez P, Soria RJ, Samama F di Maria G, Guy-Grand B, Bour H. L'association triacetyl oleandomycin-tartrate d'ergotamine. Est-elle dangereuse? Nouv Presse méd (1975) 4, 2723.
12 Vayssairat M, Fiescinger J-N, Becquemin M-H and Housset E. Association dihydroergotamine et tbiacetyloleandomycine. Role dans ene necrose digitale iatrogene. Nouv Presse méd (1978) 7, 2077.
13 Matthews NT, and Havill JH. Ergotism with therapeutic doses of ergotamine tartrate. NZ Med J.(1979) 89, 476–7.
14 Chignier E, Riou R, Descotes J. Ergotisme iatrogène aigu par association médicamenteuse diagnostiqué par exploration non invasive (vélocimétrie à effet Doppler). Nouv Presse méd (1978) 7, 2478.
15 Pessayre D, Larrey D, Funck-Brentano C, Benhamou JP. Drug interactions and hepatitis produced by some macrolide antibiotics. J Antimicrob Chemother (1985) 16, Suppl A, 181–94.
16 Grolleau JY, Martin M, De la Guerrande B, Barrier J, Peltier P. Ergotism aigu lors d'une association josamycine/tartrate d'ergotamine. Therapie (1981) 36, 319–21.
17 Bacourt F, Couffinhal J-C. Ischemie des membres par association dihydroergotamine-triacetyloleandomycine. Nouvelle observation. Nouv Presse méd (1978) 7, 1561.
18 Couet W, Mathiieu HP, Fourtillan JB. Effect of ponsinomycin on the pharmacokinetics of dihydroergotamine administered orally. Fundam Clin Pharmacol (1991) 5, 47–52.
19 Baudouy PhY, Mellat M, Velleteau de Moulliac M. Infarctus du myocarde provoqué par l'association tartrate d'ergotamine-troléandomycine. Rev Med Intern (1988) 9, 420–2.

Ergot + Methysergide

Abstract/Summary

The concurrent use of ergot alkaloids and methysergide can increase the risk of severe and persistent spasm of major arteries in some patients.

Clinical evidence

A man developed right faciobrachial thermoanaesthesia, vertigo, dyphagia and hoarseness seven days after starting combined treatment with 2 mg methysergide three times daily and 0.5 mg subcutaneous ergotamine tartrate at night. Continued use resulted in impaired pain, touch and temperature sensation over his right face, shoulder and arm. Arteriography demonstrated left vertebral artery occulsion and right vertebral arterial spasm. These, apart from the faciobrachial thermoanaesthesia, resolved when the drugs were stopped. Another man treated for cluster headaches with 2 mg methysergide, intramuscular ergotamine tartrate and pizotifen developed ischaemia of the right foot, with impalpable popliteal and pedal pulses. Arteriography showed a 22 cm spasm in the arteries of the leg.[1]

Another report describes prolonged myocardial ischaemia in a patient with cluster headaches when 2 mg ergotamine tartrate was added to 2 mg methysergide three times daily.[2]

Mechanism

Cluster headaches are associated with abnormal dilatation of the carotid arteries which can be constricted by both of these drugs. In the cases cited their combined vasoconstrictor effects caused arterial spasm elsewhere in the body, resulting in serious tissue ischaemia. Parenteral ergotamine raises the risk of arterial spasm.

Importance and management

Direct information seems to be limited to these cases. Cardiovascular complications can occur with either of these drugs given alone, but these cases suggest that concurrent use may unpredictably increase the risk in some patients. Clearly they should be used with great caution.

References

1 Joyce DA, Gubbay SS. Arterial complications of migraine treatment with methysergide and parenteral ergotamine. Br Med J (1982) 285, 260–1.
2 Galer BS, Lipton RB, Solomon S, Newman LC, Spierings ELH. Myocardial ischemia related to ergot alkaloids: a case report and literature review. Headache (1991) 31, 446–50.

Ergot + Tetracyclines

Abstract/Summary

Five patients taking ergotamine or dihydroergotamine developed ergotism when additionally treated with doxycycline or tetracycline.

Clinical evidence

A woman who had previously taken ergotamine tartrate succesfully and uneventfully for 16 years, was treated with doxycycline and dihydroergotamine methane sulfonate (DHE-Sandoz), 30 drops three times a day. Five days later her hands and feet became cold and reddened, and she was diagnosed as having developed a mild form of ergotism.[1]

Other cases of ergotism, some of them more severe, have been described in patients taking ergotamine tartrate and doxycycline (one patient) or tetracycline-trypsin-alpha chymotrypsin (three patients).[2–4]

Mechanism

Unknown. One suggestion[1] is that these antibiotics may have inhibited the activity of the liver enzymes concerned with the metabolism and clearance of the ergotamine, thereby prolonging its stay in the body and enhancing its activity. One of the patients had a history of alcoholism[2] and two of them were in their eighties[4] so that their liver function may have already been reduced.

Importance and management

Information is very limited indeed. The incidence and general importance of this interaction is uncertain, but it would clearly be prudent to be on the alert for any signs of ergotism in any patient given ergot derivatives and any of the tetracyclines. Impairment of liver function may possibly be a contributory factor.

References

1 Amblard P, Reymond JL, Franco A, Beani JC, Carpentier P, Lemonnier D,

Bessard G. Ergotism. Forme mineure par association dihydroergotamine-chlorhydrate de doxycycline, etude capillaroscopique. Nouv Presse Med. (1978) 7, 4148.
2 Dupuy JC, Lardy Ph, Seaulau P, Kervoelen P, Paulet J. Spasmes arteriels systemiques. Tartrate d'ergotamine. Arch Mal Coeur (1978) 72, 86.
3 L'Yvonnet M, Boillot A, Jacquet AM, Barale F, Grandmottet P, Zurlinden B, Gillet JY. A propos d'un cas exceptionnel d'intoxication aigue par un derive de l'ergot de seigle. Gynecologie (1974) 30, 541.
4 Sibertin-Blanc M. Les dangers de l'ergotisme a propos de deux observations. Arch Med Ouest (1977) 9, 265.

Ethylene dibromide + Disulfiram

Abstract/Summary

The very high incidence of malignant tumours in rats exposed to both ethylene dibromide and disulfiram is the basis of the recommendation that concurrent exposure of man to these compounds should be avoided.

Clinical evidence, mechanism, importance and management

The incidence of malignant tumours in rats exposed to 20 ppm ethylene dibromide (6 h daily, 5 days weekly) while receiving 0.05% disulfiram is very high indeed.[1,4] The reasons are not understood. In addition to the precautions needed to protect workers from the toxic effects of ethylene dibromide, it has been strongly recommended that disulfiram should not be given to those who may be exposed to this compound.[2–4]

References

1 Plotnick HB. Carcinogenesis in rats of combined ethylene dibromide and disulfiram. J Amer Med Ass (1978) 239, 1609.
2 Anon. Ethylene dibromide and disulfiram toxic interaction. NIOSH Current Intelligence Bulletin (1978) 23, Apr 11. US Department of Health, Education and Welfare Publication No 78–145.
3 Yodaiken RE. Ethylene dibromide and disulfiram-a lethal combination. J Am Med Ass (1978) 239, 2783.
4 Stein HP, Bahlman LJ, Leidel NA, Parker JC, Thomas AW. Ethylene dibromide and disulfiram toxic interaction. Am Ind Hyg Assoc J (1978) 39, A35–7.

Evening primrose oil + Phenothiazines or Anticonvulsants

Abstract/Summary

Although seizures have occurred in a few schizophrenics while on phenothiazines and evening primrose oil, no adverse effects were seen in others and there appears to be no firm evidence that evening primrose oil should be avoided by epileptic patients. Some epileptics even appear to be improved.

Clinical evidence

Thirteen chronic schizophrenics failed to respond in a double-blind cross-over trial when given eight capsules of evening primrose oil (*Efamol*) daily with vitamin supplements. Two developed seizures. Both were also taking fluphenazine decanoate 25–50 mg fortnightly, and one was on thioridazine, later changed to chlorpromazine. One patient in the placebo group also developed seizures. In another study, three long-stay hospitalized schizophrenics became much worse and showed EEG evidence of temporal lobe epilepsy when treated with evening primrose oil.[2]

In contrast, no seizures or epileptiform events were seen in a further cross-over study of 48 patients (most of them schizophrenics) on phenothiazines with tardive dyskinesia when additionally treated with evening primrose oil for 4 months.[5] Concurrent use was also apparently uneventful in studies in schizophrenic patients.[3]

Mechanism

Not understood. One suggestion is that evening primrose oil possibly increases the well-recognized epileptogenic effects of the phenothiazines, rather than having an epileptogenic action of its own.[1] Another idea is that it might unmask temporal lobe epilepsy.

Importance and management

The phenothiazine/evening primrose oil interaction is not well established, nor is its incidence known, but clearly some caution is appropriate during concurrent use in schizophrenic patients because seizures may develop in a few individuals. There seems to be no way of identifying the patients at particular risk, nor is it clear the extent to which the underlying disease condition might affect what happens.

No anticonvulsant/evening primrose oil interaction has been established and the reports cited above[1,2] appear to be the sole basis for the suggestion that evening primrose oil should be avoided by epileptics. No seizures have been reported in patients on evening primrose oil not taking phenothiazines. The makers of *Epogam*, an evening primrose oil preparation, claim that it is known to have improved the control of epilepsy in patients previously uncontrolled with conventional antiepileptic drugs, and other patients are said to have had no problems during concurrent treatment.[4] Even so, until the situation is formally examined it would seem prudent to monitor concurrent use.

References

1 Holman CP, Bell AFJ. A trial of evening primrose oil in the treatment of chronic schizophrenia. J Orthomolecular Psychiatry (1983) 12, 302–4.
2 Vaddadi KS. The use of gamma-linolenic acid and linoleic acid to differentiate between temporal lobe epilepsy and schizophrenia. Prostaglandins and Medicine (1981) 6, 375–9.
3 Vaddadi KS, Horrobin DF. Weight loss produced by evening primrose oil administation in normal and schizophrenic individuals. IRCS Med Sci: Clinical Pharmacology and Therapeutics; Endocrine System; Metabolism and Nutrition; Physiology; Psychology and Psychiatry (1979) 7, 52.
4 Scotia Pharmaceuticals. Personal Communication 1991.
5 Vaddadi KS, Courtney P, Gilleard CJ, Manku MS, Horrobin DF. A double-blind trial of essential fatty acid supplementation in patients with tardive dyskinesia. Psychiatry Research (1989) 27, 313–23.

Famotidine, Nizatidine and Roxatidine + other drugs

Abstract/Summary

Famotidine, nizatidine and roxatidine do not inhibit liver microsomal enzymes. What is known so far suggests that, in the context of drug interactions, they are likely to behave more like ranitidine than cimetidine.

Clinical evidence, mechanism, importance and management

Cimetidine interacts with a wide range of other drugs because it is a potent liver enzyme inhibiting agent, the effect of which is to reduce the metabolism and clearance from the body of drugs taken concurrently, thereby raising their serum levels, sometimes into the toxic range. Ranitidine on the other hand does not inhibit liver microsomal enzymes so that it interacts with far fewer drugs. Studies using antipyrine as an indicator of changes in liver enzyme activity have shown that famotidine, nizatidine and roxatidine[9] are more like ranitidine in not inhibiting the liver microsomal enzymes (cytochrome P-450 mixed function oxidase system) which are affected by cimetidine.

For example, cimetidine increases serum theophylline levels by inhibiting its metabolism by the liver whereas famotidine, nizatidine and roxatidine do not.[1,6,7] Cimetidine also interacts with diazepam in the same way whereas famotidine, nizatidine and roxatidine do not.[2–6,8] Roxatidine also does not interact with propranolol,[6] and nizatidine does not interact with chlordiazepoxide or lorazepam.

Thus in the absence of direct information about the outcome of giving famotidine, nizatidine or roxatidine with other drugs which are known to interact with cimetidine because their metabolism by the liver is reduced, the behaviour of ranitidine rather than cimetidine is likely to be the better guide.

References

1 Chremos AN, Lin JH, Yeh KC, Chiou WF, Bayne WF, Lipschutz K, Williams RL. Famotidine does not interfere with the disposition of theophylline in man: comparision with cimetidine. Clin Pharmacol Ther (1986) 39, 187.
2 Sambol NC, Upton RA, Chremos AN, Lin E, Gee W, Williams RL. Influence of famotidine and cimetidine on the disposition of phenytoin and indocyanine green. Clin Pharmacol Ther (1986) 39, 225.
3 Locniskar A, Greenblatt DJ, Harmatz JS, Zinny MA, Shader RI. Interaction of diazepam with famotidine and cimetidine, two H$_2$-receptor antagonists. J Clin Pharmacol (1986) 26, 299–303.
4 Klotz U, Arvela P, Rosenkranz B. Famotidine, a new H$_2$-receptor antagonist, does not affect hepatic elimination of diazepam or tubular secretion of procainamide. Eur J Clin Pharmacol (1985) 28, 671–5.
5 Klotz U. Lack of effect of nizatidine on drug metabolism. Scand J Gastroenterol (1987) 22 (Suppl 136) 18–23
6 Labs RA. Interaction of roxatidine acetate with antacids, food or other drugs. Drugs (1988) 35 (Suppl 3) 82–9.
7 Secor JW, Speeg KV, Meredith CG, Johnson RF, Snowdy P, Schenker S.

Lack of effect of nizatidine on hepatic drug metabolism in man. Br J Clin Pharmac (1985) 20, 710–3.

8 Pasanen M, Arvela P, Pelkonen O, Sotianemi E, Klotz U. Effect of five structurally diverse H2-receptor antagonists on drug metabolism. Biochem Pharmacol (1986) 35, 4457–4461.

9 Tanaka E, Nakamura K. The effect of roxatidine acetate and cimetidine on hepatic clearance assessed by simultaneous administration of three model substrates. Br J Clin Pharmac (1989) 28, 171–4.

Famotidine + Probenecid

Abstract/Summary

Serum famotidine levels are markedly increased by probenecid but toxicity would not be expected.

Clinical evidence, mechanism, importance and management

1500 mg probenecid increased the AUC (area under the curve over 10 h) of single 20 mg doses of famotidine in eight normal subjects by 81% (from 424 to 768 ng/h/ml) and reduced the tubular secretion clearance by 89% (from 196 to 22 ml/min).[1] The reason appears to be that probenecid inhibits the renal secretion of famotidine, thereby reducing its loss from the body, which is consistent with the way it affects some other drugs. The famotidine effects would be expected to be increased, but dose-related toxicity arising from this interaction seems unlikely. There would seem to be no reason for avoiding concurrent use.

Reference

1 Inotsume N, Nishimura M, Nakano M, Fujiyama S. The inhibitory effect of probenecid on renal excretion of famotidine in young healthy volunteers. J Clin Pharmacol (1990) 30, 50–6.

Fenfluramine + Mazindol

Abstract/Summary

An isolated case of cardiomyopathy is attributed to the use of fenfluramine and mazindol.

Clinical evidence, mechanism, importance and management

A woman of 36 developed acute cardiomyopathy while taking 40 mg fenfluramine and 1 mg mazindol daily for obesity. The problem resolved within a week of stopping both drugs and appropriate cardiac treatment with digoxin, frusemide and hydralazine.[1]

Reference

1 Gillis D, Wengrower D, Witztum E, Leitersdorf E. Fenfluramine and mazindol: acute reversible cardiomyopathy associated with their use. Int J Psychiatry Med (1985–6) 15, 197–200.

Flumazenil + miscellaneous drugs

Abstract/Summary clinical evidence, mechanism, importance and management

Flumazenil is a benzodiazepine antagonist which can reverse (oppose) the sedative and amnesic effects of benzodiazepines such as diazepam[1] and midazolam,[3] as well as related drugs such as zolpidem.[2] Normally this is a sought-for interaction.

References

1 Ghoneim MM, Dembo JB, Block RI. Time course of antagonism of sedative and amnesic effects of diazepam by flumazenil. Anesthesiology (1989) 70, 899–904.

2 Naef MM, Forster A, Nahory A, Danjou P, Rosenzweig P. Flumazenil antagonizes the sedative action of zolpidem, a new imidazopyridine hypnotic. Anesthesiology (1989) 71, A298.

3 Khalil AA, Seraj MA, Elmikkti N, Alsherbiny A, Joseph NJ. Flumazenil antagonizes most of the central effects of midazolam in short surgical procedures. Anesthesiology (1992) 77, A210.

Fluvastastin + miscellaneous drugs

Abstract/Summary, clinical evidence, mechanism, importance and management

In vitro studies with human liver microsomes show that fluvastatin has a high affinity for the cytochrome P450TB, CYP2C subfamily, and selectively inhibits 4'-hydroxylation.[1] It is therefore expected to interact like lovastatin with warfarin (causing bleeding) and possibly other drugs which undergo oxidation by the liver, but direct clinical studies are needed to confirm this.

Reference

1 Selective *in vitro* P450 inhibition profile by fluvastatin indicates its potential *in vivo* drug interactions. Clin Pharmacol Ther (1993) 53, 188.

Folic acid + Adsorbents

Abstract/Summary, clinical evidence, mechanism, importance and management

In vitro studies show that folic acid is markedly adsorbed by magnesium trisilicate and edible clay.[1] This would be expected to reduce its absorption from the gut, but the clinical importance of this awaits assessment.

Reference

1 Iwuagwu MA, Jideonwo A. Preliminary investigations into the in-vitro

interaction of folic acid with magnesium trisilicate and edible clay. Int J Pharmaceutics (1990) 65, 63–7.

Folic acid + Sulphasalazine

Abstract/Summary

Sulphasalazine can reduce the absorption of folic acid.

Clinical evidence, mechanism, importance and management

The absorption of folic acid in a group of patients with ulcerative and granulomatous colitis was reduced about a third (from 65.0% to 44.4%) by the inflammatory bowel disease when compared with normal subjects, and even further reduced (down to 32.0%) while taking sulphasalazine.[1] The clinical importance of this is uncertain, but it should be borne in mind when both compounds are given together.

Reference

1 Franklin JL and Rosenberg IH. Impaired folic acid absorption in inflammatory disease: effects of salicylazosulfapyridine (Azulfidine). Gastroenterology (1973) 64, 517.

Food + miscellaneous drugs

Abstract/Summary

Food does not interact with cholestyramine or imipramine. Fatty meals markedly increase the absorption of griseofulvin.

Clinical evidence, mechanism, importance and management

A study in 10 patients with Type IIA hyperlipoproteinaemia found that the efficacy of cholestyramine in controlling total cholesterol and low density lipoprotein levels was unaltered whether the cholestyramine was taken with or before meals.[1] The absorption of griseofulvin is approximately doubled if taken with a high fat meal.[2,3]

References

1 Sirtori M, Pazzuccconi F, Gianfranceschi G, Sirtori CR. Efficacy of cholestyramine does not vary when taken before or during meals. Atherosclerosis (1991) 88, 249–52.
2 Crounse RG. Human pharmacology of griseofulvin: the effect of fat intake on gastrointestinal absorption. J Invest Dermatol (1961) 37, 529–33.
3 Crounse RG. Effective use of griseofulvin. Arch Dermatol (1963) 87, 176–8.

Gemfibrozil + Antacids

Abstract/Summary

Antacids can reduce the absorption of gemfibrozil.

Clinical evidence, mechanism, importance and management

A study in patients with kidney and liver disease showed that the concurrent use of antacids (aluminium hydroxide, aluminium magnesium silica hydrate) reduced the maximum serum gemfibrozil levels to about 30–45%, and the AUC to 30–60%. The precise values are not given in the text. The reasons for these reductions is not known but adsorption of the gemfibrozil onto the antacids within the gut is suggested. The authors recommend that gemfibrozil is given 1–2 h before antacids.[1] More study is needed to confirm these findings.

Reference

1 Knauf H, Kölle EU, Mutschler E. Gemfibrozil absorption and elimination in kidney and liver disease. Klin Wschr (1990) 68, 692–8.

Gemfibrozil + Colestipol

Abstract/Summary

Colestipol can reduce the absorption of gemfibrozil if given at the same time, but not if given 2 h apart.

Clinical evidence

A study in 10 patients with raised serum cholesterol and triglyceride levels found that if 600 mg gemfibrozil was given alone or 2 h before or 2 h after 5 g colestipol, the serum gemfibrozil concentration curves were similar. When given at the same time, the AUC was reduced about 30% (from 62.6 to 43.6 mg/h/l).[1,2] Another study found that combined use enhanced the lipid-lowering effects of both drugs but the addition of colestipol was less effective than the addition of lovastatin.[3]

Mechanism

Uncertain. It seems probable that the colestipol binds with the gemfibrozil in the gut, thereby reducing its absorption.

Importance and management

Combined use is effective, but information is very limited about the clinical importance of the reduction in gemfibrozil bioavailability. However the interaction can be avoided by separating the administration of the two drugs by at least 2 h. More study is needed.

Reference

1 Forland SC, Feng Y, Cutler RE. Apparent reduced absorption of gemfibrozil when given with colestipol. J Clin Pharmacol (1990) 30, 29–32.
2 Forland SC, Feng Y, Cutler RE. The effect of colestipol on the oral absorption of gemfibrozil. J Clin Pharmacol (1988) 28, 931.
3 East C, Bilheimer DW, Grundy SM. Combination drug therapy for familial combined hyperlipidemia. Ann Intern Med (1988) 109, 25–32.

Gemfibrozil + Ispaghula (Psyllium)

Abstract/Summary

Psyllium causes a small, but almost certainly clinically unimportant, reduction in the absorption of gemfibrozil.

Clinical evidence, mechanism, importance and management

When 600 mg gemfibrozil was taken together with 3 g psyllium in 240 ml water or 2 h after the psyllium, the AUC in 10 normal subjects was reduced about 10%.[1] This change in bioavailability is almost certainly too small to matter. No special precautions would seem to be necessary.

Reference

1 Forland SC, Cutler RE. The effect of psyllium on the pharmacokinetics of gemfibrozil. Clin Res (1990) 38, 94A.

Gemfibrozil + Rifampicin

Abstract/Summary, clinical evidence, mechanism, importance and management

600 mg rifampicin daily for 6 days was found not to affect significantly the pharmacokinetics of 600 mg gemfibrozil in 10 normal subjects.[1] No special precautions seem necessary.

Reference

1 Forland SC, Feng Y, Cutler RE. The effect of rifampin on the pharmacokinetics of gemfibrozil. J Clin Pharmacol (1988) 28, 908–959.

Glucagon + Beta-blockers

Abstract/Summary

The hyperglycaemic effects of glucagon may be reduced by propranolol.

Clinical evidence, mechanism, importance and management

A study in five normal subjects showed that the hyperglycaemic activity of glucagon was reduced to some extent in the presence of propranolol.[1] The reason is uncertain, but one suggestion is that the propranolol inhibits the effects of the catecholamines which are released by glucagon. A similar response would be expected in patients under treatment with propranolol. Whether this is also true for other beta-blockers awaits confirmation.

Reference

1 Messerli FH, Kuchel O, Tolis G. Effects of beta-adrenergic blockage on plasma cyclic AMP and blood sugar responses to glucagon and isoproterenol in man. Int J Clin Pharmacol (1976) 14, 189.

Glutethimide + Tobacco Smoking

Abstract/Summary

The effects of glutethimide appear to be greater in smokers than in non-smokers.

Clinical evidence, mechanism, importance and management

A study in seven subjects found that glutethimide worsened the performance of a psychomotor test in smokers more than in non-smokers, possibly due to an increase in its absorption.[1] However there would seem to be no reason for smokers to avoid glutethimide.

Reference

1 Crow JW et al. Glutethimide and 4-OH glutethimide pharmacokinetics and effect on performance in man. Clin Pharmacol Ther (1978) 22, 458.

Glyceryl trinitrate (GTN) + Anticholinergics

Abstract/Summary, clinical evidence, mechanism, importance and management

Drugs with anticholinergic effects, such as the tricyclic antidepressants and disopyramide, depress salivation and most patients complain of having a dry mouth. In theory sublingual glyceryl trinitrate will dissolve less readily under the tongue in these patients, thereby reducing its absorption and its effects, however no formal studies to confirm this seem to have been carried out.

Glyceryl trinitrate (GTN, nitroglycerin) + Aspirin

Abstract/Summary

Some limited evidence suggests that analgesic doses of aspirin can increase the serum levels of glyceryl trinitrate, possibly resulting in an increase in its side-effects such as hypotension and headaches. Paradoxically, long-term aspirin use appears to reduce the effects of glyceryl trinitrate used for vasodilation in patients following coronary artery by-pass surgery.

Clinical evidence

(a) Glyceryl trinitrate effects increased

When 0.8 mg glyceryl trinitrate was given to seven normal subjects as a sublingual spray an hour after taking 1 g aspirin, the mean plasma glyceryl trinitrate levels 30 min later were increased by 54% (from 0.24 to 0.37 ng.ml^{-1}). The haemodynamic effects of the glyceryl trinitrate (reduced diastolic blood pressure, end-diastolic diameter and end-systolic diameter) were enhanced. Some changes were seen when 500 mg aspirin was given every two days (described as an antiaggregant dose) but the effects were not statistically significant.[1]

(b) Glyceryl trinitrate effects reduced

A study in patients following coronary artery by-pass surgery found that those who had been taking 150 or 300 mg aspirin daily (33 patients) for at least 3 months, needed more glyceryl trinitrate during the recovery period than those who had not taken aspirin (also 33 patients). To achieve the blood pressure criteria required, the aspirin-group needed an infusion of 8.2 µg min^{-1} glyceryl trinitrate which remained relatively high (3.3 µg min^{-1}) even after 8 hr, whereas the non-aspirin group only needed 5.5 µg min^{-1} which fell to 1.9 µg min^{-1} after 8 hr.[2]

Mechanism

Not understood. (a) Although prostaglandin-synthetase inhibitors such as aspirin can suppress the vasodilator effects of glyceryl trinitrate to some extent by blocking prostaglandin release, it seems that a much greater pharmacodynamic interaction also occurs in which aspirin reduces the flow of blood through the liver so that the metabolism of the glyceryl trinitrate is reduced, thus increasing its effects.

Importance and management

A confusing and unexplained situation. It seems possible that patients taking glyceryl trinitrate may experience an exaggeration of its side-effects such as hypotension and headaches if they are taking analgesic doses of aspirin. More study is needed to find out if this is of any practical importance. But also be aware that long-term aspirin use may reduce the vasodilatory effects glyceryl trinitrate. The anti-aggregant effects of aspirin and glyceryl trinitrate appear to be additive.[3]

Reference

1 Weber S, Rey E, Pipeau C, Lutfalla G, Richard M-O, Daoud-El-Assaf H, Olive G, Degeorges M. Influence of aspirin on the hemodynamic effects of sublingual nitroglycerin. J Cardiovasc Pharmacol (1983) 5, 874–7.
2 Key BJ, Keen M, Wilkes MP. Reduced responsiveness to nitro-vasodilatorr following prolonged low dose aspirin administration in man. Br J Clin Pharmac (1992) 34, 453–4P.
3 Karlberg K-E, Ahlner J, Henriksson P, Torfgård K, Sylvén C. Effects of nitroglycerin on platelet aggregation beyond the effects of acetylsalicylic acid in healthy subjects. Am J Cardiol (1993) 71, 361–4.

H$_2$-blockers + Antacids

Abstract/Summary

The absorption of cimetidine, ranitidine and famotidine may possibly be reduced to some extent by antacids but whether this reduces their ulcer-healing effects is uncertain. Separating the dosages by 1–2 h to reduces the possibility. Metoclopramide only interacts minimally with cimetidine.

Clinical evidence

(a) Cimetidine

A study in which 12 normal subjects were given 300 mg cimetidine orally four times a day, with and without 30 ml *Mylanta II*, indicated that the absorption of cimetidine was unaffected.[10]

The serum levels and urinary excretion of cimetidine were unaffected in six healthy subjects when given either 20 ml *Aludrox SA* (4.75 ml aluminium hydroxide gel + 100 mg magnesium hydroxide in every 5 ml) or two *Rennies* (80 mg light magnesium carbonate + 680 mg chalk per tablet).[1] No interaction was found in another study with an aluminium phosphate antacid.[5,12]

In contrast, a number of other single dose studies indicated that antacids reduce absorption: 30 ml *Novalucol* (6 g aluminium hydroxide + 2.5 g magnesium hydroxide in every 100 ml) reduced serum cimetidine levels by 22% (range 3–48%)[2]; *Maalox* and *Mylanta* were found to reduce peak serum cimetidine levels 24–50% and the 4 h AUC were similarly reduced.[3,14] Reductions have been found in other studies.[4,6] Giving the cimetidine 2 h after *Mylanta II* resulted in only a 10% reduction, and minimal changes were seen when given 2 h before 20 mg metoclopramide.[16]

(b) Famotidine

A study in 17 normal subjects showed that *Mylanta II* reduced the absorption of famotidine to some extent.[11] Another study found that this 30 ml of this antacid reduced the AUC and peak serum levels of famotidine by about a third when taken together, but no significant interaction occurred when the antacid was taken 2 h later.[15]

(c) Ranitidine

A study in six subjects showed that the concurrent use of 30 ml *Mylanta II* (aluminium/magnesium hydroxide mixture) reduced the peak ranitidine serum levels and the AUC after a single 150 mg dose by one-third.[7]

Reductions up to 59% were found in two other studies.[9,14] Another study showed that aluminium phosphate reduced the bioavailability of ranitidine by 30%.[13]

Mechanism

Not fully understood. Changes in gastric pH caused by the antacid and retarded gastric motility have been suggested.

Importance and management

A reduction in the bioavailability of cimetidine, famotidine and ranitidine can occur with some antacids, but none of these interactions is very well established and evidence that the ulcer-healing effects are reduced to a significant extent seems to be lacking. It may prove not be necessary to take any special precautions. However until the absence of an interaction is confirmed it might be prudent to follow the general recommendation that the antacid should be given 1–2 h before or after the H$_2$-blocker if fasting, or 1 h after if the blocker is taken with food, in which case no significant reduction in absorption should occur.[3,8,9,11,15]

References

1 Burland WL, Darkin DW, Mills MW. Effect of antacids on absorption of cimetidine. Lancet (1976) ii, 965.
2 Bodemar G, Norland B, Walan A. Diminished absorption of cimetidine caused by antacids. Lancet (1979) i, 444.
3 Steinberg WM, Lewis JH, Katz DM. Antacids inhibit absorption of cimetidine. N Engl J Med (1982) 307, 400–4.
4 Russell WL, Lopez LM, Normann SA, Doering PL and Guild RT. Effect of antacids on predicted steady-state cimetidine concentrations. Dig Dis Sci (1984) 29, 385–9.
5 Albin H, Vincon G, Pehoucq F, Dangoumau J. Influence d'un antacide sur la biodisponibilite de la cimetidine. Therapie (1982) 37, 563–6.
6 Gugler R, Brand M, Somogyi A. Impaired cimetidine absorption due to antacids and metoclopramide. Eur J Clin Pharmacol(1981) 20, 225–8.
7 Mihaly GW, Marino AT, Webster LK, Jones DB, Louis WJ, Smallwood RA. High dose of antacid (*Mylanta II*) reduces the bioavailability of ranitidine. Br Med J (1982) 285, 998–9.
8 Frislid K, Berstad A. High dose antacid reduced bioavailability of ranitidine. Br Med J (1983) 286, 1358.
9 Desmond PV, Harman PJ, Gannoulis N, Kamm M, Mashford ML. The effect of antacids and food on the absorption of cimetidine and ranitidine. Gastroenterology (1986) 90, 1393.
10 Shelly DW, Doering PL, Russell WL, Guild RT, Lopez LM and Perrin J. Effect of concomitant antacid administration on plasma cimetidine concentrations during repetitive dosing. Drug Intell Clin Pharm (1986) 20, 792–5.
11 Tupy-Visich MA, Tarzian SK, Schwartz S, Lin JH, Hessey GA, Kanovsky SM, Chremos AN. Bioavailability of oral famotidine when administered

with antacid or food. J Clin Pharmacol (1986) 26, 541–60.
12 Albin H, Vincon G, Demotes-Mainard F, Begaud B, Bedjaoui A. Effect of aluminium phosphate on the bioavailability of cimetidine and prednisolone. Eur J Clin Pharmacol (1984) 26, 271–3.
13 Albin H, Vincon G, Begaud B, Bistue C, Perez P. Effect of aluminium phosphate on the bioavailability of ranitidine. Eur J Clin Pharmacol (1987) 32, 97–99.
14 Desmond PV, Harman PJ, Gannoulis N, Kamm M, Mashford ML. The effect of an antacid and food on the absorption of cimetidine and ranitidine. J Pharm Pharmac (1990) 42, 352–4.
15 Barzaghi N, Gatti G, Crema F, Perucca E. Impaired bioavailability of famotidine given concurrently with a potent antacid. J Clin Pharmacol (1989) 29, 670–2.
16 Barzaghi N, Crema F, Mescoli G, Perucca E. Effects on cimetidine bioavailability of metoclopramide and antacids given two hours apart. Eur J Clin Pharmacol (1989) 37, 409–10.

H$_2$-blockers + Sucralfate

Abstract/Summary

Sucralfate normally appears not to affect the bioavailability of cimetidine or ranitidine, or only to reduce it moderately, and there is some evidence that the healing rate may possibly be increased.

Clinical evidence, mechanism, importance and management

Most *in vitro* and human studies show that sucralfate does not affect the absorption of either cimetidine or ranitidine,[1–5] but two studies found 22–30% reductions in ranitidine bioavailability.[6,8] There is no clear reason for avoiding concurrent use and there is some indication that it may possibly be valuable: sucralfate and cimetidine were not different in the rate at which they healed duodenal ulcers in eight patients and there was some evidence of a possible trend towards more rapid healing if given together.[7] More confirmatory study of this is needed.

References

1 Mullersman G, Gotz VP, Russell WL and Derendorf H. Lack of clinically significant *in vitro* and *in vivo* interactions between ranitidine and sucralfate. J Pharm Sci (1986) 75, 995–8.
2 Mullersman G, Gotz VP, Russell WL and Derendorf H. *In vitro* and *in vivo* interactions between ranitidine and sucralfate. Drug Intell Clin Pharm (1986) 20, 452.
3 Albin H, Vincon G, Lalague MC, Couzigou P, Amouretti M. Effect of sucralfate on the bioavailability of cimetidine. Eur J Clin Pharmacol (1986) 30, 493–4.
4 D'Angio R, Mayersohn M, Conrad KA, Bliss M. Cimetidine absorption in humans during sucralfate coadministration. Br J Clin Pharmac (1986) 21, 515–20.
5 Beck CL, Dietz AJ, Carlson JD, Letendre PW. Evaluation of potential cimetidine sucralfate interaction. Clin Pharmacol Ther (1987) 41, 168.
6 Maconochie JG, Thomas M, Michael MF, Jenner WR, Tannger WR. Ranitidine sucralfate interaction study. Clin Pharmacol Ther (1987) 41, 205.
7 Van Deventer G, Schneidman D, Olson C, Walsh J. Comparison of sucralfate and cimetidine taken alone and in combination for treatment of active duodenal ulcers. Gastroenterology (1984) 86, 1287.

8 Kimura K, Sakai H, Yoshida Y, Kasano T, Hirose M. Effects of concomitant drugs on the blood concentration of a histamine H2 antagonist (the second report) — concomitant or time lag administration of ranitidine and sucralfate. Jap J Gastroenterol (1986) 83, 603–7.

H$_2$-blockers + Tobacco smoking

Abstract/Summary

Duodenal ulcers treated with H$_2$-blockers heal less easily in smokers and are more likely to recur when treatment is over if smoking continues. Cimetidine, and to a lesser extent ranitidine, reduce the clearance of nicotine from the body.

Clinical evidence, mechanism, importance and management

The healing of duodenal ulcers in those on H$_2$-blockers such as cimetidine and ranitidine is slower than in non-smokers, and recurrence is more common.[1-3] One of the possible reasons appears to be that smoking reduces the serum levels of these drugs although peak levels occur sooner and are higher.[4]

It has also been found that 1200 mg cimetidine for 2 days reduced the clearance of nicotine (1 µg/kg/min IV for 30 min) in six normal subjects by 27–30%, while 600 mg ranitidine for two days reduced it by about 7–10%.[5]

Patients with ulcers should be encouraged to stop smoking, but if persuasion fails, the use of an H$_2$-blocker (cimetidine in particular) might possibly help them to reduce or give up smoking because it maintains nicotine levels with less tobacco.[5] There seems to be nothing documented about other H$_2$-blockers (famotidine, nizatidine, etc) and nicotine.

References

1 Korman MG, Hansky J, Eaves ER, Schmidt GT. Cigarette smoking and the healing of duodenal ulcer. Gastroenterology (1982) 82, 1104.
2 Korman MG, Hetzel DJ, Hansky J, Shearman DJC, Eaves ER, Schmidt GT, Hecker R, Fitch R. Oxmetidine or cimetidine in duodenal ulcer: healing rate and effect of smoking. Gastroenterology (1982) 82, 1104.
3 Boyd EJS, Wilson JA, Wormsley KG. Smoking inhibits therapeutic gastric inhibition. Lancet (1983) i, 95.
4 Boyd EJS, Johnston DA, Wormsley KG, Jenner WN, Salanson X. The effects of cigarette smoking on plasma concentrations of gastric antisecretory drugs. Aliment Pharmacol Ther (1987) 1, 57–65.
5 Bendayan R, Sullivan JT, Shaw C, Frecker RC, Sellers EM. Effect of cimetidine and ranitidine on the hepatic and renal elimination of nicotine in humans. Eur J Clin Pharmacol (1990) 38, 165–9.

Ipratropium bromide + Salbutamol (albuterol)

Abstract/Summary

Acute glaucoma developed rapidly in eight patients given nebulised ipratropium and salbutamol, and increased intra-ocular pressure has been reported in others. No interaction has been seen when the drugs were given by inhaler.

Clinical evidence, mechanism, importance and management

Five patients with acute chronic obstructive airways disease, given nebulised ipratropium and salbutamol (albuterol), developed acute angle closure glaucoma, four of them within 1–36 h of starting treatment.[1] Three other similar cases of acute glaucoma due to concurrent use are reported elsewhere.[3,4] An increase in intra-ocular pressure has also been previously reported in other patients given both drugs by nebuliser.[2]

Mechanism

The reason appears to be that the anticholinergic action of the ipratropium causes semi-dilatation of the pupil, partially blocking the flow of aqueous humour from the posterior to the anterior chamber, thereby bowing the iris anteriorly and obstructing the drainage angle. The salbutamol increases the production of aqueous humour and makes things worse. Additional factors are that higher doses of both drugs are achieved by using a nebuliser, and that some drug may escape round the edge of the mask and have a direct action on the eye.[1]

Importance and management

An established but uncommon interaction. The authors of the first report[1] advise care in the placing of the mask to avoid the escape of droplets (the use of goggles is also effective[2]) and if possible the avoidance of concurrent use by nebuliser in patients predisposed to glaucoma. They point out that no cases of glaucoma have been reported with either drug given by inhaler.[1]

References

1 Shah P, Dhurjon L, Metcalfe T, Gibson JM. Acute angle closure glaucoma associated with nebulised ipratropium bromide and salbutamol. Br Med J (1992) 304, 40–1.
2 Kalra L, Bone M. The effect of nebulised bronchodilator therapy on intraocular pressure in patients with glaucoma. Chest (1988) 93, 739–41.
3 Packe GE, Cayton TM, Mashoudi N. Nebulised ipratropium bromide and salbutamol causing closed-angle glaucoma. Lancet (1984) 2, 691.
4 Reuser T, Flanagan DW, Borland C, Bannerjee DK. Acute angle closure glaucoma occurring after nebulized bronchodilator treatment with ipratropium bromide and salbutamol. J Roy Soc Med (1992) 85, 499–500.

Iron preparations + Antacids

Abstract/Summary

The absorption of iron and the expected haematological response can be reduced by the concurrent use of antacids. Separate their administration as much as possible.

Clinical evidence

(a) Magnesium trisilicate

When oral iron failed to cause an expected rise in haemoglobin levels, a study was undertaken in nine patients who were given 5 g of isotopically labelled ferrous sulphate. 35 g magnesium trisilicate reduced the absorption from an average of 30 to 12%, the reduction being small in some patients but one individual showed a fall from 67 to 5%.[1]

(b) Aluminium and Magnesium Hydroxides, Sodium Bicarbonate and Calcium carbonate

A study in 22 healthy subjects who were mildly iron deficient (due to blood donation or menstruation) showed that one teaspoonful of *Mylanta II* had little effect on the absorption at 2 h of 10 or 20 mg ferrous sulphate, whereas 1 g sodium bicarbonate almost halved the absorption and 500 mg calcium carbonate reduced it by two-thirds. Iron absorption from a multivitamin-mineral preparation was little affected by calcium carbonate.[5] Another study found that an antacid containing aluminium and magnesium hydroxides and magnesium carbonate reduced the absorption of 15 mg ferrous sulphate and ferrous fumarate in healthy iron-replete subjects by 38 and 31% respectively.[6] Poor absorption of iron during treatment with sodium bicarbonate and aluminium hydroxide has been described elsewhere.[2,3]

Mechanism

Uncertain. One suggestion is that magnesium sulphate changes ferrous sulphate into less easily absorbed salts, or increases its polymerization.[1] Carbonates possibly cause the formation of poorly soluble iron complexes.[2] Aluminium hydroxide is believed to precipitate iron as the hydroxide and ferric ions can become intercalated into the aluminum hydroxide lattice.[4]

Importance and management

Information is limited and difficult to assess because of the many variables (different dosages, different subjects and patients), however a 'blanket precaution' to achieve maximal absorption would be to separate the administration of iron preparations and antacids as much as possible to avoid admixture in the gut. This may prove not to be necessary with some preparations.

References

1 Hall GJL and Davis AE. Inhibition of iron absorption by magnesium trisilicate. Med J Aust (1969) 2, 95.
2 Benjamin IB, Cortell S, Conrad ME. Bicarbonate-induced iron complexes and iron absorption. Gastroenterology (1967) 35, 389.
3 Rastogi SP, Padilla F, Boyd CM. Effect of aluminium hydroxide on iron absorption. Am Soc Neph (1975) 8, 21.
4 Coste JF, De Bari VA, Keil LB and Needle MA. *In vitro* interactions of oral haematinics and antacid preparations. Curr Ther Res (1977) 22, 205.

5 O'Neil-Cutting MA, Crosby WH. The effect of antacids on the absorption of simultaneously ingested iron. J Am Med Ass (1986) 255, 1468–70.
6 Ekenved G, Halvorsen L and Solvell L. Influence of a liquid antacid on the absorption of different iron salts. Scand J Haematol (1976) Suppl 28, 65–77.

Iron preparations or Vitamin B$_{12}$ + Chloramphenicol

Abstract/Summary

In addition to the serious and potentially fatal bone marrow depression which can occur with chloramphenicol, it may also cause a milder, reversible depression which can oppose the treatment of anaemia with iron or vitamin B$_{12}$.

Clinical evidence

Ten out of 20 patients on iron-dextran for iron-deficiency anaemia also given chloramphenicol failed to show the expected haematological response, and all four patients on vitamin B$_{12}$ for pernicious anaemia were similarly refractory until the chloramphenicol was withdrawn.[4]

Mechanism

Chloramphenicol can cause two forms of bone marrow depression. One is serious and irreversible and can result in fatal aplastic anaemia, whereas the other is probably unrelated, milder and reversible, and appears to occur at serum levels of 25 µg/ml or more. The reason is that chloramphenicol can inhibit protein synthesis, the first sign of which is a fall in the reticulocyte count which reflects inadequate red cell maturation. This response has been seen in animals,[1] normal individuals,[2] normal individuals receiving vitamin B$_{12}$ and folic acid,[3] and in anaemic patients being treated with iron-dextran or vitamin B$_{12}$.[4]

Importance and management

An established interaction of clinical importance. The authors of one study recommend that dosages of 25–30 mg/kg are usually adequate for treating infections without running the risk of elevating serum chloramphenicol levels to 25 µg/ml or more when marrow depression occurs.[5] Monitor the effects of using iron or B$_{12}$ concurrently. A preferable alternative would be to use a safer antibiotic. It has been claimed that the optic neuritis which sometimes occurs with chloramphenicol can be reversed with large doses of vitamins B$_6$ and B$_{12}$.[6]

References

1 Rigdon RH, Crass G, Martin A. Anemia produced by chloramphenicol (chloromycetin) in the duck. AMA Arch Pathol (1954) 58, 85.
2 McCurdy PR. Chloramphenicol bone marrow toxicity. J Amer Med Ass (1961) 176, 588.
3 Jiji RM, Gangarosa EJ and de la Marcorra F. Chloramphenicol and its

sulfamoyl analogue. Report of reversible erythropoietic toxicity in healthy volunteers. Arch InternMed (1963) 111, 70.

4 Saidi P, Wallerstein RO, Aggeler PM. Effect of chloramphenicol on erythropoiesis. J Lab Clin Med (1961) 57, 247.

5 Scott JL, Finegold SM, Belkin GA, Lawrence IS. Chloramphenicol and bone marrow depression. N Engl J Med (1965) 272, 1137.

6 Cocke JC. Chloramphenicol optic neuritis. Amer J Dis Child (1967) 114, 424.

Iron preparations + Cholestyramine

Abstract/Summary

Cholestyramine binds with ferrous sulphate in the gut, thereby reducing its absorption, but the clinical importance of this is uncertain.

Clinical evidence, mechanism, importance and management

A single case report briefly describes the development of iron-deficiency anaemia in a patient with erythropoietic proto-porphyria treated with cholestyramine.[1] Subsequent studies showed that cholestyramine binds with iron (as it does with many other drugs), and in rats this was found to halve the absorption from the gut of a single $100\,g$ dose of ferrous sulphate.[2] But nobody seems to have checked on the general clinical importance of this in patients. Until more is known it would seem prudent to separate the dosages of the iron and cholestyramine to avoid mixing in the gut, thereby minimizing the effects of this possible interaction.

References

1 Kuffin JC, Noyes WD, Porter S. Iron and cholestyramine in erythropoietic protoporphyria. Clin Res (1970) 18, 38.

2 Thomas FB, McCullough F, Greenberger NJ. Inhibition of the intestinal absorption of inorganic and hemoglobin iron by cholestyramine. J Lab Clin Med (1971) 78, 70–80.

Iron preparations + Cimetidine

Abstract/Summary

Cimetidine is alleged to have reduced the response to ferrous sulphate in three patients, but this reaction remains unconfirmed. The serum levels of cimetidine can be modestly reduced.

Clinical evidence, mechanism, importance and management

A brief report describes three patients taking 1 g cimetidine and 600 mg ferrous sulphate daily whose ulcers healed after 2 months but their anaemia and altered iron metabolism persisted. When the cimetidine was reduced to 400 mg daily but with the same dose of iron, the blood picture resolved satisfac-

torily within a month.[1] The author of the report attributed this response to the cimetidine-induced rise in gastric pH which reduced the absorption of the iron, however this suggested mechanism was subsequently disputed.[2] This interaction has never been confirmed. A later study in six normal subjects found that 300 mg cimetidine had no significant effect on the AUC of 300 mg ferrous sulphate although the peak serum cimetidine levels were reduced by 16%.[3] It seems very doubtful if this interaction is clinically relevant.

References

1 Esposito R. Cimetidine and iron-deficiency anaemia. Lancet (1977) 2, 1132.

2 Rosner F. Cimetidine and iron absorption. Lancet (1978) 1, 95.

3 Partlow ES, Chan SC, Pap KM, Campbell NRC. The effect of ferrous sulfate on cimetidine serum levels in healthy volunteers. Clin Pharmacol Ther (1993) 53, 163.

Iron preparations + Coffee or Tea

Abstract/Summary

Coffee may possibly contribute towards the development of iron-deficiency anaemia in pregnant women and reduce the levels of iron in breast milk. As a result their babies may also be iron-deficient. Tea may also possibly be associated with microcytic anaemia in children.

Clinical evidence

A controlled study among pregnant low-income women in Costa Rica found that coffee consumption was associated with reductions in the haemoglobin levels and haematocrits of the mothers during pregnancy, and of their babies shortly after birth, despite the fact that the women were taking 200 mg ferric sulphate and 0.5 mg folate daily.[1] The babies also had a slightly lower birth weight (96%). Almost a quarter of the mothers were considered as having iron-deficiency anaemia (haemoglobin levels of <110 g/l) compared with none among the control group of non-coffee drinkers. Levels of iron in breast milk were reduced about one third. The coffee drinkers drank more than 450 ml of coffee daily, equivalent to more than 10 g ground coffee.

A much higher incidence of microcytic anaemia has been described in tea-drinking infants in Israel.[2] Another report describes no change in the absorption of iron in daily doses of 2–15.8 mg/kg in 10 iron-deficient children.[3]

Mechanism

The reasons for the reduced iron levels are not understood. The inference to be drawn is that both coffee and tea interfere with the way the body handles iron.

Importance and management

The general importance of these findings is uncertain, but it highlights the need to keep a check on the haemoglobin levels and red cell counts of pregnant and lactating women who drink substantial amounts of coffee, and of their babies while being breast fed, even though iron supplements may be given. A similar check is needed in children who drink substantial amounts of tea. More study is needed.

References

1 Muñoz L M, Lönnerdal B, Keen C L, Dewey K G. Coffee consumption as a factor in iron deficiency anemia among pregnant women and their infants in Costa Rica. Am J Clin Nutr (1988) 48, 645–51.
2 Merhav H, Amitai Y, Palti H, Godfrey S. Tea drinking and microcytic anemia in infants. Am J Clin Nutr (1985) 41, 1210–3.
3 Koren G, Bolchis H, Keren G. Effects of tea on the absorption of pharmacological doses of an oral iron preparation. Isr J Med Sci (1982) 18, 547.

Isotretinoin + Alcohol

Abstract/Summary

A single case report describes a marked reduction in the effects of isotretinoin following the acute intake of alcohol.

Clinical evidence, mechanism, importance and management

A former alcoholic, who normally no longer drank, was treated for acne conglobata with some success for 3 months with 60 mg isotretinoin daily. When for a fortnight he briefly started to drink again as part of his job (he was a sherry taster) his skin lesions reappeared and the isotretinoin side-effects (mucocutaneous dryness) vanished. When he stopped drinking his skin lesions became controlled again and the drug side-effects re-emerged. The following year while on another course of isotretinoin the same thing happened when he started and stopped drinking. The reasons are not known but one suggestion is that the alcohol briefly induced the liver microsomal enzymes responsible for the metabolism of isotretinoin, thereby reducing both its therapeutic and side-effects.[1] The general importance of this apparent interaction is not known.

Reference

1 Soria C, Allegue F, Galiana J, Ledo A. Decreased isotretinoin efficacy during alcohol intake. Dermatologica (1991) 182, 203–5.

Lansoprazole + miscellaneous drugs

Abstract/Summary

Lansoprazole appears not to interact with diazepam, theophylline or warfarin, and seems unlikely to interact with other drugs normally affected by enzyme inducers and inhibitors. Both food and an antacid can reduce the bioavailability of lansoprazole.

Clinical evidence, mechanism, importance and management

A double-blind study in 14 subjects found that 60 mg lansoprazole daily for 9 days caused only a very slight reduction in their steady-state theophylline serum levels.[1] In another study on 24 subjects 60 mg lansoprazole daily for 9 days had no effect on the pharmacokinetics of either S- or R-warfarin, and no significant changes were seen in their prothrombin times.[2] 60 mg lansoprazole daily for 10 days was found to have no effect on the pharmacokinetics of a single 0.1 mg/kg dose of diazepam.[4] 60 mg lansoprazole daily for 11 days also had minimal effects on the pharmacokinetics of antipyrine (phenazole) and indocyanin green.[3] These last two compounds are used as markers of changes in drug metabolism and in liver blood flow. Another study found that 30 ml *Maalox* reduced the AUC of 30 mg lansoprazole by 13% and reduced the maximum serum level by 27%, but no changes were seen when the lansoprazole was given 1 h after the antacid.[5] Food reduced the bioavailability by 27%.[5]

These findings suggest that no special precautions will be needed if lansoprazole is given to patients taking diazepam, theophylline or warfarin, and that lansoprazole is unlikely to have a clinically significant effect on other drugs which are susceptible to the actions of enzyme inducers or inhibitors. Studies in patients are needed to confirm these findings. It is recommended that lansoprazole should not be given with food nor at the same time as antacids.[5]

References

1 Granneman G, Winters EP, Locke CS, Leese PT, Karol MD, Cavanaugh JH. Lack of effect of concomitant lansoprazole on steady-state theophylline pharmacokinetics. Gastroenterology (1991) 100, A75.
2 Cavanaugh JH, Winters EP, Cohen A, Locke CS, Braeckman R. Lack of effect of lansoprazole on steady state warfarin metabolism. Gastroenterology (1991) 100, A40.
3 Cavanaugh JH, Park YK, Awni WM, Mukherjee DX, Karol MD, Granneman GR. Effect of lansoprazole on antipyrine and ICG pharmacokinetics. Gastroenterology (1991) 100, A40.
4 Lefebrve RA, Flouvat B, Karolac-Tamisier S, Moerman E, Van Ganse E. Influence of lansoprazole treatment on diazepam plasma concentrations. Clin Pharmacol Ther (1992) 52, 458–63.
5 Delhotal-Landes B, Cournot A, Vermerie N, Dellatolas F, Benoit M, Flouvat B. The effect of food and antacids on lansoprazole absorption and disposition. Eur J Drug Metab Pharmacokinet (1991), 3 Spec No 3, 315–20.

Laxatives + miscellaneous drugs

Abstract/Summary

Sodium sulphate and castor oil used as laxatives can cause a modest but probably clinically unimportant reduction in drug absorption.

Clinical evidence, mechanism, importance and management

An experimental study of the possible effects of laxatives on drug absorption in normal subjects found that 10–20 mg oral doses of sodium sulphate reduced the absorption of sulphafurazole and aspirin by 15 and 7% respectively (as measured by drug excreted in the urine over 24 hr). The four hour excretion of isoniazid in the urine was reduced by 41%. Parallel studies using two 10 ml doses of castor oil found some changes (mostly small reductions), but the overall picture was that while these laxatives can alter the pattern of absorption, they do not seriously impair the total amount of drug absorbed.[1] More study is needed in a clinical situation.

Reference

1 Mattila MJ, Takki S, Jussila J. Effect of sodium sulphate and castor oil on drug absorption from the human intestine. Ann Clin Res (1974) 6, 19–24.

Liquorice + miscellaneous drugs

Abstract/Summary

Very large amounts of liquorice can cause pseudoaldosteronism which may adversely affect the treatment of cardiac failure and hypertension, and the control of body potassium levels.

Clinical evidence, mechanism, importance and management

The serum potassium levels of 11 out of 14 normal subjects fell by over 0.3 mmol/l after eating 100–200 g liquorice daily for 4 weeks. Four withdrew from the study because of hypokalaemia. Mild or uncomfortable oedema of the face, hands and ankles occurred in six and some of them gained weight.[1] Four patients developed pseudohyperaldosteronism after taking large amounts of liquorice laxatives in doses of 0.5 to 8 g daily for periods of 3 months to 3 years.[3] A previously healthy patient developed fulminant congestive heart failure after eating large amounts of liquorice for a week.[2] The reason is that liquorice contains glycyrrhizic acid which has potent mineralocorticoid properties. The conclusion to be drawn is that patients under treatment for hypertension or cardiac failure, or taking drugs which lower body potassium levels, should avoid large amounts of liquorice.

References

1 Epstein MT, Espiner EA, Donald RA, Hughes H. Effects of eating liquorice on the renin-antiotensin-aldosterone axis in normal subjects. Br Med J (1977) 1, 488.
2 Chamberlain TJ. Licorice poisoning, pseudoaldosteronism, and heart failure. J Amer Med Ass (1970) 213, 1343.
3 Scali M, Pratesi C, Zennaro MC, Zampollo V, Armanini D. Pseudohyper-

aldosteronism from liquorice-containing laxatives. J Endocrinol Invest (1990) 13, 847–8.

Loperamide + Cholestyramine

Abstract/Summary

An isolated report, supported by an *in vitro* study, indicates that the effects of loperamide can be reduced by cholestyramine.

Clinical evidence, mehcanism, importance and management

A man who had had extensive surgery of the gut with the creation of an ileostomy, needed treatment for excessive fluid loss. His fluid loss was observed to be 'substantially less' (not precisely quantified) when given loperamide alone (2 mg 6-hourly) than when given in combination with cholestyramine (2 g every 4 h).[1] The probable reason is that the cholestyramine binds to the loperamide in the gut, thereby reducing its activity. An *in vitro* study using 50 ml simulated gastric fluid showed that 64% of a 5.5 mg dose of loperamide was bound by 4 g of cholestyramine.[1] Direct information is limited to this report but what occurred is consistent with the way cholestyramine interacts with other drugs. It has been suggested that the two drugs should be separated as much as possible to prevent mixing in the gut, or the loperamide dosage should be increased.[1]

Reference

1 Ti TY, Giles HG, Sellers EM. Probable interaction of loperamide and cholestyramine. Can Med Ass J (1978) 119, 607.

Lovastatin + Antihypertensives

Abstract/Summary

Lovastatin normally appears not to interact adversely with ACE-inhibitors, beta-blockers, calcium channel blockers, potassium sparing or thiazide diuretics. An isolated report describes severe hyperkalaemia in a diabetic when given lisinopril and lovastatin.

Clinical evidence, mechanism, importance and management

An extensive study of 8245 patients with moderate hypercholesterolaemia found that the effects of lovastatin (20–80 mg daily for 4 years) were not altered in any group taking calcium antagonists, selective or non-selective beta-blockers, potassium-sparing diuretics or thiazides, and only slightly increased by calcium antagonists and possibly ACE-inhibitors.[3] None of the drugs was individually named. A study in normal subjects given lovastatin found that 40 mg propranolol twice daily reduced the AUC of total inhibitors by 18%, of active inhibitors by 12% and of lovastatin acid by 13%.[4] These changes are small and the results of this study would seem to confirm the previous findings[3] with beta-blockers. No special precautions would seem to be necessary if any of these drugs is given concurrently.

An isolated report describes a Type I diabetic (on insulin) with hypertension and hyperlipidaemia who developed myositis and severe hyperkalaemia when treated with lovastatin and lisinopril. The reason seemed to be a combination of the hyperkalaemic effects of the lisinopril, the release of intracellular potassium into the blood associated with the myositis caused by the lovastatin, and a proneness to hyperkalaemia due to the diabetes.[1,2] This is an unusual case and unlikely to be of general importance.

References

1 Edelman S, Witztum JL. Hyperkalaemia during treatment with HMG-CoA reductase inhibitor. N Engl J Med (1990) 320, 1219–20.
2 Grundy SM. Reply to ref 1.
3 Pool JL, Chear CL, Downton M, Schnaper H, Stinnett S, Dujovne C, Bradford RH, Chremos AN. Lovastatin and coadministered antihypertensive/cardiovascular agents. Hypertension (1992) 19, 242–8.
4 Pan HY, Triscari J, DeVault AR, Smith SA, Wang-Iverson D, Swanson BN, Willard DA. Pharmacokinetic interaction between propranolol and the HMG-CoA reductase inhibitors pravastatin and lovastatin. Br J Clin Pharmac (1991) 31, 665–70.

Lovastatin + Cyclosporin

Abstract/Summary

Although lovastatin has been successfully used to treat transplant patients on cyclosporin, the risk of muscle damage and possibly severe rhabdomyolysis with renal failure is considerably increased if the dose exceeds 20 mg daily..

Clinical evidence

Four out of a total of six heart transplant patients with marked hypercholesterolaemia and on cyclosporin developed severe rhabdomyolysis within 6 weeks to 16 months of starting lovastatin (20–40 mg twice daily). Two of them were also taking gemfibrozil. Mild to moderate myalgias were previously present for 4–21 days. One patient developed acute renal failure.[1]

Lovastatin (20 mg daily) was withdrawn from seven out of 12 heart transplant patients on cyclosporin because of side-effects. Four complained of myalgia and muscle weakness and three without symptoms had an increase in serum CPK.[3] Two other heart transplant patients on cyclosporin developed acute renal failure and rhabdomyolysis when given lovastatin. Myolosis and acute renal failure occurred in another patient on cyclosporin and lovastatin (20 mg twice daily).[5] Four out of five heart transplant patients on cyclosporin and 40–80 mg lovastatin daily developed rhabdomyolysis, and two of the four had acute renal failure. No rhabdomyolysis was seen in other patients using 20 mg or less lovastatin daily[6] Only one out of another 44

heart transplant patients on cyclosporin given 20 mg lovastatin daily had side-effects. He developed rhabdomyolysis and reversible acute renal failure when the dosage was raised to 40 mg daily.[4]

Mechanism

Not understood.

Importance and management

An established interaction of clinical importance. Myopathy with lovastatin alone was estimated in 1988 as being rare (0.2%) but as high as 30% in those taking lovastatin and immunosuppressants.[2] It has been recommended that concurrent use should be undertaken with caution and close monitoring, avoiding doses exceeding 20 mg lovastatin daily.[2,6] All patients should be advised to report promptly any unexplained muscle aches, tenderness or weakness, particularly if accompanied by malaise or fever.[2] The patient's serum creatinine kinase levels should be measured and the lovastatin stopped if necessary to avoid the risk of renal failure.[1,2] Pravastatin appears to be a safer alternative (see 'Pravastatin + Cyclosporin').

References

1 East C, Alivizatos PA, Grundy SM, Jones PH, Farmer JA, Rhabdomyolysis in patients receiving lovastatin after cardiac transplantation. N Engl J Med (1988) 318, 47–8.
2 Tobert JA. Rhabdomyolysis in patients receiving lovastatin after cardiac transplantation. N Engl J Med (1988) 318, 48–9.
3 Heroux AL, Thompson JA, Katz S, Hastillo AK, Katz M, Quigg RJ, Hess ML. Elimination of the lovastatin-cyclosporin interaction in heart transplant patients. Circulation (1989) 90, II-641.
4 Kobashigawa JA, Murphy F, Stevenson LW, Moriguchi JD, Katawa N, Chuck C, Wilmarth J, Leonard L, Drinkwater D, Laks H. Low dose of lovastatin safely lowers cholesterol after cardiac transplantation. Circulation (1989) 80, II-641.
5 Corpier CL, Jones PH, Suki WN, Lederer ED, Quinones MA, Schmidt SW, Young JB. Rhabdomyolysis and renal injury with lovastatin use. Report of two cases in cardiac transplant recipients. J Amer Med Ass (1988) 260, 239–41.
6 Ballantyne CM, Radovancevic B, Farmer JA, Frazier OH, Chandler L, Payton-Ross C, Cocanougher B, Jones PH, Young JB, Gotto AM. Hyperlipidaemia after heart transplantation: report of a 6-year experience, with treatment recommendations. J Amer Coll Cardiol (1992) 19, 1315–21.

Lovastatin + Fibre or Pectin

Abstract/Summary

Pectin and oat bran can reduce the blood cholesterol-lowering effects of lovastatin.

Clinical evidence, mechanism, importance and management

The serum low-density lipoprotein cholesterol levels of three patients on 80 mg lovastatin daily showed a marked rise when additionally given 15 g pectin daily (mean rise from 4.48 to 6.36 mmol/l). One had a 59% rise. Two other patients on lovastatin showed a rise when additionally given 50–100 g oat bran daily (from 5.02 to 6.54 mmol/l). One had a 41% rise. When the pectin and oat bran were stopped, the serum levels of the low-density lipoprotein cholesterol fell. It is presumed that both pectin and oat bran reduce the absorption of lovastatin from the gut.[1] Evidence is still very limited but patients should be advised not to take either of these two fibres at the same time as lovastatin. Separate their ingestion as much as possible.

Reference

1 Richter WO, Jacob BG, Schwandt P. Interaction between fibre and lovastatin. Lancet (1991) 338, 706.

Lovastatin + Gemfibrozil

Abstract/Summary

The risk of myopathy and/or rhabdomyolysis appears to be increased in patients given both lovastatin and gemfibrozil. Concurrent use is possible and effective provided stringent precautions are followed.

Clinical evidence

The FDA has documented 12 case reports of severe myopathy or rhabdomyolysis associated with the the concurrent use of lovastatin and gemfibrozil. The mean serum creatine kinase levels of the patients reached 15250 U/l. This is 20 times greater than the levels seen with gemfibrozil alone and 30 times greater than with lovastatin alone. Four of those tested showed myoglobinuria and five had acute renal failure.[1] Six other cases of rhabdomyolysis associated with the concurrent use of these drugs, three with renal failure, have been described.[2,3,5,8,10,12] Other cases have been seen in patients taking lovastatin and gemfibrozil with cyclosporin.[9,11]

These adverse reports contrast with others[3,4,7,13,14] describing apparently safe and effective concurrent use in large numbers of patients under very well controlled conditions, with myopathy (without rhabdomyolysis) ranging from 3–8%.

Mechanism

Not understood. Myopathy can occur with either drug alone and their effects may therefore be additive.

Importance and management

An established interaction of unknown incidence. The advice arising from the FDA study is that concurrent use should be avoided if possible, and no concomitant use in patients with compromised kidney or liver function.[1]

Other advice is that concurrent use is safe and effective provided precautionary measures are taken, namely monitor-ing every 6–8 weeks, palpation of skeletal muscles, measurements of creatinine phosphatase and liver function. Patients should be told to report any muscle pain, tenderness or weakness immediately, and to stop taking both drugs.[6]

References

1 Pierce LR, Wysowski DK, Gross TP. Myopathy and rhabdomyolysis associated with lovastatin-gemfibrozil combination therapy. J Amer Med Ass (1990) 264, 71–75.
2 Goldman JA, Fisherman AB, Lee JE, Johnson RJ. The role of cholesterol lowering agents in drug-induced rhabdomyolysis and polymyositis. Arthritis Rheum (1989) 32, 358–9.
3 Tobert JA. Reply letter. N Engl J Med (1988) 318, 48.
4 Illingworth DR, Bacon S. Influence of lovastatin plus gemfibrozil on plasma lipids and lipoproteins in patients with heterzygous familial hypercholesterolaemia. Circulation (1989) 79, 590–6.
5 Marais GE, Larson KK. Rhabdomyolysis and acute renal failure induced by combination lovastatin and gemfibrozil therapy. Ann Intern Med (1990) 112, 228–30.
6 Bilheimer DW. Long term clinical tolerance of lovastatin (Mevinolin) and simvastatin (Epistatin). An overview. Drug Invest (1990) 2 (suppl 2) 58–67.
7 Glueck CJ, Oakes N, Speirs J, Tracy T, Lang J. Gemfibrozil-lovastatin therapy for primary hyperlipoproteinemias. Am J Cardiol (1992) 70, 1–9.
8 Manoukian AA, Bhagavan NV, Hayashi T, Nestor TA, Rios C, Scottlini AG. Rhabdomyolysis secondary to lovastatin therapy. Clin Chem (1990) 36, 2145–7.
9 Norman DJ, Illingworth DR, Munson J, Hosenpud J.. Myolysis and acute renal failure in a heart transplant patient receiving lovastatin. N Engl J Med (1988) 318, 46–7.
10 Kogan AD, Orenstein S. Lovastatin-induced acute rhabdomyolysis. Postgrad Med J (1990) 66, 294–6.
11 East C, Alivizatos PA, Grundy SM, Jones PH, Farmer JA.. Rhabdomyolysis in patients receiving lovastatin after cardiac transplantation. N Engl J Med (1988) 318, 47–8.
12 Goldman JA, Fisherman AB, Lee JE, Johnson RJ. The role of cholesterol-lowering agents in drug-induced rhabdomyolysis and polymyositis. Arth Rheum (1989) 32, 358–9.
13 East C , Bilheimer DW, Grundy SM. Combination drug therapy for familial combined hyperlipidaemia. Ann Intern Med (1988) 109, 25–32
14 Wirebaught SR, Shapiro ML, McIntyre TH, Whitney EJ. A retrospective review of the use of lipid lowering agents in combination, specifically gemfibrozil and lovastatin. Pharmacotherapy (1992) 12, 445.

Lovastatin + miscellaneous drugs

Abstract/Summary

Isolated cases of rhabdomyolysis have been seen in patients on lovastatin when treated with cyclosporin, erythromycin or nicotinic acid.

Clinical evidence, mechanism, importance and management

A man on lovastatin (20 mg three times daily), diltiazem, allopurinol and aspirin developed progressive weakness and diffuse myalgias after being treated with erythromycin for 13 days (500 mg 6-hourly). When admitted to hospital his creatine kinase level was high (35200 U/l) and his urine was reddish-brown. The rhabdomyolysis was treated by stopping the lovastatin, and vigorous IV hydration and frusemide.[1] Rhabdomyolysis also developed in another patient on lovastatin which appeared to be related to the addition of nicotinic acid (2.5 g daily),[2] and in yet another also taking cyclosporin[3] (see also 'Lovastatin + Cyclosporin'). Myositis in a further patient on lovastatin and nicotinic acid is also briefly reported.[4] However no adverse effects of this kind occurred in 22 other patients concurrently treated with lovastatin, nicotinic acid and colestipol.[6]

Myopathy with lovastatin is very low (0.1%) in the absence of these other drugs.[5] Concurrent use should clearly be very well monitored and patients should be warned to report promptly any unexplained muscle aches, tenderness, cramps, stiffness or weakness.

References

1 Ayanian JZ, Fuchs CS, Stone RM. Lovastatin and rhabdomyolysis. Ann Intern Med (1988) 109, 682.
2 Reaven P, Witztum JL. Lovastatin, nicotinic acid and rhabdomyolysis. Ann Intern Med (1988) 109, 597–8.
3 Norman DJ, Illingworth DR, Munson J, Hosenpud J. Myolosis and acute renal failure in a heart-transplant recipient receiving lovastatin. N Engl J Med (1988) 318, 46–7.
4 Frost P. Personnal communication quoted in ref 2.
5 Bilheimer DW. Long term clinical tolerance of lovastatin (Mevinolin) and Simvastatin (Epistatin). An overview. Drug Invest (1990) 2 (Suppl 2) 58–67.
6 Malloy MJ, Kane JP, Kunitake ST, Tun P. Complementarity of colestipol, niacin and lovastatin in treatment of severe familial hypercholestrolemia. Ann Intern Med (1987) 107, 616–23.

Methoxsalen + Phenytoin

Abstract/Summary

The serum levels of methoxsalen (8-methoxypsoralen) can be markedly reduced by the concurrent use of phenytoin.

Clinical evidence

A patient with epilepsy failed to respond to treatment for psoriasis with PUVA (12 treatments of 30 mg 8-methoxypsoralen given orally and ultraviolet A irradiation) while taking 250 mg phenytoin daily. Methoxsalen serum levels were normal in the absence of phenytoin but abnormally low while taking phenytoin,[1] due, it is suggested, to the enzyme inducing effects of the phenytoin. This interaction could lead to serious erythema and blistering because the stimulant effects of the methoxsalen on the melanin pigmentation of the skin is reduced. Concurrent use should be avoided or very closely monitored.

Reference

1 Staberg B, Hueg B. Interaction between 8-methoxypsoralen and phenytoin. Consequence for PUVA therapy. Acta Derm Venereol (1985) 65, 552–3.

Metyrapone + Cyproheptadine

Abstract/Summary

Cyproheptadine may falsify the results of the metyrapone hypothalamic-hypophyseal function test.

Clinical evidence, mechanism, importance and management

Pretreatment with 4 mg cyproheptadine six-hourly before undergoing a standard metyrapone test (750 mg 4-hourly for six doses) reduced the metyrapone-induced urinary 17-hydroxycorticosteroid response in nine normal subjects by 32% and also reduced the serum 11-deoxycortisol response.[1] The results of metyrapone tests will therefore be unreliable in patients taking cyproheptadine.

Reference

1 Plonk J, Feldman JM, Keagle D. Modification of adrenal function by the anti-serotonin agent cyproheptadine. J Clin Endocrinol Metab (1976) 42, 291–5.

Metyrapone + Phenytoin

Abstract/Summary

The results of the metyrapone hypothalamic-hypophyseal function test are unreliable in patients taking phenytoin. Doubling the dose of metyrapone gives results which are close to normal.

Clinical evidence, mechanism, importance and management

A study in five normal subjects and three patients taking 300 mg phenytoin showed that their serum metyrapone levels 4 h after taking a regular 750 mg dose were very low indeed compared with a control group (6.5 compared with 48 g/100 ml). Their response to metyrapone was proportionately lower.[1] Other reports confirm that the urinary steroid response is subnormal in patients taking phenytoin.[3,4] The reason is that phenytoin is a potent liver enzyme inducing agent which increases the metabolism of the metyrapone, thereby reducing its biological activity,[1,2] as a result of which the results of the metyrapone test for hypothalamic-hypophyseal function are invalid. Doubling the dose of metyrapone from 750 mg 4-hourly to 2-hourly has been shown to give results similar to those in subjects not taking phenytoin.[1]

References

1 Meikle AW, Jubiz W, Matsukura S, West CD, Tyler FH. Effect of diphenylhydantoin on the metabolism of metyrapone and release of ACTH in man. J Clin Endocrinol Metab(1969) 29, 1553.

2 Jubiz W, Levinson RA, Meikle AW, West CD, Tyler FH. Absorption and conjugation of metyrapone during diphenylhydantoin therapy: mechanism of the abnormal response to oral metyrapone. Endocrinology (1970) 86, 328.

3 Krieger DT. Effect of diphenylhydantoin on pituitary-adrenal interrelations. J Clin Endocrinol (1962) 22, 490.

4 Werk EE, Thrasher K, Choi Y, Sholiton LJ. Failure of metyrapone to inhibit 11-hydroxylation of 11-deoxycortisol during drug therapy. J Clin Endocrinol (1967) 27, 1358.

Mifepristone + Sulprostone

Abstract/Summary, clinical evidence, mechanism, importance and management

An isolated report describes reversible ventricular fibrillation and cardiac arrest in a woman of 35 after being given mifepristone and sulprostone to induce an abortion. Coronary spasm may have occurred. [1]

Reference

1 Delay M, Genestal M, Carrie D, Livarek B, Boudjemaa B, Bernadet P. Arrêt cardiocirculatoire après administration de l'association mifépristone (Mifégyne) sulprostone (Nalador) pour interruption de grossesse. Arch Mal Coeur Vaiss (1992) 85, 105–7.

Nicotinic acid (niacin) + Alcohol

Abstract/Summary, clinical evidence, mechanism, importance and management

An isolated report describes delerium and lactic acidosis in a patient taking nicotinic acid for hypercholesterolaemia after ingesting about 1 litre of wine. It is suggested that the niconitic acid may have caused liver dysfunction which was exacerbated by the large amount of alcohol. [1] No general conclusions can be drawn from this single case.

Reference

1 Schwab RA, Bachhuber BH. Delerium and lactic acidosis caused by ethanol and niacin ingestion. Am J Emerg (1991) 9, 363–5.

Nicotinic acid (niacin) + Salicylates

Abstract/Summary

Aspirin can reduce the flushing reaction which often occurs with nicotinic acid, but it can also increase the nicotinic acid serum levels. The importance of this latter reaction is uncertain.

Clinical evidence, mechanism, importance and management

Six normal subjects were infused with nicotinic acid (0.075– 0.1 mg/kg/min) for 6 hours. When additionally given 1 g aspirin orally two hours after the infusion was started, the serum nicotinic acid levels rose markedly because its clearance was decreased by 45%. [1] The probable reason is that the salicylate competes with the nicotinic acid for its metabolism by the liver (glycine conjugation) so that it clearance is reduced, resulting in a rise in its levels. The clinical importance of this is not known. However if aspirin is given to reduce the annoying nicotinic acid flushing reaction, [2] check that the effects of the latter do become excessive.

References

1 Ding RW, Kolbe K, Merz B, de Vries J, Weber E, Benet LZ. Pharmacokinetics of nicotinic acid-salicylic acid interaction. Clin Pharmacol Ther (1989) 46, 642–7.

2 Kane JP, Malloy MJ, Tun P et al. Normalization of low-density lipoprotein levels in heterozygous familiar hypercholesterolemia with a combined drug regimen. N Engl J Med (1981) 304, 251–8.

Olestra + miscellaneous drugs

Abstract/Summary

Olestra appears not to affect the absorption of drugs taken orally.

Clinical evidence, mechanism, importance and management

While taking 18 g olestra daily for 28 days, the pharmacokinetics of the ethinyloestradiol and norgestrel components of a combined oral contraceptive (*Lo/Ovral-28*) in 28 women were unchanged. Serum progesterone levels also remained unaltered. [1] This confirms the findings of earlier single dose studies which found that olestra had no effect on the bioavailability of single doses of ethinyloestradiol, norethindrone, diazepam or propranolol. [2] Olestra, formerly called sucrose polyester, is a non-absorbable, noncaloric fat replacement. It is concluded that olestra is unlikely to reduce the absorption of oral drugs in general. [1]

References

1 Miller KW, Willkiams DS, Carter SB, Jones MB, Mishell DR. The effect of olestra on systemic levels of oral contraceptives. Clin Pharmacol Ther (1990) 48, 34–40.

2 Roberts RJ, Leff RD. Influence of absorbable and non-absorbable lipids and lipidlike substances on drug availability. Clin Pharmacol Ther (1989) 45, 299–304.

Omeprazole + Disulfiram

Abstract/Summary

An isolated report describes confusion and catatonia in a patient when treated with disulfiram and omeprazole.

Clinical evidence, mechanism, importance and management

A patient on 40 mg omeprazole daily for 7 months was additionally given 500 mg disulfiram daily. Six days later he gradually developed confusion, which progressed into a catatonic state with muscle rigidity and trismus after 15 days. Both drugs were withdrawn and he gradually recovered. Some months later while taking 250 mg disulfiram daily, he again developed confusion, disorientation and nightmares within 72 h of starting to take 40 mg omeprazole each morning. He recovered when both drugs were stopped.[1] The reason for this reaction is not understood, but the authors of the report postulate that the omeprazole may have allowed the accumulation of one of the metabolites of disulfiram, carbon disulphide, which could have been responsible for the toxic effects.[1]

This is the first report of a possible interaction between omeprazole and disulfiram. Other patients given both drugs are said not have shown adverse effects.[2] The general importance of the report cited is therefore uncertain, but it would now seem prudent to monitor concurrent use in any patient for any evidence of these toxic effects.

References

1 Hajela R, Cunningham GM, Kapur BM, Peachey JE, Devenyi P. Catatonic reaction to omeprazole and disulfiram in a patient with alcohol dependence. Can Med Assoc J (1990) 143, 1207–8.
2 Campbell LM (Astra Pharmaceuticals). Personal communication 1991.

Omeprazole + miscellaneous drugs

Abstract/Summary

Omprazole appears not interact to a clinically important extent with alcohol, amoxycillin, bacampicillin, caffeine, food, lignocaine (lidocaine), quinidine or theophylline, nor is omeprazole affected by the concurrent use of *Maalox* or metoclopramide. An isolated report describes prolonged atracurium effects possibly due to omeprazole. The situation with digoxin is as yet uncertain.

Clinical importance, mechanism, importance and management

Two studies have shown that antacids (such as **Maalox**) and **metoclopramide** do not affect the absorption or disposition of omeprazole.[2,3] The hypoacidity caused by omeprazole causes a few small changes in the pharmacokinetics of **bacampicillin** and **amoxycillin**, but their bioavailabilities are not reduced.[6] Omeprazole is also reported not to affect either blood **alcohol** levels[4,11,12,17,18] or the pharmacokinetics of lignocaine[8] or caffeine.[10] Yet another study found that omeprazole does not affect the pharmacokinetics or pharmacodynamics of **quinidine**.[5] The changes in the half-life and clearance of **theophylline** by omeprazole were found in three studies to be small and clinically unimportant.[1,16,19] No changes in the

steady-state pharmacokinetics of theophylline were found in another study.[7,15] No special precautions would seem necessary if any of these drugs is given with omeprazole.

In isolated report describes a prolongation of the action of atracurium possibly due to the presence of omeprazole.[13] **Food delays the absorption of omeprazole, but does not affect the total amount absorbed.**[20] **A study using 20 mg omeprazole daily for 11 days found that only minor changes occurred in the disposition of a 1 mg oral dose of digoxin.** On average the $AUC_{0-96\,h}$ showed only a 10% increase.[1,9] However later work suggests that non-selective digoxin assay methods may fail to detect an interaction, whereas selective HPLC assay methods and ECG studies provide some evidence that the bioavailability of digoxin may be increased by omeprazole.[14] Until this is confirmed and quantified it would seem reasonable to monitor concurrent use thoroughly.

References

1 Oosterhuis B, Jonkman JHG. Omeprazole: pharmacology, pharmacokinetics and interactions. Digestion (1989) 44 (Suppl 1) 9–17.
2 Tuynman HARE, Festern HPM, Röhss K, Meuwissen SGM. Lack of effect of antacids on plasma concentrations of omeprazole given as enteric-coated granules. Br J Clin Pharmac (1987) 24, 833–5.
3 Howden CW, Reid JL. The effect of antacids and metoclopramide on omeprazole absorption and disposition. Br J Clin Pharmac (1988) 25, 779–80.
4 Guram M, Holt S. Are ethanol-H2 receptor antagonist interactions 'relevant'. Gastroenterlogy (1991) 100, 5 part 2, A749.
5 Ching MS, Elliott SL, Stead CK, Murdoch RT, Devenish-Meares S, Morgan DJ, Smallwood RA. Quinidine single dose pharmacokinetics and pharmacodynamics are not affected by omeprazole. Aliment Pharmacol Therap (1991) 5, 523–31.
6 Paulsen O, Högland P, Walder M. No effect of omeprazole-induced hypoacidity on the bioavailability of amoxycillin and bacampicillin. Scand J Infect Dis (1989) 21, 219–23.
7 Genève J, Bocquentin M, Taburet AM, Simoneau G, Caulin C, Singlas E. Effect of omeprazole on theophylline metabolism in healthy subjects. Gastroenterology (1991) 100, A69.
8 Bannister J, Noble DW, Lamont M, Scott DB. Lack of effect of omeprazole on the disposition of lignocaine and its active metabolite in healthy subjects. World Congr Gastroenterol, Sydney August 1990, Abstract no PP1363.
9 Oosterhuis B, Jonkman JHG, Andersson T, Zuiderwijk PBM, Jedema JN. Minor effect of multiple dose omeprazole on the pharmacokinetics of digoxin after a single oral dose. Br J Clin Pharmac (1991) 32, 569–72.
10 Andersson T, Bergstrand R, Cederberg C, Eriksson S, Lagerström P-F, Skånberg I. Omeprazole treatment does not affect the metabolism of caffeine. Gastroenterology (1991) 101, 943–7.
11 Jönsson K-Å, Jones AW, Boström T. No influence of omeprazole on the pharmacokinetics of ethanol in healthy men. World Congr Gastroenterology, Sydney, August 1990. Abstracts II, PD201.
12 Roine R, DiPadova C, Frezza M, Hernández-Muñoz R, Baraona E, Lieber CS. Effects of omeprazole, cimetidine and ranitidine on blood ethanol concentrations. Gastroenterology (1990) 98, A114.
13 Beeley L, Cunningham H, Carmichael A. Bull W Midlands Centre for Adverse Drug Reaction Reporting (1990) 31, 9.
14 Cohen AF, Kroon R, Schoemaker HC, Hoogkamer JFW, van Vliet-Verbeek A. Effects of gastric acidity on the bioavailability of digoxin. Evidence for a new mechanism for interactions with omeprazole. Br J Clin Pharmac (1991) 31, 565P.
15 Taburet AM, Geneve J, Bocquentin M, Simoneau G, Caulin C, Singlas E. Theophylline steady state pharmacokinetics is not altered by omeprazole. Eur J Clin Pharmacol (1992) 42, 343–5.
16 Oosterhuis B, Jonkman JHG, Andersson T, Zuiderwijk PBM. No influence of single intravenous doses of omeprazole on theophylline elimination kinetics. J Clin Pharmacol (1992) 32, 470–5.
17 Roine R, Hernández-Muñoz R, Baraona E, Greenstein R, Lieber CS. Effect

of omeprazole on gastric first-pass metabolism of ethanol. Dig Dis Sci (1992) 37, 891–6.

18 Jönsson K-Å, Jones AW, Boström H, Andersson T. Lack of effect of omeprazole, cimetidine, and ranitidine on the pharmacokinetcis of ethanol in fasting male volunteers. Eur J Clin Pharmacol (1992) 42, 209–212.

19 De K Sommers, van Wyk M, Sneyman JR, Moncrieff J. The effects of omeprazole-induced hypochlorhydria on absorption of theophylline from a sustained release formulation. Eur J Clin Pharmacol (1992) 43, 141–3.

20 Rohss K, Andren K, Heggelund A, Lagerstrom P-O, Lundborg P. Bioavailability of omeprazole given in conjuction with food. III World Conf Clin Pharmacol Ther, Stockholm July-Aug 1986. Acta Pharmacol Toxicol (1986) Suppl 5, 85, Abstract 207.

Oxpentifylline + Cimetidine

Abstract/Summary

Cimetidine increases serum oxpentifylline (pentoxifylline) levels to a moderate extent.

Clinical evidence, mechanism, importance and management

1200 mg cimetidine daily for 7 days increased the mean steady-state plasma of oxpentifylline (taken as a 400 mg controlled-release tablet 8-hourly) in 10 normal subjects by 27.4%.[1] The reason is not known. Side-effects such as headaches, nausea, vomiting were said to be more common and bothersome while taking the cimetidine,[1] however there seem to be no strong reasons for avoiding concurrent use.

Reference

1 Mauro VF, Mauro LS, Hageman JH. Alteration of pentoxifylline pharmacokinetics by cimetidine. J Clin Pharmacol (1988) 28, 649–54.

Oxygen (hyperbaric) + Acetazolamide, Barbiturates, Narcotics

Abstract/Summary, clinical evidence, mechanism, importance and management

It has been suggested, but not confirmed, that because increased levels of carbon dioxide in the tissues can increase the sensitivity to oxygen-induced convulsions, drugs such as acetazolamide which are carbonic anhydrase-inhibitors are contraindicated in those given hyperbaric oxygen. Nor should oxygen be given during narcotic or barbiturate withdrawal because the convulsive threshold of such patients is already low.[1]

Reference

1 PG. HBO can interact with pre-existing patient conditions. J Amer Med Ass (1981) 246, 1177–8.

Papaverine + Benzodiazepines

Abstract/Summary

Two men given normal test doses of papaverine for the investigation of impotence had prolonged penile erections attributed to the concurrent use of diazepam.

Clinical evidence, mechanism, importance and management

Papaverine can be used for the diagnosis and treatment of impotence because, when injected into the corpus cavernosum, it causes erection of the penis. Undesirably prolonged erections (5–6 h) occurred in two patients who had been given 5–10 mg diazepam intravenously for anxiety before the papaverine (60 mg).[1] Papaverine acts by relaxing the arterioles which supply the corpora so that the pressure rises. The increased pressure in the corpora compresses the venules so that the pressure continues to maintain the erection. Diazepam also relaxes smooth muscle and this it would seem can be additive with the effects of papaverine. The authors of the report say that say that '..caution should be exercised in the choice of papaverine dosage..' (i.e. use less) '.. in patients on anxiolytics..' although these two cases involving diazepam seem to be the only ones recorded. The authors also suggest that prolonged erections of this kind can be resolved either by aspirating with a large bore needle, or an intracavernosal injection of an alpha-agonist such as phenylephrine (1 mg) or noradrenaline.[1]

Reference

1 Vale JA, Kirby RS, Lees W. Papaverine, benzodiazepines, and prolonged erections. Lancet (1991) 337, 1552.

Paraldehyde + Disulfiram

Abstract/Summary

Concurrent use should be avoided because toxic reactions seem likely.

Clinical evidence, mechanism, importance and management

It is thought that paraldehyde is depolymerized in the liver to acetaldehyde, and then oxidized by acetaldehyde dehydrogenase.[1] Since disulfiram inhibits this enzyme, concurrent use would be expected to result in the accumulation of acetaldehyde and in a modified 'antabuse' reaction,[2] but so far there appear to be no reports of this in man. In addition, alcoholics with impaired liver function are said to be sensitive to the toxic effects of paraldehyde and may show restlessness rather than sedation. These are all good reasons for avoiding concurrent use.

References

1 Hitchcock P, Nelson EE. The metabolism of paraldehyde: II. J Pharmac Exp Ther (1943) 79. 286.
2 Keplinger ML and Wells JA. Effect of antabuse on the action of paraldehyde in mice and dogs. Fed Proc (1956) 15, 445.

Piperine + miscellaneous drugs

Abstract/Summary

Piperine can increase the bioavailability of phenytoin, propranolol, rifampicin (rifampin), theophylline and other drugs.

Clinical evidence, mechanism, importance and management

A study in five normal subjects found that piperine (20 mg for seven days) increased the absorption of a single 300 mg oral dose of phenytoin (AUC +50%) and raised the peak serum levels.[1] In another study in 12 subjects, 20 mg piperine daily for seven days roughly doubled the peak serum levels and the AUC's of propranolol and theophylline.[2] 50 mg piperine was also found to increase the AUC of 450 mg rifampicin by 70% in patients with tuberculosis.[3].

Piperine is the major alkaloid of black and long peppers (*Piper nigrum* and *longum*) both of which are used in Ayurvedic formulations, the presumption being that these plant products are empirically included to increase the bioavailability of other constituents, thereby increasing their efficacy. One of the reports[1] also quotes other studies showing that the piperine increases blood levels of sulphadiazine and tetracycline. It might therefore be possible to exploit this interaction in cases where it is difficult to achieve therapeutic levels with conventional drug doses. No cases of adverse interactions seem to have been reported but it seems possible that piperine might increase some drug levels to toxic concentrations.

Reference

1 Bano G, Amla V, Raina RK, Zutshi U, Chopra CL. The effect of piperine on pharmacokinetics of phenytoin in healthy volunteers. Planta Medica (1987) 53, 568–9.
2 Bano G, Raina RK, Zutshi U, Bedi KL, Johri RK, Sharma SC. Effect of piperine on bioavailability and pharmacokinetics of propanolol and theophylline in healthy volunteers. Eur J Clin Pharmacol (1991) 41, 615–7.
3 Zutshi RK, Singh R, Zutshi U, John RK, Atal CK. Influence of piperine on rifampicin blood levels in patients with pulmonary tuberculosis. J Assoc Phys India (1985) 33, 223–4.

Pirenzepine + Cimetidine, Food, Antacid

Abstract/Summary

Food and *Mylanta* reduce the bioavailability of pirenzepine by about 30% but this is probably of little clinical importance.

Pirenzepine and cimetidine appear to interact together advantageously.

Clinical evidence, mechanism, importance and management

The pharmacokinetics of pirenzepine and cimetidine are not affected by the presence of the other drug, but pirenzepine increases the cimetidine-induced reduction in gastric acid secretion. An apparently advantageous interaction.[2]

The AUCs of a single 50 mg tablet of pirenzepine in 24 normal subjects were reduced by about 30% when taken half an hour before food, with food or with 30 ml *Mylanta*. The food and antacid reduced the peak serum levels by 30% and 45% respectively, and the food shortened the time to achieve peak levels.[1] In practical terms this modest reduction in bioavailability is probably too small to matter, and in fact the makers suggest that pirenzepine should be taken 30 min before meals with a little fluid. The authors of this report also suggest taking it with food because compliance is better if associated with a convenient daily ritual.[1]

References

1 Matzek KM, MacGregor TR, Keirns JJ, Vinocur M. Effect of food and antacids on the oral absorption of pirenzepine in man. Int J Pharmaceutics (1986) 28, 151–5.
2 Jamali F, Mahachai V, Reilly PA, Thomson AB R. Lack of pharmacokinetic interaction between cimetidine and pirenzepine. Clin Pharmacol Ther (1985) 38, 325–30.

Pravastatin + Cholestyramine, Colestipol

Abstract/Summary

Although cholestyramine and colestipol reduce serum pravastatin levels, their total lipid-lowering effects are increased by concurrent use. Separating their administration minimizes this interaction. Concurrent use appears to be safe and effective.

Clinical evidence

(a) Cholestyramine

33 patients with primary hypercholesterolaemia were given pravastatin (5,10 or 20 mg) twice daily for 4 weeks before their morning and evening meals, to which was later added 24 mg cholestyramine daily with meals for a further 4 weeks. The cholestyramine was taken at least an hour after the pravastatin. The pravastatin alone significantly reduced their blood lipid levels, and this was enhanced by the addition of the cholestyramine, despite the fact that the cholestyramine reduced the bioavailability of the pravastatin up to almost 50%.[1] A related study in 24 subjects by the same group of

workers found that cholestyramine reduced the bioavailability of the pravastatin by about 40% when given together, but only a small and clinically insignificant reduction occurred when the pravastatin was given 1 h before or 4 h after the cholestyramine.[2]

A multicentre study involving 311 patients found that combined use (40 mg pravastatin plus 12 g cholestyramine daily) was highly effective in the treatment of hypercholesterolaemia and without significant problems.[4]

(b) Colestipol

Colestipol in 18 subjects reduced the bioavailability of pravastatin by about 50%, but not when given 1 h before or with food.[3]

Mechanism

It seems probable that these bile acid binding resins bind with pravastatin in the gut, thereby reducing its absorption.

Importance and management

Established interactions but of only relatively minor importance. Despite the reduction in the bioavailability of the pravastatin caused by the cholestyramine or colestipol, the overall lipid-lowering effect is increased by concurrent use.[4] The effects of the interaction can be minimized by separating their administration by at least an hour. This can be achieved by taking the cholestyramine or colestipol with meals, and the pravastatin an hour before the meals, or possibly at bedtime.

References

1 Pan HY, DeVault AR, Swites BJ, Whigan D, Ivashki E, Willard DA, Brescia D. Pharmacokinetics and pharmacodynamics of pravastatin alone and with cholestyramine in hypercholesterolemia. Clin Pharmacol Ther (1990) 48, 201–7.

2 Pan HY, DeVault AR, Ivashkiv E, Whigan D, Brennan JJ, Willard DA. Pharmacokinetic interaction studies of pravastatin with bile-acid-binding resins. 8th Int Symp Atherosclerosis, October 9–13, Rome (1988), 711.

3 Pan HY, DeVault AR, Ivashkiv E, Whigan D, Brennan JJ, Willard DA. Pharmacokinetic interaction studies of pravastatin with bile-acid-binding resins. 8th Int Symp Atherosclerosis, October 9–13, Rome (1988), 711.

4 Pravastatin Multicenter Study Group II. Comparative efficacy and safety of pravastatin and cholestyramine alone and combined in patients with hypercholesterolaemia. Arch Intern Med (1993) 153, 1321–9.

Pravastatin + Cyclosporin(e)

Abstract/Summary

Pravastatin is an effective treatment for hypercholesterolaemia in patients on cyclosporin, and none of the severe adverse effects seen with lovastatin (e.g. muscle damage, rhabdomyolysis) appear to occur.

Clinical evidence, mechanism, importance and management

Forty-four patients with heart transplants on cyclosporin were treated with 20 mg pravastatin daily for 3 months. Eight of them were subsequently treated with 40 mg daily. Total and LDL cholesterol levels were lowered without creatinine phosphokinase (CPK) elevation, while HDL cholesterol levels were unchanged.[1] 24 patients with kidney transplants on cyclosporin (2.7 mg/kg), azathioprine and prednisolone showed no adverse effects when additionally given 10 mg pravastatin daily. Kidney function and CPK levels were unaffected.[2] None of the adverse effects observed with lovastatin (e.g. rhabdomyolysis) were seen.[1,2]

Mechanism

None. The authors of one study point out that pravastatin is water soluble and unlikely to enter non-liver cells (such as muscle) to cause damage, unlike lovastatin which is lipophilic and can enter non-liver cells.[2]

Importance and management

Information is limited but concurrent use would appear to be safe and effective, nevertheless until clinical experience is greater it would be prudent to warn patients to report any muscle pain or weakness.

References

1 Kobashigawa JA , Brownfield ED, Stevenson S, Gleeson MP, Moriguchi JD, Kawata N, Hamilton MA, Hage AS, Minkley R, Salamandra J, Ruzevitch S, Drinkwater DC, Laks H. Effects of pravastatin in hypercholesterolemia in cardiac transplant patients. J Amer Coll Cardiol (1993) 21, 141A.

2 Yoshimura N, Oka T, Okamoto M, Ohmori Y. The effects of pravastatin on hyperlipidemia in renal transplant recipients. Transplantation (1992) 53, 94–99.

Pravastatin + Gemfibrozil

Abstract/Summary

Pravastatin and gemfibrozil have additive lipid-lowering effects. Severe myopathy has not been seen but the safety of combined use is not yet established.

Clinical evidence, mechanism, importance and management

No clinically significant changes in the bioavailability of single 20 mg doses of pravastatin were seen in studies on the concurrent use of 600 mg gemfibrozil in 20 normal subjects.[1] A 12-week large scale survey of 290 patients found that 40 mg pravastatin daily and 600 mg gemfibrozil twice daily had additive lipid-lowering effects when used together. Marked abnormalities in creatine kinase concentrations (four times the pretreatment values) occurred in only eight patients: pravastatin one, placebo one, gemfibrozil two, combined treatment four. These were not statistically significant. Severe myopathy or rhabdomyolysis was not seen in any patient, although 14 patients had musculoskeletal pain which was not considered to be related to the treatment.[2]

The authors of the report point out that the rises in creatine kinase may poossibly indicate a sublinical myopathy, so that the safety of combined use is not yet fully established. They do not advise the routine use of this combination. Patients given both drugs should be monitored for evidence of muscle pain or tenderness (warn them to report this if it happens), and creatine kinase levels should be checked.

References

1 Pan HY, Glaess SR, Kassalow LM, Meehan RL and Martynowicz H. A report on the bioavailability of pravastatin in the presence and absence of gemfibrozil in healthy male subjects. Unpublished report on file of ER Squibb. Protocol No. 277, 201–18 (1988).
2 Wiklund O, Bergman M, Bondjers G, Lindén T, Ödman B, Saarinen I, Kron B, Wright I. Pravastatin and gemfibrozil alone and in combination for the treatment of hypercholesterolemia. Amer J Med (1993) 94, 13–9.

Pravastatin + miscellaneous drugs

Abstract/Summary

No clinically significant interactions have been seen in studies on pravastatin taken with antipyrine, aspirin, cimetidine, *Maalox*, nicotinic acid or probucol. No interactions were seen in clinical trials in patients taking diuretics, antihypertensives, digitalis, ACE-inhibitors, calcium channel blockers, beta-blockers or nitroglycerins.

Clinical evidence, mechanism, importance and management

No clinically significant changes in the bioavailability of single 20 mg doses of pravastatin were seen in studies on the concurrent use of 500 mg probucol in 20 normal subjects.[4] The concurrent use of *Maalox TC* (15 ml four times daily) or cimetidine (300 mg four times daily) — both given 1 h previously — was found to reduce the bioavailability of single 20 mg doses of pravastatin by 52 and 68% respectively, however the makers say that it is unlikely that these changes will affect the clinical efficacy of pravastatin.[5,6] Other studies found that neither aspirin (324 mg) nor nicotinic acid (1 g) affected the bioavailability of pravastatin.[3]

The makers also say that during clinical trials of pravastatin no noticeable drug interactions were seen in patients taking diuretics, antihypertensives, digitalis, ACE-inhibitors, calcium channel blockers, beta-blockers or nitroglycerins.[6] A study in normal subjects given pravastatin found that 40 mg propranolol twice daily reduced the AUC (area under the curve) of total inhibitors by 23%, of active inhibitors by 20% and of

pravastatin by 16%.[2] These changes are small and the results of this study would seem to confirm the previous findings[6] with beta-blockers. No special precautions would seem to be necessary if any of these drugs is given concurrently.

Antipyrine is used as a model or marker drug to find out if drugs are likely to affect the metabolism of others. A study in 24 type II hypercholesterolaemic patients given 5, 10 or 20 mg pravastatin twice daily for 4 weeks found that antipyrine saliva samples showed no changes in either its elimination half-life or its clearance.[1] Thus pravastatin appears not to induce or inhibit liver microsomal enzymes (cytochrome P450 system) and would not be expected to interact with other drugs commonly affected in this way (e.g. phenytoin, warfarin).

References

1 Pan HY, Swanson BN, DeVault AR, Willard DA, Brescia D. Antipyrine elimination is not affected by chronic administration of pravastatin (SQ31,000). A tissue-selective HMG CoA reductase inhibitor. Clin Res (1988) 36, 368A.
2 Pan HY, Triscari J, DeVault AR, Smith SA, Wang-Iverson D, Swanson BN, Willard DA. Pharmacokinetic interaction between propranolol and the HMG-CoA reductase inhibitors pravastatin and lovastatin. Br J Clin Pharmac (1991) 31, 665–70.
3 Pan HY, DeVault AR, Waclawski AP. A report on the effect of nicotinic acid alone and in the presence of aspirin on the bioavailability of SQ 31,000 in healthy male subjects. Protocol No 27, 201–6 (1987).
4 Pan HY, Glaess SR, Kassalow LM, Meehan RL and Martynowicz H. A report on the bioavailability of pravastatin in the presence and absence of gemfibrozil or probucol in healthy male subjects. Unpublished report on file of ER Squibb. Protocol No. 277, 201–18 (1988).
5 Marino MR, Pan HY, Bakry D, Glaess SR, Martyniwicz H. A report on the comparative pharmacokinetics of pravastatin in the presence and absence of cimetidine or antacids in healthy male subjects. Unpublished report on file of ER Squibb. Protocol No 27, 201–43 (1988).
6 Lipostat (Pravastatin) datasheet, ER Squibb (1990).

Prostaglandins + Alcohol

Abstract/Summary

Enprostil appears to increase, rather than decrease, the possible damage to the mucosal lining of the stomach which can be caused by alcohol whereas misoprostol appears to protect the mucosa.

Clinical evidence, mechanism, importance and management

A double blind trial cross-over study in 8 normal healthy subjects found that enprostil appears to increase rather than protect the antral mucosa of the stomach from damage by alcohol. The study was carried out by spraying the mucosa with 10 ml solutions of 70 µg enprostil or a placebo, and 100 ml of 80% ethanol. The mucosa was viewed using a gastroscope, recorded on video film, and the damage assessed by two endoscopists.[1] This study suggests that enprostil should not be used to treat alcoholic gastritis, and patients taking enprostil should be warned to avoid alcohol. More study is needed to confirm these findings. In contrast misoprostol appears to protect the mucosa against damage by alcohol.[2] Nocloprost clathrate delays the absorption of alcohol but appears not to interact adversely.[3]

References

1 Cohen M M, Yeung R, Wang H-R, Clark L. Human antral damage induced by alcohol is potentiated by enprostil. Gastroenterology (1990) 99, 45–50.
2 Agrawal N M, Godiwala T, Arimura A, Dajani E Z. Cytoprotection by a synthetic prostaglandin against ethanol-induced gastric mucosal damage. A double-blind endoscopic study in human subjects. Gastrointest Endosc (1986) 32, 67–70.
3 Siegmund W, Zschiesche M, Bohne M, Franke G, Amon I. Pharmacokinetic interactions between nocloprost, acetylsalicylic acid and ethanol. Int J Clin Pharmacol Ther Toxicol (1992) 30, 539–40.

Retinoids + Tetracyclines, Vitamin A

Abstract/Summary

The development of 'pseudotumour cerebri' has been associated with the concurrent use of isotretinoin and tetracyclines. A condition similar to vitamin A overdosage may occur if isotretinoin and vitamin A are given concurrently.

Clinical evidence, mechanism, importance and management

(a) Retinoids + Tetracyclines

The concurrent use of isotretinoin and a tetracycline has resulted in the development of 'pseudotumour cerebri' (i.e. a clinical picture of cranial hypertension with headache, dizziness and dysopia). By 1983 the FDA had received reports of 10 patients with pseudotumour cerebri and/or papilloedema associated with the use of isotretinoin. Four had retinal haemorrhages. Five of the 10 were also being treated with a tetracycline.[2] The manufacturers (Hoffman La Roche) also have similar reports on file of three patients given isotretinoin and either minocycline or tetracycline.[3] The same reaction has been seen in two patients given etretinate with minocycline or prednisolone.[4] It seems that the two drugs have an additive effect in increasing intracranial pressure. Be alert for the development of this adverse response if these drugs are used.

(b) Retinoids + Vitamin A

Combined treatment may result in a condition similar to overdosage with vitamin A, for which reason concurrent use should be avoided or very closely monitored because changes in bone structure can occur, including premature fusion of the epiphyseal disc in children.[1] Roche, the makers of isotretinoin say that high doses of vitamin A (more than 4–5000 iu daily) should be avoided.[5]

References

1 Milstone LM, McGuire J, Ablow RC. Premature epiphyseal closure in a child receiving oral 13-cis-retinoic acid. J Am Acad Dermatol (1982) 7, 663–6.
2 Adverse effects with isotretinoin. FDA Drug Bull (1983) 13, 21–3. Quoted verbatim in J Amer Acad Dermatol (1984) 10, 519–20.
3 Hoffmann La Roche, data on file. Quoted by Shalita AR, Cunningham WJ, Leyden JJ, Pochi PE, Strauss JS. Isotretinoin treatment of acne and related disorders; an update. J Amer Acad Dermatol (1983) 9, 629–38.
4 Viraben R, Matthieu C, Fonton B. Benign intracranial hypertension during etretinate therapy for mycosis fungoides. J Amer Acad Dermatol (1985) 13, 515–17.
5 Roaccutane (Roche). ABPI Datasheet Compendium 1991–2, p 1280.

Roxatidine + Antacids, Food, Sucralfate

Abstract/Summary

Neither food, *Maalox* nor sucralfate interact to an important extent with roxatidine.

Clinical evidence, mechanism, importance and management

Food slightly delayed but increased the peak serum levels in 10 normal subjects given 150 mg roxatidine, but the extent of the absorption (bioavailability) was unchanged.[1] Another study in 24 normal subjects found that two tablespoons of *Maalox* (aluminium and magnesium hydroxides) four times daily had no clinically important effects on the absorption of 150 mg roxatidine.[1] 1 g sucralfate four times daily was found not to affect the pharmacokinetics of a single 150 mg dose of roxatidine.[2] No special precautions would seem necessary.

References

1 Labs RA. Interaction of roxatidine acetate with antacids, food and other drugs. Drugs (1988) 35 (Suppl 3) 82–9.
2 Seibert-Grafe M, Pidgen A. Lack of effect of multiple dose sucralfate on the pharmacokinetics of roxatidine acetate. Eur J Clin Pharmacol (1991) 40, 637–8.

Simvastatin + miscellaneous drugs

Abstract/Summary

Simvastatin causes a small but probably clinically unimportant increase in the serum levels of digoxin. It appears not to interact with beta-blockers, calcium antagonists, diuretics or NSAID's.

Clinical evidence, mechanism, importance and management

Serum digoxin levels can be slightly raised (+ 0.3 ng/ml) by simvastatin but this appears to be of little or no clinical importance. In clinical studies no adverse interaction was seen between simvastatin and propranolol or other beta-blockers, calcium antagonists, diuretics or non-steroidal anti-inflammatory drugs. Simvastatin also has little effect on the pharmacokinetics of antipyrine (phenazone) in hypercholesterolaemic patients which suggests that simvastatin is unlikely to interact with other drugs which use the same metabolic pathway in the liver.[1-3]

References

1 ZOCOR (simvastatin) data sheet (MSD). February 1989.
2 ZOCOR information booklet (MSD) 1989.
3 Walker JF. Simvastatin: the clinical profile. Amer J Med (1989) 87, Suppl 4A, 44–46S

Sodium polystyrene sulphonate + Antacids

Abstract/Summary

The concurrent use of antacids with sodium polystyrene sulphonate can result in metabolic alkalosis.

Clinical evidence, mechanism, importance and management

A man with metabolic acidosis developed metabolic alkalosis when given 90 g sodium polystyrene sulphonate with 90 ml magnesium hydroxide mixture.[1] Alkalosis has also been described in a study on a number of patients given this cation exchange resin with *Maalox* (magnesium-aluminium hydroxides) and calcium carbonate.[2] The suggested reason is that the sodium polystyrene sulphonate and magnesium react together within the gut to form magnesium polystyrene sulphonate and sodium chloride. As a result the normal neutralization of the bicarbonate ions by the gastric juice and the resin within the gut fails to occur, resulting in the absorption of the bicarbonate leading to metabolic alkalosis. This interaction appears to be established. Concurrent use should be undertaken with caution and serum electrolytes should be closely monitored. Administration of the resin rectally as an enema can avoid the problem.

References

1 Fernandez PC, Kovnat PJ. Metabolic acidosis reversed by the combination of magnesium and a cation-exchange resin. N Engl J Med (1972) 286, 23.
2 Schroeder ET. Alkalosis resulting from combined administration of a 'non-systemic' antacid and a cation-exchange resin. Gastroenterology (1969) 56, 868.

Sodium polystyrene sulphonate + Sorbitol

Abstract/Summary

Potentially fatal colonic necrosis may occur if sodium polystyrene sulphonate is given as an enema with sorbitol.

Clinical evidence

Five patients with uraemia developed severe colonic necrosis after being given enemas containing sodium polystyrene sulphonate and sorbitol. Four of the five died as a result. Associated studies in rats (made uraemic) found that all of them died over a two-day period after being given enemas of sodium polystyrene sulphonate with sorbitol, but none died after enemas without sorbitol. Extensive haemorrhage and transmural necrosis developed.[1]

Mechanism

Not understood.

Importance and management

Information is very limited and the interaction is not firmly established, nevertheless its seriousness indicates that sodium polystyrene sulphonate should not be given as an enema in aqueous vehicles containing sorbitol. More study is needed.

Reference

1 Lillemore KD, Romolo JI, Hamilton SR, Pennington LR, Burdick JF, Williams GM. Intestinal necrosis due to sodium polystyrene (Kayexalate) in sorbitol enemas: clinical and experimental support for the hypothesis. Surgery (1987) 101, 266.

Somatropin (Human growth hormone) + miscellaneous hormones

Abstract/Summary

The glucocorticoid corticosteroids can oppose the effects of somatropin. Somatropin opposes the hypoglycaemic effects of insulin and may also reduce thyroid function.

Clinical evidence, mechanism, importance and management

Large doses of glucocorticoid corticosteroids can inhibit the growth stimulating effects of somatropin. Close monitoring of concurrent use is needed.[1] Somatropin raises blood sugar levels. The control of blood sugar levels in diabetic children will therefore need to be closely monitored if somatotropin and insulin are used concurrently.[1] Somatropin can cause the development of hypothyroidism which can reduce the growth stimulating effects of somatotropin. Monitor the thyroid function and administer thyroid hormone if necessary.[1]

Reference

1 Humatrope (somatotropin). Data sheet, Lilley (1989).

Sulphinpyrazone + Flufenamic, Meclofenamic or Mefenamic acid

Abstract/Summary, clinical evidence, mechanism, importance and management

The uricosuric effects of sulphinpyrazone are not opposed by the concurrent use of flufenamic acid, meclofenamic acid or mefenamic acid.[1,2]

References

1 Latham BA, Radcliff F, Robinson RG. The effect of mefenamic acid and flufenamic acid on plasma uric acid levels. Ann Phys Med (1966) 8, 242.
2 Robinson RG, Radcliff FJ. The effect of meclofenamic acid on plasma uric acid levels. Med J Aust (1972) 1, 1079–80.

Sulphinpyrazone + Probenecid

Abstract/Summary

Probenecid reduces the loss of sulphinpyrazone in the urine, but the uricosuria remains unaltered.

Clinical evidence, mechanism, importance and management

A study in eight gouty patients showed that while probenecid was able to inhibit the renal tubular excretion of sulphinpyrazone, reducing it by about 75%, the maximal uric acid clearance seen with each drug alone remained unchanged.[1] There would therefore seem to be no advantage in using these drugs together. Whether the toxic effects of sulphinpyrazone are increased seems not to have been studied.

Reference

1 Perel JM, Dayton PG, McMillan PG, Snell M, Yu TF, Gutman AB. Studies of interactions among drugs in man at the renal level: probenecid and sulphinpyrazone. Clin Pharmacol Ther (1969) 10, 834.

Sumatriptan + miscellaneous drugs

Abstract/Summary

Sumatriptan appears not to interact with alcohol, flunarizine, food or pizotifen, but it has been advised that ergotamine should be avoided because of the risk of coronary vasoconstriction. For the same reason sumatriptan should not be taken by patients taking nitrates, beta-blockers or other drugs used for the treatment of angina.

Clinical evidence, mechanism, importance and management

A study in 38 migraine sufferers found that 1 mg **dihydroergotamine** alone caused maximum increases in blood pressure of 13/9 mmHg, while 2 or 4 mg subcutaneous sumatriptan caused a smaller rise in blood pressure (+ 7/ + 6 mmHg). When given together the rises were no greater than with dihydroergotamine alone.[1] Another study found that sumatriptan and ergotamine had additive vasoconstrictive effects.[6] The makers advise the avoidance of concurrent use of sumatriptan and **ergotamine** because of the theoretical risk of additive vasospastic reactions.[3] CSM has received 34 reports of pain or tightness in the chest caused by sumatriptan, possibly due to coronary vasoconstriction, and they say that for this reason the concurrent use of ergotamine should be avoided.[5]

No pharmacokinetic interaction occurs with **propranolol** (80 mg twice daily for 7 days),[4] however because of the risk of coronary vasoconstriction the CSM advise that sumatriptan should not be used in patients with ischaemic heart disease or Prinzmetal's angina. Patients who are taking **nitrates** or **beta-blockers** or other drugs for angina should therefore not be given sumatriptan. There would seem to be no reason for avoiding beta-blockers when used for other conditions (eg hypertension).

Other studies found that **flunarizine** (10 mg daily for 8 days) had no effect on pharmacokinetics of single doses of sumatriptan, and no significant changes in blood pressure, ECG or heart rate occurred.[1,7] **Food** also does not affect the bioavailability of sumatriptan.[1] 16 normal subjects were given single 0.8 g/kg doses of **alcohol** followed 30 min later by 200 mg sumatriptan. No statistically significant changes in the pharmacokinetics of the sumatriptan were seen.[2] None of these drugs appears to interact adversely with sumatriptan and there would seem to be no reason for special precautions.

The makers of sumatriptan say that '..until further data are available..' sumatriptan is contraindicated with the MAOI, lithium and selective 5-HT reuptake inhibitors,[3] but there appears to be no direct evidence that any adverse interactions actually occur.

References

1 Fowler PA, Lacey LF, Thomas M, Keene ON, Tanner RJN, Baber NS. The clinical pharmacology, pharmacokinetics and metabolism of sumatriptan. Eur Neurol (1991) 31, 291–4.
2 Kempsford RD, Lacey LF, Thomas M, Fowler PA. The effect of alcohol on

the pharmacokinetic profile of oral sumatriptan. Fundam Clin Pharmacol (1991) 5, 470.

3 Imigran Injection datasheet (Glaxo) July 1991.

4 Scott AK, Walley T, Breckenridge AM, Lacey LF, Fowler PA. Lack of an interaction between propranolol and sumatriptan. Br J Clin Pharmac (1991) 32, 581–4.

5 Committee on the Safety of Medicines. Current Problems (1992) 34, 2.

6 Tfelt-Hansen P, Sperling B, Winter PDO'B. Transient additional effect of sumatriptan on ergotamine-induced constriction of peripheral arteries in man. Clin Pharmacol Ther (1992) 51, 149.

7 Van Hecken AM, Depré M, De Schepper PJ, Fowler PA, Lacey LF, Durham JM. Lack of effect of flunarizine on the pharmacokinetics and pharmacodynamics of sumatriptan in healthy volunteers. Br J Clin Pharmac (1992) 34, 82–4.

Terfenadine + Cimetidine, Ranitidine

Abstract/Summary

Cimetidine and ranitidine appear not to interact adversely with terfenadine.

Clinical evidence, mechanism, importance and management

Five days treatment with 1200 mg cimetidine was found to have no effect on the pharmacokinetics of single 120 mg doses of terfenadine in 12 normal subjects.[1] Other studies in two groups of five normal subjects confirmed the lack of effect of 600 mg cimetidine 12-hourly and also 150 mg ranitidine 12-hourly on the pharmacokinetics of 60 mg terfenadine 12-hourly. No adverse ECG changes were seen (QT_c intervals, T-U morphologies).[2] There would seem to be no good reason for avoiding concurrent use.

References

1 Eller MG, Okerholdm RA. Effect of cimetidine on terfenadine and terfenadine metabolite pharmacokinetics. Pharm Res (1991) 8 (10 Suppl) S-297.

2 Cantilena L, Wortham D, Zamani K, Conner D, Honig P. Effect of cimetidine and ranitidine on the pharmacokinetics and ECG pharmacodynamics of terfenadine. Clin Pharmacol Ther (1993) 53, 161.

Terfenadine + Imidazole antifungals

Abstract/Summary

Three reports described the development of terfenadine toxicity (torsades de pointes arrhythmias) in two patients taking ketoconazole and one taking itraconazole. Potentially serious ECG changes have been demonstrated in clinical studies in other subjects. Fluconazole appears not to interact.

Clinical evidence

(a) Fluconazole

Six normal subjects were given 60 mg terfenadine 12-hourly.

None of them showed any evidence of accumulating (unmetabolized) terfenadine when additionally given 200 mg fluconazole daily for a week, and no significant ECG changes were seen.[9] No clinically significant interactions between terfenadine and fluconazole had been reported to the FDA by January 1993.[10]

(a) Itraconazole

A woman of 26 taking 60 mg terfenadine twice daily for sinusitis began to have fainting episodes on the third evening after starting to take 100 mg itraconazole twice daily for vaginitis. When admitted to hospital next morning her ECG showed a QT interval of 580 ms and her heart rate was 67 bpm. Several episodes of torasades de pointes ventricular tachycardia were recorded, and she fainted during two of them. No arrhythmias were seen 20 h after both drugs were stopped. Her QT-interval returned to normal after three days. She was found to have 28 μg/ml terfenadine in the first sample of serum taken (normally undetectable <10 μg/ml) and she still had 12μg/ml 60 h after taking the last tablet.[6]

(b) Ketoconazole

A 39-year-old woman on 60 mg terfenadine twice daily for sinusitis developed a number of episodes of syncope and lightheadedness, preceded by palpitations, dyspnoea and diaphoresis within 2 days of starting 200 mg ketoconazole twice daily. ECG monitoring revealed a torsades de pointes rhythm abnormality. Her terfenadine serum levels were 57 ng/ml (expected levels of 10 ng/ml or less). Other drugs being taken were cefaclor (stopped 3–4 days before the problems started) and medroxyprogesterone acetate. She had had terfenadine and cefaclor on two previous occasions in the absence of ketoconazole without problems.[1,5]

Another woman, aged 22, similarly developed torsades de pointes after taking 120 mg terfenadine and 200 mg ketoconazole daily for five days.[4] The FDA's spontaneous reporting system has on record other cases of torsades de pointes arrhythmias in patients taking both drugs.[8]

400 mg ketoconzole four times daily for a week markedly increased the serum levels of terfenadine (single 120 mg doses) in 12 normal subjects (a rise from <10 to 27 ng/ml). The clearance of the active metabolite of terfenadine was reduced about 30% and its half-life prolonged almost threefold.[2] The ECG's of those given both drugs showed a prolongation (10–20 ms) of the corrected QT interval.[3] 200 mg ketoconazole 12-hourly for six days increased the QT interval in six normal subjects taking 60 mg terfenadine 12-hourly from 416 to 490 msec and raised the unmetabolized serum terfenadine levels of all of them. It increased to 81 ng/ml in one individual. Four of the subjects were given a shortened course because of the significant ECG repolarization changes.[7]

Mechanism

Itraconazole and ketoconazole appear to reduce the metabolism of the terfenadine by the liver so that it cleared more slowly.

The accumulating levels of unmetabolised terfenadine are cardiotoxic and can alter the repolarization of the cardiac muscle (reflected in an increase in the QT interval) in a way as yet not understood.

Importance and management

Established and clinically important interactions. Terfenadine can accumulate in those given itraconazole or ketoconazole, leading to the development of potentially life-threatening torsades de pointes arrhythmia in some individuals. Because of its seriousness the FDA, the CSM and the makers of terfenadine now advise the avoidance of itraconazole or ketoconazole in all patients taking terfenadine. The limited evidence available suggests that fluconazole is unlikely to interact in this way in normal dosages.[9,10]

References

1 Monahan BP, Ferguson CL, Killeavy ES, Lloyd BK, Troy J, Cantilena LR. Torsades de Pointes occurring in association with terfenadine use. J Am Med Ass (1990) 264, 2788–90.
2 Eller MG, Okerholm RA. Pharmacokinetic interaction between terfenadine and ketoconazole. Clin Pharmacol Ther (1991) 49, 130.
3 Mathews DR, McNutt B, Okerholm R, Flicker M, McBride G. Torsades de Pointes occurring in association with terfenadine use. J Amer Med Ass (1991) 266, 2375–6.
4 Zimmermann M, Duruz H, Guinand O, Broccard O, Levy P, Lacatis D, Bloch A. Torsades de Pointes after treatment with terfenadine and ketoconazole. Eur Heart J (1992) 13, 1002–3.
5 Cantilena LR, Ferguson CL, Monahan BP. Torsades de Pointes occurring in association with terfenadine use. J Amer Med Ass (1991) 266, 2375–6.
6 Pohjola-Sintonen S, Viitasalo M, Toivonen L, Neuvonen P. Torsades de pointes after terfenadine-itraconazole interaction. Br Med J (1993) 306, 186.
7 Honig PK, Wortham DC, Zamani K, Conner DP, Mullin JC, Canilena LR. Terfenadine-ketoconazole interaction. Pharmacokinetic and electrocardiographic consequences. J Amer Med Ass (1993) 269, 1513–8.
8 Peck CC, Temple R, Collins JM. Understanding consequences of concurrent therapies. J Amer Med Ass (1993) 269, 1550–2.
9 Honig PK, Wortham DC, Zamani K, Mullin JC, Conner DP, Cantilena LR. The effect of fluconazole on the steady-state pharmacokinetics and electrographic pharmacodynamics of terfenadine in humans. Clin Pharmacol Ther (1993) 53, 630–6.
10 Sevka M. Personnal Communication, January 1993, quoted in ref 9.

Terfenadine + Macrolide antibiotics

Abstract/Summary

Erythromycin causes terfenadine to accumulate in a few individuals which can prolong the QT_c interval in those with otherwise apparently normal cardiac function, increasing the risk of life-threatening torsades de pointes arrhythmias. Clarithromycin and triacetyloleandomycin (troleandomycin) appear to interact similarly, but possibly not azithromycin.

Clinical evidence

(a) Azithromycin

250 mg azithromycin four times daily for 5 days had no effect on the mean AUC of terfenadine, 60 mg twice daily, in six normal subjects.[7]

(b) Clarithromycin

500 mg clarithromycin twice daily for seven days approximately doubled the mean AUC (from 1053 to 2699 ng-hr/ml) of terfenadine, 60 mg twice daily, in six normal subjects. Four of them had detectable terfenadine in their serum (normally undetectable).[7]

(c) Erythromycin

Nine subjects on terfenadine (60 mg 12-hourly) showed a 107% rise in the maximum serum levels of the active acid metabolite of terfenadine, and a 170% rise in its AUC after additionally taking 500 mg erythromycin three times daily for a week. Three of the nine accumulated unmetabolized terfenadine in their serum (normally none can be detected if terfenadine is taken alone). These three showed a marked prolongation of the QT_c of 59 msec compared with only 12 msec in the rest of the group.[1] One of them showed pronounced notching of the T wave.[1]

Other studies have confirmed that erythromycin increases the AUC of terfenadine and/or prolongs the QT interval.[6,7] These studies contrast with another which found that 1 g erythromycin daily for five days had no effect on the serum levels of either terfenadine or its metabolite after taking a single 120 mg dose.[4]

(d) Triacetyloleandomycin (Troleandomycin)

The makers of terfenadine (Marion Merrell Dow) have on record a single case of a woman with a history of aortic valve disease who suffered an episode of torsades de pointes arrhythmia while taking triacetyloleandomycin (troleandomycin). She had taken more than the maximum recommended dose of terfenadine.[8]

Mechanism

Terfenadine is a prodrug which is metabolised firstly to an active carboxylic acid metabolite, and then further oxidised to a second inactive metabolite. The interacting macrolides can apparently inhibit the second metabolic step so that the acid metabolite accumulates, and in a small number of susceptible individuals it may also inhibit the first step too.[6,7] The accumulating unmetabolised terfenadine is cardiotoxic and can alter the repolarization of the cardiac muscle (reflected in an increase in the QT_c interval) in a way as yet not understood. Intravenous erythromycin on its own can also cause torsades de pointes.[2]

Importance and management

An established interaction with erythromycin, clarithromycin and possibly triacetyloleandomycin (troleandomycin), but probably not azithromycin, which affects some but not all individuals.[7] Only triacetyloleadomycin (troleandomycin) has been directly implicated in an adverse report, but the resulting prolongation of the QT_c interval which occurs with the other interacting macrolides is clear evidence that the risk of potentially life-threatening torsades de pointes arrhythmia is also increased with these drugs. Even though this risk may be small,[5] because of the unpredictability and seriousness of this interaction, the FDA, the CSM[3] and the makers of terfenadine now advise the avoidance of erythromycin or other macrolides in patients taking terfenadine.

Reference

1 Honig PK, Woosley RL, Zamani K, Conner DP, Cantilena LR. Changes in the pharmacokinetics and electrocardiographic pharmacodynamics of terfenadine with concomitant administration of erythromycin. Clin Pharmacol Ther (1992) 52, 231–8.
2 Lindsay J, Smith MA, Light JA. Torsades de pointes associated with antimicrobial therapy for pneumonia. Chest (1990) 98, 222–3.
3 CSM Current Problems Series (1992) 35, 1.
4 Matthews DR et al. Torsades to pointes occurring in association with terfenadine use. J Amer Med Ass (1991) 266, 2375.
5 Schoenwetter WF, Kelloway JS, Lindgren D. A retrospective evaluation of potential cardiac side-effects induced by concurrent use of terfenadine and erythromycin. J All Clin Immunol (1993) 91, 259.
6 Eller M, Russel T, Ruberg S, Okerholm R, McNutt B. Effect of erythromycin on terfenadine metabolite pharmcokinetics. Clin Pharmacol Ther (1993) 53, 161.
7 Honig P, Wortham D, Zamani K, Conner D, Cantilena L. Effect of erythromycin, clarithromycin and azithromycin on the pharmacokinetics of terfenadine. Clin Pharmacol Ther (1993) 53, 161.
8 Jarvis S (Marion Merrell Dow). Personnal Communication, August 1993.

Terodiline + miscellaneous drugs

Abstract/Summary

Terodiline has been associated with serious cardiac arrhythmias in the presence of certain predisposing factors which include antipsychotic and cardioactive drugs, diuretics, hypokalamic agents and tricyclic antidepressants.

Clinical evidence, mechanism, importance and management

On the basis of 17 'yellow card reports' of ventricular tachycardia (13 torsades de pointes) associated with the use of terodiline, The Committee on the Safety of Medicines (CSM) in the UK issued a warning that the predisposing risk factors were ischaemic heart disease, hypokalaemia, and the current use of cardio-active drugs, diuretics, tricyclic antidepressants and anti-psychotics. These conditions and drugs should be regarded as contra-indicated. Age greater than 75 is not an absolute contra-indication, but is if the other predisposing factors are present. Terodiline is also contra-indicated in patients with any heart arrhythmia or ECG evidence of QT prolongation.[1] Terodiline has now been withdrawn in the UK.

Reference

1 Asscher AW. Terodiline (Micturin) and adverse cardiac reactions. Committee on the Safety of Medicines letter, 25th July 1991.

Thyroid hormones + Amiodarone

Abstract/Summary

Amidarone may reduce the effects of thyroid hormones used in the treatment of hypothyroidism.

Clinical evidence

A retrospective study of hospital records identified two patients who had had levothyroxine for hypothyroidism and who were given amiodarone. One of them on 0.075 mg levothyroxine daily developed signs of hypothyroidism (fatigue, weakness and cold intolerance) about 10 weeks after starting to take 200 mg amiodarone daily. Her T3/T4 molar ratio fell by a third, and her TSH increased from 20 to 30 mU/l. The hypothyroidism resolved when the levothyroxine dosage was incrementally raised to 0.112 mg daily.[1] Another patient treated with levothyroxine and amiodarone remained euthyroid, but his T3/T4 molar ratio also fell by about a third, and his TSH levels rose.[1]

Mechanism

Not fully understood. Hyper- as well as hypothyroidism can occur with amiodarone. Amiodarone contains 37% iodine and has several actions on the thyroid gland. It slows the conversion of T4 to T3, inhibits their cellular uptake and the binding of T3 to receptors. This would seem to explain some of its hypothyroidic actions.

Importance and management

Information is limited, but the interaction is established. If amiodarone is added to treatment with levothyroxine, monitor the effects and be alert for any evidence of a changed response to the thyroid hormone. Increase the dosage if necessary. The makers amiodarone (Sanofi) advise avoidance of concurrent use except in life-threatening situations.

Reference

1 Figge J, Dluhy RG. Amiodarone-induced elevation of thyroid stimulating hormone in patients receiving levothyroxine for primary hypothyroidism. Ann Intern Med (1990) 113, 553–5.

Thyroid hormones + Antacids

Abstract/Summary

An isolated report describes reduced levothyroxine effects in a patient when given an aluminium-magnesium hydroxide antacid.

Clinical evidence, mechanism, importance and management

A man controlled on 0.15 mg levothyroxine daily for hypothyroidism developed high serum thyrotropin levels (a rise from 1.1 up to 36 mU/l) while taking an aluminium-magnesium hydroxide antacid, and on two subsequent occasions when rechallenged. The reasons are not understood. He remained asymptomatic throughout.[1] The rise in the thyrotropin levels indicated that the dosage of the levothyroxine had become insufficient in the presence of the antacid. The general importance of this interaction is not known, but be alert for the need to increase the thyroid dosage in any patient on replacement treatment given this type of antacid. More study is needed.

Reference

1 Sperber AD, Liel Y. Evidence for interference with the intestinal absorption of levothyroxine sodium by aluminium hydroxide. Arch Intern Med (1991) 152, 183–4.

Thyroid hormones + Anticonvulsants

Abstract/Summary

An isolated report describes a reduction in the effects of thyroxine when phenytoin was given. Both carbamazepine and phenytoin can reduce serum thyroid hormone levels but clinical hypothyroidism caused by an interaction seems to be rare.

Clinical evidence

A patient with hypothyroidism, successfully treated with 0.15 mg thyroxine daily for 4 years, became hypothyroidic again when given 300 mg phenytoin daily. Doubling the thyroxine dosage proved to be effective. Later this interaction was confirmed by stopping and restarting the phenytoin.[1]

A number of other reports describe very significant reductions in serum thyroid hormone levels in considerable numbers of subjects and patients when treated with phenytoin or carbamazepine,[3–6] but there seem to be only two cases in which hypothyroidism (reversible) has been seen, one with carbamazepine and phenytoin and the other with carbamazepine alone.[2]

There is also a report attributing arrhythmia to the use of phenytoin in a hypothyroidic patient with rheumatic heart disease,[7] but this report was later criticized by others as being inaccurate and misleading.[8,9]

Mechanism

Both phenytoin and carbamazepine can increase the metabolism of the thyroid hormones, thereby reducing their serum levels.

Importance and management

Despite very clear evidence that both carbamazepine and phenytoin can cause a marked reduction in serum thyroid hormone levels, the development of clinical hypothyroidism seems to be very rare and there seems to be only one case on record (cited above) of an interaction between administered thyroxine and phenytoin. There seems to be little reason for avoiding the concurrent use, but the outcome should be monitored. Increase the thyroid dosage if necessary. See also 'Thyroid hormones + Barbiturates'.

References

1 Blackshear JL, Schultz AL, Napier JS, Stuart DD. Thyroxine replacement requirements in hypothyroid patients receiving phenytoin. Ann InternMed (1983) 99, 341.
2 Aanderud S, Strandjord RE. Hypothyroidism induced by antiepileptic therapy. Acta NeurolScand (1980) 61, 330–2.
3 Hansen JM, Skovsted L, Lauridsen UB, Kirkegaard C, Siersbaek-Nielsen K. The effect of diphenylhydantoin on thyroid function. J Clin Endocrinol Metab(1974) 39, 785.
4 Oppenheimer JH, Fisher LV, Nelson KM, Jailer JW. Depression of the serum protein-bound iodine level by diphenylhydantoin. J Clin Endocrinol Metab(1961) 21, 252–62.
5 Rootwelt K, Ganes T, Johannessen SI. Effect of carbamazepine phenytoin and phenobarbitone on serum levels of thyroid hormones and thyrotropin in humans. Scand J Clin Lab Invest (1978) 38, 731–6.
6 Connell JMC, Rapeport WG, Gordon S, Brodie MJ. Changes in circulating thyroid hormones during short-term hepatic enzyme induction with carbamazepine. Eur J Clin Pharmacol (1984) 26, 453–6.
7 Fulop M, Widrow DR, Colmes RA, Epstein EJ. Possible diphenylhydantoin-induced arrhythmia in hypothyroidism. J Amer Med Ass (1966) 196, 454–7.
8 Farzan S. Diphenylhydantoin and arrhythmia. J Amer Med Ass (1966) 197, 63.
9 Gaspar HL. Diphenylhydantoin and arrhythmia. J Amer Med Ass (1966) 197, 63.

Thyroid Hormones + Barbiturates

Abstract/Summary

An isolated report describes a reduction in the response of a woman to thyroxine when treated with a barbiturate hypnotic.

Clinical evidence, mechanism, importance and management

An elderly woman on 0.3 mg L-thyroxine daily for hypothyroidism complained of severe breathlessness within a week of reducing her nightly dose of *Tuinal* (quinalbarbitone sodium 199 mg + amylobarbitone sodium 100 mg) from two capsules to one. She was subsequently found to be thyrotoxic. She became symptom-free once again when the dosage of the thyroxine was halved.[1] The reason is not understood, but an animal study showed that barbiturates increase the turnover of thyroxine by increasing its hepatocellular binding.[2] The general importance of this interaction is uncertain, but be alert for any evidence of changes in thyroid status if barbiturates are added or withdrawn from patients being treated for hypothyroidism.

References

1 Hoffbrand BI. Barbiturate:thyroid-hormone interaction. Lancet (1970) ii, 903.
2 Oppenheimer JH, Bernstein G, Surks MI. Increased thyroxine turnover and thyroidal function after stimulation of hepatocellular binding of thyroxine by phenobarbital. J Clin Invest (1968) 47, 1399.

Thyroid hormones + Cholestyramine

Abstract/Summary

The absorption of thyroid extract, levothyroxine and tri-iodothyronine from the gut is reduced by the concurrent use of cholestyramine. Separate the dosages by 4–6 h.

Clinical evidence

When a hypothyroidic patient taking thyroxine showed a fall in his basal metabolic rate when given cholestyramine, a further study was made on two similar patients taking 60 mg thyroid extract or 100 g levothyroxine sodium daily, and on five normal subjects. 4 g cholestyramine four times daily reduced their absorption of thyroxine[131] and the amount remaining in the faeces was roughly doubled. One of the patients showed a worsening of her hypothyroidism. Separating the dosages by 4–5 h reduced the interaction to a minimum.[1] Another report describes a patient on levothyroxine whose thyroid-stimulating hormone (TSH) levels rose when given cholestyramine, and fell again when it was stopped.[2]

Mechanism

Cholestyramine binds to thyroxine in the gut, thereby reducing its absorption. Since thyroxine probably also takes part in the entero-hepatic shunt (after absorption it is resecreted in the bile), continued contact with the cholestyramine is possible.

Importance and management

An established interaction (although the documentation is very limited) and of clinical importance. *In vitro* tests show that tri-iodothyronine interacts similarly.[1] The effects can be minimized by separating the dosages by 4–6 hr, even so the outcome should be monitored so that any necessary thyroid hormone dosage adjustments can be made.

References

1 Northcutt RC, Stiel JN, Hollifield JW, Stant EG. The influence of cholestyramine on thyroxine absorption. J Amer Med Ass (1969) 208, 1857.
2 Harmon SM, Seifert CF. Levothyroxine-cholestyramine interaction reemphasized. Ann Intern Med (1991) 115, 658–9.

Thyroid hormones + Cimetidine, Ranitidine

Abstract/Summary

Cimetidine, but not ranitidine, causes a small reduction in the absorption of levothyroxine given orally.

Clinical evidence, mechanism, importance and management

When given 400 mg of cimetidine 90 minutes before a single capsule of levothyroxine containing radio-iodine (^{125}I), the absorption of thyroxine in 20 women with simple goitre was reduced over the first four hours by 20.6%. The reasons are not understood. A single 30 mg dose of ranitidine was found not to affect the levothyroxine absorption.

The clinical importance of this interaction with cimetidine awaits assessment but it is probably not great, nevertheless it would be prudent to monitor the outcome if both drugs are used, being alert for the need to increase the thyroxine dosage.

Reference

1 Jonderko G, Jonderko K, Marcisz CZ, Kotulska A. Effect of cimetidine and ranitidine on absorption of [^{125}I] levothyroxine administered orally. Acta Pharmacol Sin (1992) 13, 391–4.

Thyroid hormones + Ferrous sulphate

Abstract/Summary

Ferrous sulphate causes a reduction in the effects of thyroxine in patients with hypothyroidism.

Clinical evidence

Fourteen patients with primary hypothyroidism showed a more than three-fold increase in TSH levels (from 1.6 to 5.4 mU/l) when given 300 mg ferrous sulphate daily with their thyroxine (T4) for 12 weeks. The symptoms of hypothyroidism in nine of the patients worsened.[1,2]

Mechanism

The addition of iron to thyroxine *in vitro* was found to produce a poorly soluble purple iron-thyroxine complex (possibly poorly absorbable?) suggesting that this might also occur in the gut.[1,2]

Importance and management

Information is limited to this study but it appears to be a clinically important interaction. Monitor the effects of concurrent use and separate the dosages by 2 h or more, on the assumption that reduced absorption accounts for this interaction. The same precautions should be applied with any other iron preparation. More study is needed.

Reference

1 Campbell NRC, Wong N, Hasinoff BB, Rao B, Stalts H. Ferrous sulfate reduces thyroxine efficacy. Clin Pharmacol Ther (1992) 51, 165.
2 Campbell NRC, Hasinoff BB, Stalts H, Rao B, Wong NCW. Ferrous sulfate reduces thyroxine efficacy in patients with hypothyroidism. Ann Int Med (1992) 117, 1010–3.

Thyroid hormones + Lovastatin

Abstract/Summary

An isolated report describes raised serum thyroid hormone levels and evidence of thyrotoxicosis in a patient on levothyroxine when given lovastatin.

Clinical evidence, mechanism, importance and management

A 54-year-old diabetic taking 20 mg levothyroxine daily and a number of other drugs (gemfibrozil, clofibrate, propranolol, diltiazem, quinidine, aspirin, dipyridamole, insulin) was started on 20 mg lovastatin daily. Weakness and muscle aches developed within 2–3 days and over a 27-day period he lost 10% of his body weight. His serum thyroxine levels rose from 11.3 to 27.2 g/dl. The reasons are not understood but the author of the report postulated that the lovastatin may have displaced the thyroid hormones from their binding sites, thereby increasing their effects and causing this acute thyrotoxic state.[1] The general importance of this interaction is uncertain, but the thyroid status should be monitored if lovastatin is added or discontinued in any patient receiving thyroid hormone treatment.

Reference

1 Lustgarten BP. Catabolic response to lovastatin therapy. Ann Intern Med (1988) 109, 171–2.

Thyroid hormones + Rifampicin (Rifampin)

Abstract/Summary

A case report suggests the possibility that rifampicin might reduce the effects of the thyroid hormones.

Clinical evidence, mechanism, importance and management

A woman with Turner syndrome who had had total thyroidectomy and who was being treated with 0.1 mg L-thyroxine daily, showed a marked fall in serum thyroxine levels and free thyroxine index with a dramatic rise in serum thyrotropin levels when given rifampicin. However no symptoms of clinical hypothyroidism developed.[1] A possible reason for the changes seen is that rifampicin is a potent enzyme inducing agent which can markedly increase the metabolism of many drugs, thereby increasing their loss from the body and reducing their effects. Rifampicin given to normal subjects also reduces endogenous serum thyroxine levels. There seem to be no reports of adverse effects in patients given both drugs but it would seem prudent to monitor the effects of concurrent use.

Reference

1 Isley WL. Effect of rifampicin therapy on thyroid function tests in a hypothyroidic patient on replacement L-thyroxine. Ann Intern Med (1987) 107, 517–18.

Thyroid hormones + Sucralfate

Abstract/Summary

An isolated report describes a marked reduction in the effects of levothyroxine in a patient taking sucralfate.

Clinical evidence, mechanism, importance and management

A woman with hypothyroidism failed to respond to levothyroxine despite taking 4.8 μg/kg daily (three times the usual dose) while on sucralfate. Her response remained inadequate (TSH levels high, T4 levels low) even when the levothyroxine was taken 2.5 h after the sucralfate, but when taken 4.5 h before the sucralfate the response gradually became normal. A later *in vitro* study demonstrated that sucralfate binds strongly to thyroxine and it is presumed that this also can occur in the gut, thereby reducing its absorption.[1] Although this seems to be the first and only report of this interaction, it would now seem prudent not to take sucralfate until a few hours after the levothyroxine. Patients should be advised accordingly and the response well monitored.

Reference

1 Havarankova J, Lahaie. Levothyroxine binding by sucralfate. Ann Intern Med (1992) 117, 445–6.

Ticlopidine + Antacids or Food

Abstract/Summary

Food causes a moderate increase in the absorption of ticlopidine, whereas *Maalox* causes a moderate reduction.

Clinical evidence, mechanism, importance and management

The extent of the ticlopidine absorption was increased (+ 20%) by food in 12 normal subjects and it occurred more quickly, whereas 30 ml *Maalox* (magnesium-aluminium hydroxides) reduced the extent of absorption by 20%.[1] These modest changes are unlikely to be of much clinical importance. It is suggested that ticlopidine is taken with food to minimize gastric intolerance.[1]

Reference

1 Shah J, Fratis A, Ellis D, Murakami S, Teitelbaum P. Effect of food and antacid on absorption of orally administered ticlopidine hydrochloride. J Clin Pharmacol (1990) 30, 733–6.

Total parenteral nutrition + Potassium-sparing diuretics

Abstract/Summary

Metabolic acidosis occurred in two patients receiving total parenteral nutrition which was attributed to the use of triamterene or amiloride.

Clinical evidence, mechanism, importance and management

Metabolic acidosis developed in two patients receiving total parenteral nutrition associated with the concurrent use of triamterene and amiloride. The cases were complicated by a number of pathological and other factors, but the suggestion is that the major reason for the acidosis was because the diuretics prevented the kidneys from responding normally to the acid load. Caution is advised during concurrent use.[1]

Reference

1 Kushner RF, Sitrin MD. Metabolic acidosis. Development in two patients receiving a potassium-sparing diuretic and total parenteral nutrition. Arch InternMed (1986) 146, 343–5.

Trimetazidine + miscellaneous drugs

Abstract/Summary

Trimetazidine appears not to interact with theophylline or digoxin.

Clinical evidence, mechanism, importance and management

After taking 20 mg trimetazidine twice daily for 24 days the pharmacokinetics of single 375 mg doses of theophylline, 0.5 mg digoxin and 500 mg antipyrine remained unchanged in 13 normal subjects.[1] These results suggest that treatment with theophylline or digoxin is unlikely to be altered in patients concurrently treated with trimetazidine, but this needs confirmation. The non-interaction with antipyrine also indicates that trimetazidine is neither an inducer nor an inhibitor of drug metabolism (hydroxylation) in the liver and therefore it is unlikely to interact with many drugs which are affected by changes in liver metabolism.

References

1 Edeke TI, Johnston A, Campbell DB, Ings RMJ, Brownsill R, Genissel P, Turner P. An examination of the possible pharmacokinetic interaction of trimetazidine with theophylline, digoxin and antipyrine. Br J Clin Pharmac (1989) 26, 675P.

Trimoprostil + Antacids

Abstract/Summary, clinical evidence, mechanism, importance and management

The bioavailability of trimoprostil is not affected by *Mylanta I, Di-Gel* or food.[1]

Reference

1 Wills RJ, Rees MMC, Rubio F, Gibson DM, Givens S, Parsonnet M, Gallo-Torres HE. Influence of antacids on the bioavailability of trimoprostil. Eur J Clin Pharmacol (1984) 27, 251–2.

Trinitrotoluene + Alcohol

Abstract/Summary, clinical evidence, mechanism, importance and management

Men exposed to trinitrotoluene in a munitions factory were found to have a greater risk of chronic liver impairment if they had a long history of drinking than non-drinkers.[1]

Reference

1 Li J, Jiang QG, Zhong WD. Persistent ethanol drinking increases liver

injury induced by trinitrotoluene exposure: an in-plant case-control study. Hum Exp Toxicol (1991) 10, 405–9.

Vinpocetine + Antacids

Abstract/Summary, clinical evidence, mechanism, importance and management

Magnesium-aluminium hydroxide gel (1 sachet four times daily) had no significant effects on the serum levels of vinpocetine (20 mg three times daily) in 18 normal subjects.[1] No special precautions seem necessary if taken together.

Reference

1 Lohmann A, Grobara P, Dingler E. Investigation of the possible influence of the absorption of vinpocetine with concomitant application of magnesium-aluminium-hydroxide gel. Arzneim.-Forsch/Drug Res (1991) 41, 1164–7.

Vitamin A + Aminoglycoside antibiotics

Abstract/Summary

Neomycin can markedly reduce the absorption of vitamin A from the gut and may have some effect on iron absorption.

Clinical evidence, mechanism, importance and management

2 g neomycin markedly reduced the absorption of a test dose of vitamin A (retinyl palmitate) in five normal subjects due, it is suggested, to a direct chemical interference between the neomycin and bile and fatty acids in the gut which disrupts the absorption of fats and fat-soluble vitamins.[1] The extent to which chronic treatment with neomycin (or other aminoglycosides) would impair the treatment of vitamin A deficiency has not been determined. A study in patients found that neomycin markedly reduced the absorption of iron (iron[59] as ferrous citrate) in four patients, but increased absorption in the other two who initially had low serum iron levels. None was anaemic.[2] The importance of this is uncertain, but monitor the outcome of concurrent use.

References

1 Barrowman JA, D'Mello A amd Herxheimer A. A single dose of neomycin impairs absorption of vitamin A (Retinol) in man. Eur J Clin Pharmacol (1973) 5, 199.
2 Jacobson ED, Chodos RB, Faloon WW. An experimental malabsorption syndrome induced by neomycin. Am J Med (1960) 28, 524–33.

Vitamin B_{12} (Cyanocobalamin) + miscellaneous drugs

Abstract/Summary

Although neomycin, aminosalicylic acid and the H_2-blockers can reduce the absorption of Vitamin B_{12} from the gut, no interaction is likely because B_{12} is usually given by injection.

Clinical evidence, mechanism, importance and management

Neomycin causes a generalized malabsorption syndrome which has been shown to reduce the absorption of vitamin B_{12}.[1] Aminosalicyclic acid (PAS) reduces vitamin B_{12} absorption for reasons which are not understood but which are possibly related to a mild generalized malabsorption syndrome.[2] The H_2-blockers (such as cimetidine[3] and ranitidine[4]) can also reduce vitamin B_{12} absorption, primarily because they reduce gastric acid production. The acid is needed to release of B_{12} from dietary protein sources. None of these drugs is likely to cause vitamin B_{12} deficiency unless treatment extends for two years or more because the body normally has enough in store for 2–5 years.

Within the context of adverse drug interactions, none of these drugs is normally likely to interact adversely because, for anaemia, vitamin B_{12} is usually given parenterally in order to by-pass the gut.

References

1 Faloon WW, Chodos RB. Vitamin B_{12} absorption studies using colchicine, neomycin and continuous ^{37}Co B_{12} administration. Gastroenterol (1969) 56, 1251.
2 Palva IP, Rytkönen V, Alatulkkila M, Palva HLA. Drug-induced malabsorption of vitamin B_{12}. V. Intestinal pH and absorption of vitamin B_{12} during treatment with para-aminosalicylic acid. Scand J Haematol (1972) 9, 5.
3 Steinberg WM, King CE, Toskes PP. Malabsorption of protein-bound cobalamin but not unbound cobalamin during cimetidine administrations. Dig Dis Sci (1980) 25, 188–92.
4 Belaiche J, Cattan D, Zittoun J, Marquet J, Yvart J. Effect of ranitidine on cobalamin absorption. Dig Dis Sci (1983) 28, 667–8.

Vitamin C (Ascorbic acid) + Salicylates

Abstract/Summary

Aspirin reduces the absorption of ascorbic acid by about a third. Serum salicylate levels do not appear to be affected by ascorbic acid.

Clinical evidence, mechanism, importance and management

Studies in guinea pigs and man have shown that 900 mg aspirin reduces the absorption of ascorbic acid (single 500 mg doses) from the gut by about a third, and reduces the urinary excretion by about a half.[1] The clinical importance of this is uncertain, but in view of the increased ascorbic acid requirements in conditions such as rheumatoid arthritis and the common cold, both of which are often treated with aspirin, there may be a case for increasing the intake of ascorbic acid. One suggestion is an increase from the normal physiological requirement of 30–60 mg to 100–200 mg daily. More study is needed. Studies in man have shown that ascorbic acid does not significantly affect serum salicylate levels given as choline salicylate.[2]

References

1 Basu TK. Vitamin C-aspirin interactions. Int J Vit Nutr Res (1982) Suppl 23, 83–90.
2 Hansten PD, Hayton WL. Effect of antacids and ascorbic acid on serum salicylate concentration. J Clin Pharmacol (1980) 24, 326.

Vitamin D + Phenytoin

Abstract/Summary

The long-term use of phenytoin and other anticonvulsants can disturb vitamin D and calcium metabolism which may result in osteomalacia. There are a few reports of patients taking vitamin D supplements who responded poorly while taking phenytoin. Serum phenytoin levels are not altered.

Clinical evidence

(a) Effect of phenytoin on vitamin D

A 16-year-old with grand mal epilepsy and under treatment for idiopathic hypoparathyroidism failed to respond adequately to daily doses of 10 μg 1-alpha-hydroxycholecalciferol and 6–12 g calcium, apparently due to the concurrent use of 200 mg phenytoin and 500 mg primidone daily. Replacement with 0.6–2.4 mg dihydrotachysterol daily produced a satisfactory response.[1] Two other reports describe patients whose response to vitamin D was poor because of concurrent anticonvulsant treatment with phenytoin.[2,5] Other reports clearly show that while taking phenytoin the serum levels of vitamin D are reduced.[6–8]

(b) Effect of vitamin D on phenytoin

A controlled trial on 151 epileptic patients on phenytoin and calcium showed that the addition of 2000 IU vitamin D2 daily over a 3-month period had no significant effect on serum phenytoin levels.[4]

Mechanism

The well-recognized enzyme-inducing effects of phenytoin and other anticonvulsants increase the metabolism of the vitamin D, thereby reducing its effects and disturbing the calcium metabolism.[3] In addition the phenytoin may possibly reduce the absorption of the calcium from the gut.[1]

Importance and management

The disturbance of calcium metabolism by phenytoin and other anticonvulsants is very well established but there are only a few reports describing a poor response to vitamin D. The effects of concurrent treatment should be well monitored. Those who need vitamin D supplements may probably need greater than usual doses.

References

1 Rubinger D, Korn-Lubetzki I, Feldman S, Popovtzer MM. Delayed response to 1-alpha-cholecalciferol therapy in a case of hypoparathyroidism during anticonvulsant therapy. Isr J Med Sci (1980) 16, 772.
2 Asherov J, Weinberger A, Pinkhas H. Lack of response to vitamin D therapy in a patient with hypoparathyroidism under anticonvulsant drugs. Helv Pediatr Acta (1977) 32, 369.
3 Chan JCM, Oldham SB, Holick MF, DeLuca HF. One alpha-hydroxyvitamin D3 in chronic renal failure. A potent analogue of the kidney hormone 1,25-dihydroxycholecalciferol. J Amer Med Ass (1975) 234, 47.
4 Christiansen D, Redbro P. Effect of vitamin D2 on serum phenytoin. A controlled therapeutic trial. Acta NeurolScand (1974) 50, 661.
5 McLaren N, Lifschitz F. Vitamin D-dependency rickets in institutionalized, mentally retarded children on long-term anticonvulsant therapy. III. The response to 25-hydroxycholecalciferol and to vitamin D2. Pediatr Res (1973) 7, 914–22.
6 Mosekilde L and Melsen F. Anticonvulsant osteomalacia determined by quantitative analyses of bone changes. Population study and possible risk factors. Acta Med Scand (1976) 199, 349–55.
7 Hahn TJ, Avioli LV. Anticonvulsant osteomalacia. Arch Intern Med (1975) 135, 997–1000.
8 Hunter J, Maxwell JD, Stewart DA, Parson V, Williams R. Altered calcium metabolism in epileptic children on anticonvulsants. Br Med J (1971) 4, 202–4.

Vitamin K + Gentamicin and Clindamycin

Abstract/Summary

Seven patients in intensive care failed to respond to intravenous vitamin K for hypoprothrombinaemia while receiving gentamicin and clindamycin.

Clinical evidence, mechanism, importance and management

Some patients, particularly those in intensive care[1,2] who are not eating, can quite rapidly develop acute vitamin K deficiency which leads to prolonged prothrombin times and possibly bleeding. This can normally be controlled by giving vitamin K parenterally. However one report[2] describes seven such patients, all with normal liver function, who unexpectedly failed to respond to vitamin K. Examination of their records showed that all were receiving gentamicin/clindamycin. Just why these antibiotics oppose the effects of vitamin K is not understood, but it would seem prudent to avoid the use of these particular antibiotics wherever possible in patients within this category. More study is needed.

References

1 Ham JM. Hypoprothrombinaemia in patients undergoing prolonged intensive care. Med J Aust (1971) 2, 716.
2 Rodriguez-Erdmann F, Hoff JV, Carmody G. Interaction of antibiotics with vitamin K. J Amer Med Ass (1981) 246, 937.

X-ray contrast media + Cholestyramine

Abstract/Summary

A single report describes poor radiographic visualization of the gall bladder in a man due to an interaction between iopanoic acid and cholestyramine within the gut.

Clinical evidence, mechanism, importance and management

The cholecystogram of a man on cholestyramine with postgastrectomy syndrome who was given oral iopanoic acid as an X-ray contrast medium, suggested that he had an abnormal and apparently collapsed gall bladder. A week after stopping the cholestyramine a repeat cholecystogram gave excellent visualization of a gall bladder of normal appearance.[1] The same effects have been observed experimentally in dogs.[2] The reason seems to be that the cholestyramine binds with the iopanoic acid in the gut so that little is absorbed and little is available for secretion in the bile. Hence the poor visualization of the gall bladder. On the basis of reports about other drugs which similarly bind to cholestyramine, it seems probable that this interaction could be avoided if the administration of the iopanoic acid and the cholestyramine were to be separated as much as possible. Whether other oral acidic X-ray contrast media such as iobenzamic acid, ioglycamic acid, iophenoxic acid, iothalamic acid and others bind in a similar way to cholestyramine is uncertain, but this possibility should be considered.

References

1 Nelson JA. Effect of cholestyramine on teleopaque oral cholecystography. Am J Roentgenol Radium Ther Nucl (1974) 122, 333.
2 Berk RN. Cited as a personal communication in ref 1.

X-ray contrast media + Papaverine

Abstract/Summary, clinical evidence, mechanism, importance and management

Thrombosis of the brachial artery occurred in a woman given 30 mg papaverine in normal saline followed by iopamidol (*Isovue 370*).[1] It appeared that the contrast medium precipitated within the blood vessels. Hexabarix is also said to be incompatible with papaverine.[2]

References

1 Pallan T, Wulkan IA, Flores L, Chandhry MR, Gintautas J, Abadir AR. Radiological contrast material and a vasodilator can produce arterial thrombosis. Proc West Pharmacol Soc (1991) 34, 315–7.
2 Shah SJ, Gerlock AJ. Radiology (1987) 162, 619.

X-ray contrast media + Phenothiazines

Abstract/Summary

Two isolated case reports describe epileptiform reactions in two patients when metrizamide was used in the presence of chlorpromazine and dixyrazine.

Clinical evidence, mechanism, importance and management

A patient on chronic treatment with 75 mg chlorpromazine daily had grand mal seizures 3½ hours after being given metrizamide (16 ml of 170 mg iodine per ml) by the lumbar route. 5 h later he had another seizure.[1] One out of 34 other patients demonstrated epileptogenic activity on the EEG when given metrizamide for lumbar myelography. He was taking 10 mg dixyrazine three times daily.[2] A clinical study of 77 patients given levomepromazine for the relief of lumbago-sciatic pain found no evidence of an increased risk of epilepsy after receiving metrizamide.[3]

References

1 Hindmarsh T, Grepe A, Widen L. Metrizamide-phenothiazine interaction. Report of a case with seizures following myelography. Acta Radiol Diag (1975) 16, 129.
2 Hindmarsh T. Lumbar myelography with meglumine locarinate and metrizamide. A double-blind investigation. Acta Radiol Diag (1975) 16, 24.
3 Standnes B, Oftedal S-I and Weber H. Effect of levopromazine on EEG and on clinical side-effects after lumbar myelography with metrizamide. Acta Radiol Diag (1982) 23, 111–14.

Index

All of the pairs of individual drugs included in the text of this book which are known to interact or not to interact are listed in this index. They may also be listed under the group names as well but **you should always look up the names of both individual drugs and their groups to ensure that you have access to all the information.** You can possibly get a lead on the way unlisted drugs behave if you look up those which are related, but bear in mind that no two drugs are absolutely identical and any conclusion you reach should only be tentative. I have also indexed an extremely small number of interactions which are only speculative or theoretical. The text shows very clearly which these are.

British and American drug names and synonyms, including spelling variations, have been used, but brand names have been avoided except for some compound preparations in order to keep the index to a manageable size. However, tables of many international brand names/generic names are included in the introductory sections of most chapters. You can find these tables by looking up the group names of the drugs in question (eg Anticoagulants, Anticonvulsants etc).